Brief Contents

P9-CDU-393

PHARMACOLOGY

for Canadian Health Care Practice

LILLEY | HARRINGTON | SNYDER

Canadian Editor **Beth Swart**

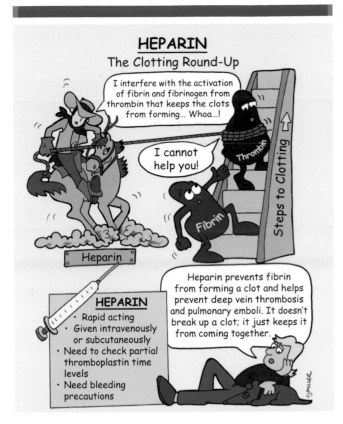

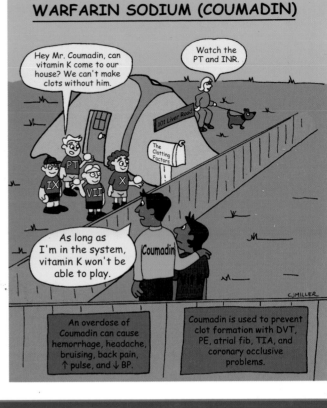

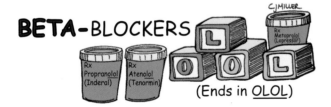

(Ends in OLOL)

Action: Blocks beta-receptors in the heart causing:
↓ Heart rate
↓ Force of contraction
↓ Rate of AV conduction

Side Effects: Bradycardia
Lethargy
GI disturbance
CHF
↓ BP
Depression

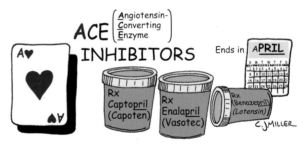

Action: ↓ Peripheral vascular resistance without:
∅ ↑ Cardiac output
∅ ↑ Cardiac rate
∅ ↑ Cardiac contractility

Side Effects: Dizziness
Orthostatic hypotension
GI distress
Cough
Headache

What You Need to Know

Warfarin Sodium (Coumadin)

CLASSIFICATION

Anticoagulant

ACTION

Antagonist of vitamin K, which is necessary for the synthesis of clotting factors VII, IX, X, and prothrombin; as a result, it disrupts the coagulation cascade.

USES

- Prevents venous thrombosis and thromboembolism associated with atrial fibrillation and prosthetic heart valves.
- Decreases risk of recurrent transient ischemic attack (TIA), cerebrovascular accident (stroke), and myocardial infarction.

CONTRAINDICATIONS

- Bleeding disorders (hemophilia, thrombocytopenia)
- Vitamin K deficiency; severe hypertension
- Pregnancy—category X; breastfeeding (crosses into breast milk)

PRECAUTIONS

- Renal or liver disease, alcoholism

SIDE EFFECTS

- Spontaneous bleeding
- Hypersensitivity reactions (e.g., dermatitis, fever, pruritus, urticaria)
- Red-orange discoloration of urine (not to be confused with hematuria); weakening of bones with long-term use

NURSING IMPLICATIONS

1. Monitor prothrombin time (PT) and international normalized ratio (INR) as ordered (2 to 3 is usually an acceptable INR).
2. Interacts with a large number of medications; consequently, monitor for drug interactions before initiating therapy.
3. Monitor for bleeding tendencies.
4. Vitamin K is an antidote.
5. Teach client to decrease intake of green, leafy vegetables.

Important nursing implications	Serious/life-threatening implications
Most frequent side effects	Patient teaching

What You Need to Know

Heparin

CLASSIFICATION

Anticoagulant

ACTION

Exerts direct effect on blood coagulation by enhancing the inhibitory actions of antithrombin III on several factors essential to normal blood clotting, thereby blocking the conversion of prothrombin to thrombin and fibrinogen to fibrin.

USES

- Prevents and treats deep vein thrombosis, pulmonary embolism, and emboli in atrial fibrillation.
- Diagnoses and treats disseminated intravascular coagulation.
- Preferred anticoagulant during pregnancy.

CONTRAINDICATIONS

- Bleeding tendencies—hemophilia, dissecting aneurysm, peptic ulcer
- Thrombocytopenia, uncontrollable bleeding
- Postoperative clients, especially eye, brain, spinal cord surgery, lumbar puncture, and regional anesthesia

SIDE EFFECTS

- Injection site reactions; heparin-induced thrombocytopenia
- Large doses may suppress renal function
- Spontaneous bleeding at mucous membranes

NURSING IMPLICATIONS

1. Monitor the partial thromboplastin time (PTT) and activated PTT (aPTT)— should be 1½ to 2 times the normal range; *watch for bleeding*.
2. Protamine sulfate is the antidote.
3. Low–molecular-weight heparins (e.g., enoxaparin [Lovenox]) do not require PTT or aPTT monitoring; used most often for preventing and treating deep vein thrombosis (DVT).
4. Administered either intravenously (IV) or subcutaneously.

Important nursing implications	Serious/life-threatening implications
Most frequent side effects	Patient teaching

What You Need to Know

Angiotensin Converting Enzyme (ACE) Inhibitors

ACTION

Suppress formation of angiotensin II from the renin-angiotensin-aldosterone system, reduce peripheral resistance, and improve cardiac output.

USES

- Hypertension
- Heart failure

CONTRAINDICATIONS

- History of angioedema
- Second and third trimesters of pregnancy
- Renal artery stenosis

PRECAUTIONS

- Renal impairment, collagen vascular disease
- Hypovolemia, salt depletion

SIDE EFFECTS

- Headache, dizziness, postural hypotension
- Rash, angioedema
- Altered sense of taste
- Nagging, nonproductive cough

NURSING IMPLICATIONS

1. Regularly monitor blood pressure, especially for 2 hours after the first dose, because severe first-dose hypotension often develops.
2. Teach client to rise slowly from a lying to a sitting position to reduce postural hypotensive effects.
3. Before administration, assess the client for history or presence of renal impairment.
4. Administer on an empty stomach for best absorption.
5. Teach client to notify health care provider if cough develops.
6. Teach client to avoid potassium supplements or potassium containing salt substitutes.

Important nursing implications	Serious/life-threatening implications
Most frequent side effects	Patient teaching

What You Need to Know

Beta-Blockers

ACTION

$Beta_1$ action is primarily on the heart—decreases rate, decreases force of contraction, and delays impulse conduction. $Beta_2$ action is primarily on the heart, but it also blocks receptors in the lungs and can cause bronchoconstriction.

USES

- Uncomplicated hypertension
- Dysrhythmias; angina

CONTRAINDICATIONS

- Bradydysrhythmias, atrioventricular (AV) block
- $Beta_2$ in chronic respiratory problems

PRECAUTIONS

- Hepatic and renal dysfunction, diabetes
- History of depression; heart failure

SIDE EFFECTS

- Headache, flushing, dizziness, fatigue, weakness
- Bradycardia, postural hypotension
- Bronchospasm, bronchoconstriction
- Decreased cardiac output, congestive heart failure (CHF)

NURSING IMPLICATIONS

1. Assess for symptoms of heart failure.
2. Instruct the client to report any weakness, dizziness, or fainting.
3. Before giving, evaluate the client's blood pressure and pulse for significant changes. Hold if systolic blood pressure is below 90 mm Hg.
4. Monitor clients with diabetes as tachycardia (a symptom of hypoglycemia) is often masked as a result of the $beta_1$ blockade.
5. Propranolol (Inderal) has both $beta_1$- and $beta_2$-receptor blocking actions and is considered nonselective; metoprolol (Lopressor) is cardioselective, which means it blocks only $beta_1$. Atenolol (Tenorim) is considered a cardioselective $beta_1$ blocker, but it blocks $beta_2$ at high doses.

Important nursing implications	Serious/life-threatening implications
Most frequent side effects	Patient teaching

Ca⁺LCIUM CHANNEL BLOCKERS

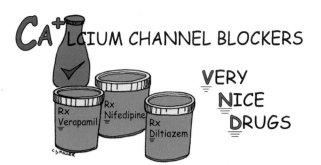

VERY
NICE
DRUGS

Action: Blocks calcium access to cells
causing: ↓ Contractility +
↓ Conductivity of the **heart**

↓ Demand for oxygen

Side Effects: ↓ BP
Bradycardia
May precipitate AV block
Headache
Abdominal discomfort
(constipation, nausea)
Peripheral edema

ANTIHYPERLIPIDEMICS

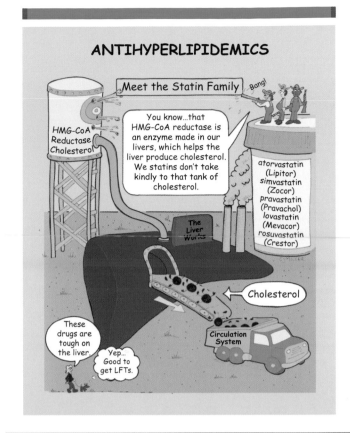

Cardiac   71

DIURETIC WATER SLIDE

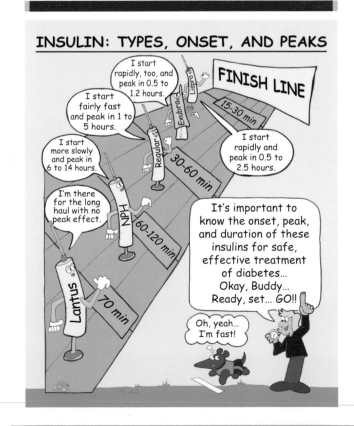

Diuretics   83

INSULIN: TYPES, ONSET, AND PEAKS

Endocrine   89

What You Need to Know

HMG-CoA Reductase Inhibitors (Statins) Beta-Adrenergic

EXAMPLES

Atorvastatin (Lipitor), simvastatin (Zocor), pravastatin (Pravachol), lovastatin (Mevacor), rosuvastatin (Crestor)

ACTION

Lower cholesterol levels by inhibiting the formation of HMG-CoA reductase, which is an enzyme that is required for the liver to synthesize cholesterol.

USES

- Hypercholesterolemia
- Primary and secondary prevention of cardiovascular events
- Clients with type 2 diabetes and coronary heart disease

CONTRAINDICATIONS

- Hepatitis, pregnancy

PRECAUTIONS

- Liver disease
- Excessive alcohol use

SIDE EFFECTS

- Myopathy—rhabdomyolysis (severe form)
- Hepatoxicity—liver injury with increases in serum transaminases

NURSING IMPLICATIONS

1. Instruct client to report unexplained muscle pain or tenderness.
2. Monitor liver function studies.
3. Inform women of childbearing age about the potential for fetal harm should they become pregnant.
4. Administer medication in the evening without regard to meals.
5. Instruct client about dietary changes to reduce weight and cholesterol.

Important nursing implications	Serious/life-threatening implications
Most frequent side effects	Patient teaching

What You Need to Know

Calcium Channel Blockers

CLASSIFICATION

Calcium channel blockers

ACTION

Block calcium access to the cells, causing decreased heart contractility and conductivity and leading to a decreased demand for oxygen.

USES

- Angina, hypertension (nifedipine), and dysrhythmias (verapamil and diltiazem)

CONTRAINDICATIONS

- *Nifedipine:* Hypersensitivity
- *Verapamil:* Severe left ventricular dysfunction, decreased blood pressure, cardiogenic shock, or heart block
- *Diltiazem:* Sick sinus syndrome, heart block, decreased blood pressure, acute myocardial infarction, or pulmonary congestion

PRECAUTIONS

- Renal or hepatic insufficiency
- Do not give verapamil or diltiazem with beta blockers

SIDE EFFECTS

- Decreased blood pressure, edema of the extremities, headache
- Constipation, nausea, skin flushing, dysrhythmias

NURSING IMPLICATIONS

1. Administer before meals; may be taken with food if needed; do not crush or allow client to chew sustained-release medication preparations.
2. Monitor vital signs and watch for low blood pressure.
3. Teach about postural hypotension.
4. Check liver and renal function studies.
5. Weigh client; report any edema or weight gain.
6. Teach client to avoid grapefruit.
7. Teach client that constipation can be minimized by increasing dietary fiber and fluid.

Important nursing implications	Serious/life-threatening implications
Most frequent side effects	Patient teaching

What You Need to Know

Types of Insulin

ACTION

	Onset	Peak	Duration
Short Duration: Rapid Acting			
Insulin lispro (Humalog)	15-30 min	0.5-2.5 hr	3.0-6.5 hr
Insulin aspart (NovoLog)	10-20 min	1.0-3.0 hr	3.0-5.0 hr
Insulin glulisine (Apidra)	10-15 min	1.0-1.5 hr	3.0-5.0 hr
Short Duration: Slow Acting			
Regular insulin (Humulin R)	30-60 min	1-5 hr	6-10 hr
Intermediate Duration			
NPH insulin (Humulin N)	60-120 min	6-14 hr	16-24 hr
Insulin detemir (Levemir)	—	6-8 hr	12-24 hr
Long Duration			
Insulin glargine (Lantus)	70 min	none	24 hr
Inhaled (Short Duration: Slow Acting)			
Exubera	15-30 min	0.5-1.5 hr	6.5 hr

From Lehne RA: *Pharmacology for nursing care*, ed 6, 2007, Philadelphia, Saunders.

NURSING IMPLICATIONS

1. U100 insulin is the most common concentration.
2. NPH is the only cloudy insulin; roll vial gently between palms to mix.
3. Draw up clear (regular, lispro—short acting) before the cloudy (intermediate) insulin to prevent contaminating a short-acting insulin with a long-acting insulin.
4. Inject subcutaneously; aspiration is not necessary.
5. Avoid massaging the site after injection.
6. Rotate sites within anatomic area; the abdomen is preferred for more rapid, even absorption.
7. Exubera is an inhaled insulin; the dose may be very different from an injected insulin.
8. Clean inhaler once a week and replace the release unit every 2 weeks.
9. Inhaled insulin can replace mealtime insulin but does not provide basal glycemic control; need to also use an intermediate or long-acting insulin.

Important nursing implications	Serious/life-threatening implications
Most frequent side effects	Patient teaching

What You Need to Know

Diuretics

ACTION

Loop diuretics inhibit sodium (Na) and chloride (Cl) reabsorption through direct action primarily in the ascending loop of Henle but also in the proximal and distal tubules. Thiazide diuretics act primarily on the distal tubules, inhibiting Na and Cl reabsorption.

USES

- Treat edema that involves fluid volume excess resulting from a number of disorders of the heart, liver, or kidney
- Hypertension

CONTRAINDICATIONS

- Pregnancy, breastfeeding
- Severe adrenocortical impairment, anuria, progressive oliguria

PRECAUTIONS

- Fluid and electrolyte depletion, gout
- Clients taking digitalis, lithium, nonsteroidal antiinflammatory drugs (NSAIDs), and other antihypertensive medications

SIDE EFFECTS

- Dehydration, hyponatremia, hypochloremia, hypokalemia
- Unusual tiredness, weakness, dizziness
- Irregular heart beat, weak pulse, orthostatic hypotension
- Tinnitus, hyperglycemia, hyperuricemia, hearing loss (Lasix)

NURSING IMPLICATIONS

1. Monitor for adequate intake and output and potassium loss.
2. Monitor client's weight and vital signs.
3. Monitor for signs and symptoms of hearing loss, which may last from 1 to 24 hours.
4. Teach client to take medication early in the day to decrease nocturia.
5. Teach client to report any hearing loss or signs of gout.

Important nursing implications	Serious/life-threatening implications
Most frequent side effects	Patient teaching

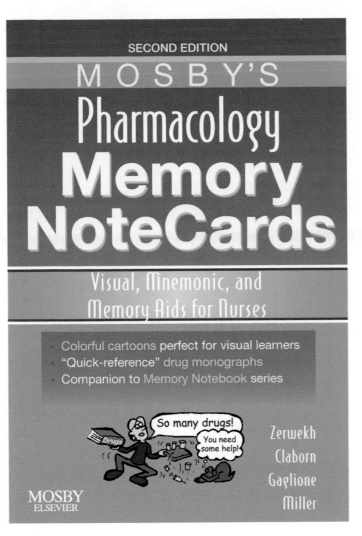
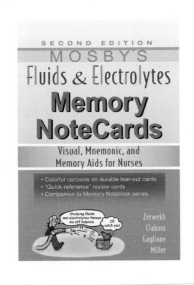
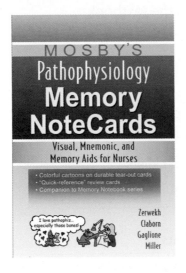
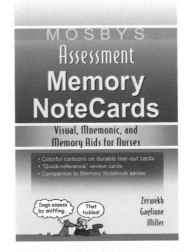
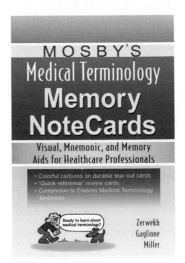

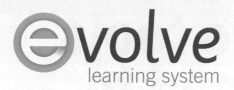

evolve
learning system

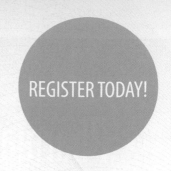

Evolve provides online access to free learning resources and activities designed specifically for the textbook you are using in your class. The resources will provide you with information that enhances the material covered in the book and much more.

Visit the Web address listed below to start your learning evolution today!

http://evolve.elsevier.com/Canada/Lilley/pharmacology/

Evolve® Student Learning Resources for Lilley/Harrington/Snyder/Swart, *Pharmacology for Canadian Health Care Practice,* **Second Canadian Edition, offer the following features:**

- Animations depicting important pharmacological concepts and administration techniques
- Answers to the Examination Review Questions, Critical Thinking Activities, and Case Studies from the textbook
- Calculators for dosages, weights, and other assessments, and Category Catcher handouts containing need-to-know information about each drug category
- Frequently Asked Questions and Content Updates
- Glossary with audio pronunciations
- IV Therapy and Medication Error Checklists
- Multiple-Choice Review Question quizzes for every chapter
- Nursing Care Plans
- Online Appendices and Supplements
- An extensive library of pharmacology Web Links carefully chosen to supplement the content of the textbook

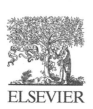

ELSEVIER

PHARMACOLOGY

for Canadian Health Care Practice

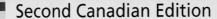

Second Canadian Edition

Linda Lane Lilley, RN, PhD
Associate Professor Emeritus and University Professor
Old Dominion University
Norfolk, Virginia

Scott Harrington, PharmD
Harrington Health Informatics, LLC
Tucson, Arizona
Director of Pharmacy, Northern Cochise Community Hospital
Willcox, Arizona

Julie S. Snyder, MSN, RN, BC
Adjunct Faculty
Old Dominion University
Norfolk, Virginia

Canadian Editor:

Beth Swart, BScN, MES
School of Nursing
Ryerson University
Toronto, Ontario

With Study Skills content by:
Diane Savoca
Coordinator of Student Transition
St. Louis Community College at Florissant Valley
St. Louis, Missouri

With special thanks to
Richard E. Lake, BS, MS, MLA
for his contribution to the first edition Study Skills content

With special thanks to
Michelle Forbes
for her contribution to the second Canadian edition
Study Skills content

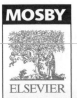

MOSBY

ELSEVIER

NOTICE

Knowledge and best practice in this field are constantly changing. As new research and expertise broaden our knowledge, changes in practice, treatment, and drug therapy may become necessary or appropriate. Readers are advised to check the most current information provided (i) on procedures featured or (ii) by the manufacturer of each product to be administered, to verify the recommended dose or formula, the method and duration of administration, and contraindications. It is the responsibility of the practitioner, relying on their own experience and knowledge of the patient, to make diagnoses, to determine dosages and the best treatment for each individual patient, and to take all appropriate safety precautions. To the fullest extent of the law, neither the Publisher nor the Authors assumes any liability for any injury and/or damage to persons or property arising out of or related to any use of the material contained in this book.

Library and Archives Canada Cataloguing in Publication

Pharmacology for Canadian health care practice / Linda Lilley, Scott Harrington,
Julie S. Snyder, U.S. editors ; Beth Swart, Canadian editor; Michelle Forbes, study skills
Canadian ed. — 2nd Canadian ed.
First Canadian ed. published under title: Pharmacology and the nursing process in Canada.
Includes bibliographical references and index.
ISBN 978-1-897422-14-4
1. Pharmacology—Textbooks. 2. Nursing—Canada—Textbooks. I. Lilley, Linda Lane I
I. Harrington, Scott III. Snyder, Julie S. IV. Swart, Beth, 1948- V. Lilley, Linda Lane.
Pharmacology and the nursing process in Canada.
RM301.P4564 2010   615'.1   C2009-903643-6

Vice President, Publishing: Ann Millar
Managing Developmental Editor: Tammy Scherer
Developmental Editor: May Look
Managing Production Editor: Roberta A. Spinosa-Millman
Copy Editor: Jerri M. Hurlbutt
Cover, Interior Design: Brett J. Miller, BJM Graphic Design & Communications
Cover Image: © doc-stock/Corbis
Typesetting and Assembly: Jansom
Printing and Binding: Transcontinental

Elsevier Canada
905 King Street West, 4th Floor, Toronto, ON, Canada M6K 3G9
Phone: 1-866-896-3331
Fax: 1-866-359-9534

Printed in Canada

5 6 7 8   17 16 15 14

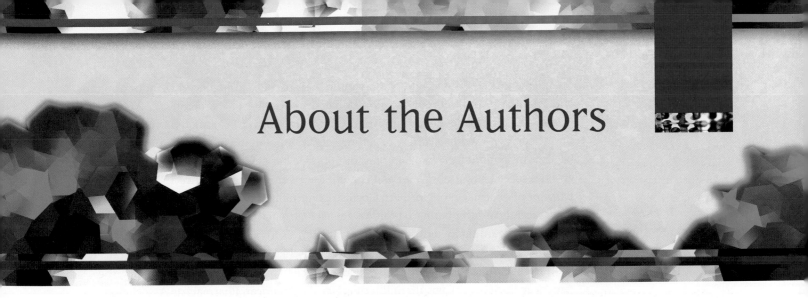

About the Authors

Linda Lane Lilley, RN, PhD

Linda Lilley received her diploma from Norfolk General School of Nursing, her BSN from the University of Virginia, her Master of Science (Nursing) from Old Dominion University, and her PhD in Nursing from George Mason University. As an Associate Professor Emeritus and University Professor at Old Dominion University, her teaching experience in nursing education spans over 25 years, including almost 20 years at Old Dominion University. Linda's teaching expertise includes drug therapy and the nursing process, adult nursing, physical assessment, fundamentals in nursing, oncology nursing, nursing theory, and trends in health care. The awarding of the University's most prestigious title of University Professor reflects her teaching excellence as a tenured faculty member. She has also been a two-time university nominee for the State Council of Higher Education in Virginia award for excellence in teaching, service, and scholarship. While at Old Dominion University, Linda mentored and taught undergraduate and graduate students as well as registered nurses returning for their BSN. She continues to serve as a member on dissertation committees with the College of Health Sciences. Since retirement in 2005, Linda has continued to be active in nursing, with involvement in the American Nurses Association, Virginia Nurses Association, Sigma Theta Tau International, Phi Kappa Phi, and other professional organizations. Linda's research interests include the identification of factors affecting recruitment and retention of minority students in baccalaureate schools of nursing. Dr. Lilley's professional service varies, having served as a consultant with school nurses in the city of Virginia Beach and as a member on the City of Virginia Beach's Health Advisory Board. Linda was also an appointed member on the national advisory panel on medication errors prevention with the U.S. Pharmacopeia in Rockville, Maryland. Linda currently serves as a member of the Community Health Services Advisory Board, City of Virginia Beach. She continues to educate nursing students and professional nurses about drug therapy and the nursing process and offers educational sessions to older adults about medication safety.

Scott Harrington, PharmD

Scott Harrington received his Associate of Science in Pharmacy Technology with High Honors from Pima Community College, Tucson, Arizona, in 1991. He then worked as both an outpatient and inpatient pharmacy technician while completing his Doctor of Pharmacy degree at the University of Arizona College of Pharmacy, which he received in 1997. He then completed two postdoctoral residency training programs. The first was a specialty residency in Pharmacocybernetics at Creighton University in Omaha, Nebraska, which he completed in 1998. The second was an additional specialty residency in Drug Information and Pharmaceutical Informatics at the University of California–San Francisco Medical Center and First DataBank in San Bruno, California, which he completed in 1999. Since that time, he has worked in a variety of settings, including outpatient retail pharmacy, where he also compounded customized prescriptions. He has since worked in hospital pharmacy and has served as a proofreader and content reviewer for Elsevier since 1999. He is now Director of Pharmacy for Northern Cochise Community Hospital in Willcox, Arizona, and most recently a staff pharmacist for Walgreens Pharmacy. Scott also regularly offers public education regarding medication use in mental illness to public outreach support groups at the office of the National Alliance for the Mentally Ill of Southern Arizona in Tucson. Scott's professional affiliations include the American Society of Health-System Pharmacy, the American Society for Consultant Pharmacists, the American Pharmacists Association, the Society for Technical Communicators, the American Medical Informatics Association, and the American College of Clinical Pharmacy. Scott is also a member of American MENSA.

Julie S. Snyder, MSN, RN, BC

Julie Snyder received her diploma from Norfolk General Hospital School of Nursing and her BSN and MSN from Old Dominion University. After working in medical-surgical nursing for over 10 years, she began working in nursing staff development and community education. After 8 years, she transferred to teaching in a school of nursing, and over the past 10 years she has taught fundamentals of nursing, pharmacology, physical assessment, gerontological nursing, and adult medical-surgical nursing. She has been certified by the American Nurses Credentialing Center (ANCC) in Nursing Continuing Education and Staff Development, and currently holds ANCC certification in Medical-Surgical Nursing. She is a member of Sigma Theta Tau International and was inducted into Phi Kappi Phi as Outstanding Alumni for Old Dominion University. She has worked for Elsevier as a reviewer and ancillary writer since 1997. Julie's professional service has included serving on the Virginia Nurses Association Continuing Education Committee, serving as Educational Development Committee chair for the Epsilon Chi chapter of Sigma Theta Tau, serving as an item writer for the ANCC, working with a regional hospital educators' group, and serving as a consultant on various projects for local hospital education departments.

Beth Swart, BScN, MES

Beth Swart, BScN, MES, is a professor in the School of Nursing, Ryerson University. She received her diploma in nursing from the Hospital for Sick Children School of Nursing, her BScN from the University of Toronto, and her MES from York University. For more than 30 years, Beth has taught nursing students at the baccalaureate level. She has also been a mentor to Masters students. Her areas of specialty are pathophysiology and epidemiology. Beth has also developed innovative Distance Education courses for RNs returning to university to pursue their degree. Research interests include differences in student learning between online and in-class teaching. Beth was for many years a board member of the Lambda-Pi Chapter-At-Large of Sigma Theta Tau International. She has served on the steering committee and the board of the National Immunization Education Initiative since 2003. In 2005, Beth received an award for teaching excellence in the faculty of Community Services. Beth has worked as a reviewer and author for Elsevier since 2004.

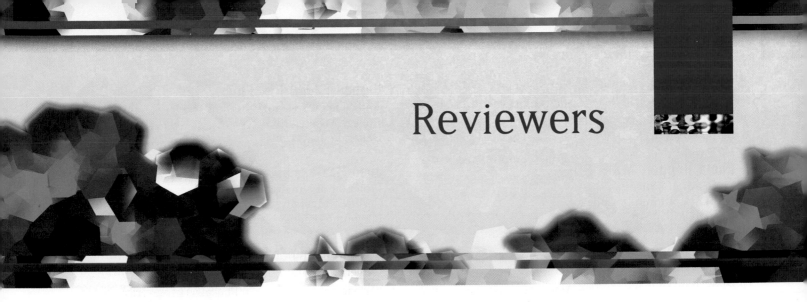

Reviewers

Reviewers for the Fifth American Edition

Barbara Allerton, RN, MSN
Assistant Professor of Nursing
Boise State University
Boise, Idaho

Diane S. Benson, RN, EdD
Associate Professor of Nursing
Humboldt State University
Arcata, California

Vivian Biggers, MSN, RN, CS
President
Dynamic Presentations
Midlothian, Virginia

Kevin Boesen, PharmD
Clinical Assistant Professor
Pharmacy Practice and Science
The University of Arizona College of Pharmacy
Tucson, Arizona

Timothy L. Brenner, PharmD
Assistant Professor
Department of Pharmacy Practice and Science
University of Arizona College of Pharmacy
Tucson, Arizona

Imad F. Btaiche, PharmD, BCNSP
Clinical Associate Professor
Department of Clinical Sciences, College of Pharmacy
Ann Arbor, Michigan

Teresa Burckhalter, MSN, RN, C
Nursing Faculty
Technical College of the Lowcountry
Beaufort, South Carolina

Nina R. Cuttler, MSN, APRN, BC
Nursing Faculty
Central Carolina Technical College
Sumter, South Carolina

Kimberly A. Deppe
Assistant Professor of Nursing
University of Dubuque
Dubuque, Iowa

Lisa M. Easterby, RNC, MSN, FN-CSA
Instructor of Nursing
Our Lady of Lourdes School of Nursing
Camden, New Jersey

Nancy Eksterowicz, RN, MSN
Pain Services Coordinator
University of Virginia Health Systems
Afton, Virginia

Dr. Penny Fairman
Dean of Nursing
Northland Pioneer College
Show Low, Arizona

Sherry D. Ferki, BSN, MSN
Adjunct Faculty
Old Dominion University School of Nursing
Norfolk, Virginia
College of the Albemarle
Elizabeth City, North Carolina

Alice J.A. Gardner, PhD
Assistant Professor
Department of Pharmaceutical Sciences
Massachusetts College of Pharmacy and
  Health Sciences
Worcester, Massachusetts

Janice Hoffman, RN, MSN
Nurse Educator
The Johns Hopkins Hospital
Baltimore, Maryland

Paula Hopper, MSN, RN
Professor of Nursing
Jackson Community College
Jackson, Michigan

Charlie Jacques, BSN, MSN, FNP
Assistant Professor of Nursing
Dixie State College
St. George, Utah

Lynn D. Kennedy, MN, RN
Assistant Professor of Nursing
Francis Marion University
Florence, South Carolina

Ujjaini Khanderia, PharmD
Clinical Assistant Professor of Pharmacy
College of Pharmacy and University of
      Michigan Health System
University of Michigan
Ann Arbor, Michigan

Dorothy Mathers, MSN, RN
Associate Professor of Nursing
Pennsylvania College of Technology
Williamsport, Pennsylvania

Lora McGuire, RN, MS
Professor of Nursing
Joliet Junior College
Joliet, Illinois

Diana King Mixon, BSN, MSN
Associate Professor of Nursing
Boise State University
Boise, Idaho

Melissa O'Neill, BSN
Nurse Practitioner
Dermatology—Division of Internal Medicine
Creighton University Medical Center
Omaha, Nebraska

Julie Painter, RN, MSN, OCN
Clinical Nurse Specialist/Adult Nurse Practitioner
Clinical Practice Education and Research
Community Health Network
Indianapolis, Indiana

Brenda Pavill, RN, PhD
Associate Professor of Nursing
College Misericordia
Dallas, Pennsylvania

Joan Reale, PhD, RN
Professor of Nursing
Carlow University
Pittsburgh, Pennsylvania

Randolph Regal, BS, PharmD
Clinical Assistant Professor/Clinical Pharmacist
College of Pharmacy, Department of Pharmacy Services
University of Michigan
Ann Arbor, Michigan

Bruce Austin Scott, MSN, APRN, BC
Nursing Instructor
San Joaquin Delta College
Stockton, California

Roberta Secrest, PhD, PharmD
Global Media Communications
Eli Lilly and Company
Indianapolis, Indiana

Sarah Steele, BSN, MSN
Assistant Professor
Allen College
Waterloo, Iowa

Darlene Thomay, RN, BA, DNC
Medical Specialties Clinics
Metrohealth
Cleveland, Ohio

Sarah Reidunn Tvedt, MS, RN
Nursing Education Specialist of Cardiac Surgery
Mayo Clinic
Rochester, Minnesota

Kathleen Dorman Wagner, RN, MSN, EdD (c)
Lecturer
College of Nursing
University of Kentucky
Lexington, Kentucky

Derek Wood, RN, BC, MS
Instructor of Nursing
Aims Community College
Greeley, Colorado

Reviewers for the Second Canadian Edition

Harrison Applin, BScN, MEd, PhD(Nurs), RN
Instructor, Nursing Program
Grant MacEwan College
Edmonton, Alberta

Julie Duff Cloutier, RN, MSc
Assistant Professor, School of Nursing
Laurentian University
Sudbury, Ontario

Kathryn Ellis, RN, BScN, MA (Ed)
Professor and Coordinator, Ryerson University/
    Centennial College/George Brown Collaborative
    Nursing Program
Centennial College
Toronto, Ontario

Trudy Hahn, RN, PhD
Senior Instructor, Department of Nursing
University of New Brunswick
Saint John, New Brunswick

Amandah Hoogbruin, RN, BScN, MScN, PhD
Instructor, Department of Nursing
Kwantlen Polytechnic University
Vancouver, British Columbia

Barbara Jamieson, MN, RN
Assistant Professor, Department of Nursing
Cape Breton University
Sydney, Nova Scotia

Brenda J. Lane, RN, BScN, Dip Ad Ed, MN
University-College Professor, Faculty of Health
    and Human Services, BScN Program
Vancouver Island University
Nanaimo, British Columbia

Pat Lewis, BScN, Med, CRCCN(C)
Instructor, Nursing Program
Camosun College
Victoria, British Columbia

June MacDonald-Jenkins, RN, BScN, MSc, PhD (cand.)
Professor, School of Health and Community Studies
Assistant Adjunct Professor, Faculty of Health Science
Collaborative Nursing Program
Durham College/University of Ontario Institute of
    Technology
Oshawa, Ontario

Tara MacKenzie, RN, BSN, MS
Instructor, School of Nursing
College of New Caledonia
Prince George, British Columbia

Christa MacLean, RN, BSN, MN
Faculty, Psychiatric Nursing Program
Saskatchewan Institute of Applied Science
    and Technology
Regina, Saskatchewan

Mary Anne Maloney, RN, BScN, MN
University-College Professor, Faculty of Health
    and Human Services, BScN Program
Vancouver Island University
Nanaimo, British Columbia

Brenda McLean, MEd, BScN, RN
Year 1 Associate Coordinator
Faculty Lecturer
Faculty of Nursing, BScN Collaborative Program
University of Alberta
Edmonton, Alberta

Kim Munich, RN, BScN, MN, PhD
Faculty, Nursing Program
British Columbia Institute of Technology
New Westminster, British Columbia

Vicki Niblett, RN, BScN
Coordinator, Brock-Loyalist Collaborative
    Nursing Program
Loyalist College
Frankford, Ontario

Gail Potter, RN, BScN, M. Div., MN (cand.)
Instructor, Department of Nursing, BScN Program
Selkirk College
Castlegar, British Columbia

Faith Richardson, BSc, MSN-FNP, DNP (cand.)
Assistant Professor, Faculty of Nursing
Trinity Western University
Langley, British Columbia

Karen Riley, BScPhm, Pharm D, BCPS, RPh
Faculty, Faculty of Nursing
University of Windsor, Sarnia Campus
Sarnia, Ontario

Karen Rowles, RN, BN, MEd
Instructor, School of Health Sciences, NESA (Nursing
    Instructor in Southern Alberta) Program
Lethbridge College
Lethbridge, Alberta

Claudia R. Seiler-Mutton, RN, BScN, MEd
Instructor, Nursing Program
Grant MacEwan College
Edmonton, Alberta

L. Gail Sheppard, RN, MSN
Graduate Nurse Instructor, Faculty of Community and
    Health Studies
Kwantlen Polytechnic University
Surrey, British Columbia

Cindy Skolud, RN, MScN
Professor, Seneca College/York University
    Collaborative BScN Program
Seneca College
Aurora, Ontario

Helen Taylor, BA, RN, DHSW, BScN, MScN
Assistant Professor, School of Nursing
McMaster University
Hamilton, Ontario

Barbara Thompson, RN, BScN, MScN, APRN, BC
Faculty, Collaborative BScN Program
Sault College of Applied Arts and Technology
Sault Ste. Marie, Ontario

Sherri Leon Torres, RN, BSN, MC
Instructor, School of Nursing
College of New Caledonia
Prince George, British Columbia

Judy Turner, RPN, RN, BScN, MS (Nrsg)
Faculty, Department of Psychiatric Nursing
Douglas College
Coquitlam, British Columbia

Sylvia van der Weg, BScN, MA (Ed), RN
Professor, Georgian College/York University
    Collaborative BScN Program
Georgian College
Barrie, Ontario

Barb Walsh, RPN (Registered Psychiatric Nurse), RN, BScN, MEd
Faculty, Department of Psychiatric Nursing
Douglas College
New Westminster, British Columbia

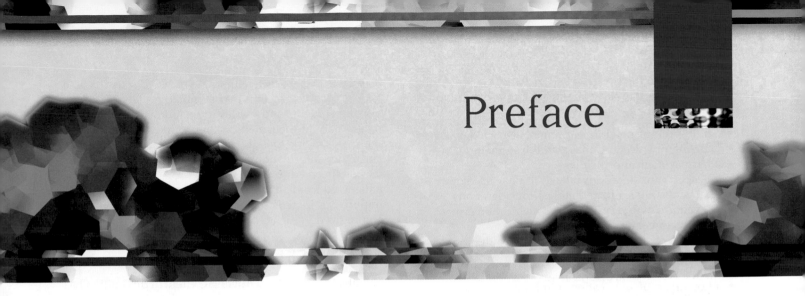

Preface

INTRODUCTION

This second edition of *Pharmacology and the Nursing Process in Canada* has been retitled *Pharmacology for Canadian Health Care Practice* to reflect a move toward a broader context incorporating both the nursing process and evidence-informed practice into Canadian nursing. This text provides the most current and clinically relevant information in an appealing, understandable, and practical format. The accessible size, readable writing style, and full-colour design are ideal for busy nursing students. This text takes a unique approach to the study of pharmacology by presenting study skills that will help students understand and learn this particularly demanding subject. Each part begins with a Study Skills Tips section, which features a discussion of researched and proven study skills and applies the discussion to the content in that part. Students are encouraged to use research-based study skills to enhance their study of pharmacology and nursing.

The text incorporates chapter-specific Canadian content relevant to Canadian students and educators that will strengthen their knowledge of the field. Also included are clinical practice guidelines produced or endorsed in Canada by national, provincial, or territorial medical or health organizations, or by professional societies, government agencies, or expert panels. Ethnocultural examples reflect the varied and complex ethnodemographic diversity of Canada.

MARKET RESEARCH

To aid in the preparation of this text, nursing instructors and students from across Canada participated in extensive, detailed reviews of the First Canadian Edition. These reviewers assessed changes that had occurred in the field of pharmacology since publication of the first edition and determined what was needed to better teach this subject to nursing students and how their evolving learning needs could be met.

On the basis of their feedback, several suggestions for improvement were incorporated:

- Streamlining the Study Skills Tips sections to better reflect student reality
- Including discussions of critical thinking and evidence-informed practice in introductory chapters
- Adding information that reflects the current trend of using clinical practice guidelines and evidence-informed practice
- Centralizing all information for each drug in a single area of the textbook
- Enhancing coverage of look-alike, sound-alike drugs and of how drugs are classified
- Incorporating a lifespan focus throughout the text
- Adding material on epidemiology and pathology at the beginning of each section

This Canadian edition maintains the philosophy of making the challenging subject of pharmacology approachable and easy to understand. Additional concerns raised and enhancements suggested by educators and nursing students who served as reviewers or consultants throughout the manuscript's development, as well by the author and editors of this text, also have been addressed.

ORGANIZATION

This book includes 59 chapters presented in 10 parts, organized by body system. Each part begins with a *Study Skills Tips* section that presents a study skills topic and relates it to the unit being discussed. Topics include time management, note taking, studying, test taking, and others. This unique approach to teaching pharmacology is intended to aid students who find pharmacology difficult and to provide a tool that may prove beneficial throughout their nursing school careers. Coverage of this study skills content is limited to the beginning of each part so that instructors who choose not to require their students to read this material can easily eliminate it. This arrangement of content may be beneficial, however, to educators who teach pharmacology through an integrated approach because it helps the student identify key content and concepts. This arrangement also facilitates location of content for required or optional reading.

The 10 introductory chapters in Part One lay a solid foundation for the subsequent drug units and address the following topics:

- Study skills applied to learning pharmacology
- Nursing practice in Canada and drug therapy
- Pharmacological principles
- Lifespan considerations related to pharmacology
- Ethnocultural, legal, and ethical considerations
- Prevention of and responses to medication errors
- Patient education and drug therapy
- Over-the-counter drugs and natural health products
- Vitamins and minerals
- Problematic substance use
- Photo atlas of medication administration techniques, including more than 100 illustrations and photographs

Parts Two through Ten present pharmacology and nursing management in a traditional body-systems and drug-function framework. This approach facilitates learning by grouping functionally related drugs and drug groups. It also provides an effective means to integrate the content into medical-surgical or adult health nursing courses or for teaching pharmacology as a separate course.

The 49 drug chapters in these parts constitute the main portion of the book. Drugs are presented in a consistent format with an emphasis on drug groups and key similarities and differences among the drugs in each group. Each chapter is subdivided into two discussions, beginning with a complete discussion of the relevant pharmacology and a brief review of the pathophysiology of disease processes to be treated, followed by a comprehensive yet succinct discussion of the associated nursing process. A new feature, *Evidence-Informed Practice* boxes, is incorporated throughout the text and includes research that affects nursing practice and pharmacology. The pharmacology for each drug group is presented in a consistent format:

- Mechanism of Action and Drug Effects
- Indications
- Contraindications
- Adverse Effects
- Interactions (often including Toxicity and Management of Overdose)
- Dosages

Drug-group discussions are followed by *Drug Profiles*, or brief narrative capsules of individual drugs in the class or group, including Pharmacokinetics tables for each drug. Key drugs, or prototypical drugs within a class, are identified with the ▶▶ symbol for easy identification. These individual drug profiles are followed by a *Nursing Process* discussion relating to the entire drug group. The nursing content is covered in the following functional, five-step format:

- Assessment
- Nursing Diagnoses
- Planning (including Goals and Outcome Criteria)
- Implementation
- Evaluation

At the end of each Nursing Process discussion is a *Patient Education* section that summarizes key points for nursing students and nurses to include when educating patients about their medications, with attention to how the drugs work, possible interactions, adverse effects, and other information related to the safe and effective use of the medication. With the role of the nurse as patient educator and advocate continuing to grow in importance in professional practice, this key content is emphasized in each chapter of this edition.

NEW TO THIS EDITION

The pharmacology and nursing content in this edition has been thoroughly revised to reflect the latest drug information and research. Such revisions include the following:

- The use of the term *health care provider* rather than *health care professional*, which reflects the regulated, unregulated, and informal members who make up the team of care providers across the country, and the specialized knowledge and education required to fulfill new roles and expanded scopes of practice
- **An increased focus on drug classes** to help students acquire a better knowledge base of how various drugs work in the body; they can then apply this knowledge to individual drugs
- **A revised and consistent order within the Dosages tables**, from smaller to larger dosages (i.e., from infants to children to adults), in order to minimize the potential for medication errors
- **The division of the antibiotics and antineoplastics chapters** into smaller chapters, in order to make the complex content easier to grasp and to more thoroughly cover the specific classes of drugs used
- **Expanded coverage of pandemic preparedness and cultural aspects of drug therapy**
- **Distribution of the former *Community Health Points* material** within the content of the chapters
  New features in this edition include the following:
- The inclusion of both **generic and brand names of drugs**
- *In My Family* boxes, written by nursing students of various ethnocultural backgrounds, describing specific cultural health beliefs and practices; these offer different perspectives and can remind nurses to be aware of and respect the wide range of cultural customs
- **Improved readability** throughout the text to make the content more understandable than ever
- *Evidence-Informed Practice* boxes, which summarize current research and emphasize findings relevant to professional nursing practice and safe and effective drug therapy
- *Lab Values Related to Drug Therapy* boxes, which highlight specific laboratory tests applicable to drug therapy, including normal ranges, values, and rationales for lab assessments
- *Preventing Medication Errors* boxes, which reinforce concepts introduced in the chapter on medication

errors and relate them to specific common errors that occur in clinical practice

- *Special Populations* boxes, focusing on the unique needs of children, adolescents, older adults, and women
- *Examination Review Questions* at the end of each chapter now feature a new focus on application and analysis.
- **A selection of tear-out note cards from** *Mosby's Pharmacology Memory NoteCards,* **Second Edition,** chosen for their frequently used content, provided as a helpful quick reference for students to use in nursing practice

FEATURES

This book includes *various pedagogical features* that prepare the student for important content covered in each chapter and encourage review and reinforcement of that content. Chapter opener pedagogy includes the following:

- *Learning Objectives*
- An *e-Learning Activities* box, listing related content and exercises on the Evolve Web site
- A *Drug Profiles* list, outlining the profiles in each chapter, with page number references and key drugs identified
- A *Glossary* of key terms, with definitions and page number references

Glossary terms are boldfaced in the narrative to emphasize this essential terminology. In addition, included at the back of the book is an index of glossary terms with page numbers for quick reference.

The following features appear at the end of each chapter:

- *Patient Education* tips related to drug therapy
- *Points to Remember,* summarizing key points
- *Examination Review Questions,* with answers provided on the Evolve Web site
- *Critical Thinking Activities,* with answers provided on the Evolve Web site

Additional special features that appear throughout the text include the following:

- *Ethnocultural Implications* boxes, which include examples, such as genetic differences and metabolic deficiencies, of how racial and ethnic populations may respond to drugs differently
- *Natural Health Products* boxes, providing up-to-date information about some of the most commonly used natural health products, including possible adverse effects and drug interactions
- *Legal and Ethical Principles* boxes, which include situations and relevant information that may influence legal and ethical principles governing nursing practice
- *Research* boxes, describing current and relevant research findings used to support nursing practice
- *Case Studies,* with answers provided on the Evolve Web site

- Alphabetized *Dosages* tables, listing generic and trade names, pharmacological class, usual dosage ranges, and indications for the drugs

For a more comprehensive listing of the special features, please refer to the final pages of the book.

Additional features found at the end of the book include the following:

- An *Appendix* of pharmaceutical abbreviations
- A *Bibliography,* listing both general and chapter-specific references for further information
- A *General Index* that highlights boxes, tables and figures, and disorders referenced in the text
- A separate *Drug Index* that lists both generic and trade drug names and page numbers, for easy reference

COLOUR

The first American edition of this book was the first full-colour pharmacology text for nursing students. In preparation for that book, nursing educators had suggested that colour be used in both a functionally and visually appealing manner to more fully engage students in this typically demanding yet important content. This Canadian edition continues to use full colour throughout to do the following:

- Highlight important content
- Illustrate how drugs work in the body through numerous anatomical and drug process colour figures
- Improve the visual appearance of the content in order to make it more engaging and appealing to visually sophisticated readers

The use of colour in these ways should significantly improve students' involvement and understanding of pharmacology.

SUPPLEMENTAL RESOURCES

A comprehensive ancillary package is available to students and instructors using *Pharmacology for Canadian Health Care Practice.* The supplemental resources described below have been thoroughly revised and can significantly assist in the teaching and learning of pharmacology.

Study Guide

The carefully prepared student workbook includes the following:

- A *Student Study Tips* section that reinforces and enhances the study skills explained in the text, and provides a "how to" guide to applying test-taking strategies
- *Worksheets* for each chapter that contain review questions, critical thinking and application questions, case studies, and other activities
- An updated *Overview of Drug Calculations* section, with helpful tips for calculating doses, sample drug labels, practice problems, and a quiz
- Answers to all questions, provided at the back of the workbook to enable self-study

Evolve Web Site

Located at **http://evolve.elsevier.com/Canada/Lilley/pharmacology**, the Evolve Web site for this book includes the following elements:

For Students

- Answers to the Examination Review Questions, Critical Thinking Activities, and Case Studies from the textbook
- State-of-the-art animations to help students understand and retain information more easily by visually depicting important pharmacological concepts (topics include agonists and antagonists, therapeutic effects of various types and classes of drugs, drug movement through the body, medication administration techniques, and many more)
- Frequently Asked Questions and Content Updates
- An updated library of pharmacology WebLinks
- Multiple-choice review questions for every chapter, including rationales for each correct answer
- IV Therapy and Medication Error checklists
- Category Catcher handouts containing need-to-know information about each drug category
- Nursing Care Plans
- Supplemental resources and appendices, including additional chapter content, and information on common weights, formulas, and equivalents
- An Audio Glossary
- Calculators for dosages, weights, and other assessments

For Instructors

Instructors have access to all student Evolve content. Additionally, the following instructor resources are available:

- An Instructor's Manual, with chapter overviews; key terms; chapter outlines; teaching strategies; and open-book quizzes and student worksheets, including answers, to provide additional review of challenging content and important concepts
- A Test Bank with over 650 multiple-choice formatted questions, coded for cognitive level. All answers include rationales. The test bank is provided in the user-friendly ExamView® program, which allows the instructor to create new tests; edit, add, and delete test questions; sort questions by cognitive level; and administer and grade online tests.
- An Image Collection with more than 230 full-colour images from the book. The images can be viewed, printed, or imported into PowerPoint®.
- Teaching tips
- An I-Clicker Question Suite, developed especially for use with audience response systems
- Expanded and updated PowerPoint® presentation slides featuring more than 2250 lecture outlines covering every chapter in the textbook. These outlines can be customized by adding or deleting text, as well as images from the Image Collection.

Evolve Select

This exciting program is available to faculty who adopt a number of Elsevier texts, including *Pharmacology for Canadian Health Care Practice*. Evolve Select is an integrated electronic study centre consisting of a collection of textbooks made available online. It is carefully designed to "extend" the textbook for an easier and more efficient teaching and learning experience. It includes study aids such as highlighting, e-note taking, and cut-and-paste capabilities. Even more importantly, it allows students and instructors to do a comprehensive search within the specific text or across a number of titles. Please check with your Elsevier Canada sales representative for more information.

ICONS AT A GLANCE

- CASE STUDY
- DRUG PROFILES
- ETHNOCULTURAL IMPLICATIONS
- EVIDENCE-INFORMED PRACTICE
- IN MY FAMILY
- LAB VALUES RELATED TO DRUG THERAPY
- LEGAL & ETHICAL PRINCIPLES
- NATURAL HEALTH PRODUCTS
- PREVENTING MEDICATION ERRORS
- RESEARCH
- SPECIAL POPULATIONS: THE ADOLESCENT
- SPECIAL POPULATIONS: CHILDREN
- SPECIAL POPULATIONS: THE OLDER ADULT
- SPECIAL POPULATIONS: WOMEN

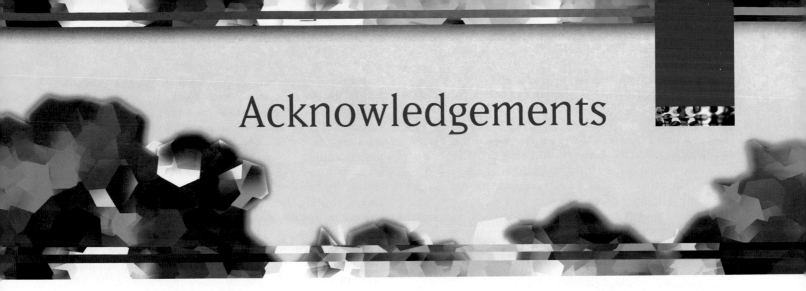

Acknowledgements

Acknowledgments for the Fifth American Edition

This book truly has been a collaborative effort. We wish to thank the instructors who provided input on an ongoing basis throughout the development of the first, second, third, and fourth editions. In addition, we would like to thank the following people: Rick Brady, Dottie Mathers, Chuck Dresner, Judith Myers, Ted Huff, Donald O'Connor, Linda Wendling, Ken Turnbough, Greg McVicar, Anthony Saranita, and Susan Orf. We thank Carolyn Duke and the Saint Louis University School of Nursing for their assistance and cooperation. Thanks also to Chesapeake General Hospital for assistance with the fourth edition photo shoot.

We thank Kristin Geen and Jamie Horn for their contributions and support throughout the fourth edition. We are also grateful to Jeff Patterson and Clay Broeker for very capably guiding the project through to publication and to Paula Ruckenbrod for her effective design. Diane Savoca lent her study skills expertise and has updated the unique and appropriate feature for students, and for her collaboration we are most grateful. Finally we thank Joe Albanese for his contributions to the first edition and Bob Aucker for his contributions to the first three editions of the book.

Linda thanks her husband Les, daughter Karen, and mother-in-law Mary Anne Lilley for their constant support and encouragement. Long hours and time spent researching and writing have pre-empted time with family, but they have been there through all five editions. Linda wishes to dedicate this book to her parents, John and Thelma Lane, who passed away during the fourth edition, and to her father-in-law, J.C. Lilley, who passed away during the last drafts of the fifth edition. Their memory continues to serve as inspiration and motivation for Linda's work with this book. Students and graduates of Old Dominion University School of Nursing have been eager to provide feedback and support, beginning with the class of 1990 and continuing through the class of 2005. Without their participation, the book would not have been so user-friendly and helpful to students beginning the study of drug therapy and subsequently applying this knowledge to nursing practice. Linda attributes

her successes and accomplishments to a strong sense of purpose, faith, family, and appreciation for the light-hearted side of life. To Jibby Baucom, Linda offers many thanks, because without her recommendation to Mosby, Inc., the book would never have been developed. Robin Carter and Kristin Geen have been constant resources and more than just editors with Elsevier; they have been sources of strength and encouragement. Working with Jamie Horn has been positive, and her calming nature and vision to succeed will forever be appreciated. The fifth edition also involved Clay Broeker, who has been a tremendous resource with editorial issues; his contributions to this edition have been strong and forward-thinking. Elsevier has shared some of its best employees with Linda beginning with day one of the first edition; for that, Linda is most thankful.

Scott extends his thanks to his fellow staff members at Northern Cochise Community Hospital: thank you for all of your consultations and questions that continuously help make me a better pharmacist. Thanks go to both hospital staff and citizens of Willcox and Tucson, Arizona, as well as family and friends, who have been kind enough to show interest in this project and to ask me how it was coming along. Your interest and enthusiasm helped me down the long road to completion. Thank you also to the staff and volunteers of the National Alliance for the Mentally Ill of Southern Arizona (NAMISA), where I continue to grow and learn through volunteer work, for your continued support and encouragement for this and other endeavors and for allowing me to be a part of your team. Very special thanks go to my dear friend Gerry Bovell, who allowed me to work on this project for many months at his home and congratulated me as I finished each chapter. Both he and my other friend, Ed Thorpe, also sometimes brought me food. Thanks go to both of them for their support and encouragement. Lastly, I offer heartfelt thanks to my mother and father, Bonnie and John Harrington, who granted me this life to begin with. My mother has an amazing heart and my father has an amazing mind. I believe that I was fortunate enough to inherit some of the best of both.

Julie thanks her husband Jonathan, her daughter Emily, and her parents, Willis and Jean Simmons, for their unfailing support and encouragement. They were all patient despite the long hours spent at the computer for revisions. Thanks also go to those who participated in the fourth edition photo shoot. At Chesapeake General Hospital, Doug Crowe in the Pharmacy Department was an unending source of answers and support. Thanks go to Kristin Geen, Jamie Horn, and others at Elsevier for keeping the project organized and on track, as well as for providing all the support needed for such a project. Thanks also to each student who provided feedback and comments on the text and study aids. Deep appreciation goes to Dr. Linda L. Lilley for her encouragement and mentoring over the years. Lastly, the support and encouragement of family and friends is vital to projects like this, so thanks and gratitude to all.

Finally, to those who teach, although your work may seem to go unnoticed or unappreciated, your impact will always be remembered in the accomplishments of your students. Your inspiration and motivation shape the future.

We always welcome comments from instructors and students who use this book so that we may continue to make improvements and be responsive to your needs in future editions. Please send any comments you may have in care of the publisher.

Linda Lane Lilley
Scott Harrington
Julie S. Snyder

Acknowledgments for the Second Canadian Edition

My part in this book would not have been possible without the original efforts of the American authors who conceptualized and wrote the first five U.S. editions of *Pharmacology and the Nursing Process*, the fifth edition of which has shaped the content of *Pharmacology for Canadian Health Care Practice*. Linda Lane Lilley, RN, PhD; Scott Harrington, PharmD; and Julie S. Snyder, MSN, RN, BC are to be commended for their thorough and expert handling of a vast and complex subject matter and for creating an excellent foundation over which the Canadian content could be easily laid.

I dedicate *Pharmacology for Canadian Health Care Practice* to my sons, Jeffrey I. and Derk, who continue to inspire me with their dedication, strength, and support; I could not have met the challenges of editing this pharmacology textbook without their encouragement and understanding. To my students, both past and present, who are a never-ending source of inspiration and who constantly challenge me to make material relevant, fun, and interesting, I give heartfelt thanks for inspiring my writing in this book. As part of a class activity, second-year students were asked to submit family stories about the use of natural health therapies for the new In My Family boxes included in this edition. While not all of their submissions could be incorporated into the text, numerous ones were, and I thank all of my students for their enthusiastic responses.

I could not have accomplished this project without the assistance of May Look, Developmental Editor, whose quirky sense of humour, dedication, attention to detail, and subtle reminders about deadlines kept me on track and made the task almost enjoyable! Many individuals at Elsevier Canada are responsible for this Canadian edition. My thanks go to Ann Millar, Publisher, who provided encouragement and ongoing support; Jerri Hurlbutt, Copy Editor, who responded almost immediately to all my calls for help, and pointed me in the right direction with a sense of humour and discussions of tennis; Tammy Scherer, Managing Developmental Editor; Roberta Spinosa-Millman, Managing Production Editor, for handling all the details involved in the final production of the book; and, finally, Brenda Kirkconnell, Director, e-Products, for her encouragement and friendship.

Thanks are due to the Canadian reviewers who reviewed content of this book and gave their invaluable comments, expertise, and editing suggestions on the draft manuscript. Thanks are also extended to Michelle Forbes, for her work in revising the Study Skills Tips sections.

As existing diseases and disorders and their treatments evolve, bringing with them new challenges and information in pharmacology, we will no doubt be looking forward to future editions of this textbook. Instructors and students are welcome to send comments to the publisher; your feedback will be invaluable to future editions.

Beth Swart

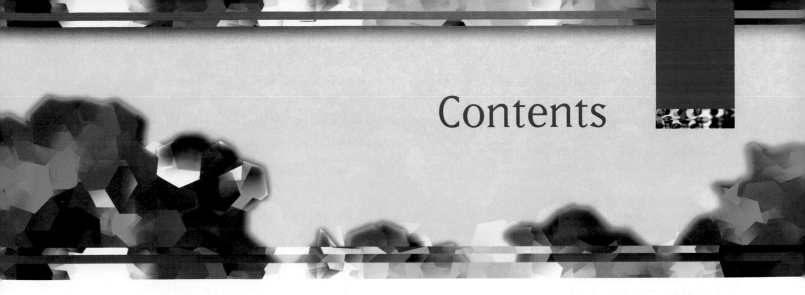

Contents

xviii CONTENTS

PART ONE

Pharmacology Basics

STUDY SKILLS TIPS:
- INTRODUCTION TO STUDY SKILLS CONCEPTS
- PURR
- PHARMACOLOGY BASICS

INTRODUCTION TO STUDY SKILLS CONCEPTS

What to study? When to study? How much to study? How to study? In the best of worlds, every student would have all the skills necessary to be effective in all academic areas. Unfortunately, many students do not know how to study effectively or have developed techniques that work well in some circumstance but not in others. The purpose of this Study Skills Tips section is to introduce you to the steps to follow in learning text and maintaining focus on the appropriate material. This section also offers some specific examples for selected chapters in Part One to help you apply the study techniques and strategies discussed here.

Extensive study skills covering time management, note taking, mastering of the text, preparation for and taking of examinations, and development of vocabulary are

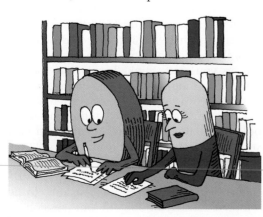

presented in the *Study Guide* that accompanies this text. These tools are important to any student, but even more valuable in challenging technical areas such as nursing and pharmacology. The techniques described here and in the *Study Guide* will not necessarily make learning easy, but they will help you achieve your goals as a student.

PURR

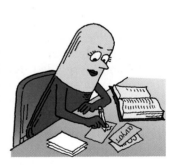

PURR is a handy mnemonic device representing a four-step process that will lead to mastery of material:
- *Prepare*
- *Understand*
- *Rehearse*
- *Review*

PURR has positive and negative aspects. The negative is that it requires that you go through every chapter four times. The good news is that you are not going to actually *read* the chapter four times. You are only going to *go through* it four times. Only one of those times is a slow, careful, intensive reading. The other trips through the chapter are much quicker. The first time you go through the chapter should only take 5 or 10 minutes. Each time you go through the chapter, you are processing the information in distinctly different ways. The PURR approach will enhance your learning, and if you use it from the first assignment on, you will find that it takes you less time than what you were spending before you adopted the PURR approach to learn what you need.

Prepare

As with any complex process, reading the text is not something to dive into without thought and planning. *Pharmacology for Canadian Health Care Practice* is organized to help you learn the material, but you have to take advantage of what the authors have done for you to facilitate this. Preparing to read means setting goals and objectives for your own learning; the tools you need to help you do this are already in place. Look at the opening pages of any chapter in the text and you will see a standard structure.

Every chapter begins with a **title**. Learn to use the title as the first step in preparing to learn. Chapter 4 is entitled "Ethnocultural, Legal, and Ethical Considerations." This instantly identifies what the chapter is about. Do not start reading immediately; instead think about the title for a few seconds. Are there any unfamiliar terms? If your answer is "no," great. If it is "yes," then you already have some focus for your reading because you know you will need to learn the unfamiliar terms and their meanings.

The next feature of every chapter is the **objectives**. You need objectives for learning, and the authors have anticipated this. Read the objectives actively. Do not just look at the words; think about the objectives. Ask yourself the following questions: What do I already know about this material? How do these objectives relate to earlier assignments? How do they relate to objectives the instructor has given? The chapter objectives identify things you should be able to do after you have read the material. Do not wait until you have read the chapter to start trying to respond. *Prepare* means getting the brain engaged from the beginning. Studying the chapter objectives establishes a direction and purpose for your reading. This will enable you to maintain concentration and focus while you read.

Another feature in the opening pages of each chapter is the **Glossary**. This is one of the most valuable tools the authors have provided. They know that there are many terms to learn and are giving you a head start on learning them. Spend a few minutes with the Glossary. Notice the terms that are also used in the chapter objectives. Go back and look at the objectives and think about what you have learned from the Glossary. As you study the Glossary, look for shared root words, prefixes, or suffixes. Words that share common elements usually also have a shared meaning. Learning the meaning of common word elements can simplify the whole process of learning vocabulary. Perhaps you remember in elementary school being told to "look for the little words in the big word." This is essentially the same technique—one that worked then and that will work now.

Now make a quick pass through the chapter or the assigned pages from the chapter. Focus on the text conventions, which are described later in this chapter. Look for anything that stands out in the chapter, such as boldfaced text, boxed material, and tables. This provides a quick overview of the chapter, which will make the next steps in the PURR process much more effective and efficient.

The **chapter headings** show the major points to be covered. Study them and notice the major headings (topics) and the subordinate headings (subtopics). This is essentially a picture of the chapter, and using the picture is an essential step in preparing to read. As you read through the chapter headings, turn the topics and subtopics into a series of questions that you want to be able to answer when you finish reading. Think about the objectives and how these headings relate to them. Finally, in the headings devoted to specific classes of agents, notice that there are elements that are common to every one. The last two headings are always "Implementation" and "Evaluation." This tells you that these are two common elements that you will be expected to know at the end of every chapter. The minutes you spend preparing will pay off in a big way when you start to read.

Preparing makes the whole approach to learning an active one. It may not make the chapters the most exciting reading you will ever do, but it will help you accomplish your personal learning objectives as well as those set by the authors.

On-the-Run Action. Preparing is great to do during "found" time. It should not take more than 5 or 10 minutes. Time between classes, time spent waiting for the coffee water to boil, or any other small block of time that usually just slips away can be used to accomplish this step.

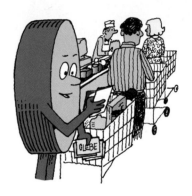

Understand

The time has now come to read the assignment. Go to your desk, the library, or wherever you have chosen for serious study. Reading the assignment is when all your preparation pays off. If you did the *Prepare* step earlier in the day, it is not a bad idea to spend a minute or two going through the chapter features again to get your focus. As you read the assignment, remember the chapter objectives and notice the chapter headings in the body of the chapter. As you read, rephrase the chapter headings as questions to help keep you focused on the task at hand. Because this is the first time you are really focusing on the concepts and the details, this is not the time to do any text notations. Read and, as you read, think. Terms from the Glossary are repeated, and their meanings are often expanded and clarified in the body of the text. Pay attention to these terms as you read. Think about what they mean and how you would define them to someone else. Read for meaning. Read to understand. Do not read just to get to the end of the assignment. That is a passive action. Ask yourself questions. Analyze, respond, and react as you read.

Often reading assignments are too long to be read with complete understanding in one session. If you find that your concentration is flagging or you do not remember anything you read on the previous page, it is time to take a break. All too often students have only one objective—to finish the assignment. You might be able to force yourself to continue reading, but you will not learn much. Mark your place and take a 5- or 10-minute break. Take a walk, read the daily comic strips, get a cold drink or a cup of coffee, and then go back to reading. When you come back to the assignment, spend the first 3 or 4 minutes reviewing. Look back at the previous chapter heading and think about what you were reading before the break. The chapter can be broken down into many small reading sessions, but it is critical that you do not lose sight of the chapter as a whole. Spending these few minutes in review may seem like time that could be better spent continuing with the reading, but this quick review will save time in the long run.

There is no quick way to read a chapter. You will not find an "on-the-run action" for this step because it cannot be done in this way. However, if you do the *Prepare* step first, you will be surprised at how much more easily you get the reading done and how much more learning you have achieved in the process.

Rehearse

Rehearsing is the third step in the process. It starts the process of consolidating learning and establishing a basis for long-term memory. Rehearsal accomplishes two things. First, it helps you find out what you understand from the reading. Knowing what you know is really important. Second, it identifies what you do not understand—this may be an even more important benefit. Knowing what you do not know before it appears during an examination is critical.

How to Rehearse. Everything you do in the *Prepare* and *Understand* steps comes into play in the *Rehearse* step. Rehearsal should begin with the features at the beginning of the chapter. Open the text to the beginning of the chapter. Start with the chapter title and begin to quiz yourself on what you have read. Compose three or four questions pertaining to the chapter title, and then try to answer them to your satisfaction. The questions you ask yourself should be both literal (asking for specific information presented in the chapter) and interpretive (testing your comprehension of concepts and relationships). An example of a literal question based on the Chapter 4 title might be, "What are the definitions of *ethnocultural*, *legal*, and *ethical*?" This question would help you determine whether you can satisfactorily define these terms in your own words. The process of asking and answering questions like these always serves to move learning from short-term to long-term memory. Literal questions are important to help you grasp the factual information and terminology contained in the reading assignment.

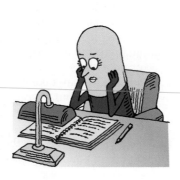

However, it is also necessary to ask questions that stimulate thought about the concepts and the relationships between the facts and concepts presented in the chapter. An example of an interpretive question regarding the Chapter 4 title might be, "What are the most important ethnocultural, legal, and ethical concepts pertaining to the use of drugs?" Sometimes you will find that, even though the question is interpretive, the authors have anticipated the question and the text contains the direct answer to your question. Other times you will need to formulate your own response by pulling together bits and pieces of information from the entire reading assignment.

Once you have exhausted the question potential for the chapter title, move on to the chapter objectives. Use the same process here. Rephrase the objectives as questions and try to answer them. Remember that the object of rehearsal is to reinforce what you have learned and to identify areas where you need to spend additional time (review).

Go to the Glossary. Cover the definitions, and try to define each term in your own words. Another method is to cover the term, and on the basis of the definition, name the term. Do not just memorize the definition because you may find the information presented differently on an examination and you will then be unable to respond.

Now proceed to the chapter or assigned pages. The chapter headings are the main tools for rehearsal. Apply the same question-and-answer technique used for the title and objectives to test what you may already know about the chapter content. Turn the headings into questions and answer them. Look at the text for boldfaced and italicized items, lists, and other text conventions. These too can become the basis for questions. The tables and diagrams should also be used for this purpose. Keep in mind the importance of asking both literal and interpretive questions. Some of the questions you ask yourself should also tie different topic headings together. Ask yourself how topic A relates to topic B.

As you proceed through the chapter, do not worry if you cannot answer the questions you ask. As stated earlier, one of the goals of the rehearsal process is to identify what you need to spend more time on. If you cannot respond to a particular question, put a mark in the margin of the

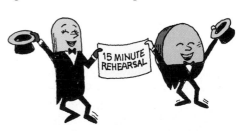

pertinent place in the text to remind yourself to come back and spend more time on this material, but move on at this point. Rehearsal should be a relatively quick procedure. Once you become accustomed to the PURR method, it should take no more than 15 or 20 minutes to rehearse 15 pages after doing the *Prepare* and *Understand* steps.

As you reach the end of the chapter, skim the Implementation and Evaluation sections. Make sure that the relationship between these sections and the information in the rest of the chapter is clear. If you have questions or concerns, note them in the margins and ask your instructor to clarify these points. Although the objective is to master the chapter content as an independent learner, sometimes it is essential to ask questions of the instructor to facilitate the process.

When to Rehearse. Ideally rehearsal should take place almost immediately after you finish reading the material. Take a 10- to 15-minute break, and then start the process. The longer the gap between reading and rehearsal, the more you will forget and the longer it will take to rehearse. If you are breaking a reading assignment down into smaller segments, do the rehearsal for each segment before you begin reading the new material. This helps maintain the sense of continuity in the chapter. This seems like a lot of work to do in a study session, but with practice it will go quickly and you will be pleasantly surprised at the quality and quantity of your learning.

Review

Review is the fourth and final step in the PURR process, and it is an essential step. No matter how well you have learned material in the preceding steps, forgetfulness will always occur. Reviewing is the only way to store what you have learned in long-term memory. The good news is that, using the PURR model, the review can be done for small segments of material and can be done relatively quickly.

How to Review. The basic review process is essentially the same as the rehearsal process, with some limited rereading as the only difference. When you cannot immediately answer a question, read the pertinent material again. *This does not mean you should read the entire chapter again.* Often the answer to the question will pop into your mind after you have read only a few lines. When this happens, stop reading and go back to responding to your question. The idea is to reread only as much material as is necessary to make the answer clear. One or two words or one or two sentences may trigger personal recall, but it may also take two or three paragraphs for this to happen.

Frequency of Review. How many times should you review material in this way? This actually depends on many factors, such as the difficulty of the material, the length of the assignment, and your personal background. Only you can determine how often you need to review, but some guidelines will help you decide this for yourself.

First, consider the difficulty of the material. If it is complex, contains many new terms and difficult concepts, and seems difficult to grasp, then you should review frequently. On the other hand, if the material is straightforward and you are able to relate it well to what you have already learned, then less frequent reviews will serve to keep the material in your memory.

Second, consider how well the review went. If you had difficulty answering many questions to your satisfaction or had to do a lot of rereading, you should schedule another review soon (a day or two later at most).

Use the success of each review session to help you determine when to schedule another session. The review step is a means of monitoring the success of the learning process. If reviews go well, with limited rereading being necessary, and you are able to give clear answers to your questions, then you can wait several days (4 or 5) before reviewing this material again. A mediocre review, with more extensive rereading and poor answers, indicates that you should let only 2 or 3 days go by before reviewing the material again. If the review goes poorly, you should plan to review the material again the next day. It is up to you to judge the success of each review and to decide how often you need to review. The nice thing about PURR is that it enables you to monitor your success and easily regulate the learning process.

Technique for Rehearsal and Review. Both rehearsal and review foster active learning, which helps you maintain interest in the material and strengthens your memory. For these benefits to occur, it is essential to review and rehearse orally. Simply talk aloud as you go through the material. Ask questions and give your answers out loud. This forces you to think about the material and helps you organize it and translate it into your own words. The object is not to memorize everything you have read but to understand and be able to explain it. Eventually you will need to answer questions on an examination. Framing questions as a part of the learning process is a way to anticipate examination questions. The more questions you ask yourself during study time, the more likely it is that some of the questions on the examination will be ones you have asked yourself. Furthermore, by doing the rehearsal and review orally, you will find it easier to recall the answers during the examination because this oral model requires more than just remembering seeing the material; you will actually be able to hear the rehearsed answers in your mind. Another advantage of doing the rehearsal and review processes orally is, as stated earlier, that it helps to identify what needs further study. When your oral answer is fragmentary, contains many "uh's," and is really disorganized, then you know that you need to devote more time to learning that particular term, fact, or concept.

The PURR system may seem like a lot of work at first. Understandably, the idea of going through a chapter four times seems daunting. Add to this the need for several review sessions, and the first reaction is likely to be, "This won't work" or "I don't have the time to do this." Don't take that attitude. This system does work. It cultivates interest, aids concentration, fosters mastery of the material, and ensures long-term retention of the material, which is important not just for doing well on examinations but also for doing well as a nurse—the safe care of patients is at stake. The PURR system will work if you use it. It may take 3 or 4 weeks to get comfortable with the system, but if you keep at it, pretty soon it will become a good habit. After a while you will not be able to imagine studying in any other way.

Like all study systems, the PURR method is a model. As you use it, you may discover ways of changing it that work better for you. That is okay. Do not hesitate to make adjustments that better suit your learning style and strategies. Just remember as you start out that *Preparation, Understanding, Rehearsal,* and *Review* are solid learning principles and cannot be ignored.

Study skills tips are included on the two pages at the beginning of each part. These hints are directly applied to the content found within the chapters contained in that part. Detailed information on specialized study skills, such as time management, note taking, 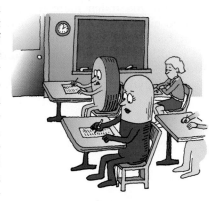 examination preparation, and vocabulary building, are present in the *Study Guide* that accompanies this text.

PHARMACOLOGY BASICS

Prepare

As you begin to work with individual chapters, consider how the first step in the PURR system can be used to help you set a purpose and become an active learner.

Chapter 1 Objectives

Consider Objective 1: "List the five phases of the nursing process as applicable to drug therapy." Now turn the objective into a question: *What are the five phases of the nursing process?* Now move to Objective 2 and make it a question: *What are the components of the assessment process for patients receiving medications, including the collection and analysis of subjective and objective data?*

You might recognize that this question relates to Objective 1 because assessment is one phase of the nursing process. By putting Objective 2 into a question format, you begin to expand on the focus of the first objective, and you begin focusing on active learning with a clear purpose.

When you begin to read Chapter 1, you will discover that the five phases of the nursing process are repeated as topic headings, and you have the Objective 2 question on which to focus your reading. Begin now to develop the habit of applying this strategy to the objectives in every chapter assigned before you begin to read. Remember to look at the chapter headings at this point as well. It is amazing how much can be learned by using the text structures provided.

Vocabulary Development

Turn to Chapter 2. Objective 1 makes an important point: "Define common terms used in pharmacology." Success depends heavily on knowledge of the language used in the field. The objective makes it clear that this chapter contains a number of terms that the author views as important to be mastered. Starting particularly with Chapter 2, it is time to start mastering the language of this content. Look at the Glossary. There are six terms that share the common element *pharmaco*. Although each of these six words has a different meaning, they all have something in common. *Pharmaco* is an example of a group word. No matter what prefixes, group words, or suffixes are added to it, a part of the meaning of any word containing *pharmaco* will be "drug" or "medicine." Look up *pharmaco* in any dictionary and you will find "drug" or "medicine" as the definition. Although you probably already knew that, it is always beneficial when working on a new technique to start with something that is familiar. Look at four of the words that begin with *pharmaco*, and consider the rest of the words:

dynamics   genetics   gnosy   kinetics

What do each of these word parts mean? The meaning of *pharmacodynamics* is simply the combination of the meaning of *pharmaco* and *dynamics*. The definition, according

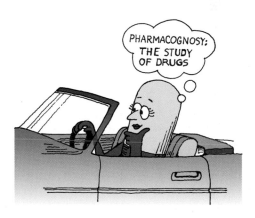

to the Glossary, begins, "the study of the biochemical and physiological interactions of drugs at their sites of activity." You could simply memorize this definition, which would seem to accomplish Objective 1. However, memorization does not always equal understanding. Try another approach. What does *dynamics* mean? Think about the word, and relate it to your own experience and background. It appears to deal with movement or action. After looking it up in the dictionary, all the meanings given seem to relate in some fashion to the idea of motion or action. A simplistic definition of *pharmacodynamics* would be "drugs in action." Certainly this is not a technical or medical definition, but it contributes a great deal to an understanding of the definition provided in the Glossary. This is the object of learning vocabulary. Do not memorize words without understanding. Apply a little thought, and relate the term and definition in a way that makes the meaning personal for you. When you do that, you will find that you understand the Glossary definition better, and your ability to retain the meaning will be significantly improved. This means that the test item that asks you to select the definition for *pharmacodynamics* from a list of similar definitions will be much easier because you will remember action and movement and look for the choice that best represents that concept.

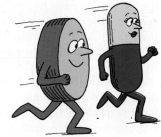

Apply this same strategy to *genetics*. You already know what genetics means. Now you must determine how to connect that to the meaning in the text. After you have the definitions of *gnosy* and *kinetics*, you can apply the same procedure. When you have done this with all four words, you will discover that you will not need to spend a great amount of time trying to memorize esoteric definitions; you will have personalized the meanings. Those meanings will stay with you much more readily than those learned by rote memorization. And by the way, do you know what *biochemical* and *physiological* mean? These terms are used in the Glossary definition of *pharmacodynamics*. You need to know what they mean to fully understand pharmacodynamics.

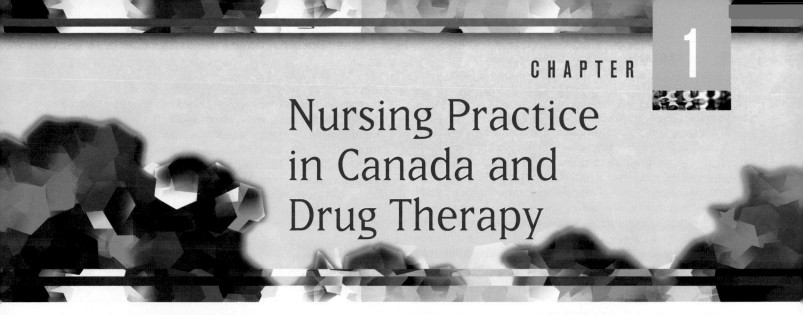

Nursing Practice in Canada and Drug Therapy

Learning Objectives

After reading this chapter, the successful student will be able to do the following:

1 List the five phases of the nursing process as applicable to drug therapy.

2 Identify the components of the assessment process for patients receiving medications, including the collection and analysis of subjective and objective data.

3 Discuss the process of formulating nursing diagnoses for patients receiving medications.

4 Identify goals and outcome criteria for patients receiving medications.

5 Discuss the key elements of implementation in the administration of medications.

6 Discuss the evaluation process involved in the administration of medications and reflected in the goals and outcome criteria.

7 Develop a collaborative plan of care using the nursing process and medication administration.

8 Identify the "Ten Rights" of drug administration and the related professional responsibility to patients for safe medication practice.

e-Learning Activities

Web site
(http://evolve.elsevier.com/Canada/Lilley/pharmacology/)

- Animations
- Answers to chapter questions, activities, and case studies
- Calculators and Category Catchers
- Glossary with audio pronunciations
- IV Therapy and Medication Error Checklists
- Multiple-Choice Review Question quizzes
- Nursing Care Plans
- Online Appendices and Supplements
- WebLinks

Glossary

Critical thinking Major component of the nursing process and often considered to be the underpinning of providing the best possible patient care supported by current and progressive approaches. (p. 8)

Goals Statements that are time specific and describe generally what is to be accomplished to address a specific nursing diagnosis. (p. 12)

Medication error Any preventable adverse drug event involving inappropriate medication use by a patient or health care provider. (p. 13)

Nursing process An organizational framework for the practice of nursing that encompasses all steps taken by the nurse in caring for a patient: assessment, nursing diagnoses, planning (with goals and outcome criteria), implementation of the plan (with patient teaching), and evaluation. (p. 8)

Outcome criteria Descriptions of specific patient behaviours or responses that demonstrate the meeting or achievement of goals related to each nursing diagnosis. (p. 12)

OVERVIEW

The nursing practice environment in Canada is increasingly demanding due in part to the increased acuity and complexity of patient care and the aging population. Nurses are expected to keep up-to-date with the rising use of intricate pharmacological therapies including natural health products and over-the-counter drugs. In addition to rising costs, other factors, such as professional shortages, advances in treatment modalities, and new technologies continue to challenge the health care system. In such an environment, knowledge of drugs, their adverse effects, and interactions is critical for nurses to provide safe, competent care. Greater accountability is expected of nurses with increased attention focused on safe medication practices. Evaluating and promoting therapeutic effects, as well as reducing the harm associated with adverse effects, adverse interactions, and drug toxicity, and making decisions about *prn* (*pro re nata* or "as needed") medications require excellent critical thinking and decision-making skills.

The **nursing process** is a well-established, research-supported framework for professional nursing practice. It is a flexible, adaptable, and adjustable five-step process consisting of *assessment*, *nursing diagnoses*, *planning* (including the establishment of **goals** and **outcome criteria**), *implementation* (including patient education), and *evaluation*. As such, the nursing process ensures the delivery of thorough, individualized, and quality nursing care to patients, regardless of age, gender, ethnicity or culture, medical diagnosis, or setting. When use of the nursing process is combined with knowledge and skills, the professional nurse is well equipped to develop effective solutions to meet patient needs. Although the use of the nursing process is seen as controversial in some educational and health care institutions, it is still the major systematic framework for professional nursing practice. The nursing process is usually discussed within nursing courses and in textbooks on the fundamentals of nursing practice, nursing theory, physical assessment, adult and pediatric nursing, and other nursing specialty areas. However, because the nursing process is so important in the care of patients, the nursing process is addressed in this textbook and applied in the chapters as it relates to drug therapy and patient education. Along with evidence-informed practice, the process, with all five phases, will be included in each chapter of this book as related to specific drug groups and classifications.

Box 1-1 provides a sample collaborative plan of care based on drug therapy and the nursing process. Examples of collaborative plans of care for specific disorders are located online at http://evolve.elsevier.com/Canada/Lilley/pharmacology/.

ASSESSMENT

Importance of Critical Thinking to the Nursing Process

Critical thinking is a major component of the nursing process and often considered to be the underpinning to provide the best possible patient care supported by current and progressive approaches. It involves using the mind to develop conclusions, make decisions, draw inferences, and reflect on all aspects of the patient. These aspects include the physical, emotional, spiritual, sexual, financial, ethnocultural, and cognitive parts of a patient. Attention to these many aspects allows a more *holistic* approach to patient care. Thus, higher-level thinking and decision-making skills are requisite for nurses to enable them to deliver quality care, including medication administration. The Canadian Nurses Association (CNA, 2002) recognizes critical thinking as a "complex, active, and purposeful process encompassing the essential skills of interpretation and evaluation and requiring the RN [registered nurse] to go beyond the role of performance of skills and interventions" (p. 18). Critical thinking "compels the RN to identify and challenge assumptions, use an organized approach to assessment, check for accuracy and reliability of information, distinguish relevant from irrelevant, normal from abnormal and recognize inconsistencies, cluster related information, identify patterns and missing information and draw valid conclusions based on evidence, identify different concurrent conclusions and underlying causes, set priorities, and evaluate and correct thinking" (CNA, 2002, p. 18).

According to Wilkinson (2006), critical thinkers have the following characteristics: (1) the ability to generate ideas rapidly; (2) flexibility and spontaneity (i.e., ability to discard one viewpoint for another or change directions in thinking quickly and easily); (3) the ability to provide original solutions to problems; (4) they prefer complex thought processes to simple and easily understood ones; (5) they demonstrate independence and self-confidence, even when under pressure; and (6) they exhibit distinct individualism (p. 41).

The professional nurse critically thinks, processes, and integrates all of the points of information about the patient and develops and coordinates patient care.

Assessing the Patient and Drugs

During the initial assessment phase of the nursing process, data are collected, reviewed, and analyzed. Performing a comprehensive assessment allows the nurse to formulate a nursing diagnosis related to the patient's needs and, specifically, for the purposes of this textbook, needs related to drug administration. Information about the patient and environment may come from a variety of sources, including the patient, the patient's family, caregiver, or significant other, and the patient's chart. Methods of data collection include interviewing, direct and indirect questioning, observation, medical records review, and head-to-toe physical examination (nursing assessment). Data are categorized into *objective* and *subjective data*. *Objective data* may be defined as any information gathered through the senses (that which is seen, heard, felt, or smelled). Objective data may also be obtained through a nursing physical

BOX 1-1	Sample Collaborative Plan of Care Related to Drug Therapy Using the Nursing Process

This sample presents information useful for developing a nursing process–focused care plan for patients receiving medications. Brief listings and suggestions of what should be presented in each phase of the nursing process are included. The sample may be used as a template for formatting plans of care in a variety of patient care situations. Only one nursing diagnosis will be presented with each plan throughout the book.

Assessment

Objective Data
Objective data include information available through the senses, such as what is seen, felt, heard, and smelled. Among the sources of data are the chart, laboratory test results, reports of diagnostic procedures, health history, physical assessment, and examination findings. Other examples include age, height, weight, allergies, medication profile, and health history.

Subjective Data
Subjective data include all spoken information shared by the patient such as complaints, problems, or stated needs (e.g., patient complaints of "dizziness, headache, vomiting, and feeling hot for 10 days").

Nursing Diagnosis

Once the assessment phase has been completed, the nurse analyzes the objective and subjective data about the patient and the drug and formulates nursing diagnoses. The following is an example of a nursing diagnosis statement: "Deficient knowledge related to lack of experience with medication regime and second-grade reading level as an adult as evidenced by inability to perform a return demonstration and inability to state adverse effects to report to the physician." This statement can be broken down into three parts, as follows:
- Part 1: "Deficient knowledge"
  This part of the statement reflects the patient's human response to illness, injury, medications, or significant change. This can be an actual response, an increased risk, or an opportunity to improve the patient's health status.
- Part 2: "Related to lack of experience with medication regime and second-grade reading level as an adult."
  This statement identifies factors related to the response; it often includes multiple factors with some degree of connection between them. The nursing diagnosis statement does not necessarily claim that there is a cause-and-effect link between these factors and the response, only that there is a connection.
- Part 3: "As evidenced by inability to perform a return demonstration and inability to state adverse effects to report to the physician."

This statement lists clues, cues, evidence, and data that support the nurse's claim that the nursing diagnosis is accurate.

Nursing diagnoses are prioritized in order of critically based patient needs or problems. The ABCs of care (airway, breathing, and circulation) are used as a basis for prioritization. Prioritizing always begins with the most important, significant, or critical need of the patient. Nursing diagnoses that involve actual responses are always ranked above nursing diagnoses that involve only risks.

Planning: Goals and Outcome Criteria

The planning phase includes the identification of goals and outcome criteria, provides time frames, and is patient oriented. Goals are objective, verifiable, realistic, and measurable patient-centred statements with time frames and are broad, whereas outcome criteria are more specific descriptions of patient goals. For examples of goal and outcome criteria for select disorders, see the Collaborative Care Plans available at http://evolve. elsevier.com/Canada/Lilley/pharmacology/.

Implementation

In the implementation phase, the nurse intervenes on behalf of the patient to address specific patient problems and needs. This is done through independent nursing actions; collaborative activities such as physical therapy, occupational therapy, and music therapy; and implementation of medical orders. Family, the significant other, and other caregivers assist in carrying out this phase of the collaborative care plan. Specific interventions that relate to particular drugs (e.g., giving a particular cardiac drug only after monitoring the patient's pulse and blood pressure), nonpharmacological interventions that enhance the therapeutic effects of medications, and patient education are major components of the implementation phase. See the discussion of the nursing process in the main text of this chapter for more information on nursing interventions.

Evaluation

Evaluation is the part of the nursing process that includes monitoring whether patient goals and outcome criteria related to the nursing diagnoses are met. Monitoring includes observing for therapeutic effects of drug treatment as well as for adverse effects and toxicity. Many indicators are used to monitor these aspects of drug therapy and the results of appropriately related nonpharmacological interventions. If the goals and outcome criteria are met, the plan of care may or may not be revised to include new nursing diagnoses; such changes are made only if appropriate. If goals and outcome criteria are not met, then revisions are made to the entire plan of care with further evaluation.

assessment, nursing history, past and present medical history, laboratory reports, results of diagnostic studies and procedures, vital signs, weight, height, and

medication profile. A comprehensive medication profile should include, but not be limited to, collection of data about the following:

- Any and all drug use
- Use of natural health products
- Intake of alcohol, tobacco, and caffeine
- Use of over-the-counter (OTC) medications, including, but not limited to, aspirin or acetaminophen products, vitamins, laxatives, cold preparations, sinus medications, antacids, acid reducers, antidiarrheals, minerals, and elements
- Use of hormonal drugs (e.g., testosterone, estrogens, progestins, and oral contraceptives)
- Past and present health history and associated drug regimen
- Family history and any racial, ethnic, or cultural differences, with attention to specific and different responses to medications
- Any unusual responses to medications
- Growth and developmental stages (e.g., Erikson's Developmental Tasks) and related issues to the patient's age and medication use

A holistic nursing assessment would include gathering data about religious preferences, health beliefs, sociocultural profile, race, ethnicity, lifestyle, stressors, socioeconomic status, educational level, motor skills, cognitive ability, support systems, lifestyle, and use of any alternative or complementary therapies. *Subjective data* include information shared by the spoken word from any reliable source (e.g., patient, spouse, family member, significant other, and caregiver).

Assessment of the drug is also important. Specific information about use of prescribed, OTC, natural health products should be obtained, including signs and symptoms of allergic reactions; administration routes; recommended dosages; actions; contraindications; drug incompatibilities; drug–drug, drug–food, and drug–laboratory test interactions; and adverse effects and toxic effects. Nursing pharmacology textbooks provide a more nursing-specific knowledge base regarding drug therapy (and the nursing process) and use of current references (e.g., references dated within the previous 5 years). Some examples of authoritative resources include the *Compendium of Pharmaceuticals and Specialties* (*CPS*; a subscription-based e-CPS is also available online), the drug manufacturer's insert, drug handbooks, and a licensed pharmacist. Some reliable online resources include the following (although this is not a comprehensive listing):

- Health Canada's Drug Product Database (http://www.hc-sc.gc.ca/dhp-mps/prodpharma/databasdon/index-eng.php)
- Objective Comparisons for Optimal Drug Therapy (http://www.rxfiles.ca/).

Data gathering about the patient and drug may be done through asking simple questions, such as the following:

- What is the patient's oral intake and tolerance of fluids? What is the patient's swallowing ability for pills, tablets, capsules, and liquids? If there is difficulty swallowing, what is the degree of difficulty? Are there solutions to the problem (e.g., "thickening" of fluids for some patients) or are there other dosage forms needed?

- What laboratory and diagnostic tests are related to organ functioning and drug therapy? What do the renal panel tests such as blood urea nitrogen level or serum creatinine level show? What are the results of liver function tests such as total protein level and serum levels of bilirubin, alkaline phosphatase, alanine aminotransferase, and other liver enzymes? What are the patient's red blood cell count, hemoglobin level, hematocrit, and white blood cell count?
- What have been the patient's previous and current experiences with health, illness, prescription drug use, and use of natural health products and other alternative medications? How were the patient's previous relationships with health care professionals, and what is the patient's previous experience with hospitalization?
- What are past and present values for blood pressure, pulse rate, temperature, and respiratory rate?
- In addition to the medication profile, how is the patient taking medications, and how is the patient tolerating them? Are there adherence issues? Is there any application of folklore?
- What does the given drug do? Is it really helping the patient? What is the patient's understanding of this information?
- What are a given drug's adverse effects, contraindications, appropriate dosages, routes of administration, therapeutic levels, and toxicity and any antidotes?
- What emotional, physical, cognitive, ethnocultural, and socioeconomic factors are influencing drug therapy and the nursing process for the patient (for a holistic framework)?
- Are there any age-specific medication concerns?

These are just a few sample questions that may be posed to patients, family members, significant others, and caregivers.

Once assessment of the patient and of the drug has been completed, the specific prescription or medication order from the physician or other professional licensed or certified prescriber must be checked for the following six elements:

1. Patient's full name
2. Date and time the order was written
3. Generic and trade name of the drug to be administered
4. Dosage of the drug (includes size, frequency, and number of doses)
5. Route of administration
6. Signature of the prescriber

The essential components of a prescription include the following elements:

- Descriptive information about the patient: name, address, and sometimes age, health insurance number (or identification number)
- Date on which the prescription was written
- The Rx symbol, meaning "take thou"
- Medication name, dosage, and strength
- Route of administration
- Dispensing instructions for the pharmacist; for example, "Dispense 30 capsules"

- Directions for administration to be given to the patient; for example, "Sig. Tab 1 with meals"
- Refill or special labelling, for example, "Refill 3×"
- Prescriber's signature

During assessment it is important to consider the traditional, nontraditional, expanded, and collaborative roles of the nurse. Physicians and dentists are no longer the only health care providers prescribing and writing medication orders. Nurse practitioners have gained the professional privilege to legally prescribe medications. Nurses should always be aware of these roles and be familiar with the specific provincial/territorial standards for nursing practice. For nurses in Canada, standards are based on professional values articulated in the Code of Ethics for Registered Nurses.

Analysis of Data

Once data about the patient and drug have been collected and reviewed, the nurse must critically analyze and synthesize the information. All information should be verified and documented appropriately, and it is at this point that the sum of the information about the patient and drug are used in the development of nursing diagnoses.

NURSING DIAGNOSES

Nursing diagnoses are developed by professional nurses and are used as a means of communicating and sharing information about the patient and the patient experience. Nursing diagnoses are the result of critical thinking, creativity, and accurate data collection about the patient and the drug.

Nursing diagnoses related to drug therapy will most likely develop out of data associated with the following: deficient knowledge; risk of injury; nonadherence; and various disturbances, deficits, excesses, or impairments in bodily functions and other problems or concerns as noted by the North American Nursing Diagnosis Association (NANDA).

NANDA is a formal organization recognized by professional groups such as the Canadian Nurses Association (CNA) and the American Nurses Association as being the major contributor to the development of nursing knowledge and is considered the leading authority in the development and classification of nursing diagnoses. The purpose of NANDA is to increase the visibility of nursing's contribution to the care of patients and to further develop, refine, and classify the information and phenomena related to nurses and professional nursing practice. The use of a standardized language of nursing diagnoses documents the analysis, synthesis, and accuracy required in making a nursing diagnosis and establishes nursing's contribution to cost-effective, efficient, quality health care.

More recently, a long-term project of the International Council of Nurses (ICN) to provide a unified language system was initiated. The International Classification for Nursing Practice (ICNP) is a framework that can be cross-mapped with other health care classification systems such as NANDA to create multidisciplinary health vocabularies or lexicons within information systems. The overall intent is that nursing diagnoses, nursing interventions, and nursing outcomes within the ICNP would be used in health care record documentation. The Canadian Nurses Association has recommended that the ICNP be the foundational framework for Canadian nursing practice (CNA, 2002). The objectives of the ICNP are as follows: (1) to establish a common language for describing nursing practice in order to improve communication among nurses and between nurses and others; (2) to describe the nursing care of people (individuals, families, and communities) in a variety of settings, both institutional and noninstitutional; (3) to enable comparison of nursing data across clinical populations, settings, geographic areas, and time; (4) to demonstrate or project trends in the provision of nursing treatments and care and the allocation of resources to patients according to their needs based on nursing diagnoses; (5) to stimulate nursing research through links to data available in nursing information systems and health information systems; and (6) to provide data about nursing practice in order to influence health policymaking.

Formulation of nursing diagnoses is usually a three-step process. The first part of the nursing diagnosis statement is the human response of the patient to illness, injury, or significant change. This response can be an actual problem, an increased risk of developing a problem, or an opportunity or intent to increase the patient's health. The second part of the nursing diagnosis statement identifies the factor or factors related to the response, and more than one factor is often named. The nursing diagnosis statement does not necessarily claim a cause–effect link between those factors and the response, but only indicates that there is a connection between them. The third part of the nursing diagnosis statement lists clues, cues, evidence, or other data that support the nurse's claim that this diagnosis is accurate.

Some tips for writing a nursing diagnosis are as follows:
- Start with a statement of a *human response*.
- Connect the first part of the statement or human response with the second part, the cause, using the phrase *related to.*
- Be sure that the first two parts are not restatements of one another.
- Several factors may be included in the second part of the statement (i.e., the etiology).
- Select a cause for the second part of the statement that can be changed by nursing interventions.
- Avoid negative wording or language.
- List clues or cues that led to the nursing diagnosis in the third part of the statement, which may also include more defining characteristics (e.g., *as evidenced by*).

There are currently more than 170 nursing diagnoses. See http://evolve.elsevier.com/Canada/Lilley/pharmacology for a list of NANDA-approved diagnoses. These nursing diagnoses, as well as all other phases of the nursing process, will be presented in the chapters to follow because of the framework of practice that the nursing process provides to all professional nurses.

PLANNING

After data are collected and nursing diagnoses formulated, the planning phase begins; this includes identification of goals and the outcome criteria. The major purposes of the planning phase are to prioritize the nursing diagnoses and to specify goals and outcome criteria, including time frames for their achievement. The planning phase provides time to obtain special equipment for interventions, review the possible procedures or techniques to be used, and gather information either for the nurse or for the patient. This step leads to the provision of safe care if professional judgement is combined with the acquisition of knowledge about the patient and the medications to be given.

Goals and Outcome Criteria

Goals are objective, measurable, and realistic, with an established time period for achievement of the outcomes, which are specifically stated in the outcome criteria. Patient goals reflect expected changes through nursing care. The **outcome criteria** (concrete descriptions of patient goals) should be succinct, well thought out, and patient focused. They should include expectations of behaviour (something that can be changed) that are to be met by certain deadlines. The ultimate aim of these criteria is the safe and effective administration of medications, and they should relate to each nursing diagnosis and guide implementation of the nursing care. Formulation of outcome criteria begins with the analysis of the judgements made about all of the patient data and subsequent nursing diagnoses and ends with the development of a collaborative care plan. Outcome criteria provide a standard for measuring movement toward goals. They may address special storage and handling techniques, administration procedures, equipment needed, drug interactions, adverse effects, and contraindications. In this textbook, specific time frames generally are *not* provided in the discussion of the nursing process because each patient care situation is individualized. Patient-oriented outcome criteria must apply to any medications the patient will receive. For example, the outcome criteria for a 43-year-old male with diabetes mellitus might be focused on the administration of insulin and general aspects of insulin therapy. In this situation, the patient-oriented outcome criteria revolve around specific patient education regarding insulin, adverse effects, contraindications, and injection techniques. It is also during the planning phase that planning for the unexpected must occur as well as planning to allow the nurse to be ready for any status or order changes.

IMPLEMENTATION

Implementation involves the use of nursing interventions to activate the plan and is guided by the preceding phases of the nursing process (e.g., assessment, nursing diagnoses, planning). Implementation requires constant communication and collaboration with the patient and with members of the health care team involved in the patient's care, including any family members, significant other, or other caregivers. Implementation consists of initiation and completion of specific actions by the nurse as defined by nursing diagnoses, goals, and outcome criteria. Nursing interventions or actions may be independent, collaborative, or dependent upon a physician's order.

With medication administration, the nurse needs to know and understand all of the information about the patient and about each medication prescribed (see assessment questions on p. 10). Implementation is based on the nurse's clinical judgement and knowledge. The Standards for Nursing Practice and Indicators and the Code of Ethics are upheld at all times.

The nurse must also adhere to safe administration practices to prevent errors. Such practices are often referred to as the "rights" of medication administration. The traditional "Five Rights" include *right drug, right dose, right time, right route,* and *right patient.* However, there are additional rights that also must be considered when administering medications (summarized in Box 1-2). *Right reason* and *right documentation* as well as *patient education,* the *patient's right to refuse* a drug, and *evaluation* of the drug's effects are additional rights to be considered when administering drugs. These Ten Rights are discussed in the next sections of this chapter.

Right Drug

Administration of the right drug begins with the nurse's valid license to practice. Some provinces and territories allow practical nurses to administer medications; they should also hold a current license. Unregulated care providers (UCPs) may also assist with medication administration. Nurses may teach UCPs medication administration and documentation, but the nurse remains ultimately accountable for the process of medication administration. The registered nurse should check all medication orders and prescriptions. To ensure that the correct drug is given, the nurse must check the specific medication order against the medication label or profile three times prior to giving the medication, beginning with the first check of the right drug and drug name while preparing medications for administration (see Box 1-3 on p. 14). At this time, the nurse should also consider whether the drug is appropriate for the patient; if in doubt or an error is deemed possible, the physician should be contacted immediately. At this time it would also be appropriate to note the drug's indication and be aware that a drug may have multiple indications.

All medication orders or prescriptions must be signed by the physician, nurse practitioner, or other health care provider. If there is a verbal order, the prescriber should sign the order within 24 hours or as per facility protocol. Verbal or telephone orders are often used in emergency

BOX 1-2   "Rights" of Medication Administration: The Five, Seven, or Ten Rights

In discussing the "rights" of medication administration, the literature tends to vary on the number of rights there are to consider, and students will notice references to "Five," "Seven," or "Ten" rights. Traditionally, the following five points (in no particular order of importance) are considered to be the basic Five Rights of medication administration (see the main text in this chapter for a detailed discussion of these rights):

- *Right Drug (or Right Medication):* Ensuring that the drug to be administered is the right medication that was ordered.
- *Right Dose:* Ensuring that the dose ordered is correct for the patient's age and body parameters, and questioning doses that do not seem correct or are outside the patient's usual dose range.
- *Right Time:* Ensuring that the drug is administered at the time ordered, and at the right frequency and according to institutional policy.
- *Right Route:* Ensuring that the drug is administered by the route ordered, as well as verifying that the route is safe and appropriate for the patient.
- *Right Patient:* Ensuring the drug is being administered to the patient it was intended for, by checking the drug order information against the patient's identification band.

When referring to Seven Rights, the following two points are usually included:

- *Right Reason:* Ensuring that the drug ordered is being given for the right reason, thus necessitating prior knowledge of the drug's actions and adverse effects.
- *Right Documentation:* Ensuring that documentation of the medication administration is done after the drug has been administered, not before; moreover, ensuring that any unusual variances in time, dose, and drug reactions are properly recorded, as well as if the patient has refused the drug.

Finally, the next three points round out the total Ten Rights:

- *Right Evaluation (or Right Assessment):* Ensuring that any special assessment requirements have been made prior to the drug administration, such as specific pulse rate and blood pressure readings, and laboratory results; moreover, ensuring that appropriate monitoring of the patient has been done following drug administration and that follow-up measures are taken if the drug has not achieved its desired effect.
- *Right Patient Education:* Ensuring that the patient has been given proper explanation of the drug being given, the reason for its administration, and what to expect in terms of the drug's effects and possible adverse effects.
- *Right to Refuse:* Ensuring that patients know they have a right to refuse the drug being administered and informing them properly of the potential consequences of refusal.

situations or time-sensitive patient care situations. To ensure that the right drug is given, the nurse must obtain information about the patient and drug (see previous discussion under Assessment) to ensure that all factors have been considered. Information about prescribed drugs should come from authoritative sources (see previous discussion under Assessment). Relying upon knowledge from peers is discouraged. The professional nurse should be familiar with the *generic* (nonproprietary) drug name as well as the *trade name* (proprietary name that is registered by a specific drug manufacturer); however, use of the drug's generic name is now preferred in clinical practice to reduce the risk of **medication errors** (preventable adverse drug events involving inappropriate medication use by a patient or health care provider). Trade names for drugs are often numerous, and similarly spelled names occur across drug classifications, leading to possible medication errors. If the nurse has any questions at any time during the process, the nurse should contact the physician to clarify the order. The nurse should never *assume* anything when it comes to drug administration and, as previously emphasized in this chapter, the nurse should check for adherence with all of the rights before giving the medication.

There are literally thousands of pharmaceutical drugs available. To learn about each drug individually would be an impossible task. Typically, drugs are usually systematically grouped into categories or classifications according to the action on the organ or system in the body, therapeutic use or relief of symptoms, or the desired effect, making the task of learning about drugs a little less daunting. Understanding how a class of drugs affects the cellular, tissue, organ, and functional system levels enables the nurse to gain knowledge about a wide range of drugs. For example, the classification of all drugs used for hypertension is *antihypertensives* and may include diuretics, angiotensin converting enzyme inhibitors, or calcium channel blockers. Each of the classes may also be used to treat other conditions (e.g., diuretics are also used to manage heart failure).

Within this textbook, a key drug within a classification will be highlighted and discussed thoroughly. One key drug will also be compared with other drugs within the classification. Common characteristics of the drug classification will be profiled such as its major uses, mechanisms of action, absorption, distribution, metabolism and excretion, onset and duration of action, and adverse effects.

Right Dose

Whenever a medication is ordered, a dosage is also identified from the order. The nurse must always check the dose and confirm that it is appropriate to the patient's age and size and check the prescribed dose against what is available and against what the normal dosage range is. Always *recheck* any mathematical calculations and pay

BOX 1-3

Check Three Times for Safe Medication Administration

First Check

- Read the medication administration record (MAR) and remove the medication(s) from the patient's drawer. Verify that the patient's name and hospital number match the MAR.
- Compare the label of the medication against the MAR.
- If the dosage does not match the MAR, determine if you need to do a math calculation.
- Check the expiration date of the medication.

Second Check

- While preparing the medication (e.g., pouring, drawing up, or placing unopened package in a medication cup), look at the medication label and check against the MAR.

Third Check

- Recheck the label on the container (e.g., vial, bottle, or unused unit-dose medications) before returning it to its storage place.
  or
- Check the label on the medication against the MAR before opening the package at the bedside.

From Przybycien, P. (2005). *Safe meds.* St. Louis, MO: Mosby. Adapted with permission.

careful attention to decimal points, which could lead to a tenfold or even greater overdose. Leading zeros, or zeros placed before a decimal point, are allowed, but trailing zeros, or zeros following the decimal point, should not be used. For example, 0.2 milligrams is allowed but 2.0 milligrams is not acceptable. Pay special attention if the calculation indicates multiple pills or tablets or a large quantity of a liquid medication. This can be a "cue" that the math calculation may be incorrect.

Patient variables (e.g., vital signs, age, gender, weight, height) should be noted because of the need for dosage change because of specific parameters. Remember that children and the older adult are more sensitive to medications than adolescents and the middle-aged; thus, extra caution is needed with drug dosage amounts in children and the older adult.

Right Time

Each health care agency or institution has a policy regarding routine medication administration times; therefore, the nurse must always check this policy. However, when giving a medication at the prescribed time, the nurse may be confronted with a dilemma between the timing suggested by the physician and specific pharmacokinetic and pharmacodynamic drug properties, concurrent drug therapy, dietary influences, laboratory or diagnostic testing, and specific patient variables. For example, the prescribed right time for administration of antihypertensive drugs may be four times a day, but for an active, professional 42-year-old male patient working 13 to 14 hours a day, taking a medication four times a day may not be feasible and may lead to nonadherence and subsequent complications. The nurse should contact the physician and inquire about another drug with different dosing frequency (e.g., once or twice daily).

For routine medication orders, the medications must be given no more than a half hour before or after the actual time specified in the physician's orders (i.e., if a medication is ordered to be given at 0900 every morning, it may be given anytime between 0830 and 0930); the exception is medications designated to be given *stat* (immediately), which must be administered within a half hour of the time the order is written. The nurse should always check the hospital or facility policy and procedure for any other specific information concerning the "half hour before or after" rule. For medication orders with the annotation *prn* (*pro re nata*, or "as needed"), the medication should be given at special times and under certain circumstances. For example, suppose that an analgesic is ordered every 4 to 6 hours prn for pain; after one dose of the medication, the patient complains of pain. After assessment, intervention with another dose of analgesic would occur, but only 4 to 6 hours after the previous dose. Military time is used when medication and other orders are written into a patient's chart (Table 1-1). Nursing judgement may lead to some variations in timing, but the nurse should be sure to document any change and rationale for the change. If medications are ordered to be given once every day, twice daily, three times daily, or even four times daily, the times of administration may be changed if this is not harmful to the patient, if the medication or patient's condition does not require adherence to an exact schedule, and only if approved by the physician. For example, suppose that an antacid is ordered to be given three times daily at 0900, 1300, and 1700, but the nurse has misread the order and gives the first dose at 1100. Depending on the hospital or facility policy, the medication, and the patient's condition, such an occurrence may not be considered an error because the dosing may be changed, once the physician is contacted, so the drug may be given at 1100, 1500, and 1900 without harm to the patient and without incident to the nurse. If this were an antihypertensive medication, however, the patient's condition and well-being could be compromised by one late or missed dose. Thus, falling behind in dosing times is not to be taken lightly or ignored. A change in the dosing or timing of medication should never be underestimated because one missed dose of certain medications can be life-threatening.

TABLE 1-1	
Conversion of Standard Time to Military Time	
Standard Time	**Military Time**
1 AM	0100
2 AM	0200
3 AM	0300
4 AM	0400
5 AM	0500
6 AM	0600
7 AM	0700
8 AM	0800
9 AM	0900
10 AM	1000
11 AM	1100
12 PM (noon)	1200
1 PM	1300
2 PM	1400
3 PM	1500
4 PM	1600
5 PM	1700
6 PM	1800
7 PM	1900
8 PM	2000
9 PM	2100
10 PM	2200
11 PM	2300
12 AM (midnight)	2400

Other factors must be considered in determining the right time. These include multiple-drug therapy, drug–drug or drug–food compatibility, scheduling of diagnostic tests, bioavailability of the drug (e.g., the need for consistent timing of doses around the clock to maintain blood levels), drug actions, and any biorhythm effects such as those that occur with steroids. It is also critical to patient safety to *avoid* using abbreviations for *any* component of a drug order (i.e., dose, time, route). The nurse should always be careful to spell out all terms (e.g., "three times daily" instead of "tid") because the possibility of miscommunication or misinterpretation poses a risk to the patient.

Right Route

As previously stated, the nurse must know the particulars about each medication before administering it to ensure that the right drug, dose, and route are being used. A complete medication order includes the route for administration. If a medication order does not include the route, the nurse must ask the physician to clarify it. The nurse must never *assume* the route of administration.

Right Patient

Checking the patient's identity before giving each medication dose is critical to the patient's safety. The nurse should ask the patient to state the patient's own name and then check the patient's identification band to confirm the patient's name, identification number, age, and allergies. With children, the parents or legal guardians are often the ones who identify the patient for the purposes of giving prescribed medications. With newborns and labour and delivery situations, the mother and baby have identification bracelets with matching numbers that should be checked before giving medications. With the older adult or patients with altered sensorium or level of consciousness, asking them for their name or having them state their name is not realistic, nor is it safe. Thus checking identification bands against the medication profile or medication order is important to avoid errors.

Right Documentation

The nurse is responsible for accurate documentation in electronic form, narrative form, SOAP (*s*ubjective, *o*bjective, *a*ssessment, *p*lanning) notes format, or other form. The nurse should document medication administration during or after (not before) administration in the patient's record according to documentation standards. Documentation consists of clear, concise, abbreviation-free charting related to the meeting of goals and outcome criteria as well as noting of therapeutic effects versus adverse effects and toxic effects of anything related to the medication process. If the time of administration varies from the prescribed time, the time should be noted on the patient's record with the reason for the altered time. Appropriate follow-through activities should also be documented (e.g., pharmacy states medication will be available in 2 hours). Medications should be observed being swallowed and not left at the bedside. If a medication is not given or taken, the nurse must follow the agency's policy for documenting the reason for this. Adult patients have the right to refuse a medication. The nurse's role is to inform the patient of the potential consequences of refusal and to inform the appropriate health care provider.

Many provinces are moving to implement electronic health records. The *electronic health record* (EHR) is a health record of an individual that is accessible online from many separate, interoperable automated systems within an electronic network. It provides an online profile of a patient's drug prescription history. The system also notifies of drug interactions.

Right Reason

The nurse must ensure that the drug is being given for the right reason. If the nurse administers an unfamiliar drug and remains unknowledgeable about its action and intended effect, the drug may cause harm, although unintended, to the patient. Sometimes a medication may be administered for a reason that is not obvious, as the classification is not the reason for the administration. For example, lactulose, although classified as a laxative, is also used for the treatment of hepatic encephalopathy to bind with ammonia to reduce toxic levels.

Medication Errors

When the "rights" of drug administration are discussed, medication errors must be considered. Medication errors are a major problem in health care, regardless of the setting. The National Coordinating Council for Medication Error Reporting and Prevention (2008) defines *medication error* as "any preventable event that may cause or lead to inappropriate medication use or patient harm while the medication is in the control of the health-care provider, patient, or consumer. Such events may be related to professional practice, health-care products, procedures, and systems including prescribing; order communication; product labelling, packaging, and nomenclature; compounding; dispensing; distribution; administration; education; monitoring; and use" (http://www.nccmerp.org/aboutMedErrors.html).

It is important for the nurse to understand the definition of medication errors because it emphasizes that, in evaluating contributors to a medication error, the nurse must look at all the "rights" of medication administration and at the systems (i.e., ordering, dispensing, preparing, administering, and documenting) involved in the medication administration process, which may include health care providers and ancillary personnel, as well as unit stocking, transcription of orders, and how the medication order is verified and interpreted. Indeed, pharmacists are responsible for their own actions, but nurses also have to check the actions of other health care providers (such as UCPs), never assume that all is correct and appropriate, and be responsible for their own actions. For further discussion of medication errors and their prevention, see Chapter 5.

EVALUATION

Evaluation occurs after the collaborative plan of care has been implemented. It is a systematic, ongoing, and dynamic part of the nursing process as related to drug therapy. It includes monitoring the patient's therapeutic response to the drug and its adverse effects and toxic effects. Documentation is also an important component of evaluation and should include charting related to the medication administration process (see Legal and Ethical Principles). Charting should be done at the time of an event or as close to it as is prudently possible. Charting should also be consistent with and follow the existing written policy on charting of your current employer (see Box 1-4).

Evaluation also includes the process of monitoring the standards for nursing practice. Several standards of care are in place to help in the evaluation of outcomes of care, such as those standards established by nursing provincial governing bodies and the Canadian Council on Health Services Accreditation (CCHSA). Within the CCHSA, guidelines are established for nursing services,

---

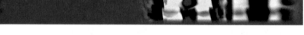

⚖ LEGAL & ETHICAL PRINCIPLES

Charting "Don'ts"

Charting is a critical component of the nursing process. The following is a list of charting don'ts:

- Don't record staffing problems (don't mention them in a patient's chart but instead talk to the appropriate nurse manager).
- Don't record a peer's conflicts such as charting possible disputes between a patient and a nurse.
- Don't mention incident reports in charting because they are confidential and are filed separately and not in the patient's chart. The facts of an incident may be documented, but don't mention the terms (e.g., that it was an error).
- Don't use the following terms: "by mistake," "by accident," "accidentally," "unintentional," or "miscalculated."
- Don't chart other patients' names because this is a violation of confidentiality.

- Don't chart anything but facts.
- Don't chart casual conversations with peers, physicians, or other members of the health care team.
- Don't use abbreviations, as a general rule of thumb. Some agencies or facilities may still use a list of approved abbreviations, but overall they are discouraged.

Note: Although this is taken from an American reference, institutions in Canada follow similar rules.

Data from the Institute for Safe Medication Practices. (2003, February 20). *ISMP medication safety alert,* available at http://www.ismp.org/Newsletters/acutecare/archives.asp; and *Nursing* (2000, revised 2004). Incredibly easy!: Charting "don'ts". Retrieved July 23, 2009, from http://findarticles.com/p/articles/mi_qa3689/is_200007/ai_n8911410/.

policies, and procedures. The CNA Code of Ethics (Canadian Nurses Association, 2008) and specific medication practice standards regarding nurses' accountability for medication administration were established to protect both the patient and the nurse.

In summary, the nursing process is an ongoing and constantly evolving process (see Box 1-1). The nursing process, as it relates to drug therapy, is the way in which the nurse gathers, analyzes, organizes, provides, and acts on data about the patient within the context of prudent nursing care and standards of care. The nurse's ability to make astute assessments, formulate sound nursing diagnoses, establish goals and outcome criteria, correctly administer drugs, and continually evaluate the patients' responses to drugs increases with additional experience and knowledge.

BOX 1-4   Ten Rules for Good Charting

1 Record the facts—what you can see, hear, smell, and touch.
2 Record information as closely as possible to the time you deliver care. Don't document in advance, and don't leave important notes until the end of the shift.
3 Chart in chronological order, writing on every line so that the chronology cannot be altered.
4 Eliminate bias from your notes. Labelling a patient can alter patient care: In one situation, nurses caring for a patient in labour labelled her a "complainer" and missed the clues to her abdominal obstruction.
5 Use flow sheets to record routine care. Keep them in the patient's room, if possible, so you can chart immediately after giving a treatment.
6 Consider using a problem-oriented approach. Identify and describe the problem, how it was resolved, and the patient's response.
7 Ensure continuity. Note problems as they occur and the interventions that followed.
8 Document all medical visits and consultations, whether in person or by phone. Note the discussion of the patient's condition, any abnormal findings, directions the physician gave, and the actions you took. Also note the time and date of the visit or consultation.
9 Document discussions about concerns with medical orders and directions the physician gave confirming, cancelling, or modifying the orders. Include the time and date of the discussion and your actions as a result of the orders—for example: 5/12 1930—Discussed morphine dose order and pt.'s pain level ratings over the past 24 hr with Dr. Donhauser. PCA doses changed and pain control improved (see pain-flow sheet). B. Haldeman, RN
10 Prepare a discharge plan that lists instructions for the patient and follow-up. Send a copy of the plan home with the patient and keep a copy in the record. Good charting takes time and effort, but in return it offers protection for you and your patient.

Source: Philpott, M. (1985). *Legal liability and the nursing process*. Toronto, ON: Saunders. Adapted and updated with the permission of the publisher. 10 rules for good charting obtained from *Nursing 2008* (1998 May), *28*(5): 27. Reprinted with permission of Wolters Kluwer Health.

POINTS TO REMEMBER

❖ Nurses are entrusted with confidential information and with the lives of their patients during all facets of patient care, including drug therapy.

❖ Safe, therapeutic, and effective medication administration is a major responsibility of professional nurses in the care of patients of all ages and in a wide variety of facilities.

❖ Nurses are responsible for safe and prudent decision making in the nursing care of their patients, including the provision of drug therapy and use of the Ten Rights, and must always adhere to legal and ethical standards related to medication administration and documentation.

❖ Nurses need to document in clear, concise language and avoid the use of abbreviations.

EXAMINATION REVIEW QUESTIONS

1 An 86-year-old patient is being discharged home on digitalis therapy and has little information regarding the medication. Which of the following statements best reflects a realistic goal or outcome of patient teaching activities?
   a. The patient will call the physician if adverse effects occur.
   b. The patient will state all the symptoms of digitalis toxicity.
   c. The nurse will provide teaching about the drug's adverse effects.
   d. The patient and patient's daughter will state the correct dosing and administration of the drug.

2 What is the most appropriate response to a patient who informs the nurse that she does not want to share information about the drugs she takes at home?
   a. "We're just asking to make sure that you do not have any drug allergies."
   b. "It sounds like something you are taking is something that you do not want us to know about."
   c. "This information will not become part of your medical record, but we need to know so that we can monitor your responses to therapy while you are here."
   d. "Information about the drugs that you take at home, including any natural health products, is important for safe administration of drugs while you are here and will be kept confidential."

3 A patient's chart includes an order that reads as follows: Lanoxin 0.025 mcg once daily at 0900. Which of the following statements regarding the dosage route for this drug is correct?
   a. The drug should only be given orally.
   b. The drug should be given intravenously.
   c. The drug should be given via the transdermal route.
   d. The dosage route should never be assumed when an order does not specify a route.

4 Which of the following questions is most effective in compiling a drug history for a patient?
   a. "What childhood diseases did you have?"
   b. "Do you have a family history of heart disease?"
   c. "Do you depend on sleeping pills to get to sleep?"
   d. "When you take your pain medicine, does it relieve the pain?"

5 A 77-year-old male who has been diagnosed with an upper respiratory infection tells the nurse that he is allergic to penicillin. Which of the following would be the nurse's most appropriate response?
   a. "That is to be expected—lots of people are allergic to penicillin."
   b. "What type of reaction did you have when you took penicillin?"
   c. "This allergy is not of major concern because the drug is given so commonly."
   d. "Drug allergies don't usually occur in older individuals because they have built up resistance."

For answers see http://evolve.elsevier.com/Canada/Lilley/pharmacology/.

CRITICAL THINKING ACTIVITIES

1 What are the crucial responsibilities of the nurse when implementing drug therapy?

2 When medications were administered during the night shift, a patient refused to take his 0200 dose of an antibiotic, claiming that he had just taken it. What actions by the nurse would ensure sound decision making and maintain patient safety?

3 During a busy shift, you note that the chart of your newly admitted patient has few orders for medications and diagnostic tests, taken by telephone by another nurse. You were on the way to the patient's room to do your assessment when the unit secretary tells you that one of the orders reads as follows: "Lasix, 20 mg, stat." What should you do first? How do you go about giving this drug? Explain.

For answers see http://evolve.elsevier.com/Canada/Lilley/pharmacology/.

CHAPTER 2

Pharmacological Principles

Learning Objectives

After reading this chapter, the successful student will be able to do the following:

1 Define common terms used in pharmacology (see the listing of terms in the Glossary).

2 Describe the role of pharmaceutics, pharmacokinetics, and pharmacodynamics in drug administration.

3 Discuss the application of the four principles of pharmacotherapeutics to nursing practice as they relate to a variety of patients in different health care settings.

4 Discuss the use of natural drug sources in the development of new drugs.

5 Describe evidence-informed nursing practice.

6 Discuss the role of evidence-informed practice as it relates to pharmacology and medication administration.

7 Develop a collaborative plan of care that considers the phases of pharmacokinetics in carrying out drug therapy.

e-Learning Activities

Web site
(http://evolve.elsevier.com/Canada/Lilley/pharmacology/)

- Animations
- Answers to chapter questions, activities, and case studies
- Calculators and Category Catchers
- Glossary with audio pronunciations
- IV Therapy and Medication Error Checklists
- Multiple-Choice Review Question quizzes
- Nursing Care Plans
- Online Appendices and Supplements
- WebLinks

Glossary

Additive effects Drug interactions in which the effect of a combination of two or more drugs with similar actions is equivalent to the sum of the individual effects of the same drugs given alone (compare with *synergistic effects*). (p. 37)

Adverse drug event (ADE) Any undesirable occurrence related to administering or failing to administer a prescribed drug. (p. 38)

Adverse drug reaction (ADR) Any unexpected, unintended, undesired, or excessive response to a medication given at therapeutic dosages; one type of ADE. (p. 38)

Adverse effects Any undesirable bodily effects that are a direct response to one or more drugs. (p. 22)

Agonist A drug that binds to and stimulates the activity of one or more biochemical receptor types in the body. (p. 34)

Allergic reaction An immunological hypersensitivity reaction resulting from the unusual sensitivity of a patient to a particular medication; a type of ADE. (p. 38)

Antagonist A drug that binds to and inhibits the activity of one or more biochemical receptor types in the body, resulting in inhibitory or antagonistic drug effects; also called *inhibitors*. (p. 34)

Antagonistic effects Drug interactions in which the effect of a combination of two or more drugs is less than the sum of the individual effects of the same drugs given alone. (p. 37)

Bioavailability A measure of the extent of drug absorption for a given drug and route (can vary from 0% to 100%). (p. 23)

Biotransformation One or more biochemical reactions involving a *parent* drug. (p. 30)

Chemical name The name that describes the chemical composition and molecular structure of a *drug*. (p. 21)

Contraindication Any condition, especially one related to a disease state or other patient characteristic, including current or recent drug therapy, that renders a particular form of treatment improper or undesirable. (p. 35)

Cytochrome P450 General name for a large class of enzymes (found especially in the liver) that play a significant role in drug metabolism. (p. 30)

Dissolution The process by which solid forms of drugs disintegrate in the gastrointestinal tract, become soluble, and are absorbed into the circulation. (p. 22)

Drug Any chemical that affects the physiological processes of a living organism. (p. 21)

Drug actions The cellular processes involved in the interaction between a drug and cell (e.g., the action of a drug on a receptor); also referred to as *mechanism of action*. (p. 22)

Drug effects The physiological reactions of the body to a drug. (p. 33)

Drug-induced teratogenesis The development of congenital anomalies or defects in the developing fetus that are caused by the toxic effects of drugs. (p. 39)

Drug interaction Alteration of the pharmacological activity of a given drug caused by the presence of one or more additional drugs; it is usually related to effects on the enzymes required for metabolism of the involved drugs. (p. 37)

Duration of action The length of time in which the concentration of a drug in the blood or tissues is sufficient to elicit a therapeutic response. (p. 33)

Enzymes Protein molecules that catalyze one or more of a variety of biochemical reactions, including those related to the body's own physiological processes as well as those related to drug metabolism. (p. 34)

Evidence-informed practice (EIP) Continuous interactive process involving the explicit, conscious, and judicious consideration of the best research evidence available to make collaborative decisions between the health care team and the patient and family when providing patient care. (p. 41)

First-pass effect The initial metabolism in the liver of a drug absorbed from the gastrointestinal tract before the drug reaches the systemic circulation through the bloodstream. (p. 24)

Generic name The name given to a drug approved by Health Canada; also called the *nonproprietary name* or the *official name*. (p. 21)

Half-life In *pharmacokinetics*, the time required for one half of an administered dose of drug to be eliminated by the body; also called *elimination half-life*. (p. 32)

Idiosyncratic reaction An abnormal and unexpected response to a drug, other than an allergic reaction, that is peculiar to an individual patient. (p. 38)

Incompatibility The quality of two parenteral drugs or solutions that leads to a reaction resulting in chemical deterioration of at least one of the drugs when the two substances are mixed together. (p. 37)

Medication error (ME) Any *preventable* ADE involving inappropriate drug use by a patient or health care provider; it may or may not cause patient harm. (p. 38)

Medication use process The prescribing, dispensing, and administering of drugs, and the monitoring of their effects. (p. 38)

Metabolite A chemical form of a drug that is the product of one or more biochemical (metabolic) reactions involving the *parent drug*. (p. 22)

Onset of action The time required for a drug to elicit a therapeutic response after dosing. (p. 33)

Parent drug The chemical form of a drug that is administered before it is metabolized by the body's biochemical reactions into its active or inactive metabolites. (p. 22)

Peak effect The time required for a drug to reach its maximum therapeutic response in the body. (p. 33)

Peak level The maximum concentration of a drug in the body after administration, usually measured in a blood sample for *therapeutic drug monitoring*. (p. 33)

Pharmaceutics The science of preparing and dispensing drugs, including dosage form design (e.g., tablets, capsules, injections, patches, etc.). (p. 22)

Pharmacodynamics The study of the biochemical and physiological interactions of drugs at their sites of activity. (p. 22)

Pharmacogenetics The study of the influence of genetic factors on drug response, including the nature of genetic aberrations that result in the absence, overabundance, or insufficiency of drug-metabolizing enzymes; also called *pharmacogenomics*. (p. 38)

Pharmacognosy The study of drugs that are obtained from natural plant and animal sources. (p. 22)

Pharmacokinetics The rate of drug distribution among body compartments after a drug has entered the body. (p. 22)

Pharmacology Broadest term for the study or science of drugs. (p. 21)

Pharmacotherapeutics The treatment of pathological conditions through the use of drugs. (p. 22)

Prodrug An inactive drug dosage form that is converted to an active metabolite by biochemical reactions once it is inside the body. (p. 22)

Receptor A molecular structure within or on the outer surface of cells to which specific substances (e.g., drug molecules) bind. One or more corresponding cellular effects (drug effects) occur as a result of this drug–receptor interaction. (p. 22)

Steady state The physiological state in which the amount of drug removed via elimination is equal to the amount of drug absorbed with each dose. (p. 33)

Substrate A substance (e.g., drug or natural biochemical in the body) on which an enzyme acts. (p. 30)

Synergistic effects Drug interactions in which the effect of a combination of two or more drugs with similar actions is *greater than* the sum of the individual effects of the same drugs given alone (compare with *additive effects*). (p. 37)

Therapeutic drug monitoring The process of measuring drug *peak* and *trough levels* to gauge the level of a patient's drug exposure and allow adjustment of dosages with the joint goals of maximizing *therapeutic effects* and minimizing *toxicity*. (p. 34)

Therapeutic effect The desired or intended effect of a particular drug. (p. 34)

Therapeutic index The ratio between the toxic and therapeutic concentrations of a drug. (p. 36)

Toxic The quality of being poisonous (i.e., injurious to health or dangerous to life). (p. 22)

Toxicity The condition of producing adverse bodily effects because of poisonous qualities. (p. 33)

Toxicology The study of the effects of drugs, poisons, and other chemicals in living systems, their detection, and treatments to counteract their poisonous effects. (p. 22)

Trade name The commercial name given to a drug product by its manufacturer; also called the *proprietary name*. (p. 21)

Trough level The lowest concentration of a drug reached in the body after it falls from the *peak level*, usually measured in a blood sample for *therapeutic drug monitoring*. (p. 33)

OVERVIEW

Any chemical that affects the processes of a living organism can broadly be defined as a **drug.** The study or science of drugs is known as **pharmacology.** This study may incorporate knowledge from a variety of areas:

- Absorption
- Biochemical effects
- Biotransformation (metabolism)
- Distribution
- Drug history
- Drug origin
- Drug receptor mechanisms
- Excretion
- Mechanisms of action
- Physical and chemical properties
- Physical effects
- Therapeutic (beneficial) effects
- Toxic (harmful) effects

Knowledge of these areas of pharmacology enables the nurse to better understand how drugs affect humans. Without a sound understanding of basic pharmacological principles, the nurse cannot fully appreciate the therapeutic benefits and potential toxicity of drugs.

Pharmacology is an extensive science that incorporates several interrelated sciences: *pharmaceutics, pharmacokinetics, pharmacodynamics, pharmacotherapeutics, pharmacognosy,* and *toxicology.* The drugs discussed in each chapter of this text are described from the standpoint of one or more of these six areas.

Throughout the process of development, a drug will acquire at least three different names. The **chemical name** describes the drug's chemical composition and molecular structure. The **generic name,** or nonproprietary name, is given to the drug and approved by Health Canada under the Food and Drugs Act and Food and Drug Regulations. It is often much shorter and simpler than the chemical name. The generic name is used in most official drug compendiums to list drugs. The **trade name,** or proprietary name, indicates that the drug has a registered trademark and that its commercial use is restricted to the owner of the patent for the drug until the patent expires. The owner is usually the manufacturer of the drug. Trade names are generally created by the manufacturer with marketability in mind. For this reason, trade names are usually shorter and easier to pronounce and remember than generic names. The company that researches and manufactures the drug retains sole rights to sell the drug without competition for a specified number of years owing to patent protection. The patent life of a newly discovered drug molecule in Canada is 20 years from the time of filing. After the patent period expires, competing manufacturers may produce and sell *generic* versions of the drug with the same active ingredients. At this point, the price of the drug usually falls substantially, which offers many patients and third-party payers the benefits of savings on the generic (versus the original brand-name) drug (Figure 2-1).

Three basic phases of drug activity—pharmaceutics, pharmacokinetics, and pharmacodynamics—describe

Chemical name
(+/−)-2-(p-isobutylphenyl) propionic acid

Generic name
ibuprofen

Trade name
Motrin, others

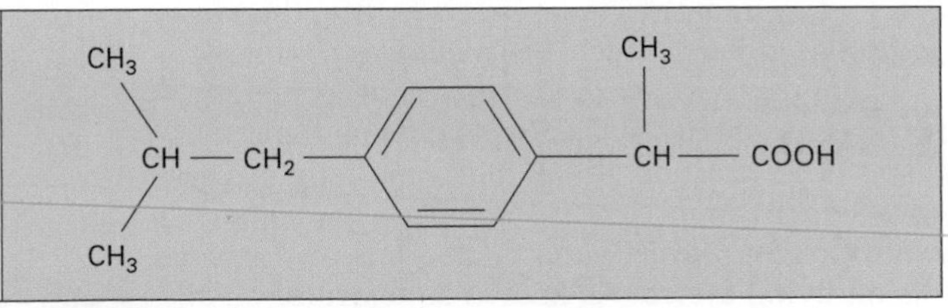

FIG. 2-1 Chemical structure of the common analgesic ibuprofen and the chemical, generic, and trade names for the drug.

the relationship between the dose of a drug given to a patient and the effectiveness of that drug in treating the patient's disorder. **Pharmaceutics** includes the study of how different dosage forms (e.g., injection, capsule, controlled-release tablet) influence the way in which the body metabolizes a drug and the way in which the drug affects the body. **Pharmacokinetics** includes the study of what the body does to the drug molecules. It includes the phases of absorption, distribution, metabolism, and excretion of drugs. These four phases and their relationship to drug and drug metabolite concentrations are determined for different body sites over specified periods. A **metabolite** is the product of one or more biochemical (metabolic) reactions involving the **parent drug** (the original drug administered). A parent drug that is not pharmacologically active is called a **prodrug**. A prodrug is then metabolized to pharmacologically *active metabolites*. Often, a prodrug is more readily absorbed than its active metabolite, hence the need for its development. *Inactive metabolites* lack pharmacological activity and are simply drug waste products awaiting excretion from the body (e.g., via the urinary, gastrointestinal, or respiratory tract). The onset of action, the peak effect of a drug, and the duration of action of a drug are all part of the drug's pharmacokinetics.

Pharmacodynamics, on the other hand, is the study of what the drug does to the body. It examines the physicochemical properties of drugs and their pharmacological interactions with body receptors. **Receptors** are specialized protein molecules embedded in the outer surfaces of cells or within cells to which drug molecules bind to exert their effects. *Receptor theory* assumes that all drugs perform their unique actions at chemically specific *receptor sites* in various tissues. Not all mechanisms of action, however, have been identified for all drugs. Thus, a drug may be said to have an unknown or unclear mechanism of action, even though it has observable therapeutic effects in the body. Figure 2-2 illustrates the three phases that affect drug activity, starting with the pharmaceutical phase, proceeding to the pharmacokinetic phase, and finishing with the pharmacodynamic phase.

Pharmacotherapeutics (also called *therapeutics*) focuses on the use of drugs and the clinical indications for administering drugs to prevent and treat diseases. It defines the principles of **drug actions**—the cellular processes that change in response to the presence of drug molecules. Therefore, an understanding of pharmacotherapeutics is essential for nurses when implementing drug therapy. *Empirical therapeutics* refers to drug therapy that is effective but for which the mechanism of drug action is unknown. *Rational therapeutics* is drug therapy in which specific evidence has been obtained for the mechanisms of drug action. Recall that some drug mechanisms of action are more clearly understood than others.

The study of the adverse effects of drugs and other chemicals on living systems is known as **toxicology.** An **adverse effect** is a direct response to one or more drugs that results in an undesirable effect. These effects are generally considered to be relatively minor but are expected to occur in a percentage of the population receiving a given drug. The severity of effects occurs on a continuum. More serious adverse effects may result in changes in prescribed drug therapy after weighing the risk-to-benefit ratio of a drug in a specific clinical situation. **Toxic** effects are often an extension of a drug's therapeutic action. Therefore, toxicology often involves overlapping principles of both pharmacotherapy and toxicology.

The study of *natural* (versus *synthetic*) drug sources (both plants and animals) is called **pharmacognosy.** This science was formerly called *materia medica* (medicinal materials) and is concerned with the botanical or zoological origin, biochemical composition, and therapeutic effects of *natural* drugs, their derivatives, and their constituents.

In summary, pharmacology is a dynamic science incorporating several different disciplines. Traditionally, chemistry has been seen as the primary basis of pharmacology, but pharmacology also relies heavily on physiology and biology.

PHARMACEUTICS

Different drug dosage forms have different pharmaceutical properties. Dosage form design determines the rate at which a drug undergoes **dissolution** (dissolving of solid dosage forms and their absorption [e.g., from

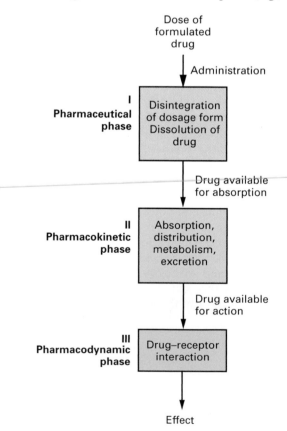

FIG. 2-2 Phases of drug activity. From McKenry, L. M., Tessier, E., & Hogan, M. (2006). *Mosby's pharmacology in nursing* (22nd ed.). St. Louis, MO: Mosby.

gastrointestinal tract fluids]). A drug to be ingested orally may be taken in either a solid form (tablet, capsule, or powder) or a liquid form (solution or suspension). Table 2-1 lists some drug preparations and the relative rate at which they are absorbed. Oral drugs that are liquids (e.g., elixirs, syrups) are already dissolved and are usually absorbed more quickly than solid dosage forms. Enteric-coated tablets, by contrast, have a coating that prevents them from being broken down in an acidic pH environment and thus are not absorbed until they reach the higher (more alkaline) pH of the intestines. This pharmaceutical property results in slower dissolution and slower absorption. Sometimes the size of the particles within a capsule can make different capsules containing the same drug dissolve at different rates, become absorbed at different rates, and thus have different onsets of action. A prime example of this is the difference between micronized (meaning tiny particles) and nonmicronized forms of a drug. The micronized formulation of the lipid-modifying drug fenofibrate, for example, reaches a maximum concentration peak faster than would a nonmicronized formulation because of how the dosage form is pharmaceutically engineered.

A variety of dosage forms exist to provide both accurate and convenient drug delivery systems (Table 2-2). These delivery systems are designed to achieve a desired therapeutic response with minimal adverse effects. Many dosage forms have been developed to encourage patient adherence with the medication regime. Convenience of administration correlates strongly with medication adherence. Many of the extended-release oral dosage forms were designed with this in mind as they often require fewer daily doses.

The specific characteristics of the different dosage forms have a large impact on how and to what extent the drug is absorbed. If a drug is to work at a specific site in the body, it must either be applied directly at that site in an active form or have a way of getting to that site. *Enteral* (systemic) administration refers to drugs administered via the gastrointestinal tract. Oral dosage forms rely on gastric and intestinal enzymes and pH environments to break the medication down into particles that are small enough to be absorbed into the circulation. Once absorbed through the mucosa of the stomach or intestines, the drug is then transported to the site of action by blood or lymph.

Many *topically* applied dosage forms work directly on the surface of the skin. Therefore, when the drug is applied, it is already in a dosage form that allows it to act immediately. With other topical dosage forms, the skin acts as a barrier through which the drug must pass to get to the circulation; once there, the drug is carried to the site of action (e.g., fentanyl transdermal patch for pain).

Dosage forms administered via injection are called *parenteral* forms. They must have certain characteristics to be safe and effective. The arteries and veins that carry drugs throughout the body can easily be damaged if the drug is too concentrated or corrosive. The pH of injections must be similar to the blood to be safely administered. Parenteral dosage forms that are injected intravenously or intra-arterially are immediately placed into solution in the bloodstream and do not have to be dissolved in the body. Therefore, 100% absorption is assumed to occur immediately upon intravenous or intra-arterial injection. The intra-arterial route is used much less commonly than the intravenous route but may be used in critical care units and oncology care settings.

PHARMACOKINETICS

A particular drug's onset of action, peak effect, and duration of action are all characteristics defined by pharmacokinetics. *Pharmacokinetics* is the study of what actually happens to a drug from the time it is put into the body until the parent drug and all metabolites have left the body. Thus, drug absorption into, distribution and metabolism within, and excretion from a living organism represent the combined focus of pharmacokinetics.

Absorption

Absorption is the movement of a drug from its site of administration into the bloodstream for distribution to the tissues. A term used to express the extent of drug absorption is **bioavailability**. For example, a drug that is absorbed from the gastrointestinal tract travels via the venous portal system to the liver before it reaches the systemic circulation. If the drug is metabolized in

TABLE 2-1

Drug Absorption of Various Oral Preparations

Liquids, elixirs, and syrups	Fastest
Suspension solutions	
Powders	
Capsules	
Tablets	
Coated tablets	
Enteric-coated tablets	Slowest

TABLE 2-2

Dosage Forms

Route	Forms
Enteral	Tablets, capsules, pills, timed-release capsules, sublingual or buccal tablets, elixirs, suspensions, syrups, timed-release tablets, enteric-coated tablets, emulsions, solutions, lozenges or troches, caplets, suppositories (rectal), pessary (vaginal)
Parenteral	Injectable forms, solutions, suspensions, emulsions, powders for reconstitution
Topical	Aerosols, sprays, ointments, creams, pastes, powders, solutions, foams, gels, transdermal patches, inhalers

the liver or excreted in the bile, some of the active drug will be inactivated or diverted before it can reach the general circulation and its intended sites of action. This is known as the **first-pass effect,** and it reduces the bioavailability of the drug to less than 100%. Many drugs administered by mouth have a bioavailability of less than 100%, whereas drugs administered by the intravenous route are 100% bioavailable. If two medications have the same bioavailability and same concentration of active ingredient, they are said to be bioequivalent (e.g., a brand-name drug and the same generic drug).

Several factors affect the rate of drug absorption. These include the presence of food or fluids ingested with the drug, the dosage formulation, the status of the absorptive surface, the rate of blood flow to the small intestine, the acidity of the stomach, and GI motility. How a drug is administered, or its route of administration, also affects the rate and extent of absorption of that drug (see Preventing Medication Errors: Does IV = PO?). Although a number of dosage formulations are available for delivering medications to the body, they can all be categorized into three routes of administration: *enteral* (gastrointestinal tract), *parenteral*, and *topical*. Various administration routes and their effects on absorption are examined in detail in the following sections. Drug distribution, metabolism, and excretion are then discussed.

Route

Enteral. In enteral drug administration, the drug is absorbed into the systemic circulation through the mucosa of the stomach or small intestine. The enteral route involves *oral* ingestion of the drug. Two subtypes of the enteral route are *sublingual* (under the tongue) and *buccal* (through the cheek and gums) drug administration; these routes are considered partly enteral and partly parenteral because they also allow direct transfer of the drug into the blood via blood vessels in the mouth. The rate of absorption of enterally administered drugs can be altered by many factors. Depending on the particular drug, it may be extensively metabolized in the liver before it reaches the systemic circulation. Normally,

orally administered drugs are absorbed from the intestinal lumen into the mesenteric blood system and conveyed by the portal vein to the liver. Once the drug is in the liver, the liver microsomal P450 enzyme system metabolizes it, and it is passed into the general circulation. As noted previously, this initial metabolism of a drug and its passage from the liver into the circulation is called the *first-pass effect* (Figure 2-3). If a large proportion of a drug is chemically processed into inactive metabolites in the liver, then a much less active drug will make it into circulation. Such a drug would have a high first-pass effect. Consequently, the oral dose has to be calculated to compensate for the lower bioavailability. For example, nitroglycerin administered orally undergoes rapid liver metabolism and, as a result, has almost no pharmacological effect. If administered sublingually, the drug is absorbed into the system circulation via the rich supply of blood vessels under the tongue and is carried to its site of action prior to circulating through the liver.

The same drug given intravenously will bypass the liver altogether. This prevents the first-pass effect from taking place, therefore, all of the drug reaches the circulation. For this reason, parenteral doses of drugs with a high first-pass effect are much smaller than enterally (oral) administered doses, yet they produce the same pharmacological response. See Table 2-3 (p. 26) for further discussion of the advantages, disadvantages, and nursing considerations related to the different routes of administration.

Many factors can alter the absorption of enterally administered drugs, including acid changes within the stomach and absorption changes in the intestines. Factors that affect the acidity of the stomach include the time of day; the age of the patient; and the presence and types of any medications, foods, or beverages. If food is in the stomach when an orally administered medication is taken, this may interfere with the drug's dissolution and absorption and delay its transit from the stomach to the small intestine. On the other hand, food may enhance the absorption of some lipid-soluble drugs (depending on the fat content of the food) or drugs that are more easily broken down in an acidic environment. (Food in the

✋ PREVENTING MEDICATION ERRORS

Does IV = PO?

The physician writes an order for *"furosemide (Lasix) 80 mg IV STAT"* for a patient who is short of breath because of pulmonary edema. When the nurse prepares to administer the drug, only the PO (per os or "by mouth") form is immediately available. Someone needs to go to the pharmacy to pick up the intravenous (IV) dose. Another nurse says, "Go ahead and give the pill. He needs it fast. It's all the same!" But is it?

Remember, the oral forms of medications must be processed through the gastrointestinal tract, absorbed through the small intestines, and undergo the first-pass effect in the liver before the drug can reach the intended site of action.

However, IV forms are injected directly into the circulation and can act almost immediately because the first-pass effect is bypassed. The time of onset of action for the PO form is 30 to 60 minutes; for the IV form, this time is 5 minutes. This patient is in respiratory distress, and the immediate effect of the diuretic is desired. In addition, because of the first-pass effect, the available amount of orally administered drug that actually reaches the site of action would actually be less than the available amount of intravenously administered drug. Therefore, IV does NOT equal PO! Never change the route of administration of a medication; if questions come up, always check with the prescriber.

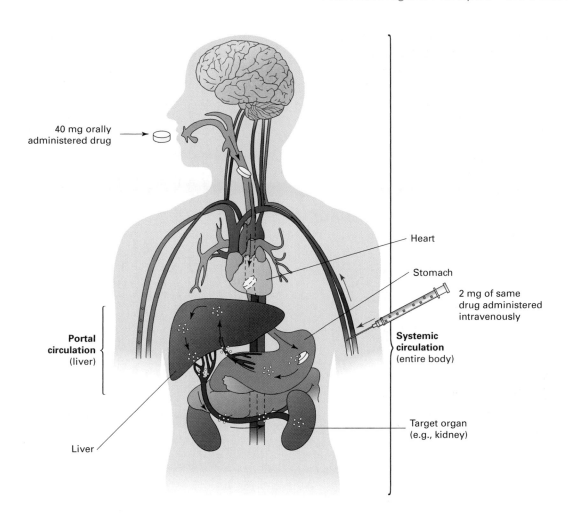

40 mg orally
administered drug

Heart

Stomach

2 mg of same
drug administered
intravenously

**Portal
circulation**
(liver)

**Systemic
circulation**
(entire body)

Target organ
(e.g., kidney)

Liver

FIG. 2-3 First-pass effect of a drug by the liver before its systemic availability.

stomach increases gastric acid production.) Before orally administered drugs pass into the portal circulation of the liver, they are absorbed in the small intestine, which has an enormous surface area. Drug absorption may be altered in patients who have had portions of their small intestine removed because of disease. Anticholinergic drugs may slow down the gastrointestinal *transit time*, or the time it takes substances in the stomach to be dissolved and passed into the intestines. This may allow more time for an acid-susceptible drug to be in contact with the acid in the stomach and subsequently be broken down, which reduces the drug absorption. Examples of drugs to be taken on an empty stomach and those to be taken with food are provided in Box 2-1 on p. 28. The stomach and small intestine are highly vascularized. When blood flow to that area is decreased, absorption may also be decreased. Sepsis and exercise are examples of circumstances under which blood flow to the gastrointestinal tract is often reduced. In both cases, blood tends to be routed to the heart and other vital organs. In exercise, blood is also routed to the skeletal muscles.

Sublingual and Buccal. Drugs administered by the *sublingual* route are absorbed rapidly into the highly vascularized tissue under the tongue (the oral mucosa), an area that has a large blood supply. Sublingually administered drugs therefore bypass the liver and yet are systemically bioavailable. The same concepts apply for drugs administered by the *buccal* route (the oral mucosa between the cheek and the gum). Through these routes, drugs like sublingual nitroglycerin are absorbed directly into the bloodstream and delivered rapidly to their site of action (e.g., coronary arteries).

Parenteral. For most medications, the parenteral route is the fastest route by which a drug can be absorbed, followed by the enteral and the topical routes. *Parenteral* is a general term meaning any route of administration other than the GI tract. Most commonly it refers to injection by any method, although topical and transdermal medications can also be considered parenteral dosage forms (see Topical section, below), as can sublingual and buccal medications. An intravenous injection delivers the drug directly into the circulation, where it is distributed

TABLE 2-3

Routes of Administration and Related Nursing Considerations

Route	Advantages	Disadvantages	Nursing Considerations
Inhalant (nebulizer, metered-dose inhaler [MDI], dry powder inhaler [DPI])	Delivers precisely measured dose of drug directly into airways of lungs. Acts quickly and minimizes the dose required, minimizes adverse effects, and avoids first-pass effect. Easily used by child, adult, and older adult. Portable. Use of a spacer provides increased dead air space for improved penetration and deposition of the drug into the lungs. DPIs in general are easier to use than MDIs and cause fewer irritant effects. The DPI inhaler contains 200 doses of drug; a dose counter is included so that the patient knows how many doses are remaining.	Less than 20% drug delivery with MDIs. Inhaled drug may be systemically absorbed. Patients often do not use MDIs optimally. DPIs cannot be used with spacers. Nebulizers are generally larger in size, inconvenient, and complex to use.	The inhaler must be used correctly to ensure optimal effect of the drug. Newer devices (flow-triggered MDIs) eliminate the requirement of hand–breath coordination to deliver medication; the drug is automatically dispersed in response to the patient's inspiratory effort. When administering a bronchodilator and corticosteroid, the bronchodilator is given first to open the airways for optimum delivery of the corticosteroid. Some specific inhalant drugs may be contraindicated (e.g., bronchodilator drugs in a patient with cardiac arrhythmias).
Intramuscular (IM); subcutaneous (SC)	IM injections are good for poorly soluble drugs, which are often given in "depot" preparation form and are then absorbed over a prolonged period; onsets of action differ depending on route (e.g., IM injections often produce more rapid onset than SC injections).	Discomfort of injection; inconvenience; bruising; inconvenience; slower onset of action compared with IV, although quicker than oral in most situations	Use of landmarks to identify correct IM and SC sites is always required and is recommended as a nursing standard of care. Ventral gluteal site is IM site of choice with use of 38 mm (sometimes 25 mm in thin or emaciated patients) and 21–25 gauge needle, given at a 90-degree angle. It is recommended that SC injections be given at a 90-degree angle with proper-sized syringe and needle (13- to 16-millimetre needle); in emaciated or thin patients, SC angle should be 45 degrees. Selection of correct size of syringe and needle is key to safe administration by these routes and is based on thorough assessment of the patient as well as drug characteristics.
Intravenous (IV)	Provides rapid onset (drug delivered immediately to bloodstream); allows more direct control of drug level in blood; gives option of larger fluid volume, thus diluting irritating drugs; avoids first-pass metabolism	Higher cost; inconvenience (e.g., not self-administered); irreversibility of drug action in most cases and inability to retrieve medication; risk of fluid overload; greater likelihood of infection; possibility of embolism	Continuous IV infusions require frequent monitoring to be sure that the correct volume and amount are administered and that the drug reaches safe, therapeutic blood levels. IV drugs and solutions should be checked for compatibilities. IV sites should be monitored for redness, swelling, heat, and drainage—all are indicative of complications, such as thrombophlebitis. If intermittent IV infusions are used, clearing or flushing of the line with normal saline before and after is generally indicated to keep the IV site patent and minimize incompatibilities.

TABLE 2-3 (cont'd)

Routes of Administration and Related Nursing Considerations (cont'd)

Route	Advantages	Disadvantages	Nursing Considerations
Oral	Usually easier, more convenient, and less expensive; safer than injection; dosing more likely to be reversible in cases of accidental ingestion (e.g., through induction of emesis, administration of activated charcoal)	Variable absorption; inactivation of some drugs by stomach acid or pH; problems with first-pass effect or presystemic metabolism; greater dependence of drug action on patient variables	Enteral routes include oral administration and involve a variety of dosage forms; e.g., liquids, solutions, tablets, and enteric-coated pills or tablets. Some medications should be taken with food and some should not be taken with food; oral forms should always be taken with at least 180–240 mL of fluid, such as water. Other factors to consider include other medicines being taken at the same time and concurrent use of dairy products or antacids. If oral forms (liquids are preferred; tablets should be crushed well) are given via nasogastric tube or gastrostomy tube, tube should be assessed for placement in stomach and head should remain elevated; at least 30–60 mL of water or carbonated fluids should be used to flush tube prior to and after drug has been given to keep tube patent.
Sublingual, buccal (subtypes of oral, but more parenteral than enteral)	Absorbed more rapidly from oral mucosa and leads to more rapid onset of action; avoids breakdown of drug by stomach acid; avoids first-pass metabolism because gastric absorption is bypassed	Patients may swallow pill instead of keeping under tongue until dissolved; pills often smaller to handle	Drugs given via sublingual route should be placed under the tongue; once dissolved, drug may then be swallowed. In the buccal route, medication is placed between the cheek and gum. Both of these dosage forms are relatively nonirritating; drug is usually without flavour and is water soluble.
Rectal	Provides relatively rapid absorption; good alternative when oral route not feasible; useful for local or systemic drug delivery; usually leads to mixed first-pass and non–first-pass metabolism	Possible discomfort and embarrassment to patient; often higher cost than oral route	Absorption via this route is erratic and unpredictable, but it provides a safe alternative whenever nausea or vomiting prevents oral dosing of drugs. Patient should lie on the left side for insertion of rectal dosage form. Suppositories are inserted using the index finger of a gloved hand and water-soluble lubricant. Drug should be administered exactly as ordered.
Topical	Delivers medication directly to affected area; decreases likelihood of systemic drug effects	Sometimes awkward to self-administer (e.g., eye drops); can be messy; usually higher cost than oral route	Most dermatological drugs are given via topical route in form of a solution, ointment, spray, or drops. Skin should be clean and free of debris; if measurement of ointment is necessary, such as with topical nitroglycerin, it should be done carefully and per instructions (e.g., apply 25 millimetres of ointment). The nurse should wear gloves to minimize cross contamination and prevent absorption of drug into the skin. If patient's skin is not intact, sterile technique is needed.
Transdermal (subtype of topical)	Provides relatively constant rate of drug absorption; one patch can last 1–7 days, depending on drug; avoids first-pass metabolism	Rate of absorption can be affected by excessive perspiration and body temperature; patch may peel off; cost is higher.	Transdermal drugs should be placed on alternating sites, on a clean and nonirritating area, and only after the previously applied patch has been removed and the area cleansed and dried. Transdermal drugs generally come in a single-dose, adhesive-backed drug application system. Used patches must be disposed of safely.

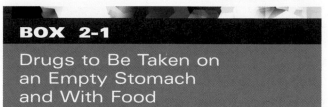

BOX 2-1

Drugs to Be Taken on an Empty Stomach and With Food

Many medications are taken on an empty stomach with at least 180 mL of water. The nurse must give patients specific instructions regarding those medications *not* to be taken with food and that should be taken on an empty stomach. Examples include alendronate sodium and risedronate sodium.

Medications that are generally taken with food include carbamazepine, iron and iron-containing products, hydralazine, lithium, propranolol, spironolactone, nonsteroidal anti-inflammatory drugs, and theophylline.

Erythromycins, tetracyclines, and theophylline are often taken with food (even though they are specified to be taken with a full glass of water and on an empty stomach) to minimize the gastrointestinal irritation associated with these drugs.

If doubt exists, a licensed pharmacist or a current authoritative drug resource should be consulted. An Internet source to use is Shopper's Drug Mart HealthWATCH Medication Library (http://www.shoppersdrugmart.ca/english/health_wellness/medication_library/index.html).

with the blood throughout the body. An intravenous drug formulation is thus absorbed the fastest. Transdermal patches, intramuscular injections, and subcutaneous injections are usually absorbed over a period of several hours, days, or weeks.

Drugs can be injected *intradermally*, *subcutaneously*, *intra-arterially*, *intramuscularly*, *intrathecally*, *intra-articularly*, or *intravenously*. Medications given by the parenteral route also have the advantage of bypassing the first-pass effect of the liver. The parenteral route of administration offers an alternative route of delivery for those medications that cannot be given orally. The problems posed by acid changes within the stomach, absorption changes in the intestines (e.g., following intestinal surgery), and the presence or absence of food and fluid are no longer a concern. There are fewer obstacles to absorption with parenteral administration than with enteral administration of drugs. However, drugs administered by the parenteral route must still be absorbed into cells and tissues before they can exert their pharmacological effect (see Table 2-3).

Subcutaneous, Intradermal, and Intramuscular. Parenteral injections into the fatty subcutaneous tissues under the dermal layer of the skin are referred to as *subcutaneous injections*, whereas injections under the more superficial skin layers immediately underneath the epidermal layer of skin and into the dermal layer are known as *intradermal injections*. Parenteral injections given into the muscle beneath the subcutaneous fatty tissue are

referred to as *intramuscular* injections. Muscles have a greater blood supply than that of the skin; therefore, drugs injected intramuscularly are typically absorbed faster than drugs injected subcutaneously. Absorption from either of these sites may be increased by applying heat to the injection site or by massaging the site; both methods increase blood flow to the area, thereby enhancing absorption. Most intramuscularly injected drugs are absorbed over several hours. However, specially formulated long-acting intramuscular dosage forms known as *depot* drugs are designed for slow absorption and may be absorbed over a period of several days to a few months or longer. The intramuscular corticosteroid methylprednisolone acetate (Depo-Medrol) can provide anti-inflammatory effects for several weeks. The intramuscular contraceptive medroxyprogesterone acetate (Depo-Provera) normally prevents pregnancy for 3 months per dose. The subcutaneously administered drug insulin glargine is a long-acting insulin product that is now commonly used. In contrast, the presence of cold, hypotension, or poor peripheral blood flow compromises the circulation, reducing drug activity by reducing drug delivery to the tissues.

Topical. Topical routes of drug administration involve the application of medications to body surfaces. Several different topical drug delivery systems exist. Topically administered drugs can be applied to the skin, eyes, ears, nose, lungs, rectum, or vagina. As with the enteral and parenteral routes, there are both benefits and drawbacks to use of the topical route of administration. Topical application delivers a more uniform amount of drug over a long period, but the effects of the drug are usually slower in their onset and prolonged in their duration of action. This can be a problem if the patient begins to experience adverse effects from the drug and a considerable amount of drug has already been absorbed in the subcutaneous tissues or mucosal tissues. All topical routes of drug administration also avoid first-pass effects of the liver, with the exception of rectal drug administration. Because the rectum is part of the gastrointestinal tract, some drug will be absorbed into the capillaries that feed the portal vein to the liver. However, some drugs will also be absorbed locally into the perirectal tissues. Therefore, rectally administered drugs are said to have a mixed first-pass and non–first-pass absorption and metabolism. Box 2-2 lists the drug routes and indicates whether they are associated with first-pass effects in the liver.

Topical ointments, gels, and creams are common types of topically administered drugs. Examples include sunscreens, antibiotics, and nitroglycerin ointment. The drawback to their use is that their systemic absorption is often erratic and unreliable. Generally, these medications are used for local effects, but some are used for systemic effects (e.g., nitroglycerin ointment for maintenance treatment of angina). Topically applied drugs can also be used in the treatment of illnesses of the eyes, ears, and sinuses. Eye, ear, and nose drops are administered primarily for local and not systemic effects, whereas nasal sprays may

BOX 2-2

Drug Routes and First-Pass Effects

First-Pass Routes

Hepatic arterial
Oral
Portal venous
Rectal*

Non–First-Pass Routes

Aural (instilled into the ear)
Buccal
Inhaled
Intra-arterial
Intramuscular
Intranasal
Intraocular
Intravaginal
Intravenous
Subcutaneous
Sublingual
Transdermal

*Leads to both first-pass and non–first-pass effects.

Inhalation. Inhalation is another type of topical drug administration. Inhaled drugs are delivered to the lungs as micrometre-sized drug particles. This small drug size is necessary for the drug to be transported to the small air sacs within the lungs (alveoli). Once the small particles of drug are in the alveoli, drug absorption is fairly easy. At this site the thin-walled pulmonary alveolus is in contact with the capillaries, where the drug can be absorbed quickly. Many pulmonary and other types of diseases can be treated with such topically applied (inhaled) drugs. Examples of inhaled drugs are zanamivir, which is used for the prevention of influenza; salbutamol sulfate, which is used to treat bronchial constriction in individuals with asthma; and beclomethasone, which is used to prevent inflammation associated with asthma.

Distribution

Once a drug enters the bloodstream (circulation), it is distributed throughout the body. At this point, it is also beginning to be eliminated by the organs that metabolize and excrete drugs—primarily the liver and the kidneys. *Distribution* refers to the transport of a drug in the body by the bloodstream to its site of action (Figure 2-4). The areas to which the drug is distributed first are those that are most extensively supplied with blood. Areas of rapid distribution include the heart, liver, kidneys, and brain. Areas of slower distribution include muscle, skin, and fat. Drug molecules can be freely distributed to *extravascular* (outside the blood vessels) tissue to reach their site of action only if they are not bound to plasma proteins. If a drug is bound to plasma proteins, the drug–protein complex is generally too large to pass through the walls of blood capillaries into tissues. There are three primary proteins that bind to and carry drugs in the bloodstream throughout the body: *albumin*, α_1-*acid glycoprotein*, and *corticosteroid-binding globulin*. By far the most important of these is albumin. If a given drug binds to plasma proteins as part of its chemical attributes, then there is only a limited amount of drug that is *not* bound to protein. This unbound portion is pharmacologically active and is considered "free" drug, whereas "bound" drug is pharmacologically inactive. Certain conditions that cause low albumin levels, such as extensive burns, malnourished states, and negative nitrogen balance, result in the presence of a larger fraction of free (unbound and active) drug. This can raise the risk of drug toxicity.

When an individual is taking two drugs that are highly protein bound, the drugs may compete for binding sites on plasma proteins. Because of this competition, less of one or both of the drugs binds to the proteins. Consequently, there is more free, unbound drug. This can lead to an unpredictable drug response called a *drug–drug interaction*, which occurs when the presence of one drug decreases or increases the action of another drug administered concurrently (given at the same time).

A theoretical volume, called the *volume of distribution*, is sometimes used to describe the areas where drugs may be distributed. These areas, or *compartments*, may be the blood (*intravascular space*), total body water, body fat,

be used for both (e.g., oxymetazoline for nasal sinus congestion, sumatriptan for migraine headaches). Rectally administered drugs are often given for systemic effects (e.g., antinausea, analgesia), but they are also used to treat disease within the rectum or adjacent bowel (e.g., anti-inflammatory ointment for hemorrhoids, corticosteroid enemas for colitis). Vaginal medications may also be given for systemic effects (e.g., progestational hormone therapy) but are more commonly used for local effects (e.g., treatment of vaginal infection).

Transdermal. Transdermal drug delivery through adhesive drug patches is a more elaborate topical route of drug administration that is commonly used for systemic drug effects. Some examples of drugs administered by this route are fentanyl (for pain), nitroglycerin (for angina), nicotine (for smoking cessation), estrogen (for menopausal symptoms), and rivastigmine (for Alzheimer's disease). Transdermal patches are usually designed to deliver a constant amount of drug per unit of time for a specified time period. For example, a nitroglycerin patch may deliver 0.2 mg or 0.4 mg of drug in a 24-hour period, whereas a fentanyl patch may deliver 25 to 100 mcg/hr of fentanyl for a 72-hour period. Transdermal drug delivery also offers the advantage of bypassing the liver and its first-pass effects. It is suitable for patients who cannot tolerate orally administered medications and in other situations provides a convenient method for drug delivery. The design of the drug delivery system in a specific transdermal patch determines its duration of action.

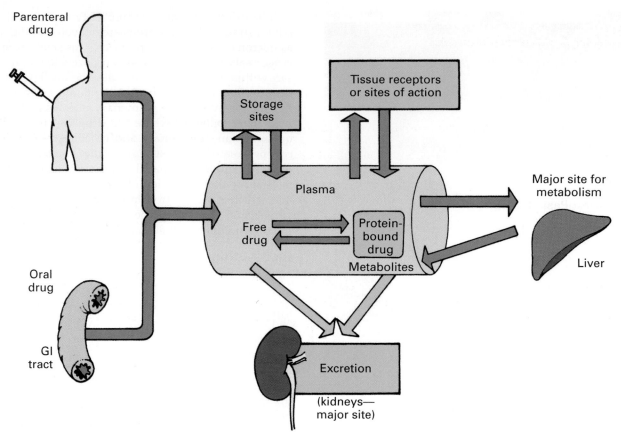

FIG. 2-4   Drug transport in the body. From McKenry, L. M., & Salerno, E. (1995). *Mosby's pharmacology in nursing* (19th ed.). St. Louis, MO: Mosby.

or other body tissues and organs. Typically a drug that is highly water soluble will have a small volume of distribution and high blood concentrations. In other words, the drug tends to stay within the blood because of its high water content. The opposite is true for drugs that are highly fat soluble. Fat-soluble drugs have a large volume of distribution and low blood concentrations. This is because they tend to be chemically repelled by the high water content of the blood and more attracted by the relatively low water content and higher fat content of the tissues. Drugs that are water soluble and highly protein bound are more strongly bound to proteins in the blood and are less likely to be absorbed into tissues. Because of this, their distribution and onset of action can be slow. Drugs that are highly lipid soluble and poorly bound to protein are more easily taken up into tissues and distributed throughout the body. They may even be reabsorbed back into the circulation from tissue. There are some sites in the body into which it may be difficult to distribute a drug. These sites typically either have a poor blood supply (e.g., bone) or have physiological barriers that make it difficult for drugs to pass through (e.g., the brain because of the blood–brain barrier).

Metabolism

Metabolism is also referred to as **biotransformation** because it involves the biochemical alteration of a drug

into an inactive metabolite, a more soluble compound, or a more potent metabolite (as in the conversion of an inactive prodrug to its active form). Metabolism is the next step after absorption and distribution. The organ most responsible for the biotransformation or metabolism of drugs is the liver. Other metabolic tissues include the skeletal muscle, kidneys, lungs, plasma, and intestinal mucosa.

Liver biotransformation involves the activity of a large class of enzymes known as **cytochrome P450** enzymes (or simply P450 enzymes), also known as microsomal enzymes. These enzymes control a variety of biochemical reactions that aid in the metabolism of medications and are largely targeted against lipid-soluble, nonpolar (no charge) drugs, which are typically difficult to eliminate. This includes the majority of medications. Those medications with water-soluble (polar) molecules may be more easily metabolized by simpler metabolic reactions such as *hydrolysis* (splitting by water molecules). Some of the chemical reactions by which the liver can metabolize drugs are listed in Table 2-4. Drug molecules that are the metabolic targets of specific enzymes are said to be **substrates** of those enzymes. Specific P450 enzymes are identified by standardized number and letter designations. Some of the most common P450 enzymes and common drug substrates are listed in Table 2-5.

The biotransformation capabilities of the liver can vary considerably from patient to patient. Factors that

TABLE 2-4

Mechanisms of Biotransformation

Type of Biotransformation	Mechanism	Result
Oxidation Reduction Hydrolysis	Chemical reactions	Increased polarity of chemical, making it more water soluble and more easily excretable. Often this results in a loss of pharmacological activity.
Conjugation (e. g., glucuronidation, glycination, sulphation methylation, alkylation)	Combination with another substance (e.g., glucuronide, glycine, sulfate, methyl groups, alkyl groups)	

can alter the biotransformation of a drug, including genetics, diseases, and the concurrent use of other medications, are listed in Table 2-6.

Delayed drug metabolism results in the accumulation of the drug in the body and prolongation of the effects of or responses to drugs. Stimulating drug metabolism can thus cause diminishing pharmacological effects. This often occurs with the repeated administration of some drugs that can stimulate the formation of new microsomal enzymes. Such drugs are said to be enzyme *inducers.* Conversely, many other drugs inhibit various classes of drug-metabolizing enzymes and are called enzyme *inhibitors. Such inhibition can lead to drug toxicity.*

Excretion

Whether they are parent compounds or are active or inactive metabolites, all drugs must eventually be removed from the body. *Excretion* is the process through which drugs are eliminated; the primary organ responsible for this is the kidney. Two other organs that play an important role in the excretion of drugs are the liver and the bowel. Most drugs are metabolized in the liver by glucuronidases and by hydroxylation and acetylation. Therefore, by the time most drugs reach the kidneys, they have been extensively metabolized and only a relatively small fraction of the original drug is excreted

as the original compound. Other drugs may circumvent metabolism and reach the kidneys in their original form.

Drugs that have been metabolized by the liver become more polar and water soluble. This makes their elimination by the kidney much easier because the urinary tract is water based. The kidneys are also capable of forming glucuronides and sulfates from various drugs and their metabolites, although usually to a lesser extent than the liver.

The act of kidney excretion is accomplished through *glomerular filtration, active tubular reabsorption,* and *active tubular secretion.* Free (unbound) water-soluble drugs and metabolites go through passive glomerular filtration, which takes place between the blood vessels of the afferent arterioles and the glomeruli. Many substances present in the nephrons go through active reabsorption at the level of the tubules, where they are taken back up into the circulation and transported away from the kidney. This process is an attempt by the body to retain needed substances. Some substances are actively resorbed back into the systemic circulation. Some substances may also be secreted into the nephron from the vasculature surrounding it. The processes of filtration, reabsorption, and secretion in urinary elimination are shown in Figure 2-5.

TABLE 2-5

Common Liver Cytochrome P450 Enzymes and Corresponding Drug Substrates

Enzyme	Common Drug Substrates
1A2	acetaminophen, caffeine, theophylline, warfarin
2C9	ibuprofen, phenytoin
2C19	diazepam, naproxen, omeprazole, propranolol
2D6	clozapine, codeine, fluoxetine, haloperidol, hydrocodone, metoprolol, oxycodone, paroxetine, propoxyphene, risperidone, selegiline, tricyclic antidepressants
2E1	acetaminophen, enflurane, ethanol, halothane
3A4	acetaminophen, amiodarone, cocaine, cyclosporine, diltiazem, ethinyl estradiol, indinavir, lidocaine, macrolides, progesterone, spironolactone, sulfamethoxazole, testosterone, verapamil

TABLE 2-6

Examples of Conditions and Drugs That Affect Drug Metabolism

Category	Example	Drug Metabolism Increased	Drug Metabolism Decreased
Diseases	Cardiovascular dysfunction		X
	Kidney insufficiency		X
Condition	Genetic constitution		
	Obstructive jaundice		X
	Starvation		X
	Fast acetylator	X	
	Slow acetylator		X
Drugs	Barbiturates	X	
	erythromycin (P450 inhibitor)		X
	ketoconazole (P450 inhibitor)		X
	rifampin (P450 inducer)	X	

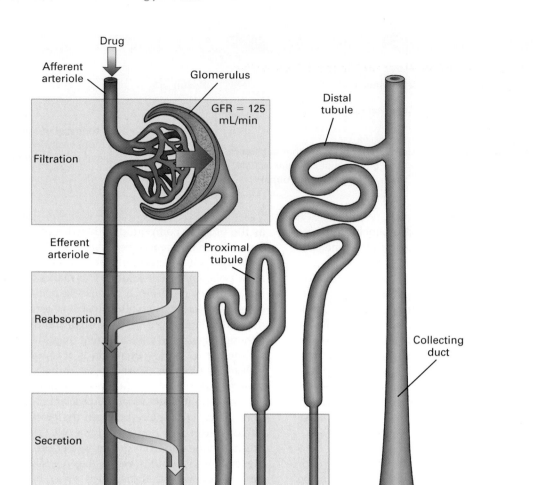

FIG. 2-5 Renal drug excretion. The primary processes involved in drug excretion and the approximate location where these processes take place in the kidney are illustrated. *GFR*, glomerular filtration rate.

The excretion of drugs by the intestines is another common route of elimination. This process is referred to as *biliary excretion*. Drugs eliminated by this route are taken up by the liver, released into the bile, and eliminated in the feces. Once certain drugs, such as fat-soluble drugs, are in the bile, they may be reabsorbed into the bloodstream, returned to the liver, and again secreted into the bile. This process is called *enterohepatic recirculation*. Enterohepatically recirculated drugs are often associated with multiple peaks and a longer half-life (see Half-Life section, below) of a drug. For example, estrogen, a fat-soluble drug, undergoes enterohepatic recycling; as a result, estrogen has a longer half-life and duration of action. Another example is the common laxative Ex-Lax Chocolate, a sennoside, which takes approximately 12 hours to take effect. Because the drug undergoes enterohepatic recycling, in another 12 hours there is likely to be further effect from the drug.

Less common routes of elimination are the lungs and the sweat, salivary, and mammary glands. Depending on the drug, these organs and glands can be highly effective eliminators.

Half-Life

Another pharmacokinetic variable is the drug's **half-life,** which is the time it takes for one half of a given amount of a drug in the body to be removed and is a measure of the rate at which the drug is eliminated from the body. For instance, if the maximum level that a particular dosage could achieve in the body is 100 mg/L and in 8 hours the measured drug level is 50 mg/L, then the estimated half-life for that drug is 8 hours. The concept of drug half-life viewed from several perspectives is illustrated in Table 2-7.

After about five half-lives, most drugs are considered removed from the body. At that time approximately 97%

TABLE 2-7					
Example of a Drug Half-Life Viewed from Different Perspectives					
Different Perspectives			**Changing Values**		
Drug concentration (mg/L)	100 (peak)	50	25	12.5	6.25	3.125 (trough)
Hours after peak concentration	0	8	16	24	32	40
Number of half-lives	0	1	2	3	4	5
Percentage of drug removed	0	50	75	88	94	97

of the drug has been eliminated, and what little amount remains is too small to have a therapeutic or toxic effect.

The concept of half-life is clinically useful for determining when a patient taking a particular drug will be at steady state. **Steady state** with regard to blood levels of a drug refers to the physiological state in which the amount of drug removed via elimination (e.g., kidney clearance) is equal to the amount of drug absorbed with each dose. This physiological-plateau phenomenon typically occurs after four to five half-lives of administration of a drug. Therefore, if a drug has an extremely long half-life, it will take much longer for the drug to reach steady-state blood levels. This commonly occurs, for example, when patients are started on certain antidepressants such as fluoxetine (Chapter 16). Once steady-state blood levels have been reached, there are consistent levels of drug in the body that correlate with maximum therapeutic benefits.

Onset, Peak, and Duration

The pharmacokinetic terms *absorption, distribution, metabolism,* and *excretion* are all used to describe the movement of drugs through the body. *Drug actions* are the cellular processes involved in the interaction between a drug and a cell (e.g., a drug's action on a receptor). In contrast, **drug effects** are the physiological reactions of the body to the drug. The terms *onset, peak,* and *duration* are used to describe drug effects. *Peak* and *trough* are also used to describe drug concentrations, which are usually measured from blood samples.

A drug's **onset of action** is the time required for the drug to elicit a therapeutic response. A drug's **peak effect** is the time required for a drug to reach its maximum therapeutic response. Physiologically, this corresponds to increasing drug concentrations at the site of action. The **duration of action** of a drug is the length of time that the drug concentration is sufficient (without more doses) for the drug to elicit a therapeutic response. These concepts are illustrated in Figure 2-6.

The amount of time of the onset and peak of action, and the duration of action often plays an important part in determining the **peak level** (highest blood level) and **trough level** (lowest blood level) of a drug. If the peak blood level is too high, then drug **toxicity** may occur; that is, the drug may become poisonous. The toxicity

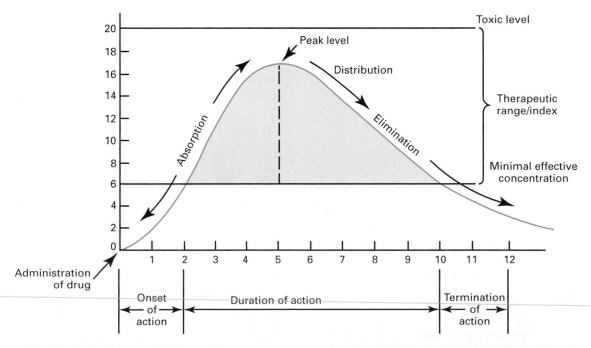

FIG. 2-6 Characteristics of drug effects and relationship to the therapeutic window. From McKenry, L. M., Tessier, E., & Hogan, M. (2006). *Mosby's pharmacology in nursing* (22nd ed.). St. Louis, MO: Mosby Elsevier.

may be mild, such as extension of the effects of the given drug (e.g., excessive sedation resulting from overdose of a drug with sedative properties). However, it can also be severe (e.g., damage to vital organs or cessation of vital signs due to excessive drug exposure). If the trough blood level is too low, then the drug may not be at a therapeutic level. (A common example is antibiotic drug therapy with aminoglycoside antibiotics; see Chapter 39). Therefore, peak and trough levels are important monitoring parameters for some medications and are used in **therapeutic drug monitoring** of some medications. In therapeutic drug monitoring, peak and trough values are measured to verify adequate drug exposure, maximize therapeutic effects, and minimize drug toxicity. This monitoring is often carried out by a clinical pharmacist working with other members of the health care team.

PHARMACODYNAMICS

Anatomy and physiology are the study of how the body is structured and why the body functions the way it does. Drug-induced alterations in these normal physiological functions are explained by the principles of *pharmacodynamics*, which is concerned with the mechanisms of drug action in living tissues. A positive change in a faulty physiological system is called a **therapeutic effect** of a drug. Such an effect is the goal of drug therapy. Understanding the pharmacodynamic characteristics of a drug can aid in assessing the drug's therapeutic effect.

Mechanism of Action

Drugs can produce actions (therapeutic effects) in several ways. The effects of a particular drug depend on the cells or tissue targeted by the drug. Once the drug is at the site of action, it can modify (increase or decrease) the rate at which that cell or tissue functions, or the drug can modify the strength of function of that cell or tissue. A drug cannot, however, cause a cell or tissue to perform a function that is not part of its natural physiology.

Drugs can exert their actions in three basic ways: through *receptors*, through *enzymes*, and through *nonselective interactions*. These mechanisms are discussed in the following sections.

Receptor Interactions

If the mechanism of action of a drug involves a receptor interaction, then the molecular structure of the drug is critical. Drug–receptor interaction entails the selective joining of the drug molecule with a reactive site on the surface of a cell or tissue. Most commonly, this site is a macromolecular protein structure within the cell membrane. This binding of the drug molecule to the receptor molecule in turn elicits a biological effect. Therefore, a receptor can be defined as a reactive site on the surface or inside of a cell. Once a drug binds to and interacts with the receptor, a pharmacological response is produced (Figure 2-7). The degree to which a drug attaches and binds with a receptor is called its *affinity*. The drug with the best "fit" and strongest affinity for the receptor will elicit the greatest response from the cell or tissue. A drug becomes bound to the receptor through the formation of chemical bonds between the receptor on the cell and the *active site* on the drug molecule. A drugs that binds to receptors and stimulates a physiological response is called an **agonist**; one that blocks or inhibits a response is an **antagonist**. Table 2-8 describes the different types of drug–receptor interaction. The drugs that are most effective at eliciting a response from a receptor are those drugs that most closely resemble the body's endogenous substances (e.g., hormones, neurotransmitters) that normally bind to that receptor.

Enzyme Interactions

Enzymes are substances that catalyze nearly every biochemical reaction in a cell. The second way drugs can produce effects is by interacting with these enzyme systems. For a drug to alter a physiological response in this way, it may either inhibit (more common) or enhance (less common) the action of a specific enzyme. This process is called *selective interaction*. A drug–enzyme interaction occurs when the drug chemically binds to an enzyme molecule in such a way that alters (inhibits or enhances) the enzyme's interaction with its normal target molecules in the body. For example, angiotensin-converting enzyme (ACE) causes a chemical reaction that results in the production of a substance called *angiotensin II*, which is a potent vasoconstrictor and mediator of several other processes. Drugs called *ACE inhibitors* attract ACE to bind to them rather than to angiotensin I, the usual substrate of ACE, and thereby prevent the formation of angiotensin II. This in turn causes vasodilation and helps reduce blood pressure.

Nonselective Interactions

Drugs with nonselective mechanisms of action do not interact with receptors or enzymes to alter a physiological or biological function of the body. Instead, cell membranes and cellular processes such as metabolic

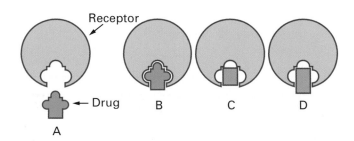

FIG. 2-7 **A,** Drugs act by forming a chemical bond with specific receptor sites, similar to a key and lock. **B,** The better the "fit," the better the response. Drugs with complete attachment and response are called *agonists*. **C,** Drugs that attach but do not elicit a response are called *antagonists*. **D,** Drugs that attach, elicit some response, and also block other responses are called *partial agonists* or *agonist–antagonists.* From Clayton, B. D., & Stock, Y. N. (2004). *Basic pharmacology for nurses* (13th ed.). St. Louis, MO: Mosby.

TABLE 2-8

Drug–Receptor Interactions

Drug Type	Action
Agonist	Drug binds to the receptor; there is a response.
Partial agonist (agonist–antagonist)	Drug binds to the receptor; the response is diminished compared with that elicited by an agonist.
Antagonist	Drug binds to the receptor; there is no response. Drug prevents binding of agonists.
Competitive antagonist	Drug competes with the agonist for binding to the receptor. If it binds, there is no response.
Noncompetitive antagonist	Drug combines with different parts of the receptor and inactivates it; agonist then has no effect.

activities are their main targets. Such drugs can either physically interfere with or chemically alter these cellular structures or processes. Some cancer drugs and antibiotics have this mechanism of action. By incorporating themselves into the normal metabolic process, they cause a defect in the final product or state. This defect may be an improperly formed cell wall that results in cell death through cell lysis or it may be the lack of a needed energy substrate, which leads to cell starvation and death.

PHARMACOTHERAPEUTICS

Before drug therapy is initiated, an end point or expected outcome of therapy should be established. This desired therapeutic outcome should be patient specific, should be established in collaboration with the patient, and, if appropriate, should be determined with other members of the health care team. Outcomes must be clearly defined and either measurable or observable by the patient or caregiver. A time line for these outcomes should also be specified. The progress being made toward the targeted objective should be monitored. Goal outcomes should be realistic and prioritized so that drug therapy begins with interventions that are essential to the patient's acute well-being or interventions that the patient perceives to be important. Examples of such outcomes are curing a disease, eliminating or reducing a pre-existing symptom, arresting or slowing a disease process, preventing a disease or other unwanted condition, or otherwise improving the quality of life. These goals and outcomes are not the same as nursing goals and outcomes.

Patient therapy assessment is the process by which practitioners integrate their knowledge of medical and drug-related facts with information about a specific patient's medical and social history. Items that should be considered in the assessment are drugs currently used (prescription, over-the-counter, and illicit or street drugs), pregnancy and breastfeeding status, and concurrent illnesses that could contraindicate starting a given medication. A **contraindication** to a medication is any characteristic of the patient, especially a disease state, which makes the use of a given medication dangerous for the patient. Careful attention to this assessment process helps to ensure an optimal therapeutic plan for the patient.

The implementation of a treatment plan can involve delivery of several types and combinations of therapies. The type of therapy can be categorized as acute, maintenance, supplemental (or replacement), palliative, supportive, prophylactic, or empiric.

Types of Therapy

Acute Therapy

Acute therapy often involves more intensive drug therapy and is implemented in the acutely ill (those with a rapid onset of illness) or even the critically ill. It is often needed to sustain life or treat disease. Examples are the administration of vasopressors to maintain blood pressure and cardiac output after open-heart surgery, the use of volume expanders in a patient who is in shock, the use of antibiotics in a trauma patient at high risk of infection, and intensive chemotherapy for a patient with newly diagnosed cancer.

Maintenance Therapy

Maintenance therapy typically does not eradicate problems the patient may have but does prevent progression of a disease or condition. It is used for the treatment of chronic illnesses such as hypertension. In such a case, maintenance therapy maintains the patient's blood pressure within given limits, which prevents certain end-organ damage. Another example of maintenance therapy is the use of oral contraceptives for birth control.

Supplemental Therapy

Supplemental or replacement therapy supplies the body with a substance needed to maintain normal function. This substance may be needed because it either cannot be made by the body or is produced in insufficient quantity. Examples are the administration of insulin to diabetic patients and of iron to patients with iron-deficiency anemia.

Palliative Therapy

The goal of palliative therapy is to make the patient as comfortable as possible. It is typically used in the end stages of an illness when all attempts at curative therapy have failed. Examples are the use of high-dose opioid analgesics to relieve pain in the final stages of cancer and the use of oxygen in end-stage pulmonary disease.

Supportive Therapy

Supportive therapy maintains the integrity of body functions while the patient is recovering from illness or trauma. Examples are provision of fluids and electrolytes to prevent dehydration in a patient with influenza who is vomiting and has diarrhea, and administration of fluids, volume expanders, or blood products to a patient who has lost blood during surgery.

Prophylactic Therapy and Empirical Therapy

Prophylactic therapy is drug therapy provided to *prevent* illness or other undesirable outcome. Its use is based on scientific knowledge often acquired during years of observation of a disease and its causes. For example, a surgeon knows that when an incision is made through the skin there is the possibility that skin bacteria are present that can later infect the incision. Thus the surgeon administers an antibiotic before making the incision. Prophylactic therapy is also used in dental procedures for patients with mitral valve prolapse and in patients with prosthetic valves or joints or Teflon grafts. Intravenous antibiotic therapy may also be used to prevent infection during a high-risk surgery and is considered prophylactic.

Unlike most prophylactic therapy, empiric therapy does not have a scientific basis but instead is based on experience. It is the administration of a drug when a certain pathological process is suspected, based on the patient's symptoms, because the drug has been found in the past to be beneficial in such cases. For example, acetaminophen is given to a patient who has a fever. The cause of the fever may not be known, but empirically the patient is given acetaminophen because it has been demonstrated to lower the body temperature.

Monitoring

Once the appropriate therapy has been implemented, the effectiveness of that therapy—that is, the *clinical response* of the patient to the therapy—must be evaluated. Evaluating the clinical response requires that the evaluator be familiar with both the drug's intended therapeutic action (beneficial effects) and its unintended possible adverse effects (predictable adverse drug reactions). It should be noted that this text generally highlights only the most common adverse effects of a given drug; the drug may have many other less commonly reported adverse effects. One must always keep in mind that patients may sometimes experience less common, and therefore less readily identifiable, adverse drug effects. The nurse should consult comprehensive references, pharmacists, or poison and drug information centre staff whenever there is uncertainty regarding adverse effects that a patient may be experiencing. All drugs are potentially toxic and can have cumulative effects. Recognizing these toxic effects and knowing their manifestations in the patient are integral components of the monitoring process. A drug accumulates when it is absorbed more quickly than it is eliminated or when it is administered before the previous dose has been metabolized or cleared from the body.

Knowledge of the function of the organs responsible for metabolizing and eliminating a drug, combined with knowledge of how a particular drug is metabolized and excreted, enables the nurse to anticipate problems and treat them appropriately if they occur.

Therapeutic Index

The ratio of a drug's toxic level to the level that provides therapeutic benefits is referred to as the drug's **therapeutic index.** The safety of a particular drug therapy is determined by this index. A low therapeutic index means that the difference between a therapeutically active dose and a toxic dose is small. A drug with a low therapeutic index has a greater likelihood than other drugs of causing an adverse reaction, thus its use requires closer monitoring. Examples of such drugs are warfarin and digoxin.

Drug Concentration

Drug concentration in patients can be an important tool for evaluating the clinical response to a drug. Certain drug levels are associated with therapeutic responses, whereas other drug levels are associated with toxic effects. Toxic drug levels are typically seen when the body's normal mechanisms for metabolizing and excreting drugs are impaired. This commonly occurs when liver and kidney functions are impaired or when the liver or kidneys are immature (as in neonates). Dosages should be made in these patients to appropriately accommodate their impaired metabolism and excretion.

Patient's Condition

Another patient-specific factor to be considered when monitoring drug therapy is the patient's concurrent diseases or other medical conditions. A patient's response to a drug may vary greatly depending on physiological and psychological demands. Disease of any kind, infection, cardiovascular function, and GI function are just a few of the physiological elements that can alter a patient's therapeutic response. Stress, depression, and anxiety are some of the psychological factors affecting response.

Tolerance and Dependence

The monitoring of drug therapy requires knowledge of tolerance and dependence and an understanding of the difference between the two. *Tolerance* is a decreasing response to repeated drug doses. *Dependence* is a physiological or psychological need for a drug. *Physical dependence* is the physiological need for a drug to avoid physical withdrawal symptoms (e.g., tachycardia in an opioid-addicted patient). *Psychological dependence*, also known as *addiction,* is the obsessive desire for the euphoric effects of a drug. Addiction typically involves the recreational use of drugs such as benzodiazepines, narcotics, and amphetamines. See Chapter 9 for further discussion of dependence.

Interactions

Drugs may interact with other drugs, with foods, or with agents administered as part of laboratory tests.

Alteration of the action of one drug by another is referred to as a **drug interaction.** A drug interaction can either increase or decrease the actions of one or both of the involved drugs and can be either beneficial or harmful. Knowledge of drug interactions is vital for the appropriate monitoring of drug therapy, and understanding the mechanisms by which drug interactions occur can help prevent them. Concurrently administered drugs that do interact with each other alter the pharmacokinetics of one another during the four phases of pharmacokinetics discussed previously: absorption, distribution, metabolism, and excretion. Table 2-9 provides examples of drug interaction during each of these phases. It also illustrates how some drug interactions can be beneficial.

Careful patient care combined with knowledge of all drugs being administered can decrease the likelihood of a harmful drug interaction. The more drugs a patient receives, the more likely it is that a drug interaction will occur. This is especially true in older adults, who typically have an increased sensitivity to drug effects and are receiving several medications. In addition, over-the-counter drugs and natural health products can interact significantly with prescribed medications.

Many terms are used to categorize drug interactions. When two drugs with similar actions are given together they can have **additive effects.** This means simply that the combined effects of the drugs summate such that if two or more drugs are administered at the same time, the action of one plus the action of the other results in an action as if just one drug had been given. This can be represented by 1 + 1 = 2. Examples are the many combinations of analgesic products, such as acetylsalicylic acid and opioid combinations (acetylsalicylic acid and codeine) or acetaminophen and opioid combinations (acetaminophen and oxycodone).

Often drugs are used together for their additive effects so that smaller doses of each drug can be given; toxic effects are thus avoided while adequate drug action is maintained. An example would be a barbiturate and a tranquilizer given together before surgery to relax the patient.

Synergistic effects are different from simple additive effects and occur when two drugs administered together interact in such a way that their combined effects exceed that predicted by the individual actions of these compounds (i.e., the resulting effect is more than additive). The combination of hydrochlorothiazide with enalapril maleate for the treatment of hypertension is one example. If two drugs are taken together that are similar in action, such as barbiturates and alcohol, both depressants, an effect exaggerated out of proportion to that of each drug taken separately at the given dose may occur. This can be represented by 1 + 1 = 5. Another example is an individual who takes one dose of alcohol and one dose of a barbiturate. Normally, when taken alone, neither substance would cause serious harm, but if taken together the combination could cause coma or death. Drug effects that are almost the opposite of synergistic effects are known as **antagonistic effects.** Antagonistic effects are said to occur when the combination of two drugs results in drug effects that are less than the sum of the effects for each drug given separately. Such an interaction is seen when antacids are given with tetracycline, which results in decreased absorption of tetracycline.

Incompatibility is a term most commonly used with parenteral drugs. Drug incompatibility occurs when two parenteral drugs or solutions are mixed together and the result is a chemical deterioration of one or both of the drugs. The combination of two such drugs usually produces a precipitate, haziness, or colour change in the solution. An example of incompatible drugs is the combination of parenteral furosemide and heparin.

Adverse Drug Events

The recognition of the potential hazards and actual detrimental effects of medication use is a topic that continues to receive much attention in the literature. This focus has contributed to an increasing body of knowledge regarding this topic as well as the development of new terminology. Health care institutions are also under increasing pressure to put into practice effective

| TABLE | 2-9 |

Examples of Drug Interactions and Their Effects on Pharmacokinetics

Pharmacokinetic Phase	Drug	Mechanism	Result
Absorption	antacids with ketoconazole	Increases gastric pH, preventing the breakdown of ketoconazole	Decreased effectiveness of ketoconazole, resulting from decreased blood levels (harmful)
Distribution	warfarin with amiodarone	Both drugs compete for protein-binding sites	Higher levels of free (unbound) warfarin and amiodarone, which increases actions of both drugs (harmful)
Metabolism	erythromycin with cyclosporine	Both drugs compete for the same liver enzymes	Decreased metabolism of cyclosporine, possibly resulting in toxic levels of cyclosporine (harmful)
Excretion	amoxicillin with probenecid	Inhibits the secretion of amoxicillin into the kidneys	Elevates and prolongs the plasma levels of amoxicillin (can be beneficial)

strategies for preventing adverse effects of drugs and addressing them when they do occur.

Adverse drug event (ADE) is a broad term for any undesirable occurrence involving medications. A similarly broad term seen in the literature is *drug misadventure*. Patient outcomes associated with ADEs vary from no effects to mild discomfort to life-threatening complications, permanent disability, disfigurement, or death. ADEs can be preventable (see discussion of medication errors below) or nonpreventable. Fortunately, many ADEs result in no measurable patient harm. For example, a nurse may mistakenly give a single dose of an unprescribed drug (medication error) that is simply metabolized and excreted by the patient's body with no resultant injury. The most common causes of ADE *external* to the patient are errors by caregivers (both professional and nonprofessional) and malfunctioning equipment (e.g., intravenous infusion pumps). However, an ADE can also be *patient induced*, such as when a patient fails to take medication as prescribed or drinks alcoholic beverages despite being advised not to consume alcohol while taking a given medication. In such situations as well, the patient may experience no ill effects or may suffer varying degrees of harm. An ADE that is noticed before it actually occurs should be considered a *potential* ADE (and appropriate steps should be taken to avoid such a "near miss" in the future). A less common situation, but one still worth mentioning, is an *adverse drug withdrawal event*. This is an adverse outcome associated with discontinuation of drug therapy, such as hypertension caused by abruptly discontinuing blood pressure medication or return of infection caused by stopping antibiotic therapy too soon. Of course, these situations can also result from either patient or caregiver actions.

The two most common broad categories of ADE are medication errors and adverse drug reactions. A **medication error (ME)** is a *preventable* situation in which there is a compromise in the *Ten Rights* of medication use: *right patient, right drug, right time, right route, right dose, right documentation, right reason, right patient education, right to refuse, right assessment, and right evaluation.* MEs are more common than adverse drug reactions but can also be the direct cause of such reactions. MEs occur during the *prescribing, dispensing, administering,* or *monitoring* of drug therapy. These four phases are collectively known as the **medication use process.** MEs are discussed in more detail in Chapter 5.

An **adverse drug reaction (ADR)** is any reaction to a drug that is unexpected and undesirable and occurs at therapeutic drug dosages. ADRs may or may not be caused by MEs. ADRs may result in hospital admission, prolongation of hospital stay, change in drug therapy, initiation of supportive treatment, or complication of a patient's disease state. ADRs are caused by processes inside the patient's body. They may or may not be preventable, depending on the situation. Milder ADRs (e.g., drug adverse effects—see later discussion) usually do not require a change in the patient's drug therapy or

other interventions. More severe ADRs, however, are likely to require changes to a patient's drug regimen. Severe ADRs can be permanently or significantly disabling, life threatening, or fatal. They may require or prolong hospitalization, lead to organ damage (e.g., to the liver, kidneys, bone marrow, skin), cause congenital anomalies, or require specific interventions to prevent permanent impairment or tissue damage.

ADRs that are specific to particular drug groups are discussed in the corresponding drug chapters in this book. Four general categories of ADR are discussed here: pharmacological reaction, hypersensitivity (allergic) reaction, idiosyncratic reaction, and drug interaction.

A *pharmacological reaction* is an extension of the drug's normal effects in the body. For example, a drug used to lower blood pressure in a patient with hypertension causes a pharmacological ADR when it lowers the blood pressure to the point at which the patient becomes unconscious.

Pharmacological reactions also include adverse effects. *Adverse effects* are predictable, well-known ADRs resulting in minor or no changes in patient management. They have predictable frequency and intensity, and their occurrence is related to the dose. They also usually resolve upon discontinuation of drug therapy.

An **allergic reaction** (also known as a *hypersensitivity reaction*) involves the patient's immune system. Immune system proteins known as *immunoglobulins* (Chapter 47) recognize the drug molecule, its metabolite(s), or another ingredient in a drug formulation as a dangerous foreign substance. At this point, an *immune response* may occur in which immunoglobulin proteins bind to the drug substance in an attempt to neutralize the drug. Chemical mediators, such as *histamine,* as well as *cytokines* and other inflammatory substances (e.g., *prostaglandins* [Chapter 45]) usually are released during this process. This response can result in reactions ranging from mild (e.g., skin erythema or mild rash) to severe, even life-threatening reactions such as constriction of bronchial airways and tachycardia.

An **idiosyncratic reaction** is not the result of a known pharmacological property of a drug or patient allergy but instead occurs unexpectedly in a particular patient. Such a reaction is a genetically determined abnormal response to ordinary doses of a drug. Genetically inherited traits that result in the abnormal metabolism of drugs are distributed throughout the population. The study of such traits, which are solely revealed by drug administration, is called **pharmacogenetics** (see Chapter 51). Idiosyncratic drug reactions are usually caused by a deficiency or excess of drug-metabolizing enzymes. Many pharmacogenetic disorders exist. A more common one is glucose-6-phosphate dehydrogenase (G6PD) deficiency. This pharmacogenetic disease is transmitted as a sex-linked trait and affects approximately 100 million people (see Ethnocultural Implications). People who lack proper levels of G6PD have idiosyncratic reactions to a wide range of drugs. There are more than 80 variations of the disease, and all produce some degree of drug-induced

ETHNOCULTURAL IMPLICATIONS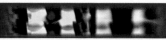

Glucose-6-Phosphate Dehydrogenase Deficiency

Glucose-6-phosphate dehydrogenase (G6PD) is an enzyme found in abundant amounts in the tissues of most individuals. It reduces the risk of hemolysis of red blood cells when they are exposed to oxidizing agents such as acetylsalicylic acid and Chinese remedies such as naphthalene, henna, and fava. G6PD deficiency is inherited as an X-linked, recessive condition, which means the condition usually occurs in boys. There is an increased prevalence of G6PD deficiency in descendants of immigrants to Canada. Approximately 13% of Black males carry the gene that results in G6PD deficiency, and it is prevalent in people of Mediterranean heritage, including Italians, Greeks, Sardinians, Arabs, and Sephardic and Kurdish Jews. The condition tends to be milder in Blacks and more severe in individuals of Mediterranean descent. When exposed to agents such as sulfonamides, antimalarials, acetylsalicylic acid, and some Chinese herbal products, patients with this deficiency may suffer life-threatening hemolysis of the red blood cells, whereas individuals with adequate quantities of the enzyme have no problems in taking these drugs.

---

hemolysis. Drugs capable of inducing hemolysis in G6PD-deficient patients are listed in Box 2-3.

Drug interaction can also lead to an ADR. As described earlier, drug interaction occurs when the simultaneous presence of two (or more) drugs in the body produces an unwanted effect. This unwanted effect can result when one drug either accentuates or reduces the effects of another drug to an undesirable degree. In some instances drug interactions are intentional and beneficial (see Table 2-9).

Other Drug Effects

Other drug-related effects that must be considered during therapy are *teratogenic*, *mutagenic*, and *carcinogenic* effects. These can result in devastating patient outcomes and can be prevented in many instances by appropriate monitoring.

Teratology is the science that studies abnormal fetal development due to different factors. *Teratogenesis* refers to abnormal development of fetal organ(s). Drugs or other chemicals can result in structural defects in the fetus, otherwise known as *teratogenic effects*. Compounds that produce such effects are called *teratogens*. Viral diseases (e.g., measles) and radiation can also have teratogenic effects. Prenatal development involves a delicate programmed sequence of interrelated embryological events. Any significant disruption in this process of embryogenesis can have a teratogenic effect. The period during which the fetus is most vulnerable to teratogenic effects begins with the third week of fetal development and usually ends after the third month. Drugs administered during pregnancy can produce different types of congenital anomalies. Drugs capable of crossing the placenta can act as teratogens and cause **drug-induced teratogenesis**. Chapter 3 describes the safety classification for drugs used by pregnant women.

Mutagenic effects are permanent changes in the genetic composition of living organisms and consist of alterations in the chromosome structure, the number of chromosomes, or the genetic code of the deoxyribonucleic acid (DNA) molecule. Drugs capable of inducing mutations are called *mutagens*. Radiation, viruses, chemicals, and drugs can all act as mutagenic agents in human beings. The largest genetic unit that can be involved in a mutation is a *chromosome* (large DNA strand in all cells); the smallest is a base pair in a DNA molecule. Drugs that affect genetic processes are active primarily during cell reproduction *(mitosis)*.

Carcinogenic effects are the cancer-causing effects of drugs, other chemicals, radiation, and viruses. Entities that produce such effects are called *carcinogens*. Some exogenous causes of cancer are listed in Box 2-4.

BOX 2-3

Drugs to Avoid in Patients With Glucose-6-Phosphate Dehydrogenase Deficiency

acetylsalicylic acid
chloramphenicol
chloroquine
nitrofurantoin
oxidants (all)
primaquine
probenecid
sulfonamides
sulfones

BOX 2-4

Exogenous Carcinogens

Carcinogenic drugs
Dietary customs
Drug misuse
Environmental pollution
Food-processing procedures
Food production procedures
Oncogenic viruses
Radiation
Smoking
Workplace chemicals

PHARMACOGNOSY

The source of all early drugs was nature, and the study of these natural drug sources (plants and animals) is called *pharmacognosy*. Although many drugs in current use are synthetically derived, most were first isolated in nature. By studying the composition of natural substances and their physiological effects in living systems, researchers can identify the chemical features of a substance that produce the desired clinical response. Once identified and isolated, these natural substances are often synthesized in a laboratory for mass production of synthetic drugs. Isolation of a specific natural compound may also alleviate undesirable effects that may occur from other compounds in the natural source (e.g., a plant). Although most new drug products are synthetic, the underlying principle of pharmacognosy is that an understanding of the actions and effects of natural drug sources is essential to new drug development. As one important example, pharmacognosy enabled the isolation of the naturally occurring hormone insulin from animal sources, determination of its exact genetic sequence, modification of this sequence to "humanize" the insulin, and large-scale synthesis of that modified product in the laboratory. This led to the commercial production of synthetic human insulin, one of the world's most widely used drugs.

The four main sources for drugs are plants, animals, minerals, and laboratory synthesis. An example of a plant from which a drug is derived is foxglove. Foxglove is the source of cardiac glycosides and has yielded the present-day drug digoxin. Plants provide many weak acids and weak bases (*alkaloids*) that are useful and potent drugs. Alkaloids are more common. Examples include atropine (belladonna plant), caffeine (coffee bean), and nicotine (tobacco leaf). Animals are the source of many hormone drugs. Conjugated estrogen is derived from the urine of pregnant mares (hence the drug trade name Premarin). Insulin available in Canada comes from two sources: pigs (pork) and humans. Human insulin is either semi-synthetic (pork insulin is converted to human insulin by changing one amino acid) or is made from human sources. Both types are now mass-produced using recombinant DNA techniques. Heparin is another commonly used drug that is derived from cows and pigs (bovine and porcine heparin). Some common mineral sources of currently used drugs are acetylsalicylic acid, aluminum hydroxide, and sodium chloride. Recombinant DNA techniques provide many other synthetic drug products, such as erythropoietin and the granulocyte-colony stimulating factor (filgrastim), both used to stimulate formation of blood components (Chapter 50).

TOXICOLOGY

The study of poisons and unwanted adverse effects of both drugs and other chemicals on living organisms is known as *toxicology*. *Clinical toxicology* deals specifically with the care of the poisoned patient. Poisoning can result from a variety of causes, ranging from prescription drug overdose to ingestion of household cleaning agents to snakebite. Poison control centres (PCCs) are health care institutions equipped with sufficient personnel who have specific expertise in the provision of drug and poison information services to recommend appropriate treatment for the poisoned patient. They are usually staffed with specially trained pharmacists, nurses, and physicians who triage incoming calls and refer complex cases to clinical toxicologists. Telephone contact with a PCC is usually an important early step in aiding the poisoned patient. Computerized drug and chemical information databases are often searched to quickly determine the most effective known treatment for a particular case of poisoning. Many cases can be managed over the telephone with advice from the PCC pharmacist, nurse, or physician. As noted, treatment of more severe poisonings is overseen by clinical toxicologists, who are usually specially trained physicians.

Effective treatment of the poisoned patient is based on a system of priorities, the first of which is to preserve the patient's vital functions by maintaining airway, ventilation, and circulation. The second priority is to prevent absorption of the toxic agent and to speed its elimination from the body using one or more clinical methods available. These methods include adsorption of the agent from the stomach using activated charcoal and cathartics (laxatives) to speed fecal elimination of the charcoal–toxin complex. Syrup of ipecac has been used for several decades as a means to induce vomiting to clear the stomach. However, there is currently a clinical trend away from its use in favour of other treatments for most types of poisoning because of frequent misuse by patients and caregivers and its limited efficacy. Whole bowel irrigation, using solutions of polyethylene glycol 3350 (e.g., Colyte), for example, may also be helpful in eliminating some drugs. In more severe cases, hemodialysis or peritoneal dialysis may be effective in removing certain types of drugs that have already been absorbed into the bloodstream. Hemoperfusion is similar to dialysis and involves pumping the patient's blood through a charcoal column, clearing certain drugs from the blood by adsorption (as when charcoal is used in the GI tract). Diuretic drugs may also be administered to force elimination of the toxic substance from the kidneys. In this instance, acid or alkaline diuresis involves administering weak acids or bases to speed elimination of basic or acidic drugs from the kidneys, respectively, by altering the chemistry of the urine. Oral or intravenous solutions of ascorbic acid (vitamin C) or sodium bicarbonate (a base) are often used for this purpose. In the case of snakebite, a drug product known as *antivenin* (also called *antivenom*) is often administered intravenously. This compound chemically binds to venom molecules to reduce tissue damage. Radiation poisoning requires decontamination using specially trained personnel and equipment. Several common poisons and their specific antidotes are listed in Table 2-10.

TABLE 2-10

Common Causes of Poisoning and Their Antidotes

Substance	Antidote
acetaminophen	acetylcysteine
Benzodiazepines	flumazenil
β-blockers	glucagon
Calcium channel blockers	Intravenous calcium
Carbon monoxide (by inhalation)	Oxygen (at high concentration), known as bariatric therapy
digoxin and other cardiac glycosides	digoxin antibodies
Ethylene glycol (e.g., automotive antifreeze solution), methanol	Ethanol (same as alcohol used for drinking), administered intravenously
heparin	protamine sulfate
Iron salts	deferoxamine
Opiates, opioid drugs	naloxone
Organophosphates (e.g., insecticides)	atropine
Tricyclic antidepressants, quinidine	sodium bicarbonate
warfarin	vitamin K

EVIDENCE-INFORMED PRACTICE AND DRUG THERAPY

In this information era, nurses encounter a plethora of health conditions and possible treatments, which include pharmacotherapeutics. In order to stay informed and current, **evidence-informed practice** ([EIP], also referred to as *evidence-based practice*) has emerged in the past 10 years as the "gold standard" for using current, valid, and relevant information when making clinical decisions. When applying EIP, results include more accurate diagnoses, effective and efficient interventions, and improved patient outcomes. Evidence derived from systematic reviews of randomized clinical trials (RCTs) is often considered the strongest level of evidence; however, descriptive and qualitative studies as well as expert opinions may be considered when making decisions (Melnyk and Fineout-Overholt, 2005). The development of clinical practice guidelines based on scientific evidence helps to integrate the best research evidence into practice. Within this textbook, Evidence-Informed Practice boxes will be used to identify current, clinically relevant research evidence about specific prescription drugs as well as natural health products.

CONCLUSION

A thorough understanding of the interrelated pharmacological principles of pharmacokinetics, pharmacodynamics, pharmacotherapeutics, pharmacognosy, and toxicology is essential to the implementation of drug therapy in the nursing process and to safe, quality nursing practice. Medications may be helpful in treating disease, but without an adequate, up-to-date knowledge base and clinical skills combined with critical thinking and good decision making, this useful treatment modality may become a harmful one in the nurse's hands. Application of pharmacological principles enables the nurse to provide safe and effective drug therapy while always acting on behalf of the patient and respecting the patient's rights. Nursing considerations associated with different routes of drug administration are summarized in Table 2-3.

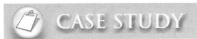

CASE STUDY

Nitroglycerin Therapy

Four patients with angina are receiving a form of nitroglycerin, as follows:

Mrs. A., age 88, takes 10 mg twice a day to prevent angina.

Mr. B., age 63, takes a form that delivers 0.2 mg/hr, also to prevent angina.

Mrs. C., age 58, takes 0.4 mg only if needed for chest pain.

Mr. D., age 62, is in the hospital with severe, unstable angina and is receiving 20 mcg/hr.

You may refer to the section on nitroglycerin in Chapter 24 or to a nursing drug handbook to answer the following questions:

1 State the route or form of nitroglycerin that each patient is receiving. In addition, specify the trade name(s) for each particular form.

2 For each patient, state the rationale for the route or form of drug that was chosen. Which forms have immediate action? Why would this be important?

3 Which form or forms are most affected by the first-pass effect? Explain.

4 What would happen if Mrs. A. chewed her nitroglycerin dose? If Mrs. C chewed her nitroglycerin dose?

For answers see http://evolve.elsevier.com/Canada/Lilley/pharmacology/.

POINTS TO REMEMBER

❖ The nurse's role in drug therapy and the nursing process as it relates to pharmacological treatment is more than just memorizing the names of drugs, their uses, and associated interventions. It involves a thorough comprehension of all aspects of pharmaceutics, pharmacokinetics, and pharmacodynamics and the sound application of this drug knowledge to a variety of clinical situations. Refer to Chapter 1 for more detailed discussion of drug therapy in relation to the nursing process.

❖ Drug actions are related to the pharmacological, pharmaceutical, pharmacokinetic, and pharmacodynamic properties of a given medication, and each of these has a specific influence on the overall effects produced by the drug in a patient. Selection of the route of administration is based on patient variables and the specific characteristics of a drug.

EXAMINATION REVIEW QUESTIONS

1 An older adult woman took a prescription medicine to help her to sleep; however, she felt restless all night and did not sleep at all. Which term below best describes this patient's response to the drug?
a. Allergic reaction
b. Mutagenic effect
c. Synergistic effect
d. Idiosyncratic reaction

2 In which phase of pharmacokinetics may patients with cirrhosis or hepatitis have abnormalities?
a. Absorption
b. Distribution
c. Metabolism
d. Excretion

3 A patient who has advanced cancer is receiving opioid medications around the clock to "keep him comfortable" as he nears the end of his life. Which term best describes this type of therapy?
a. Palliative therapy
b. Maintenance therapy
c. Supportive therapy
d. Supplemental therapy

4 The nurse is giving medications to a patient in cardiogenic shock. The intravenous route is chosen instead of the intramuscular route. Which patient factor most influences this decision?
a. Altered biliary function
b. Diminished circulation
c. Reduced liver metabolism
d. Increased glomerular filtration

5 A patient has just received a prescription for an enteric-coated stool softener. Which of the following statements is most important to include when teaching the patient?
a. "Take the tablet with 60 to 90 mL of orange juice."
b. "Be sure to swallow the tablet whole without chewing it."
c. "Avoid taking all other medications with any enteric-coated tablet."
d. "Crush the tablet before swallowing if you have problems with swallowing."

For answers see http://evolve.elsevier.com/Canada/Lilley/pharmacology/.

CRITICAL THINKING ACTIVITIES

1 Your patient tells you during the nursing assessment that he experiences some "strange" problem with drug metabolism that he was born with, so he is not to take certain medications. What type of disorder do you think this patient is referring to, and what problems can it cause in the patient when specific medications are taken?

2 Mr. L. is admitted to the trauma unit with multisystem injuries as a result of an automobile accident. He arrived at the unit with multiple abnormal findings including shock, decreased cardiac output, and urinary output of less than 30 mL/hr. Which route of administration would be indicated for any medications for this patient? Explain your reasoning.

3 Explain the difference between a medication's action and its effect.

4 Explain the importance of each phase of pharmacokinetics.

For answers see http://evolve.elsevier.com/Canada/Lilley/pharmacology/.

CHAPTER 3

Considerations for Special Populations

Learning Objectives

After reading this chapter, the successful student will be able to do the following:

1 Discuss the influence of a patient's age on the effects of drugs and drug responses.

2 Identify drug-related concerns during pregnancy and lactation.

3 Explain the physiological basis for drug-related concerns during pregnancy and lactation.

4 Discuss the process of pharmacokinetics and associated changes in different patient age groups, such as in children, pregnancy, and the older adult in relation to lifespan considerations as well as related physiological concerns.

5 Summarize the impact of age-related changes on pharmacokinetics in drug therapy.

6 Calculate a drug dosage for a child by using a variety of formulas.

7 Identify the importance of a body surface area (BSA) nomogram for children.

8 Develop a collaborative plan of care for drug therapy and the nursing process for patients across the lifespan.

e-Learning Activities

Web site
(http://evolve.elsevier.com/Canada/
Lilley/pharmacology/)

- Animations
- Answers to chapter questions, activities, and case studies
- Calculators and Category Catchers
- Glossary with audio pronunciations
- IV Therapy and Medication Error Checklists
- Multiple-Choice Review Question quizzes
- Nursing Care Plans
- Online Appendices and Supplements
- WebLinks

Glossary

Active transport The active (energy-requiring) movement of a substance between different tissues via biomolecular pumping mechanisms contained within cell membranes. (p. 44)

Diffusion The passive movement of a substance (e.g., a drug) between different tissues from areas of higher concentration to areas of lower concentration. (p. 44)

Nomogram A graphical tool for estimating drug dosages using body measurements. (p. 46)

Older adult A person who is 65 years of age or older. (Note: Some sources consider older adults to be 55 years of age or older.) (p. 48)

Polypharmacy The use of many different drugs concurrently in treating a patient, who often has several health problems. (p. 48)

OVERVIEW

Most of the experience with drugs and pharmacology has been gained from the adult population, and by far, the greater majority of drug studies and articles on drugs have focused on the population between the ages of 13 and 65 years. It has also been identified that 75% of currently approved drugs lack Health Canada's Food and Drugs Directorate approval for use in neonates and children and therefore lack specific dosage guidelines for use in this special population. Drug usage, however, extends far beyond patients between the ages of 13 and 65 years. Most drugs are also effective in younger and older patients, but drugs often behave differently in these patients at the opposite ends of the age spectrum. It is therefore vitally important from the standpoint of safe and effective drug administration to understand what these differences are and how to adjust for them.

From the beginning to the end of life, the human body changes in many ways. These changes have a dramatic effect on the four phases of pharmacokinetics—*drug absorption, distribution, metabolism,* and *excretion.* Children, the older adult, and pregnant and lactating women have special needs, which are discussed in this chapter. Drug therapy at the two ends of the spectrum of life is more likely to result in adverse effects and toxicity. This is especially true if certain basic principles are not understood and followed. However, response to drug therapy does change in a reasonably predictable manner in younger and older patients. Knowing the effect that age has on the pharmacokinetic characteristics of drugs helps in predicting these changes.

DRUG THERAPY DURING PREGNANCY

Exposure to drugs occurs across the entire lifespan, which begins before birth. A fetus is exposed to many of the same substances as the mother, including any drugs that she takes—prescription, nonprescription, or street drugs. Therefore, it is important to know and understand drug effects during gestational life. The first trimester of pregnancy is generally the period of greatest danger for drug-induced developmental defects. According to the U.S. Food and Drug Administration's Office of New Drugs, Center for Drug Evaluation and Research, an average of three to five drugs is taken by the typical pregnant woman. The World Health Organization (WHO) also completed an international survey on drug use during pregnancy involving 14,778 pregnant women from 22 countries on four continents. Eighty-six percent of these women took medication during pregnancy, receiving an average of 2.9 prescriptions. No comparable Canadian statistics are available.

Transfer of both drugs and nutrients to the fetus occurs primarily by **diffusion** across the placenta, although not all drugs cross the placenta. **Active transport** plays a lesser role. Recall from chemistry studies that diffusion is a passive process based on differences in concentration between different tissues, whereas active transport requires the expenditure of energy to move a substance between different areas and often involves some sort of cell-surface protein pump. The factors that contribute to the safety or potential harm of drug therapy during pregnancy can be broadly broken down into three areas: drug properties, fetal gestational age, and maternal factors.

Factors that impact drug transfer to the fetus include the drug's chemical properties, drug dosage, and concurrently administered drugs. Examples of relevant chemical properties are molecular weight, protein binding, lipid solubility, and chemical structure. Important drug dosage variables are dose and duration of therapy.

Fetal gestational age is an important factor in determining the potential for harmful drug effects to the fetus. As noted earlier, the fetus is at the greatest risk for drug-induced developmental defects during the first trimester of pregnancy. During this period, the fetus undergoes rapid cell proliferation, and the skeleton, muscles, limbs, and visceral organs are developing at their most rapid rate. Self-treatment of any minor illness should be strongly discouraged anytime during pregnancy, but particularly during the first trimester. Gestational age is also important in determining when a drug can most easily cross the placenta to the fetus. During the last trimester, the greatest percentage of maternally absorbed drug gets to the fetus. This is the result of enhanced blood flow to the fetus, increased fetal surface area, and an increased amount of free drug in the mother's circulation.

Maternal factors can also play a role in determining drug effects on the fetus. Any change in the mother's physiology that could impact the pharmacokinetic characteristics of drugs (absorption, distribution, metabolism, and excretion) can also affect the amount of drug to which the fetus may be exposed. Maternal kidney and liver functions play a major role in drug metabolism and excretion and are critical factors, especially if the drug crosses the placenta. Impairment in either kidney or liver function may result in higher drug levels than normal or prolonged drug exposure. Maternal genotype may also affect how and to what extent certain drugs are metabolized (pharmacogenetics), which in turn affects drug exposure of the fetus. The lack of certain enzyme systems, as seen in the pharmacogenetic disease glucose-6-phosphate dehydrogenase deficiency, may result in adverse drug effects to the fetus when the mother is exposed to a drug that is normally metabolized by this enzyme, including the commonly used over-the-counter (OTC) drug aspirin.

As important as it is to judiciously use drugs during pregnancy, there are certain situations that require their use. Without drugs, such maternal conditions as hypertension, epilepsy, diabetes, and infection could seriously endanger both the mother and the fetus. The U.S. Food and Drug Administration (FDA) classifies drugs according to their safety for use during pregnancy. The basis for this system of drug classification lies primarily in animal studies and less so in limited human studies. This greater dependence on animal studies is in part because of ethical dilemmas surrounding the study of potential adverse effects on fetuses. We have also learned from some unfortunate mistakes, such as the maternal use of thalidomide, which induces birth defects, and diethylstilbestrol (DES), which causes a high incidence of gynecological malignancy in female offspring. Currently the best method in Canada for determining the potential fetal risk of a drug is to note the FDA's pregnancy safety category for the drug. The five safety categories are described in Table 3-1.

Motherisk, Canada's teratogen research and counselling program based in The Hospital for Sick Children, Toronto, Ontario, is considered an international authority in maternal–fetal toxicology. Since 1985, this program has provided evidence-informed research and education about the safety or risk for the developing fetus of maternal exposure to drugs. Four help lines are available on the Motherisk Web site to give women and health care providers information on risk or safety of prescription and OTC drugs as well as natural health products. Their Web site with the hotline numbers is http://www.motherisk.org/women/index.jsp.

DRUG THERAPY DURING BREASTFEEDING

Breastfed infants are also at risk for exposure to drugs consumed by the mother. A wide variety of drugs easily cross from the mother's circulation to the breast milk and subsequently to the breastfeeding infant. Drug properties similar to those discussed in the previous section on drug therapy during pregnancy influence the exposure of infants to drugs taken by mothers who breastfeed. The primary drug characteristics that increase the likelihood that a drug given to a breastfeeding mother will end up in the breast milk include fat solubility, low molecular weight, nonionization, and high concentration.

Fortunately, breast milk is not the primary route for maternal drug excretion. Drug levels in breast milk are usually lower than those in the maternal circulation. The actual amount of drug to which a breastfeeding infant is exposed depends largely on the volume of milk consumed. The ultimate decision as to whether a breastfeeding mother should take a particular drug depends on the harm-to-benefit ratio. The harm of transfer of maternal medication to the infant in relation to the benefits of continuing breastfeeding and the therapeutic benefits to the mother must be considered on a case-by-case basis.

CONSIDERATIONS FOR CHILDREN

In terms of age, a child is defined differently from a neonate or an infant. Therefore, the term *child* should not be mistakenly used to refer to a patient younger than 1 year of age. The age ranges that correspond to the terms applied to young patients are shown in Table 3-2. This classification is used throughout this chapter.

Physiology and Pharmacokinetics

The anatomy and physiological characteristics unique to children account for most of the differences in the pharmacokinetic and pharmacodynamic behaviour of drugs in their bodies (as is the case with other age-related anatomic and physiological differences between neonates and adults). The immaturity of organs is the physiological factor most responsible for these differences. The physiological characteristics of the neonatal population are seen in the overall child population, but to a lesser extent. In both groups, anatomic structures and physiological systems and functions are still in the process of developing. Special Populations: Children: Pharmacokinetic Changes in Children lists those physiological factors that alter the pharmacokinetic properties of drugs in young patients.

Pharmacodynamics

As previously mentioned, drug actions (or pharmacodynamics) are altered in young patients, and the maturity of organs plays a role in how drugs act in the body. In young patients, certain drugs may be more toxic and others less toxic than they are in adult patients. Drugs that are more toxic in children include phenobarbital, morphine, and acetylsalicylic acid. Drugs that children tolerate as well as or better than adults include atropine,

TABLE	3-1

Pregnancy Safety Categories

Category	Description
Category A	Studies indicate no risk to the human fetus.
Category B	Studies indicate no risk to animal fetus; information in humans is not available.
Category C	Adverse effects reported in animal fetus; information in humans is not available.
Category D	Possible fetal risk in humans reported; however, consideration of potential benefit versus risk may, in selected cases, warrant use of these drugs in pregnant women.
Category X	Fetal abnormalities reported and positive evidence of fetal risk in humans is available from animal or human studies or both. These drugs should not be used in pregnant women.

TABLE	3-2

Classification of Young Patients

Age Range	Classification
Younger than 38 wk gestation	Premature or preterm infant
Younger than 1 mo	Neonate or newborn infant
1 mo to younger than 1 yr	Infant
1 yr to younger than 12 yr	Child

Note: The meaning of the term *pediatric* may vary with the individual drug and clinical situation. Often the maximum age for a pediatric patient may be identified as 16 years of age. Consult manufacturer's guidelines for specific dosing information.

SPECIAL POPULATIONS: CHILDREN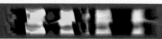

Pharmacokinetic Changes in Children

Absorption
- Gastric pH is less acidic because acid-producing cells in the stomach are immature until approximately 1–2 years of age.
- Gastric emptying is slowed because of slow or irregular peristalsis.
- First-pass elimination by the liver is reduced because of liver immaturity and reduced levels of microsomal enzymes.
- Intramuscular absorption is faster and irregular.

Distribution
- Total body water is 70% to 80% in full-term infants, 85% in premature newborns, and 64% in children 1 to 12 years of age.
- Fat content is lower in young patients because of greater total body water.
- Protein binding is decreased because of decreased production of protein by the immature liver.
- More drugs enter the brain because of an immature blood–brain barrier.

Metabolism
- Levels of microsomal enzymes are decreased because the immature liver has not yet started producing enough.
- Older children may have increased metabolism and require higher doses once liver enzymes are produced.
- Many variables affect metabolism in premature infants, infants, and children, including the status of liver enzyme production, genetic differences, and what the mother has been exposed to during pregnancy.

Excretion
- Glomerular filtration rate and tubular secretion and reabsorption are all decreased in young patients because of kidney immaturity.
- Perfusion to the kidneys may be decreased and results in reduced kidney function, concentrating ability, and excretion of drugs.

---

codeine, digoxin, and phenylephrine. The sensitivity of receptor sites may also vary with age; thus higher or lower doses may be required depending on the drug. In addition, rapidly developing tissues may be more sensitive to certain drugs and therefore smaller doses may be required. Because of this, certain drugs are generally contraindicated during the growth years. For instance, tetracycline may discolour a young person's teeth; corticosteroids may suppress growth if given systemically (but not when delivered via asthma inhalers, for example); and fluoroquinolone antibiotics may damage cartilage, which can lead to deformities in gait.

Dose Calculations for Children

Many drugs commonly used in adults have not been sufficiently investigated to ensure their safety and effectiveness in children. Most drugs administered in children are given on an empirical basis. Because children (especially premature infants and neonates) are small and have immature organs, they are particularly susceptible to many drug interactions, toxicity, and unusual drug responses and thus require different dosage calculations. Characteristics of children that play a significant role in dosage calculation include the following:
- Skin is thinner and more permeable.
- Stomach lacks acid to kill bacteria.
- Lungs have weaker mucous barriers.
- Body temperature is less well regulated and dehydration occurs easily.
- Liver and kidneys are immature and so drug metabolism and excretion are impaired.

Many formulas for child dosage calculation have been used throughout the years. Formulas involving age, weight, and body surface area (BSA) are most commonly employed as the basis for calculations. BSA is the most accurate of these dosage formulas. For the BSA method, the nurse needs the following information:
- Drug order with drug name, dose, route, time, and frequency
- Information regarding available dosage forms
- Child's height in centimetres (cm) and weight in kilograms (kg)
- BSA **nomogram** for children a graphical tool for estimating dosages (e.g., West nomogram [see Figure 3-1])
- Recommended adult drug dosage

The West nomogram uses a child's height and weight to determine the child's BSA. This information is then inserted into the BSA formula to obtain a drug dosage for a specific child (see Box 3-1 on p. 48). Consider the following example:

$$\frac{\text{BSA of child}}{\text{BSA of adult}} \times \text{adult dose} = \text{estimated child's dose}$$

$$\text{BSA of child (m}^2) \times \frac{\text{manufacturer recommended dose}}{\text{m}^2} = \text{estimated child's dose}$$

Note: the normal adult BSA is 1.7 m².

Calculating the drug dosage according to the body weight method is appropriate when the child is of usual stature for age and gender, and most drug references recommend dosages based on milligrams per kilogram of body weight. The following information is needed to calculate the child dosage:

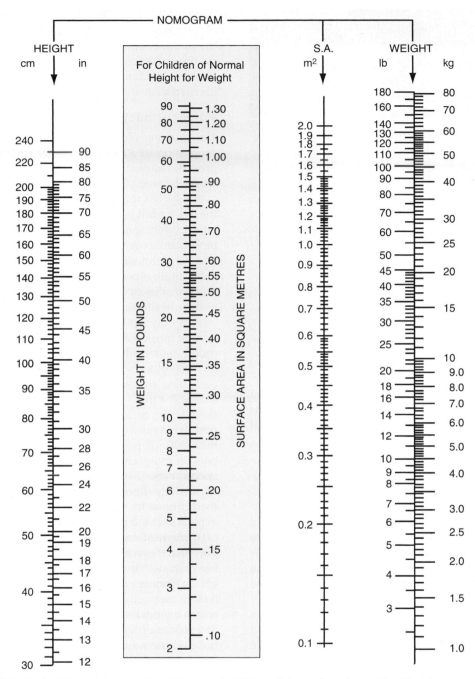

FIG. 3-1   West nomogram for infants and children. *S.A.*, surface area. Modified from data by Boyd, E., & West, C. D. (2004). In R. E. Behrman, R. M. Kliegman, & H. B. Jensen (Eds.) *Nelson textbook of pediatrics* (17th ed.). Philadelphia: Saunders.

- Drug order (as discussed previously)
- Child's weight in kilograms (1 kg = 2.2 pounds)
- Child dosage as per manufacturer or drug formulary (provides drug and regimen monographs) guidelines
- Information regarding available dosage forms

When using either of the previous methods, the nurse does the following:

- Determines the child's weight in kilograms
- Uses a current drug reference to determine the usual dosage range per day in milligrams per kilogram
- Determines the dose parameters by multiplying the weight by the minimum and maximum daily doses of the drug (the safe range)
- Determines the total amount of the drug to administer per dose and per day
- Compares the drug dosage prescribed with the calculated safe range
- If the drug dosage raises any concerns or varies from the safe range, contacts the health care provider or prescriber immediately and does not administer the drug

BOX 3-1

Example of Using the West Nomogram to Calculate Dosage

If a child weighs 15.5 kg (34 lb) and is 95 cm (37 inches) tall and the adult dosage for a medication is 500 mg, using the West nomogram, place and hold one end of a straight edge on the first column at 95 cm and move it so that it lines up with 15.5 kg in the far right column. On the surface area (S.A.) column, the straight edge falls across 0.64 m². Using the formula, calculate the child's BSA: 0.64 over 1.7 = 0.38. The child's BSA is 0.38 that of the average adult. To calculate the child drug dose, multiply 0.38 by 500 mg (0.38 × 500 = 190). Therefore, the child's dosage is 190 mg.

The nurse should never underestimate the importance of organ maturity along with BSA, age, and weight in calculating child dosage. If all of these physical developmental factors are considered, the likelihood of safe and effective drug administration is increased. Emotions-related developmental considerations must also be a part of the decision-making process in drug therapy with children (see Special Populations: Children).

CONSIDERATIONS FOR THE OLDER ADULT

In this book, the term *older adult* is used instead of the words *geriatric* or *elderly*; however, these terms are synonymous. An **older adult** is defined as one who is 65 years of age or older. At the beginning of the twentieth century, the older adult constituted a mere 5% of the total population in Canada. At that time, more people died of infections than of degenerative, chronic illnesses such as heart disease, cancer, and diabetes. As medical and health care technology has advanced, so has the ability to prolong life, often by treating and controlling, or even curing, illnesses from which people commonly died in the past. Life expectancy in Canada is currently approximately 80.4 years. Patients over 65 years of age will constitute 15% of the population by 2011. The older-adult segment of the population is growing at a dramatic pace, increasing by about 2% a year, with those aged 80 years and over being the fastest growing age group. It is estimated that by the year 2020, 20% of the estimated 7.8 million population will be over 65 years of age (see Special Populations: The Older Adult: Percentage of Population Over 65 Years of Age). These trends are expected to continue as new disease prevention and treatment methods are developed, but with this trend also comes the challenge for governments and health care institutions to meet the growing special needs of this population (see Special

Populations: The Older Adult: Alzheimer's Disease). The older adult has special needs because of the decline in organ function, which contributes to pharmacokinetic changes. Therefore, drug therapy is much more likely to result in adverse effects and toxicity at this end of the lifespan than at other times.

Polypharmacy and Drug Use

The growing older-adult population consumes a larger proportion of all medications than do other population groups. The older-adult patient population consumes anywhere between 20% to 40% of all prescription drugs and over 40% of OTC drugs. Commonly prescribed drugs for the older adult include antihypertensives, β-blockers, digitalis, diuretics, insulin, and potassium supplements. The most commonly used OTC drugs are analgesics, laxatives, and nonsteroidal anti-inflammatory drugs (NSAIDs). The older adult, especially those of certain ethnicities, may use folk remedies of unknown composition that are unfamiliar to their health care providers.

Not only do older adults consume a greater proportion of prescription and OTC medications, they commonly take multiple medications on a daily basis. One in three older adults takes more than 8 different drugs each day, and some take as many as 15 or more. One reason for this age population's use of so many medications is the occurrence of more chronic diseases, which now have even more drug options for treatment. More than 80% of patients taking eight or more drugs have one or more chronic illnesses. In this age of medical specialization, patients may see several physicians for their many illnesses. These specialists may all prescribe medications for the disorder(s) they are treating, which explains why a patient can be taking 8 to 15 drugs plus OTC medications. This situation is called **polypharmacy.** Polypharmacy leads to what is known as the "prescribing cascade," in which an older adult develops adverse effects from one or more of the medications taken and the health care provider then prescribes yet another drug, which creates the potential for even more adverse effects. The risk of drug interactions, adverse effects, and potentially a hospitalization (possibly prolonged) is far greater in this situation. As the number of medications a person takes increases, so does the risk of drug interaction. For example, the chance of a drug interaction is approximately 6% for a patient receiving two medications. For a patient taking five medications, the risk of a drug interaction dramatically increases to 50%. This likelihood rises to 100% if the patient is taking eight medications. Some drugs in a regimen may even be given specifically to counteract the adverse effects of other drugs (e.g., a potassium supplement to counteract the potassium loss caused by certain diuretic medications). While Canadian older adults make up 15% of the total population, these adults account for 44% of the adverse drug reactions causing death (as many as 3300 deaths) according to Health Canada's Adverse Drug Reaction database (see more discussion in Chapter 5).

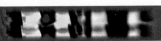

 SPECIAL POPULATIONS: CHILDREN

Age-Related Considerations for Medication Administration from Infancy to Adolescence

General Interventions
- Always come prepared for the procedure (e.g., prepare for injections with needleless syringe and gather all needed equipment).
- Ask the parent or child (if age appropriate) if the parent should or should not remain for the procedure (for in-hospital administration).
- Assess comfort methods that are appropriate before and after drug administration.

Infants
- While maintaining safe and secure positioning of the infant (e.g., with parent holding, rocking, cuddling, soothing the child), perform the procedure (e.g., injection) swiftly and safely.
- Allow self-comforting measures as age appropriate (e.g., use of pacifier, fingers in mouth, self-movement).

Toddlers
- Offer a brief, concrete explanation of the procedure but with realistic expectations of the child's actual understanding of the information. Parents, caregivers, or other legal guardians must be part of the process. Hold the child securely while administering the medication.
- Accept aggressive behaviour as a healthy response, but only within reasonable limits.
- Provide comfort measures immediately after the procedure (e.g., touching, holding).
- Help the child understand the treatment and his or her feelings through puppet play or play with stuffed animals or hospital equipment such as empty, needleless syringes.
- Provide for healthy ways to release aggression such as age-appropriate, supervised playtime.

Preschoolers
- Offer a brief, concrete explanation of the procedure at the patient's level and with the parent or caregiver.
- Provide comfort measures after the procedure (e.g., touching, holding).
- Identify and accept aggressive responses and provide age-appropriate outlets.

- Make use of magical thinking (e.g., using ointments or "special medicines" to make discomfort go away).
- Note that the role of the parent is important for providing comfort and understanding.

School-Age Children
- Explain the procedure, allowing for some control over body and situation.
- Provide comfort measures.
- Explore feelings and concepts through the use of therapeutic play. Art may be used to help the patient express fears. Use of age-appropriate books and realistic hospital equipment may also be helpful.
- Set appropriate behaviour limits (e.g., it is okay to cry or scream, but not to bite).
- Provide activities for releasing aggression and anger.
- Use the opportunity to teach about the relationship between getting medication and body function and structure (e.g., what a seizure is and how medication helps prevent the seizure).
- Offer the complete picture (e.g., need to take medication, relax with deep breaths, medication will help prevent pain).

Adolescents
- Prepare the patient in advance for the procedure but without scare tactics.
- Allow for expression in a way that does not cause losing face, such as giving the adolescent time alone after the procedure (e.g., once a seizure is controlled) and giving the adolescent time to discuss his or her feelings.
- Explore with the adolescent any current concepts of self, hospitalization, and illness, and correct any misconceptions.
- Encourage self-expression, individuality, and self-care.
- Encourage participation in the procedures and as appropriate.

Modified from McKenry, L. M., Tessier, E., & Hogan, M. (2006). *Mosby's pharmacology in nursing* (22nd ed.), St. Louis, MO: Elsevier Mosby; Blaber, M. Related to nursing intervention in pain. *Newington's Children's Hospital manual for global pediatric nursing assessment* (unpublished).

 SPECIAL POPULATIONS: THE OLDER ADULT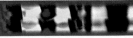

Percentage of Population Over 65 Years of Age

Year	Percentage Over Age 65
1900	5%
2001	13%
2011	15%
2021	20%
2041	22% to 25%

SPECIAL POPULATIONS: THE OLDER ADULT

Alzheimer's Disease

- Alzheimer's disease affects approximately 300,000 Canadians, and the figure may reach 480,000 by 2031. It is presently the fourth leading cause of death in adults, preceded by heart disease, cancer, and stroke. Unfortunately, approximately 17% of Canadians have someone with Alzheimer's disease in their family. This disease affects one in four Canadians over 85.
- The disease process has a major impact on the patient's mental and physical abilities. Because of

deterioration of mental status and chronic physical decline, these patients require assistance in performing the activities of daily living, including assistance with medication administration.

- Caregivers and family members need to be informed of the short-term and long-term characteristics of the illness, and resources need to be provided in either a private care setting or through special-needs units in assisted living settings or nursing homes.

Along with the risk of drug interaction come other risks. More hospitalizations for the treatment of adverse drug effects, greater likelihood of drug-induced falls that lead to hip fractures, and heightened risk of addiction are just a few. Many of these are preventable. Recognizing polypharmacy in a patient and taking steps to reduce it whenever possible by decreasing the number or dosages of drugs taken can dramatically reduce the incidence of these undesirable drug effects and adverse outcomes.

Physiological Changes

The physiological changes associated with aging also affect how drugs act. Having an understanding of these physiological changes and how they affect pharmacokinetics and pharmacodynamics in the older adult helps ensure the provision of safe and effective drug therapy. The body ages and the function of several organ systems slowly deteriorates after many years of wear and tear. The collective physiological changes associated with the aging process have a major effect on the disposition of drugs. Table 3-3 lists some of the body systems most affected by the aging process.

Because the sensitivity of the older adult to many drugs is altered as a result of physiological changes, drug usage should be adjusted to accommodate these changes. For instance, with aging there is a general decrease in

body weight. However, the drug doses administered to the older adult are often the same as those administered to younger adults. The criteria for drug doses in older adults should thus include consideration of kilograms of body weight and organ functioning, as well as hepatic, renal, cardiovascular, and central nervous systems function (similar to the criteria for child dosages).

It is important for the nurse to monitor the results of laboratory tests that have been ordered in the older adult. These values serve as a gauge of organ function. The most important organs from the standpoint of the breakdown and elimination of drugs are the liver and the kidneys. Kidney function is assessed by measuring serum creatinine and blood urea nitrogen levels. A more thorough but also more cumbersome and expensive test that is sometimes ordered is creatinine clearance. This test involves collecting a patient's entire urine output for 24 hours and measuring the actual amount of creatinine excreted. The test is usually only ordered for more complicated clinical cases. Liver function is assessed by testing liver enzymes such as aspartate aminotransferase (AST) and alanine aminotransferase (ALT). These laboratory values can help in the assessment of an older patient's ability to metabolize and eliminate medications and can aid in anticipating the risk of toxicity, drug accumulation, or both. Laboratory assessments should ideally be conducted at least annually for most older adults, both for preventive health monitoring and for screening for possible toxic effects of drug therapy. Such assessments may be indicated more frequently (e.g., every 1, 3, or 6 months) in those patients requiring higher-risk drug regimens.

Pharmacokinetics

What happens during the pharmacokinetic phases of absorption, distribution, metabolism, and excretion may be different in the older adult than in the younger adult. Awareness of these differences helps the nurse ensure appropriate administration of drugs and monitoring of the older adult taking medications. Special Populations: The Older Adult: Pharmacokinetic Changes lists the four pharmacokinetic phases and summarizes how they are altered by the aging process.

TABLE 3-3

Physiological Changes in the Older Adult

System	Physiological Change
Cardiovascular	↓ Cardiac output = ↓ absorption and distribution
	↓ Blood flow = ↓ absorption and distribution
Gastrointestinal	↑ pH (alkaline gastric secretions) = altered absorption
	↓ Peristalsis = delayed gastric emptying
Liver	↓ Enzyme production = ↓ metabolism
	↓ Blood flow = ↓ metabolism
Kidney	↓ Blood flow = ↓ excretion
	↓ Function = ↓ excretion
	↓ Glomerular filtration rate = ↓ excretion

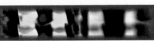

SPECIAL POPULATIONS: THE OLDER ADULT

Pharmacokinetic Changes

Absorption
- Gastric pH is less acidic because of a gradual reduction in the production of hydrochloric acid in the stomach.
- Gastric emptying is slowed because of a decline in smooth muscle tone and motor activity.
- Movement throughout the gastrointestinal (GI) tract is slower because of decreased muscle tone and motor activity.
- Blood flow to the GI tract is reduced by 40% to 50% because of decreased cardiac output and decreased blood flow.
- The absorptive surface area is decreased because the aging process blunts and flattens villi.

Distribution
- In adults 40 to 60 years of age, total body water is 55% in males and 47% in females; in those over 60 years of age, total body water is 52% in males and 46% in females.

- Fat content is increased because of decreased lean body mass.
- Protein (albumin) binding sites are reduced because of decreased production of proteins by the aging liver and reduced protein intake.

Metabolism
- The levels of microsomal enzymes are decreased because the capacity of the aging liver to produce them is reduced.
- Liver blood flow is reduced by approximately 1.5% per year after 25 years of age, which decreases liver metabolism.

Excretion
- Glomerular filtration rate is decreased by 40% to 50% primarily because of decreased blood flow.
- The number of intact nephrons is decreased.

Absorption

Advancing age results in reduced absorption of both dietary nutrients and drugs in the older person. Several physiological changes account for this. There is a gradual reduction in the ability of the stomach to produce hydrochloric acid, which results in a decrease in gastric acidity and may alter the absorption of weakly acidic drugs such as barbiturates and acetylsalicylic acid. In addition, the combination of decreased cardiac output and advancing atherosclerosis results in a general reduction in the flow of blood to major organs, including the stomach. By 65 years of age, there is an approximately 50% reduction in blood flow to the gastrointestinal tract. Absorption, whether of nutrient or drug, is dependent on good blood supply to the stomach and intestines. The absorptive surface area of an older adult person's gastrointestinal tract is often reduced by flattening and blunting of the villi. These age-related changes reduce overall gastrointestinal absorptive capabilities, including drug absorption. Once absorbed, drugs must be carried by the bloodstream to their eventual site of action (i.e., to receptors in tissues). The speed and intensity with which this happens depends on the quality of the circulation, which in turn depends on cardiac output, blood pressure, and patency of both central and peripheral blood vessels.

Gastrointestinal motility is important not only for moving substances out of the stomach but also for moving them throughout the gastrointestinal tract. Muscle tone and motor activity in the gastrointestinal tract are reduced in older adults. This often results in constipation, for which older adults frequently take laxatives. This use of laxatives may accelerate gastrointestinal motility enough to actually reduce the absorption of drugs. One particular category of laxatives, bulk-forming laxatives, has been shown to reduce the absorption of certain medications such as cardiac glycosides (e.g., digoxin). Bran and high-fibre foods may have the same effect on this group of medications.

Distribution

The distribution of medications throughout the body is vastly different in older adults than it is in younger adults. There seems to be a gradual reduction in the total body water content with aging. Therefore, the concentrations of highly water-soluble drugs may be higher in older adults because they have less body water in which the drugs can be diluted. The composition of the body also changes with aging. As the lean muscle mass decreases, body fat increases. In both men and women there is an approximately 20% reduction in muscle mass between the ages of 25 and 65 years and a corresponding 20% increase in body fat. Drugs such as hypnotics and sedatives that are primarily distributed to the fat will therefore have a prolonged effect.

Many drugs distributed by means of the blood are carried by proteins. By far the most important of these proteins is albumin. Reduced protein concentrations are seen with aging, due in part to reduced liver function. In addition, reduced dietary intake, or poor gastrointestinal protein absorption even with adequate dietary intake, also contributes to reduced blood protein levels. Whatever the cause, the reduced number of protein-binding sites for highly protein-bound drugs results in higher levels of unbound drug in the blood. Drugs that are not bound to proteins are active. Therefore, the effects of highly protein-bound drugs may be enhanced if their doses are not adjusted to accommodate any reduced serum albumin concentrations, as measured in blood samples. Highly protein-bound drugs include warfarin and phenytoin, among many others.

Metabolism

Metabolism declines with advancing age. The transformation of active drugs into inactive metabolites is performed primarily by the liver; however, the liver slowly loses its ability to metabolize drugs effectively because the production of microsomal enzymes is reduced. There is also a reduction in blood flow to the liver because of reduced cardiac output and atherosclerosis. A reduction in the liver blood flow of approximately 1.5% per year occurs after 25 years of age. All of these factors contribute to prolonging the half-life of many drugs (e.g., warfarin), which can potentially result in drug accumulation if serum drug levels are not closely monitored.

Excretion

The excretion of drugs is reduced in the older adult population. A reduction in the glomerular filtration rate of 40% to 50% in older adults, combined with a reduction in blood flow (for the same reasons as in the liver), can result in extremely delayed drug excretion and hence drug accumulation. Kidney function should be monitored frequently in the older adult through laboratory studies such as measurement of serum creatinine level, blood urea nitrogen level, or creatinine clearance to prevent drug accumulation. Appropriate dose and interval adjustments may be determined on the basis of results of a patient's renal and liver panels as well as the presence of therapeutic levels of the drug in the serum. If a decrease in liver function is a known variable, the drug dosage should be altered—as ordered—so that accumulation of the drug and possible toxicity may be minimized.

Problematic Medications for the Older Adult

Drugs in certain classes are more likely to cause problems in the older adult because of many of the physiological alterations and pharmacokinetic changes already discussed. Table 3-4 lists some of the more common medications that are problematic. Knowledge of the physiological changes in older adults and an understanding of accompanying pharmacokinetic changes are extremely useful in optimizing drug therapy for the older adult. Some of the drugs that should be avoided in the older adult have been identified by professional organizations such as the Institute for Safe Medication Practices–Canada, as

TABLE 3-4

Problematic Medications and Conditions to Consider for the Older Adult

Medication	Common Complications
Analgesics and opioids	Confusion, constipation, urinary retention, nausea, vomiting, respiratory depression, decreased level of consciousness, falls
Anticholinergics and antihistamines	Blurred vision, dry mouth, constipation, confusion and sedation, urinary retention, tachycardia
Anticoagulants (heparin, warfarin)	Major and minor bleeding episodes, many drug interactions, dietary interactions
Antidepressants	Sedation and strong anticholinergic adverse effects (see above)
Antihypertensives	Nausea, hypotension, diarrhea, bradycardia, heart failure, impotence
Cardiac glycosides (e.g., digoxin)	Visual disorders, nausea, diarrhea, dysrhythmias, hallucinations, decreased appetite, weight loss
CNS depressants (muscle relaxants, narcotics)	Sedation, weakness, dry mouth, confusion, urinary retention, ataxia
Nonsteroidal anti-inflammatory drugs (NSAIDs)	Edema, nausea, abdominal distress, gastric ulceration, bleeding, kidney toxicity
Sedatives and hypnotics	Confusion, daytime sedation, ataxia, lethargy, forgetfulness, increased risk of falls
Thiazide diuretics	Electrolyte imbalance, rashes, fatigue, leg cramps, dehydration

Condition	Common Drugs to Avoid
Bladder flow obstruction	Anticholinergics, anithistamines, decongestants, antidepressants
Chronic constipation	Calcium channel blockers, tricyclic antidepressants, anticholinergics
Chronic obstructive pulmonary disease (COPD)	Long-acting sedatives and hypnotics, narcotics, β-blockers
Clotting disorders	NSAIDs, aspirin, antiplatelet drugs
Depression	Some anithypertensives: methyldopa, reserpine, quanethidine
Heart failure and hypertension	Sodium, decongestants, amphetamines, OTC cold products
Insomnia	Decongestants, bronchodilators, MAO inhibitors
Parkinson's disease	Antipsychotics, phenothiazines
Syncope and falls	Sedatives, hypnotics, narcotics, CNS depressants, muscle relaxants, antidepressants, antihypertensives

CNS, central nervous system; MAO, monoamine oxidase; OTC, over-the-counter.

well as by other authoritative sources. Since the 1990s, an effective tool, the Beers criteria, has been used to identify drugs that may be inappropriately prescribed, ineffective, or cause adverse drug reactions in the older adult (see Evidence-Informed Practice). Research has been conducted using these criteria and was updated in 2002. The Beers criteria are useful and help determine risk-associated situations for the older adult and specific drugs that may be problematic. The 2003 Beers criteria include 48 drugs or classes considered inappropriate, regardless of diagnosis, as well as drugs and classes considered inappropriate in 20 conditions.

NURSING PROCESS

Assessment

Before any medication is administered to a child, a thorough health history and medication history should be obtained with assistance from parents or caregivers, or legal guardian; these include the following:

- Age
- Age-related concerns about organ functioning
- Allergies to drugs and food
- Baseline vital signs
- Fears
- Head-to-toe physical assessment findings
- Height in feet/inches and centimetres
- Weight in kilograms and pounds
- Level of growth and development and related developmental tasks
- Medical and medication history (including adverse drug reactions); current medication and related dosage forms and routes and the patient's tolerance of the forms and routes
- State of anxiety of the patient and of family members or caregiver
- Use of prescription and OTC medications in the home setting
- Usual method of medication administration, such as use of a calibrated spoon or needleless syringe
- Usual response to medications
- Motor and cognitive responses and their age appropriateness
- Resources available to the patient and family

EVIDENCE-INFORMED PRACTICE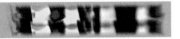

The Beers Criteria for Drug Use in the Older Adult

Background
The Beers criteria have been published since the 1990s, being one of the first tools to suggest a positive association between adverse drug reactions (ADRs) and drug prescribing policies in older adults, especially in those who take fewer than five drugs. The Beers criteria establish basic guidelines for identifying medications that may be inappropriate for the older adult. These criteria define drugs that have been determined by a panel of experts to have "potential risks" that outweigh the possible benefits of their use in this age group. Chang et al. (2005) applied the Beers criteria to evaluate drug therapy in patients 65 years or older with the purpose of predicting ADRs in older adults managed in an outpatient clinic.

Type of Evidence
The research method was a prospective study of some 500 or more participants through use of a follow-up telephone survey. Statistical analysis focused on the possible relationship between ADRs and inappropriate drug prescribing in the older adult.

Results of the Study
The study provided evidence that the Beers criteria may be used to predict ADRs among older adult outpatients and to examine the possible impact of potentially inappropriate drug prescribing. Of the 500 patients, 64 had potentially inappropriate drugs prescribed and 126 experienced ADRs. Statistical analysis confirmed an association between ADRs and potentially inappropriate drug prescribing. The results of this study have been extremely beneficial because few studies have focused on investigation of drug-related problems experienced by the older adult.

Link of Evidence to Nursing Practice
This study showed a positive association between potentially inappropriate drug prescriptions, as defined by the Beers criteria, and ADRs. This study alerts clinicians to the possibility of ADRs in the older adult and raises concerns specific to certain medications. Developing and publishing these criteria for professional nursing practice is important because of the increase in serious problems and concerns caused by inappropriate drug use in the older adult as well as in other age groups. With education, awareness, more research, and subsequent evidenced-informed nursing practice, medication-related risks may be decreased and safety may be increased. The Beers criteria may be applied to other patient care and medication-related issues as well and is a useful resource for nurses.

Based on Chang, C. M., Liu, P.Y., Yang, Y. H., Yang, Y., Wu, C., & Lu, F. (2005). Use of the Beer's criteria to predict adverse drug reactions among first-visit older adult outpatients. *Pharmacotherapy* 25(6), 831–838. Retrieved August 10, 2008, from http://www.medscape.com/viewarticle/507059; Molony, S. (2004). Beers criteria for potentially inappropriate medication use in the elderly. *Dermatology Nursing, 16*(6), 547–548. Available at http://www.medscape.com/viewarticle/496383; Sloane, P. D., Zimmerman, S., Brown, L. C., Ives, T. J., & Walsh, J. F. (2002). Inappropriate medication prescribing in residential care/assisted living facilities. *Journal of the American Geriatrics Society, 50*(6), 1001–1011.

In addition, the prescriber's orders should be checked and rechecked by the nurse because there is no room for error when working with children (or any patient). The medication dosage should be calculated and rechecked several times for accuracy. Calculations for dosages should take into account a variety of information and variables that may affect patient response, and should use BSA formulas and body weight formulas (milligrams per kilogram). If any doubts exist regarding the calculation, time should always be taken to have the calculations rechecked. In addition to an assessment of the patient, an assessment of the drug should be performed, focusing specifically on information about the drug's purpose, dosage ranges, routes of administration, and cautions and contraindications. The saying that children are just "small adults" is incorrect, because in these patients every organ is anatomically and physiologically immature and not fully functioning. As children grow older, their body surface areas and weights are still smaller; thus, children must be treated with extreme caution. Organ function may be determined through laboratory testing. Hepatic and renal panels, red and white blood cell counts, and measurement of hemoglobin levels, hematocrit, and protein levels are just a few examples of tests needed before initiation of drug therapy. Immature organ and system development will influence pharmacokinetics and thus affect the way the patient responds to a drug.

General assessment data to be gathered in the older adult include the following:

- Age
- Allergies to drugs and food
- Dietary habits
- Financial status and any limitations
- History of smoking and use of alcohol with notation of amount, frequency, and years of use
- Laboratory testing results, especially those indicative of kidney and liver function
- List of all health-related care professionals, including physicians, dentists, optometrists and ophthalmologists, podiatrists, alternative medicine health care practitioners such as osteopathic physicians, chiropractors, and nurse practitioners
- Listing of medications, past and present, including prescription drugs, OTC medications, and natural health products
- Polypharmacy
- Present and past medical history
- Risk situations related to drug therapy identified by the Beers criteria (see Evidence-Informed Practice on p. 53)
- Self-medication practices
- Sensory, visual, hearing, cognitive, and motor skill deficits

One way to collect data about the medications or drugs being taken is to obtain that information from the patient or caregiver using the *brown-bag technique*. It is an effective means of identifying drugs that the patient is taking, regardless of the patient's age, and should be used in conjunction with a complete review of the patient's medical history or record. The brown-bag technique requires the patient or caregiver to collect all medications in a bag and bring them to the health care provider. All medications should be kept within their original containers. A list of medications with generic names, dosages, routes of administration, and frequencies is compiled. The list of medications should be compared with what is prescribed or with what the patient states is actually being taken. In addition, the patient's insight into his or her own medical problems is beneficial in developing a plan of care. It is also important for the nurse to realize that although older adults may be able to provide the required information themselves, many may be confused or poorly informed about their medications. In such cases, a more reliable historian, such as a significant other, family member, or caregiver, should be used. The older adult may also have sensory deficits that require the nurse to speak slowly, loudly, and clearly while facing the patient. In Canada, some physicians and pharmacists have electronic access to the patient's prescription drugs records (e.g., Pharmanet in British Columbia).

With the older adult, as with a patient of any age, the nurse should always assess support systems and the patient's ability to take medications safely. Whenever possible, with the older adult and different age groups, health care providers should always opt to use a nonpharmacological approach to treatment first if appropriate. Other data the nurse should gather include information about acute or chronic illnesses, nutritional problems, heart problems, respiratory illnesses, and gastrointestinal tract disorders. Laboratory tests related to special-populations considerations that should be completed include the following: hemoglobin and hematocrit levels, red and white blood cell counts, blood urea nitrogen level, serum and urine creatinine levels, urine-specific gravity, serum electrolyte levels, and protein and serum albumin levels.

▨ Nursing Diagnoses

- Risk for injury related to adverse effects of medications or to the method of drug administration
- Imbalanced nutrition, less than body requirements, related to age or drug therapy and possible drug adverse effects
- Risk for injury related to idiosyncratic reactions to drugs due to age-related drug sensitivity
- Deficient knowledge related to information about drugs and their adverse effects or about when to contact the physician

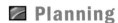 Planning

◼ Goals

- Patient will state measures to minimize complications and adverse effects associated with the drugs taken during the therapeutic regimen.
- Patient will state the importance of adhering to drug regimen (or takes medication as prescribed with assistance).
- Patient will contact the physician when appropriate (such as when unusual effects occur) during drug therapy.

◼ Outcome Criteria

- Patient (or parent, legal guardian, or caregiver) states the importance of taking the medication as prescribed (e.g., improved condition, decreased symptoms) for the duration of the recommended drug therapy.
- Patient (or parent, legal guardian, or caregiver) follows instructions specific to administration of the medication ordered (e.g., the special application of an ointment, proper administration of a liquid, correct dosage) for the duration of treatment.
- Patient (specifically the older adult) states reason for taking a specific medication and identifies what the drug looks like and when the drug is to be taken during the duration of drug treatment.
- Patient shows improvement in the condition being treated that is related to adherence with the medication regimen and successful medication therapy during the treatment period.
- Patient takes or receives medications safely and without injury over the duration of therapy.
- Patient (or parent, legal guardian, or caregiver) states specific situations in which the physician must be contacted (e.g., occurrence of fever, pain, vomiting, rash or diarrhea; worsening of the condition being treated; bronchospasms; dyspnea; intolerable adverse effects; signs of major adverse effects).

◪ Implementation

In general, it is always important to emphasize and practise the "Ten Rights" of medication administration (see Chapter 1) and follow the physician's order and medication instructions. All drugs should be checked three times against the physician's order diligently to following the appropriate "rights" before giving the drug to the patient (for inpatient situations). For the child, some specific nursing actions are as follows:

- If necessary, mix medications in a substance or fluid other than essential foods such as milk, orange juice, or cereal because the child may develop a dislike for the food in the future. Instead of such foods, find a liquid or food item that can be used to make the medications taste better, such as sherbet or another form or flavour of ice cream. This intervention should be used only if the patient is not able to swallow the dosage form.
- Do not add drug(s) to the fluid in a cup or bottle because the amount consumed is difficult to calculate if the entire amount is not taken.
- Always document special techniques of drug administration so that others involved in the care of the patient may use the same technique. For example, if having the child eat a frozen Popsicle before giving an unpleasant-tasting pill, liquid, or tablet helps to get the medication administered, then share that information.
- Unless contraindicated, add small amounts of water or fluids to elixirs so that the child may tolerate the medication. Remember, however, that it is essential that the child take the entire volume, so be cautious with this practice.
- Avoid using the word *candy* in place of *drug* or *medication*. Medications should be called medicines and their dangers made known to children, and no games should be played with this information.
- Keep all medications out of the reach of children of all ages and be sure that parents and other family members understand this information and know to request child-protective lids or tops for medication containers.
- Always ask about how the child is used to taking medications (e.g., liquid versus pill or tablet dosage forms) and if there are any methods that the family or caregiver have found to be helpful in administering distasteful drugs.

See Special Populations: Children, on page 49, for recommendations regarding medication administration in children from infancy through adolescence.

The older adult should be encouraged to take medications as directed and not to discontinue them or double up on doses. Regardless of the patient's age, the nurse should ensure that the patient, parent, legal guardian, or caregiver understands treatment- and medication-related instructions and understands safety measures related to drug therapy, such as keeping all medications out of the reach of children. Written and oral instructions should be provided concerning the drug name, action, purpose, dose, time of administration, route, adverse effects, safety of administration, storage, interactions, and any cautions about or contraindications to its use. Remember that simple is always best. Always try to find ways to simplify the patient's therapeutic regimen and be especially alert to polypharmacy. If a nurse advocate or a nurse practitioner with prescription privileges has the opportunity to review the patient's chart, this individual should take the time to simplify and write down the use or purpose of the drug, how to best take the drug, and a list of adverse effects. This information needs to be provided on paper in bold, large print. Some specific interventions proving to be helpful in promoting medication safety in the older adult include use of the Beers criteria (see Evidence-Informed Practice on p. 53). These criteria provide a systematic way of identifying prescription medications that are potentially harmful to the older adult. The prescriber and nurse must constantly remember that clinical judgement and knowledge base are important in making critical decisions about a patient's care and drug therapy. In addition, evidence-informed nursing practice, as seen with the Beers criteria, is important for the nurse to remain current in clinical nursing practice. Specific guidelines for medication administration by different routes are presented in detail in Chapter 10.

In summary, drug therapy across the lifespan must be well thought out, with full consideration to the patient's age, gender, ethnocultural background, medical history, and medication profile. With inclusion of all phases of the nursing process and the specific lifespan considerations discussed in this chapter, there is a better chance of decreasing adverse effects, reducing risks to the patient, and increasing drug safety.

Evaluation

In general, when the nurse is dealing with lifespan issues and drug therapy, the nurse's observation and monitoring for therapeutic effects and adverse effects are critical to safe and effective therapy. Nurses must know a patient's profile and history just as well as they know the drug and related information. The drug's purpose, specific use in the patient, simply stated action, dose, frequency of dosing, adverse effects, cautions, and contraindications should be listed and kept on the nurse's person. This information will allow more comprehensive monitoring of drug therapy, regardless of the age of the patient.

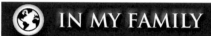

IN MY FAMILY

Special Diet for the Adolescent Girl
(as told by T.A., from Sri Lanka)

"When a young girl first starts her menstrual period, she is required by elders of her family to maintain a strict diet, lasting about a month from her first period. Her diet consists of mild spices, mild spiced coffee, red rice that replaces white rice, mild spiced curry, raw and fried egg, fried eggplant, mild spiced shark, dried fish curry, rice porridge, use of sesame oil (nalanai) which replaces other traditional oils, minimal water intake, minimal milk intake, etc.... By maintaining this diet it is supposed to minimize menstrual cramps, other menstrual-related pain such as leg pain, stomach pain, back pain, etc. This diet is also supposed to completely remove the uterine lining if implantation does not occur.... This diet is thought to help regulate future menstruation.... Following a 1-month period after a young girl's first menstruation, she is slowly allowed to consume and return back to her regular diet."

POINTS TO REMEMBER

- ❖ There are many age-related pharmacokinetic effects that lead to dramatic differences in drug absorption, distribution, metabolism, and excretion. At one end of the lifespan is the child and at the other end is the older adult, both of whom are very sensitive to the effects of drugs.
- ❖ Most common dosage calculations use the milligrams per kilogram formula related to age; however, BSA is also used for drug calculations, as is consideration of organ maturity. It is important for the nurse to know that many variables besides the mathematical calculation itself contribute to safe dosage calculations. Safety should be the number one concern,

with full consideration of the Ten Rights of medication administration.
- ❖ The percentage of the population over the age of 65 years continues to grow; therefore, nurses will continue to be exposed to an increasing number of older adults. Polypharmacy raises many concerns for the older adult, thus there is a need for a current listing of all medications with the patient at all times!
- ❖ The nurse's responsibility is to act as a patient advocate as well as to be informed about growth and development principles and the effects of drugs throughout the lifespan and in the phases of illness.

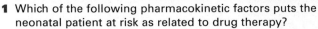

EXAMINATION REVIEW QUESTIONS

1 Which of the following pharmacokinetic factors puts the neonatal patient at risk as related to drug therapy?
   a. Immature renal system
   b. Hyperperistalsis in the gastrointestinal tract
   c. Functional temperature regulation
   d. Smaller circulatory capacity

2 Which of the following is one of the main physiological differences in infants that affects the amount of drug needed to produce a therapeutic effect?
   a. Increased protein in circulation
   b. Fat composition less than 0.001%
   c. More muscular body composition
   d. Water composition of approximately 75%

3 Which of the following alterations in pharmacokinetics best explains why the nurse encourages 76-year-old Mr. Y. to keep a journal of adverse effects experienced from his medications?
   a. Less adipose tissue to store fat-soluble drugs
   b. Increased kidney excretion of protein-bound drugs
   c. More alkaline gastric pH, resulting in more adverse effects
   d. Decreased blood flow to the liver with altered metabolism

4 When the nurse is reviewing a list of medications taken by an 88-year-old patient, the patient notes, "I get dizzy when I stand up," and has nearly fainted in the afternoon. Her systolic blood pressure drops 15 points when she stands up. Which of the following types of medications may be responsible for these effects?
   a. NSAIDs
   b. Anticoagulants
   c. Antihypertensives
   d. Cardiac glycosides

5 A patient who is at 32 weeks' gestation has a cold and calls the office to ask about taking an OTC medication that is rated as pregnancy category A. Which answer by the nurse is correct?
   a. "This drug causes problems in the human fetus, so you should not take this medication."
   b. "Studies indicate there is no risk to the human fetus, so it is okay to take this medication, as directed, if you need it."
   c. "This drug has not caused problems in animals, but no testing has been done in humans. It is probably safe to take."
   d. "This drug may cause problems in the human fetus, but nothing has been proven in clinical trials. It is best not to take this medication."

For answers see http://evolve.elsevier.com/Canada/Lilley/pharmacology/.

CRITICAL THINKING ACTIVITIES

1 Select either phenytoin or tetracycline and discuss the potential risks to the fetus or breastfeeding newborn in relation to the benefits to the mother.

2 A 73-year-old nursing home resident is experiencing problems that the nurse thinks are indicative of absorption problems with his oral medications (he is currently taking warfarin sodium). Specifically, the nurse notices that he has been experiencing unusual "bleeding" tendencies over the past few days; however, he tolerated the medication "very well" over the "last 3 years."

Which of the following physiological changes is *most* likely the basis of his untoward reaction to the warfarin?
   a. Increased cardiac output and cardiac volume
   b. Increased glomerular filtration and renin excretion
   c. Decreased gastrointestinal pH with increased peristalsis
   d. Decreased liver enzyme production and altered liver perfusion

3 List medications that have a high risk for causing problems (e.g., adverse effects or toxicity) for the older adult. Discuss the problems or complications associated with these drugs or drug classifications.

For answers see http://evolve.elsevier.com/Canada/Lilley/pharmacology/.

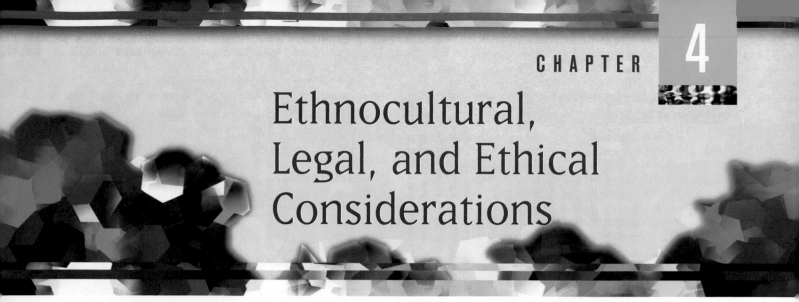

CHAPTER 4

Ethnocultural, Legal, and Ethical Considerations

Learning Objectives

After reading this chapter, the successful student will be able to do the following:

1 Discuss the racial and ethnocultural factors that may influence an individual's response to medications.

2 Identify ethnocultural phenomena affecting health care and the use of medications.

3 List the drugs more commonly affected by racial and ethnocultural factors.

4 Develop a collaborative plan of care that addresses the ethnocultural care of patients in drug therapy and the nursing process.

5 Briefly discuss the important components of drug legislation at the provincial and federal levels.

6 Identify the impact of drug legislation on drug therapy and the nursing process.

7 Discuss the categories of controlled substances and provide specific drug examples.

8 Identify the process involved in the development of new drugs, including the investigational new drug application, phases of investigational drug studies, and the process for informed consent.

9 Discuss the nurse's role in the development of new and investigational drugs and the informed consent process.

10 Discuss the ethical aspects of drug administration as they relate to drug therapy and the nursing process.

11 Identify the principles involved in making an ethical decision.

12 Develop a collaborative care plan that addresses the legal and ethical care of patients, drug therapy, and the nursing process.

e-Learning Activities

Web site
(http://evolve.elsevier.com/Canada/Lilley/pharmacology/)

- Animations
- Answers to chapter questions, activities, and case studies
- Calculators and Category Catchers
- Glossary with audio pronunciations
- IV Therapy and Medication Error Checklists
- Multiple-Choice Review Question quizzes
- Nursing Care Plans
- Online Appendices and Supplements
- WebLinks

Glossary

Benzodiazepines and Other Targeted Substances Regulations Implemented in 2000, these regulations specify the requirements for producing, assembling, importing, exporting, selling, providing, transporting, delivering, or destroying benzodiazepines and other targeted substances. (p. 61)

Blinded investigational drug study A research design in which, to eliminate bias on the part of the subject reporting the substance's effects, subjects in the study are purposely unaware of whether the substance they are administered is the drug under study or a placebo. (p. 64)

Canada Health Act Canada's federal legislation for publicly funded health care insurance. (p. 66)

Controlled Drug and Substances Act A Health Canada Act that makes it a criminal offence to possess, traffic, produce, import, or export controlled substances. (p. 61)

Controlled substances Any drugs listed on one of the "schedules" of the Controlled Drug and Substances Acts (also a called *scheduled drug* if it is an item under the Food and Drug Regulations Part G). (p. 61)

Double-blind, investigated drug study A research design in which, to eliminate bias on the part of both the investigator and the subject, both the study investigator(s) and the study subject are purposely unaware if the substance administered to a given subject is the drug under study or a placebo. (p. 64)

Drug Identification Number (DIN) A number, assigned by the Drugs Directorate, that is placed on the label of prescription and over-the-counter drug products that have been evaluated by the Therapeutic Products Directorate (TPD) and approved for sale in Canada. (p. 64)

Drug polymorphism Variation in response to a drug because of a patient's age, sex, size, and body composition. (p. 68)

Ethnopharmacology The study of the health beliefs and health practices of different ethnocultures, particularly in relation to their use of medicines and natural health products. (p. 67)

Food and Drugs Act The main piece of drug legislation in Canada that protects consumers from contaminated, adulterated, and unsafe drugs and labelling practices, and addresses appropriate advertising and selling of drugs, foods, cosmetics, and devices. (p. 60)

Food and Drug Regulations An adjunct to the Food and Drugs Act, these regulations clarify terms used in the Act, and state the processes that companies must carry out to comply with the Act in terms of importing, preparing, treating, processing, labelling, advertising, and selling foods, drugs, cosmetics, natural health products including herbal products, and medical devices. (p. 61)

Generic drug A chemically identical equivalent of a brand name drug. (p. 65)

Informed consent Permission obtained from a patient or legal guardian consenting to the performance of a specific test or procedure, as well as from ill and healthy research subjects consenting to participation in a research study. (p. 63)

Investigational new drug (IND) A drug not approved for marketing by Health Canada's Therapeutic Products Directorate (TPD) but available for use in experiments to determine its safety and efficacy; also, the actual name of the category of application that the drug manufacturer submits to the TPD to obtain permission for human (*clinical*) studies following successful completion of animal (*preclinical*) studies. (p. 63)

Marihuana Medical Access Regulations Implemented in 2001, these regulations clearly define the circumstances and the manner in which access to marihuana for medical purposes is permitted. (p. 62)

Narcotic Control Act This 1961 Health Canada Act addressed the possession, sale, manufacture, production, and distribution of narcotics; replaced by the CDSA 1997. (p. 61)

New drug submission The type of application that a drug manufacturer submits to the TPD of Health Canada following successful completion of required human research studies. (p. 64)

Notice of Compliance A notification issued when Health Canada decides that the drug and the manufacturing process are safe and effective, allowing the pharmaceutical company to sell the product by prescription to the Canadian population. (p. 64)

Over-the-counter (OTC) drugs Drugs that are available to consumers without a prescription; also called *nonprescription drugs*. (p. 61)

Patent Act A Canadian Act created in 1987 that allows pharmaceutical companies intellectual property and a time frame in which a drug can be marketed without competition from generic drugs. (p. 65)

Patented Medicine Prices Review Board An independent tribunal that limits the prices set by pharmaceutical manufacturers for all patented medicines, prescription or over the counter, to ensure that both existing and new drugs are not sold at excessive prices in Canada. (p. 65)

Placebo An inactive (inert) substance (e.g., saline, distilled water, starch, sugar) given to select patients to satisfy an unnecessary medication request and that can also be used in some drug studies (termed *placebo controlled*) as a control to compare against the effects of an experimental drug. (p. 63)

Precursor Control Regulations A scheme intended to allow Canada to fulfill its international obligations and meet its domestic needs with respect to the monitoring and control of precursor chemicals such as methamphetamine, γ-hydroxybutyrate (GHB), and other drugs listed in Schedules I, II, and III of the Controlled Drugs and Substances Act, across Canadian borders and within Canada. (p. 61)

Priority Review of Drug Submission A Health Canada policy that allows for earlier review of drug products for serious, life-threatening, or severely debilitating diseases or conditions for which there is no effective drug on the Canadian market. (p. 65)

Romanow Commission A commission on the future of health care in Canada, headed by Commissioner Roy J. Romanow; Romanow's report focused on health care reform. (p. 66)

Special Access Programme A program that allows practitioners to apply for access to drugs currently unavailable for sale in Canada. (p. 65)

CANADIAN DRUG LEGISLATION

In Canada, concerns over the sale and use of foods, drugs, cosmetics, and medical devices began long before these concerns arose in the United States. Canadian drug legislation began in 1875 when the Parliament of Canada passed an act to prevent the sale of adulterated foods, drinks, and drugs. Since that time, foods and drugs have been controlled on a national basis. The Health Protection Branch (HPB) of Health Canada is the federal regulator responsible for the administration and enforcement of the Food and Drugs Act and Food and Drug Regulations and the Controlled Drugs and Substances Act, the two Acts that form the underlying foundation for the drug laws in Canada. The Therapeutic Products Directorate (TPD) is the Canadian federal authority that regulates these Acts. These Acts are designed to protect the Canadian consumer from potential health hazards and fraud or deception in the sale and use of foods, drugs, cosmetics, and medical devices.

Canadian Food and Drugs Act

The Canadian **Food and Drugs Act** is the primary piece of legislation governing foods, drugs, cosmetics, and medical devices in Canada. The Act has been amended several times since its inception in 1953 (Table 4-1). Schedule A of the Act lists the diseases for which treatments may not be promoted to the public. Section 3(1) and 3(2) of the Food and Drugs Act prohibit any label claim or advertisement that is both directed to the general public and contains treatment, preventative or cure claims for Schedule A diseases. Revisions to Schedule A came into force on June 1, 2008. The updated Schedule A generally includes life-threatening diseases such as cancer and acute forms of specific diseases. For example, "liver disease," which covers all liver diseases, disorders and abnormalities, is now listed as "hepatitis," which is a more specific disease. The legend *Canadian Standard Drug*, or CSD, must appear on the inner and outer labels of the drug packaging to show that a drug meets the standards for which it is prescribed.

According to the Act, and to protect the consumer, drugs must comply with official prescribed standards stated in recognized pharmacopoeias and formularies listed in Schedule B of the Act. Recognized pharmacopoeias and formularies include the following:

- *Pharmacopée française*
- *Pharmacopoeia Internationalis*
- *The British Pharmacopoeia*
- *The Canadian Formulary*
- *The National Formulary*
- *The Pharmaceutical Codex: Principles and Practices of Pharmaceuticals*
- *The United States Pharmacopoeia*

Drugs listed in Schedule C are radiopharmaceuticals and drugs listed in Schedule D include allergenic substances, immunizing agents (vaccines), insulin, anterior pituitary extracts, drugs obtained by recombinant DNA technology, and blood derivatives. The distribution of *drug samples*, defined as trial packages of medication, is also regulated, with the exception of the distribution under

TABLE 4-1	
Additions to the Food and Drugs Act	
Schedule	**Description**
Schedules C and D	Drugs in these schedules must list where the drug was manufactured and the process and conditions of manufacturing.
Schedule F	This is a list of drugs that can be sold and refilled only on prescription; refills cannot exceed 6 months; labels on these drugs are marked *Pr*, or prescription required. *Examples:* Antibiotics, hormones, and tranquilizers.
Part G	These drugs, also known as controlled drugs, affect the central nervous system (CNS); labels on these drugs are marked *C*. Controlled drugs are categorized into three parts: Part I: designated controlled drugs with misuse potential that may be used for designated medical conditions outlined in Food and Drug Regulations. *Examples:* amphetamines, methylphenidate, pentobarbital, and preparations containing one controlled drug and one or more active noncontrolled drug. Part II: controlled drugs with misuse potential prescribed for medical conditions. *Examples:* sedatives such as barbiturates and derivatives (secobarbital), thiobarbiturates (pentothal sodium). Part III: controlled drugs with misuse potential. *Examples:* anabolic steroids (androstanolone), weight reduction drugs (anorexiants).
Narcotic Drugs and Preparations	Drugs with high misuse potential. *Examples:* morphine, codeine >8 mg, amidones (methadone), coca and derivatives (cocaine), benzazocines (analgesics such as pentazocine), fentanyls
Part J	These are restricted drugs with high misuse potential, dangerous physiological and psychological adverse effects, and no recognized medical use. *Examples:* lysergic acid diethylamide (LSD), mescaline (peyote), harmaline, psilocin and psilocybin (magic mushrooms).
Benzodiazepines and Other Targeted Substances Regulations	A "targeted substance" is either a controlled substance that is included in Schedule I, or a product or compound that contains a controlled substance that is included in Schedule I. These are drugs with misuse potential. *Examples:* benzodiazepine tranquilizers such as diazepam, lorazepam, flumitrazepam, and zolpidem.

prescribed conditions to physicians, dentists, or pharmacists. Schedule F is a list of medicinal ingredients, the sale of which legally requires a prescription for use in Canada. Examples are amoxicillin, antihypertensives, and thyroid replacement drugs. The recommended degree of regulatory control is based on the risk factors associated with each specific drug and each drug's potential for abuse. Prescription status helps to ensure that consumers receive adequate risk and benefit information from a health care provider before taking the drug. The *Pr* symbol on the label of Schedule F drugs identifies the product as a prescription drug. The symbol appears in the upper left quarter of the label as a black box with the letters *Pr* in white inside. The Food and Drugs Act also regulates the information manufacturers may put on a drug label including directions for use. A Schedule F prescription may be refilled as often as indicated by the subscriber. Prescriptions may be written (including facsimiles) or transmitted orally (via telephone to the pharmacist) by a qualified health care professional.

The **Food and Drug Regulations** are an adjunct to the Food and Drugs Act. These regulations clarify terms used in the Act and state the processes that companies must carry out to comply with the Act in terms of importing, preparing, treating, processing, labelling, advertising, and selling foods, drugs, cosmetics, natural health products, including herbal products, and medical devices.

Controlled drugs of the Food and Drug Regulations are listed in Part G of the Food and Drugs Act. Part G defines and provides an appropriate level of control for controlled drugs, which have a significant potential for abuse. Drugs listed in Part I of the schedule to Part G include amphetamines, certain barbiturates, and other psychoactive substances; these substances have a significant abuse potential. Controlled drugs are dispensed only by prescription. A controlled drug must be marked with the symbol *C* in a clear manner and a conspicuous colour and size on the upper left quarter of the label. The proper name of the drug must also appear on the label and either precedes or follows the brand name of the drug.

The Food and Drug Regulations (Parts G and J) outline similar regulations for controlled and restricted drugs, respectively. The Narcotic Control Regulations (discussed further in the next section) apply to *narcotics*, defined as "any substance set out in the schedule or anything that contains any substance set out in the schedule" (Department of Justice, Canada, 2004). The letter *N* is printed on the label of all narcotic agents.

Controlled Drug and Substances Act

The **Controlled Drug and Substances Act (CDSA)** was passed in 1997, replacing the Narcotic Control Act and Parts III and IV of the Food and Drugs Act. The first **Narcotic Control Act**, passed in 1961, was enacted in response to the growing use and misuse of drugs in the middle and late 1960s. It replaced the previous Act, the Canadian Opium and Narcotic Act of 1952. The Narcotic Control Act and Parts III and IV of the Food and Drugs

Act prohibited activities such as possession; possession for the purpose of trafficking; trafficking; importing and exporting; and cultivation of narcotics or controlled and restricted drugs.

The CDSA provides a framework for the control of certain drugs, their precursors, and other substances classified as controlled. The Act prohibits the import and export, production, distribution, and, in some cases, possession of substances that can alter mental processes and that may produce harm to health and to society when distributed or used without supervision. A **controlled substance** is anything scheduled under the CDSA, whereas a *controlled drug* includes Schedule G items under the Food and Drug Regulations. Controlled drugs and substances for medical treatment may be legally obtained only with a prescription from a licensed medical practitioner. The *Narcotic Control Regulations* apply to narcotics and specify the requirements for licensing for the import or export, sale, manufacture, and production or distribution of narcotics and for the cultivation of cannabis; the requirements for prescriptions for products containing narcotics; and the required record keeping. The CDSA is based on eight schedules that list controlled drugs and substances in order of misuse or harm potential. For nonprescription or **over-the-counter (OTC) drugs** (drugs that do not require a prescription) in Canada, there are three CDSA categories that regulate the conditions of sale, with the scheduling being overseen by the National Drug Scheduling Advisory Committee (NDSAC). A detailed discussion of the regulation and scheduling of nonprescription or OTC drugs is given in Chapter 7.

Schedule I contains the most dangerous drugs, including opiates (opium, heroin, morphine, cocaine) and methamphetamine. Schedule II contains cannabis-related drugs, including marihuana and its derivatives. Schedule III contains the more dangerous drugs such as amphetamines and lysergic acid diethylamide (LSD). Schedule IV contains drugs such as barbiturates and anabolic steroids, which are dangerous but have therapeutic uses. A prescription is required for possession of drugs listed in Schedule IV. Schedules V and VI contain precursors required to produce controlled substances. Schedules VII and VIII contain amounts of cannabis and cannabis resin required for charge and sentencing purposes. The factors that determine the schedule under which a controlled substance should be placed are international requirements, the dependence potential and likelihood of abuse of the substance, the extent of its abuse in Canada, the danger it represents to the safety of the public, and the usefulness of the substance as a therapeutic agent. The **Benzodiazepines and Other Targeted Substances Regulations** specify similar restrictions with regard to benzodiazepines, their salts and derivatives, and other targeted substances mentioned in Schedules I and II. The **Precursor Control Regulations**, introduced in 2003, address the need for the control of essential and precursor chemicals routinely used in clandestine labs for the production of methamphetamine, ecstasy, and other Schedule III drugs. The **Marihuana Medical Access Regulations** deal with the production, distribution, sale, destruction, record keeping, and licensing issues concerning marihuana for medical use. The *Controlled Drugs and Substances Act (Police Enforcement) Regulations* apply to the members of a police force. The Royal Canadian Mounted Police (RCMP) are responsible for enforcing the CDSA and related sections of the Criminal Code and exempt members of police forces from sections of the CDSA for the purpose of performing their duties.

NEW DRUG DEVELOPMENT

The research into and development of new drugs is an ongoing process. The pharmaceutical industry is a multibillion-dollar industry, and pharmaceutical companies must continuously develop new and better drugs to maintain a competitive edge. The research required for the development of these new drugs may take several years. Hundreds of substances are isolated that never make it to market. Once a potentially beneficial drug has been identified, the pharmaceutical company must follow a regulated, systematic process before the drug can be sold on the open market. This highly sophisticated process is regulated and carefully monitored by Health Canada. The primary purpose of Health Canada's TPD is to protect the patient and ensure the safety, efficacy, and quality of the drug. This system of drug research and development is one of the most stringent in the world, and there are many benefits and drawbacks to it. It was developed out of concern for patient safety and drug efficacy. To ensure that these two important objectives are met with some degree of certainty, much time and paperwork are required—this is the downside to the system. Many drugs are marketed and used in foreign countries long before they get approval for use in Canada. However, drug-related tragedies are more likely to be avoided by this more stringent drug approval system. For example, thalidomide was a widely used sedative-hypnotic that was originally marketed in Europe and made available for distribution in Canada in 1961. It was later found to cause severe deformities in the babies of mothers who took the drug during pregnancy. It was never approved in the United States because a Canadian pharmacologist working for the U.S. Food and Drug Administration (FDA) as a medical officer convinced authorities that the drug was not proven to be safe for use during pregnancy. As a result of the thalidomide tragedy, many governments, including Canada's, tightened their drug approval process. It now takes approximately 5 years of animal and human testing for a drug to be approved in Canada.

A balance must be achieved between making new lifesaving therapies available and protecting consumers from potential drug-induced adverse effects. In 2003, Canada introduced the *Natural Health Products Regulations*. These regulations cover natural health products such as vitamins and minerals, herbal remedies, homeopathic medicines, traditional medicines (e.g., traditional Chinese medicines), probiotics, and other products such as amino acids and essential fatty acids (e.g., omega-3). The manufacturers' primary obligation regarding such products was to not make "false or misleading" claims about their efficacy. For example, a product label may read "For depression," but cannot read "Known to cure depression." In 2008, Bill C-51 was drafted to complement and support the current policies for foods and health products, including natural health products. Reliable, objective information about these kinds of products is limited but is growing as more formal research studies are conducted. Consumer demand for and interest in alternative medicine products continues to drive this process. Patients should be advised to exercise caution in using such products and to communicate regularly with their health care professionals regarding their use.

Naming Drugs

All medications have a *chemical* name, a *generic* name, and a *trade* name. A drug's *chemical name* is used by the chemists who first discover and work with the drug. This is usually the very first name used to identify a particular chemical compound, often before it is classified as a "drug" with known therapeutic properties. The chemical name is based on the standard chemical nomenclature recommended by the International Union of Pure and Applied Chemists (IUPAC). For this reason, it is also known as the *IUPAC name*. *Generic names* are usually shorter and less complex than chemical names, and their spelling is typically loosely based on the chemical structural features of the drug. The generic name is assigned to a chemical compound after a pharmaceutical manufacturer has determined that it is worthy of continued clinical research because of apparent therapeutic properties.

The first evidence of therapeutic properties often appears in the laboratory setting. For example, a research scientist may discover that a given chemical compound destroys or inhibits the growth of cancer cells in a live cell culture. It is at this point that the chemical compound becomes an investigational drug per se. In clinical practice, at the time the drug is undergoing clinical research, the drug is referred to by its *investigational* or *protocol name*, especially in the case of cancer drugs. The protocol name may be the same as the generic name; it is a code name that consists of a combination of letters and numbers separated by one or more dashes. One of the purposes of this name is to protect the code of a blinded study so that neither research staff nor study patients know who is (or is not) receiving the actual drug under investigation. This helps in distinguishing real drug effects from *placebo* effects when a placebo-controlled study format is used (which is not always the case). Protocol names tend to be used more commonly in patient care settings for cancer drugs than for other drug classes. The following are two typical examples that illustrate these concepts:

Investigational Name	Generic Name	Trade Name
STI-571 (protocol name)	imatinib	Gleevec
5-fluorouracil* (chemical name)	fluorouracil	Fluouracil

*The "5" refers to the position of a fluorine atom in the cyclic ring structure of the uracil molecule.

The *trade name* is a marketing name used by the manufacturer of a given drug primarily to advertise the drug to prescribers and even to patients themselves. The trade name is frequently strategically chosen to be shorter and easier to pronounce and remember than the chemical, protocol, or generic names. Some pharmaceutical companies identify themselves as the manufacturer of the drug in the drug's trade name. For example, an APO- in front of the trade name reflects Apotex Incorporated (e.g., APO-divalproex); DOM-[trade name] reflects Dominion Pharmacal.

Investigational New Drug Application

A pharmaceutical company must prove both the safety and efficacy of a newly isolated drug before it can be used in the general population. It has been noted that, on average, approximately 12 years are needed for a drug to go from application to actual availability for prescribing. The new medication must be tested for its pharmacological effects, dosage ranges, and possible toxic effects. Testing begins in animal subjects. After extensive animal testing that proves the safety and efficacy of the new drug, the pharmaceutical company can then submit an application to have it accepted as an **investigational new drug (IND)**. Only after the Health Products and Food Branch Inspectorate of Health Canada reviews and approves this application can the pharmaceutical company proceed with investigational studies of the IND in human subjects.

Informed Consent

Informed consent is required before most invasive procedures can be performed and before a patient can be admitted into a research study. Informed consent involves the careful explanation to the human test patient or *research subject* of the purpose of the study in which the individual is being asked to participate, the procedures to be used, the possible benefits, and the risks involved. The document must be written in a language understood by the patient and be dated and signed by the patient and at least one witness. Included in the document are clear, rational descriptions of the procedure or test. Should the patient decide *not* to participate in the research at any time, the patient should be informed that this decision will not have a negative effect on the patient's ongoing nursing or health care. Informed consent is voluntary. The principles of medical ethics dictate that informed consent must be obtained from all patients (or their legal guardians) more than a given number of days or hours before certain procedures are performed or before they can be enrolled in an IND study and must always be obtained when the patient or research subject (or legal guardian) is fully mentally competent.

Some patients may have unrealistic expectations of the IND's usefulness. Often they have the misconception that because an investigational drug is new it must automatically be better than existing forms of therapy. Other volunteers may be reluctant to enter the study because they think they will be treated like "guinea pigs." Whatever the circumstances of the study, the research subjects must be informed of all potential hazards as well as the possible benefits of the new therapy. It should be stressed that involvement in IND studies is truly voluntary and that the subject can quit the study at any time. To enhance objectivity, many studies are designed to incorporate a placebo. A **placebo** is an inert substance that is not a drug (e.g., normal saline, distilled water, starch, sugar). In some drug studies (termed *placebo controlled*), a placebo is given to some subjects so that the effects of this inactive substance can be compared with the effects of the experimental drug. (See also Legal and Ethical Principles: Use of Placebos.)

Health Canada Drug Approval Process

The Therapeutic Products Directorate (TPD) of Health Canada is responsible for approving drugs for clinical safety and efficacy before they are brought to the market.

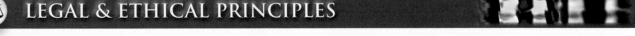

 LEGAL & ETHICAL PRINCIPLES

Use of Placebos

Use of placebo therapy may be one of the legal–ethical dilemmas within the context of research studies and clinical trials and should never be taken lightly. All aspects of research studies (e.g., drug trials) are to be clearly identified within the informed-consent documents. Informed consent should clearly identify the research subject's rights, such as the right to (1) leave the study at any time without any pressure or coercion to stay, (2) leave the study without consequences to medical care, (3) have full and complete information about the study, and (4) be aware of all alternative options, with information on all options, including placebo therapy, being made available in the study. It is important to know that placebo therapy is randomly assigned and that even the researchers have no say in the decision or assignment of patients. Use of randomization does not guarantee what a person will get when entering a drug trial; however, if patients inquire about the specifics of the drug(s) offered, including use of a placebo, the information must be shared truthfully but within the confines of the trial or research study.

The approval process begins with *preclinical* testing phases, which includes in vitro studies (using tissue samples and cell cultures) and animal studies. *Clinical* (human) testing follows the preclinical phase. There are four clinical phases. The drug is put on the market after Phase 3 is completed if an investigational **new drug submission (NDS)** submitted by the manufacturer is approved by the TPD. Phase 4 consists of postmarketing studies. The collective goal of these phases is to provide information on the safety, toxicity, efficacy, potency, bioavailability, and purity of the NDS. A **Notice of Compliance** is issued when Health Canada decides that the drug and the manufacturing process are safe and effective, allowing the pharmaceutical company to sell the product by prescription to the Canadian population. Once a drug is approved for sale, it is assigned a **Drug Identification Number (DIN)** by the Drugs Directorate. The DIN is placed on the label of prescription and OTC drug products.

Preclinical Investigational Drug Studies

Current medical ethics still require that all new drugs undergo laboratory testing using both *in vitro* (cell or tissue) and animal studies before any testing in human subjects can be done. In vitro studies include testing the response of mammalian (including human) cells and tissues to different concentrations of the investigational drug. Cells and tissues used for this purpose are collected from living or dead animal or human subjects (e.g., surgical or autopsy specimens). These cell samples may then be grown synthetically in the laboratory for several generations of continuous research. These in vitro studies help researchers to determine early on if a substance might be too toxic for human patients. Many prospective new drugs are ruled out for human use during this preclinical phase of drug testing. However, a small percentage of the many drugs tested in this manner are referred on for further clinical testing in human subjects. At this stage, an application is made to Health Canada with a protocol of the objectives, methods, and rules under which the sponsor will operate during the trial.

Four Clinical Phases of Investigational Drug Studies

Phase 1

Phase 1 studies usually involve small numbers of healthy subjects (normally fewer than 100) rather than those who have the disease or ailment that the new drug is intended to treat. An exception might be a study involving a toxic drug used to treat a life-threatening illness. In this case, the only study subjects might be those who already have the illness and for whom other viable treatment options may not be available. The purpose of Phase 1 studies is to determine the potential adverse effects, optimal dosage range, and the pharmacokinetics of the drug (i.e., absorption, distribution, metabolism, and excretion) and to ascertain if further testing is needed. Blood tests, urinalyses, assessments of vital signs, and specific monitoring tests are also performed. These trials usually last a few days to a few weeks.

Phase 2

Phase 2 studies involve larger numbers of volunteers (usually around 100 to 500) who have the disease or ailment that the drug is designed to diagnose or treat. This is usually a randomized control study composed of patients of similar age, sex distribution, and medical history. Study participants are closely monitored for the drug's effectiveness and short-term adverse effects. This is also the phase during which the ideal therapeutic dosage ranges are refined. Phase 2 trials normally last 6 months to 1 year. If no serious adverse effects occur, the study can progress to Phase 3.

Phase 3

Phase 3 studies involve larger numbers of patients (normally 1000 to 3000), who are followed by medical research centres and other types of health care facilities. The patients may be treated at the centre or may be spread over a wider geographic area and be followed at a local inpatient or outpatient facility. The purpose of this larger sample size is to provide information about infrequent or rare adverse effects that may not have been observed during previous smaller studies. To enhance objectivity, many studies are designed to incorporate a placebo. The rationale for administering a placebo to a portion of the research subjects is to separate out the real benefits of the investigational drug from the apparent benefits arising out of researcher or subject bias regarding expected or desired results of the drug therapy. A study incorporating a placebo is called a *placebo-controlled study*. If the study subject does not know whether the drug he or she is administered is a placebo or the IND but the investigator does know, then the study is referred to as a **blinded investigational drug study**. In most studies neither the research staff nor the subjects being tested know which subjects are being given the real drug and which are receiving the placebo. This further enhances the objectivity of the study results and is known as a **double-blind, investigated drug study** because both the researcher and the subject are "blinded" to the actual identity of the substance administered to a given subject. Both drug and placebo dosage forms given to patients often look identical except for a secret code that appears on the medication itself or its container. At the completion of the study, this code is revealed or broken to determine which study patients received the drug and which were given the placebo. The code can also be broken before study completion by the principle investigator in the event of a clinical emergency that requires a determination of what individual patients received. The three objectives of Phase 3 studies are to establish the drug's clinical effectiveness, safety, and dosage range. After Phase 3 is completed, Health Canada's TPD and Biologics and Genetic Therapies Directorate (BGTD) receive a report from the manufacturer as well as an NDS. The approval of an NDS paves the way for the pharmaceutical company to market the new drug exclusively until the patent for the drug molecule expires. As mandated by the Canadian Patent Act, this is normally 20 years after discovery of the molecule and includes the 10- to 12-year period generally required to complete drug research. Therefore, a new drug manufacturer typically has 8 to 10 years after drug marketing to recoup research costs, which are usually in the hundreds of millions of dollars for a single drug.

Phase 4

Phase 4 studies are postmarketing studies voluntarily conducted by pharmaceutical companies to obtain further proof of the therapeutic effects of the new drug. Data from such studies are usually gathered for at least 2 years after the drug's release. Often these studies compare the safety and efficacy of the new drug with that of another drug in the same therapeutic category. An example would be a comparison of a new nonsteroidal anti-inflammatory drug (NSAID) with ibuprofen in the treatment of osteoarthritis. Some medications make it through all phases of clinical trials without causing any problems among study patients. When they are used in the larger general population, however, severe adverse effects may appear for the first time. If a pattern of severe reactions to a newly marketed drug begins to emerge, Health Canada may request that the manufacturer of the drug issue a voluntary recall. If the drug manufacturer refuses to recall the medication, and if the number or severity of reactions reaches a certain level, then the Health Products and Food Branch Inspectorate of Health Canada will seek court action to condemn the product and allow it to be seized by legal authorities. Such an action, in effect, becomes an involuntary recall on behalf of the manufacturer.

There are three designated types of drug recall based on Health Canada's response to postmarketing data for a given drug:

Type I: a situation in which there is a reasonable probability that the use of, or exposure to, a product will cause serious adverse health consequences or death.

Type II: a situation in which the use of, or exposure to, a product may cause temporary adverse health consequences or where the probability of serious adverse health consequences is remote.

Type III: a situation in which the use of, or exposure to, a product is not likely to cause any adverse health consequences.

Health Canada issues warnings and advisories in the form of press releases, Web site announcements (http://www.hc-sc.gc.ca/dhp-mps/medeff/advisories-avis/index-eng.php), or letters to health professionals.

Priority Review Process

Health Canada has attempted to make lifesaving investigational drug therapies available to the population sooner by offering a **Priority Review of Drug Submission** process. This policy applies to New Drug Submissions (NDS) or Supplemental New Drug Submissions (S/NDS) and allows for earlier review of drug products for serious, life-threatening, or severely debilitating diseases or conditions (e.g., cancer, AIDS, Parkinson's disease) for which there is no effective drug on the Canadian market.

Special Access Programme

Health Canada has attempted to make lifesaving investigational drug therapies available on an individual basis through the **Special Access Programme (SAP)**. The SAP provides compassionate access to drugs not approved for sale in Canada and is limited to those with serious or life-threatening conditions (e.g., intractable depression, epilepsy, transplant rejection, hemophilia and other blood disorders, terminal cancer, and AIDS) who may require experimental drugs for compassionate reasons or on an emergency basis when other conventional therapies have failed. It can also respond to an emergency health crisis. One example is when the drinking water in Walkerton, Ontario, became contaminated with *Escherichia coli* 0157:H7. Doctors in Walkerton applied to Health Canada for access to a drug not yet approved for use for seriously ill patients with *Escherichia coli* bacteria infections. Because of the urgent need, Health Canada approved the application.

This program is not intended to get around the clinical-trial approval process. The physician is responsible for initiating the request on the patient's behalf and for ensuring that the request is supported by reliable evidence. Health Canada then reviews the request and upon approval delivers a Letter of Authorization to both the drug manufacturer and the physician. The drug company makes the final decision of whether the patient may receive the drug and under which conditions. The physician is responsible for informing the patient of all possible risks and benefits of the drug.

Patent Protection

Early in the research and development stage, drug manufacturers of newly discovered or invented drugs apply for patent protection. The **Patent Act** allows brand name drug companies to extend their exclusive market rights of patented medicine to 20 years. Regulations also link the issuing of notices of compliance for *generic* drugs (discussed in the next section) to the expiry of the patent protection period for the innovator drug. The Act also established the **Patented Medicine Prices Review Board (PMPRB)** to monitor and control the price of patented medicine (see Legal and Ethical Principles: Patient Access to and Costs of Prescription Drugs). Twice yearly, patentees must file price and sales information for all patented medicine. If a price is deemed excessive, the PMPRB can order it reduced (this has only happened eight times since 1999). When patents expire, competing pharmaceutical companies can manufacture and sell generic forms of the drug.

Generic Drugs

A **generic drug** is a chemically identical equivalent of a brand (trade) name drug. A manufacturer will develop a generic version in 2 to 3 years, at a cost of approximately $1 million. Once a generic drug is developed, the manufacturer submits an Abbreviated New Drug Submission (ANDS) to Health Canada TPD, with evidence that the generic formulation is bioequivalent to the brand formulation.

The consumer cost of a generic drug is generally about 45% less than that of the brand name equivalent drug.

LEGAL & ETHICAL PRINCIPLES

Patient Access to and Costs of Prescription Drugs

The twenty-first century in Canada has seen rapid growth in prescription drug use and costs. In 2004, prescription drugs for Canadians cost $562 per capita (not including drugs provided in hospital). Almost half of this cost (approximately $268) was paid directly out of patients' pockets. Prescription drug costs are increasing at 9% annually. In 2006, Canadian pharmacists filled 400 million retail prescriptions. According to the Canadian Institute for Health Information, costs of prescription-only medicines accounted for $25 billion in 2006. The increased costs are attributed not only to the increase in numbers of prescriptions, some of which can be attributed to Canada's aging population, but also to more costly drugs. Costs of prescription drugs are determined by ingredient costs (manufacturer cost), pharmacy retail mark-up, and the dispensing fee. Dispensing fees are the additional fee pharmacists charge for dispensing prescription drugs to patients. Such costs can vary from $2 to over $10, depending on the pharmacy.

Prescription drugs are not covered under the **Canada Health Act.** Patients must pay for a drug unless the drug is covered by a private drug plan or a federal, provincial, or territorial (F/P/T) drug plan. Most provincial plans provide for the costs of drugs to the poor, the older adult, those with catastrophic drug costs, and those with certain conditions (e.g., cancer, HIV/AIDS). The federal government provides coverage for Aboriginal peoples. Each Canadian province and territory has a formulary committee that decides which drugs are listed on a provincial formulary and reimbursed by the drug benefit health plan, which have restricted access, and which are not covered. There is a wide variety of access to prescription drugs across the country: provincial and territorial drug plans vary in eligibility criteria, drugs covered, and financing. Provinces base the decision to list a drug on a variety of factors such as effectiveness analyses, cost, government priorities, and patient advocacy. Some drugs may be restricted if they require special monitoring or if the cost is high.

Because of discrepancies in drug coverage among F/P/T drug plans, the Common Drug Review Directorate was established in 2002 at the Canadian Coordinating Office for Health Technology Assessment. An independent advisory body, the Canadian Expert Drug Advisory Committee (CEDAC), has members from all jurisdictions except Quebec. CEDAC makes evidence-informed recommendations regarding the listing of drugs to the F/P/T formularies. This process is intended to provide equal access to all drugs, reduce duplication between formularies, and streamline the review process for new drugs. However, the drug plans make the decision on which drugs will make the final formulary listing.

In 2002, Roy Romanow, the head of the **Romanow Commission**, presented a report, *Building on Values: The Future of Health Care in Canada,* which recommended extensive changes to protect the long-term sustainability of the Canadian health care system. One recommendation was to establish a national pharmacare program. One aspect of the national program would be the Catastrophic Drug Transfer Program (CDTP), under which the federal government would assist the provinces to cover those who have extremely high drug costs. In addition, a national formulary administered by a National Drug Agency would be formed in an effort to control costs and to evaluate safety and cost-effectiveness of all new and existing prescription drugs. Romanow also recommended a review of the Canadian patent legislation regarding new prescription drugs and better access to generic drugs. A full discussion of the report is available at http://www.hc-sc.gc.ca/hcs-sss/hhr-rhs/strateg/romanow-eng.php.

Generic drug (and all nonpatented drugs) prices are not regulated by the PMPRB but are determined provincially. For example, in Ontario, the Ontario Drug Benefit Act and the Ontario Drug Interchangeability and Dispensing Fee Act allow the Ontario government to establish generic drug prices for the drugs that it will reimburse. Basically there is a "70/90" rule: a new generic drug is priced at no higher than 70% of the price of the brand name; succeeding generic drugs are priced no higher than 90% of the price of the initial generic drug. Generic and existing or revised drugs do not have to go through the Common Drug Review to receive a listing recommendation as new drugs do, but requests are submitted directly to the drug plans.

Drug Advertising in Canada

Drug advertising in Canada is regulated by Health Canada. Direct-to-consumer advertising (such as ads in consumer magazines and on subways) is restricted to simply giving the names of prescription drugs, but these ads do not make claims for product effectiveness. (This is not the case in the United States.) Advertisements in professional health care journals contain claims and prescribing information. Advertising Standards Canada (ASC) and the Pharmaceutical Advertising Advisory Board (PAAB) review and clear advertisements according to standards set by the Food and Drugs Act. Although the clearance procedure is voluntary, most companies comply with the regulations.

ETHICAL NURSING PRACTICE

Ethical nursing practice is based on basic ethical principles such as *beneficence, autonomy, justice, veracity,* and *confidentiality* (see Legal and Ethical Principles: Common Legal and Ethics-Related Terms). The Canadian Nurses Association (CNA) *Code of Ethics for Registered Nurses* (2008) should be a familiar framework of practice to all nurses and serve as an ethical guideline for nursing care. It is a statement of the ethical values of nurses and of nurses' commitments to persons with health care needs and persons receiving care. The *Code of Ethics* is intended for nurses in all contexts and domains of nursing practice and at all levels of decision making. Developed by nurses for nurses, it can assist nurses in practising ethically and working through ethical challenges that arise in their practice with individuals, families, communities, and public health systems.

These ethical principles and codes of ethics ensure that the nurse is acting on behalf of the patient and with the patient's best interests at heart. As a professional, the nurse has the responsibility to provide safe nursing care to patients regardless of the setting, person, group, community, or family involved. Although it is not within the nurse's realm of ethical and professional responsibility to impose his or her values or standards on the patient, it is within the nurse's realm to provide information and to assist the patient in facing decisions regarding health care.

The nurse also has the right to refuse to participate in any treatment or aspect of a patient's care that violates the nurse's personal ethical principles. However, this should be done without deserting the patient, and in some facilities the nurse may be transferred to another patient care assignment only if the transfer is approved by the nurse manager or nurse supervisor. The nurse must always remember, however, that the *Code of Ethics* and professional responsibility and accountability require the nurse to provide nonjudgemental nursing care from the start of the patient's treatment until the time of the patient's discharge. If transferring to a different assignment is not an option because of institutional policy and because of the increase in the acuteness of patients' conditions and the high patient-to-nurse workload, then the nurse must always act in the best interest of the patient while remaining an objective patient advocate.

It is always the nurse's responsibility to provide the highest quality nursing care and practice within the professional standards of care. The CNA *Code of Ethics*, the *ICN Code of Ethics for Nurses*, standards of nursing practice, federal and provincial codes, ethical principles, and the previously mentioned legal principles are readily accessible and provide nurses with a sound, rational framework for professional nursing practice.

ETHNOCULTURAL CONSIDERATIONS

Because the health care system overall emphasizes cure, prescribed drugs tend to be a major part of a patient's therapeutic regimen. The Canadian health care system often advocates a "one-size-fits-all" treatment approach. However, Canada is an ethnoculturally diverse nation, thus a more multicultural, holistic approach to alterations in health status could help in meeting the needs of such a diverse patient population. According to the 2006 Canada Census, the Canadian population was 31,612,897 (as of August 2009, the population was 33,716,731); of this total, 16.2% were members of a visible minority (Statistics Canada, 2006). Canada's minority population is ethnoculturally diverse, with some groups being more so than others. Population growth among Canada's visible minority was five times the rate of growth of the total population between 2001 and 2006. The three largest self-identified visible minorities, accounting for approximately two-thirds of the visible minority population, are South Asian (e.g., East Indian, Pakistani, Sri Lankan), Chinese, and Black. These groups are followed in population size by Filipino, Latin American, and Southeast Asian (Vietnamese, Cambodian, Malaysian, Laotian). Aboriginal people account for 3.8% of Canada's total population. It is estimated that by 2017, one in every five Canadian residents will be a member of a visible minority.

The new and expanding field of **ethnopharmacology** (the study of the health beliefs and practices of different ethnocultures) holds much promise for understanding the specific impact of ethnicity on drug effects and responses. It is hampered, however, by the lack of clarity in terms such as *race*, *ethnicity*, and *ethnoculture*. Although some researchers have used the term *Hispanic* to encompass groups as diverse as Puerto Ricans, Mexicans, and Peruvians, other researchers have used it to denote a specific racial group. This lack of clarity in terminology and lack of consistency in the use of terms in research raises questions about the validity of the data collected. One thing is certain, however: it is impossible to know a patient's genotype simply by looking at the patient or at the patient's health care history and documentation.

 ## LEGAL & ETHICAL PRINCIPLES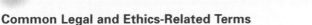

Common Legal and Ethics-Related Terms

Autonomy: Self-determination and ability to act on one's own; implications include promoting a patient's decision-making process, supporting informed consent, and assisting in decisions or making a decision when a patient poses harm to himself or herself.

Beneficence: The doing or active promotion of good; implications include determining how the patient can best be served.

Confidentiality: The duty to respect privileged information about a patient; implications include not talking about a patient in public or outside the context of the health care setting.

Justice: Being fair or equal in one's actions; implications include the fair distribution of resources for the care of the patient and determination of when to treat.

Nonmaleficence: The duty to do no harm to a patient; implications include avoiding doing any deliberate harm while rendering nursing care.

Veracity: Duty to tell the truth; implications include telling the truth with regard to placebos, investigational new drugs, and informed consent.

The ever-changing national demographics require the nurse to be ethnoculturally competent while administering holistic and individualized nursing care involving both nonpharmacological and pharmacological therapies. To ensure this competence, the nurse must be up to date in basic knowledge of the nursing process and in the art and science of professional nursing practice. Acknowledgement and acceptance of the influences of a patient's ethnocultural beliefs, values, and customs is necessary to promote optimal health and wellness. Some related terms and examples of ethnocultural influences are presented below in Ethnocultural Implications: Ethnocultural Terms Related to Nursing Practice, and Ethnocultural Implications: Common Practices of Select Ethnocultural Groups.

Influence of Ethnicity and Genetics

Medication response depends greatly on the level of the patient's adherence to the therapy regimen. Given multiple ethnocultural factors, adherence may vary according to the patient's ethnocultural beliefs, experiences with medications, personal expectations, family expectations, family influence, and level of education. Adherence is not the only issue, however. Health care providers must also be aware that some patients use alternative therapies, such as herbal and homeopathic remedies, that can inhibit or accelerate drug metabolism and therefore alter a drug's response.

In reference to specific drug therapy and a patient's response, the important concept of *polymorphism* is critical to understanding how the same drug can result in different responses in different individuals. **Drug polymorphism** refers to the effect of a patient's age, sex, size, body composition, and other characteristics on the pharmacokinetics of specific drugs. For example, why does a Chinese patient require lower doses of an anti-anxiety drug than a White patient? Why do Black patients respond differently to antihypertensives than do White patients? Factors contributing to drug polymorphism may be loosely categorized into environmental factors (e.g., diet and nutritional status), ethnocultural factors, and genetic (inherited) factors. For example, a diet high in fat has been documented to increase the absorption of the agent griseofulvin (an antifungal agent). Malnutrition with deficiencies in protein, vitamins, and minerals may modify the functioning of metabolic enzymes, which may alter the body's ability to absorb or eliminate a medication.

 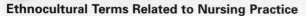

ETHNOCULTURAL IMPLICATIONS

Ethnocultural Terms Related to Nursing Practice

Ethnicity: Ethnic affiliation based on shared ethnoculture, genetic heritage, or both.

Ethnoculture: An integrated system of beliefs, values, and customs that are associated with an ethnically distinct group of people and are generally handed down from generation to generation.

Ethnocultural competence: The ability to work with patients with proper consideration for the ethnocultural context, which includes patients' belief systems and values regarding health, wellness, and illness. It also involves learning about patients of distinct ethnicity and their specific responses to treatment, including drug therapies.

Ethnopharmacology: The study of the effect of ethnicity on drug responses, specifically drug absorption, metabolism, distribution, and excretion (i.e., pharmacokinetics; see Chapter 2) as well as the study of genetic variations to drugs (i.e., pharmacogenetics).

Race: Often defined as a class of individuals with a common lineage. In genetics, a race is considered to be a population having a somewhat different genetic composition or gene frequencies. Race is also used to refer to geographic origins of ancestry.

ETHNOCULTURAL IMPLICATIONS

Common Practices of Select Ethnocultural Groups

Ethnoculture	Common Practices
African	Practise folk medicine; employ "root workers" as healers
Asian	Believe in traditional medicine
Hispanic	View health as a result of good luck and living right, and illness as a result of doing a bad deed; use heat and cold as remedies
European	Hold traditional health beliefs; some still practise folk medicine
Aboriginal	Believe in harmony with nature; view ill spirits as causing disease
Filipino	Believe in and practise traditional and Western medicine; illness results from an imbalance in the body
South Asian	Believe dietary imbalance is a source of illness
Western	Show increased participation in health care; demand more explanation about diseases and treatment, as well as the prevention of diseases

Note: The above are generalizations. It is important for the nurse to conduct a thorough assessment of individual patients.

As indicated above, genetic factors also influence how different racial or ethnic groups respond to drugs. Some European and African patients are slow acetylators and metabolize drugs at a slower rate, which results in elevated drug level concentrations. Some Japanese and Inuit patients are more rapid acetylators and metabolize drugs more quickly, which leads to decreased drug concentrations. The Chinese, Japanese, Malaysians, and Thais are poor metabolizers of debrisoquine; therefore, drugs such as codeine are likely to be *more* effective at lower dosages in these individuals than in a European person. Several major drug classifications are relatively well researched with regard to differential responses in different ethnocultural groups; these are outlined in Table 4-2.

Individuals throughout the world share many common views and beliefs regarding health practices and medication use. However, specific ethnocultural influences, beliefs, and practices related to medication administration do exist. Awareness of ethnocultural differences is critical for the care of patients in Canada today because Canadian demographics are constantly changing. As previously mentioned, the minority composition of Canada is expected to continue to change drastically. In addition, the White majority is not only shrinking but also aging, whereas the Asian and Aboriginal groups are not only growing but are also young. As a result of these changes, nurses need to attend to and be concerned with each patient's ethnocultural background to ensure safe and quality nursing care, including medication administration.

For example, some people in the Black and Caribbean communities have health beliefs and practices that include an emphasis such as proper diet and rest; the use of herbal teas, laxatives, and protective bracelets; and the use of folk medicine, prayer, and the "laying on of hands." Reliance on home remedies can also be an important component of their health practices. (See Ethnocultural Implications: Common Practices of Select Ethnocultural Groups, on page 68).

Some Asian patients, especially the Chinese, believe in traditional medicines and healing such as yin and yang. Ying and yang are opposing forces that lead to illness or health, depending on which force is dominant in the individual and whether the forces are balanced; balance produces healthy states. Yin represents the female and the negative energies of darkness and cold; yang represents the male and the positive energies of light and warmth. Beliefs in yin and yang must be respected by all who participate in the care of Chinese patients. Other common health practices of Asians include acupuncture, use of herbal remedies, and use of heat. All such beliefs and practices need to be considered—especially when the patient values their use more highly than the use of medications. Many of these beliefs are strongly grounded in religion. The Asian and Pacific Islander racial–ethnic group also includes Thais, Vietnamese, Filipinos, Koreans, and Japanese, among others.

Some Aboriginals believe in preserving harmony with nature or keeping a balance between the body and mind and the environment to maintain health. Ill spirits are seen as the cause of disease. The traditional healer for this ethnoculture is the medicine man, and treatments vary from massage and application of heat to acts of purification. "Smudging" is a common ceremony used to cleanse the body spiritually and physically. An herb such as sage or sweetgrass is burned and the smoke is rubbed or brushed over the body.

Some South Asian individuals follow a variety of traditional health practices. Illness is seen as an imbalance in the body humours, bile, wind, and phlegm, and treatment is seen to restore these imbalances. Treatment may consist of home remedies, dietary regimens, prayers, rituals, and consultation with hakims, veds, babajis, pundits, homeopaths, and jyotshis.

Some Hispanic individuals view health as a result of good luck and living right and illness as a result of bad luck or committing a bad deed. To restore health, these individuals seek out a balance between the body and mind through use of cold remedies or foods for "hot" illnesses (of blood or yellow bile) and hot remedies for "cold" illnesses (of phlegm or black bile). Hispanics may use a variety of religious rituals for healing (e.g., lighting of candles), which may also be practised by adherents of other religions and belief systems.

It is important to remember that these beliefs vary from patient to patient. Therefore, the nurse should

TABLE 4-2

Examples of Varying Responses of Different Ethnocultural Groups to Major Drug Classes

Racial or Ethnic Group	Drug Classification	Response
Blacks	Antihypertensive agents	Respond better to diuretics than to β-blockers and ACE inhibitors Respond less effectively to β-blockers Respond best to calcium channel blockers, especially diltiazem Respond less effectively to single-drug therapy
Asians and Hispanics	Antipsychotic and antianxiety agents	Asians need lower doses of certain drugs such as haloperidol. Japanese and Chinese are more prone to rapid buildup of mephenytoin and, as a result, are at risk for sedation and overdosage. Asians and Hispanics respond better to lower doses of antidepressants. Chinese require lower doses of antipsychotics. Japanese require lower doses of antimanic agents.

Note: The comparative group for these responses comprises Whites. *ACE,* angiotensin-converting enzyme.

always consult with the patient rather than assuming that the individual holds certain beliefs.

Barriers to adequate health care for the ethnoculturally diverse Canadian patient population include language, poverty, access, pride, and beliefs regarding medical practices. Medications may have a different meaning to different ethnocultures, as would any form of medical treatment. Thus, before any medication is administered, a thorough ethnocultural assessment should be completed, which should include questions regarding the following:
- Health beliefs and practices
- Past uses of medicine
- Use of folk remedies
- Use of home remedies
- Use of over-the-counter (OTC) drugs and natural health products, including herbal remedies
- Usual responses to illness
- Responsiveness to medical treatment
- Religious practices and beliefs (e.g., many Christian Scientists believe in taking no medications at all)

In addition, the legal and ethical guidelines and principles mentioned earlier must be taken into account in developing and implementing each patient's collaborative plan of care and drug therapy.

NURSING PROCESS

▰ Assessment

A thorough ethnocultural assessment is needed for the provision of ethnoculturally competent nursing care. A variety of assessment tools and resources are available for the professional nurse to incorporate into nursing care, including Madeline Leininger's 2002 book, *Transcultural Nursing: Concepts, Theories, Research, and Practice*.

To identify different racial and ethnocultural influences, the following areas should be assessed (Specter, 2000, pp. 24–25). (The questions provided are only examples of those that can be used to identify the patient's methods for maintaining, protecting, and restoring physical, mental, and spiritual health.)

▰ Maintaining Health

- *For physical health:* Where are special foods and clothing items purchased? What types of health education are of the patient's ethnoculture? Where does the patient usually obtain information about health and illness? From folklore? Where are health services obtained? Who does the patient rely on for health care (e.g., physicians, nurse practitioners, community services, health departments, healers)?
- *For mental health:* What are examples of ethnoculturally specific activities for the mind and for maintaining mental health, as well as beliefs about reducing stress, rest, and relaxation?

- *For spiritual health:* What resources are used to meet spiritual needs?

▰ Protecting Health

- *For physical health:* Where are special clothing and everyday essentials purchased? What are examples of the patient's symbolic clothing, if any?
- *For mental health:* Who within the family and community teaches the roles in the patient's specific ethnoculture? Are there rules about avoiding certain persons or places? Are there special activities that must be performed?
- *For spiritual health:* Who teaches spiritual practices and where can special protective symbolic objects such as crystals or amulets be purchased? Are they expensive and how available are they for the patient when needed?

▰ Restoring Health

- *For physical health:* Where are special remedies purchased? Can individuals produce or grow their own remedies and herbs? How often are traditional and nontraditional services obtained?
- *For mental health:* Who are the traditional and nontraditional resources for mental health? Are there ethnoculture-specific activities for coping with stress and illness?
- *For spiritual health:* How often and where are traditional and nontraditional spiritual leaders or healers accessed?

▰ Nursing Diagnoses

- Risk for injury related to interruption of daily activities and ethnocultural patterns of health and wellness
- Risk for injury and falls related to decreased sensorium and confusion caused by unfamiliar hospital environment
- Insomnia related to a lack of adherence to ethnocultural practices for encouraging stress release and sleep induction
- Risk for injury or adverse drug reactions related to drug therapy and impact of ethnocultural and racial factors on pharmacokinetics (ethnopharmacology)
- Deficient knowledge related to lack of experience with and information about drug therapy

▰ Planning
▰ Goals

- Patient will state the need for assistance while in the hospital or while health status is altered.
- Patient will request assistance in implementing ethnocultural practices.

- Patient will state specific needs related to performance of activities of daily living (ADLs), relaxation, healing, sleep, or rest.
- Patient will state the importance of racial and ethnocultural influences on nonpharmacological and pharmacological treatment regimens.

Outcome Criteria

- Patient experiences minimal or no difficulty in obtaining assistance with special needs and ADLs.
- Patient identifies specific ethnocultural practices such as use of herbal teas and other herbal preparations, yin and yang balancing, aromatherapy, crystal therapy, and healing bracelets that will help with healing during illness.
- Patient implements ethnocultural practices as an integral part of a holistic collaborative plan of care and treatment regimen.

Implementation

There are numerous interventions for implementation of ethnoculturally competent nursing care, but one important requirement is that the nurse remain current in the knowledge of ethnocultures and related ADL practices, health beliefs, and emotional and spiritual health practices and beliefs. The nurse's knowledge about drugs that may elicit varied responses in specific racial and ethnic groups must remain current, and critical thinking must be used in applying the concepts of ethnoculturally competent care and ethnopharmacology to each patient care situation. For example, one group of enzymes, cytochrome P450, or CYP, enzymes, are responsible for certain phases of the metabolism of many drugs, including antipsychotics and antidepressants. Genetic differences in certain CYP enzymes affect the rate of drug metabolism and thus influence drug levels and dosages. People with more than two functioning copies of *CYP2D6* genes have faster than normal enzyme activity and are quick metabolizers and will thus have lower serum drug concentrations; those with two nonfunctional copies of *CYP2D6* genes have slower enzyme activity and are slow metabolizers, thus attaining higher serum concentrations of certain drugs. Consequently, these genetic differences will affect specific treatment of individuals from different groups. Hispanic patients may be treated effectively using lower dosages of antipsychotics than usual. Black patients taking lithium need closer monitoring for toxicity, and Japanese and Taiwanese patients may also require lower dosages of lithium. In treatment for hypertension, Black patients have been found to respond less favourably to some angiotensin-converting enzyme inhibitors, such as captopril, than do Whites. Thiazide diuretics have been found to be more effective in Black patients than in White patients. Additional factors to consider during implementation are lifestyle and health belief systems. For example, with regard to adherence to the treatment regimen, Hispanic patients with hypertension have been found in some studies to be less likely than Black or White patients to continue to take medication as prescribed, a finding that may reflect the patients' health belief systems. Other lifestyle decisions (e.g., use of tobacco or alcohol) may also affect responses to drugs and must be considered during drug administration.

Evaluation

The impact of ethnocultural, legal, and ethical factors on the therapeutic effects of drug therapy should be evaluated for the duration of therapy. Evaluation should also include monitoring of goals and outcome criteria as well as therapeutic versus adverse effects and toxic effects.

POINTS TO REMEMBER

- ❖ Federal legislation, provincial law, provincial nursing practice acts, and institutional policies have been established to ensure the safety and efficacy of drug therapy and the nursing process.
- ❖ The Food and Drugs Act and the Controlled Drugs and Substances Act provide nurses and other health care providers with information on drugs that cause little to no dependence as well as those with a high level of misuse and dependency.
- ❖ Informed consent should always be obtained as needed and nurses must thoroughly understand their responsibilities as patient advocates in obtaining such consent.
- ❖ A nurse's role in the IND process should be one of adhering to the research protocol while also acting as a patient advocate and honouring the patient's right to safe, ethical nursing care.

- ❖ The "rights" of medication administration include the right drug, dose, time, route, patient, reason, and documentation. There are other rights to consider, such as the right to a "system analysis" (see Chapter 1), the right to proper functioning of equipment for administration of specific medications (i.e., intravenous [IV] pump, patient-controlled analgesia [PCA]), and the right to know about the medications for safe and efficient use.
- ❖ Adherence to legal guidelines, ethical principles, and the CNA *Code of Ethics for Registered Nurses* ensures that the nurse's actions are based on a solid foundation.
- ❖ There are a variety of ethnoculturally based assessment tools available for use in patient care and drug therapy.
- ❖ In relation to racial and ethnic variables, drug therapy and subsequent patient responses may be affected by specific enzymes and metabolic pathways of drugs.

EXAMINATION REVIEW QUESTIONS

1 During a home visit, an older adult woman tells the home care nurse that she has been taking six or more acetylsalicylic acid tablets per day for her "bad bones." The nurse continues with a thorough assessment and makes the decision to double the prescribed dose to help minimize this patient's "bad bones." Which of the following statements correctly describes this scenario?
   a. The "right" to the right dosage of drug is being violated in this situation.
   b. The nurse should make her own decision to change the specific dosage of the drug.
   c. The nurse is following one of the "Ten Rights" of drug administration—specifically the right to fairly safe standards of care.
   d. The nurse is planning to give medications within the guidelines of professional autonomy, such as deciding on a dosage not ordered.

2 Which of the following ethnocultural beliefs would most likely influence health care for a 59-year-old female Chinese patient?
   a. X-rays are seen as a break in the soul's integrity.
   b. Hospital diets are interpreted as being healing and healthful.
   c. The use of heat may be an important practice for this patient.
   d. Being hospitalized is a source of peace and socialization for this ethnoculture.

3 A patient is being counselled for possible participation in a clinical trial for a new medication. After meeting with the physician, the nurse is asked to obtain the patient's signature on the consent forms. Which of the following does this "informed consent" indicate?
   a. Once therapy has begun, the patient cannot withdraw from the clinical trial.
   b. The patient has been informed of all potential hazards and benefits of the therapy.
   c. No matter what happens, the patient will not be able to sue the researchers for damages.
   d. The patient has received only the information that will help to make the clinical trial a success.

4 A new drug has been approved for use and the drug manufacturer has made it available for sale. During the first 6 months, Health Canada receives reports of severe adverse effects that were not discovered during the testing and considers whether to withdraw the drug. Which phase of investigational drug studies does this illustrate?
   a. Phase 1
   b. Phase 2
   c. Phase 3
   d. Phase 4

5 A Japanese patient describes a family trait that manifests frequently: she says that members of her family often have "strong reactions" after taking certain medications, but her White friends have no problems with the same dosages of the same medications. Because of this trait, which of the following statement applies?
   a. She may need lower dosages of the medications prescribed.
   b. She may need higher dosages of the medications prescribed.
   c. She should not receive these medications because of potential problems with metabolism.
   d. These situations vary greatly, and her accounts may not indicate a valid cause for concern.

For answers see http://evolve.elsevier.com/Canada/Lilley/pharmacology/.

CRITICAL THINKING ACTIVITIES

1 Discuss the impact of ethnocultural practices as they relate to safe and effective drug therapy.

2 Choose at least two of the terms in Legal and Ethical Principles: Common Legal and Ethics-Related Terms on page 67 and apply the concepts to an example of drug administration and nursing.

3 Interview someone who is not in your racial or ethnic group about their ethnocultural practices and drug therapy. Compare their family practices with those of your family.

For answers see http://evolve.elsevier.com/Canada/Lilley/pharmacology/.

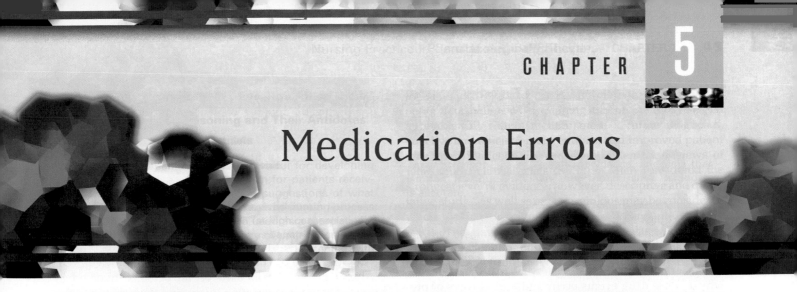

CHAPTER 5

Medication Errors

Learning Objectives

After reading this chapter, the successful student will be able to do the following:

1 Differentiate between the following terms related to drug therapy in the context of professional nursing practice: adverse drug event, adverse drug reaction, medication error, and the new term, medication reconciliation.

2 Discuss the importance of the Safer Healthcare Now! campaign to drug therapy.

3 Describe the medication errors that are most common to nurses and other health care providers.

4 Develop a framework for professional nursing practice that includes specific measures to prevent medication errors in patients of all ages.

5 Identify the possible consequences of a medical error on a patient's physiological and psychological well-being.

6 Discuss the impact of medication errors in patients of different ages.

7 Discuss the impact of medication errors in relation to the nursing process.

8 Discuss the role of advocacy for political action related to drug therapy and the prevention of medication errors.

e-Learning Activities

Web site
(http://evolve.elsevier.com/Canada/
Lilley/pharmacology/)

- Animations
- Answers to chapter questions, activities, and case studies
- Calculators and Category Catchers
- Glossary with audio pronunciations
- IV Therapy and Medication Error Checklists
- Multiple-Choice Review Question quizzes
- Nursing Care Plans
- Online Appendices and Supplements
- WebLinks

Glossary

Adverse drug event (ADE) Any undesirable occurrence related to administration of or failure to administer a prescribed medication. (p. 74)

Adverse drug reaction (ADR) Any unexpected, unintended, undesired, or excessive response to medication given at therapeutic dosages (as opposed to overdose); one type of ADE. (p. 74)

Adverse effects Any undesirable bodily effects that are a direct response to one or more drugs. (p. 74)

Allergic reaction An immunological hypersensitivity reaction resulting from an unusual sensitivity of a patient to a particular medication. (p. 74)

Idiosyncratic reaction An abnormal and unexpected response to a medication, other than an allergic reaction, that is peculiar to an individual patient. (p. 74)

Medical error Broad term commonly used to refer to any error in any phase of clinical patient care that causes or has the potential to cause patient harm. (p. 74)

Medication error (ME) Any *preventable* ADE involving inappropriate medication use by a patient or health care provider. (p. 74)

Medication reconciliation A procedure implemented by health care providers to continually maintain an accurate and up-to-date list of medications for all patients at every phase of health care that is communicated in a timely manner to all applicable members of the health care team, with the overall goal of dramatically reducing the number of medication errors. (p. 81)

Safer Healthcare Now! A collaborative effort aimed at reducing the number of injuries and deaths related to adverse events, a key strategy of which is the implementation of medication reconciliation (MedRec) in institutions across Canada. (p. 81)

OVERVIEW

In 2004, The World Health Organization launched the World Alliance for Patient Safety to learn more about why adverse drug events occur and to find ways of preventing them. According to a landmark study of adverse events in Canadian hospitals, between 9000 and 24,000 patients die each year because of adverse events or errors. Another Canadian study found that adverse drug–related events are responsible for 12% of emergency department visits. Of these, 68% were considered preventable.

Although **medical error** is often used as an umbrella term in the published literature, errors can occur during all phases of health care delivery and involve errant actions by all categories of health professionals. Some of the more common types of errors are incorrect actions related to medication errors, medical- or surgical-procedure errors such as misdiagnosis or wrong-site surgery, patient misidentification errors, and patient-monitoring errors (errors of commission), or the error may involve failure to implement an intervention when it would normally be indicated (error of omission). Intangible losses resulting from such adverse outcomes include dissatisfaction with and loss of trust in the health care system. This chapter focuses on the issues related to medication errors and ways to prevent and respond to these errors. Included is an overview of institutional, educational, and sociological issues that may contribute to such errors.

MEDICATION ERRORS

As discussed in Chapter 2, **adverse drug event (ADE)** is a general term that includes *all* types of clinical problems encountered regarding medications. These include **medication errors (MEs)** and **adverse drug reactions (ADRs).** Such errors may or may not cause the patient harm. The subsets of ADEs and their interrelationships are illustrated in Figure 5-1. Two major types of ADR are **allergic reaction** (often predictable) and **idiosyncratic reaction** (usually unpredictable). An **adverse effect** is a direct response to one or more drugs that results in an undesirable effect. These effects are generally considered to be relatively minor but are expected to occur in a percentage of the population receiving a given drug. The severity of effects varies, appearing on a continuum. More severe adverse effects may result in changes in prescribed drug therapy after weighing the risk-to-benefit ratio of a drug in a specific clinical situation.

It is important to consider the processes of medication administration and system analysis when discussing MEs. In order to identify, respond to, and ultimately prevent MEs, more than just use of the Ten Rights of drug administration or consideration of the nurse is required. Attention must be focused on all persons involved in medication administration, including the prescriber, the transcriber of the order to the chart, nurses, pharmacy staff, and any other ancillary staff taking part in this process. A system analysis takes the rights one step further and examines the entire health care system, the health care providers involved, and any other factor that has an impact on the error.

MEs are a particularly important segment of ADEs because, by definition, any error is potentially preventable. MEs are a common cause of adverse health care outcomes and can range in severity from having no significant effect on the patient to directly causing patient disability or death. Children and the older adult are particularly vulnerable. U.S. figures estimate MEs as the eighth leading cause of death. Approximately five MEs occur for every 100 medication administrations, and an estimated 30% of patients with drug-related injuries are disabled for more than 6 months or die as a result of the ME. According to The Institute for Safe Medication Practices Canada (ISMP Canada), it is estimated that 39% of MEs occur during prescribing, 12% occur during transcription, 11% occur during dispensing, and 38% occur during administration. MEs can occur with any type of drug, but certain classifications of medications are associated with a higher likelihood of adverse outcomes because of pharmacological properties or narrow therapeutic indices or simply because of the frequency of prescribing. Chemotherapeutic agents,

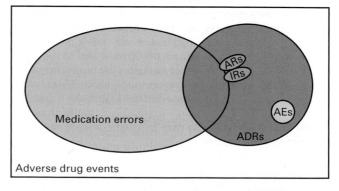

FIG. 5-1 Diagram illustrating the classes and subclasses of adverse drug events. *ADRs,* adverse drug reactions; *AEs,* adverse effects; *ARs,* allergic reactions; *IRs,* idiosyncratic reactions.

central nervous system drugs, antibiotics, and vaccines are the top causative drugs for drug-induced disability. The ISMP Canada independently reviews voluntary reports of MEs and regularly composes a list (see Box 5-1) of "high-alert" medications, a small number of drugs that have a high risk of causing injury if misused. The errors from misuse of these drugs may or may not be more common than with other drugs, but the consequences of these errors are devastating. Many of these errors result from the fact that the number of drugs on the market is increasing, thus there are more drug names to keep track of, some of which have similarities in spelling, pronunciation, or both (i.e., look-alike or sound-alike names). The most dangerous situation is when two drugs from different therapeutic classes have similar names. Inadvertent use of a similar-sounding but wrong drug can result in effects on the patient that are grossly different from those intended as part of the prescribed drug therapy. Table 5-1 lists examples of commonly confused drug names.

It is widely recognized that the majority of MEs result from weaknesses in the systems within health care organizations rather than from individual shortcomings. Such weaknesses include failure to create a "just culture" or nonpunitive work atmosphere for reporting errors, excessive workload with minimal time for preventive education for staff, and lack of interdisciplinary communication and collaboration.

Nursing Measures to Prevent Medication Errors

The first step toward preventing errors is to assess and document information about drug allergies. Nurses may reduce the likelihood of MEs by also taking the following precautions:

- Minimize the use of verbal and telephone orders. If such an order must be taken, repeat the order to confirm with prescriber, spelling the drug name aloud and speaking slowly and clearly.
- List the indication (reason for use) next to each drug order on the medication administration record, patient materials, and any other educational materials.
- Avoid the use of abbreviations, medical shorthand, and acronyms because they can lead to confusion, miscommunication, and risk for error (see Legal and Ethical Principles: Use of Abbreviations, Symbols and Dose Designations).
- Never assume anything about a drug order or prescription, including medication route.
- If questioning a medication order for any reason (e.g., dose, drug, indication), do not assume that the prescriber is correct. Resist any fear of challenging prescriber authority when in doubt or when the situation clearly warrants such action. Prescribers may and often do make errors. Remember your important role as patient advocate and seek support from colleagues and superiors wherever available and whenever appropriate.

BOX 5-1

Some Common High-Alert Medications Involved in Serious Errors

Intravenous (IV) adrenergic agonists and antagonists
IV calcium
Chemotherapeutic drugs
Chloral hydrate and midazolam syrups in children
IV digoxin
IV heparin and oral warfarin
Insulin
Lidocaine and local anesthetics in large vials
IV magnesium sulfate
Neuromuscular blocking agents
Opiates
IV potassium (phosphate and chloride)
Sodium chloride injection in greater than 0.9% concentration
Thrombolytics

Source: Institute for Safe Medication Practices (2008). *ISMP's list of high-alert medications*. Retrieved June 25, 2009, from http://www.ismp.org/tools/highalertmedications.pdf

---

- Do not try to decipher illegibly written orders. Instead, contact the prescriber for clarification. Illegible orders fall below applicable standards for quality medical care and can endanger patient well-being.
- If in doubt about the correctness of a legibly written order, always double-check with the prescriber, pharmacist, or other acceptable authoritative resource.
- Check the medication order and what is available, while using the Ten Rights of medication administration.
- *Never* use trailing zeros (e.g., 1.0 mg). Use of trailing zeros is associated with increased occurrence of overdose. For example, "1.0 mg warfarin sodium" could be misread as "10 mg warfarin," a 10-fold dose increase. Instead, use "1 mg."
- *Do* use a leading zero for decimal dosages (e.g., 0.25 mg). Failure to use leading zeros can also lead to overdose. For example, ".25 mg digoxin" could be misread as "25 mg digoxin," a potentially lethal dose that is 100 times the dose ordered. Instead, write "0.25 mg."
- The numeral 7 can be confused with the numeral 1. Always write a numeral 7 with a line through the middle (7̶).

Other measures to prevent MEs include the following:

- *Carefully* read all labels for accuracy, expiration dates, and dilution requirements.
- Be familiar with new techniques of administration and new equipment (e.g., use of Diskus inhaled dosage forms or transdermal or transbuccal forms of drugs).
- Encourage the use of both trade names and generic names in drug orders and prescriptions and include

TABLE 5-1

Selected Examples of Commonly Confused Generic Drug Names

Drug Products	Recommended Revision, Comments
Accupril vs. Monopril	Two different antihypertensive drugs (although both are ACE inhibitors)
Avandia vs. Amaryl	Two different antidiabetic drugs
Cardura vs. Coumadin	Antihypertensive vs. anticoagulant
chlorpropamide vs. chlorpromazine	Oral antidiabetic vs. antipsychotic
chlorpromazine vs. prochlorperazine	Antipsychotic drug vs. antiemetic drug
Claritin-D 24-Hour vs. Claritin-D	24-hr vs. 12-hr duration of action
clomiphene vs. clomipramine	Estrogen agonist–antagonist vs. norepinephrine reuptake inhibitor.
Cytovene vs. Cytosar	Antiviral drug vs. antineoplastic (anticancer) drug
daunorubicin vs. doxorubicin	Two different antineoplastic drugs with possibly different indications for use
Depo-Estradiol vs. Depo-Testadiol	Female vs. male hormonal injection
dopamine vs. dobutamine	β-1-adrenergic agonists
Elavil vs. Plavix	Antidepressant vs. antiplatelet agent
Epivir vs. Combivir	Single-drug anti-HIV agent vs. double-drug combination anti-HIV agent
fentanyl vs. sufentanil	Both are injectable anesthetics but with a significant difference in potency and duration of action
glipizide vs. glyburide	Two different antidiabetic agents
Lacrilube vs. Surgilube	Ophthalmic lubricant vs. skin or orifice lubricant
Micronase vs. Micro-K	Antidiabetic agent vs. potassium supplement
Narcan vs. Norcuron	Opiate antidote vs. skeletal muscle paralyzing agent for operating room use
Ocuflox vs. Ocufen	Ophthalmic antibiotic vs. ophthalmic anti-inflammatory agent
paclitaxel vs. Paxil	Antineoplastic agent vs. antidepressant
Paxil vs. Plavix	Antidepressant vs. antiplatelet agent
quinine vs. quinidine	Antimalarial agent vs. cardiac antidysrhythmic agent
Reminyl vs. Amaryl	Cholinesterase inhibitor for mild to moderate Alzheimer's disease vs. antidiabetic agent for type 2 diabetes
Soma Compound vs. Soma	Combination muscle relaxant with acetylsalicylic acid vs. muscle relaxant alone
Tamiflu vs. Theraflu	Prescription antiviral agent vs. nonprescription (OTC) cold remedy
Tegretol vs. Toradol	Anticonvulsant vs. anti-inflammatory agent
TobraDex vs. Tobrex	Combination ophthalmic antibiotic and anti-inflammatory agent vs. ophthalmic antibiotic alone
Vancenase vs. Vanceril	Nasal steroid inhaler vs. oral steroid inhaler
Viagra vs. Allegra	Male sexual stimulant vs. antihistamine allergy drug
Xanax vs. Zantac	Antianxiety agent vs. anti–stomach acid agent
Zocor vs. Cozaar vs. Zoloft	Anticholesterol agent vs. antihypertensive agent vs. antidepressant
Zofran vs. Zyban	Antiemetic agent vs. smoking cessation aid

LEGAL & ETHICAL PRINCIPLES

Use of Abbreviations, Symbols, and Dose Designations

Medication errors often occur as a result of misinterpretation of abbreviations, symbols, and dose designations. The Institute for Safe Medication Practices Canada (ISMP Canada), Accreditation Canada, and the Canadian Patient Safety Institute support the elimination of dangerous abbreviations, symbols, and dose designations in health care to enhance the safety of Canadian patients and recommend that abbreviations be written out *in full*. As part of Accreditation Canada Required Organizational Practices, organizations are required to identify and implement a list of abbreviations, dose designations, and symbols

that are not to be used in the organization. This list is inclusive of the following Institute for Safe Medication Practices Canada "Do Not Use" chart on page 77.

Note: In Canada, the trend is now toward using "mcg" in practice, so it is important to note the difference between "mcg" and "mg" in orders.

Source: Adapted from Institute for Safe Medication Practices (2006). *List of error-prone abbreviations, symbols, and dose designations.* Retrieved June 26, 2009, from http://www.ismp.org/tools/errorproneabbreviations.pdf. Used with permission from ISMP Canada.

DO NOT USE

DANGEROUS ABBREVIATIONS, SYMBOLS AND DOSE DESIGNATIONS

The abbreviations, symbols, and dose designations found in this table have been reported as being frequently misinterpreted and involved in harmful medication errors. They should NEVER be used when communicating medication information.

Abbreviation	Intended Meaning	Problem	Correction
U	unit	Mistaken for "0" (zero), "4" (four), or cc.	Use "unit".
IU	international unit	Mistaken for "IV" (intravenous) or "10" (ten).	Use "unit".
Abbreviations for drug names		Misinterpreted because of similar abbreviations for multiple drugs; e.g., MS, MSO_4 (morphine sulphate), $MgSO_4$ (magnesium sulphate) may be confused for one another.	Do not abbreviate drug names.
QD QOD	Every day Every other day	QD and QOD have been mistaken for each other, or as 'qid'. The Q has also been misinterpreted as "2" (two).	Use "daily" and "every other day".
OD	Every day	Mistaken for "right eye" (OD = oculus dexter).	Use "daily".
OS, OD, OU	Left eye, right eye, both eyes	May be confused with one another.	Use "left eye", "right eye" or "both eyes".
D/C	Discharge	Interpreted as "discontinue whatever medications follow" (typically discharge medications).	Use "discharge".
cc	cubic centimetre	Mistaken for "u" (units).	Use "mL" or "millilitre".
µg	microgram	Mistaken for "mg" (milligram) resulting in one thousand-fold overdose.	Use "mcg".
Symbol	**Intended Meaning**	**Potential Problem**	**Correction**
@	at	Mistaken for "2" (two) or "5" (five).	Use "at".
> <	Greater than Less than	Mistaken for "7"(seven) or the letter "L". Confused with each other.	Use "greater than"/"more than" or "less than"/"lower than".
Dose Designation	**Intended Meaning**	**Potential Problem**	**Correction**
Trailing zero	X.0 mg	Decimal point is overlooked resulting in 10-fold dose error.	Never use a zero by itself after a decimal point. Use "X **mg**".
Lack of leading zero	. X mg	Decimal point is overlooked resulting in 10-fold dose error.	Always use a zero before a decimal point. Use "0.X mg".

Adapted from ISMP's List of Error-Prone Abbreviations, Symbols, and Dose Designations 2006

Report actual and potential medication errors to ISMP Canada via the web at https://www.ismp-canada.org/err_report.htm or by calling 1-866-54-ISMPC. ISMP Canada guarantees confidentiality of information received and respects the reporter's wishes as to the level of detail included in publications.

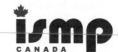

Institute for Safe Medication
Practices Canada
Institut pour l'utilisation sécuritaire
des médicaments du Canada

the purpose whenever posssible. Relying too heavily on trade names especially increases the likelihood of MEs because many trade names sound alike and have similar spellings and syllabic structure.

- Listen to and honour any concerns expressed by patients. Should the patient state that he or she is allergic to a medication, that a pill has already been taken, or that the medication is not what the patient usually takes, stop, listen, and investigate. Remain alert, in good health, and educated and never be too busy to stop, learn, and inquire.
- If working conditions are a problem, join organizations with other nurses to advocate for improved working conditions (see Political Action section on p. 83) and to stand up for nurses' and patients' rights.
- Always double-check a medication's product labelling; often there are different formulations of the same active ingredient.
- Remember that generic names are preferred.
- Never crush, open, or allow the patient to chew extended-released or long-release dosage forms.
- Safeguard any medications that the patient had on admission or transfer so that additional doses are not given. In such situations, safeguarding is accomplished by compiling a current medication history and resolving any discrepancies rather than ignoring them.

There are other significant interventions that may help to decrease the risk of MEs. The following measures address aspects of the system in order to prevent errors:

- Always verify new medication administration records if they have been rewritten or re-entered for any reason. Make sure that all nurses and staff are alerted to carry out this process.
- Always compare the pharmacy label against the initial medication administration record before giving the first dose.
- Use computerized prescriber order entry and have that order entry system integrated with the computer in the pharmacy, because this can help eliminate the need for yet another person (pharmacist, technician, etc.) to enter an order. Fewer entries mean fewer errors!
- Provide for mandatory entry of the weight of every patient into the medication administration record before the first medication order goes to the pharmacy; this practice can help reduce dosage errors.
- Institute mandatory recalculation of every drug dosage for patients taking high-risk drugs, for children, and for the older adult and in any other situation in which there is a narrow margin between therapeutic serum drug levels and toxic levels (e.g., administration of chemotherapeutic drugs or digitalis drugs, or presence of altered liver or kidney function in an older adult or any other patient).
- Always suspect an error whenever an adult dosage form is dispensed for a child (see Evidence-Informed Practice).
- Be sure to provide a translator for patients who speak a language other than English.

- Use simple, sans serif fonts and a font size appropriate to reading distance and lighting levels to substantially improve the readability of labels.
- Use "tall-man lettering" (i.e., combinations of uppercase and lowercase letters, rather than all uppercase or all lowercase lettering) as an effective strategy of differentiating look-alike drug names. Tall-man lettering creates a mental alert by changing the shape of words that look similar when seen in uppercase letters only. One example of tall-man lettering is VINCRISTINE VinCRIStine; VINBLASTINE VinBLAStine.

PSYCHOSOCIAL FACTORS THAT CONTRIBUTE TO ERRORS

Organizational Factors

Increasingly, the literature is directing attention away from the nurse, who is often the primary focus of MEs, toward a broader context. Studies suggest that systemic organizational factors contribute to MEs. Such factors include "nurse staffing adequacy, hours worked per week, overtime, staffing mix (professional versus unregulated) and other factors reflecting how the work system is designed" (Wilkins & Shields, 2008, p. 2).

The 2005 National Survey of the Work and Health of Nurses (NSWHN) examined 19,000 Canadian nurses' perceptions of patient safety, specifically the frequency of ME, and work organization and workplace conditions. The researchers found numerous factors related to ME in Canadian hospitals, including working overtime, feeling overloaded, perceiving that staffing or resources are inadequate, poor relations with physicians, unsupportive co-workers, and low job security (Shields & Wilkins, 2006).

One half of all preventable ADRs begin at the medication ordering (prescribing) stage. A study published in the *Archives of Internal Medicine* also stated that prescribers are involved in "most" errors (LaPointe & Jollis, 2003). This particular study focused on cardiovascular medications, the most commonly used general category of prescription drugs. It concluded that the presence of a pharmacist during medical rounds reduced the incidence of errors. This finding illustrates an important issue in modern health care practice: both nurses and pharmacists have a vested interest in rational drug therapy, yet normally, neither acts independently in health care delivery. This points to the value of developing collaborative relationships between these two groups of professionals and between these groups and all other health care providers in the health care system. Such relationships can be especially helpful when approaching prescribers regarding questionable orders or when advocating for workplace improvements that benefit both patients and staff.

Effective use of technologies such as computerized prescriber order entry and bar coding of medication packages has also been shown to reduce MEs. Computerized order entry eliminates handwriting and standardizes many prescribing functions, especially dosage

EVIDENCE-INFORMED PRACTICE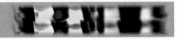

Factors Associated with Preventable Medication Errors

Review

The purpose of this study was to evaluate the steps involved in preparing an intravenous morphine infusion to determine the circumstances associated with preventable medication errors. The study took place at the Hospital for Sick Children in Toronto, Ontario.

Type of Evidence

This was a direct observational study conducted in a structured, nonclinical environment. The participants were 118 health care professionals, with the majority being registered nurses. Participants were either self-selected or approached informally.

Participants completed a survey describing their individual characteristics; a registered nurse then "read the instructions aloud for the infusion-preparation tasks and for preparation of the morphine infusions." Participants performed a variety of tasks associated with preparing an intravenous drug infusion, such as drug-volume calculations, rounding calculations, and syringe-volume measurements, as well as preparing morphine infusions. Calculators were available to the participants.

Results of Study

A medication error was determined if a participant's response or prepared morphine infusion was outside pharmaceutical standards. Errors were found in 1.5% to 4.9% of the infusion-preparation tasks and in 34.7% of the prepared infusions. The researchers identified four factors that were positively associated with the occurrence of a concentration error: fewer infusions prepared in the previous week, increased number of years of professional experience, the use of the more concentrated stock solution, and the preparation of smaller dose volumes. A reduction in the hours of sleep in the previous 24 hours, the use of more concentrated solutions, and smaller doses were identified as factors that negatively influenced error occurrence.

Link of Evidence to Nursing Practice

Although the researchers suggest that this study has limited generalization, there are several significant observations. They found that clinical expertise and years of experience did not ensure fewer errors; in fact, the opposite was true. Fatigue played a significant role in making errors. However, the main factor that resulted in errors was the use of the more concentrated stock solution to prepare smaller (pediatric) doses. These findings increase the awareness of factors that need to be considered in medication-preparation practices and the creation of strategies to reduce errors.

Source: Based on Parshuram, C. S., To, T., Seto, W., Trope, A., Koren, G., & Laupacis, A. (2008). Systematic evaluation of errors occurring during the preparation of intravenous medication. *Canadian Medical Association Journal, 178*(1), 42–48.

specifications. With bar coding of medications, nurses can use electronic devices for verification of correct medication at the patient's bedside. Error reporting systems that offer the option of anonymity can also improve practice safety. Internal, facility-based systems of error tracking may generate data to help customize policy and procedure development. Computer programs are often used in the pharmacy to screen for potential drug interactions when prescriber orders are being entered into the patient's computer profile. As noted previously, however, the workload at many institutions may prevent adequate staff education on the use of such technology. Also, technology that is difficult to use may itself present a barrier to medication safety. This often happens when patient care staff has insufficient input into the design of patient care–related technology. Interestingly, self-medication by patients (e.g., patient-controlled analgesia) has been shown to reduce errors, provided patients have adequate cognitive ability and mental alertness.

Educational-System Factors

Because of the rigorous cognitive and even physical challenges of health care study and practice, the health professions tend to attract strong-willed, intelligent people. However, the constant expectation that one be "smart" and "on top of things" with regard to clinical knowledge often leads to denial, fear, or shame about being wrong or simply not remembering a piece of information. Instead of making guesses in clinical situations about medications, nurses need to stop and check the order and be sure they have a thorough knowledge about the drug and its route, dosage, and indications *before* administering the drug. Authoritative sources for finding information about drugs include current (less than 5 years old) drug reference guides such as *Mosby's Drug Consult for Health Professionals*, the *Compendium of Pharmaceuticals and Specialties (CPS)*, and others written by experts. Even the most capable health care provider cannot know everything or have immediate recall of every fact ever read. This is especially true given the increasing complexity of health care practice. Forward-thinking faculty members recognize that learning is a lifelong process. Adopting a philosophy of "no question is a stupid question" helps clinical instructors teach error prevention habits to their students as they begin their careers. In contrast, berating or otherwise penalizing a student for not immediately recalling a given fact or for simply asking questions instills fear and shame. It also discourages dialogue that would otherwise promote and enhance student learning and mastery of concepts. In general, it is important to endorse routine competency evaluation of professional registered nurses and their knowledge of drugs and measures to reduce MEs. The level of nurses' knowledge and understanding of drugs must be boosted to ensure safety and prevent harm to patients.

Medication Errors and Related Sociological Factors

Health care practice has a long and ingrained tradition of disparate social and economic class structures among different categories of professionals. The most recognized differences are those among nurses, physicians, and administrators. At their worst, these differences have fostered maltreatment of nurses, especially by physicians, whose inappropriate behaviour has often not been challenged or corrected by administrators. A 2005 study, published in the *American Journal of Nursing* (Rosenstein & O'Daniel), assessed nurses' perceptions of the effects of disruptive behaviour on relationships between disciplines and on patient care. *Disruptive behaviour* is defined in this study as "any inappropriate behaviour, ranging from rudeness, intimidating manner, shouting, to physical or sexual harassment" (p. 55). This survey revealed a significant level of disruptive behaviour among nurses as well as among physicians, suggesting a sobering problem within and across disciplines. The respondents reported that disruptive behaviour contributed to stress, frustration, and lack of concentration and undermined team collaboration, information transfer, communication, and nurse–physician relationships. This type of behaviour, when not met with corrective action by the institution, is felt to contribute strongly to nursing shortages in health care facilities. Thirty percent of surveyed nurses stated that they knew of one or more colleagues who had resigned their position because of this problem. With regard to possible impact on MEs, this study pointed out that the quality of nurse–physician communication was one of the strongest predictors of patient outcomes. Fortunately, communication between prescribers and other members of the health care team has improved somewhat over the years with newer generations of physicians. This change has come about in large part because of more progressive approaches in medical education that emphasize a team orientation, which is recognized as more realistic given the ever-increasing complexities of health care delivery and the undeniable fact that no one team member can master every fact and skill.

PREVENTING AND RESPONDING TO ERRORS

Reporting and Responding to Medication Errors

The reporting of MEs is a professional responsibility shared by nurses and all members of the health care team. Steps for the nurse to take to prevent and respond to MEs include the following:

- Check the patient by assessing all relevant parameters (e.g., vital signs, latest laboratory values) and document accordingly.
- Assess the patient for effects of the drug, and consult reference materials or colleagues as needed.
- Perform medication reconciliation to verify all of the patient's correct medications at each point of care (e.g., transfer from critical care unit to general nursing unit), and prepare a complete list of medications for the next health care provider upon patient discharge.
- Take a "time-out" when appropriate for all staff to collectively verify medications, especially during high-risk procedures.
- Regularly ask the patient for identity verification and date of birth.
- Check the patient's identification bracelet and cross-reference with the medication administration record.
- Complete ME reporting forms after contacting the physician, charge nurse, nurse supervisor, or, for a student nurse, the patient's nurse and the instructor.
- Monitor the progress of the patient's condition closely.
- Think and act critically and modify nursing practice to prevent further errors.
- Conduct detailed root-cause analyses to learn from errors and avoid repeating an error.
- Coordinate and participate in educational sessions to discuss errors and strategies for their prevention.
- Analyze methods to reduce the complexity of drug administration and develop consistent, easy-to-read procedures related to medication administration.
- Suggest needed changes in policy and procedures related to safe medication administration and the provision of simple ME-related policies.
- Participate in the development of user-friendly technology such as computerized prescriber order entry systems and systems for bar coding of medications that enable nurses to verify medications at bedside before administering them.
- Encourage the reporting of "near-misses" to identify areas for improvement before an incident occurs.
- Focus efforts on specific high-alert drugs and error-prone situations.
- Join political efforts to advocate for safer nurse–patient staffing ratios and for improved quality assurance protocols in the handling of MEs.
- Support a change in culture in organizations from a suppressive and closed error-reporting culture to a more open and nonpunitive culture.

Error reporting systems that offer the option of anonymity can also help to foster improved practice safety. Internal, facility-based systems of error tracking may generate data to help customize policy and procedure development. All institutional pharmacy departments are required to have an ADE monitoring program. Nurses should be aware of and be comfortable with reporting suspected ADEs to this department for evaluation and follow-up. In addition, there are nationwide confidential reporting programs that collect and disseminate safety information on a larger scale. One such program is the Canadian Medication Incident Reporting and Prevention System, which collects incident reports of MEs. The Canada Vigilance Program (formerly the Canadian Adverse Drug Reaction Monitoring Program) is Health Canada's postmarket surveillance program that collects and assesses reports of suspected adverse reactions to health products marketed in Canada. The Health Canada Web site is a valuable source of adverse reaction information (Table 5-2). Anyone, a health care provider or consumer, can report an adverse reaction online or by telephone, or receive Health Canada's MedEffect e-Notice to obtain the *Canadian Adverse Reaction Newsletter* and health product advisories free by e-mail (http://www.healthcanada.gc.ca/medeffect). The ISMP-Canada, Safer Heathcare Now!, and Accreditation Canada also provide useful information to health care providers aimed at safety enhancement. See the Evolve Web site (http://evolve.elsevier.com/Canada/Lilley/pharmacology/) for addresses of these and other helpful organizations (see Table 5-2).

Medication Reconciliation

Drug and fluid-related events are the second most common type of adverse events (Baker et al., 2004). Forster et al. (2004) found that 23% of hospitalized patients discharged from an internal medicine service experienced an adverse event. Of the 23%, 72% were adverse events. Cornish et al. (2005) found that 53.6% had at least one unintended discrepancy, of which 38.6% had the potential to cause moderate to severe discomfort or clinical deterioration. Of these discrepancies, 46.4% occurred because of the omission of a regularly used drug. Most errors happen at the interface of care.

In 2005, the **Safer Healthcare Now!** campaign (http://www.saferhealthcarenow.ca/) was launched. Similar to its U.S. model, the Institute for Healthcare Improvement's 100,000 Lives campaign, the primary focus of the Safer Healthcare Now! campaign is the implementation of 10 targeted interventions to improve patient care. It is a collaborative effort aimed at reducing the number of injuries and deaths related to adverse events. Accreditation Canada's (http://www.cchsa.ca/) implementation

of the Safer Healthcare Now! campaign in 2008 has made a good patient safety record a requirement of accreditation for all health care facilities. This campaign promotes specific strategies through which health care facilities can dramatically improve their patient safety records. One of these strategies focuses on preventing MEs through medication reconciliation (called Med Rec). **Medication reconciliation** is a procedure with the aim of preventing MEs through ongoing assessment and updating of every patient's list of medications throughout the health care process and the timely communication of such information to both patients and their health care providers. This procedure involves three steps (additional information can be found on either of the Web sites mentioned previously):

1 Verification: Collection of the most complete or best possible medication history of all medications currently used by the patient (including prescription drugs as well as over-the-counter medications and supplements)
2 Clarification: Professional review of this information to ensure that all medications and dosages are appropriate for the patient
3 Reconciliation: Further investigation of any discrepancies and documentation of relevant communications and changes in medication orders

To ensure ongoing accuracy of medication use, the steps listed should be repeated at each stage of health care delivery (see Figure 5-2):

a Admission
b Status change (e.g., from critical to stable)
c Patient transfer within or between facilities or health care provider teams
d Discharge (the latest medication list should be provided to the patient to take to the next health care provider or this information should be otherwise forwarded to the provider; applicable confidentiality guidelines should be followed)

Some applicable assessment and education tips regarding medication reconciliation are the following:

1 Ask the patient open-ended questions and gradually progress to yes–no questions to help determine specific

TABLE	5-2	

Organizations and Web Sites With Information Pertaining to Medication Safety

Name of Organization	Internet Address
Accreditation Canada	http://www.cchsa.ca/
Canadian Institute for Health Information	http://secure.cihi.ca/cihiweb/splash.html
Canadian Institutes of Health Research	http://www.cihr-irsc.gc.ca/e/193.html
Canadian Medication Incident Reporting and Prevention System (CMIRPS)	http://secure.cihi.ca/cihiweb/
Canadian Patient Safety Institute (CPSI)	http://www.patientsafetyinstitute.ca/index.html
Health Canada	http://www.hc-sc.gc.ca/dhp-mps/medeff/vigilance-eng.php
Institute for Safe Medication Practices (ISMP) Canada	http://www.ismp-canada.org/
Medication Error Report: Voluntary Medication Incident and Near-Miss Reporting Program	https://www.ismp-canada.org/err_report.htm
Safer Healthcare Now!	http://www.saferhealthcarenow.ca/

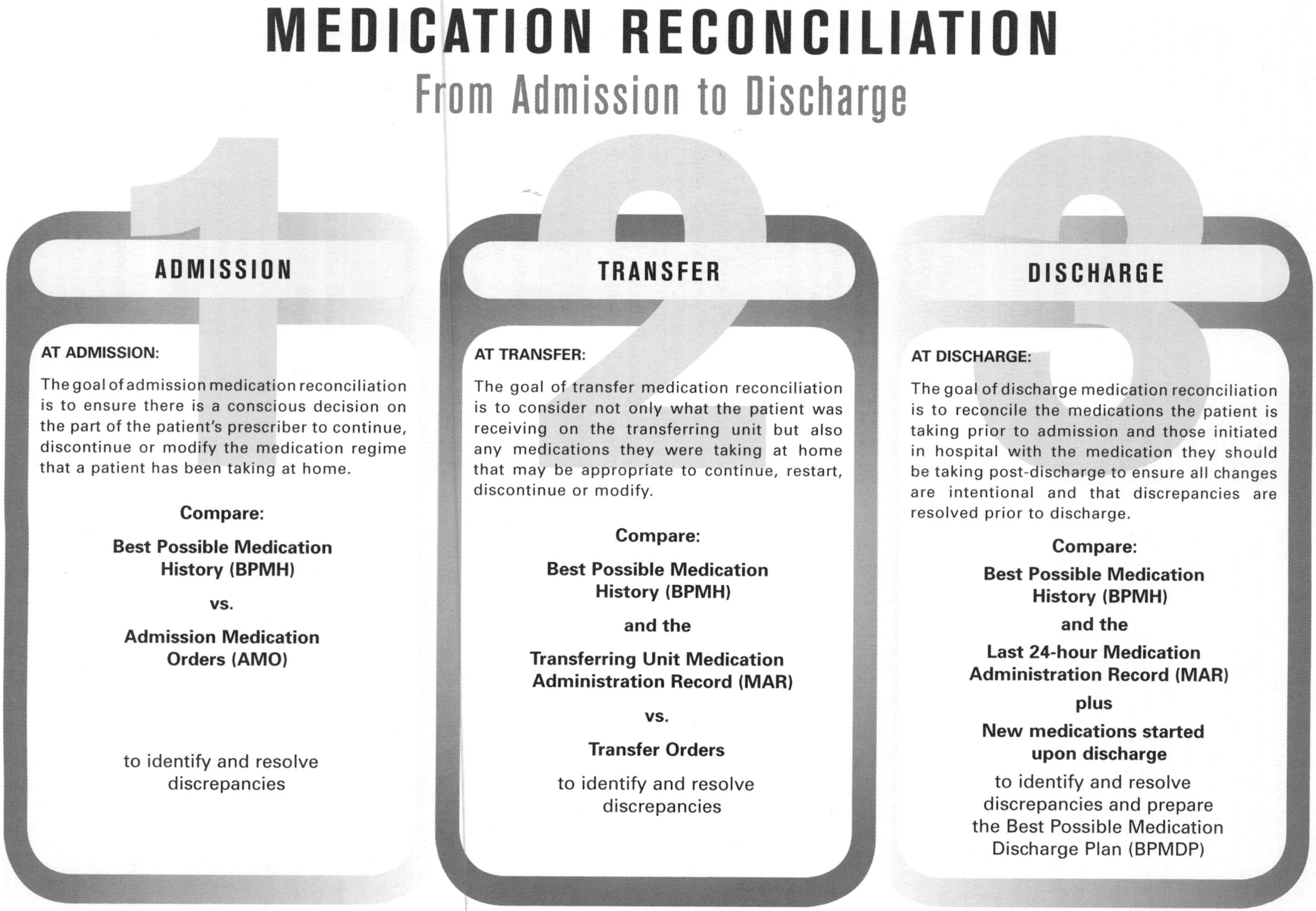

MEDICATION RECONCILIATION
From Admission to Discharge

ADMISSION

AT ADMISSION:

The goal of admission medication reconciliation is to ensure there is a conscious decision on the part of the patient's prescriber to continue, discontinue or modify the medication regime that a patient has been taking at home.

Compare:

Best Possible Medication History (BPMH)

vs.

Admission Medication Orders (AMO)

to identify and resolve discrepancies

TRANSFER

AT TRANSFER:

The goal of transfer medication reconciliation is to consider not only what the patient was receiving on the transferring unit but also any medications they were taking at home that may be appropriate to continue, restart, discontinue or modify.

Compare:

Best Possible Medication History (BPMH)

and the

Transferring Unit Medication Administration Record (MAR)

vs.

Transfer Orders

to identify and resolve discrepancies

DISCHARGE

AT DISCHARGE:

The goal of discharge medication reconciliation is to reconcile the medications the patient is taking prior to admission and those initiated in hospital with the medication they should be taking post-discharge to ensure all changes are intentional and that discrepancies are resolved prior to discharge.

Compare:

Best Possible Medication History (BPMH)

and the

Last 24-hour Medication Administration Record (MAR)

plus

New medications started upon discharge

to identify and resolve discrepancies and prepare the Best Possible Medication Discharge Plan (BPMDP)

FIG. 5-2   Medication reconciliation. Created by the Institute for Safe Medication Practices Canada (ISMP Canada) for the Safer Healthcare Now! campaign. Graphic adapted from St. Mary's Hospital & Medical Center, Grand Junction, Colorado, USA. Adapted by the ISMP from Barnsteiner, J. H. (2005). Medication reconciliation: Transfer of medication information across settings—keeping it free from error. *American Journal of Nursing, 105* (3), 31–36. Retrieved February 22, 2010, from http://www.safer-healthcarenow.ca/EN/Interventions/medrec/Documents/Med Rec (Acute Care) One Pager.pdf.TS

medication information. (Details are important and perhaps critical.)

2 Avoid the use of medical jargon unless it is clear that the patient understands and is comfortable with such language.

3 Prompt the patient to try to remember all applicable medications (e.g., patches, creams, eye drops, inhalers, professional samples, injections, dietary supplements). If the patient does provide a medication list, make a copy for the patient's chart as part of this process.

4 Clarify unclear information to the extent possible (e.g., by talking with the home caregiver or the out-patient pharmacist who fills the patient's prescriptions, if needed).

5 Record the aforementioned information in the patient's chart as the first step in the medication reconciliation process.

6 Emphasize to the patient the importance of always maintaining a current and complete medication list and bringing it to each health care encounter (e.g., as a wallet card or other list).

OTHER ETHICAL ISSUES

Notification of Patients Regarding Errors

In an article published in the *Journal of Clinical Outcomes Management,* McCleave (2001) recognized the obligation of institutions and health care providers to notify patients when errors have occurred in their care. The article not only emphasized the ethical basis for this practice but also addressed the legal implications and was a starting point for understanding the issue of notification of patients about medication errors. The point was made that patients who seek attorney services are often motivated primarily by a perceived imbalance in power between themselves and their health care providers and by fear of financial burden. Health care organizations can choose to apologize and accept responsibility for obvious errors and even offer needed financial support (e.g., for travel expenses, temporary loss of wages). Research indicates that such actions help health care organizations to avoid litigation and potentially much larger financial settlements.

Whistle-Blowing

In clinical settings, *whistle-blowing* refers to a disclosure made outside a health care facility regarding patient care errors when the organization's internal chain of command has failed to correct significant problems within the facility. Such a disclosure may be made to a regulatory or investigative agency or to the public through the news media. One view is that whistle-blowing results from a failure of organizational ethics. Virtually all practising nurses will eventually witness situations involving significant lapses in patient care. Although a student or an inexperienced nurse may not realistically be in a viable position to challenge an institution's hierarchy, every nurse should consider, preferably in advance, how to choose to respond to such a situation. In the Canadian

Code of Ethics for Registered Nurses (Canadian Nurses Association [CNA], 2008), described in Chapter 4, several moral imperatives are identified for the practising nurse that may ultimately justify whistle-blowing action, even in the face of termination of employment. All health care providers should familiarize themselves with their institution's usual procedures for error reporting, including how and when to approach levels of leadership above their immediate supervisor. When the usual systems fail, disclosure may be the most ethical course of action.

POLITICAL ACTION

An Ounce of Prevention: Nurse Advocacy for Safer Health Care Organizations

Since its inception, one of the Canadian Nurses Association's objectives has been legislative advocacy on behalf of nurses and their patients. A 2001 Canadian study (Baumann et al.) found that nurses are stressed, are vulnerable to injury, and have one of the highest professional absentee and disability rates, undermining quality of patient care and overall patient satisfaction. Increased workloads and unsupportive workplace environments contribute to nurses choosing to leave the profession or their practice setting. Even new graduates report high levels of emotional distress. Almost every study conducted in the past 15 years has emphasized the need for improvement in the work life of nurses. The need to retain and recruit nurses is critical not only in Canada but also internationally. Projected shortages of 78,000 registered nurses by 2011 and 113,000 by 2016 are anticipated in Canada (CNA, 2002). Of particular concern is that the ageing experienced nursing workforce is retiring in increasing numbers.

In the 1990s, nurses in Alberta, Saskatchewan, Quebec, and Nova Scotia went on strike to protest working conditions and cuts to health care spending. Provincial governments refused to negotiate and nurses were legislated back to work. Canada's Office of Nursing Policy was developed in 1999 in an attempt to bring more attention to nursing policy issues. One of the initiatives was to develop six *Healthy Work Environment Best Practice Guidelines (BPG)*, which were completed in 2008 (Registered Nurses Association of Ontario, 2008).

There is a growing advocacy movement among several groups of nurses in various regions of the Canada. The Canadian Federation of Nurses Unions (CFNU) provides a national action-oriented voice for nurses, campaigning to improve the working conditions for nurses and the quality of patient care. Specifically, the CFNU advocates for nurses by aggressively pressuring the federal government to recognize the professional skills and knowledge of nurses and to ensure that nurses' and patients' priorities are reflected in health and budgetary policies.

SUMMARY

The increasing complexity of nursing practice also increases the risk for medication errors. Widely recognized and common causes of errors include misunderstanding of abbreviations, illegibility of prescriber handwriting, miscommunication during verbal or telephone orders, and confusing drug nomenclature. The structure of the organizational, educational, and sociological systems involved in health care delivery may also contribute directly or indirectly to the occurrence of medication errors. Understanding these influences can help the nurse take proactive steps to improve these systems. Such actions can range from fostering improved communication with other health care team members, including students, to advocating politically for safer conditions for both patients and staff. The first priority when an error does occur is to protect the patient from further harm whenever possible. All errors should serve as red flags that warrant further reflection, detailed analysis, and future preventive actions on the part of nurses, other health care providers, and possibly even patients themselves.

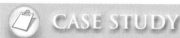

CASE STUDY

Medication Errors

During your busy clinical day as a student nurse, the staff nurse assigned to your patient comes to you and says, "Would you like to give this injection? We have a 'now' order for Sandostatin (octreotide) 200 mcg subcutaneously. I've already drawn it up; 200 mcg equals 2 mL. It needs to be given as soon as possible, so I drew it up to save time." She hands you a syringe that has 2 mL of a clear fluid in it, and the patient's medication administration record (MAR).

1 Should you give this medication "now," as ordered? Why or why not?

You decide to check the order that is handwritten on the MAR with the order written on the chart. The physician wrote, "Octreotide, 200 mcg now, SC, then 100 mcg every 8 hours as needed." Before you have a chance to find your instructor, the nurse returns and says, "Your instructor probably won't let you give the injection unless you can show the medication ampoules. Here are the ampoules I used to draw up the octreotide. Be quick—your patient needs it now!" You take the order, the MAR, the two ampoules, and the syringe to your instructor. Together you read the order, then check the ampoules. Each ampoule is marked "Sandostatin (octreotide) 500 mcg/mL."

2 If the nurse drew up 2 mL from those two ampoules, how much octreotide is in the syringe? How does that amount compare with the order?

The nurse is astonished when you point out that the ampoules read "500 mcg/mL." She goes into the automated medication dispenser and sees two identical boxes of Sandostatin next to each other in the refrigerated section. One box is labelled "100 mcg/mL" and the other box is labelled "500 mcg/mL." She then realizes she chose an ampoule of the wrong strength of drug and drew up an incorrect dose.

3 What would have happened if you had given the injection?

4 What should be done at this point? What contributed to this potential medication error, and how can it be prevented in the future?

Note: High-alert drugs include adrenal drugs (corticosteroids), analgesics (acetaminophen), anti-infectives and antibiotics, antihistamines, antineoplastics, asthma drugs, bronchodilators, heart drugs, electrolytes, vitamins, minerals, insulin, opioids, and sedatives.

For answers see http://evolve.elsevier.com/Canada/Lilley/pharmacology/.

POINTS TO REMEMBER

❖ *Medical error* is a broad term used to address any error that occurs within any phase of clinical patient care. Medical errors *may* involve medications.

❖ Medical errors may or may not lead to adverse drug events. Medical errors specific to medication errors include giving the drug to the wrong patient; confusing sound-alike and look-alike drugs, giving the wrong drug or the wrong dose, giving a drug by the wrong route, and giving the drug at the wrong time.

❖ There are several measures that nurses can implement to help prevent medication errors. Being prepared and knowledgeable and taking the time always to triple-check the Ten Rights of medication administration are important. It is also important for nurses always to be aware of the entire medication administration process and to take a system analysis approach to prevent medication errors.

❖ Nurses should always encourage patients to ask questions about their medications and to let their health care provider know if they are questioning the drug or any component of the medication administration process.

❖ Nurses should encourage patients always to keep drug allergy information on their person and a current list of medications in their wallet or purse and on their refrigerator. This list should include the following information:
  • Drug name
  • Reason the drug is being used
  • Usual dosage range and the dosage the patient is taking
  • Expected adverse effects and toxic effects of the drug
  • Physician's name and phone number

EXAMINATION REVIEW QUESTIONS

1 Which of the following nursing measures should be included to reduce the risk of medication errors?
   a. If questioning a drug order, always assume that the prescriber is correct.
   b. Be careful about questioning the drug order a surgeon has written for a patient.
   c. Always double-check the many drugs with sound-alike and look-alike names because of the high risk of error.
   d. Always go with your gut reaction and if you think a drug route has been incorrectly prescribed, use the oral route.

2 Which of the following is an important medication administration process to remember?
   a. When in doubt about an order, ask a colleague about the drug.
   b. Stop, listen, and investigate any concerns expressed by the patient.
   c. Contact the patient and ask what the patient knows about the medication and whether it was taken prior to this hospitalization.
   d. If you are too busy, ask the charge nurse about the drug, then research the drug once you have given it to the patient at the right time.

3 If a student nurse realizes that a drug error has been committed, which of the following should be emphasized to the student?
   a. The student bears no legal responsibility when giving medications.
   b. The major legal responsibility for drug errors lies with the faculty members.
   c. The major legal responsibility lies with the health care institution at which the student is placed for nursing practice experience.
   d. Once the student has committed a medication error, the responsibility is to the patient and to being honest and accountable.

4 The nurse is giving medications to a newly admitted patient who is to receive nothing by mouth (NPO) and finds an order written as follows: "Digoxin, 250 mcg stat." Which action is appropriate?
   a. Ask the charge nurse what route the physician meant to use.
   b. Clarify the order with the prescribing physician before giving the drug.
   c. Give the medication immediately (stat) by mouth because the patient has no intravenous (IV) access at this time.
   d. Start an IV line, then give the medication IV so that it will work faster, because the patient's status is NPO at this time.

5 Which of the following is an acceptable authoritative resource for information about medications?
   a. Drug information pulled from Internet sites for lay persons
   b. An experienced professional nurse colleague
   c. The faculty person supervising the student during clinical rotations
   d. Drug information obtained from Internet sites such as http://www.hc-sc.gc.ca/dhp/ or http://www.rxlist.com/

For answers see http://evolve.elsevier.com/Canada/Lilley/pharmacology/.

CRITICAL THINKING ACTIVITIES

1 Medication errors have been occurring with increasing frequency on the unit on which you are employed. A committee has been appointed to investigate why the medication errors occur and how to resolve the problem. Considering this situation and the drug administration process, is it always safe to follow only the guideline of checking the Ten Rights of drug administration? Why or why not?

2 You are a charge nurse at a small community hospital. The physician ordered a STAT IV vancomycin infusion, but when the bag comes up from the pharmacy, you notice that the dose is incorrect. It takes 2 hours for the pharmacy to send up an IV bag with the correct dose. As you check the medication, you note that it is the right drug, right dose, and so on, yet it has been 2 hours since it was ordered STAT. What, if anything, should you do before you give this medication?

3 List several Internet sources for information on medication safety and briefly discuss how this information could be shared with patients in a community outpatient setting where the patients are primarily indigent.

For answers see http://evolve.elsevier.com/Canada/Lilley/pharmacology/.

Patient Education and Drug Therapy

Learning Objectives

After reading this chapter, the successful student will be able to do the following:

1 Discuss the importance of patient education in the safe and efficient administration of drugs (e.g., prescription drugs, over-the-counter drugs, natural health products).

2 Discuss some of the teaching and learning principles related to patient education and drug therapy across the lifespan that are applicable to any health care setting.

3 Identify the impact of the developmental phases (according to Erikson) on patient education and drug therapy.

4 Develop a complete patient education plan as part of a collaborative plan of care for drug therapy.

e-Learning Activities

Web site
(http://evolve.elsevier.com/Canada/
Lilley/pharmacology/)

- Animations
- Answers to chapter questions, activities, and case studies
- Calculators and Category Catchers
- Glossary with audio pronunciations
- IV Therapy and Medication Error Checklists
- Multiple-Choice Review Question quizzes
- Nursing Care Plans
- Online Appendices and Supplements
- WebLinks

OVERVIEW

Given the continual change in health care and the increasing emphasis on consumer awareness, the role of nurses as educators is expanding. Because the frequency with which patients are being managed in the home setting is increasing, patient education is an essential component of health care. Without it, high-quality patient care cannot be provided. Patient education is crucial for helping patients adapt to illness, prevent illness, maintain wellness, and provide self-care. Patient education is a process in which patients are assisted in learning and assimilating healthy behaviours into their lifestyle. *Learning* is defined as a change in behaviour, and *teaching* is defined as a sharing of knowledge. Although nurses can never be certain that patients will take medications as prescribed, they can be sure to carefully assess, plan, implement, and evaluate the teaching they provide to patients about their medications. When discussing patient education, remember that family members often are important participants to be included in the education process. The nursing process (discussed in Chapter 1) as applied to patient education is presented

in this chapter using the following format: assessment; nursing diagnoses; planning, including goals and outcome criteria; implementation; and evaluation.

ASSESSMENT OF LEARNING NEEDS RELATED TO DRUG THERAPY

The patient education process is similar to the nursing process. An important facet of the patient education process is a thorough assessment of learning needs, and this assessment must be completed before patients begin any form of drug therapy, whether it involves a prescription drug, over-the-counter (OTC) drug, or natural health products. Performing a thorough assessment includes gathering subjective and objective data about the following variables and factors:

- Adaptation to any illnesses
- Cognitive abilities
- Coping mechanisms
- Developmental status for age group with attention to cognitive and mental processing abilities
- Emotional status
- Environment at home and at work

- Ethnocultural background (see Ethnocultural Implications: Patient Education)
- Family relationships
- Financial status
- Health beliefs
- Information the patient understands about past and present medical condition, medical therapy, and medications
- Language(s) spoken
- Level of education (including literacy levels)
- Limitations (physical, psychological, cognitive, and motor)
- Medications currently taken (including OTC drugs, prescription drugs, and natural health products)
- Mobility
- Motivation
- Nutritional status
- Past and present health behaviours
- Past and present experience with drug regimens and other forms of therapy
- Psychosocial growth and development level according to Erikson's stages (Box 6-1)
- Race and ethnicity
- Readiness to learn
- Self-care ability
- Sensory status
- Social support

In addition, the assessment is an appropriate time to probe for any misinformation regarding drug therapy or related health care and to identify practices that might be contraindicated given the current drug regimen (e.g., use of folk medicine or home remedies, or alternative therapies such as chiropractic and osteopathic medicine and aromatherapy). Other questions posed to the patient may need to focus on the patient's belief system about health, wellness, and illness as well as any experiences with health care regimens and therapies and history of adherence to drug and

BOX 6-1

Erikson's Stages of Development

American psychoanalyst Erik Erikson (1902–1994) believed that the interaction between internal drives and cultural demands causes people to develop through eight crises, or psychosocial stages (Erikson, 1959).

Infant (birth–1 year of age): Trust versus mistrust. Infant learns to trust self, others, and the environment; learns to love and be loved.

Toddler (1–3 years of age): Autonomy versus shame and doubt. Toddler learns independence; learns to master the physical environment and maintain self-esteem.

Preschooler (3–6 years of age): Initiative versus guilt. Preschooler learns basic problem solving; develops conscience and sexual identity; initiates activities, as well as imitates.

School-age child: Industry versus inferiority. School-age child learns to do things well; develops a sense of self-worth.

Adolescent: Identity versus role confusion. Adolescent integrates many roles into self-identity through role models and peer pressure.

Young adult: Intimacy versus isolation. Young adult establishes deep and lasting relationships; learns to make commitment as spouse, parent, partner.

Middle-aged adult: Generativity versus stagnation. Adult learns commitment to community and world; is productive in career, family, civic interests.

Older adult: Integrity versus despair. Older adult appreciates life role and status; deals with loss and prepares for death.

 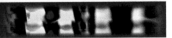

ETHNOCULTURAL IMPLICATIONS

Patient Education

The nurse must research ethnocultures to enhance the individualized approach to nursing care. For example, with the Somali patient, aspects of nursing care need to be approached in a sensitive manner with strong consideration for the family, communication needs, and religion. The majority of Somalis are Sunni Muslims. Islamic religion is a significant part of Somali life. Islamic religious teachings provide meaning for living, dying, family life, child-rearing, and the maintenance of health. In Islam, prayer is performed five times a day; before prayer, the hands, face, and feet are washed. Islam forbids the eating of pork, drinking alcohol, or touching (or being near) dogs. Attitudes, social customs, and gender roles in Somalia are based primarily on Islamic tradition. Married Somali women cover their bodies and veil their

faces in a hijab. Elders are treated with respect. Health is considered a gift from Allah (God), so it is an expectation to maintain health. Taking preventative medications is not within the traditional Somali view. Illness prevention occurs because of the use of prayer and living a life according to Islam. Traditionally, men and women do not touch members of the opposite sex, except for close family members.

Somalis believe that spirits reside within each individual. When the spirits become angry, illnesses such as fever, headache, dizziness, and weakness can result. The cure involves a healing ceremony including reading from the Koran, eating special foods, and burning incense. To help meet the needs of Somali patients, it is important to assess and include their beliefs in their care.

other therapies. Other barriers to learning may include language, finances, ethnocultural beliefs, previous negative or limited experiences with the health care system or team, and denial of illness or need for health care intervention.

During the assessment of learning needs, the nurse must be astutely aware of the patient's verbal and nonverbal communication. Often a patient will not divulge true feelings to the nurse. A seeming discrepancy is an indication that the patient's emotional or physical state may need to be further assessed in relation to readiness for learning and motivation to learn. The nurse should use open-ended questions when assessing patients because this type of question encourages greater clarification and more discussion from the patient. Closed-ended questions that require only a "yes" or "no" answer provide limited information and insight about the patient. The patient's level of anxiety must also be assessed, because a mild anxiety level is usually motivating, but a moderate or severe level may be an obstacle.

NURSING DIAGNOSES RELATED TO LEARNING NEEDS AND DRUG THERAPY

Some of the most common nursing diagnoses related to patient education and drug therapy include deficient knowledge, ineffective health maintenance, ineffective therapeutic regimen management, risk for injury, impaired memory, and nonadherence. *Deficient knowledge* refers to a situation in which the patient (or caregiver or significant other) has a limited knowledge base or skills with regard to the medication. A nursing diagnosis of deficient knowledge grows out of collected data indicating that the patient has limited or no understanding of the medication and its action, adverse effects, or cautions, and any related administration techniques. Deficient knowledge may also pertain to the lack of motor skills needed to safely self-administer the medication. Deficient knowledge differs from *nonadherence,* which means that the patient does not take the medication as prescribed or at all; in other words, the patient does not adhere to the instructions given about the medication. Nonadherence is the patient's choice. A nursing diagnosis of nonadherence is made when data collected from the patient show that the condition or symptoms for which the patient is taking the medication have recurred or were never resolved because the patient did not take the medication per the physician's orders or did not take the medication at all. Other nursing diagnoses, listed by the North American Nursing Diagnosis Association (NANDA) (see Chapter 1), may also be used in relation to medication administration, when applicable.

PLANNING RELATED TO LEARNING NEEDS AND DRUG THERAPY

The planning phase of the teaching and learning process occurs as soon as a learning need has been identified in a patient or caregiver. With mutual understanding, the nurse and patient identify goals and outcome criteria that are associated with the identified nursing diagnosis and relate to the specific medication the patient is taking. For example, for a patient who is self-administering an oral antihyperglycemic drug and has many questions about the medication therapy, a measurable goal with an outcome criterion related to a nursing diagnosis of deficient knowledge could be established. The *goal* would be that the patient will safely self-administer the prescribed oral antihyperglycemic drug. The *outcome criterion* would be that the patient remains without signs and symptoms of overmedication with an oral antihyperglycemic drug, such as hypoglycemia with tachycardia, palpitations, diaphoresis, hunger, and fatigue. When drug therapy goals and outcome criteria are developed, appropriate time frames for meeting outcome criteria should also be identified (see Chapter 1 for more information on the nursing process). Goals and outcome criteria should be realistic, based on patient needs, stated in patient terms, and include terms that are measurable, such as *list, identify, demonstrate, self-administer, state, describe,* and *discuss.*

IMPLEMENTATION RELATED TO DRUG THERAPY

After the nurse has completed the assessment phase, identified nursing diagnoses, and created a plan of care, the nurse begins the implementation phase of teaching–learning, which includes conveying specific information about the medication to the patient. Teaching sessions should include clear, simple, concise written instructions; oral instructions; and pamphlets, films, or any other learning aids that will help ensure patient learning. The nurse may have to conduct several short teaching sessions with multiple strategies, depending on the needs of the patient. (Table 6-1 lists educational strategies for accommodating changes related to aging that may influence learning.) Teaching may need to focus on either the cognitive, affective, or psychomotor domain or a combination of all three. The cognitive domain includes thought processes and problem-solving abilities and may involve recall for synthesis of facts. The affective domain includes values and beliefs and behaviours such as responding, valuing, and organizing. The psychomotor domain includes gross motor movements, speech, and nonverbal communication and involves behaviours such as learning how to perform a procedure. The nurse may also need to identify aids to help the patient in the safe administration of medications at home, such as the use of medication day and time calendars, pill reminder stickers, daily medication containers with alarms, and/or a method of documenting doses taken to avoid over-dosage or omission of doses.

Special considerations arise when the patient speaks little or no English. The nurse should communicate with the patient in the patient's native language if at all possible. If the nurse is not able to speak the patient's native language, a translator should be made available if possible to prevent communication problems, minimize errors, and help boost the patient's level of trust and understanding of the nurse.

In practice, this translator is often a lay family member (perhaps even a child) or a nonclinical staff member, and the nurse should keep in mind that these individuals may not be competent at or comfortable with communicating technical clinical information. As well, technical information may be difficult to interpret as the native language may not have words to describe the terms.

In response to the rapidly growing population of non-English-speaking Chinese in Canada, a number of publications have appeared containing patient education materials printed in both English and Chinese. Similar materials for other languages are often also available. These publications may enable the nurse to speak a sufficient amount of the patient's language to effectively educate the patient and can be given to the patient and family members to read on their own. The publishers of these patient education materials have generally granted permission to photocopy them for educational purposes.

Health care professionals who work in a geographic area where a variety of non-English languages are widely spoken should consider learning one or more of these languages. Adult foreign language education is available in many Canadian cities, often at colleges or universities. Many classes are designed for working professionals and are scheduled at a variety of convenient times during the day and evening to accommodate demanding work schedules. Many employers will pay for job-related courses, and some courses may be used as professional continuing education (CE) credits. Language courses provide a means for networking and developing friendships with other highly motivated, empathetic individuals, both within and outside the health care profession.

TABLE 6-1

Educational Strategies to Address Common Changes Related to Aging That May Influence Learning

Changes Related to Aging	Educational Strategy
DISTURBED THOUGHT PROCESSES	
Slowed cognitive functioning	Slow the pace of the presentation and attend to verbal and nonverbal patient cues to verify understanding.
Decreased short-term memory	Provide smaller amounts of information at one time. Repeat information frequently. Provide written instructions for home use.
Decreased ability to think abstractly	Use examples to illustrate information. Use a variety of methods, such as audiovisuals, props, videos, large-printed materials, materials with vivid colours, return demonstrations, and practice sessions.
Decreased ability to concentrate. Increased reaction time (slower to respond)	Decrease external stimuli as much as possible. Always allow sufficient time and be patient. Allow more time for feedback.
DISTURBED SENSORY PERCEPTION	
Hearing	
Diminished hearing	Perform a baseline hearing assessment. Use tone- and volume-controlled teaching aids; use bright, large-printed material to reinforce learning.
Decreased ability to distinguish sounds (e.g., words beginning with *S, Z, T, D, F,* and *G*)	Speak distinctly and slowly, and articulate carefully.
Decreased conduction of sound	Sit on the side of the learner's "best" ear.
Loss of ability to hear high-frequency sounds	Do not shout; speak in a normal voice but lower voice pitch.
Partial to complete loss of hearing	Face the patient so that lip-reading is possible. Use visual aids to reinforce verbal instruction. Reinforce teaching with easy-to-read materials. Decrease extraneous noise. Use community resources for the hearing impaired.
Vision	
Decreased visual acuity	Ensure that the patient's glasses are clean and in place and that the prescription is current.
Decreased ability to read fine detail	Use large-print, clear, brightly coloured material.
Decreased ability to discriminate among blue, violet, and green: tendency for all colours to fade, with red fading the least	Use high-contrast materials, such as black on white. Avoid the use of blue, violet, and green in type or graphics; use red instead
Thickening and yellowing of the lenses of the eyes, with decreased accommodation	Use nonglare lighting and avoid contrasts of light (e.g., darkened room with single light).
Decreased depth perception	Adjust teaching to allow for the use of touch to gauge depth.
Decreased peripheral vision	Keep all teaching materials within the patient's visual field.
Touch and Vibration	
Decreased sense of touch	Increase the time allowed for the teaching of psychomotor skills, the number of repetitions, and the number of return demonstrations.
Decreased sense of vibration	Teach patient to palpate more prominent pulse sites (e.g., carotid and radial arteries).

Modified from Weinrich, S. P., Boyd, M., & Nussbaum, J. (1989). Continuing education: Adapting strategies to teach the elderly. *Journal of Gerontology Nursing, 15*(11), 17; McKenry, L. M., Tessier, E., & Hogan, M. (2006). *Mosby's pharmacology in nursing* (22nd ed.). St. Louis, MO: Mosby.

Native English speakers may also have problems learning about their medications and treatment regimens because of learning deficits or difficulties, hearing and speech deficits, lack of education, or minimal previous exposure to treatment regimens and medication use. The teaching of manual skills for specific medication administration is also part of the teaching and learning session. Sufficient time (each patient has different needs) should be allowed for the patient to become familiar with any equipment and to perform several return demonstrations to the nurse or other health care provider. Family members, significant others, or caregivers should also be included in this session or sessions for reinforcement purposes. Audiovisual aids may be incorporated.

Resources for information about medications include the Shopper's Drug Mart medication library, which provides information for the public. This type of resource may be helpful to the patient when seeking information about a medication (e.g., purpose, adverse effects, method of administration, drug interactions) and helpful to the nurse in developing a patient teaching plan. The nurse should be sure to create a safe, nonthreatening, nondistracting environment for learning and to be receptive to the patient's questions.

The nurse should do the following to ensure the effectiveness of the teaching–learning session:
- Individualize the teaching session.
- Provide positive rewards or reinforcement for accurate return demonstration of the procedure or technique during the teaching session.

- Complete a medication calendar that includes medications to take and dosage schedule.
- Use audiovisual aids.
- Involve family members or significant others.
- Keep the teaching on a level that is most meaningful to the given patient; general research on reading skills has shown that materials should be written at an eighth-grade reading level.

Box 6-2 lists some general teaching and learning principles for the nurse to keep in mind.

Documentation of learning, including specific information about what was taught (content), strategies used, patient response, and evaluation of learning, should be carried out after the teaching–learning process has been completed. The nurse also should remember that patient teaching begins with admission to the health care setting and should be documented in the appropriate area of the patient's chart (for information on discharge teaching, see Legal and Ethical Principles on page 91). Throughout this textbook, patient education is integrated into each chapter in the Implementation subsection under Nursing Process.

EVALUATION OF PATIENT LEARNING RELATED TO DRUG THERAPY

Evaluation of patient learning is critical to safe patient drug administration. Nurses should always verify whether learning has occurred by asking the patient questions related to the teaching session and having

---

BOX 6-2   General Teaching and Learning Principles

- Make learning patient centred and individualized to each patient's needs, including the patient's learning needs. This involves assessment of the patient's ethnocultural beliefs, educational level, previous experience with medications, level of growth and development (to best match a teaching–learning strategy), age, gender, family support system, resources, ability to learn and the way the patient learns best, and level of sophistication with health care and health care treatment
- Assess the patient's motivation and readiness to learn.
- Assess the patient's ability to use and interpret label information on medication containers.
- Remember that a patient's ability to interpret drug instructions is ethnoculturally based and, therefore, somewhat consistent regardless of age, sex, or educational background.
- Some studies have shown that as much as 22% of the Canadian population is functionally illiterate. Ensure that the educational strategies and materials are at a level the patient is able to understand, while taking care to not embarrass the patient.
- Regardless of the patient's literary skills, all patients still need to be instructed on safe medication administration. Use pictures, demonstrations, and return demonstrations to emphasize instructions.

- Consider, assess, and appreciate language and ethnicity during patient teaching. Make every effort to educate non-English-speaking patients in their native language. Ideally the patient should be instructed by a health professional familiar with the patient's clinical picture who also speaks the patient's native language. At the least, provide the patient detailed written instructions in the patient's native language if possible.
- Assess the family support system for adequate patient teaching. Family living arrangements, financial status, resources, communication patterns, the roles of family members, and the power and authority of different family members should always be considered.
- Make the teaching–learning session simple, easy, fun, thorough, effective, and interesting. Make it applicable to daily life and schedule it at a time when the patient is ready to learn.
- Remember that learning occurs best with repetition and periods of demonstration and with the use of audiovisuals and other educational aids.
- Patient teaching should focus on the processes and actions within the cognitive, affective, or psychomotor domains.
- Consult online resources for help in obtaining the most up-to-date and accurate patient teaching materials and information.

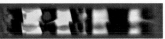

LEGAL & ETHICAL PRINCIPLES

Discharge Teaching

The safest practices for discharge teaching include the following:

- Always follow the health care facility's policy on discharge teaching regarding how much information to provide to the patient.
- Do not assume that any patient has received adequate teaching before interacting with you.
- Always begin discharge teaching as soon as possible when the patient is ready.
- Minimize any distractions during the teaching session.
- Evaluate any teaching of the patient and significant others by having the individuals repeat the instructions you have given to them.

- Contact the institution's social service department or the discharge planner if there are any concerns regarding the learning capacity of the patient.
- Document what you have taught, who was present with the patient during the teaching, what specific written instructions were given, what the actions were of the patient or significant other or caregiver, and what your own nursing actions were, such as specific demonstrations or referrals to community resources.
- Document teaching–learning strategies, such as use of videos and pamphlets.

Modified from the U.S. Pharmacopeia Safe Medication Use Expert Committee Meeting, Rockville, MD, May 2003. Available at http://www.usp.org.

the patient provide a return demonstration of any skills taught. The patient's behaviour, such as adherence to the schedule for medication administration with few or no complications of therapy, is the key to determining whether the teaching was successful and learning occurred. If a patient's behaviour suggests nonadherence or an inadequate level of learning, a new plan of teaching should be developed and implemented.

SUMMARY

Patient education is a critical part of patient care, and education concerning medication administration is no exception. From the time of initial contact with the patient throughout the time the nurse works with the patient, the patient is entitled to all information about the medication as well as all aspects of patient care. Evaluation of learning and adherence with the medication regimen should

be a continual process, and the nurse should always be willing to listen to the patient about any aspects of the drug therapy. The Institute of Safe Medication Practices (ISMP) Canada (http://www.ismp-canada.org/) and the Canadian Patient Safety Institute (http://www.patient-safetyinstitute.ca) advocate for patient safety and medications, and the Canadian Patient Safety Institute has taken on the challenge of reducing injuries and deaths due to medication errors. These organizations are also a tremendous resource for patients as well as for the health care profession, ensuring that quality patient education can be provided.

Patient education is a means of enhancing patient safety and decreasing medication errors in the hospital setting or at home. Health care providers must continue to be patient advocates and take the initiative to plan, design, create, and implement discharge teaching regarding drug therapy and other parts of the therapy regimen.

POINTS TO REMEMBER

- ❖ A thorough assessment of the patient and the patient's spouse, significant other, family members, or caregivers and their readiness to learn is crucial to effective patient education.
- ❖ Realistic patient teaching goals should be established and the patient should be involved in setting these goals.
- ❖ The importance to the patient of knowing about the medications to prevent errors and maximize therapeutic benefits should be emphasized to the patient.
- ❖ Patient teaching is an important and necessary part of the nursing function during the implementation phase of the nursing process to ensure safe and effective drug therapy.

- ❖ Patient teaching should occur after the nurse has thoroughly assessed the patient's readiness to learn, and a comprehensive, holistic approach should be adopted.
- ❖ Patient teaching may need to focus on either the cognitive, affective, or psychomotor domain or a combination of all three.
- ❖ Patients need to receive information through as many senses as possible, such as aurally and visually (as with pamphlets, videos, diagrams), to maximize learning. Information should also be on the patient's reading level, in the patient's native language (if possible), and suitable for the patient's level of cognitive development (see Erikson's stages in Box 6-1).
- ❖ Both the patient and any significant others should always be involved in the teaching process.

EXAMINATION REVIEW QUESTIONS

1 A 47-year-old patient with diabetes is being discharged home on insulin injections twice a day. Which of the following statements is most accurate regarding proper teaching for this patient?
   a. The majority of the teaching can be done with pamphlets that the patient can share with family members.
   b. A thorough and comprehensive teaching plan designed for an eighth-grade reading level should be developed.
   c. Teaching should begin at the time of diagnosis or admission and should be individualized to the patient's reading level.
   d. The nurse can assume that because the patient is in his 40s he will be able to read any written or printed documents provided.

2 Which of the following strategies about discharge teaching and medications is correct?
   a. Teaching should be done right before the patient leaves the hospital or doctor's office.
   b. Teaching should be individualized and based on the patient's level of cognitive development.
   c. Teaching should be reserved for when the patient is comfortable or after narcotics are administered.
   d. Teaching should include videos, demonstrations, and instructions written at least at the fifth-grade level.

3 A nurse is responsible for the preoperative teaching for a patient who is mildly anxious about receiving narcotics postoperatively. The nurse acknowledges that this level of anxiety may result in which of the following effects?

   a. Impede learning because anxiety is helpful
   b. Lead to major unsteadiness of emotional status
   c. Result in learning by increasing the patient's willingness to learn
   d. Reorganize the patient's thoughts and lead to inadequate potential for learning

4 What action by the nurse is the best way to assess a patient's learning needs?
   a. Quiz the patient daily on all medications.
   b. Begin with validation of the patient's present level of knowledge.
   c. Assess family members' knowledge of the medication even if they are not involved in the patient's care.
   d. Question other caregivers about their level of experience with the drug regimen and assume lack of interest if no answers are given.

5 Which of the following techniques would be most appropriate for teaching a patient with a possible language barrier?
   a. Provide only written instructions.
   b. Use detailed and lengthy explanations, speaking slowly and clearly.
   c. Obtain an interpreter who can speak in the patient's native tongue for teaching sessions.
   d. If the nurse notes that there are no questions, it can be assumed that the patient understands the information.

For answers see http://evolve.elsevier.com/Canada/Lilley/pharmacology/.

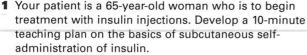

CRITICAL THINKING ACTIVITIES

1 Your patient is a 65-year-old woman who is to begin treatment with insulin injections. Develop a 10-minute teaching plan on the basics of subcutaneous self-administration of insulin.

2 Formulate a teaching plan for a 69-year-old male patient who has experienced a left-sided stroke, is aphasic, and is paralyzed on the right side. He is going to be returning home where his wife will care for him. Your discharge teaching will be directed to the patient and his wife, and you are to teach them about safety measures for the patient, who has slight difficulty in

swallowing and will be taking oral medications when he returns home. He tolerates liquids, soft foods, and thickened liquids fairly well.

3 Your patient does not speak English or understand any of your communication techniques thus far. Develop a plan of care that addresses the patient's need for medication information on the heart drug cardiazem (Diltiazem) and also focuses on the potential for toxicity. (Note: You may need to look the drug up in the textbook if you are not familiar with it.)

For answers see http://evolve.elsevier.com/Canada/Lilley/pharmacology/.

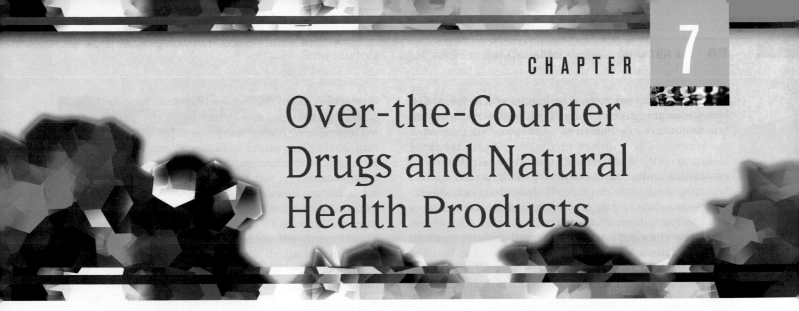

CHAPTER 7

Over-the-Counter Drugs and Natural Health Products

Learning Objectives

After reading this chapter, the successful student will be able to do the following:

1 Differentiate between prescription drugs, over-the-counter (OTC) drugs, and natural health products.

2 Briefly discuss the differences between the federal legislation governing the promotion and sale of prescription drugs and that governing OTC drugs and natural health products.

3 Describe the advantages and disadvantages of the use of OTC drugs and natural health products.

4 Explain the proper use of OTC drugs and natural health products.

5 Discuss the potential dangers associated with the use of OTC drugs and natural health products.

6 Develop a collaborative plan of care for the patient who uses OTC drugs or natural health products.

e-Learning Activities

Web site
(http://evolve.elsevier.com/Canada/
Lilley/pharmacology/)

- Animations
- Answers to chapter questions, activities, and case studies
- Calculators and Category Catchers
- Glossary with audio pronunciations
- IV Therapy and Medication Error Checklists
- Multiple-Choice Review Question quizzes
- Nursing Care Plans
- Online Appendices and Supplements
- WebLinks

Glossary

Alternative medicine Herbal medicine, natural health approaches, chiropractic, acupuncture, reflexology, and any other therapies not taught in a Western medical school but used for health care. (p. 97)

Commission E Monographs Comprehensive, published herbal recommendations from the German equivalent of Health Canada's Natural Health Products Directorate. (p. 97)

Compendium of Monographs Comprehensive, published herbal recommendations from Health Canada's Natural Health Products Directorate. (p. 98)

Complementary medicine Wide variety of health care practices that may be used simultaneously with standard Western medicine. (p. 98)

Conventional medicine The practice of medicine as taught in a Western medical school. (p. 97)

Dietary supplement A product taken by mouth that contains an ingredient intended to supplement the diet, including vitamins, minerals, herbs or other botanicals, amino acids, and substances such as enzymes, organ tissues, glandular preparations, metabolites, extracts, and concentrates. (p. 97)

Herbal medicine The practice of using herbs to heal. (p. 97)

Herbs Herbaceous plants as well as the bark, roots, leaves, seeds, flowers, and fruit of trees, shrubs, and woody vines and extracts of these plants and materials that are valued for their savoury, aromatic, or medicinal qualities. (p. 97)

Iatrogenic effects Unintentional adverse effects caused by the actions of a physician or other health care provider or by a specific treatment. (p. 97)

Marihuana Medical Access Regulations Guidelines that allow special access to marihuana for medical purposes and define the circumstances and the manner in which such access is permitted. (p. 100)

Natural health products (NHPs) Umbrella term that includes vitamins and minerals, herbal remedies, homeopathic medicines, traditional medicines such as traditional Chinese medicines, probiotics, and other products such as amino acids and essential fatty acids. (p. 96)

Over-the-counter (OTC) drugs Medications that are legally available to consumers without a prescription; also called *nonprescription drugs*. (p. 94)

Phytochemicals The pharmacologically active ingredients in herbal remedies. (p. 97)

Prebiotics Carbohydrates that may help to stimulate and support the intestinal bacteria. (p. 97)

Probiotics Live microorganisms which, when administered in adequate amounts, confer a health benefit on the host. (p. 97)

OVER-THE-COUNTER DRUGS

The Internet allows access to medical information that was unavailable to the Canadian population only a decade ago. As a result, health care consumers are increasingly involved in their own diagnosis and treatment of common ailments. This has led to a great increase in the use of *nonprescription*, or **over-the-counter (OTC), drugs**. A 2004 survey revealed that approximately 66% of Canadians had used OTC drugs in the previous 6 months and as many as 12% take OTC drugs daily (Be Medwise, 2005). The daily usage of OTC drugs increases with age, with 26% of Canadians aged 65 years and older using OTC drugs daily. OTC, or nonprescription, drugs play a significant role in health care and generated in excess of $2.4 billion in sales in Canada in 2007. The share of nonprescribed drugs in total drug expenditure reached 16.7% in 2006 and 16.4% in 2007 according to the Canadian Institute for Health Information (2008).

For nurses to understand current OTC classification, it is helpful to have some background information on the scheduling and approval process for OTC drugs. (A detailed discussion of the acts and government bodies regulating all types of controlled medications and natural health products is presented in Chapter 4.) The Drug Strategy and Controlled Substances Program (DSCSP) manages the 1997 *Controlled Drugs & Substances Act*, which controls the import, production, export, distribution, and possession of narcotics and controlled substances. All provinces in Canada (excluding Quebec) use a drug scheduling model to align the provincial drugs schedules and ensure consistent sale conditions across Canada. Factors such as potential for drug dependency, drug adverse reactions, and drug interactions determine the schedule under which a drug is sold. At the request of the drug manufacturer, scheduling recommendations are made to the provincial regulatory authorities by the National Drug Scheduling Advisory Committee (NDSAC). In Canada, there are three categories that regulate the conditions of sale for nonprescription drugs. *Schedule I* drugs are available only by prescription. A *Schedule II* drug is a restricted-access drug that is available only from a pharmacist and is retained in an area behind the counter where there is no opportunity for consumer self-selection. Examples include insulin, loperamide (an antidiarrheal agent), and acetaminophen with codeine 8 mg. This strategy ensures that the consumer

is not self-medicating inappropriately and that the use of these drugs is subject to counselling by the pharmacist. *Schedule III* includes pharmacy-only nonprescription drugs. The consumer has open access to Schedule III drugs and a pharmacist is available to answer questions. Examples are antihistamines and ulcer medications. *Unscheduled drugs* covers nonprescription drugs such as ibuprofen, acetaminophen, and nicotine gum that can be sold in any store without professional supervision. The National Association of Pharmacy Regulatory Bodies (NAPRA) sets out the level of professional intervention and advice necessary for the safe and effective use of drugs by consumers. OTC drugs may also be prescribed but legally do not require a prescription. Although OTC drugs are usually paid for by the consumer, sometimes they are covered by public or private drug plans.

The NDSAC of the Therapeutic Products Programme reviews the status of chemical entities proposed for marketing. This advisory group makes recommendations to provincial and territory regulatory authorities about the conditions under which and where drugs can be sold in Canada. Drug ingredients can be descheduled from prescription to nonprescription status following the thorough review of data accompanying the submission of a "switch" application. The application must contain information about the safety and efficacy of the ingredient. The ingredient usually has been marketed in Canada and other countries long enough to demonstrate that it can be used safely by consumers on their own. Generally, to be switched from prescription to nonprescription status, a drug must meet the three criteria listed in Box 7-1. This information is obtained from clinical-trial results and postmarketing safety surveillance data, which are submitted to Health Canada by the manufacturer. Once the review is completed, it is the active ingredient that is switched rather than the product for which market authorization is sought. Once Health Canada's Therapeutic Products Directorate has completed its review and approved the ingredient for nonprescription status, the ingredient must then be removed from Schedule F of the Food and Drug Regulations before the product can be marketed. Before this happens, the public's opinion is sought through the *Canada Gazette* process. The *Canada Gazette* is an official newspaper of the government of Canada in which all laws and Orders-in-Council issued by the government are published. The *Canada Gazette* process typically takes 14 to 24 months from proposing a

BOX 7-1

Criteria for Over-the-Counter Status

I: Indications for Use

The consumer must be able to easily
• Diagnose condition
• Monitor effectiveness

II: Safety Profile

The drug should have
• Favourable adverse event profile
• Limited drug-interaction profile
• Low potential for misuse

III: Practicality for Over-the-Counter Use

The drug should be
• Easy to use
• Easy to monitor

regulatory amendment to removing the ingredient from Schedule F. Although this procedure has been criticized as overly time consuming, it is structured to ensure that products classified to OTC status are safe and effective when used by the average consumer.

Over the past few years in Canada, a number of drugs have been switched to OTC status (see Box 7-2). For example, vaginal antifungals, nonsedating antihistamines, and H_2 receptor antagonists are now available without a prescription, as is the nicotine patch. The OTC H_2 receptor antagonists are at a lower dose than the prescription version and the higher dose is still available by prescription.

OTC status has many advantages over prescription status. Patients can conveniently and effectively self-treat many minor ailments. Some professionals argue that allowing patients to self-treat minor illnesses enables physicians to spend more time caring for patients with serious health problems. Others argue that it delays patients from seeking medical care until they are quite ill. The financial effect of this status change is enormous.

Reclassifying a prescription drug to an OTC drug may increase out-of-pocket costs for many patients. The reason for this is that most third-party health insurance plans will not pay for OTC products. However, overall health care costs tend to decrease when reclassification occurs because of a direct reduction in drug costs, elimination of physician office visits, and avoidance of pharmacy dispensing fees. For example, one study, conducted by the Queen's Health Policy of Queen's University in Kingston, Ontario in 1994 cited by the Nonprescription Drug Manufacturers Association of Canada (1995) investigated the impact of the switch from prescription to nonprescription status of nonsedating antihistamines. The conclusion was that this switch saved the health care system $16 million, including $12 million in the reduction of office visits to doctors and the elimination of the

pharmacy dispensing fee. Interestingly, the study also found no change in health outcomes. Because it is the active ingredient rather than the brand that gets changed to OTC status in Canada, manufacturers do not benefit as they do in the United States from prolonged market exclusivity without generic competition. This difference allows competing manufacturers to also market their drugs as OTC once approval is gained via Health Canada. In addition, all clinical data are on public record for 12 months, which provides competitor access to the proprietary details, leading to the immediate introduction of private-label OTC drugs.

The importance of patient education cannot be overstated. Many patients are inexperienced in interpreting medication labels, which results in misuse of the products (Figure 7-1). The lack of experience and possibly deficient knowledge about the medications may lead to adverse events or drug interactions with prescription medications, other OTC medications, or natural health products. Another common problem associated with OTC drugs is that their use may postpone effective

BOX 7-2

Reclassified OTC Products

Analgesics

acetaminophen, codeine 8 mg, caffeine (Tylenol No.1)
acetylsalicylic acid, codeine 8 mg, caffeine (222, A. C. & C)
ibuprofen (Advil, Motrin)

Histamine Blockers

H_1 Receptor Antagonists
cetirizine (Aller-Relief, Reactine)
chlorpheniramine maleate (Advil Cold & Sinus, Chlor-Tripolon)
clemastine (Tavist)
desloratadine (Aerius)
diphenhydramine (Allerdyl, Benadryl)
fexofenadine (Allegra-D)
loratine (Claritin)

H_2 Receptors
famotidine (Pepsid)
ranitidine (Zantac)

Mast Cell Stabilizers

cromolyn sodium (Rhinaris) nasal mist

Smoking Deterrents

nicotine gum (Nicorette)
nicotine transdermal patch (Nictrol)

Topical Medications

clotrimazole (Canesten)
miconazole (Micazole)
minoxidil solution and hydrocortisone acetate 1% cream (Rogaine, Loniten)

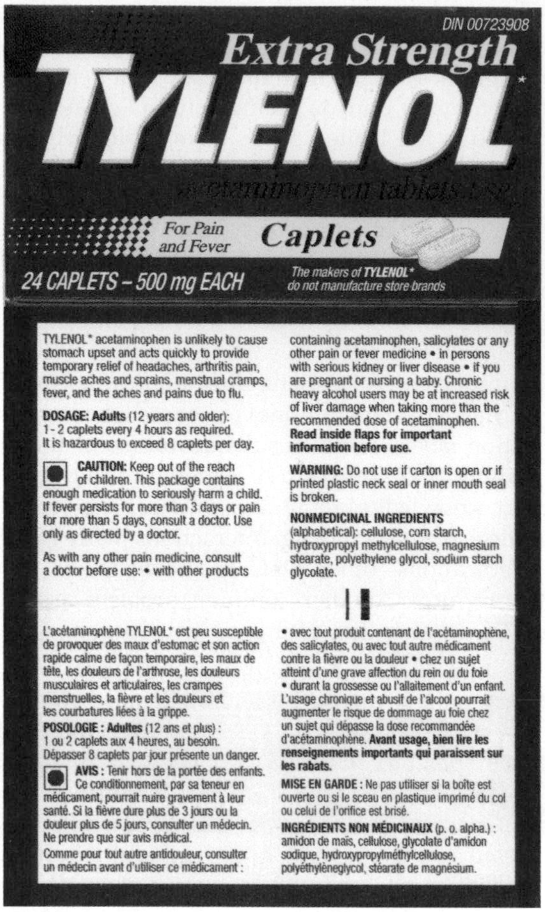

FIG. 7-1 Example of an over-the-counter (OTC) drug label. Reproduced by permission of McNeil Consumer Healthcare. All rights reserved.

management of serious or life-threatening disorders. The OTC medication may relieve symptoms without necessarily addressing the cause of the disorder.

Normally, OTC medications should be used only for short-term treatment of common minor illnesses. An appropriate medical evaluation should be sought for all chronic health conditions, even if the final decision is to prescribe OTC medications. Patient assessment

should definitely include questions regarding OTC drug use, including what conditions OTC medications are being used to treat. Such questions may help uncover more serious ongoing medical problems that require further evaluation. Patients should be informed that OTC medications, including natural health products (NHPs), are still medications. Because of this, their use may have associated risks depending on the specific OTC drugs used, concurrent prescription medications, and the patient's overall health status and disease states.

Health care providers have an excellent opportunity to prevent common problems associated with the use of reclassified drugs. Up to 60% of patients consult a health care provider when selecting an OTC product. Patients should be provided with verbal information about choice of an appropriate product, correct dosing, common adverse effects, and drug interactions with other medications For specific information on OTC drugs, see the appropriate drug chapters later in this text (see Table 7-1 for a cross-reference to these chapters).

NATURAL HEALTH PRODUCTS

Regulation and Types of Natural Health Products

Canadians use natural health products in many forms. Under the Natural Health Products Regulations, **natural health products (NHPs)** are defined as vitamin and mineral supplements, herbal remedies, homeopathic preparations, traditional Chinese, Ayurvedic, and other traditional medicines, probiotics, and other products such as amino acids and essential fatty acids. The effectiveness of natural health products is often supported by traditional use and anecdotal reports. More recently, this anecdotal evidence is being measured by science. Many controversies remain about the safety and the control of natural health products. They are freely available in Canada and their uses and advantages are widely publicized. These products are marketed and placed in grocery stores, pharmacies, health food stores, and fitness gyms and can even be ordered through television and radio ads

TABLE 7-1

Common OTC Drugs Discussed in This Book

Type of OTC Drug	Examples	Where Discussed in This Book
Acid-controlling agents (H_2 blockers) and antacids	famotidine (Pepsid), ranitidine (Zantac); aluminum- and magnesium-containing products (Maalox, Mylanta), calcium-containing products (Tums)	Chapter 52: Acid-Controlling Drugs
Antifungal agents (topical)	clotrimazole (Canesten), miconazole (Monistat)	Chapter 57: Dermatological Drugs
Antihistamines and decongestants	diphenhydramine hydrochloric acid (HCl) (Benadryl), loratadine (Claritin), desloratidine (Aerius), pseudoephedrine HCl (Sudafed)	Chapter 36: Antihistamines, Decongestants, Antitussives, and Expectorants
Eye drops	Artificial tears (Murine)	Chapter 58: Ophthalmic Drugs
Hair growth drugs (topical)	minoxidil (Rogaine)	Chapter 57: Dermatological Drugs
Pain-relieving drugs (analgesics)	acetaminophen (Tylenol)	Chapter 11: Analgesic Drugs
Pain-relieving drugs (NSAIDs)	aspirin, ibuprofen (Advil, Motrin)	Chapter 45: Anti-Inflammatory, Antiarthritic, and Related Drugs

and over the Internet. With greater use, their therapeutic effects have been acknowledged, and they have been believed by some to be more beneficial than existing synthetic and natural prescription drugs. Adverse effects are considered to be minimal by the public as well as by the companies and businesses that sell these supplements. A false sense of security has been created by their widespread use, however, and the view of the public tends to be that if a product is "natural," then it is safe.

The language surrounding natural health products can be confusing, so a brief discussion of the forms and history of natural health products follows. **Herbs** come from nature and include the leaves, bark, berries, roots, gums, seeds, stems, and flowers of plants. They have been used for thousands of years to help maintain good health. The many different herbs that make up these herbal remedies contain a wide variety of active **phytochemicals** (plant compounds). Herbs have been an integral part of society because of their culinary and medicinal properties. **Herbal medicine** has made many contributions to commercial drug preparations that are currently manufactured (Table 7-2). About 30% of all modern drugs are derived from plants.

In the early nineteenth century, scientific methods became more advanced and became preferred. At this time, the practice of botanical healing was dismissed as quackery. Herbal medicine lost ground to new synthetic medicines as the development of patent medicines took off in the early part of the twentieth century. These new synthetically derived medicines were hailed by scientists and physicians as being more effective and reliable.

Dietary supplement is a broad term for orally administered alternative medicines and includes the category of herbal supplement. Basic definitions are provided here to ensure complete understanding and to prevent confusion in how these terms are used. *Dietary supplements* are products taken by mouth that contain ingredients intended to augment the diet; they include vitamins, minerals, herbs or other botanicals, amino acids, and substances such as enzymes, organ tissues, glandular products, metabolites, extracts, and concentrates. Dietary supplements may also be extracts or concentrates and may be produced in many forms, such as tablets, capsules, softgels, gelcaps, liquids, or powders. These supplements may also be found in nutritional, breakfast, snack, or health food bars and drinks or shakes. Labelling must be provided but must *not* represent the product as a conventional food item.

Probiotics are a type of dietary supplement defined by the Natural Health Products Regulations as a "monoculture or mixed-culture of live microorganisms that benefit the microbiota indigenous to humans. A probiotic is limited to nonpathogenic microorganisms." One example is *Lactobacillus acidophilus*. The normal human digestive tract contains about 400 types of probiotic bacteria that reduce the growth of harmful bacteria and promote a healthy digestive system. Probiotic knowledge was brought into popular scientific awareness by a Russian researcher in the early 1900s. More recently, the use of probiotics has gained popularity. The largest group of probiotic bacteria in the intestine is lactic acid bacteria, of which *Lactobacillus acidophilus*, found in yogurt, is the best known. Yeast is also a probiotic substance. In Canada, the majority of probiotic products have not been clinically tested. It has been suggested that probiotics be used to treat conditions such as inflammatory bowel disease and the diarrhea that results from antibiotic use.

Prebiotics are carbohydrates that may help to stimulate and support the intestinal bacteria. Examples of prebiotics are flora soybeans, artichokes, jicama, raw oats, unrefined wheat and barley, and breast milk.

In the 1960s, concerns were expressed over the **iatrogenic effects** (i.e., unintentional adverse effects) of **conventional medicine** (that taught in the West). These concerns, along with a desire for more self-reliance, led to a renewed interest in "natural health," and as a result, the use of natural health products, including the use of herbal products, increased. In 1974, the World Health Organization encouraged developing countries to use traditional plant medicines to "fulfill a need unmet by modern systems" (Winslow & Kroll, 1998). In 1978, the German equivalent of Health Canada published a series of herb recommendations known as the **Commission E Monographs** (Blumenthal, Goldberg, & Busse, 2001). These monographs focus on herbs whose effectiveness is supported by the research literature. Worldwide use of natural health products, in particular herbal medicines, again became popular. Recognition of the rising use of herbal medicines and other nontraditional remedies, known as **alternative medicine**, led to the establishment in the U.S. by the National Institutes of Health of the Office of Alternative Medicine in 1992. This office was later renamed the National Center for Complementary and Alternative Medicine (NCCAM). **Complementary medicine** refers to the simultaneous use of both traditional and alternative medicine. NCCAM classifies complementary and alternative medicine into five categories: (1) alternative medical systems; (2) mind–body interventions; (3) biologically based therapies; (4) manipulative and body-based methods; and (5) energy therapies.

TABLE 7-2

Conventional Medicines Derived From Plants

Medicine*	Plant
acetylsalicylic acid	*Salix alba*
atropine	*Atropa belladonna*
capsaicin	*Capsicum frutescens*
cocaine	*Erythroxylon coca*
codeine, morphine	*Papaver somniferum*
digoxin	*Digitalis purpurea*
quinine	*Cinchona officinalis*
reserpine	*Rauwolfia serpentina*
scopolamine	*Datura fastuosa*
senna	*Cassia acutifolia*
paclitaxel	*Taxus brevifolia*
vincristine	*Catharanthus roseus*

*Includes both over-the-counter and prescription drugs.

Concerns over the accessibility and regulation of all natural health products led the Health Canada Directorate to establish the Advisory Panel on Natural Health in 1997. After consultations with interested stakeholders, the Minister of Health tabled *Natural Health Products: A New Vision*, which provided the framework for the development of the Office of Natural Health Products. This office would later be renamed the Natural Health Products Directorate (NHPD). The NHPD's role is "to ensure that Canadians have ready access to natural health products that are safe, effective and of high quality while respecting freedom of choice and philosophical and cultural diversity"(NHPD, 2009). In 2004, the Natural Health Products Regulations came into effect. Manufacturers must obtain a product license from Health Canada to sell their products in Canada. If the product meets the NHPD criteria, then a Natural Product Number will be issued. The Licensed Natural Health Products Database (LNHPD), managed by Health Canada, provides information on licensed natural health products. These include vitamin and mineral supplements, herb and plant-based remedies, traditional medicines (such as traditional Chinese medicines or Ayurvedic [Indian] medicines), omega-3 and essential fatty acids, probiotics and homeopathic medicines, and many everyday consumer products, such as certain toothpastes, antiperspirants, shampoos, facial products, and mouthwashes. This database can be accessed at http://www.hc-sc.gc.ca/dhp-mps/prodnatur/applications/licen-prod/lnhpd-bdpsnh-eng.php.

Homeopathic medicines (HMs) receive a Drug Identification Number (DIN)-HM followed by a product number. Extensive product labelling must meet specific requirements regarded as essential to risk management. On the basis of information from the World Health Organization, the European Scientific Cooperative on Phytotherapy, and the German Commission E, the NHPD developed the **Compendium of Monographs**. The NHPD classifies natural health products into six risk categories from highest to lowest (see Box 7-3). The risk classification scheme is an "evidence-based approach that classifies a product into a level of risk based on relevant information from published and unpublished sources such as, but not limited to, journals, textbooks, or reports from regulatory bodies" (Health Canada, 2007). The regulations also impose standard labelling requirements to ensure that consumers can make informed choices about natural health products. Labels contain such things as the product name, the quantity of the product in the bottle, and the recommended conditions for use, which include recommended use or purpose and dose, warnings, cautionary statements, contraindications, and possible adverse reactions. With such regulations, Canada, like Germany, France, and the United Kingdom, enforces standards for the assessment of natural-product quality and safety.

Consumer Use of Natural Health Products

A 2005 Health Canada survey showed that 71% of Canadians regularly take NHPs in the forms of vitamins and minerals, herbal products, and homeopathic medicines. Thirty-eight percent use NHPs on a daily basis, with 37% usage during certain seasons or weekly (11%). Individuals often select NHPs to gain more control over and positively influence their health. Most Canadians associate NHPs with vitamins and minerals, herbal remedies and teas, additive-free foods, organic foods, and plants or plant products. When used appropriately, NHPs can be an integral part of an individual's health management. Other NHPs may be used to treat minor conditions and illnesses (e.g., coughs, colds, stomach upset) in much the same manner as conventional OTC drugs approved under the Food and Drugs Regulations. As the number of NHPs in the market increases, nurses will have more opportunities for patient education about these products.

Safety

Complementary and alternative medicines (CAMs) can benefit from a strong research base from which evidence-informed practice and research may be derived. As mentioned previously, natural health products, especially herbal medicines, are often perceived as being natural and therefore harmless; however, this is not always the case. Any substance, whether natural or synthetic, that has an effect on the body has the potential to be a risk to health. Because of underreporting, present knowledge may represent but a small fraction of potential safety concerns. Children, pregnant or breastfeeding women, the older adult, those diagnosed with a serious disease, or those scheduled for an operation are particularly susceptible to risk.

BOX 7-3

Risk Classification of Natural Health Products

High Risk

- Level 1: Natural health products on the Therapeutic Products Directorate's listing of drugs currently regulated as new drugs
- Level 2: Isolates, amino acids, fatty acids, concentrated volatile (essential) oils indicated for internal use, and extracts other than those prepared by traditional methods
- Level 3: Algal, bacterial, probiotic, fungal, and non-human animal materials
- Level 4: Plants, plant materials, extracts prepared by traditional methods, and volatile (essential) oils other than those concentrated and indicated for internal use
- Level 5: Vitamins and minerals
- Level 6: Homeopathic medicines

Low Risk

Source: Health Canada (2003b). Natural health products regulations. Note: Review of risk classification to be finalized pending revisions from the HPFB (Risk Classification) Working Group.

Some herbs have been shown to have possible mutagenic effects and to interact with drugs (see Natural Health Products and Their Possible Drug Interactions). Recent examples of some of the growing concerns with herbal remedies include Health Canada warnings about possible liver toxicity with the use of kava and possible cardiovascular and stroke risks with the use of ephedra. In July 2005, Health Canada warned consumers to avoid the use of certain Ayurvedic medicinal products because they contain high levels of heavy metals such as lead, mercury, and arsenic. As a result, of knowing that there are potential risks associated with the use of natural health products, the public attitude is beginning to change.

Goldman, Rogovik, Lai, and Vohra (2008) investigated the use of NHPs with medications in children arriving at an emergency department of a large children's hospital in Canada. The researchers interviewed 1804 families and found that one in five children was administered medications concurrent with NHPs and 15% were receiving more than one NHP simultaneously. The researchers estimated that 16% of the children had taken a combination of medication and NHP that could result in pharmacodynamic or pharmacokinetic interactions. Eight percent of the cohort had more than one pair of possible medication–NHP or NHP–NHP interactions.

Although still in the beginning stages, there is a body of evidence on NHP–medication interactions that is rapidly developing. The Canadian Interdisciplinary Network for CAM Research (IN-CAM) is a new research community established by Dr. Heather Boon, a pharmacist and medical sociologist at the University of Toronto's Faculty of Pharmacy with an interest in CAM, and Dr. Marja Verhoef, a social scientist and epidemiologist who holds a Canada Research Chair in Complementary Medicine at the University of Calgary's Department of Community Health Sciences. To address the gaps that exist in the CAM evidence base, IN-CAM's mission is to "create a sustainable, well-connected, highly trained Complementary and Alternative Medicine (CAM) research community in Canada that is internationally recognized and known for both its excellence in research and its contributions to understanding CAM and its use" (Canadian Interdisciplinary Network for Complementary & Alternative Medicine Research, 2009). The National Center for Complementary and Alternative Medicine/National Institutes of Health (NCCAM/NIH) and the International Society for Complementary Medicine Research (ISCMR) are other organizations involved in generating high-quality research. In

NATURAL HEALTH PRODUCTS

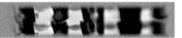

NATURAL HEALTH PRODUCTS AND THEIR POSSIBLE DRUG INTERACTIONS

Natural Health Product	Possible Drug Interaction
Chamomile	Increased risk for bleeding with anticoagulants
Cranberry	Decreased elimination of many drugs excreted by the kidneys
Echinacea	Possible interference with or counteraction to immunosuppressant drugs
Evening primrose	Possible interaction with antipsychotic drugs
Garlic	Possible interference with hypoglycemic therapy
	Alters bleeding time of warfarin
Ginger root	At high dosages, possible interference with heart, antidiabetic, or anticoagulant drugs
Grapefruit	Increases blood levels of some calcium channel blockers (e.g., felodipine, nimodipine, verapamil), which can result in an increase in the effect and adverse effects of these drugs
	Increases blood levels and absorption of some statins (atorvastatin, lovastatin and simvastatin, and ezetimibe/simvastatin)
	Decreases metabolism of drugs used for erectile dysfunction
	Decreases metabolism of estrogens, some psychotherapeutic drugs (sertraline)
	Increases risk of toxicity of immunosuppressants and of some psychotherapeutic drugs (pimozide, escitalopram)
	Increases intensity and duration of effects of caffeine
Hawthorn	May lead to toxic levels of cardiac glycosides (e.g., digitalis)
Kava	May increase the effect of barbiturates and alcohol
Saw palmetto	May change the effects of hormones in oral contraceptive drugs, patches, or hormonal replacement therapies
St. John's wort	If other serotonergic drugs are also used (such as selective serotonin reuptake inhibitors), may lead to serotonin syndrome
Valerian	Increases central nervous system depression if used with sedatives

Modified from Mertens-Talcott, S. U., Zadezensky, I., De Castro, W. V., Derendorf, H., & Butterweck, V. (2006). Grapefruit–drug interactions: Can interactions with drugs be avoided? *Journal of Clinical Pharmacology, 46*(12), 1390–1416; Skalli, S., Zaid, A., & Soulaymani, R. (2007). Drug interactions with herbal medicines. *Therapeutic Drug Monitoring, 29*(6), 679–686; McCloskey, W. W., Zaiken, K., & Couris, R. R. (2008). Clinically significant grapefruit juice–drug interactions. *Nutrition Today, 43*(1), 19–28.

addition, journals such as *Evidence-Based Complementary and Alternative Medicine* (eCAM) and *The Journal of Alternative and Complementary Medicine* provide researchers with a peer-reviewed forum in which to publish their findings. It is important that this trend continue, as one of the criticisms levelled at CAM is the lack of evidence for efficacy.

Health care providers should be aware of literature about the safe and effective use of herbal remedies and reported adverse effects. For some herbal remedies the risk may be less than that for conventional drugs. The discriminate and proper use of some herbal products is safe and may provide some therapeutic benefits, but the indiscriminate or excessive use of herbs can be unsafe and even dangerous. In order to improve the NHP vigilance system, several initiatives have been put in place by Health Canada that are available to both consumers and health care providers. The Canada Vigilance Program maintains an online database of suspected adverse reactions submitted by both consumers and health care providers. The database provides information only. MedEffect e-Notice is a free e-mail service that provides advisories, warnings, and recalls for health products that Canadians use. Also available is the *Canadian Adverse Reaction Newsletter*, published quarterly, with facts and safety information about marketed health products and reported adverse reactions that are suspected to be associated with specific health products. To identify and track serious and life-threatening reactions associated with natural health products in children there is a Canadian pediatric surveillance program. In addition, Health

Canada maintains a public information Web site, *It's Your Health,* to reinforce the safe use of natural health products. Specific natural health products are discussed in greater detail in the Natural Health Products boxes that appear in various chapters on specific drugs (see the inside back cover for a complete listing of these special-feature boxes with page numbers).

Medical Use of Marihuana

Marihuana is an herb with a long history of use for its therapeutic and medicinal qualities. In Canada, marihuana remains an illegal and controlled substance. In 2003, Health Canada implemented the **Marihuana Medical Access Regulations** to allow access to and possession of marihuana for individuals suffering from specific grave and debilitating illnesses. Marihuana seeds and dried product are made available to those authorized to use marihuana for medicinal purposes from a company under contract to Health Canada. Marihuana is produced for clinical trials to determine the safety and efficacy of marihuana for medical purposes. However, in January 2008, a Federal Court judge declared the Marihuana Medical Access Regulations invalid because they limited licensed producers to growing marihuana for only one patient. This was deemed a violation of the charter rights of patients and their ability to rightfully access the drug. In April 2009, Health Canada appealed the ruling but this was denied. See Box 7-4 for discussion of the use of marihuana (also known as *cannabis*) for medical purposes.

BOX 7-4 | Cannabis

Cannabis sativa, or cannabis from the hemp plant, is widely used for recreational purposes. After tobacco, it is the most frequently smoked substance worldwide. Cannabinoids are the psychoactive ingredients of marihuana, of which $1-\Delta^9$-trans-tetrahydrocannabinol (THC), concentrated in the bud of the female plant, is the main psychoactive substance. When marihuana is smoked, the effect is almost immediate and lasts for 1 to 3 hours. THC is absorbed by most tissues and organs in the body; however, it is primarily found in fat tissues. The body attempts to eliminate the foreign chemical by chemically transforming THC into metabolites. THC metabolites can be found in the urine for up to 1 week after smoking marihuana. THC acts on cannabinoid receptors on brain cells and triggers a series of chemical reactions that ultimately lead to the "high" that users experience. Cannabinoid receptors are found in areas of the brain that influence pleasure, memory, thought, concentration, sensory and time perception, and coordinated movement. There is evidence that THC acts on neurotransmitters and exerts either excitatory or inhibitory effects.

While there is sociopolitical concern around the medical use of marihuana and the clinical therapeutic potential

for marihuana has not yet been proven in controlled clinical trials beyond 6 weeks, there is anecdotal evidence that marihuana may be beneficial in a variety of disorders. In Canada, there are four cannabinoid products available for medical use. Three cannabinoids are available by prescription. One product is *Cannabis sativa* L. extract (Sativex), a buccal spray, which has been issued marketing authorization on the basis of promising clinical evidence for use as an adjunctive treatment for neuropathic pain in adults with multiple sclerosis and as adjunctive analgesic treatment in adult patients with advanced cancer. A synthetic derivative of dronabinol (Marinol) is available in capsules for AIDS-related anorexia associated with weight loss, as well as for severe nausea and vomiting associated with cancer chemotherapy. The third product, nabilone (Cesamet), is a synthetic derivative of THC and is available in capsules for severe nausea and vomiting associated with chemotherapy. The medical use of the herbal form of cannabis for smoking is available through the Medical Marihuana Access Regulations. It is estimated that over 2200 patients are legally authorized to use herbal cannabis for medical purposes; however, only approximately 20% access the government-endorsed supplier.

NURSING PROCESS

Assessment

 ### Over-the-Counter Drugs

Assessment of patients taking any type of OTC drugs should include consideration of allergies to any of the ingredients. A medication history must be taken that documents *all* medications and substances used (including prescription drugs, OTC drugs, natural health products such as vitamins and minerals, and alcohol and tobacco). Also needed is a past and present medical history so that possible drug interactions, contraindications, and cautions may be identified. Patients should be screened carefully before an OTC drug is recommended because patients may assume that if a drug is sold OTC then it must be completely safe and without negative consequences. This assumption is not true; OTC drugs can be just as lethal or problematic as prescription drugs if they are not taken properly or are taken in high dosages and without regard to product directions. Consumer safety begins with education. The preferred way for patients to help themselves as consumers is for them to learn how to assess each situation, weigh all the factors, and find out all they can about any OTC product they consider using.

Although complete nursing assessments should be performed, this may be difficult to carry out as in many situations the patient is self-medicating. The nurse should be aware of ethnocultural factors that could affect patient assessment (see Ethnocultural Implications: Ethnocultural Factors and Drug Responses). Reading level, cognitive level, motor abilities, previous use of OTC drugs, successes and failures with drug therapies and self-medication, and caregiver support are just a few of the variables to be assessed as the nurse deems appropriate.

Assessment of a patient's knowledge about the components of self-medication, including the positive and negative consequences of the use of a given OTC drug, is important to carry out. Determination of the patient's (or caregiver's or family member's) level of knowledge and experience with OTC self-medication is critical to the patient's safety, as is assessment of attitudes toward and beliefs about drug therapy, such as having an attitude that is too casual or a lack of respect for and concern about the use of OTC drugs. Such beliefs can result in overuse, overdosage, and potential complications. The patient's level of readiness and developmental stage must also be assessed to tailor individualized teaching.

Generally speaking, laboratory tests are not ordered before OTC drugs are taken because OTC drugs are self-administered and self-monitored. However, there are situations in which patients may be taking certain medications that react adversely with OTC drugs and such testing may be deemed necessary. Certain patient groups are also at higher risk for adverse reactions to OTC drugs (as well as to all drugs), such as the older adult, children, patients with single or multiple acute and chronic illnesses, those who are frail or in poor health, debilitated and nutritionally deficient patients,

---

ETHNOCULTURAL IMPLICATIONS

Ethnocultural Factors and Drug Responses

Responses to drugs, including over-the-counter (OTC) drugs and natural health products, may be affected by beliefs, values, and genetic factors as well as by ethnoculture and race. For example, Japanese patients experiencing nausea, vomiting, and bowel changes as adverse effects of OTC drugs or natural health products often do not mention these effects. In this ethnoculture it is unacceptable to complain about gastrointestinal symptoms, thus symptoms may go unreported to the point of causing risk to the patient.

Natural health products, specifically herbal and alternative therapies, may also be used more extensively in some ethnocultures than in others. Wide acceptance of herbal use without major concern for the effects on other therapies may be problematic because of the many interactions of conventional drugs with herbs and dietary supplements. For example, the Chinese herb ginseng may inhibit or accelerate the metabolism of a specific medication and significantly affect the drug's absorption or elimination.

Genetic factors having an influence on drug response include acetylation polymorphism—that is, prescription drugs, OTC drugs, and natural health products may be metabolized in different ways that are genetically determined and that vary with race or ethnicity. The way in which ethnicity affects drug response is challenging because of the many variations that exist within ethnocultural groups. For example, European or African populations have approximately equal numbers of individuals showing rapid or slow acetylation (which affects drug metabolism), whereas Japanese and Inuit populations may contain more rapid acetylators. Chinese and Japanese patients are more likely to respond favourably to codeine than are European patients. In addition, factors such as diet and the use of tobacco can influence the expression of a gene, which can consequently alter a drug's effect.

Modified from Munoz, C., & Hilgenberg, C. (2006). Ethnopharmacology: Understanding how ethnicity can affect drug response is essential to providing culturally competent care. *Holistic Nursing Practice, 105*(8), 40–49.

and those who are immunocompromised. Other groups for whom there may be cautions and contraindications for OTC drug use are patients with a history of kidney, liver, heart, or vascular disorders. More assessment information for OTC drugs and natural health products is provided in chapters that have corresponding drug and pharmacology content (see Table 7-1). The patient should be aware of contraindications, cautions, and drug interactions.

Natural Health Products

Many natural health products, including herbs, probiotics, and dietary supplements, are readily available in drug, health food, and grocery stores as well as in gardens, kitchens, and medicine cabinets. The most commonly used herbal and dietary supplements discussed in this book are aloe, echinacea, garlic, ginkgo, ginseng, St. John's wort, saw palmetto, and valerian. Although patients generally self-administer these products and do not perform an assessment, in various settings the nurse may be able to assess the patient through a head-to-toe physical examination, medical and nursing history, and medication history. Assessment data as well as factors and variables to consider should be shared with the patient for the patient's safety. Through this sharing of assessment information, the health care provider can be more confident that the patient who is taking any natural health products is taking them in as safe a manner as possible. Many natural health products can potentially cause a variety of adverse effects. For example, some products cause dermatitis when used topically and others are associated with nephritis. Therefore, patients with existing skin problems or renal dysfunction, for example, should seek medical advice before using certain herbal products. Contraindications, cautions, and drug interactions should be considered by the patient and nurse. See the Natural Health Products box on page 99 for potential drug interactions with specific herbal products and dietary supplements.

Nursing Diagnoses

Nursing diagnoses appropriate for the patient who is taking an OTC drug or natural health product include the following:
- Acute pain related to disease processes
- Persistent pain related to tissue injury
- Impaired physical mobility related to disease processes or injury
- Deficient knowledge related to first-time drug therapy with OTC drugs or natural health products

- Risk for injury related to potential drug interactions and adverse reactions of OTC drugs and natural health products
- Risk for injury related to possible nicotine withdrawal (applies to patients using a smoking deterrent system)

Planning

Goals

- Patient will describe use of the drug in relation to symptoms or complaints.
- Patient will experience pain relief or relief of symptoms of the disease process or injury within the expected time period.
- Patient will report both adverse effects and therapeutic responses to the appropriate health care provider.
- Patient will state the rationale for and proper use of the drug.
- Patient will state the adverse effects, cautions, and contraindications associated with use of the drug.
- Patient will have minimal complaints and experience minimal adverse effects related to use of the drug.
- Patient will remain free from injury caused by improper use of the drug.
- Patient will avoid adverse effects from improper self-administration (e.g., is able to properly apply a transdermal patch).

Outcome Criteria

- Patient states the actions of the OTC drug or natural health product as well as a method to minimize adverse effects and enhance therapeutic effects.
- Patient identifies factors that aggravate or alleviate symptoms for which the drug is being taken.
- Patient describes nonpharmacological approaches to the treatment of symptoms, such as the use of hot or cold packs, physical therapy, massage, relaxation therapy, biofeedback, imagery, and hypnosis.
- Patient states the importance of immediately reporting any severe adverse effects or complications associated with the OTC drug or natural health product, such as changes in blood pressure, clotting, or lack of clotting.
- Patient experiences relief of symptoms (the actual indication for the use of the OTC drug or natural health product) such as a decrease in itching, pain, swelling, cold symptoms, or cough.
- Patient takes the OTC drug or natural health product as indicated, using proper dosage and technique (using no more than is directed), and knows to stop medication if certain untoward effects occur.

- Patient contacts health care provider or local poison control hotline should toxicity or complications occur.
- Patient demonstrates correct technique for using the transdermal route or any other route of administration, including the specific steps required.

Implementation

The most important determinant of safe patient self-administration with OTC drugs is whether the patient receives thorough and individualized patient education. Patients need to receive as much information as possible and should understand that, although these drugs are nonprescription, they are *not* completely safe and without toxicity. Instructions should include information about safe use, dose and frequency of dosing specifics of how to take the medication (e.g., with food or at bedtime), and steps the patient may take to prevent complications and toxic effects. Another consideration is the dosage form, because a variety of dosage forms are available, from liquids, tablets, and enteric-coated tablets to patches and gum. Instructions must be provided and the need to recheck dosage emphasized. With many of the patches used today for smoking cessation and for other indications, it is crucial to emphasize the proper use and application of the transdermal patch systems. For patients using natural health products (as with other OTC medications), education is of utmost importance for safe and effective use. The health care provider must inform the patient that Health Canada now requires the manufacturers of all natural health products, including herbal remedies, to provide evidence of safety and effectiveness. Unfortunately, many patients believe that no risks exist if a medication is herbal and "natural." It is important for patients to realize that even if a product is natural, it must be taken as cautiously as any other medication. Health Canada requires standard labelling of all natural health products with the product name, the quantity of product in the bottle, recommended conditions of use (including such things as its recommended use or purpose, dosage form, route of administration, recommended dose, and any cautionary statements, warnings, contraindications, and possible adverse reactions associated with the product), as well as any special storage conditions. The fact that a drug is a natural health product does not mean that it can be safely administered to children, infants, pregnant or lactating women, or patients with certain health conditions that put them at risk.

Evaluation

Patients taking OTC drugs or natural health products should carefully monitor themselves for unusual or adverse reactions and therapeutic responses to the medication to prevent overuse. The range of therapeutic responses will vary, depending on the specific drug and the indication for which it is used. These responses may include decreased pain; decreased stiffness and swelling in joints; increased ability to carry out activities of daily living; the ability to move around with more ease; increased hair growth; decreased asthma-related, gastrointestinal, or allergic symptoms; decreased vaginal itching and discharge; increased healing; increased sleep; decreased fatigue; improved energy; and others.

For specific nursing diagnoses, planning, outcome criteria, nursing implementation, and evaluation information related to OTC drugs, see the appropriate drug chapters in this book (see Table 7-1 for cross-references to these chapters).

🌐 IN MY FAMILY

"Spicy" Indian Cures (as told by S.H., of Indian descent)

"Spices are used when medical treatment is not available or in combination with [medical] treatment.
- Tumeric powder is a natural antibiotic.
  - Apply on cuts.
  - Mix with water to make a paste to apply on sprains.
  - Add spice while preparing foods to aid digestion.
  - Mix with milk, saffron, and honey for coughs and colds.

- Fennel seeds are for ulcers and digestion.
- Dill water is for gassy babies.
- Cumin seeds are mixed with yogourt for diarrhea.
- Cinnamon powder is for diabetes.
- Garlic is for cholesterol and heart."

PATIENT EDUCATION

- ❖ Patients should be provided with verbal and written information about how to choose an appropriate over-the-counter (OTC) drug or natural health product (NHP) as well as information about appropriate dosing, common adverse effects, and possible interactions with other medications.
- ❖ Patients should be made aware that Health Canada requires manufacturers of NHPs to provide evidence of safety and effectiveness.
- ❖ Many patients believe that no risks exist if a medication is herbal and "natural" or if it is sold OTC, so patients should be educated about the drug or product as well as all of the pros and cons of its use because this is crucial to patient safety.
- ❖ Patients should be instructed on how to read OTC and NHP labels. Emphasize the importance of taking OTC drugs and NHPs with extreme caution, being aware of all of the possible interactions and concerns associated with the use of these products, and informing all health care providers about their use.
- ❖ Patients should be encouraged to keep a journal of any improvement of symptoms noted with the use of a specific OTC drug or NHP.
- ❖ Patients should be encouraged to use appropriate and authoritative resources for patient information.
- ❖ Patients should be instructed that all medications, whether OTC drug or NHP, or prescription drug, should be kept out of the reach of children and pets.
- ❖ Patients should be provided thorough instructions for the dosage forms of OTC drugs and NHPs, such as how to mix powders and how to properly use transdermal patches, inhalers, ointments, lotions, nose drops, eye drops, elixirs, suppositories, vaginal suppositories or creams, and all other dosage forms (Chapter 10). They should also receive information about proper storage and cleansing of any equipment.

POINTS TO REMEMBER

- ❖ Consumers use natural health products therapeutically as agents for the treatment and cure of diseases and pathological conditions, prophylactically for the long-term prevention of disease, and proactively as agents for the maintenance of health and wellness.
- ❖ Health Canada has established the Canada Vigilance postmarket surveillance program that collects and assesses adverse reaction (AR) reports to NHPs and other drug therapy. Health care providers and consumers may report adverse events anonymously and without consequence. The toll-free number is 1-866-234-2345. Some of the more commonly used herbal remedies are aloe, echinacea, garlic, ginkgo, ginseng, grapefruit extract, grapefruit juice, St. John's wort, saw palmetto, and valerian. The nurse needs to be informed about these products so that adequate patient education can be provided regarding potential risks and adverse drug reactions and so that drug interactions can be prevented or minimized.
- ❖ Natural health products are approved by Health Canada with specific labelling requirements to provide adequate instructions for use and warnings.
- ❖ The fact that a drug is a natural health product or an OTC medication is no guarantee that it can be safely administered to children, infants, pregnant or lactating women, or patients with certain health conditions that may put them at risk.

EXAMINATION REVIEW QUESTIONS

1 When reviewing a list of OTC drugs taken by a patient, the nurse recalls that the most commonly used OTC products currently available include which types of drugs?
   a. Diuretics
   b. Mild antihypertensives
   c. Acid-controlling drugs
   d. Drugs for bladder control

2 Which of the following points concerning natural health products is important for the nurse to communicate to patients?
   a. Natural health and OTC products are not approved by Health Canada and are under strict regulation.
   b. These products are scrutinized for safety and tested repeatedly by Health Canada.
   c. No adverse effects are associated with these agents because they are "natural" and may be purchased without a prescription.
   d. Labelling is not 100% reliable for the provision of proper instructions or warnings, and the products should be taken with caution.

3 When taking a patient's drug history, the nurse asks about use of OTC drugs. The patient responds by saying, "Oh, I frequently take something for my headaches, but I didn't mention it because aspirin is nonprescription." What is the best response from the nurse?
   a. "Aspirin is one of the safest drugs out there."
   b. "That's true, over-the-counter drugs are generally not harmful."
   c. "Although aspirin is over the counter, it is still important to know why you take it, how much you take, and how often."
   d. "We need you to be honest about the drugs you are taking—are there any others that you have not told us about?"

4 When making a home visit to a patient who was recently discharged from the hospital, the nurse notes that she has a small pack over her chest and that the pack has a strong odour. She also is drinking herbal tea. When asked about the pack and the tea, she says, "Oh, my grandmother never used medicines from the doctor. She told me that this plaster and tea were all I would need to fix things." Which of the following responses by the nurse is most appropriate?
   a. "What's in the plaster and the tea? When do you usually use them?"
   b. "You really should listen to what the doctor told you if you want to get better."
   c. "These herbal remedies rarely work, but if you want to use them, then it is your choice."
   d. "It's fine if you want to use this home remedy, as long as you use it with your prescription medicines."

5 Which of the following is true about current legislation regarding natural health products?
   a. Herbals were regulated in the early 1900s in reference to their efficacy and toxicity.
   b. The Natural Health Products Directorate (NHPD) regulates the safety, efficacy, and quality of natural health products.
   c. The Marihuana Medical Access Regulations allow access to and possession of marihuana for individuals.
   d. The NHPD was specifically designed to encourage the freedom of choice and philosophical and ethnocultural diversity of natural health products.

For answers see http://evolve.elsevier.com/Canada/Lilley/pharmacology/.

CRITICAL THINKING ACTIVITIES

1 Is the following statement true or false? Provide a rationale for your answer.
   OTC drugs and natural health products may be safely taken in the recommended amounts without concern for adverse effects.

2 Explain how the current laws regulating OTC medications have evolved.

3 Discuss important points to include when teaching patients about analgesia and use of OTC products for pain control at home.

4 Your neighbour, who tells you that he has been taking warfarin, a "blood thinner," for several months, calls you to ask your opinion about taking ginkgo to prevent memory loss. He says his sister uses it and it "works wonders." He also thinks it is safe because he can buy it at the local grocery store. What should you tell him? (You may need to look up the drug warfarin and the product ginkgo elsewhere in the text.)

For answers see http://evolve.elsevier.com/Canada/Lilley/pharmacology/.

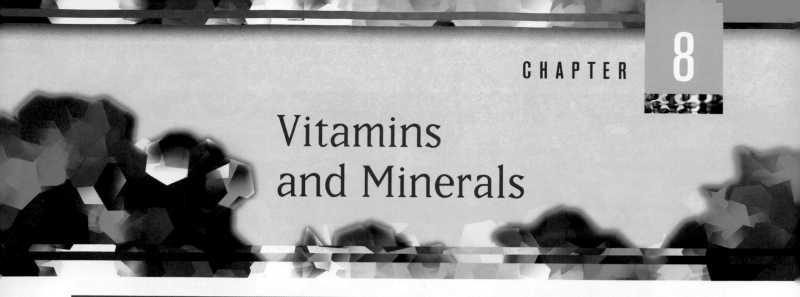

CHAPTER 8

Vitamins and Minerals

Learning Objectives

After reading this chapter, the successful student will be able to do the following:

1 Discuss the importance of vitamins and minerals to the normal functioning of the human body.

2 Briefly describe the disease states, conditions, and acute or chronic illnesses that may lead to imbalances with vitamins and minerals.

3 Discuss the pathologies that result from vitamin and mineral imbalances.

4 Discuss the treatment of these vitamin and mineral imbalances.

5 Identify mechanisms of action, indications, cautions, contraindications, drug interactions, dosages, recommended daily allowances (RDAs), and routes of administration associated with each of the vitamins and minerals.

6 Develop a collaborative plan of care encompassing all phases of the nursing process related to the use of vitamins and minerals.

e-Learning Activities

Web site
(http://evolve.elsevier.com/Canada/Lilley/pharmacology/)

- Animations
- Answers to chapter questions, activities, and case studies
- Calculators and Category Catchers
- Glossary with audio pronunciations
- IV Therapy and Medication Error Checklists
- Multiple-Choice Review Question quizzes
- Nursing Care Plans
- Online Appendices and Supplements
- WebLinks

Drug Profiles

alfacalcidol (Vitamin D analogue), p. 115
ascorbic acid (vitamin C), p. 123
calcitriol (vitamin D analogue), p. 115
calcium, p. 125
cholecalciferol (vitamin D_3), p. 115
cyanocobalamin (vitamin B_{12}), p. 122
doxercalciferol (vitamin D analogue), p. 115
ergocalciferol (vitamin D_2), p. 115
magnesium, p. 126
niacin (vitamin B_3), p. 120
paricalcitol (vitamin D analogue), p. 115
phosphorus, p. 127
pyridoxine (vitamin B_6), p. 121
riboflavin (vitamin B_2), p. 119
thiamine (vitamin B_1), p. 118
vitamin A, p. 110
vitamin E, p. 116
vitamin K_1, p. 117
zinc, p. 127

Glossary

Beriberi A disease of the peripheral nerves caused by an inability to assimilate thiamine (vitamin B_1). (p. 118)

Coenzyme A nonprotein substance that combines with a protein molecule to form an active enzyme. (p. 107)

Enzyme A specialized protein that catalyzes chemical reactions in organic matter. (p. 107)

Fat-soluble vitamin A vitamin that can be dissolved (i.e., is soluble) in fat. (p. 108)

Mineral An inorganic substance that is ingested and attaches to enzymes or other organic molecules. (p. 107)

Pellagra A disease resulting from a niacin deficiency or a metabolic defect that interferes with the conversion of tryptophan to niacin (vitamin B_3). (p. 118)

Rhodopsin The purple-pigmented compound in the rods of the retina, formed by a protein, opsin, and a derivative of retinol (vitamin A). (p. 109)

Rickets   A condition caused by a vitamin D deficiency. (p. 113)

Scurvy   A condition resulting from an ascorbic acid (vitamin C) deficiency. (p. 123)

Tocopherols   Biologically active chemicals that make up vitamin E compounds. (p. 114)

Vitamin   An organic compound essential in small quantities for normal physiological and metabolic functioning of the body. (p. 107)

Water-soluble vitamin   A vitamin that can be dissolved (i.e., is soluble) in water. (p. 108)

OVERVIEW

For the body to grow and maintain itself, it needs the essential building blocks provided by carbohydrates, fats, and proteins. Vitamins and minerals are needed to efficiently utilize these nutrients. **Vitamins** are organic molecules needed in small quantities for normal metabolism and other biochemical functions, such as growth or repair of tissue. Equally important are **minerals,** inorganic elements, or salts found naturally in the earth. **Enzymes** are proteins secreted by cells; they act as catalysts to induce chemical changes in other substances, but they themselves remain chemically unchanged by the process. A **coenzyme** is a substance that enhances or is necessary for the action of enzymes. Many enzymes are totally useless without the appropriate vitamins and minerals that chemically bind with them and cause them to function properly. Both vitamins and minerals function primarily as coenzymes, binding to enzymes (or other organic molecules) to activate anabolic (tissue-building) processes in the body. This helps regulate many body functions. For example, the collagen, hormone, and enzyme syntheses that are needed to heal wounds require the presence of certain vitamins and minerals. As another example, coenzyme A (CoA) is an important carrier molecule associated with the *citric acid cycle*, one of the body's major energy-producing metabolic reactions. CoA requires pantothenic acid (vitamin B_5), however, to complete its function in the citric acid cycle.

Vitamins and minerals are essential in our lives, whether we make conscious food choices or consume whatever we desire. Under most circumstances, daily requirements of vitamins and minerals are met by ingestion of fluids and regular, balanced meals. Ingesting food helps us maintain adequate stores of essential vitamins and minerals and serves to preserve the intestinal mass and structure, provide chemicals for hormones and enzymes, and prevent harmful overgrowth of bacteria.

Life events can occur that cause acute or chronic deficiencies in vitamins, minerals, electrolytes, and fluids. In these conditions the body requires replacement or supplementation of these nutrients. Excessive loss of vitamins and minerals may be the result of poor dietary intake, an inability to swallow after cancer chemotherapy or radiation, or mental health disorders such as anorexia nervosa. Poor dietary absorption is also attributable to some gastrointestinal malabsorption syndromes. Drug and alcohol misuse are frequently associated with inadequate nutritional intake that warrants vitamin and mineral supplementation.

In this chapter, we discuss vitamins and minerals and their therapeutic effects. Deficiencies in dietary protein, fat, and carbohydrates are also common. These nutrients are discussed in Chapter 55. Because of some of their relatively distinct properties and functions in the body that are related to blood formation, the mineral iron and the vitamin folic acid (vitamin B_9) are discussed separately in Chapter 56.

VITAMINS

Vitamin sources occur naturally in both plant and animal foods. The human body requires vitamins on a daily basis in specific minimum amounts and can obtain them from plant and animal food sources. In some cases, the body synthesizes some of its own vitamin supply. Supplemental amounts of vitamin B complex and vitamin K are synthesized by normal bacterial flora in the gastrointestinal tract. Vitamin D can be synthesized by the skin when exposed to sunlight.

An inadequate diet will cause nutrition-related vitamin deficiencies. As a result of extensive food content studies, in 1942, the Nutrition Division of the federal government in collaboration with the Canadian Council on Nutrition published Canada's Official Food Rules. Based on six food groups, a list of *Recommended Daily Allowances (RDAs)* of essential nutrients was identified. In 1944, the RDAs became Canada's Food Rules. There have since been six revisions of the RDAs, with the latest revision in 1992. A newer published standard is the list of *Dietary Reference Intakes (DRIs)*, published by the National Academy of Sciences (NAS) and the Institute of Medicine (IOM). Whereas the RDAs represented *minimum* nutrient requirements, the DRIs are designed to represent *optimal* nutrient requirements for good health. The *Estimated Average Requirement (EAR)* and the *Tolerable Upper Intake Level (UL)* within the DRIs provide improved tools for use in dietary assessment and planning for individuals and for groups. In Canada, vitamins and minerals are considered natural health products (NHPs) and are governed under the Natural Health Products Regulations. In December 2007, Health Canada required mandatory nutrition labelling for all prepackaged foods. The Nutrition Facts table, the nutrition claims, and the ingredient list provide Canadians with more information to make informed food choices. The *percentage Daily Values (DVs)* are the values that appear on the mandatory labels of commercial food products and indicate what percentage of the DRI for a specific nutrient is met by a single serving of the food product. Information regarding DRIs and nutrition labelling is available at the following Web sites:

- Health Canada Food and Nutrition
  http://www.hc-sc.gc.ca/fn-an/nutrition/reference/table/index-eng.php
- Dietary Reference Intakes for Vitamins
  http://www.hc-sc.gc.ca/fn-an/nutrition/reference/table/ref_vitam_tbl-eng.php
- Nutrition Labelling
  http://www.hc-sc.gc.ca/fn-an/label-etiquet/nutrition/cons/inl_flash-eng.php

Vitamins are classified as either fat or water soluble. **Water-soluble vitamins** can be dissolved in water and are easily excreted in the urine. **Fat-soluble vitamins** are dissolvable in fat and, in contrast to water-soluble vitamins, are not readily excreted in the urine but rather via feces.

Because water-soluble vitamins (the B-complex group and vitamin C) cannot be stored in the body in large amounts over long periods, daily intake is required to prevent the development of deficiencies. Conversely, fat-soluble vitamins (vitamins A, D, E, and K) do not need to be taken daily to maintain good health because they are stored in the liver and fatty tissues in large amounts. Deficiency in these vitamins occurs only after prolonged deprivation from an adequate supply or from disorders that prevent their absorption. Table 8-1 lists fat-soluble and water-soluble vitamins.

One controversial topic related to vitamins is that of nutrient "megadosing," as a strategy both for health promotion and maintenance and for treating illnesses. Some cancer patients elect to use supplemental megadosing of specific nutrients in hopes of strengthening their body's response to more conventional cancer treatments, such as surgery, radiation, and chemotherapy. Megadosing is considered doses of a nutrient that are 10 or more times the customary recommended amount. A related term was coined in 1968 by the Nobel prize–winning chemist Linus Pauling, who defined *orthomolecular medicine* as "the preventive or therapeutic use of high-dose vitamins to treat disease." Probably the best-known claim of Dr. Pauling was that megadoses of vitamin C (at more than 100 times Canadian RDA) could prevent or cure the common cold and cancer. Many studies since have

not substantiated this claim. However, there are some situations in which nutrient megadosing is known to be helpful, including the following:

- When concurrent long-term drug therapy depletes vitamin stores or otherwise interferes with the function of a vitamin. A common clinical example is the use of vitamin B_6 (pyridoxine) supplementation in patients receiving the drug isoniazid (INH) for tuberculosis (TB; Chapter 41).
- For gastrointestinal malabsorption syndromes such as those seen in patients with severe colitis and cystic fibrosis (all major nutrient classes, including protein, fat, carbohydrates, vitamins, and minerals).
- For the treatment of pernicious anemia, which results from vitamin B_{12} (cyanocobalamin) deficiency. The gastrointestinal tract uses a quite complex mechanism to drive cyanocobalamin absorption. Specifically, a glycoprotein known as *intrinsic factor* is secreted by the parietal cells of the gastric glands (Chapter 52). Intrinsic factor serves to facilitate absorption of cyanocobalamin, primarily in the intestine. When this process is compromised (e.g., by disease), megadoses of cyanocobalamin can bypass this absorption mechanism by allowing a small amount of the vitamin to diffuse on its own through the intestinal mucosa.
- When the vitamin acts as a drug when megadosed. The most common example is niacin (vitamin B_3, also called *nicotinic acid*). At doses of up to 20 mg daily, it functions as a vitamin; at doses 50 to 100 times higher, it reduces blood levels of both triglycerides and low-density lipoprotein (LDL) cholesterol, thus acting more as a drug than as a vitamin (Chapter 29).

In contrast with the above examples, there are some situations in which nutrient megadosing is known to be harmful. For example, any excess of one or more nutrients can result in deficiencies of other nutrients because of chemical "competition" for sites of absorption through the intestinal mucosa. This is more likely to be the case with mineral megadosing, such as with calcium, copper, iron, and zinc, and is less likely to result from vitamin megadosing.

Vitamin megadosing can also lead to toxic accumulations known as *hypervitaminosis*, primarily with the fat-soluble vitamins A, D, and K, since, as mentioned, the

TABLE 8-1

Fat- and Water-Soluble Vitamins

Fat Soluble		Water Soluble	
Designation	Name	Designation	Name
vitamin A	retinol	vitamin B_1	thiamine
vitamin D	D_3, cholecalciferol	vitamin B_2	riboflavin
	D_2, ergocalciferol	vitamin B_3	niacin
vitamin E	tocopherols	vitamin B_5	pantothenic acid
vitamin K	K_1, phytonadione	vitamin B_6	pyridoxine
	K_2, menaquinone	vitamin B_9	folic acid
		vitamin B_{12}	cyanocobalamin
		biotin	
		vitamin C	ascorbic acid

fat-soluble vitamins are already stored in large amounts in the liver and fatty tissues. Another reason for accumulation is that fat-soluble vitamins exhibit slow metabolism or breakdown. Vitamin E appears safer, however, even at doses 10 to 20 times the recommended DRI. Hypervitaminosis is much less likely to occur with the water-soluble vitamins (B-complex and C) because they are readily excreted through the urinary system. Megadosing with vitamin B_6 (pyridoxine) at 50 to 100 times the DRI can nonetheless cause nerve damage.

Persons with illnesses may be the least able to tolerate nutrient megadosing, although megadosing regimens are often prescribed to them. For example, megadosing may be more of a strain on the gastrointestinal tract that is already weakened by illness. Megadosing can interfere with other treatments for illnesses, such as drug therapy. For example, in cancer patients, many chemotherapy drugs, as well as radiation treatments, work to destroy cancer cells through oxidation processes. Nutritional supplementation with antioxidants may hinder such treatment mechanisms. Patients should be advised to share with their health care provider any unusual nutritional regimens that they plan to try, especially if they have serious illnesses.

VITAMIN A

Vitamin A (retinol) is derived from animal fats such as those found in dairy products (butter and milk), eggs, meat, liver, and fish liver oils. The vitamin A stored in animal tissues is derived from carotenes, which are found in plants (green and yellow vegetables, yellow fruits). Therefore, vitamin A is an exogenous substance for humans because it must be obtained from either plant or animal foods.

There are over 600 naturally occurring carotenoid compounds in plant-based foods. Of these, 40 to 50 commonly occur in the human diet. Beta-carotene is the most prevalent of these, followed by alpha-carotene and cryptoxanthin. These are known as *provitamin A carotenoids* because they are all metabolized in the body to various forms of vitamin A.

The sources of vitamin A can be outlined as follows:

Vitamin A (retinol) → animal source, for example, dairy products, meat, liver

Provitamin A (carotenoids) → plant source, for example, green and yellow vegetables, yellow fruit

Table 8-2 lists sources of several specific nutrients.

Mechanism of Action and Drug Effects

Vitamin A is essential for night vision and for normal vision because it is part of one of the major retinal pigments called **rhodopsin**. Specifically, one molecule of *beta-carotene* is metabolized in the body to two molecules of the aldehyde compound *retinaldehyde,* often shortened to the name *retinal*. The *cis* isomer of retinal combines with the protein *opsin* to form *rhodopsin*, the visual pigment required for normal "rod vision" in the retina. This is the vision that results from stimulation (by light) of the retinal visual cells known as *rods*, enabling both black-and-white vision and peripheral vision. These are the predominant types of vision that are operative at night, when the colours of objects are not as visible. Other retinal cells known as *cones* are chiefly involved in colour and central vision (see Chapter 58).

Some of the retinal from beta-carotene is also reduced to the alcohol compound known as *retinol*. The term *vitamin A*, in the strictest sense, refers to this alcohol

TABLE 8-2	
Food Sources of Vitamins and Minerals	
Vitamin or Mineral	**Food Sources**
vitamin A	Liver; fish; dairy products; egg yolks; dark green, leafy, yellow–orange vegetables and fruit
vitamin D	Dairy products, fortified cereals and fortified orange juice, liver, fish liver oils, saltwater fish, butter, eggs
vitamin E	Fish, egg yolks, meats, vegetable oils, nuts, fruits, wheat germ, grains, fortified cereals
vitamin K	Cheese, spinach, broccoli, brussels sprouts, kale, cabbage, turnip greens, soybean oils
vitamin B_1 (thiamine)	Yeast, liver, enriched whole-grain products, beans
vitamin B_2 (riboflavin)	Meats, liver, dairy products, eggs, legumes, nuts, enriched whole-grain products, green leafy vegetables, yeast
vitamin B_3 (niacin)	Liver, turkey, tuna, peanuts, beans, yeast, enriched whole-grain breads and cereals, wheat germ
vitamin B_6 (pyridoxine)	Organ meats, meats, poultry, fish, eggs, peanuts, whole-grain products, vegetables, nuts, wheat germ, bananas, fortified cereals
vitamin B_{12} (cyanocobalamin)	Liver, kidney, shellfish, poultry, fish, eggs, milk, blue cheese, fortified cereals
vitamin C (ascorbic acid)	Broccoli, green peppers, spinach, brussels sprouts, citrus fruits, tomatoes, potatoes, strawberries, cabbage, liver
calcium	Dairy products, fortified cereals and calcium-fortified orange juice, sardines, salmon
magnesium	Meats, seafood, milk, cheese, yogourt, green leafy vegetables, bran cereal, nuts
phosphorus	Milk, yogourt, cheese, peas, meat, fish, eggs
zinc	Red meats, liver, oysters, certain seafood, milk products, eggs, beans, nuts, whole grains, fortified cereals

From Medline Plus. Retrieved August 29, 2008, from http://www.nlm.nih.gov/medlineplus/vitamins.html

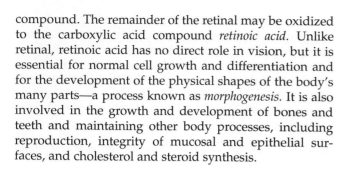

compound. The remainder of the retinal may be oxidized to the carboxylic acid compound *retinoic acid*. Unlike retinal, retinoic acid has no direct role in vision, but it is essential for normal cell growth and differentiation and for the development of the physical shapes of the body's many parts—a process known as *morphogenesis*. It is also involved in the growth and development of bones and teeth and maintaining other body processes, including reproduction, integrity of mucosal and epithelial surfaces, and cholesterol and steroid synthesis.

Indications

Supplements of vitamin A may be used to satisfy normal body requirements or an increased demand such as in infants and in pregnant and nursing women. A normal diet should provide adequate amounts of vitamin A, but in cases of excessive need or inadequate dietary intake, vitamin A supplementation is indicated to avoid problems associated with deficiency. Symptoms of vitamin A deficiency include night blindness; xerophthalmia; keratomalacia (softening of the cornea); hyperkeratosis of both the stratum corneum (outermost layer) of the skin and the sclera (outermost layer of eyeball); retarded growth in infants; generalized weakness; and increased susceptibility of mucous membranes to infection. Vitamin A–related compounds, such as isotretinoin, are also used to treat skin conditions, including acne, psoriasis, and *keratosis* follicularis (Chapter 57).

Contraindications

The only usual contraindications to vitamin A supplementation are known allergy to the individual vitamin product; known current state of hypervitaminosis; and excessive supplementation beyond recommended guidelines, especially during pregnancy. See Drug Profiles for further detail.

Adverse Effects

There are few acute adverse effects associated with normal vitamin A ingestion. Only after long-term, excessive ingestion of vitamin A do symptoms appear. Adverse effects are usually noticed in bones, mucous membranes, the liver, and the skin. Table 8-3 lists some of the symptoms of long-term, excessive ingestion of vitamin A.

Toxicity and Management of Overdose

The major toxic effects of vitamin A result from ingestion of excessive amounts, which occurs most commonly in children. A few hours after administration of an excess dose of vitamin A (over 7500 RE or 25,000 units/kg), irritability, drowsiness, vertigo, delirium, coma, vomiting, diarrhea, or both may occur. In infants, excessive amounts of vitamin A can cause an increase in cranial pressure, resulting in symptoms such as bulging fontanelles, headache, papilledema, exophthalmos (bulging eyeballs), and visual disturbances. *Papilledema* is the presence of edematous fluid, often including blood, in the optic disc. The *optic disc* is the portion of the eye in the back of the retina, where nerve fibres converge to form the optic nerve.

Over several weeks, a generalized peeling of the skin and erythema (skin reddening) may occur. These symptoms usually disappear a few days after discontinuation of the drug, which is the only treatment necessary in situations of overdose. For an acute overdose, the use of activated charcoal achieves gastrointestinal decontamination.

Interactions

Vitamin A is absorbed to a lesser extent with the simultaneous use of lubricant laxatives cholestyramine. In addition, the use of isotretinoin concurrently with vitamin A supplementation can result in additive effects and possibly toxicity. Orlistat reduces the absorption of all fat-soluble vitamins, including vitamin A. Supplementation with a multivitamin preparation is often recommended; to avoid interference with absorption, separate the doses of orlistat and vitamin A by 2 hours.

Dosages

For the recommended dosages for vitamin A, see the Dosages table on p. 112.

 DRUG PROFILES

vitamin A

There are three forms of vitamin A: retinol, retinyl palmitate, and retinyl acetate. Medications containing vitamin A may require a prescription, but many over-the-counter products, such as multivitamins, are also available. All vitamin A products are classified as pregnancy category A drugs and are contraindicated in patients who have a hypersensitivity to vitamin A and in those with oral malabsorption syndromes.

Vitamin A is available in a variety of oral forms as well as an injectable form. Doses for vitamin A are expressed in microgram retinol activity equivalents, or RAE (i.e., mcg all-*trans* retinol), irrespective of the source material used. International units may be provided as optional additional information on product labels.

One RAE is approximately equal to the following:
- 1 mcg of retinol (either dietary or supplemental)
- 2 mcg of supplemental β-carotene
- 12 mcg of dietary β-carotene
- 24 mcg of dietary carotenoids

PHARMACOKINETICS

Half-Life	Onset	Peak	Duration
PO: 50–100 days*	PO: 42 days	PO: 4 hr	PO: Unknown

*Rate of elimination of liver reserves upon eating a retinol-free diet.

TABLE 8-3

Vitamin A: Adverse Effects

Body System	Adverse Effects
Central nervous	Headache, increased intracranial pressure, lethargy, malaise
Gastrointestinal	Nausea, vomiting, anorexia, abdominal pain, jaundice
Integumentary	Drying of skin, pruritus, increased pigmentation, night sweats
Metabolic	Hypomenorrhea, hypercalcemia
Musculoskeletal	Arthralgia, retarded growth, bone pain

VITAMIN D

Vitamin D, also called the *sunshine vitamin,* is responsible for the proper utilization of calcium and phosphorus in the body. The term *vitamin D* designates a group of analogue steroid structural chemicals with vitamin D activity. The two most important members of the vitamin D family are vitamin D_2 (ergocalciferol) and vitamin D_3 (cholecalciferol). They have different sites of origin but similar functions in the body. Ergocalciferol (vitamin D_2) is plant vitamin D and is therefore obtained through dietary sources. The natural form of vitamin D produced in the skin by ultraviolet irradiation (sun) is chemically known as 7-dehydrocholesterol. It is commonly referred to as *cholecalciferol* (vitamin D_3). This endogenous synthesis of vitamin D_3 usually produces sufficient amounts to meet daily requirements. Chemically the two vitamin D compounds are different, but physiologically they produce the same effect.

Vitamin D_2 → ergocalciferol → plant vitamin D

Vitamin D_3 → cholecalciferol → human vitamin D

Vitamin D is obtained both through endogenous synthesis and through vitamin D_2 containing foods such as fish oils, salmon, sardines, and herring; fortified milk, bread, and cereals; and animal livers, tuna fish, eggs, and butter.

Mechanism of Action and Drug Effects

The basic function of vitamin D is to regulate the absorption and subsequent utilization of calcium and phosphorus. It is also necessary for the normal calcification of bone. Vitamin D, in coordination with parathyroid hormone and calcitonin, regulates serum calcium levels by increasing calcium absorption from the small intestine and extracting calcium from the bone when needed. As ergocalciferol and cholecalciferol, vitamin D is inactive and requires transformation into active metabolites for biological activity. Both vitamin D_2 and vitamin D_3 are biotransformed, primarily in the liver, by the actions of the parathyroid hormone. The resulting compound, calcifediol, is then transported to the kidney, where it is converted to calcitriol, which is believed to be the most physiologically active vitamin D analogue. Calcitriol promotes the intestinal absorption of calcium and phosphorus and the deposition of calcium and phosphorus into the structure of teeth and bones.

The drug effects of vitamin D are similar to those of vitamin A and essentially all vitamin and mineral compounds. It is used as a supplement to satisfy normal daily

DOSAGES Selected Vitamins*

Agent	Pharmacological Class	Usual Dosage Range	Indications
VITAMIN D–ACTIVE COMPOUNDS			
alfacalcidol	Fat-soluble	*Adult and children* PO: 1.0 mcg/day; increase 0.5 mcg every 2–4 wk; maintenance 0.25–1.0 mcg/day	Hypocalcemia and osteodystrophy in patients with chronic kidney failure on dialysis
calcitriol	Fat-soluble	*Adult* PO/IV: 0.25 mcg/day; increase by 0.25 mcg q4–6 wk as necessary followed by 0.5–1.0 mcg/day *Children* PO/IV: 0.01–0.05 mcg/kg/day	Management of hypocalcemia and osteodystrophy in patients receiving regular hemodialysis; rickets, hypoparathyroidism
cholecalciferol (vitamin D_3)	Fat-soluble	*Adult* 12,000–50,0000 units/day *Children* 5000 units/day	Vitamin D deficiency
doxercalciferol	Fat-soluble	*Adult* PO: 10 mcg × 3/week Secondary hypoparathyroidism	Vitamin D–resistant rickets
paricalcitol	Fat-soluble	*Adult and children* 0.04–0.1 mcg/kg bolus every other day	Secondary hyperparathyroidism of chronic kidney failure

Continued

DOSAGES Dosages Selected Vitamins* (cont'd)

Agent	Pharmacological Class	Usual Dosage Range	Indications
VITAMIN B–ACTIVE COMPOUNDS			
vitamin B$_1$ (thiamine HCl)	Water-soluble, B complex	*Adult* PO/IM/IV: 5–30 mg/day × 1 mo *Infant or child* PO/IM/IV: 10–50 mg/day	Nutritional supplement; nutritional deficiency
vitamin B$_{12}$ (cyancobalamin, hydroxocobalamin)	Water-soluble, B complex	*Adult* IM/deep SC: 30–100 mcg/day × 5–10 days, then 100–200 mcg/mo PO: 1000–2000 mcg/day then 1000 mcg/day *Children* IM/SC: 100 mcg/day until 1–5 mg, then 60 mcg/mo	Deficiency; megaloblastic anemia
vitamin B$_2$ (riboflavin)	Water-soluble, B-complex	*Adult* PO: 5–30 mg/day *Children* 3–10 mg/day	Deficiency
vitamin B$_3$ (niacin, niacinamide)	Water-soluble, B-complex	*Adult* PO: 1.5–4 g/day 300–500 mg/day *Children* PO: 100–300 mg/day	Dyslipidemia; deficiency (pellagra)
vitamin B$_6$	Water-soluble, B complex	*Adult* PO/IV/IM/SC: 2.5–10 mg/day then 2–5 mg/day for several wk (use multivitamin product) *Children* PO/IV: 5–25 mg/day for 3 wk, then 1.5–2.5 mg/day (use a multivitamin product)	Deficiency
		Adult PO/IV: 10–50 mg/day *Children* PO: 1–2 mg/kg/day	Drug-induced neuritis (e.g., isoniazid for TB)
VITAMINS A, C, E, AND K			
vitamin A	Fat-soluble	**Adult and children over 19 yr* PO: 150,000 RE (5,000,000 units × 3 days; then 15,000 RE (50,000 units) daily × 2 wk; then 3000–6000 RE (10,000–20,000 units) daily × 2 mo *Children 1–8 yr* PO: 1500–3000 RE (5000–10,000 units) / kg/day for 5 days, then 5100–10,500 RE (17,000–35,000 units) /day for 10 days	Deficiency
vitamin C (ascorbic acid)	Water-soluble	*Adult* PO/IV/IM/SC: 100–250 mg daily–bid × 3 wk *Children* PO/IV: 100–300 mg/day	Deficiency (scurvy)
vitamin E	Fat-soluble	*Adult* PO: 60–75 units/day	Deficiency
vitamin K (phytonadione)	Fat-soluble	*Adult* PO: 5–25 mg/day IV: 10 mg single dose *Infants and Children* PO/IV/SC: 2.0–10 mg single dose *Infant* IM/SC: 1 mg single dose	Deficiency; warfarin-induced hypoprothrombinemia Hemorrhagic disease of newborn

*Adequate dietary intake is always preferred over supplementation to prevent vitamin deficiencies.

requirements or an increased demand, as in infants and in pregnant and nursing women.

Indications

Vitamin D can be used either to supplement the present daily intake of vitamin D or to treat a deficiency of vitamin D (see also Ethnocultural Implications: Vitamin D Deficiency). In the case of supplementation, it is given as a prophylactic measure to prevent deficiency-related problems. Vitamin D is also used therapeutically to treat and correct the result of a long-term deficiency that leads to such conditions as infantile rickets, tetany (involuntary sustained muscular contractions), and osteomalacia (softening of bones). **Rickets** is specifically a vitamin D deficiency state. Symptoms include soft, pliable bones, causing such deformities as bow legs and knock knees; nodular enlargement on the ends and sides of the bones; muscle pain; enlarged skull; chest deformities; spinal curvature; enlargement of the liver and spleen; profuse sweating; and general tenderness of the body when touched. Vitamin D can also help promote the absorption of phosphorus and calcium. For this reason, its use is important in preventing osteoporosis. Because of the role of vitamin D in the regulation of calcium and phosphorus, it may be used to correct deficiencies of these two elements. Other uses include as a dietary supplement and to treat osteodystrophy, hypocalcemia, hypoparathyroidism, pseudohypoparathyroidism, and hypophosphatemia. There is growing body of research regarding vitamin D's benefits in disease prevention, including that of cancer, heart disease, autoimmune diseases, and neuromuscular disorders. See Evidence-Informed Practice: The Role of Vitamin D in Disease Prevention, on p. 114.

Contraindications

The only usual contraindications to vitamin D supplements are known allergy to a given vitamin product or known hypervitaminosis D state.

Adverse Effects

As with vitamin A, few acute adverse effects are associated with normal vitamin D ingestion. Only after long-term, excessive ingestion of vitamin D do symptoms appear. Such effects are usually noticed in the gastrointestinal tract or the central nervous system; these are listed in Table 8-4.

Toxicity and Management of Overdose

The major toxic effects from ingesting excessive amounts of vitamin D occur most commonly in children. Discontinuation of vitamin D and reduced calcium intake reverse the toxic state. The amount of vitamin D considered to be too much varies considerably among individuals but is generally thought to be 1.25 to 2.5 mg of ergocalciferol daily in adults and 25 mcg daily in infants and children.

The toxic effects of vitamin D are those associated with hypertension, such as weakness, fatigue, headache, anorexia, dry mouth, metallic taste, nausea, vomiting, ataxia (loss of muscular coordination), and bone pain. If not recognized and treated, these symptoms can progress to impairment of renal function and osteoporosis.

Interactions

Reduced absorption of vitamin D occurs with the simultaneous use of lubricant laxatives and cholestyramine. Patients taking digitalis preparations can develop cardiac dysrhythmias as a result of vitamin D intake.

 # ETHNOCULTURAL IMPLICATIONS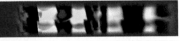

Vitamin D Deficiency

Recently, vitamin D, specifically vitamin D deficiency, has garnered much interest in the research community. Vitamin D plays a significant role in the regulation of cell growth, immunity, and cell metabolism. Vitamin D receptors are found in most tissues and cells in the body. People who live in Canada's north experience lack of sunlight for much of the year and dress for intense cold, which reduces the opportunity for taking in vitamin D. In addition, the availability and dependence on traditional vitamin D–rich foods has diminished. Consequently, low levels of vitamin D are common in the northern hemispheres.

Maternal deficiency of vitamin D is a major risk factor for vitamin D deficiency in infants that may play a role in the future health status of the child. Between 2002 and 2004, the Canadian Paediatric Surveillance Program confirmed 104 cases of rickets in Canada; 13% were of First Nations peoples and 12% were Inuit while 14% were of Middle-Eastern origin (those who wear clothing that covers most of their skin). Several other conditions have been linked to low vitamin D levels during fetal life, including lower bone density, increased severity of asthma, and the susceptibility to type 1 diabetes. Maternal deficiency is thought to contribute to newborn hypocalcemia and rickets, as well as smaller size, decreased vitamin D in breast milk, and dental malformations. The Canadian Paediatric Society recommends that breastfed infants receive 400 units (10 mcg) of vitamin D daily beginning at birth and lasting until the infant's diet includes at least 400 units a day from other dietary sources or until 1 year of age. Breastfed infants living in northern communities should receive 800 units (20 mcg) daily, whereas formula-fed infants require a supplement of 400 units daily. The Canadian Paediatric Society also recommends a higher dose of 2000 units of vitamin D daily for pregnant and lactating mothers, particularly during the winter months.

Source: First Nations, Inuit and Métis Health Committee, Canadian Paediatric Society (CPS). (2007). Vitamin D supplementation: Recommendations for Canadian mothers and infants. *Paediatrics & Child Health, 12*(7): 583–589; Gordon, C. M., Feldman, H. A., Sinclair, L., Williams, A. L., Kleinman, P. K., Perez-Rossello, J., et al. (2008). Prevalence of vitamin D deficiency among healthy infants and toddlers. *Archives of Pediatrics & Adolescent Medicine, 162*(6), 505–512.

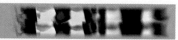

EVIDENCE-INFORMED PRACTICE

The Role of Vitamin D in Disease Prevention

Vitamin D is receiving much attention in the research community because of its potential role in reducing the risk of many chronic illnesses, including cancer, autoimmune diseases, infectious diseases, and cardiovascular disease. Specifically, vitamin D has been hypothesized to reduce cancer mortality.

In a randomized double-blind study of 1500 women over 55 years of age, women who took vitamin D and calcium had 60% less breast, lung, and colon cancer (Lappe et al., 2007) at the end of the trial than in the placebo group.

Based on the promising results of research studies, the Canadian Cancer Society and the Canadian Paediatric Society have recommended that Canadians increase their daily intake of vitamin D (cholecalciferol) to 1000 units. Some advocate for 2000 units daily; however, further research must be conducted to determine what amount of vitamin D will ensure positive health benefits.

Based on: Lappe, J. M., Travers-Gustafson, D., Davies, K. M., Recker, R. R., & Heaney, R. P. (2007). Vitamin D and calcium supplementation reduces cancer risk: Results of a randomized trial. *American Journal of Clinical Nutrition, 85*(6), 1586–1591.

Dosages

For the recommended dosages for vitamin D, see the Dosages table on p. 111. The recommended total daily intake of vitamin D for the general adult population varies. The 2006 Canadian Consensus Conference on Osteoporosis recommends a total daily intake of 800 units of vitamin D from all sources, simultaneous with calcium to prevent osteoporosis. The Canadian Cancer Society recommends 1000 units daily for all adults during the fall and winter months. Those individuals at higher risk of lower levels of vitamin D, such as the older adult, those with dark skin, or those with minimal sun exposure, should take 1000 units of vitamin D daily throughout the year. Health Canada has not altered the recommended dosages given the lack of assessment of long-term safety in the current research.

The Canadian Dermatology Association, the World Health Organization, and the Canadian Cancer Society warn against the use of tanning beds to increase levels of vitamin D because of the risk for skin cancer from exposure to harmful ultraviolet rays.

VITAMIN E

Vitamin E exists in eight different forms, each with its own biological activity. The degree of biological activity determines the measure of potency in the body.

TABLE 8-4

Vitamin D: Adverse Effects

Body System	Adverse Effects
Cardiovascular	Hypertension, dysrhythmias
Central nervous	Fatigue, weakness, drowsiness, headache
Gastrointestinal	Nausea, vomiting, anorexia, cramps, metallic taste, dry mouth, constipation
Genitourinary	Polyuria, albuminuria, increased BUN
Musculoskeletal	Decreased bone growth, bone pain, muscle pain

BUN, blood urea nitrogen.

Biologically active chemicals, **tocopherols**, make up the vitamin E compounds. α-Tocopherol is the most biologically active natural form of vitamin E. There are four isomers of α-tocopherol that exist in human blood: RRR-, RRS-, RSR-, and RSS-α-tocopherol. These four isomers of α-tocopherol are all found in fortified foods and dietary supplements. The exact biological function of vitamin E is unknown, but it is believed to act as an antioxidant. Vitamin E is found naturally in vegetable oils (sunflower, safflower, canola, and olive), seeds and nuts (sunflower, almonds, hazelnuts, peanuts), wheat germ, and in small amounts in some leafy green vegetables.

Mechanism of Action and Drug Effects

Although vitamin E is thought to be a powerful biological antioxidant and an essential component of the diet, its exact nutritional function has not been fully demonstrated. The only significant deficiency syndrome for vitamin E has been recognized in premature infants. In this situation, vitamin E deficiency may result in irritability, edema, thrombosis, and hemolytic anemia.

The drug effects of vitamin E are not as well defined as those of the other fat-soluble vitamins. It is believed to protect polyunsaturated fatty acids, a component of cellular membranes. It has also been shown to hinder the deterioration of substances such as vitamin A and ascorbic acid (vitamin C), two substances that are highly oxygen sensitive and readily oxidized, thus acting as an antioxidant. Vitamin E is absorbed from the gastrointestinal tract and depends on the presence of bile. Approximately 20% to 40% is absorbed from dietary sources. As the dosage increases, less vitamin E is absorbed. Vitamin E is transported to the general circulation by chylomicrons and lipoproteins.

Indications

Vitamin E is most commonly used as a dietary supplement to augment current daily intake or to treat a deficiency. Those at greatest risk of complications from vitamin E deficiency are premature neonates. Vitamin E has recently received much attention as an antioxidant. Preventing the

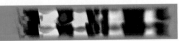

vitamin D

There are six forms of vitamin D: alfacalcidol, calcitriol, cholecalciferol, doxercalciferol, ergocalciferol, and paricalcitol. Vitamin D is available in over-the-counter (OTC) medications, such as a multivitamin product, or by prescription. Contraindications to vitamin D products include known drug product allergy, hypercalcemia, renal dysfunction, or hyperphosphatemia.

alfacalcidol

Alfacalcidol (One-Alpha) is a potent derivative of cholecalciferol (vitamin D_3). This vitamin D analogue does not require metabolic conversion by the kidney to be activated. It is used for the management of hypocalcemia, secondary hyperparathyroidism, and osteodystrophy of patients with chronic kidney disease. It is available for oral (capsule or drops) and parenteral use.

PHARMACOKINETICS

Half-Life	Onset	Peak	Duration
3 hr	3 hr	3-4 hr	48 hr

calcitriol

Calcitriol (Calcijex, Rocaltrol) is the 1,25-dihydroxylated form of cholecalciferol (vitamin D_3). It is a vitamin D analogue used for the management of hypocalcemia in patients with chronic kidney failure on dialysis. Calcitriol is available for oral and parenteral use.

PHARMACOKINETICS

Half-Life	Onset	Peak	Duration
3–6 hr	Under3 hr	3–6 hr	3–5 days

cholecalciferol

Cholecalciferol is vitamin D_3. It is used for vitamin D deficiency due to reduced dietary intake, hypoparathyroidism, and vitamin D–resistant rickets. It is available in oral form in combination with other vitamins and minerals.

PHARMACOKINETICS

Half-Life	Onset	Peak	Duration
12–30 days	Unknown	4 hr	Unknown

doxercalciferol

Doxercalciferol (Hecterol) is a vitamin D analogue that is administered orally once daily three times a week after dialysis for reduction of elevated parathormone levels to manage secondary hyperparathyroidism in patients undergoing chronic kidney dialysis. Capsules are available for oral use.

PHARMACOKINETICS

Half-Life	Onset	Peak	Duration
32–37 hr	Unknown	11–12 hr	Unknown

ergocalciferol

Ergocalciferol is vitamin D_2. It is available in combination with other vitamins and minerals as a supplement.

paricalcitrol

Paricalcitol (Zemplar), a synthetic vitamin D analogue of calcitriol, is used for the prevention and treatment of secondary hyperparathyroidism associated with chronic kidney disease in patients on hemodialysis or peritoneal dialysis. It is available in injectable form. Paricalcitol injection contains propylene glycol, which interacts with heparin and neutralizes its effect.

PHARMACOKINETICS

Half-Life	Onset	Peak	Duration
5–7 hr in healthy adults; 11–15 hr in hemodialysis patients	< 3 hr	30 minutes	3 days

oxidation of substances prevents the formation of toxic chemicals within the body, some of which are believed to cause cancer. There is a popular but unproved theory that vitamin E has beneficial effects for patients with cancer, heart disease, Alzheimer's disease, premenstrual syndrome (PMS), and sexual dysfunction. Some health care practitioners support the use of vitamin E supplementation as part of a regime to slow the progression of age-related macular degeneration. It is also thought to promote wound healing and inhibit platelet aggregation.

Contraindications

Contraindications for vitamin E include known allergy to a specific vitamin E product.

Adverse Effects

As with vitamin D, few acute adverse effects are associated with normal vitamin E ingestion because it is relatively nontoxic. Adverse effects are usually noticed in the gastrointestinal tract or central nervous system and are listed in Table 8-5.

Dosages

For the recommended dosages for vitamin E, see the Dosages table on p. 112.

TABLE 8-5

Vitamin E: Adverse Effects

Body System	Adverse Effects
Central nervous	Headache, blurred vision
Gastrointestinal	Nausea, diarrhea, intestinal cramps
Genitourinary	Creatinuria, increased serum cholesterol and triglycerides
Musculoskeletal	Weakness

DRUG PROFILES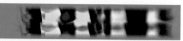

vitamin E

Vitamin E (tocopherol) is available as an OTC medication. It exists in eight different forms. The α-tocopherol RRR-α-tocopherol refers to supplements made from natural sources. The synthetic form of vitamin E has one half the activity of the natural form of vitamin E. The synthetic form is labelled "dl" or "all racemic (all rac)," while the natural form is labelled "d" or "RRR."

Vitamin E is available in many multivitamin preparations. Vitamin E products are usually contraindicated only in cases of known drug allergy.

The quantity of vitamin E is generally expressed in units. This method is currently changing to α-tocopherol equivalents (α-TE or mg RRR-α-tocopherol) but the majority of available products and dosages still express quantity in international units. See Table 8-6 for conversion of vitamin E source material quantity into vitamin E quantity, as well as conversion of vitamin E source material activity into vitamin E quantity. Vitamin E is available for oral, injection, and topical use.

PHARMACOKINETICS

Half-Life	Onset	Peak	Duration
Variable	Unknown	Unknown	Variable

VITAMIN K

Vitamin K is the last of the four fat-soluble vitamins (A, D, E, and K). There are three types of vitamin K: phytonadione (vitamin K_1), menaquinone (vitamin K_2), and menadione (vitamin K_3). The body does not store large amounts of vitamin K; however, vitamin K_2 is synthesized by the intestinal flora, thus providing an endogenous supply.

Vitamin K_1 = phytonadione → green leafy vegetables
(exogenous)
Vitamin K_2 = menaquinone → intestinal flora
(endogenous)

Vitamin K is essential for the synthesis of blood coagulation factors, which takes place in the liver. Vitamin K–dependent blood coagulation factors are factors II, VII, IX, and X. Other names for these clotting factors are as follows:

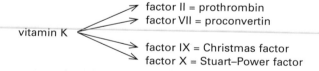

vitamin K
factor II = prothrombin
factor VII = proconvertin
factor IX = Christmas factor
factor X = Stuart–Power factor

Mechanism of Action and Drug Effects

As previously mentioned, vitamin K activity is essential for effective blood clotting because it facilitates the liver biosynthesis of factor II (*prothrombin*), factor VII (*proconvertin*), factor IX (*Christmas factor*), and factor X (*Stuart–Power factor*). Vitamin K deficiency results in coagulation disorders caused by hypoprothrombinemia.

The drug effects of vitamin K are limited to its action on the vitamin K–dependent clotting factors produced in the liver (II, VII, IX, and X). Coagulation defects affecting these clotting factors can be corrected with administration of vitamin K. Vitamin K deficiency is rare because the intestinal flora are normally able to synthesize sufficient amounts. If a deficiency develops, it can be corrected with vitamin K supplementation.

Indications

Vitamin K is indicated for dietary supplementation and for treating deficiency states. Although rare, deficiency states can develop with inadequate dietary intake or broad-spectrum inhibition of the intestinal flora resulting from the administration of broad-spectrum antibiotics. Deficiency states can also be seen in newborns because of malabsorption attributable to inadequate amounts of bile or selected drugs. For this reason, infants born in hospitals are often given a prophylactic intramuscular dose of vitamin K on arrival in the nursery. Vitamin K deficiency can also result from the administration and pharmacological action of specific anticoagulants that inhibit liver vitamin K activity. Coumarin- and indanedione-derivative anticoagulants (e.g., warfarin) thin the blood by inhibiting vitamin K–dependent clotting factors in the liver. Administration of vitamin K overrides the mechanism by which the anticoagulants inhibit production of vitamin K–dependent clotting factors.

Contraindications

The only usual contraindication to treatment with vitamin K is known drug allergy.

Adverse Effects

Vitamin K is relatively nontoxic and thus causes minimal adverse effects. Severe reactions limited to hypersensitivity or anaphylaxis have occurred rarely during or immediately after intravenous administration. Adverse effects are usually related to injection-site reactions and hypersensitivity. See Table 8-7 for a list of such major effects by body system.

Toxicity and Management of Overdose

Toxicity is primarily limited to use in the newborn. Hemolysis of red blood cells (RBCs) can occur, especially in infants with low levels of glucose-6-phosphate dehydrogenase (G6PD). In severe cases, replacement with blood products may be indicated.

TABLE 8-6

Conversion of Vitamin E Source Material Quantity

Conversion of Vitamin E Source Material Quantity into Vitamin E Quantity in Terms of α-Tocopherol (AT) and Vitamin E Activity in Terms of International Units

Source Material (1 mg)	Vitamin E Quantity (mg AT)	Vitamin E Activity (units)
RRR-α-tocopherol	1.00	1.49
RRR-α-tocopheryl acetate	0.91	1.36
RRR-α-tocopheryl succinate	0.81	1.21
All *rac*-α-tocopherol	0.50	1.10
All *rac*-α-tocopheryl acetate	0.46	1.00
All *rac*-α-tocopheryl succinate	0.41	0.89

Conversion of Vitamin E Source Material Activity into Vitamin E Quantity in Terms of α-Tocopherol (AT)

Source Material (1 unit)	Vitamin E Quantity (mg AT)
RRR-α-tocopherol	0.67
RRR-α-tocopheryl acetate	0.67
RRR-α-tocopheryl succinate	0.67
All *rac*-α-tocopherol	0.45
All *rac*-α-tocopheryl acetate	0.45
All *rac*-α-tocopheryl succinate	0.45

Source: Institute of Medicine. (2006). *Dietary reference intakes*. Reprinted with permission from The National Academies Press, Copyright 2006, National Academy of Sciences. Tables available online through Health Canada's Web site at http://www.hc-sc.gc.ca/dhp-mps/prodnatur/applications/licen-prod/monograph/mono_borage-bourrache-eng.php.

Dosages

Oral vitamin K is only available through the Special Access Programme (Health Canada). For the recommended dosages see the Dosages table on p. 112.

WATER-SOLUBLE VITAMINS

The water-soluble vitamins include the vitamin B complex and vitamin C (ascorbic acid). They are present in a variety of plant and animal food sources. The vitamin B complex is a group of 10 vitamins that are often found together in food, although they are chemically dissimilar and have different metabolic functions. Because the B vitamins were originally isolated from the same sources, primarily liver and yeast, they were grouped together as B-complex vitamins. Vitamin C (ascorbic acid), the other principal water-soluble vitamin, is concentrated more heavily in different food sources (primarily citrus fruits) than the B-complex vitamins and thus is not classified as part of the B complex. The numeric subscripts associated with B vitamins reflect the sequential order in which they were discovered. In clinical practice, some B vitamins are more often referred to by their "common" name, whereas others are more often referred to by their numeric designation. For example, "vitamin B_{12}" is used more often in clinical practice than its corresponding common name, "cyanocobalamin." However, "folic acid" is rarely referred to as "vitamin B_9," although this would also be correct. The most commonly used B-complex vitamins, as well as vitamin C, are listed in the Dosages for Selected Vitamins on p. 112. Folic acid (vitamin B_9) has a special role in hematopoiesis and therefore is discussed further in Chapter 56.

Water-soluble vitamins are a chemically diverse group sharing only the characteristic of being dissolvable in water. Similar to fat-soluble vitamins, they act primarily as coenzymes or oxidation-reduction agents in important metabolic pathways. Unlike fat-soluble vitamins, water-soluble vitamins are not stored in the body in appreciable amounts. Their water-soluble properties promote urinary excretion and reduce their half-life in the body. Therefore, dietary intake must be adequate and regular or deficient states will develop. Because these vitamins are water soluble, excess amounts are excreted in the urine. The body excretes what it does not need, which makes toxic reactions to water-soluble vitamins rare.

TABLE 8-7

Vitamin K: Adverse Effects

Body System	Adverse Effects
Central nervous	Headache, brain damage (large doses)
Gastrointestinal	Altered sensations of taste, decreased liver function tests
Hematological	Hemolytic anemia, hemoglobinuria, hyperbilirubinemia
Integumentary	Rash, urticaria

 DRUG PROFILES

vitamin K_1

The most commonly used form of vitamin K is phytonadione (vitamin K_1). Phytonadione is available by prescription only in parenteral form. Oral vitamin K is available as 5 mg tablets through the Special Access Programme. It is a category C agent. Phytonadione is contraindicated in patients who have shown a hypersensitivity reaction to it. Its use is also contraindicated during the last few weeks of pregnancy and in patients with severe hepatic disease.

PHARMACOKINETICS

Half-Life	Onset	Peak	Duration
Unknown	Variable	1–2 hr	12–14 hr

VITAMIN B₁

A deficiency of vitamin B₁ (thiamine) results in the classic disease **beriberi** or Wernicke's encephalopathy (cerebral beriberi). Common findings in beriberi include brain lesions, polyneuropathy of peripheral nerves, serous effusions (abnormal collections of fluids in body tissues), and cardiac anatomical changes. Vitamin deficiency can result from poor diet, extended fever, hyperthyroidism, hepatic disease, alcoholism, malabsorption, or pregnancy and breastfeeding.

Mechanism of Action and Drug Effects

Thiamine is an essential precursor for the formation of *thiamine pyrophosphate*. When thymine combines with *adenosine triphosphate (ATP)*, the result is *thiamine pyrophosphate coenzyme*. This is required for the *Krebs cycle (citric acid cycle)*, a major part of carbohydrate metabolism and several metabolic pathways. Additionally, thiamine plays a key role in the integrity of the peripheral nervous system, cardiovascular system, and the gastrointestinal tract.

Indications

The beneficial drug effects and the essential role of thiamine in so many metabolic pathways make it useful in treating a variety of metabolic disorders. These include subacute necrotizing encephalomyelopathy, maple syrup urine disease, and lactic acidosis associated with pyruvate carboxylase enzyme deficiency and hyper-β-alaninemia. Some of the deficiency states treated by thiamine are beriberi, Wernicke's encephalopathy syndrome, peripheral neuritis associated with **pellagra** (niacin deficiency), and neuritis of pregnancy. Thiamine is used as a dietary supplement to prevent or treat deficiency in cases of malabsorption such as that induced by alcoholism, cirrhosis, or gastrointestinal disease.

Other areas in which thiamine may have therapeutic value are the management of poor appetite, ulcerative colitis, chronic diarrhea, and cerebellar syndrome or ataxia (impaired muscular coordination). Studies do not support the use of oral vitamin B as an insect repellant.

Contraindications

The only usual contraindication to any of the B-complex vitamins is known allergy to a specific vitamin product.

Adverse Effects

Adverse effects are rare but include hypersensitivity reactions, nausea, restlessness, pulmonary edema, pruritus, urticaria, weakness, sweating, angioedema, cyanosis, and cardiovascular collapse. Administration by intramuscular injection can produce local tenderness, and intravenous injections can produce anaphylaxis.

Interactions

Thiamine is incompatible with alkaline-and sulfite-containing solutions.

Dosages

See the Dosages table on p. 112.

⬭ DRUG PROFILES

thiamine

Thiamine (vitamin B₁) is contraindicated only in individuals with a history of a hypersensitivity reaction. Thiamine is available for both oral and parenteral use. It is pregnancy category A.

PHARMACOKINETICS

Half-Life	Onset	Peak	Duration
Unknown	Unknown	Unknown	24 hr

VITAMIN B₂

A deficiency of vitamin B₂ (riboflavin) results in cutaneous, oral, and corneal changes that include seborrheic dermatitis, cheilosis, and keratitis.

Mechanism of Action and Drug Effects

Riboflavin has several important functions. In the body, riboflavin is converted into two coenzymes (flavin mononucleotide [FMN] and flavin adenine dinucleotide [FAD]) that are essential for tissue respiration. Riboflavin also plays an important part in transfer reactions, especially in carbohydrate catabolism. Another B vitamin, vitamin B₆ (pyridoxine), requires riboflavin for activation. It is also needed to convert tryptophan into niacin and to maintain erythrocyte integrity. The drug effects of riboflavin are mainly limited to replacement therapy for deficiency states. Deficiency is rare and does not usually occur in healthy people, but it may occur as a result of malnutrition or intestinal malabsorption or because of alcoholism or other diseases or infections.

Indications

Riboflavin is primarily used as a dietary supplement and to treat deficiency states. Patients who may suffer from riboflavin deficiency are those with long-standing infections, hepatic disease, alcoholism, or malignancy and those taking probenecid. Riboflavin supplementation may also be beneficial in treating microcytic anemia; acne; migraine headache; congenital methemoglobinemia (presence in the blood of an abnormal, nonfunctional hemoglobin [Hgb] pigment); muscle cramps; and

Gopalan's syndrome, a symptom of suspected riboflavin (and possibly pantothenic acid [vitamin B_5]) deficiency that involves a sensation of tingling in the extremities. For this reason, it is also called "burning feet syndrome."

Contraindications

The only usual contraindication to riboflavin is known allergy to a given vitamin product.

Adverse Effects

Riboflavin is a safe and effective vitamin; to date, no adverse effects or toxic effects have been reported. In large doses, riboflavin will discolour urine to yellow–orange.

Dosages

Commonly recommended dosages for riboflavin are listed in the Dosages table on p. 112.

DRUG PROFILES

riboflavin

Riboflavin (vitamin B_2) is needed for normal respiratory reactions. It is a safe, nontoxic water-soluble vitamin with almost no adverse effects. It is available for oral and parenteral use. It is pregnancy category A.

PHARMACOKINETICS

Half-Life	Onset	Peak	Duration
66–84 min	Unknown	Unknown	24 hr

VITAMIN B₃

The body is able to produce a small amount of vitamin B_3 (niacin) from dietary tryptophan, an essential amino acid occurring in dietary proteins and some commercially available nutritional supplements.

A dietary deficiency of niacin will produce the classic symptoms of pellagra:

- *Mental:* psychotic symptoms
- *Neurological:* neurasthenic syndrome
- *Cutaneous:* crusting, erythema, desquamation, scaly dermatitis
- *Mucous membrane:* inflammation of oral, vaginal, and urethral mucosa, including glossitis (inflamed tongue)
- *Gastrointestinal:* diarrhea or bloody diarrhea

Mechanism of Action and Drug Effects

Generally speaking, the metabolic actions of niacin (vitamin B_3) are not because of niacin in the ingested form but rather its metabolic product, *nicotinamide*. Nicotinamide is required for numerous metabolic reactions, including those involved in carbohydrate, protein, purine, and lipid metabolism, as well as tissue respiration (Figure 8-1). A key example involves two compounds, *nicotinamide adenosine dinucleotide (NAD)* and *nicotinamide adenosine dinucleotide phosphate (NADP)*, both of which are necessary for the carbohydrate pathway known as *glycogenolysis* (the breakdown of stored glycogen to usable glucose). The parent compound, niacin itself, also has a pharmacological role as an *antilipemic* drug (see Chapter 29). The doses of niacin required for this pharmacological effect are substantially higher than those required for the nutritional and metabolic effects described earlier. Niacin lowers serum cholesterol and triglyceride levels by reducing very low–density lipoprotein (VLDL) synthesis. The principal carrier of cholesterol in the blood is LDL. Because VLDL is the precursor to LDL, reducing VLDL will result in reduction of LDL and, consequently, cholesterol.

Indications

Niacin is indicated for the prevention and treatment of pellagra, a condition caused by a deficiency of vitamin B_3 that is most commonly the result of malabsorption. As previously indicated, niacin is used for certain types of hyperlipidemia. It also has a beneficial effect in peripheral vascular disease.

Contraindications

Niacin, unlike certain other B-complex vitamins, has a few additional contraindications besides drug allergy.

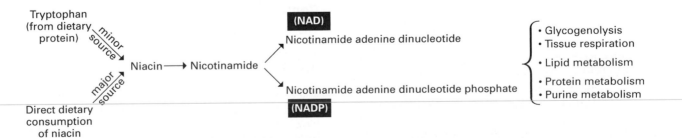

FIG. 8-1 Niacin, once in the body, is converted to NAD and NADP, which are coenzymes needed for many metabolic processes.

These include hepatic disease, severe hypotension, arterial hemorrhage, and active peptic ulcer disease.

Adverse Effects

The most frequent adverse effects associated with the use of niacin are flushing, pruritus, and gastrointestinal distress. These usually subside with continual use. They are most frequently seen when larger doses of niacin are used in the treatment of hyperlipidemia. Table 8-8 lists adverse effects by body system.

Dosages

Commonly recommended dosages for niacin are listed in the Dosages table on p. 112.

TABLE 8-8

Niacin: Adverse Effects

Body System	Adverse Effects
Cardiovascular	Postural hypotension, dysrhythmias, atrial fibrillation
Central nervous	Headache, dizziness, anxiety, sensation of warmth
Gastrointestinal	Nausea, vomiting, diarrhea, peptic ulcer
Genitourinary	Hyperuricemia
Hepatic	Abnormal liver function tests, hepatitis
Integumentary	Flushing, dry skin, rash, pruritus, keratosis
Metabolic	Decreased glucose tolerance

 DRUG PROFILES

niacin

Niacin (vitamin B_3) is used to treat pellagra, hyperlipidemias, and peripheral vascular disease. Its use should be monitored closely in patients who have a history of coronary artery disease, gallbladder disease, jaundice, hepatic disease, or arterial bleeding. Niacin is available for oral use. It is pregnancy category A.

PHARMACOKINETICS

Half-Life	Onset	Peak	Duration
45 min	Variable	Serum: 45 min	Variable

VITAMIN B$_6$

Vitamin B_6 (pyridoxine) is composed of three compounds: pyridoxine, pyridoxal, and pyridoxamine. Deficiency of vitamin B_6 can lead to a type of anemia known as *sideroblastic anemia*, neurological disturbances, seborrheic dermatitis, cheilosis (chapped or fissured lips), and xanthurenic aciduria (formation of xanthine crystals or "stones" in urine). It may also result in epileptiform convulsions, especially in neonates and infants; hypochromic microcytic anemia; and glossitis (inflamed tongue) and stomatitis (inflamed oral mucosa). Pyridoxine deficiency also affects the peripheral nerves, skin, mucous membranes, and the hematopoietic system. Inadequate intake or poor absorption of pyridoxine causes the development of these conditions. Vitamin B_6 deficiency may occur as a result of uremia, alcoholism, cirrhosis, hyperthyroidism, malabsorption syndromes, or heart failure. It may also be induced by drugs, such as isoniazid, hydralazine, penicillamine, and pyrazinamide.

Mechanism of Action and Drug Effects

Pyridoxine, pyridoxal, and pyridoxamine are all converted in erythrocytes to the active coenzyme forms of vitamin B_6, *pyridoxal phosphate* and *pyridoxamine phosphate*. These compounds are necessary for many metabolic functions, such as protein, carbohydrate, and lipid utilization in the body. They also play an important part in the amino acid conversion of tryptophan to niacin (vitamin B_3) and the neurotransmitter *serotonin*. They are essential in the synthesis of γ-aminobutyric acid (GABA), an inhibitory neurotransmitter in the central nervous system (CNS). They are important in the synthesis of heme and the maintenance of the hematopoietic system. Additionally, these substances are necessary for the integrity of the peripheral nerves, skin, and mucous membranes, as well as the hematopoietic system.

Indications

Pyridoxine is used to prevent and treat vitamin B_6 deficiency. This includes deficiency that can result from therapy with certain medications, including isoniazid (for TB), hydralazine (for hypertension), and oral contraceptives. Although deficiency of vitamin B_6 is rare, it can occur in conditions of inadequate intake or poor absorption of pyridoxine. Seizures that are unresponsive to usual therapy, morning sickness during pregnancy, and metabolic disorders may respond to pyridoxine therapy.

Contraindications

The only usual contraindication to pyridoxine use is drug allergy.

Adverse Effects

Adverse effects with pyridoxine use are rare and usually do not occur with normal doses; high doses and chronic usage may produce CNS adverse effects such as paraesthesia, flushing, warmth, headache, and lethargy, or integumentary adverse effects such as pain at the injection side. Toxic effects are a result of large doses sustained for several months. Neurotoxicity is the most likely result, but this will subside upon discontinuation of the pyridoxine.

Interactions

Pyridoxine exhibits several significant interactions with selected drugs. Pyridoxine will reduce the activity of levodopa; therefore, vitamin formulations containing B_6

should be avoided in patients taking levodopa. Drugs that have an antivitamin effect on pyridoxine include isoniazid, pyrazinamide, and oral contraceptives.

Dosages

Commonly recommended dosages for vitamin B_6 are listed in the Dosages table on p. 112.

 DRUG PROFILES

pyridoxine

Pyridoxine (vitamin B_6) is a water-soluble B-complex vitamin composed of three components: pyridoxine, pyridoxal, and pyridoxamine. It has several vital roles in the body but is primarily responsible for the integrity of peripheral nerves, skin, mucous membranes, and the

hematopoietic system. It is available for oral and parenteral use. It is pregnancy category A.

PHARMACOKINETICS

Half-Life	Onset	Peak	Duration
15–20 days	Unknown	Unknown	Unknown

VITAMIN B_{12}

Vitamin B_{12} (cyanocobalamin) is a cobalt-containing (hence, its name; and *cyano-* means "blue"), water-soluble B-complex vitamin. It is synthesized by microorganisms and is present in the body as two different coenzymes: adenosylcobalamin and methylcobalamin. Cyanocobalamin is a required coenzyme for many metabolic pathways, including fat and carbohydrate metabolism and protein synthesis. It is also required for growth, cell replication, hematopoiesis, and nucleoprotein and myelin synthesis (Figure 8-2).

Vitamin B_{12} deficiency results in gastrointestinal lesions, neurological symptoms that can result in degenerative CNS lesions, and megaloblastic anemia. The major cause of cyanocobalamin deficiency is malabsorption. Other possible but less likely causes are poor diet, chronic alcoholism, and chronic hemorrhage.

Mechanism of Action and Drug Effects

Humans must have an exogenous source of cyanocobalamin because it is required for nucleoprotein and myelin synthesis, cell reproduction, normal growth, and the maintenance of normal erythropoiesis. The cells that have the greatest requirement for vitamin B_{12} are those that divide rapidly, such as epithelial cells, bone marrow, and myeloid cells.

Reduced sulfhydryl (-5H) groups are required to metabolize fats and carbohydrates and to synthesize protein. Cyanocobalamin is involved in maintaining 5H groups in the reduced form that is required by many 5H-activated enzyme systems. Cyanocobalamin deficiency can lead to neurological damage that begins with an inability to produce myelin and is followed by gradual degeneration of the axon and nerve head.

Cyanocobalamin activity is identical to the activity of the antipernicious anemia factor present in liver extract called the *extrinsic factor* or *Castle's factor*. As previously mentioned, the oral absorption of cyanocobalamin (extrinsic factor) requires the presence of the *intrinsic factor*, which is a glycoprotein secreted by gastric parietal cells. A complex is formed between the two factors, which is then absorbed by the intestines. This is depicted in Figure 8-3.

Indications

Cyanocobalamin is used to treat deficiency states that develop because of an insufficient intake of the vitamin. It is also included in a multivitamin formulation used as a dietary supplement. As previously mentioned, deficiency states are most often the result of malabsorption or poor dietary intake. Poor dietary intake is most common in vegetarians because the primary source of cyanocobalamin is foods of animal origin.

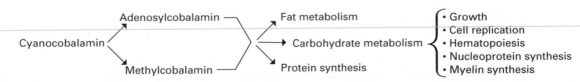

FIG. 8-2 Cyanocobalamin is a required coenzyme for many body processes.

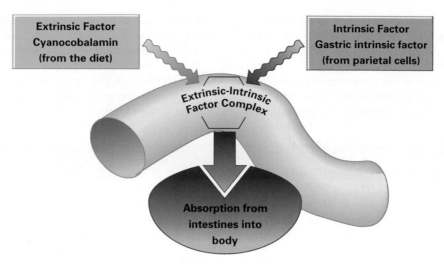

FIG. 8-3 The oral absorption of cyanocobalamin requires the presence of the intrinsic factor secreted by gastric parietal cells.

The most common manifestation of untreated cyanocobalamin deficiency is pernicious anemia leading to megaloblastic anemia and irreversible neurological damage. The use of vitamin B_{12} to treat pernicious anemia and other megaloblastic anemias results in a rapid conversion of a megaloblastic bone marrow to a normoblastic bone marrow. The preferred route of administration of vitamin B_{12} in treating megaloblastic anemias is by deep intramuscular injection. Cyanocobalamin is also useful in the treatment of pernicious anemia caused by an endogenous lack of intrinsic factor.

Contraindications

The only usual contraindication to administration of extrinsic cyanocobalamin (vitamin B_{12}) is known drug product allergies. This may include sensitivity to the chemical element cobalt, which is part of the structure of cyanocobalamin. Other contraindications include hereditary optic nerve atrophy (Leber's disease).

Adverse Effects

Vitamin B_{12} is nontoxic and large doses must be ingested to produce adverse effects, which include itching, transitory diarrhea, and fever. Other adverse effects are listed by body system in Table 8-9.

Interactions

Use with anticonvulsants, aminoglycoside antibiotics, or long-acting potassium preparations decreases the oral absorption of vitamin B_{12}. In addition, chloramphenicol may antagonize the hematological response of vitamin B_{12}.

Dosages

Current recommended dosages for vitamin B_{12} are listed in the Dosages table on p. 112.

TABLE 8-9

Cyanocobalamin: Adverse Effects

Body System	Adverse Effects
Cardiovascular	Heart failure, peripheral, vascular
Central nervous	thrombosis, pulmonary edema
	Flushing, optic nerve atrophy
Gastrointestinal	Diarrhea
Integumentary	Itching, rash, pain at injection site
Metabolic	Hypokalemia

 DRUG PROFILES

cyanocobalamin

Cyanocobalamin (vitamin B_{12}) is a water-soluble B-complex vitamin required for maintaining body fat and carbohydrate metabolism and protein synthesis. It is also needed for growth, cell replication, blood cell production, and the integrity of normal nerve function. Cyanocobalamin is available both as OTC preparations and by prescription. Most of the OTC cyanocobalamin-containing products are multivitamin preparations, whereas many of the sole cyanocobalamin-containing products contain large doses for parenteral injection and are available by prescription only. Cyanocobalamin is pregnancy category A.

PHARMACOKINETICS

Half-Life	Onset	Peak	Duration
6 days	Unknown	Plasma: 8–12 hr	Unknown

VITAMIN C

Vitamin C (ascorbic acid) can be synthesized for use as a drug and is used in many therapeutic situations. Prolonged ascorbic acid deficiency results in the nutritional disease **scurvy**, which is characterized by weakness, edema, gingivitis and bleeding gums, loss of teeth, anemia, subcutaneous hemorrhage, bone lesions, delayed healing of soft tissues and bones, and hardening of leg muscles. Scurvy was recognized for several centuries, especially among sailors. In 1795, the British navy ordered ingestion of limes to prevent the disease.

Mechanism of Action and Drug Effects

Vitamin C is reversibly oxidized to dehydroascorbic acid in the body, and it acts in oxidation-reduction reactions. It is required for several important metabolic activities, including collagen synthesis and the maintenance of connective tissue; tissue repair; maintenance of bone, teeth, and capillaries; and folic acid metabolism (specifically, the conversion of folic acid into its active metabolite). It is also essential for erythropoiesis. Vitamin C enhances the absorption of iron and is required for the synthesis of lipids, proteins, and steroids. It has also been shown to aid in cellular respiration and resistance to infections.

Indications

Vitamin C is used to treat diseases associated with vitamin C deficiency and as a dietary supplement. It is most beneficial in patients who require larger daily requirements because of pregnancy, lactation, hyperthyroidism, fever, stress, infection, trauma, burns, smoking, exposure to cold temperatures, and the consumption of certain drugs (e.g., estrogens, oral contraceptives, barbiturates, tetracyclines, and salicylates). Because vitamin C is an acid, it can also be used as a urinary acidifier. The benefits

of other uses of vitamin C are less well documented. For example, taking vitamin C to prevent or treat the common cold is common practice. However, most large controlled studies have shown that ascorbic acid has little or no value as a prophylactic for the common cold.

Contraindications

The only usual contraindication for vitamin C use is known allergy to a specific vitamin product.

Adverse Effects

Vitamin C is usually nontoxic unless excessive dosages are consumed. Megadoses can produce nausea, vomiting, headache, and abdominal cramps and will acidify the urine, resulting in the formation of cystine, oxalate, and urate kidney stones. Furthermore, individuals who discontinue taking excessive daily doses of ascorbic acid can suffer from scurvy-like symptoms.

Interactions

Ascorbic acid has the potential to interact with many classes of drugs. However, clinical experience concerning many interactions is inconclusive. For example, it has been reported that ascorbic acid can decrease the effectiveness of oral anticoagulants. This does not always happen, but practitioners should be aware of this possibility. Coadministration with acid-labile drugs such as penicillin G or erythromycin should be avoided. As previously mentioned, vitamin C can acidify the urine. This usually requires large doses for a significant effect but can enhance the excretion of basic drugs and delay the excretion of acidic drugs. Either outcome may sometimes be desirable.

Dosages

Commonly recommended dosages for vitamin C are listed in the Dosages table on p. 112.

DRUG PROFILES

ascorbic acid

Ascorbic acid (vitamin C) is a water-soluble vitamin required for the prevention and treatment of scurvy. As previously explained, it is also required for erythropoiesis and the synthesis of lipids, protein, and steroids. It is available both in OTC preparations such as multivitamin products and by prescription. Ascorbic acid is available in

many oral dosage forms and as an injectable form. It is pregnancy category A.

PHARMACOKINETICS

Half-Life	Onset	Peak	Duration
PO: Unknown	PO: Unknown	PO: Unknown	PO: Unknown

MINERALS

Minerals are essential nutrients that are classified as inorganic compounds. They act as building blocks for many body structures and thus are necessary for a variety of physiological functions. They are also needed for intracellular and extracellular body fluid electrolytes. Iron is

essential for the production of hemoglobin, which is necessary for oxygen transport throughout the body (Chapter 56). Minerals are required for muscle contraction, nerve transmission, and the makeup of essential enzymes.

Mineral compounds are composed of metallic and nonmetallic elements that are chemically combined with ionic bonds. When these compounds are dissolved in water, they separate (dissociate) into positively charged metallic cations and electrolytes or negatively charged nonmetallic anions and electrolytes (Figure 8-4).

Ingestion of mineral nutrients provides essential elements necessary for vital bodily functions. Elements required in larger amounts are called *macrominerals*; those required in smaller amounts are called *microminerals* or *trace elements*. Table 8-10 lists the classification of nutrient elements as either macrominerals or microminerals and as metal or nonmetal.

CALCIUM

Calcium is the most abundant mineral element in the human body, accounting for approximately 2% of the total body weight. The highest concentration of calcium is in bones and teeth. The efficient absorption of calcium requires adequate amounts of vitamin D.

Calcium deficiency results in hypocalcemia and affects many bodily functions. Causes of calcium deficiency include inadequate calcium intake and insufficient vitamin D to facilitate absorption; hypoparathyroidism; and malabsorption syndrome, especially in older adults. Calcium deficiency–related disorders include infantile rickets, adult osteomalacia, muscle cramps, osteoporosis (especially in postmenopausal women), hypothyroidism, and renal dysfunction. Table 8-11 lists the possible causes of calcium deficiency and the resulting disorders.

Mechanism of Action and Drug Effects

Calcium is essential for the normal maintenance and function of the nervous, muscular, and skeletal systems and for cell membrane and capillary permeability. Calcium participates in a variety of essential physiological

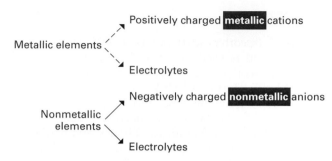

FIG. 8-4 When mineral compounds are dissolved in water, they separate into positively charged metallic cations or negatively charged nonmetallic anions and electrolytes.

functions, including transmission of nerve impulses; contraction of heart, smooth, and skeletal muscles; and enzymatic reactions. Calcium is essential in many physiological processes, including transmission of nerve impulses, renal function, respiration, and as a catalyst for many of the coagulation pathways in the blood. It acts as a cofactor in clotting reactions involving the intrinsic and extrinsic pathways of thromboplastin. It is also a cofactor in the conversion of prothrombin to thrombin by thromboplastin and the conversion of fibrinogen to fibrin. Calcium plays a regulatory role in the release and storage of neurotransmitters and hormones, in white blood cell (WBC) and hormone activity, in the uptake and binding of amino acids, and in intestinal absorption of cyanocobalamin (vitamin B_{12}) and gastrin secretion.

Indications

Calcium salts are used as a source of calcium cations for the treatment or prevention of calcium depletion in patients for whom dietary measures are inadequate.

TABLE 8-10

Mineral Elements

Element	Symbol	Type	Ionic/Electrolyte Form
MACROMINERALS			
Calcium*	Ca	Metal	Ca^{12} calcium cation
Chlorine	Cl	Nonmetal	Cl^{1-} chloride anion
Magnesium*	Mg	Metal	Mg^{2+} magnesium cation
Phosphorus*	P	Nonmetal	PO_4^{3-} phosphate anion
Potassium	K	Metal	K^{1+} potassium cation
Sodium	Na	Metal	Na^{1+} sodium cation
Sulfur	S	Nonmetal	SO_4^{2-} sulfate anion
MICROMINERALS			
Chromium	Cr	Metal	Cr^{3-} chromium cation
Cobalt	Co	Metal	Co^{2+} cobalt cation
Copper	Cu	Metal	Cu^{2+} copper cation
Fluorine	F	Nonmetal	F^{1-} fluoride anion
Iodine*	I	Nonmetal	I^{1-} iodide anion
Iron*	Fe	Metal	Fe^{2+} ferrous cation
Manganese	Mn	Metal	Mn^{2+} manganese cation
Molybdenum	Mo	Metal	Mo^{6+} molybdenum cation
Selenium*	Se	Metal	Se^{14+} selenium cation
Zinc*	Zn	Metal	Zn^{2+} zinc cation

*Mineral elements that have a current recommended daily allowance (RDA).

TABLE 8-11

Calcium Deficiency: Causes and Disorders

Cause	Disorder
Hypoparathyroidism	Muscle cramps
Inadequate intake	Infantile rickets
Insufficient vitamin D	Adult osteomalacia
Malabsorption syndrome	Osteoporosis

TABLE 8-12

Calcium Salts: Calcium Content

Calcium Salt	Calcium Content (per gram)
Phosphate tribasic	400 mg (5.8 mmol)
Carbonate	400 mg (10 mmol)
Phosphate dibasic anhydrous	290 mg (7.3 mmol)
Chloride	270 mg (6.8 mmol)
Acetate	253 mg (6.3 mmol)
Phosphate dibasic dihydrate	230 mg (5.8 mmol)
Citrate	210 mg (5.3 mmol)
Lactate	130 mg (3.3 mmol)
Gluconate	90 mg (2.3 mmol)
Glucoheptonate	82 mg (2.1 mmol)

Calcium requirements are also high for growing children and for women who are pregnant or breastfeeding. Many conditions may be associated with calcium deficiency:

- Achlorhydria alkalosis
- Chronic diarrhea
- Hyperphosphatemia
- Hypoparathyroidism
- Menopause
- Pancreatitis
- Pregnancy and lactation
- Premenstrual syndrome (PMS)
- Renal failure
- Sprue steatorrhea
- Vitamin D deficiency

Calcium is also used to treat manifestations of established deficiency states, including adult osteomalacia, hypothyroidism, infantile rickets or tetany, muscle cramps, osteoporosis, and renal insufficiency. It is used as a dietary supplement for women during pregnancy and lactation.

There are many different selected calcium salts available for treatment or nutritional supplementation. Each calcium salt contains a different amount of elemental calcium per gram of calcium salt. Table 8-12 lists the available salts and their associated calcium contents.

Contraindications

Contraindications for administration of exogenous calcium include hypercalcemia, ventricular fibrillation of the heart, and known allergy to a specific calcium drug product.

Adverse Effects

Although adverse effects and toxicity are rare, hypercalcemia can occur. Symptoms include anorexia, nausea, vomiting, and constipation. In addition, when calcium salts are administered by intramuscular or subcutaneous injection, mild to severe local reactions may occur, including burning, necrosis and sloughing of tissue, cellulitis, and soft tissue calcification. Venous irritation may occur with intravenous administration. Other adverse effects associated with both oral and parenteral use of calcium salts are listed in Table 8-13.

Toxicity and Management of Overdose

Chronic and excessive calcium intake can result in severe hypercalcemia, which can cause heart irregularities, delirium, and coma. Management of acute hypercalcemia may require hemodialysis, whereas milder cases will respond to discontinuation of calcium intake.

Interactions

Calcium salts will chelate (bind) with tetracyclines to produce an insoluble complex. If hypercalcemia is present in patients taking digitalis preparations, serious cardiac dysrhythmias can occur.

TABLE 8-13

Calcium Salts: Adverse Effects

Body System	Adverse Effects
Cardiovascular	Hemorrhage, rebound hypertension
Gastrointestinal	Constipation, obstruction, nausea, vomiting, flatulence
Genitourinary	Renal dysfunction, renal stones, renal failure
Metabolic	Hypercalcemia, metabolic alkalosis

 DRUG PROFILES

calcium

Calcium salts are minerals that are used primarily in the treatment or prevention of calcium depletion in patients in whom dietary measures are inadequate. Many calcium salts are available, all with a different content of elemental calcium per gram of salt. Calcium is available in both oral and parenteral (injectable) forms. There are numerous dosages and names of calcium preparations. Consult manufacturer's instructions for recommended dosages.

The pharmacokinetics of calcium are highly variable and depend on individual patient physiology and the characteristics of the specific drug product used. Calcium is pregnancy category C.

MAGNESIUM

Magnesium is one of the principal cations present in the intracellular fluid. It is an essential part of many enzyme systems associated with energy metabolism. Magnesium deficiency (hypomagnesemia) is usually caused by malabsorption, especially in the presence of high calcium intake; alcoholism; long-term intravenous feeding; diuretics; and metabolic disorders, including hyperthyroidism and diabetic ketoacidosis. Symptoms associated with hypomagnesemia include cardiovascular disturbances, neuromuscular impairment, and mental health disorders. Dietary intake from vegetables and other foods will usually prevent magnesium deficiency. However, magnesium is required in greater amounts in individuals with diets high in protein-rich foods, calcium, and phosphorus.

Mechanism of Action and Drug Effects

The precise action mechanism for magnesium has not been fully determined. Magnesium is a known cofactor for many enzyme systems. It is required for muscle contraction and nerve physiology. Magnesium produces an anticonvulsant effect by inhibiting neuromuscular transmission for selected convulsive states.

Indications

Magnesium is used to treat magnesium deficiency and as a nutritional supplement in total parenteral nutrition (TPN) and multivitamin preparations. It is used as an anticonvulsant in magnesium deficiency–induced seizures; for complications of pregnancy, including pre-eclampsia and eclampsia; as a tocolytic drug for inhibition of uterine contractions in premature labour; in acute nephropathy in children; for cardiac dysrhythmias; and for short-term treatment of constipation.

Contraindications

Contraindications to magnesium administration include known drug product allergy, heart block, renal failure, adrenal gland failure (Addison's disease), and hepatitis.

Adverse Effects

Adverse effects of magnesium are due to hypermagnesia, which results in tendon reflex loss, difficult bowel movements, CNS depression, respiratory distress and heart block, and hypothermia.

Toxicity and Management of Overdose

Toxic effects are extensions of symptoms caused by hypermagnesemia, a major cause of which is the long-term use of magnesium products (especially antacids in patients with renal dysfunction). Severe hypermagnesemia is treated with a calcium salt administered intravenously in doses up to 10 mmol. The diuretic furosemide (Lasix) may also be prescribed.

Interactions

The use of magnesium with neuromuscular blocking agents and CNS depressants produces additive effects.

DRUG PROFILES

magnesium

Magnesium is a mineral that has a variety of dosage forms and uses. It is an essential part of many enzyme systems. When absent or diminished in the body, cardiovascular, neuromuscular, and mental health disorders can occur. Magnesium sulfate is the most common form of magnesium used as a mineral replacement. It is pregnancy category B.

PHOSPHORUS

Phosphorus is widely distributed in foods, thus a dietary deficiency is rare. Deficiency states are usually nondietary and are primarily due to malabsorption, extensive diarrhea or vomiting, hyperthyroidism, hepatic disease, or long-term use of aluminum or calcium antacids.

Mechanism of Action and Drug Effects

Phosphorus in the form of the phosphate group or anion (PO_4^{-3}) is a required precursor for the synthesis of essential body chemicals. In addition, the mineral is an important building block for body structures. Phosphorus is required as a structural unit for the synthesis of nucleic acid and the adenosine phosphate compounds (adenosine monophosphate [AMP], adenosine diphosphate [ADP], and adenosine triphosphate [ATP]) responsible for cellular energy transfer. It is also necessary for the development and maintenance of the skeletal system and teeth. The skeletal bones contain up to 85% of the phosphorus content of the body. In addition, phosphorus is required for the proper utilization of many B-complex vitamins, and it is an essential component of physiological buffering systems.

Indications

Phosphorus is used to treat deficiency states and as a dietary supplement in many multivitamin formulations.

Contraindications

Contraindications to phosphorus or phosphate administration include hyperphosphatemia and hypocalcemia.

Adverse Effects

Adverse effects are usually associated with phosphorus replacement products. Effects include diarrhea, nausea, vomiting, and other gastrointestinal disturbances. Other adverse effects include confusion, weakness, and breathing difficulties.

Toxicity and Management of Overdose

Toxic reactions to phosphorus are extremely rare and are usually restricted to the ingestion of the pure element.

Interactions

Antacids can reduce the oral absorption of phosphorus.

 DRUG PROFILES

phosphorus

Phosphorus is a mineral that is essential to our well-being. It is needed to make energy in the form of ADP and ATP for all bodily processes. Phosphorus is present in a large number of drug formulations and appears as a phosphate salt (PO_4). Phosphorus should be used with caution in patients with renal impairment. It is available in both oral and parenteral formulations.

zinc

The metallic element zinc is often taken orally as a mineral supplement and is available as a sulfate salt for this purpose. Normally a dietary trace element, zinc plays a crucial role in the enzymatic metabolic reactions of both proteins and carbohydrates. This serves to make it especially important for normal tissue growth and repair. It therefore also has a major role in wound repair.

NURSING PROCESS

Assessment

Before administering vitamins, the nurse needs to assess the patient for nutritional disorders through a survey of laboratory tests such as Hgb, hematocrit (Hct), WBC and RBC counts, and serum albumin and protein levels. The patient's dietary intake, dietary patterns, menu planning, grocery shopping, food and meal practices and habits, and ethnocultural influences should be assessed prior to giving any supplemental therapy. Contraindications, cautions, and drug interactions should also be noted.

For vitamin A deficiencies, a baseline assessment of the patient's vision, including night vision, and examination of the skin and mucous membranes should be completed and documented. Serum vitamin A levels less than 0.7 mcmol/L (adults) indicates a deficiency.

Patients who are deficient in vitamin D should have a baseline assessment of skeletal formation with attention to any deformities. Serum calcium levels should also be drawn as ordered. During the assessment phase for vitamin D, it is important to remember that patients with a serum calcium level of less than 2.25 mmol/L may have deficient vitamin D levels. In addition, baseline levels of inorganic phosphorus and serum citrate levels may prove helpful.

Before administering vitamin E, patients should be assessed for hypoprothrombinemia because this condition may occur secondary to vitamin E deficiency. Any baseline bleeding or hematological problems need to be documented with a thorough skin assessment noting its integrity, presence of any edema, muscle weakness, easy bruising, or bleeding.

The last of the fat-soluble vitamins, vitamin K, is associated with clotting function, thus prior to its use, the patient's prothrombin time, international normalized ratio (INR), and platelet counts should be documented. Assessment of the skin for bruises, petechiae, and erythema should be completed as well as assessment of the gums for gingival bleeding. Urine and stool should also be assessed for bleeding prior to the use of this drug. Vital signs with attention to blood pressure and pulse rate should be noted. If intravenous (IV) dosage forms are used, it is important to assess baseline skin colour, temperature, and vital signs because of the associated risk for facial flushing, chest pain, weak pulse rate, profuse diaphoresis, and hypotension with possible progression to shock and cardiac arrest. It is also important to remember that the fat-soluble vitamins are all stored in the body tissue when excessive quantities are consumed and may become toxic if taken in large doses; baseline values of vitamins A, D, E, and K should always be known prior to beginning any ordered or recommended therapy.

Vitamin B_1 (thiamine) hypersensitivity may cause skin rash and wheezing; therefore, presence of any allergic reactions to vitamin B compounds needs to be documented. Because it is rare that only one vitamin B_1 deficiency occurs, deficiencies of all forms of vitamin B must be ruled out before treatment. Baseline assessments of vital signs, mental status, and urinary thiamine levels may also be ordered. When dietary intake is inadequate, little or no thiamine is excreted in urine. When the diet contains an excess of the minimal requirement, the excess is excreted in urine as intact thiamine or as pyrimidine. Vitamin C is usually well tolerated; however, assessment should include a history of nutritional deficits or problems with dietary intake, with notation of any allergies.

With trace elements, a baseline assessment should include contraindications, cautions, and drug interactions, as well as assessment of nutritional status and nutrition-related laboratory studies (Hgb, Hct, RBC, and

WBC counts; trace-elemental laboratory values). Before calcium and magnesium are administered, the patient's serum levels should be obtained and recorded. Calcium interacts with many medications, so a review of previously stated interactions is important. If there is a history of heart disease, a baseline electrocardiogram (ECG) may be ordered prior to calcium therapy; if decreased QT wave and T wave inversion are observed, calcium may be discontinued or given in reduced dosages as ordered. Magnesium is also associated with several drug interactions and should be reviewed prior to drug therapy being initiated. Because magnesium may be given for a desired systemic effect, the patient's renal status should be assessed. It is also important to assess the physician's order for completeness and rationale for use so that it is fully understood as to why the drug is being given (e.g., replacement, antacid, or laxative purposes). In addition, it is also important to assess the order for use of trace elements (e.g., calcium, magnesium, zinc) in total parenteral nutritional infusions or hyperalimentation.

Nursing Diagnoses

- Disturbed sensory perception (visual) related to night blindness from vitamin A deficiency
- Acute pain related to bone or skeletal deformities resulting from vitamin D deficiency
- Impaired physical mobility related to poorly developed muscles from vitamin D or vitamin E deficiency
- Diarrhea related to vitamin E adverse effects
- Risk for injury (e.g., bruising, bleeding) related to deficient levels of vitamin K and potential for bleeding disorders
- Disturbed thought processes related to vitamin B_1 deficiency
- Impaired physical mobility related to fatigue from poor nutrition and B vitamin deficiencies
- Acute pain in joints related to disease from vitamin C deficiency
- Impaired tissue integrity related to vitamin C deficiency and subsequent decreased healing

Planning

Goals

- Patient will maintain sensory, perceptual, and skin and mucosal integrity during therapy.
- Patient will experience minimal complaints and adverse effects related to vitamin and mineral therapy.
- Patient will regain or maintain normal bowel elimination patterns during therapy.
- Patient will report improved comfort levels during drug therapy.
- Patient will report improved thought processes and cognitive ability with therapy.
- Patient will regain and maintain activity at expected level considered normal for age, weight, and height.

Outcome Criteria

- Patient expresses fears and anxieties about possible visual, perceptual, and bodily changes due to vitamin and mineral deficiencies with positive reports of adherence to therapies.
- Patient states measures to minimize injury and maximize intactness of skin and mucous membranes, such as frequent mouth care and keeping skin clean and dry with moisturizers as needed with at least 180 mL to 240 mL of water/day.
- Patient states measures to help prevent falls and injury on a daily basis (e.g., minimizing obstacles in the home; removing excess furniture or small, loose rugs; adding night lights).
- Patient uses dietary measures (e.g., increase in bulk, fibre), hydration, and progressive exercise to assist with regaining normal bowel patterns.
- Patient increases stamina and energy to enhance tolerance of performing activities of daily living and progressive exercise, as tolerated.

Implementation

Before administering vitamin A, the nurse should document the patient's dietary intake for the last 24 hours. Any signs and symptoms of hypervitaminosis and hypercarotenemia (excess vitamin A) should be documented.

Vitamin D should be given with concurrent evaluations of renal function and serum calcium levels. The nurse should assess growth measurements in children, and all patients should be informed of signs and symptoms to report to their health care provider, such as constipation, anorexia, nausea, vomiting, metallic taste, and dry mouth. Vitamin B_1 (thiamine) therapy should be given as ordered. Niacin should be administered with milk or food to decrease gastrointestinal upset. If pyridoxine is ordered to be given intravenously, the proper infusion rate and dilutional solutions need to be verified. Cyanocobalamin should be given orally, and oral effervescent forms should be dissolved in at least 180 mL of water or juice.

Should vitamin C be used for acidification of the urine, it is important for the nurse to frequently assess urinary pH.

Because of problems with venous irritation, calcium should be given via an IV infusion pump and with proper dilution. Giving IV calcium too rapidly may precipitate heart irregularities or cardiac arrest, thus the need to give it slowly, as ordered, and within the manufacturer guidelines (e.g., usually less than 1 mL/min). Patients should be kept recumbent for 15 minutes after the infusion to prevent further problems. Should extravasation of the IV solution with calcium occur, the nurse should discontinue the infusion immediately and leave the IV catheter in place. The physician may then order an injection of 1% procaine or other antidotes or fluids to reduce vasospasm at the site and dilute the effects of calcium on surrounding tissue.

However, all facility policies and procedural guidelines and manufacturer insert information should be followed as deemed appropriate. In addition, appropriate documentation should include appearance of the IV site (e.g., erythema, swelling, and any drainage). If oral dosage forms of calcium are used, it should be given 1 to 3 hours after meals.

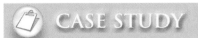 Evaluation

Evaluation should always include monitoring of goals and outcome criteria as well as therapeutic responses and adverse effects of each vitamin or mineral. Therapeutic responses to vitamin A therapy include restoration of normal vision and intact skin. Adverse effects of vitamin A include lethargy, night blindness, skin and corneal changes, and, in infancy, failure to thrive. Therapeutic responses to vitamin D include improved bone growth or formation and an intact skeleton with decreased or no pain compared to baseline musculoskeletal deformity, weakness, and discomfort. Adverse effects include constipation, anorexia, metallic taste, and dry mouth. Therapeutic responses to vitamin E include improved muscle strength, improved skin integrity, and α-tocopherol levels within normal limits. Adverse effects include blurred vision, dizziness, drowsiness, breast enlargement, and flulike symptoms. Therapeutic responses to vitamin K include a return to normal clotting. Adverse effects are presented in the Adverse Effects section of the text on vitamin K. Therapeutic response to vitamin B_1 (thiamine) includes improved mental status with less confusion. Therapeutic responses to riboflavin, niacin, pyridoxine, and cyanocobalamin include improved skin integrity; normal vision; improved mental status; and normal RBC, Hgb, and Hct levels. Therapeutic responses to vitamin C include improved capillary intactness, skin and mucous membrane integrity, healing, and energy and mental health state. An adverse reaction associated with vitamin C is precipitate formation in the urine with possible stone formation. Therapeutic responses to trace elements include resolution of the deficient state and associated signs and symptoms, depending on the specific element or mineral.

CASE STUDY

Magnesium Sulfate Therapy

D.C., a 68-year-old female, was admitted to a small community hospital (100 beds with a 6-bed CCU) for exacerbation of heart failure. After 2 days of diuretic treatment with furosemide (Lasix), the physician ordered serum potassium and magnesium levels, which showed a serum magnesium level at 0.45 mmol/L and a potassium level of 2.6 mmol/L. The physician ordered 20 mEq of magnesium sulfate in 50 mL of a 5% dextrose solution q6h × 2 doses, with the first dose stat. The night supervisor has to retrieve the medication because the pharmacy is closed. She returns to your unit with the medication. Because you are aware of many medication errors with magnesium sulfate, you are extra cautious in checking and double-checking the order. You notice that the magnesium is available in solution for intravenous injection as 20 mg/mL in 5% dextrose.

1 What are the normal serum levels for magnesium?

2 What are some of the indications for magnesium sulfate as a medication? What are some manifestations of overdosage with magnesium sulfate? What patients are especially prone to toxic effects of magnesium?

3 Because you are aware that $MgSO_4$ is a high-alert medication, you want to make sure that you administer the correct dosage. What steps should you follow to ensure that the correct amount of $MgSO_4$ is given? (NOTE: 1 g $MgSO_4$ = 4 mmol = 8 mEq)

CCU, critical care unit.
For answers see http://evolve.elsevier.com/Canada/Lilley/pharmacology/.

IN MY FAMILY

Seaweeds (Sea Mustard)
(as told by J.O., of Korean descent)

"Seaweeds are a commonly eaten food in Asia. The sea mustard contains proteins, vitamin A, B_1, B_2, C, calcium, phosphorus, and iron, etc. It has been known to have an effect on constipation, obesity, metabolic acceleration, and hematopoiesis. Also, it has been reported to affect thyroid function because of its iodine content, and it reduces cholesterol (LDL) and symptoms of hypertension. In Korea, seaweed soup is a traditional birthing dish, and every woman who gives birth eats this soup because it is believed that seaweed soup helps with breastfeeding."

PATIENT EDUCATION

❖ Patients should be educated about the best dietary sources of both water- and fat-soluble vitamins (vitamins A, B, C, D, E, and K), as well as about the best sources of elements and minerals. See Table 8-2 for the nutrient content of select food items.

❖ Patients taking vitamins, minerals, or elements should be closely monitored for therapeutic and adverse effects. Encourage patients to monitor their own progress on how well they feel, noting any improvement in their condition and health status. Encourage intake of fluids with all vitamin and mineral therapy.

❖ Patients should be informed about signs and symptoms of any related adverse effects. Vitamin E adverse effects include diarrhea, blurred vision, dizziness, and flulike symptoms.

❖ Patients who have had a gastrectomy or ileal resection or who have pernicious anemia should be informed of the need for cyanocobalamin (vitamin B_{12}) in their diet.

❖ Patients taking up to 600 mg/day of vitamin C should be informed that there may be a slight increase in daily urination frequency and that diarrhea is associated with more than 1 g of vitamin C per day.

❖ Patients taking trace elements (e.g., zinc, copper, magnesium, iodine, chromium) should be instructed to take the medication as prescribed and with adequate amounts of fluids. They should also know to call the physician if any unusual reactions occur.

❖ Patients should be educated about calcium therapy and about food items and drugs that will chelate or bind with it. For example, calcium chelates (binds) with tetracycline antibiotics and leads to a decreased or negated effect of the antibiotic.

POINTS TO REMEMBER

❖ Use of OTC vitamins and minerals may lead to serious problems and adverse effects; therefore, a physician should be consulted before supplements are taken.

❖ Nurses must incorporate the nutritional status of patients into the collaborative plan of care to provide comprehensive care during medication therapy.

❖ The nurse's participation in health promotion and wellness includes providing information about dietary needs and the body's need for vitamins and minerals.

❖ Patient education related to vitamin and mineral replacement must focus on dietary sources of the specific nutrient, drug and food interactions, and adverse effects. Patients must be instructed about when it is necessary to contact the physician.

❖ Vitamins and minerals can be dangerous to the patient if given without concern for the patient's overall condition and underlying disease processes.

❖ It should never be assumed that because the drug is a vitamin or a mineral it does not have adverse reactions or toxicity. Most vitamins and minerals can become toxic.

EXAMINATION REVIEW QUESTIONS

1 When giving IV calcium, the nurse needs to give it slowly. Which of the following is caused by rapid IV administration of calcium?
a. Tetany
b. Ototoxicity
c. Kidney damage
d. Cardiac dysrhythmias

2 Which laboratory tests should be assessed before administration of vitamin K?
a. Prothrombin time and INR
b. Red and white blood cell counts
c. Phosphorus and calcium levels
d. Total protein and albumin levels

3 For a patient who has had severe intestinal damage because of a gastrointestinal infection, which vitamin or mineral deficiency will the nurse need to assess for signs of damage?

a. Magnesium
b. Vitamin A (retinol)
c. Vitamin E (tocopherols)
d. Vitamin B_{12} (cyanocobalamin)

4 Which vitamin known to help with wound healing will a patient with a stage IV pressure ulcer probably receive?
a. Vitamin K
b. Vitamin B_1
c. Vitamin C
d. Vitamin D

5 While caring for a newly admitted patient who has a long history of alcoholism, which of the following vitamins should the nurse anticipate will be part of the patient's medication regimen?
a. Vitamin D
b. Vitamin C
c. Vitamin B_1 (thiamine)
d. Vitamin B_6 (pyridoxine)

For answers see http://evolve.elsevier.com/Lilley/pharmacology/.

CRITICAL THINKING ACTIVITIES

1 Explain why patients with a cardiac history need a baseline ECG and serum calcium assessment performed before initiation of calcium supplemental therapy.

2 Your patient is experiencing constipation and abdominal pain since beginning calcium therapy. Your assessment reveals a distended abdomen and diminished bowel sounds. What could be occurring, and what should your nursing actions be at this time?

3 Zinc oxide is often used as a skin protectant in cases of diaper rash or even sun exposure, but why would a patient with a surgical wound or a pressure ulcer benefit from doses of oral zinc during recovery?

For answers see http://evolve.elsevier.com/Lilley/pharmacology/.

Problematic Substance Use

Learning Objectives

After reading this chapter, the successful student will be able to do the following:

1 Define problematic substance use.

2 Discuss the significance of the problem of substance use and misuse in Canada and in health care settings.

3 Identify the drugs that are most frequently misused and their drug classifications.

4 Differentiate among the signs and symptoms of drug misuse for specific drugs.

5 Compare the symptoms of and treatments for drug withdrawal for the most commonly misused narcotics and opioids, amphetamines, other stimulants, and depressants, as well as alcohol and nicotine.

6 Describe alcohol misuse syndrome, its signs and symptoms, its withdrawal symptoms (mild to severe), and its treatment regimen.

7 Develop a collaborative plan of care, encompassing all phases of the nursing process, for the patient undergoing treatment for substance misuse and dependency.

e-Learning Activities

Web site
(http://evolve.elsevier.com/Canada/
Lilley/pharmacology/)

- Animations
- Answers to chapter questions, activities, and case studies
- Calculators and Category Catchers
- Glossary with audio pronunciations
- IV Therapy and Medication Error Checklists
- Multiple-Choice Review Question quizzes
- Nursing Care Plans
- Online Appendices and Supplements
- WebLinks

Glossary

Addiction Strong psychological or physical dependence on a drug or other psychoactive substance that is beyond normal voluntary control. (p. 133)

Amphetamines A drug that stimulates the central nervous system. (p. 135)

Enuresis Urinary incontinence. (p. 137)

Habituation Development of a tolerance to a substance following prolonged medical use, but without psychological or physical dependence (addiction). (p. 133)

Illicit drug use The use of a drug or substance that is not intended to be used in the manner in which it is being used, or the use of a drug that is not legally approved for human consumption. (p. 135)

Intoxication Stimulation, excitement, or stupefaction produced by a chemical substance. (p. 133)

Korsakoff's psychosis A syndrome of anterograde and retrograde amnesia with confabulation (making up of stories) associated with chronic alcohol misuse; it often occurs together with *Wernicke's encephalopathy*. (p. 140)

Micturition Urination, the desire to urinate, or the frequency of urination. (p. 137)

Narcolepsy A sleep disorder characterized by sleeping during the day, disrupted night-time sleep, cataplexy, sleep paralysis, and hypnagogical hallucinations. (p. 137)

Narcotics Drugs that produce insensibility or stupor (narcosis); the term is applied most commonly to the opioid analgesics. (p. 134)

Opioid analgesics Synthetic pain-relieving substances that were originally derived from the opium poppy. Naturally occurring opium derivatives are called *opiates*. (p. 134)

Physical dependence A condition characterized by physiological reliance on a substance; it is usually indicated by tolerance to the effects of the substance and withdrawal symptoms that develop when use of the substance is terminated. (p. 133)

Psychoactive properties Drug properties that affect mood, behaviour, cognitive processes, and mental status. (p. 136)

Psychological dependence A pattern of compulsive use of any addictive substance that is characterized by a continuous craving for the substance and the need to use it for effects other than pain relief (also called *addiction*). (p. 133)

Raves Increasingly popular all-night parties that typically involve dancing, drinking, and the use of illicit drugs. (p. 136)

Roofies Pills classified as benzodiazepines. They have recently gained popularity as a recreational drug; chemically known as flunitrazepam. (p. 138)

Substance misuse The use of a mood- or behaviour-altering substance in a maladaptive manner that often compromises health, safety, and social and occupational functioning and causes legal problems. (p. 133)

Wernicke's encephalopathy A neurological disorder characterized by apathy, drowsiness, ataxia, nystagmus, and ophthalmoplegia; it is caused by thiamine (vitamin B_1) deficiency secondary to chronic alcohol misuse. (p. 140)

Withdrawal A substance-specific mental health disorder that follows the cessation or reduction in use of a psychoactive substance that has been taken regularly to induce a state of intoxication. (p. 133)

OVERVIEW

Substance use and misuse (also called *problematic substance use*) affects men and women of all ages and ethnic and socioeconomic groups. Health Canada regards problematic substance use as a serious health issue that often results in social, economic, and public safety consequences for Canadians. According to Health Canada, "problematic substance use" best captures the range of consequences that can result from drug use. **Physical dependence** and **psychological dependence** on a substance are chronic disorders with remissions and relapses such as with any other chronic illness. Exacerbations should not be seen as failures but as indications to intensify treatment. Recognizing physical or psychological dependence and understanding the basis and guidelines for treatment are important skills for the individual caring for these patients. **Habituation** refers to situations in which a patient becomes accustomed to a certain drug (develops tolerance) and may have mild psychological dependence on it, but does not show compulsive dose escalation, drug-seeking behaviour, or major withdrawal symptoms upon drug discontinuation. This might occur, for example, in a postsurgical patient who receives opioid pain therapy regularly for only a few weeks.

According to the *Canadian Community Health Survey*, in 2002, more than 600,000 (approximately 2.6%) Canadians were dependent on alcohol, and nearly 200,000 (approximately 0.8%) were dependent on illicit drugs (Tjepkema, 2002). Sixty percent of illicit drug users were between the ages of 15 and 24. One out of every 10 Canadians aged 15 and over (approximately 2.6 million people) reported symptoms consistent with alcohol or illicit drug dependence. Based on the most current data available from the Canadian Institute for Health Information (CIHI), 27,084 hospital admissions involved alcohol-related conditions in 2000–2001 (Thomas, 2006). Another study estimated the total social costs (death, illness, and economic cost) of substance misuse in Canada to be $39.8 billion in 2002 (Relm et al., 2006). Alcohol accounted for 36.6% ($14.6 billion) of the total estimate, whereas illegal drugs accounted for 20.7% ($8.2 billion) (Relm et al., 2006). In 2002, the costs of alcohol misuse in Canada were estimated at $14.6 billion in additional health care, law enforcement, and loss of productivity in the workplace or at home (Thomas, 2004). Thomas also identified that the vast majority of these patients were men (19,067), and the majority were hospitalized for alcohol-related conditions (15,447).

Substance use and misuse is also strongly associated with many types of mental health illness. Treatment of both disorders concurrently is often very difficult, in part because of the much greater risk of drug interactions with the substances (Chapter 16). Assessment, intervention, prescription of medications, collaboration in implementing specific **addiction** (drug dependence) treatment strategies, and monitoring of recovery are essential to the care of this patient population. The focus of this chapter is the three major classes of commonly misused substances and two commonly misused individual drugs. Provided here is a description of the category or the individual drug, along with its possible effects, signs and symptoms of **intoxication** (stimulation, excitement, or stupefaction from use of drug) and **withdrawal** (mental health disorders arising from cessation of use of the drug), peak period and duration of withdrawal symptoms, and drugs used to treat withdrawal. The list of substances of misuse in Box 9-1 is not all inclusive, but it contains some of the substances most commonly misused at this time.

The specific drugs used to treat withdrawal symptoms are discussed in the sections covering the major drug category or the individual drug whose withdrawal symptoms they are intended to treat. Pharmacological therapies are indicated for patients with addictive disorders to prevent life-threatening withdrawal complications, such as seizures and delirium tremens, and to increase adherence to psychosocial forms of addiction treatment.

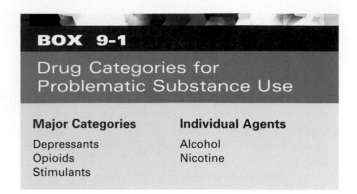

BOX 9-1

Drug Categories for Problematic Substance Use

Major Categories	Individual Agents
Depressants	Alcohol
Opioids	Nicotine
Stimulants	

OPIOIDS

Opioid analgesics are synthetic pain-relieving substances that were originally derived from the opium plant. Similar substances that occur in nature are called *opiates.* More than 20 different alkaloids are obtained from the unripe seed of the opium poppy plant, only a few of which are clinically useful. Morphine and codeine are the only two that are useful as analgesics. The multitude of other opioid analgesics that are currently used in medical practice are synthetic or semisynthetic derivatives of these two drugs.

Diacetylmorphine (better known as *heroin*) and opium are also opioids. Heroin and opium are covered by Schedule I of the Controlled Drugs and Substances Act (CDSA) and the Food and Drug Regulations (FDR) and are not available in Canada for therapeutic use. Heroin is a potent analgesic whose use is allowed for medical pain control purposes in Europe, where governmental programs also exist to provide addicts with the drug to reduce crime. Heroin was banned in Canada in 1908 because of its high potential for misuse and the increasing number of heroin addicts. Heroin addiction afflicts an estimated 60,000 to 90,000 Canadians. Some of the other commonly misused substances in the opioid category are codeine, hydrocodone, hydromorphone, meperidine, morphine, opium, oxycodone, and propoxyphene.

Heroin is one of the most commonly misused opioids in Canada and often is used in combination with the stimulant drug cocaine (discussed later in the section on stimulants). When heroin is injected (mainlining or skin-popping), sniffed (snorting), or smoked, it binds with opiate receptors found in many regions of the brain. The result is intense euphoria, often referred to as a "rush." This rush lasts only briefly and is followed by a period of a relaxed, contented state that lasts for a couple of hours. In large doses, heroin, like other opioids, can reduce or stop respiration.

Mechanism of Action and Drug Effects

Opioids work by blocking receptors in the central nervous system (CNS). When these receptors are blocked, the perception of pain is blocked. There are three main receptor types to which opioids bind. These receptors and their physiological effects when stimulated are discussed in

Chapter 11. The unique mixture of receptor affinities that a specific opioid possesses determines its therapeutic and toxic effects. One of the reasons that opioids are misused is their ability to produce euphoria, which is mediated by the μ (mu) subset of opioid receptors in the brain.

The drug effects of opioids are primarily centred in the CNS. However, these drugs also act outside the CNS, and many of their unwanted effects stem from these actions. In addition to analgesia, opioids produce drowsiness, euphoria, tranquility, and other alterations of mood. The mechanism by which opioids produce these latter effects is not entirely clear. The effects of opioids can be collectively referred to as *narcosis* or *stupor,* which involves reduced sensory response, especially to painful stimuli. For this reason, opioid analgesics, along with other classes of drugs that produce similar effects, are also referred to as **narcotics,** especially by law enforcement authorities. Areas outside the CNS that are affected by opioids include the skin, gastrointestinal tract, and genitourinary tract.

Indications

The intended drug effects of opioids are to relieve pain, reduce cough, relieve diarrhea, and induce anaesthesia. Many have a high potential for problematic use and are therefore classified as Schedule I controlled substances under the CDSA. Relaxation and euphoria are the most common drug effects that lead to misuse and psychological dependence. Sustained-release oxycodone is one example of an opioid narcotic that is controversial because it is often overprescribed and grossly misused.

Certain opioid drugs are themselves used to treat opioid dependence. Historically, methadone has been used most commonly for this purpose. Its long half-life of up to 12 to 24 hours allows patients to be dosed once daily at federally approved methadone maintenance clinics. One drug used for the same purpose is buprenorphine/naloxone (Suboxone). In theory, the ultimate goal of such programs is to reduce the patient's dosage gradually so that eventually the patient can live permanently drug free. Unfortunately, relapse rates are often high in these programs. However, patients who remain on long-term opioid maintenance therapy in a medical setting still benefit by avoiding the hazards associated with obtaining and using illegal street drugs.

Contraindications

Contraindications to the therapeutic use of opioid medications include known drug allergy, pregnancy (high dosage or prolonged use is contraindicated), respiratory depression or severe asthma without available resuscitative equipment, and paralytic ileus (bowel paralysis).

Adverse Effects

The adverse effects of opioids can be broken down into two groups: CNS and non-CNS. The primary adverse effects of opioids are related to their actions in the CNS. These include diuresis, miosis, convulsions, nausea, vomiting, and respiratory depression. Many of the non-CNS adverse effects are secondary to the release of histamine caused by opioids. This histamine release can cause vasodilation leading to hypotension; spasms of the colon leading to constipation; increased contractions of the ureter resulting in decreased urine flow; and dilation of cutaneous blood vessels leading to flushing of the skin of the face, neck, and upper thorax. The release of histamine is also thought to cause sweating, urticaria, and pruritus.

Toxicity and Management of Overdose

Listed in Box 9-2 are the signs and symptoms of opioid drug withdrawal, as well as the period when these symptoms are most likely to occur with intensity and their duration. See Chapter 11 for a detailed discussion of physical dependence and the management of acute intoxication. Withdrawal symptoms include nausea, dysphoria, muscle aches, lacrimation, rhinorrhea, pupillary dilation, piloerection (hair standing on end) or sweating, diarrhea, yawning, fever, and insomnia. The medications, listed in Box 9-3, are intended to help decrease the desire for the misused opioid and reduce the severity of these withdrawal symptoms.

Medications are sometimes used to prevent relapse to drug use once an initial remission is secured. These medications are only useful when used with concurrent counselling and offer additional insurance against return to illicit drug use. For opioid misuse or dependence, naltrexone, an opioid antagonist, is administered (50 mg/day). Naltrexone works by blocking the opioid receptors so that use of opioid drugs does not produce euphoria. When euphoria is eliminated, the reinforcing effect of the drug is lost. The patient should be free from opioids for at least 1 week before beginning this medication because naltrexone can produce withdrawal symptoms if given too soon. Naltrexone is also approved for use with alcohol-dependent patients. The same dose of naltrexone given to opioid-dependent patients, 50 mg/day, decreases craving for alcohol and reduces the likelihood of a full relapse if a slip occurs. Refer to Chapter 11 for information on management of toxicity and overdose.

STIMULANTS

The stimulants category of drugs includes the amphetamines, cocaine, benzedrine, benzphetamine, butyl nitrite, methylphenidate, and phenmetrazine. Although these drugs have many therapeutic benefits, they are often misused and can lead to physical and psychological dependence. Some of the effects of stimulants that have led to their misuse are elevation of mood, reduction of fatigue, a sense of increased alertness, and invigorating aggressiveness. Amphetamine and cocaine are two of the most commonly misused stimulants, both producing strong CNS stimulation.

Amphetamines

Chemically, three classes of amphetamine exist: salts of racemic amphetamine, dextroamphetamine, and methamphetamine. These classes vary with respect to their potency and peripheral effects, with methamphetamine having a much stronger effect on the CNS than the other two classes of amphetamines. Multiple slight chemical derivations of methamphetamine exist. Table 9-1 is a list of the common misused forms of amphetamine (and cocaine) and their street names.

BOX 9-2
Signs and Symptoms of Opioid Drug Withdrawal

Peak Period

1–3 days

Duration

5–7 days

Signs

Drug seeking, mydriasis, piloerection, diaphoresis, rhinorrhea, lacrimation, diarrhea, insomnia, elevated blood pressure and pulse

Symptoms

Intense desire for drugs, muscle cramps, arthralgia, anxiety, nausea, vomiting, malaise

BOX 9-3
Medications for Treatment of Opioid Withdrawal

Clonidine (Catapres) Substitution

Clonidine, 0.1 or 0.2 mg orally, is given every 4-6 hr as needed for signs and symptoms of withdrawal for 5–7 days. Days 2–4 are typically the toughest days in detoxification. Check blood pressure before each dose, and do not give medication if patient is hypotensive.

Methadone Substitution

Methadone test dose of 10 mg is given orally in liquid or crushed tablet. Additional 10–30 mg doses are given daily for the first 3 days. Patients at high risk for methadone toxicity should be administered 10–20 mg. Range for daily dose is 15–30 mg. Repeat total first-day dose in two divided doses (stabilization dose) for 2–3 days, then reduce dosage by 5–10 mg/day until medication is completely withdrawn. This process may be completed within 1 month or can take up to 6 months. Some individuals prefer to continue with the treatment rather than taper off.

TABLE 9-1

Various Forms of Amphetamine and Cocaine and Street Names

Chemical Name	Street Names
Dimethoxymethylamphetamine	DOM, STP
Methamphetamine (crystallized form)	Ice, crystal, glass, jibb, tina
Methamphetamine (powdered form)	Speed, meth, crank
Methylenedioxyamphetamine	MDA, love drug
Methylenedioxymethamphetamine	MDMA, ecstasy or E
Cocaine (powdered form)	Coke, dust, snow, flake, blow, girl

These "designer drugs" have **psychoactive properties** (affecting mood, behaviour, cognitive processes, and mental status) along with their stimulant properties, which further enhance their misuse potential (see Special Populations: The Adolescent: Substance Use and Misuse). Widespread misuse of methamphetamine exists. Methamphetamine is generally used orally in pill form or in powder form by snorting or injecting (known as "banging it"). The favourite injection site is at the base of the skull, which delivers the drug directly to the brain. Methamphetamine has 15 to 20 times the potency of amphetamine sulfate, the original drug in this class. Crystallized methamphetamine, known as "ice," "crystal," "glass", "jibb," or "tina," is a smokable and more powerful form of the drug. Crystal meth is more likely to cause dependence than the other forms of

methamphetamine (Buxton & Dove, 2008). It can also be ingested by wrapping the drug in a tissue to dull the harshness of the drug. Methamphetamine users who inject the drug and share needles are at risk for human immunodeficiency virus (HIV) infection and acquired immune deficiency syndrome (AIDS), as well as hepatitis B and C. Marihuana and alcohol are commonly listed as additional drugs of misuse in those admitted for treatment of methamphetamine misuse. Most of the methamphetamine-related deaths involve methamphetamine used in combination with at least one other drug, most often alcohol, heroin, or cocaine (spiking cocaine with methamphetamine is common practice). The over-the-counter (OTC) decongestant pseudoephedrine is now commonly used to synthesize methamphetamine in clandestine drug laboratories, often in private homes. This practice has led to dramatic increases in the misuse of this drug. For these reasons, many retail pharmacies now sell pseudoephedrine tablets only from behind the pharmacy counter and in limited quantities.

Another synthetic amphetamine derivative is methylenedioxymethamphetamine (MDMA, "ecstasy," or "E"), which is also usually prepared in secret home laboratories. This drug tends to have more calming effects than those of other amphetamine drugs. It is usually taken in pill form but can also be snorted or injected. Users often feel a strong sense of social bonding with and acceptance of other people, hence the nickname "love drug." The drug can also be energizing, which makes it popular at **raves** (all-night dance parties). Originally synthesized by Merck Pharmaceuticals in 1914, it was studied by the U.S. Army

 SPECIAL POPULATIONS: THE ADOLESCENT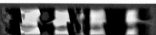

Substance Use and Misuse

Since 1977, the Centre for Addiction and Mental Health (CAMH) school survey has investigated the nature and scope of drug use among high school students in Ontario. Initially the survey was conducted among Toronto, Ontario, students in grades 7, 9, 11, and 13. In 1999, the survey was expanded to include students in grades 7 through 13. The recent trends from the 16th biannual study (2007) revealed that the rates of use of most drugs have decreased or remained the same. Survey data indicated that 64.7% of youth in grades 7 to 12 reported lifetime use of alcohol, 29.9% used cannabis, 4.3% used cocaine, and less than 4% used other drugs, including heroin, ketamine, and crystal methamphetamine. Other provinces have carried out surveys that revealed similar prevalence and trends, with few regional variations. Rates of drug use (with the exception of inhalant use) increased with age during adolescence and were similar among boys and girls. Twenty-six percent of students in grades 7 to 12 reported binge drinking (5 or more drinks at one time) in the 4 weeks before the survey. A small percentage of youth reported the misuse of stimulant medication, including methylphenidate (Ritalin). Recent data also suggested

that the misuse of prescription opiate medication, such as oxycodone and hydrocodone plus acetaminophen, in the year before the survey was as high as 24% among grade 9 students.

It is important to note that surveys such as the Ontario survey do not capture substance use and misuse by street youth, youth not attending school, those in correctional facilities, or Aboriginal youth residing on reserves, all of whom have higher reported rates of substance use than those of youth in the general population. In particular, street youth have significantly higher rates of use of methamphetamine, methylenedioxymethamphetamine ("ecstasy"), cocaine, and ketamine than those of youth in the general population. They are also more likely to be involved with injection drug use, which magnifies the potential for adverse health outcomes.

Source: Adlaf, E. M., & Paglia-Boak, A. (2007). *Drug use among Ontario students, 1977–2007: Detailed OSDUS findings* [CAMH Research Document series no. 20]. Toronto: Centre for Addiction and Mental Health. Retrieved September 7, 2008, from www.camh.net/Research/Areas_of_research/Population_Life_Course_Studies/OSDUS/OSDUHS2007_DrugDetailed_final.pdf

as a "brainwashing" drug in the 1950s. In 2005, methamphetamine was reclassified from a Schedule III drug to a Schedule I drug of the *Controlled Drugs and Substances Act* on the basis of harms caused by methamphetamine production, trafficking, and misuse, bringing offences in line with those of cocaine. A product sold as "herbal ecstasy" does not contain MDMA. It usually has ephedrine in it.

Cocaine

Cocaine is a white powder that is derived from leaves of the South American coca plant. The powder is either snorted or injected intravenously. Cocaine tends to give a temporary illusion of limitless power and energy that, when it ends, leaves the user feeling depressed, edgy, and craving more. Crack is a smokable form of cocaine that has been chemically altered. Cocaine and crack are highly addictive. The psychological and physical dependence can erode physical and mental health and can become so strong that these drugs dominate all aspects of an addict's life.

Cocaine was originally classified as a narcotic with the passage of the Opium and Drug Act of 1911. Since then, it has continued to be considered a narcotic by the penal system and has been treated as a narcotic in terms of secured storage in health care facilities. However, unlike the opioid analgesics, cocaine does not normally induce a state of narcosis or stupor and is therefore more correctly categorized as a stimulant drug, which is its current classification.

Mechanism of Action and Drug Effects

Stimulants work by releasing *biogenic amines* from their storage sites in the nerve terminals. The primary biogenic amine released is norepinephrine. This release results in stimulation of the CNS. The drug effects of stimulants are typically cardiovascular stimulation, which results in increased blood pressure and heart rate and possible cardiac dysrhythmias. The effect on smooth muscle is primarily seen in the urinary bladder and results in contraction of the sphincter. This is helpful in treating **enuresis** (urinary incontinence) but results in pain and difficulty in **micturition** (voiding or urination). Stimulants, particularly amphetamines, act potently on the CNS. This CNS stimulation commonly results in wakefulness, alertness, and a decreased sense of fatigue; elevation of mood, with increased initiative, self-confidence, and ability to concentrate; often elation and euphoria; and an increase in motor and speech activity. Physical performance in athletes may be improved because of both enhanced alertness and reduction of fatigue. This quality leads to misuse of these agents by many athletes, especially those under intense pressure to perform. However, these performance enhancement effects may reach a plateau and may even result in a personal or professional crisis for an athlete who misuses these agents on a long-term basis.

Indications

Many therapeutic uses of stimulants exist. Currently their most common use is in the treatment of attention deficit disorder or attention deficit hyperactivity disorder. Stimulants may be used to prevent or reverse fatigue and sleep, such as when they are used to treat **narcolepsy** (episodes of acute sleepiness). They may also be used to enhance the analgesic effects and limit the CNS-depressant effects of stronger analgesics, such as opioids. Another therapeutic effect of amphetamines is their ability to stimulate the respiratory centre. Occasionally, they are used after anaesthesia in individuals whose respirations are slowed. Stimulants are also used to reduce food intake and treat obesity. This therapeutic effect is limited because of rapid development of tolerance.

Contraindications

Contraindications to the therapeutic use of stimulant medications include drug allergy, diabetes, cardiovascular disorders, states of agitation, hypertension, known history of problematic drug use, and Tourette's syndrome.

Adverse Effects

The adverse effects of stimulants are commonly an extension of their therapeutic effects. The CNS-related adverse effects are restlessness, syncope (fainting), dizziness, tremor, hyperactive reflexes, talkativeness, tenseness, irritability, weakness, insomnia, fever, and sometimes euphoria. Confusion, aggression, increased libido, anxiety, delirium, paranoid hallucinations, panic states, and suicidal or homicidal tendencies occur, especially in mentally ill patients. Fatigue and depression usually follow the CNS stimulation. Cardiovascular effects are common and include headache, chilliness, pallor or flushing, palpitations, tachycardia, cardiac dysrhythmias, anginal pain, hypertension or hypotension, and circulatory collapse. Excessive sweating can also occur. Gastrointestinal effects include dry mouth, metallic taste, anorexia, nausea, vomiting, diarrhea, and abdominal cramps. A sometimes fatal hyperthermia can also occur, driven partly by excessive drug-induced muscular contractions.

Management of Withdrawal, Toxicity, and Overdose

Box 9-4 is a list of the signs, symptoms, and timing of withdrawal from stimulants. Also indicated within the box is the peak period when these symptoms are most likely to occur as well as their duration. Death because of poisoning or toxic levels is usually a result of convulsions, coma, or cerebral hemorrhages and may occur during periods of intoxication or withdrawal.

DEPRESSANTS

Depressants are drugs that relieve anxiety, irritability, and tension when used as intended. They are also used to treat seizure disorders and induce anaesthesia. The two main pharmacological classes of depressants are benzodiazepines and barbiturates. Both of these drug classes are discussed further in Chapter 13. Benzodiazepines are relatively safe. They offer many advantages over older drugs used to relieve anxiety and insomnia.

However, they are often intentionally and unintentionally misused. Ingestion of benzodiazepines together with alcohol can be lethal. Another depressant that is neither a benzodiazepine nor a barbiturate is marihuana. Derived from the cannabis plant ("pot," "grass," "weed"), marihuana is the most commonly misused drug worldwide. The United Nation's 2007 World Drug Report found that 16.8% of Canadians between the ages of 15 and 64 had used the drug at some time in 2004. This is the highest rate among developed nations. It is generally smoked as a cigarette ("joint") or in a pipe ("bong") but can be mixed in food or tea.

A benzodiazepine that has recently gained popularity as a recreational drug is flunitrazepam. Flunitrazepam is not legally available for prescription in Canada, but it is legal in more than 60 countries for treatment of insomnia. Flunitrazepam is sold under the trade name Rohypnol, from which the street name "rophy" was derived and modified to "roofy." Street names include **roofies**, roachies, La Roche, rope, rophies, and ruffies. Being under the influence of the drug is referred to as being "roached out." Flunitrazepam is similar in appearance to an acetylsalicylic acid tablet and has 10 times the potency of diazepam. The drug creates a sleepy, relaxed, drunk feeling that lasts 2 to 8 hours. A single dose costs from $2 to $6.50. Roofies are commonly used in combination with alcohol and other drugs. They are sometimes taken to enhance a heroin high or to mellow or ease the experience of coming down from a cocaine or crack high. Used with alcohol, roofies produce disinhibition and amnesia.

Roofies have recently gained a reputation as the "date rape" drug. Girls and women around the country have reported being raped after being involuntarily sedated with roofies, which were often slipped into their drink by their attackers. Since 1997, the tablets have been made to dissolve more slowly in liquid, turn clear beverages bright blue, and turn darker beverages murky, making it much easier to detect the presence of the drug in a drink. The drug has no taste or odour so the victims often do not realize what is happening. About 10 minutes after ingesting the drug, the woman may feel dizzy and disoriented, simultaneously too hot and too cold, and nauseous. She may experience difficulty speaking and moving and then pass out. Such a victim will have no memories of what happened while under the influence of the drug. Another popular date rape drug used in similar fashion is γ-hydroxybutyric acid (GHB). GHB works by mimicking the natural inhibitory brain neurotransmitter γ-aminobutyric acid (GABA). It is also known as "liquid Ecstasy." These drugs are also used simply for their depressant and hallucinogenic effects.

Mechanism of Action and Drug Effects

Benzodiazepines and barbiturates work by increasing the action of GABA. GABA is an amino acid in the brain that inhibits nerve transmission in the CNS. The alteration of GABA in the CNS results in relief of anxiety, sedation, and muscle relaxation, and it can also induce amnesia and unconsciousness. The effects of depressants are primarily limited to the CNS. They have moderate effects outside the CNS, causing slight blood pressure decreases.

The active ingredients of the marihuana plant are known as cannabinoids, the most active of which is Δ-9-trans-tetrahydrocannabinol (abbreviated THC). THC exerts its effects on the body by chemically binding to and stimulating two cannabinoid receptors in the CNS (CB1 and CB2). Smoking the drug leads to acute sensorial changes that start within 3 minutes, peak in 20 to 30 minutes, and last for 2 to 3 hours. Effects are longer when the drug is taken via the oral route. Specific effects include mild euphoria, memory lapses, dry mouth, enhanced appetite, motor awkwardness, and distorted sense of time and space. THC also stimulates sympathetic receptors and inhibits parasympathetic receptors in heart tissue, which leads to tachycardia. Other effects include hallucinations, anxiety, paranoia, and unsteady gait.

Indications

Many therapeutic uses of depressants exist. Benzodiazepines are more widely used and misused than barbiturates, and they are more commonly prescribed because they are felt by many to be safer than barbiturates. Benzodiazepines are used primarily to relieve anxiety, to induce sleep, to sedate, and to prevent seizures. Barbiturates are used as hypnotics, sedatives, and anticonvulsants and to induce anaesthesia. Controversial medical uses for marihuana (see Chapter 7 for further discussion) include treatment of persistent pain, reduction of nausea and vomiting associated with cancer treatment, and appetite stimulation in those with wasting syndromes, such as patients with cancer or AIDS. Dronabinol (Marinol) is a synthetic Health Canada–approved THC prescription capsule used for these indications (see Chapter 54 for further discussion of this drug). However, it is often not popular with those who claim it is not as effective as inhaled marihuana.

Contraindications

Contraindications to the therapeutic use of depressant medications include known drug allergy, dyspnea or airway obstruction, narrow-angle glaucoma, and porphyria (a metabolic disorder).

Adverse Effects

The most common undesirable effect of benzodiazepines and barbiturates is an overexpression of their therapeutic effects. The CNS is the primary area of the body adversely affected by these drugs. Drowsiness, sedation, loss of coordination, dizziness, blurred vision, headaches, and paradoxical reactions (insomnia, increased excitability, hallucinations) are the primary CNS adverse effects. Occasional gastrointestinal effects include nausea, vomiting, constipation, dry mouth, and abdominal cramping. Other possible adverse effects include pruritus and skin rash. Long-term use of marihuana may result in chronic respiratory symptoms (similar to those of tobacco misuse) and memory and attention deficit problems. A chronic, depressive "amotivational" syndrome has also been observed, especially among younger users.

Toxicity and Management of Overdose

Box 9-5 lists the signs and symptoms of withdrawal from depressants. The peak periods of when these symptoms are most likely to occur and their duration are also included within the box. Fatal poisoning is unusual with benzodiazepines when they are ingested alone. When benzodiazepines are ingested with alcohol or barbiturates, however, the combination can be lethal. Death is typically due to respiratory arrest. Abrupt withdrawal of benzodiazepines when they have been taken for several months to years has resulted in autonomic withdrawal symptoms, seizures, delirium, rebound anxiety, myoclonus (involuntary muscle contractions), myalgia, and sleep disturbances.

Table 9-2 shows the conversion from several barbiturates to phenobarbital, which is less addicting and from which withdrawal is easier. To use this table, the nurse determines the total dose of the barbiturate on which the patient is dependent, multiplies this dose by the conversion factor to get the equivalent dose of phenobarbital, and then tapers the phenobarbital as described in Box 9-5. Of course, a prescriber's order is required to implement this regimen.

Flumazenil can be used to acutely reverse the sedative effects of benzodiazepines. Flumazenil antagonizes the action of benzodiazepines on the CNS by directly competing for binding at the benzodiazepine receptor in the CNS. Flumazenil has a stronger affinity for the receptor and knocks the benzodiazepine off the receptor, which reverses the sedative action of the benzodiazepine. The dosage regimen to be followed for the reversal of conscious sedation or general anesthesia induced

---

BOX 9-5

Signs, Symptoms, and Treatment of Depressant Withdrawal

Peak Period

2–4 days for short-acting agents
4–7 days for long-acting agents

Duration

4–7 days for short-acting agents
7–12 days for long-acting agents

Signs

Increased psychomotor activity; agitation; muscular weakness; hyperpyrexia; diaphoresis; delirium; convulsions; elevated blood pressure, pulse rate, and temperature; tremors of eyelids, tongue, and hands

Symptoms

Anxiety; depression; euphoria; incoherent thoughts; hostility; grandiosity; disorientation; tactile, auditory and visual hallucinations; suicidal thoughts

Treatment of Benzodiazepine Withdrawal

A 7–10 day taper (10–14 day taper with long-acting benzodiazepines). Treat with diazepam (Valium) 10–20 mg orally four times daily on day 1, then taper until the dosage is 5–10 mg orally on last day. Avoid giving the drug "as needed." Adjustments in dosage according to the patient's clinical state may be indicated.

Treatment of Barbiturate Withdrawal

A 7–10 day taper or 10–14 day taper. Calculate barbiturate equivalence and give 50% of the original dosage (if actual dosage is known before detoxification); taper. Avoid giving the drug "as needed."

---

by benzodiazepines and the management of suspected benzodiazepine overdoses are summarized in Table 13-6 (Chapter 13, p. 245).

Limiting depressant misuse is important. Barbiturates and benzodiazepines are commonly implicated in

TABLE 9-2

Barbiturate Equivalencies

Drug	Dose (mg)	Phenobarbital Dose (mg)	Conversion Factor
BARBITURATES			
butalbital	100	30	0.3
phenobarbital sodium	100	30	0.3
OTHERS			
meprobamate	2400	180	0.075

suicides, especially in combination with alcohol. Generally speaking, depressants should not be regularly prescribed over a long period. Relatively safe hypnotic agents such as benzodiazepines are preferred whenever possible, especially in emotionally disturbed patients. Combinations of sedative–hypnotic compounds and the use of a single drug with alcohol should be avoided. Long-term use of hypnotic drugs leads to ineffective control of insomnia, decreased rapid eye movement sleep, dependence, and drug withdrawal symptomatology.

Effects of marihuana use are usually self-limiting and resolve within a few hours.

ALCOHOL

Alcoholic beverages have been consumed since the beginning of human civilization. The Arabian people introduced the technique of distillation to Europe in the Middle Ages. Alcohol has been termed the "elixir of life" and has been touted as a remedy for practically all diseases, which led to the term *whisky*, Gaelic for "water of life." Over time, it has been determined that the therapeutic value of ethanol is extremely limited, and chronic ingestion of excessive amounts is a major social as well as medical problem.

Mechanism of Action and Drug Effects

Alcohol, more accurately known as *ethanol* (abbreviated as ETOH), causes CNS depression by dissolving in lipid membranes in the CNS. The latest hypothesis is that ethanol causes a local disordering in the lipid matrix of the brain. This has been termed *membrane fluidization*. Ethanol may also augment GABA-mediated synaptic inhibition and fluxes of chloride. This enhancement of the action of GABA, an inhibitory neurotransmitter in the brain, causes CNS depression. Ethanol has many effects. The CNS is continuously depressed in the presence of ethanol. Moderate amounts of ethanol may stimulate or depress respirations. Effects of ethanol on the circulation are relatively minor. In moderate doses, ethanol causes vasodilation, especially of the cutaneous vessels, and produces warm, flushed skin. Ingestion of ethanol causes a feeling of warmth because it enhances cutaneous and gastric blood flow. Increased sweating may also occur. Heat is therefore lost more rapidly, and the internal body temperature consequently falls. The acute (versus chronic) ingestion of ethanol, even in intoxicating doses, probably produces little lasting change in liver function. Ethanol exerts a diuretic effect by virtue of its inhibition of antidiuretic hormone secretion and the resultant decrease in renal tubular reabsorption of water.

Indications

Few legitimate medical uses of ethanol and alcoholic beverages exist. Ethanol is an excellent solvent for many drugs and is commonly employed as a vehicle for medicinal mixtures. When applied topically to the skin, ethanol acts as a coolant. Ethanol may also be used in liniments (oily medications used on the skin). Applied topically, ethanol is the most popular skin disinfectant. More commonly, however, the type of alcohol used on the skin is isopropyl alcohol, which is similar in structure to ethanol but is more toxic and not drinkable.

Ethanol is still widely employed for its hypnotic and antipyretic effects in several cold and cough products. Dehydrated alcohol is injected very close to nerves or sympathetic ganglia for relief of long-lasting pain that occurs in trigeminal neuralgia, inoperable carcinoma, and other conditions. Systemic uses of ethanol are primarily limited to the treatment of methyl alcohol and ethylene glycol intoxication (e.g., from drinking automotive antifreeze solution). However, small amounts of ethanol preparations (such as red wine) have been shown to have cardiovascular benefits.

Adverse Effects

Chronic excessive ingestion of ethanol is directly associated with serious neurological and mental health disorders. These neurological disorders can result in seizures. Nutritional and vitamin deficiencies, especially of the B vitamins, can occur, resulting in **Wernicke's encephalopathy**, **Korsakoff's psychosis**, polyneuritis, and nicotinic acid deficiency encephalopathy.

Moderate amounts of ethanol may stimulate or depress respirations. Large amounts produce dangerous or lethal depression of respiration. Although circulatory effects of ethanol are relatively minor, acute severe alcoholic intoxication may cause cardiovascular depression. Long-term excessive use of ethanol has largely irreversible effects on the heart, such as cardiomyopathy.

When consumed on a regular basis in large quantities, ethanol produces a constellation of dose-related negative effects or serious sequelae, such as alcoholic hepatitis or its progression to cirrhosis. Teratogenic effects can be devastating and are caused by the direct action of ethanol, which inhibits embryonic cellular proliferation early in gestation. This often results in a condition known as *fetal alcohol syndrome*, which is characterized by craniofacial abnormalities, CNS dysfunction, and both prenatal and postnatal growth retardation in the infant. Pregnant women should therefore be strongly advised not to consume alcohol during pregnancy, and appropriate treatment and counselling should be arranged for pregnant women addicted to alcohol or any other drug of problematic use.

Toxicity and Management of Overdose

Box 9-6 lists the common signs and symptoms of ethanol withdrawal. Signs and symptoms may vary depending on the individual's pattern of use, preferred type of ethanol, and presence of concurrent disorders.

One pharmacological option for the treatment of alcoholism is disulfiram, an antidipsotropic drug. Disulfiram is not a cure for alcoholism; it helps patients who have a sincere desire to stop drinking. The rationale for its use

BOX 9-6 Signs, Symptoms, and Treatment of Ethanol Withdrawal

Mild Withdrawal

Signs and Symptoms

Systolic blood pressure higher than150 mm Hg, diastolic blood pressure higher than 90 mm Hg, pulse rate greater than 110 beats/min, temperature above 37.7°C, tremors, insomnia, agitation

Treatment

diazepam (Valium), 5–10 mg PO prn
lorazepam (Ativan), 1–2 mg PO q4–6h prn for 1–3 days
chlordiazepoxide, taper 5–25 mg PO q6–8h prn for 1–3 days

Moderate Withdrawal

Signs and Symptoms

Systolic blood pressure 150–200 mm Hg, diastolic blood pressure 100–140 mm Hg, pulse 110–140 beats/min, temperature 37.7–38.3°C, tremors, insomnia, agitation

Treatment

diazepam (Valium)
Day 1: 15–20 mg PO qid
Day 2: 10–20 mg PO qid
Day 3: 5–15 mg PO qid
Day 4: 10 mg PO qid
Day 5: 5 mg PO qid

lorazepam (Ativan)
Days 1 and 2: 2–4 mg PO qid
Days 3 and 4: 1–2 mg PO qid
Day 5: 1 mg PO bid

chlordiazepoxide, taper 5–25 mg PO q6–8h prn for 1–3 days

Severe Withdrawal (Delirium Tremens)*

Signs and Symptoms

Systolic blood pressure higher than 200 mm Hg, diastolic blood pressure higher than 140 mm Hg, pulse higher than 140 beats/min, temperature higher than 38.3°C, tremors, insomnia, agitation

Treatment

diazepam, 10–25 mg PO prn q1h while awake until sedation occurs
lorazepam, 1–2 mg IV prn q1h while awake for 3–5 days
chlordiazepoxide, 50–100 mg IV prn q2–4h, maximum 300 mg/day

IV, intravenously; *IM*, intramuscularly; *PO*, orally

*Monitoring in a critical care unit for heart and respiratory function, fluid and nutrition replacement, vital signs, and mental status is recommended. Restraints are indicated for a patient who is confused or agitated to protect the patient from self and to protect others (delirium tremens can be a terrifying and life-threatening state). Thiamine (100 mg IM or PO daily for 3–7 days), hydration, and magnesium replacement may be indicated depending on the severity of the withdrawal state.

---

is that patients know that if they are to avoid the devastating experience of *acetaldehyde syndrome*, they cannot drink for at least 3 or 4 days after taking disulfiram. Table 9-3 provides a description of the acetaldehyde syndrome. These adverse effects are obviously uncomfortable and even potentially dangerous for someone with any other major illnesses. For this reason, disulfiram is usually reserved as the treatment of last resort for the "hard-core" alcoholic patients for whom other treatment options (e.g., Alcoholics Anonymous, psychotherapy) have failed but who still hope to avoid continued alcohol misuse. A less noxious drug therapy option is the use of naltrexone, as mentioned previously in the section on opioids in this chapter.

Disulfiram works by altering the metabolism of alcohol. When ethanol is given to an individual previously treated with disulfiram, the blood acetaldehyde concentration rises 5 to 10 times higher than that in an untreated individual. Within about 5 to 10 minutes of ingesting alcohol, the face feels hot, and soon afterward it is flushed and scarlet. After this, throbbing in the head and neck, nausea, copious vomiting, diaphoresis, dyspnea, hyperventilation, vertigo, blurred vision, and confusion appear. As little as 7 mL of alcohol will cause mild symptoms in

a sensitive person. The effects last from 30 minutes to several hours. After the symptoms wear off, the patient is exhausted and may sleep for several hours. Most of the signs and symptoms observed after the ingestion of disulfiram plus alcohol are attributable to the resulting increase in the concentration of acetaldehyde in the body. There have even been a few published reports of localized disulfiram–alcohol skin reactions when alcohol preparations—even beer-containing shampoo—were

TABLE 9-3

Acetaldehyde Syndrome

Body System Affected	Body System Result
Cardiovascular	Vasodilation over the entire body, hypotension, orthostatic syncope, chest pain
Central nervous	Intense throbbing of the head and neck leading to a pulsating headache, sweating, marked uneasiness, weakness, vertigo, blurred vision, confusion
Gastrointestinal	Nausea, copious vomiting, thirst

placed on the skin. The usual dosage of disulfiram is 250 mg per day, or 125 mg per day in patients who experience adverse effects such as sedation, sexual dysfunction, and elevated liver enzyme levels.

NICOTINE

Nicotine was first isolated from tobacco leaves by Posselt and Reiman in 1828. The medical significance of nicotine grows out of its toxicity, presence in tobacco, and propensity for eliciting dependence in its users. The chronic effects of nicotine and the untoward effects of the chronic use of tobacco are considerable. Although many people smoke because they believe cigarettes calm their nerves, smoking releases epinephrine, a hormone that creates physiological stress in the smoker rather than relaxation. The apparent calming effects may be related to the increased deep breathing associated with smoking. The use of tobacco is addictive. Most users develop tolerance for nicotine and need greater amounts to produce the desired effect. Smokers become physically and psychologically dependent and will suffer withdrawal symptoms. Smoking is particularly dangerous in adolescents because their bodies are still developing and changing. The 4000 chemicals, including 200 known poisons, present in cigarette smoke can adversely affect their maturation. One third of young people who are just "experimenting" end up being addicted by the time they are 20 years of age.

Mechanism of Action

Nicotine works by directly stimulating the autonomic ganglia of the nicotinic receptors. Its site of action is the ganglion rather than the preganglionic or postganglionic nerve fibre. The organs throughout the body that are innervated by nerves stimulated by nicotine actually contain nicotinic receptors. These receptors are so named because they were originally tested with nicotine to measure their responses. Nicotine can have multiple unpredictable and dramatic effects on the body because nicotinic receptors are found in several organ systems, including the adrenal glands, skeletal muscles, and the CNS.

The major action of nicotine is transient stimulation, followed by more persistent depression of all autonomic ganglia. Small doses of nicotine stimulate the ganglion cells directly and facilitate the transmission of impulses. When larger doses of the drug are applied, the initial stimulation is followed quickly by a blockade of transmission.

Nicotine markedly stimulates the CNS. Respiratory stimulation is also common. This stimulation of the CNS is followed by depression. Nicotine can have dramatic effects on the cardiovascular system as well, resulting in increases in heart rate and blood pressure. The gastrointestinal system is generally stimulated by nicotine, which produces increased tone and activity in the bowel. This often leads to nausea and vomiting and occasionally diarrhea.

Indications

The nicotine found in nature (i.e., tobacco plants) has no therapeutic uses. It is medically significant because of its addictive and toxic properties. However, nicotine that is formulated into drug products to reduce cravings and promote smoking cessation can be considered a therapeutic drug. It is available for this purpose as chewing gum, transdermal patches, and nasal spray.

Adverse Effects

Nicotine primarily affects the CNS. Large doses can produce tremors and even convulsions. Respiratory stimulation is also common. The initial stimulation of the CNS induced by nicotine is quickly followed by depression. Death can even result from respiratory failure, which is thought to occur because of both central paralysis and peripheral blockade of respiratory muscles.

The cardiovascular effects of nicotine are an increase in heart rate and blood pressure. Nicotine stimulates sympathetic ganglia with the discharge of catecholamines from the sympathetic nerve endings.

The effects of nicotine on the gastrointestinal system are largely due to parasympathetic stimulation, which results in increased tone and motor activity of the bowel. Nicotine induces vomiting by both central and peripheral actions. Centrally, nicotine's emetic effects result from stimulation of the *chemoreceptor trigger zone* in the brain.

Management of Withdrawal, Toxicity, and Overdose

Smoking cessation is the primary cause for nicotine withdrawal, although discontinuation of any tobacco product can lead to this syndrome. An important and often overlooked problem in hospitalized patients is nicotine withdrawal, which manifests largely as cigarette craving. Irritability, restlessness, and a decrease in heart rate and blood pressure occur. Heart symptoms resolve over 3 to 4 weeks, but cigarette craving may persist for months or even years.

The nicotine transdermal system (patch) and nicotine polacrilex (gum) can be used to provide nicotine without the carcinogens in tobacco and are now available over the counter. The patch uses a stepwise reduction in subcutaneous delivery to gradually decrease the nicotine dose. Patient adherence seems to be higher than with the gum because rapid chewing releases an immediate dose of nicotine. The dose is approximately one half the dose that the average smoker receives in one cigarette, however, and the onset of action is 30 minutes instead of 10 minutes or less from smoking. These pharmacological changes in delivery minimize the immediate reinforcement and self-reward effects that are prominent with the rapid nicotine delivery of cigarette smoking.

A sustained-release form of the antidepressant bupropion, called Zyban, has been approved as first-line therapy to aid in smoking cessation treatment. Zyban is an innovative treatment because it is the first nicotine-free prescription medicine to treat nicotine dependence. A list of the currently available agents for nicotine withdrawal is provided in Table 9-4.

NURSING PROCESS

Assessment

The nurse's responsibility in treating substance misuse includes having excellent interpersonal communication skills and a strong knowledge base regarding the culture of misuse, drugs that are misused, misuse prevention, and development of an action plan that is individualized for the patient. A thorough patient assessment and history taking must be carried out that includes specific questions about the substance(s) being used, the duration of misuse, related physical and mental health concerns, and withdrawal potential. In patients with suspected or confirmed substance misuse, lack of honesty—on the part of the patient as well as the family or significant other—may be an issue when it comes to answering questions about drug use. Therefore, the nurse should use open-ended questions and maintain a nonjudgemental approach during the nursing process and in all contacts with the patient. In taking a medication history, the nurse should also ask the patient about all drugs being used, including prescription drugs, OTC drugs, natural health products, and illegal drugs. The names of the drugs, doses, and frequency and duration of use should be noted. The nurse must also be attentive to any clues the patient, family, or significant other may be sending, including behavioural and mood changes. A patient's reported use of multiple prescribed drugs as well as contact with multiple prescribers may well be a sign of drug misuse. Laboratory findings are important to assess, especially results of renal panel and liver function studies and any drug screening studies. Baseline vital signs should also be measured and documented.

The most dangerous substances to be aware of in terms of withdrawal are CNS depressants such as alcohol, barbiturates, and benzodiazepines. Delirium tremens (DTs) may begin with tremors and agitation and progress to hallucinations and sometimes death. Careful assessment of mental status is critical to the safe care of the patient because early withdrawal symptoms may begin with an increase in blood pressure and pulse rate, with subsequent altered mental status.

Assessment of opioid misuse, in addition to the assessment data mentioned earlier, includes determination of the route being used for drug delivery, such as oral versus intravenous. The use of some routes may give rise to other concerns (e.g., HIV/AIDS or hepatitis transmission with needle use). Respiratory status and breathing rate and rhythm are important to assess because of the risk for respiratory depression. Assessment for marihuana use includes appraisal of cognitive and motor function and assessment for the inability to carry out minor tasks. Hallucinogen misuse requires assessment of neurological status, cognitive dysfunction, bizarre changes in mood and demeanor, feelings of paranoia or dysphoria, and a feeling of unreality. The nurse should also assess for and document flashbacks, irrational behaviour, psychosis, combativeness, and violent tendencies.

With alcohol misuse, the nurse should assess for interactions with other drugs, including other CNS depressants such as narcotics, sedatives, and hypnotics. Because alcohol use (long-term) impacts the patient's nutritional status and liver function, assessment of vitamin and mineral levels, iron, clotting and platelet studies, and protein and albumin levels are needed. Also, blood alcohol levels should be obtained as ordered because the problems that appear are directly proportional to the blood alcohol level. If the blood alcohol level is less than 2.8 mmol/L, the patient may have euphoria, excitement, impaired judgement, lack of coordination, and loss of inhibitions. If the level is 2.8 to 5.6 mmol/L, the patient may show unstable gait, impaired cognitive and

TABLE 9-4		
Nicotine Withdrawal Therapies		
Drug	**Dosage per Patch**	**Recommended Duration of Use**
TRANSDERMAL NICOTINE SYSTEMS		
Nicorette Patch	5 mg/16 hr, 10 mg/16 hr, 15 mg/16 hr	2–4 wk, 2–4 wk, 4–12 wk
Prostep Patch	15 mg/24 hr, 30 mg/24 hr	
NICORETTE GUM/ NICORETTE GUM PLUS		
	When the patient has a strong urge to smoke, a stick of gum is chewed; use is gradually reduced over a 2–3 mo period.	
ANTIDEPRESSANT		
bupropion HCl (Zyban)	150 mg sustained-release tabs	150 mg once daily for 3 days, then 150 mg bid for 7–12 wk. To prevent relapse, treatment may be continued for up to 1 year and is well tolerated and efficacious.

motor function, and further impairment of judgement and speech. At 5.8 to 6.9 mmol/L, ataxia, worsening cognitive and motor function, and worsening memory are seen. At 6.9 to 9.9 mmol/L, the patient is unable to drive a vehicle. At 9.9 to 14.9 mmol/L, the patient will experience blackouts and possibly death if alcohol is mixed with other CNS depressants or the patient has altered health status. Finally, at more than 14.9 mmol/L, cardiac and respiratory arrest may occur. It is important to understand that chronic alcohol use is associated with the following health problems: cirrhosis, ascites, esophageal varices, portal hypertension, heart irregularities, enlarged heart (cardiomyopathy), gastrointestinal bleeding, liver dysfunction, hypertension, impotence, malnutrition, ulcer disease, pancreatitis, and neurological complications with neuropathies and seizures. This list is by no means complete; at the very least, these systems need thorough assessment.

Misuse of CNS depressants is manifested by confusion; decreased blood pressure, pulse rate, and respiration rate; poor concentration; and excessive sedation. Thus, assessment in these areas is necessary for a thorough history. Misuse of CNS stimulants, however, leads to increased blood pressure, increased pulse rate, and feelings of total exhilaration but with reduced appetite, gastrointestinal problems, heart irregularities, and heart failure. Assessment should also include a head-to-toe physical examination (as for misuse of any drug) and documentation of any vomiting, agitation, tremors, seizures, hyperactive reflexes, flushing, headache, high temperatures, and mydriasis (pupil dilation). Nicotine

is a CNS stimulant, so assessment in these areas is also appropriate for this substance. If the patient has a history of malnutrition, chronic lung disease, stroke, cancer, heart disease, or kidney or liver dysfunction, associated laboratory test results must also be thoroughly examined (see Special Populations: The Older Adult: Substance Misuse).

 ## Nursing Diagnoses

* Risk for injury and falls related to substance misuse or abrupt withdrawal
* Self-concept disturbance with low self-esteem related to the influence of substance misuse
* Disturbed thought processes related to biochemical changes as a result of the chemical misuse
* Risk for other-directed violence related to drug misuse or alcohol misuse
* Ineffective health maintenance related to substance misuse
* Deficient knowledge related to lack of information about abusive, addictive behaviours and their long-term management

Planning

Goals

* Patient will remain without injury during treatment for substance misuse.
* Patient will gain improved self-esteem during treatment.

SPECIAL POPULATIONS: THE OLDER ADULT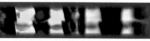

Substance Misuse

* The proportion of older adults in Canadian society is increasing, with projections by 2021 that older adults will represent 18.9% of the total population. Alcohol remains the main substance of misuse among older adults. Approximately 58% of women and 75% of men over 65 years of age use alcohol. Problematic alcohol use occurs in approximately 6% to 10% of people over 65 years of age and leads to significant alcohol-related hospitalization.
* Alcohol may alter the effects of other medications that the older adult is taking (such as CNS depressants), leading to lethargy, confusion, hypotension, and dizziness. This interaction may also occur with over-the-counter alcohol-containing products such as cough and cold syrups.
* Health risks associated with heavy alcohol use include fractures from falls, liver disease, cardiovascular and gastrointestinal problems, and malnutrition.
* The misuse of prescription and over-the-counter medications is recognized as a problem.

* The use of illicit drugs among seniors is not considered a major issue currently. However, challenges in the future may begin as baby boomers reach the age of 65. Also, baby boomers may have experiences with marihuana, cocaine, heroin, and illicitly purchased prescription medications.
* Nicotine addiction from lifelong smoking is problematic in older adults. It may alter drug metabolism and cause increased peripheral vasoconstriction, stimulation of antidiuretic hormone (ADH) release, and increased gastric acid levels.
* Caffeine use is found in older adults and can result in gastrointestinal irritation, medication-induced changes in drug metabolism, increased lithium excretion, increased CNS stimulation, and heart irregularities.

CNS, central nervous system.

Source: Health Canada. (2002). *Best practices: Treatment and rehabilitation for seniors with substance use problems.* Retrieved September 7, 2008, from http://www.hc-sc.gc.ca/hl-vs/pubs/adp-apd/treat_senior-trait_ainee/index-eng.php

- Patient will discuss the drug misuse problem and its management openly with the health care team.
- Patient will regain control of behaviour with assistance from the health care team.
- Patient will identify any barriers to effective health maintenance and healthy self-image.

■ Outcome Criteria

- Patient is safely withdrawn from drug use with stabilization of physical state that was aggravated by the substance misuse (see the specific drug and related signs and symptoms).
- Patient receives appropriate referrals and humane treatment for the substance misuse problem in a safe, nonthreatening, healthy environment
- Patient has a decreased number of violent responses and identifies possible preventative measures.
- Patient has appropriate verbalization of increased positive feelings and healthy adaptation and coping skills.

✐ Implementation

Nurses working with patients who misuse substances need a special understanding and empathy, beginning with knowledge of the problematic substance use process and understanding of the patient's lifestyle. In general, nursing interventions involve maximizing all of the therapeutic plans and minimizing those factors contributing to the abusive behaviours. Once a therapeutic rapport has been established and a patient–nurse–physician contract has been agreed upon, the plan is maximizing recovery. Interventions will be based on the patient's specific physical and emotional problems and carried out accordingly and in order of priority of basic needs. For example, if the patient is experiencing hallucinations from either the substance or withdrawal, the nurse must manage the ABCs of care (airway, breathing, circulation) and monitor vital signs and neurological and mental status while providing a calm, quiet, nonjudgemental, and nonthreatening environment. Seizures may occur, so safety precautions are also necessary, with attention to airway, padding of side rails, and implementation of other seizure precautions.

Substance withdrawal symptoms may be treated with other drugs, and thorough knowledge of the misused substance and treatment is critical to patient safety. For example, with alcohol withdrawal, diazepam may be used to help ease the symptoms of withdrawal, but there are also concerns and specific interventions regarding its use; for example, diazepam given intravenously is compatible with NaCl and should be given slowly to prevent cardiovascular collapse. Clonidine is sometimes used to treat opioid or cocaine withdrawal, and disulfiram may be used to treat alcohol misuse. With misuse, the nurse and members of the health care team need to remain informed on all treatment approaches, both pharmacological and nonpharmacological.

Family members and significant others should be encouraged to lend their support and assistance during treatment. Lifelong treatment is often indicated; the need for support during the long-term process of recovery should be emphasized and support recommended. Methods to encourage recovery and minimize relapse should be individualized for each patient and draw on all available resources, whether private or public. Communication techniques must be reinforcing and firm, yet sensitive to the patient's values and beliefs. Family members must be an integral part of all treatment and must participate in all educational sessions.

✐ Evaluation

The patient should experience a feeling of safety and security during treatment and should understand the symptoms that may be experienced during withdrawal of the drug and associated substance misuse treatment. Any change in mental status or in any parameter (vital signs) should be reported.

PATIENT EDUCATION

- ❖ Patients and their family or significant others should receive current and accurate information about the treatment regimen to make a more informed and individualized decision about the treatment plan.
- ❖ Patients' family or significant others should be educated about support groups and community resources that are important for success during and after a treatment program.

- ❖ Patients should be informed by the health care provider about any medication they may be receiving, with an emphasis on timing of doses, consequences of missed doses, and toxic effects.
- ❖ Patients should be properly educated by the health care provider about the danger of multiple drug use and of combining drugs with alcohol.

POINTS TO REMEMBER

❖ Nurses and all other health care providers continually encounter a variety of substance use and misuse problems in patients and may play a significant part in patient recovery.

❖ A thorough assessment of a patient's medical history, including medication history, is crucial to the successful treatment of patients with substance misuse problems.

❖ Drug withdrawal symptoms vary with the class of drug and may even be the opposite of the drug's action, such as with alcohol (a CNS depressant),

which produces withdrawal symptoms that are typically characterized by hyperactivity.

❖ The nurse must understand the pathology of substance use and misuse, addictive behaviours, and the way in which these behaviours dominate all aspects of the patient's life as the patient "lives for the drug" every minute of the day.

❖ Including family members or other supportive persons in the treatment regimen results in more successful treatment.

EXAMINATION REVIEW QUESTIONS

1 A patient is experiencing withdrawal from opioids. Which of the following is most commonly associated with acute withdrawal from opioids and opioid-like drugs?
   a. Lethargy
   b. Constipation
   c. Elevated blood pressure
   d. Decreased blood pressure

2 During treatment for withdrawal from opioids, which agent may be used for opioid drug withdrawal?
   a. diazepam (Valium)
   b. clonidine (Catapres)
   c. disulfiram (Antabuse)
   d. amphetamine (Dexedrine)

3 A patient being admitted from the emergency department is a young female adolescent of unknown age. She is being transferred to the critical care unit after a suicide attempt. The initial assessment shows the following: blood pressure 80/40 mm Hg, pulse 118 beats/min, and respiratory rate 8 breaths/min; thought processes are altered, and she is responsive to some verbal

commands. Which of the following drugs did the overdose probably involve?
   a. Alcohol
   b. Marihuana
   c. Barbiturates
   d. Amphetamines

4 A patient taking disulfiram as part of an alcohol treatment program accidentally takes a dose of cough syrup that contains a small percentage of alcohol. What symptom may he experience as a result of acetaldehyde syndrome?
   a. Lethargy
   b. Hypertension
   c. Copious vomiting
   d. No ill effect because of the small amount of alcohol in the cough syrup

5 When a patient is assessed for possible substance misuse, which of the following would indicate the possible use of amphetamines?
   a. Lethargy and fatigue
   b. Cardiovascular depression
   c. Talkativeness and euphoria
   d. Difficulty swallowing and constipation

For answers see http://evolve.elsevier.com/Canada/Lilley/pharmacology/.

CRITICAL THINKING ACTIVITIES

1 Your patient has been admitted to the labour and delivery department. She has a history of heavy use of alcohol and appears to be intoxicated. What are the potential complications of alcohol use on a fetus, and what would be some concerns during the first few months of the newborn's life?

2 A friend of yours reveals that she has used crack cocaine often in the past few months and tells you that even though she enjoys the sensations, she can "stop at any time." What should you do?

3 A patient is admitted to the hospital for major abdominal surgery, and the physician has ordered that a transdermal nicotine patch be used while the patient is hospitalized because the patient was a heavy smoker until recently. While applying the patch, the patient asks, "Why in the world would you want to give me nicotine when I'm trying to stop smoking?" How do you answer him?

For answers see http://evolve.elsevier.com/Canada/Lilley/pharmacology/.

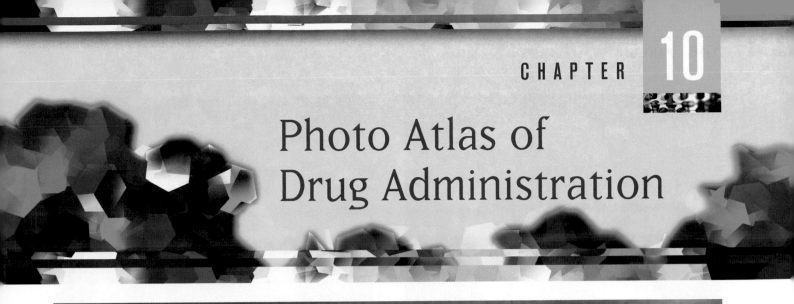

CHAPTER 10

Photo Atlas of Drug Administration

PREPARING FOR DRUG ADMINISTRATION

When giving medications, the nurse must remember safety measures and correct administration techniques to avoid errors and to ensure optimal drug actions. Keep in mind the "Ten Rights":

1 Right drug
2 Right dose
3 Right time
4 Right route
5 Right patient
6 Right reason
7 Right documentation
8 Right assessment
9 Right patient education
10 Right to refuse

Refer to Chapter 1 for a discussion of the rights regarding drug administration. Other things to keep in mind when preparing to give medications include the following:

- Remember to wash your hands before preparing or giving medications.
- If unsure about a drug or dosage calculation, do not hesitate to double-check with a drug reference or with a pharmacist. **DO NOT** give a medication that you are unsure about!
- Be punctual when giving drugs. Some medications must be given at regular intervals to maintain therapeutic blood levels.
- Figure 10-1 shows an example of a computer-controlled drug-dispensing system. To prevent errors, obtain the drugs for one patient at a time.
- Remember to check the drug at least three times before giving it. The nurse is responsible for checking medication labels against the transcribed medication order. In Figure 10-2, the nurse is checking the drug against the medication administration record (MAR) after removing the drug from the dispenser drawer. The drug

should also be checked before opening the container, and again after opening the container but before giving the drug to the patient.

- Health care facilities have means of checking the MAR when a new one is printed, so be sure that you are working from an MAR that has been checked or verified before giving the oral medication. If the patient's MAR has a new drug order on it, the best practice is to double-check that order against the patient's chart.
- Check the expiration date of all medications. Medications used past the expiration date may be less potent or even harmful.
- Before administering any medication, check the patient's identification bracelet. In addition, the patient's drug allergies should be assessed (Figure 10-3). Some hospitals use a bar code system, shown in Figure 10-4.
- Be sure to take the time to explain to the patient and caregiver the purpose of each medication, its

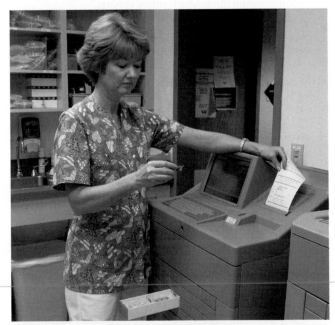

FIG. 10-1 Using a computer-dispensing system to remove unit-dose medication.

Note: This photo atlas is designed to illustrate general aspects of drug administration. For detailed instructions, please refer to a nursing fundamentals or skills book.

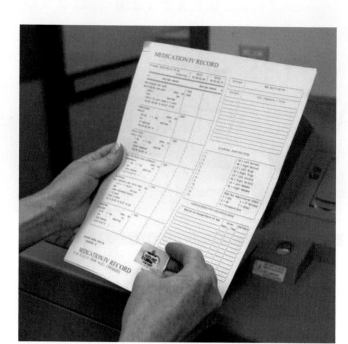

FIG. 10-2 Checking the medication against the order on the medication administration record.

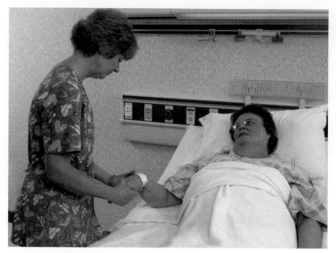

FIG. 10-3 Always check the patient's identification and allergies before giving medications.

action, possible adverse effects, and any other pertinent information, especially drug–drug or drug–food interactions.

- Open the medication at the bedside into the patient's hand or into the medicine cup. Try not to touch the drugs with your hands. Leaving the drugs in their packaging until you get to the patient's room helps avoid contamination and prevent waste should the patient refuse the drug.
- Discard any medications that fall to the floor or become contaminated by other means.
- Chart the medication on the MAR as soon as it is given and before going to the next patient (Figure 10-5). Be sure to also document therapeutic responses, adverse effects (if any), and other concerns in the nurse's notes.
- Return to evaluate the patient's response to the drug. Remember that the expected response time will vary

according to the drug route. For example, responses to sublingual nitroglycerin or intravenous push medications should be evaluated within minutes, but it may take 1 hour for a response to be noted after an oral medication is given.

- See Special Populations: Children: Pharmacokinetic Changes in Children on page 46 in Chapter 3 for age-related considerations when adminstering medication to infants and children.

TTH / PMH / OCI		Run from 06/03/17 07:31 to 06/03/18 07:30			
24 Hour Check Done Date: _____ Time: _____ RN: _____		*Location:* TEST *Name:* Test, Patient *Diagnosis:* *Allergies:* No Known Allergy	*Physician:* Doctor, John Q. *MRN #:* 0012457 *Age:* 49 *Visit #:* 000012457		
US/RN	START STOP	MEDICATION		07:31 – 19:30	19:31 – 07:30
		***** ROUTINE MEDS *****			
/	06/03/16 07/03/16	ENOXaparin Sodium Inj 80 MG/0.8 ML SYRINGE 80 MG = 0.8 ML SC every 12 hours	Q12H	10:00	22:00
/	06/03/16 07/03/16	Famotidine Inj 20 MG in Dextrose Inj 5% 50 ML Baxter Batch Infuse IV over 15–30 min	Q12H	10:00	22:00
/	06/03/16 07/03/16	Mycophenolate Susp 1000MG/5ML 1000 MG = 5 ML PO/NG 2 times a day	BID	10:00	22:00
		***** PREMEDS *****			
/	06/03/16 07/03/16	Acetaminophen Tab 325 MG 650 MG = 2 Tab orally as directed (For Tylenol) pre platelets infusion	UD		
		***** ANTIMICROBIAL PREMIXED INJECTABLES *****			
/	06/03/16 06/04/15	Ampicillin Inj 1 GM Sodium Chloride Inj 0.9% Infuse IV over 15 min	Q6H	12:00 18:00	00:00 06:00
		***** CHEMO & MISC. INJECTABLES *****			
/	06/03/16 06/03/18	Doxorubicin HCl Inj 100 MG For IV use **VESICANT** Total number of syringes: ____ Each syringe contains: ____MG per ____mL	Q24H	17:00	–
/	06/03/16 06/03/18	Granisetron HCl Inj 1 MG in Dextrose Inj 5% 25 ML Baxter Batch Infuse IV over 5 min	Q24H	15:00	–
		***** PRN ORDERS *****			
/	06/03/16 07/03/16	Docusate Sodium Cap 100 MG 100 MG = 1 Cap orally 2 times a day as needed (For Colace) Give with plenty of water	BIDPO		

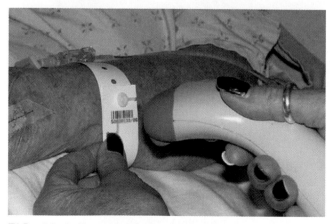

FIG. 10-4 Example of a hospital bar code.

FIG. 10-5 Example of a medication administration record (MAR).

ENTERAL DRUGS

Administering Oral Drugs

Always begin by washing your hands, and maintain Standard Precautions (see Box 10-1). When administering oral drugs, keep in mind the points outlined in the sections below.

Oral Medications

- Administration of some oral medications (and medications by other routes) requires special assessments. For example, the apical pulse should be auscultated for 1 full minute before any digitalis preparation is given (Figure 10-6). Administration of other oral medications may require blood pressure monitoring. Be sure to document all parameters on the MAR. In addition, do not forget to check your patient's identification and allergies before giving any medication (or medication by any other route).
- If the patient is experiencing difficulty swallowing (dysphagia), some tablets can be crushed with a clean mortar and pestle (or other device) (Figure 10-7) for easier administration. Crush one type of pill at a time

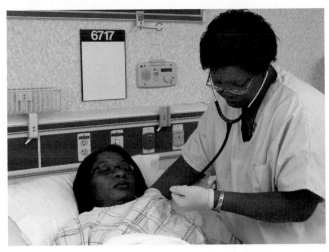

FIG. 10-6 Some medications require special assessment before administration, such as measuring the apical pulse rate.

because if you mix together all of the medications before crushing (instead of crushing them one at a time) and then spill some, there is no way to tell which drug has been wasted. Also, if all are mixed together, you cannot check the "Ten Rights" three times before giving the drug. Mix the crushed medication in a small amount of soft food, such as apple sauce or pudding. Be sure that the pill-crushing device is clean before and after you use it.

- *Caution:* Be sure to verify whether a medication can be crushed, by consulting a drug reference book or a pharmacist. Some oral medications, such as capsules, enteric-coated tablets, and sustained-release or long-acting drugs, should *not* be crushed, broken, or chewed (Figure 10-8). These medications are formulated to protect the gastric lining from irritation or to protect the drug from destruction from gastric acids, or are designed to break down gradually to slowly release the medication. If these drugs, designated with labels such as *sustained-release* or *extended-release*, are crushed or opened, then the intended action of the dosage form is destroyed. As a result, gastric irritation may

---

BOX 10-1

Standard Precautions

Always adhere to Standard Precautions, including the following:

- Wear clean gloves when exposed to or there is potential exposure to blood, body fluids, secretions, excretions, or any items that may contain these substances. Always wash hands immediately when there is direct contact with these substances or any item contaminated with blood, body fluids, secretions, or excretions. Gloves should be worn when giving injections. Be sure to assess for latex allergies and use nonlatex gloves if indicated.
- Wash hands after removing gloves and between patient contacts.
- Wear a mask, eye protective gear, and face shield during any procedure or patient care situation with the potential for splashing or spraying of blood, body fluids, secretions, or excretions. Use of a gown may also be indicated for these situations.
- When administering medications, once the exposure or procedure is completed and exposure is no longer a danger, remove soiled protective garments or gear.
- Never remove, cap, recap, bend, or break any used needle or needle system. Be sure to discard any disposable syringes and needles in the appropriate puncture-resistant container.
- If, during drug administration, you are handling or transporting soiled and contaminated items from the patient, dispose of them in the appropriately labeled containers for contaminated wastes.

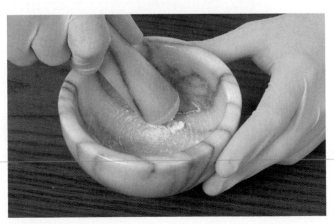

FIG. 10-7 Crushing tablets with a mortar and pestle.

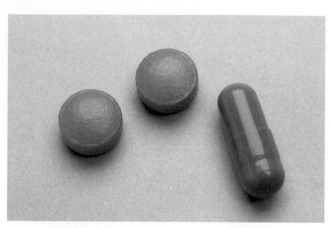

FIG. 10-8 Enteric-coated tablets and long-acting medications should not be crushed.

occur, the drug may be inactivated by gastric acids, or the immediate availability of a drug that was supposed to be released slowly may cause toxic effects. Check with the health care provider to see if an alternate form of the drug is needed.

- Be sure to position the patient in a sitting or side-lying position to make it easier to swallow oral medications and to avoid the risk of aspiration (Figure 10-9). Always take aspiration prevention measures as needed.
- Offer the patient a full glass of water; 120 to 180 mL of water or other fluid is recommended for the best dissolution and absorption of oral medications. Young patients and older adults may not be able to drink a full glass of water but should take enough fluid to ensure that the medication reaches the stomach. If the patient prefers another fluid, be sure to check for interactions between the medication and the fluid of choice. If fluid restriction is ordered, be sure to follow the guidelines.
- If the patient requests it, you may place the pill or capsule in his or her mouth with your gloved hand.
- Lozenges should not be chewed unless this is specifically instructed.

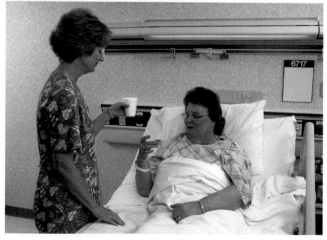

FIG. 10-9 Giving oral medications.

- Effervescent powders and tablets should be mixed with water and then given immediately after they are dissolved.
- Remain with the patient until all medication has been swallowed. If you are unsure whether a pill has been swallowed, ask the patient to open his or her mouth so that you can inspect to see if it is gone. Assist the patient to a comfortable position after the medication has been taken.
- Document the medication given on the MAR and monitor the patient for a therapeutic response as well as for adverse reactions.

Sublingual and Buccal Medications

The sublingual and buccal routes prevent destruction of the drugs in the gastrointestinal tract and allow for rapid absorption into the bloodstream through the oral mucous membranes. These routes are not often used. Be sure to provide instruction to the patient before giving these medications.

- Sublingual tablets should be placed under the tongue (Figure 10-10). Buccal tablets should be placed between the upper or lower molar teeth and the cheek.
- Be sure to wear gloves if you are placing the tablet into the patient's mouth. Adhere to Standard Precautions (see Box 10-1).
- Instruct the patient to allow the drug to dissolve completely before swallowing it.
- Fluids should not be taken with these drug forms. Instruct the patient not to drink anything until the tablet has dissolved completely.
- Be sure to instruct the patient not to swallow the tablet.
- When using the buccal route, alternate sides with each dose to reduce possible oral mucosal irritation.
- Document the medication given on the MAR (see Figure 10-5) and monitor the patient for a therapeutic response as well as for adverse reactions.

Liquid Medications

- Liquid medications may come in a single-dose (unit-dose) package, be poured into a medicine cup from a

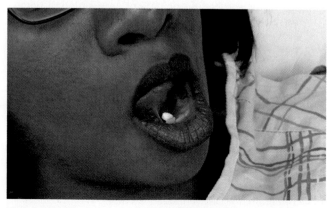

FIG. 10-10 Proper placement of a sublingual tablet.

multi-dose bottle, or be drawn up in an oral-dosing syringe (Figure 10-11). For young children, liquid forms are preferred because children may aspirate pills.

- When pouring a liquid medication from a container, first shake the bottle gently to mix the contents if indicated. Remove the cap and place it on the counter, upside down. Hold the bottle with the label against the palm of your hand to keep any spilled medication from altering the label. Place the medication cup at eye level and fill to the proper level on the scale (Figure 10-12). Pour the liquid so that the base of the meniscus is even with the appropriate line measure on the medicine cup.

- If you overfill the medication cup, discard the excess in the sink. Do not pour it back into the multidose bottle. Before replacing the cap, wipe the rim of the bottle with a paper towel.

- For small doses of liquid medications, draw liquid into a calibrated oral syringe. Do not use a hypodermic syringe or a syringe with a needle or syringe cap. If hypodermic syringes are used, the drug may be inadvertently given parenterally, or the syringe cap or needle, if not removed from the syringe, may become dislodged and accidentally aspirated by the patient when the syringe plunger is pressed.

Oral Medications and Infants

- Because infants cannot swallow oral pills or capsules, liquids are usually ordered.

- A plastic disposable oral-dosing syringe is recommended for measuring small doses of liquid medications. Using an oral-dosing syringe prevents the inadvertent parenteral administration of a drug once it is drawn up into the syringe.

- Position the infant so that the head is slightly elevated to prevent aspiration. Not all infants will be cooperative, and many may need to be partially restrained (Figure 10-13).

- Place the plastic dropper or syringe inside the infant's mouth, beside the tongue, and administer the liquid in

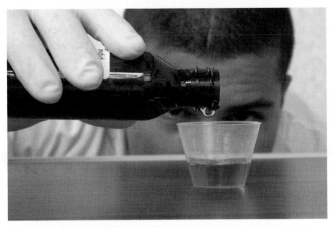

FIG. 10-12   Measuring liquid medication.

small amounts while allowing the infant to swallow each time.

- An empty nipple may be used to administer the medication. Place the liquid inside the empty nipple and allow the infant to suck the nipple. Add a few milliliters of water to rinse any remaining medication into the infant's mouth, unless contraindicated.

- Take great care to prevent aspiration. A crying infant can easily aspirate the medication.

- Do not add medication to a bottle of formula; the infant may refuse the feeding or may not drink all of it.

- Make sure that all of the oral medication has been taken, and then return the infant to a safe, comfortable position.

Administering Drugs Through a Nasogastric or Gastrostomy Tube

Always begin by washing your hands, and maintain Standard Precautions (see Box 10-1). Gloves should be

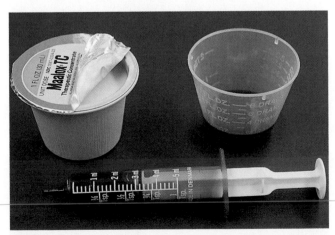

FIG. 10-11   **A,** Liquid medication in a unit-dose package. **B,** Liquid measured into a medicine cup from a multidose container. **C,** Liquid medicine in an oral-dosing syringe.

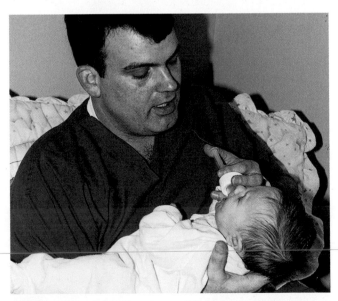

FIG. 10-13   Administering oral liquid medication to an infant.

worn for these procedures. When administering drugs via these routes, keep in mind the following points:

- Before giving drugs via these routes, position the patient in a semi-Fowler's or Fowler's position, and leave the head of the bed elevated for at least 30 minutes afterward to reduce the risk of aspiration (Figure 10-14).
- Assess whether fluid restriction or overload is a concern. It will be necessary to give water along with the medications to flush the tubing.
- Check to see if the drug should be taken on an empty or full stomach. If the drug is to be taken on an empty stomach, the feeding may need to be stopped before and after giving the medication. Follow the guidelines for the specific drug if this is necessary.
- Whenever possible, give liquid forms of the drugs to prevent clogging the tube.
- If tablets must be given, crush the tablets individually into a fine powder. Administer the drugs separately (Figure 10-15). Keeping the drugs separate allows for accurate identification if a dose is spilled. Be sure to check whether the medication should be crushed; enteric-coated and sustained-release tablets or capsules should not be crushed. Check with a pharmacist if you are unsure.
- Before administering the drugs, follow the institution's policy for verifying tube placement and checking gastric residual. Reinstill gastric residual per institutional policy, then clamp the tube (Figure 10-16).
- Dilute a crushed tablet or liquid medication in 15 to 30 mL of warm water. Some capsules may be opened and dissolved in 30 mL of warm water; check with a pharmacist.

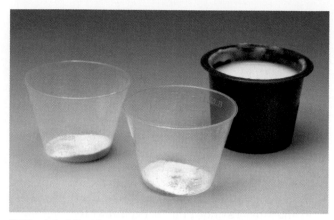

FIG. 10-15 Medications given through gastric tubes should be administered separately. Dilute crushed pills in 15 to 30 mL of water before administration.

- Remove the piston from an adaptable-tip syringe and attach it to the end of the tube. Unclamp the tube and pinch the tubing to close it again. Add 30 mL of warm water, and release the pinched tubing. Allow the water to flow in by gravity to flush the tube, and then pinch the tubing closed again before all the water is gone to prevent excessive air from entering the stomach.
- Pour the diluted medication into the syringe, and release the tubing to allow it to flow in by gravity. Flush between each drug with 10 mL of warm water (Figure 10-17). Be careful not to spill the medication mixture. Adjust fluid amounts if fluid restrictions are ordered, but sufficient fluid must be used to dilute the medication and to flush the tubing.

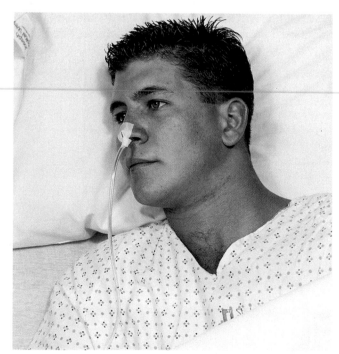

FIG. 10-14 Elevate the head of the bed before administering medications through a nasogastric tube.

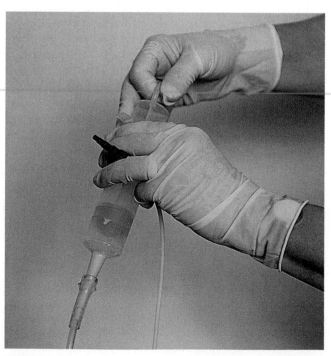

FIG. 10-16 Check the gastric residual before administering medications.

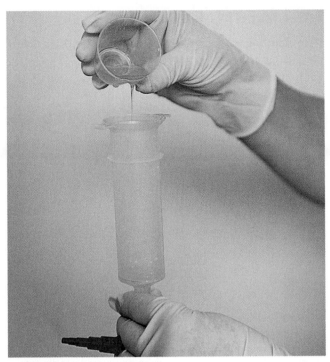

FIG. 10-17 Pour liquid medication into the syringe, then unclamp the tubing and allow it to flow in by gravity.

- If water or medication does not flow freely, you may apply gentle pressure with the plunger of the syringe or the bulb of an Asepto syringe. Do not try to force the medicine through the tubing.
- After the last drug dose, flush the tubing with 30 mL of warm water, and then clamp the tube. Resume the tube feeding when appropriate.
- Have the patient remain in a high Fowler's or slightly elevated right-side-lying position to reduce the risk of aspiration.
- Document the medications given on the MAR, the amount of fluid given on the patient's intake and output record, and the patient's response.

Administering Rectal Drugs

Always begin by washing your hands, and maintain Standard Precautions (see Box 10-1). Gloves should be worn for these procedures. When administering rectal drugs, keep in mind the following points:
- Assess the patient for the presence of active rectal bleeding or diarrhea, which generally are contraindications for rectal suppositories.
- Suppositories should not be divided to provide a smaller dose. The active drug may not be evenly distributed within the suppository base.
- Position the patient on the left side, unless contraindicated. The uppermost leg should be flexed toward the waist (Sims' position). Provide privacy, and drape the patient.
- The suppository should not be inserted into stool. Gently palpate the rectal wall for presence of feces. If possible, have the patient defecate. DO NOT

palpate the patient's rectum if the patient has had rectal surgery.
- Remove the wrapping from the suppository and lubricate the rounded tip with water-soluble jelly (Figure 10-18).
- Insert the tip of the suppository into the rectum while having the patient take a deep breath and exhale through the mouth. With your gloved finger, quickly and gently insert the suppository into the rectum, alongside the rectal wall, at least 2.5 cm beyond the internal sphincter (Figure 10-19).
- Have the patient remain lying on the left side for 15 to 20 minutes to allow absorption of the medication. With children it may be necessary to gently but firmly hold the buttocks in place for 5 to 10 minutes until the urge to expel the suppository has passed. Older adults with loss of sphincter control may not be able to retain the suppository.
- If the patient prefers to self-administer the suppository, the nurse should give specific instructions on the correct procedure and its purpose. Be sure to tell the patient to remove the medication wrapper.
- Use the same procedure for medications administered by a retention enema, such as sodium polystyrene sulfonate (see Chapter 27). Drugs given by enema are diluted in the smallest amount of solution possible.

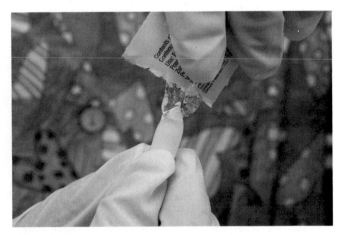

FIG. 10-18 Lubricate the suppository with a water-soluble lubricant.

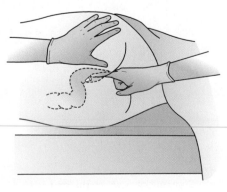

FIG. 10-19 Inserting a rectal suppository.

Retention enemas should be held for 30 minutes to 1 hour before expulsion, if possible.

- Document the medication on the MAR, and monitor the patient for the therapeutic effects of the rectal medication.

PARENTERAL DRUGS

Preparing for Parenteral Drug Administration

Figures 10-20 through 10-31 show equipment used for administering parenteral drugs.

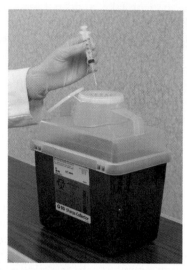

FIG. 10-20 NEVER RECAP A USED NEEDLE! Always dispose of *uncapped* needles in the appropriate sharps container. Refer to Box 10-1 for Standard Precautions.

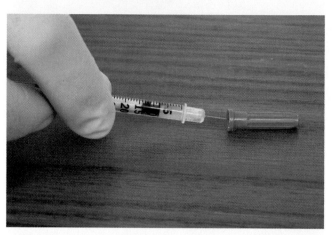

FIG. 10-21 An UNUSED needle may need to be recapped before the medication is given to the patient. The "scoop method" is one way to recap an unused needle safely. Several devices are also available for recapping needles safely. Be sure not to let the needle touch the counter top or the outside of the needle cap.

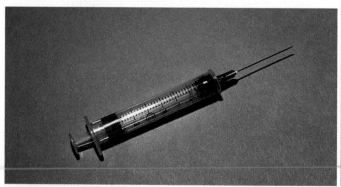

FIGS. 10-22 AND 10-23 There are several types of needle-stick prevention syringes. This example (Fig. 10-22) has a guard over the unused syringe. After the injection, the nurse pulls the guard up over the needle until it locks into place (Fig. 10-23).

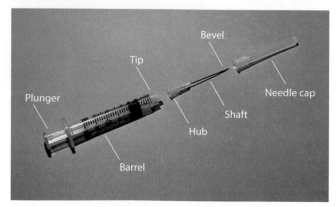

FIG. 10-24 The parts of a syringe and hypodermic needle.

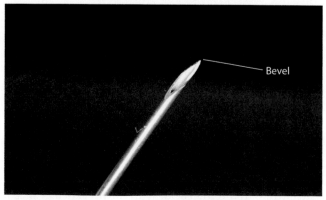

FIG. 10-25 Close-up view of the bevel of a needle.

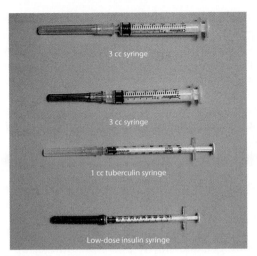

FIG. 10-26 Be sure to choose the correct size and type of syringe for the drug ordered.

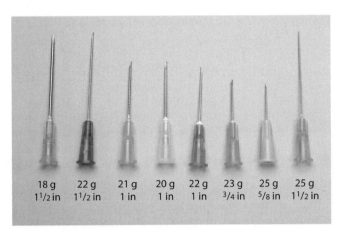

FIG. 10-27 Needles come in various gauges and lengths. The larger the gauge, the smaller the needle and often the shorter in length. Be sure to choose the correct needle—gauge and length—for the type of injection ordered.

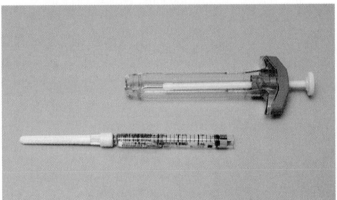

FIGS. 10-28 AND 10-29 Some medications come in prefilled, sterile medication cartridges that fit into a syringe. These figures show the Carpuject prefilled cartridge and syringe system. Follow the manufacturer's instructions for assembling prefilled syringes. After use, the syringe is disposed of in a sharps container.

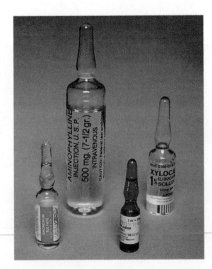

FIG. 10-30 Ampoules containing medications come in various sizes. The ampoules must be broken carefully to withdraw the medication.

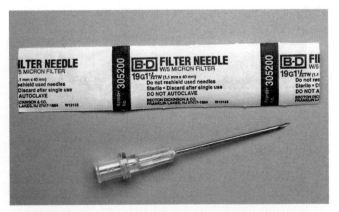

FIG. 10-31 A filter needle should be used when withdrawing medication from an ampoule. Filter needles help remove minute glass particles that may result from breaking the ampoule. DO NOT USE A FILTER NEEDLE for injecting medication into a patient! Filter needles should also be used to withdraw medication from a vial if a needleless system is not used.

Removing Medications from Ampoules

Always begin by washing your hands, and maintain Standard Precautions (see Box 10-1). Gloves may be worn for these procedures. When performing these procedures, keep in mind the following points:

- When removing medication from an ampoule, use a sterile filter needle (see Figure 10-31). These needles are designed to filter out glass particles that may be present inside the ampoule after it is broken. The filter needle IS NOT intended for administration of the drug to the patient.
- Medication often rests in the top part of the ampoule. Tap the top of the ampoule lightly and quickly with your finger until all fluid moves to the bottom portion of the ampoule (Figure 10-32).
- Place a small gauze pad or dry alcohol swab around the neck of the ampoule to protect your hand. Snap the neck quickly and firmly and break the ampoule *away* from your body (Figures 10-33 and 10-34).

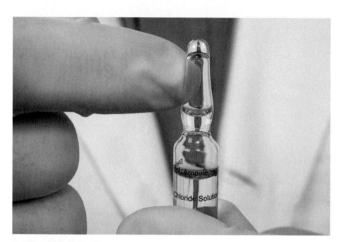

FIG. 10-32 Tapping the ampoule to move the fluid below the neck.

- To draw up the medication, either set the open ampoule on a flat surface or hold the ampoule upside down. Insert the filter needle (attached to a syringe) into the centre of the ampoule opening. Do not allow the needle tip or shaft to touch the rim of the ampoule (Figure 10-35).
- Gently pull back on the plunger to draw up the medication. Keep the needle tip below the fluid within the vial; tip the ampoule to bring all of the fluid within reach of the needle.
- If air bubbles are aspirated do not expel them into the ampoule. Remove the needle from the ampoule, hold the syringe with the needle pointing up, and tap the side of the syringe with your finger to cause the bubbles to rise toward the needle. Draw back slightly on the plunger, and slowly push the plunger upward to eject the air. Do not eject fluid.
- Excess medication should be disposed in the sink. Hold the syringe vertically with needle tip upward and slanted toward the sink. Slowly eject the excess fluid into the sink, and then recheck the fluid level by holding the syringe vertically.
- Remove the filter needle and replace with the appropriate needle for administration.
- Dispose of the glass ampoule pieces and the used filter needle into the appropriate sharps container.

Removing Medications from Vials

Always begin by washing your hands, and maintain Standard Precautions (see Box 10-1). Gloves may be worn for these procedures. When performing these procedures, keep in mind the following points:

- Vials can contain either a single dose or multiple doses of medications. Follow the institution's policy for using opened multidose vials. Many facilities require that multidose vials be marked with the date and time of opening and the discard date (per institution

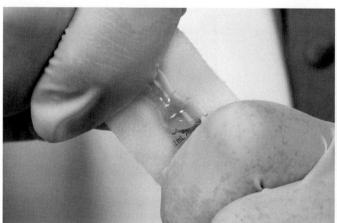
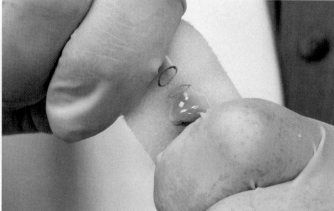

FIGS. 10-33 AND 10-34 Breaking an ampoule.

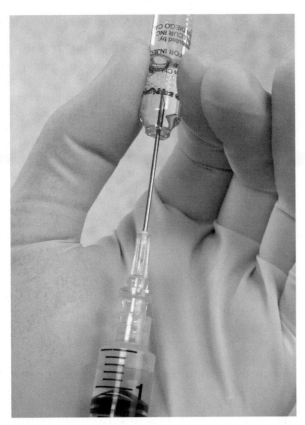

FIG. 10-35 Using a filter needle to draw medication from an ampoule.

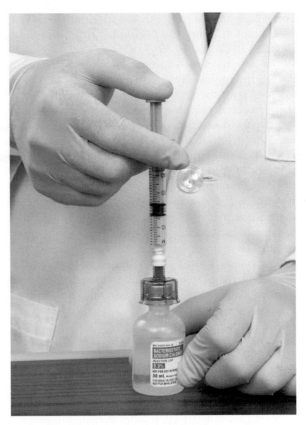

FIG. 10-36 Insert air into a vial before withdrawing medication (needleless system shown).

policy). If you are unsure about the age of an opened vial of medication, discard it and obtain a new one.

- Check institutional policies regarding which drugs should be prepared using a filter needle.
- If the vial is unused, remove the cap from the top of the vial.
- If the vial has been previously opened and used, wipe the top of the vial vigorously with an alcohol swab.
- Air must first be injected into a vial before fluid can be withdrawn. The amount of air injected into a vial should equal the amount of fluid that needs to be withdrawn.
- Determine the volume of fluid to be withdrawn from the vial. Pull back on the syringe's plunger to draw the amount of air into the syringe that is equivalent to the volume of medication to be removed from the vial. Insert the syringe into the vial, preferably using a needleless system. Figure 10-36 shows a needleless system of vial access. Inject the air into the vial.
- While holding onto the plunger, invert the vial, and remove the desired amount of medication (Figure 10-37).
- Gently but firmly tap the syringe to remove air bubbles. Excess fluid, if present, should be discarded into a sink.

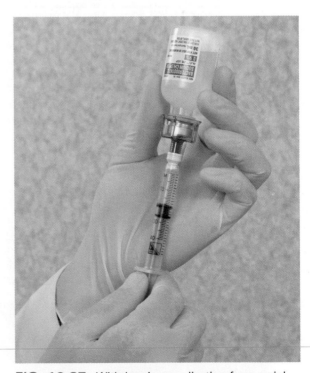

FIG. 10-37 Withdrawing medication from a vial (needleless system shown).

- Some vials are not compatible with needleless systems and therefore require a needle for fluid withdrawals (Figures 10-38 and 10-39).
- When an injection requires two medications from two different vials, begin by injecting air into the first vial (without touching the fluid in the first vial), and then inject air into the second vial. Immediately remove the desired dose from the second vial. Change needles (if possible), and then remove the exact prescribed dose of drug from the first vial. Take great care not to contaminate the drug in one vial with the drug from the other vial.
- For injections, if a needle has been used to remove medication from a vial, always change the needle before administering the dose. Changing needles ensures that a clean and sharp needle is used for the injection. Medication that remains on the outside of the needle may cause irritation to the patient's tissues. In addition, the needle may become dull if used to puncture a rubber stopper.

Injections Overview

Needle Insertion Angles for Intramuscular, Subcutaneous, and Intradermal Injections

- For intramuscular (IM) injections, insert the needle at a 90-degree angle (see Figure 10-40). Intramuscular injections deposit the drug deep into muscle tissue, where the drug is absorbed through blood vessels within the muscle. The rate of absorption of medication with the intramuscular route is slower than with the intravenous route but faster than with the subcutaneous route. Intramuscular injections generally require a longer needle to reach the muscle tissue, but shorter needles may be needed for older patients, children, and adults who are malnourished. The site chosen will also determine the length of the needle needed. In general, aqueous medications can be given with a 22- to 27-gauge needle but oil-based or more viscous medications are given with an 18- to 25-gauge needle. Average needle lengths for children range from 16 mm to 25 mm, and needles for adults range from 25 mm to 38 mm.
- For subcutaneous (SC or SQ) injections, insert the needle at either a 90- or a 45-degree angle. Subcutaneous injections deposit the drug into the loose connective tissue under the dermis. This tissue is not as well supplied with blood vessels as is the muscle tissue; as a result, drugs are absorbed more slowly than when given intramuscularly. In general, use a 25-gauge, 12-mm to 16-mm needle. A 90-degree angle is used for an average-sized patient; a 45-degree angle may be used for thin, emaciated, or cachectic patients and for children. To ensure correct needle length,

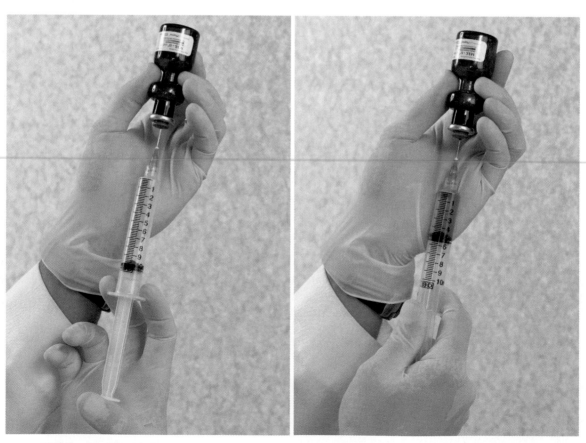

FIGS. 10-38 AND 10-39 Using a needle and syringe to remove medication from a vial.

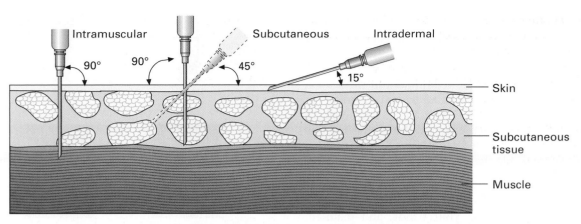

FIG. 10-40   Various needle angles.

grasp the skinfold with the thumb and forefinger, and choose a needle that is approximately one half the length of the skinfold from top to bottom.

- Intradermal (ID) injections are given into the outer layers of the dermis in tiny amounts, usually 0.01 to 0.1 mL. These injections are used mostly for diagnostic purposes, such as testing for allergies or tuberculosis, and for local anaesthesia. Little of the drug is absorbed systemically. In general, choose a tuberculin or 1-mL syringe with a 26- or 27-gauge needle that is 10 mm to 16 mm long. The angle of injection is 5 to 15 degrees with the bevel angled upward.

Z-Track Method

- The Z-track method is used for injections of irritating substances such as iron dextran and hydroxyzine (Figures 10-41 and 10-42). This technique reduces pain, irritation, and staining at the injection site. Some facilities recommend this method for *all* intramuscular injections.
- After choosing and preparing the site for injection, use your nondominant hand to pull the skin laterally and hold it in this position while giving the injection. Insert the needle at a 90-degree angle, aspirate for 5 to 10 seconds to check for blood return, and then inject the medication slowly. After injecting the medication, wait 10 seconds before withdrawing the needle. Withdraw the needle slowly and smoothly, maintaining the 90-degree angle.
- Release the skin immediately after withdrawing the needle in order to seal off the injection site. This technique forms a Z-shaped track in the more sensitive subcutaneous tissue, which prevents the medication from leaking through the tissue from the muscle site of injection. Apply gentle pressure to the site with a dry gauze pad.

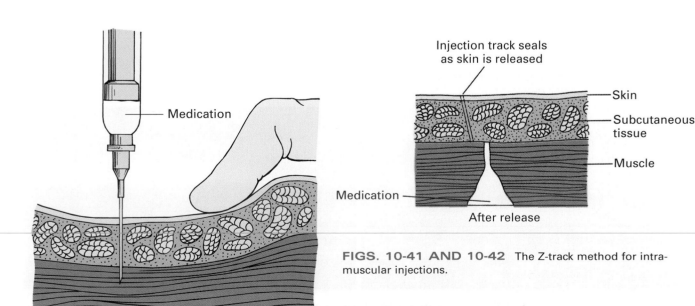

FIGS. 10-41 AND 10-42   The Z-track method for intramuscular injections.

Air-Lock Technique

- Some facilities recommend administering intramuscular injections using the air-lock technique (Figure 10-43). Check institutional policy.
- After withdrawing the desired amount of medication into the syringe, withdraw an additional 0.2 mL of air. Be sure to inject at a 90-degree angle. The small air bubble that follows the medication during the injection may help prevent the medication from leaking through the needle track into the subcutaneous tissues.

Intradermal Injection

Always begin by washing your hands, and maintain Standard Precautions (see Box 10-1). Gloves should be worn for these procedures. When giving an intradermal injection, keep in mind the following points:

- Be sure to choose an appropriate site for the injection. Avoid areas of bruising, rashes, inflammation, edema, or skin discolorations.
- Help the patient to a comfortable position. Extend and support the elbow and forearm on a flat surface.
- In general, three to four finger-widths below the antecubital space and one hand-width above the wrist are the preferred locations on the forearm. Areas on the back that are also suitable for subcutaneous injection may be used if the forearm is not appropriate.
- After cleansing the site with an alcohol swab and allowing it to dry, stretch the skin over the site with your nondominant hand.
- With the needle almost against the patient's skin, insert the needle, bevel UP, at a 5- to 15-degree angle until resistance is felt, and then advance the needle through the epidermis, approximately 3 mm (Figures 10-44 and 10-45). The needle tip should still be visible under the skin.
- Do not aspirate. This area under the skin contains a minimal number of blood vessels.
- Slowly inject the medication. It is normal to feel resistance, and a bleb that resembles a mosquito bite (about 6 mm in diameter) should form at the site.
- Withdraw the needle slowly while gently applying a gauze pad at the site, but do not massage the site.

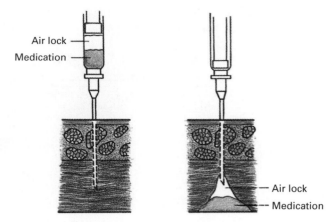

FIG. 10-43 Air-lock technique for intramuscular injections.

- Dispose of the syringe and needle in the appropriate container. DO NOT RECAP the needle. Wash your hands after removing gloves.
- Provide instructions to the patient as needed for a follow-up visit for reading the skin testing.
- Document in the MAR the date of the skin testing and the date that results should be read, if applicable.

Subcutaneous Injections

Always begin by washing your hands, and maintain Standard Precautions (see Box 10-1). Gloves should be worn for these procedures. When giving a subcutaneous injection, keep in mind the following points:

- Be sure to choose an appropriate site for the injection (Figure 10-46). Avoid areas of bruising, rashes, inflammation, edema, or skin discolorations.
- Ensure that the needle size is correct. Grasp the skinfold between your thumb and forefinger and measure from top to bottom. The needle should be approximately one half of this length.
- Cleanse the site with an alcohol or antiseptic swab (Figure 10-47), and let the skin dry (occurs almost immediately). NOTE: Some facilities discourage the use of alcohol for insulin injections (some use saline, whereas others may use nothing).
- Tell the patient that he or she will feel a "stick" as you insert the needle.

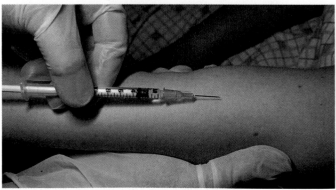
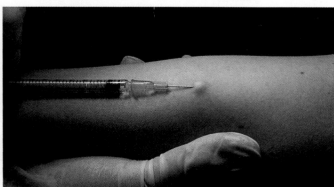

FIGS. 10-44 AND 10-45 Intradermal injection.

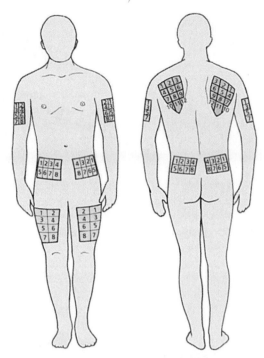

FIG. 10-46 Potential sites for subcutaneous injections.

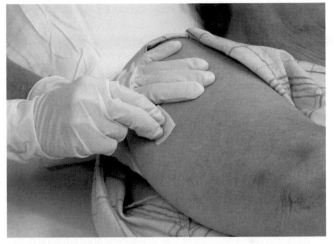

FIG. 10-47 Before giving an injection, cleanse the skin with an alcohol or antiseptic swab.

- For an average-sized patient, pinch the skin with your nondominant hand, and insert the needle quickly at a 90-degree angle (Figure 10-48).
- For an obese patient, pinch the skin, and insert the needle at a 90-degree angle. Be sure the needle is long enough to reach the base of the skinfold.
- For a thin patient or a child, pinch the skin gently, then insert the needle at a 45-degree angle.
- Injections given in the abdomen should be given at least 5 cm away from the umbilicus because of the surrounding vascular structure (Figure 10-49).
- After the needle enters the skin, grasp the lower end of the syringe with your nondominant hand. Move your dominant hand to the end of the plunger—be careful not to move the syringe.

- Aspiration of medication to check for blood return is not necessary for subcutaneous injections, but some institutions may require it. Check institutional policy. Heparin injections and insulin injections are NOT aspirated before injection.
- With your dominant hand, slowly inject the medication.
- Withdraw the needle quickly, and place a swab or sterile gauze pad over the site.
- Apply gentle pressure, but do not massage the site. If necessary, apply a bandage to the site.
- Dispose of the syringe and needle in the appropriate container. DO NOT RECAP the needle. Wash your hands after removing gloves.

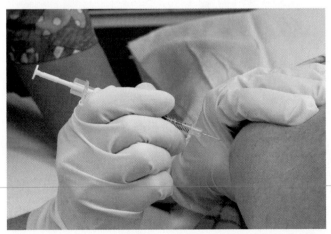

FIG. 10-48 Giving a subcutaneous injection at a 90-degree angle.

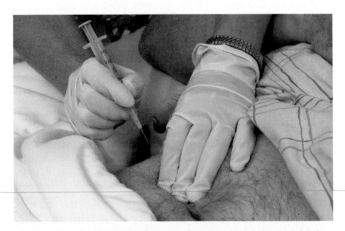

FIG. 10-49 When giving a subcutaneous injection in the abdomen, be sure to choose a site at least 5 cm away from the umbilicus.

- Document the medication given on the MAR and monitor the patient for a therapeutic response as well as for adverse reactions.
- For heparin or other subcutaneous anticoagulant injections, follow the manufacturers' recommendations for injection technique as needed. DO NOT ASPIRATE before injecting, and DO NOT MASSAGE the site after injection. These actions may cause a hematoma at the injection site.

Insulin Syringes

- Always use an insulin syringe to measure and administer insulin. When giving small doses of insulin, use an insulin syringe that is calibrated for smaller doses. Figure 10-50 shows insulin syringes with two different calibrations. Note that on the 100-unit syringe, each line represents 2 units; on the 50-unit syringe, each line represents 1 unit. NOTE: One unit of insulin is NOT equivalent to one millilitre of insulin.
- Figure 10-51 shows several examples of devices that can be used to help the patient self-administer insulin. These devices feature a multidose container of insulin and easy-to-read dials for choosing the correct dose. The needle is changed with each use.
- When two different types of insulin are drawn up into the same syringe, always draw up the clear, rapid-acting insulin into the syringe first (Figure 10-52). An easy way to remember which insulin is drawn up first is thinking "Fast/First."

Intramuscular Injections

Always begin by washing your hands, and maintain Standard Precautions (see Box 10-1). Gloves should be worn for these procedures. When giving an intramuscular injection, keep in mind the following points:

- Choose the appropriate site for the injection by assessing not only the size and integrity of the muscle but also the amount and type of injection. Palpate potential sites for areas of hardness or tenderness and note the presence of bruising or infection.
- Assist the patient to the proper position and ensure the patient's comfort.
- Locate the proper site for the injection and cleanse the site with an alcohol swab. Keep the swab or a sterile gauze pad nearby and allow the alcohol to dry before injection.
- With your nondominant hand, pull the skin taut. Follow the instructions for the Z-track method (p. 159), if appropriate.
- Grasp the syringe with your dominant hand as if holding a dart and hold the needle at a 90-degree angle to the skin. Tell the patient to expect a "stick" feeling as you insert the needle.
- Insert the needle quickly and firmly into the muscle. Grasp the lower end of the syringe with the non-

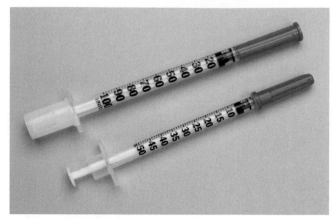

FIG. 10-50 Insulin syringes are available in 100-unit and 50-unit calibrations.

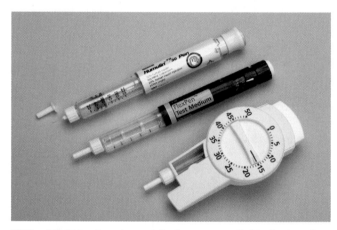

FIG. 10-51 A variety of devices are available for insulin injections.

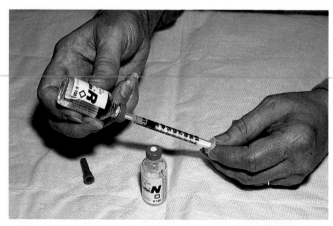

FIG. 10-52 Mixing two types of insulin in the same syringe.

dominant hand while still holding the skin back, to stabilize the syringe. With the dominant hand, pull back on the plunger for 5 to 10 seconds to check for blood return.

- If no blood appears in the syringe, inject the medication slowly, at the rate of 1 mL every 10 seconds. After the drug is injected, wait 10 seconds, and then withdraw the needle smoothly while releasing the skin.
- Apply gentle pressure at the site and watch for bleeding. Apply a bandage if necessary.
- If blood does appear in the syringe, remove the needle, dispose of the medication and syringe, and prepare a new syringe with the medication.
- Dispose of the syringe and needle in the appropriate container. DO NOT RECAP the needle. Wash your hands after removing gloves.
- Document the medication given on the MAR and monitor the patient for a therapeutic response as well as for adverse reactions.

Ventrogluteal Site

- The ventrogluteal site is the *preferred* site for adults and for children as well as infants. It is considered the safest of all the sites because the muscle is deep and away from major blood vessels and nerves (Figure 10-53).

- The patient should be positioned on one side, with knees bent and upper leg slightly ahead of the bottom leg. If necessary, the patient may remain in the supine position.
- Palpate the greater trochanter at the head of the femur and the anterosuperior iliac spine. As in Figure 10-54, use the left hand to find landmarks when injecting into the patient's right ventrogluteal, and use the right hand to find landmarks when injecting into the patient's left ventrogluteal site. Place the palm of your hand over the greater trochanter and your index finger on the anterosuperior iliac spine. Point your thumb toward the patient's groin and your fingers toward the patient's head. Spread the middle finger back along the iliac crest, toward the buttocks, as much as possible.
- The injection site is the centre of the triangle formed by your middle and index fingers (see arrow in Figure 10-54).
- Before giving the injection, you may need to switch hands so that you can use your dominant hand to give the injection.
- Follow the general instructions for giving an intramuscular injection (Figure 10-55).

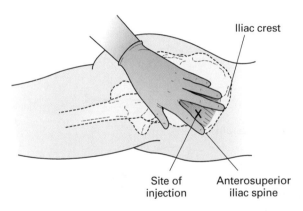

Iliac crest

Site of injection

Anterosuperior iliac spine

FIG. 10-53 Finding landmarks for a ventrogluteal injection.

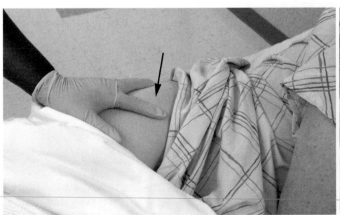
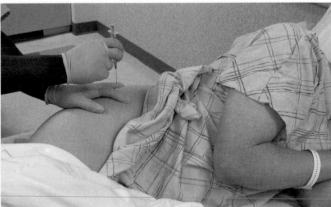

FIGS. 10-54 AND 10-55 Ventrogluteal intramuscular injection.

Vastus Lateralis Site

- Generally, the vastus lateralis muscle is well developed and not located near major nerves or blood vessels. It is the preferred site of injection of drugs such as immunizations for infants (Figure 10-56).

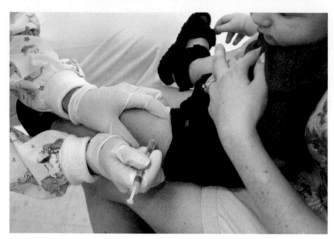

FIG. 10-56 Vastus lateralis intramuscular injection in an infant.

- The patient may be sitting or lying supine; if supine, have the patient bend the knee of the leg in which the injection will be given.
- To find the correct site of injection, place one hand above the knee and one hand below the greater trochanter of the femur. Locate the midline of the anterior thigh and the midline of the lateral side of the thigh. The injection site is located within the rectangular area (Figures 10-57, 10-58, and 10-59).

Deltoid Site

- The deltoid injection site is easily accessible but should only be used for small volumes of medication (0.5 to 1 mL). Assess the site carefully—this muscle may not be well developed in some adults (Figure 10-60). In addition, the axillary nerve lies beneath the deltoid muscle. Always check medication administration policies, because some facilities do not use deltoid intramuscular injections. The deltoid site is used for giving immunizations to toddlers, older children, and adults, but not to infants.
- The patient may be sitting or lying down. Remove clothing to expose the upper arm and shoulder.

FIGS. 10-57, 10-58, AND 10-59 Vastus lateralis intramuscular injection.

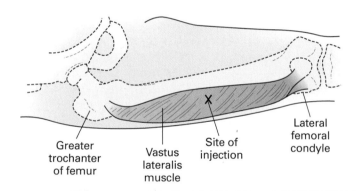

Greater trochanter of femur

Vastus lateralis muscle

Site of injection

Lateral femoral condyle

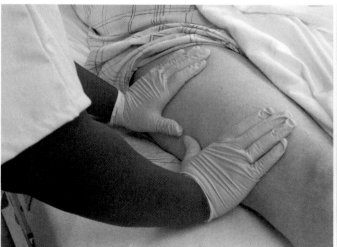

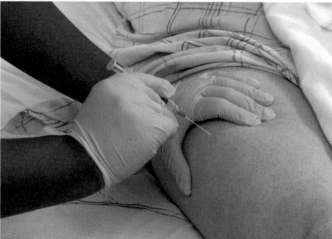

Tight-fitting sleeves should not be rolled up. Have the patient relax the arm and slightly bend the elbow.

- Palpate the lower edge of the acromion process. This edge becomes the base of an imaginary triangle (Figure 10-61).
- Place three fingers below this edge of the acromion process. Find the point on the lateral arm in line with the axilla. The injection site will be in the centre of this

triangle, three finger-widths (2.5 to 5 cm) below the acromion process.

- In children and smaller adults it may be necessary to bunch the underlying tissue together before giving the injection and use a shorter (16 mm) needle (Figure 10-62).
- To reduce patient anxiety, have the patient look away before you give the injection.

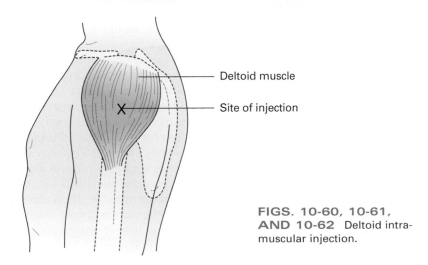

Deltoid muscle

Site of injection

FIGS. 10-60, 10-61, AND 10-62 Deltoid intramuscular injection.

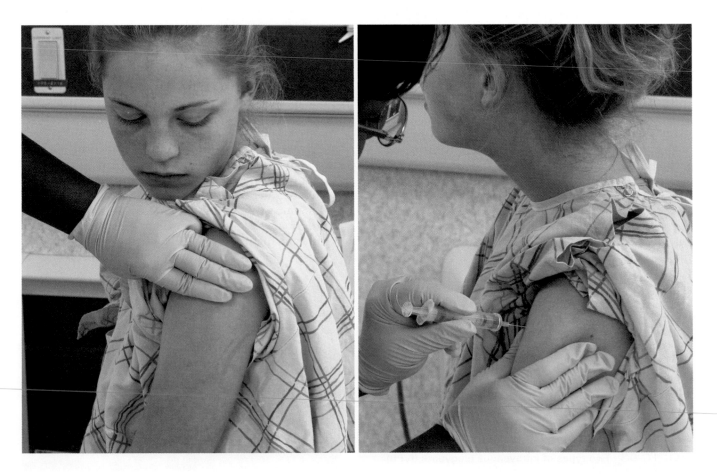

Preparing Intravenous Medications

Always begin by washing your hands, and maintain Standard Precautions (see Box 10-1). Gloves should be worn for most of these procedures. When administering intravenous drugs, keep in mind the following points:

- The intravenous route for medication administration provides for rapid onset and faster therapeutic drug levels in the blood than other routes. However, the intravenous route is also potentially more dangerous. Once an intravenous drug is given, it begins to act immediately and cannot be removed. The nurse must be aware of the drug's intended effects and possible adverse effects. In addition, hypersensitivity (allergic) reactions may occur quickly.
- Many provinces in Canada have made safety-engineered needles or needleless systems mandatory for all infusion lines.
- Before giving an intravenous medication, assess the patient's drug allergies, assess the intravenous line for patency, and assess the site for signs of phlebitis or infiltration.
- When more than one intravenous medication is to be given, check with the pharmacy for compatibility if medications are to be infused at the same time.
- Check the expiration date of both the medication and infusion bags.
- In many institutions, the pharmacy is responsible for preparing intravenous solutions and intravenous piggy-back (IVPB) admixtures for administration under a special laminar air-flow hood. If you are mixing the IVPB medications, be sure to verify which type of fluid to use and the correct amount of solution for the dosage.
- Most IVPB medications are provided with a system that allows the intravenous medication vial to be attached to a small-volume minibag for administration. Figure 10-63 shows two examples of IVPB medications attached to small-volume infusion bags.
- These IVPB medication setups allow for mixing of the drug and diluent immediately before the medication is given. Remember that if the seals are not broken and the medication is not mixed with the fluid in the infusion bag, the medication stays in the vial! As a result, the patient does not receive the ordered drug dose; instead, the patient receives a small amount of plain intravenous fluid.

- One type of IVPB that needs to be activated before administration is illustrated in Figure 10-64. To activate this type of IVPB, snap the connection area between the intravenous infusion bag and the vial (Figure 10-65). Gently squeeze the fluid from the infusion bag into the vial and allow the medication to dissolve (Figure 10-66). After a few minutes, rotate the vial gently to ensure that all of the powder is dissolved. When the drug is fully dissolved, hold the IVPB apparatus by the vial and squeeze the bag; fluid will enter the bag from the vial. Make sure that all of the medication is returned to the IVPB bag.
- When hanging these IVPB medications, take care NOT to squeeze the bag. This may cause some of the fluid to leak back into the vial and alter the dose given.
- Always label the IVPB bag with the patient's name and room number, the name of the medication, the dose, the date and time mixed, your initials, and the date and time it was given.
- Some intravenous medications must be mixed using a needle and syringe. After checking the order, and the compatibility of the drug with the intravenous fluid, wipe the port of the intravenous bag with an alcohol swab (Figure 10-67).
- Carefully insert the needle into the centre of the port and inject the medication (Figures 10-68 and 10-69). Note how the medication remains in the lower part of the intravenous infusion bag. To infuse an even concentration of medication, gently shake the bag after injecting the drug (Figure 10-70).
- Always label the intravenous infusion bag when a drug has been added (Figure 10-71). Label per institution policy and include the patient's name and room number, the name of the medication, the date and time mixed, your initials, and the date and time the infusion was started. In addition, label all intravenous infusion tubing per institution policy.

FIG. 10-63   Two types of intravenous piggyback (IVPB) medication delivery systems. These IVPB medications must be activated before administration to the patient.

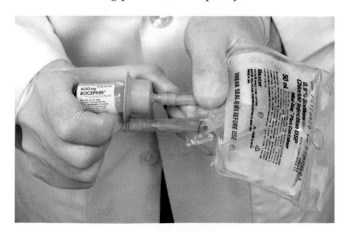

FIG. 10-64   Activating an IVPB infusion bag (step 1).

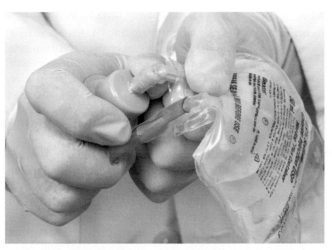

FIG. 10-65 Activating an IVPB infusion bag *(step 2).*

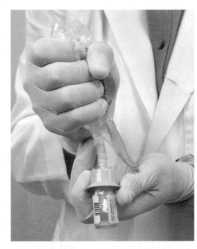

FIG. 10-66 Activating an IVPB infusion bag *(step 3).*

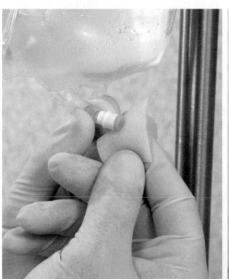
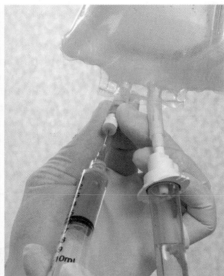
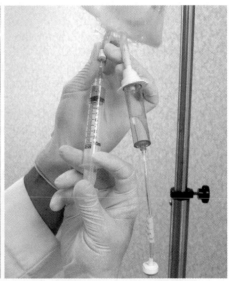

FIGS. 10-67, 10-68, AND 10-69 Adding a medication to an intravenous infusion bag with a needle and syringe.

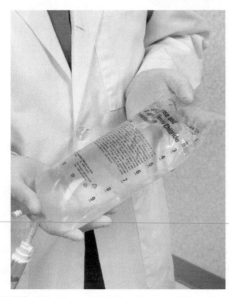

FIG. 10-70 Mix the medication thoroughly before infusing.

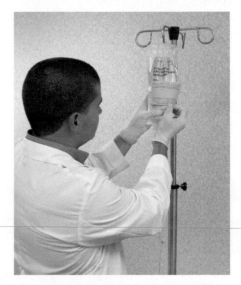

FIG. 10-71 Label the intravenous infusion bag when medication has been added.

Infusions of Intravenous Piggyback Medications

Always begin by washing your hands, and maintain Standard Precautions (see Box 10-1). Gloves should be worn for these procedures.

- Figure 10-72 shows an IVPB medication infusion with a primary gravity infusion. When the IVPB bag is hung higher than the primary intravenous infusion bag, the IVPB medication will infuse until empty, and then the primary infusion will take over again.
- When beginning the infusion, attach the IVPB tubing to the upper port on the primary intravenous tubing. A back-check valve above this port prevents the medication from infusing up into the primary intravenous infusion bag.
- Fully open the clamp of the IVPB tubing and regulate the infusion rate with the roller clamp of the primary infusion tubing. Be sure to note the drip factor of the tubing and calculate the drops per minute to count to set the correct infusion rate for the IVPB.
- Monitor the patient during the infusion. Observe for hypersensitivity and for adverse reactions. In addition, observe the intravenous infusion site for infiltration. Have the patient report if pain or burning occurs.
- Monitor the rate of infusion during the IVPB administration. Changes in arm position may alter the infusion rate.

- When the infusion is complete, clamp the IVPB tubing, and check the primary intravenous infusion rate. If necessary, adjust the clamp to the correct infusion rate.
- Figure 10-73 shows an IVPB medication infusion with a primary infusion that is running through an electronic infusion pump.
- When giving IVPB drugs through an intravenous infusion by a pump, attach the IVPB tubing to the port on the primary intravenous tubing *above* the pump. Open the roller clamp of the IVPB bag. Make sure that the IVPB bag is higher than the primary intravenous infusion bag.
- Following the manufacturer's directions, set the infusion pump to deliver the IVPB medication. Entering the volume of the IVPB bag and the desired time frame of the infusion (such as over a 60-minute period) will cause the pump to automatically calculate the IVPB rate. Start the IVPB infusion as indicated by the pump.
- Monitor the patient during the infusion, as described earlier.
- When the infusion is complete, the primary intravenous infusion will automatically resume.
- Be sure to document the medication given on the MAR and continue to monitor the patient for adverse reactions and therapeutic effects.
- When giving IVPB medications through a saline (heparin) lock, follow the facility's guidelines for the

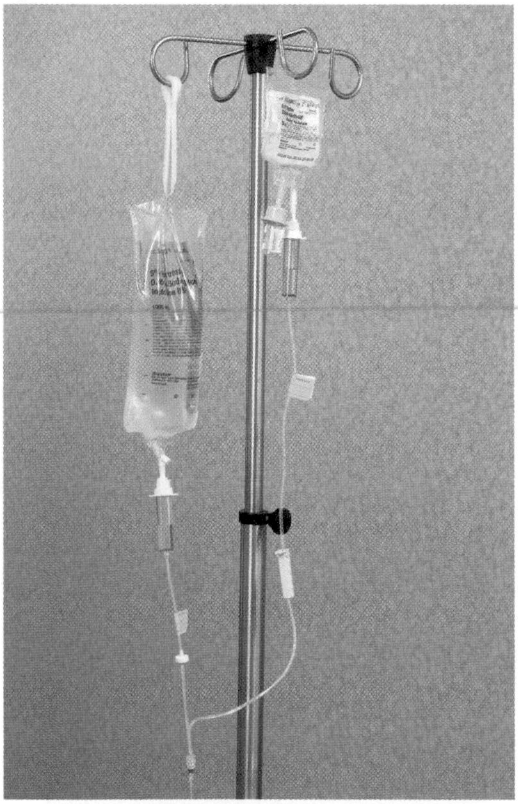

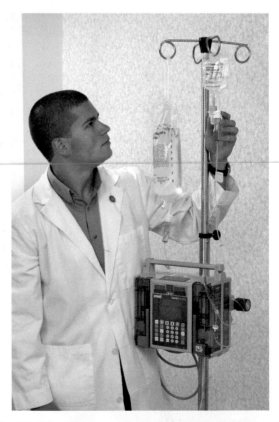

FIG. 10-72 Infusing an IVPB medication with a primary gravity intravenous infusion.

FIG. 10-73 Infusing an IVPB medication with the primary intravenous infusion on an electronic infusion pump.

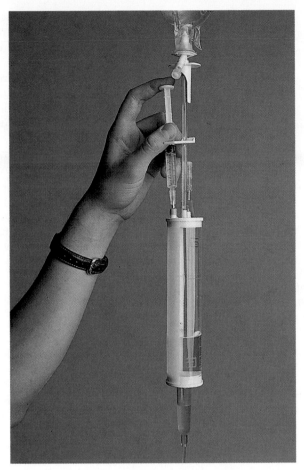

FIG. 10-74 Adding a medication to a volume-controlled administration set.

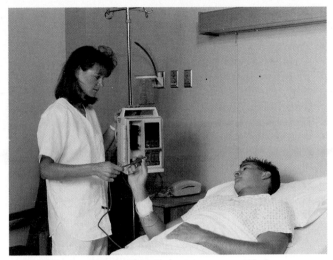

FIG. 10-75 Instructing the patient on the use of a patient-controlled analgesia (PCA) pump.

Intravenous Push Medications

Always begin by washing your hands, and maintain Standard Precautions (see Box 10-1).

When administering intravenous push (or bolus) medications, keep in mind the following points:

- Registered nurses are usually the only nursing staff members allowed to give intravenous push medications, and they may do so only under specified conditions.
- Intravenous push injections allow for rapid intravenous administration of a drug. The term *bolus* refers to a dose given all at once. Intravenous push injections may be given through an existing intravenous line, through an intravenous (saline or heparin) lock, or directly into a vein.
- Because the medication may have an immediate effect, monitor the patient closely for adverse reactions, as well as for therapeutic effects.
- Follow the manufacturer's guidelines carefully when preparing an intravenous push medication. Some drugs require careful dilution. Consult a pharmacist if unsure about the dilution procedure. Improper dilution may increase the risk of phlebitis and other complications.

Most drugs given by intravenous push injection should be given over a period of 1 to 5 minutes to reduce local or systemic adverse effects. Always time the dosage with your watch because it is difficult to estimate the time accurately. However, adenosine (Adenocard) must be given rapidly, within 2 to 3 seconds, for optimal action. ALWAYS check packaging information for guidelines because many errors and adverse effects have been associated with too-rapid intravenous drug administration. Many institutions have a Parenteral Drug Guide manual that provides guidelines regarding dilution, time of infusion, and key information such as action, adverse effects, and compatibilities.

flushing protocol before and after the medication is administered.

- Figure 10-74 illustrates a volume-controlled administration set that can be used for intravenous medications. The chamber is attached to the infusion between the intravenous infusion bag and the intravenous tubing. Fill the chamber with the desired amount of fluid, and then add the medication via the port above the chamber, as shown in the photo. Be sure to cleanse the port with an alcohol swab before inserting the needle in the port. The chamber should be labelled with the medication's name, dosage, and time added and your initials. Infuse the drug at the prescribed rate.
- In patient-controlled analgesia (PCA), a specialized pump is used to allow patients to self-administer pain medications, usually opiates (Figure 10-75). These pumps allow the patient to self-administer only as much medication as needed to control the pain by pushing a button for intravenous bolus doses. Safety features of the pump prevent accidental overdoses. A patient receiving PCA pump infusions should be monitored closely for response to the drug, excessive sedation, hypotension, and changes in mental and respiratory status. Follow the facility's guidelines for setup and use.

Intravenous Push Medications Through an Intravenous Lock

- Prepare two syringes of 0.10% normal saline (NS); both syringes should contain 2 mL. (NOTE: Some extension tubings require 3 mL). Prepare medication for injection. (Facilities may differ in protocol for intravenous lock flushes; follow institutional policy.) If ordered, prepare a syringe with heparin flush solution.
- Follow the guidelines for a needleless system, if used.
- Cleanse the injection port of the intravenous lock with an antiseptic swab after removing the cap, if present (Figure 10-76).
- Insert the syringe of 2–3 mL NS to the injection port (Figure 10-77; needleless system shown). Open the clamp of the intravenous lock tubing, if present.
- Gently aspirate and observe for blood return. Absence of blood return does not mean that the intravenous line is occluded; further assessment may be required.

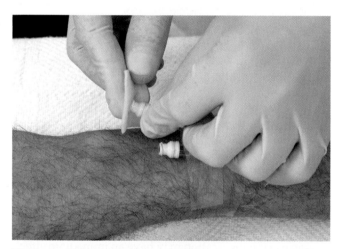

FIG. 10-76 Cleanse the port before attaching the syringe.

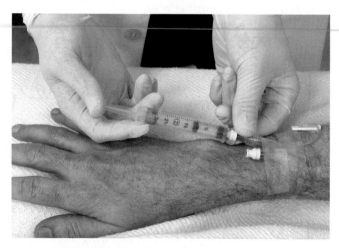

FIG. 10-77 Attaching the syringe to the intravenous lock.

- Flush gently with saline while assessing for resistance. If resistance is felt, do not apply force. Stop and reassess the intravenous lock. Observe for signs of infiltration while injecting saline.
- Reclamp the tubing (if a clamp is present), and remove the NS syringe. Repeat cleansing of the port, and attach the medication syringe. Open the clamp again.
- Inject the medication over the prescribed length of time. Measure time with a watch or clock (Figure 10-78).
- When the medication is infused, clamp the intravenous lock tubing (if a clamp is present), and remove the syringe.
- Repeat cleansing of the port; attach a 2–3 mL NS syringe and inject the contents into the intravenous lock slowly. If a heparin flush is ordered, attach the syringe containing heparin flush solution and inject slowly (per the institution's protocol).

Intravenous Push Medications Through an Existing Infusion

- Prepare the medication for injection. Follow the guidelines for a needleless system, if used.
- Check compatibility of the intravenous medication with the existing intravenous solution.
- Choose the injection port that is closest to the patient.
- Remove the cap (the syringe should be capped during transportation), and cleanse the injection port with an antiseptic swab.
- Occlude the intravenous line by pinching the tubing just above the injection port (Figure 10-79). Attach the syringe to the injection port.
- Gently aspirate for blood return.
- While keeping the intravenous tubing clamped, slowly inject the medication according to administration

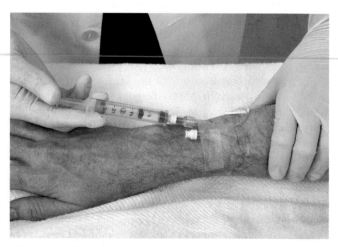

FIG. 10-78 Slowly inject the intravenous push medication through the intravenous lock; use a watch to time the injection.

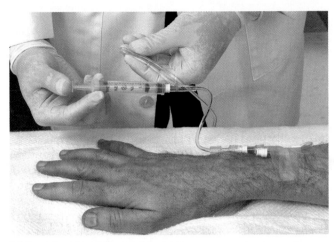

FIG. 10-79 When giving an intravenous push medication through an intravenous line, pinch the tubing just above the injection port.

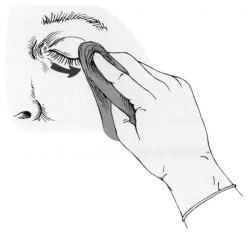

FIG. 10-80 Cleanse the eye, washing from the inner canthus to the outer canthus, before giving eye medications.

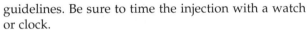

guidelines. Be sure to time the injection with a watch or clock.
- After the injection, flush with normal saline. Then release the intravenous tubing, remove the syringe, and check the infusion rate of the intravenous fluid. The flush should be administered at the same rate as the drug; this prevents the drug in the extension tubing from being administered too quickly.

For example, if an IV is infusing at 250 mL/hr, the possibility of infusing the drug (e.g., morphine) at a rate greater than that desired (1 mg/min) exists. In contrast, if an IV is infusing at a rate to keep the vein open (TKO) such as 30 mL/hr, then the drug would be infused at a slower rate. If the drug was morphine, the nurse may not be able to assess respirations immediately following administration.

After Injecting an Intravenous Push Medication
- Monitor the patient closely for adverse effects. Monitor the intravenous infusion site for signs of phlebitis and infiltration.
- Document medication given on the MAR, and monitor for therapeutic effects.

TOPICAL DRUGS

Administering Eye Medications
Always begin by washing your hands, and maintain Standard Precautions (see Box 10-1). Gloves should be worn for these procedures. When administering eye preparations, keep in mind the following points:
- Assist the patient to the supine or sitting position. The patient's head should be tilted back slightly.
- Remove any secretions or drainage with a sterile gauze pad; be sure to wipe from the inner canthus to the outer canthus (Figure 10-80).

- Have the patient look up and, with your nondominant hand, gently pull the lower lid open to expose the conjunctival sac.

Eye Drops
- With your dominant hand resting on the patient's forehead, hold the eye medication dropper 1 to 2 cm above the conjunctival sac. Do not let the tip of the dropper touch the eye or your fingers (Figure 10-81).
- Drop the prescribed number of drops into the conjunctival sac. Never apply eye drops to the cornea.
- If the drops land on the outer lid margins (if the patient moved or blinked), repeat the procedure.
- Infants often shut the eyes tightly to avoid the eye drops. To give drops to an uncooperative infant, restrain the head gently, and place the drops at the corner where the eyelids meet the nose. When the eye opens, the medication will flow into the eye.

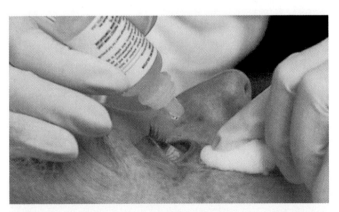

FIG. 10-81 Insert the eye drop into the lower conjunctival sac.

Eye Ointment

Gently squeeze the tube of medication to apply an even strip (about 1 to 2 cm) of medication along the border of the conjunctival sac. Start at the inner canthus, and move toward the outer canthus (Figure 10-82).

After Instilling Eye Medications

- Ask the patient to close the eye gently. Squeezing the eye shut may force the medication out of the conjunctival sac. A tissue may be used to blot liquid that runs out of the eye, but the patient should be instructed not to wipe the eye.
- You may apply gentle pressure to the patient's nasolacrimal duct for 30 to 60 seconds with a gloved finger wrapped in a tissue. This will help reduce systemic absorption of the drug through the nasolacrimal duct and may also help to reduce the taste of the medication in the nasopharynx (Figure 10-83).
- Assist the patient to a comfortable position.
- Document the medication given on the MAR and check the patient for a therapeutic response or adverse reactions.

Administering Ear Drops

Always begin by washing your hands, and maintain Standard Precautions (see Box 10-1). Gloves may be worn for these procedures. When administering ear medications, keep in mind the following points:

- After explaining the procedure to the patient, assist the patient to a side-lying position with the affected ear facing up. If cerumen (earwax) or drainage is noted in the outer ear canal, remove it carefully without pushing it back into the ear canal. Remove excessive amounts of cerumen before instilling medication.
- If refrigerated, the ear medication should be taken out of refrigeration at least 30 minutes before administration to warm it up. Instillation of cold ear drops can cause nausea, dizziness, and pain.
- With an adult (Figure 10-84) or a child older than 3 years of age, pull the pinna up and back.
- With an infant or a child younger than age 3 years of age, pull the pinna down and back (Figure 10-85).
- Administer the prescribed number of drops. Direct the drops along the sides of the ear canal rather than directly onto the eardrum.
- Instruct the patient to lie on one side for 5 to 10 minutes. Gently massaging the tragus of the ear with a finger will help distribute the medication down the ear canal.
- If ordered, a loose cotton pledget can be gently inserted into the ear canal to prevent the medication from flowing out. The cotton should still be loose enough to allow any discharge to drain out of the ear canal. To prevent the dry cotton from absorbing the ear drops that were instilled, moisten the cotton with a small amount of medication before inserting the pledget. Insertion of cotton too deeply may result in increased pressure within the ear canal and on the eardrum. Remove the cotton after about 15 minutes.
- If medication is to be administered in the other ear as well, wait 5 to 10 minutes after instillation of the ear drops in the first ear.
- Document the medication given on the MAR, and observe the patient for a therapeutic response or adverse reactions.

Administering Nasal Medications

Always begin by washing your hands, and maintain Standard Precautions (see Box 10-1). Patients may self-administer some of these drugs, after proper instruction. The nurse should wear gloves for these procedures. When administering nasal medications, keep in mind the points that follow on the next page:

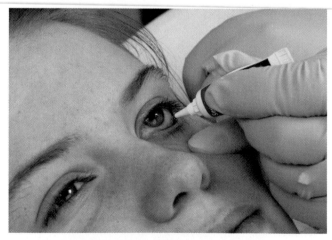

FIG. 10-82 Applying eye ointment.

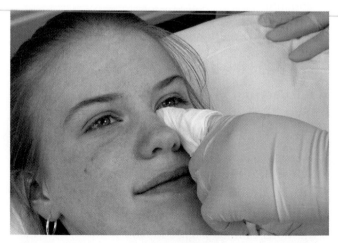

FIG. 10-83 Applying gentle pressure against the nasolacrimal duct after giving eye medications.

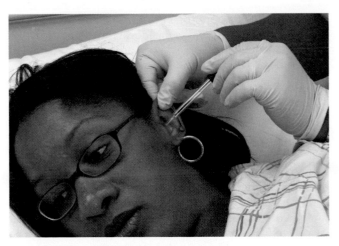

FIG. 10-84 With adults, pull the pinna up and back.

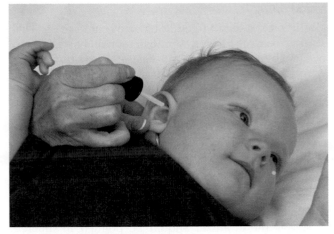

FIG. 10-85 With infants and children under 3 years of age, pull the pinna down and back.

- Before giving nasal medications, explain the procedure to the patient. Explain to the patient that temporary burning or stinging may occur. Instruct the patient that it is important to clear the nasal passages by blowing of the nose, unless contraindicated (e.g., with increased intracranial pressure or nasal surgery), before administering the medication.
- Figure 10-86 illustrates delivery forms for nasal medications: sprays, drops, and dose-measured sprays.
- Assist the patient to the supine position. Support the patient's head as needed.
- If specific areas are targeted for the medication, position the patient's head as follows:
- For the posterior pharynx, position the head backward.

- For the ethmoid or sphenoid sinuses, place the head gently over the top edge of the bed or place a pillow under the shoulders, and tilt the head back.
- For frontal or maxillary sinuses, place the head back and turned toward the side that is to receive the medication.

Nasal Drops

- Hold the nose dropper approximately 1 cm above the nostril. Administer the prescribed number of drops toward the midline of the ethmoid bone (Figure 10-87).
- Repeat the procedure as ordered, instilling the indicated number of drops per nostril.
- Keep the patient in the supine position for 5 minutes.
- Infants are nose breathers, and the potential congestion caused by nasal medications may make it difficult for them to suck. If nose drops are ordered, give them 20 to 30 minutes before a feeding.

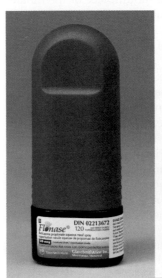
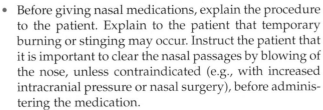

FIG. 10-86 Nasal medications in various delivery forms.

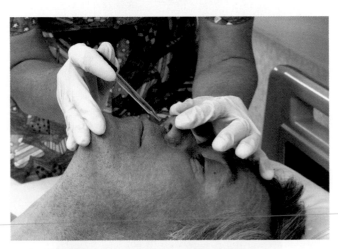

FIG. 10-87 Administering nose drops.

Nasal Spray

- The patient should gently blow the nose to clear the nasal passage prior to administration of the nasal spray.
- The patient should be sitting upright with the head tilted slightly forward. The patient then closes one nostril with a finger, and after gently shaking the atomizer, gently inserts the tip into the other nostril. As the patient inhales through the open nostril, the atomizer is pumped into the nostril at the same time, using a firm and rapid pumping action (Figure 10-88). The patient's head must be tilted backward after removing the atomizer, allowing the medication to spread over the back of the nose.
- If more than one spray is prescribed, for subsequent sprays the atomizer should be pointed in different directions within the nose in order for the mist to cover a wider area of the nasal passages.
- Keep the patient in the supine position for 5 minutes.

After Administration of Nasal Medicines

- Offer the patient tissues for blotting any drainage, but instruct the patient to avoid blowing his or her nose for several minutes after instillation of the drops.
- Assist the patient to a comfortable position.
- Document the medication administration on the MAR and document drainage, if any. Monitor for adverse reactions and a therapeutic response.

Administering Inhaled Drugs

Always begin by washing your hands, and maintain Standard Precautions (see Box 10-1). Patients with asthma should monitor their peak expiratory flow rates by using a peak flowmeter. A variety of inhalers are available

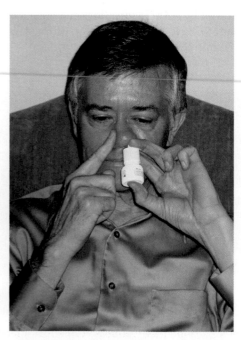

FIG. 10-88 Before self-administering the nasal spray, the patient should occlude the other nostril.

(Figure 10-89). Be sure to check for specific instructions from the manufacturer as needed. Improper use will result in inadequate dosing. When administering inhaled preparations, keep in mind the following points.

Metered-Dose Inhalers

- Shake the metered-dose inhaler (MDI) gently before using it; failure to shake the canister can reduce the amount of medication delivered by 33%.
- Remove the cap; hold the inhaler upright and grasp with the thumb and first two fingers.
- Tilt the patient's head back slightly.
- If the MDI is used without a spacer, do the following:
  1 Have the patient open his mouth; position the inhaler 3 to 5 cm away from the mouth (Figure 10-90). The patient must begin to inhale slowly prior to actuation of the MDI and continue to full inhalation at a relatively low flow. This technique allows vaporization of the aerosol and reduced impaction as the particle size of the inhalant is reduced, and more of the drug is likely to reach the lower airways. However, this technique is difficult and can be almost impossible for older adults and children, or patients in respiratory distress.
  2 Have the patient exhale, then press down once on the inhaler to release the medication; immediately have the patient breathe in slowly and deeply for 5 seconds.
  3 Have the patient hold his breath for approximately 10 seconds, and then exhale slowly through pursed lips.
- Spacers should be used with children and adults who have difficulty coordinating inhalations with activation of MDIs. If the MDI is used with a spacer, do the following:
  1 Attach the spacer to the mouthpiece of the inhaler after removing the inhaler cap (Figures 10-91 and 10-92).
  2 Place the mouthpiece of the spacer in the patient's mouth.
  3 Have the patient exhale.
  4 Press down on the inhaler to release the medication, and have the patient inhale deeply and slowly through the spacer. The patient should breathe in and out slowly for 2 to 3 seconds, and then hold her breath for 10 seconds (Figure 10-93).
- If a second puff of the same medication is ordered, wait 20 to 30 seconds between puffs.
- If a second type of inhaled medication is ordered, wait 2 to 5 minutes between medication inhalations or as prescribed.
- If both a bronchodilator and a steroid inhaled medication are ordered, the bronchodilator should be administered first so that the air passages will be open for the second medication.
- Patients should be instructed to rinse their mouth with water after inhaling a steroid medication to prevent the development of an oral fungal infection.

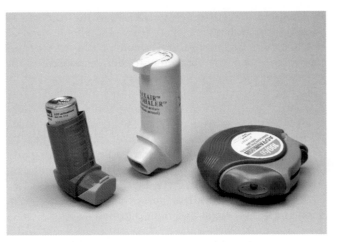

FIG. 10-89   **A,** Metered-dose inhaler (MDI). **B,** Automated MDI. **C,** "Disk-type" MDI that delivers powdered medication.

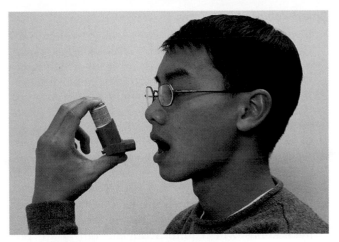

FIG. 10-90   Using an MDI without a spacer.

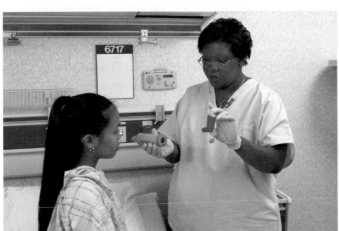

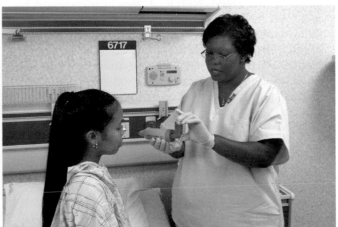

FIGS. 10-91 AND 10-92   Instructing the patient on how to use a spacer device.

- Document the medication given on the MAR, and monitor the patient for a therapeutic response and adverse reactions.
- It is important to teach the patient how to calculate the number of doses in the inhaler and to keep track of uses. Simply shaking the inhaler to "estimate" whether it is empty is not accurate and may result in its being used when it is empty. The patient should be taught to count the number of puffs needed per day (doses) and divide this amount into the actual number of actuations (puffs) in the inhaler to estimate the number of days the inhaler will last. Then, a calendar can be marked a few days before this date with a note that it is time to obtain a refill. In addition, the date can be marked on the inhaler with a permanent marker. For example, an inhaler with 200 puffs, ordered to be used 4 times a day (2 puffs per dose, 8 puffs per day), would last for 25 days (200 divided by 8).
- Dry powder inhalers (DPIs) have varied instructions, so the manufacturer's directions should be followed closely. Patients should be instructed to cover the mouthpiece

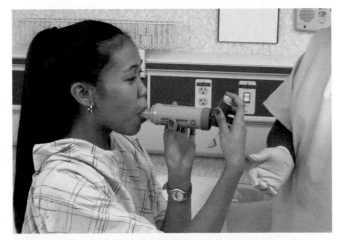

FIG. 10-93   Using a spacer device with an MDI.

completely with their mouths. Capsules intended for use with DPIs should NEVER be taken orally. Some DPIs have convenient built-in dose counters.

Small-Volume Nebulizers

- In some facilities, the air compressor is located in the wall unit of the room. In other facilities and at home, a small, portable air compressor is used. Be sure to follow the manufacturer's recommendations for use.
- If the patient is receiving oxygen, the oxygen should not be turned off during administration of the nebulizer; also, some facilities do not have air compressors, so the nebulizer must be administered using oxygen.
- Be sure to take the patient's baseline heart rate, especially if a β-adrenergic agent is used. Some drugs may increase the heart rate.
- After gathering the equipment, add the prescribed medication to the nebulizer cup (Figure 10-94). Some medications will require a diluent; others are pre-mixed with a diluent. Be sure to verify before adding a diluent.
- Have the patient hold the mouthpiece between his lips (Figure 10-95). NOTE: A face mask should be used for a child or an adult who is too fatigued to hold the mouthpiece. Special adaptors are available if the patient has a tracheostomy.
- Before starting the nebulizer treatment, the patient should take a slow, deep breath, hold it briefly, then exhale slowly. Patients who are short of breath should be instructed to hold their breath every fourth or fifth breath.
- Turn on the small-volume nebulizer machine (or turn on the wall unit), and make sure that a sufficient mist is forming.
- Instruct the patient to repeat the breathing pattern mentioned previously during the treatment.
- Occasionally tap the nebulizer cup during the treatment and toward the end to move the fluid droplets back to the bottom of the cup.
- Monitor the patient's heart rate during and after the treatment.
- If inhaled steroids are given, instruct the patient to rinse his or her mouth afterward.

- After the procedure, clean and store the tubing per institution policy.
- Document the medication given on the MAR, and monitor the patient for a therapeutic response and for adverse reactions.
- If the patient will be using a nebulizer at home, instruct the patient to rinse the nebulizer parts daily after each use with warm, clear water and allow to air dry. Once a week, the nebulizer parts should be soaked in a solution of vinegar and water (four parts water and one part white vinegar) for 30 minutes, rinsed thoroughly with clear, warm water, and air dried. Storing nebulizer parts that are still wet will encourage bacterial and mould growth.

Administering Medications to the Skin

Always begin by washing your hands, and maintain Standard Precautions (see Box 10-1). Gloves should be worn for these procedures. Avoid touching the preparations to your own skin. When administering skin preparations, keep in mind the following points:

Lotions, Creams, Ointments, and Powders

- Before administering any dose of a topical skin medication, ensure that the site is clean and dry. Thoroughly remove previous applications using soap and water, if appropriate for the patient's condition, and dry the area thoroughly. Also, rotate application sites.
- When applying powder, have the patient turn the head to the other side during application to avoid inhalation of powder particles.
- With lotion, cream, or gel, obtain the correct amount with your gloved hand (Figure 10-96). If the medication is in a jar, remove the dose with a sterile tongue depressor and place on your gloved hand. Do not contaminate the medication in the jar.
- Apply the preparation with long, smooth, gentle strokes that follow the direction of hair growth (Figure 10-97). Avoid excessive pressure.

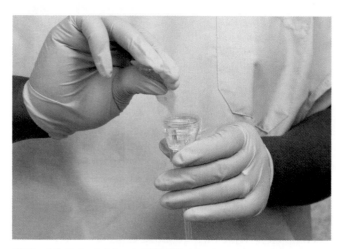

FIG. 10-94 Adding medication to the nebulizer cup.

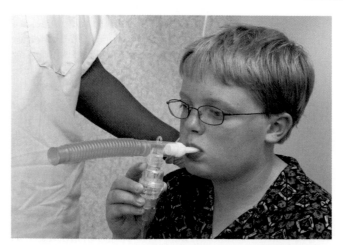

FIG. 10-95 Administering a small-volume nebulizer treatment.

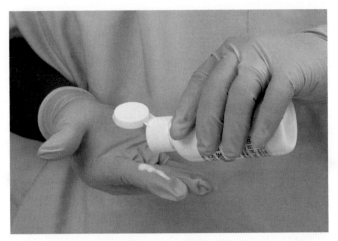

FIG. 10-96 Use gloves to apply topical skin preparations.

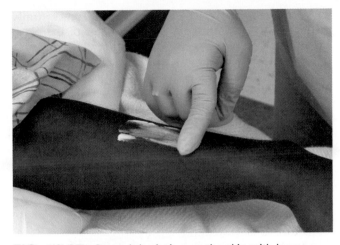

FIG. 10-97 Spread the lotion on the skin with long, smooth, gentle strokes.

- Be particularly careful with the skin of the older adult because age-related changes may result in increased capillary fragility and tendency to bruise.
- Some ointments and creams may soil the patient's clothes and linens. If ordered, cover the affected site with gauze or a transparent dressing.
- Nitroglycerin ointment in a tube is measured carefully on clean, ruled application paper before it is applied to the skin (Figure 10-98). Unit-dose packages should not be measured. Do not massage nitroglycerin ointment into the skin. Apply the measured amount onto a clean, dry site and then secure the application paper with a transparent dressing or a strip of tape. Always remove the old medication before applying a new dose.

Transdermal Patches

- Be sure that the used patch is removed as ordered. Some patches may be removed before the next patch

is required—check the order. Clear patches may be difficult to find, and patches may be overlooked in obese patients with skinfolds. Cleanse the site of the used patch thoroughly. Observe for signs of skin irritation at the used patch site.
- Transdermal patches should be applied at the same time each day if ordered daily.
- The used patch should be pressed together, and then wrapped in a glove as you remove the glove from your hand. Dispose in the proper container according to the facility's policy.
- Select a new site for application and ensure that it is clean and without powder or lotion. The site should be hairless and free from scratches or irritation. If it is necessary to remove hair, clip the hair instead of shaving to reduce irritation to the skin.
- Remove the backing from the new patch (Figure 10-99). Take care not to touch the medication side of the patch with your fingers.

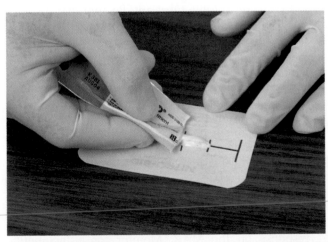

FIG. 10-98 Measure nitroglycerin ointment carefully before application.

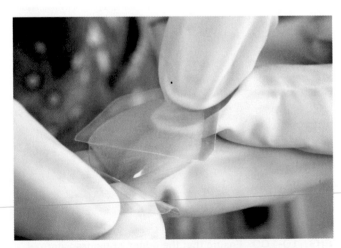

FIG. 10-99 Opening a transdermal patch medication.

- Place the patch on the skin site and press firmly (Figure 10-100). Press around the edges of the patch with one or two fingers to ensure that the patch is adequately secured to the skin. Rotate sites of application with each dose.
- Document the site of administration on the MAR.

After Administering Topical Skin Preparations

- Chart the medication given on the MAR, and monitor the patient for a therapeutic response and adverse reactions.
- Provide instruction on administration to the patient or caregiver, as appropriate.

Administering Vaginal Medications

Always begin by washing your hands, and maintain Standard Precautions (see Box 10-1). Gloves should be worn for these procedures. When administering vaginal preparations, keep in mind the following points:

- Vaginal suppositories are larger and more oval than rectal suppositories (Figure 10-101).
- Figure 10-102 shows examples of a vaginal suppository in its applicator and vaginal cream in an applicator.
- Before giving these medications explain the procedure to the patient, and have her void.
- If possible, administer vaginal preparations at bedtime to allow the medications to remain in place for as long as possible.
- Some patients may prefer to self-administer vaginal medications. Provide specific instructions if necessary.
- Position the patient in the lithotomy position, and elevate the hips with a pillow, if tolerated. Be sure to drape the patient to provide privacy.

Creams, Foams, or Gels Applied with an Applicator

- Fit the applicator to the tube of the medication, and then gently squeeze the tube to fill the applicator with the correct amount of medication.

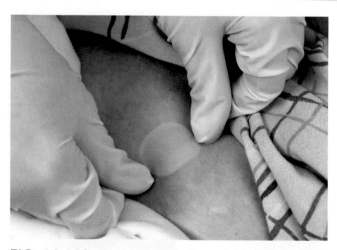

FIG. 10-100 Ensure that the edges of the transdermal patch are secure after applying.

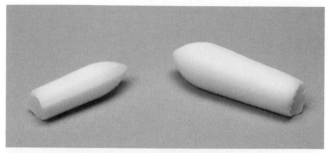

FIG. 10-101 Vaginal suppositories *(right)* are larger and more oval than rectal suppositories *(left)*.

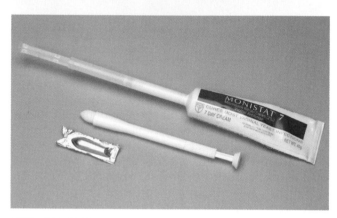

FIG. 10-102 Vaginal cream and suppository, with applicators.

- Lubricate the tip of the applicator with a water-soluble lubricant.
- Use your nondominant hand to spread the labia and expose the vagina. Gently insert the applicator as far as possible into the vagina (Figure 10-103).
- Push the plunger to deposit the medication. Remove the applicator, and wrap it in a paper towel to be cleaned later.

Suppositories

- Remove the wrapping, and lubricate the suppository with a water-soluble lubricant. Be sure that the suppository is at room temperature.
- Using the applicator, insert the suppository into the vagina, and then push the plunger to deposit the suppository.
- If no applicator is available, use your dominant index finger to insert the suppository about 5 cm into the vagina (Figure 10-104).
- Have the patient remain in the supine position with hips elevated for 5 to 10 minutes to allow the suppository to dissolve and the medication to spread.
- If the patient so desires, apply a perineal pad.
- If the applicator is to be reused, wash with soap and water, and store in a clean container for the next use.
- Document the medication given and the patient's response on the MAR. Monitor for a therapeutic response and adverse reactions.

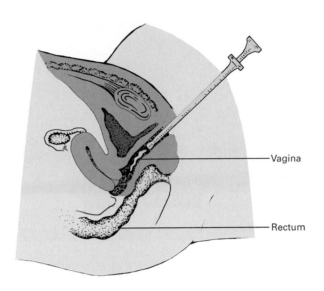

FIG. 10-103 Administering vaginal cream with an applicator.

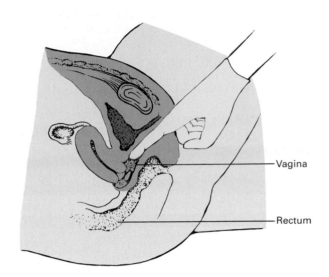

FIG. 10-104 Administering a vaginal suppository.

ILLUSTRATION CREDITS

Figures 10-1, 10-2, 10-3, 10-6, 10-7, 10-8, 10-9, 10-10, 10-15, 10-18, 10-20, 10-21, 10-27, 10-31, 10-32, 10-33, 10-34, 10-35, 10-36, 10-37, 10-38, 10-39, 10-42, 10-47, 10-48, 10-49, 10-50, 10-51, 10-54, 10-55, 10-56, 10-58, 10-59, 10-61, 10-62, 10-63, 10-64, 10-65, 10-66, 10-67, 10-68, 10-69, 10-70, 10-71, 10-72, 10-73, 10-76, 10-77, 10-78, 10-79, 10-82, 10-83, 10-84, 10-85, 10-87, 10-88, 10-89, 10-91, 10-92, 10-93, 10-94, 10-95, 10-96, 10-97, 10-98, 10-99, 10-100, 10-101and 10-102: from Rick Brady, Riva, MD. Figure 10-4: Interior Health (2005). Meds check at bedside. *Interior Health, 50* (November 2005): 3. Retrieved October 6, 2009, from www.llbc.leg.bc.ca/public/PubDocs/bcdocs/359084/2005/50_November_2005.pdf. Reproduced by permission of Interior Health. All rights reserved. Figure 10-5: courtesy Princess Margaret Hospital, Toronto, ON. Figures 10-11, 10-12, 10-17, 10-41, 10-43, 10-81, 10-90, 10-103, and 10-104: from Elkin, M. K., Perry, A. G., & Potter, P. A. (2004). *Nursing interventions and clinical skills* (3rd ed.). St. Louis, MO: Mosby. Figure 10-13: courtesy Oscar H. Allison, Jr. (2004).

In Clayton, B. D., & Stock, Y. N. (Eds.). *Basic pharmacology for nurses* (13th ed.). St. Louis, MO: Mosby. Figure 10-19: modified from Perry, A. G., & Potter, P. A. (2006). *Clinical nursing skills and techniques* (6th ed.). St. Louis, MO: Mosby. Figures 10-22, 10-23, 10-24, 10-25, 10-44, 10-45, and 10-52: courtesy Chuck Dresner. Figures 10-30 and 10-74: from Potter, P. A., & Perry, A. G. (2001). *Fundamentals of nursing* (5th ed.). St. Louis, MO: Mosby. Figure 10-40: courtesy Nadine Sokol. Figure 10-46: from Potter, P. A., & Perry, A. G. (1997). *Fundamentals of nursing: concepts, process, and practice* (4th ed.). St. Louis, MO: Mosby. Figures 10-53, 10-57, and 10-60: modified from Potter, P. A., & Perry, A. G. (1993). *Fundamentals of nursing: concepts, process, and practice* (3rd ed.). St. Louis, MO: Mosby. Figure 10-80: from Perry, A. G., & Potter, P. A. (2006). *Clinical nursing skills and techniques* (6th ed.). St. Louis, MO: Mosby. Figure 10-86: Flonase® photo reproduced with permission from GlaxoSmithKline Inc., Canada. All rights reserved. Nasonex® photo reproduced with permission from Schering Canada, Inc. All rights reserved.

PART **TWO**

Drugs Affecting the Central Nervous System

STUDY SKILLS TIPS:

- VOCABULARY
- TEXT NOTATION
- LANGUAGE CONVENTIONS

VOCABULARY

In a complex, technical subject such as nursing pharmacology, it is necessary to master the vocabulary in order to understand the content. Most chapters in this text begin with a glossary of related terms, and it is helpful to spend time on the vocabulary in the glossary. The terms are further defined and explained in the body of the chapter. When you read the chapter you should expect to fully master the vocabulary.

Consider the terms *agonist* and *antagonist* in the Chapter 11 glossary. What does *agonist* mean? What is the similarity between *agonist* and *antagonist* and what is the difference? Asking these questions as you start is a valuable technique for mastering the language of the content. Do not simply memorize the terms—learn what they mean, and link relationships between words with common elements.

The Chapter 11 glossary has another group of words that should be viewed together. The first of these words, *pain*, has a definition that is clear and relatively easy to understand and learn. But your focus should not be on simply learning that single word because there are 14 other words that relate to pain: *acute, cancer, central,* *persistent, neuropathic, phantom, psychogenic, referred, somatic, superficial, threshold, tolerance, vascular,* and *visceral.* Each of these words defines and categorizes pain in a specific way. Thus instead of focusing on only the meaning of each term, ask what the similarities and differences are and how these words relate to one another.

TEXT NOTATION

The Study Skills Tips for Part One discussed a method for text underlining. The object of text underlining is to pick out important terms, ideas, and key information so you can come back to them later for quick review. The three key elements in successful text notation are as follows:

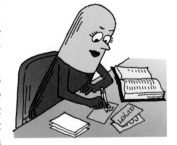

1 Read the material once before attempting any underlining.
2 Be aware of the author's language.
3 Be highly selective. The most common fault in underlining is to mark too much material.

Following is a paragraph from Chapter 11 that has been underlined. Each reader will mark the text somewhat differently on the basis of his or her background and experience. As you study this example, ask yourself *why* that material was chosen.

"A full understanding of how analgesics work requires knowledge of what pain is and what its characteristics are. <u>**Pain** is most commonly defined as an unpleasant sensory and emotional experience</u> associated with either actual or potential tissue damage. It is also associated with many diseases or health conditions. Pain can be <u>further classified in terms of its onset and duration as being either acute pain or persistent pain</u>, and different treatments are prescribed for each type. <u>**Acute pain** is sudden and usually subsides when treated;</u> for example, postoperative pain or the sudden onset of a headache. <u>**Persistent pain** is long-lasting or recurring,</u> lasting 6 weeks or longer. The patient presentation becomes more complex and often with more psychological features. Persistent pain is frequently more challenging to treat because changes occur in the nervous system (tolerance) that often require increasing drug doses. Table 11-1 lists the different characteristics of acute and persistent pain and diseases and conditions associated with each."

LANGUAGE CONVENTIONS

Certain words and phrases are like signal lights at an intersection. They serve to tell the reader that something special, important, or noteworthy is happening.

The text following the topic heading *Opioid Analgesics: Chemical Structure* contains several examples. The second sentence contains the phrase *classified according to*. Whenever an author says that something is being classified, it means there are at least two (and perhaps several more) elements of the term or idea that are being classified. This means that you should ask the question: "What is being classified? How many classifications are there for this?"

As you read this chapter, or any other chapter, pay attention to words and phrases like these that are intended to draw your attention to something the author especially wanted to emphasize. The more aware you are, the easier it will become to select from the mass of information those concepts and terms that the writers tried to stress.

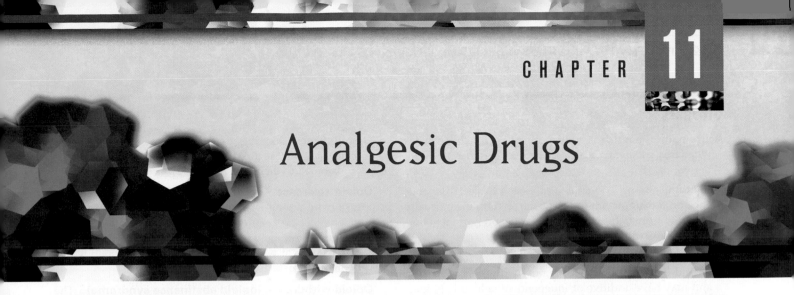

CHAPTER **11**

Analgesic Drugs

Learning Objectives

After reading this chapter, the successful student will be able to do the following:

1 Define analgesia.

2 Describe pharmacological and nonpharmacological approaches for the management and treatment of acute and persistent (chronic) pain.

3 Discuss the use of nonopioids, nonsteroidal anti-inflammatory drugs (NSAIDs), and opioids (opioid agonists and partial opioid agonists and antagonists) in the management of acute and persistent pain.

4 Identify the drugs that are classified within the non-narcotic and narcotic drug groups. (NSAIDs are discussed in Chapter 45, Anti-Inflammatory, Antiarthritic, and Related Drugs.)

5 Discuss the difference between opioid agonist, agonist–antagonist, and antagonist drugs and their specific use in the management of acute and persistent pain.

6 Compare the mechanisms of action, drug effects, indications, adverse effects, cautions, contraindications, drug–drug and drug–food interactions, dosages, and routes of administration for non-narcotic and narcotic drugs (agonist and partial agonist–antagonist narcotics).

7 Contrast the management of acute and persistent pain with the management of pain associated with cancer and pain experienced in terminal conditions.

8 Describe briefly the special pain situations as well as specific standards of pain management as defined by the World Health Organization and the Canadian Pain Society.

9 Develop a collaborative plan of care related to the use of non-narcotic and narcotic drugs and the nursing process for patients experiencing pain.

10 Identify resources, agencies, and professional groups involved in establishing standards for the management of all types of pain and for a holistic approach to the care of patients with acute or persistent pain and those in special pain situations.

e-Learning Activities

Web site
(http://evolve.elsevier.com/Canada/
Lilley/pharmacology/)

- Animations
- Answers to chapter questions, activities, and case studies
- Calculators and Category Catchers
- Glossary with audio pronunciations
- IV Therapy and Medication Error Checklists
- Multiple-Choice Review Question quizzes
- Nursing Care Plans
- Online Appendices and Supplements
- WebLinks

Drug Profiles

▸▸ **acetaminophen**, p. 201
   codeine (codeine sulfate)*, p. 195
   fentanyl, p. 195
   meperidine (meperidine hydrochloride)*,
      p. 196
   methadone (methadone hydrochloride)*,
      p. 196
▸▸ **morphine (morphine sulfate)***, p. 195
▸▸ **naloxone (naloxone hydrochloride)***, p. 197
   naltrexone (naltrexone hydrochloride)*,
      p. 197
   oxycodone (oxycodone hydrochloride)*,
      p. 196
   tramadol (tramadol hydrochloride)*, p. 201

▸▸ Key drug.

*Full generic name is given in parentheses. For the purposes of this text, the more common shortened name is used.

Glossary

Acute pain Pain that is sudden in onset, usually subsides when treated, and typically occurs over less than a 6-week period. (p. 185)

Addiction Strong psychological or physical dependence on a drug or other psychoactive substance, usually resulting from habitual use, that is beyond normal voluntary control. (p. 189)

Adjuvant analgesic drugs Drugs that are added as a second drug for combined therapy with a primary drug and may have additive or independent analgesic properties, or both. (p. 192)

Agonist A substance that binds to a receptor and causes a response. (p. 191)

Agonist–antagonist A substance that binds to a receptor and causes a partial response that is not as strong as that caused by an agonist (also known as a *partial agonist*). (p. 194)

Analgesic ceiling effect A phenomenon that occurs when a given pain drug no longer effectively controls a patient's pain despite the administration of the highest safe dosages. (p. 190)

Analgesics Medications that relieve pain without causing loss of consciousness (sometimes referred to as *painkillers*). (p. 185)

Antagonist An agent that binds to a receptor and prevents (blocks) a response, resulting in inhibitory or antagonistic drug effects; also called an *inhibitor*. (p. 191)

Breakthrough pain Pain that lingers despite doses of a long-acting dosage form for every 12 hours. (p. 189)

Gate theory A common and well-described theory of pain transmission and pain relief. It uses a gate model to explain how impulses from damaged tissues are sensed in the brain. (p. 186)

Neuropathic pain Pain that results from a disturbance of function or pathological change in a nerve. (p. 186)

Nociceptive pain Pain that arises from mechanical, chemical, or thermal irritation of peripheral sensory nerves (e.g., after surgery or trauma or associated with degenerative processes). (p. 185)

Nonopioid analgesics Analgesics that are not classified as opioids. (p. 186)

Nonsteroidal anti-inflammatory drugs (NSAIDs) A large, chemically diverse group of drugs that are analgesics and possess anti-inflammatory and antipyretic activity but are not steroids. (p. 185)

Opiate analgesic A natural narcotic drug containing or derived from opium that binds to opiate receptors in the brain to relieve pain. (p. 190)

Opioid analgesic A synthetic narcotic drug that binds to opiate receptors in the brain to relieve pain. (p. 190)

Opioid-naïve Describes patients who are receiving opioid analgesics for the first time and who therefore are not accustomed to their effects. (p. 192)

Opioid tolerance A normal physiological condition that results from long-term opioid use, in which larger doses of opioids are required to maintain the same level of analgesia and in which abrupt discontinuation of the drug results in withdrawal symptoms (same as physical dependence). (p. 193)

Opioid withdrawal (opioid abstinence syndrome) The signs and symptoms associated with abstinence from or withdrawal of an opioid analgesic when the body has become physically dependent on the substance. (p. 194)

Pain An unpleasant sensory and emotional experience associated with actual or potential tissue damage. (p. 185)

Pain threshold The level of stimulus that results in the perception of pain. (p. 188)

Pain tolerance The amount of pain an individual can endure without its interfering with normal function. (p. 188)

Partial agonist A drug that binds to a receptor and causes an activation response and that is less than that caused by a full agonist. (p. 191)

Persistent pain Persistent or recurring pain that is often difficult to treat. Typically it is pain that lasts longer than 3 months. (p. 185)

Phantom pain Pain experienced in a body part that has been surgically or traumatically removed. (p. 186)

Physical dependence The physical adaptation of the body to an addictive substance; it is usually indicated by tolerance to the effects of the substance and withdrawal symptoms that develop when use of the substance is terminated. (p. 193)

Psychogenic pain Pain that is of psychological origin in nature but is actual pain in the sense that pain impulses travel through nerve cells. (p. 186)

Psychological dependence A pattern of compulsive use of any addictive substance that is characterized by a continuous craving for the substance and the need to use it for effects other than pain relief (also called *addiction*). (p. 193)

Referred pain Pain occurring in an area away from the organ of origin. (p. 186)

Somatic pain Pain that originates from skeletal muscles, ligaments, or joints. (p. 185)

Special pain situation General term for a pain control situation that is complex and whose treatment typically involves multiple medications, different health care personnel, and nonpharmacological therapeutic modalities (e.g., massage, chiropractic care, surgery). (p. 188)

Superficial pain   Pain that originates from the skin or mucous membranes. (p. 186)

Vascular pain   Pain that results from pathology of the vascular or perivascular tissues. (p. 186)

Visceral pain   Pain that originates from organs or smooth muscles. (p. 185)

World Health Organization (WHO)   An international body of health care professionals, including clinicians and epidemiologists among many others, that studies and responds to health needs and trends worldwide. (p. 189)

OVERVIEW

The management of patients experiencing acute or persistent pain (the terms *persistent pain* and *chronic pain* are often used interchangeably in the literature) is a significant aspect of nursing care in a variety of settings and across the lifespan. Pain remains one of the more common reasons for patients to seek out the care of a physician. Eighty percent of physician office visits in Canada involve a pain-related component. Surgical and diagnostic procedures often require pain management, and there are many diseases and pathological conditions that also require pain management, such as arthritis, diabetes, multiple sclerosis, cancer, and AIDS. Pain leads to much suffering and is a tremendous economic burden as a result of lost productivity, workers' compensation, and related health care costs. Because of the personal suffering involved and the prevalence and scope of the problem (e.g., overall, 30% to 45% of cancer patients have pain; this figure increases to 75% of patients in advanced stages), it is critical for nurses to be well informed about pain management, including both nonpharmacological (e.g., massage, acupuncture, therapeutic touch, spirituality, relaxation techniques, imagery) and pharmacological means, so that they can provide high-quality patient care.

Medications that relieve pain without causing loss of consciousness (commonly referred to as *painkillers*) are considered **analgesics**. There are several classes of analgesics. These classes are determined by the chemical structures and mechanisms of action of the drugs. The focus of this chapter is on those drugs commonly used to relieve moderate to severe pain—opioid analgesics. The next most common analgesic class consists of

nonsteroidal anti-inflammatory drugs (NSAIDs), which are discussed in Chapter 45.

PHYSIOLOGY AND PSYCHOLOGY OF PAIN

Definition and Classification of Pain

A full understanding of how analgesics work requires knowledge of what pain is and what its characteristics are. **Pain** is most commonly defined as an unpleasant sensory and emotional experience associated with either actual or potential tissue damage. It is also associated with many diseases or health conditions. Pain can be further classified in terms of its onset and duration as being either acute pain or persistent pain, and different treatments are prescribed for each type. **Acute pain** is sudden and usually subsides when treated—for example, postoperative pain or the sudden onset of a headache. **Persistent pain** is long-lasting or recurring, lasting 3 months or longer. The patient presentation becomes more complex and often with more psychological features. Persistent pain is frequently more challenging to treat because changes occur in the nervous system (tolerance) that often require increasing drug doses. Table 11-1 lists the different characteristics of acute and persistent pain and the diseases and conditions associated with each.

Pain can be further classified according to its sources, the two main ones being *nociceptive* and *neuropathic*. Acute **nociceptive pain** is classified as either somatic or visceral pain. **Somatic pain** originates from skin, bone, muscle, connective tissue, or joints and is often described as well-localized and throbbing. **Visceral pain** originates from internal organs and can be well-localized or referred.

TABLE 11-1

Acute versus Persistent Pain

Type of Pain	Onset	Duration	Examples
Acute	Sudden (minutes to hours); usually sharp, localized; physiological response (SNS: tachycardia, sweating, pallor, increased blood pressure)	Limited (has an end)	Myocardial infarction, appendicitis, dental procedures, kidney stones, surgical procedures
Persistent	Slow (days to months); long duration; dull, long-lasting aching	Long-lasting or recurring (endless)	Arthritis, cancer, lower back pain, peripheral neuropathy

SNS, sympathetic nervous system.

Referred pain occurs because visceral nerve fibres synapse at a level in the spinal cord close to fibres that supply specific subcutaneous tissues in the body. One example is the pain associated with cholecystitis, which often affects the back and scapula areas. Sometimes pain is described as superficial. **Superficial pain** originates from the skin and mucous membranes. Another type of pain is **vascular pain**, which possibly originates from some pathology of the vascular or perivascular tissues and is thought to account for a large percentage of migraine headaches. Pain treatment may be more appropriately selected when the source of the pain is known. For example, visceral pain usually requires opioids for relief, whereas somatic pain (including bone pain) usually responds better to **nonopioid analgesics** such as NSAIDs (see Chapter 45).

Neuropathic pain affects approximately 2% to 3% of the population and results from injury or damage to peripheral nerve fibres or to central neurological damage to the central nervous system (CNS) rather than stimulation of nerve receptors. It may be present in the absence of disease or pathological processes that generally result in pain. Neuropathic pain is usually severe, persistent, and resistant to over-the-counter analgesics. Reorganization or abnormal processing of sensory input by the peripheral or central nervous system causes nerve dysfunction, resulting in numbness, weakness, and loss of deep tendon reflexes in the affected nerve area. Neuropathic conditions also cause atypical symptoms of spontaneous and stimulus-evoked pain. Spontaneous pain (continuous or intermittent) is commonly described as burning, shooting, or shock-like. **Phantom pain** is a type of neuropathic pain that occurs in the area of a body part that has been removed, surgically or traumatically, and is characterized as burning, itching, tingling, or stabbing. It can also occur in attached limbs following spinal cord injury.

Cancer pain can be acute, persistent, or both. It stems from causes such as pressure on nerves, organs, or tissues. Other causes of cancer pain include hypoxia; blockage to an organ; metastasis; pathological fractures; muscle spasms; and adverse effects of radiation, surgery, and chemotherapy. **Psychogenic pain** is pain that originates from psychological factors, not physical conditions or disorders. However, this definition assumes that all physical causes of pain can be determined. Because the physical basis for many persistent pain syndromes is unknown, physiological sources can never be completely ruled out. A diagnosis of psychogenic pain can lead to the assumption that the patient is not experiencing "real" pain, and the patient may receive a psychiatric diagnosis despite the presence of a medical cause for the pain.

Theories of Nociceptive Pain Transmission and Relief

Several theories have been developed to attempt to explain pain development, transmission, and relief. One common and well-described one is the **gate theory**. Proposed by Melzack and Wall in 1965, they used the analogy of a gate to describe how impulses from damaged tissues are sensed in the brain. Four distinct processes, all of which operate simultaneously, are required for nociceptive pain to occur and are widely believed to determine the perception of and response to acute pain. These processes are described in the next sections below.

Transduction

The first process, *transduction*, begins in the periphery (skin, subcutaneous tissue, somatic structures) where primary afferent neurons (*nocireceptors*) are scattered. These free nerve endings are preferentially sensitive to noxious or potentially noxious or tissue-damaging chemical, mechanical, or thermal stimuli. Such stimuli cause the release of numerous chemicals (prostaglandins, bradykinin, serotonin, substance P, histamine, leukotrienes). These substances initiate the conversion of the stimulus to an *impulse* (or *action potential*). Some current pain management strategies are aimed at altering the actions and levels of these substances.

The *action potential* is created on the neuron cell surface. The intracellular surface of the neuron carries a negative charge compared with the positive charge of the extracellular surface (called *resting membrane potential*). The substance(s) released by the noxious stimulus causes the receptor membrane to become permeable to extracellular sodium (Na^+) ions. These ions rush into the cell and create a temporary positive charge inside relative to outside (called *depolarization*). Potassium (K^+) leaves the cell, causing *repolarization*. "If enough depolarization and repolarization occur, the action potential is created and the stimulus is converted to an impulse" (McCaffery & Pasero, 1999, p. 18).

Transmission

The next process, *transmission*, involves the transmittal of the pain impulses along pain fibres, as well as other sensory nerve fibres, to activate pain receptors in the spinal chord and brain. There are two types of nociceptor pain fibres: A-delta (A-δ) and C. The *C fibres* are sensitive to mechanical, thermal, and chemical stimuli, and transmit poorly localized, dull, and aching pain. The *A-delta fibres* are sensitive to mechanical and thermal stimuli and transmit well-localized, sharp, cutting, or stabbing pain. A-delta fibres also result in activation of the sympathetic nervous system (fight-or-flight response), allowing the individual to react; however, this response is time limited. Table 11-2 summarizes further characteristic differences between the A and C fibres.

The spinothalamic tract is the most important pathway for transmission. The site where the nociceptive fibres enter the spinal cord is called the *dorsal (posterior) horn* of the spinal cord. Here, neurotransmitters glutamate and substance P continue the pain impulse across the synaptic cleft between nociceptors and dorsal horn neurons. From the dorsal horn, numerous different *ascending fibre tracts* within the larger spinothalamic tract transmit pain. These originate in the spinal cord and terminate in the brain stem and thalamic regions.

TABLE 11-2

A and C Nerve Fibres

Type of Fibre	Myelin Sheath	Fibre Size	Conduction Speed	Type of Pain
A	Yes	Large	Fast	Sharp and well localized
C	No	Small	Slow	Dull and nonlocalized

It is at the dorsal horn that the so-called *gates* are located and control pain transmission. Activation of A fibres closes the gates, thus inhibiting transmission of pain impulses to the brain. As a result, no pain is perceived. Conversely, opening of the gate is affected by the stimulation of the C fibres. This allows impulses to be transmitted to the brain and pain to be perceived. Figure 11-1 depicts the gate theory of pain transmission.

Perception

Perception, the third process, is less an actual physiological event than a subjective phenomenon of pain (how it feels) that encompasses complex behavioural, psychological, and emotional factors.

The μ-receptors in the dorsal horn appear to play a crucial role. Pain perception and, conversely, emotional well-being, are closely linked to the number of μ-receptors. This number is controlled by a single gene, the μ-opioid receptor gene. Pain sensitivity is diminished when the receptors are present in relative abundance. When the receptors are reduced in number or missing altogether, relatively minor noxious stimuli may be perceived as painful.

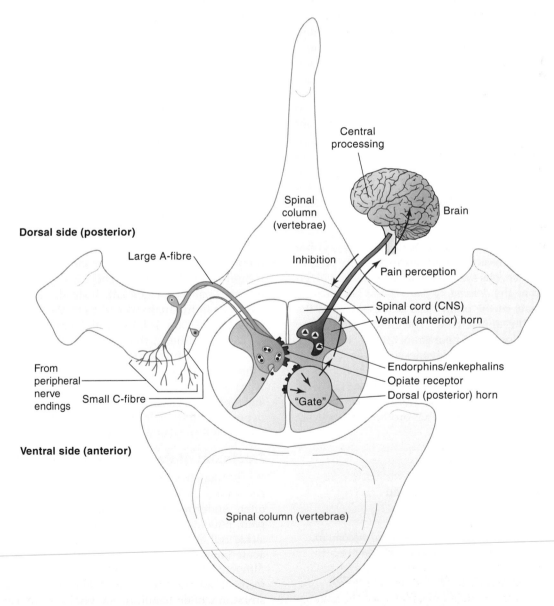

FIG. 11-1   Gate theory of pain transmission. *CNS*, central nervous system.

Pain always carries unpleasantness and desire to escape. The exact location of pain perceived is unclear, as are individual differences in subjective experience of pain. It is thought that the reticular system is responsible for the autonomic response to pain and for warning the individual to attend to it. The somatosensory cortex localizes and characterizes pain. The limbic system is responsible for emotional and behavioural responses. It is also thought that pain perception occurs in cortical structures. This is why cognitive–behavioural strategies can be applied to reduce the sensory and affective components of pain. The level of stimulus needed to produce a painful sensation is referred to as the **pain threshold**. Because this is a measure of the physiological response of the nervous system, it is similar for most persons. Variations in sensitivity to pain may be a result of genetic regulation.

The patient's emotional response to the pain is also moulded by that individual's age, gender, ethnocultural background, personality, previous pain experience, and anxiety level as well the environmental conditions under which the individual lives. This psychological element of pain is called **pain tolerance**, or the amount of pain a patient can endure without it interfering with normal function. Pain tolerance can vary from patient to patient because it is a subjective response to pain. A constant pain threshold exists in all people under normal circumstances. However, pain tolerance varies widely. It can vary within the same person depending on the circumstances involved. Table 11-3 lists the conditions that can cause a person's pain threshold to be altered.

Modulation

Modulation, the fourth process, is a neural activity that controls pain transmission to neurons in both the peripheral and central nervous systems. The pathways involved are referred to as the *descending pain system* because the neurons originate in the brain stem and descend to the distal horn of the spinal cord. The descending nerve fibres release endogenous neurotransmitters known as *enkephalins* and *endorphins* (endogenous opiods, serotonin [5-HT], norepinephrine [NE], gamma [γ]-aminobutyric acid [GABA], neurotensin). These substances bind with opioid receptors and inhibit the transmission of pain impulses by closing the gates, thus producing analgesia (McCaffery & Pasero, 1999).

TABLE 11-3

Conditions That Alter Pain Threshold

Pain Threshold	Conditions
Lowered	Anger, anxiety, depression, discomfort, fear, isolation, persistent pain, sleeplessness, tiredness
Raised	Diversion, empathy, rest, sympathy, medications (analgesics, antianxiety drugs, antidepressants)

Endogenous pain modulation helps explain the wide variations in perception of pain seen from one person to another. These endogenous analgesic substances are responsible for the phenomenon of "runner's high." Figure 11-1 showing the gate theory depicts this entire process. Just like exogenous opioids, endogenous opioids bind to opioid receptor sites and prevent the release of neurotransmitters (like substance P), inhibiting the transmission of pain impulses. However, they usually break down too quickly to be useful as analgesics.

Another phenomenon of pain relief that may be explained by the gate theory is the fact that massaging the affected area often decreases the pain. When an area is rubbed or liniment applied, large sensory "A" fibres from peripheral receptors carry impulses to the spinal cord, thus causing impulse transmission to be inhibited and the gate to be closed. This, in turn, reduces the recognition of the pain impulses arriving by means of the small fibres. This is the same pathway used by opioid analgesics to alleviate pain.

The cells that control the gate have a threshold. Impulses that reach these cells must rise above this threshold before an impulse is permitted to travel up to the brain.

Psychology of Pain and Pain Management

Pain involves physical, psychological, and emotional factors. It is a subjective and individual experience; it can be defined as whatever the experiencing person says it is, and it exists whenever the person says it does. It cannot be quantified. Although the mechanisms of pain and the nature of pain pathways are becoming better understood, an individual patient's perception of pain and appreciation of its meaning are complex processes.

To effectively care for a patient suffering from pain, the nurse must culitvate a relationship with the patient that is built on trust and faith. There is no single approach to effective pain management. Instead, pain management has to be individualized and must take into account the cause of the pain, if known; the existence of concurrent medical conditions; the characteristics of the pain; and the psychological and ethnocultural characteristics (see Ethnocultural Implications: The Patient Experiencing Pain). It also requires ongoing reassessment of the pain and the effectiveness of treatment. The emotional response depends on the psychological experiences resulting from the physiological stimulation (or *nociception*).

Treatment of Pain in Special Situations

It is estimated that one of every three Canadians experiences pain and that this pain is poorly understood and often undertreated. In addition to baseline persistent pain, patients with illnesses such as cancer, AIDS, and sickle cell anemia may also experience crisis periods of acute pain. Effective management of acute pain is often different from management of persistent pain in terms of medications and dosage used. Patients with **special pain situations** often benefit from a holistic clinical approach and well-informed health care providers. Therapy in

ETHNOCULTURAL IMPLICATIONS

The Patient Experiencing Pain

- Each ethnoculture has its own beliefs, thoughts, and ways of approaching, defining, and managing pain. Attitudes, meanings, and perceptions of pain vary with each ethnoculture.

- Many Black and Caribbean Canadians believe in the power of healers who rely strongly on the religious faith of the people and often use prayer and the laying on of hands.

- Many Somali Canadians believe in Quranic readings, the wearing of amulets, and the use of a wide variety of herbs. Illness and healing are often viewed as the will of Allah. The evil eye "al-ayn," spirits called Jinn, or curses may also cause illness. Ritual scarification and fumigation are common, as is cauterization, in which a thin burning stick or heated metal is applied on an affected part.

- For some Hindus, pain must be endured. It is part of preparing for a better life in the next cycle. The devout Hindu who senses imminent death prepares for a "good death" by remaining conscious in order to experience the events to come. Asking for pain medication, especially with somnolent adverse effects, is generally avoided.

- Many members of the Jewish culture express their pain openly. The pain experience is to be shared, recognized, and validated by others. Intense complaining that may be expressed by Jewish patients does not necessarily mean intense pain; it may relate to the need for the presence of others to listen to them and affirm their experience.

- Traditional methods of healing for the Chinese include acupuncture, acupressure, herbal remedies, balancing the yin and yang, and cold treatment. Moxibustion, in which cones or cylinders of pulverized wormwood are burned on or near the skin over specific meridian points, is another form of healing.

- For many Aboriginal people, treatments include massage, the application of heat, sweat baths, herbal remedies, and being in harmony with nature.

- In the Arab culture, patients are expected to openly express their pain and anticipate immediate relief, preferably through injections or intravenous drugs.

Nurses should be aware of ethnocultural influences on health-related behaviours and on patients' attitudes toward medication therapy and thus, ultimately, on its effectiveness. Nurses interpret pain behaviour through their own cultural lens and often make culturally learned judgements about patients by the behaviour they display. Although there are helpful generalizations about the influence of culture on the expression of pain and this information provides a reservoir of information, nurses are cautioned not to use this background knowledge to fit everyone into a mould, stereotyping people. A thorough assessment with questions about the patient's ethnocultural background and practices is important to the effective and individualized delivery of nursing care.

such situations may include use of opioid or nonopioid drugs (or both) as well as nonpharmacological treatments such as transcutaneous electric nerve stimulation, massage, meditation, biofeedback, relaxation therapy, and psychological counselling.

In situations such as pain associated with malignancies, the main consideration in pain management is patient comfort and not prevention of drug **addiction**. Often this means aggressive treatment with gradually increasing scheduled doses of opioid analgesics to relieve the pain and prevent it from recurring. As the disease progresses, the patient may require even larger doses and more frequent medication administration using oral, injectable, rectal, transdermal, or parenteral routes. This is primarily because of increasing pathology, but tolerance may also be a factor. For long-term use, as with cancer patients, however, injectable forms are not the first choice because of the break in skin integrity and possible infections, especially with multiple intramuscular injections. Also, if a patient is taking long-acting narcotic analgesics, then **breakthrough pain** (pain that lingers despite the patient receiving doses of a long-acting dosage form every 12 hour) can be problematic and must be treated with shorter-acting or fast-acting forms on a

regular schedule. In this case, if the patient is requiring larger doses for breakthrough pain, the baseline dose of the narcotic may need to be titrated upward (that is, increased in increments). Other adjuvant medications may be added. Antiemetics and laxatives may also be used to prevent or relieve the constipation, nausea, and vomiting because all of these adverse effects are commonly associated with opioid drugs (Box 11-1).

Before specific drug classes and recommended approaches to pain management in a variety of clinical situations are discussed, the standards established by the **World Health Organization (WHO)** should be mentioned. For safe and efficient use of analgesics, the health care practitioner should be knowledgeable about standards of pain management and should remain current on all forms of and protocols for pain management (for mild to severe pain). The three-step analgesic ladder defined by the WHO is often applied as the pain management standard for the use of nonopioid and opioid drugs. Step 1 is the use of nonopioids (with or without adjuvant medications) once the pain has been identified and assessed. If pain persists or increases, treatment moves to step 2, which is defined as the use of opioids with or without nonopioids and with or without adjuvants.

BOX 11-1 — Potential Opioid Adverse Effects and Their Management

Constipation

Opioids decrease gastrointestinal tract peristalsis because of their central nervous system (CNS) depression, with subsequent constipation as an adverse effect. Stool becomes excessively dehydrated because it remains in the gastrointestinal tract longer.

Preventive measures: Constipation may be managed with increased intake of fluids; a regimen of stool softeners such as docusate sodium at the onset of treatment; possible use of mild osmotic drugs such as 70% sorbitol solution; use of bulk-forming laxatives (psyllium) with fluids; and use of mild cathartics such as senna.

Nausea and Vomiting

Opioids decrease gastrointestinal tract peristalsis, and some also stimulate the vomiting centre in the CNS, so nausea and vomiting are often experienced.

Preventive measures: Nausea and vomiting may be managed with the use of antiemetics such as phenothiazines or metoclopramide.

Sedation and Mental Clouding

Always evaluate any change in mental status to be sure that causes other than drug-related CNS depression are ruled out.

Preventive measures: Persistent drug-related sedation may be managed with a decrease in the dosage of opioid, and the physician may order CNS stimulants.

Respiratory Depression

Long-term opioid use is generally associated with tolerance to respiratory depression but can occur because opioids can inhibit brainstem respiratory pathways.

Preventive measures: For severe respiratory depression, narcotic antagonists may be used to improve respiratory status and, if titrated in small amounts, the respiratory depression may be reversed without analgesia reversal.

Subacute Overdose

Subacute overdose may be more common than acute respiratory depression and may progress slowly (over hours to days), with somnolence and respiratory depression. Before analgesic dosages are changed or reduced, advancing disease must be considered, especially in the dying patient.

Preventive measures: Often, holding one or two doses of an opioid analgesic is enough to judge if the mental and respiratory depressions are associated with the opioid. If there is improvement with this measure, the opioid dosage is often decreased by 25%.

Other Opioid Adverse Effects

Dry mouth, urinary retention, pruritus, myoclonus, dysphoria, euphoria, sleep disturbances, sexual dysfunction, and inappropriate secretion of antidiuretic hormone may occur but are less common than the previously mentioned adverse effects.

Preventive measures: Ongoing assessment is needed for each of the adverse effects so that appropriate measures may be implemented (e.g., sucking sugar-free hard candy or using artificial saliva drops or gum for dry mouth; use of diphenhydramine for pruritus).

Should pain persist or increase, management then rises to step 3, which is the use of opioids indicated for moderate to severe pain, administered with or without nonopioids or adjuvant medications. The ultimate goal for patients, as confirmed by the WHO, is freedom from pain.

It is also important to understand that opioids and agonists are classified into mild agonists (codeine and hydrocodone) and strong agonists (morphine, hydromorphone, levorphanol, oxycodone, oxymorphone, meperidine, fentanyl, and methadone). Meperidine is not recommended for long-term use because of the accumulation of a neurotoxic metabolite, normeperidine. The opiate agonists–antagonists such as pentazocine and nalbuphine are associated with an **analgesic ceiling effect,** a phenomenon that occurs when a drug at a specific dosage produces a maximal analgesic effect that does not improve even if the dosage is increased; raising the dosage beyond this level is dangerous, has unpredictable effects, and provides no further therapeutic benefit

for the patient (see Drug Profiles). They are useful only in patients who have not been previously exposed to opioids and can be used for nonescalating moderate to severe pain. Finally, because of associated bruising and bleeding risks, as well as injection discomfort, there is now a strong trend away from intramuscular injections in favour of intravenous (IV), oral, and transdermal routes of drug administration.

OPIOID DRUGS

The synthetic pain-relieving drugs currently known as **opioid analgesics** originated from the opium plant. The natural narcotic containing or derived from opium is known as an **opiate analgesic.** The word *opium* is a Greek word that means "juice." More than 20 different alkaloids are obtained from the unripe seed of the opium poppy plant. The properties of opium and its many alkaloids have been known for centuries. As early as the third century BC, reference to poppy juice is found in the writings of Theophrastus. Arabian physicians were well versed in the uses of opium as well. It was Arabian traders who introduced the drug to East Asia. Opium-smoking immigrants brought opium to Canada, where unrestricted availability of opium prevailed until the early twentieth century.

Chemical Structure

Opioid analgesics are strong pain relievers. They can be classified according to their chemical structure or their action at specific receptors. Of the 20 different natural alkaloids available from the opium poppy plant, only three are clinically useful: morphine, codeine, and papaverine. Of these three, only morphine and codeine are pain relievers; papaverine is a smooth muscle relaxant. Relatively simple chemical modifications of these opium alkaloids have produced the three different chemical classes of opioids: morphine-like drugs, meperidine-like drugs, and methadone-like drugs. Table 11-4 lists the opioid analgesics and their respective chemical categories.

Mechanism of Action and Drug Effects

Opioid analgesics can also be characterized according to their mechanism of action. They can be agonists, partial agonists, or antagonists (nonanalgesic). These same designations also apply to many other pharmacological classes of medications and their respective sites of action (receptor proteins) in the tissues. In the case of opioid analgesics, an **agonist** binds to an opioid pain receptor in the brain and causes an analgesic response resulting in the reduction of pain sensation. A **partial agonist**, also called an *agonist–antagonist* or a *mixed agonist*, binds to a pain receptor but causes a weaker neurological response than that of a full agonist. These three terms may present some confusion. For the practical purposes and scope of this textbook, the terms mixed agonist and agonist–antagonist are synonymous with partial agonist. Some advanced references used by pharmacological researchers further distinguish a mixed agonist as a drug with varying levels of agonist (not antagonist) potency among the different opiate receptor subtypes. These drugs are sometimes useful in pain management in opioid-addicted patients. An **antagonist** binds to a pain receptor but does not reduce pain signals. It also functions as a *competitive antagonist* because it competes with

and reverses the effects of agonist and partial-agonist drugs at the receptor sites. The nurse must keep in mind that the body also has its own internal biochemicals that stimulate various receptors. In the case of opioid receptors, these are known as *endorphins*, which stands for "endogenous morphine." The endorphins are a natural bodily mechanism of pain control.

Five types of opioid receptors have been identified to date: μ, κ, σ, δ, and ε. The μ, κ, and δ receptors are the most responsive to drug activity and are the receptors to which opioids bind to relieve pain; their characteristics are summarized in Table 11-5.

Many of the characteristics of a particular opioid, such as its ability to sedate, its potency, and its ability to cause hallucinations, can be attributed to the particular opioid's relative affinity for these receptors. Opioid analgesics achieve their beneficial effects by their actions in the CNS. However, they also act outside the CNS, and many of their unwanted effects stem from these actions.

Indications

The main use of opioids is to alleviate moderate to severe pain. The degree to which pain is relieved or unwanted adverse effects occur depends on the specific drug, the receptors to which it binds, and its chemical structure. Strong opioid analgesics such as fentanyl, sufentanil, and alfentanil are commonly used in combination with anaesthetics during surgery. Use of fentanyl injection for postoperative and procedural pain has become popular because of its rapid onset and short duration. Transdermal fentanyl comes in a patch formulation for use in long-term pain management; however, this dosage form poses titration difficulties and should not be used for postoperative pain (see Preventing Medication Errors: Fentanyl Transdermal Patches).

Similarly strong opioids such as morphine, meperidine, hydromorphone, and oxycodone are often used to control postoperative and other types of pain. Because morphine, meperidine, and hydromorphone are available in injectable forms, they are first-line analgesics in the immediate postoperative setting. All available oxycodone dosage forms are orally administered. The brand name product OxyContin is a sustained-release form of oxycodone that is designed to last up to 12 hours. The

TABLE 11-4

Chemical Classification of Opioids

Chemical Category	Opioid Drugs
meperidine-like drugs	meperidine, fentanyl, sufentanil, alfentanil
methadone-like drugs	methadone
morphine-like drugs	morphine, heroin, hydromorphone, codeine, hydrocodone, oxycodone

TABLE 11-5

Opioid Receptors and Their Characteristics

Receptor Type	Prototypical Agonist	Effects
μ	morphine	Supraspinal analgesia, respiratory depression, euphoria, ++sedation
κ	butorphanol	Spinal analgesia, ++++sedation, miosis
δ	enkephalins	Analgesia

++, moderate; ++++, severe.

PREVENTING MEDICATION ERRORS

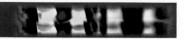

Fentanyl Transdermal Patches

When applying fentanyl (Duragesic) transdermal patches, the nurse needs to keep in mind several important points to avoid improper administration:

- These patches should only be used in patients who are considered opioid tolerant. To be considered opioid tolerant, a patient should have been taking, for a week or longer, morphine 60 mg daily, oral oxycodone 30 mg daily, or oral hydromorphone 8 mg daily (or an equianalgesic dose of another opioid). Giving fentanyl transdermal patches to non–opioid-tolerant patients may result in severe respiratory depression. Thorough assessment is important.

- Patients should be taught that heat, such as from a sauna, hot tub, heating pad or heated water bed, or an electric blanket, should never be used with a fentanyl transdermal patch. The increased circulation that results from the application of heat may result in increased absorption of medication, resulting in an overdose.

- Patients should be taught to dispose of patches properly. Children have retrieved used patches from the trash, which led to deaths because of exposure to the drug. Used patches should be folded with sticky sides together and flushed down the toilet.

Health Canada and the manufacturer issued a safety alert to consumers and health professionals about deaths in Canada from inappropriate use of the patches. It is essential for the patient's safety to read the product labelling and follow instructions precisely.

"Contin" in the product name stands for "continuous-release," a synonym for long action in any drug product. There are also immediate-release forms of oxycodone in tablet, capsule, and liquid forms. Similarly, the drug product MS Contin is a long-acting or sustained-release form of morphine that is also designed to provide about 12 hours of pain relief. The "MS" stands for the salt name, morphine sulfate. Morphine is also available in injectable forms, suppository, and oral syrup, as well as immediate-release and controlled-release tablets. Meperidine is available only in immediate-release dosage forms, both oral and injectable. The analgesic effects of immediate-release tablets of all three drugs typically last for about 4 hours. In the event of breakthrough pain, the patient's medication may be supplemented with immediate-release drugs (e.g., morphine, oxycodone). If the relief period for the long-acting drug continues to be inadequate, then the dosage of the long-acting drug may itself be increased.

Opioids also suppress the medullary cough centre, which results in cough suppression. The most commonly used opioid for this purpose is codeine. Hydrocodone has also been used in many cough suppressants, either alone or in combination with other drugs. Sometimes the opioid-related cough suppressants have a depressant effect on the CNS and cause sedation. To avoid this problem, dextromethorphan, a nonopioid cough suppressant, is often given instead (see Chapter 36).

Constipation from decreased gastrointestinal (GI) motility is often an unwanted adverse effect of opioids related to their anticholinergic effects. However, these effects are sometimes helpful in treating diarrhea. One of the most common opioid-containing antidiarrheal preparations is diphenoxylate/atropine tablets.

Often drugs from other chemical categories are added to the opioid regimen as **adjuvant analgesic drugs** (or adjuvants). These assist the primary drugs in relieving pain. Such adjuvant drug therapy may include NSAIDs, antidepressants, anticonvulsants, and corticosteroids, all of which are discussed further in their corresponding chapters. This therapy allows the use of smaller dosages of opioids, which accomplishes two important functions. First, it diminishes some of the adverse effects seen with higher dosages of opioids, such as respiratory depression, constipation, and urinary retention. Second, it approaches the pain stimulus by another mechanism of drug action and has a beneficial synergistic effect in reducing the pain.

Contraindications

Contraindications to the use of opioid analgesics include known drug allergy and severe asthma. Although they are not absolute contraindications, extreme caution should be used in cases of respiratory insufficiency, especially when resuscitative equipment is not available; conditions involving elevated intracranial pressure (e.g., severe head injury); morbid obesity or sleep apnea; myasthenia gravis; paralytic ileus (bowel paralysis); and pregnancy, especially with long-term use or high doses.

Adverse Effects

As previously mentioned, many of the unwanted effects of opioid analgesics are related to their effects on parts of the body other than the CNS. Some of these unwanted effects can be explained by the respective drug's selectivity for the receptors listed in Table 11-5. The body systems that the opioids affect and the corresponding adverse effects are summarized in Table 11-6.

All opioid drugs have a strong abuse potential. Opioids that have an affinity for μ-receptors and have rapid onset of action produce marked euphoria. These are the opioids that are most likely to be misused and used recreationally by the lay public as well as by health care providers who often have relatively easy access to them. A patient receiving opioid analgesics who does not normally take such medication is said to be **opioid-naïve** and is therefore not accustomed to the powerful effects

TABLE 11-6

Opioid-Induced Adverse Effects by Body System

Body System	Adverse Effect
Cardiovascular	Hypotension, palpitations, flushing
Central nervous	Sedation, disorientation, euphoria, lightheadedness, dysphoria, lowered seizure threshold, tremors
Gastrointestinal	Nausea, vomiting, constipation, biliary tract spasm
Genitourinary	Urinary retention
Integumentary	Itching, rash, wheal formation
Respiratory	Respiratory depression and aggravation of asthma

of opioid drugs. Such a patient typically requires lower drug dosages for adequate therapeutic effects. In contrast, the person taking opioids to deliberately achieve an altered mental status will soon become psychologically dependent on the drugs.

Psychological dependence is also known as addiction. It is defined by the Centre for Addiction and Mental Health (2008) as a primary, chronic, neurobiological disease with genetic, psychosocial, and environmental factors influencing its development and manifestations. Addiction is characterized by behaviours that include one or more of the following: impaired control over drug use, compulsive use and craving, and continued use despite harm.

In contrast, **physical dependence** is a state of physiological adaptation manifested by a drug-class-specific withdrawal syndrome that can be produced by abrupt cessation, rapid dose reduction, decreasing blood level of the drug, and administration of an antagonist. Typical withdrawal symptoms include rebound pain, mental agitation, tachycardia, elevated blood pressure, and seizures. In severe cases, these symptoms can become life threatening. Treatment of withdrawal is discussed in Chapter 9.

Opioid tolerance is a state of adaptation in which exposure to a drug (legally or otherwise) for an extended period of time induces changes that result in a diminution of one or more of the drug's effects over time. The opioid-tolerant patient is more likely to require higher drug dosages for desired therapeutic effects and is also at greater risk of opioid withdrawal syndrome upon dosage reduction or drug discontinuation. This is obviously a common problem with patients addicted to opioids, but it can also result from legitimate control of severe pain in patients with serious illnesses such as cancer. A patient who becomes addicted to pain medication under the latter circumstance is sometimes called a "medical addict." It should be noted, however, that patients who become addicted to opiate drug therapy most often have some initial predisposition toward addiction in general. Nonetheless, fear of creating a medical addict may lead well-meaning prescribers to undertreat pain, which is generally considered inhumane and unethical. Under these circumstances, control of the patient's pain takes ethical and even clinical priority over concerns regarding drug addiction (see Legal and Ethical Principles: The North American Opiate Medication Initiative). All opioids cause some histamine release. It is thought that this histamine release is responsible for many of the drugs' unwanted adverse effects, such as itching or pruritus, rash, and hemodynamic changes. The histamine release causes peripheral arteries and veins to dilate, which leads to flushing and orthostatic hypotension. The amount of histamine release that an opioid analgesic causes is related to its chemical class. The naturally occurring opiates elicit the most histamine release; the synthetic opioids (e.g., meperidine) elicit the least histamine release. (See Table 11-4 for a list of the opioids and their respective chemical classes.)

The most serious adverse effect of opioid use is CNS depression, which may lead to respiratory depression. When opioids are given, care should be taken to titrate

 LEGAL & ETHICAL PRINCIPLES

The North American Opiate Medication Initiative

Currently in Canada, it is estimated that 60,000 to 90,000 people are addicted to illicit opiates. While methadone is a successful strategy for some people, it is not effective for many higher-risk patients. Although these individuals represent approximately 10% to 20% of the heroin-addicted population, they account for a disproportionately large percentage of the drug-related problems undermining public health, the criminal justice system, and public order. The North American Opiate Medication Initiative (NAOMI), funded by the Canadian Institutes of Health Research and approved by Health Canada, is a controlled clinical trial that tests whether medically supervised injectable pharmaceutical-grade heroin benefits individuals suffering from persistent opiate addictions who have not benefited

from other treatments such as methadone maintenance and abstinence programs. Two sites in Canada, Vancouver and Montreal, are being used for the trials. The study has generated some controversy from researchers who believe that it is better to treat heroin addiction with methadone and that providing free heroin is not cost-effective, safe, or practical. In addition, there are ethical issues associated with providing free heroin to addicts. Proponents argue that the NAOMI study may answer questions that could result in improvements in the health of those with persistent addictions and identify new ways of reintegrating this population into society. The researchers hypothesize that heroin maintenance therapy could also help to reduce both the use of illicit drugs and drug-related crime.

the dose so that the patient's pain is controlled without respiratory functions being affected. Individual responses to opioids vary, and patients may occasionally suffer respiratory compromise or the loss of airway reflexes despite careful dose titration. Respiratory depression can be prevented in part by using drugs with short duration of action and no active metabolites. Respiratory depression seems to be more common in patients with a pre-existing condition causing respiratory compromise, such as asthma or chronic obstructive pulmonary disease. Respiratory depression is strongly related to the degree of sedation. Stimulation of the patient may be adequate to reverse mild hypoventilation. If this is unsuccessful, ventilatory assistance using a bag and mask or by endotracheal intubation may be needed to support respiration. Administration of naloxone hydrochloride, an opioid reversal drug, will reverse severe respiratory depression. However, the nurse should keep in mind that naloxone will reverse not only the patient's respiratory depression but also the pain control. Careful, slow titration of naloxone (until the patient is responding) will prevent an over-reversal of the opioid-induced respiratory depression and pain relief. The effects of naloxone are short-lived and usually last about 1 hour. With long-acting opioids the respiratory depressant effects can reappear after the naloxone has worn off, and redosing may be needed.

Gastrointestinal tract adverse effects are common in patients receiving opioids. Nausea, vomiting, and constipation are the most common adverse effects associated with opioid analgesics. Opioids can irritate the gastrointestinal tract, stimulating the chemoreceptor trigger zone in the CNS, which, in turn, may cause nausea and vomiting. Opioids slow peristalsis and increase water absorption from intestinal contents. These two actions combine to produce constipation. This is more pronounced in a hospitalized patient who is nonambulatory because of lack of daily activity.

Urinary retention, or the inability to void, is another unwanted adverse effect of opioid analgesics. They cause this by increasing bladder tone. This is sometimes prevented by giving low dosages of an opioid **agonist–antagonist** or an opioid antagonist. An alternative drug is a cholinergic agonist (Chapter 20) such as bethanechol.

Severe hypersensitivity or anaphylactic reaction to opioid analgesics is rare. Most patients will experience gastrointestinal discomforts or histamine-mediated reactions to

opioids and call these allergic reactions. However, true anaphylaxis is rare, even with intravenously administered opioids. Some patients may complain of flushing, itching, or wheal formation at the injection site, but this is usually local and histamine mediated. Refer to Box 11-1 (p. 190) for additional information on opioid adverse effects and their management.

Toxicity and Management of Overdose

Opioid analgesics produce both beneficial effects and toxic or unwanted effects by means of receptors. These receptors and the positive and negative effects they bring about are listed in Table 11-5. The opioid antagonists naloxone and naltrexone bind to and occupy all of these receptor sites (μ, κ, and δ). They are competitive antagonists with a strong affinity for these binding sites. Through such binding, they can reverse the adverse effects induced by the opioid, such as respiratory depression. These drugs are used in the management of both opioid overdose and opioid addiction. The commonly used opioid antagonists (reversal drugs) are listed in Table 11-7.

For effective management of opioid overdose or toxicity, it is important for the nurse to recognize the signs and symptoms of withdrawal. Opioid tolerance and physical dependence are expected in patients undergoing long-term opioid treatment and should not be confused with physiological dependence, as seen with drug abuse behaviour. Confusing these concepts in relation to opioid therapy sometimes leads to ineffective pain management and contributes to the problem of undertreatment. The extent of physical dependence on opioids becomes most visible to the nurse when an opioid drug is discontinued abruptly or when an opioid antagonist is administered. This physiological response is referred to as **opioid withdrawal** (**opioid abstinence syndrome**) and is manifested by anxiety, irritability, chills and hot flashes, joint pain, lacrimation (tearing), rhinorrhea, diaphoresis, nausea, vomiting, and abdominal cramps and diarrhea. Drug therapy for acute withdrawal from opioids and other drugs of misuse is described in Chapter 9.

The timing of the onset of withdrawal symptoms is directly related to the half-life of the opioid analgesic being used. The withdrawal symptoms resulting from the discontinuance or reversal of short-acting opioid therapy (codeine, hydrocodone, morphine, and hydromorphone) will arise within 6 to 12 hours and peak

TABLE 11-7

Opioid Antagonists (Reversal Drugs)

Generic Name	Trade Name	Dosage	Cautions
naloxone hydrochloride (IV)	Naloxone hydrochloride injection	0.4–2 mg q2–3 min; IV infusion: 2 mg in 500 mL (titrate to response)	Raised or lowered blood pressure, dysrhythmias, pulmonary edema, withdrawal
naltrexone (PO)	ReVia	25–50 mg daily	Nervousness, headache, nausea, vomiting, pulmonary edema, withdrawal

IV, intravenous; *PO*, oral.

at 24 to 72 hours. The withdrawal symptoms associated with drugs with long half-lives (methadone and transdermal fentanyl) may not appear for 24 hours or more after drug discontinuation and may be milder. The appearance of abstinence syndrome indicates physical dependence on the opioid, which may occur after as little as 2 weeks of therapy. It does not, however, imply the existence of psychological dependence or addiction. Most patients with cancer take opioid analgesics for longer than 2 weeks, and only rarely do they exhibit the drug abuse behaviour and psychological dependence that characterize addiction. Gradual dosage reduction, when possible, after persistent opioid use generally helps minimize the severity of withdrawal symptoms.

Interactions

Potential drug interactions with opioids are significant. Coadministration of opioids with alcohol, antihistamines, barbiturates, benzodiazepines, phenothiazine, and other CNS depressants can result in additive respiratory depressant effects. The combined use of opioids (such as meperidine) with monoamine oxidase inhibitors (MAOIs) can result in respiratory depression, seizures, and hypotension.

Laboratory Test Interactions

Opioids can cause an abnormal increase in the serum levels of amylase, alanine aminotransferase, alkaline phosphatase, bilirubin, lipase, creatinine kinase, and lactate dehydrogenase. Other abnormal results include a decrease in urinary 17-ketosteroid levels and an increase in the urinary alkaloid and glucose concentrations.

Dosages

For the recommended initial dosages of selected analgesic drugs in opioid-naive patients, see the Dosages table on p. 198. Drug pharmacokinetics for selected drugs are provided in the Drug Profiles table.

 ## DRUG PROFILES

▶▶ *morphine sulfate*

Morphine sulfate, a naturally occurring alkaloid derived from the opium poppy, is the drug prototype for opioids and narcotics. Opium is the dried juice of the poppy plant *Papaver somniferum* and is a mixture of opioid and nonopioid alkaloids. As with other narcotics, there is a strong potential for misuse and abuse with morphine. For this reason, morphine is classified as a Schedule I controlled substance.

Morphine is highly constipating and stool softeners or laxatives are often required as adjunct medications. Although it is not as dangerous as meperidine, morphine also has a potentially toxic metabolite known as morphine-6-glucuronide. Accumulation of this metabolite is more likely to occur in patients with kidney impairment. For this reason, other opioids such as hydromorphone (Dilaudid) and fentanyl may be safer analgesic choices for these patients. Drug profile information for hydromorphone is similar to that for morphine and meperidine. For dosage information, see the Dosages table on p. 198.

PHARMACOKINETICS

Half-Life	Onset	Peak	Duration
IM: 1.7–4.5 hr	IM: Rapid	IM: 30–60 min	IM: 6–7 hr

codeine sulfate

Codeine sulfate (methylmorphine) is another natural opiate alkaloid obtained from opium. The plant yield of this drug is too low to meet the high medical consumption needs for codeine. Therefore, it is most often prepared synthetically in the laboratory by methylation of morphine. Codeine is similar to morphine in terms of its pharmacokinetic and pharmacodynamic properties. However, codeine is less effective as an analgesic and is more widely used as an antitussive drug in an array of cough preparations. For example, codeine combined with acetaminophen (tablets or elixir) is classified as a Schedule II controlled substance and is commonly used for control of mild to moderate pain as well as cough. Codeine alone is still classified as Schedule I, which implies a high misuse and addiction potential. There is also an associated analgesic ceiling effect. For dosage information, see the Dosages table on p. 198.

PHARMACOKINETICS

Half-Life	Onset	Peak	Duration
PO: 2.5–4 hr	PO: 15–30 min	PO: 35–45 min	PO: 4–6 hr

fentanyl

Fentanyl is a synthetic opioid used to treat moderate to severe pain. Like other opioids, it also has a high abuse potential. It is also used as an adjunct to general anaesthetics. It is available in several dosage forms: parenteral injections and transdermal patches. In the United States, a "lollipop" lozenge on a stick (Actiq) has recently become available. The injectable form of fentanyl is used most commonly in perioperative settings (e.g., induction of general anaesthesia) and in critical care unit settings for sedation during mechanical ventilation. The oral and transdermal forms are used primarily for long-term control of both malignant and nonmalignant persistent pain. Fentanyl is a potent analgesic. The equianalgesic doses of some of the more common opioids compared with both 10 mg of intramuscular and 30 mg of oral morphine are listed in Table 11-8. Fentanyl at a dose of 0.1 mg given intravenously is roughly equivalent to 10 mg of morphine given intravenously.

The transdermal delivery system (patch) has been shown to be highly effective in the treatment of persistent types of pain syndrome such as cancer-induced pain, especially in patients who cannot take oral medications.

Continued

DRUG PROFILES (cont'd)

This route should never be used in opiate-naive patients. Generally, fentanyl patches are best employed for non-escalating pain because of the difficulty of titrating doses. Table 11-9 is provided to aid in converting from morphine to fentanyl in the treatment of pain. To perform the conversion using the table, first the daily (24-hour) opioid requirement of the patient should be determined. Second, if the opioid is not morphine, its dose should be converted to the equianalgesic dose of morphine using Table 11-8. Finally, the equipotent transdermal fentanyl dose can be calculated using Table 11-9. These tables are conservative in their dosages for achieving pain relief, and supplemental short-acting opioid analgesics should be added as needed. Nurses should be aware that after the first patch is applied it will take 6 to 12 hours to reach steady-state pain control again, thus supplemental short-acting therapy is required. Most patients will experience adequate pain control for 72 hours with this method of fentanyl delivery.

PHARMACOKINETICS

Route	Half-Life	Onset	Peak	Duration
Intravenous	1.5–6 hr	Rapid	Minutes	30–60 min
Intramuscular	1.5–6 hr	7–15 min	20–30 min	1–2 hr
Transdermal	Delayed	12–24 hr	48–72 hr	13–40 hr

meperidine hydrochloride

Meperidine hydrochloride (Demerol, Pethidine) is a widely used synthetic opioid analgesic. Meperidine should be used with caution, if at all, in the older adult and in patients who require long-term analgesia or who have kidney dysfunction. A metabolite, normeperidine, can accumulate and lead to seizures. After 48 hours, meperidine accumulates in the body and is toxic. Use of the drug is contraindicated in patients showing a hypersensitivity to it and in patients currently or recently treated with MAOIs. The concurrent use of MAOIs and meperidine can lead to deep coma and death. Meperidine is available in tablet and injectable form. For dosage information, see the Dosages table on p. 198.

PHARMACOKINETICS

Half-Life	Onset	Peak	Duration
IM: 3–5 hr	IM/PO: Rapid	IM/PO: 30–60 min	IM/PO: 2–4 hr

methadone hydrochloride

Methadone hydrochloride (Metadol) is a synthetic opioid analgesic. It is the opioid of choice for the detoxification treatment of persons addicted to opioids in methadone maintenance programs. Use of agonist–antagonist opioids (e.g., pentazocine) in patients addicted to heroin or those in methadone-maintenance programs can induce significant withdrawal symptoms. There has been renewed interest in the use of methadone for persistent (e.g., neuropathic) and cancer-related pain. Methadone is readily absorbed through the gastrointestinal tract with peak plasma concentrations at 4 hours for single dosing. Multiple daily dosing (e.g., every 8 hours) slows down elimination of the drug, providing a longer duration of

effect. However, 24-hour dosing is more common in methadone maintenance programs for addicted patients. Methadone is eliminated through the liver, which makes it a safer choice than some other opioids for kidney-impaired patients. For dosage information, see the Dosages table on p. 198.

PHARMACOKINETICS

Half-Life	Onset	Peak	Duration
PO: 25 hr	PO: 30–60 min	PO: 1.5–2 hr	PO: 24–48 hr

oxycodone hydrochloride

Oxycodone hydrochloride (OxyContin, Oxy-IR, Supeudol) is an analgesic drug that is structurally related to morphine and has comparable analgesic activity. Like morphine, it is a Schedule I drug. It is available in tablet, controlled-release tablet, and suppository oral solution forms but not in injectable form. It is also commonly combined in tablets with acetaminophen (Endocet, Percocet) and with aspirin (Endodan, Percodan). A somewhat weaker but commonly used opioid is hydrocodone (Hycodan), which is available in immediate-release and controlled-release tablet forms, as a syrup, rectally, parenterally, and as an expectorant. For dosage information, see the Dosages table on p. 198.

PHARMACOKINETICS (IMMEDIATE RELEASE)

Half-Life	Onset	Peak	Duration
PO: 2–3 hr	PO: 10–15 min	PO: 1 hr	PO: 3–6 hr

OPIOIDS AGONISTS–ANTAGONISTS

Opioids with mixed actions, often called agonists–antagonists, bind to the μ-receptor and can therefore compete with other substances for these sites. However, they either exert no action (i.e., they are competitive antagonists) or have only limited action (i.e., they are partial agonists).

PARTIAL OPIOID AGONISTS

The partial opioid agonists, or, more simply, partial agonists, are a group of analgesic drugs that have varying degrees of agonistic and antagonistic effects on the different opioid receptor subtypes. These drugs are similar to the agonist opioid drugs in their therapeutic indications. They are potent synthetic analgesics, but their misuse potential and addiction risk are both lower than those of the pure agonist opioids. The antagonistic activity of this group can produce withdrawal symptoms in patients who are opioid-dependent. Their use is also contraindicated in patients who have shown hypersensitivity reactions to the drugs. These drugs are normally used in situations requiring short-term pain control, such as after surgery and for obstetric procedures. They are sometimes chosen for patients who have a history of opioid addiction. These medications can both help prevent overmedication and reduce post-treatment addictive cravings in these patients. These drugs are normally not strong enough for management of longer-term persistent pain (e.g., cancer

Continued

DRUG PROFILES (cont'd)

pain, persistent low-back pain). They should also not be given concurrently with full opioid agonists because they can both reduce analgesic effects and cause withdrawal symptoms in opioid-tolerant patients. Four partial agonists are currently available: buprenorphine hydrochloride, butorphanol (Apo-Butorphanol), nalbuphine hydrochloride (Nubain), and pentazocine hydrochloride (Talwin). They are available in oral, injectable, and intranasal dosage forms as indicated in the Dosages table. Buprenorphine hydrochloride is also available in combination with the opioid antagonist naloxone (Suboxone) to enhance its opioid antagonistic effects, which is usually weaker than the agonistic effects of the drugs.

OPIOID ANTAGONISTS

Opioid antagonists are synthetic derivatives of oxymorphone, a potent semisynthetic opioid. They produce their opioid antagonistic activity by competing with opioids for CNS receptor sites.

▶▶ naloxone hydrochloride

Naloxone hydrochloride is a pure opioid antagonist because it possesses no agonist morphine-like properties and works as a blocking agent to the opioid drugs. Accordingly, the drug does not produce analgesia or respiratory depression. Naloxone is the drug of choice for the complete or partial reversal of opioid-induced respiratory depression. It is also indicated in cases of suspected acute opioid overdose. Failure of its administration to significantly reverse the effects of the presumed opioid overdose indicates that the condition may be caused by an overdose of nonopioid drugs or the dosing process. Naloxone is available only in injectable dosage forms. Use of the drug is contraindicated in patients with a history of hypersensitivity to it. For dosage information, see the Dosages table on p. 198.

PHARMACOKINETICS

Half-Life	Onset	Peak	Duration
IV: 64 min	IV: < 2 min	IV: Rapid	IV: Variable depending on dose and route

naltrexone hydrochloride

Naltrexone hydrochloride (ReVia) is an opioid antagonist used as an adjunct for the maintenance of an opioid-free state in former opioid addicts. It has been recognized as a safe and effective adjunct to psychosocial treatments of alcoholism. It is also recommended for reversal of postoperative opioid depression. It is available only in tablet form. Use of naltrexone hydrochloride is contraindicated in patients with hepatitis or liver dysfunction or failure and is also contraindicated in those with drug hypersensitivity. Nausea and tachycardia are the most common adverse effects and are related to reversal of the opioid effect. For dosage information, see the Dosages table on p. 199.

PHARMACOKINETICS

Half-Life	Onset	Peak	Duration
PO: 3.9–12.9 hr	PO: Rapid	PO: 1 hr	PO: 24–72 hr

TABLE 11-8

Equianalgesic Opioid Potencies (Based on Morphine 10 mg Intramuscularly and 30 mg Orally)

Opioid Analgesic	Equianalgesic Dose (mg)	
	Intramuscular	Oral
codeine	120	75
hydromorphone	1.5	7.5
meperidine	75	300
methadone	10	20
morphine	10 (standard)	30 (standard)
oxycodone	Injection not available	30
oxymorphone	1	10 (rectal)

Note: Fentanyl is most commonly given intravenously or transdermally (patch). See Table 11-9.

TABLE 11-9

Transdermal Fentanyl Dosages

Oral 24-Hour Morphine (mg/day)	Duragesic Dose (mcg/hr)
45–59	12
60–134	25
135–179	25 + 12
180–224	50
225–269	50 + 12
270–314	75
315–359	75 + 12
360–404	100
405–494	125
495–584	150
585–674	175
675–764	200
765–854	225
855–944	250
945–1034	275
1035–1124	300

DOSAGES Selected Analgesic Drugs and Related Drugs

Drug (Pregnancy Category)	Pharmacological Class	Usual Dosage Range	Indications
OPIOIDS			
codeine sulfate (D)	Opioid; opiate; opium alkaloid	*Children (2–5 yr)* 2.5–5 mg q4–6h—do not exceed 30 mg/day	Cough relief
		Children (6–11 yr) 6–11 yr, 5–10 mg q4–6h	Cough relief
		Adult/Children (older than 12 yr) 10–20 mg q4–6h—do not exceed 120 mg/day	Opioid analgesia
		Adult 15–60 mg tid–qid All doses titrated to response, starting with lowest effective dose	Cough relief
fentanyl (Duragesic, Ran-Fentanyl Transdural system) (D)	Opioid analgesic	IV/IM doses available in 50 mcg/mL ampoule or premixed infusion of varying strengths *Children (2–12 yr)* IV/IM: 2–3 mcg/kg/dose *Adult*	Procedural sedation or adjunct to general anaesthesia
		Epidural: 100 mcg diluted in 8 mL 0.9% sodium chloride IV: continuous infusion 1 mcg/kg/hr Duragesic (transdermal patch): 12.5–200 mcg/hr q72h;	Relief of moderate to severe acute pain; relief of persistent pain, including cancer pain
meperidine hydrochloride (Demerol, Pethidine) (D)	Opioid analgesic	*Children* PO: 1.1–1.8 mg/kg q3–4h prn IM/SC: 1–1.5 mg/kg q2–3h prn (max 100 mg/dose) IM/SC: 0.5–1 mg/kg 30–90 min before anaesthesia (max 100 mg/day) *Adult* PO: 50–150 mg q3–4h prn IM/SC: 50–100 mg 30–90 min before anaesthesia IV: 50–150 mg q3–4h	Relief of moderate to severe pain. Meperidine use should be restricted because of the unpredictable effects of neurometabolites at analgesic doses and risk for seizures Obstetric analgesia, preoperative sedation
methadone hydrochloride (Metadol) (D)	Opioid analgesic	*Adult* PO for pain 5–10 mg q3–4h; 40 mg or more daily, reduced doses every few days; 40–120 mg or more once daily	Opioid analgesic, relief of persistent pain, opioid detoxification, opioid addiction maintenance
⤞morphine sulfate (Doloral, Kadian, M-Eslon, M. O. S., Statex) (D)	Opioid; opiate; opium alkaloid	*Children* SC: 0.1–0.2 mg/kg dose—do not exceed a 15 mg single dose	Opioid analgesia
		Adult PO/IM/SC: 5–30 mg q4h Rectal: 10–20 mg q4h IV: 2.5–15 mg IV: 2.5–20 mg q2–6h PCA pump, epidural: titrate to effect	Opioid analgesia
morphine sulfate, continuous release (MS Contin) (D)	Opiate analgesic; opium alkaloid	*Adult only* PO: 15 mg q8h to 200 mg q12h	Relief of moderate to severe pain
oxycodone hydrochloride (OxyContin, Oxy-IR, Supeudol) (D)	Opioid, synthetic	*Children* PO: 1.25–2.5 mg q6h prn *Adult* PO: 5–20 mg q4–6h prn	Relief of moderate to severe pain
OPIOID ANTAGONISTS			
⤞naloxone hydrochloride	Opioid antagonist	*Children* IM/IV/SC: 0.01 mg/kg IV followed by 0.1 mg/kg if needed; 0.005–0.01 mg/kg IV—repeat in 2–3 min intervals	Relief of moderate to severe pain
		Adult IM/IV/SC: 0.4–2 mg IV—repeat in 2–3 min if needed; 0.1–0.2 mg IV—repeat in 2–3 min intervals	Treatment of opioid overdose, postoperative anaesthesia reversal

Continued

DOSAGES   Selected Analgesic Drugs and Related Drugs (cont'd)

Drug (Pregnancy Category)	Pharmacological Class	Usual Dosage Range	Indications
naltrexone hydrochloride (ReVia)	Opioid antagonist	*Adult* PO: 50 mg daily or 100 mg every other day	Maintenance of opioid-free state
OPIOID/ACETAMINOPHEN* COMBINATION PRODUCTS NOTE: There are many others on the market, including combinations with aspirin			
Percocet ratios various strengths of OXY/APAP ratios: 2.5 mg/ 325 mg (Percocet-Demi); 5 mg/325 mg (Percocet) (D)	Opioid combination Analgesic	*Children (6–12 yr)* PO: 0.25 tab q6h (Percocet-Demi) *Children (12 yr and older)* PO: 0.5 tab q6h (Percocet-Demi) *Adult* PO: 1–2 tab q6h (Percocet-Demi); 1 tab q6h (Pecocet) (Percocet) (not to exceed 4000 mg APAP/24h, assuming normal liver function)	Combination opioid/ nonopioid analgesic
Tylenol with various ratios of APAP, caffeine/codeine and caffeine OR APAP and codeine: 300 mg/15 mg / 8 mg (Tylenol No. 1); 500 mg/ 15 mg / 8 mg codeine (Tylenol No.1 Forte)	Opioid combination Analgesic	1–2 caplets q4h (not to exceed 12 caplets in 24 hr) 1–2 caplets 3–4× daily (not to exceed 8 caplets in 24 hr)	Analgesia
300 mg / 15 mg / 15 mg (Tylenol No. 2)	Opioid combination analgesic	1–2 tablets q4h	Analgesia
300 mg / 15 mg / 30 mg (Tylenol No. 3)	Opioid combination analgesic	1–2 tablets q4h	Analgesia
300 mg/ 15 mg / 60 mg (Tylenol No. 4)	Opioid combination analgesic	1–2 tablets q4h	Analgesia
PARTIAL AGONISTS **buprenorphine (single entity available only through Special Access Programme) (D)**	Partial opioid agonist	SL: individualized	Management opioid dependence
butorphanol (Apo-butorphanol) (D)	Partial opioid agonist	Intranasal: 1 spray/nostril q3–4h (maximum, 16 mg)	Relief of moderate to severe pain
nalbuphine (Nubain) (D)	Partial opioid agonist	*Adult* SC/IV/IM: 10–20 mg q3–6h (maximum single dose 20 mg; not to exceed 160 mg daily)	Opioid analgesic
pentazocine (Talwin) (D)	Partial opioid agonist	*Adult* PO: 50–100 mg q3–4h	Relief of persistent or acute pain of moderate to severe degree
NONOPIOID ▸▸**acetaminophen (Tylenol, others) (B)**	Nonopioid analgesic, antipyretic	*Children* PO/PR: 0–3 mo, 40 mg q4–6h 4–11 mo, 80 mg q4–6h 12–23 mo, 120 mg q4–6h 2–3 yr, 160 mg q4–6h 4–56 yr, 240 mg q4–6h 6–8 yr, 320 mg q4–6h 9–10 yr, 400 mg q4–6h 11–12 yr, 480 mg q4–6h *Adult* PO/PR: 325–650 mg q4–6h; do not exceed 4 g/day In alcoholics do not exceed 2 g/day	Relief of mild to moderate pain Relief of mild to moderate pain

IM, intramuscular; *IV*, intravenous; *PCA*, patient-controlled analgesia; *PO*, oral; *PR*, rectal; *SC*, subcutaneous; *SL*, sublingual; *APAP*, acetaminophen; *ES*, extra strength; *HC*, hydrocodone bitartrate; *HP*, high potency; *OXY*, oxycodone hydrochloride.

*The maximum recommended daily dose of acetaminophen for a typical adult patient with *normal* liver function is 4000 mg per 24-hr period. For liver compromised patients, this dosage may be 2000 mg or even lower. If in doubt, check with a pharmacist or prescriber regarding a particular patient. The Canadian Pediatric Association recommends consultation with a physician for infants under 6 months.

NONOPIOID ANALGESICS

The most widely used nonopioid analgesic is acetaminophen. All drugs in the NSAID class, which includes aspirin, and the cyclooxygenase-2 (COX-2) inhibitors (e.g., Celebrex) are also nonopioid analgesics; these drugs are discussed in greater depth in Chapter 45. These medications are commonly used for management of pain, especially pain associated with inflammatory conditions such as arthritis, because they have significant anti-inflammatory effects in addition to their analgesic effects. Acetaminophen is available in a variety of dosage formulations, both over the counter (OTC) and by prescription. It is also a component of many combination products with opioids.

Mechanism of Action and Drug Effects

The mechanism of action of acetaminophen is similar to that of the salicylates. It blocks peripheral pain impulses by inhibition of prostaglandin synthesis. Acetaminophen also lowers the febrile body temperature by acting on the hypothalamus, the structure in the brain that regulates body temperature. Heat is dissipated through resulting vasodilation and increased peripheral blood flow. In contrast to NSAIDs, acetaminophen has only weak anti-inflammatory effects and thus is not used to treat inflammation (e.g., arthritic inflammation). Although acetaminophen shares the analgesic and antipyretic effects of the salicylates and other NSAIDs, it does not have many of the unwanted effects of these drugs. For example, acetaminophen products are not usually associated with cardiovascular effects (e.g., edema) or platelet effects (e.g., bleeding) and have no effect on platelets (such as a tendency to cause bleeding) as do aspirin and other NSAIDs. They cause none of the aspirin-related gastrointestinal tract irritation or bleeding or any of the aspirin-related acid–base changes.

Indications

Acetaminophen is indicated for the treatment of mild to moderate pain and fever. It is an appropriate substitute for aspirin because of its analgesic and antipyretic properties. Acetaminophen is a valuable alternative for those patients who cannot tolerate aspirin or for whom aspirin may be contraindicated. Acetaminophen is also the antipyretic (antifever) drug of choice in children and adolescents with flu syndromes because the use of aspirin in such populations is associated with a brain-wasting condition known as Reye's syndrome.

Contraindications

Contraindications to acetaminophen use include known drug allergy, severe liver disease, and the genetic disease known as *glucose-6-phosphate dehydrogenase (G6PD) enzyme deficiency.*

Adverse Effects

Acetaminophen is an effective and relatively safe drug. It is therefore available OTC and in many combination prescription drugs. Acetaminophen is generally well tolerated. Possible adverse effects include rash, nausea, and vomiting. Much less common but more severe are the adverse effects of blood disorders or dyscrasias (e.g., anemias) and nephrotoxicities, especially if the manufacturer guidelines for dosage ranges are not followed.

Toxicity and Management of Overdose

Many people do not realize that acetaminophen, despite its OTC status, is a potentially lethal drug when taken in overdose. Depressed patients (especially adolescents) may intentionally overdose on the drug as an attention-seeking gesture without realizing the grave danger involved.

The ingestion of large amounts of acetaminophen, as in an acute overdose, or even persistent unintentional misuse can cause liver necrosis. This is the most serious acute toxic effect. Acute ingestion of acetaminophen doses of 150 mg/kg or more may result in liver toxicity.

The standard maximum daily dose of acetaminophen for healthy adults is 4000 mg. For most patients, nurses, physicians, and patients should be careful to avoid doses in excess of this amount. Excessive dosing may occur inadvertently with the use of combination drug products such as tablets that include a fixed ratio of an opioid drug plus acetaminophen (e.g., hydrocodone plus acetaminophen).

The long-term ingestion of large doses of acetaminophen is more likely to result in nephropathy. Because the reported or estimated quantity of drug ingested is often inaccurate and not a reliable guide to the therapeutic management of the overdose, serum acetaminophen concentration should be determined for this purpose no sooner than 4 hours after the ingestion. If a serum acetaminophen level cannot be determined, it should be assumed that the overdose is potentially toxic and treatment with acetylcysteine (the recommended antidote for acetaminophen toxicity) should be started. Acetylcysteine works by preventing the hepatotoxic metabolites of acetaminophen from forming. The treatment regimen consists of an initial loading dose of 140 mg/kg orally, followed by 70 mg/kg every 4 hours for 17 additional doses. If the patient vomits within 1 hour of receiving a dose of acetylcysteine, that dose should be given again immediately. All 17 doses must be given to prevent hepatotoxicity, regardless of the subsequent acetaminophen serum levels.

Interactions

A variety of substances may interact with acetaminophen. Alcohol is potentially the most dangerous. Persistent heavy alcohol abuse may increase the risk of liver toxicity from excessive acetaminophen use. Most reports are of cases in which individuals with severe, persistent alcoholism took large doses of acetaminophen and exceeded recommended dosages, which led to possible overdose. Health care providers should alert patients with regular intake of moderate to large amounts of alcohol not to exceed recommended doses of acetaminophen because of the risk of liver dysfunction and possible liver

DRUG PROFILES

▸▸ *acetaminophen*

Acetaminophen (Tylenol) is an effective and relatively safe nonopioid analgesic used for mild to moderate pain relief. It is contraindicated in patients with a hypersensitivity to it or intolerance of tartrazine (yellow dye no. 5), alcohol, sugar, or saccharin. Its use should be avoided in patients who are anemic or who have kidney or liver disease. Acetaminophen is provided in many oral and rectal dosage formulations. It is available in the form of caplets, liquid drops, suspension, granules, immediate-release and extended-release tablets, chewable tablets, and rectal suppositories and in numerous strengths, depending on whether it is for use in children or adults.

PHARMACOKINETICS

Half-Life	Onset	Peak	Duration
PO: 1–4 hr	PO: 10–30 min	PO: 0.5–2 hr	PO: 3–4 hr

tramadol hydrochloride

Tramadol hydrochloride (Ralivia, Tridural, Zytram XL) is categorized as a miscellaneous analgesic because of its unique properties. It is a centrally acting analgesic with a dual mechanism of action. It creates a weak bond to the μ-opioid receptors and inhibits the reuptake of both norepinephrine and serotonin. Both these neurotransmitters are known as monoamines because they have a single amino group (–NH3) as part of their chemical structure.

In the spinal cord, their presence in the nerve synapses promotes what is known as monoaminergic inhibition of pain impulses. Although it does have weak opioid receptor activity, tramadol is not currently classified as a controlled substance. Tramadol is indicated for the treatment of moderate to moderately severe pain. Tramadol is rapidly absorbed and its absorption is unaffected by food. It is metabolized in the liver to an active metabolite (O-dimethyl tramadol) and eliminated via renal excretion. Adverse effects are similar to those of opioids and include drowsiness, dizziness, headache, nausea, constipation, and respiratory depression. Use of the drug is contraindicated in patients who have previously demonstrated hypersensitivity to tramadol, any other component of this product, or opioids. It is also contraindicated in cases of acute intoxication with alcohol, hypnotics, centrally acting analgesics, opioids, or psychotropic drugs. Seizures have been reported in patients taking tramadol. These seizures have occurred in patients taking normal dosages as well as dosages exceeding the normal recommended dosages. Patients who may be at risk are those taking tricyclic antidepressants, selective serotonin reuptake inhibitor antidepressants, MAOIs, neuroleptics, or other drugs that reduce the seizure threshold.

PHARMACOKINETICS

Half-Life	Onset	Peak	Duration
PO: 5–8 hr	PO: 30 min	PO: 2 hr	PO: Unknown

failure. Ideally, alcohol consumption should not exceed three drinks daily. Other hepatotoxic drugs should also be avoided. Other drugs that potentially can interact with acetaminophen include phenytoin, barbiturates, isoniazid, rifampin, β-blockers, and anticholinergic drugs, all of which are discussed in greater detail in later chapters. Drug pharmacokinetics for selected drugs are provided in the Drug Profiles table.

NURSING PROCESS

Patients experiencing pain pose many challenges to the nurse and other health care providers involved in their health and nursing care, as well as to significant others or family members. This challenge requires astute nursing assessment with appropriate intervention based on the specific individual as well as the specific type of pain and related disease processes and health status. Adequate analgesia (providing pain relief without complications, toxicity, or a diminished level of consciousness) with thorough patient teaching is the goal of all those involved in the care of these patients. Nurses need to adequately and accurately assess the nature of the patient's pain (Box 11-2). Pain has been accepted as the fifth vital sign that must be assessed (along with blood pressure, pulse

rate, temperature, and respirations) to ensure that pain management is adequate and effective. Pain assessment has also been established as a standard by the Canadian Council on Health Services Accreditation. Nurses need to assess and reassess the patient's response to the pain management regimen, regardless of of the medications involved—non-narcotics, narcotics, a combination of both, or NSAIDs (see Chapter 45).

There are several organizations and professional groups that establish standards for pain management (e.g., the Agency for Healthcare Research and Quality) or identify assessment tools such as the Numeric Pain Intensity Scale (a 0 to 10 pain rating scale) and the Visual Analogue Scale. Other reliable resources include age-appropriate pain-rating tools from the Canadian Pain Society. These tools have proved to be valid if the patients are capable of answering questions and are alert enough to participate in their care. With children, use of the Visual Analogue Scale as an "ouch" scale, along with other objective and subjective indicators, is helpful. On the opposite end of the age spectrum, older adults also require special assessment and consideration of medications they are taking and of pre-existing health problems. Because kidney and liver function may be decreased in the older adult, lower doses of drugs may be needed or ordered. For analgesics, this may mean giving the lowest but most effective dosage amount ordered. In addition,

BOX 11-2 Assessment of Pain

- Assess factors influencing pain, such as individual reaction, pain tolerance, underlying cause, individual pain threshold; age; physical factors (e.g., stress), and psychological factors (family roles, spiritual system, meaning of pain, stereotypes. Also take into account gender, societal influences, and general state of health.
- Use an age-appropriate scale to assess pain. In children younger than 5 years of age, consider level and stage of growth and development (e.g., Erikson's stages). Use pictures with happy faces (no pain with a rating of 0) and sad faces (bad pain with a rating 5) and tools that the child can relate to, such as a 15-cm ruler, to assess the level of pain.
- When assessing the older adult, never assume that these patients do not feel pain the same way that they did when they were younger. Although they may have barriers to verbal or nonverbal expression of pain (e.g., dementia, cognitive impairment), older adults still experience pain.
- When assessing for persistent pain, consider that pain can occur with or without evident tissue damage and serves no useful purpose. It is a complex, multifactorial problem that requires a holistic approach to patient care, with consideration of not only physical factors but also psychological factors (insomnia, depression, withdrawal, anxiety, personality changes, and changes

in lifestyle), because persistent pain is generally characterized more by psychological and functional-ability changes than by physical changes.
- Assessing for persistent pain is challenging; nonetheless, health care providers must go beyond what is expected to assess and then act. Remember that persistent pain is difficult to describe and manage and often is not responsive to conventional measures.
- When assessing for cancer pain, remember that management of this pain should be as individualized as all other aspects of patient care with full belief in the patient's pain and suffering. Treatment may include narcotics, possibly at high dosages; however, quality of life for the patient, rather than addiction, should be the concern in this situation.
- Ask the patient with acute or persistent pain (or any type of pain) to keep a daily journal of his or her pain experience, including information on precipitating and aggravating factors; measures that alleviate or help the pain; duration and intensity of pain; referred pain; character, onset, and pattern; the meaning of pain to the patient; and psychological factors.
- Remember that persistent pain and cancer pain (in addition to the pain experience) may be perceived as an actual or potential loss to the patient, including loss of control.

drug accumulation and toxicity may occur with any patient with decreased kidney or liver functioning.

▨ Assessment

Adequate analgesia, pain relief without complications, and patient teaching are goals of all health care providers. Nurses need to thoroughly assess the nature of the pain and whether the pain occurring is acute, persistent, or represents a special pain situation (see Evidence-Informed Practice: Strategies of Pain Assessment Used by Nurses on Surgical Units). The management of acute or persistent pain in patients is a common part of clinical practice and a challenging part of nursing and health care.

Before the nurse administers *any* analgesic, a thorough health history, medication history, and nursing assessment must be obtained. This ensures that these medications are used safely—that is, that analgesic treatment is free of complications or injury to the patient. The nurse should obtain and document information regarding the following (also see Box 11-2):

- Allergies to nonopioids (acetaminophen, aspirin, and other NSAIDs) including COX-2 inhibitors (Chapter 45), opioids, or partial or mixed agonists
- Drug history with identification of any interactions with other drugs, herbals, foods, and home remedies
- Underlying level of any CNS depression because of drug therapy or other physical conditions or diseases

- Adjunctive use of other nonopioids, NSAIDs, or opioids as well as their routes of administration, which should be assessed even more cautiously because of the risk of toxicity and overdosage
- Use of alcohol, street drugs, or any illegal drug or substance
- Pain intensity and character: onset, location, quality (stabbing, throbbing, dull ache, sharp, diffuse, localized, referred, or knifelike); intensity or severity (rated on a scale of 1 to 10, with 10 being the worst, and assessed using validated age-appropriate tools); precipitating, aggravating, and relieving factors; previous treatment; and effect of pain on physical and social function
- Type of pain being experienced, such as acute pain, persistent pain, or pain due to cancer. Each type of pain will require a different approach to treatment, with cancer pain and bone metastasis pain being most difficult to manage; opioid drugs, along with NSAIDs or COX-2 inhibitors, and a variety of routes of administration and dosage forms (transdermal, parenteral [intramuscular, subcutaneous, IV, or patient-controlled analgesia], oral, transmucosal, suppository, and epidural) may be used.
- Other pain treatments (both pharmacological and nonpharmacological)
- Laboratory values reflective of liver function (levels of alanine aminotransferase, alkaline phosphatase,

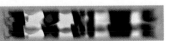

EVIDENCE-INFORMED PRACTICE

Strategies of Pain Assessment Used by Nurses on Surgical Units

Background

The purpose of this study was to identify criteria that nurses use in the assessment of patients who are experiencing postoperative pain. In addition, the study looked at the kind of knowledge the nurses applied from previous experiences. Phenomenology research design was used for this study. Data were analyzed using a qualitative approach to studying pain assessment in an attempt to describe the differences and similarities in individual conceptions of the pain experience.

Type of Evidence

Ten nurses and 30 postsurgical patients were involved in this study, which was conducted at a large urban hospital in New England. Strategic sampling was used to identify five nurses with fewer than 6 years of experience (categorized as the least experienced group) and five nurses with more than 6 years of experience (the more experienced group). It was anticipated that the number of years of nursing experience on a surgical unit might be important in differentiating the types of criteria nurses used to assess pain. All patients had undergone surgery within the previous 24 hours and were experiencing pain but were not connected to a patient-controlled analgesia pump, had not been diagnosed with metastatic cancer, and were not experiencing confusion or an altered level of consciousness. The research method included a series of five highly interactive, semistructured, audiotaped interviews with each nurse. Interviews focused on what the nurse's conception of the patient's situation was and how and on what basis the nurse judged the patient's pain.

Results of Study

Data from 30 clinical pain assessments performed by the 10 nurses identified multiple criteria used in each nurse's assessment of a patient. These criteria related to the patient's appearance and other observational data as well as to the content of communication between the nurse and the patient. These criteria were used as the framework from which the nurses developed and implemented variations in pain assessment. Nurses were also found to draw on their past experiences in several ways when working with their patients, including how to focus on listening to patients, what to look for, and what to do for the patient in pain. This study was one of the first to empirically identify criteria and types of past knowledge that nurses use when assessing patients for pain on a postoperative unit. Because it was a qualitative, descriptive study, the sample size was small and the strategies identified became saturated. The criteria used by the nurses to assess pain were both objective and subjective. Objective criteria concerned how the patient looked, whereas subjective criteria were more concerned with what the patient said. The facility in which the research took place has now changed its pain assessment guidelines to provide a more subjective orientation and has identified the patient's self-report as one of the single most reliable indicators of the existence and intensity of pain.

Link of Evidence to Nursing Practice

This study had a major impact on the assessment of pain in the facility in which the data were collected, and major policy changes were made in the criteria to be used in assessing patients' pain. As a qualitative approach to studying pain assessment, this study provided significant data identifying the criteria and types of past knowledge that nurses used while actually assessing patients for pain on a postoperative nursing unit. Questions that remain to be answered include the following: Does the strategy used for assessment influence the nurse's perception of the intensity of pain and the need for pain management? Does the assessment strategy used have an influence on pain management decisions? Quantification of the use of different pain assessment strategies in a large sample of nurses will allow the findings of this particular study to be extended to identify the strategies actually used in contemporary nursing practice and the resulting pain management techniques implemented by nurses.

Based on Kim, H. S., Schwartz-Barcott, D., Tracy, S. M., Fortin, J. D., & Sjostrom, B. (2005). Strategies of pain assessment used by nurses on surgical units. *Pain Management Nursing 6*(1), 3–9.

γ-glutamyl transferase, 5′-nucleotidase, and bilirubin) and kidney function (blood urea nitrogen and creatinine levels)
- Level of orientation, status of bowel sounds and urine output (e.g., possible confusion from narcotics and from CNS depression with resultant constipation or urinary retention)
- Ethnocultural and religious beliefs about the experience of pain and its management; use of alternative measures to relieve pain by Asian and other ethnocultural groups should be accepted

Objective and subjective findings of a thorough nursing assessment of patients who are being newly treated for pain or whose pain is being undermanaged are important to efficient and effective therapy. Psychosocial assessment includes obtaining information regarding the following influences on the pain experience: family and occupational roles, past experiences with pain, spiritual beliefs, meaning of pain, ethnocultural and societal influences, sexual identity, communication skills, level of growth and development in terms of Erikson's stages of development and related tasks, personality, attitude toward pain, level of anxiety, fatigue, motivations, and fears. Other factors or influences for which to assess include pain threshold, general state of health, sleep patterns and stressors, pain intensity and frequency, pain tolerance, prior experience of pain, CNS intactness, and age. The nurse should always remember, however, that each patient is an individual and should approach the patient from that perspective.

Vital signs (blood pressure, pulse, and respirations) should also be assessed and documented. The nurse should remember that during the acute pain response, stimulation of the sympathetic nervous system may result in elevated values for vital signs (blood pressure over 120/80 mm Hg, pulse rate over 100 beats/min, respiration rate over 20 breaths/min), and use of analgesics, especially narcotics will depress vital signs because of the CNS-depressive effects. The nurse should always document all data and findings related to a total system assessment and continue to monitor (and document) all basic system-related assessment parameters.

It is essential that the nurse check the route and time of administration of any previous analgesic and the patient's response before administering another analgesic dose, regardless of whether it is a nonopioid or opioid analgesic. The route of administration may also be dictated by considerations such as avoiding intramuscular dosage routes in persistent pain and cancer pain management. The nurse must always check the patient's chart, physician's order, nurses' notes, and medication administration record before administering any additional doses of an analgesic. Patients taking *any* type of analgesic should be reassessed at regular intervals before and during treatment.

For nonopioid analgesics, specifically acetaminophen and tramadol hydrochloride (NSAIDs and COX-2 inhibitors are discussed in Chapter 45), assessment parameters are similar to those for opioids, but there are some differences because of the nonopioid status of the analgesics. With acetaminophen, assessment should include all of the parameters mentioned earlier as well as determination of whether the patient is pregnant or breastfeeding. There are no age-related precautions for children or the older adult, and all other contraindications, cautions, and drug interactions should also be thoroughly assessed. Liver and kidney function tests should be assessed, especially if long-term therapy is indicated. Once therapy has been initiated, the nurse must be cautious to assess for symptoms of persistent acetaminophen poisoning, such as rapid, weak pulse; dyspnea; and cold and clammy extremities. Persistent daily use of the drug may also lead to increased risk of permanent liver damage, and so liver function should continue to be monitored. Children rarely experience liver damage; however, adults who ingest more than 2.6 g within a 24-hour period may be at higher risk of varying degrees of loss of appetite, jaundice, nausea, and vomiting.

Use of tramadol hydrochloride requires assessment of contraindications, cautions, drug interactions, and liver and kidney function (information presented previously).

The older adult and children may need age-related dosage adjustments (as for other non-narcotic and narcotic analgesics). CNS stimulation may occasionally occur, so tramadol is not a drug of choice (analgesic) if there is a history of seizures.

For narcotic analgesics, assessment data include all the previously mentioned information as well as respiratory status, kidney status, and presence of head injury. Because narcotics are CNS depressants, respiratory depression is of major concern; therefore, assessing respiratory rate, depth, and pattern and listening to breath sounds are important. Decreased kidney function can lead to possible drug accumulation and toxicity, thus the patient's blood urea nitrogen and creatinine levels should be assessed. Urinary output may need to be assessed as well because of possible urinary retention. With head injuries of undiagnosed cause, the administration of narcotics is not recommended because of the masking of changes in level of consciousness. Contraindications, cautions, and drug interactions also need to be assessed. The use of opioids in patients with disorders such as dementia, Alzheimer's disease, head injuries, increased intracranial pressure, multiple sclerosis, muscular dystrophy, myasthenia gravis, and cerebrovascular accident or a stroke may lead to an alteration of symptoms of the disease process with possible masking or worsening of the clinical presentation without actual pathological changes. With opioids it is also important to be aware that the older adult, although potentially more sensitive to the effects of these drugs, may also exhibit paradoxical excitement and excitatory behaviour even though a CNS depressant drug has been given (thus the term "paradoxical"). Children are also more susceptible to the CNS-depressant effects, especially respiratory depression. See Special Populations: Children and Special Populations: The Older Adult for use of opioids in both of these age groups.

In patients taking partial agonists such as buprenorphine hydrochloride, it is important to assess for pain and to assess for all of the parameters discussed earlier for opioids; these drugs are still considered narcotics because of their effect at the opioid receptors. It is also important in the assessment to remember that these drugs are effective analgesics and still have CNS-depressant effects. They are subject to the analgesic ceiling effect.

For opioid agonist–antagonist drugs, it is important for the nurse to determine whether the patient is in an addictive state or not because if these drugs are given to a patient who is taking a narcotic (whether by self-administration or addiction or on an order from the physician), withdrawal will occur in the addicted patient, with reversal of the effects of the narcotic. Other assessment data include vital signs, particularly respirations. Use in children younger than 18 years of age is not recommended, and effects of these medications are more unpredictable in the older adult. These drugs also cause spasms of the sphincter of Oddi in the gallbladder and are not recommended for those who have biliary ductal

ⓘ SPECIAL POPULATIONS: CHILDREN

 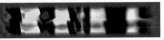

Use of Opioids

- Assessment of children is challenging, and all types of behaviour that may indicate pain, such as muscular rigidity, restlessness, screaming, fear of moving, and withdrawn behaviour, must be carefully considered.

- Pain management in children is complex because it is more difficult to determine their pain, especially in infants. Frequently the reason older children do not verbalize their pain is their fear of the treatment, such as shots. Compassionate and therapeutic communication skills will help the nurse in these situations.

- The "ouch scale" is often used to determine the level of pain in children. This scale is used to obtain the child's rating of the intensity of pain from 0 to 5 by means of simple face diagrams, from a happy face for level 0 (no pain) to a sad, tearful face for level 5 pain. Parents and caregivers play an important role in pain management in the child and in noting any crying or distress.

- Assessment of pain is important in children because they are often undermedicated. The nurse should always thoroughly assess the child and not underestimate the child's complaints.

- Always know the child's age, weight, and height because drug calculations are often based on these variables. With children, all mathematical calculations should be checked and double-checked for accuracy to avoid excessive dosages; this is especially true for opioids.

- Always give analgesics before pain becomes severe, with use of oral dosage forms first if appropriate.

- If suppositories are used, the nurse must be careful to administer the exact dose and not to split, halve, or divide an adult dose into a child's dose. This may result in the administration of an unknown amount of medication and possible overdose.

- When subcutaneous, intramuscular, and intravenous medications are used, the principle of nontraumatic care in the delivery of nursing care is being followed. One method to ensure atraumatic care is the use of EMLA (eutectic mixture of local anaesthetics) on the site before the actual injection. EMLA is a topical cream that anaesthetizes the site of the injection if applied 1 to $2\frac{1}{2}$ hours prior to the injection. Once the EMLA is applied to the site, the site is covered with a transparent dressing to keep the medication on the skin. A physician's order is needed.

- For neonatal infants, randomized controlled trials have shown that a nonpharmacological approach such as using a pacifier or syringe to deliver an oral sucrose solution is effective in reducing pain during minor painful procedures (e.g., injections, heel lancing). For the best analgesic effect, small amounts of the sucrose solution should be administered 2 minutes prior to the procedure, immediately upon beginning the procedure, and every 2 minutes throughout the procedure.

- Distraction and creative imagery may be used for older children such as toddlers or preschool-aged children. An example would be to have the child blow on a pinwheel. Not only does it distract the child, but it also encourages the child to take deep breaths, which relaxes the child.

- Children should always be monitored closely for any unusual behaviour while they are receiving opioids.

- The following signs and symptoms should be reported to the physician immediately if they occur: CNS changes such as dizziness, lightheadedness, drowsiness, hallucinations, changes in the level of consciousness, or sluggish pupil reaction. No further medication should be given until the nurse receives further orders from the physician. Always monitor and document vital signs before, during, and after the administration of opioid analgesics. Medication is withheld if the respiration rate is less than 12 breaths/min or if there are any changes in the level of consciousness.

- Carefully assess respiratory status—respiratory rate, rhythm, and character (rate, and difficulty).

- Generally speaking, smaller doses of opioids (with close and frequent monitoring) are indicated for children.

- Give medications with meals to help decrease gastrointestinal tract distress.

---

disease or are scheduled for biliary surgery. (Morphine is usually indicated in this situation.)

If, during assessment, overdose, toxicity, or respiratory depression is suspected, narcotic antagonists are available for reversal of CNS depression. Analgesia will also be reversed. The pure opioid antagonists (e.g., naltraxone) will bind at opioid receptors and reverse the opioid's action.

The nurse must remember that the narcotic antagonists are effective only in reversing respiratory depression secondary to opioid overdosage. Naloxone may be used in patients of all ages, including neonates and children. Vital signs should be assessed and documented just before, during, and after the use of the antagonist so that the therapeutic effects can be further noted. Also, the nurse must remember that the antagonist drug may not work with just one dosing and that repeated doses are generally needed to reverse the effects of the opioid. This helps ensure effective treatment of the overdosage and CNS depression as well as safe patient recovery.

SPECIAL POPULATIONS: THE OLDER ADULT

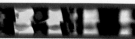

Use of Opioids

- Assess the patient carefully before administering opioids, because a dose and interval adjustment may be necessary if undesirable adverse reactions such as confusion, decreased respiration, and excessive central nervous system (CNS) depression have developed.
- Note and record height and weight before the start of opioid treatment.
- Carefully monitor and document any changes in older adults who are receiving opioids because they are generally more sensitive to these drugs. This includes frequent monitoring of vital signs, respiratory function, and CNS status.
- Many institutionalized older adult patients are stoic about pain and may also have altered presentations of common illnesses, so the pain experience presents in a different manner. For example, the older adult may have silent myocardial infarctions or even painless abdominal or intra-abdominal emergencies.
- It is a myth that aging increases the pain threshold. The problem is that cognitive impairment and dementia are often major barriers to pain assessment. Many older adults are nonetheless still reliable in their reporting of pain, even with moderate to severe cognitive impairment.
- Over time, the older adult may lose reliability in recalling and accurately reporting persistent pain.
- The older adult, especially those older than 75 years of age, are at higher risk for too much or too little pain management, and it is important to remember that there is a higher peak and longer duration of action of drugs in these patients than in their younger counterparts. Smaller dosages of narcotics are generally indicated for the older adult because of their increased sensitivity to the CNS-depressant effects of the drugs as well as their diminished kidney and liver functions. Paradoxical (opposite) reactions and unexpected reactions may be more likely to occur in patients of this age group as well.
- In older adult male patients, benign prostatic hypertrophy or obstructive urinary diseases should be considered because of the urinary retention associated with the use of narcotics. Urinary outflow can become further diminished in these patients and result in adverse reactions or complications. Dosage adjustments may need to be made by the physician.
- Polypharmacy is often a problem in older adults; therefore, it is important for the nurse to have a complete list of all medications that the patient is currently taking and to assess for drug interactions and treatment (drug) duplication.
- The nurse should conduct frequent assessments of patients for level of consciousness, alertness, and cognitive ability while ensuring that the environment is safe and that a call bell or light is kept at the bedside; bed alarms are indicated where available.
- Decreased circulation causes variation in the absorption of intramuscular or intravenous dosage forms and often results in the slower absorption of parenteral forms of opioids.
- Encourage the older adult to ask for medications if needed. They often hesitate to ask for pain medication because they do not want to bother the nurse or give in to pain.
- Health Canada (2006) has recommended that nonsteroidal anti-inflammatory drugs (NSAIDs) be used with caution because of their potential for renal and gastrointestinal toxicity. Acetaminophen is the drug of choice for relieving mild to moderate pain but with cautious dosing because of liver and kidney concerns. Adverse reactions tend to increase with dose and duration of treatment; consideration should be given to a starting dose lower than the one usually recommended, with individual adjustment when necessary and under close supervision. The oral route of administration is preferred. The regimen should be as simple as possible to enhance adherence, and the nurse should be sure to note, report, and document any unusual reactions to the opioid drugs.
- Hypotension and respiratory depression may occur more often in the older adult who is taking opioids for pain management, thus the need for even more astute vital-sign monitoring.

Nursing Diagnoses

- Acute pain related to specific disease processes or conditions and other pathologies leading to the different levels and types of pain (acute pain is pain of less than 3 months' duration)
- Persistent pain related to disease processes, conditions, or syndromes causing pain (pain is usually considered persistent if it occurs over more than 3 months—e.g., migraine headaches, rheumatoid arthritis)
- Risk for injury related to decreased sensorium or level of consciousness from analgesics with use of either non-narcotic or narcotic or opioid drugs
- Risk for injury related to possible overdosage and severe adverse reactions or drug interactions with the various classes of analgesics
- Impaired gas exchange related to possible respiratory depression secondary to CNS-depressive effects of narcotics or opioids
- Constipation related to the use of narcotics or opioid causing CNS depression and decreased peristalsis

- Risk for infection related to the adverse effect of urinary retention and subsequent urinary stasis from the use of narcotics or opioids
- Deficient knowledge related to lack of unfamiliarity with opioids, their use, and their adverse effects

Planning

Goals

- Patient will state measures that will enhance the effectiveness of the analgesic regimen.
- Patient will identify the rationale for use, therapeutic effects, and adverse effects associated with all types of analgesics.
- Patient will state measures to help minimize the occurrence of common adverse effects of non-narcotics as well as of narcotics and opioids.

Outcome Criteria

- Patient demonstrates increased comfort levels as seen by decreased use of analgesics, increased activity and performance of activities of daily living (ADLs), decreased complaints of pain, and decreased levels of pain as rated on a scale of 0 to 10.
- Patient experiences minimal adverse effects and complications such as nausea, vomiting, and constipation associated with the use of analgesics, especially narcotics and opioids.
- Patient uses nonpharmacological measures such as relaxation therapy, distraction, and music therapy to improve comfort and enhance any pharmacological regimens.
- Patient manages adverse effects associated with analgesics through fluid intake and possible antiemetic therapy when necessary.

Implementation

Once the cause of pain has been diagnosed, pain management should begin immediately and aggressively in conformity with each individual situation and the needs of each individual patient. Pain management is varied and multifaceted; it incorporates pharmacological and nonpharmacological approaches to pain relief (see Box 11-3 and Natural Health Products: Feverfew). Negotiate with patients by integrating religious ceremonies and traditional healing practices into pain care, rather than imposing Western cultural approaches. Pain management strategies should include an emphasis on the type of pain and its rating as well as pain quality, duration, precipitating factors, and interventions that help the pain. Some general principles of pain management include the following:

1. Management of mild to moderate pain often begins with the use of non-narcotic drugs such as acetaminophen, tramadol, and NSAIDs (Chapter 45) unless contraindicated.
2. Moderate to severe pain is generally not managed with non-narcotics but is usually treated with narcotics; such treatment requires a knowledge of the drugs used for acute versus persistent pain; drug action, adverse effects, and toxicity; and other drug- and patient-related information.
3. Drug selection for treatment of moderate to severe pain should be based on variables such as the characteristics of the individual patient, ethnocultural influences (see Ethnocultural Implications on p. 189), the disease process, and the use of other therapies such as homeopathic or folk remedies or natural health products.

Nonpharmacological measures for pain management should always be used, either as a beginning mode of treatment or as an adjuvant to pharmacological therapy, and include relaxation therapy, guided imagery, music

---

CASE STUDY

Opioid Administration

Ms. M.B. is 67 years of age and has recently undergone surgery, chemotherapy, and irradiation for breast cancer. She has been in pain after her therapy, for which she has been taking oxycodone/acetaminophen, which has 5 mg of oxycodone and 325 mg of acetaminophen per tablet. Ms. M.B. has been taking two tablets orally (PO) every 4 hours as needed for pain. She has also been taking MS Contin 200 mg SR every 12 hours but remains in pain. Oral thrush has also developed as a result of her chemotherapy and she can no longer tolerate swallowing. The oncology nurse recommends to the physician that Ms. M.B.'s oral medications need to be adjusted or even changed altogether. The physician wants to know her total daily dose of opioids so that the accurate conversion

to an equivalent dose of transdermal fentanyl may be made. Answer the following questions using the information provided in the chapter:

1. What is the patient's total daily dose of oxycodone and morphine?

2. What type of adverse effects and possible complications may occur with the patient taking both these medications, and what information can you share with the patient to help decrease these adverse effects?

3. What dose of transdermal fentanyl should this patient receive, and why?

For answers see http://evolve.elsevier.com/Lilley/pharmacology/.

distraction, exercise, transcutaneous electrical stimulation, and massage.

Nonopioid analgesics, such as acetaminophen, should be given as ordered or as indicated for fever or pain. Acetaminophen should be taken as prescribed by all patients, especially in children and the older adult. Patient teaching should emphasize taking the medication as indicated to avoid liver damage and acute toxicity. If a patient is taking other OTC medications with acetaminophen, the patient should read the labels carefully to identify other drug–drug interactions. The patient should also be taught the signs of acetaminophen overdose, which include bleeding, malaise, fever, sore throat, and easy bruising (because of hepatotoxicity). The nurse should also instruct the patient to report pain lasting longer than 3 days, because further evaluation by a health care provider is then indicated.

The wrapped suppository dosage forms of acetaminophen should be placed in a medicine cup of ice, and once the suppository is unwrapped, cold water should be run over it to moisten it for insertion into the rectum using a gloved finger and water-soluble lubricating gel if necessary. Tablets may be crushed if needed. Adult patients who take more than 2.6 g in 24 hours are at risk for mild liver damage; those taking 10 g or more (e.g., deliberate overdoses) are at high risk for severe liver damage, and death is possible after ingestion of more than 15 g. Liver damage from acetaminophen may be minimized by timely dosing with acetylcysteine (see p. 200). Should acetylcysteine be ordered, an important point to remember is that it has the flavour of rotten eggs and is better tolerated if it is disguised by mixing with a drink such as cola or flavoured water to increase its palatability. Use of a straw will help minimize contact with mucous membranes of the mouth and is recommended. This antidote may be given through a nasogastric or orogastric tube, if necessary.

Tramadol may cause nausea and vomiting. The patient should be offered cola or dry crackers to help relieve the nausea, as taking tramadol with food or a snack may help to decrease gastrointestinal upset. If dizziness,

BOX 11-3

Nonpharmacological Treatment Options for Pain

- Acupressure
- Acupuncture
- Art therapy
- Behavioural therapy
- Comfort measures
- Counselling
- Distraction
- Hot or cold packs
- Hypnosis
- Imagery
- Massage
- Meditation
- Music therapy
- Pet therapy
- Reduction of fear
- Relaxation
- Surgery
- Therapeutic baths
- Therapeutic communication
- Therapeutic touch
- Transcutaneous electric nerve stimulation
- Yoga

blurred vision, or drowsiness occurs, the nurse should be sure to assist the patient with ambulation (as with any analgesic that may lead to dizziness or lightheadedness). Educate the patient about injury prevention, such as the need to move and change positions slowly and to avoid any tasks that require mental clarity and alertness. The patient should be encouraged to report any heart palpitations, seizures, tremors, difficulty breathing, chest pain, or muscle weakness.

With use of narcotics (and other analgesics), the nurse should administer it as ordered after checking for the "rights" of medication administration (right drug, right

 NATURAL HEALTH PRODUCTS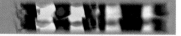

FEVERFEW *(Chrysanthemum parthenium)*

Overview
A member of the marigold family known for its anti-inflammatory properties

Common Uses
Treatment of migraine headaches, menstrual problems, arthritis, fever

Adverse Effects
Nausea and vomiting, anorexia, hypersensitivity reactions, muscle stiffness, muscle and joint pain

Potential Drug Interactions
Possible increase in bleeding with use of aspirin, dipyridamole, and warfarin

Contraindications
Contraindicated in those allergic to ragweed, chrysanthemums, and marigolds, and those about to undergo surgery

dose, right patient, right route, and right time) as with any medication. Documentation is stricter, however, with controlled substances such as opioids. Documents should be checked for the last time the medication was given before another dose is administered. The medication profile should always be double-checked against the original physician's order and signed with a full signature once the medication has been administered. The nurse should always return at the appropriate time (taking into consideration the onset and peak effect times of the drug and the route) and assess for effects of the drug on the pain and the presence of any adverse effects. When administering analgesics, whether pure, mixed, or partial, the nurse must always be sure to give the patient the medication before the pain becomes severe or when the pain is beginning to return, to provide adequate analgesia. It is recommended that oral forms of narcotics be used first, if ordered, and if there is no nausea or vomiting. Taking the dose with food may help minimize gastrointestinal upset. Antiemetic therapy may be needed if nausea and vomiting from the narcotic occurs or is present prior to dosing. Safety measures such as keeping the side rails up (if used in the facility), turning the bed safety alarm on, and making sure the call bell is within the patient's reach are all crucial measures to prevent falls stemming from the use of narcotics (or other analgesics) and from the adverse effects of these drugs, including confusion, hypotension, and decreased sensorium. The older adult is at higher risk for falls and adverse effects (see Box 11-1).

When managing pain with morphine, meperidine, and similar opioid drugs, the nurse should withhold the dose and contact the physician if there is any decline in the patient's condition or if vital signs are abnormal (see normal values given earlier), and especially if the respiratory rate is less than 12 breaths/min. Intramuscular injections should be used only if there is no other route available. Intramuscular injections of analgesics are rarely given because of the availability of newer dosage forms such as patient-controlled analgesic (PCA) pumps, transdermal patches, and constant subcutaneous or epidural infusions. For cancer patients, intramuscular injections may not be an option because of trauma at the site and possible thrombocytopenia and leucopenia with resulting bleeding or infection at the injection site.

For transdermal patches (e.g., transdermal fentanyl) two systems are used. The older type of patch contains a reservoir system consisting of four layers beginning with the adhesive layer and ending with the protective backing. Between these two layers are the permeable rate-controlling membrane and the reservoir layer, which holds the drug in a gel or liquid form. The newer patch has a matrix system consisting of two layers: one layer containing the active drug with the releasing and adhesive mechanisms and the other comprising the protective impermeable backing layer. The advantages of the matrix system over the reservoir system are that the patch is slimmer and smaller, thus more comfortable; it is worn for up to 7 days (the older reservoir system patch is worn for up to 3 to 4 days); and it appears to result in more constant serum drug levels. In addition, the matrix system is alcohol free; the alcohol in the reservoir system often irritates the patient's skin. It is important for the nurse to know what type of delivery system is being used in order to follow proper guidelines to enhance the system's and drug's effectiveness.

Transdermal patches can be applied to intact, nonirritated, and nonirradiated skin on a flat surface such as the chest, back, flank, or upper arm. Hair at the application site should be clipped (not shaved) prior to patch attachment. The patch should be changed as ordered and placed on a new site only after the old site has been cleansed of any residual medication using clear water. Do not use soaps, oils, lotions, alcohol, or any other agents that may irritate the skin or alter its characteristics. The skin must be dry before applying the patch. Rotation of sites helps decrease irritation and enhance drug effects. Transdermal systems are beneficial for delivery of many types of medications, especially analgesics, and have the benefits of allowing multiday therapy with a single application, avoiding first-pass metabolism, improving patient adherence, and minimizing frequent dosing. However, the patient should be watched carefully for the development of any type of contact dermatitis (the physician or health care provider should be contacted immediately if this occurs) and should maintain a pain journal when at home. Journal entries are a valid source of information for the nurse, other health care providers, the patient, and family members to assess the patient's pain control and to monitor the effectiveness of not only transdermal analgesia but also any medication regimen.

With the intravenous administration of narcotic agonists, the nurse should always follow the manufacturer's guidelines and institutional policies regarding specific dilutional amounts and solution as well as the time period for infusion. When PCA is used, the amounts and times of dosing should be noted in the appropriate records and tracked by appropriate personnel. The fact that a PCA pump is being used, however, does not mean that it is 100% reliable. To be sure that all is stable, the nurse should monitor pain levels, response to medication, and vital signs just as frequently as with other parenteral opioid administration. The nurse should follow dosage ranges for all opioid agonists and agonists–antagonists and pay special attention to the dosages of morphine and morphine-like drugs. For intravenous infusions, the nurse is responsible for monitoring the intravenous needle site and infusion rates and documenting any adverse effects or complications. Another point for the nurse to remember when administering narcotic and non-narcotic analgesics is that each medication has a different onset of action, peak, and duration of action. These differences apply to the route of administration as well; onset of action is immediate with intravenous administration (Table 11-10).

There are several important points to emphasize in discussing the use of opioids and related nursing

TABLE 11-10	

Opioid Administration Guidelines

Narcotic	Nursing Administration
buprenorphine and butorphanol	When giving IV, infuse over the recommended time (usually 3–5 min). Always assess respirations. Give IM butorphanol in deep gluteal muscle mass.
codeine	Give PO doses with food to minimize GI tract upset; there are analgesic ceiling effects with oral codeine.
fentanyl	Administer parenteral doses as ordered and per manufacturer's guidelines in regard to mg/min to prevent to prevent CNS depression and possible cardiac or respiratory arrest. Transdermal patches come in a variety of dosages. Be sure to remove residual amounts of the old patch prior to application of a new patch. Dispose of patches properly to avoid inadvertent contact with children or pets. Fentanyl may also soon be available in lozenge form for anaesthetic premedication for children and adults and an inhalation form is currently in trials for use in breakthrough pain. A fentanyl lollypop is also available in the United States but not in Canada.
hydromorphone	May be given IV, IM, rectally, or PO
meperidine	Given by a variety of routes: IV, IM, or PO; highly protein bound so watch for interactions and toxicity. Monitor the older adult for increased sensitivity.
morphine	Available in a variety of forms: SC, IM, IV, rectal, PO, extended, sustained, and immediate release, and for epidural infusion; morphine sulfate (Kadian) now available in a 200 mg sustained-release tab. Always monitor respiratory rate.
nalbuphine	IV dosages of 10 mg undiluted over 5 min
naloxone	Antagonist given for opioid overdose; 0.4 mg usually given IV over 15 sec or less. Reverses analgesia as well.
oxycodone	Often mixed with acetaminophen or aspirin; PO and dosage forms. It is now available in both immediate- and extended-release tabs.
pentazocine	PO, SC, IV, and IM forms; mixed agonist/antagonist; 5 mg IV to be given over 1 min
sufentanil	Epidural, IV form; used as adjunct to anaesthesia

CNS, central nervous system; *GI*, gastrointestinal; *IM*, intramuscular; *IV*, intravenous; *PO*, oral; *SC*, subcutaneous.

interventions, including watching for adverse effects. Urinary output and bowel status should be monitored. The patient should have a urinary output of at least 600 mL/24 hr and bowel movements of normal patterns and consistency for that patient—even if stool softeners must be ordered (see Box 11-1 for adverse effects related to persistent opioid use and related interventions). The patient's pupils should be monitored along with vital signs because pinpoint pupils may indicate overdosage. Naloxone should be kept available should respiratory depression or overdosage occur.

To reverse an opioid overdose or opioid-induced respiratory depression, an opioid antagonist such as naloxone must be administered. If naloxone is used, 0.4 to 2 mg should be given intravenously in its undiluted form and should be administered over 15 seconds (or as ordered); if reconstitution is needed, 0.9% NaCl or 5% dextrose injection should be used (see Table 11-7). However, the guidelines in the package insert should also be followed. Emergency resuscitative equipment should be nearby in the event of respiratory or cardiac arrest.

The nurse must remember when giving agonists–antagonists that they are effective analgesics when administered alone, but when they are given with other opioids or are given to a patient with long-term opioid use, their administration may lead to reversal of analgesia and acute withdrawal. If partial agonist drugs are given to a patient who is opioid naive and is not currently taking opioids in any form, the patient will experience effective analgesia, but analgesia reversal will occur with the co-administration of other opioids.

With opioid agonist–antagonist drugs the nurse must be careful always to check the dosages and routes as well as to perform the interventions mentioned previously. If a pure opioid is used with a mixed narcotic, the analgesic effects will be reversed; when a mixed narcotic is used alone, respirations and other vital signs must be monitored, just as with pure narcotic agonists. Patient education regarding mixed opiate agonists should emphasize the need for careful dosing to avoid CNS and respiratory depression and should include information on nonpharmacological measures to manage pain. Patients should report any dizziness, constipation, difficulty with urination, blurred vision, hallucinations, or tachycardia. The nurse should remember that opioid agonist–antagonist drugs act similarly to the pure opioids when given by themselves; however, when a partial agonist–antagonist is used with a pure opioid, there will be reversal of analgesia, thus the same nursing interventions apply. The nurse must be careful to always check the dosages and routes. Mixed narcotic agonists also have the potential for misuse and addiction. The nurse should remember that withdrawal symptoms could manifest in individuals who are opioid dependent.

Regardless of whether nonopioid, opioid, or combination drug therapy is used, it is always important to be up to date on all forms and protocols of pain management, whether for moderate to severe pain or for the management of cancer pain. The WHO's three-step analgesic ladder is often accepted as the standard for guiding the use of nonopioids and opioids and serves as a reminder for the stepped approach to pain management when this is appropriate. Dosing of medications for pain management is important to the treatment regimen. Once a thorough assessment has been performed, it is best to treat the patient's pain before it becomes severe—as noted earlier, pain needs to be added as the fifth vital sign. When pain is present, analgesic doses are best administered around the clock rather than as needed but always within dosage guidelines for each drug used. Round-the-clock (or scheduled) dosing maintains steady-state levels of the medication and prevents drug troughs and escalation of pain. No given dosage of an analgesic will provide the same level of pain relief for every patient, thus titration upward or even titration downward should be handled individually and should be implemented as long as the analgesic is needed. Aggressive titration may be necessary in difficult pain control cases and in cancer pain situations. Patients with severe pain, metastatic pain, or bone metastasis pain may need increasingly higher doses of analgesic, so an opiate such as morphine should be titrated until the desired response is achieved or until adverse effects occur. A patient-rated pain level of 4 out of 10 is considered to indicate effective pain relief. If pain is not managed adequately by monotherapy, other drugs or adjuvants may need to be added to enhance analgesic efficacy. This includes the use of NSAIDs (for analgesic, anti-inflammatory effects), acetaminophen (for analgesic effects), corticosteroids (for mood elevation and anti-inflammatory, antiemetic, and appetite stimulation effects), anticonvulsants (for treatment of neuropathic pain), tricyclic antidepressants (for treatment of neuropathic pain and for innate analgesic properties and opioid-potentiating effects), neuroleptics (for treatment of persistent pain syndromes), local anaesthetics (for treatment of neuropathic pain), hydroxyzine (for mild antianxiety properties as well as sedating effects and antihistamine and mild antiemetic actions), and psychostimulants (for reduction of opioid-induced sedation when opioid dosage adjustment is not effective). See Table 11-11 for a list of drugs that should not be used in patients experiencing cancer pain.

Dosage forms are also important, especially with persistent pain and cancer pain. Oral administration is always preferred but is not always tolerated by the patient and may not even be a viable option for pain control. If oral dosing is not appropriate, less invasive routes of administration include rectal and transdermal routes. Rectal dosage forms are safe, inexpensive, effective, and helpful if the patient is experiencing nausea or vomiting or altered mental status; this route would not be suitable for those with diarrhea, stomatitis, or low blood cell counts. Transdermal patches may provide up to 72 hours of pain control but are not for rapid dose titration and are used only when stable analgesia has been previously achieved. In fact, long-acting forms of morphine and fentanyl may be delivered via transdermal patches when a longer duration of action is needed. Intermittent injections or continuous infusions via the intravenous or subcutaneous routes are often used for opioid delivery and may be administered at home in special pain situations, such as in hospice care and in persistent cancer pain

TABLE 11-11

Drugs Not Recommended for Treatment of Cancer Pain

Class	Drug	Rationale for not Recommending
Antagonists	naloxone naltrexone	Reverses analgesia
Anxiolytics (as monotherapy) or sedatives–hypnotics (as monotherapy)	Benzodiazepines (e.g., alprazolam)	Analgesic properties not associated with these drugs except in some situations of neuropathic pain; common risk of sedation, which may put some patients at higher risk for neurological complications
	Barbiturates Benzodiazepines	Analgesic properties not demonstrated; sedation is problematic and limits use
Combination preparations	Brompton's cocktails	No evidence of analgesic benefit over use of single opioid analgesic
	DPT* (meperidine, promethazine, and chlorpromazine)	Efficacy poor compared with that of other analgesics; associated with a higher incidence of adverse effects
Miscellaneous	Cannabinoids	Adverse effects of dysphoria, drowsiness, hypotension, and bradycardia, which preclude its routine use as an analgesic; may be more appropriate for use in treating severe chemotherapy-induced nausea and vomiting
Opioid agonists–antagonists	pentazocine butorphanol nalbuphine	May precipitate withdrawal in opioid-dependent patients; analgesic ceiling effect; possible production of unpleasant psychological adverse effects, including dysphoria, delusions, and hallucinations
Opioids with dosing round the clock	meperidine	Short (2–3 hr) duration of analgesia; administration may lead to CNS toxicity (tremor, confusion, or seizures)
Partial agonist	buprenorphine	Analgesic ceiling effect; can precipitate withdrawal if given with a narcotic

*DPT is the abbreviation for the trade names Demerol, Phenergan, and Thorazine.

management. Subcutaneous infusions are often used when there is no intravenous access. Patient-controlled analgesia pumps may be used to help deliver opioids intravenously, subcutaneously, or even intraspinally and can be managed in home health care or hospice care for the patient at home. Use of the intrathecal or epidural route requires special skill and expertise, and delivery of pain medications using these routes is available only from certain home health care agencies for at-home care. The main reason for long-term intraspinal opioid administration is intractable pain. Transnasal dosage forms are approved only for butorphanol, an agonist–antagonist drug, and this dosage form is generally not used or recommended. Regardless of the specific drug or dosage form used, a fast-acting rescue drug should always be ordered for the patient with cancer pain and patients presenting other special challenges in pain management.

In summary, regardless of the drug(s) used for the pain management regimen, the nurse must always remember that individualization of treatment is one of the most important considerations for effective and quality pain control. The nurse should always do the following:

- At the initiation of pain therapy, conduct a review of all relevant histories, laboratory test values, and diagnostic study results in the patient's medical record.
- If there are underlying problems, be sure to consider them but do not forget to treat the patient. Do not let these problems overshadow the fact that there is a patient who is in pain.
- Always develop goals for pain management in conjunction with the patient and any family members or significant others.
- Collaborate with other members of the health care team to select a regimen that will be easy for the patient to follow while in the hospital and, if necessary, at home (e.g., with cancer patients and other patients experiencing persistent pain).
- Be aware that most regimens for acute pain include management with short-acting opioids plus the addition of other medications such as NSAIDs.
- Be familiar with equianalgesic doses of opioids, because lack of knowledge of equivalencies may lead to inadequate analgesia or overdose.
- Use an analgesic appropriate for the situation (e.g., short-acting opioids for severe pain secondary to a myocardial infarction, surgery, or kidney stones). For cancer pain, the regimen usually begins with short-acting opioids with eventual conversion to controlled-release formulations. Preventative measures should be used to manage adverse effects. In addition, a switch is made to another opioid as soon as possible if the patient finds that the medication is not controlling the pain adequately.

- Consider the option of using adjuvants to analgesia, especially for persistent pain or cancer pain. These might include other prescribed drugs such as corticosteroids, antidepressants, anticonvulsants, and muscle relaxants. OTC drugs, natural health products, and NSAIDs are also helpful.
- Be alert to patients with special needs, such as patients with breakthrough pain. Generally, the drug used is a short-acting form of the longer-acting opioid (e.g., immediate release for breakthrough pain while also using sustained-release morphine).
- Identify community resources for assistance to the patient and any family members or significant others. These resources may include Web-based sites such as http://www.canadianpainsociety.ca, http://www.WebMD.com, http://www.pain.com, http://www.persistentpaincanada.com, and http://www.mayohealth.org. Many other pain management sites may be found on the Internet by searching using the term pain or pain clinic.
- Because patient falls and the resulting injuries are common, when analgesics of any type—but especially opioids—are used, be sure to assess the patient's potential for falls. Take great care to prevent falls, whether by simply checking on the patient frequently after the patient has received analgesics, placing the patient on a frequent watch program, using bed alarms, or obtaining an order for restraints (but only in extreme circumstances).
- Restraints may cause many injuries; therefore, follow the appropriate procedures. Assess, monitor, evaluate, and document the reason for the restraint; also document the patient's behaviour, type of restraint, and the assessment of the patient after the placement of restraints. Use of restraints has been replaced in most facilities by a bed watch system and the use of bed and wheelchair alarms as well as by instruction of the patient and family members regarding alternatives to restraints. Restraints are not used in long-term care facilities.

For more specific information regarding patient teaching, see Patient Education.

Evaluation

Positive therapeutic outcomes of acetaminophen use are decreased symptomatology, fever, and pain. Adverse reactions for which the nurse should monitor include anemia and the previously mentioned liver problems with hepatotoxicity. In addition, abdominal pain and vomiting should be reported to the physician. During and after the administration of non-narcotic analgesics, tramadol, opioids, and mixed narcotic agonists, the nurse

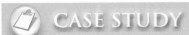

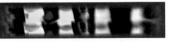

CASE STUDY

Pain Management for Terminal Illness

You are assigned to care for a patient who is in the terminal stage of breast cancer. As a community health care nurse, you have many responsibilities; however, you have not cared for many patients who are in the terminal stages of their illness. In fact, most of your patients are postoperative and have only required assessments, dressing changes, and wound care.

Ms. D. is 48 years of age and underwent bilateral mastectomy 4 years ago. She had lymph node involvement at the time of surgery, and recently metastasis to the bone has been diagnosed. She has been taking sustained-release oxycodone (one 10 mg tab every 12 hours) at home but is not sleeping through the night and is now complaining of increasing pain to the point that her quality of life has decreased significantly. She wants to stay at home during the terminal stage of her illness but needs to have adequate and safe pain control. Her husband of 18 years is supportive. They have no children. They are both university graduates and have medical insurance.

1. Ms. D's recent increase in pain has been attributed to bone metastasis in the area of the lumbar spine. At this time the oxycodone is not beneficial, and you need to advocate for Ms. D. to receive adequate pain relief. When discussing her pain medications with her physician, what type of medication would you expect to be ordered to relieve the bone pain, and what is the rationale for this recommendation? Provide references from within this chapter for the selection of the specific opioid drug.

2. Ms. D.'s husband confides in you that he is worried that she will become addicted to the new medication. He is not sure he agrees with round-the-clock dosing. How do you address his concerns?

3. What should Mr. D. do if he feels that Ms. D. has had an overdose?

For answers see http://evolve.elsevier.com/Lilley/pharmacology/.

---

should monitor the patient for both therapeutic effects and adverse effects. Therapeutic effects include decreased complaints of pain and increased periods of comfort, with improvements in performance of activities of daily living, appetite, and sense of well-being. Adverse effects vary with each drug but often consist of nausea, vomiting, constipation, dizziness, headache, blurred vision, decreased urinary output, drowsiness, lethargy, sedation, palpitations, bradycardia, bradypnea, dyspnea, and hypotension. Should vital signs change, the patient's condition decline, or pain continue, the physician should be contacted immediately and the patient closely monitored. Respiratory depression may be manifested by a rate of less than 12 breaths/min, dyspnea, diminished breath sounds, or shallow breathing.

Although many patients benefit from the administration of prescribed opioids alone, additional medications or complementary therapies may be needed to help enhance comfort. During the evaluation process, the nurse should evaluate multimodal approaches to pain management such as relaxation, imagery, art therapy, pet therapy, massage, acupuncture, and music therapy. The nurse should evaluate the effectiveness of pain management by determining the degree, duration, and nature of pain experienced with drug therapy and by evaluating and reassessing for any new or different complaints of pain.

IN MY FAMILY

Clove Oil
(as told by H.I., from Somalia)

"Clove is grown on the island of Zanzibar in Tanzania, Africa. . . . Clove oil is a natural analgesic and antiseptic and is used to relieve pain in various locations of the body. Its first use is to treat pain from arthritis and muscle aches. . . . Its second use includes using it as a remedy for pain from toothaches. Clove oil specifically decreases infection due to its antiseptic–antibacterial properties. The oil is applied directly to the site of pain in the mouth. . . . The idea for the use of clove oil as a pain reliever came from the Middle East. Somalia is greatly influenced by the Middle Eastern countries through culture, religion, and dress."

PATIENT EDUCATION

- ❖ Patients should be informed of the adverse effects of analgesics: GI tract upset, constipation, drowsiness, dizziness, headache, sleepiness, tinnitus (ringing in the ears), blurred vision, palpitations, bradycardia, and hypotension.
- ❖ Patients should be encouraged to report any wheezing or difficulty breathing; itching, rash, or hives; low blood pressure; excessive sleepiness (sedation); or CNS changes such as weakness, dizziness, fainting, confusion, or loss of memory to their health care providers.
- ❖ Patients taking an opioid drug should be instructed to ambulate and perform activities of daily living with caution. If experiencing any drowsiness or sedation, activities requiring mental clarity or alertness should be avoided.
- ❖ Patients should be instructed that opioids should not be used with alcohol or other CNS depressants because of worsening of CNS-depressant effects.
- ❖ Patients should be instructed to change positions slowly to prevent possible orthostatic hypotension.
- ❖ Patients should be encouraged to report any nausea or vomiting because these are adverse effects of opioids that may be prevented with the appropriate dosing of medications with food or use of antiemetics.
- ❖ Patients should be encouraged to drink fluids at up to 3 L/day, unless contraindicated, and increase of fibre and bulk consumption and exercise as tolerated is recommended to prevent problems with constipation.
- ❖ Patients should be encouraged to share any history of addiction with health care providers. But when such a patient experiences pain and is in need of opioid analgesia, the nurse must understand that the patient has a right to comfort. Any further issues with addiction may be managed during and after use of opioids. Keeping an open mind regarding the use of resources, counselling, and other treatment options is important in dealing with addictive behaviours.
- ❖ Patients should be made to understand that if pain is problematic and is not managed by monotherapy, then a combination of a variety of medications may be needed. It is not uncommon to see use of opioids, nonopioids, antianxiety drugs, sedatives or hypnotics, and NSAIDs. Most importantly, however, the patient must remain in communication with the physician or health care provider about alternative and combination drug therapy options.
- ❖ Patients or their caregiver(s) must be instructed to carefully read the directions on all prescription containers as well as on any OTC medications for possible contraindications or drug interactions.
- ❖ Patients should be informed that a holistic approach to pain management may be appropriate, with the use of complementary modalities. Some complementary and alternative therapies include biofeedback, imagery, relaxation, deep breathing, humour, pet therapy, music therapy, massage, use of hot or cold compresses, and use of natural health products including herbal products.
- ❖ Patients should be informed that most hospitals have inpatient and outpatient resources such as pain clinics. Many hospitals have pain management teams. Patients should seek out these options and remain active in their own care for as long as possible.
- ❖ Cancer patients should be informed that the health care provider will monitor pain control and the need for other options for therapy or dosing of drugs. For example, the use of transdermal patches, buccal tablets, and continuous infusions while the patient remains mobile or at home is often helpful in pain management. It is also important to understand that if morphine or morphine-like drugs are being used, the addictive potential is present; however, in specific situations, the concern for quality of life and pain management is more important than the concern for addiction.
- ❖ Patients should be informed that should bone pain become moderate to severe with cancer patients, the physician may order NSAIDs or other anti-inflammatory drugs.
- ❖ Patients should be informed that tolerance does occur with opioid use, so if the level of pain increases while the patient remains on the prescribed dosage, the patient should contact the physician or health care provider for assistance. The patient should never change dosages of or double up on medication of any type.
- ❖ Patients should be informed that narcotic agonists–antagonists work well as analgesics when given by themselves. Use with a pure narcotic agonist would lead to reversal of analgesia. CNS depression is also experienced.

POINTS TO REMEMBER

❖ Pain is individual and involves senses and emotions. It is influenced by age, ethnoculture, race, spirituality, and all other aspects of the person.

❖ Pain is associated with actual or potential tissue damage and may be exacerbated or alleviated depending on the treatment and type of pain.

❖ Types of analgesics are as follows:
  • Nonopioids including acetaminophen and aspirin and other NSAIDs
  • Opioids, which are natural or synthetic drugs that either contain or are derived from morphine (opiates) or have opiate-like effects or activities (opioids); pure opioid agonists and partial opioid agonist–antagonist drugs are available.

❖ Special-populations considerations are an important aspect in medication administration. A few examples are as follows:
  • Child dosages of morphine should be calculated cautiously with close attention to the dose and kilograms of body weight.
  • The older adult generally tolerates morphine well but seem less tolerant of other opioids such as meperidine.
  • In treating the older adult, the nurse should remember that these patients experience pain the same as the general population does, but they may be reluctant to report pain. They metabolize opiates at a slower rate and thus are at increased risk for adverse effects such as sedation and respiratory depression. The best rule is to start with low dosages, re-evaluate often, and go slowly during upward titration.

EXAMINATION REVIEW QUESTIONS

1 When treating severe pain associated with pathological spinal fractures related to metastatic bone cancer, which type of pain medication dosage schedule should be used for best results?
  a. As needed
  b. Round the clock
  c. On schedule during waking hours only
  d. Round the clock, with additional doses as needed for breakthrough pain

2 A patient is receiving an opioid via a PCA pump as part of his postoperative pain management program. During rounds, the nurse notices that his respirations are 8 breaths/min and he is extremely lethargic. After stopping the opioid infusion, what should the nurse do next?
  a. Notify the charge nurse
  b. Administer oxygen
  c. Administer an opiate antagonist per standing orders
  d. Perform a thorough assessment, including mental status examination

3 Which of the following is a benefit of using transdermal fentanyl patches in the management of bone pain from metastatic cancer?

  a. More analgesia for longer time periods
  b. Less constipation and minimal dry mouth
  c. Greater CNS stimulation than with oral narcotics
  d. Lower dependency potential and no major adverse effects

4 The nurse suspects that a patient is showing signs of respiratory depression. Which of the following drugs could be the cause of this complication?
  a. naloxone
  b. hydromorphone (Dilaudid)
  c. acetaminophen (Tylenol)
  d. naltrexone (ReVia)

5 Several patients have standard prn orders for acetaminophen as needed for pain. When the nurse reviews their histories and assessments, it is discovered that one of the patients has a contraindication to acetaminophen therapy. Which of the following patients should receive an alternate medication?
  a. A patient who has a fever of 39.7°C
  b. A patient admitted with severe hepatitis
  c. A patient admitted with a deep vein thrombosis
  d. A patient who had abdominal surgery 1 week earlier

For answers see http://evolve.elsevier.com/Canada/Lilley/pharmacology/.

CRITICAL THINKING ACTIVITIES

1 The nurse administers 5 mg morphine sulfate IV to a patient with severe postoperative pain, as ordered. What assessment data should be gathered before and after the administration of this drug? Explain your answer.

2 The patient complains that the drugs he is receiving for severe pain are not really helping. What would be the most appropriate response to this patient?

3 Compare the effectiveness of the following routes of opioid administration, including their ease of self-preparation and administration, onset of therapeutic serum concentrations, degree of sedation, adverse effects, and ease of management in the home setting: oral, intramuscular, transdermal.

For answers see http://evolve.elsevier.com/Canada/Lilley/pharmacology/.

General and Local Anaesthetics

Learning Objectives

After reading this chapter, the successful student will be able to do the following:

1 Define anaesthesia.

2 Discuss the basic differences between general and local anaesthesia.

3 List the most commonly used general and local anaesthetics and their associated risks.

4 Discuss the differences between depolarizing neuromuscular blocking drugs and nondepolarizing blocking drugs.

5 Compare the mechanisms of action, indications, adverse effects, routes of administration, cautions, contraindications, and drug interactions of general anaesthesia and local anaesthesia, and for drugs used for moderate or conscious sedation.

6 Develop a collaborative plan of care for patients before anaesthesia (preanaesthesia), during anaesthesia, and after anaesthesia (postanaesthesia) as related to general anaesthesia.

7 Develop a collaborative plan of care for patients undergoing local anaesthesia or moderate or conscious sedation.

e-Learning Activities

Web site
(http://evolve.elsevier.com/Canada/Lilley/
pharmacology/)

- Animations
- Answers to chapter questions, activities, and case studies
- Calculators and Category Catchers
- Glossary with audio pronunciations
- IV Therapy and Medication Error Checklists
- Multiple-Choice Review Question quizzes
- Nursing Care Plans
- Online Appendices and Supplements
- WebLinks

Drug Profiles

halothane, p. 221
isoflurane, p. 221
▸▸ lidocaine (lidocaine hydrochloride)*, p. 224
nitrous oxide, p. 221
pancuronium (pancuronium bromide)*, p. 228
▸▸ propofol, p. 221
▸▸ rocuronium (rocuronium bromide)*, p. 228
sevoflurane, p. 221
▸▸ succinylcholine, p. 228
▸▸ vecuronium, p. 228

▸▸ Key drug.

*Full generic name is given in parentheses. For the purposes of this text, the more common shortened name is used.

Glossary

Adjunctive anaesthetic drugs Drugs used in combination with anaesthetic drugs to control the adverse effects of anaesthetics or to help maintain the anaesthetic state in the patient. (See *balanced anaesthesia*) (p. 218)

Anaesthesia Loss of the ability to feel pain, resulting from the administration of an anaesthetic drug or other medical intervention. (p. 217)

Anaesthetics Drugs that depress the central nervous system (CNS) to produce diminution of consciousness, loss of responsiveness to sensory stimulation, or muscle relaxation. (p. 217)

Balanced anaesthesia The practice of using combinations of drugs rather than a single drug to produce anaesthesia. A common combination is a mixture of a sedative–hypnotic, an antianxiety drug, an analgesic, an antiemetic, and an anticholinergic. (p. 218)

General anaesthesia A drug-induced state in which the CNS is altered to produce varying degrees of pain relief thoughout the body as well as depression of consciousness, skeletal muscle relaxation, and diminished or absent reflexes. (p. 217)

General anaesthetic A drug that induces a state of anaesthesia. Its effects are global in that it involves the whole body, with loss of consciousness being one of those effects. (p. 217)

Local anaesthetics Drugs that render a specific portion of the body insensitive to pain at the level of the peripheral nervous system, normally without affecting consciousness; also called *regional anaesthetics.* (p. 220)

Malignant hyperthermia A genetically linked major adverse reaction to general anaesthesia, characterized by a rapid rise in body temperature, as well as tachycardia, tachypnea, and sweating. (p. 226)

Minimum alveolar concentration The minimal concentration of the gas in the lungs that is needed to provide anaesthesia in 50% of subjects. (p. 219)

Moderate sedation A form of anaesthesia induced by combinations of parenteral benzodiazepines and an opiate; also called *conscious sedation.* (p. 229)

Overton-Meyer theory A theory that describes the relationship between the lipid solubility of anaesthetic drugs and their potency. (p. 219)

Parenteral anaesthetics Any anaesthetic drugs that can be administered by injection via any route (e.g., intravenously, spinally/epidurally) as a local nerve block. (p. 220)

Topical anaesthetics A class of local anaesthetics consisting of solutions, ointments, gels, creams, powders, ophthalmic drops, and suppositories that are applied directly to the skin and mucous membranes. (p. 220)

OVERVIEW

Anaesthetics are drugs that depress the central nervous system (CNS), the peripheral nervous system (PNS), or both, which, in turn, produces depression of consciousness, loss of responsiveness to sensory stimulation (including pain), or muscle relaxation. This state of depressed CNS or PNS activity is called **anaesthesia.** There are many mechanisms by which anaesthetics accomplish these responses, but in general they do so by interfering with nerve conduction. They can produce any or all of the actions just mentioned, depending on the drug. Anaesthetics are most commonly classified as either general anaesthetics or local anaesthetics, depending on where in the CNS or PNS the particular anaesthetic drug works. Functions of the autonomic nervous system, which is a branch of the PNS, may also be affected.

GENERAL ANAESTHETICS

A **general anaesthetic** is a drug that induces a state in which the CNS is altered so that varying degrees of pain relief, depression of consciousness, skeletal muscle relaxation, and reflex reduction are produced. This condition is known as **general anaesthesia.** General anaesthesia can be achieved by the use of one drug or a combination of drugs. Often a combination of drugs is used to produce general anaesthesia, which allows less of each drug to be used and a more balanced, controlled state of anaesthesia to be achieved. General anaesthetic drugs are used most commonly to produce deep muscle relaxation and loss of consciousness during surgical procedures. For a historical perspective on general anaesthesia, see Box 12-1.

There are two main categories of general anaesthetics based on their route of administration: inhaled and injectable. Inhaled anaesthetics are volatile liquids or gases that are vaporized in oxygen and inhaled to induce anaesthesia. Injectable anaesthetics are administered intravenously. The different inhaled gases and volatile liquids used as general anaesthetics are listed in Table 12-1.

Intravenously administered anaesthetic drugs are used for induction or maintenance of general anaesthesia, induction of amnesia, and as an adjunct to

BOX 12-1 General Anaesthesia: A Historical Perspective

Until recently, general anaesthesia was described as having several definitive stages. This was especially true of the use of many of the ether-based inhaled anaesthetic drugs. Features of these distinctive stages were easily observable to the trained eye. They included specific physical and physiological changes that progressed gradually and predictably with the depth of the patient's anaesthetized state. Gradual changes in pupil size, progression from thoracic to diaphragmatic breathing, vital-sign changes, and several other changes all characterized the various stages. Newer inhalational and intravenous general anaesthetic drugs, however, often have a much

more rapid onset of action and body distribution. As a result, the stages of anaesthesia once observed with older drugs are no longer sufficiently well defined to be observable. Thus the concept of stages of anaesthesia is an outdated one in most modern surgical facilities.

Registered nurses who pursue advanced training to become a certified registered nurse anaesthetist often find this to be a rewarding and interesting area of nursing practice. Some nurses also find that this type of work offers greater flexibility in their work schedule than do other practice areas.

TABLE 12-1

Inhaled General Anaesthetic Drugs

Generic Name	Trade Name
INHALED GAS	
nitrous oxide ("laughing gas")	
INHALED VOLATILE LIQUID	
desflurane	Suprame
halothane	Halothane
isoflurane	Forane
sevoflurane	Sevorane VF

TABLE 12-2

Intravenous Anaesthetic Drugs

Generic Name	Trade Name	Dosage
ketamine	Ketalar	1–4.5 mg/kg IV; 6.5–13 mg/kg IM
▶▶ propofol*	Diprivan	2–2.5 mg/kg IV (induction); 0.1–0.2 mg/kg/min IV (maintenance)
thiopental	Pentothal	25–280 mg IV as needed

IV, intravenous; *IM*, intramuscular.

*Dosages for propofol are typically 5–50 mg/kg/min for initiation and maintenance of sedation in the critical care unit.

inhalation-type anaesthetics. Common intravenous anaesthetic drugs include the following:

- General anaesthetics, such as etomidate and propofol
- Sedatives–hypnotics, such as barbiturates (e.g., etomidate) and benzodiazepines (e.g., diazepam, midazolam)
- Narcotics (e.g., morphine sulfate, fentanyl, sufentanil, propofol)
- Neuromuscular blocking agents (NMBAs), both depolarizing (e.g., succinylcholine) and nondepolarizing, or competitive (e.g., pancuronium, vecuronium)

The term for the practice of using such combinations of drugs is **balanced anaesthesia,** which is the administration of minimal doses of multiple anaesthetic drugs to achieve the desired level of anaesthesia for the given surgical procedure. Other than the inhaled drugs, almost all of the drugs used in balanced anaesthesia are administered intravenously. Although propofol is an example of a true general anaesthetic in the sense that it is used not only to induce but also to maintain the state of anaesthesia, most of the other drugs previously mentioned serve a

more limited function, such as anaesthesia induction, sedation, amnesia, and reduction of anxiety. These drugs are commonly called **adjunctive anaesthetic drugs** because they are administered in addition to a general anaesthetic drug. Common adverse effects include dry mouth, bradycardia, nausea, and vomiting. The combining of several different drugs makes it possible for general anaesthesia to be accomplished using smaller amounts of anaesthetic gases, which reduces the adverse effects.

General anaesthetics and their usual dosages are presented in Table 12-2. Table 12-3 lists the adjunctive anaesthetic drugs. These drugs are discussed in greater detail in chapters covering the respective classes of drugs.

Mechanism of Action and Drug Effects

Many theories have been proposed to explain the actual mechanism of action of general anaesthetics. The drugs vary widely in their chemical structures, thus their mechanisms of action are not easily explained by a

TABLE 12-3

Adjunctive Anaesthetic Drugs

Drug	Pharmacological Class	Usual Dosage Range	Indications
alfentanil (Alfenta)	Opioid analgesic	Initial loading dose: 5–75 mcg/kg IV (increments as needed)	Anaesthesia induction
fentanyl		0.5–100 mcg/kg IV	
remifentanil (Ultiva)		0.05–2 mcg/kg IV	
sufentanil		25–50 mcg/kg IV	
diazepam	Benzodiazepine	2–20 mg PO/IV/IM	Amnesia and anxiety reduction
lorazepam		0.05–0.35 mg/kg IV	
midazolam		0.1–0.6 mg IV/IV/SC	
atropine	Anticholinergic	0.02–0.6 mg/kg IV/IM/SC	Drying up of excessive secretions
glycopyrrolate		0.005 mg/kg IM	
scopolamine		**Children:** 0.006 mg/kg IV/IM/SC	
		Adults: 0.3–0.6 mg IV/IM/SC	
meperidine (Demerol)	Opioid analgesic	50–100 mg IM/SC	Pain prevention and pain relief
morphine		5–20 mg IM/SC	
promethazine	Sedative–hypnotic	25–50 IV/IM	Amnesia and sedation

IM, intramuscular; *IV*, intravenous; *PO*, oral; *SC*, subcutaneous.

structure–receptor relationship. The concentrations of anaesthetics required to produce a given state of anaesthesia also differ greatly. The **Overton-Meyer theory** explains some of the properties of anaesthetic drugs that may make the mechanism of action of these drugs easier to understand. This theory implies that there is a relationship between the lipid solubility of an anaesthetic drug and its potency: the greater the solubility of the drug in fat, the greater is the effect. Nerve cell membranes have a high lipid content, as does the blood–brain barrier. Anaesthetic drugs can therefore easily cross this blood–brain barrier and concentrate in nerve cell membranes. Initially this produces a loss of the senses of sight, touch, taste, smell, and hearing and a loss of awareness, and usually the patient becomes unconscious. Although the heart and lungs (the vital organs responsible for blood pressure and breathing) are controlled by the medulla, they can usually be spared because the medullary centre is depressed last during anaesthetic procedures.

The overall effect of general anaesthetics is an orderly and systematic reduction of sensory and motor CNS functions. They produce a progressive depression of cerebral and spinal cord functions. Therapeutic (anaesthetic) doses cause minimal depression of the medullary centres that govern vital functions. However, an anaesthetic overdose paralyzes the medullary centres. This can lead to death from circulatory and respiratory failure. The progressive paralysis of nervous system functions produced by general anaesthetics and the level of decreased CNS functioning depend on the anaesthetic used and the dosage and route of administration. The reactions of the CNS (and other systems) to these general anaesthetics are presented in Table 12-4. The previously distinct and identifiable stages of anaesthesia now exist more on a continuum with the newer-generation anaesthetics discussed in this chapter. This is especially the case with the now standardized use of balanced anaesthesia and moderate sedation. Therefore, rather than structuring patient assessment in terms of the older concept of stages of anaesthesia, the nurse should focus on each of the drug types used, including their characteristics, actions, and adverse effects, and toxicities.

The **minimum alveolar concentration (MAC)** measures the anaesthetic potency of volatile anaesthetics. This value represents the minimum amount of alveolar air concentration of an inhaled anaesthetic that is required to prevent movement in 50% of the patients in response to pain. By knowing the MAC, the anaesthesiologist will know how much anaesthetic must be in the inspired air to produce anaesthesia. Generally, the alveolar concentration of the gas equals the blood concentration and, a short time later, equals the brain concentration so it can indicate anaesthetic potency. MAC is age dependent; it is lowest in newborns, peaks in infants, and then decreases progressively with increasing age. MAC values for inhaled anaesthetic are additive; the addition of nitrous oxide (the MAC of nitrous oxide is high) will decrease the MAC of another volatile anaesthetic. The MAC can also be altered following administration of other drugs such as opioids and lithium.

Indications

General anaesthetics are used to produce unconsciousness, skeletal muscular relaxation, and visceral smooth muscle relaxation for surgical procedures.

Contraindications

Contraindications to the use of anaesthetic drugs include known drug allergy and, depending on the drug type, may include pregnancy, narrow-angle glaucoma, and known susceptibility to malignant hyperthermia from prior experience with anaesthetics.

Adverse Effects

The adverse effects of general anaesthetics are dose dependent and vary with the individual drug. The heart, peripheral circulation, liver, kidneys, and respiratory tract are the sites primarily affected. Myocardial depression is a common adverse effect. All of the halogenated anaesthetics are capable of causing hepatotoxicity.

With the development and use of newer drugs, many of the unwanted adverse effects characteristic of the older drugs (such as hepatotoxicity and myocardial depression) are now in the past. In addition, many of the

TABLE 12-4

Effects of Inhaled and Intravenous General Anaesthetics

Organ/System	Reaction
Cardiovascular	Depressed myocardium; hypotension and tachycardia; bradycardia in response to vagal stimulation
Central nervous system	CNS depression; blurred vision; nystagmus; progression of CNS depression to decreased alertness and sensorium as well as decreased level of consciousness
Cerebrovascular	Increased intracranial blood volume and increased intracranial pressure
Cutaneous circulation	Vasodilation
Gastrointestinal	Reduced liver blood flow and thus reduced liver clearance
Renal	Decreased glomerular filtration
Respiratory	Depressed muscles and patterns of respiration; altered gas exchange and impaired oxygenation; depressed airway-protective mechanisms; airway irritation and possible laryngospasms
Skeletal muscles	Skeletal muscle relaxation

bothersome adverse effects such as nausea, vomiting, and confusion have become less common since balanced anaesthesia has become more widely used. This practice prevents many of the unwanted, dose-dependent adverse effects and toxicity associated with the anaesthetic drugs while also achieving a more balanced general anaesthesia. One medication with a long history of use for prevention or control of postoperative nausea and vomiting is droperidol. Its common dosage range is 0.625 to 1.25 mg intravenously or intramuscularly every 4 to 6 hours as needed. Substance misuse (e.g., alcohol) can also predispose a patient to anaesthetic-induced complications (e.g., liver toxicity). A positive determination of substance misuse during the anaesthetist's history-taking interview may lead to dosage adjustments in one or more of the drugs used. The anaesthetist may reduce drug dosages in cases of known liver or kidney damage, regardless of whether it is a consequence of substance misuse or not. However, a substance-misusing patient with a high tolerance for street drugs may also require larger doses of anaesthesia-related drugs (e.g., benzodiazepines) to achieve the desired sedative effects. Again, the anaesthetist makes these decisions based on the best knowledge of each patient's social history.

Toxicity and Management of Overdose

In large doses all anaesthetics are potentially life threatening, with cardiac and respiratory arrest as the ultimate causes of death. However, these drugs are almost exclusively administered in a controlled environment by personnel trained in advanced cardiac life support. These drugs are also quickly metabolized. In addition, the medullary centre, which governs the vital centres, is the last area of the brain to be affected by anaesthetics and the first to regain function if it is lost. These factors combined make an anaesthetic overdose rare and easily reversible. Symptomatic and supportive therapy, primarily of circulatory and respiratory functions, is usually all that is needed in the event of an anaesthetic overdose.

Interactions

Because general anaesthetics produce both desired and adverse effects on so many body systems, they are associated with a wide array of drug interactions that also vary widely in severity. Some of the more common drug–drug interactions occur with antihypertensives, β-blockers, and tetracycline. These drugs have additive effects when given with general anaesthetics. When given with antihypertensives, general anaesthetics may lead to increased hypotensive effects; with β-blockers, to increased myocardial depression; and with tetracycline, to increased kidney toxicity. No significant laboratory test interactions have been reported.

Dosages

For the recommended dosages of selected general anaesthetic drugs, see the Dosages table below.

LOCAL ANAESTHETICS

Local anaesthetics are the second class of anaesthetics. They are also called *regional anaesthetics* because they render a specific portion of the body insensitive to pain without major reduction of CNS function and level of consciousness. They do this by interfering with nerve transmission in specific areas of the body, blocking nerve conduction only in the area in which they are applied without causing loss of consciousness. They are most commonly used in those clinical settings in which loss of consciousness, whole body muscle relaxation, and loss of responsiveness are either undesirable or unnecessary (e.g., during childbirth). Other uses for local anaesthetics include dental procedures, the suturing of skin lacerations, spinal anaesthesia, and diagnostic procedures such as lumbar puncture or thoracentesis.

Most local anaesthetic belong to one of two major groups of organic compounds, esters or amides, and are classified as either topical or parenteral (injectable) anaesthetics. **Topical anaesthetics** are applied directly to the skin and mucous membranes. They are available in the form of solutions, ointments, gels, creams, or powders, and their dosage strengths are listed in Table 12-5. **Parenteral anaesthetics** can be administered intravenously or by spinal injection techniques. Depending on the specific site of injection, the drug may anaesthetize all or parts of the central or peripheral nervous system or both. The injection of certain anaesthetic drugs into the area near the spinal cord is known as spinal anaesthesia. This type of anaesthesia is generally used to block all peripheral nerves that branch out below a selected level of the spinal cord. The result is temporary skeletal and smooth muscle paralysis and anaesthesia within the anatomical areas of the body that are ultimately innervated by these nerve tracts lying between this

DOSAGES Selected General Anaesthetic Drugs			
Drug	Pharmacological Class	Usual Dosage Range	Indications
halothane	Inhalation general anaesthetic (halogenated hydrocarbon)	0.5%–1.5% concentration	General anaesthesia
isoflurane (Forane)	Inhalation general anaesthetic (enflurane isomer)	0.1%–2% concentration with appropriate drugs	General anaesthesia
nitrous oxide ("laughing gas")	Inorganic inhalation general anaesthetic	20%–40% with oxygen (e.g., 70% with 30% oxygen)	Analgesia Anaesthesia

DRUG PROFILES

All of the drugs used for general anaesthesia are, of course, prescription-only drugs. Desflurane, sevoflurane, halothane, and isoflurane are all volatile liquids; nitrous oxide is a gas. The dose of each drug depends on the surgical procedure to be performed and the physical characteristics of the patient. All of the general anaesthetics have a rapid onset of action, and action is maintained for the duration of the surgical procedure by continuous administration of the drug. Propofol is chemically unrelated to the other intravenous anaesthetic drugs. Its favourable pharmacokinetics and the quick onset of anaesthesia and quick recovery associated with it have popularized its use.

halothane

Halothane is a halogenated hydrocarbon (containing three atoms of fluorine and one each of chlorine and bromine) that is commonly used with nitrous oxide. It was a mainstay of general anaesthesia for many years and is still on the Canadian market. However, it causes considerable cardiac sensitivity to catecholamines and produces poor muscular relaxation when used alone, and its high halogen content can result in significant liver toxicity. Because of these limitations and toxicities, halothane is now less commonly used than the newer, less toxic inhalational anaesthetics. Dosage information is given in the Dosages table on p. 220.

isoflurane

Isoflurane (Forane) has a more rapid onset of action, causes less cardiovascular depression, and overall has been associated with little or no toxicity. Dosage information is given in the Dosages table on p. 220.

nitrous oxide

Nitrous oxide, also known as "laughing gas," is the only inhaled gas currently used as a general anaesthetic. It is the weakest of the general anaesthetic drugs and is primarily used for dental procedures or as a useful supplement to other more potent anaesthetics. Dosage information is given in the Dosages table on p. 220.

▶▶ propofol

Propofol (Diprivan) is an intravenous general anaesthetic drug used for the induction and maintenance of anaesthesia or sedation in the critical care unit (CCU) and other critical care settings. Propofol has many favourable characteristics that have led to its widespread use. It produces its effects rapidly, and when its delivery is halted, its effects subside quickly. Propofol also is typically well tolerated, producing few undesirable effects. Propofol can be used to induce and maintain monitored anaesthesia care sedation during diagnostic procedures in adults. It is also used in intubated, mechanically ventilated adult patients in the CCU to provide continuous sedation and control of stress responses. When used in the CCU, typical doses are 5 to 50 mg/kg/min. At higher doses it can be used for induction and maintenance of general anaesthesia. Dosage information is provided in Table 12-2 on p. 218.

sevoflurane

Sevoflurane (Sevorane AF) is another fluorinated ether that is becoming more widely used in Canada following several years of successful use in Japan. Its rapid onset and recovery pharmacokinetics make it especially useful in outpatient surgery settings. It is nonirritating to the airway, which greatly facilitates induction of an unconscious state, especially in children.

selected spinal cord location and the affected organs and tissues. Because spinal anaesthesia does not normally depress the CNS in a way that causes loss of consciousness, spinal anaesthesia can be thought of as a large-scale type of local rather than general anaesthesia. Some of the common types of local anaesthesia are described in Box 12-2. The parenteral anaesthetic drugs and their pharmacokinetics are summarized in Table 12-6.

TABLE 12-5

Topical Anaesthetics

Drug	Route	Dosage Strength
benzocaine (Comfortcaine, Dermoplast, Lanacane, Solarcaine)	Topical, aerosol, and spray	0.5%–20% ointment or cream
butamben (Cetacaine)	Topical	2% solution or spray
cocaine	Topical	4%–10% solution
dibucaine (Nupercanal)	Topical	0.5%–1% ointment or cream
dyclonine (Cepacol Sore Throat Spray, Sucrets)	Topical	0.1% spray, lozenges
lidocaine (Lidodan, Lidomax 5)	Topical	Jelly, ointment, cream, spray
pramoxine (Dermoplast)	Topical	1% jelly, cream, lotion
prilocaine/lidocaine (EMLA)	Topical	2.5% prilocaine and 2.5% lidocaine cream, patch
tetracaine (Pontocaine)	Injection, topical, and ophthalmic	0.5%–2% solution, gel, ointment, or cream

BOX 12-2 — Types of Local Anaesthesia

Central

Spinal or intraspinal anaesthesia: Anaesthetic drugs are injected into the area near the spinal cord within the vertebral column. Intraspinal anaesthesia is commonly accomplished by one of two injection techniques: intrathecal or epidural.

- Intrathecal anaesthesia involves injection of anaesthetic into the subarachnoid space. Intrathecal anaesthesia is commonly used for patients undergoing major abdominal or limb surgery for whom the risks of general anaesthesia are too high or for patients who prefer this technique over complete loss of consciousness during their surgical procedure. More recently, intrathecal injection of anaesthetics through implantable drug pumps is being used on an outpatient basis in patients with severe persistent pain syndromes, such as those resulting from occupational injuries.
- Epidural anaesthesia involves injection of the anaesthetic via a small catheter into the epidural space without puncturing the dura. Epidural anaesthesia is commonly used to reduce maternal discomfort during labour and delivery and to manage postoperative acute pain after major abdominal or pelvic surgery. This route

is becoming more popular for the administration of opioids for pain management.

Peripheral

Infiltration: Small amounts of anaesthetic solution are injected into the tissue that surrounds the operative site. This approach to anaesthesia is commonly used for procedures such as wound suturing and dental surgery. Often drugs that cause constriction of local blood vessels (e.g., epinephrine, cocaine) are also administered to limit the site of action to the local area.

Nerve block: Anaesthetic solution is injected at the site where a nerve innervates a specific area such as tissue. This allows large amounts of the anaesthetic drug to be delivered to a very specific area without affecting the whole body. This method is often reserved for more difficult-to-treat pain syndromes such as cancer pain and chronic orthopedic pain.

Topical anaesthesia: The anaesthetic drug is applied directly onto the surface of the skin, eye, or any other mucous membrane to relieve pain or prevent it from being sensed. It is commonly used for diagnostic eye examinations and skin suturing.

Intraspinal anaesthesia is accomplished by the insertion of a needle into the subarachnoid space to achieve intrathecal dose administration. The subarachnoid space surrounds the spinal cord and is filled with cerebrospinal fluid that continually bathes the spinal cord. The dura mater membrane separates the epidural space from the subarachnoid space. The epidural space is filled with a network of nerve extensions. Analgesic and anaesthetic drugs are injected into the epidural space into the twelfth thoracic vertebral space, or through the first lumbar space in the vertebral column. If the needle is aimed at the subarachnoid space it is termed *intrathecal administration*. Distinguishing between these terms and understanding the spinal column and spinal nerves is very important for the nurse. If the epidural space is the desired site of administration, the needle must stop before penetrating the dura; otherwise, it will enter into the subarachnoid space and free-flowing cerebrospinal fluid may be aspirated. Some of the medications that

may be used for intraspinal anaesthesia and analgesia include morphine, hydromorphone (Dilaudid), fentanyl, and meperidine (Demerol).

Finally, anaesthesia of specific areas of the peripheral nervous system is accomplished either by injecting the drugs adjacent to major nerves (to produce anaesthesia in a large body area) or by infiltrating the area with multiple small injections (for a more limited area of anaesthesia). Like spinal anaesthesia, this type of anaesthesia is also a local (rather than a general) type of anaesthesia, but unlike spinal anaesthesia, it is focused on a much smaller ("local") region of the body (e.g., hand, part of face, teeth, skin wound). For this reason, it is what is usually meant by the term *local anaesthesia*. Some of the common types of local anaesthesia are described in Box 12-2. Yet another option is the injection or topical application of a local anaesthetic (e.g., lidocaine) near the most distal peripheral nerves at a surgical site (e.g., eye, mucous membrane) as needed to further enhance patient comfort.

TABLE 12-6

Parenteral Anaesthetic Drugs*

Generic Name	Trade Name	Potency	Onset	Duration	Dose
lidocaine		Moderate	Immediate	60–90 min	0.4%–4% injection
mepivacaine	Carbocaine, Isocaine	Moderate		120–150 min	1%, 2%, 3% injection
procaine	Novocain	Lowest	2–5 min	30–60 min	2% injection
tetracaine	Pontocaine	Highest	5–10 min	90–120 min	0.5% injection

*Other common parenteral anaesthetic drugs include bupivacaine (Marcaine, Sensorcaine), chloroprocaine (Nesacaine), and ropivacaine (Naropin).

Mechanism of Action and Drug Effects

Local anaesthetics work by rendering a specific portion of the body insensitive to pain by interfering with nerve transmission in that area. Nerve conduction is blocked only in the area in which the anaesthetic is applied, and there is no loss of consciousness. Local anaesthetics block both the generation and conduction of impulses through all types of nerve fibres (sensory, motor, and autonomic) by blocking the movement of certain ions (sodium, potassium, and calcium) important to this process. They do this by making it more difficult for these ions to move in and out of the nerve fibre. For this reason, some of these drugs are also described as *membrane stabilizing* because they alter the cell membrane of the nerve so that the free movement of ions is inhibited. The membrane-stabilizing effects occur first in the small fibres, then in the large fibres. In terms of paralysis, usually autonomic activity is affected first, then pain and other sensory functions are lost. Motor activity is the last to be lost. When the effects of the local anaesthetic wear off, recovery occurs in reverse order: motor activity returns first, then sensory functions, and finally autonomic activity.

Possible systemic effects of the administration of local anaesthetics include effects on circulatory and respiratory functions. The systemic adverse effects depend on where and how the drug is administered (e.g., injection at a certain level in the spinal cord or topical application of a drug that gains access to the circulation). Such adverse effects are somewhat unlikely, unless large quantities of a drug are injected, which increases the likelihood of significant systemic absorption. Local anaesthetics produce sympathetic blockade: that is, they block the action of the two neurotransmitters of the sympathetic nervous system, norepinephrine and epinephrine. The cardiac effects of such a sympathetic blockade include a decrease in stroke volume, cardiac output, and peripheral resistance. The respiratory effects include reduced respiratory function and altered breathing patterns, but complete paralysis of respiratory function is unlikely because of the large amount of drug that would have to be absorbed. Some local anaesthetics used for either infiltration or nerve block anaesthesia are combined with vasoconstrictors such as epinephrine, phenylephrine, and norepinephrine to help confine the local anaesthetic to the injected area and prevent systemic absorption.

Indications

Local anaesthetics are used for surgical, dental, or diagnostic procedures, as well as for the treatment of certain types of persistent pain. They are administered by two techniques: infiltration anaesthesia and nerve block anaesthesia. *Infiltration anaesthesia* is commonly used for minor surgical and dental procedures. It involves the injection of the local anaesthetic solution by intradermal, subcutaneous, or submucosal routes and across the path of nerves supplying the area to be anaesthetized. The local anaesthetic may be administered in a circular pattern around the operative field. *Nerve block anaesthesia* is used for surgical, dental, and diagnostic procedures and for the therapeutic management of persistent pain. It involves injection of the local anaesthetic directly into or around the nerve trunks or nerve ganglia that supply the area to be numbed.

Contraindications

Contraindications of local anaesthetics include known drug allergy. Only specially designed dosage forms are intended for ophthalmic use.

Adverse Effects

The adverse effects of the local anaesthetics are limited and of little clinical importance in most circumstances. The undesirable effects usually occur with high plasma concentrations of the drug, which result from inadvertent intravascular injection, an excessive dose or rate of injection, slow metabolic breakdown, or injection into highly vascular tissue. When a local anaesthetic is absorbed into the circulation, it may lead to adverse reactions similar to those produced by general anaesthetics. One particular complication of spinal anaesthesia is "spinal headache," which occurs in varying numbers of patients. Spinal headache is most often self-limiting with bed rest and conventional analgesic medications. However, severe cases may be treated by the anaesthetist injecting a small volume (roughly 15 mL) of a venous blood sample from the same patient into the patient's epidural space. The exact mechanism of this "epidural blood patch" is unknown, but it has shown efficacy against spinal headache in over 90% of cases.

True allergic reactions to local anaesthetics are rare. However, allergic reactions can occur. They may appear as skin lesions, urticaria, or edema, or they may be acutely anaphylactic. These rare allergic reactions are generally limited to a particular chemical class of anaesthetics called the *ester type*. Box 12-3 separates the local anaesthetic drugs into these two chemical families. Different enzymes are responsible for the breakdown of these two groups of anaesthetics in the body. Anaesthetics belonging to the ester family are metabolized by cholinesterase in the plasma and liver. They are converted into a para-aminobenzoic acid (PABA) compound. This compound is

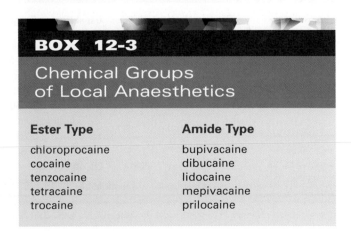

BOX 12-3

Chemical Groups of Local Anaesthetics

Ester Type	Amide Type
chloroprocaine	bupivacaine
cocaine	dibucaine
tenzocaine	lidocaine
tetracaine	mepivacaine
trocaine	prilocaine

mainly responsible for the allergic reactions. The amide type of anaesthetics is metabolized in the liver by other enzymes to active and inactive metabolites. Often when an individual has an undesirable experience after the administration of one of the local anaesthetics, changing from one chemical class to another helps to decrease the chance of future problems.

Toxicity and Management of Overdose

Local anaesthetics have little opportunity to cause toxicity under most circumstances. As mentioned, however, they can become just as toxic as general anaesthetics if they are systemically absorbed. To prevent this from occurring, a vasoconstrictor such as epinephrine is often coadministered with the local anaesthetic at its site of action. Another reason for the lower incidence of toxic effects with local anaesthetics is that doses are, on average, much smaller than those of general anaesthetics. This property of epinephrine also serves to reduce local

blood loss during minor surgical procedures. If for some reason significant amounts of the locally administered anaesthetic are absorbed systemically, cardiovascular and respiratory function may be compromised. Symptomatic and supportive therapy is usually all that is needed to reverse the toxic effects stemming from systemic absorption of the drug until it is eventually metabolized by the body.

Interactions

Few clinically significant drug interactions occur with the local anaesthetics. Some of the more important drug–drug interactions are seen with bupivacaine and chloroprocaine. When given with enflurane, halothane, or epinephrine, they can lead to dysrhythmias.

Dosages

For the recommended dosages of local anaesthetic drugs, see the Dosages table below.

DRUG PROFILES

Besides lidocaine, profiled here, local anaesthetics include bupivacaine, chloroprocaine, mepivacaine, prilocaine, procaine, and tetracaine. As noted earlier, there are two major types of local anaesthetics as determined by their chemical structure: amides and esters. These designations refer to the type of linkage between the aromatic ring and the amino group of the drug, two of the structural components that make an anaesthetic an anaesthetic. Lidocaine belongs to the amide class of local anaesthetics. Some patients may report that they have allergic or anaphylactic reactions to "caines," as they may refer to lidocaine and the other amide drugs. In these situations, it may be wise to try a local anaesthetic of the amide type.

 lidocaine hydrochloride

Lidocaine hydrochloride (Xylocaine) is one of the most commonly used local anaesthetics. It is available in

several strengths, both alone and in different concentrations with epinephrine, and is used for both infiltration and nerve block anaesthesia. The epinephrine reduces blood loss from minor surgical procedures because of its vasoconstrictive properties, and it reduces systemic absorption of lidocaine for the same reason. Lidocaine is also available in combination with prilocaine as a 2.5% patch (the EMLA patch) used in children for relief from the pain of vaccinations. A mixture consisting of lidocaine 1% and methylprednisolone acetate 40 mg/mL is also available for soft-tissue injection to manage localized musculoskeletal pain. Lidocaine is contraindicated in those who have a hypersensitivity to it. It is classified as pregnancy category B. Commonly recommended dosages are listed in the Dosages table below.

DOSAGES Local Anaesthetic

Drug	Pharmacological Class	Usual Dosage Range	Indications
▸▸lidocaine hydrochloride (Xylocaine)	Amide local anaesthetic	1%, 2% solution: 5–200 mg	Percutaneous infiltration
		1% solution: 200–300 mg	Caudal obstetric analgesia, thoracic nerve block
		1% solution: 100 mg each side	Paracervical obstetric analgesia
		1% solution: 50–100 mg	Sympathetic lumbar nerve block
		1% solution: 30–50 mg	Paravertebral nerve block
		1% solution: 30 mg	Intercostal nerve block
		1% solution: 50 mg	Sympathetic cervical nerve block
		2% solution: 225–300 mg	Brachial nerve block, caudal surgical anaesthesia
		2% solution: 20–100 mg	Dental procedures
		2% solution: 200–300 mg	Lumbar anaesthesia

NEUROMUSCULAR BLOCKING DRUGS

Neuromuscular blocking drugs or agents (NMBAs) prevent nerve transmission in certain muscles, leading to paralysis of the muscles. They are often used with anaesthetics for surgical procedures. Use of NMBAs requires mechanical ventilation, as these drugs paralyze the respiratory and skeletal muscles. The patient is rendered unable to breathe independently. The drugs do not cause sedation or relieve pain; therefore, the health care provider should assume that the paralyzed patient is in pain and anxious and should take steps to relieve this with analgesics and anxiolytics.

Snakes and plants played a large role in the identification of the chemical structure of substances that cause paralysis and in the discovery of the related receptor. The beginning steps in identification of the receptor involved study of the seemingly irreversible inhibition of nerve transmission in muscles by venoms of krait snake species (e.g., *Bungarus multicinctus*) and the venoms of certain varieties of cobra (e.g., *Naja naja* or king cobra). Once the receptor at which these venoms work was identified, pharmacological drugs that would mimic the venoms and produce paralysis were developed.

Curare, a nondepolarizing NMBA, has a long and romantic history. It has been used for centuries by natives of South America along the Amazon and Orinoco rivers and in other parts of that continent for killing wild animals for food. Animals shot with arrows soaked in this plant substance normally die from paralysis of the respiratory muscles. Curare is actually a generic term for South American arrow poisons. The most potent of all curare alkaloids are the toxiferines, obtained from *Strychnos toxifera*. The seeds of the trees and shrubs of the genus *Erythrina*, widely distributed in tropical and subtropical areas, also contain substances with curare-like activity.

NMBAs are traditionally classified as *depolarizing* or *nondepolarizing* drugs. Succinylcholine is now the only commonly used depolarizing NMBA. Nondepolarizing NMBAs prevent acetylcholine (ACh) from acting at neuromuscular junctions. Consequently, the nerve cell membrane is not depolarized, the muscle fibres are not stimulated, and skeletal muscle contraction does not occur. Nondepolarizing NMBAs are typically classified into three groups based on their duration of action: short-, intermediate-, and long-acting drugs (Table 12-7).

Mechanism of Action and Drugs Effects

The original prototypical depolarizing NMBA was d-tubocurarine, the active ingredient of curare. It is a naturally occurring plant alkaloid that causes skeletal muscle relaxation or paralysis. It is no longer available on the Canadian market, however, and has been replaced by newer synthetic drugs. Succinylcholine, a synthetic drug, works similarly to the neurotransmitter ACh. Succinylcholine is metabolized much more slowly than ACh. Because of this slower metabolism, succinylcholine combines with cholinergic receptors at the motor endplate of muscle nerves to produce ongoing depolarization and muscle contraction. Repolarization and further muscle contraction are then inhibited. As long as sufficient succinylcholine concentrations are present, the muscle is unable to contract, and a flaccid muscle paralysis results. This muscle paralysis is sometimes preceded by muscle spasms, which may damage muscles. These muscle spasms are termed *muscle fasciculations* and are most pronounced in the muscle groups of the hands, feet, and face. Injury to muscle cells may cause postoperative muscle pain and release potassium into the circulation. Small doses of nondepolarizing NMBAs are sometimes administered with succinylcholine to minimize these muscle fasciculations. This reduces the muscle pain caused by depolarizing drugs such as succinylcholine. Nondepolarizing NMBAs prevent ACh from acting at neuromuscular junctions. They behave as antagonists, blocking ACh from binding to the postsynaptic receptors. Consequently, the nerve cell membrane is not depolarized, the muscle fibres are not stimulated, and skeletal muscle contraction does not occur.

If hyperkalemia develops, it is usually mild and insignificant. Rarely, cardiac dysrhythmias or even cardiac arrest has occurred. Succinylcholine is normally deactivated by plasma cholinesterase. This enzyme breaks down succinylcholine, freeing up the receptor site and allowing repolarization of the motor endplate. The duration of action of succinylcholine after a single intubating dose is about 5 to 9 minutes because of the rapid breakdown of the drug by this enzyme.

Anticholinesterase drugs, such as neostigmine, pyridostigmine, and edrophonium, are antidotes and are used to reverse muscle paralysis. They work by preventing the enzyme cholinesterase from breaking down ACh. This causes ACh to build up at the muscle endplate, and it eventually displaces the nondepolarizing NMBA molecule, returning the nerve to its original state.

To summarize the drug effects of the NMBAs, the first sensation that is typically felt is muscle weakness. This is usually followed by a total flaccid paralysis. Small, rapidly moving muscles such as those of the fingers

TABLE	12-7

Classification of Neuromuscular Blocking Drugs

Drug	Structure
INTERMEDIATE-ACTING	
atracurium (Nimbex)	Benzylisoquinolinium
rocuronium (Zemeron)	Steroid
veruronium	Steroid
LONG-ACTING	
pancuronium	Steroid

Currently no short-acting drugs are available in Canada.

and eyes are typically the first to be paralyzed. The next are those of the limbs, neck, and trunk. Finally, the intercostal muscles and the diaphragm are paralyzed. Respirations stop as a result; the patient can no longer breathe independently. Recovery of muscular activity after discontinuation of anaesthesia usually occurs in the reverse order to the initiation of paralysis during anaesthesia induction, and thus the diaphragm is ordinarily the first to regain function. Before causing paralysis, depolarizing drugs such as succinylcholine often evoke transient muscular fasciculations. For this reason, when succinylcholine is administered, muscle soreness may occur when the patient wakes up from anaesthesia. One general anaesthetic drug that helps alleviate this common but undesirable effect is the newer inhalational drug sevoflurane. CNS effects are usually minimal because of the chemical structure of most of the nondepolarizing drugs. They are quaternary ammonium compounds and are not able to penetrate the blood–brain barrier. The effects on the cardiovascular system vary depending on the NMBA used and the individual patient. Increases and decreases in blood pressure and heart rate have been seen. Some NMBAs cause a release of histamine, which can result in bronchospasm, hypotension, and excessive bronchial and salivary secretion. The gastrointestinal tract is seldom affected by NMBAs. When it is affected, decreased tone and motility typically result, which can lead to constipation or even ileus.

Indications

The main therapeutic use of NMBAs is for maintaining controlled ventilation during surgical procedures. When respiratory muscles are paralyzed by an NMBA, mechanical ventilation is easier because the body's desire to control respirations is eliminated by the NMBA; this allows the ventilator to have total control of respirations.

Because NMBAs reduce muscle contractions, they are also helpful when the muscle tissue itself is part of the surgical site in an area that needs surgery. Short-acting NMBAs are often used to facilitate intubation with an endotracheal tube. This is commonly done to facilitate a variety of diagnostic procedures such as laryngoscopy, bronchoscopy, and esophagoscopy. When used for this purpose, NMBAs are often combined with anxiolytics or anaesthetics. Additional nonsurgical applications include reduction of laryngeal or general muscle spasms, reduction of spasticity from tetanus and neurological diseases such as multiple sclerosis, and prevention of bone fractures during electroconvulsive therapy. These drugs are also used for the diagnosis of myasthenia gravis.

Contraindications

Contraindications to NMBAs include known drug allergy and also may include previous history of malignant hyperthermia, penetrating eye injuries, and narrow-angle glaucoma.

Adverse Effects

The key to limiting adverse effects with most NMBAs is to use only enough of the drug to block the neuromuscular receptors. If too much is used, the risk is increased that other ganglionic receptors will be affected. Blockade of these other ganglionic receptors leads to most of the undesirable effects of NMBAs. The effects of ganglionic blockade in various areas of the body are listed in Table 12-8.

Nondepolarizing NMBAs have relatively few adverse effects when used appropriately. Their cardiovascular effects include blockade of autonomic ganglia, resulting in hypotension; blockade of muscarinic receptors, resulting in tachycardia; and release of histamine, resulting in hypotension. Use of the depolarizing drug succinylcholine has been associated with hyperkalemia; dysrhythmias; fasciculations; muscle pain; myoglobinuria; and increased intraocular, intragastric, and intracranial pressure, as well as malignant hyperthermia. **Malignant hyperthermia** (MH) is an uncommon, genetically linked adverse metabolic reaction to general anaesthesia that includes a rapid rise in body temperature, tachycardia, tachypnea, and muscular rigidity. Patients known statistically to be at greater risk for MH include children, adolescents, and those with such musculoskeletal abnormalities as hernias, strabismus, ptosis, scoliosis, and muscular dystrophy. MH is treated with cardiorespiratory supportive care as needed to stabilize heart and lung function (e.g., β-blockers to slow heart rate, supplemental oxygen to reduce respiratory intensity), as well as with the skeletal muscle relaxant dantrolene (see Chapter 13).

Toxicity and Management of Overdose

The primary concern when NMBAs are overdosed is prolonged paralysis requiring prolonged mechanical ventilation (see Preventing Medication Errors: Neuromuscular Blocking Drugs). Cardiovascular collapse may also be seen and is thought to be the result of histamine release. Multiple medical conditions can predispose an

TABLE 12-8

Effects of Ganglionic Blockade by Neuromuscular Blocking Drugs

Site	Part of Nervous System Blocked	Physiological Effect
Arterioles	Sympathetic	Vasodilation and hypotension
Veins	Sympathetic	Dilation
Gastrointestinal tract	Parasympathetic	Reduced tone and motility; constipation
Heart	Parasympathetic	Tachycardia
Salivary glands	Parasympathetic	Dry mouth
Urinary bladder	Parasympathetic	Urinary retention

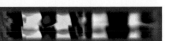

 PREVENTING MEDICATION ERRORS

Neuromuscular Blocking Drugs

Neuromuscular blocking drugs are considered high-alert drugs because improper use may lead to severe injury or death. The Institute for Safe Medication Practice–Canada has published several examples of patient death or injury as a result of medication errors involving neuromuscular blocking drugs. Because these drugs paralyze the respiratory muscles, incorrect administration without sufficient ventilator support has resulted in patient deaths. Medication errors have also occurred because of "sound-alike" drug names (e.g., vancomycin and vecuronium). Most facilities have followed recommendations to restrict access to these drugs, provide warning labels and reminders, and increase staff awareness of the dangers of neuromuscular blocking drugs.

For more information, visit http://www.ismp-canada.org/download/ISMPCSB2004-07.pdf.

---

individual to toxicity, increasing the sensitivity of the individual to NMBAs and prolonging their effects. These predisposing conditions are listed in Box 12-4. Some conditions make it more difficult for NMBAs to work and thus require higher doses of NMBAs. Although these conditions do not result in toxicity or overdose, they are worthy of mention and are listed in Box 12-5.

Interactions

Many drugs can interact with NMBAs, which can lead to either synergistic or opposing effects. Some antibiotics, when given concomitantly with an NMBA, can have additive effects. The aminoglycoside antibiotics are a common example. They produce neuromuscular blockade by inhibiting ACh release from the preganglionic terminal. The tetracycline antibiotics can also produce neuromuscular blockade, possibly by chelation of calcium, and calcium channel blockers have been shown to enhance neuromuscular blockade. Some of the more notable drugs that interact with NMBAs are listed in Box 12-6.

Dosages

For the recommended dosages of selected neuromuscular blocking drugs, see the Dosages table on p. 229.

BOX 12-4

Conditions That Predispose Patients to Toxic Effects from Neuromuscular Blocking Drugs

Acidosis
Amyotrophic lateral sclerosis
Hypermagnesemia
Hypocalcemia
Hypokalemia
Hypothermia
Myasthenia gravis
Myasthenic syndrome
Neonatal status
Neurofibromatosis
Paraplegia
Poliomyelitis

BOX 12-5

Conditions That Oppose the Effects of Neuromuscular Blocking Drugs

Cirrhosis with ascites
Clostridial infections
Hemiplegia
Hypercalcemia
Hyperkalemia
Peripheral nerve transection
Peripheral neuropathies
Thermal burns

BOX 12-6

Drugs That Interact with Neuromuscular Blocking Drugs

Additive Effects	Opposing Effects
Aminoglycosides	carbamazepine
Calcium channel blockers	Corticosteroids
clindamycin	phenytoin
cyclophosphamide	
cyclosporine	
dantrolene	
furosemide	
Inhalation anaesthetics	
Local anaesthetics	
magnesium	
polymyxin	
procainamide	
quinidine	

DRUG PROFILES

NMBAs are one of the most commonly used classes of drugs in the operating room. They are given primarily with general anaesthetics to facilitate endotracheal intubation and to relax skeletal muscles during surgery. In addition to their use in the operating room, NMBAs commonly are administered in the CCU to paralyze mechanically ventilated patients. As noted earlier, the two basic types of NMBAs are depolarizing and nondepolarizing drugs. The only depolarizing drug is succinylcholine. Nondepolarizing drugs can be classified in a variety of ways but are typically classified by their chemical structure or their duration of action. Table 12-8 lists some nondepolarizing drugs currently in use.

DEPOLARIZING NEUROMUSCULAR BLOCKING DRUGS

As mentioned previously, succinylcholine is the only drug in this subclass of NMBAs. Succinylcholine has a structure similar to that of the parasympathetic neurotransmitter ACh. It stimulates the same neurons as ACh and produces the same physiological responses initially. Unlike ACh, succinylcholine is metabolized slowly. Because of this slower metabolism, succinylcholine subjects the motor endplate to ongoing depolarizing stimulation. Repolarization cannot occur. As long as sufficient succinylcholine concentrations are present, the muscle loses its ability to contract, and flaccid muscle paralysis results. Because of its quick onset of action, succinylcholine is most commonly used to facilitate endotracheal intubation. It is seldom used over long periods because of the unwanted effects that develop with continuous infusions.

▸▸ succinylcholine

Succinylcholine (Quelicin) is the only currently available depolarizing NMBA. It is an ultra–short-acting, depolarizing skeletal muscle relaxant for intravenous administration and is used primarily during procedures of short duration such as endoscopic examinations. Succinylcholine is used as an adjunct to general anaesthesia to facilitate tracheal intubation and to provide skeletal muscle relaxation during surgery or mechanical ventilation or endoscopic examinations. It is contraindicated in patients with personal or familial history of malignant hyperthermia, skeletal muscle myopathies, and known hypersensitivity to the drug. It is available as 20 mg/mL and 100 mg/mL solutions and is classified as pregnancy category C. The recommended dosage is given in the Dosages table on p. 229.

PHARMACOKINETICS

Half-Life	Onset	Peak	Duration
Seconds	Rapid, <1 min	Rapid	4–6 min

NONDEPOLARIZING NEUROMUSCULAR BLOCKING DRUGS

Nondepolarizing NMBAs are commonly used to facilitate endotracheal intubation, reduce muscle contraction in an area that needs surgery, and facilitate a variety of diagnostic procedures. They are often combined with anxiolytics or anaesthetics. They may also be used to induce respiratory arrest in patients on mechanical ventilation.

pancuronium bromide

Pancuronium bromide is a long-acting nondepolarizing NMBA. It is used as an adjunct to general anaesthesia to facilitate tracheal intubation and to provide skeletal muscle relaxation during surgery or mechanical ventilation. It is most commonly employed for long surgical procedures that require prolonged muscle paralysis. Use of pancuronium is contraindicated in patients with known hypersensitivity to the drug. It is available as 1 g/mL and 2 mg/mL solutions. It is classified as pregnancy category C. The recommended dosage is given in the Dosages table on p. 229.

PHARMACOKINETICS

Half-Life	Onset	Peak	Duration
80–120 min	3–5 min	Rapid	60–100 min

▸▸ rocuronium bromide

Rocuronium bromide (Zemeron), a newer nondepolarizing muscle relaxant (NDMR), is an intermediate-acting nondepolarizing NMBA. It has a rapid to intermediate onset of action, depending on the dosage. It is indicated as an adjunct to general anaesthesia to facilitate both routine tracheal intubation and *rapid-sequence intubation (RSI)* and to provide skeletal muscle relaxation during surgery or mechanical ventilation. RSI is used in patients requiring emergency surgery. In order to rapidly intubate the larynx, a high degree of muscle relaxation is required. This is achieved using rocuronium. Rocuronium is one of the most commonly used NMBAs. Rocuronium is contraindicated in patients with known hypersensitivity to it. It is available as a 10 mg/mL soultion, and it is calssified as pregnancy category C. The recommended dosage is given in the Dosages table on p. 229.

PHARMACOKINETICS

Half-Life	Onset	Peak	Duration
14–18 min	1–3 min	2.5 min	25–40 min

▸▸ vecuronium

Vecuronium (Norcuron) is an intermediate-acting nondepolarizing NMBA. It is used as an adjunct to general anaesthesia to facilitate tracheal intubation and to provide skeletal muscle relaxation during surgery or mechanical ventilation and is one of the most commonly used NMBAs. Long-term use in the CCU setting has resulted in prolonged paralysis and consequent difficulty weaning from mechanical ventilation. This result is thought to stem from an active metabolite, 3-desacetyl vecuronium, which tends to accumulate with prolonged use. Use of vecuronium is contraindicated in patients with known hypersensitivity to the drug. It is available as 10-mL and 20-mL solutions, and it is classified as pregnancy category C. The recommended dosage is given in the Dosages table on p. 229.

PHARMACOKINETICS

Half-Life	Onset	Peak	Duration
65–75 min	2.5–3 min	3–5 min	25–40 min

DOSAGES Selected Neuromuscular Blocking Drugs

Drug	Pharmacological Class	Usual Dosage Range	Indications
pancuronium bromide	Nondepolarizing NMBA (long acting)	*Children* IV: 0.02 mg/kg *Adult* IV: 0.04–0.1 mg/kg Continuous infusion: 0.1 mg/kg/hr	Intubation Mechanical ventilation
▸▸rocuronium bromide (Zemeron)	Nondepolarizing NMBA (intermediate acting)	*Children* IV: 0.6 mg/kg *Adult* IV: 0.6–1.2 mg/kg Continuous infusion: 0.01–0.012 mg/kg/ min; 0.1 mg/kg/hr	Intubation Mechanical ventilation
▸▸succinylcholine (Quelicin)	Depolarizing NMBA (short acting)	*Children* IV: 1–2 mg/kg IM: 2.5–4 mg/kg *Adult* IV: 0.3–1.1 mg/kg over 10–30 sec IM: 2.5–4 mg/kg	Intubation Mechanical ventilation
▸▸vecuronium (Norcuron)	Nondepolarizing NMBA (intermediate acting)	*Children* IV: 0.08–0.1 mg/kg *Adult* IV: 0.08–0.1 mg/kg Continuous infusion: 0.1 mg/kg/hr	Intubation Mechanical ventilation

MODERATE SEDATION

Many types of procedures, including diagnostic and minor surgical procedures, do not require as great a depth of anaesthesia as do more extensive procedures. **Moderate sedation**, conscious sedation, and procedural sedation are terms that all mean the same thing, namely, an anaesthesia that does not lead to loss of consciousness. This technique uses combinations of several drugs that may be classified differently. For example, one or more benzodiazepines may be used with one or several narcotic agonists or opioids. Drugs may be given by intravenous, intramuscular, or spinal routes. The net effect is a type of anaesthesia that allows the patient to remain conscious, respond verbally to commands, relax, and maintain an open airway. Mild amnesia related to the procedure may occur. All types of moderate sedation have a more rapid recovery time than that of general anaesthesia and a better safety profile because of lower cardiorespiratory risks.

In children, moderate sedation may be accomplished using an oral syrup form of midazolam, with or without concurrent use of injected medications such as opiates. This technique can be especially helpful for children who must undergo uncomfortable procedures such as wound suturing or diagnostic procedures requiring reduced movement such as computed tomography and magnetic resonance imaging. See Special Populations: Children: Moderate or Conscious Anaesthesia for other considerations regarding this type of anaesthesia.

PHARMACOKINETIC BRIDGE TO NURSING PRACTICE

With moderate (conscious or procedural) sedation or anaesthesia, it is always important to understand the pharmacokinetic properties of the drugs used. For example, the intravenous form of diazepam has an onset of action of 1 to 5 minutes, peak effect time of 15 minutes, duration of action of 15 to 60 minutes, and half-life of 20 to 70 hours. (Half-life is the time it takes for 50% of the drug to be excreted from the body.) Therefore, if diazepam is used for sedation or anaesthesia, the drug could be present in the body and cause effects for up to 70 hours. In the care of patients receiving drugs for anaesthesia (whether for conscious or moderate anaesthesia, or general or local anaesthesia), these drug profile properties help the nurse to predict the drugs' onset of action, peak effect, and duration of action.

NURSING PROCESS

▨ Assessment

Associated with each drug used in general and local anaesthesia are some broad assessment parameters and some specific ones. First, for general anaesthesia, once assessment for any drug or food allergies has been

SPECIAL POPULATIONS: CHILDREN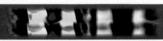

Moderate or Conscious Anaesthesia

The American Academy of Pediatrics (no Canadian-specific guidelines exist to date) recommends that moderate or conscious sedation (anaesthesia) be used to reduce anxiety, pain, and fear in children. The use of moderate anaesthesia in children allows a procedure to be performed restraint-free in most situations while keeping the patient responsive.

Child dosing often conforms to the following guidelines:

- Hydromorphone—child dosing is at 0.015 to 0.02 mg/kg.

- Fentanyl—child dosing may be 0.5 to 1 mcg/kg with increments over 3 minutes to a maximum of three doses. Too rapid intravenous (IV) injection may result in chest rigidity, which may need to be treated with muscle relaxants and possibly mechanical ventilation. Fentanyl is used often for short procedures.

- Meperidine—child dosing is at 0.5 to 1 mg/kg over 2 minutes.

- Morphine—child dosing may be at 0.05 to 0.1 mg/kg IV over a 2-minute period and is ideal for long procedures or cases in which pain is anticipated after the procedure.

Discharge status of the child depends on the type of drugs and drug combinations used. Discharge after conscious or moderate sedation is based mainly on whether the following criteria are met:

- Patient is alert and oriented compared with the baseline neurological assessment.

- Protective swallowing and gag reflexes are intact.

- Vital signs are stable and consistent with baseline values for at least 30 minutes after the last dosing. Different health care facilities set different criteria that must be met and documented (blood pressure and pulse rate within normal limits or within 20 points of baseline, temperature lower than 38.3°C).

- Oxygen saturation is at least 95% on room air 30 minutes after the last dose.

- Pain rating is at baseline levels or less.

- Ambulation is at baseline.

- An adult is present to get the patient home and remain with the patient for at least two half-lives of the drugs used for the anaesthesia.

- If a reversal drug was administered, there has been time for the drug to be excreted.

performed, the next group of major parameters to be assessed is the ABCs (airway, breathing, and circulation). Assessment should also include a thorough survey of the patient's physical and mental status before, during, and after the administration of the drugs used for general anaesthesia. The nurse's responsibility is to assess and document previous reactions, positive or negative (adverse), to general anaesthetics and related drug, so that the appropriate health care professionals such as the anaesthesiologist, nurse anaesthetist, registered nurse, physician, and any other health care professional involved in the patient's care can be notified.

For general anaesthesia, it is important to identify and document any problems or areas of concern in the patient's profile. A patient's profile includes subjective and objective data. One important area in the profile is drug use, including prescription drugs, over-the-counter drugs, natural health products (see Natural Health Products: Possible Effects of Popular Natural Health Products When Combined with Anaesthetics), and social and illegal drugs. Unusual and adverse reactions to any previously used drugs should be noted. Another important area to consider is the use of alcohol and nicotine. Excessive use of alcohol or illicit substances can alter the patient's response to general anaesthesia. Also, if the patient has a history of alcohol misuse, withdrawal symptoms may occur during recovery from surgery. The patient's history of smoking is important because nicotine has an adverse effect on the cilia in

the respiratory system. The cilia become paralyzed and unable to perform the function of clearing foreign bodies from the airways.

Other objective data include physical assessment, weight, height, electrocardiogram, chest X-ray (as ordered), and laboratory tests, including hemoglobin, hematocrit, complete blood count, blood urea nitrogen level, creatinine level, alkaline phosphate level, prothrombin time, partial thromboplastin time, and platelet count. Results of tests for serum electrolytes (such as potassium, sodium, chloride, phosphorus, magnesium, and calcium), urinalysis with specific gravity, and a pregnancy test (indicated if a female patient is of childbearing age) should be assessed and the findings documented. Results of these laboratory studies are important in establishing baseline organ function prior to the use of any form of anaesthetic or related drugs.

Neurological assessment should include motor assessments with bilateral and upper extremity versus lower extremity comparisons of strength, reflexes, grasp, and ability to move on command. Sensory assessment includes the same anatomical areas with comparison of response to the types of stimuli such as sharp, dull, soft, and cold versus warm. Swallowing ability and gag reflexes are also important to assess and document for baseline status and comparison. In addition, the patient's level of consciousness, alertness, and orientation to person, place, and time should be assessed. These motor, sensory, and cognitive parameters, when

NATURAL HEALTH PRODUCTS

Possible Effects of Popular Natural Health Products

When Combined with Anaesthetics

Ephedra: Changes in blood pressure; exaggerated responses to blood pressure medications; increased risk of acute myocardial infarction and cerebrovascular accident (stroke)

Feverfew: Migraine headaches, insomnia, anxiety, joint stiffness, risk of increased bleeding times with increased risk of bleeding

Garlic: Changes in blood pressure, risk of increased bleeding

Ginger: Sedating effects; risk of bleeding, especially if taken with either aspirin or ginkgo

Ginseng: Irritability and insomnia, risk of cardiac adverse effects

Kava: Sedating effects, potential liver toxicity, risk of additive effects with medications

St. John's Wort: Sedation, blood pressure changes, risk of interaction with other medications that prolong the effects of anaesthesia.

For more information, see http://www.hc-sc.gc.ca/dhp-mps/pubs/complement/interaction_drug-medicament_11-01/interaction_drug-medicament_11-01_9-eng.php

---

within normal limits, indicate an intact neurological system. Other baseline parameters include the patient's intake and output as well as oxygen saturation levels.

One significant reaction to assess for patients receiving general anaesthesia is that of malignant hyperthermia. This is a rapid progression of hyperthermia that may be fatal if not promptly recognized and aggressively treated. It is an inherited condition, so questions about related signs and symptoms in the family and patient medical history would be important. These signs and symptoms include tachycardia, tachypnea, muscle rigidity, cyanosis, irregular heartbeat, fever, mottling of the skin, diaphoresis (profuse sweating), and an unstable blood pressure. Astute and careful monitoring for the slightest change in vital signs and the parameters listed previously and for the occurrence of any abnormality associated with the anaesthesia is crucial to patient safety. Regardless of the degree of altered sensorium, constant and intense assessment is necessary. Whether the assessment occurs during the preanaesthesia, intra-anaesthesia, or postanaesthesia period, the nurse should remember that no matter how intense and critical the situation, use of the basic ABCs will always be the starting point for prioritizing and organizing patient care. Other areas of assessment include drug interactions, cautions, and contraindications (see previous discussion in the pharmacology section earlier in this chapter).

Intravenously administered anaesthetic drugs are usually combined with sedatives–hypnotics, antianxiety drugs, opioid and nonopioid analgesics, antiemetics, and anticholinergics. These drugs are used to decrease some of the undesirable after-effects of inhaled anaesthetics. With any form of adjuvant drug (a drug given at the same time) use, the patient should be assessed for any problems in liver, kidney, or heart functioning because of the risk for complications or adverse events. Generally speaking, the use of general anaesthetics (either intravenous or inhaled) carries a greater potential for more systemic adverse effects in the patient related to overall CNS depression that affects all body systems.

With the use of conscious sedation, as with any anaesthesia technique, assessment for cautions, contraindications, and drug interactions is important. Cautions and contraindications are similar to those for all other types of anaesthesia, as are drug interactions. Because moderate sedation is often used in children, there should be close assessment of organ function and diseases or conditions that could lead to excessive levels of the drug in the child's body. Even with the use of local anaesthesia, there are concerns about complications. Just because an anaesthetic is local, it does not mean that adverse reactions will not occur—they do occur and may be rather severe. Adverse reactions to or complications with local anaesthesia and intraspinal anaesthesia include the following: reduced respiratory function and altered breathing patterns, hypotension, tachycardia, decreased respiratory rate, diminished sensation, and decreased motor responses. "Spinal headaches" may also be associated with intraspinal anaesthesia and occur because of the leakage of cerebrospinal fluid from the insertion site. This type of headache is often severe and occurs when the patient stands or ambulates once the initial bed rest has ended. An assessment of blood pressure and other vital parameters, including respiratory function, provides important baseline data, and a history of any previous headaches is important information for the patient profile. See Special Populations: Children and Special Populations: The Older Adult, respectively, for points to consider when administrating anaesthetics to these groups.

Local-topical anaesthetics used for either infiltration or nerve block anaesthesia may be combined with other medications such as vasoconstrictors (e.g., epinephrine, phenylephrine, or norepinephrine). The vasoconstrictors are used to help confine the local anaesthetic to the injected area, prevent systemic absorption, and reduce bleeding. Systemic absorption of the vasoconstrictors results in hypertensive episodes that may be

SPECIAL POPULATIONS: CHILDREN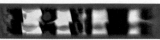

Anaesthesia

- Premature infants, neonates, and children are more adversely affected by anaesthesia than are the young or middle-aged adult patients. The reason for this difference in response is the increased sensitivity of the child to anaesthetics and related drugs. Immature functioning of the liver and kidneys leads to possible drug accumulation and toxicity and subsequent complications. The central nervous system of children is more sensitive to the effects of anaesthetics. Because of the risk of toxicity and complications with all forms of anaesthesia, the nurse must take all precautions to ensure that the patient remains safe and free from harm.

- The child's cardiac and respiratory systems are not fully developed or not yet fully functional. Patients in this age group are thus more susceptible to problems such as central nervous system depression accompanied by respiratory and cardiac depression, which can result in atelectasis, pneumonia, and heart abnormalities.

- Documentation of a thorough head-to-toe assessment with additional focus on the patient profile (such as results of laboratory studies, chest radiography, and other tests of organ function) is key to preventing complications and to identifying patients potentially

at risk. Thorough assessment for the presence of any diseases of the heart, kidney, liver, lung, and central nervous systems is important in identifying patients at risk and preventing complications during anaesthesia.

- Neonates in particular (see age-group definitions in Chapter 3) are at higher risk of upper airway obstruction during general anaesthesia. During the anaesthetic process, the risk of laryngospasm, which often occurs with intubation in patients of any age, may be increased for neonates because of the specific airway physical characteristics of the larynx and respiratory structures. Their higher metabolic rate and small airway diameter also put neonates at greater risk of experiencing complications during general anaesthesia.

- All drugs used in preanaesthesia and postanaesthesia phases require careful checks of mathematical drug calculations. The patient's weight, body surface area, and laboratory test results that indicate organ function or dysfunction should always be taken into consideration.

- Resuscitative equipment should be readily available on any neonatal or pediatric nursing unit for postanaesthesia care.

life threatening, especially in patients who are at high risk (e.g., those with underlying arterial disease). When local-topical anaesthetics such as lidocaine are used (e.g., when lacerations are sutured), the patient must be assessed for any pre-existing illnesses and allergies. Blood pressure, pulse rate, respiration rate, and temperature also must be assessed and documented. In addition, information about any illnesses or conditions

as well as a list of prescription medications, natural health products, and over-the-counter medications taken should be obtained and recorded. There is always concern about possible drug interactions or adverse effects that may be exacerbated by use of anaesthetics or other drugs in combination with the topical-local anaesthetic drug. One example is the use of topical lidocaine with epinephrine. If this topical-local anaesthetic

SPECIAL POPULATIONS: THE OLDER ADULT

Anaesthesia

- Older adults are affected more adversely by anaesthesia than are young or middle-aged adult patients. With aging comes organ system deterioration. A decline in the function of the liver results in decreased metabolism of drugs. A decline in kidney functioning leads to decreased drug excretion so that unsafe levels of the drug may be reached. If either of these organ systems are not functioning properly, drug toxicity may occur because of inadequate drug metabolism and excretion. Because of this decline in organ functioning, the older adult becomes more sensitive to the effects of anaesthetics. In addition, the central nervous system is more sensitive to the effects of anaesthetics and other drugs.

- The older adult's cardiac and respiratory systems are also affected by aging. These age-related changes

make the older adult more susceptible to problems such as respiratory depression, atelectasis, pneumonia, and heart abnormalities.

- With the older individual, it is important to assess for the presence of any disease of the cardiovascular, renal, hepatic, or respiratory systems because these would put the patient at higher risk for complications related to the anaesthesia and adjunct drugs.

- Another concern regarding anaesthesia in the older adult is polypharmacy. Because of the presence of age-related diseases, the older patient is generally taking more than one or two drugs. The more drugs a patient is taking, the higher is the risk of adverse reactions and drug–drug interactions, including those with anaesthesia.

combination gains access to the systemic circulation, the epinephrine may lead to hypertension, creating an even greater risk for hypertensive emergency than if plain lidocaine (without epinephrine) was used. There is a higher risk of such a crisis occurring if the patient has hypertension or is taking medications or natural health products that elevate blood pressure.

For patients about to undergo anaesthesia with NMBAs, a complete head-to-toe assessment should be performed and thorough medical and medication history taken. The specific drug being used and its status as depolarizing or nondepolarizing will guide nursing assessment and practices because of the NMBAs' action on the patient's neuromuscular functioning. All cautions, contraindications, and drug interactions must also be assessed (see previous discussion under NMBAs). Another concern with the use of NMBAs is that they are associated with an increase in intraocular pressure and intracranial pressure. Therefore, these anaesthetic drugs should not be used at all or should be used with extreme caution (close monitoring of these pressures) in patients with glaucoma or closed head injuries. Patients receiving NMBAs should also receive a thorough respiratory assessment because of the impact of these drugs on the respiratory system, including a paralyzing effect on the muscles used for breathing. In fact, some of the NMBAs are often used to induce paralysis of respiratory muscles in patients requiring mechanical ventilation. Paralysis of respiratory muscles is necessary so that patients will relax and not fight the machine and work against the breaths that the machine delivers. If an NMBA is indicated for other uses, it is critical to make sure that mechanical ventilation is available because of the potential for respiratory arrest.

Also indicated with the use of NMBAs is careful assessment of serum electrolyte levels, specifically potassium and magnesium levels. Imbalances in these electrolytes may lead to increased action of the NMBA with exacerbation of the drug's actions and adverse effects. Allergic reactions to NMBAs are most commonly characterized by rash, fever, respiratory distress, and pruritus. Drug interactions with natural health products are outlined in Natural Health Products on p. 231.

Once any type of anaesthesia is discontinued, patient assessment continues with further notation of the patient's ABCs, vital signs, and other critical parameters (e.g., pulse oximetry, neurological assessment, and urinary output). The nurse's responsibility is to provide continual assessment and care.

Nursing Diagnoses

- Impaired gas exchange related to the anaesthetic's CNS-depressant effects with altered respiratory rate and effort (decreased rate, decreased depth)
- Decreased cardiac output related to systemic effects of anaesthesia
- Risk for injury related to the impact of anaesthesia on the CNS (i.e., decreased sensorium)

- Anxiety related to the use of anaesthesia and the possibility of surgery
- Deficient knowledge related to lack of information about anaesthesia

Planning

Goals

- Patient will state the adverse effects of general or local anaesthesia, including decreased sensorium.
- Patient will state potential complications of anaesthesia involving the cardiac system.
- Patient will experience minimal to no respiratory complications related to anaesthesia.
- Patient will adhere to postanaesthesia care to help decrease the chance of complications.
- Patient will follow instructions regarding his or her care during the postoperative period.
- Patient will communicate (as needed) anxiety regarding preanaesthesia and postanaesthesia care.
- Patient will communicate anxiety, fears, and concerns regarding anaesthesia.
- Patient will understand the purpose, adverse effects, and complications of anaesthesia.

Outcome Criteria

- Patient experiences minimal to no adverse effects from anaesthesia, such as myocardial depression, during and after anaesthesia.
- Patient remains free of complications such as injury, falls, cardiac and respiratory depression, and hepatotoxicity during the preanaesthesia, intra-anaesthesia, and postanaesthesia periods.
- Patient experiences minimal anxiety or fear, as a result of specific interventions and education.
- Patient is adherent to all interventions, measures, and treatments such as turning, coughing, and deep breathing once the anaesthesia has been terminated.

Implementation

Regardless of the type of anaesthesia used, one of the most important nursing considerations during the preanaesthesia, intra-anaesthesia, and postanaesthesia periods is close and frequent observation of all body systems, with specific attention to the ABCs of nursing care (vital signs) and arterial oxygen saturation by pulse oximetry (SpO$_2$). These observations and interventions should be performed as frequently as needed depending on the patient's status and in keeping with the standard of care for anaesthesia. Sudden elevation in the patient's body temperature (e.g., higher than 40°C) while a patient is receiving general anaesthesia may indicate malignant hyperthermia, and immediate intervention is needed to protect the patient from injury and possible death. Other nursing interventions include monitoring all body systems, implementing safety measures, and carrying out the physician's orders.

Oxygen is often administered after a patient has received general anaesthesia to compensate for the respiratory depression that occurred during surgery and to elevate oxygen levels. Because oxygen is a drug, a doctor's order is needed for its administration. Continuous monitoring of SpO_2 is usually performed. In addition, hypotension and orthostatic hypotension are possible problems after anaesthesia, so postural blood pressure measurements (supine and standing) are needed. Should the patient require pain medication once the anaesthesia has been terminated, the nurse must remember that the anaesthetic and any adjuvant drugs used will continue to have an effect on the patient. Therefore, administration of any sedatives–hypnotics, narcotics, non-narcotics, analgesics, and other CNS depressants for pain relief should be done cautiously and only with close monitoring of vital signs. If the patient has received other medications (such as narcotics or CNS depressants) in a recovery area, dosages of drugs used in the postanaesthesia period and on the general nursing unit may be decreased by one half to one fourth as ordered. This reduction will help prevent any further CNS depression. For those patients receiving anaesthetics that are quick acting and whose effects are reversed quickly, dosages of analgesics may not need to be altered.

For intravenous anaesthesia, all resuscitative equipment—as well as a drug antidote—is usually readily available in case of cardiorespiratory distress or arrest. Neurological indicators (e.g., reflexes, response to commands, level of consciousness), electrocardiogram, pulse oximetry readings, and vital signs are some of the parameters that need to be monitored frequently. Additional nursing interventions with anaesthesia include assessing the status of breath sounds by means of auscultation (hypoventilation may be a complication of general anaesthesia). Neurological changes and status (no matter how small) and any change in sensations, such as those noted with nerve blocks (local anaesthesia), should also be documented and reported. If changes occur in body parts distal to the site of local anaesthesia or in locations where restraints were placed, the body part should be assessed for temperature, colour, and presence or absence of pulses, and the findings should be documented and reported to the physician. Improper positioning during surgery may lead to the injury of arteries and nerves and should be reported immediately.

Patients undergoing moderate sedation as the method of anaesthesia should receive education about the technique. As noted earlier, recovery from this type of anaesthesia is more rapid, and the safety profile is better than with general anaesthesia, which has inherent cardiorespiratory risks. As with general anaesthesia, the nurse should monitor the ABCs, vital signs, pulse oximetry readings, and patient's level of consciousness. See Box 12-7 for more information on conscious sedation.

With regard to the use of topical or local anaesthetics (e.g., lidocaine with or without epinephrine), solutions that are not clear and appear cloudy or discoloured should not be used. Some anaesthesiologists mix the solution with sodium bicarbonate to minimize local pain during infiltration, but this also causes a more rapid onset of action and a longer duration of sensory analgesia. If an anaesthetic ointment or cream is used, the nurse should thoroughly cleanse and dry the area to be anaesthetized before application of the drug.

If a topical or local anaesthetic is being used in the nose or throat, the nurse must remember that it may cause paralysis or numbness of the structures of the upper respiratory tract, which can lead to aspiration. Exact amounts of the drug should be used, and it should be administered only at the prescribed times. Local anaesthetics are not to be swallowed unless the physician has so instructed. Should this occur, the nurse must closely observe the patient, check the patient's gag reflex, and expect to withhold food or drink until the patient's sensation and gag reflex have returned.

A patient who receives an NMBA should be monitored closely during and after anaesthesia or initiation of mechanical ventilation. Vital signs and other parameters should be constantly monitored, with measurement of blood pressure, pulse, respirations (rate, depth, pattern, quality), SpO_2, and hand grasp strength (for neuromotor assessment). Intake and output are also monitored. Recovery from NMBAs is manifested by a decrease in paralysis of the face, diaphragm, legs, arms, and remainder of the body. The health care provider must reassure the patient of his or her condition at the beginning of the recovery process because the patient may become frightened if communication is difficult later during the recovery process.

Once anaesthesia and procedures are completed and the patient is to be discharged or transferred, some general areas of patient teaching must be completed. One major focus is sharing information regarding health care resources available to the patient at home should assistance be necessary. Home health care is often required and ordered by the physician; if it is not ordered, there may be a need for additional resources for assistance at home. Education about home health care resources and assistance-in-living programs should be guided by the findings of an at-home nursing assessment and the needs identified. Assistance with activities of daily living and assistance with health care–related procedures

BOX 12-7 Moderate or Conscious Sedation: What to Expect

- What questions should the patient or caregiver ask about the technique of moderate or conscious sedation?
  - Who will be providing this type of anaesthesia?
  - Who will be monitoring me or my loved one?
  - Will there be constant monitoring of blood pressure, pulse rate, respiratory rate, and temperature?
  - Will there be emergency equipment in the room, if needed?
  - Are the personnel qualified to administer these drugs? To administer advanced cardiac life support?
  - What do I need to know about care at home? Will I need help? Can I drive after having the procedure?
- What are the adverse effects of moderate or conscious sedation?
  - Brief periods of amnesia (loss of memory)
  - Headache
  - Hangover
  - Nausea and vomiting
- What should be expected immediately following the procedure?
  - Frequent monitoring
  - Written postoperative instructions and care
  - No driving, if the patient is driving age, for at least 24 hours after undergoing moderate sedation
  - A follow-up contact by phone to check on the patient

- Who can administer the conscious sedation?
  - Moderate or conscious sedation is safe when administered by qualified providers. Certified registered nurse anaesthetists, anaesthesiologists, other physicians, dentists, and oral surgeons are qualified to administer conscious sedation.
- Which procedures generally require moderate sedation?
  - Breast biopsy
  - Vasectomy
  - Minor foot surgery
  - Minor bone fracture repair
  - Plastic or reconstructive surgery
  - Dental prosthetic or reconstructive surgery
  - Endoscopy (such as diagnostic studies and treatment of stomach, colon, and bladder cancer)
- What are the overall benefits of this type of anaesthesia?
  - It is a safe and effective option for patients undergoing minor surgeries or diagnostic procedures.
  - It allows patients to recover quickly and resume normal activities in a shorter period of time.

Data from American Association of Nurse Anesthetists. (2005). Conscious sedation: what patients should expect. For more information, see http://www.aana.com/uploadedFiles/For_Patients/sedation_brochure03.pdf

or interventions may be required. Some examples of health care procedures for which help might be needed are wound care, dressing changes, surgical site care, drawing of samples for laboratory studies, intravenous infusions, and administration of medications through the intravenous, intramuscular, or subcutaneous route. Pain management may also need to be addressed (Chapter 11) with thorough teaching of the patient and those involved in the patient's care at home. Simple instructions using age-appropriate teaching strategies are always important (Chapter 6). Sharing of information about community resources is also important, especially for those who may need transportation, assistance with meals and housekeeping during recovery, and rehabilitation at home. Some of these community resources may be agencies supported by city or state social service programs, Meals on Wheels, senior citizen support groups, or church-sponsored support resources. Many of these resources are free or have income-based fees. Teaching tips important for patients receiving general or local anaesthesia are given in Patient Education.

⬛ Evaluation

The therapeutic effects of any general or local anaesthetic include loss of sensation during a procedure (such as loss of sensation in the eye for corneal surgery) and loss of consciousness and other reflexes (such as insensitivity to pain during abdominal or other major procedures). The patient who has received general anaesthesia should be constantly monitored for the occurrence of adverse effects of the anaesthesia. These effects include myocardial depression, convulsions, respiratory depression, allergic rhinitis, and decreased kidney or liver function. Patients who have received a local anaesthetic also need to be constantly monitored for adverse effects (mostly stemming from the systemic absorption of the specific drug). These effects include bradycardia, myocardial depression, hypotension, and dysrhythmias. As mentioned earlier in the chapter, significant overdoses of local anaesthetic drugs or direct injection into a blood vessel may result in cardiovascular collapse or cardiac or respiratory depression.

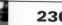

PATIENT EDUCATION

General Anaesthesia

❖ Patients should be informed that it is important to know whether any medications he or she is taking may need to be discontinued or tapered before the anaesthesia administration.

❖ Patient should be educated about the route of administration and the specific anaesthetic being used. Include information about the action, use, adverse effects, and special precautions associated with that specific anaesthetic after the anaesthesia has been discontinued.

❖ Patients and their family members should be encouraged to openly discuss any fears or anxieties about anaesthesia and related procedures or surgery.

❖ Patients should be instructed about the postanaesthesia process, especially if there is a need to turn, cough, and deep breathe (which helps prevent atelectasis and pneumonia).

❖ Patients should be encouraged to ambulate with assistance as needed. This helps increase circulation and improve ventilation to the alveoli of the lungs; consequently, circulation to the legs will be improved (which helps prevent stasis of blood and possible blood clot formation in the leg veins).

❖ Patients should be encouraged to request pain medication if needed before the pain becomes severe. Inform the patient that even though anaesthesia had been administered, he or she may experience discomfort or pain resulting from the procedure or surgery.

❖ Patients should be encouraged to rate pain on a scale of 0 to 10, with 0 being no pain and 10 being the worst pain.

❖ Patients should be instructed about the rationale for any other treatments or procedures related to the anaesthesia (such as epidural catheter placement; delivery of oxygen; administration of a gas; or use of tubes, catheters, or intravenous lines).

❖ Patients should be informed that frequent measurement of vital signs and pulse oximetry monitoring are a standard of care and do not necessarily mean that a problem or complication exists.

❖ Family members or caregivers of a patient with diminished sensorium should be instructed to ensure that the bed's side rails are up and that a call button at the bedside is critical to patient safety. (Note that bed alarms are now generally used instead of side rails, but the alarms may not always be available.)

❖ Patients receiving NMBAs for mechanical ventilation should be informed that although they may not be able to move (due to the paralyzing effects of the NMBA), they will still be able to hear.

Local Anaesthesia

❖ Patients should be educated about how local anaesthetics work, what the adverse effects are, and why the specific local drug was selected.

❖ Patients receiving local (spinal) anaesthesia should be informed about the need for frequent assessments, measurement of vital signs, and system assessments during and after the procedure to monitor for and assess any complications.

❖ Patients should be informed that even though the anaesthesia is local, concerns regarding the procedure and adverse effects exist.

Miscellaneous

❖ Patients should receive clear wound care instructions, and return demonstrations from the patient or caregiver should be ensured.

POINTS TO REMEMBER

❖ Anaesthesia is a drug-induced state of altered nerve conduction and may be used for general, local, or moderate sedation.

❖ Anaesthesia allows surgeons to carry out specific and often sophisticated procedures.

❖ The CNS is profoundly altered with general anaesthesia so that pain perception and consciousness are lost; drug effects also include skeletal muscle relaxation and loss of reflexes.

❖ General anaesthetics induce a state of anaesthesia; the effects are global, influencing the entire body.

❖ NMBAs, if given in high doses, may block neuromuscular receptors and other ganglionic receptors, leading to hypotension, tachycardia, decreased GI and genitourinary (GU) tone, and dry mouth.

❖ Moderate sedation often uses a combination of drugs to produce anaesthesia while maintaining a level of consciousness. It often includes the administration of sedatives, hypnotics, anxiolytics, analgesics, antiemetics, anticholinergics, or an NMBA.

❖ Local anaesthetics, also termed *regional anaesthetics*, render specific portions of the body essentially insensitive to pain without affecting consciousness.

❖ Local anaesthetics may be applied to the skin and mucous membranes or injected locally. They are available as parenteral (injectable) solutions, ointments, gels, creams, powders, ophthalmic drops, and suppositories.

❖ Nursing considerations related to the perioperative phase include all nursing actions with a client before (preoperative stage), during (intraoperative stage), and after (postoperative stage) anaesthesia and the surgical process. Each phase demands often complex and specific nursing actions.

❖ NMBAs have many cautions and contraindications and should be used only if mechanical ventilation is being used or is on hand. They should *not* be kept on hand on any nursing unit because of the potential for careless use and the possible induction of apnea.

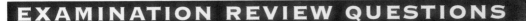

EXAMINATION REVIEW QUESTIONS

1 Your patient is in the hospital for removal of a lymph node from his arm under local anaesthesia. The physician has requested "lidocaine *with* epinephrine." Which of the following is the most accurate rationale for adding epinephrine?
a. It helps reduce local bleeding.
b. It enhances the effect of the local lidocaine.
c. It helps calm the patient before the procedure.
d. It helps minimize the risk of an allergic reaction.

2 Which of the following patients is more prone to complications from general anaesthesia?
a. A 49-year-old male athlete who quit heavy smoking 12 years ago
b. A 79-year-old woman who is about to have her gallbladder removed
c. A 30-year-old woman who is in perfect health but has never had anaesthesia
d. A 50-year-old woman scheduled for outpatient laser surgery for vision correction

3 Which of the following may occur in a patient who has been under general anaesthesia for 3 to 4 hours for abdominal–thoracic surgery?
a. Decreased urine output from use of vasopressors for anaesthesia
b. Increased cardiac output related to the effects of general anaesthesia

c. Risk for injury (fall) related to decreased sensorium for 2 to 4 days postoperatively
d. Decreased gaseous exchange because of the CNS-depressant effect of general anaesthesia

4 Which of the following should be the nurse's main concern for a patient recovering from general anaesthesia during the immediate postoperative period?
a. Airway
b. Pupillary reflexes
c. Return of sensations
d. Level of consciousness

5 A patient is recovering from surgery during which he received an NMBA. As he wakes up during recovery, he looks as if he is panicking, and yet is unable to speak. Which of the following should be the nurse's reaction?
a. Re-administer the NMBA to help the patient calm down
b. Increase oxygen administration and monitor oxygenation
c. Call the anaesthesia department for reintubation because of an impaired airway
d. Reassure the patient that he is recovering and that the medication is still wearing off

For answers see http://evolve.elsevier.com/Canada/Lilley/pharmacology/.

CRITICAL THINKING ACTIVITIES

A 53-year-old woman is scheduled to have a colonoscopy this morning, and she is anxious. The nurse anaesthetist has explained the conscious sedation that is planned, but the patient says after the anaesthetist leaves the room, "I'm so afraid of feeling it during the test. Why don't they just put me to sleep?"

1 How does conscious sedation differ from general anaesthesia?
2 How do you answer her question?
3 What is important to assess before this procedure is performed?

For answers see http://evolve.elsevier.com/Canada/Lilley/pharmacology/.

CHAPTER 13

Central Nervous System Depressants and Muscle Relaxants

Learning Objectives

After reading this chapter, the successful student will be able to do the following:

1 Describe the impact of central nervous system (CNS) depressants on all body systems.

2 Differentiate between the following terms: sedative–hypnotic drugs, barbiturates, benzodiazepines, muscle relaxants, and non-benzodiazepine drugs.

3 Identify the specific drugs within each category of CNS depressants.

4 Contrast the mechanism of action, indications, adverse effects, toxic effects, cautions, contraindications, dosage forms, routes of administration, and drug interactions of barbiturates, benzodiazepines, muscle relaxants, nonbenzodiazepines, and miscellaneous sedative–hypnotic drugs.

5 Discuss nonpharmacological approaches to the treatment of sleep disorders.

6 Develop a collaborative plan of care related to the use of CNS depressants.

e-Learning Activities

Web site
(http://evolve.elsevier.com/Canada/Lilley/pharmacology/)

- Animations
- Answers to chapter questions, activities, and case studies
- Calculators and Category Catchers
- Glossary with audio pronunciations
- IV Therapy and Medication Error Checklists
- Multiple-Choice Review Question quizzes
- Nursing Care Plans
- Online Appendices and Supplements
- WebLinks

Drug Profiles

▸▸ **baclofen**, p. 249
▸▸ **cyclobenzaprine (cyclobenzaprine hydrochloride)***, p. 249
   dantrolene (dantrolene sodium)*, p. 249
   flurazepam (flurazepam hydrochloride)*, p. 246
   lorazepam, p. 246
   pentobarbital (pentobarbital sodium)*, p. 242
   phenobarbital (phenobarbital sodium)*, p. 242
▸▸ **temazepam**, p. 246
▸▸ **thiopental (thiopental sodium)***, p. 243
   triazolam, p. 246
▸▸ **zopiclone**, p. 246

▸▸ Key drug.

*Full generic name is given in parentheses. For the purposes of this text, the more common shortened name is used.

Glossary

Anxiolytic A medication that relieves anxiety. (p. 243)

Barbiturates A class of drugs that are chemical derivatives of barbituric acid. They can induce sedation and sleep. (p. 240)

Benzodiazepines A chemical category of drugs most frequently prescribed as sedative–hypnotic and anxiolytic drugs; the most common group of psychotropic drugs currently prescribed to alleviate anxiety. (p. 243)

Gamma-aminobutyric acid (GABA) An inhibitory neurotransmitter found in the brain that functions to inhibit nerve transmission in the central nervous system (CNS). (p. 241)

Hypnotics Drugs that, when given at low to moderate doses, calm or soothe the central nervous system (CNS) without inducing sleep but when given at high doses may cause sleep. (p. 239)

Non–rapid eye movement (non-REM) sleep One of the stages of the sleep cycle. It characteristically has four stages and precedes REM sleep. Most of a normal sleep cycle consists of non-REM sleep. (p. 240)

Rapid eye movement (REM) sleep One of the stages of the sleep cycle. Some of the characteristics of REM sleep are rapid movement of the eyes, vivid dreams, and irregular breathing. (p. 240)

REM interference A drug-induced reduction of REM sleep time. (p. 240)

REM rebound Excessive REM sleep following discontinuation of a sleep-altering drug. (p. 240)

Sedatives Drugs that have an inhibitory effect on the CNS to the degree that they reduce nervousness, excitability, and irritability without causing sleep. (p. 239)

Sedative–hypnotics Drugs that can act in the body either as sedatives or hypnotics. (p. 239)

Sleep A transient, reversible, and periodic state of rest in which there is a decrease in physical activity and consciousness. (p. 239)

Sleep architecture The structure of the elements involved in the sleep cycle, including normal and abnormal patterns of sleep. (p. 239)

Tachyphylaxis The rapid appearance of a progressive decrease in response to a drug after repetitive administration of the drug. (p. 249)

Therapeutic index The ratio between the toxic and therapeutic concentrations of a drug. If the index is low, the difference between the therapeutic and toxic drug concentrations is small, and use of the drug is more hazardous. (p. 240)

OVERVIEW

Drugs that have a calming effect or that depress the central nervous system (CNS) are referred to as *sedatives* and *hypnotics.* A drug is classified as either a sedative or a hypnotic drug depending on the degree to which it inhibits the transmission of nerve impulses to the CNS. **Sedatives** reduce nervousness, excitability, and irritability without causing sleep, but a sedative can become a hypnotic if it is given in large enough doses. **Hypnotics** cause sleep. They have a much more potent effect on the CNS than do sedatives. Many drugs can act in the body as either a sedative or a hypnotic, and for this reason are called **sedative–hypnotics.** Listed in Table 13-1 are some points of interest relating to sedative–hypnotics.

Sedative–hypnotics can be classified chemically into three main groups: barbiturates, benzodiazepines, and miscellaneous drugs. Before the sedative–hypnotic drugs are discussed in depth, it is important that the physiology of normal sleep be understood because of the significant effects these drugs can have on sleep patterns.

SLEEP

Sleep is defined as a transient, reversible, and periodic state of rest in which there is a decrease in physical activity and consciousness. Normal sleep is cyclic and repetitive, and a person's responses to stimuli are markedly reduced during sleep. During waking hours the body is bombarded with stimuli that provoke the senses of sight, hearing, touch, smell, and taste. These stimuli elicit voluntary and involuntary movements or functions. During sleep a person is no longer aware of the sensory stimuli within the immediate environment.

Sleep research involves study of the patterns of sleep, or what is sometimes referred to as **sleep architecture.**

TABLE 13-1

Sedative–Hypnotic Drugs: Points of Interest

Drug	Point
flurazepam	Causes less REM rebound than the other benzodiazepines; use cautiously in the older adult; give 15–30 min before bedtime.
pentobarbital	Short acting; can be given PO, by rectal suppository, or IM; IM injection given deep in large muscle mass. As with any of these drugs, patients should avoid caffeine intake 4 hr before or after the time of dosing because of the decreased effectiveness that results.
phenobarbital	Long acting (up to 16 hr); in the body longer and thus can react with other medications such as alcohol and other CNS depressants. Because of its long duration, use cautiously in the older adult with decreased liver and kidney function.
temazepam	Induces sleep within 20–40 min; give 20–30 min before bedtime.
triazolam	Short-term use only; try other medications in this category, as ordered by a physician. Use cautiously in the older adult—it causes confusion, so protect the patient from injury.

CNS, central nervous system; *GI,* gastrointestinal; *IM,* intramuscular; *PO,* orally; *REM,* rapid eye movement.

The architecture of sleep consists of two basic stages that occur cyclically: **rapid eye movement (REM) sleep** and **non–rapid eye movement (non-REM) sleep**. The normal cyclic progression of the stages of sleep is summarized in Table 13-2. Sedative–hypnotics affect different stages of the normal sleep pattern. If usage is prolonged, emotional and psychological changes can occur. An appreciation of this fact will help prevent the inappropriate use of long-term sleeping drugs. For example, prolonged sedative–hypnotic use may reduce the cumulative amount of REM sleep; this is known as **REM interference**. This can result in daytime fatigue since REM sleep provides a certain component of the "restfulness" of sleep. Upon discontinuing a sedative–hypnotic drug, **REM rebound** can occur during which the patient has an abnormally large amount of REM sleep, often leading to frequent and vivid dreams. Misuse of sedative–hypnotic drugs is common and discussed in Chapter 9. In Ethnocultural Implications, sleep aids used by different ethnocultural groups are listed.

BARBITURATES

Barbiturates were first introduced into clinical use in 1903 and were the standard drugs for treating insomnia and producing sedation. Chemically they are derivatives of barbituric acid. Although there are close to 35 different barbiturates approved for clinical use in Canada, only a handful are in common clinical use today. This is, in part, because of the favourable safety profile and proven efficacy of the class of drugs commonly referred to as *benzodiazepines*. Barbiturates can produce many unwanted adverse effects. They are habit forming and have a low **therapeutic index** (the ratio between the toxic and therapeutic concentrations of a drug; there is only a narrow dosage range within which the drug is effective, and above that range the drug is rapidly toxic). Barbiturates can be classified into four groups based on their onset and duration of action. Table 13-3 lists the drugs in each category and summarizes their pharmacokinetic characteristics.

Mechanism of Action and Drug Effects

Barbiturates are CNS depressants that act primarily on the brainstem in an area called the *reticular formation*. Their sedative and hypnotic effects are dose related, and they act by reducing the nerve impulses travelling to the area of the brain called the *cerebral cortex*. Their ability to inhibit nerve impulse transmission comes, in part, from their ability to potentiate the action of an inhibitory amino acid

TABLE	13-2

Stages of Sleep

Stage	Characteristics	Average Percentage of Time in Each Stage (for Young Adults)
NON-REM SLEEP		
1	Dozing, or feeling of drifting off to sleep; person can be easily awakened; insomniacs have longer stage 1 periods than normal	2%–5%
2	Relaxed, but person can be easily awakened; person has occasional REMs and also slight eye movements	50%
3	Deep sleep; difficult to wake person; respiratory rates, pulse, and blood pressure may decrease	5%
4	Difficult to wake person; person may be groggy if awakened; dreaming, especially about daily events; sleepwalking or bedwetting may occur	10%–15%
REM SLEEP		
	REMs occur; vivid dreams occur; breathing may be irregular	25%–33%

Modified from McKenry, L., Tessier, E., & Hogan, M. (2006). *Mosby's pharmacology in nursing* (22nd ed.). St. Louis, MO: Mosby.

 ## ETHNOCULTURAL IMPLICATIONS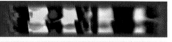

Sleep Aids Used by Different Ethnocultural Populations

- The nurse should question a patient of another ethno-culture about what the patient's usual sleep patterns and habits are and what is accepted and practised to promote sleep.
- The Hispanic culture depends on many food rituals for resolving problems such as insomnia. The hot and cold theory of balancing foods is most common.
- People from Africa and Asia as well as Aboriginal peoples have a high incidence of lactose intolerance, so use of warm milk may lead to gastrointestinal

distress, abdominal cramping, and bloating unless a lactose-free milk is used.

- Some Jewish people are less accepting of therapeutic touch, and the nurse should be aware of this if this therapy is planned to promote relaxation.
- A thorough health, medication, and diet history is important to collect in order to identify food and herbal practices used to manage common everyday problems, such as insomnia.

TABLE 13-3

Barbiturates: Onset and Duration

Category	Pharmacokinetics		Barbiturates
	Onset	Duration	
Ultrashort	IV: 1 min	IV: 10-30 min	thiopental, pentobarbital
Short	PO: 60 min	PO: 2–4 hr	pentobarbital
Intermediate	PO: 15–60 min	PO: 4–6 hr	butalbital
Long	PO: 30–60 min	PO: 10–12 hr	phenobarbital, primidone
	N/A	PO: 10–12 hr	

IV, intravenous; *PO*, oral.

known as **gamma-aminobutyric acid (GABA)**, which is found in high concentrations in the CNS. Barbiturates are capable of raising the convulsive or seizure threshold and are therefore also effective in treating status epilepticus and tetanus- or drug-induced convulsions. In addition, selected barbiturates are used as prophylaxis for epileptic seizures.

At low doses, barbiturates act as sedatives. Increasing the dosage produces a hypnotic effect but also decreases the respiratory rate. At normal dosages they have little effect on the circulation. Barbiturates as a class are notorious enzyme inducers. They stimulate the action of enzymes in the liver that are responsible for the metabolism or breakdown of many drugs. By stimulating the action of these enzymes, they cause many drugs to be metabolized more quickly, which usually shortens their duration of action. Other drugs that are enzyme inducers are warfarin, theophylline, and phenytoin.

Indications

All barbiturates have the same sedative–hypnotic efficacy but differ in their potency, onset, and duration of action. They are used as hypnotics, sedatives, and anticonvulsants and also for anaesthesia during surgical procedures. The categories of barbiturates are used for the following therapeutic purposes:

Ultrashort acting: Anaesthesia for short surgical procedures, anaesthesia induction, control of convulsions, narcoanalysis, and reduction in intracranial pressure in neurosurgical patients

Short acting: Sedative–hypnotic and control of convulsive conditions

Intermediate acting: Sedative–hypnotic and control of convulsive conditions

Long acting: Sedative–hypnotic, epileptic seizure prophylaxis, and treatment of neonatal hyperbilirubinemia

Contraindications

Contraindications to barbiturate use include known drug allergy, pregnancy, significant respiratory difficulties, and severe liver disease.

Adverse Effects

The main adverse effects of barbiturates affect the CNS and include drowsiness, lethargy, dizziness, hangover (prolongation of drowsiness, lethargy, and dizziness), and paradoxical restlessness or excitement. Their chronic effects on normal sleep architecture can be detrimental. Sleep research has shown that adequate rest is obtained from the sleep process only when there are proper amounts of REM sleep, which is sometimes referred to as *dreaming sleep*. Barbiturates deprive people of REM sleep, which can result in agitation and an inability to deal with normal stress. When the barbiturate is stopped and REM sleep once again takes place, a rebound phenomenon can occur. During this rebound the proportion of REM sleep is increased, the patient's dream time constitutes a larger percentage of total sleep, and the dreams are often nightmares. The adverse effects of barbiturates and the body systems affected are listed in Table 13-4. As is the case with most sedative drugs, barbiturates are associated with an increased incidence of falls when used in the older adult. If they are recommended at all, the usual dose is reduced by one half whenever possible.

Toxicity and Management of Overdose

Overdose frequently results in respiratory depression, leading to respiratory arrest. Often this is done therapeutically to induce anaesthesia. In this situation, however, the patient is ventilated mechanically, and respiration is controlled or assisted mechanically. Another situation in which intentional overdoses are given for therapeutic reasons is the management of uncontrollable seizures. Patients in such a seizure state are sometimes put into what is called a *phenobarbital coma*. Because of the inhibitory effects of barbiturates on nerve transmission in the brain (possibly GABA mediated), the uncontrollable seizures can be stopped until appropriate serum levels of anticonvulsant drugs are reached.

An overdose of barbiturates produces CNS depression ranging from sleep to profound coma and death. Respiratory depression progresses to Cheyne–Stokes respiration, hypoventilation, and cyanosis. Affected patients often have cold, clammy skin or are hypothermic. Later, patients can exhibit fever, areflexia, tachycardia, and

TABLE 13-4

Barbiturates: Adverse Effects

Body System	Adverse Effects
Cardiovascular	Vasodilation and hypotension, especially if administered too rapidly
Gastrointestinal	Nausea, vomiting, diarrhea, constipation
Hematological	Agranulocytosis, thrombocytopenia, megaloblastic anemia
Nervous	Drowsiness; lethargy; vertigo; headache; depression; myalgic, neuralgic, or arthralgic pain
Respiratory	Respiratory depression, apnea, laryngospasm, bronchospasm, coughing
Other	Hypersensitivity reactions: urticaria, angioedema, rash, fever, serum sickness, Stevens–Johnson syndrome

hypotension. Pupils are usually slightly constricted but may be dilated in cases of severe drug toxicity.

Treatment of an overdose is mainly symptomatic and supportive. The mainstays of therapy are maintenance of an adequate airway, assisted respiration, and oxygen administration, if needed, along with fluid and vasopressor support as indicated. Multiple-dose (every 4 hours) nasogastric administration of activated charcoal is highly effective in removing barbiturates from the stomach and the circulation. Barbiturates are highly metabolized by the liver, and they increase enzyme activity there. In an overdose, however, the amount of barbiturate may overwhelm the liver's ability to metabolize it; in this situation, activated charcoal may be helpful. Activated charcoal assists in pulling the drug from the circulation and eliminating it by means of the gastrointestinal (GI) system. Some of the barbiturates (e.g., phenobarbital) can be eliminated more quickly by the kidneys when the urine is alkalized. This keeps the drug in the urine and prevents it from being reabsorbed back into the circulation. Alkalization, along with forced diuresis, can hasten elimination of the barbiturate.

Interactions

The drug interactions possible with barbiturates can be intense and often dramatic. The risk encountered in the coadministration of barbiturates with alcohol, antihistamines, benzodiazepines, opioids, and tranquilizers is additive CNS depression. Most of the drug–drug interactions involving barbiturates are secondary to the effects of barbiturates on the liver enzyme system. As mentioned previously, barbiturates increase the activity of liver microsomal enzymes. This process is called *enzyme induction*. Induction of this enzyme system results in increased drug metabolism and breakdown. However, if the two drugs are competing in the same enzyme system for metabolism, this can lead to inhibited drug metabolism or breakdown. Examples are the administration of monoamine oxidase inhibitors (MAOIs), anticoagulants, glucocorticoids, tricyclic antidepressants, quinidine, and oral contraceptives with barbiturates. Coadministration of MAOIs and barbiturates can result in prolonged barbiturate effects. Coadministration of anticoagulants with barbiturates can result in decreased anticoagulation response and possible clot formation. Coadministration of barbiturates with oral contraceptives can result in accelerated metabolism of the contraceptive drug and possible unintended pregnancy. Women taking both types of medication concurrently should be advised to consider an additional method of contraception as a backup.

Laboratory Test Interactions

Barbiturates can also interact with body substances and affect the results of laboratory tests. Barbiturates can cause an increase in the serum levels of bilirubin, glutamic pyruvate transaminase (alanine aminotransferase [ALT]), serum glutamic-oxaloacetic transaminase (aspartate aminotransferase [AST]), and alkaline phosphatase.

Dosages

As previously mentioned, barbiturates can act as either sedatives or hypnotics depending on their dosage. Selected barbiturates and their recommended sedative and hypnotic dosages are listed in the Dosages table on p. 243.

 DRUG PROFILES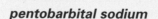

Barbiturates are available in a variety of dosage forms, including tablets, capsules, elixirs, injections, and suppositories. They are all rated as pregnancy category D drugs. All barbiturates are considered prescription-only drugs because of their potential for misuse and the severe effects that result if they are not used appropriately. From a legal standpoint, they are considered controlled substances. As discussed in Chapter 4, controlled substances are medications that Health Canada within the Controlled Drugs and Substances Act has identified as drugs that have an abuse potential. Provincial laws may place further restrictions on the way these drugs are dispensed; therefore, health care providers must be careful to comply with both federal and provincial laws. The controlled-substance schedule classifications of selected barbiturates are as follows:

- C-III: pentobarbital
- C-IV: phenobarbital, butalbital

Use of barbiturates is contraindicated in patients with known hypersensitivity reactions to them, latent porphyria, significant liver dysfunction, and known previous addiction.

pentobarbital sodium

Pentobarbital sodium formerly prescribed as a sedative–hypnotic for insomnia, is now principally used preoperatively to relieve anxiety and provide sedation. It is used in certain cases of increased intracranial pressure. Pentobarbital is available only through the Special Access Programme, Health Canada. It is classified as pregnancy category D. The sedative and hypnotic dosages are given in the Dosages table on p. 243.

PHARMACOKINETICS

Half-Life	Onset	Peak	Duration
IV: 15–48 hr	IV: < 1 min	IV: < 30 min	IV: 15 min

phenobarbital sodium

Phenobarbital sodium is the barbiturate most commonly prescribed, either alone or in combination with other drugs. It is considered the prototypical barbiturate and is classified as a long-acting drug. Phenobarbital is used for the prevention of generalized tonic–clonic seizures, simple partial seizures, and fever-induced convulsions. It may sometimes be used in the treatment of acute alcohol

Continued

DRUG PROFILES (cont'd)

withdrawal. Phenobarbital in solution for injection or intravenous use is available only through the Special Access Programme, Health Canada. It is available orally as tablets and elixir, as well as in tablet form in combination with belladona and ergotamine for treatment of migraine. It is classified as pregnancy category D. See the Dosages table below for dosages.

PHARMACOKINETICS

Route	Half-Life	Onset	Peak	Duration
PO	80–120 hr	60 min	8–12 hr	10–12 hr
IV	80–120 hr	5 min	30 min	4–10 hr

▸▸ *thiopental sodium*

Thiopental sodium (Pentothal) is used for the induction of sleep, either as a supplementation to or as the sole anaesthetic drug. It is also used for the emergency control of certain convulsive states. It may be used in neurosurgical patients with increased intracranial pressure and for narcoanalysis and narcosynthesis in patients with psychiatric disorders. It is classified as pregnancy category D. See the Dosages table below for dosages.

DOSAGES Selected Barbiturates

Drug	Onset and Duration	Usual Dosage Range	Indications
pentobarbital sodium*	Short acting	*Children* IV: 2.5 mg/kg (max 50 mg) over 1 min; increased in increments if necessary *Adult* IM: 150–200 mg	Preoperative sedation Procedural sedation
phenobarbital sodium*	Long acting	*Neonatal* PO: 5–10 mg/kg/day *Children* PO: 2–6 mg/kg/day in 1 or 2 divided doses PO/IM: 1–3 mg/kg 60–90 min before surgery IV: 20 mg/kg over 20 min *Adult* PO: 90–120 mg HS IM: 100–200 mg 60–90 min before surgery IV: 20 mg/kg at rate of 50–75 mg/min	Seizure disorders Preoperative sedation Status epilepticus Seizure disorders Preoperative sedation Status epilepticus
▸▸thiopental sodium (Pentothal)	Individualized dosage		Induction or maintenance of anaesthesia; management of increased intracranial pressure

HS, at bedtime; *IM,* intramuscular; *IV,* intravenous; *PO,* orally.

*Only available through Special Access Programme, Health Canada.

BENZODIAZEPINES

Benzodiazepines are the most commonly prescribed sedative–hypnotic drugs and one of the most commonly prescribed classes of drugs. This is directly attributable to their favourable adverse effect profiles, efficacy, and safety. Even when a drug in this class is taken as the sole drug in an overdose (e.g., not with alcohol), it is relatively benign, causing little more than sedation. Benzodiazepines are classified as either anxiolytics or sedative–hypnotics depending on their primary usage. An **anxiolytic** relieves anxiety. The benzodiazepines discussed in Chapter 16 work primarily to produce sedation or sleep. There are five such commonly used benzodiazepines as sedative–hypnotic drugs. They are listed in Table 13-5 and can be further classified on the basis of their duration of action as either long acting or short acting.

Mechanism of Action and Drug Effects

As mentioned previously, the sedative and hypnotic action of benzodiazepines is related to their ability to depress activity in the CNS. Benzodiazepines exhibit an affinity for benzodiazepine receptors, which act as specific binding sites for the major CNS inhibitory neurotransmitter gamma-aminobutyric acid (GABA), the major inhibitory neurotransmitter in the CNS. It is thought that benzodiazepines produce their CNS effects by interacting with a macromolecular protein complex in the neuronal membrane, which includes GABA receptors, high-affinity benzodiazepine receptors, and chloride channels. Different types of benzodiazepine receptors in different areas of the CNS are believed to produce the pharmacological actions of the drugs. The specific areas they affect in the CNS appear to be the hypothalamic, thalamic, and limbic systems of

TABLE 13-5

Sedative–Hypnotic Benzodiazepines Available in Canada

	Trade Name
LONG ACTING	
chlordiazepoxide hydrochloride	Apo-Chlordiazepoxide
diazepam	Diastat, Diazemuls, Valium
flurazepam hydrochloride	Apo-Flurazepam
INTERMEDIATE ACTING	
alprazolam	Zanax
bromazepam	Lectopam
clobazam	Apo-Clobazam
clonazepam	Rivotril, Clonapam
lorazepam	Ativan
nitrazepam	Nitrazadon
oxazepam	Apo-Oxazepam
temazepam	Restoril
SHORT ACTING	
midazolam hydrochloride (IM/IV only)	
triazolam	Halcion

Note: The benzodiazepines discussed in Chapter 16 and those discussed here all have similar pharmacological properties. They all act as anxiolytics and sedative–hypnotics. Different benzodiazepines are just more effective at producing one or the other pharmacological effect.

the brain. Their depressant action on the CNS may be related to their ability to inhibit stimulation of the brain. They have many favourable characteristics compared with barbiturates. They do not suppress REM sleep to the same extent as barbiturates. They also do not induce liver microsomal enzyme activity and are therefore safe to administer to patients who are taking medications that are metabolized by this enzyme system.

In terms of patient experience, benzodiazepines have a calming effect on the CNS. As the dose of benzodiazepine is increased, anxiolytic effects are first produced, followed by anticonvulsant effects, a reduction in muscle tonus, and finally sedation and hypnosis. The calming effect causes the inhibition of hyperexcitable nerves in the CNS that might be responsible for initiating seizure activity. Similarly, this calming effect on the CNS makes benzodiazepines useful in controlling agitation and anxiety. It also reduces excessive sensory stimulation and induces sleep. In addition, benzodiazepines have been shown to induce skeletal muscle relaxation. Their receptors in the CNS are in the same area where those that play a role in alcohol addiction are found. Therefore, benzodiazepines are used in the treatment and prevention of the symptoms of alcohol withdrawal (see Chapter 16).

Indications

Benzodiazepines have a variety of therapeutic applications. Benzodiazepines with similar chemical structures can differ in their potency, rate of absorption, and other pharmacokinetic parameters. The potency of a benzodiazepine is correlated with its affinity for its binding site, the benzodiazepine receptor. In therapeutic use, the

benzodiazepines, while differing in potency, have similar pharmacological profiles. Benzodiazepines are most commonly used for sedation, sleep induction, skeletal muscle relaxation, and anxiety relief. They have also been used in the treatment of alcohol withdrawal, agitation, depression, and epilepsy. They are often combined with anaesthetics, analgesics, and neuromuscular blocking drugs in what is called *balanced anaesthesia* and also moderate or "conscious" sedation (see Chapter 12). They are used in this setting mostly for their amnesiac properties because most persons undergoing surgery would rather not remember the events of their procedure.

Contraindications

Contraindications to the use of benzodiazepines include known drug allergy, narrow-angle glaucoma, and pregnancy.

Adverse Effects

As a class, benzodiazepines have a relatively safe adverse-effect profile. The adverse effects associated with their use are usually mild and primarily involve the CNS. The more commonly reported undesirable effects are headache, drowsiness, paradoxical excitement or nervousness, dizziness or vertigo, cognitive impairment, and lethargy. Benzodiazepines can create a significant risk for falls in the frail older adult, however, and their use should be avoided, when possible, in this patient population. To help prevent adverse effects, the lowest effective dosages are recommended for all patients, especially older adults. Because of the effect of the benzodiazepines on the normal sleep cycle, a hangover effect is sometimes reported. Other less common adverse effects are palpitations, dry mouth, nausea, vomiting, hypokinesia, and occasional nightmares.

Toxicity and Management of Overdose

An overdose of benzodiazepines may result in one or all of the following symptoms: somnolence, confusion, coma, or diminished reflexes. An overdose of benzodiazepines alone rarely results in hypotension and respiratory depression. These symptoms are more commonly seen when benzodiazepines are taken with other CNS depressants such as alcohol or barbiturates. The same is true for their lethal effects. In the absence of the concurrent ingestion of alcohol or other CNS depressants, benzodiazepine overdose rarely results in death.

The treatment of benzodiazepine intoxication is generally symptomatic and supportive. If ingestion is recent, decontamination of the gastrointestinal system is indicated. Ordinarily, drugs that have been orally ingested may be absorbed by activated charcoal (approximately 1 g/kg). Activated charcoal is beneficial if it can be administered within 2 to 4 hours of ingestion, if the patient is sufficiently alert to adequately protect the airway, and the risk of aspiration is minimal. Hemodialysis is not useful in the treatment of benzodiazepine overdose. Flumazenil, a benzodiazepine antagonist, can be used to acutely reverse the sedative effects of benzodiazepines, although this is normally done extremely cautiously in cases of excessive overdose or sedation. Flumazenil antagonizes the action of benzodiazepines on the CNS by directly competing for binding at the benzodiazepine receptor in the CNS. However, it has a stronger affinity for the receptor and knocks the benzodiazepine off the receptor, reversing the sedative action of the benzodiazepine. Sudden reversal by flumazenil in patients who persistently take benzodiazepines can induce withdrawal and precipitate seizures. In addition, in patients who may have also ingested a tricylcic antidepressant, it may result in increased sympathetic tone and enhanced cardiac electrical instability, causing cardiac arrest. The dosage regimen to be followed for the reversal of conscious sedation or general anaesthesia induced by benzodiazepines and the management of suspected benzodiazepine overdose are summarized in Table 13-6.

Interactions

The potential drug interactions with the benzodiazepines are significant because of their intensity, particularly when they involve other CNS depressants (e.g., alcohol, analgesics). These drugs may result in further CNS-depressant effects (including decreased blood pressure, respiratory rate, sedation, confusion, and diminished reflexes). Natural health product interactions include those with kava and valerian, which may also lead to further CNS depression (see Natural Health Products: Kava and Valerian). Food–drug interactions include grapefruit or grapefruit juice, which alters drug absorption. Prior to the use of any drugs within the category of CNS depressants, it is always important to remember that when combined with other drugs affecting the CNS, there is a 90% chance of causing adverse drug reactions. The risks associated with the coadministration of these and some other drugs are described in Table 13-7.

TABLE 13-6

Flumazenil Treatment Regimen

Indication	Recommended Regimen	Duration
Reversal of conscious sedation or general anaesthesia	0.2 mg (2 mL) given IV over 15 sec, then give 0.1 mg if consciousness does not occur; may be repeated at 60-sec intervals prn up to 8 additional times (maximum total dose, 1 mg; usual dose is 0.3–0.6 mg)	1–4 hr
Management of suspected benzodiazepine overdose	0.3 mg (3 mL) given IV over 30 sec; wait 30 sec, then give 0.3 mg (3 mL) over 30 sec if consciousness does not occur; further doses of 0.5 mg (5 mL) can be given over 30 sec at intervals of 1 min up to a cumulative dose of 2 mg	1–4 hr

Important note: Flumazenil has a relatively short half-life and duration of effect of 1–4 hr; therefore if using flumazenil to reverse the effects of a long-acting benzodiazepine, the dose of the reversal drug may wear off and the patient may become sedated again, requiring more flumazenil.

 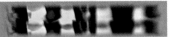

NATURAL HEALTH PRODUCTS

KAVA AND VALERIAN

Kava *(Piper methysticum)*

Overview
Kava rhizome consists of the dried rhizomes of *Piper methysticum.* The drug contains kavapyrones (kawain). Extended continuous intake can cause a temporary yellow discoloration of skin, hair, and nails.

Common Uses
Relief of anxiety, stress, restlessness; promotion of sleep

Adverse Effects*
Skin discoloration, possible accommodative disturbances and papillary enlargement, scaly skin (with long-term use)

Potential Drug Interactions
Alcohol, barbiturates, psychoactive drugs

Contraindications
Contraindicated in patients with Parkinson's disease, liver disease, or alcoholism; in those operating heavy machinery; and in pregnant and breastfeeding women

Valerian *(Valeriana officinalis)*

Overview
Valerian root, consisting of fresh underground plant parts, contains essential oil with monoterpenes and sesquiterpenes (valerianic acids).

Common Uses
Relief of anxiety, restlessness, sleep disorders

Adverse Effects
Central nervous system (CNS) depression, hepatotoxicity, nausea, vomiting, anorexia, headache, restlessness, insomnia

Potential Drug Interactions
CNS depressants, monamine oxidase inhibitors, phenytoin, warfarin; may have enhanced relative and adverse effects when taken with other drugs (including other natural health products) that have known sedative properties (including alcohol)

Contraindications
Contraindicated in patients with heart disease or those operating heavy machinery

TABLE 13-7

Benzodiazepines: Drug Interactions

Drug	Mechanism	Result
cimetidine	Decreased benzodiazepine metabolism	Prolonged benzodiazepine action
CNS depressants	Additive effects	Increased CNS depression
MAOIs	Decreased metabolism	Increased benzodiazepine effects
Protease inhibitors	Decreased metabolism	Increased benzodiazepine effects

CNS, central nervous system; *MAOI*, monoamine oxidase inhibitor.

Laboratory Test Interactions

There are no laboratory test interactions that occur with the benzodiazepines typically used as either sedatives or hypnotics.

Dosages

The benzodiazepines discussed in this chapter are those that are commonly used to treat insomnia. Therefore, the dosage recommendations given in the Dosages table

 DRUG PROFILES

The benzodiazepines are all prescription-only drugs and are designated as Schedule IV controlled substances. All five benzodiazepines discussed here have active metabolites that can accumulate during long-term use, especially in patients who have altered metabolic function (liver dysfunction) or altered excretion capabilities (kidney dysfunction). There are several other benzodiazepines, but they are more commonly used to treat anxiety or agitation, to produce amnesia, and to relax skeletal muscles. These other benzodiazepines are discussed in detail in Chapters 14 and 16.

flurazepam hydrochloride

Flurazepam hydrochloride (Apo-Flurazepam) is available in 15 and 30 mg capsules. It is considered a long-acting hypnotic drug and is indicated for the short-term treatment of insomnia for periods of up to 4 weeks. Flurazepam has two active metabolites that account for its hypnotic effects. These active metabolites have also been shown to be responsible for inducing a hangover effect, causing lethargy or grogginess the morning after the medication has been taken. Flurazepam is classified as pregnancy category X. The recommended dosages for adults and the older adult are given in the Dosages table on p. 247.

PHARMACOKINETICS

Half-Life	Onset	Peak	Duration
100 hr	15–45 min	30–60 min	7–8 hr

lorazepam

Lorazepam (Ativan) is available in 0.5, 1, and 2 mg oral and sublingual tablets as well as a parenteral solution. It is considered an intermediate-acting hypnotic drug and is indicated for the short-term treatment of insomnia for periods of up to 4 weeks. Because of its short duration, morning drowsiness is not a problem. Lorazepam is classified as pregnancy category X. The recommended dosages for adults and the older adult are given in the Dosages table on p. 247.

PHARMACOKINETICS

Half-Life	Onset	Peak	Duration
10–20 hr	30–60 min	2–4 hr	up to 8 hr

▸▸ temazepam

Temazepam is available in 15 and 30 mg capsules. It is contraindicated in patients who have narrow-angle glaucoma because it can exacerbate the glaucoma. It is indicated for the short-term treatment of insomnia. It is classified as pregnancy category X. The common dosages are given in the Dosages table on p. 247.

PHARMACOKINETICS

Half-Life	Onset	Peak	Duration
10–20 hr	60 min	2–4 hr	7–8 hr

triazolam

Triazolam (Halcion) is available in 0.125 and 0.25 mg tablets and is indicated for the short-term treatment of insomnia. The best approach with this drug is for the nurse to give the smallest effective dose for the shortest possible duration. Triazolam is classified as pregnancy category X. The common dosages are given in the Dosages table on p. 247.

PHARMACOKINETICS

Half-Life	Onset	Peak	Duration
1.5–5 hr	15–30 min	1–2 hr	6–7 hr

▸▸ zopiclone

Zopiclone (Immovane, Rhovane) is a short-acting non-benzodiazepine hypnotic drug. It is indicated for the short-term treatment of insomnia and, as with all benzodiazepines, should be limited to 7 to 10 days of treatment. Zopiclone belongs to a novel chemical class of hypnotics that are structurally unrelated to the existing benzodiazepines. However, the pharmacological profile of zopiclone is similar to that of the benzodiazepines. It is available in 7.5 mg tablets and is classified as pregnancy category B. The recommended dosage is given in the Dosages table on p. 247.

PHARMACOKINETICS

Half-Life	Onset	Peak	Duration
3.8–6.5 hr	30 min	90 min	4–6 hr

below are those for achieving hypnotic effects. All drugs administered for the treatment of insomnia should be limited to short-term use of 2 to 4 weeks or less. With long-term usage, rebound insomnia and severe withdrawal can develop. The older adult should also be started on lower dosages because they generally experience a more pronounced effect from benzodiazepines.

MUSCLE RELAXANTS

A variety of conditions such as trauma, inflammation, anxiety, and pain can be associated with acute muscle spasms. Although there is no completely satisfactory form of therapy available for relief of skeletal muscle spasticity, muscle relaxants are capable of providing some relief. The muscle relaxants are a group of compounds that act predominantly within the CNS to relieve pain associated with skeletal muscle spasms. Most muscle relaxants are called *central-acting skeletal muscle relaxants* because their site of action is the CNS. Central-acting skeletal muscle relaxants are similar in structures and action to other CNS depressants such as diazepam. It is believed that the muscle-relaxant effects of these drugs are related to this CNS-depressant activity. Only one of these compounds, dantrolene, acts directly on skeletal muscle. It belongs to a group of relaxants known as *direct-acting skeletal muscle relaxants*. It closely resembles GABA.

These drugs are most effective when used in conjunction with rest and physical therapy. When muscle relaxants are taken with alcohol, other CNS depressants, or opioid analgesics, enhanced CNS-depressant effects are seen. In such cases, close monitoring and dosage reduction of one or both drugs should be considered.

Mechanism of Action and Drug Effects

As noted earlier, most the muscle relaxants work within the CNS. Their effects are the result of CNS depression in the brain primarily at the level of the brainstem, thalamus, and basal ganglia but also at the spinal cord. With the exception of dantrolene, which works directly on skeletal muscle, all the other muscle relaxants have no direct effects on muscles, nerve conduction, or muscle–nerve junctions. One of the more effective drugs in this class of drugs, baclofen, is a derivative of GABA. It is believed to work by depressing nerve transmission in the spinal cord. The other drugs in this class are not derivatives of GABA but act by enhancing GABA's central inhibitory effects at the level of the spinal cord. These drugs are generally less effective than baclofen. Dantrolene acts by decreasing the response of the muscle to stimuli. It acts on the excitation–contraction coupling of muscle fibres and not at the level of the CNS. It appears to exert its action by decreasing the amount of calcium released from storage sites in the sarcoplasmic reticulum.

The beneficial effects of muscle relaxants are believed to come from their sedative effects rather than from direct muscle relaxation. The effects of muscle relaxants are relaxation of striated muscles, mild weakness of skeletal muscles, decreased force of muscle contraction, and muscle stiffness. Other drug effects that may be experienced are generalized CNS depression manifested as sedation, somnolence, ataxia, and respiratory and cardiovascular depression.

Indications

Muscle relaxants are used primarily for the relief of painful musculoskeletal conditions such as muscle spasms. They are most effective when used in conjunction with

DOSAGES	Benzodiazepines: Selected Hypnotic Drugs			
Drug	**Onset and Duration**	**Usual Dosage Range**		**Indications**
flurazepam hydrochloride (Apo-Flurazepam)	Long acting	*Adult* PO: 15–30 mg at bedtime		
lorazepam (Ativan)	Intermediate acting	*Adult* PO: 0.5 – 1 mg at bedtime		
nitrazepam (Nitrazadon)	Intermediate acting	*Adult* PO: 5–10 mg at bedtime		
oxazepam (Apo-Oxazepam)	Short acting	*Adult* PO: 15 mg, 30–60 min before bedtime		
▸▸temazepam (Restoril)	Intermediate acting	*Adult* PO: 15 mg at bedtime *Older adult* PO: 7.5 mg at bedtime		Insomnia
triazolam (Halcion)	Short acting	*Adult* PO: 0.125–0.25 mg at bedtime *Older adult* PO: 0.125–0.25 mg at bedtime		
▸▸zopiclone (Imovane, Rhovane)	Short acting	*Adult* PO: 5–7.5 mg at bedtime *Older adult* PO: 3.75 mg initial dose at bedtime, may be increased to 5 or 7.5 mg		

physical therapy. They may also be used in the management of spasticity associated with severe chronic disorders such as multiple sclerosis and other types of cerebral lesions, cerebral palsy, and rheumatic disorders. Some relaxants are used to reduce choreiform movement in patients with Huntington's chorea, to reduce rigidity in patients with parkinsonian syndrome, or to relieve the pain associated with trigeminal neuralgia. Intravenous dantrolene is used for the management of full-blown hypermetabolism of skeletal muscle that is characteristic of a malignant hyperthermia crisis. Baclofen has been shown to be effective in relieving hiccups.

Contraindications

The only usual contraindication to the use of muscle relaxants is known drug allergy, but severe kidney impairment may also be a contraindication.

Adverse Effects

The primary adverse effects of muscle relaxants are an extension of their effects on the CNS and skeletal muscles. Euphoria, lightheadedness, dizziness, drowsiness, fatigue, and muscle weakness are often experienced early in treatment. These adverse effects are generally short-lived, with patients growing tolerant to them over time. Less common adverse effects seen with muscle relaxants include diarrhea, gastrointestinal upset, headache, slurred speech, muscle stiffness, constipation, sexual problems in men, hypotension, tachycardia, and weight gain. Dantrolene has a strong potential to cause hepatotoxicity. However, this is rare, occurring in 0.1% to 0.2% of patients treated with the drug for more than 60 days.

Toxicity and Management of Overdose

The toxicities and consequences of an overdose of muscle relaxants involve primarily the CNS. There is no specific antidote or reversal drug for muscle relaxant overdoses. They are best treated with conservative supportive measures. More aggressive therapies are generally needed when muscle relaxants are taken along with other CNS-depressant drugs as an overdose. Gastric lavage and close observation of the patient are recommended. An adequate airway should be maintained and means of artificial respiration should be readily available. Electrocardiographic monitoring should be instituted, and large quantities of intravenous fluids should be administered to avoid crystalluria.

Interactions

When muscle relaxants are administered along with other depressant drugs such as alcohol and benzodiazepines, caution should be used to avoid overdosage. The combination of propoxyphene and orphenadrine has resulted in additive CNS effects. Mental confusion, anxiety, tremors, and additive hypoglycemic activity have been reported with this combination as well. A dosage reduction or discontinuance of one or both drugs is recommended.

Laboratory Test Interactions

A reducing substance in the urine of patients receiving methocarbonal may produce false-positive results for glucose determination using cupric sulfate (Benedict's solution, Clinitest, Fehling's solution) but does not interfere with glucose tests using glucose oxidase (Clinistix, Diastix, TesTape). Although these types of testing are somewhat outdated, they are still used in some patient care scenarios.

Dosages

For an overview of dosages for the more commonly used muscle relaxants see the Dosages table below.

DOSAGES　Selected Muscle Relaxants

Drug	Pharmacological Class	Usual Dosage Range	Indications
▸▸baclofen (Lioresal)	Central acting	*Adult* PO: 5 mg tid daily ×3 days, then 10 mg daily tid ×3 days, then 15 mg daily tid ×3 days, then 20 mg tid daily ×3 days, then titrated to response to max of 80 mg daily Intrathecal: 300–800 mcg/day maintenance	Spasticity
▸▸cyclobenzaprine hydrochloride (Novo-Cycloprine, Riva-Cycloprine)	Central acting	*Adult* PO: 5–10 mg tid	Acute musculoskeletal system spasticity
dantrolene sodium (Dantrium)	Direct acting	*Children* PO: 0.5 mg/kg/ bid/day up to 3 mg/kg/day given in divided doses bid–qid *Adult* PO: 25 mg/day; may increase to 25–100 mg bid–qid *Children/Adult* IV: 1 mg/kg, may repeat to total dose of 10 mg/kg	Chronic spasticity and malignant hyperthermia Malignant hyperthermia
tizanidine hydrochloride (Zanaflex)	Central acting	*Adult* PO: 2 mg increased by 2–4 mg to optimum effect up to 36 mg/day divided tid	Spasticity

DRUG PROFILES

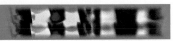

Muscle relaxants are all (except for dantrolene) centrally acting relaxants because of their site of action in the CNS. These include baclofen (Lioresal), cyclobenzaprine, methocarbamol (Robaxin), and orphenadrine citrate (Norflex). Use of all muscle relaxants is contraindicated in patients who have shown a hypersensitivity reaction to them or have compromised pulmonary function, active liver disease, or impaired myocardial function.

▶▶ *baclofen*

Baclofen (Lioresal) is available in 10 and 20 mg tablets and as a 0.5 and a 2 mg/mL concentration for intrathecal injection. To determine baclofen's optimum dosage individualized titration is required. The recommendation is to begin with a low oral dosage such as 5 mg 3 times a day for 3 days. It is then recommended that the dose be increased by 5 mg every 3 days until a maximum of 20 mg 3 times a day is reached. The total daily dose should not be greater than 80 mg. When the drug is given via the intrathecal route, a compatible pump must be implanted. With this administration route a test dose should be administered initially to test for a positive response. The injection is diluted before infusion. Baclofen is classified as pregnancy category C.

PHARMACOKINETICS

Half-Life	Onset	Peak	Duration
2–4 hr	0.5–1 hr	2 hr	> 8 hr

▶▶ *cyclobenzaprine hydrochloride*

Cyclobenzaprine hydrochloride (Novo-Cycloprine, Riva-Cycloprine) is available in a 10 mg dose. Cyclobenzaprine is a central-acting muscle relaxant that is structurally and pharmacologically related to the tricyclic antidepressants. The usual oral dosage is 10 mg 3 times daily for 1 week. Dosage can be increased to a maximum of 60 mg daily.

In the older adult and those with mild liver dysfunction, a dose of 5 mg 3 times daily is recommended. Cyclobenzaprine is recommended for use for short periods (2 to 3 weeks). It is classified as pregnancy category B.

PHARMACOKINETICS

Half-Life	Onset	Peak	Duration
1–3 days	1 hr	3–8 hr	12–24 hr

dantrolene sodium

Dantrolene sodium (Dantrium) is available in 25 and 100 mg capsules and as a 20 mg parenteral injection. Dantrolene is a direct-acting muscle relaxant that is pharmacologically different from the central-acting relaxants in that it can work directly on the skeletal muscles. It is important that the dosage is titrated and individualized. Dantrolene can be administered orally to children beginning with a dosage of 1 mg/kg/day in two divided doses; this dose can be titrated up to 3 mg/kg four times daily. The adult dosage begins with 25 mg once daily. In adults, dantrolene dosage can be increased to 25 to 100 mg 2 to 4 times daily when given orally. Malignant hyperthermia can occur on its own or as a complication of general anaesthesia. When dantrolene is given intravenously for an acute crisis of malignant hyperthermia, it is given at a dosage of 1 mg/kg and may be repeated until a total dose of 10 mg/kg has been given. Oral dantrolene may also be used for the prophylactic preoperative management of malignant hyperthermia in susceptible patients and for post-crisis follow-up management for those patients stabilized intravenously. Dantrolene is classified as pregnancy category C.

PHARMACOKINETICS

Half-Life	Onset	Peak	Duration
8 hr	0.5–1 hr	5 hr	12–24 hr

MISCELLANEOUS DRUGS

There are several other sedative–hypnotic medications that do not fall into the barbiturate or benzodiazepine drug class. These drugs include buspirone, chloral hydrate, tizanidine, and paraldehyde. These are all prescription-only drugs. Of these four sedative–hypnotic drugs, chloral hydrate and tizanidine are most commonly prescribed because paraldehyde is associated with severe adverse effects and is extremely toxic if taken inappropriately or in an overdose.

Chloral hydrate (Chlorinum, Chlorum) is one of the oldest nonbarbiturate, miscellaneous-category sedative–hypnotic drugs. It has the favourable characteristic of not suppressing REM sleep at the usual therapeutic doses, and the incidence of hangover effects associated with its use is low because of its relatively short duration of action. One potential disadvantage is that tachyphylaxis can develop rather quickly. **Tachyphylaxis** is the rapid appearance of a progressive decrease in response to a

pharmacologically or physiologically active substance after its repetitive administration. This makes chloral hydrate useful only for short-term therapy. High doses lead to dependence and cause gastrointestinal tract irritation. The combination of alcohol and chloral hydrate leads to rapid loss of consciousness. This combination is commonly referred to as a "Mickey Finn" because of its rapid "knockout" ability.

Tizanidine (Zanaflex) is a short-acting, centrally active α-adrenergic receptor agonist similar to clonidine. Tizanidine is a muscle relaxant but is not chemically classified with the other major drug categories in this chapter. It has been shown to reduce spastic muscle tone and decrease the frequency of daytime muscle spasms and night-time awakenings caused by spasms. It is indicated for increased muscle tone associated with spasticity. It has been used in Europe and Japan for over a decade and was recently approved for use in Canada. It is most commonly used in patients with multiple sclerosis or spinal cord injury. The typical starting dose is 2 mg. It is then slowly titrated by 2 to 4 mg steps to optimum effect, not to exceed 36 mg/day. Patients are less likely to suffer from hypotension and bradycardia when it is slowly titrated.

NURSING PROCESS

Assessment

Before administering any CNS-depressant drug, whether a barbiturate, benzodiazepine, muscle relaxant, non-benzodiazepine, or miscellaneous drug, the nurse needs to determine allergies and whether the patient has any conditions that would be contraindications or cautions to receiving the drug. The patient's mental status (mood, affect, level of consciousness, and memory) should be assessed and documented, because a lack of sleep itself may lead to confusion, mood changes, and restlessness. A sleep diary or journal with a description of the patient's sleep habits, patterns, and any related problems may be available and would provide insight into a patient's insomnia. The nurse must also assess the patient's vital signs, including supine and erect blood pressures, respirations, and temperature, especially if the intravenous use of any of these drugs is planned. For example, if an intravenous dosage form of any of these drugs is administered, a rapid drop could occur in blood pressure and other vital parameters such as respiratory rate, so administering the drug per protocol is critical to patient safety. Also, the drug may need to be withheld if the blood pressure and other vital signs are below normal limits and are unable to sustain further decreases. In addition, a neurological assessment should be performed and documented before initiation of therapy.

Cautions, contraindications, and drug interactions for barbiturates are as discussed earlier in the chapter. Other assessment data include kidney and liver function and lifespan considerations (e.g., because barbiturates rapidly cross the placenta and pass into breast milk; respiratory depression may be problematic in neonates during labour; withdrawal symptoms may appear in neonates born to women who have taken barbiturates during their last trimester). Barbiturates may produce paradoxical excitement in children and confusion and mental depression in the older adult, so baseline neurological assessment is needed.

Patients taking benzodiazepines and other chemically related drugs (benzodiazepine-like drugs) should be assessed for previous allergic reactions to these drugs. Cautious use with close monitoring of the patient's response to the drug and of vital signs is indicated in patients who are anemic, suicidal, and have a history of alcohol or other substance misuse. Cautious use is also indicated in the older adult and in those who are younger than the age of 18 years because of their increased sensitivity to these drugs, as well as in those who are pregnant or are lactating. In addition, before initiating drug therapy with the benzodiazepines and most other sedative–hypnotic drugs, the physician may order blood studies such as hematocrit, hemoglobin level, and red blood cell count. Tests of kidney function (blood urea nitrogen or creatinine levels) or liver function (alkaline phosphatase) may be ordered to rule out any potential problems from organ dysfunction, such as a decreased excretion capability with kidney dysfunction and decreased metabolic abilities with liver dysfunction. Lifespan assessment considerations regarding placental crossing and distribution of the drug into breast milk are similar to those for the barbiturates, and fetal abnormalities may occur if these drugs are used during the first trimester of pregnancy. Other assessment data related to lifespan include the possible reduction in drug dosage that may be needed for children and the older adult to avoid ataxia and excessive sedation. Potential drug interactions, discussed and presented in Table 13-7, need to be noted, as well as the fact that use of any other CNS-depressant drug may lead to severe decreases of blood pressure, respiratory rate, reflexes, and level of consciousness.

For muscle relaxants, drug allergies should also be noted before use. A head-to-toe assessment, with focus on the neurological system, should be completed. Cautions, contraindications, and drug interactions are as discussed earlier in the chapter under Muscle Relaxants. In the older adult, there is increased risk of CNS toxicity with possible hallucinations, confusion, and excessive sedation. Assessment associated with the use of miscellaneous drugs (e.g., chloral hydrate) includes taking a thorough health and medication history and examining the complete patient profile with associated laboratory studies. Cautions, contraindications, and drug interactions for miscellaneous drugs are as discussed earlier in the sections under Miscellaneous Drugs.

Nursing Diagnoses

- Impaired gas exchange related to the respiratory depression associated with CNS depressants
- Deficient knowledge related to inadequate information about the CNS-depressant drugs
- Disturbed sleep pattern related to the drug's interference with REM sleep
- Risk for injury and falls as related to drug-related decreased sensorium
- Risk for injury as related to possible drug overdose or adverse reactions related to drug–drug interactions (e.g., combined use of the drug with alcohol, tranquilizers, analgesics, or all three agents)
- Risk for injury, addiction, related to physical or psychological dependency on CNS drugs

Planning

Goals

- Patient will remain free of respiratory depression.
- Patient will remain free of further sleep deprivation.

- Patient will experience little or no rebound insomnia.
- Patient will remain free of injury and falls related to decreased sensorium.
- Patient will adhere to drug therapy and will keep follow-up appointments with the physician or other health care provider.
- Patient will regain normal sleep patterns.
- Patient will remain free of or experiences minimal adverse effects and toxic effects from sedative–hypnotic drugs, muscle relaxants, and other CNS depressants.
- Patient will remain free of drug interaction effects.
- Patient will experience no problems with addiction.

▮ Outcome Criteria

- Patient states the common adverse effects, toxic effects, and symptoms related to sedative–hypnotic drugs to be reported to the physician, such as drowsiness, confusion, and respiratory depression.
- Patient states ways to minimize injury and falls related to decreased sensorium, such as changing positions slowly.
- Patient states risk for REM interference from sedative–hypnotic drugs with associated sleep hangovers and uses nonpharmacological measures as appropriate.
- Patient states the common adverse effects related to muscle relaxants such as euphoria, dizziness, drowsiness, and fatigue.
- Patient minimizes adverse effects and toxic effects by taking medications as prescribed.
- Patient states the common drug interactions with alcohol and other medications (e.g., tranquilizers and analgesics) that may be life threatening.
- Patient states the importance of taking measures to minimize problems with addiction, such as taking medication only as needed.
- Patient, family, or significant other states the need to contact physician about possible complications, such as respiratory depression.
- Patient demonstrates increased knowledge related to inadequate information about pharmacological and nonpharmacological treatment and regimen for sleeping disturbance.

▨ Implementation

For management of sleep disorders, the benzodiazepines and nonbenzodiazepines are generally used because the barbiturates have a greater addiction potential and more CNS-depressant adverse effects. However, barbiturates may be indicated in specific situations. Short-acting barbiturates (e.g., secobarbital) should be given 15 to 30 minutes before bedtime, as should some of the intermediate-acting drugs (e.g., butabarbital). The longer-acting drugs such as phenobarbital have an onset of action of 60 minutes. Oral dosage forms are tolerated better when given with a light snack, crackers, or milk. Intramuscular injections should not be used unless absolutely

necessary. With phenobarbital, the intramuscular route may be ordered, but the injection must be into the lateral aspect of the thigh and into an adequate muscle mass.

Intravenous use requires dilution with normal saline (NaCl) and other recommended solutions. Rates of administration are important for safe use, and most of the drugs should not be administered any faster than 1 mg/kg/min with a maximum amount per minute. Guidelines for maximum amounts per minute are outlined in any authoritative drug source, such as a current drug handbook, or in the manufacturer's insert. Too rapid an infusion of a barbiturate may produce profound hypotension and marked respiratory depression. Should there be intravenous infiltration, the site may become red and tender, with tissue necrosis to follow. Some intravenous barbiturates have antidote protocols. With phenobarbital intravenous infiltration, 0.5% procaine solution should be injected into the affected area and moist heat applied. Protocol for management of intravenous infiltrations of a given drug should always be checked before intervening. Intravenous incompatibilities include amphotericin B, hydrocortisone, and hydromorphone, so these drugs should be given only after the intravenous line has been adequately flushed with NaCl. With intramuscular injection, the solution should be given deep into a large muscle mass to prevent tissue sloughing. However, this route should be avoided and used only when absolutely necessary. Administration of barbiturates also requires frequent CNS monitoring, with observation for level of consciousness, sedation, reflexes, and excessive drowsiness. Use of a bed alarm system or raising of side rails and assistance with ambulation are important for prevention of injury. If the patient is in the post-anaesthesia care unit or other hospital setting, the nurse should monitor blood pressure, pulse, and respiratory rate. Abrupt withdrawal of barbiturates after prolonged therapy may produce adverse effects ranging from nightmares, hallucinations, and delirium to seizures. In addition, while the patient is taking barbiturates it is important to monitor the patient's red blood cell count, hemoglobin, and hematocrit because of the possible adverse effect of anemia.

Long-term use of barbiturates also requires monitoring of therapeutic blood levels of the drug. For example, the level of phenobarbital should be 10 to 30 mcg/mL. Patients with serum levels above 40 mcg/mL may experience toxicity. Toxicity and overdosage are manifested by cold clammy skin, respiratory rate less than 12 breaths/min, and severe CNS depression.

Patients taking benzodiazepines may become sedated and sleepy, so safety precautions are important. If the patient is in the hospital setting, bed alarms should be used and side rails kept up (per hospital policy or physician's order), and assistance with ambulation should be provided. Safety at home should also be emphasized if any of the CNS-depressant drugs are used. In addition, dependence may be a problem with the benzodiazepines, but not to the same degree as with the barbiturates. While taking these drugs, patients should avoid driving or participating in any activities that require mental alertness. These drugs should be taken on an empty stomach for faster onset; however, this often results in gastrointestinal upset, so they can be taken with meals or a snack. Orally administered benzodiazepines have an onset of action of 30 minutes to 6 hours, depending on the drug (see the pharmacokinetics information in the Drug Profiles). These drugs should be given at the appropriate interval before bedtime to maximize the drug's effectiveness for sleep induction. In addition, it is crucial for patient adherence and safety to understand that drug tolerance may develop to many of the CNS-depressant drugs. This means that the body develops physiological tolerance to the drug so that larger dosages are required to produce the same therapeutic effect. Interrupting therapy helps to decrease such tolerance, not only with these drugs but with other drugs as well.

Most of the benzodiazepines (and other CNS depressants) actually interfere with REM sleep instead of aiding it. This is an important concept to understand because REM sleep is the restful and nurturing part of the sleep cycle. With REM interference, REM rebound may occur, especially if the drug is taken long term and withdrawn abruptly. REM rebound is manifested by vivid dreams and nightmares. Of the benzodiazepines, REM interference is less problematic with flurazepam, primarily because it produces fewer active metabolites. In addition, patients should be informed that REM interference and rebound may occur with just a 3- to 4-week regimen of drug therapy. To minimize REM interference, benzodiazepines and other drugs should be used only when nonpharmacological methods fail and should be used with caution in all patients with sleep disorders. Other recommendations include use of these drugs for the specific period associated with each drug class (e.g., some are to be used for only short periods). Gradual weaning-off periods are recommended with benzodiazepines and all CNS depressants. Hangover effects are also associated with many of the CNS depressants but occur less frequently with benzodiazepines and non-benzodiazepines than with barbiturates. The hangover effect is a residual drowsiness that results in impaired reaction times and occurs upon awakening. The intermediate- and long-acting hypnotics are often the culprits in this adverse effect. The nurse should also be vigilant to avoid medication errors arising from confusion of drug names (see Preventing Medication Errors: Sound-Alike/Look-Alike Benzodiazepines).

Muscle relaxants have indications different from those of the barbiturates and benzodiazepines and are not indicated for insomnia, unlike other sedative–hypnotic drugs. Toxicities associated with these drugs are usually treated with support measures to airway, breathing, and circulation. Early identification of toxicity is critical to prompt treatment and prevent respiratory and other CNS-depressant effects. Close monitoring of all vital parameters and level of consciousness is needed with use of these muscle relaxants, and assistance with ambulation, moving, and changing positions is needed to prevent syncope or dizziness. Purposeful and slow movements should be encouraged with these (and other) drugs. The greatest risk for hypotension is usually within 1 hour of dosing, so it is important for the patient to be more cautious with activity in this time frame.

The miscellaneous drug chloral hydrate should be given with fluids (e.g., 180 to 240 mL of water or juice). Capsule dosage forms should not be altered in any way and should be swallowed whole. Activities requiring mental alertness or driving a vehicle should be avoided while taking any of the miscellaneous drugs or the other CNS depressants discussed in this chapter. Gradual weaning off the drug is also recommended.

Nonbenzodiazepines should be taken for the prescribed time and with attention to any special instructions. As with any CNS-depressant drug, tasks requiring mental alertness should be avoided until the patient's response to the drug is known. Tolerance and dependence are possible with prolonged use, and no drug should be discontinued without gradual weaning.

Evaluation

Some of the criteria by which to confirm a patient's therapeutic response to a CNS depressant include an increased ability to sleep at night, fewer awakenings, shorter sleep induction time, few adverse effects such as hangover effects, and an improved sense of well-being

---

⊘ PREVENTING MEDICATION ERRORS

Sound-Alike/Look-Alike Benzodiazepines

Some benzodiazepines as well as most drug groups that are "sound alike/look alike" in nature are associated with medication errors. Assessing the drug order for the right drug is important in order to prevent this potential error as well as the negative consequences to the patient. Sound-alike benzodiazepine drugs that could be confused with other medications include the following:

- clonazepam and clonidine
- diazepam and ditropan
- lorazepam and alprazolam

Clonazepam is a highly potent anticonvulsant, muscle relaxant, and anxiolytic within the class of benzodiazepines. Clonidine is an antihypertensive.

because of improved sleep. Therapeutic effects related to muscle relaxants include decreased spasticity, reduction of choreiform movements in patients with Huntington's chorea, decreased rigidity in parkinsonian syndrome, and relief of pain from trigeminal neuralgia. The nurse must constantly watch for and document the occurrence

of any of the adverse effects of benzodiazepines, barbiturates, and muscle relaxants. See the previous discussion on adverse effects for each type of drug. Toxic effects to evaluate for with the CNS depressants may range from severe CNS depression of all body systems to respiratory and circulatory collapse.

BOX 13-1   Sleep Diaries and Nonpharmacological Treatment of Sleep Disorders

Information for a Sleep Diary

- What time do you usually go to bed and wake up?
- How long and how well do you sleep?
- When were you awake during the night and for how long?
- How easy was it to go to sleep?
- How easy was it to wake up in the morning?
- How much caffeine or alcohol do you consume?
- What time did you last eat or drink (if after dinner)?
- Did you have any bedtime snacks?
- What emotions or stressors are present?
- What medications do you take daily?
- Do you smoke? How much and for how long?
- Do you consume alcohol? How much and for how long?
- Do you take any over-the-counter drugs? If so, what drug and for what reason? How much and for how long?
- Do you take any natural health products? If so, which one? For what and for how long?

Nonpharmacological Sleep Interventions

- Establish a set sleep pattern with a time to go to bed at night and a regular time to get up in the morning and stick to it. This will help reset your internal clock.

- Sleep only as much as you need to feel refreshed and renewed. Too much sleep may lead to fragmented sleep patterns and shallow sleep.
- Keep the bedroom temperature moderate, if possible.
- Avoid caffeine-containing beverages and food within 6 hours of bedtime.
- Decrease exposure to loud noises.
- Avoid daytime napping.
- Avoid exercise late in the evening (i.e., not past 7 pm).
- Avoid alcohol in the evening. Rather than helping you sleep, it actually causes fragmented sleep.
- Avoid tobacco at bedtime because it disturbs sleep.
- Try to relax before bedtime with soft music, yoga, relaxation therapy, deep breathing, or light reading on a topic that is not intense or anxiety provoking.
- Drink a warm decaffeinated beverage, such as warm milk or chamomile tea, 30 minutes to 1 hour before bedtime.
- If you are still awake 20 minutes after going to bed, get up and engage in a relaxing activity (as noted previously) and go back to bed once you feel drowsy. Repeat as necessary.

PATIENT EDUCATION

- ❖ Patients should be encouraged to keep a journal of sleep habits and response to both drug and nondrug therapies (see Box 13-1).
- ❖ Patients should be encouraged to always try non-pharmacological measures first in an attempt to enhance sleep (see Box 13-1) because use of CNS depressants often leads to interference with the REM stage of sleep, hangover effects, and tolerance.
- ❖ Patients should be cautioned about the addictive qualities of the use of benzodiazepines.
- ❖ Patients should be informed to always check with the physician or pharmacist before taking any over-the-counter medications because of the many drug interactions associated with CNS depressants and, more specifically, with sedative–hypnotic drugs.
- ❖ Patients should be educated to keep all medications out of the reach of children.
- ❖ Patients should be informed to take the medication only as prescribed. Usually the patient is informed

that if one dose does not work, he or she is not to double up on the dosage unless otherwise prescribed or directed.
- ❖ Patients should be fully informed of time constraints related to driving, operating heavy machinery or equipment, and participating in activities requiring mental alertness while taking these medications.
- ❖ Patients should be informed that they should never stop taking these medications abruptly, to avoid possible withdrawal and rebound insomnia.
- ❖ Patients should be educated that sedative–hypnotic drugs (used for sleep) are not intended for long-term use because of their adverse effects, interference with REM sleep, and addictive properties.
- ❖ Patients should be warned that hangover effects may occur with most of these drugs and that this is more problematic in the older adult.
- ❖ Patients should be educated to avoid smoking in bed or when lounging.

POINTS TO REMEMBER

❖ Nonpharmacological measures for sleep disorders should always be tried before resorting to treatment with medications.

❖ Nurses should understand the classification and pharmacokinetic properties of barbiturates. The short-acting barbiturate is pentobarbital sodium.

❖ The pharmacokinetics of each group of barbiturates lends specific characteristics to the drugs in that group. The nurse also needs to understand how these drugs are absorbed orally and used parenterally, as well as their onset, peak, and duration of action. In addition, the life-threatening potential of these drugs should never be minimized by the nurse or other health care provider administering the drug(s) because too rapid an infusion may precipitate respiratory or cardiac arrest.

❖ Nursing interventions for barbiturates include careful consideration of parenteral injection with complete knowledge about incompatibilities with other drugs in solution as well as dilutional fluid incompatibilities.

❖ Most sedative–hypnotic drugs suppress REM sleep and should only be used for the recommended period. This time frame varies according to the specific drug used.

❖ Muscle relaxants are often used for the treatment of muscle spasms, spasticity, and rigidity. They result in varying levels of decreased sensorium and CNS depression depending on the specific drug, dosage, and route of administration. Nurses need to understand that even though muscle relaxants are discussed in this chapter, they are not used as sedative–hypnotic drugs.

EXAMINATION REVIEW QUESTIONS

1 Which of the following is an important nursing consideration regarding the administration of a benzodiazepine as a sedative–hypnotic drug?
 a. A benzodiazepine is intended for the long-term management of insomnia.
 b. A benzodiazepine should be used as a first choice for treatment of sleeplessness.
 c. Benzodiazepines can be administered safely with other CNS depressants for insomnia.
 d. The patient should be evaluated for the drowsiness that may occur the morning after a benzodiazepine is taken.

2 An older adult had been given a barbiturate for sleep induction, but the night nurse noted that the patient was awake most of the night, watching television and reading in bed. Which of the following options describes this type of reaction?
 a. An allergic reaction
 b. A teratogenic reaction
 c. A paradoxical reaction
 d. An idiopathic reaction

3 Which of the following interventions applies to the administration of a nonbenzodiazepine, such as buspirone?

 a. These drugs are less likely to interact with alcohol.
 b. These drugs are meant for long-term treatment of insomnia.
 c. Because of their rapid onset, they should be taken just before bedtime.
 d. The patient should be cautioned about the high incidence of morning drowsiness that may occur after taking these drugs.

4 In a patient taking a muscle relaxant, which adverse effect should the nurse monitor for?
 a. CNS depression
 b. Hypertension
 c. Peripheral edema
 d. Blurred vision

5 A patient on a cardiac medical-surgical unit is complaining of having difficulty sleeping. Which action should the nurse take first to address this problem?
 a. Administer a sedative–hypnotic drug if ordered.
 b. Offer tea made with the herbal preparation valerian.
 c. Provide an environment that is restful and reduce loud noises.
 d. Encourage the patient to exercise by walking up and down the hall a few times if tolerated.

For answers see http://evolve.elsevier.com/Canada/Lilley/pharmacology/.

CRITICAL THINKING ACTIVITIES

1 Explain the difference between a drug that is a sedative and a drug that is a hypnotic.

2 One of your patients has been told to discontinue the use of flurazepam, which she has been taking for about 1 year. The health care provider gave her no other instructions. As her home health nurse, does this cause you concern? Why, or why not?

3 a. A patient has undergone conscious sedation with benzodiazepine for a brief diagnostic procedure. What drug can be given to reverse the effects of the benzodiazepine? How is it administered?
 b. The patient woke up after the procedure, and vital signs have been stable. However, 3 hours after the procedure, the patient gradually becomes sleepy. Is this a concern, or is the patient just tired? What should the nurse expect to do at this time?

For answers see http://evolve.elsevier.com/Canada/Lilley/pharmacology/.

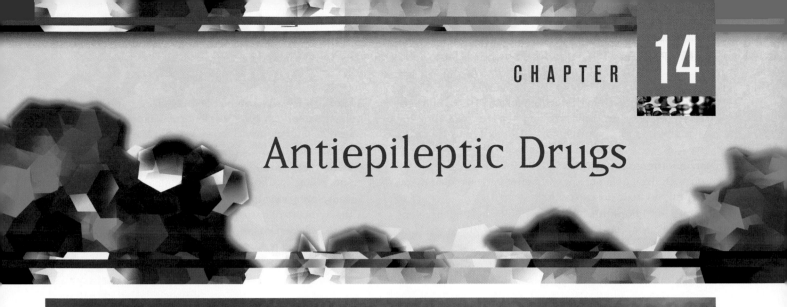

CHAPTER 14

Antiepileptic Drugs

Learning Objectives

After reading this chapter, the successful student will be able to do the following:

1 Discuss the rationale for the classes of antiepileptic drugs used in management of the different forms of epilepsy.

2 Identify the antiepileptic drugs within each of the following drug classes: iminostilbenes, benzodiazepines, barbiturates, hydantoins, and miscellaneous.

3 Identify the mechanisms of action, indications, cautions, contraindications, dosages, routes of administration, adverse effects, toxic effects, any related serum therapeutic levels, and drug interactions for the drugs within the different classifications of antiepileptic drugs.

4 Develop a collaborative plan of care, including patient education related to the nursing process for patients receiving antiepileptic drugs.

e-Learning Activities

Web site
(http://evolve.elsevier.com/Canada/Lilley/pharmacology/)

- Animations
- Answers to chapter questions, activities, and case studies
- Calculators and Category Catchers
- Glossary with audio pronunciations
- IV Therapy and Medication Error Checklists
- Multiple-Choice Review Question quizzes
- Nursing Care Plans
- Online Appendices and Supplements
- WebLinks

Drug Profiles

▸▸ **carbamazepine**, p. 263
▸▸ **gabapentin**, p. 263
    lamotrigine, p. 263
    levetiracetam, p. 263
    oxcarbazepine, p. 263
▸▸ **phenobarbital (phenobarbital sodium)***, p. 261
▸▸ **phenytoin (phenytoin sodium)***, p. 262
    pregabalin, p. 264
    topiramate, p. 264
▸▸ **valproic acid**, p. 262

▸▸ Key drug.

*Full generic name is given in parentheses. For the purposes of this text, the more common shortened name is used.

Glossary

Anticonvulsant A substance or procedure that prevents or reduces the severity of epileptic or other convulsive seizures. (p. 257)

Antiepileptic drug A substance that prevents or reduces the severity of epilepsy and different types of epileptic seizures, not just convulsive seizures. (p. 257)

Autoinduction A metabolic process that occurs when a drug increases its own metabolism over time, leading to lower than expected drug concentrations. (p. 263)

Convulsion A type of seizure involving excessive stimulation of neurons in the brain and characterized by the spasmodic contraction of voluntary muscles. (See also *seizure.*) (p. 256)

Epilepsy General term for any of a group of neurological disorders characterized by recurrent episodes of convulsive seizures, sensory disturbances, abnormal behaviour, loss of consciousness, or any combination of these. (p. 256)

International Classification of Seizures The most extensively used system of classifying seizures, including the symptoms and characteristics of each type of seizure. (p. 256)

Narrow therapeutic index (NTI) drugs Drugs that are characterized by a narrow difference between their therapeutic and toxic doses. (p. 261)

Primary or idiopathic epilepsy Epilepsy that develops without an apparent cause. More than 50% of cases of epilepsy are of unknown origin. (p. 256)

Secondary epilepsy Epilepsy that has a distinct cause (e.g., trauma). (p. 256)

Seizure Excessive stimulation of neurons in the brain leading to a sudden burst of abnormal neuron activity that results in temporary changes in brain function. (p. 256)

Status epilepticus A common seizure disorder characterized by generalized tonic–clonic convulsions that occur in succession. (p. 256)

Tonic–clonic seizure Formerly called *grand mal seizure*, this type of epilepsy is characterized by a series of generalized movements of tonic (stiffening) and clonic (rapid, synchronized jerking) muscular contraction. (p. 256)

Unclassified seizures Seizures that are not described by any of the seizure classifications. (p. 256)

EPILEPSY

A seizure disorder, or what is more commonly referred to as *epilepsy*, is not as specific a disease as, say, cancer or diabetes. It is a broad syndrome of central nervous system (CNS) dysfunction that can manifest in many ways, from momentary sensory disturbances to convulsive seizures. More likely, it involves the generation of excessive electrical discharges from nerves located in the area of the brain known as the *cerebral cortex*.

The terms *convulsion, seizure,* and *epilepsy* are often used interchangeably, but they do not have the same meaning. A **seizure** is a brief episode of abnormal electrical activity in the nerve cells of the brain. A **convulsion** is characterized by involuntary spasmodic contractions of any or all voluntary muscles throughout the body, including skeletal and facial muscles. **Epilepsy** is a chronic, recurrent pattern of seizures. These excessive electrical discharges can often be detected by an electroencephalogram (EEG), which is commonly obtained to help diagnose epilepsy. Other diagnostic aids that are helpful in the diagnosis of epilepsy are computed tomography (CT) and magnetic resonance imaging (MRI). The information yielded by these diagnostic aids in conjunction with the common symptoms of the particular seizure disorder help establish the diagnosis. In particularly severe cases, patients may be observed in a hospital setting or sleep study laboratory with continuous EEG and video monitoring to determine detailed patterns of seizure activity in hopes of tailoring an effective treatment. Commonly reported symptoms are abnormal motor function, loss of consciousness, altered sensory awareness, and psychic changes.

The cause of more than 50% of the cases of epilepsy is unknown. That type of epilepsy for which a cause cannot be identified is called **primary** or **idiopathic epilepsy.** Other types of epilepsy have a distinct cause such as trauma, infection, cerebrovascular disorder, or other illness. These types of epilepsy are termed **secondary epilepsy.** The chief causes of secondary epilepsy in children and infants are developmental defects, metabolic disease, or injury at birth. Acquired brain disorder is the major cause of secondary epilepsy in adults. Some examples are head injury, disease or infection of the brain and spinal cord, stroke, metabolic disorder, a primary or metastatic brain tumour, or some other recognizable neurological disease. Interestingly, among all age groups, the older adult has the highest incidence of new-onset epilepsy. Fortunately, seizures in the older adult are often well controlled with drug therapy. The accurate diagnosis of a seizure disorder requires careful patient observation, a reliable patient history, and an EEG. Other diagnostic tests often used in revealing structural lesions of the CNS as the cause of the seizure disorder are CT and MRI (which are superior to the clinical examination) and routine skull radiographs. Between the MRI and CT, MRI is more sensitive than CT and is now preferred in the evaluation of a patient with seizures.

Seizures can be classified into distinct categories based on their characteristics. In traditional classifications, seizures were categorized as grand mal seizures **(tonic–clonic seizures),** petit mal seizures, Jacksonian epilepsy, and psychomotor attacks. Currently, the **International Classification of Seizures** involves a more systematic approach that divides seizures into two main types: partial and generalized. This system is more extensively used because it more adequately describes the symptoms and characteristics of each type of seizures (Box 14-1). Under this new nomenclature, two other classifications of seizures also exist: status epilepticus and unclassified. **Status epilepticus** seizures begin as either partial or generalized seizures and become status epilepticus when there is no recovery between attacks. **Unclassified seizures** are those that do not clearly fit into any of the other categories. It should also be noted that seizure episodes can sometimes start off as partial and then become generalized. If the partial component is not noticed, the patient may be given drug therapy that is more suitable for generalized seizures and possibly not receive optimal treatment.

Seizure activity is characterized by paroxysmal, hypersynchronous excessive electrical neuronal discharges in the neurons of the cerebral cortex. A seizure occurs as a

BOX 14-1   International Classification of Seizures

I. Partial Seizures (seizures begin locally)

Description

Short alterations in consciousness, repetitive unusual movements (chewing or swallowing movements), psychological changes, and confusion occur.

A. Simple Partial Seizures (without impairment of consciousness)

- Symptoms determined by the brain region involved
- Discrete motor symptoms (most commonly face, arm, or leg)
- Hallucinations of sight, hearing, or taste along with somatosensory changes (tingling)
- Autonomic nervous system responses such as nausea, flushing, salivation, or urinary incontinence
- Personality changes
- Seizures last for 20 to 60 seconds

B. Complex Partial Seizures (with impairment of consciousness)

- Memory impairment
- Behavioural effects such as random walking, mumbling, head turning, or pulling at clothing
- Repetitive, purposeless behaviours (lip smacking, hand wringing) called automatisms

- Aura, chewing and swallowing movements, unreal feelings, bizarre behaviour
- Tonic, clonic, or tonic–clonic seizures
- Seizures last 45 to 90 seconds

II. Generalized Seizures

Description

These seizures are most often seen in children and commonly characterized by temporary lapses in consciousness lasting a few seconds. Staring off into space, daydreaming, and inattentive look are common symptoms. Patients may exhibit rhythmic movements of their eyes, head, or hands but do not convulse. They may have several attacks per day.

- Both cerebral hemispheres involved
- Tonic, clonic, myoclonic, atonic, or tonic–clonic seizures and infantile spasms possible
- Brief loss of consciousness for a few seconds with no confusion
- Head drop or falling-down symptoms

III. Unclassified seizures

IV. Status epilepticus

result of changes in the excitation of a single neuron or a network of cortical neurons. The clinical manifestations depend on the area of excitability, the degree of irritability of the surrounding area, and the intensity of the impulse. For example, if the affected cortical network is in the visual cortex, the clinical manifestations are visual phenomena. Other affected areas of primary cortex give rise to sensory, gustatory, or motor manifestations.

ANTIEPILEPTIC DRUGS

Antiepileptic drugs (or antiepileptics) are also called anticonvulsants. The term **antiepileptic drugs** (or antiepileptics) is a more appropriate term because many of these medications are indicated for the management of all types of epilepsy, not just with convulsions. **Anticonvulsants,** by contrast, are medications used to prevent the seizures typically associated with epilepsy. In practice, however, there is significant overlap between these two terms, and both are often used interchangeably.

The combined goal of antiepileptic drug therapy is to control or prevent seizures while maintaining a reasonable quality of life. Approximately 70% of patients can expect to become seizure-free with modern drug therapy, and most will only take one antiepileptic drug. The remaining 30% of cases are more complicated, often requiring additional medications. Many antiepileptic drugs have adverse effects, and balancing seizure control with adverse effects is often a difficult task. In most

cases, the therapeutic goal is not to eliminate seizure activity but rather to maximally reduce the incidence of seizures as much as possible while minimizing drug-induced toxicity. Many patients must take antiepileptic drugs for their entire lives. Treatment may eventually be stopped in some patients, but others will suffer repeated seizures if constant levels of antiepileptic drugs are not maintained in their blood. In both children and adults there is only a 40% chance of recurrence after the first partial or generalized seizure; therefore, many physicians choose not to initiate treatment after the first seizure. However, it is the consensus that antiepileptic drug therapy should be implemented in patients who have had two or more seizures.

There are several antiepileptic drugs available, and most seizure disorders can be controlled with their use. Sometimes, a combination of drugs must be used to control the disorder. To optimize drug selection for each patient, neurologists consider the efficacy of the drug for seizure types, adverse effect profile, likelihood of drug interactions, cost, ease of use, and availability of child dosage forms. In addition, a number of antiepileptic drugs are also used for other types of illnesses, including psychiatric disorders, migraine headaches, and neuropathic pain syndromes. Generally, single-drug therapy must fail before two-drug and then multiple-drug therapy is implemented. A patient should always be started on a single antiepileptic drug and the dosage slowly increased until the seizures are controlled or until clinical toxicity occurs. If the first antiepileptic drug does not work, the drug should be tapered slowly while a second antiepileptic drug is introduced. Antiepileptic drugs should never be stopped abruptly unless a severe adverse effect occurs. Although it is sometimes difficult to control a patient's seizures using a single antiepileptic drug monotherapy is likely to result in higher serum drug concentrations, fewer adverse effects, and better control.

Serum drug concentrations are useful guidelines in assessing the effectiveness of therapy. They should, however, be only guidelines. Maintaining serum drug levels within therapeutic ranges helps to not only control seizures but also reduce adverse effects. There are established normal therapeutic ranges for many antiepileptic drugs, but these are useful only as guidelines. Each patient should be monitored individually and the dosages adjusted on the basis of the individual case. Many patients are maintained successfully below or above the usual therapeutic range. The goal should be to slowly titrate to the lowest effective serum drug level that controls the seizure disorder. This decreases the risk for medication-induced adverse effects and interactions. The serum concentrations of phenytoin, phenobarbital, carbamazepine, and primidone correlate better with seizure control and toxicity than do those of valproic acid, ethosuximide, and clonazepam. Emphasis should be placed primarily on the clinical symptoms and patient's history rather than on strict adherence to established drug concentration ranges.

There are six traditional classes of antiepileptic drugs, and many new drugs have been marketed. These newer drugs were developed with the goal of eliminating many of the drug interactions and adverse effects associated with the older drugs. There is current debate in the literature as to whether patients benefit more from newer drugs than from older drugs. Prescribers must consider all pertinent nuances of the drugs used and the patient. Some newer antiepileptic drugs may be less likely than older drugs to cause undesirable drug interactions. This may especially benefit older adults, who are more likely to be on multiple medications and thus more prone to drug interactions. Successful control of a seizure disorder hinges on selecting the appropriate drug class and drug dosage, the patient adhering to the treatment regimen, and limiting toxicity.

The underlying cause of most cases of epilepsy is an excessive electrical discharge from abnormally functioning nerve cells (neurons) within the CNS. Therefore, the object of antiepileptic drug therapy is to prevent the generation and spread of these excessive discharges while simultaneously protecting surrounding normal cells.

Mechanism of Action and Drug Effects

As with many classes of drugs, the exact mechanism of action of the antiepileptic drugs is not known with certainty. However, strong evidence shows that they alter the movement of sodium, potassium, calcium, and magnesium ions. The changes in the movement of these ions induced by antiepileptic drugs result in stabilized and less responsive cell membranes. This ion theory may explain how antiepileptic drugs decrease the excitability and responsiveness of brain neurons (nerve cells).

Theoretically, the primary pharmacological effects of antiepileptic drugs are threefold. First, they increase the threshold of activity in the brain motor cortex. In other words, they make it more difficult for a nerve to be excited or they reduce the nerve's response to incoming electrical or chemical stimulation. Second, they act to depress or limit the spread of a seizure discharge from its origin. They do this by suppressing the transmission of impulses from one nerve to the next. Third, they can decrease the speed of nerve impulse conduction within a given neuron. Antiepileptic drugs may also have effects on the neuron, indirectly affecting the area in the brain responsible for the problem by altering, for instance, the blood supply to that area. However, the overall effect is that antiepileptic drugs stabilize neurons and keep them from becoming hyperexcited and generating excessive nerve impulses to adjacent neurons.

Indications

The major therapeutic indication for antiepileptic drugs is the prevention or control of seizure activity. They are especially useful for maintenance therapy in patients with the chronic recurring seizures commonly associated with epilepsy. As evidenced by the wide range of seizure disorders listed in Box 14-1, epilepsy is a diverse disorder. Consequently, no one drug can control all types of epilepsy. Although the understanding of epilepsy is still growing, there is some understanding of the primary causes of many of the seizure disorders. Each involves a distinct area of dysfunction and has certain characteristics that make particular drugs more effective than others in treating it. Therefore, specific drugs are indicated for the control of specific seizures. Some of the antiepileptic drugs and the seizure disorders they are used to treat are listed in Table 14-1.

Antiepileptic drugs are chiefly used for the long-term maintenance treatment of epilepsy. However, antiepileptic drugs are also useful for the acute treatment of convulsions and status epilepticus. Status epilepticus is a common seizure disorder that is a life-threatening emergency; it is characterized by generalized tonic–clonic convulsions that occur in succession. Affected patients typically do not regain consciousness between the many convulsions. Hypotension, hypoxia, and cardiac dysrhythmias complicate the disorder, and brain damage and death quickly ensue if prompt, appropriate therapy is not started. Therapy is typically diazepam or lorazepam, considered first-line anticonvulsant medications by the Canadian Pediatric Society. The Canadian Pediatric

TABLE 14-1

Antiepileptic Drugs of Choice

Simple	Complex	GTC	Absence	Myoclonic	Clonic	Tonic	Atonic
FIRST CHOICE							
carbamazepine	carbamazepine	carbamazepine	ethosuximide	valproic acid	valproic acid	valproic acid	valproic acid
phenobarbital	phenobarbital	phenobarbital	phenobarbital				
phenytoin	phenytoin	phenytoin	valproic acid				
primidone	primidone	primidone					
valproic acid	valproic acid	valproic acid					
SECOND CHOICE							
clonazepam	clonazepam	clonazepam	acetazolamide	clonazepam	clonazepam	clonazepam	clonazepam
levetiracetam	pregabalin	oxcarbazepine	clonazepam	lamotrigine	lamotrigine	topiramate	lamotrigine
clorazepate	tiagabine	levetiracetam		topiramate	topiramate	oxcarbazepine	levetiracetam
lamotrigine	clorazepate	lamotrigine				clonazepam	topiramate
topiramate	lamotrigine	topiramate				lamotrigine	
oxcarbazepine	topiramate					levetiracetam	
	oxcarbazepine					phenytoin	

GTC, Generalized tonic–clonic

TABLE 14-2

Antiepileptic Drugs Used for Treatment of Status Epilepticus

Drug	Dose (mg/kg)	Onset	Duration	Half-Life	Adverse Effects
diazepam	0.3–0.5 (less than 30 mg)	3–10 min	Minutes	35 hr	Apnea, hypotension, somnolence
fosphenytoin	(75 mg IV fosphenytoin = 50 mg phenytoin)	15–30 min	12–24 hr	12–30 hr	Comparable to phenytoin (see below)
lorazepam	0.05–0.1	1–20 min	Hours	12–15 hr	Apnea, hypotension, somnolence
phenobarbital	10–20	10–30 min	4–10 hr	53–140 hr	Apnea, hypotension, somnolence
phenytoin	15–20	5–30 min	12–24 hr	10–60 hr	Cardiac dysrhythmias, hypotension

Society also recommends the use of longer-acting phenytoin for children in status epilepticus who will require long-term anticonvulsant therapy but are not already on it. Other drugs useful for the treatment of status epilepticus are listed in Table 14-2.

Once status epilepticus is controlled, long-term drug therapy is started with other drugs for the prevention of future seizures. Patients who undergo brain surgery or who have suffered severe head injuries may receive prophylactic antiepileptic drug therapy. These patients are at high risk for acquiring a seizure disorder and often severe complications will arise if seizures are not controlled.

Contraindications

The only usual contraindication to antiepileptic drugs is known drug allergy. Pregnancy is also a common contraindication, but the prescriber must consider the risks to mother and infant of untreated maternal epilepsy and the increased risks for seizure activity.

Adverse Effects

Antiepileptic drugs are plagued by many adverse effects, which often limit their usefulness. Drugs must be withdrawn from many patients because of some of these effects. In addition, although some medications are safer than others, antiepileptic drugs do appear to be responsible for many birth defects in the offspring of epileptic women. Each antiepileptic drug is associated with its own diverse set of adverse effects, which makes it difficult to categorize all of the classes of antiepileptic drugs according to their common adverse effects. The antiepileptic drugs and their most common adverse effects are listed in Table 14-3.

Interactions

The drug interactions that can occur with the antiepileptic drugs are many and varied, and these are summarized in Table 14-4. Significant drug interactions for selected drugs are also listed in Table 14-4.

TABLE   14-3

Adverse Effects of Antiepileptic Drugs

Drug or Drug Class	Adverse Effects
Barbiturates	**CNS:** Drowsiness, dizziness, lethargy, paradoxical restlessness, excitement
	Gastrointestinal: Nausea, vomiting
	Other: Rash, Stevens–Johnson syndrome, urticaria
carbamazepine	**Heart:** Dysrhythmias, heart failure
	Hematological: Bone marrow suppression (aplastic anemia, agranulocytosis, thrombocytopenia)
	Integumentary: Exfoliative dermatitis, erythema multiforme, Stevens–Johnson syndrome
	Other: Thrombophlebitis, vision and hearing disturbances, acute urinary retention, dyspnea, pneumonitis, pneumonia
divalproex (valproic acid)	**Children:** Fever, purpura, nervousness, somnolence
	Hematological: Thrombocytopenia
	Other: Pancreatitis, irregular menses, secondary amenorrhea, galactorrhea, rare breast enlargement, weight gain
gabapentin	Dizziness, somnolence, peripheral edema, NVD, visual changes
Hydantoins	**Cardiovascular:** Dysrhythmias, hypotension
	Hematological: Bone marrow suppression (agranulocytosis, thrombocytopenia, megaloblastic anemia)
	Integumentary: Exfoliative dermatitis, lupus erythematosus, Stevens–Johnson syndrome
	Other: Neuropathies, gingival hyperplasia
lamotrigine	Headache, dizziness, somnolence, rash, nausea, rhinitis, pharyngitis, diplopia, fever
levetiracetam	Somnolence, headache, dizziness, asthenia, pharyngitis
oxcarbazepine	Headache, dizziness, somnolence, NVD, fatigue, visual changes
pregabalin	Dizziness, somnolence, dry mouth, edema, blurred vision, weight gain, difficulty concentrating
topiramate	**Integumentary:** Dermatitis, rash, alopecia
	Other: Cognitive impairment, fatigue or somnolence, anorexia

CNS, central nervous system; *NVD,* nausea, vomiting, diarrhea.

TABLE   14-4

Drug Interactions of Selected Antiepileptic Drugs

Drug or Drug Class	Mechanism	Results
CARBAMAZEPINE		
Bone marrow depressants	Additive effect	Increased bone marrow toxicity
doxycycline, phenytoin, theophylline, warfarin	Alters metabolism	Significant decrease in half-life
Grapefruit juice	Inhibits liver enzymes	Increased carbamazepine levels
DIVALPROEX (valproic acid)		
Barbiturates	Additive effect	Increased CNS depression
clonazepam	Not determined	May produce absence status
phenytoin	Not determined	May produce breakthrough seizures
GABAPENTIN		
Antacids		Reduced gabapentin absorption
cimetidine, hydrocodone, morphine		Increased gabapentin levels
pregabalin		None reported to date
HYDANTOINS		
disulfiram, isoniazid, valproic acid	Inhibits liver enzymes	Increased hydantoin levels
Tricyclic antidepressants	Not determined	Possible seizures
LAMOTRIGINE		
acetaminophen, carbamazepine, oral contraceptives, progestins, oxcarbazepine, phenytoin	Uncertain	Reduced lamotrigine levels
valproic acid	Uncertain	Increased lamotrigine levels
OXCARBAZEPINE		
phenytoin, phenobarbital	Uncertain	Reduced oxcarbazepine levels and increased phenytoin/phenobarbital levels
TOPIRAMATE		
Alcohol	Synergism	Increased CNS depression
carbamazepine, phenytoin, valproic acid	Enzymatic induction	Reduced topiramate levels
digoxin	Uncertain	Reduced digoxin levels
metformin	Uncertain	Increased topiramate and metformin levels
Oral contraceptives (OC), estrogens	Uncertain	Reduced OC/estrogen levels

TABLE 14-5

Therapeutic Plasma Levels of NTI Antiepileptic Drugs

Antiepileptic Drug	Therapeutic Plasma Level (mmol/L)
carbamazepine	17–50
clonazepam	40–230
divalproex	350–690
ethosuximide	280–710
phenobarbital	65–170
phenytoin	40–80
primidone	23–55
valproic acid	350–700

NTI, narrow therapeutic index.

Dosages

With certain antiepileptic drugs, the safe and toxic levels are close. Drugs that have a narrow difference between safe and toxic levels are called **narrow therapeutic index (NTI) drugs.** Table 14-5 lists the antiepileptic drugs that require monitoring of therapeutic plasma levels and their corresponding therapeutic levels. For an overview of dosages, see the Dosages table on p. 264.

It is important for the safe use of the various classes of drugs used in the management of seizure disorders that the nurse understands the nursing process. The discussion in this chapter focuses on the different groups of the barbiturates, benzodiazepines, and hydantoins. Some of these antiepileptic drugs, such as the barbiturates and benzodiazepines, are also discussed with the sedative–hypnotic drugs (Chapter 13).

DRUG PROFILES

All antiepileptic drugs are prescription-only drugs. These drugs are associated with many characteristics that make it undesirable for patients to take them without the supervision of a qualified medical specialist. They are available in many oral, injectable, and rectal formulations. The U.S. Food and Drug Administration (FDA) uses a pregnancy risk classification of antiepileptic drugs, summarized in Table 14.6. As Canada has no comparable list, the U.S. FDA classifications are also used as a reference guide.

In most children and adults, epilepsy can be controlled with a first-line antiepileptic drug such as carbamazepine, ethosuximide, phenobarbital, primidone, phenytoin, or valproic acid. For patients who do not respond to the first-line antiepileptic drugs, there are a number of second-line antiepileptic drugs that are used occasionally, such as the benzodiazepines, clonazepam, clorazepate; methsuximide; and acetazolamide. These are often used as first-line drugs for status epilepticus.

After valproic acid was introduced in 1978, no major new drugs for the treatment of epilepsy were introduced in Canada until the 1990s. Gabapentin and lamotrigine were approved during this decade. Gabapentin and lamotrigine are primarily used as add-on drugs in adults who have partial seizures alone or with secondary generalized seizures.

Antiepileptic drugs that have more recently been approved are levetiracetam (Keppra), topiramate (Topamax), and pregabalin (Lyrica). These drugs fall under the miscellaneous category of antiepileptic drugs and have greatly expanded the options currently available to patients with seizure disorders. Dosage, pregnancy category, and specific indication information appears in the corresponding table. The following general information applies to most antiepileptic drugs as a group. If a given drug is to be replaced with another antiepileptic drug, the prescriber will often recommend gradual tapering off of the first drug and gradual tapering up of the new one. For those drugs available in both tablet and suspension forms, switching from tablet to suspension will often result in more frequent, but smaller, doses for an equivalent total daily dose. Extended-release forms are usually given in one to two divided daily doses. These dosage forms normally should not be crushed. In contrast, immediate-release tablets can usually be crushed, but neither of these rules is absolute. Check with a pharmacist when in doubt.

BARBITURATES

▶▶ *phenobarbital sodium*

Originally, two of the most commonly used antiepileptic drugs were the barbiturates phenobarbital and primidone. Primidone is metabolized in the liver to phenobarbital and phenylethylmalonamide, both of which have anticonvulsant properties. Phenobarbital has been used since 1912, principally for controlling tonic–clonic and partial seizures. Phenobarbital is still one of the first-line drugs for the management of status epilepticus and is an effective prophylactic drug for the control of febrile seizures. Although the use of phenobarbital for seizure emergencies is still common even in the more advanced societies, its use by the oral route for seizure prevention is much less so. However, in developing countries, oral phenobarbital is often the drug of choice for routine seizure prophylaxis because of its significantly lower cost than that of the newer antiepileptic drugs more common in developed countries. By far, the most common adverse effect is sedation, but tolerance to this effect usually develops with continued therapy. In children the most common adverse effects are irritability, hyperactivity, depression, sleep disorders, and cognitive abnormalities. Therapeutic effects are generally seen at serum drug levels of 15 to 40 mcg/mL. It interacts with many drugs because it is a major "inducer" of liver enzymes, causing more rapid clearance of some drugs. Its major advantage is that it has the longest half-life of all the standard antiepileptic drugs, which allows for once-a-day dosing. This can be a substantial advantage for patients who have a hard time remembering to take their medication or for those who have erratic schedules. A patient may take a dose 12 or even 24 hours too late and still have therapeutic blood levels at that time. In addition,

Continued

DRUG PROFILES (cont'd)

phenobarbital is the most inexpensive antiepileptic drug, costing only pennies a day compared with several dollars a day for other antiepileptic drugs.

PHARMACOKINETICS

Half-Life	Onset	Peak	Duration
PO: 53–118 hr	PO: 20–60 min	PO: 8–12 hr	PO: 6–12 hr

HYDANTOINS

▶▶ phenytoin sodium

Phenytoin sodium (Dilantin) has been used as a first-line antiepileptic drug for many years. It is primarily indicated for the management of tonic–clonic and partial seizures. The most common adverse effects are lethargy, abnormal movements, mental confusion, and cognitive changes. Therapeutic drug levels are usually 40–80 μmol/L. At toxic levels, phenytoin can cause nystagmus, ataxia, dysarthria, and encephalopathy. Long-term phenytoin therapy can cause gingival hyperplasia, acne, hirsutism, and hypertrophy of subcutaneous facial tissue, resulting in an appearance known as "Dilantin facies." Scrupulous dental care can help to prevent gingival hypertrophy. Another long-term consequence of phenytoin therapy is osteoporosis. Vitamin D therapy may be necessary to prevent this, particularly in women. Phenytoin can interact with other medications, for two main reasons. First, it is highly bound to plasma proteins and competes with other highly protein-bound medications for binding sites. Second, it induces liver microsomal enzymes, primarily the cytochrome P450 system, thereby increasing the metabolism of other drugs and decreasing their levels.

Exaggerated phenytoin effects can be seen in patients with low serum albumin concentrations. This scenario is most commonly seen in patients who are malnourished or have chronic kidney failure. In these patients, it may be necessary to maintain phenytoin levels well below 80 μmol/L. With lower levels of albumin in a patient's body, more free, unbound, pharmacologically active phenytoin will be present. Phenytoin has many advantages from the standpoint of long-term therapy. It is usually well tolerated, highly effective, and relatively inexpensive. It can also be given intravenously if needed. Phenytoin's long half-life allows it to be given only twice a day, and in some cases once a day. As stressed earlier, adherence to antiepileptic drug treatment is important to seizure control. If a patient has to remember to take medication only once or twice a day, adherence will be increased and thus the likelihood of therapeutic drug levels being reached is increased, leading to better seizure control.

Parenteral phenytoin is adjusted chemically to a pH of 12 for drug stability. It is irritating to veins when injected and should be given slowly (not exceeding 50 mg/min in adults), directly into a large vein through a large-gauge needle (or needleless system, preferably larger than 20 gauge) or intravenous (IV) catheter. Each injection should be followed by an injection of sterile saline through the same needle or intravenous catheter to avoid local venous irritation caused by the alkalinity of the solution. Continuous infusion should be avoided.

Soft-tissue irritation and inflammation can occur at the site of injection with and without extravasation of intravenous phenytoin. Soft-tissue irritation may vary from slight tenderness to extensive necrosis, sloughing, and, in rare instances, amputation. Improper administration, including subcutaneous (SC) or perivascular injection, should be avoided to help prevent these occurrences. Local irritation, inflammation, tenderness, necrosis, and sloughing have been reported with or without extravasation of intravenous phenytoin.

Fosphenytoin (Cerebyx) was developed in an attempt to overcome some of the physical shortcomings of phenytoin sodium. Fosphenytoin is a water-soluble, phosphorylated phenytoin derivative that can be given intramuscularly or intravenously without causing the burning on injection associated with phenytoin. Fosphenytoin is dosed in phenytoin equivalents (PE) as indicated in Table 14-7. The conversion factor is as follows: 1.5 mg of fosphenytoin is equivalent to 1 mg of phenytoin. Therefore, for a patient requiring a 100 mg injection dose of phenytoin, 150 mg would be the correct dose of fosphenytoin. Concentrations for IV dosages range from 1.5 to 25 mg phenytoin equivalent (PE)/mL and at a rate of 150 mg PE/min or less to avoid hypotension or cardiorespiratory depression. Should arrhythmias or hypotension occur, the infusion should be discontinued. Safety measures are to be implemented post-infusion because of ataxia and dizziness, and vital signs should be taken consistently up to 2 hours after infusion. Fosphenytoin (Cerebyx) should not be confused with Celebrex. Intravenous incompatabilities are numerous, so always check for in-syringe and in-solution incompatibilities (as is the case with any intravenously administered drug) (see Table 14-7).

PHARMACOKINETICS

Half-Life	Onset	Peak	Duration
7–42 hr	2–24 hr	1.5–3 hr	6–12 hr

▶▶ valproic acid

Valproic acid (Apo-Valproic, Depakene, Divalproex, Epival ECT, others) is used primarily in the treatment of generalized seizures (absence, myoclonic, and tonic–clonic). It has also been shown to be effective for controlling partial seizures. It is indicated for the management of manic episodes associated with bipolar disorder. The main adverse effects are drowsiness; nausea, vomiting, and other gastrointestinal disturbances; tremor; weight gain; and transient hair loss. The most serious adverse effects, hepatotoxicity and pancreatitis, can be fatal. Valproic acid can interact with many medications primarily because of protein binding and liver metabolism. Valproic acid is highly bound to plasma proteins and competes with other highly protein-bound medications for binding sites. It is also highly metabolized by liver microsomal enzymes and competes for metabolism. This drug is available in both oral and injectable forms.

PHARMACOKINETICS

Half-Life	Onset	Peak	Duration
6–16 hr	15–30 min	1–4 hr	4–6 hr

Continued

DRUG PROFILES (cont'd)

IMINOSTILBENES

▶▶ carbamazepine

Carbamazepine (Mazepine, Tegetrol, others) is the second most commonly prescribed antiepileptic drug in Canada, after phenytoin. It was marketed in the late 1960s for the treatment of epilepsy in adults after its efficacy and safety for the treatment of trigeminal neuralgia were proved. It was granted approval for use in children in 1976. It is chemically related to the tricyclic antidepressants and is considered a first-line antiepileptic drug for the treatment of simple partial, complex partial, and generalized tonic–clonic seizures. It is also used as montherapy or as an adjunct to lithium in the management of acute mania or prophylaxis management of bipolar disorders in patients who may be resistant to the tradional antimania drugs. It is contraindicated in patients with absence and myoclonic seizures and those who have shown previous hypersensitivity to the drug. Carbamazepine is available in numerous oral forms including a suspension, chewable tablet, and extended-release tablets. The typical therapeutic serum carbamazepine drug level is 17 to 50 µmol/mL, but as with all antiepileptic drugs, the therapeutic concentrations should be used only as a guideline. Carbamazepine is metabolized to carbamazepine epoxide, which has both anticonvulsant and toxic effects. Carbamazepine undergoes **autoinduction,** the process whereby a drug increases its own metabolism over time, leading to lower than expected drug concentrations. With carbamazepine this process usually occurs within the first 2 months after the start of therapy.

PHARMACOKINETICS

Half-Life	Onset	Peak	Duration
14–16 hr	Slow	2–24 hr	12–24 hr

oxcarbazepine

Oxcarbazepine (Trileptal) is a keto-analogue of carbamazepine. Its precise mechanism of action is unknown, though it is known to block voltage-sensitive sodium channels, which aids in stabilizing excited neuronal membranes. It is indicated for monotherapy or adjunctive therapy in the management of partial seizures in adults and children ages 6 to 16. It should be used with caution in the older adult over the age of 65.

PHARMACOKINETICS

Half-Life	Onset	Peak	Duration
2–9 hr	2–4 hr	2–3 days	Unknown

MISCELLANEOUS DRUGS

▶▶ gabapentin

Gabapentin (Neurontin, others) is an adjunctive drug for the management of partial seizures, including secondary generalized tonic–clonic seizures. The drug is ineffective for or worsens absence, myoclonic, or tonic–atonic type seizures. It is also commonly used to treat neuropathic pain. Low-dose gabapentin has recently been introduced as an off-label treatment for hot flashes. The exact mechanism of action of gabapentin is unknown, although it is structurally related to the inhibitory neurotransmitter gamma-aminobutyric acid (GABA). Many believe that it works by increasing the synthesis and accumulation of the inhibitory neurotransmitter GABA between neurons, hence the drug name. It may also bind to undiscovered receptor sites in the brain to produce anticonvulsant activity. Abrupt discontinuation of gabapentin can lead to withdrawal seizures. The drug's only usual contraindication is known drug allergy.

PHARMACOKINETICS

Half-Life	Onset	Peak	Duration
5–7 hr	Unknown	2–3 hr	Unknown

lamotrigine

Lamotrigine (Lamictal) is indicated as adjunctive therapy for partial seizures (with or without generalized tonic-clonic seizures) in adults whose condition is not well controlled using conventional therapy, as monotherapy following the withdrawal of concomitant drugs, and as adjunctive therapy for the management of generalized seizures associated with Lennox–Gastaut syndrome in both children and adult patients. There is evidence that lamotrigine is also useful in treating resistant depression, rapid-cycling bipolar affective disorder, depressive episodes in bipolar affective disorder, and in the maintenance phase or prophylaxis of bipolar affective disorder. It stabilizes neuronal cell membranes by blocking voltage-sensitive sodium channels and inhibiting the release of excitatory neurotransmitters (e.g., glutamate, aspartate), although its precise mechanism of action is unknown. It has no known contraindications other than drug allergy. Its pharmacokinetic parameters can vary widely when taken concurrently with other antiepileptic drugs. Lamotrigine is available in oral tablet form.

PHARMACOKINETICS

Half-Life	Onset	Peak	Duration
25–32 hr	Variable	1.7–2.2 hr	Unknown

levetiracetam

Levetiracetam (Keppra) is indicated as adjunctive managament for adults with partial-onset seizures with or without secondary generalization. Its mechanism of action is unknown. However, it is generally well tolerated, with the most common adverse effects being somnolence, asthenia, dizziness, and infection. New studies support levetiracetum use in children with seizures resistant to conventional antiepileptic drug therapy. Child dosing information should be determined for each patient by a pediatric neurologist.

PHARMACOKINETICS

Half-Life	Onset	Peak	Duration
6–8 hr	Rapid	1.3 hr	Unknown

Continued

DRUG PROFILES (cont'd)

pregabalin

Pregabalin (Lyrica), like gabapentin, is structurally related to GABA, a major neurotransmitter that inhibits brain activity. However, the drug does not bind to GABA receptors but rather to the α_2-δ receptor sites, which affect calcium channels in CNS tissues. This is believed to be related to its mechanism of action, although the full mechanism is still uncertain. The drug may be indicated as adjunctive therapy for complex seizure disorders in adult patients; however, in Canada, the drug is used primarily for the management of neuropathic pain associated with diabetic peripheral neuropathy or post-herpetic neuralgia in adults.

PHARMACOKINETICS

Half-Life	Onset	Peak	Duration
5–6.5 hr	Rapid; affected by food	1 hr	Unknown

topiramate

Topiramate (Topamax) is a structurally unique drug chemically related to fructose, classified as a sulfamate substituted monosaccharide. Topiramate is indicated for management of patients (adults and children over 6 years of age) with newly diagnosed epilepsy and as adjunctive therapy for partial seizures in adults and children 2 years of age and older. It is also indicated for the prophylaxis of migraine headache in adults. Its exact mechanism of action is unknown. However, it is believed to work by blocking sodium channels in neurons, blocking glutamate activity, and enhancing GABA activity.

PHARMACOKINETICS

Half-Life	Onset	Peak	Duration
21 hr	Rapid; unaffected by food	2–3 hr	Unknown

TABLE 14-6

Antiepileptic Drugs: FDA Risk Classification

Pregnancy Category	Anticonvulsant
C	acetazolamide, ethosuximide, gabapentin, lamotrigine, levetiracetam, oxcarbazepine, topiramate
D	Barbiturates (e.g., phenobarbital), carbamazepine, clonazepam, clorazepate, diazepam, divalproex, phenytoin, primidone, valproic acid

FDA, U.S. Food and Drug Administration.

TABLE 14-7

Phenytoin Sodium Versus Fosphenytoin Sodium

	phenytoin sodium (Dilantin) IV	fosphenytoin sodium (Cerebyx) IM/IV
pH	12	8.6–9
Maximum infusion rate	50 mg/min	150 mg PE*/min
Admixtures	0.9% saline	0.9% saline or 5% dextrose

IM, intramuscular; *IV,* intravenous; *PE,* phenytoin sodium equivalents.

*150 mg fosphenytoin sodium = 100 mg phenytoin sodium.

DOSAGES   Selected Antiepileptic Drugs

Drug (Pregnancy Category)	Pharmacological Class	Usual Dosage Range	Indications
▸▸carbamazepine (Mazepine, Tegetrol) (D)	Iminostilbene	*Children* PO: 6–12 yr, 200–1000 mg/day *Children/Adult* PO: over 12 yr, 800–1200 mg/day	Partial seizures with complex symptoms; tonic–clonic, mixed seizures; trigeminal—glossopharyngeal neuralgia
clobazam (ratio-Clobazam) (D)	Benzodiazepine	*Adult* PO: Initial: 5–15 mg/day at bedtime; maintenance: 20–4 mg/day	Adjunctive for tonic-clonic, complex partial, myoclonic seizures
clonazepam (Clonapam, Rivotril) (D)	Benzodiazepine	*Children* PO: under 10 yr or 30 kg, 0.1–0.2 mg/kg/day divided tid *Adult* PO: 20 mg/day	Lennox–Gastaut syndrome; absence, akinetic, and myoclonic seizures
clorazepate dipotassium (Novoclopate) (D)	Benzodiazepine	*Children* PO: 9–11 yr, 22.5–60 mg/day	Partial seizures
ethosuximide (Zarontin) (D)	Succinimide	*Children* PO: 3–6 yr, 250 mg/day then adjust; over 6 yr, 500 mg/day then adjust *Adult* PO: 500 mg/day then adjust	Absence seizures

Continued

DOSAGES   Selected Antiepileptic Drugs (cont'd)

Drug (Pregnancy Category)	Pharmacological Class	Usual Dosage Range	Indications
fosphenytoin (Cerebyx) (D)	Hydantoin	*Children* IV: 10–20 PE*/kg loading dose; may begin maintenance dosing 8–12 hr later using child phenytoin dosing guidelines (see below) *Adult* IV: 15–20 PE*/kg loading dose; maintenance dose 4–6 mg/kg/day	Tonic–clonic seizures; psychomotor seizures, convulsions
▸gabapentin (Neurontin) (C)	GABA analogue	*Children* PO: not recommended *Adult* PO: over 18 yr, 900–1800 mg/day	Adjunctive therapy for partial seizures and neuropathic pain
lamotrigine (Lamictal) (C)	Miscellaneous	*Children* PO: 2–12 yr, 5–15 mg/kg/day depending on other antiepileptic drugs used *Adult* PO: 75–400 mg/day	Partial seizures, Lennox–Gastaut syndrome
levetiracetam (Keppra) (C)	Miscellaneous	*Children* (per neurologist) *Adult* PO: 500 mg bid–3000 mg/day	Partial seizures
oxcarbazepine (Trileptal) (C)	Iminostilbene	*Children* PO: 6–16 yr, 8–10 mg/kg/day divided bid; max 600 mg/day *Adult* 300–600 mg bid	Adjunctive therapy, monotherapy of partial seizures
▸phenobarbital (D)	Barbiturate	*Children* PO: 2–6 mg/kg/day IV available through Special Access Programme: 20 mg/kg over 20 min *Adult* PO: 90–120 mg at bedtime IV Available through Special Access Programme: 20 mg/kg at 50–75 mg/min	Partial, tonic–clonic seizures Status epilepticus Partial, tonic–clonic seizures Status epilepticus
▸phenytoin (Dialantin) (D)	Hydantoin	*Children* PO: 4–8 mg/kg/day individualized IV: 14–18 mg/kg *Adult* PO: 300–600 mg/day IV: 14–18 mg/kg	Tonic–clonic; psychomotor seizures Status epilepticus Tonic–clonic; psychomotor seizures Status epilepticus
pregabalin (Lyrica) (C)	Miscellaneous	*Adult* PO: 150–600 mg/day divided	Off-label for partial seizures
primidone (D)	Barbiturate	*Children* PO: 10–25 mg/kg/day divided *Children/Adult* PO: 500–1000 mg/day divided	Partial seizures Tonic–clonic seizures
topiramate (Topamax) (C)	Miscellaneous	*Children* PO: 2–16 yr, 5–9 mg/kg/day divided *Adult (over 17 yr)* PO: 200–400 mg/day divided *Children/Adult* PO: over 6 yr: 100–400 mg/day divided	Adjunctive therapy partial seizures Monotherapy partial seizures
▸valproic acid (Depakene, Epival ECT) (D)	Miscellaneous	*Children/Adult* PO: 15–60 mg/kg/day divided	Multiple seizures

IM, intramuscular; *IV*, intravenous; *PO,* oral.

*PE = phenytoin equivalent: 1.5 mg fosphenytoin to be given for each milligram of phenytoin desired. One PE = 1.5 mg fosphenytoin = 1 mg phenytoin.

NURSING PROCESS

◪ Assessment

When any of the antiepileptic drugs are to be administered, the nurse should first obtain a thorough health and medication history so that any possible allergies, drug interactions (see Table 14-4), and untoward reactions, concerns, contraindications, or cautions to any of these medications can be known in advance. Review of the patient's history of seizure disorders is important to assess and document, with emphasis on precipitating events, duration and frequency, and intensity of the seizure activity. The nurse also needs to gather results from diagnostic studies and serum laboratory tests—especially those associated with heart, respiratory tract, kidney, liver, hematological, and CNS functioning.

Topiramate is a more recently approved miscellaneous antiepileptic drug that has significant contraindications, cautions, and drug interactions (previously discussed in the pharmacology section of this chapter and presented in Tables 14-3 and 14-4). In addition, assessment of mental status with attention to the patient's sensorium and level of consciousness before, during, and after drug therapy and seizure activity needs to be completed.

If barbiturates have been ordered, astute assessment of vital signs is particularly important because of their CNS depression. Assess the room for safety measures (e.g., side rails up or use of a bed alarm system depending on facility policy), noise level (keeping control of it), and the presence of seizure precautions (keeping oxygen, suctioning equipment, and airway nearby; use of padded side rails; and IV access per facility policy). With barbiturates and phenytoins, assessment of complete blood count (CBC) levels and serum chemistry before initiating drug therapy and after the physician's order is also important, with intervals of blood testing about every 2 weeks, should maintenance therapy continue.

Other assessment data include questioning the patient about possible "panic attacks" because high levels of anxiety or stress may precipitate seizure activity. Assess for autonomic nervous system responses to anxiety and "panic," such as cold, clammy hands, excessive sweating (diaphoresis), agitation, trembling of extremities, and complaints of "tension." Patients who are taking oral contraceptives with the drug topiramate should receive education about other means of contraception because of decreased effectiveness. It is also important to be aware of all other uses of antiepileptic drugs, such as with valproic acid in manic episodes and migraine prevention, so that an appropriate assessment is done.

◪ Nursing Diagnoses

- Risk for injury related to decreased sensorium from drug-related CNS depression and adverse effects of antiepileptic drugs

- Deficient knowledge related to lack of familiarity with and information concerning the use of antiepileptic drugs
- Nonadherence (therapeutic regimen) related to patient's misuse of drugs or lack of understanding about the seizure disorder and its treatment

◪ Planning

◼ Goals

- Patient will experience little or no adverse effects associated with nonadherence or with overtreatment or undertreatment.
- Patient will identify therapeutic effects of antiepileptic drugs.
- Patient will remain adherent with therapy and without major harm to self during antiepileptic drug treatment.

◼ Outcome Criteria

- Patient states the therapeutic drug effects and adverse effects of the antiepileptic drug (e.g., sedation, confusion, CNS depression).
- Patient (or family members) states the importance of taking the medication exactly as prescribed (e.g., same time every day).
- Patient states the dangers associated with sudden withdrawal of the medication, such as rebound convulsions.
- Patient maintains a protective environment at home and at work to minimize injury.

◪ Implementation

Oral antiepileptic drugs should be taken regularly at the same time of day at the recommended dose and with meals to diminish gastrointestinal upset. Oral suspensions should be shaken thoroughly, and capsules should not be crushed, opened, or chewed, especially if they are extended- or long-release forms. Extended-release drugs are usually taken once a day, so be cautious with their use if more frequent dosing is ordered—always check and double-check. If there are any questions about the medication order or the medication prescribed, the physician should be contacted for clarification. It is best to give oral antiepileptic drugs with water and not with juices, milk, or carbonated beverages. Do not mix valproate sodium oral solution with carbonated beverages, as valproic acid will be generated in the carbonated beverage and may cause mouth and throat irritation. Topiramate and valproic acid, in particular, should be taken in the original oral dosage form. The "capsule" forms (not the delayed/extended-release forms) may be opened and sprinkled in 30 mL of soft food such as apple sauce. See also Special Populations: Children: Antiepileptic Drugs.

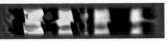

SPECIAL POPULATIONS: CHILDREN

Antiepileptic Drugs

- Should a skin rash develop in a child or infant taking phenytoin, the drug should be discontinued immediately and the physician notified.
- Chewable dosage forms of antiepileptic drugs should not be used for once-a-day administration, and intramuscular injections of barbiturates or phenytoin should not be used in any patient.
- Family members, parents, guardians, or caregivers should be encouraged to keep a journal with a record of the signs and symptoms before, during, and after the seizure, and before, during, and after the treatment with an antiepileptic drug.
- Patients should be encouraged to wear a medical alert bracelet or necklace at all times with information about the diagnosis and medication therapy.
- Suspension forms of antiepileptic drugs should always be shaken thoroughly before use, and a graduated device or oral syringe used for more accurate dosing.

- Children are more sensitive to barbiturates and may respond to doses at lower levels than expected. They may also show more profound CNS-depressive effects related to the antiepileptic drug or show depression, confusion, or excitement (a paradoxical reaction).
- Any excessive sedation, confusion, lethargy, hypotension, bradypnea, tachycardia, or decreased movement in children taking any antiepileptic drug should be reported to the health care provider immediately.
- Carbamazepine is to be given with meals to reduce risk of gastrointestinal distress. All suspension forms should be shaken well before use.
- Oral forms of valproic acid should not be given with milk because this may cause the drug to dissolve early and irritate local mucosa. Do not give with carbonated beverages.

CNS, central nervous system.

The following interventions are more drug specific or drug class specific:

- Carbamazepine: This drug should not be given with grapefruit because of increased toxicity of the antiepileptic drug. Grapefruit inhibits intestinal enzymes CYP3A4; consequently, grafefruit can significantly increase serum levels of carbamazepine because of its high first-pass metabolism. If the drug is to be replaced with another antiepileptic drug, there should be a plan to decrease one drug prior to beginning low doses (at first) of the new antiepileptic drug. Serum therapeutic levels are presented in Table 14-5.
- Clonazepam: Tablets may be crushed, as needed, if they are regular release.
- Fosphenytoin: As a point of reference, 150 mg of this drug yields 100 mg of phenytoin, and the dose, concentration solution, and infusion rate of fosphenytoin would be expressed as a phenytoin equivalent (PE). Dilutional fluids include D5W or 0.9% normal saline (NaCl), and rates of infusion should reflect manufacturer guidelines and are usually given at a rate of 150 mg PE/min or less to avoid hypotension or cardiorespiratory depression. Should arrhythmias or hypotension occur, the infusion should be discontinued, patient vital signs monitored, and the physician contacted immediately. Safety measures (e.g., help with ambulation, moving slowly and purposefully) should be implemented with this drug (as with all other antiepileptic drugs) and especially with intravenous infusions because of the adverse effects of ataxia and dizziness.
- Phenytoin: Intravenous dosage forms should be given cautiously, only with 0.9% NaCl (to avoid precipitation

of the solution), and administered slowly or as ordered because of possible cardiovascular and respiratory collapse. CNS depression is always a concern, thus the patient's vital signs need to be frequently monitored. If existing intravenous lines are used that contain D5W or other solutions, the line should be flushed with NaCl before and after dosing to avoid precipitate formation. If infiltration of the intravenous site leads to subcutaneous tissue access, ischemia and sloughing may occur because of the high alkalinity of the drug (as with other antiepileptic drugs) and hospital or facility policy as well as manufacturer guidelines should be reviewed for use of possible antidotes. If infiltration occurs, discontinue the solution, but leave the needle in place until all orders from the physician have been received. Oral dosage forms that are sustained or extended release should never be opened, punctured, chewed, or broken or halved. Other regular forms of the drug may be crushed as needed. For the adverse effect of gingival hyperplasia, the patient needs to perform frequent oral care on a daily basis and have frequent dental checkups. CBC levels are often monitored very closely within the first year of therapy (e.g., monthly for 1 year, then every 3 months).
- Barbiturates: Avoid abrupt withdrawal, as with all antiepileptic drugs, and mix elixir dosage forms with fruit juice, milk, or water. Too-rapid infusion of intravenous dosage forms may lead to cardiovascular collapse and respiratory depression; therefore, vital signs and intravenous infusion rates should be frequently monitored.
- Valproic acid: Oral dosage forms are not to be given with carbonated beverages.

In addition to the above drug- and drug class–related nursing interventions, it is also important to maintain patient safety, particularly airway maintenance.

A clenched jaw, poorly coordinated respirations, and production of secretions and vomitus may be responsible for varying degrees of blockage of the airway and ineffective ventilation. Breathing usually stops only for a few seconds. The patient should be positioned to one side (if possible). Secretions that are easily accessible may be suctioned. The teeth should never be pried apart nor should a flexible suction catheter be placed between clenched teeth. Airway problems usually improve rapidly once the seizure is over. Also important is maintaining seizure precautions according to hospital policy (e.g., making sure the patient is gently kept in bed or kept from falling, and maintaining quick access to oxygen and suctioning equipment). The dosage frequency of antiepileptic drugs is important as well, so if such a medication is ordered to be taken, for example, every 6 hours, it should be given around the clock so that drug levels are maintained. See Patient Education for more information.

Evaluation

A therapeutic response to antiepileptic drugs means that seizure activity is decreased or absent, not that the patient is cured of the seizures. Any response to the medication should be documented appropriately. Because antiepileptic drugs have other indications, such as for chronic pain and migraines, the existing problem, condition, or disorder should show improvement with minimal adverse effects. In addition, when monitoring and evaluating the effects of antiepileptic drugs, the nurse needs to constantly assess the patient for mental status, mood and mood changes, sensorium, behavioural changes, changes in the level of consciousness, affect, eye problems or visual disorders, sore throat, and fever (blood dyscrasia is an adverse effect of the hydantoins). The occurrence of vomiting, diplopia (double vision), cardiovascular collapse, and Stevens–Johnson syndrome indicates toxicity of the bone marrow. The physician should be contacted immediately and no further doses administered if these adverse and toxic effects occur. Therapeutic serum levels of the specific antiepileptic drug are ordered at baseline or at the start of therapy and frequently thereafter to monitor the amount of drug in the blood and to see if subsequent serum levels are subtherapeutic, therapeutic, or toxic. Subtherapeutic levels would mean that the drug may need to be increased in dosage amount by the physician or health care provider and toxic levels would require withholding or decreasing the dose. Specific antiepileptic drug blood levels are listed with each drug profile, as appropriate to the specific drug.

PATIENT EDUCATION

- Patients should be informed of the sedating effects of drug therapy so that appropriate steps can be taken to ensure patient safety.
- Patients should be encouraged to avoid tasks requiring alertness to prevent harm to self until a steady state of the drug is achieved (takes 4–5 half-lives).
- Patients should be encouraged to avoid alcohol and smoking while taking antiepileptic drugs.
- Patients should be informed to not abruptly discontinue antiepileptic drugs. Abrupt withdrawal may precipitate rebound seizure activity.
- Patients should be informed that the adverse effect most common with antiepileptic drugs is drowsiness, and that this often decreases after several weeks of being on the drug.
- Patients should be informed to contact the physician if any unusual reactions such as glandular swelling, fever, sore throat, tarry stools, back pain, hematuria, easy bruising, lethargy, or mouth ulcers occur.
- Patients should be informed that the reason for a recurrence of seizure activity is usually lack of adherence.

- Patients should know that some antiepileptic drugs cause photosensitivity (e.g., lamotrigine), so exposure to sunlight or tanning beds should be avoided. Patients should be instructed on use of sunscreen and protective clothing.
- Patients should be encouraged to avoid any form of stimulants (e.g., caffeine) because of the higher risk for seizure activity.
- Patients taking topiramate should be instructed to force fluids, unless contraindicated, to avoid renal calculi (kidney stone) formation.
- Patients should be presented with age-appropriate instructions regarding backup contraception, which is recommended with topiramate.
- Patients should be clearly informed that treatment of epilepsy is usually lifelong and that adherence is important to the effectiveness of drug therapy. Community and other appropriate resources (e.g., national and local support groups) should be discussed with the patient.

POINTS TO REMEMBER

❖ The terms for epilepsy (i.e., *seizure* and *convulsion*) have different meanings and should not be used interchangeably:
  • *Epilepsy:* Disorder of the brain manifested as a chronic, recurrent pattern of seizures
  • *Seizure:* Abnormal electrical activity in the brain
  • *Convulsion:* A type of seizure (spasmodic contractions of involuntary muscles)

❖ Specific drugs are indicated for the different classifications of seizure disorders. The more common classifications are as follows:
  • *Partial:* Short alterations in consciousness, repetitive unusual movements, psychological changes, and confusion
  • *Generalized:* Most common in childhood; temporary lapses in consciousness (seconds); rhythmic movement of eyes, head, or hands; person does not convulse; may have several a day
  • *Status epilepticus:* A common seizure disorder; a life-threatening emergency characterized by tonic–clonic convulsions and may result in brain damage and death if not treated immediately

❖ Nursing considerations include the following:
  • The nurse must distinguish between the type of seizures: focal, primary, secondary, status, tonic–clonic, grand mal, and petit mal, and describe exactly what has occurred before, during, and after the seizure event.
  • Nonadherence is the most notable factor leading to treatment failure.
  • Therapeutic blood levels should be monitored at all times, and abrupt withdrawal of the antiepileptic drug should be avoided.
  • Intravenous infusions of antiepileptic drugs are very dangerous and should be managed cautiously and through adhering to hospital or facility policy and manufacturer guidelines.
  • There are many drug interactions, and there are also many intravenous incompatibilities.

EXAMINATION REVIEW QUESTIONS

1 Which of the following reflects the most appropriate nursing action for intravenous (IV) phenytoin (Dilantin)?
a. Ensure continuous infusion of drug.
b. Give IV doses via rapid IV push.
c. Administer in dextrose solutions.
d. Administer in normal saline solutions.

2 The nurse is reviewing the current drugs taken by a patient who will be starting drug therapy with carbamazepine. Which of the following drugs may be a concern regarding interactions?
a. digoxin (Lanoxin)
b. diazepam (Valium)
c. warfarin (Coumadin)
d. acetaminophen (Tylenol)

3 Which of the following would you expect in a patient with a phenytoin level of 60 μmol/L?
a. Ataxia
b. Seizures
c. Hypertension
d. No unusual response; this level is therapeutic.

4 Which of the following is the most appropriate when administering an antiepileptic drug?
a. Take on an empty stomach.
b. Take at the same time every day.
c. Crush tablets if unable to swallow.
d. Stop if seizure activity disappears.

5 During assessment of a patient with a history of epilepsy, which question would be most important to ask the patient about epilepsy and its treatment?
a. "Do you have a family history of seizures?"
b. "Do your seizures interfere with your appetite?"
c. "Do you have severe migraines with the seizure?"
d. "Do you experience any unusual sensations or perceptions before the seizure occurs?"

For answers see http://evolve.elsevier.com/Canada/Lilley/pharmacology/.

CRITICAL THINKING ACTIVITIES

1 Why is assessment of patients important in determining the most appropriate antiepileptic drug?

2 Why is it important to be aware of concurrent medication administration, including over-the-counter drugs, with patients taking antiepileptic drugs?

3 A 21-year-old woman was brought to the emergency room in status epilepticus. She weighs 63 kg. The physician has decided to treat the woman as follows: intravenous diazepam (Valium) 0.3 mg/kg IV push; if no response, phenytoin (Dilantin), 15 mg/kg IV push.
a. Calculate the dose for each of these drugs and how they will be given.
b. Specify what assessments are important when these drugs are given. How do you measure therapeutic response?

For answers see http://evolve.elsevier.com/Canada/Lilley/pharmacology/.

CHAPTER 15

Antiparkinsonian Drugs

Learning Objectives

After reading this chapter, the successful student will be able to do the following:

1 Briefly discuss the pathophysiology related to Parkinson's disease (PD).

2 Identify the different classes of medications used as antiparkinsonian drugs, including first and second line of drugs used in the management of PD.

3 Discuss the mechanisms of action, dosages, indications, routes of administration, contraindications, cautions, adverse effects, and toxic effects associated with the use of antiparkinsonian drugs.

4 Develop a collaborative plan of care that includes all phases of the nursing process related to antiparkinsonian drugs.

e-Learning Activities

Web site
(http://evolve.elsevier.com/Canada/Lilley/pharmacology/)

- Animations
- Answers to chapter questions, activities, and case studies
- Calculators and Category Catchers
- Glossary with audio pronunciations
- IV Therapy and Medication Error Checklists
- Multiple-Choice Review Question quizzes
- Nursing Care Plans
- Online Appendices and Supplements
- WebLinks

Drug Profiles

amantadine, p. 277
▸▸ benztropine (benztropine mesylate)*, p. 279
bromocriptine (bromocriptine mesylate)*, p. 277
entacapone, p. 278
▸▸ levodopa–carbidopa, p. 277
▸▸ ropinirole (ropinirole hydrochloride)*, p. 277
▸▸ selegiline (selegiline hydrochloride)*, p. 275

▸▸ Key drug.

*Full generic name is given in parentheses. For the purposes of this text, the more common shortened name is used.

Glossary

Akinesia Reduction or lack of psychomotor activity of voluntary muscles. (p. 272)

Anticholinergic drugs Drugs that block or impede the activity of the neurotransmitter acetylcholine (ACh) at cholinergic receptors in the brain. (p. 278)

Catechol ortho-methyltransferase (COMT) inhibitors A class of indirect-acting dopaminergic drugs that work by inhibiting the enzyme COMT, which catalyzes the breakdown of dopamine. (p. 276)

Chorea A condition characterized by involuntary, purposeless, rapid motions such as flexing and extending the fingers, raising and lowering the shoulders, or grimacing. (p. 284)

Dopaminergic drugs Drugs used to replace the deficiency of dopamine at dopamine receptors in the nerve endings, especially in the brain when treating Parkinson's disease (can be direct- or indirect-acting or replacement drugs). (p. 275)

Dyskinesia An impaired ability to execute voluntary movements. (p. 272)

Dystonia Impaired or distorted voluntary movement because of a disorder of muscle tone. (p. 272)

Endogenous Describes any substance produced by the body's own natural biochemistry (e.g., hormones, neurotransmitters). (p. 275)

Exogenous Describes any substance produced out of the body that may be taken into the body (e.g., a medication, food, or an environmental toxin). (p. 275)

On–off phenomenon A phenomenon seen in patients taking levodopa long term, in which patients have periods of good control ("on" time) and those when they have bad control or breakthrough Parkinson's disease ("off" time). (p. 277)

Parkinson's disease (PD) A slowly progressive, degenerative neurological disorder characterized by resting tremor, pill-rolling of the fingers, masklike facies, shuffling gait, forward flexion of the trunk, loss of postural reflexes, and muscle rigidity and weakness. (p. 271)

Presynaptic drugs Drugs that exert their antiparkinsonian effects before the nerve synapse. (p. 275)

Wearing-off phenomenon A gradual worsening of parkinsonian symptoms as a patient's medications begin to lose their effectiveness, despite maximal doses with a variety of medications. (p. 276)

PARKINSON'S DISEASE

Parkinson's disease (PD) is a chronic, progressive, degenerative disorder affecting the dopamine-producing neurons in the brain. PD was initially recognized in 1817, when it was referred to as "shaking palsy." James Parkinson first described the symptoms of both the early and advanced stages of the disease, along with the treatment options. It was not until the 1960s, however, that the underlying pathological defect was discovered. It was then believed that Parkinson's disease was caused by a dopamine deficit in the area of the brain called the *substantia nigra,* which is contained within another brain structure known as the basal ganglia. The substantia nigra and basal ganglia are parts of the brain that are included in the extrapyramidal system, which is involved in the coordination of movement and the regulation of motor function, including posture, locomotion, muscle tone, and smooth muscle activity.

It is now recognized that PD results from an imbalance in two neurotransmitters, dopamine (DA) and acetylcholine (ACh), in the *basal ganglia.* This imbalance is caused by failure of the nerve terminals in the substantia nigra to produce the essential neurotransmitter dopamine. This neurotransmitter acts in the basal ganglia to control movements. Destruction of the substantia nigra leads to dopamine depletion. Because dopamine is an inhibitory neurotransmitter and ACh is an excitatory neurotransmitter in this area of the brain, a correct balance between these two neurotransmitters is needed for the proper regulation of posture, muscle tone, and voluntary movement. This imbalance between dopamine and ACh results in cholinergic activity because of the lack of a normal dopaminergic balancing effect. Figure 15-1 illustrates the difference in neurotransmitter concentrations in persons with normal balance and in patients with PD. PD is a prominent cause of disability because of the common accompanying motor complications.

A significant advance in the understanding of the etiology and pathogenesis of PD came in 1983 when the potent neurotoxin 1-methyl-4-phenyl-1,2,3,6-tetrahydropyridine (MPTP) and its metabolic breakdown product 1-methyl-4-phenylpyridine (MPP) were discovered. This illegal substance was produced in home laboratories and used for recreational purposes. MPTP and MPP selectively destroy the substantia nigra, the same area of the brain that is dysfunctional in PD. It has been shown that a parkinsonian syndrome almost identical to idiopathic PD develops in laboratory animals injected with this neurotoxin. Other researchers theorize

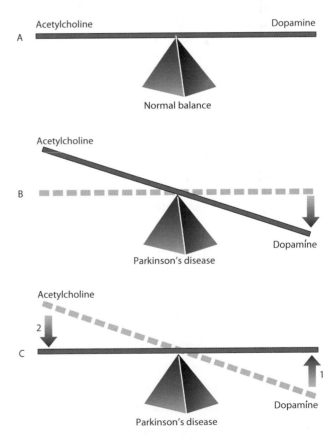

A, Normal balance of acetylcholine and dopamine in the CNS.
B, In Parkinson's disease, a decrease in dopamine results in an imbalance.
C, Drug therapy in Parkinson's disease is aimed at correcting the imbalance between acetylcholine and dopamine. This can be accomplished by either
  1. increasing the supply of dopamine or
  2. blocking or lowering acetylcholine levels.

FIG. 15-1 The neurotransmitter abnormality of Parkinson's disease.

that PD is the result of an earlier head injury or of excess iron in the substantia nigra, which undergoes oxidation and causes the generation of toxic free radicals. In still another theory, it is thought that because dopamine levels naturally decrease with age, PD represents a premature aging of the nigrostriatal cells of the substantia nigra resulting from environmental or intrinsic biochemical factors, or both. More recently, researchers have focused on a genetic connection. It seems most likely that a combination of factors contributes to the neuron loss associated with PD, potentially environmental factors with the possibility of genetic predispositions. It is also theorized that different genetic or environmental factors may be responsible for different types of PD.

Over 100,000 Canadians have Parkinson's disease. In most patients, the disease becomes apparent between 45 and 65 years of age, with a mean age of onset of 56 years. Approximately 20% of people with PD are under the age of 50 and one half of those affected in Canada are under the age of 65. The number of patients with PD is expected to continue to increase as our older adult population grows. It occasionally occurs in younger people, especially after acute encephalitis and carbon monoxide or metallic poisoning. It is usually idiopathic (of no known cause). Overall, there is a 2% lifetime chance of developing PD. Males may be affected more often than females up to a ratio of 3 to 2.

There are no readily available laboratory tests that can detect or confirm PD. Results of computerized tomography (CT), magnetic resonance imaging (MRI), cerebrospinal fluid analysis, and electroencephalography are usually normal and of little diagnostic value. A positron emission tomography (PET) scan may offer additional information. This new type of scanning involves intravenous injections of deoxyglucose with radioactive fluorine. The shades of colours that become visible indicate areas of abnormalities and assist in the diagnosis of neurological disorders, including PD. CT, MRI, and PET may be useful tools for ruling out other possible diseases as causes of the symptoms. The diagnosis of PD is usually made on the basis of the classic symptoms and physical findings. The classic symptoms of PD are listed in Table 15-1.

Unfortunately, PD is a progressive condition. With time, the number of surviving dopaminergic terminals that can take up exogenously administered levodopa and convert it into dopamine decreases. Rapid swings in the response to levodopa (known as the **on–off phenomenon**) also occur. The result is worsening PD when too little dopamine is present, or dyskinesias when too much is present. The general term **dyskinesia** refers to the difficulty in performing voluntary movements. **Akinesia** is the slowness or loss of voluntary motor function. *Akatheisia* is the feeling of inner restlessness and the urge to move as well as rocking while standing or sitting, lifting feet as if marching on the spot, and crossing and uncrossing the legs while sitting. **Dystonia** is a movement disorder that commonly involves the head, neck, and tongue and often occurs as an adverse effect of a medication. Symptoms of PD do not appear until approximately 80% of the dopamine store in the substantia nigra of the basal ganglia has been depleted. This means that by the time PD is diagnosed, only approximately 20% of the patient's original nigral dopaminergic terminals are functioning normally.

Nerve terminals can take up substances, store them, and release them for use when needed. It is this factor that forms the basis for antiparkinsonian treatment. As long as there are functioning nerve terminals that can take up dopamine, the symptoms of PD can be at least partially controlled. The blood–brain barrier does not allow exogenously supplied dopamine to enter the brain; however, it does allow levodopa, a naturally occurring dopamine precursor, to do so. After levodopa has been taken up by the dopaminergic terminal, it is converted into dopamine and then released as needed. Levodopa therapy can thus correct the neurotransmitter imbalance in patients with early PD who still have functioning nerve terminals.

The first step in the treatment of PD is a full explanation of the disease to the patient and family members or significant others. Physical therapy, speech therapy, and occupational therapy are almost always needed when the patient is in the later stages of the disease. As previously discussed, drug therapy is aimed at increasing the levels of dopamine as long as there are functioning nerve terminals. It is also aimed at antagonizing or blocking the effects of ACh and slowing the progression of the disease. The drugs available for the treatment of PD and their respective categories are listed in Table 15-2.

TABLE 15-1

Classic Parkinsonian Symptoms

Symptom	Description
Bradykinesia	Slowness of movement
Postural instability	Danger of falling, hesitation in gait as patient starts or stops walking
Rigidity	"Cogwheel" rigidity, resistance to passive movement
Tremor	Pill rolling: tremor of the thumb against the forefinger, seen mostly at rest, is less severe during voluntary activity; starts usually on one side then progresses to the other; is the presenting sign in 70% of cases

TABLE 15-2

Antiparkinsonian Drugs

Drug Category	Drugs
Anticholinergic drugs	benztropine, procyclidine, trihexyphenidyl
Antihistamines (used for their anticholinergic effects)	diphenhydramine, orphenadrine
Dopamine receptor agonists (direct-acting)	bromocriptine, levodopa, levodopa–carbidopa, pramipexole, ropinirole
INDIRECT-ACTING DOPAMINE RECEPTOR AGONISTS	
COMT inhibitor	entacapone
MAO-B inhibitor	selegiline
Miscellaneous drugs	amantadine

COMT, catechol ortho-methyltransferase; *MAO,* monoamine oxidase

SELECTIVE MONOAMINE OXIDASE INHIBITOR THERAPY

There are two subclasses of monoamine oxidase (MAO) in the body: MAO-A and MAO-B. As early as 1965, non-selective monoamine oxidase inhibitors (MAOIs), which inhibit both MAO-A and MAO-B, were being used to improve the therapeutic effect of levodopa in patients with PD. They were also among the first medications used to treat depression, but their use for this purpose has been widely supplanted by newer drug categories (see Chapter 16). However, a major adverse effect of these nonselective MAOIs has been that they interact with tyramine-containing foods (cheese, red wine, beer, and yogourt) because of their inhibitory activity against MAO-A, called the "cheese effect." One hazardous result of this effect can be severe hypertension. This has considerably restricted the therapeutic use of MAOIs. In 1974, selegiline, an amphetamine derivative, was introduced as an investigational option for PD. As a selective MAO-B inhibitor, selegiline is much less likely to elicit the classic cheese effect with daily doses of 10 mg or less. In the years that followed, many investigational studies were conducted, and in October 1989, selegiline received approval from Health Canada's Therapeutic Product Directorate for use in conjunction with levodopa therapy in the treatment of PD. There was earlier speculation by researchers that selegiline, as well as possibly vitamins E (tocopherol) and C (ascorbic acid), might have antiparkinsonian effects because of "neuroprotective" activity at the neuronal (nerve cell) level. The results of some animal studies suggested this as a possibility. However, no human or animal studies to date have conclusively demonstrated this to be the case for any of these three substances.

Mechanism of Action and Drug Effects

MAOs are widely distributed throughout the body. The areas where concentrations are high are the liver, kidney, stomach, intestinal wall, and brain. As mentioned previously, there are two subclasses of MAOs: A and B. Most of MAO-B is in the central nervous system (CNS), primarily in the brain. The primary role of MAOs is the catabolism or breakdown of the catecholamines (e.g.,

dopamine, norepinephrine, and epinephrine) as well as the breakdown of serotonin. Therefore, an MAO-B inhibitor such as selegiline causes an increase in the levels of dopaminergic stimulation in the CNS (see Figure 15-2). This helps counter the dopaminergic deficiency that arises from the PD pathology. Selegiline allows the dose of levodopa (see Dopaminergic Therapy in this chapter) to be decreased. Improvement in functional ability and decreased severity of symptoms are common after selegiline is added. However, only approximately 50% to 60% of patients show a positive response.

Indications

Selegiline is currently approved for use in combination with levodopa or levodopa–carbidopa. It is an adjunctive drug used when a patient's response to levodopa is fluctuating. Selegiline may also be somewhat beneficial as a prophylactic drug. Selegiline administration before exposure to the neurotoxin MPTP has been shown to delay patients' reduced responses to levodopa. Several studies have shown that selegiline-treated patients required levodopa therapy 1.8 times less than control patients. One challenge that patients with PD experience is that as their disease progresses, it becomes more and more difficult to control it with levodopa. Ultimately, levodopa no longer controls the PD, and the patient becomes

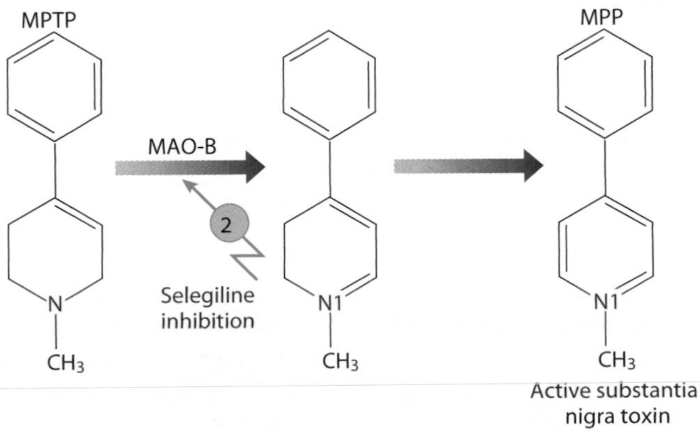

FIG. 15-2 Mechanism of action of selegiline. *MAO-B,* monoamine oxidase type B; *MPP,* 1-methyl-4-phenylpyridine; *MPTP,* 1-methyl-4-phenyl-1,2,3,6-tetrahydropyridine.

seriously debilitated. This generally occurs between 5 and 10 years after the initiation of levodopa therapy. Prophylactic selegiline use may delay the development of serious debilitating PD for 9 to 18 years. Because the average age of patients at the onset of PD is between 55 and 65 years, such a delay can prevent functional disability during the patient's life span, depending on the age at death.

Contraindications

Selegiline is normally contraindicated in cases of known drug allergy. Concurrent use of the opioid drug meperidine is contraindicated because of the likelihood of introducing a dangerous condition known as *serotonin syndrome* (see Chapter 16).

Adverse Effects

The most common adverse effects associated with selegiline use are mild and consist of nausea, lightheadedness, dizziness, abdominal pain, insomnia, confusion, and dry mouth. The adverse effects seen with selegiline use as they relate to the body systems are listed in Table 15-3. Reactions seen when the dosage exceeds 10 mg/day include a hypertensive crisis (with the consumption of tyramine-containing food), memory loss, muscular twitches and jerks, and grinding of teeth.

Interactions

The number of drugs with which selegiline interacts is relatively small, and the degree of interaction is dose dependent. At recommended doses of 10 mg/day, the drug maintains its selective MAO-B inhibition. However,

TABLE 15-3

Selegiline: Adverse Effects

Body System	Adverse Effects
Cardiovascular	Hypotension, dysrhythmia, tachycardia, palpitations, angina, edema
Central nervous	Altered sensation, pain, dizziness, drowsiness, irritability, anxiety, extrapyramidal adverse effects, CNS depression and unresponsiveness, tremors, seizures
Gastrointestinal	Nausea, vomiting, constipation, diarrhea, anorexia
Respiratory	Asthma, shortness of breath, apnea

at doses that exceed 10 mg/day, selegiline becomes a nonselective MAOI, contributing to the development of the cheese effect. Meperidine is contraindicated in patients receiving nonselective MAOIs because this combination has been associated with the occurrence of fatal hypertensive episodes. It is suggested that meperidine, as well as other opioids, be avoided in patients taking more than 10 mg/day of selegiline. For the same reasons, combinations with other drugs including dextroamphetamine, methylphenidate, dextromethorphan, sibutramine, and serotonin-selective reuptake inhibitors (SSRIs) (see Chapter 16) should also be avoided.

Dosage

For the recommended dosage of selegiline see the Dosages table below.

DOSAGES Selegiline and Selected Dopaminergic Drugs

Drug (Pregnancy Category)	Pharmacological Class	Usual Dosage Range	Indications
amantadine (Symmetrel) (C)	Indirect-acting dopamine agonist	*Adult* PO: 100–300 mg/day divided q12h	Parkinson's disease
bromocriptine mesylate (D)	Direct-acting dopamine agonist	*Adult* PO: 2.5–40 mg/day divided	Parkinson's disease
entacapone (Comptan, Stalevo) (C)	Indirect-acting dopamine agonist	*Adult* PO: 200 mg with each dosage of levodopa	Parkinson's disease
levodopa–benserazide hydrochloride (Prolopa) (C)	Combination direct-acting dopamine agonist/ replacement and decarboxylase inhibitor	*Adult* PO: 100–125, 400–800 mg/day based on levodopa divided into 4–6 doses	Parkinson's disease
▸▸levodopa–carbidopa (Sinemet, Sinemet CR)) (C)	Direct-acting dopamine agonist/replacement	*Adult* PO: 100–10, 100–25, 250–25; titrated to optimum dosage (1500 mg levodopa max/day; 70–100 mg carbidopa max/day) CR: 200–50, 1–2 tab bid; up to 8 tabs/day; 100–25: 1–4 tab bid	Parkinson's disease
pramipexole (Mirapex) (C)	Direct-acting dopamine agonist	*Adult* PO: 1.5–4.5 mg/day divided tid	Parkinson's disease
▸▸ropinirole hydrochloride (ReQuip) (C)	Direct-acting dopamine agonist	*Adult* PO: 0.25 mg tid slowly titrating to max dose of 24 mg/day	Parkinson's disease
▸▸selegiline hydrochloride (Anipril) (C)	Indirect dopamine agonist	*Adult* PO: 5 mg bid with breakfast and lunch	Parkinson's disease

CR, controlled release.

DRUG PROFILES

▸▸ *selegiline hydrochloride*

Selegiline hydrochloride (Anipril) is a selective MAO-B inhibitor used as adjunctive therapy in patients with a diminished response to levodopa–carbidopa. Selegiline has also been used as monotherapy for initial treatment of PD. When selegiline is added to ongoing drug management with levodopa–carbidopa, it reduces the amount of "off-time," decreases the required dose of levodopa, and may have other beneficial effects such as decreased end-of-dose akinesia, tremor and sialorrhea, and improved speech and dressing ability.

PHARMACOKINETICS

Half-Life*	Onset	Peak	Duration
1.2–1.8 hr	1 hr	0.5–0.9 hr	1–3 days

*Selegiline has three active metabolites with long half-lives of 18–21 hours.

DOPAMINERGIC THERAPY

In PD, little or no **endogenous** dopamine is produced; as a result, ACh becomes the predominant neurotransmitter in the brain, creating a state of imbalance. **Dopaminergic drugs** are used to provide **exogenous** replacement of the lost dopamine or to enhance the function of the few neurons that are still producing their own dopamine. Dopaminergic drugs can be broken down into three categories based on their underlying mechanisms of action: those that release dopamine from remaining functional dopamine vesicles in presynaptic fibres of neurons or that inhibit dopamine-metabolizing enzymes (indirect-acting), those that increase brain levels of dopamine by providing exogenous dopamine in tablet form (direct-acting/replacement), and dopaminergic agonists that act as dopamine substitutes and stimulate dopamine receptors directly in place of dopamine (direct-acting). The ultimate goal is to increase the levels of dopamine in the brain. By doing so and creating a balance with ACh, akinesias, the most detrimental complications of PD, can be reversed. Akinesias, are symptoms, such as a masklike facial expression and impaired postural reflexes, which eventually render patients unable to care for themselves.

Mechanism of Action and Drug Effects

The combination products levodopa–carbidopa and levodopa–benserazide hydrochloride provide exogenous sources of dopamine that directly replace the deficient neurotransmitter dopamine in the substantia nigra. Levodopa is the biological precursor of dopamine required by the brain for dopamine synthesis. Considered the cornerstone of the treatment of PD, these drugs are also referred to as **presynaptic drugs** or *replacement drugs*. This is because they work presynaptically to increase brain levels of dopamine. Dopamine must be administered in this form because, as mentioned previously, exogenously administered dopamine cannot pass through the blood–brain barrier, whereas levodopa can. Once it does, it is converted directly into dopamine by the enzyme dopa-decarboxylase (DDC). Traditionally, large doses of levodopa had to be administered to provide sufficient dopamine to the brain, as much of the levodopa administered was broken down outside the CNS by DDC. Such large doses resulted in high peripheral levels of dopamine and many unwanted adverse effects such as confusion, involuntary movements, gastrointestinal distress, and hypotension. These adverse effects can be avoided when levodopa is combined with carbidopa or benserazide hydrochloride, peripheral DDC inhibitors that do not cross the blood–brain barrier. These inhibitors prevent levodopa breakdown in the periphery. Consequently, levodopa is allowed to reach and cross the blood–brain barrier, whereas carbidopa and benserazide do not cross this barrier. Once in the brain, the levodopa is converted to dopamine, which can then exert its therapeutic antiparkinsonian effects by offsetting the dopamine–ACh imbalance.

Originally developed and used for the prophylaxis and treatment of viral disorders, amantadine (Symmetrel) has proved to be a valuable adjunct to the traditional antiparkinsonian drugs. Amantadine appears to exert its antiparkinsonian effect by causing the release of dopamine and other catecholamines from their storage sites in the ends of nerve cells that are still intact and have not yet been destroyed by the disease process. Amantadine also blocks the reuptake of dopamine into the nerve endings, which allows more dopamine to accumulate both centrally and peripherally. Therefore, its dopaminergic effects are the result of its indirect actions on the nerve because amantadine does not directly stimulate dopamine receptors as do certain other types of PD drugs. Amantadine also possesses some anticholinergic properties that may further assist by controlling symptoms of dyskinesias.

Bromocriptine is a dopaminergic agonist that directly stimulates the dopamine receptors. Chemically, bromocriptine is an ergot alkaloid similar to ergotamine in its chemical structure. Its antiparkinsonian effects stem from its ability to activate dopamine receptors and stimulate the production of more dopamine. This helps correct the imbalance between ACh and dopamine in the CNS. Bromocriptine is a D2 dopamine agonist. Pramipexole (Mirapex) and ropinirole (ReQuip) are two new highly specific D2–3 dopamine agonists that were released in 1997. They are both nonergot drugs that are effective in early and late stages of PD.

Entacapone (Comtan) belongs to a totally new class of antiparkinsonian drugs, the **catechol ortho-methyl-transferase (COMT) inhibitors.** COMT inhibitors help patients with PD by inhibiting COMT, the enzyme responsible for the breakdown of levodopa, the dopamine precursor. In this way, COMT inhibitors are also indirect-acting dopaminergic drugs. Entacapone cannot cross the blood–brain barrier and therefore can act only peripherally. The main positive effect of entacapone is that it prolongs the duration of levodopa benefit. Patients have less of a **wearing-off phenomenon** and experience prolonged benefits. A "wearing-off" effect is what many Parkinson's patients experience as medications gradually begin to lose their effectiveness and disease symptoms consequently worsen. Along with amantadine, COMT inhibitors are also considered to be indirect-acting drugs and work as presynaptic drugs.

Indications

All three of these classes of dopaminergic drugs are used to treat various stages of Parkinson's disease, either alone or in combination with other drugs. Bromocriptine also inhibits production of the hormone prolactin, which stimulates normal lactation. For this reason, it is used to treat women with excessive or undesired breast milk production (galactorrhea) and is also used for treatment of prolactin-secreting tumours.

Contraindications

Contraindications to dopaminergic drugs include known drug allergy, history of melanoma or any undiagnosed skin condition, and narrow-angle glaucoma. In addition, these drugs should not be used until at least 14 days after MAOI therapy (except selegiline) is stopped.

Adverse Effects

There are many potential adverse effects associated with the dopaminergic drugs. The most common of these are listed in Table 15-4. Effects that may occur with any of these drugs include syncope, rhinorrhea, and abdominal pain.

Interactions

The drug interactions involving dopaminergic drugs can cause significant adverse reactions, including a decrease in the efficacy of the dopaminergic drug, a hypertensive crisis, and reversal of the dopaminergic drug's effect. Hydantoins, when given with levodopa, increase the metabolism of levodopa, decreasing its effects. Haloperidol and phenothiazines, when given with levodopa, block dopamine receptors in the brain, resulting in decreased levodopa levels. Nonselective MAOIs taken concomitantly with dopaminergic drugs can result in inhibited metabolism, leading to a possible hypertensive crisis. Pyridoxine (vitamin B_6) promotes levodopa breakdown and may reverse levodopa effects. Carbidopa may help prevent this adverse outcome. The selective MAO-B inhibitor selegiline may be safely taken concurrently with COMT inhibitors.

Dosages

For the recommended dosages of the dopaminergic drugs, see the Dosages table on p. 274.

TABLE 15-4

Dopaminergic Drugs: Adverse Effects

Body System	Adverse Effects
AMANTADINE	
Central nervous	Impaired concentration, dizziness, increased irritability, nervousness, blurred vision
Gastrointestinal	Anorexia, nausea, constipation, vomiting
Other	Purple–red skin spots; dryness of mouth, nose, and throat; increased weakness
ENTACAPONE	
Central nervous	Involuntary movements (dyskinesias)
Gastrointestinal	Nausea, abdominal pain, diarrhea, decreased appetite
Other	Urine discoloration (brownish orange)
LEVODOPA–CARBIDOPA	
Hematological	Hemolytic anemia, agranulocytosis
Cardiovascular	Palpitations, orthostatic hypotension
Central nervous	Agitation; anxiety; psychotic and suicidal episodes; choreiform, dystonic, and other involuntary movements; headache and blurred vision
ROPINIROLE	
Cardiovascular	Syncope sometimes associated with bradycardia, symptomatic orthostatic hypotension
Central nervous	Hallucinations; somnolence; uncontrolled movements of body, face, tongue, arms, hands, and head
Gastrointestinal	Nausea

DRUG PROFILES

▶▶ *levodopa–carbidopa*

The peripheral decarboxylase inhibitor carbidopa does not cross the blood–brain barrier. However, it does prevent metabolism of levodopa to dopamine in the periphery (i.e., outside the CNS). This, in turn, limits peripheral dopamine-induced adverse effects, such as those described in the main text. Instead, the levodopa can reach its site of action in the brain without being broken down. As a result, much lower daily doses of levodopa are needed. Levodopa–carbidopa (Sinemet, Sinemet CR) has become the cornerstone in the treatment of PD. It also appears to limit the on–off phenomenon that some patients taking levodopa experience. This phenomenon is seen in patients taking levodopa long term. Such patients may experience periods when they have good control ("on" time) and periods when they have bad control or breakthrough PD ("off" time). A variety of studies have shown that the controlled-release product Sinemet CR (or generic levodopa–carbidopa) increases "on" time and decreases "off" time. When converting patients from conventional levodopa–carbidopa preparations, the dosage of levodopa–carbidopa CR should include 10% to 30% more levodopa per day. The interval between dosages of Sinemet CR should be 4 to 8 hours during the waking day. Sinemet CR should not be crushed.

Levodopa–carbidopa is contraindicated in patients who have shown a hypersensitivity reaction to it, those with narrow-angle glaucoma or a history of melanoma, and those concurrently taking MAOIs.

PHARMACOKINETICS

Half-Life	Onset	Peak	Duration
1–3 hr	2–3 wk* for therapeutic effect	1–3 hr	< 5 hr

*Therapeutic effect.

amantadine

Amantadine (Symmetrel) is believed to work in the CNS by eliciting the release of dopamine from nerve endings, resulting in higher concentrations of dopamine in the CNS. It is most effective in the earlier stages of PD when there are still significant numbers of nerves to act on and dopamine to be released. As the disease progresses, however, the population of functioning nerves diminishes, and so does amantadine's effect. Amantadine is usually effective for only 6 to 12 months. After amantadine fails to relieve the hypokinesia and rigidity, a dopamine agonist such as bromocriptine is usually tried next.

Amantadine is contraindicated in patients who have shown a hypersensitivity reaction to it, women who are lactating, and children younger than 1 year of age (amantadine is also an antiviral drug).

PHARMACOKINETICS

Half-Life	Onset	Peak	Duration
15 hr	48 hr	4 hr	6–12 wk

DOPAMINE AGONISTS

The traditional role of dopamine agonists (bromocriptine, pramipexole, ropinirole, and cabergoline) has been as an adjunct to levodopa for management of motor fluctuations only. These drugs differ from levodopa in that they do not replace dopamine but still act by stimulation of dopaminergic receptors in the brain. The drugs have been evaluated as initial monotherapy and as combination therapy with low-dose levodopa–carbidopa in an attempt to delay levodopa therapy or reduce total exposure to the drug and associated motor complications. The newer drugs pramipexole, ropinirole, and cabergoline are more specific for the receptors associated with parkinsonian symptoms, the dopamine 2 (D2) family (D2, D3, and D4). This, in turn, may have more specific antiparkinsonian effects with fewer adverse effects associated with generalized dopaminergic stimulation. The newer dopamine agonists have a promising role in the early treatment of PD. They appear to delay the start of levodopa therapy. Another benefit is that they have less ergot-like effects and dyskinesias. Bromocriptine is structurally similar to ergot derivatives and has some of their unwanted effects. The newer drugs have also shown efficacy in patients with advanced PD.

bromocriptine mesylate

Once amantadine becomes ineffective, a dopamine agonist such as bromocriptine may be prescribed in its place. Bromocriptine stimulates only the dopamine 2 (D2) receptors and antagonizes or blocks the dopamine 1 (D1) receptors. Eventually levodopa–carbidopa is needed to control the patient's symptoms, but by using amantadine until it fails and then a dopamine agonist until it fails, the need for levodopa therapy may be postponed for up to 3 years. Bromocriptine may also be given with levodopa–carbidopa so that lower doses of the levodopa are needed. This often results in prolonging the "on" periods, when PD is controlled, and decreasing the "off" periods, when PD is not controlled.

Bromocriptine is contraindicated in patients who have shown a hypersensitivity reaction to any of the ergot alkaloids, patients with severe ischemic disease, and those with severe peripheral vascular disease. This is primarily because of bromocriptine's ability to stimulate dopamine receptors.

PHARMACOKINETICS: BROMOCRIPTINE

Half-Life	Onset	Peak	Duration
3–5 hr	0.5–1.5 hr	1–3 hr	4–8 hr

▶▶ *ropinirole hydrochloride*

Ropinirole hydrochloride (ReQuip) is a newer nonergot dopamine agonist indicated for monotherapy for PD and adjunctive therapy with levodopa–carbidopa. It is highly selective for the D2 family of dopamine receptors. It is contraindicated in patients who have shown a hypersensitivity reaction to it.

Continued

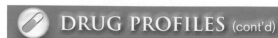

DRUG PROFILES (cont'd)

PHARMACOKINETICS

Half-Life	Onset	Peak	Duration
3–5 hr	30 min	1–2 hr	6–10 hr

COMT INHIBITORS

Inhibition of the enzyme in the body known as COMT is a new strategy for prolonging the duration of action of levodopa. As mentioned in the main text, COMT is a naturally occurring enzyme in the body that breaks down dopamine molecules and is responsible for breaking down levodopa. One compound is currently available for this enzyme inhibition purpose: entacapone (Comptan, Stalevo). Entacapone is a reversible inhibitor of COMT. The main positive effect of entacapone in patients with PD is the prolongation of levodopa benefit. Entacapone cannot cross the blood–brain barrier and therefore can act only peripherally. Patients have less wearing-off effects and experience prolonged benefits. Along with amantadine, this COMT inhibitor is considered to be an indirect-acting drug and works as a presynaptic drug.

entacapone

Entacapone (Comptan) is a potent COMT inhibitor indicated for the adjunctive treatment of PD. Entacapone is taken with levodopa–carbidopa and should be effective from the first dose. A patient with PD can feel the benefit of entacapone within 1 to 2 days. Entacapone is particularly effective in patients who are experiencing wearing-off fluctuations. Entacapone, used with levodopa–carbidopa, can reduce the daily "off" and increase the daily "on" times. The levodopa–carbidopa dose and dosing frequency can also be reduced in many cases. Entacapone is contraindicated in patients who have shown a hypersensitivity reaction to it. This drug is also now available in a combination tablet that contains various dosages of entacapone, carbidopa, and levodopa (Stalevo).

PHARMACOKINETICS

Half-Life	Onset	Peak	Duration
1.5–3.5 hr	1 hr	0.5–1.5 hr	6 hr

ANTICHOLINERGIC THERAPY

Anticholinergic drugs, or drugs that block the effects of ACh, are sometimes useful in treating the muscle tremors and muscle rigidity associated with PD. These two symptoms are caused by excessive cholinergic activity, which occurs because of lack of the normal dopamine balance. Anticholinergics do little, however, to relieve the bradykinesia associated with PD. The rationale for the use of anticholinergics is to reduce excessive cholinergic activity in the brain. The first drugs in this category to be used were the belladonna alkaloids, atropine, and scopolamine. However, the anticholinergic adverse effects of dry mouth, urinary retention, and blurred vision can be excessive; therefore, new synthetic anticholinergics and antihistamines with better adverse-effect profiles (e.g., benztropine and trihexyphenidyl) were developed.

Mechanism of Action and Drug Effects

All anticholinergics work in some way to block ACh, central cholinergic excitatory pathways. Because of the reduced number of dopamine-producing nerves associated with PD, the ACh-producing nerves are left unchecked and ACh accumulates. This results in overstimulation of the cholinergic excitatory pathways, causing muscle tremors and muscle rigidity. This is sometimes described as *cogwheel rigidity*. The muscle tremors are usually worse while the patient is at rest and consist of a pill-rolling movement and bobbing of the head. Anticholinergic drugs have either the opposite effect or oppose the effects of the neurotransmitter ACh, which is responsible for causing increased salivation, lacrimation (tearing of the eyes), urination, diarrhea, increased gastrointestinal motility, and possibly emesis (vomiting). The acronym SLUDGE is often used to describe these cholinergic-induced effects. The effects of anticholinergics are the opposite of the SLUDGE symptoms—effects such as antisecretory effects (dry mouth or decreased salivation), urinary retention, decreased gastrointestinal motility (constipation), dilated pupils (mydriasis), and smooth muscle relaxation. These drugs readily cross the blood–brain barrier and thus can arrive at the site of imbalance in the CNS, the substantia nigra. Because of their ability to directly relax smooth muscles, the muscle rigidity and akinesia (lack of movement) are reduced.

Indications

Anticholinergic drugs are indicated as antidyskinetic drugs in PD. They are also used for the treatment of drug-induced extrapyramidal reactions such as those related to selected antipsychotic drugs.

Contraindications

Contraindications to anticholinergic drugs include known drug allergy, any type of gastrointestinal or bladder outlet obstruction, heart disease, glaucoma, and myasthenia gravis.

Adverse Effects

The adverse effects associated with anticholinergic drug use are many. The most common adverse effects are listed in Table 15-5. They occur more commonly when the drugs are given in high doses. Anticholinergic-induced adverse effects are also more common in the older adult. However, wise and judicious use of such drugs can lead to effective treatment that is free of the unwanted adverse effects.

Interactions

The interactions that occur between anticholinergic drugs and other drugs and drug classes can be damaging. Alcohol, CNS depressants, amantadine, phenothiazines, tricyclic antidepressants, and antihistamines can have an additive effect with anticholinergic drugs, resulting in enhanced CNS depressant effects. Antacids, when taken with anticholinergic drugs, alter gastric pH and reduce the absorption and decrease the therapeutic effects of anticholinergic drugs.

TABLE 15-5

Anticholinergic Drugs: Adverse Effects

Body System	Adverse Effects
Central nervous	Drowsiness, confusion, disorientation, hallucinations
Gastrointestinal	Constipation, nausea, vomiting
Genitourinary	Urinary retention, pain on urination
Other	Blurred vision, dilated pupils (mydriasis), photophobia, dry skin

Dosages

For information on the dosages of benztropine and trihexyphenidyl in the treatment of PD, see the Dosages table below.

DOSAGES Selected Anticholinergic Drugs

Drug (Pregnancy Category)	Pharmacological Class	Usual Dosage Range	Indications
▸▸benztropine mesylate (C)	Anticholinergic	*Adult* PO: 0.5–6 mg/day	Parkinson's disease; drug-induced extrapyramidal symptoms
procyclidine hydrochloride (C)	Anticholinergic	*Adult* PO: 2.5 mg tid titrate to max 60 mg/day	Parkinson's disease; drug-induced extrapyramidal symptoms
trihexyphenidyl (Trihexyphen) (C)	Anticholinergic	*Adult* PO: 6–10 mg/day	Parkinson's disease; drug-induced extrapyramidal symptoms

DRUG PROFILES

Anticholinergics are helpful in alleviating the muscle tremors and rigidity commonly seen in patients with PD. They are not, however, as effective as the other drug classes used in the treatment of PD in correcting the underlying problem. They are effective for the relief of only minimal symptoms and for treatment of those patients who cannot tolerate or do not respond to dopamine replacement drugs such as levodopa or to dopaminergics such as amantadine and bromocriptine. Anticholinergics are also useful as adjuncts to these primary drugs. Treatment is usually started with small doses, which are gradually increased until the benefits or adverse effects appear. The most commonly used drugs are the synthetic anticholinergics, which are associated with fewer of the adverse effects seen with the belladonna alkaloid derivatives atropine and scopolamine. Some of the more commonly used drugs are trihexyphenidyl (Trihexyphen), diphenhydramine (Allerdyl, Allernix, Benadryl), and benztropine mesylate. A newer drug is procyclidine. These drugs must be used cautiously in older adults because significant adverse effects such as confusion, urinary retention, visual blurring, palpitations, and increased intraocular pressure can develop.

▸▸ benztropine mesylate

Benztropine mesylate is a synthetic anticholinergic drug that resembles both atropine and diphenhydramine (Allerdyl, Allernix, Benadryl) in its chemical structure. Procyclidine hydrochloride is also a synthetic anticholinergic drug used in the treatment of PD. All have anticholinergic and antihistaminic properties and are used primarily as adjuncts in the treatment of all forms of PD. They are also useful in the treatment of all antipsychotic-induced extrapyramidal reactions (see Chapter 16). Their use is contraindicated in cases of known drug allergy; in those who have narrow-angle glaucoma, myasthenia gravis, urinary retention, a history of peptic ulcer disease, megacolon, or prostate hypertrophy; and in children under 3 years of age.

PHARMACOKINETICS

Half-Life	Onset	Peak	Duration
4–8 hr	1–2 hr	2–4 hr	6–10 hr

NURSING PROCESS

☑ Assessment

As discussed in the earlier part of this chapter, antiparkinsonian drugs are used to treat Parkinson's disease to reduce the symptoms; however, some of the drugs have other indications that require additional assessment. For example, amantadine is used for PD but is also used to treat respiratory infections and control extrapyramidal reactions that occur as adverse effects to groups of drugs such as the phenothiazines. Bromocriptine, another antiparkinsonian drug, is also indicated to suppress milk "let-down" process for those new mothers who choose not to breastfeed.

After a patient is diagnosed with PD, the patient soon learns how the disease can affect every movement and alter activities of daily living (ADLs). This may be physically and emotionally stressful, and assessment of support systems and the patient's status as a whole is needed throughout the period between diagnosis and treatment. In addition, it may take weeks before therapeutic improvement is seen. As soon as the disease process and associated diagnoses are understood, the patient becomes aware of the significance of drug therapy that is not without challenges. The nurse must begin with a thorough head-to-toe assessment with a medical and medication history. A nursing history should include questions about the following:

- Central nervous system (CNS): Have there been any changes or alterations in activities of daily living, gait, balance, tremors, weakness, lethargy, and level of consciousness?
- Gastrointestinal (GI) and genitourinary (GU) systems: Have there been any changes in the patient's appetite? Changes in bowel or bladder patterns or habits?
- Psychological and emotional status: Have any recent or past changes in mood, affect, depression, or any personality changes occurred?
- Specific disease process: Have signs and symptoms of PD been apparent in the patient such as masklike expression; speech problems; dysphagia; rigidity of arms, legs, and neck; tremors; insomnia; inability to perform daily activities; or inability to maintain emotional stability?
- Neurological system and motor control and movements: What is the usual state of muscle movement and state of voluntary versus involuntary motor control? Are muscle movements coordinated and smooth or uncoordinated and rigid or with tremors? (These movements are of particular importance to note because of the tremors that occur with purposeful movements with PD.)

With dopaminergic drugs such as amantadine, levodopa–carbidopa, and ropinirole, a patient assessment should include vital signs, height, weight, medication and medical history, nursing history, nursing assessment, and a journal of presenting symptoms. All contraindications, cautions, and drug interactions should be noted. Drugs that can interact with these drugs include MAOIs. Given in combination with the dopaminergic medications, these drugs may result in a hypertensive crisis. Other drug interactions include tricyclic antidepressants, anticholinergics, alcohol, vitamin B_6, and antipsychotic drugs. Motor skills, abilities, and deficiencies should also be assessed—specifically the presence of akinesia, tremors, staggering gait, rigidity, and drooling. Vital signs should be assessed, with attention to blood pressure because of the adverse effects of hypotension and risk for syncope. Assessment of urinary patterns is also important because of the possibility of urinary retention associated with several of the drugs. If ordered, make sure to assess for blood urea nitrogen (BUN) and creatinine as indicators of kidney function and alkaline phosphatase levels as indicators for liver function. For women, it is also important to know the gynecological history of the patient and if she is pregnant or lactating, as some of the dopaminergic agents cross into the placenta and into breast milk and have unknown actions in children. Drug interactions related to the dopaminergics are presented in Table 15-4.

When anticholinergic drugs are prescribed, the nurse should assess the patient carefully to determine gross level of organ functioning (for those systems most affected by PD), such as with the gastrointestinal, genitourinary, and cardiac systems, and visual stability. Assessment of these systems is important because any pre-existing heart irregularities, tachycardia, urinary retention, bladder difficulties or obstruction, myasthenia gravis, or acute narrow-angle glaucoma (mydriasis leads to an increase in intraocular pressure) may be worsened or exacerbated with the use of anticholinergic drugs. Mental status, occurrence of agitation, confusion, or psychotic-like behaviour needs to be assessed for, especially in those 60 years of age or older because these patients are at higher risk for these problems. Age is also a significant factor to consider because of the increased likelihood of adverse effects or toxicity with increased age. The older adult experiences physiological changes of most organ functions and thus the increased risk for adverse or untoward reactions to drugs. Note their cautions, contraindications, and drug interactions as discussed earlier in this chapter.

For the dopamine agonist drugs that are also antivirals (e.g., amantadine), baseline assessment of underlying viral or other infectious disease processes is important. In fact, if the drug is used for antiviral indications, therapy is usually not begun until a positive influenza test is obtained. For use in patients with PD, the benefits of the drug may not be seen for several days after initiation of drug therapy. If used as a dopamine agonist for PD, it is always important to continue to monitor and assess the baseline functioning of the patient and degree of PD-related symptoms with this group of drugs because of the possible decline in its effectiveness within 3 to 6 months of the initial therapy.

If a dopamine agonist/prolactin inhibitor is used, it is important to understand that this drug is also used for suppression of lactation; however, for those with PD, it is crucial to be aware of its action on the symptoms of the disease. If the drug is being used for other indications, such as hyperprolactinemia or infertility, an entirely different assessment is indicated (see Chapter 34). The older adult requires additional assessment of the CNS because of the adverse effects related to that system (such as headache, lightheadedness, and visual or auditory changes). Also, if the patient with PD is taking this medication long term, assessment of the potential adverse effects is crucial to patient safety; these include rhinorrhea, fainting (syncope), peptic ulcers, severe abdominal pain, and gastrointestinal hemorrhage. The occurrence of any of these conditions should be reported to the patient's health care provider immediately.

The antiparkinsonian drugs classified as MAO type B inhibitors (e.g., selegiline hydrochloride) are associated with many of the same assessment parameters, as discussed earlier. In addition, heart status is important to know because of the problems with heart irregularities and hypotension associated with this drug class. Assessment of dosing is important because, as with other antiparkinsonian drugs, the lowest dose should be started initially with gradual increases over an approximately 3- to 4-week period. These drugs also require astute neurological assessment because of the possibility of serious reactions such as CNS depression (see Table 15-3 and discussion under Selective Monoamine Oxidase Inhibitor Therapy for more information on CNS-related adverse effects).

The COMT inhibitors (e.g., entacapone) also require assessment of baseline vital signs, especially because of the adverse effect of orthostatic hypotension and syncope, and these occur with more frequency than with the other antiparkinsonian drugs. As entacapone has no antiparkinsonian effect on its own, assessment of dosing time is also important; if not given 1 hour before or 2 hours after levodopa, the bioavailability of the drug is adversely affected. Serum transaminase levels should be assessed prior to and during drug therapy. If the patient's serum glutamic pyruvic transaminase SGPT (also called alanine aminotransferase [ALT]) is elevated, even to the upper range of normal or higher, the drug will most likely be discontinued by the physician owing to the risk of onset of liver failure. With use of entacapone, the older adult also suffers from a higher incidence of hallucinations than that among the general population.

Nursing Diagnoses

- Impaired physical mobility related to the disease process and adverse effects of the medications
- Disturbed body image related to changes in appearance and mobility because of the disease process
- Urinary retention related to effects of the disease on the bladder with incomplete emptying
- Constipation related to the disease process with decreased peristalsis
- Risk for injury related to the physical limitations produced by the disease process

- Imbalanced nutrition, less than body requirements, related to pharmacotherapy and associated adverse effects
- Deficient knowledge related to lack of exposure to treatment regimen

Planning

Goals

- Patient will remain free of injury.
- Patient will state the purpose of the specific medications prescribed for the disease.
- Patient will state the adverse effects and toxic effects of medications.
- Patient will regain bowel and bladder elimination patterns that are as normal as possible.
- Patient will maintain adequate nutritional status.
- Patient will remain as independent as possible.
- Patient will report feeling less anxious and fearful.
- Patient will regain a positive self-concept.
- Patient will remain adherent to therapy.

Outcome Criteria

- Patient (with significant others) states ways of preventing injury, such as the use of assistive devices.
- Patient states purposes, adverse effects, and toxic effects associated with specific antiparkinsonian medications, such as emesis, nausea, instability, and palpitations.
- Patient states ways to prevent some of the adverse effects and toxic effects of antiparkinsonian medication such as frequent mouth care and increased fluids.
- Patient discusses ways to minimize problems associated with drug-induced alterations in bowel and bladder elimination patterns through changes in diet and fluid intake.
- Patient discusses measures to ensure an adequate nutritional status with possible antiemetic therapy.
- Patient begins to perform activities of daily living more independently.
- Patient openly expresses fears, anxieties, and changes in self-image with members of the health care team and supportive staff.

Implementation

Nursing interventions associated with the antiparkinsonian drugs will vary somewhat depending on the drug class, but all will require close monitoring and comprehensive patient education. During the start of dopaminergic drug therapy, the patient should be assisted when walking because of dizziness caused by these drugs. Oral doses should be given with food to help minimize gastrointestinal upset. It is also important for the nurse to remember that pyridoxine (vitamin B$_6$) in doses greater than 10 mg will reverse the effects of levodopa. Foods high in vitamin B$_6$ should therefore also be avoided. Protein should be supplemented in the diet, but in divided amounts, with small, frequent meals, so that minimal protein is ingested during the actual dose of drug taken. The patient should be encouraged to drink extra fluids of at least 2000 mL/day, unless contraindicated, and to consume an adequate amount of food high in roughage and fibre. The doses of dopaminergics should be given as a single dose or in divided doses and may be given with or without food. Doses should be given several hours before bedtime to decrease the incidence of insomnia. Should edema, nausea, or vomiting occur, the patient should be encouraged to contact his or her health care provider immediately.

With the dopamine agonists, it is crucial to review (with the patient and family members) the concept of "drug holidays" with long-term use of levodopa. A *drug holiday* (usually a 10-day period) is sometimes used by physicians when drug therapy is not working. The patient is generally hospitalized so that when the drug is withdrawn, the patient can be taken care of appropriately and have needs met. Depending on the severity of the disease process, a patient may be totally dependent on others for basic care and nutritional and elimination needs. A patient may even be immobilized by a contracted physical state and unable to turn in bed, thus requiring a controlled environment with round-the-clock medical and nursing care. The purpose of the drug holiday is to obtain more therapeutic effectiveness once the levodopa is "reinitiated," with the additional hope that the patient will respond to a lower dose of the drug.

The newer COMT inhibitors have been shown to be more effective in patients with advanced forms of PD. After use of the various dosage forms of levodopa–carbidopa, a COMT inhibitor may be added, having a quicker onset of therapeutic effects. With anticholinergic drugs, patients should take the medication as prescribed but after meals or at bedtime and avoid other medications that do not have the consent or advice of a physician.

It is most important in the care of patients with PD to be aware of all other forms of therapies that may be beneficial, such as support groups, water aerobics, occupational and physical therapy, and use of community resources. Some community resources that may be helpful include community-wide recreation facilities, transportation services and assistance, Meals on Wheels, and alternative therapies. Consultation with an osteopathic physician or chiropractor may also be beneficial. Educational materials and emotional support resources should be shared with the patient and family members because of the long-term and progressive nature of the disease process. Contacting research institutes about new treatment protocols may be a viable option for patients and family members along the continuum of the disease process, and information should be made available as appropriate. Patient education tips associated with the antiparkinsonian drugs are discussed below.

Evaluation

Monitoring the patient's response to any of the antiparkinsonian medications is crucial to documenting treatment success or failure. Therapeutic responses to the antiparkinsonian drugs include an improved sense of well-being; improved mental status; increased appetite; ability to perform activities of daily living, to concentrate, and to think clearly; and less intense parkinsonism manifestations such as tremor, shuffling of gait, muscle rigidity, and involuntary movements. In addition to monitoring for therapeutic responses, the nurse must also watch for the occurrence of adverse effects such as confusion, anxiety, irritability, depression, paranoia, headache, weakness, lethargy, nausea, vomiting, anorexia, palpitations, postural hypotension, tachycardia, dry mouth, constipation, urinary retention, blurred vision, dark urine, difficulty swallowing, and nightmares.

Therapeutic effects of the COMT inhibitor entacapone may be noticed within a few days, whereas other antiparkinsonian drugs may take weeks. Adverse effects to monitor for with COMT inhibitors include those mentioned previously, but with fewer dyskinesias than with dopamine agonists. See Special Populations: The Older Adult for points related to PD in the older adult.

 SPECIAL POPULATIONS: THE OLDER ADULT

Antiparkinsonian Drugs

- Levodopa should be used cautiously, with close monitoring of the older adult, especially if there is a history of heart, kidney, liver, endocrine, pulmonary, ulcer, or mental health illness.

- The older adult taking levodopa is at an increased risk for experiencing adverse effects, especially confusion, loss of appetite, and orthostatic hypotension.

- Levodopa–carbidopa is often started at a low dose because of the increased sensitivity of the older patient to these medications and to salvage higher dosages for another point in time during treatment.

- Overheating is a problem in patients taking anticholinergics, and the older adult needs to be very careful and avoid excessive exercise during warm weather and excessive heat exposure.

- One of the main problems with the long-term use of levodopa is that its duration of effectiveness decreases over time; this is even more problematic for the older adult.

- COMT inhibitors hold much promise for the older adult who is experiencing the "wearing-off" phenomenon; they help turn the "off" times into "on" times so that the drug begins to work through the entire day.

PATIENT EDUCATION

- Patients should take their medication as ordered. Round-the-clock dosing is usually the regimen in order to achieve steady blood levels, especially with dopamine agonists.
- Patients should be instructed to avoid alcohol and to seek advice about taking any other medications, over-the-counter drugs, or natural health products.
- Patients should be encouraged to change positions slowly to avoid dizziness and possible syncope.
- Patients should be instructed to take sustained-release forms of drugs in their whole form and never crush or chew them.
- Patients should use alternative methods of contraception if taking oral contraceptives.
- With dopamine agonists or anticholinergic drugs, patients should be warned about dry mouth , an adverse effect. This may be managed with artificial saliva through drops or gum, frequent mouth care, forced fluids, and use of sugarless gum or hard candy.
- If a combination of levodopa–carbidopa is used, patients should be warned of a darkening in the colour of sweat and urine, but with the emphasis that this change is harmless.
- Patients should be instructed to contact their health care providers should vision become blurred or mental alertness diminished, or if there is confusion and lethargy with any of the antiparkinsonian drugs.
- Patients should be informed about other adverse effects associated with antiparkinsonian drugs that should be reported should they occur. These include difficulty urinating; irregular pulse rate; and severe, uncontrolled movements of arms, legs, mouth, and tongue.
- Patients should be clearly educated about potential blood pressure problems, whether they are the adverse effect of postural hypotension or the occurrence of hypertensive crisis if a MAOI is taken mistakenly. MAOIs should not be used with these drugs, and, if needed, 2 weeks should pass between the time the MAOI is discontinued and the levodopa is initiated.
- It is important for the patient and family to understand that dopaminergics are often titrated to the patient's response. It may take 3 to 4 weeks before a therapeutic response is seen.
- Patients taking newer dopamine agonists (pramipexole and ropinirole) should be educated about the "sleep attacks" that may occur without warning.

- Patients should be encouraged to always use caution with any activity. Some of these drugs may be associated with lightheadedness.
- Patients should be educated that drugs like bromocriptine may cause constipation, so measures to avoid this adverse effect need to be taken, including forcing fluids, increasing bulk and fibre in the diet, and using stool softeners as prescribed.
- Patients taking COMT inhibitors should be informed about how to minimize nausea and vomiting, such as taking the drug with food. Other instructions for COMT inhibitors should include information about adverse effects such as dizziness, drowsiness, and even nausea that may occur in the beginning of therapy but diminish as therapy continues.
- Patients taking COMT inhibitors should be encouraged to avoid tasks that require mental clarity or intact motor skills, to prevent injury with the initial onset of therapy. COMT inhibitors may result in hallucinations within the first 2 weeks of therapy.
- Patients taking entacapone should be warned about the possibility of the urine turning brownish-orange and that the therapeutic effects may take only a few days instead of the few weeks associated with other antiparkinsonian drugs.
- Patients should be informed to contact their health care provider if any abnormal contractions of the head, neck, or trunk are experienced, as well as syncope, falls, itching, or jaundice.
- Patients should be educated about the goal of therapy, especially if entacapone is being used to help the patient with the "wearing-off" phenomenon. This is a "waning" of the effects of a dose of levodopa before the scheduled time of the next dose, resulting in diminished motor ability and performance and the patient experiencing more "symptoms." If a COMT inhibitor is added to the levodopa or levodopa–carbidopa, the "wearing-off" phenomenon is minimized, and the therapeutic effects of the regimen are maximized. The patient can then expect the "off" time to go away and the drugs to work through the whole day, which is the goal in the treatment of patients with PD.
- Patients should be encouraged to never come off their medications abruptly and to contact a physician for further instructions should they accidentally skip a dose or make an error in dosage.

POINTS TO REMEMBER

❖ The neurotransmitting abnormalities with PD include a chronic, progressive, degenerative disorder of dopamine-producing neurons in the brain. Patients with PD have elevated ACh levels and lowered dopamine levels.

❖ Signs and symptoms of PD include bradykinesia (slow movements), rigidity (cogwheel), tremor (pill-rolling), postural instability, and dyskinesias (difficulty performing voluntary movements). There are two common signs or symptoms: **chorea** (irregular, spasmodic, involuntary movements of limbs or facial muscles) and dystonia (abnormal muscle tone in any tissue).

❖ Drug therapy for PD includes the following mechanisms: dopamine agonism, MAO inhibition, dopaminergic and anticholinergic effects, and COMT inhibition.

❖ COMT inhibitors are also associated with fewer "wearing-off" effects and prolonged therapeutic benefits.

❖ Nursing care considerations include thorough patient care, including providing information on the therapies involved and the variety of resources available in the community.

❖ Patient considerations include much family support, along with options for care of the family member with PD. This is a long-term process and a chronic, debilitating disease. Patients and families should be given excellent patient care, including the "holistic" approach, and patient rights should be honoured at all times.

❖ Patient care also requires much support and education about the disease process and the drugs indicated. The newer COMT inhibitors have a quicker onset of a few days compared with the several weeks required for onset by traditional drugs used for PD.

❖ Sleep attacks may occur with the newer dopamine agonists (pramipexole and ropinirole), and brownish-orange discoloration of the urine occurs with entacapone.

EXAMINATION REVIEW QUESTIONS

1 Which of the following should alert the nurse to a potential caution or contraindication with use of a dopaminergic drug for treatment of mild PD?
a. Diarrhea
b. Tremors
c. Unstable gait
d. Narrow-angle glaucoma

2 A patient is taking entacapone as part of the therapy for Parkinson's disease. Which intervention is appropriate at this time?
a. Force fluids to prevent dehydration.
b. Limit the patient's intake of tyramine-containing foods.
c. Notify the patient that this drug causes discoloration of the urine.
d. Monitor liver studies as this drug can seriously affect liver function.

3 Which of the following statements should patient teaching for antiparkinsonian drugs include?
a. Notify the physician if the urine turns brownish-orange in colour.
b. The drug should be stopped when tremors and weakness are relieved.
c. Change positions slowly to prevent falling due to postural hypotension.
d. If a dose is missed, take two doses to avoid significant decreases in blood levels.

4 Which of the following statements is true regarding new drug therapy for a patient who has PD and is not responding well to levodopa therapy?
a. Adding haloperidol will reduce adverse effects of levodopa.
b. Taking amantadine (Symmetrel) improves the effectiveness of levodopa.
c. Taking methyldopa will increase available dopamine levels in the brain.
d. Adding carbidopa will prevent the peripheral destruction of levodopa and result in increased amounts in the brain.

5 Which of the following statements should be emphasized and explained during patient teaching about the use of levodopa–carbidopa?
a. There are few, drug interactions with levodopa–carbidopa.
b. Therapeutic effects may take up to several weeks to a few months.
c. Notify the physician immediately if darkening of urine or sweat occurs.
d. Pyridoxine (vitamin B6) helps protect the action of levodopa–carbidopa.

For answers see http://evolve.elsevier.com/Canada/Lilley/pharmacology/.

CRITICAL THINKING ACTIVITIES

1 Mr. P. has been diagnosed with PD and is taking levodopa–carbidopa. He also has Alzheimer's disease and is taking donepezil (Aricept). What do you think of the use of these two medications together?

2 You discover that your patient with PD is taking levodopa–carbidopa and is also being given some of his wife's phenothiazine medication to make him "feel even better." Why is this combination unsafe and not rational?

3 Your patient has been placed on a dopaminergic for the management of PD. She tells you during the nursing history taking that her diet is high in meats, poultry, and whole-grain cereals. She also takes a "megadose multi-vitamin" daily. What would be a concern you may have with this patient's diet, and why?

4 How does levodopa help improve the function of the patient diagnosed with PD?

5 After long-term treatment, patients with PD are often placed on a "drug holiday." Explain the rationale for this approach to treatment.

6 Explain the physiology behind the "on-again/off-again" appearance of symptoms that occurs with long-term levodopa treatment.

For answers see http://evolve.elsevier.com/Canada/Lilley/pharmacology/.

CHAPTER 16

Psychotherapeutic Drugs

Learning Objectives

After reading this chapter, the successful student will be able to do the following:

1   Briefly discuss the prevalence and pathophysiology of anxiety disorders, major depression, bipolar disorder, and schizophrenia.

2   Identify psychotherapeutic drugs, such as antianxiety drugs, antidepressants, antimanic drugs, and antipsychotics.

3   Discuss the mechanisms of action, indications, therapeutic effects, adverse effects, toxic effects, drug interactions, contraindications, and cautions associated with psychotherapeutic drugs.

4   Develop a collaborative plan of care that includes all phases of the nursing process related to the administration of psychotherapeutic drugs.

5   Develop patient education guidelines for patients receiving psychotherapeutic drugs.

e-Learning Activities

Web site
(http://evolve.elsevier.com/Canada/Lilley/pharmacology/)

- Animations
- Answers to chapter questions, activities, and case studies
- Calculators and Category Catchers
- Glossary with audio pronunciations
- IV Therapy and Medication Error Checklists
- Multiple-Choice Review Question quizzes
- Nursing Care Plans
- Online Appendices and Supplements
- WebLinks

Drug Profiles

▸▸ alprazolam, p. 294
▸▸ amitriptyline (amitriptyline hydrochloride)*, p. 304
▸▸ bupropion (bupropion hydrochloride)*, p. 301
   buspirone (busipirone hydrochloride)*, p. 295
▸▸ chlordiazepoxide (chlordiazepoxide hydrochloride)*, p. 294
   clozapine, p. 311
▸▸ diazepam, p. 294
▸▸ fluoxetine (fluoextine hydrochloride)*, p. 301
   fluphenazine (fluphenazine hydrochloride)*, p. 310
   haloperidol, p. 310
   hydroxyzine (hydroxyzine hydrochloride)*, p. 295
▸▸ lithium (lithium carbonate)*, p. 297
▸▸ lorazepam, p. 295
▸▸ mirtazapine, p. 302
▸▸ olanzapine, p. 312
▸▸ paliperidone, p. 311
   quetiapine (quetiapine fumarate)*, p. 312
▸▸ risperidone, p. 311
   trazodone (trazodone hydrochloride)*, p. 301
   valproic acid, p. 297
   venlafaxine (venlafaxine hydrochloride)*, p. 301
   ziprasidone (ziprasidone hydrochloride monohydrate)*, p. 312

▸▸ Key drug.

*Full generic name is given in parentheses. For the purposes of this text, the more common shortened name is used.

Glossary

Adjunct therapy   Combination drug therapy used when a patient's condition does not respond adequately to a single drug (monotherapy), or used when a given combination of medications is known to have therapeutic benefits over a single drug. (See *monotherapy*.) (p. 298)

Affective disorders   Emotional disorders that are characterized by changes in mood. (p. 289)

Agoraphobia   Fear of leaving the familiar setting of home. (p. 289)

Akathisia   Motor restlessness. A distressing experience of uncontrollable muscular movements that can occur as an adverse effect of many psychotropic medications. (p. 308)

Antihistamine Any substance capable of reducing the physiological and pharmacological effects of histamine, including a wide variety of drugs that block histamine receptors. (p. 292)

Antipsychotic A medication that counteracts or diminishes symptoms of psychosis; also called a *neuroleptic.* (p. 306)

Anxiety The unpleasant state of mind in which real or imagined dangers are anticipated or exaggerated. (p. 289)

Anxiolytic Capable of reducing anxiety; usually said of a medication. (p. 292)

Benzodiazepine A chemical category of drugs most frequently prescribed as sedative–hypnotic and anxiolytic drugs; the most common group of psychotropic drugs currently prescribed to alleviate anxiety. (p. 292)

Biogenic amine hypothesis (BAH) Theory suggesting that depression and mania result from alterations in neuronal and synaptic amine concentrations, primarily the catecholamines dopamine and norepinephrine, as well as the indolamines serotonin and histamine. (p. 291)

Bipolar disorder (BPD) A major psychological disorder characterized by episodes of mania or hypomania, cycling with depression. (p. 289)

Depression An abnormal emotional state characterized by exaggerated feelings of sadness, melancholy, dejection, worthlessness, emptiness, and hopelessness that are inappropriate and out of proportion to reality. (p. 289)

Dopamine hypothesis Theory that dopamine dysregulation in certain parts of the brain is one of the primary contributing factors to the development of psychotic disorders (psychoses). (p. 308)

Dysregulation hypothesis Theory that depression and affective disorders are not simply the result of decreased or increased catecholamine and serotonin activity but failures of the regulation of these systems. (p. 291)

Extrapyramidal symptoms Symptoms arising adjacent to the pyrimidal portions of the brain. (p. 308)

Gamma-aminobutyric acid (GABA) An inhibitory amino acid in the brain that functions to inhibit nerve transmission in the central nervous system (CNS). (p. 289)

Mania A state characterized by an expansive emotional state; extreme excitement; excessive elation; hyperactivity; agitation; overtalkativeness; flight of ideas; increased psychomotor activity; fleeting attention; and sometimes violent, destructive, and self-destructive behaviour. (p. 289)

Monoamine oxidase inhibitor (MAOI) Any of a heterogeneous group of drugs used primarily in the treatment of depression. (p. 294)

Monotherapy Pharmacological therapy involving a single medication for a specific condition. (See *adjunct therapy.*) (p. 298)

Neurotransmitter Endogenous chemical in the body that serves to conduct nerve impulses between nerve cells (neurons). (p. 289)

Psychosis (Plural: psychoses) A syndrome consisting of a cluster of manifestations commonly associated with one or more mental health disorders. (p. 288)

Psychotherapeutics The therapy of emotional and mental health disorders, which may involve drug therapy (pharmacotherapy), a variety of counselling techniques, recreational therapy, and, in extreme cases, electroconvulsive therapy (ECT). (p. 287)

Psychotropic Capable of affecting mental processes; usually said of a medication. (p. 287)

Selective serotonin reuptake inhibitor (SSRI) Any of a heterogeneous group of newer medications used to treat depression and certain mental health disorders and that work by selectively reducing postsynaptic reuptake of the neurotransmitter serotonin in the brain; also called *serotonin selective reuptake inhibitor.* (p. 298)

Stigma Widespread negative perceptions of and prejudice toward a specific group of people such as those with mental health disorders. (p. 288)

Tardive dyskinesia A serious drug adverse effect involving disordered body movements and muscle tension that is associated with antipsychotic medications. (p. 308)

Tricyclic antidepressants (TCAs) A chemical class of antidepressant drugs with a distinctive three-ring segment in their chemical structure and that are used to block reuptake of the amine neurotransmitters serotonin and norepinephrine. (p. 298)

OVERVIEW

The treatment of emotional and mental health disorders is called **psychotherapeutics.** When a person's ability to cope with the environment to carry out the activities of daily living (ADLs) and to interact with others is seriously impaired, a **psychotropic** drug may be a treatment option. These drugs are among the most commonly prescribed drugs in Canada today. Because of the inherent subjectivity in the description and reporting of symptoms of mental health disorders, the effects of these drugs are less easily quantified than those of many other types of medications. For example, it is usually not known with certainty how long a given psychotropic drug works in the body (duration of action). Thus the effectiveness of psychotropic drug therapy is often measured by verbal reports from patients regarding the level of improvement (if any) in their social and occupational functioning. There are also several established tools that attempt to quantify patient response to psychotropic drug therapy, such as the Hamilton Depression Rating Scale (HAM-D). Of even newer interest is the rapidly expanding area of study known as *pharmacogenomics* (Chapter 51). One objective of this field is to map genetic factors (genetic polymorphisms) that contribute to different patterns of activity of drug-metabolizing enzymes across different ethnic groups (see Ethnocultural Implications: Psychotherapeutic Drugs for a discussion on psychotropic drug metabolism in different ethnocultural groups). To better understand the nature and goals of this treatment, the types and definitions of the different mental health disorders are presented first.

OVERVIEW OF MENTAL HEALTH DISORDERS

Most people experience emotions such as anxiety, depression, and grief; these are normal human emotions. However, the effect of these emotions on a person's ability to engage in normal activities of daily living (ADLs) and to interact with others can vary considerably. The duration and intensity of these emotions can range from occasional depression or anxiety to a state of constant emotional distress that interferes with a person's ability to carry out normal ADLs. For example, *seasonal affective disorder* is a recurrent episode of depressive illness that occurs most often during the winter months.

There is often considerable overlap between the symptoms of the many different psychiatric disorders, which can make it difficult to accurately diagnose a disorder. Complicating this issue further is the inherent subjectivity with which different patients experience their symptoms. Often a patient will have ongoing symptoms that meet several criteria for several mental health disorders. Such patients may be said to have a spectrum disorder. For example, research indicates that more than one half

of chronically depressed adults also have a concurrent personality disorder, and one third have a concurrent anxiety disorder, a concurrent substance use disorder, or both. People with mental health disorders may also be more susceptible to physical health problems than the general population. For example, obesity is significantly more common in patients with mental health disorders. Because of the variety of economic, educational, and psychosocial issues that may preclude a person with a mental health disorders from seeking health care, many patients self-medicate with alcohol, tobacco, and illegal drugs. This generally worsens the problem.

Despite newer, more effective treatments for mental health disorders, a long-held societal **stigma** continues to be an obstacle for diagnosed patients. The Canadian Alliance on Mental Illness and Mental Health (CAMIMH) is one major organization that advocates reducing this stigma. CAMIMH seeks to promote consumer well-being and autonomy through research funding, legislative advocacy, and public education and awareness to reduce stigma.

Ideal mental health care usually involves many factors, including a carefully detailed patient interview (to help ensure accurate and complete diagnosis); carefully chosen and regularly monitored drug therapy (if indicated); and significant emotional support, which may range from formal psychotherapy to informal support groups, social and family support systems, and spiritual support systems that the patient values.

There are three main emotional and mental health disorders: *psychoses*, *affective disorders*, and *anxiety*. A **psychosis** is a severe emotional disorder that often impairs mental function to the point of significant disability with

---

 ETHNOCULTURAL IMPLICATIONS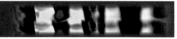

Psychotherapeutic Drugs

Many racial and ethnic groups respond to drugs differently. For example, Asians have a lower activity of drug metabolism compared with Whites as a result of various enzyme deficiencies. Asians often require lower doses of benzodiazepines and tricyclic antidepressants (TCAs) because they have lower levels of metabolizing enzymes (e.g., CYP2D6) and are thus more sensitive to these drugs. β-Blockers, specifically propranolol, are also problematic for the Asian population.

The commonly used antianxiety drug diazepam undergoes different metabolic pathways in the Chinese and Japanese populations. These two groups are found to be poor "mephenytoin pathway" metabolizers. Approximately 20% of these individuals metabolize mephenytoin poorly, resulting in rapid drug accumulation. To prevent possible toxicity, lower doses are generally required. Nurses may thus need to watch these individuals more closely for sedation, overdosage, and other adverse reactions (to diazepam).

Researchers have also identified genetic factors that help predict a response to antidepressants. In one study,

depressed and highly anxious patients with certain variant genes had a 70% greater "reduction" in anxiety and a 30% greater "reduction" in depression in response to treatment with fluoxetine and desipramine than did other racial ethnic groups without the specific gene variation. In another study, researchers examined the serotonin transporter gene (called *SLC6A4*) in 1914 study participants. Two variations in this serotonin transporter gene have a direct bearing on how individuals might respond to citalopram. *SLC6A4* produces a protein that plays an important role in achieving an antidepressant response. These two studies join a growing body of evidence suggesting that different responses to antidepressant drugs may be intimately influenced by genetic variations among patients. More and more genes such as the *HTR2A* gene, linked to serotonin, and *GR1K4*, linked to glutamate, are found to influence the pathology of depression and the efficacy and safety of treatments. Treatment decisions may ultimately be guided by genetic markers that identify individuals at high risk for treatment failure or particular adverse effects.

ADLs. A hallmark of psychosis is the loss of contact with reality. An individual experiencing psychosis tends to adhere to a set of false beliefs arising from disordered thinking. Psychoses can include hallucinatory experiences that are processed and interpreted as real, as well as delusions that persist in the face of proof to the contrary. Psychosis often results in significant disability. Psychotic disorders primarily include schizophrenia and depressive and drug-induced psychoses. **Affective disorders,** also called *mood disorders*, are characterized by changes in mood and range from **mania** (abnormally pronounced emotions) to **depression** (abnormally reduced emotions). Some patients may exhibit both mania and depression, experiencing periodic swings in emotions, from extremely negative emotions to intense, hyperactive emotions. This is referred to as **bipolar disorder (BPD)**. **Anxiety** is the unpleasant emotional state of mind chiefly characterized by the perception of a real or perceived danger that threatens the security of an individual.

The exact causes of mental health disorders are not fully understood. Many theories have been advanced in an attempt to explain the causes and pathophysiology of mental dysfunction. In the biochemical-imbalance concept, mental health disorders are thought to arise as the result of abnormal levels of endogenous chemicals in the brain known as **neurotransmitters**. This type of neurotransmission occurs in both the central nervous system (CNS) and the peripheral nervous system. However, the proposed mechanisms of both the pathology of and drug therapy for mental health disorders centre around neurotransmitter function between neurons in various regions of the brain. There is strong evidence indicating that the brain levels of catecholamines (especially dopamine and norepinephrine) and indolamines (serotonin and histamine) play an important role in maintaining mental health. Other biochemicals that seem necessary for the maintenance of normal mental function are **gamma-aminobutyric acid (GABA)**; acetylcholine (ACh); and inorganic ions such as sodium, potassium, and magnesium. Knowledge of these etiologies, especially the biochemical-imbalance theory, can aid in understanding psychotherapeutic drug action because many of the drugs used to treat psychoses, affective disorders, and anxiety work by blocking or stimulating the release of these endogenous neurotransmitters.

Anxiety Disorders

Anxiety disorders are among the most common mental health disorders encountered. Anxiety is an adaptive response that allows an individual to prepare for or react to a stressful situation or environmental changes. However, when anxiety becomes excessive, the individual will not only experience psychological and physiological responses but may also possess irrational fears in response to imaginary negative situations or to common everyday experiences that may significantly interfere with normal ADLs. Persistent anxiety is divided clinically into several distinct disorders that have been classified in the fourth edition (Text Revision) of the *Diagnostic and Statistical Manual for Mental Disorders* (DSM-IV-TR) published by the American Psychiatric Association. This reference delineates the demographic features and diagnostic criteria for the major psychiatric disorders and has categorized anxiety as follows: *obsessive–compulsive disorder* (OCD), *post-traumatic stress disorder* (PTSD), *generalized anxiety disorder* (GAD); *panic disorder* (PD) *with or without agoraphobia; agoraphobia; social anxiety disorder* (SAD), *acute stress disorder*, and *specific phobia.*

Anxiety disorders are heterogenous disorders that are more common in women and often develop before the age of 30. They affect approximately 10.4% to 28.8% of the Canadian population aged 15 to 64 years with a 12-month prevalence rate of 18% (see Box 16-1 for Canadian prevalence rates of anxiety disorders). Anxiety may occur as a result of a wide range of medical illnesses (e.g., cardiovascular or pulmonary disease, hypothyroidism, hyperthyroidism, pheochromocytoma, and hypoglycemia). Up to 75% of individuals diagnosed with an anxiety disorder have at least one other concurrent psychiatric disorder.

Having a specific phobia (i.e., fear of a situation or object such as spiders, bugs, mice, snakes, and heights) is most common, although a specific phobia is less likely than other anxiety disorders to result in significant impairment. However, these individuals will often have several phobias and thus experience considerable distress and disability. Specific phobias to animals or injections often begin in childhood; situational phobias often begin in adolescence and early adulthood.

Panic disorder is a chronic and recurrent disorder. It is associated with significant functional disability, higher rates of suicide ideation and suicide attempts, and high rates of substance misuse and concurrent depression. It is estimated that approximately one third to one half of patients with panic disorder also have symptoms of **agoraphobia**, the fear of leaving the familiar setting of home. Panic disorder and agoraphobia are more common in women and usually begin in late adolescence or early adulthood.

BOX 16-1

Anxiety Disorders: Prevalence in Canada

Type of Anxiety Disorder	Lifetime Prevalence	12-Month Prevalence
Specific phobia	12.5%	8.7%
Panic disorder	4.7%	2.7%
Obsessive–compulsive disorder	1.6%	0.7%–2.1%
Social anxiety disorder	8% –12%	3%
Generalized anxiety disorder	6%	1%–3%
Post-traumatic stress disorder	9.2%	2.4%

SAD is one of the more common anxiety disorders, affecting 750,000 adult Canadians. It is more common in women, peaking between 0 and 5 years of age and 11 and 15 years. Onset after age 25 years is rare. It is associated with significant functional impairment and distress.

OCD was thought to be rare but is now observed to be twice as common as schizophrenia. OCD is defined by obsessions that cause great anxiety or compulsions consisting of repetitive behaviours or rituals to reduce the anxiety. The age of onset of OCD is 19 years, although it can occur in childhood or in later years. It is associated with a high prevalence of functional impairment and concurrent mental health disorders.

Generalized anxiety disorder is a chronic anxiety disorder diagnosed more frequently in women. It is characterized by chronic, difficult-to-control worry often accompanied by numerous physiological and somatic symptoms.

PTSD generally occurs more frequently in women with onset in the mid- to late 20s. It is associated with a high risk of suicide. This disorder is a consequence of exposure to traumatic events, particularly motor vehicle crashes, war, and violence. The World Health Organization predicts PTSD to be a significant cause of disability by 2020.

The development of anxiety disorders appears to result from a complex interplay of genetic, biological, developmental, and other factors such as socioeconomic and workplace stress. A variety of theories have been proposed to explain how these factors contribute to the development of the disorder.

Many of the anxiety disorders are situational. They arise because of a specific event and subside with time. The treatment of these disorders should be limited to psychotherapy and, possibly, short-term drug therapy. However, when the anxiety disorder markedly affects a person's quality of life and relationships or interferes with the ability to function normally over a prolonged period (at least several months), longer-term pharmacotherapy in conjunction with psychotherapy is usually recommended.

Bipolar Disorder

Bipolar disorder is a cyclic disorder characterized by recurrent fluctuations of mood and activity. Indeed, bipolar disorder is often not diagnosed for many years because of this fluctuating course and episodic nature of mood states. Approximately 440,000 Canadian adults or 2.6% of the population have bipolar disorder. The average age of onset of a manic episode is 21 years for both men and women. Women are more likely to first experience a major depressive episode, whereas men often first experience a manic episode.

Although the etiology of bipolar disorder is unknown, numerous theories that explain its pathophysiology have been suggested. An environmental trigger such as a stressful life event, alcohol or substance misuse, or sleep–wake cycle alterations may signal the expression of an underlying genetic or biological vulnerability resulting in dysregulation of neurotransmitters, neurohormone

pathways, and secondary messenger systems. Evidence suggests that increased activity of the catecholamines, dopamine and norepinephrine, may play an important pathophysiological role in the development of hyperactivity and psychosis associated with mania, whereas reduced levels may contribute to depression. Serotonin may stabilize the catecholamine system and inhibit dopamine release. Serotonin levels are low in mania and depression. GABA (inhibitory for norepinephrine and dopamine) may also be deficient and play a role in the development of mania. Other excitatory neurotransmitters such as glutamate and aspartate may be overactive and contribute to mania.

Bipolar disorder is divided into four main subtypes based on the specific mood episodes. A discussion of these categories is beyond the scope of this book; the reader is referred to the *DSM-IV–TR* for details of the mood disorders. *Bipolar disorder type I* is associated with major depressive disorder and manic or mixed episode. *Bipolar type II disorder* is associated with major depressive disorder and hypomania disorder. Bipolar depression is often misdiagnosed as major depressive disorder. Bipolar depression occurs more frequently and lasts longer than manic episodes. Hallucinations, delusions, and suicide attempts are more common in bipolar depression. A manic episode includes symptoms of grandiosity, decreased need for sleep or food, pressured speech, flight of ideas, distractibility, and involvement in pleasurable activities often resulting in negative consequences. Hypomania is a less severe form of mania and does not result in the same impairment associated with mania. A *mixed episode* is defined as the simultaneous occurrence of both manic and depressive symptoms.

Major Depression

The World Health Organization predicts that major depressive disorders (MDDs) will be the second leading cause of disability by the year 2020. Depression is reported to have prevalence rates of approximately 6% to 8% among Canadians 18 years of age and older and up to 10% in youths. Women are at increased risk of depression from early adolescence until their mid-50s (see Special Populations: Women: Women and Depression). The highest incidence rates are in adults aged 25 to 44 years. Approximately 20% of older adults over age 65 suffer mild to severe depression, ranging from 5% to 10% of older adults in the community to as many as 30% to 40% of those in institutions. The findings of an international study conducted over 5 years of 1758 children born in Quebec and their mothers revealed that 15% of preschoolers experienecd abnormally high levels of depression and anxiety (Côté et al., 2009). Difficult temperaments at 5 months of age and maternal lifetime depression were the most significant risk factors for developing depression and anxiety. Prevention of depression in childhood may be the best way to prevent depression in adulthood.

It is estimated that the average major depressive episode persists approximately 9 months in the absence of

SPECIAL POPULATIONS: WOMEN

Women and Depression

Women are approximately twice as likely as men to experience depression. The highest rates of depression are seen among women of reproductive age, with estimates of 13% of mothers experiencing postpartum depression. The increased vulnerability of women to depression is thought to be linked to hormonal imbalances of estrogen and progesterone that occur during puberty, menopause, and pregnancy and with the use of oral contraceptives and hormone replacement therapy.

Women with a history of depression are at greater risk for postpartum depression. Psychosocial factors likely mediate the risks for depression incurred by biological influences. The effects of stress, violence, poverty, inequality, and low self-esteem may increase women's susceptibility to depression. Immigrant, asylum-seeking, and refugee women report higher levels of symptoms than Canadian-born women, possibly because of lower education, inadequate income, and fewer contacts with a health professional, and are less likely to receive adequate prenatal care, social support, or treatment for their depression.

treatment, and approximately 50% of individuals who have one episode will experience a recurrence.

The etiology of major depression is complex and incompletely understood. Several factors appear to work together to cause or precipitate depression. The symptoms of individuals with major depression reflect alterations in the brain monoamine neurotransmitters, specifically norepinephrine (NE) and serotonin (5-HT). This deficiency of neuronal and synaptic catecholamines is known as **biogenic amine hypothesis (BAH)**, a widely supported hypothesis. The cause of this deficiency, however, remains unknown. This hypothesis is shown in Figure 16-1. The role of dopamine (DA) remains unclear, although increased dopamine neurotransmission may play a role in the action of antidepressant drugs.

Another theory concerns the downregulation or desensitization of NE receptors. These changes in postsynaptic receptor sensitivity could explain the delayed onset of antidepressant effects. In a new leading theory, **dysregulation hypothesis**, depression and affective disorders are viewed not simply in terms of decreased or increased catecholamine activity but as a failure of the regulation of these systems.

Common depressive symptoms include feelings of worthlessness, loss of interest or pleasure in most or all normal daily activities, frequent reduced energy level, drastic increase or decrease in appetite, insomnia or hypersomnia, and recurrent thoughts of death or suicide. In addition to often drastic reductions in quality of life and occupational and psychosocial functioning, depression is also associated with the occurrence of major sleep disturbances in up to 80% of patients with depression. Some sleep researchers report that an 1½-hour loss of sleep on any given night may reduce alertness on the following day by 33%; therefore, insomnia associated with depression has even more far-reaching adverse effects on the patient. This loss in the patient's state of alertness may then be associated with accidents and increased risk of suicide. Despite recent advances in pharmacotherapy for depression, depression remains unrecognized,

misdiagnosed, and undertreated, particularly in the older adult and those with chronic diseases.

Schizophrenia

Schizophrenia is a chronic, complex, and challenging disorder of thought and affect. It is considered a heterogeneous syndrome consisting of disorganized and bizarre thoughts, delusions, hallucinations, inappropriate affect, and impaired psychosocial functioning. It affects approximately 1% of the population with onset in early adulthood. Although males and females are affected equally, onset of schizophrenia occurs earlier in males, during their early twenties, compared with the late twenties to early thirties in females. This disorder often has a significant impact on the affected individual's ability to engage in interpersonal relationships and daily functioning in society.

Schizophrenia is likely a multifactorial disorder. Abnormalities in brain structure and function exist. It is thought that an in utero disturbance may contribute

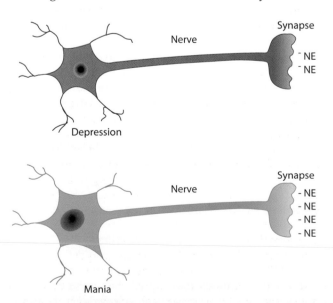

FIG. 16-1 Biogenic amine hypothesis. *NE*, norepinephrine.

to these brain abnormalities. Genetics is also thought to play a role, although a specific abnormality has not yet been identified.

Current thought is that a primary pathophysiological abnormality probably occurs in one of the numerous neurotransmitters (dopaminergic, glutaminergic, or serotoninergic systems) with changes occurring secondarily in other neurotransmitters such as GABA.

ANTIANXIETY DRUGS

Medications are only one therapeutic option for people diagnosed with one of the anxiety disorders. Other therapeutic options include nonpharmacological treatment modalities of psychotherapy, exercise, and meditation. Although benzodiazepines are generally the first-line drug treatment for anxiety disorders, there are other classes of drugs that are also effective. The efficacy of certain classes of medications in the treatment of certain anxiety disorders and their superiority over other drug classes have been documented. These drug classes are listed in Table 16-1 according to the anxiety disorders they effectively treat.

Mechanism of Action and Drug Effects

Of the several drug classes shown to be effective in the treatment of anxiety disorders, all reduce anxiety by diminishing overactivity in the CNS. There are, however, differences among the drug classes.

Benzodiazepines seem to exert their **anxiolytic** effects by depressing activity in the *brainstem* and the *limbic system*. Benzodiazepines are believed to increase the action of GABA, a neurotransmitter in the brain that functions to inhibit nerve transmission in the CNS. Benzodiazepines have specific receptor proteins (also referred to as *specific receptor binding sites*) in the same areas of the brain that govern the release of GABA. The binding of benzodiazepines with these receptor sites produces their anxiolytic effects as well as the effects of sedation and muscle relaxation.

Antihistamines (see Chapter 36) have also been used as anxiolytics because of their ability to depress the CNS by sedating the patient. The antihistamine most commonly used for the relief of anxiety is hydroxyzine. Its

significant sedative effects are related to its antihistaminic properties. This can be advantageous for patients with comorbid insomnia, often associated with both depression and antidepressant therapy. However, sedative effects of any medication can also be hazardous, and patients should be warned to use caution when driving or operating dangerous machinery. There is one salt form of hydroxyzine, hydroxyzine hydrochloride (Atarax), which is an effective anxiolytic. However, benzodiazepines, antidepressants, and buspirone (described later in this chapter) have emerged as the most effective, safe, and commonly prescribed drugs for treatment of ongoing anxiety disorders.

Miscellaneous anxiolytic drugs are the third class of anxiolytics and include the single drug buspirone (BuSpar, BusTab). It has the advantage of being both nonsedating and non–habit-forming. It is described in more detail later in this chapter.

Besides their anxiolytic effects, antianxiety drugs also produce several other effects throughout the body, including sedative, hypnotic, appetite stimulating, analgesic, and anticonvulsant effects.

Indications

Both carbamates and barbiturates were used for many years to treat anxiety, but this practice is now unusual with the introduction of newer drugs. Some antihistamines are used to treat anxiety because of their sedative adverse effects, but their primary pharmacological effect is to block the actions of histamine released during exacerbations of allergic conditions.

Benzodiazepines are the most commonly prescribed anxiolytic drug class for the rapid relief of acute anxiety symptoms. The benzodiazepenes offer several advantages over the other drug classes used to treat anxiety. At therapeutic doses, they have little effect on consciousness, they are safe because of their low adverse-effect profile, and they do not interact with many other drugs. Six commonly prescribed anxiolytic benzodiazepines are diazepam (Valium), lorazepam (Ativan), alprazolam (Xanax), clonazepam (Clonapam), chlordiazepoxide, and midazolam. In addition to treating anxiety, these drugs are used for sedation, to produce muscle relaxation, to control seizures, to treat alcohol withdrawal, and as

TABLE 16-1

Various Anxiety Disorders: Drugs of Choice

Disorder	TCAs	Benzodiazepines	MAOIs	Buspirone	SSRIs
Generalized anxiety disorder	+	++++	++	+++	
Obsessive–compulsive disorder	+++	+	+	0	++++
Panic disorder	+++	++++	+++	0	++++
Post-traumatic stress disorder	+	+	+	+	
Simple phobia	0	+	0	0	
Social phobia	+	+	+	0	

MAOI, monoamine oxidase inhibitor; *SSRI*, selective serotonin reuptake inhibitor; *TCA*, tricyclic and tetracyclic antidepressants; 0, no efficacy or use; ?, has shown some efficacy but limited use; + limited use and efficacy; ++, some use and efficacy; +++, frequent use, good efficacy; ++++, most frequent use, best efficacy.

adjuvant drug therapy for sleep disturbances associated with depression. Midazolam is available only in injectable form and is limited to use as a sedative and anaesthetic during invasive medical or surgical procedures. One of its desirable qualities is that it reduces the patient's anxiety during, and memory of, painful medical procedures that do not require general anaesthesia. This is known as *moderate sedation* (see Chapter 12). It is also used to provide sedation and to control acute anxiety and agitation in critical care unit (CCU) patients when excessive movement might be harmful (e.g., spinal cord injury in a confused patient or a patient requiring mechanical ventilation). Benzodiazepines commonly used as sedative–hypnotics, in contrast to anxiolytics, are discussed with other CNS depressants (see Chapter 13). These drugs have slightly different therapeutic actions and pharmacokinetics from those of the benzodiazepines used to treat anxiety. Because of their wide range of effects, anxiolytic drugs are sometimes used for certain other indications in addition to anxiety, such as seizure disorders, insomnia, agitation, and pain control. The commonly used anxiolytic benzodiazepines and their approved indications are listed in Table 16-2.

Contraindications

Contraindications to anxiolytic drugs include known drug allergy, narrow-angle glaucoma, and pregnancy. A positive seizure history is a relative contraindication.

Adverse Effects

The most common undesirable effect of the anxiolytic drugs is an overexpression of their therapeutic effects.

All of these classes of drugs decrease CNS activity, and many of the unwanted effects of these drugs are related directly to this action. Both antihistamines and benzodiazepines can cause hypotension. Benzodiazepines are by far more commonly used, and some adverse effects are listed in Table 16-3. Of particular note are *paradoxical* (opposite of what would normally be expected) reactions to the benzodiazepines and antihistamines, including hyperactivity and aggressive behaviour. Although these reactions are relatively uncommon, they are more likely to occur in children and adolescents as well as in patients with psychiatric disorders. There are also case reports of increasing seizure frequency in epileptic patients receiving benzodiazepines. All benzodiazepines are potentially habit forming and addictive. Although they can provide significant symptom relief, they should be used judiciously and at the lowest effective dosages and frequencies needed for symptom control.

Toxicity and Management of Overdose

Overdose of antihistamines is usually not severe but may be associated with excessive sedation, hypotension, and seizures. There is no specific antidote, but in extreme cases a cholinergic drug (see Chapter 21), may be used to treat anticholinergic adverse effects associated with antihistamines.

There is a potential for benzodiazepines to cause serious life-threatening toxicities, but when taken alone in normal doses in otherwise healthy patients, they are safe, effective anxiolytics. When taken with other sedating medications or with alcohol, life-threatening respiratory depression or arrest can occur. This serious consequence

---

TABLE   16-2

Benzodiazepines: Approved Indications

Approved Indications	Benzodiazepines
Alcohol withdrawal	clorazepate, diazepam, lorazepam, oxazepam
Anxiety	alprazolam, bromazepam, chlordiazepoxide, clorazepate, diazepam, lorazepam, oxazepam
Depression (adjunct)	alprazolam, oxazepam
Insomnia	flurazepam, nitrazepam, tenazepam, trazolam
Panic disorder	alprazolam, clorazepate
Perioperative sedation	diazepam, lorazepam, midazolam
Seizure disorders	clobazam, clonazepam, clorazepate, diazepam, lorazepam, nitrazapam
Skeletal muscle spasticity	diazepam

TABLE   16-3

Benzodiazepines: Common Adverse Effects

Body System	Adverse Effects
Cardiovascular	Hypotension
Central nervous	Drowsiness, sedation, loss of coordination, dizziness, blurred vision, headaches, paradoxical reactions (insomnia, increased excitability, hallucinations)
Gastrointestinal	Nausea, vomiting, constipation, dry mouth, abdominal cramping
Hematological	Blood dyscrasias, including anemia, leukopenia, thrombocytopenia
Integumentary	Pruritis, skin rash

can also occur in patients whose metabolism or elimination capabilities are impaired because of hepatic or renal dysfunction. In such cases, benzodiazepines can accumulate and not be eliminated. This further accentuates their therapeutic and toxic actions. An overdose of benzodiazepines may result in one or any combination of the following symptoms: somnolence, confusion, coma, or respiratory depression. However, coma and respiratory depression are much less likely with benzodiazepines taken alone than with barbiturates or meprobamate.

The treatment for benzodiazepine intoxication is generally symptomatic and supportive. If ingestion is recent (within 4 hours), decontamination of the gastrointestinal system is indicated. Gastric lavage is generally the best and most effective means of gastric decontamination. Activated charcoal and a saline cathartic may be administered after gastric lavage to remove any remaining drug. Activated charcoal is an odourless and tasteless wood powder activated to increase its adsorbency. Hemodialysis is usually not needed or useful in the treatment of benzodiazepine overdose but may be used in more extreme cases, especially those involving multiple types of drugs. A more likely treatment in such severe cases may also be the use of the benzodiazepine-specific antidote flumazenil (Anexate). This drug is a benzodiazepine receptor blocker (antagonist) that is used to reverse the effects of benzodiazepines. Although it has been approved for benzodiazepine overdose, flumazenil has not been shown to reduce mortality or length of hospital stay. For this reason, its use for this indication is more limited. Instead, this drug is more commonly used to reverse benzodiazepine effects following procedures involving moderate sedation (described earlier and in Chapter 12). It opposes the actions of benzodiazepines by directly competing with benzodiazepines for binding at the benzodiazepine receptors in the CNS. It has a stronger affinity for these receptors and thus chemically forces the benzodiazepine drug molecules off

---

BOX 16-2

Flumazenil Treatment Regimen for Benzodiazepine Overdose

Recommended Regimen

0.3 mg (3 mL) of flumazenil intravenously over 30 seconds followed by a series of 0.3 mg injections, each administered over a 30-second period, at 60-second intervals, for a total dose of 2 mg.

Duration of Action

Usually 1 hour. If reversing the effects of a long-acting benzodiazepine, you may need to re-administer flumazenil as it wears off and the effects reappear (e.g., resedation). An intravenous infusion of 0.1–0.4 mg/hr may be useful but should be individually adjusted to desired level of arousal.

---

the receptor, reversing their CNS-depressant effects. The treatment regimen for the reversal of benzodiazepine overdose is summarized in Box 16-2.

Interactions

There are a few notable drug interactions that occur with the use of anxiolytics, particularly benzodiazepines. Alcohol and CNS depressants, when coadministered with benzodiazepines, can result in additive CNS depression and subsequent death. Cimetidine, disulfiram **monoamine oxidase inhibitors (MAOIs),** and tobacco can decrease the metabolism of benzodiazepines and result in increased CNS depression.

Dosages

For the recommended dosages of selected antianxiety drugs, see the Dosages table on p. 295.

 ## DRUG PROFILES

BENZODIAZEPINES

Benzodiazepines are targeted substances under the Controlled Drugs and Substances Act. They are contraindicated in patients who have shown a hypersensitivity reaction to them and in patients who have narrow-angle glaucoma. Dosage and indication information appears in the corresponding table.

▶▶ alprazolam

Alprazolam (Xanax) is most commonly used as an anxiolytic and as an adjunct for the treatment of depression.

PHARMACOKINETICS

Half-Life	Onset	Peak	Duration
9.5–15 hr	< 1 hr	0.9–2.4 hr	6–12 hr

▶▶ chlordiazepoxide hydrochloride

Chlordiazepoxide hydrochloride is used most commonly for the relief of anxiety. A combination of chlordiazepoxide hydrochloride and clidinium bromide (Librax), an anticholinergic drug, is available as an adjunctive treatment for peptic ulcer and irritable bowel syndrome when associated with excessive anxiety and tension.

PHARMACOKINETICS

Half-Life	Onset	Peak	Duration
9–34 hr	1–3 hr	0.5–4 hr	12–24 hr

▶▶ diazepam

Diazepam (Valium) is one of the most commonly prescribed benzodiazepines. It is indicated for the relief of

Continued

DRUG PROFILES (cont'd)

anxiety, alcohol withdrawal, and seizure disorders (e.g., status epilepticus); for sedation; and as an adjunct for the relief of skeletal muscle spasms. Diazepam has active metabolites that can accumulate in patients who have liver dysfunction because it is metabolized primarily in the liver. This can result in additive, cumulative effects that may be manifested as prolonged sedation, respiratory depression, or coma.

PHARMACOKINETICS

Half-Life	Onset	Peak	Duration
20–80 hr	Less than 1 hr	0.5–2 hr	12–24 hr

▶▶ lorazepam

Lorazepam (Ativan) is another widely used benzodiazepine. It is currently approved for use in the management of anxiety disorders, for the short-term relief of acute anxiety, for insomnia, and as a preoperative medication to provide sedation and light anaesthesia and to diminish patient recall (amnesia). As well as oral forms, lorazepam is available sublingually (SL). When administered in this fashion, its onset of action is similar to that associated with intravenous administration. The injectable form requires refrigeration.

PHARMACOKINETICS

Half-Life	Onset	Peak	Duration
IV: 12–16 hr	IV: Rapid	IV: 15–20 min	IV: 4 hr
PO: 12–16 hr	PO: 1–3 hr	PO: 2–4 hr	PO: 11–20 hr

MISCELLANEOUS DRUGS

Several categories of drugs can be used in the treatment of anxiety disorders. Although benzodiazepines are by far the most widely prescribed anxiolytics, often drugs in other categories may be prescribed because of certain advantages they offer. Some of the more commonly used drugs are described in this section. The efficacy of the carbamates in treating anxiety disorders, with meprobamate the prototype, has been shown. The antihistamine hydroxyzine and the nonbenzodiazepine anxiolytic buspirone are also effective antianxiety drugs. Dosage and indication information appears in the corresponding table.

buspirone hydrochloride

Buspirone hydrochloride (BuSpar, BusTab) is a psychotropic drug with anxiolytic properties that belongs to a class of drugs known as the azaspirodecanediones, which are distinctly different both chemically and pharmacologically from the benzodiazepines. Its precise mechanism of action is unknown, but it appears to have agonist activity at a subset of both serotonin and dopamine receptors. It is indicated for short-term symptomatic relief of anxiety in patients with generalized anxiety disorder. Its only reported contraindication is drug allergy. The advantages of buspirone hydrochloride over benzodiazepines include its lack of sedative properties and of dependency potential. It does not prevent or treat benzodiazepine withdrawal symptoms, so although it may be used concurrently with benzodiazepines, they still need to be withdrawn gradually if they are to be discontinued. An additional advantage of buspirone hydrochloride is that it does not require dose adjustment for the older adult because age has not been shown to affect the pharmacokinetics of the drug in the body. It is recommended, however, that the daily dose for the older adult not exceed 30 mg for no longer than 4 weeks. The drug is not currently approved for use in children. It is recommended that MAOIs not be used concurrently with buspirone because of a risk of hypertension. A washout period of at least 14 days after discontinuation of MAOI therapy should occur before starting buspirone. See Preventing Medication Errors: Look-Alike Drugs: Bupropion and Buspirone for a note of caution using buspirone.

PHARMACOKINETICS

Half-Life	Onset	Peak	Duration
2–3 hr	Up to 2–3 wk	40–60 min	Unknown

hydroxyzine hydrochloride

Hydroxyzine hydrochloride (Atarax) is used to treat anxiety disorders. Hydroxyzine is an antihistamine that suppresses activity in the CNS, which makes it useful as both an anxiolytic and an antiemetic drug.

PHARMACOKINETICS

Half-Life	Onset	Peak	Duration
3–7 hr	15–30 min	15–30 min	4–6 hr

DOSAGES Selected Anti-Anxiety Drugs

Drug (Pregnancy Category)	Pharmacological Class	Usual Dosage Range	Indications
▶▶ alprazolam (Xanax) (D)	Benzodiazepine	*Adult* PO: 0.25–0.5 mg bid– tid; do not exceed 3 mg/day	Anxiolytic
		Older adult PO: 0.125–0.25 mg bid–tid	Anxiolytic
buspirone hydrochloride (BuSpar, BusTab) (B)	Miscellaneous	*Adult* PO: 15–45 mg/day in 2–3 divided doses	Anxiolytic

Continued

DOSAGES Selected Anti-Anxiety Drugs (cont'd)

Drug (Pregnancy Category)	Pharmacological Class	Usual Dosage Range	Indications
▸▸chlordiazepoxide hydrochloride (B)	Benzodiazepine	*Children* PO: older than 6 yr, 5 mg bid–tid	Anxiolytic
		Adult PO: 5–25 mg tid–qid	Anxiolytic
hydroxyzine hydrochloride (C)	Antihistamine	*Children* PO: 30–50 mg/day divided Under 6 yr, PO: 30–50 mg/day divided Over 6 yr, PO: 50–100 mg/day divided IM: 1 mg/kg	Anxiolytic/pruritus Pre- and postoperative adjunctive sedation Nausea/vomiting
		Adult PO: 25–100 mg tid–qid PO: 25 mg tid–qid IM: 25–100 mg	Anxiolytic Pruritus Pre- and postpartum sedation; pre- and postoperative adjunctive sedation Nausea/vomiting
▸▸lorazepam (Ativan) (D)	Benzodiazepine	*Adult* PO: 2–6 mg/day divided PO: 0.5–1 mg at bedtime SL: 0.05 mg/kg to a max of 4 mg IV: 0.044 mg/kg or 2 mg	Anxiolytic Preoperative sedation

PREVENTING MEDICATION ERRORS

Look-Alike Drugs: Bupropion and Buspirone

Is it bupropion or buspirone? These two CNS drugs have sound-alike names but different uses. Bupropion (Wellbutrin) is an antidepressant that is used to relieve depression. Bupropion (Zyban) is used to help with nicotine withdrawal symptoms. Wellbutrin is available in extended- or sustained-release formulations of 100 mg, 150 mg, and 300 mg tablets. Buspirone hydrochloride (BuSpar, BusTab) is an antianxiety drug used for short-term management of anxiety disorders. It is available in tablets ranging from 5 mg to 10 mg.

Tall Man lettering is a safety strategy recommended by the Institute of Safe Medication Practice (ISMP). Using a mix of upper and lower case letters to accentuate key parts of the drug name, this strategy is intended to limit errors associated with look-alike drug names. Some centres are using this type of labelling on pharmacy-produced packaging labels, patient medication labels, and medication administration records (MARs). For example, buspirone and bupropion are labelled busPIRone and buPROPion to accentuate key parts of the drug name.

Drugs Used to Treat Affective Disorders

Several classes of drugs are used in the treatment of affective disorders. The two main drug categories are antimanic drugs and antidepressant drugs.

ANTIMANIC DRUGS

Pharmacotherapy is critical for the acute and chronic maintenance of bipolar disorder. Drug management of bipolar disorder involves three therapeutic domains: acute mania, acute depression, and maintenance. Lithium is the drug of choice to effectively alleviate the major symptoms of mania and in maintenance treatment of BPD. There are numerous proposed mechanisms of action. Lithium may potentiate serotonergic neurotransmission,

inhibit dopamine synthesis and decrease the number of β-adrenergic receptors, and enhance GABA activity. Quetiapine fumarate, a novel antipsychotic, is also indicated as monotherapy for the acute management of manic episodes. A variety of drugs may be used in conjunction with lithium to regulate mood or stabilize patients experiencing mania. Some of these adjunctive medications are high-potency benzodiazepines, the antiepileptic drugs carbamazepine and divalproex sodium, dopamine receptor agonists, the amino acid L-tryptophan, and calcium channel antagonists. More recently, medications used for acute manic episodes include third-generation anticonvulsant valproic acid (see Chapter 14) and the novel antipsychotic drug olanzapine. Valproic acid is often a better choice than lithium in frail older adult patients because of the narrow therapeutic index and the closer monitoring requirements associated with lithium therapy.

Lithium, valproic acid, and carbamazepine are also commonly referred to as "mood stabilizers" regarding their use in treating BPD.

Antidepressants are often also required to control the depression associated with bipolar disorder. A pharmacological challenge is to choose antidepressants that are less likely to evoke manic responses secondary to the expected stimulating effects of the antidepressant medication. Several of the newer third-generation anticonvulsants (see Chapter 14) have also become more firmly established in treating mania and hypomania and, to a lesser degree, depressive symptoms. These include lamotrigine, oxcarbazepine, and topiramate. Other recent studies have shown the atypical antipsychotic drugs risperidone, olanzapine, quetiapine, and ziprasidone to be effective for acute mania or hypomania. Currently, more data support olanzapine for bipolar depression and prophylaxis.

ANTIDEPRESSANT DRUGS

Antidepressants are the pharmacological treatment of choice for major depressive disorders. Not only are they effective in treating depression, they are also useful for treating other disorders, such as dysthymia, schizophrenia (as an adjunct), eating disorders, and personality disorders.

Many of the drugs currently used to treat affective disorders increase the levels of monoamine neurotransmitter

---

 DRUG PROFILES

▸▸ lithium carbonate

The antimanic effect of lithium carbonate is not fully understood but it has a "stabilizing" effect in the body. Lithum competes at cellular sites with cations involved in the synthesis, storage, release, and reuptake of neurotransmitters. Lithium ions alter sodium ion transport in nerve and muscle cells, resulting in reduced concentrations of catecholamine neurotransmitters. The therapeutic levels of lithium that are required are close to the toxic levels, but there is increasingly greater tolerance to these toxic levels during acute manic phases. For the management of acute mania, a lithium serum level of 0.8 to 1.2 mmol/L, measured before the first lithium dose of the day, is usually required. Desirable long-term maintenance levels range between 0.6 and 0.8 mmol/L and are best measured 8 to 12 hours (roughly the midpoint of the drug half-life) after the last dose because the half-life usually ranges between 18 and 24 hours. A level of 0.4 to 0.6 mmol/L is desirable for maintenance in the older adult. Both sodium and lithium are monovalent positive ions; one can affect the other. Therefore, the patient's serum sodium levels should also be monitored. A sodium level kept in the normal range (135–145 mmol/L) helps maintain therapeutic lithium levels.

Lithium carbonate capsules (Carbolith, Lithane) and lithium citrate liquid are two currently available salts of lithium. There are no absolute contraindications to lithium therapy, although lithium toxicity is increased in patients with significant kidney or cardiovascular disease, severe debilitation or dehydration, or sodium depletion. The adverse effects are dependent on the serum levels. Lithium toxicity is usually associated with lithium levels greater than 2 mmol/L including gastrointestinal

discomfort, tremor, confusion, somnolence, seizures, and possibly death. Earlier signs to watch for include diarrhea, vomiting, muscle weakness, and lack of coordination. The most serious adverse effect is cardiac dysrhythmia. Other effects include drowsiness, slurred speech, epileptic-type seizures, choreoathetotic movements (involuntary wave-like movements of extremities), ataxia (generalized disturbance of muscular coordination), and hypotension. Long-term treatment may cause hypothyroidism.

The concurrent use of thiazides, angiotensin-converting enzyme inhibitors, calcium channel blockers, and nonsteroidal anti-inflammatory drugs can increase lithium toxicity.

PHARMACOKINETICS

Half-Life	Onset	Peak	Duration
24 hr	10–21 days*	1–3 hr	24 hr

*Therapeutic benefit for controlling mania.

valproic acid

The anticonvulsant valproic acid (Depakene, Divalproex, Epival) has been used for seizure disorders for many years (see Chapter 14). More recently, it has become one of the major drugs of choice for mania. Although lithium can be effective in both acute mania and for prevention of manic episodes, valproic acid is normally reserved for preventive drug therapy maintenance against manic episodes.

PHARMACOKINETICS

Half-Life	Onset	Peak	Duration
6–16 hr	1–3 days	1–4 hr	2–4 days

DOSAGES   Selected Antimanic Drugs

Drug (Pregnancy Category)	Pharmacological Class	Usual Dosage Range	Indications
▸▸lithium carbonate (D) (Carbolith, Lithane)	Mood stabilizer	450–1200 mg/day	Mania, acute and hypomanic, maintenance of bipolar disorder
valproic acid (Divalproex, Depakote) (D)	Anticonvulsant, mood stabilizer	750–1500 mg/day (max 60 mg/kg/day)	Mania, prevention of mania

concentrations in the CNS. Recent research data indicate that early and aggressive antidepressant treatment increases the chances for full remission. The first 6 to 8 weeks of therapy constitute the acute phase. The primary goals during this time are to obtain a response to drug therapy and improve the patient's symptoms. It is currently recommended that antidepressant drug therapy be maintained at the effective dose for an additional 8 to 14 months after remission of depressive symptoms. In choosing an antidepressant for a patient, the patient's previous psychotropic drug response history (if any) should be considered. Information regarding any family history of depression with known drug responses may also be helpful. Therapeutic response is measured primarily by subjective patient feedback. In addition, there are measurement tools that attempt to quantify response to drug therapy, such as the Hamilton Depression Rating Scale (HAM-D) and the Symptom Checklist-90 (SCL-90) anxiety factor score. A therapeutic nonresponse to antidepressant drug therapy is defined as failure to respond to adequate doses of at least 6 weeks of therapy. Twenty to 30 percent of patients who do not respond to the usual dose of a given antidepressant drug will respond to higher doses. Therefore, dose optimization, involving careful upward titration of medication dose for several weeks, is recommended before concluding that a given drug is ineffective. If the decision is to switch to a different pharmacological class of antidepressant, research indicates that 40% to 60% of patients will respond to the second drug class attempted.

Nonresponse to at least two trials, including at least two different classes of antidepressants, is classified as *treatment-resistant depression (TRD)*. Such cases can be treated by either switching to a different drug from the same or a different class or augmenting the initial drug therapy by adding a second drug. There is currently limited controlled research data regarding drug combination augmentation strategies, but more research is anticipated in this area. In the meantime, clinicians choosing drug combinations rely on trial-and-error experience, their previous clinical experience in general, and considerations of specific patient factors (e.g., concurrent anxiety). Antipsychotic drugs (discussed later in this chapter) may also be used concurrently with antidepressants in treating some cases of TRD. This practice is currently well established for cases of MDD that also involve psychotic symptoms. Two issues currently under research include the use of antipsychotic drugs as **monotherapy** for psychotic forms of MDD, and the potential use of antipsychotic drugs as **adjunct therapy** for nonpsychotic TRD. The most severe cases of TRD may warrant a treatment attempt with electroconvulsive therapy (ECT). Current ECT techniques are greatly refined from similar treatments in past decades and are usually carried out in a postanaesthesia care unit (PACU) or recovery room setting under general anaesthesia. Seizure activity is induced in the anaesthetized patient via externally applied electric shocks to the brain.

Treatment failure in cases of depression may be due to a misdiagnosis or failure to treat concurrent mental health disorder (e.g., anxiety disorder, substance misuse) or comorbid nonpsychiatric illness (e.g., hypothyroidism). It may also stem from nonadherence to drug therapy, which is the cause in an estimated 20% of TRD cases. Thus, careful choice of drug therapy to minimize adverse effects may improve adherence to treatment and therapeutic outcome. An additional reason for treatment failure may be the discouragement associated with depression itself. This alone may cause patients to give up prematurely on their drug therapy, especially because antidepressants often take several weeks to reach their full effect. Effective psychotherapy and support groups can help encourage patients to be consistent with prescribed psychotropic drug therapy.

The drug categories most commonly used in the treatment of affective disorders are the **selective serotonin reuptake inhibitors (SSRIs)** and the second- and third-generation antidepressants. Less commonly used are what are considered to be, although not formally classified as, the classes informally known as first-generation antidepressants. These include the **tricyclic antidepressants (TCAs)** and MAOIs. In 2004, Health Canada issued special warnings regarding the use of all classes of antidepressants in both adult and child populations (in the United States these are known as black box warnings; Health Canada uses a "box warning" on product monographs). Most patients do not experience severe adverse effects with these medications, and many patients experience significant relief from depressive symptoms while on these medications. However, a meta-analysis combining data from 24 small studies of child and adolescent subjects indicated a higher risk for suicide in up to 4% of patients receiving these medications, compared with 2% receiving placebo (Mosholder & Willy, 2006). Later in the same year, Health Canada expressed similar concerns regarding adult patients. As a result, current recommendations for all patients receiving antidepressants include regular monitoring for signs of worsening depressive symptoms, especially when starting or changing the dose of medication. Patients should be evaluated by their health care provider immediately if they report, or others observe, signs of worsening depression or other emotional instability.

SELECTIVE SEROTONIN REUPTAKE INHIBITORS AND SECOND- AND THIRD-GENERATION ANTIDEPRESSANTS

Selective serotonin reuptake inhibitors and second- and third-generation antidepressant drug classes are considered newer-generation antidepressants (NGAs) and are generally considered superior to TCAs and MAOIs because of their adverse effect profiles. As a result, they largely replaced TCAs and MAOIs as first-line drug therapy for depression in the 1980s following the introduction of the first SSRI, fluoxetine. The SSRIs include citalopram hydrobromide (Celexa, Cipralex), escitalopram oxalate (Cipralex), fluoxetine hydrochloride (Prozac), fluvoxamine maleate (Luvox), paroxetine hydrochloride (Paxil), and sertraline hydrochloride (Zoloft). Escitalopram is one of the two stereoisomers that make up citalopram. This chemical property provides for greater receptor specificity and thus reduces the likelihood of adverse effects. Second-generation antidepressants include bupropion hydrochloride (Wellbutrin) and trazodone hydrochloride (Desyrel). Third-generation antidepressants include mirtazapine (Remeron) and venlafaxine (Effexor). Mirtazapine along with the much less commonly used second-generation drug maprotiline are also known as *tetracyclic drugs* because of the four connected rings that form the basis of their chemical structure; thus, the tetracyclic drugs actually span more than one generation of antidepressants. In contrast, the TCAs are all solely first-generation drugs. For this reason, the terms *second-* and *third-generation* are more precise and less ambiguous when speaking of the tetracyclic antidepressants. Because maprotiline is rarely used, only mirtazapine is discussed in detail in this chapter.

These newer antidepressants offer several attractive advantages over the traditional TCAs and MAOIs. They are associated with significantly fewer and less severe systemic adverse effects, especially those to which older adults have little tolerance—anticholinergic and cardiovascular adverse effects. They are safe and have few drug–drug or drug–food interactions. However, it does take approximately the same amount of time for them to reach maximum clinical effectiveness as it does the TCAs and MAOIs, typically 4 to 6 weeks.

SSRIs were developed to slow or inhibit the reuptake of serotonin into presynaptic terminals (nerve endings) and thus to increase the levels of serotonin for neurotransmission at the postsynaptic nerve endings. Sertraline is the most selective of the three drugs in inhibiting serotonin more than norepinephrine reuptake, and fluoxetine is the least selective. Fluoxetine is the only SSRI that has an active metabolite. Fluoxetine, along with its active metabolite, has an elimination half-life of 2 to 4 days in contrast to a 1-day half-life for sertraline and paroxetine.

A newer antidepressant in its own unique category is reboxetine (Vestra). It is a norepinephrine-selective reuptake inhibitor (NSRI). Currently, reboxetine is still being researched for its antidepressant qualities and is only available through the Special Access Programme for patients with refractory depressive disorders. A still newer drug, more closely related to the SSRIs, is duloxetine hydrochloride (Cymbalta). Approved by Health Canada in 2007, this drug works as a strong inhibitor of both serotonin and norepinephrine and as a weaker reuptake inhibitor of dopamine.

Mechanism of Action and Drug Effects

The inhibition of serotonin reuptake seems to be the primary clinically significant mechanism of action for the SSRIs, although SSRIs may also have weak effects on norepinephrine and dopamine reuptake. Second- and third-generation drugs are less selective and have activity at brain serotonin as well as norepinephrine and dopamine receptors. They are also referred to as *multimodal* or *multireceptor* drugs and have greater receptor specificity than that of first-generation drugs and a generally improved adverse-effect profile compared with that of first-generation drugs. The second- and third-generation drugs have chemical structures that differ from that of the SSRIs, and there is significant overlap between the pharmacological activities of these two generations of medications. Trazodone is primarily a serotonin-reuptake inhibitor but it also has a smaller inhibitory effect on norepinephrine reuptake. Mirtazapine has both noradrenergic (norepinephrine) and serotonergic (serotonin) effects but works by promoting presynaptic release of these two neurotransmitters and does not inhibit either their pre- or postsynaptic reuptake. The antidepressant activities of bupropion and venlafaxine are believed to affect all three major neurotransmitters: serotonin, norepinephrine, and, to a lesser degree, dopamine. The latest research is starting to suggest that these newer-generation multireceptor drugs may offer significant improvement outcomes in depression treatment over even the highly acclaimed SSRI drugs. Larger clinical studies are anticipated with these newer drugs, either alone or in combination with SSRI therapy.

The increase in serotonin, norepinephrine, or dopamine reuptake causes increased concentrations of these neurotransmitters at nerve endings in the CNS, resulting in numerous functional changes associated with enhanced amine neurotransmission. This increased neurotransmitter concentration in the CNS also seems to lead to a decrease in REM sleep. In addition, it has a potentiating effect when given with opioid analgesics in that the increased serotonin concentration at nerve endings appears to work synergistically with the opioid analgesic in relieving pain.

Although all NGAs are associated with varying degrees of weight gain or loss, SSRIs are more commonly associated with anorectic activity and weight loss. This appetite-inhibiting action may result from the blocking of serotonin reuptake and the attendant increase in the serotonin concentration at the nerve endings. For this reason, SSRIs are sometimes used to treat eating disorders, such as bulimia nervosa, that involve compulsive overeating. Patients should be educated that antidepressant drugs commonly require several weeks before full therapeutic effects are realized. This requires some patience and faithful dosing on the part of patients.

Indications

All three classes of NGAs have been used to treat many affective disorders. Depression, BPD, obesity, eating disorders, OCD, panic attacks or disorders, social anxiety disorder, PTSD, premenstrual dysphoric disorder, and the neurological disorder myoclonus are only some of the many disorders that this highly effective drug class can be used to treat. This list is expanding with continued research. These newer antidepressant classes have also shown some beneficial effects in the treatment of substance misuse problems such as alcohol dependence.

Contraindications

Contraindications to NGA use include known drug allergy and use sooner than 14 days after stopping MAOI therapy. Additionally, a significant cardiac or seizure history may also be a contraindication because of relatively uncommon, but reported, heart effects and alterations in seizure threshold (see Adverse Effects). Bupropion is also contraindicated in cases of eating disorder and in seizure disorder because it can lower the seizure threshold.

Adverse Effects

Despite their advantage over TCAs and MAOIs in terms of safer adverse-effect profiles, up to two thirds of all depressed patients may discontinue NGA therapy because of drug adverse effects. Some of the most common and bothersome adverse effects include insomnia, weight gain, and sexual dysfunction. Less commonly reported cardiac effects include chest pain, palpitations, and QT-prolongation (on electrocardiogram). NGAs may also lower the seizure threshold in susceptible patients (i.e., those with previous seizure history). Bupropion and mirtazapine are both associated with a reduced incidence of sexual adverse effects, and may serve as effective substitute or adjuvant (second) drugs. The sexual dysfunction primarily involves male impotence in terms of erectile dysfunction. Other drug alternatives to treat this condition (e.g., Viagra) are discussed in the chapter pertaining to men's health (Chapter 35). One potentially hazardous adverse effect of any drug or combination of drugs that have serotonergic activity is known as *serotonin syndrome*. Fortunately, it is usually self-limiting on discontinuation of the causal drugs. The adverse effects that can occur in patients taking second-generation antidepressants are listed in Table 16-4.

TABLE 16-4

Newer-Generation Antidepressants: Adverse Effects

Body System	Adverse Effect
Central nervous	Headache, dizziness, tremor, nervousness, insomnia, fatigue
Gastrointestinal	Nausea, diarrhea, constipation, dry mouth, weight loss or gain
Other	Sweating, sexual dysfunction

Interactions

NGAs are highly bound to plasma proteins such as albumin. When given with other drugs that are also highly bound to protein (e.g., warfarin and phenytoin), both compete for binding sites on the surface of albumin. This results in a more free, unbound drug and, therefore, a greater, more pronounced drug effect.

NGAs also have the capacity to inhibit cytochrome P450. The cytochrome P450 system is an enzyme system in the liver that is responsible for the metabolism of several drugs. Inhibition of this enzyme system results in higher levels of drugs because they accumulate rather than break down to their inactive metabolites. This also prolongs the action of drugs metabolized by the cytochrome P450 system. The SSRIs fluoxetine and paroxetine seem to be more potent inhibitors of this enzyme system than sertraline. There is still controversy over whether the cytochrome P450 system is inhibited. Many studies have shown that this event is minimal or even nonexistent. The most common and significant drug interactions are listed in Table 16-5. To prevent the potentially fatal pharmacodynamic interactions that can occur between NGAs and MAOIs, a 2- to 5-week washout period is recommended between uses of the two classes of medications. NGAs that have a longer half-life, such as fluoxetine, require the longer washout period.

Dosages

For the recommended dosages of selected NGAs, see the Dosages table on p. 302.

TABLE 16-5

Newer-Generation Antidepressants: Drug Interactions

Drug	Mechanism	Result
carbamazepine	Decreases carbamazepine metabolism	Increased carbamazepine levels, carbamazepine toxicity, ocular changes, vertigo, tremor
MAOIs	Enhances serotonin activity	Hyperthermia, diaphoresis, shivering, tremor, seizures, ataxia, autonomic instability
TCAs	Increases TCA toxicity	Sedation, decreased energy, lightheadedness, dry mouth, constipation, elevated TCA levels
warfarin	Possible displacement of warfarin by NGAs from protein-binding sites	Increased warfarin effects

MAOIs, monoamine oxidase inhibitors; *NGAs*, newer-generation antidepressants; *TCAs*, tricyclic antidepressants.

DRUG PROFILES

During the 1980s and 1990s, the development of psychotropic pharmacotherapy expanded. Several new classes of antidepressants were introduced during this period. TCAs and MAOIs are considered first-generation antidepressants. Two drugs introduced in the 1980s, now classified as second-generation antidepressants, were trazodone and bupropion, both still commonly used. There are six currently available SSRIs, five introduced during the 1980s and 1990s and one more recently in 2004. In chronological order, they are fluoxetine, sertraline, paroxetine, fluvoxamine, citalopram, and escitalopram. In the 1990s, another major class of antidepressants, the third-generation antidepressants, was introduced: venlafaxine and mirtazapine. Both drugs have proven to be valuable new antidepressants. They are highly effective as antidepressants and are associated with few serious adverse effects, especially when compared with first-generation antidepressants. They are now considered first-line drugs in the treatment of depression, especially for patients with concurrent symptoms of anxiety, patients with depression with suicidal ideations, and patients unable to tolerate adverse reactions to other drugs. One notable hazard of the first-generation drugs, especially the TCAs, is their tendency to cause fatal cardiac dysrhythmias following overdose. Because depressed patients are generally at greater risk for suicide attempt, the newer generations of antidepressant drugs usually provide a safer drug choice. Dosage and indication information for selected NGAs appears in the corresponding table.

trazodone hydrochloride

Trazodone hydrochloride (Desyrel, Trazorel) was the first of the second-generation antidepressants that could selectively inhibit serotonin reuptake but that negligibly affected norepinephrine reuptake. This allowed for one advantage of trazodone over TCAs in terms of its minimal adverse effect on the cardiovascular system. It is, however, sedating. The sedating effects can be severe and impair cognitive function in older adults. However, the sedating effect of trazodone is often advantageous in assisting depressed patients, who commonly have concurrent anxiety and insomnia, obtain effective sleep. Trazodone has also been associated rarely with transient nonsexual priapism. This is reportedly the result of α-adrenergic blockade. The use of trazodone is contraindicated in patients who have shown a hypersensitivity reaction to it.

PHARMACOKINETICS

Half-Life	Onset	Peak	Duration
6–9 hr	1–2 wk*	2–4 wk*	Weeks*

*Therapeutic effects.

▶▶ bupropion hydrochloride

Bupropion hydrochloride (Wellbutrin SR, Zyban), a second-generation antidepressant, is a unique antidepressant in terms of both its structure and mechanism of action. It has relatively weak, but measurable, effects on brain serotonin activity, with little to no activity on MAO. Its strongest therapeutic effects appear to be primarily dopaminergic and noradrenergic in nature.

Bupropion is available in both immediate-release (for multiple daily dosing) and sustained-release (for single or double daily dosing) dosage forms. Bupropion is sometimes added as a second antidepressant for male patients experiencing sexual adverse effects (e.g., erectile dysfunction) secondary to SSRI therapy. The mechanism for this is unclear, but the drug is often effective in this situation. A new sustained-release form of bupropion, Zyban, has recently been approved as first-line therapy as an aid in smoking cessation treatment. Zyban is an innovative new treatment because it is the first nicotine-free prescription medicine used to treat nicotine dependence. Its exact mechanism of action in treating nicotine dependence is unknown, but it is believed to be related to the drug's ability to modulate dopamine and norepinephrine levels in the brain. Both of these neurotransmitters are thought to play an important role in maintaining nicotine addiction.

Bupropion is contraindicated in patients who have shown a hypersensitivity reaction to it, those with a seizure disorder (bupropion can lower the seizure threshold), those who are currently suffering or have previously suffered from anorexia nervosa or bulimia, and those currently on MAOI treatment.

PHARMACOKINETICS

Half-Life	Onset	Peak	Duration
10–14 hr	Up to 4 wk*	3 hr	Weeks to months

*Therapeutic effects.

▶▶ fluoxetine hydrochloride

Fluoxetine hydrochloride (Prozac) was the first SSRI marketed for the treatment of depression in 1988. Since that time, it has become the number one prescribed antidepressant in Canada and one of the most commonly prescribed of all drugs. It is contraindicated in patients who have shown a hypersensitivity reaction to it and in those taking MAOIs.

PHARMACOKINETICS

Half-Life	Onset	Peak	Duration
1–3 days	1–4 wk*	6–8 hr	2–4 wk

*Therapeutic effects.

venlafaxine hydrochloride

Venlafaxine hydrochloride (Effexor XR), a third-generation antidepressant, is unique in that it is chemically unrelated to all other available antidepressants and has a trimodal mechanism of action on the activity of the three major brain neurotransmitters. Specifically, it has potent inhibitory effects on both serotonin and norepinephrine

Continued

DRUG PROFILES (cont'd)

reuptake and weaker, although still significant, inhibitory effects on dopamine reuptake. Given this multi-neurotransmitter activity, it is not surprising that venlafaxine, along with many other newer antidepressants, is often associated with activating adverse effects such as nervousness and insomnia. However, patients often report rapid improvement in depressive symptoms. The drug is available in both immediate-release (for multiple daily dosing) and sustained-release (for single or double daily dosing) dosage forms. Venlafaxine does have significant metabolic effects on cytochrome P450 enzyme systems and is contraindicated in cases of drug allergy and in combination with MAOIs. Concurrent use with other serotonergic drugs carries the risk of serotonin syndrome and is generally not recommended.

PHARMACOKINETICS

Half-Life	Onset	Peak	Duration
3–11 hr	1–7 days	1–2 hr	Unknown

►► mirtazapine

Mirtazapine (Remeron, Remeron RD), the newest of the third-generation antidepressants, is unique in that it promotes the presynaptic release in the brain of both serotonin and norepinephrine because of its antagonist activity in the presynaptic α_2-adrenergic receptors (see Chapter 18) but does not inhibit the reuptake of either of these neurotransmitters. It is strongly associated with sedation in more than 50% of patients because of its histamine (H_1) receptor activity and, therefore, is usually dosed once daily at bedtime. However, it has demonstrated significant improvement of symptoms in depressed patients, including frail older adult patients in the nursing home setting. Furthermore, although clearance of the drug may be somewhat reduced in the older adult, no dosage adjustment is currently recommended. Mirtazapine is also sometimes helpful (mechanism unknown) in reducing the sexual adverse effects in male patients receiving SSRI therapy. Mirtazapine is contraindicated in cases of drug allergy and concurrent use of MAOIs.

PHARMACOKINETICS

Half-Life	Onset	Peak	Duration
20–40 hr	1–3 wk	2 hr	Unknown

DOSAGES   Selected NGAs

Drug (Pregnancy Category)	Pharmacological Class	Usual Dosage Range*	Indications
►► bupropion hydrochloride (Wellbutrin SR, Zyban) (B)	Second generation	PO: 100–300 mg once/day	Depression (Wellbutrin SR), smoking cessation (Zyban)
►► citalopram hydrochloride (Celexa) (C)	SSRI	20–40 mg once/day, AM or PM	Depression
duloxetine hydrochloride (Cymbalta) (C)	SNRI	30–60 mg once/day	Depression, pain from diabetic neuropathy
escitalopram oxalate (Cipralex) (C)	SSRI	10–20 mg once/day	Depression, GAD
►► fluoxetine hydrochloride (Prozac) (B)	SSRI	PO: 20–80 mg once/day	Depression, OCD, bulimia nervosa
fluvoxamine maleate (Luvox) (C)	SSRI	50–300 mg once/day, larger doses divided bid	Depression, OCD
►► mirtazapine (Remeron, Remeron RD) (C)	Third generation	15–45 mg/day at bedtime	Depression
paroxetine hydrochloride (Pavix) (B)	SSRI	PO: 20–60 mg, once/day	Depression, OCD, panic disorder, social anxiety disorder, GAD, PTSD
sertraline hydrochloride (Zoloft) (B)	SSRI	PO: 25–200 mg, once/day	Depression, OCD, panic disorder
trazodone hydrochloride (Desyrel, Trazorel) (C)	Second generation	PO: 150–600 mg/day, divided	Depression
venlafaxine hydrochloride (Effexor XR) (C)	Third generation	PO: 75–225 mg once/day	Depression, panic disorder, SAD

GAD, generalized anxiety disorder; *OCD*, obsessive–compulsive disorder; *NGA*, newer-generation antidepressant; *PTSD*, post-traumatic stress disorder.

*All dosages reflect usual adult dosage ranges. Child doses may be more variable and should be specified by a pediatric practitioner.

TRICYCLIC ANTIDEPRESSANTS

Among the original, first-generation antidepressants, TCAs have largely been superseded as first-line antidepressant drug therapy following the introduction of the SSRIs. Today, TCAs are generally considered second-line drug therapy for patients who fail NGAs or as adjunct therapy with NGAs.

Mechanism of Action and Drug Effects

TCAs are believed to work by correcting the imbalance in the neurotransmitter concentrations of serotonin and norepinephrine at the nerve endings in the CNS (the biogenic amine hypothesis). This is accomplished by blocking the reuptake of the neurotransmitters and thus causing these neurotransmitters to accumulate at the nerve endings. Some investigators also believe that these drugs may help regulate malfunctioning nerves (the dysregulation hypothesis). TCAs have several advantageous therapeutic effects, but their use is also associated with many adverse effects. Both the advantageous and adverse effects can be explained by the functions of the receptors these drugs affect. Aside from their ability to inhibit the reuptake of norepinephrine and serotonin at the nerve endings, TCAs also block muscarinic, histaminergic, adrenergic, dopaminergic, and serotonergic receptors. This nonselective antagonism of multiple receptor types contributes to their adverse effects. The therapeutic and undesirable effects as they relate to the receptors affected are presented in Table 16-6.

Indications

TCAs are used to treat depression. They have been available for more than 40 years. Overall, they have demonstrated a remarkable efficacy, and their adverse effect profiles are well established. They are also considerably less expensive than most of the newer drugs, with the majority available in generic formulations. Some of the TCAs have additional specific indications other than depression. For example, imipramine is used as an adjunct in the treatment of childhood enuresis (bedwetting), and clomipramine is useful in the treatment of OCD. As well as their beneficial antidepressant effects, TCAs are also useful as adjunctive analgesics in the treatment of persistent pain syndromes, especially neuropathic pain (trigeminal neuralgia).

Contraindications

Contraindications for TCAs include known drug allergy, use prior to 14 days of stopping MAOI therapy, and pregnancy. They are also not recommended in patients with any acute or chronic heart problems or seizure history. It is this effect that usually results in death when these medications are taken in an overdose by a patient who is suicidal.

Adverse Effects

The most common undesirable effects of TCAs stem from their effects on receptors, primarily the muscarinic receptors. Blockade of these receptors by TCAs results in many undesirable anticholinergic adverse effects. The most common adverse effects are sedation, erectile dysfunction, and orthostatic hypotension. The older adult tends to experience more dizziness, postural hypotension, constipation, delayed micturition, edema, and muscle tremors. The undesirable effects according to body systems are listed in Table 16-7 on the next page.

Toxicity and Management of Overdose

TCA overdoses are notoriously lethal. It is estimated that 70% to 80% of patients who die of TCA overdose do so before reaching the hospital. The primary organ systems affected are the CNS and cardiovascular system, and death usually results from either seizures or dysrhythmias. There is no specific antidote for TCA poisoning. Consultation with a Poison Control Centre is recommended. Treatment is symptomatic and supportive. Management efforts are aimed at decreasing drug absorption through the administration of multiple doses of activated charcoal. Administration of an alkaline drug such as sodium bicarbonate speeds up elimination of the TCA by alkalinizing the urine to a pH of greater than 7.55. CNS damage may also be minimized through the administration of diazepam, and cardiovascular dyrhythmias and resulting heart failure may be minimized by giving antidysrhythmics. Other care includes basic life support in an intensive care setting to maintain vital organ functions. These processes must continue until enough of the TCA is eliminated to permit restoration of normal organ function.

TABLE 16-6

Tricyclic Antidepressants: Therapeutic and Undesirable Drug Effects by Receptor Site

Blockade of	Drug Effect*
Adrenergic receptors	Orthostatic hypotension, antihypertensive effects
Dopaminergic receptors	Extrapyramidal and endocrine adverse effects
Histaminergic receptors	Sedation, weight gain
Muscarinic receptors	Dry mouth, constipation, blurred vision, tachycardia, urinary retention, confusion
Norepinephrine reuptake	*Antidepressant,* tremors, tachycardia, additive pressor effects with sympathomimetic drugs
Serotonergic receptors	*Alleviation of rhinitis,* hypotension
Serotonin reuptake	*Antidepressant,* nausea, headache, anxiety, sexual dysfunction

*Italicized effects are the therapeutic ones.

TABLE 16-7	

Tricyclic Antidepressants: Adverse Effects

Body System	Adverse Effects
Cardiovascular	Tremors, tachycardia, orthostatic hypotension, dysrhythmias
Central nervous	Anxiety, confusion, extrapyramidal effects, sedation
Gastrointestinal	Nausea, constipation, dry mouth
Other	Blurred vision, urinary retention, weight gain, impotence

Interactions

When taken with TCAs, adrenergics may result in increased sympathetic stimulation. Anticholinergics and phenothiazines taken with TCAs may result in increased anticholinergic effects. CNS depressants, when taken with TCAs, will have additive CNS depressant effects. MAOIs, when taken with TCAs, may result in increased therapeutic and toxic effects, including hyperpyretic crisis (excessive fever). TCAs can inhibit the metabolism of warfarin, resulting in increased anticoagulation effects.

 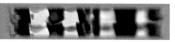

DRUG PROFILES

TCAs are effective drugs in the treatment of affective disorders, but they are also associated with serious adverse effects. Therefore, patients taking them need to be monitored closely. For this reason, all antidepressants are available only with a prescription, with the exception of some natural health products such as St. John's wort (see Natural Health Products: St. John's Wort below). Many drugs in this class are rated as pregnancy category D drugs, making their use by pregnant women relatively more hazardous than most of the NGAs.

There are many drugs in the TCA drug class, including the secondary-amine and tertiary-amine TCAs. The secondary-amine TCAs have a stronger noradrenergic (norepinephrine) receptor effect and may have a structural advantage over the tertiary-amine TCAs in augmenting drug therapy with SSRIs in TRD. Box 16-3 lists the cyclic antidepressants according to their respective categories.

▶▶ *amitriptyline hydrochloride*

Amitriptyline hydrochloride (Elavil, Levate) is one of the oldest and most widely used of all the TCAs. It is the prototypical tertiary-amine TCA and is also used in the treatment of pain disorders such as fibromalgia, migraine prophylaxis, rheumatoid arthritis, and neuropathies (postherpetic neuralgia, diabetic peripheral neuropathy). It has potent anticholinergic properties, which can lead to many adverse effects such as dry mouth, constipation, blurred vision, urinary retention, and dysrhythmias. There is one combination product that contains amitriptyline—Apo-Peram, PMS-Levazine, which also contains perphenazine.

PHARMACOKINETICS

Half-Life	Onset	Peak	Duration
10–50 hr	7–21 days*	2–12 hr	6–12 hr

*Therapeutic antidepressant effect.

NATURAL HEALTH PRODUCTS

ST. JOHN'S WORT (*Hypericum perforatum*)

Overview

St. John's wort consists of the dried, above-ground parts of the plant species *Hypericum perforatum* gathered during flowering season. St. John's wort contains several compounds that may be responsible for their pharmacological effects, although it is not clear how exactly St. John's wort exhibits its action. It may inhibit the reuptake of serotonin, norepinephrine, and dopamine. It is available over the counter in numerous oral dosage forms. St. John's wort is sometimes referred to as the "herbal Prozac," although its usefulness is limited to mild to moderate symptoms of depression and has minimal benefits for major depression. Recently, a randomized double-blind controlled trial showed that 900 or 1800 mg/day of St. John's wort was similarly effective as 20 and 40 mg/day of parexotine in preventing relapse in a 6-week continuation treatment after recovery from an episode of moderate to severe depression. As a result, St. John's wort may be an important alternative treatment option for long-term use in the prevention of depression relapse.

Common Uses

Depression, attention deficit hyperactivity disorder, anxiety, sleep disorders, nervousness

Adverse Effects

Gastrointestinal upset, allergic reactions, fatigue, dizziness, confusion, dry mouth, possible phototoxicity (especially in fair-skinned individuals)

Potential Drug Interactions

St John's wort may potentiate the serotonergic effects of SSRIs, reduce the anticonvulsive effects of carbamazepine and phenytoin, and reduce the bronchodilator effects of theophylline. It reduces the serum blood levels of contraceptives, digoxin, immunosuppressants, clarithromycin, erythromycin, cyclosporine, tacrolimus, protease inhibitors, and certain chemotherapeutic drugs.

Contraindications

St. John's wort is contraindicated in patients with BPD, schizophrenia, Alzheimer's disease, or dementia.

BOX 16-3

Cyclic Antidepressant Categories

Tertiary-Amine TCAs
amitriptyline
doxepin
imipramine
trimipramine

Secondary-Amine TCAs
desipramine
nortriptyline

Tetracyclic Antidepressants
maprotiline
mirtazapine

TCA, tricyclic antidepressant.

Dosages

For the recommended dosages for selected TCA drugs, see the Dosages table below.

MONOAMINE OXIDASE INHIBITORS

MAOIs, along with TCAs, represent the first generation of antidepressant drug therapy. Although MAOIs are potent drugs, they are now considered to be second- or third-line drugs for the treatment of depression that is not responsive to other pharmacological therapies such as the SSRIs or TCAs. As mentioned previously, such cases are known as treatment-resistant depression. The adverse effects of MAOIs are listed in Table 16-8.

A serious disadvantage to MAOI use is their potential to cause a hypertensive crisis when taken with a substance containing tyramine, which is found in many common foods and beverages (Table 16-9 on the next page). Another chemical with a similar name is tyrosine. Tyrosine is an amino acid that is a biochemical precursor of dopamine and is not to be confused with tyramine, which comes from exogenous food and beverage sources.

Two available MAOI antidepressants, phenelzine sulfate (Nardil) and tranylcypromine sulfate (Parnate), are nonselective inhibitors of both MAO-A and MAO-B. Both types of MAO are widely distributed throughout the body, including the brain. MAO-A preferentially metabolizes serotonin, norepinephrine, and tyramine. MAO-B preferentially metabolizes dopamine. By inhibiting the MAO enzyme system in the CNS of patients who have depression, amines such as dopamine, serotonin, and norepinephrine are not broken down and, therefore, higher levels occur. This, in turn, alleviates the symptoms of depression. However, higher levels of tyramine can also result in the hazardous drug–food interaction associated with MAOIs (see Table 16-9). This interaction is described in the following section on MAOI toxicity. There is also an MAO type B–selective inhibitor called selegiline hydrochloride (Anipriyl) (see Chapter 15). This medication is used primarily for treating Parkinson's disease. As with other antidepressants, MAOIs might take 1 to 4 weeks or more to reach their full therapeutic effects. However, patients vary widely in the timing of their responsiveness. Furthermore, a variety of over-the-counter drugs can interact with MAOIs to cause adverse cardiovascular effects. The following drugs must be avoided while taking MAOIs and for 2 weeks after discontinuing use: cold and cough preparations (including those containing dextromethorphan), nasal decongestants (tablets, drops or spray), hay fever medications, sinus medications, asthma inhalant medications, antiappetite medicines, weight-reducing preparations, and L-tryptophan–containing preparations. The patient taking MAOIs should always read labels and consult the pharmacist when using any such products.

DOSAGES Selected Tricyclic Antidepressants

Drug (Pregnancy Category)	Usual Dosage Range	Indications
▸▸amitriptyline hydrochloride (Elavil, Levate) (C)	*Adolescents* PO: 10–100 mg/day divided or at bedtime *Adult* PO: 25–200 mg/day divided *Older Adult* PO: 10–150 mg/day divided	Depression, atypical analgesic (unlabelled)

TABLE 16-8

MAOIs: Adverse Effects

Body System	Adverse Effects
Cardiovascular	Orthostatic hypotension, tachycardia, palpitations, other dysrhythmias, edema
Central nervous	Dizziness, drowsiness, restlessness, insomnia, headache, ataxia, hallucinations, seizures, tremors, confusion
Gastrointestinal	Anorexia, abdominal cramps, nausea, dry mouth
Other	Blurred vision, impotence, skin rashes, respiratory depression

TABLE 16-9

Food and Drink to Avoid When Taking MAOIs

Food/Drink	Examples
HIGH TYRAMINE CONTENT—NOT PERMITTED	
Aged mature cheeses	Cheddar, blue, Swiss
Aged or fermented meats	Chicken or beef liver paté, game fish, or poultry
Red wines	Chianti, burgundy, sherry, vermouth
Smoked or pickled meats	Pickled herring, dry sausage (including Genoa salami, pepperoni, and Lebanon bologna)
Vegetables	Broad bean pods (fava beans), sauerkraut
Yeast extracts	Brewer's yeast
MODERATE TYRAMINE CONTENT— LIMITED AMOUNTS ALLOWED	
Meat extracts	Bouillon, consommé
Pasteurized light and pale beer	
Ripe avocado	
LOW TYRAMINE CONTENT—PERMISSIBLE	
Canadian and mozzarella cheese	Cottage cheese, cream cheese
Chocolate and caffeinated beverages	
Distilled spirits	Vodka, gin, rye, scotch (in moderation)
Fruit	Figs, bananas, raisins, grapes, pineapple, oranges
Soy sauce	
Yogourt, sour cream	

MAOI, monoamine oxidase inhibitor.

Toxicity and Management of Overdose

Clinical symptoms of MAOI overdose generally do not appear until about 12 hours after ingestion. The primary signs and symptoms are cardiovascular and neurological in nature. The most serious cardiovascular effects are tachycardia and circulatory collapse, and the neurological symptoms of major concern are seizures and coma. Hyperthermia and miosis are also generally present in overdose. Consultation with a Poison Control Centre is recommended. The recommended treatment is aimed at eliminating the ingested toxin and protecting the brain and heart, organs at greatest risk for damage. Recommended treatments are gastric lavage with instillation of activated charcoal, urine acidification to a pH of 5, and hemodialysis.

MAOIs are one of the few drug classes that are capable of interacting with food, leading to a severe reaction. In this case, food containing the amino acid tyramine is the primary culprit, and a hypertensive crisis is the reaction. It is essential for both the patient and the nurse to know the foods and drinks that should be avoided; these are listed in Table 16-9. Treatment of hypertensive crisis resulting from consumption of tyramine-containing foods or beverages may require intravenous administration of hypotensive drugs along with careful monitoring in an intensive care setting.

Interactions

A wide variety of drug interactions can occur with MAOIs. Sympathomimetic drugs can also interact with the MAOIs and together cause a hypertensive crisis. MAOIs can markedly potentiate the effects of meperidine, and, therefore, concurrent use is contraindicated. In addition, concurrent use of MAOIs and SSRIs carries the risk of serotonin syndrome. A washout period of at least 2 weeks after discontinuation of sertraline, paroxetine, or citalopram should occur before initiation of MAOI therapy. A 5-week washout period is necessary if switching to MAOIs from fluoxetine.

Dosages

For recommended dosages for selected MAOI drugs, see the Dosages table below.

ANTIPSYCHOTIC DRUGS

Antipsychotic drugs are used to treat serious mental health disorderes such as depressive and drug-induced psychoses, schizophrenia (see Box 16-4), and autism. Antipsychotics are also used to treat extreme mania (as an adjunct to lithium), BPD, certain movement disorders (e.g., Tourette's syndrome), and certain other medical conditions (e.g., nausea, intractable hiccups). Antipsychotics have been referred to as *tranquilizers* or *neuroleptics* because they produce a state of tranquility and work on abnormally functioning nerves. However, these are both older terms that are now less commonly used.

Constituting about two thirds of all antipsychotics, phenothiazines are the largest group of antipsychotic drugs. As with many other drugs, phenothiazines were discovered by chance, in this case, during research for new antihistamines. In 1951, chlorpromazine was the first phenothiazine to be discovered in this way. Although phenothiazines can provide much relief to the patient with a mental health disorder, they are associated with a

DOSAGES Selected MAOIs

Drug (Pregnancy Category)	Usual Dosage Range	Indications
phenelzine sulfate (Nardil) (C)	PO: Initial dose 45–90 mg/day divided tid, followed by dose reduction to minimal effective dose after therapeutic effect achieved	Depression
tranylcypromine sulfate (Parnate) (C)	20–30 mg/day divided bid	Psychotic depressive states

BOX 16-4   Schizophrenia and the Metabolic Syndrome

The introduction of second-generation (atypical) anti-psychotic drugs for the treatment of schizophrenia has offered advantages to individuals with this mental health disorder. These include the lower incidence of extrapyramidal adverse effects of typical antipsychotics as well as improved efficacy in managing both negative and positive symptoms of psychoses. However, the atypical antipsychotics have been associated with metabolic effects such as an increased risk of type 2 diabetes, abdominal or visceral weight gain, and dyslipidemia. These metabolic adverse effects are associated with a reduced life expectancy of 9 to 12 years less than that of the general population. Nurses have an important role to play in the assessment, education, and monitoring of at-risk patients. Recommendations for the management of individuals with schizophrenia taking atypical antipsychotics are as follows:

1. Prior to the initiation of therapy, assess for personal and family history of cardiovascular disease, hypertension, and dyslipidemia, obesity, diabetes, and smoking.
2. Check body mass index and weight at baseline, and at 4, 8, and 12 weeks after initiating therapy and every

4 months thereafter. If a patient gains 2.5 kg or more, a switch to another antipsychotic should be considered. Waist circumference should be measured at baseline and yearly thereafter.
3. Blood pressure, fasting blood glucose, and fasting lipid profile should be checked at baseline, 12 weeks, and then annually. (NOTE: Variations may occur with follow-up blood work.)
4. Nutrition and exercise counselling should be provided to all patients who are overweight or obese.
5. Education should be provided to all patients, family members, and caregivers about the possibility of weight gain and diabetes with antipsychotic use.

Sources: Usher, K., Foster, K., & Park, T. (2006). The metabolic syndrome and schizophrenia: The latest evidence and nursing guidelines for management. *Journal of Psychiatric and Mental Health Nursing, 14*, 730–734; Woo, V., & Harris, S. B. (2005). Canadian Diabetes position paper: Antipsychotic medications and associated risk of weight gain and diabetes. *Canadian Journal of Diabetes, 29*(2), 111–112.

high incidence of anticholinergic adverse effects because they are so closely related to antihistamines. Therefore, since the early 1950s, researchers have been working on developing phenothiazines with fewer adverse effects. Phenothiazines can be divided into three groups based on structural differences: aliphatic, piperidine, and piperazine. In addition to the phenothiazine antipsychotics, there are four other categories of drugs that are commonly used to treat mental health disorders: thioxanthenes, butyrophenones, dihydroindolones, and dibenzoxazepines. Many of the therapeutic and toxic effects of the antipsychotics are the consequence of their chemical structures.

There is little difference between traditional antipsychotics in their mechanisms of action; therefore, selection of an antipsychotic is based primarily on the least undesirable drug adverse effect and the patient's type of psychosis. Of the currently available antipsychotic drugs, no single drug stands out as more or less effective in the treatment of symptoms of psychosis. Also, antipsychotic drug therapy does not provide a cure for mental health disorder; it is only a way of chemically controlling the symptoms of the illness. These drugs represent a significant advance in our treatment of mental health disorders, given that the early treatment of mental health disorder (prior to the 1950s) consisted of such extreme measures as isolation, physical restraint, shock therapy, and even lobotomy.

Over the last 6 or 7 years, a new class of antipsychotic medications has evolved, the *atypical antipsychotics (AAPs)* or *second-generation antipsychotics*. AAPs differ from first-generation drugs in both their mechanisms of action and their adverse-effect profiles.

Mechanism of Action and Drug Effects

All antipsychotics block to some degree dopamine receptors in the brain, thus decreasing the dopamine concentration in the CNS. Specifically, the older phenothiazines block the receptors to which dopamine normally binds postsynaptically in certain areas of the CNS, such as the limbic system and the basal ganglia. These are the areas associated with emotions, cognitive function, and motor function. This blocking action results in a tranquilizing effect in psychotic patients. Both the therapeutic and toxic effects of these drugs are the direct result of the dopamine blockade in these areas.

The newer AAPs block specific dopamine 2 (D_2) receptors, the dopamine receptors, as well as specific serotonin 2 (5-HT_2) receptors in the brain. The different mechanisms of action of the AAPs are responsible for their improved efficacy and improved safety profiles.

Antipsychotics have many effects throughout the body. In addition to blocking the dopamine receptors in the CNS, they also block α receptors, which can result in hypotension and other cardiovascular effects. Many of the adverse effects of antipsychotics stem from their ability to block histamine receptors, resulting in anticholinergic effects. They also block serotonin receptors. This, in combination with their ability to block dopamine receptors in the chemoreceptor trigger zone and peripherally, along with their ability to inhibit neurotransmission in the vagus nerve in the gastrointestinal tract, accounts for the ability of certain antipsychotics to function as antiemetics. Additional blockage of dopamine receptors in the brainstem reticular system also allows AAPs to have antianxiety effects. The older first-generation drugs such as phenothiazines and haloperidol can also augment prolactin release, which can result in swelling of the breasts and milk secretion in women taking these drugs. Gynecomastia (breast tissue enlargement) can also be a distressing adverse effect in male patients.

All antipsychotics show some efficacy for the positive symptoms of schizophrenia, and, over time, the improvement may even increase. These so-called positive symptoms include hallucinations, delusions, and conceptual disorganization. Unfortunately, first-generation antipsychotics are much less effective for the negative symptoms such as apathy, social withdrawal, blunted affect, poverty of speech, and catatonia. These negative symptoms account for most of the social and vocational disability caused by schizophrenia. Fortunately, newer-generation antipsychotic drugs often have improved efficacy against the negative symptoms. Another drawback to first-generation antipsychotics is that they all cause extrapyramidal symptoms (see Adverse Effects below). To summarize, first-generation antipsychotics such as haloperidol are effective for controlling symptoms, but not all symptoms, not in all patients, and not without serious adverse effects. However, there is recent debate in the literature regarding the level of overall improvement between older and newer antipsychotic drugs.

Indications

The major therapeutic effect of antipsychotic drugs is the result of blockade of dopamine receptors in certain areas of the CNS. These are the areas where regulation of dopamine activity tends to be dysfunctional in psychotic patients. The extent to which such antidopaminergic drug therapy has been shown to control psychotic symptoms is one of the major factors supporting the **dopamine hypothesis** regarding the origins of the psychotic disorders. Note that this type of drug therapy is in direct contrast to that for panic disorder, where dopaminergic activity needs to be enhanced instead of reduced. The areas within the CNS where antipsychotics have a major effect are listed in Table 16-10.

Contraindications

Contraindications to the use of antipsychotic drugs include known drug allergy; comatose state; and possibly significant CNS depression, brain damage, liver or kidney disease, blood dyscrasias, and uncontrolled epilepsy.

Adverse Effects

The adverse effects of the individual antipsychotic drugs are numerous and are important to remember. The goal of treatment is to choose a drug with the least bothersome adverse-effect profile for a given patient. Individual patients may vary widely in their responses to, and tolerance of, a given medication. Such individual variances are usually not predictable, and often the medications that best help a given patient are discovered through a trial-and-error process. The common adverse effects caused by blockade of the dopamine, muscarinic (synonymous with cholinergic), histamine, and α-adrenergic receptors are listed in Table 16-11. These undesirable effects can also be classified according to the body system affected. Severe hematological effects may include agranulocytosis (lack of granulocytes in the blood) and hemolytic anemia. Integumentary effects may include exfoliative dermatitis. CNS effects include drowsiness, neuroleptic malignant syndrome, extrapyramidal symptoms, and **tardive dyskinesia**. *Neuroleptic malignant syndrome* is a potentially life-threatening adverse effect related to acute dopamine depletion associated with antipsychotic drugs. The symptom complex includes high fever, unstable blood pressure (BP), and myoglobinemia. **Extrapyramidal symptoms** involve involuntary motor symptoms similar to those associated with Parkinson's disease and are an adverse effect associated with the use of antipsychotic drugs (see Chapter 15). This drug-induced state is known as pseudoparkinsonism and includes the symptoms of akinesia, akatheisia, dyskinesia, dystonia, Pisa syndrome, and the Rabbit syndrome. *Akinesia* is the slowness or loss of voluntary motor function. **Akathisia** is the feeling of inner restlessness and the urge to move as well as rocking while standing or sitting, lifting the feet as if marching on the spot, and crossing and uncrossing the legs while sitting. *Dyskinesia*, associated with antipsychotics, is involuntary movements of the tongue, lips, face, trunk, and extremities. *Dystonia* is a movement disorder that commonly involves the head, neck, and tongue and often occurs as an adverse effect of a medication. *Pisa syndrome* is a rare

TABLE 16-10		
Major Dopamine Systems in the Brain		
DA System	**DA-Related Function**	**Effects of DA-Receptor Blockade**
Hypothalamic–pituitary	Regulates prolactin secretion, temperature, appetite, emesis	Increased prolactin levels resulting in galactorrhea, amenorrhea, and decreased libido; loss of temperature regulation, increased appetite, and antiemetic effects
Mesocortical	Regulates behaviour	Therapeutic antipsychotic effects
Mesolimbic	Regulates stereotypical and other behaviours	Therapeutic antipsychotic effects
Nigrostriatal	Mediates function of the extrapyramidal motor system (EPS movement)	Reversible: dystonia, pseudoparkinsonism, akathisia
		Irreversible: TD (must catch early to reverse!)

DA, dopamine; *EPS*, extrapyramidal symptoms; *TD*, tardive dyskinesia.

dystonic reaction commonly associated with prolonged antipsychotic medication. It involves sustained involuntary flexion of the body and head to one side and slight rotation of the trunk so the person appears to lean like the Leaning Tower of Pisa. *Rabbit syndrome,* also uncommon, is associated with the long-term use of antipsychotics. This extrapyramidal adverse effect is characterized by fine, rapid, rhythmic movements of the mouth. Two anticholinergic medications, benztropine and trihexyphenidyl (Apo-Trihex), are commonly used to treat these symptoms. These drugs were introduced in Chapter 15 on Parkinson's disease.

Tardive is a word that means "late-appearing." Tardive dyskinesia involves involuntary contractions of oral and facial muscles (e.g., involuntary tongue-thrusting) and choreoathetosis (wavelike movements of extremities) that usually appear only after continuous long-term antipsychotic therapy. Ocular adverse effects include blurred vision, corneal lens changes, epithelial keratopathy, and pigmentary retinopathy. Cardiovascular effects include postural hypotension. Additionally, electrocardiogram (ECG) changes, notably prolonged QT interval, are associated to varying degrees with all classes of antipsychotic drugs. Baseline and periodic ECGs, as well as serum potassium and magnesium levels, can help determine if a patient is at risk for such effects or diagnose newly acquired cardiac dysrhythmias. In such cases, another drug choice may still control symptoms without causing cardiac effects. The older first-generation drugs such as

phenothiazines and haloperidol can also augment prolactin release, which can result in swelling of the breasts and milk secretion in women taking these drugs. Gynecomastia can also be a distressing adverse effect in male patients.

The common adverse effects caused by antipsychotic drugs are listed in Table 16-12.

Low-potency antipsychotic drugs generally have a low incidence of extrapyramidal symptoms and a high incidence of sedation, anticholinergic adverse effects, and cardiovascular adverse effects. The opposite is true for high-potency antipsychotic drugs. They have a high incidence of extrapyramidal symptoms and a low incidence of sedation, anticholinergic adverse effects, and cardiovascular adverse effects.

Interactions

Antacids and tannic acids (also known as tannins; e.g., in tea, grapes, wine) can decrease antipsychotic absorption when taken with these drugs. Antihypertensives may have additive hypotensive effects, and CNS depressants may have additive CNS-depressant effects when taken with antipsychotics. Clozapine effects, in particular, can be enhanced by grapefruit juice (by reducing its metabolism) and nicotine can reduce its effects (by speeding its metabolism).

Dosages

For recommended dosages for selected antipsychotic drugs, see the Dosages table on p. 313.

TABLE 16-11

Antipsychotics: Receptor-Related Adverse Effects

Receptor	Adverse Effect	Drug Category
α-Adrenergic	Postural hypotension, lightheadedness, reflex tachycardia	Low-potency drugs
Dopamine	Extrapyramidal movement disorders, dystonia, pseudoparkinsonism, akathisia, tardive dyskinesia	High-potency drugs
Endocrine	Prolactin secretion (galactorrhea, gynecomastia), menstrual changes, sexual dysfunction	Low-potency drugs
Histamine	Sedation, drowsiness, hypotension, weight gain	Low-potency drugs
Muscarinic (cholinergic)	Blurred vision, worsening of narrow-angle glaucoma, dry mouth, tachycardia, constipation, urinary retention, decreased sweating	Low-potency drugs

TABLE 16-12

Antipsychotics: Adverse Effects

Body System	Adverse Effects
Cardiovascular	Orthostatic hypotension, syncope, dizziness, ECG changes, conduction abnormalities
Central nervous	Sedation, delirium, neuroleptic malignant syndrome
Gastrointestinal	Dry mouth, constipation, paralytic ileus, hepatotoxicity, weight gain
Genitourinary	Urinary hesitancy, urinary retention, impaired erection, priapism, ejaculatory problems
Hematological	Leukopenia and agranulocytosis
Integumentary	Photosensitivity, hyperpigmentation, rash, pruritus
Metabolic and endocrine	Galactorrhea, irregular menses, amenorrhea, decreased libido, increased appetite, polydipsia, impaired temperature regulation

DRUG PROFILES

The first-generation antipsychotic drugs are currently still available on the Canadian market. However, their use in common clinical practice has been largely supplanted by the second-generation or "atypical" antipsychotic drugs, which generally have better adverse-effect profiles. All antipsychotics are prescription-only medications that are indicated for the treatment of psychotic disorders. No single drug stands out as more or less effective in the treatment of the symptoms of psychosis. Some of the factors that should be considered before selecting an antipsychotic drug are the patient's history of response to a drug and the possible adverse-effect profile. Patients should always be started with a low dose and titrated to the lowest effective dose, balancing between symptom relief and adverse effects, if any. Dosage and indication information appears in the corresponding table. Selected drugs are profiled in more detail below.

Table 16-13 on page 312 lists compatible and incompatible liquids for dosing the liquid dosage forms of both older and newer generations of selected antipsychotic drugs.

PHENOTHIAZINES

fluphenazine hydrochloride

Fluphenazine hydrochloride is available in three different salt forms, providing for varying degrees of antipsychotic potency. The decanoate and enanthate (the latter not available in Canada) salt forms have the longest durations of action, and the hydrochloride salt form is fairly short in duration. Fluphenazine has the greatest potency of all the phenothiazines: 1 mg of the drug has the antipsychotic potency of 200 mg of chlorphenazine. It is used primarily to treat psychotic disorders and schizophrenia. It is considered to be a high-potency antipsychotic and is, therefore, associated with a high incidence of extrapyramidal symptoms; however, the associated incidence of sedative, anticholinergic, and cardiovascular effects is low. It is contraindicated in patients who have shown a hypersensitivity reaction to phenothiazines and in those patients with circulatory collapse, liver dysfunction, blood dyscrasias, comatose state, bone marrow depression, or alcohol or barbiturate withdrawal.

PHARMACOKINETICS

Half-Life	Onset	Peak	Duration
PO: 15–16 hr*	PO (hydrochloride): 1 hr	PO (hydrochloride): 1.5–2 hr	PO (hydrochloride): 6–8 hr
SC/IM: Up to 2 wk†	SC/IM (decanoate): 24–72 hr	SC/IM (decanoate): Unknown	SC/IM (decanoate): ≥4 wk

*Following single dose.
†Following multiple injections.

BUTYROPHENONES

haloperidol

Haloperidol is structurally different from the phenothiazines but has similar antipsychotic properties. It is a high-potency neuroleptic drug that has a favourable cardiovascular, anticholinergic, and sedative adverse-effect profile but it can often cause extrapyramidal symptoms. Haloperidol is available in three salt forms: base, decanoate, and lactate (not available in Canada). Haloperidol decanoate has an extremely long duration of effect. It is used primarily for the long-term treatment of psychosis and is especially useful in patients who are nonadherent with their drug treatment. It is contraindicated in patients who have shown a hypersensitivity reaction to it, those in a comatose state, those taking large amounts of CNS depressants, and those with Parkinson's disease.

PHARMACOKINETICS

Half-Life	Onset	Peak	Duration
PO: 20 hr	PO: 2 hr	PO: 2–6 hr	PO: 8–12 hr
IM (deconate): 3 weeks	IM (lactate): 20–30 min	IM (lactate): 10–20 min	IM (lactate): 4–8 hr
	IM (decanoate): 3–9 days	IM (decanoate): 1 week	IM (decanoate): 1 mo

ATYPICAL ANTIPSYCHOTICS

Between 1975 and 1990 not even one single new antipsychotic drug was approved in Canada. Then, in 1991 came the approval of clozapine (Clozaril), the first of the atypical antipsychotics (AAPs). Clozapine was followed in quick succession by risperidone (Risperdal), olanzapine (Zyprexa), quetiapine (Seroquel), ziprasidone (Zeldox), zuclopenthixal (Clopixol), aripiprazole (Abilify) available through the Special Access Programme, and paliperidone (Invega). Newer antipsychotics gaining approval and showing great promise include sertindole and zotepine. The term *atypical antipsychotics* refers to the advantageous properties of these drugs, including reduced effect on prolactin levels, compared with older drugs, and improvement in the negative symptoms associated with schizophrenia. Although they are still fairly new compared with their first-generation counterparts, they also show a lower risk for neuroleptic malignant syndrome, extrapyramidal symptoms, and tardive dyskinesia. These new drugs, plus several more in clinical trials, are revolutionizing the treatment of psychosis and schizophrenia. For these reasons, AAPs are also referred to and recognized as *second-generation antipsychotic drugs.*

All of the currently available AAPs have several pharmacological properties in common. Antagonist activity at the dopamine D_1 receptor is believed to be the mechanism of antimanic activity. Serotonergic (serotonin agonist) activity at various serotonin (5-HT) receptor subtypes and α_2-adrenergic (agonist) activity are both associated with antidepressant activity. α_1-Adrenergic receptor antagonist activity is associated with orthostatic effects, and histamine H_1 receptor antagonist activity is associated with both sedative and appetite-stimulating effects. This last effect accounts for a common adverse effect of weight gain that is associated to various degrees with AAP drugs. This can cause or worsen obesity and even result in diabetes (see Box 16-4). Clozapine and olanzapine are associated with the most weight gain (which

Continued

DRUG PROFILES (cont'd)

often occurs during the first few months of therapy and ranges from 0.5 to 5 kg) and risperidone and quetiapine with less; ziprasidone is considered weight neutral. Sedative effects may diminish over time and can actually be helpful to patients with insomnia.

Although these drugs all have similar pharmacological properties, they vary in the degree of affinity that each may have for the various types of receptors. These subtle pharmacological differences, along with often unknown and unpredictable physiological patient differences, help explain why some patients respond better to one medication than to another. In 2005, Health Canada issued a special Public Health Advisory concerning the use of atypical antipsychotic drugs in the older adult for "off-label" (non–Health Canada–approved) uses. These medications are currently approved to treat schizophrenia and mania. In practice, however, they are also commonly used to control agitative behavioural symptoms in the older adult with dementia, including dementia related to Alzheimer's disease. A meta-analysis combining the data of 17 smaller placebo-controlled studies reviewed by the U.S. Food and Drug Administration (2005) found that the older adult given AAPs for this reason were up to 1.7 times more likely to die during treatment. More recently, researchers conducted a retrospective cohort study using population-based data from Ontario and found a statistically significant increase in the risk for death with the new use of atypical antipsychotic drugs (Gill et al., 2007). Such research reinforces the Health Canada announcement and is a reminder to prescribers that AAPs are not officially indicated for dementia-related behavioural symptoms. The health care provider must also consider the potential benefits and risks before prescribing AAPs, and consider nondrug alternatives.

Dosage and indication information appears in the corresponding table. Also, Table 16-13 on the next page lists compatible and incompatible liquids for dosing the liquid dosage forms of both older and newer generations of selected antipsychotic drugs.

clozapine

Clozapine (Clozaril) is a unique antipsychotic drug. It is similar to loxapine in its chemical structure in that it is a piperazine-substituted tricyclic antipsychotic; however, pharmacologically it is different from all other currently available antipsychotics in its mechanism of action. It also more selectively blocks the dopaminergic receptors in the mesolimbic system. Other antipsychotic drugs block dopamine receptors in an area of the brain called the neostriatum, but blockade in this area of the brain is believed to give rise to unwanted extrapyramidal symptoms. Because clozapine has weak dopamine-blocking abilities in this area, it is associated with minor or no extrapyramidal symptoms. In fact, although newer AAPs may be better tolerated and are not associated with the hematological adverse effects associated with clozapine, clozapine is currently the AAP with the lowest reported incidence of such effects. This often makes clozapine the drug of choice for psychotic disorders in patients with comorbid panic disorder because it will not worsen motor symptoms.

Clozapine has been extremely useful for the treatment of patients who have failed treatment with other antipsychotic drugs, especially patients with schizophrenia. Patients taking clozapine must be monitored closely for the development of agranulocytosis, a dangerous lack of white blood cell (WBC) production that is drug induced. The risk of agranulocytosis developing as the result of clozapine therapy is 1% to 2% after the first year; this compares with a risk of 0.1% to 1% for phenothiazines. For this reason, patients beginning clozapine therapy require weekly monitoring of WBC count for the first 6 months of therapy. The drug should be withheld if the count falls below 3×10^9/L, until it rises above this value. It is also recommended that weekly WBC counts be evaluated for 4 weeks after discontinuation of the drug. In addition, Health Canada mandates that any pharmacological distributor of clozapine must have a national patient risk-management monitoring system to ensure the optimal safety of all patients using the drug. This monitoring system must register patients and their respective physicians, pharmacists, and laboratories, as well as monitor for adverse effects of the drug, including neutropenia and agranulocytosis. Clozapine use is contraindicated in patients who have shown a hypersensitivity reaction to it and in those with myeloproliferative disorders, severe granulocytopenia, CNS depression, or narrow-angle glaucoma or those who are in a comatose state.

PHARMACOKINETICS

Half-Life	Onset	Peak	Duration
12 hr	1–6 hr	Weeks	4–12 hr

▶▶ risperidone

Risperidone (Risperdal) was the second atypical antipsychotic to receive Health Canada approval. It is even more active than clozapine at the serotonin (5-HT$_{2A}$ and 5-HT$_{2C}$) receptors. It also has high affinity for α_1- and α_2-adrenergic receptors and histamine H$_1$ receptors. It has lower affinity for the serotonin 5-HT$_{1A}$, 5-HT$_{1C}$, and 5-HT$_{1D}$ receptors and the dopamine D$_1$ receptor. It is effective for refractory schizophrenia, including negative symptoms, and causes minimal extrapyramidal symptoms at therapeutic dosages (1 to 6 mg/day). It is also not associated with the hematological hazards and need for frequent WBC count monitoring that is necessary with clozapine. However, it can cause mild to moderate elevation of serum prolactin levels. The use of risperidone is contraindicated in patients who have shown a hypersensitivity reaction to it. It is available in both oral and long-acting injectable forms.

PHARMACOKINETICS

Half-Life	Onset	Peak	Duration
20–24 hr	1–2 wk*	1–3 hr	7 days

*Therapeutic effects.

▶▶ paliperidone

Paliperidone (Invega), the major plasma active metabolite of risperidone, is the newest available atypical antipsychotic. It is also active at the central dopamine D$_2$ and

Continued

DRUG PROFILES (cont'd)

serotonin 5-HT$_{2A}$ receptors. Paliperidone binds less tightly to D$_2$ receptors than risperidone and has no antagonistic activity against cholinergic receptors. This may account for the different adverse effects, particularly the extrapyramidal adverse effects, including cognitive decline, associated with risperidone. There appears to be no associated weight gain with the use of paliperidone. Because paliperidone has a long half-life, there will be a reduction in the peaks and troughs normally associated with oral antipsychotics. The drug is associated with a rise in prolactin levels that results in amennorhea in female patients. Paliperidone improves both the positive and negative symptoms of schizophrenia. The drug is available as extended-release tablets.

PHARMACOKINETICS

Half-Life	Onset	Peak	Duration
23 hr	4–5 days*	24 hr	24 hr

*Therapeutic effects.

▶▶ olanzapine

Olanzapine (Zyprexa) is the third of the AAPs to receive Health Canada approval. It interacts with dopamine D$_{1-4}$ and serotonin 5-HT$_{2A}$ and 5-HT$_{2C}$ receptors. As with clozapine, it has blocking action on a variety of other receptors such as other serotonin receptors, α_1-adrenergic receptors, and histamine receptors. Olanzapine is a thienobenzodiazepine derivative. It was designated *1S* (new molecular entity) by the Notice of Compliance to Health Canada and approved to speed its availability to patients with schizophrenia. Many previous patients with disabilties as a result of schizophrenia experienced dramatic improvement in their level of day-to-day functioning. Olanzapine has only minor effects on the liver cytochrome P450 enzyme systems, greatly reducing the likelihood of significant drug interactions. It also lacks the requirement for frequent monitoring of WBC count that is necessary with clozapine. However, it is associated with both weight gain and sedation. Its only absolute contraindication is drug allergy. In 2004, Health Canada issued a safety information warning about the use of olanzapine in the older adult with dementia. In clinical trials, the use of olanzapine is associated with increased incidence of cerebrovascular adverse events (brain attack and transient ischemic attacks), including fatalities.

PHARMACOKINETICS

Half-Life	Onset	Peak	Duration
21–54 hrs	Greater than1 wk	6 hr	Unknown

quetiapine fumarate

A fourth AAP is quetiapine fumarate (Seroquel). Quetiapine is a dibenzothiazepine antipsychotic similar in structure to clozapine, but it appears to be much safer, especially from a hematological profile. Quetiapine has affinity for dopamine D$_2$ and D$_1$ receptors; serotonin 5-HT$_{1A}$, 5-HT$_{2A}$ and 5-HT$_{2C}$ receptors; muscarinic (cholinergic) M$_1$ receptors; histamine H$_1$ receptors; and α_1- and α_2-adrenergic receptors. It also has minor effects on liver cytochrome P450 enzyme systems, thus reducing the likelihood of serious drug interactions. The drug also blocks histamine and α-adrenergic receptors. This medication can cause ocular cataracts, so patients should have eye examinations every 6 months.

PHARMACOKINETICS

Half-Life	Onset	Peak	Duration
6–7 hr	2 days	1–2 hr	Unknown

ziprasidone hydrochloride monohydrate

Ziprasidone hydrochloride monohydrate (Zeldox) is the fifth of the atypical antipsychotics, approved in 2007. It is chemically classified as a benzothiazolylpiperazine. Its pharmacological activity is comparable with that of quetiapine. It has antagonist activity at several serotonin-receptor subtypes, including 5-HT$_{2A/2C}$, 5-HT$_{1D}$, 5-HT$_7$, and the D$_2$ dopamine receptors. It has agonist activity at the 5-HT$_{1A}$ serotonin receptors. It has also been shown to cause what is considered to be a mild electrocardiographic change—slight prolongation of the QT interval. It is recommended that ziprasidone be taken with food to enhance its absorption. However, as grapefruit and grapefruit juice have been shown to increase its blood concentration, it is recommended that both be avoided while taking this drug.

PHARMACOKINETICS

Half-Life	Onset	Peak	Duration
7 hr	2–3 days	6–8 hr	Unknown

TABLE 16-13

Compatibility of Select Liquid Antipsychotic Dosage Forms with Beverages for Dosing Purposes*

Drug	Compatible with	Not Compatible with
fluphenazine	Water, saline, homogenized milk, carbonated orange beverage, pineapple, apricot, prune, orange, tomato, and grapefruit juice	Beverages containing caffeine, tannics (e.g., tea), or pectinates (e.g., apple juice)
haloperidol	Water, juice	None listed
perphenazine	Water, saline, 7-Up, homogenized milk, carbonated orange beverages, pineapple, apricot, prune, orange, V-8, tomato, and grapefruit juice	Beverages containing caffeine, tannics (e.g., tea), or pectinates (e.g., apple juice)
risperidone	Water, coffee, orange juice, low-fat milk	Cola, tea

*When in doubt, the nurse should consult the manufacturer's package insert or pharmacist for information about a specific drug product.

DOSAGES   Selected First-Generation Antipsychotic Drugs

Drug (Pregnancy Category)	Pharmacological Class	Usual Dosage Range	Indications
chlorpromazine hydrochloride (Novo-Chlorpromazine) (C)	Aliphatic phenothiazine	*Children >6 months* PO, IM, IV: 0.5–1 mg/kg/dose q6–8 h *Adult* PO, IM: 25–400 mg/day with larger doses divided; IM is usually for acute care only	Psychotic disorders, mania
fluphenazine hydrochloride (generic) fluphenazine deconate (Modecate Concentrate) (c)	Piperidine phenothiazine	*Adult only* PO: 2.5–20 mg/day with larger doses divided tid–qid IM : 1.25–10 mg/day with larger doses divided tid–qid	
haloperidol deconate LA (generic) (C)	Butyrophenone	*Children 3–12 years* PO: 0.25–1.5 mg/kg/day bid–tid IM (acute care only): 2–5 mg q1h to maximum of 20 mg prn Depot: 10–15 × normal oral dose, q4weeks *Adult* PO, IM: 1.5–20 mg bid–tid	Psychotic disorders
loxapine (Apo-loxapine, Dom-loxapine)	Dibenzoxazepine dipenzepine	*Adult only* PO: 10 mg bid up to 100 mg/day divided bid–qid IM: 12.5–50 mg q4–6h	

DOSAGES   Selected Antipsychotic Drugs

Drug (Pregnancy Category)	Pharmacological Class	Usual Dosage Range*	Indications
aripiprazole (Abilify), (C) Special Access Programme	Quinolinone	10–30 mg once daily	Schizophrenia, bipolar mania
clozapine (Clozaril) (B)	Dibenzodiazepine	12.5–900 mg/day divided	Treatment-resistant schizophrenia
▶▶ olanzapine (Zyprexa), (C)	Thienobenzodiazepine	5–20 mg/day	Schizophrenia, bipolar mania
▶▶ paliperidone (Invega) (C)	Benzisoxazole	PO: 3–12 mg once daily	Schizophrenia
quetiapine fumarate (Seroquel), (C)	Dibenzothiazepine	25–800 mg/day at bedtime	Schizophrenia, bipolar mania
▶▶ risperidone (Risperdal) (C)	Benzisoxazole	PO: 1–6 mg/day–bid IM depot (Risperdal Consta): 25–50 mg every 2 wk	Schizophrenia and related psychotic disorders; severe dementia; bipolar disorder—mania
ziprasidone hydrochloride monohydrate (Zeldox), (C)	Benzisothiazolylpiperazine	20–80 mg bid	Schizophrenia
zuclopenthixol acetate (Clopixol-Acuphase) (C)	Thioxanthene	IM: 50–150 mg q2–3 days (not to exceed 2 wk)	Acute psychoses and exacerbation of schizophrenia
zuclopenthixol decanoate (Clopixol Depot) (C)		IM: 150–300 m g q 2–4 wk	Maintenance of chronic schizophrenia
zuclopenthixol dihydrochloride (Clopixol), (C)		10–100 mg/day	Acute psychoses and maintenance of schizophrenia

*All dosages reflect usual adult dosage ranges. Child doses may be more variable and should be specified by a pediatric practitioner.

Antipsychotic Drugs Summary

All of these drugs have a place in the treatment of schizophrenia. The lack of traditional neurological adverse effects is a tremendous benefit of the newer-generation atypical drugs and encourages the early use of antipsychotics when therapy is most beneficial. In the past, physicians were reluctant to prescribe drugs early in therapy. With the evolution of the AAPs, early therapy is not only possible but also safe and well tolerated.

NURSING PROCESS

Assessment

Both the physical and emotional status of patients taking psychotherapeutic drugs should be thoroughly assessed before, during, and after initiation of therapy. The potential for drug interactions, drug toxicity, drug overdose, and other adverse effects associated with these drugs is great, thus the need for an ongoing assessment. Constant assessment for any suicidal ideations or tendencies is important because patients may have covert, as well as overt, related cues or thoughts. The potential for suicide with psychotherapeutic drugs with or without the combination or other drugs or alcohol should always be considered a risk. Many of the patients needing these medications are so mentally distressed that their physical needs may be neglected, resulting in a complexity of other problems such as insomnia, poor health status, and weight loss or gain. Baseline blood pressure (BP), pulse rate, body temperature, and weight should be assessed and documented before, during, and after drug therapy. Postural (supine, then standing) BP readings are particularly important because of the postural hypotension associated with psychotherapeutics. The more potent, first-generation drugs, such as the MAOIs and TCAs, may lead to a significant drop in BP and warrant even more astute assessment.

The patient's neurological functioning should be assessed, including level of consciousness, mental alertness, and level of motor and cognitive functioning. The Mini-Mental Status Examination (MMSE) is one tool that may be used to assess the cognitive impairment found with mental health disorders. It is simple, cost efficient, and can be completed in about 20 minutes by the nurse or clinician. The procedure for conducting an MMSE is usually found in nursing assessment textbooks as well as psychiatric–mental health nursing textbooks. It includes an assessment with scoring of points in four major areas: level of orientation, attention and calculation ability, recall testing, and language skills. Other assessment tools include the six-item Blessed Orientation-Memory-Concentration Test; Clock Drawing Tasks; Functional Activities Questionnaire (for those with dementia), Alzheimer's Disease Assessment Scale; Mattis Dementia Rating Scale; Severe Impairment Battery; and Hamilton Rating Scale (HAM-D) previously discussed in this chapter. To complete assessment of the neurological system, baseline levels of motor responses and reflexes, presence of any tremors, agitation, as well as cold, clammy hands, sweating, and pallor (indicative of autonomic responses) should be assessed for and documented. It is also important to assess laboratory studies performed, which are usually ordered before, during, and after psychotropic drug therapy. It is particularly important in those who are in long-term therapy to prevent or identify early any possible complications and toxicity. Laboratory tests may include, but are not limited to, serum therapeutic levels and ranges of the specific drug, and, if appropriate, a complete blood cell count (CBC), erythrocyte sedimentation rate (ESR), serum electrolytes, glucose levels, blood urea nitrogen (BUN), liver function studies, serum vitamin B_{12}, and thyroid studies. If the patient is experiencing forms of dementia, other types of testing may be needed, such as genetic studies, computed tomography (CT) scan, or magnetic resonance imaging (MRI).

With psychotherapeutic drugs, the nurse should always assess the patient's mouth to make sure the patient has swallowed the entire oral dosage. This helps prevent "hoarding" or "cheeking" of medications, a form of nonadherence that may lead to drug toxicity or overdose. If the assessment shows that this is a potential risk, use of liquid dosage forms, when available, may minimize such problems. Appetite, sleeping patterns, addictive behaviours, elimination difficulties, hypersensitivity, and other complaints also need to be watched for and documented. Assessment of motor responses, such as trembling and agitation, and of autonomic responses (cold, clammy hands, sweating and pallor) is also important to establishing baseline information.

Antianxiety Drugs

Antianxiety drugs are associated with many contraindications, cautions, and drug interactions; specific concerns related to children and older adults are presented in Special Populations: Children and Special Populations: the Older Adult on p. 315. The older adult needs to be closely assessed and observed for oversedation and profound CNS depression for the duration of therapy. Older adults are often more sensitive to drugs, so there is constant concern for their safety. It is also critical for nurses to document these assessment findings and make safety a top priority in all phases of the nursing process. Specific serum studies that may be ordered include complete blood count (CBC), lactate dehydrogenase (LDH), creatinine, alkaline phosphatase, and BUN. In addition, blood pressure (BP) readings are important because of drug-related postural hypotension as an adverse effect. Pulse rate and temperature should also be assessed.

Ocular symptoms may occur with benzodiazepines; therefore, baseline visual testing should be determined with a basic Snellen chart examination or by the appropriate health care provider, for example, an ophthalmologist, optometrist, or nurse practitioner. Allergic reactions to some of these medications, such as clonazepam, are characterized by a red, raised rash. A significant reduction in bone marrow functioning may occur with possible blood dyscrasias, fever, sore throat, bruising, and jaundice. These "at-risk" patients for complications would require closer assessment. In addition, patients who are obese may become toxic within a shorter period of time than those who are not obese. This toxicity occurs because several antianxiety drugs are lipid soluble and most obese patients have a higher percentage of lipids; the lipid-soluble drug would have greater affinity for these tissues and stay in the body longer than anticipated, with a resultant prolonged half-life (and increased toxicity).

SPECIAL POPULATIONS: CHILDREN

Psychotherapeutic Drugs

- Children are more likely to experience adverse effects from psychotropic drugs, especially extrapyramidal symptoms. Close monitoring is required.
- The incidence of Reye's syndrome and other adverse effects is greater in children who have had chickenpox, CNS infections, measles, acute illnesses, or dehydration and are taking psychotherapeutic drugs.
- Lithium may lead to decreased bone density or bone formation in children; therefore, children taking lithium should be closely monitored for signs and symptoms of lithium toxicity and bone disorders.
- TCAs are generally not prescribed for patients under 12 years of age. However, some antidepressants are used in children with enuresis, attention deficit disorders, and major depressive disorders and may be associated with adverse effects such as changes in the ECG, nervousness, sleep disorder, fatigue, elevated BP, and gastrointestinal upset.
- Children are generally more sensitive to the effects of most drugs, and this group of drugs is no exception. Be aware of the toxicity risk, which can be fatal. Should confusion, lethargy, visual disturbances, insomnia, tremors, palpitations, constipation, or eye pain occur, report this to the physician immediately.

BP, Blood pressure; *CNS*, central nervous system; *ECG*, electrocardiogram; *TCAs*, tricyclic antidepressants.

SPECIAL POPULATIONS: THE OLDER ADULT

Psychotherapeutic Drugs

- Older adults have higher serum levels of psychotherapeutic drugs because of changes in the drug distribution and metabolism processes, less serum albumin, decreased lean body mass, less water in tissues, and increased body fat. Because of these changes, the older adult generally requires lower doses of antipsychotic and antidepressant drugs.
- Orthostatic hypotension, anticholinergic adverse effects, sedation, and extrapyramidal symptoms are more common in the older adult taking psychotherapeutic drugs.
- Careful evaluation and documentation of baseline values, including neurological findings, are important to the safe use of psychotherapeutic drugs.
- Increased anxiety is often associated with the use of TCAs.
- Patients with a history of heart disease may be at greater risk for experiencing dysrhythmias, tachycardia, stroke, myocardial infarction, or heart failure.
- Lithium is more toxic in the older adult and lower doses are often necessary. Close monitoring is important to its safe use in this age group. CNS toxicity, lithium-induced goitre, and hypothyroidism are more common in the older adult.

CNS, Central nervous system; *EPS*, extrapyramidal symptoms; *TCAs*, tricyclic antidepressants.

Some benzodiazepines, as well as most drug groups, are associated with medication errors that are "sound alike/look alike" in nature. Assessing the drug order for the right drug is important in order to prevent this potential error and the negative consequences to the patient. Sound-alike benzodiazepine drugs that could be confused with other medications include the following:
- clonazepam and clonidine
- diazepam and ditropan
- lorazepam and alprazolam

Other important assessment-related parameters for some of the specific benzodiazepines include the following:
- Lorazepam should be given cautiously (under close supervision) if the patient is suicidal because it is often used in suicide attempts.
- Alprazolam should be administered only after assessment of mental status, anxiety, mood, sensorium, sleep patterns, and dizziness.
- Chlordiazepoxide has significant assessment parameters such as monitoring for blood dyscrasias (altered blood counts) or evidence of ataxia.
- Clonazepam is commonly associated with blood dyscrasias; therefore, blood studies, such as red blood cell (RBC) count, hematocrit (Hct), hemoglobin (Hgb), and reticulocytes should be performed every week for the first 4 weeks and then monthly.

Antimanic Drugs

Prior to administering antimanic drugs, such as lithium, neurological factors, BP, pulse, intake and output, hydration status, dietary intake, skin tone, and presence of edema are important to assess and document. Baseline assessment of levels of consciousness, gait and mobility levels, and assessment of neuromotor functioning are also important to assess because poor coordination, tremors, and weakness may be symptoms of toxicity to antimanic drugs. Laboratory studies often include measurement of the sodium, albumin, and uric acid. Specific gravity and a urinalysis may also be ordered. Serum levels of sodium are important to assess because hyponatremia and hypovolemia place the patient at risk for lithium toxicity. In addition, serum lithium levels need to be assessed once drug therapy is initiated and usually every 3 to 4 days, especially during the initial phase of therapy. Generally, with lithium, it is best to have the levels assessed 8 to 12 hours after taking the dose of drug (therapeutic levels: 0.8–1.2 mmol/L with toxic levels above 2 mmol/L).

 Antidepressants

There are many cautions, contraindications, and drug interactions to assess prior to giving antidepressants. The potential for suicide with psychotherapeutic drugs, with or without the combination of other drugs or alcohol, should always be considered a risk, whether with an antidepressant or other drug group. Many of the patients needing these medications are so mentally distressed that their physical needs go unmet, resulting in a complexity of other problems, including insomnia, poor health status, and weight loss or gain. Baseline BP, pulse rate, body temperature, and body weight should be assessed and documented before, during, and after drug therapy. Postural (supine, then standing) BP readings are important because of postural hypotension. The more potent, older drugs, such as MAOIs and TCAs, may lead to a significant drop in BP and warrant even more astute assessment.

Serotonin syndrome may occur with the use of SSRIs, especially when combining two or more such drugs. Any of the following drugs may also result in hazardous adverse effects, such as MAOIs, tryptophan, and natural health products such as ephedra, ginseng (see Natural Health Products: Ginseng), and St. John's wort. See Box 16-3 for common symptoms of serotonin syndrome.

Because the newer antidepressants are associated with fewer and less potent adverse effects, only a few MAOIs are used today in psychiatric mental health settings. Patients receiving MAOIs who have a history of suicide attempts or suicidal ideations or have seizure disorders, hyperactivity, diabetes, or psychosis need to be closely monitored. Suicidal thoughts and attempts are important to consider because "hoarding" these drugs may then be used by the patient to carry out suicide. These patients should be under the care of a health care professional (such as a psychiatrist, physician, or nurse practitioner) so that they may be closely monitored for destructive behaviours. MAOIs are known for their potentiation of hypertensive crisis when used with SSRIs, meperidine, or TCAs; thus it is imperative to monitor for the risk of complications to the patient that are associated with this hypertensive event. Assess for dietary intake of tyramine if the patient is taking an MAOI (see the foods high in tyramine in Table 16-9).

Other parameters to assess with the MAO inhibitors include BP readings and postural BP. These are important for the nurse to obtain because of postural hypotension, an MAOI adverse effect, and subsequent risk of dizziness and fainting. If the patient is hospitalized, the nurse should assess supine and standing or sitting BP levels at least with each shift or more frequently, if needed. The nurse needs to wait 1 to 2 minutes after taking supine BP before taking standing or sitting BP and pulse rate. Laboratory values such as those indicative of liver functioning (alanine aminotransferase [ALT], aspartate aminotransferase [AST], bilirubin) as well as CBCs are needed to rule out any further contraindications or cautions.

Contraindications to the use of TCAs are numerous and have been previously discussed in this chapter. In addition, the older adult should be given these drugs *only* if absolutely necessary and only with careful monitoring. The older adult's BP, pulse, CBCs, weight, and liver and kidney studies should also be assessed.

NATURAL HEALTH PRODUCTS

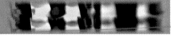

GINSENG

Overview
Ginseng comes from the Panax quinquefolius plant in North America (American ginseng), the Panax ginseng plant in the Orient (Panax ginseng), and the Acanthopanax senticosus plant in Russia (Siberian ginseng). All three are different herbs, with Siberian ginseng being markedly different from the other two, but often less expensive. Used for more than 5000 years, to be medicinally useful, ginseng needs to be at least 6 years old. The root is dried before processing and then sold in various forms.

Common Uses
Ginseng has an overall stimulant effect; however, when the chemical components are fractionated, it appears that the active compound contains both stimulant and sedative effects, giving rise to the ancient Chinese terminology translated as "balance." Ginseng is thought to improve physical endurance and concentration and to reduce stress. Ginseng's healthful effects stem from a mechanism involving the hypothalamic–pituitary–adrenal axis and the immune system. It is possible that ginseng enhances phagocytosis, natural killer cells, and the upregulation of interferon to stimulate vasodilatation and increase resistance to exogenous stress, which, in turn, affects hypoglycemic activity. More recently, ginseng has received attention for its ability to improve erectile function in some men. This is thought to occur because of its regulatory action on nitric oxide and stimulation of vasodilatation (NOTE: This is a very abbreviated list of uses for these products.)

Adverse Effects
Elevated blood pressure, chest pain or palpitations, anxiety, insomnia, headache, nausea, vomiting, diarrhea.

Potential Drug Interactions
May reduce effectiveness of anticoagulants and immunosuppressants, but enhances the effectiveness of anticonvulsants and antidiabetic drugs.

Contraindications
Hypertension, ischemic heart disease, pregnancy, child use.

The extrapyramidal adverse effects are often worse in the older adult (e.g., worsening of tremors, inability to carry out ADLs). This syndrome may lead to progressive deterioration of motor activities, so baseline motor abilities are important to assess and document. The drug interaction between TCAs and MAOIs can produce serious effects: a hyperpyretic crisis may occur if TCAs are used with MAOIs and clonidine or with patients exhibiting high fever, convulsions, or a hypertensive crisis.

With second-generation antidepressants, cautious use in the older adult and the heart patient is important. Bupropion may be preferred over other antidepressants because it has fewer anticholinergic, antiadrenergic, and cardiotoxic effects. However, the therapeutic effect of bupropion may not be reached for up to 4 weeks (as with many antidepressants); therefore, it is critical for the nurse to assess the patient for suicidal tendencies and support systems to ensure patient safety. Many of the antidepressants take weeks to have full therapeutic effect, thus close monitoring and observation of the patient are important until the drug begins to work. Because of the risk for seizures associated with second-generation antidepressants, an assessment should help to identify those patients with a history of seizures so that another medication may be used.

Third-generation antidepressants have several advantages over the older classes of antidepressants but still have contraindications, cautions, and drug interactions. The older adult with decreased kidney functioning should not take these drugs if at all possible. Concurrent use of third-generation antidepressants with any of the serotonergic (SSRIs) drugs carries the risk for serotonin syndrome and should be avoided.

Antipsychotics

The antipsychotics require careful assessment of all body systems. Different antipsychotics are associated with different adverse effects. For example, olanzapine may cause an increase in total cholesterol, and the phenothiazines are associated with extrapyramidal symptoms and a high incidence of anticholinergic effects. Therefore, assessment of cardiovascular, cerebrovascular, neurological, gastrointestinal, genitourinary, kidney, liver, and hematological functioning is important to safe and efficacious drug therapy. If there are significant diseases of one or several organ systems, the response to a drug may be more adverse and even dose limiting, thus the need for close and astute assessment of the patient prior to and during drug therapy. Weight gain may occur, and if the patient is experiencing adverse health conditions because of gaining weight, another drug may need to be ordered. Changes in sex drive, oversedation, suicidal ideations, orthostatic changes in BP, and insomnia related to some of these drugs need to be assessed thoroughly and reported as appropriate for the option of another drug. The common "anticholinergic" adverse effects of the phenothiazines (e.g., dry mouth, urinary hesitancy, constipation) and the extrapyramidal symptoms may be bothersome for some patients and lead to the use of other drugs (as ordered by the physician) for long-term treatment. It is essential that the nurse use careful and astute assessment skills to enable the most effective and high-quality therapeutic regimen for each patient in need of psychotherapeutic drug therapy and for each drug therapeutic regimen.

Haloperidol is similar to other high-potency antipsychotics because its sedating effects are low but the incidence of extrapyramidal symptoms is high. Assessment of baseline motor, sensory, and neurological functioning is, therefore, important to patient safety. With some of the antipsychotic drugs, patients may experience adverse effects of tremors and muscle twitching from the drug's blockade of dopamine receptors (dopamine generally has an inhibitory effect on specific motor movements in the musculoskeletal system). These extrapyramidal movements are manifested as parkinsonism-like and are irritating and uncomfortable for the person experiencing them. Therefore, it is important to know if there are underlying motor movement disturbances so that the best drug for the situation may be ordered.

Movement assessments are recommended for patients who are started on antipsychotic medications symptoms to assess for any movement disorders. A general recommendation is to do an assessment before a patient is started on a new medication and then every 6 months for patients who receive a first-generation antipsychotic and every 12 months for those receiving a second-generation antipsychotic. More frequent monitoring is advocated for individuals at high risk, such as older adult patients. In doing this assessment, patients can be better managed with changes or a reduction in dosage of medications and reducing the need for antiparkinsonian medications that can increase adverse effects. It is important with patients who have significant CNS disorders or symptoms or are taking medications that impact the CNS that antipsychotic drugs, such as haloperidol, be used with extreme caution and close monitoring.

Atypical antipsychotics (AAPs), such as quetiapine or clozapine, have many contraindications, cautions, and drug interactions with newer drugs in this group showing great promise, as previously discussed. A thorough mental status examination should be performed and documented appropriately before initiation of these and other antipsychotic drugs. An assessment of musculoskeletal functioning and monitoring for any extrapyramidal symptoms reactions is also important, as is assessment of the following laboratory studies: bilirubin and other liver function studies, CBC, and urinalysis. BP readings, with postural BP readings, should be assessed and documented; a drop of 20 mmHg or more should be reported to the physician immediately. In addition, the health care provider may order reduced doses to avoid toxicity in the older adult. These drugs are also associated with a high degree of sedation and should be used cautiously in the older adult and other patients who are at risk for personal injury or harm or have limited motor and sensory capabilities. With risperidone use in the older adult, it is important to assess for any unusual adverse effects, such as excessive sedation and sleepiness, that may lead to significant problems (e.g., safety concerns, falls, injury) for the patient; another drug may then be indicated. Patients taking nonphenothiazine antipsychotics or miscellaneous drugs require careful monitoring of BP as well as assessment for liver or heart disease because of drug-related drops in BP and tachycardia.

As noted earlier, antipsychotic drugs, in general, interact with many medications, natural health products, and over-the-counter drugs. These drugs include oral contraceptives, MAOIs, TCAs, SSRIs, erythromycin, quinolone antibiotics, the antibiotic ciprofloxacin (Cipro), nicotine, alcohol, antihistamines (e.g., diphenhydramine), antiepileptics, and narcotics. In addition, antipsychotic drugs may interact with foods grilled over charcoal. Using these drugs with alcohol, antihistamines, antianxiety drugs, barbiturates, meperidine, or morphine may result in additive antipsychotic effects and cause further CNS depressive effects. Antipsychotic drugs are potent drugs that deserve close monitoring and attention to detail. It is crucial for nurses to update their knowledge about these drugs so that they can be proactive in the care of patients needing these medications.

In summary, all health care providers who prescribe or administer psychotherapeutic drugs must remain current, competent, and cautious in their administering and monitoring of the use of these drugs. While safety is a major concern for any patient, the concern is much greater when the drug being administered has significant adverse effects, contraindications, cautions, and drug interactions. The nurse must always take the time to assess the patient thoroughly before administering any psychotherapeutic drug and continue to assess the needs of the patient on an ongoing basis while using all resources to be sure the patient has all of his or her needs met.

Nursing Diagnoses

- Risk for injury related to disease state and possible adverse effects of medications
- Disturbed thought processes related to neurochemical imbalance or cognitive processing problems
- Impaired social interaction related to inadequacies felt by patient due to illnesses or isolation from others
- Imbalanced nutrition, less than body requirements, related to consequences of illness, its treatment, or both
- Disturbed sleep patterns related to the mental health disorder or related drug therapy
- Situational low self-esteem related to illness and disease process, adverse effects of medication including sexual dysfunction
- Deficient knowledge related to lack of information about the specific psychotherapeutic drugs and their adverse effects
- Constipation related to adverse effects of psychotherapeutic drugs
- Urinary retention related to adverse effects of psychotherapeutic drugs
- Sexual dysfunction related to possible adverse effect of psychotherapeutic drugs

Planning

Goals

- Patient will not sustain injury while on medication.
- Patient will experience no further deterioration in thought processes.
- Patient will exhibit improved nutritional status.
- Patient will regain normal sleep patterns.
- Patient will exhibit (overtly and covertly) a more positive self-image.
- Patient will remain adherent to therapy.
- Patient will remain free of any alterations in urinary elimination patterns.
- Patient will remain free of altered bowel elimination patterns.
- Patient will be free of problems with sexual function.
- Patient will be free of complications associated with the drug and with food and drug interactions.

Outcome Criteria

- Patient does not experience falls, dizziness, or fainting attributable to adverse effects.
- Patient demonstrates improved or no deterioration in thought processes and is less hostile, withdrawn, and delusional once medication has reached a steady state.
- Patient demonstrates more open and appropriate behaviour and communication with health care team and significant others.
- Patient shows healthy nutrition habits with appropriate weight gain (if needed) and a diet that includes foods recommended by Canada's Food Guide.
- Patient reports improved sleep patterns and feeling more rested.
- Patient openly discusses feelings of poor self-image and self-concept with staff.
- Patient states the importance of taking medications exactly as prescribed at the same time every day and without omissions.
- Patient reports any problems with urinary retention.
- Patient reports any difficulty with constipation if not manageable by fluids and dietary changes.
- Patient reports any problems with sexual function.
- Patient states the importance of appointments with the physician or other health care providers to monitor therapy and improvement.
- Patient states the common adverse effects of the medication and those adverse effects (e.g., confusion and changes in level of consciousness) to be reported to the physician.
- Patient lists those medications and foods to be avoided while taking any psychotherapeutic medication.

Implementation

Regardless of the psychotherapeutic drug prescribed, several general nursing actions are important for safe administration. First and foremost is a firm but patient attitude combined with therapeutic communication. Simple explanations about the drug, action, and the length of time before therapeutic effects can be expected should be given after the patient's reading level and an effective means of teaching and learning have been established. Once a thorough psychosocial and holistic approach has been implemented, vital signs should be monitored during therapy, especially in the older adult and in patients with a history of hypertension and heart disease. Any of these drugs should be taken exactly as prescribed and at the same time every day without failure. If omission occurs, the physician should be contacted immediately. Abrupt withdrawal of any of these medications should be avoided because of the negative consequences to the patient and the patient's mental status. Soliciting help from family members or other support systems should occur so that there are options for assistance with drug administration.

Antianxiety Drugs

Specific nursing interventions and actions and patient education related to antianxiety drugs include the following:

- Frequent checks of vital signs (e.g., BP) should be done because of orthostatic hypotension that can occur.
- The patient should wear elastic compression stockings and change positions slowly if orthostatic hypotension occurs.
- Encourage communication of all disturbing thoughts (e.g., suicidal ideations, because these drugs and other psychotherapeutics should be dispensed only in small amounts to help minimize the risk for suicide attempt).
- Intravenous routes of administration of these drugs should be only as prescribed, given over the recommended time with the proper diluent, and at a rate indicated by the manufacturer and as ordered by the physician.
- Always administer intramuscular dosage forms in a large muscle mass and only as ordered or indicated.

See Patient Education for more information.

Antimanic Drugs

The antimanic drug lithium is used mainly for patients who are in a manic state. Crucial to its safe use is the patient being adequately hydrated and in a state of electrolyte balance. Lithium may become toxic if excretion is decreased or if there is dehydration or hyponatremia present. See Patient Education for more information.

Antidepressants

Antidepressants must be administered carefully and exactly as ordered. It is important (with antidepressants as well as other psychotherapeutic drugs) to emphasize that it may take several weeks before therapeutic effects are evident. The nurse must ensure that patients understand this and that they continue to take the medication as prescribed, even if they feel their condition is not improving. Careful monitoring of the patient, ready availability of staff, and supportive care during this time are critical to the therapeutic approach. The time lapse before therapeutic effects are seen may put the patient at the highest risk for self-harm or suicide. Other nursing considerations include the following:

- Most of these drugs are better tolerated if taken with food and at least 120 mL to 180 mL of water.
- Encourage assistance with ambulation and other activities if this is the patient's first time on antidepressants or if the patient is older adult or weakened, to prevent falls and subsequent injury.
- Postural hypotension, as an adverse effect, may also lead to dizziness or falls, thus caution with regular activities is recommended.
- If the patient is receiving an SSRI, remember that these are somewhat safer antidepressants, but they still need to be taken as prescribed.
- Counsel the patient about potential sexual dysfunction if related to the particular medication. If sexual dysfunction occurs, explain that there are options, such as waiting to see if the adverse effect resolves, reducing the current dose of the drug (by the health care provider, not the patient), or using a "drug holiday" as ordered by the physician. In the latter case, the patient is monitored closely, sometimes in a hospital setting, while the drug is discontinued and reinitiated. Open discussion about other medications or treatment options is encouraged if the adverse effect continues or worsens. See Patient Education for more information.

Specific nursing interventions for MAOIs and TCAs are as follows:

- Remember that MAOIs are potent antidepressants and are reserved for patients who do not respond to TCAs or other modes of therapy.
- Adverse effects to report to the physician include orthostatic hypotension, dysrhythmias, ataxia, hallucinations, seizures, tremors, dry mouth, and impotence.
- Encourage the patient to report this medication to all health care providers.
- If an MAOI or TCA is prescribed and the patient requires some sort of surgical procedure, the drug will most likely need to be weaned carefully by the physician several weeks prior to the procedure because of known interactions with anaesthesia.
- With TCAs, it is important to know that blurred vision, excessive drowsiness or sleepiness, urinary retention, or constipation need to be reported to the physician immediately.
- With some of the second- and third-generation antidepressants, it is important to inform patients that it may take up to 6 weeks for therapeutic effects and that tolerance to sedation will occur.
- Bupropion and venlafaxine come in sustained-release forms and, therefore, have a convenient once- or twice-a-day dosing, and bupropion and mirtazapine may be used as antidotes for SSRI-induced sexual dysfunction.

Antipsychotics

Patients need to be aware that all antipsychotic drugs have to be taken exactly as prescribed to be effective. Different levels of paranoia or delusions may lead to suspicion and subsequent mistrust of the nurse or physician and their treatment, so maintaining the level of trust through a therapeutic relationship is vital to adherence. Adherence is a key issue with psychotic illnesses because these patients are at higher risk for not taking medications and may not even attend follow-up or seek further medical advice. This is of major concern because the serum drug levels, such as those of haloperidol, need to be within a therapeutic range for the patient to feel better and be functional. If serum drug levels of haloperidol are less than 4 ng/mL, the patient may show symptoms of the mental health disorder, whereas levels greater than 22 ng/mL may result in toxicity. Therefore, selection of an antipsychotic, its dosage, route of administration, risk for toxicity and suicidal potential, as well as patient education and therapeutic support are all important factors to successful therapy. Because most antipsychotic drugs are quite potent, the nurse must be sure that oral dosage forms have actually been swallowed and not "tucked" in the side of the mouth or under the tongue to be discarded at a later time or taken with other dosages with a potentially lethal outcome. Oral forms of the antipsychotics are generally well absorbed and will cause less gastrointestinal upset if taken with food or a full glass of water, and use of hard candy or gum may help to relieve dry mouth. With any of the dosage forms, perspiration may be increased; therefore, patients should be warned about engaging in excessive activity or being exposed to hot or humid climates. Excessive sweating could lead to dehydration and then drug toxicity.

Haloperidol may not necessarily be the best drug to use because of the risk for under- or overmedicating; other antipsychotics may be preferred. Nurses need to understand, however, that the older, more traditional drugs, such as chlorpromazine, are highly protein-bound and, as such, have many drug interactions and even more adverse effects that are often severe in nature, such as anticholinergic effects. Anticholinergic adrenal effects include photophobia, dry mouth, mydriasis with increased intraocular pressure, sedation, constipation, and urinary retention. Antiadrenergic effects include hypotension as well as the increased risk for dysrhythmias, decreased cardiac output, and tachycardia. Other significant characteristics of the more traditional antipsychotics include extrapyramidal symptoms (occur in up 90% of the patients), dystonias, tardive dyskinesias, and neuroleptic malignant syndrome (occurs in 50% of the patients). Sore throat, malaise, fever, and bleeding, due to drug-induced blood dyscrasias, should be reported to the physician immediately.

The development of psychotherapeutic drugs is ever growing. Currently, there are a variety of atypical or newer drugs, such as clozapine, risperidone, paliperidone, olanzapine, and quetiapine, that may be preferred in treatment because of the minimal risk for tardive dyskinesia, lower incidence of extrapyramidal symptoms, and increase in cognition. With the newer antipsychotic drug quetiapine, the nurse should assist patients with ambulation until they have been stabilized on the medication. Patients should be taught to change positions slowly to avoid fainting caused by postural hypotension. Increasing fluids may help avoid constipation, and sips of water or chewing candy or gum may help with dry mouth. Some of the other atypical antipsychotic drugs have the characteristics of fewer extrapyramidal symptoms, increased cognition, and reduction of tardive dyskinesia and, therefore, may be used more commonly. The newer drugs, whether AAPs (dibenzodiazepine [clozapine], benzisoxazole [risperidone], thienobenzodiazepine [olanzapine], dibenzothiazepine [quetiapine], or benzisothiazolyl [ziprasidone]) or other atypical drugs, may be the ones used more commonly. It is important for the nurse to remember that although these drugs have different qualities and fewer of the most serious adverse effects, there are still adverse effects and concerns associated with their use. These newer drug appear to be more efficient for those individuals who are treatment resistant or who exhibit many adverse effects from other drugs. However, lethal blood dyscrasias, extrapyramidal symptoms, and anticholinergic, antiadrenergic, and antihistamine adverse effects may occur with the use of clozapine, limiting its use.

Once therapy has been initiated, it is important for the nurse and other health care members involved in the patient's care to monitor drug therapy closely, including serum drug levels during follow-up visits. If the patient is suspected of being nonadherent and serum drug levels are subtherapeutic, it is important to have the patient re-evaluated by the prescribing physician and a possible switch to a parenteral dosage form carried out. The parenteral dosage form is usually a depot (longer-releasing preparation) intramuscular injection that remains in the serum for up to 1 month, which may increase adherence and have a better therapeutic outcome. Antipsychotic drugs available for injection include chlorpromazine, fluphenazine, haloperidol, loxapine, and zuclopenthixol.

Patient education (see Patient Education) and adherence are the keys to successful treatment. Often it is the mental health disorder itself that causes patient nonadherence. Patients must be taught that overdoses can occur when these drugs are mixed with alcohol and other CNS depressants, leading to respiratory or cardiovascular collapse, which is often fatal. However, even in the best of circumstances, a lapse in therapy is possible and should always be considered. Keeping communication open with the patient and family or caregiver is important to developing trust and a sense of empathy. Although patient education may have been thorough, it is always best to emphasize that the patient can call the physician or clinic hotline 24 hours a day. Phone numbers should be updated and shared frequently with the patient, and professional counselling should be available as needed with a mental health care provider (psychiatrist or nurse practitioner) or a licensed clinical worker so that the patient's progress is consistently monitored. Group therapy and support groups are also available for the patient and significant others.

🔲 Evaluation

Both the therapeutic effects of psychotropic medications and the patient's progress within the treatment regimen must be monitored at all times during and even after therapy. Mental alertness, cognition, mood, ability to carry out ADLs, appetite, and sleep patterns are all areas that need to be closely monitored and documented. In addition to drug therapy, the patient must continue with other forms of therapy, with the goal of acquiring more effective coping skills. Along with psychotherapy, relaxation therapy, stress reduction, and other positive lifestyle changes may be needed to help with the holistic treatment of the patient. Before evaluation of the specific psychotherapeutic drugs is discussed, it is important to mention that blood levels are often drawn with these drugs so that therapeutic levels are maintained and toxic levels or undermanagement prevented. The therapeutic effects of antianxiety drugs are evidenced by improved mental alertness, cognition, and mood; fewer anxiety and panic attacks; improved sleep patterns and appetite; more interest in self and others; less tension and irritability; and fewer feelings of fear, impending doom, and stress. Adverse effects to watch for in patients taking antianxiety drugs include hypotension, lethargy, fatigue, drowsiness, confusion, constipation, dry mouth, blood dyscrasias, lightheadedness, and insomnia. Adverse reactions to antidepressants, in general, consist of drowsiness, dry mouth, constipation, dizziness, postural hypotension, sedation, blood dyscrasias, and tremors. Overdose is evidenced by irritability, agitation, CNS irritability, and seizures, with progression to CNS depression leading to respiratory or cardiac depression.

Lithium's therapeutic effects are characterized by less mania and a "stabilizing" of the patient's mood. It is usually during the manic phase that lithium is better tolerated by the patient. Therapeutic levels of lithium range from 0.8 to 1.2 mmol/L and should be determined frequently—every few days initially and then at least every few months while the patient is on the drug. The nurse should also monitor the patient's mood, affect, and emotional stability. Adverse reactions to lithium include dysrhythmias, hypotension, sedation, slurred speech, slowed motor abilities, and weight gain. Gastrointestinal symptoms such as diarrhea and vomiting, drowsiness, weakness, and unsteady gait are indicative of overdose. The physician should be consulted immediately if these occur. Patients taking clozapine should exhibit improvement in their schizophrenic state. When evaluating for adverse effects, such as development of agranulocytosis,

it is important for the nurse to remember that it is associated with minor or no extrapyramidal symptoms.

As antidepressants, SSRIs may take up to 8 weeks to reach a full therapeutic effect. They are also associated with the therapeutic effects of improved depression and mental status; improved ability to carry out ADLs; less insomnia; and improved mood disorder without an overproduction of adverse effects such as weight gain, sedation, headache, insomnia, gastrointestinal upset and complaints, dizziness, agitation, and sexual dysfunction. Be sure to monitor for symptoms of serotonin syndrome. Other therapeutic effects of the SSRIs and other antidepressants are improved sleep patterns and nutrition, increased feelings of self-esteem, decreased feelings of hopelessness, and an increased interest in self and appearance. The MAOIs and TCAs may take up to 4 weeks for full therapeutic effects. Adverse effects include sedation, dry mouth, constipation, postural hypotension, blurred vision, seizures, and tremors. Toxic reactions may be manifested by confusion or hypotension and possibly by respiratory or cardiac distress.

The therapeutic effects of haloperidol, another antipsychotic drug, are similar to those of the other drugs, but the nurse should monitor the patient for adverse reactions that are particular to haloperidol. These include sedation; tic-like trembling movements of the hands, face, neck, and head; hypotension; and dry mouth. Overdose is manifested by severe sedation, hypotension, respiratory depression, and coma. It takes approximately 3 weeks for the therapeutic effects of haloperidol to appear, but it is still important for the nurse to watch the patient for possible dyskinesia and trembling during this early period. Should these occur, the nurse should consult the physician immediately to discuss possible action. The therapeutic effects of antipsychotic drugs (e.g., phenothiazines, nonphenothiazines, and quetiapine; AAPs) should include improvement in mood and affect and alleviation of the psychotic symptoms and episodes. Emotional instability, hallucinations, paranoia, delusions, garbled speech, and inability to cope should begin to abate once the patient has been on the medication for several weeks. It is critical that the nurse carefully monitor a patient's potential to injure himself or herself or others during the delay between the start of therapy and symptomatic improvement. It is also important that the nurse watch the patient for the development of adverse reactions to phenothiazines. These include dizziness and syncope stemming from orthostatic hypotension, tachycardia, confusion, drowsiness, insomnia, hyperglycemia, blood dyscrasias, and dry mouth. Overdose is manifested by excessive CNS depression, severe hypotension, and extrapyramidal symptoms such as dyskinesias and tremors. These symptoms should be reported immediately to the physician. Other adverse effects to monitor with the AAPs include anticholinergic-, antiadrenergic-, antihistaminic-, and prolactin-related adverse effects, as well as the risk for extrapyramidal adverse effects.

PATIENT EDUCATION

Antianxiety Drugs

❖ Patients should be encouraged to change positions slowly, especially from a sitting or reclining position, to avoid dizziness or fainting, and also to avoid operating heavy machinery or driving until the adverse effects of sedation or drowsiness have resolved.

❖ Patients should be informed that tolerance often develops to the sedating properties of benzodiazepines, so drowsiness should improve taking over time.

❖ Patients should be informed to avoid over-the-counter drugs and natural health products without seeking advice from their health care provider.

❖ Patients should be informed that any psychotherapeutic drug (and all medications) should be kept out of the reach of children.

❖ Patients should avoid the use of alcohol and other CNS depressants while taking these medications.

❖ Patients should be encouraged to wear an ID bracelet or necklace showing the diagnosis and any drugs they are taking.

❖ Patients should be encouraged to always keep a list of medications on their person at all times.

❖ Patients should be informed to take medications exactly as ordered and never go off the medications suddenly.

❖ Patients should report a lack of improvement or any fears, anxiety, or feelings of despair.

Antimanic Drugs

❖ Patients should be instructed to take lithium at the same time every day and also how to handle missed doses. (If in doubt, encourage patients to contact their health care provider immediately should they miss a dose.)

❖ Patients should be informed that adverse effects of lithium (e.g., fine hand tremors, increased thirst and urination, nausea, diarrhea, anorexia) are usually transient but that they should report any excessive adverse effects.

❖ Patients should know to report the following adverse effects: extreme hand tremors, sedation, muscle weakness, vomiting, and vertigo.

❖ Patients should be instructed to maintain adequate hydration, with up to 240 mL to 300 mL of water daily (if not contraindicated).

❖ Patients need to be informed and reminded of follow-up visits with their health care provider so that serum drug levels and fluid and electrolyte status can be monitored to help decrease toxicity and maximize therapeutic effects.

Antidepressant Drugs

❖ Patients should be encouraged to increase dietary fibre and fluids to help minimize constipation.

❖ Patients should be educated on measures to help with dry mouth, such as use of saliva substitutes and chewing gum and allowing hard candy to dissolve. Diet forms of candy and gum are available.

❖ Patients should be encouraged to contact the physician if sedation and drowsiness continue past 2 to 3 weeks.

❖ Patients should be encouraged to openly discuss any concerns about their medication and adverse effects such as gastrointestinal upset, sexual dysfunction, and weight gain.

❖ Patients taking these medications should be aware to not abruptly stop them. SSRIs require a tapering period of up to 1 to 2 months. Discontinuation syndrome may occur without a tapering period; this includes symptoms of dizziness, diarrhea, movement disorders, insomnia, irritability, visual disturbance, lethargy, anorexia, and lowered mood.

❖ Patients should know about all drug interactions, such as the strong interaction between SSRIs and MAOIs, St. John's wort (a natural health product), and tryptophan (a serotonin precursor found in foods). This interaction may pose a risk for the occurrence of serotonin syndrome.

❖ Patients should be encouraged to seek medical advice about self-treating a cold or flu because of possible drug interactions.

MAOIs and TCAs

❖ Patients should be encouraged to contact their health care provider if they experience the following signs and symptoms of overdosage or toxicity: increased pulse rate, seizure activity, changes in breathing, memory, or alertness, and restlessness.

❖ Patients should be aware that it takes approximately 1 to 4 weeks for the therapeutic effects of an MAOI to be seen; therefore, medication should be continued as prescribed.

❖ If taking an MAOI, patients should be told to avoid over-the-counter cold or flu products as well as foods high in tyramine (aged cheese, wine, beer, avocados, bananas, canned meats, yogourt, soy sauce, packaged soups, and sour cream). The concern for combining MAOIs and tyramine is that this interaction leads to serious elevations in BP, heart palpitations and racing heartbeat, neck stiffness, nausea and vomiting, and severe headache. Should these problems occur, the patient must seek medical care immediately because of possible stroke from hypertensive crisis.

❖ If taking TCAs, patients should be encouraged to report any blurred vision, excessive drowsiness or sleepiness, urinary retention, or constipation to their health care provider.

❖ With all medications, patients should be advised of the importance of wearing a medic alert necklace or bracelet with a list of diagnoses and current drugs.

Haloperidol

❖ Patients should be told of the importance of avoiding hot baths, saunas, or hot climates because of the risk of further drop in BP, especially upon standing (postural hypotension). Injury may occur because of dizziness or fainting.

❖ Patients should be advised to never stop medication abruptly because of the high risk for inducing a withdrawal psychosis.

❖ Patients should be advised to avoid sun exposure and, if outdoors, apply sunscreen liberally as per instructions and wear protective clothing.

❖ Patients should report immediately any sore throat, malaise, fever, and bleeding to their health care provider.

Paliperidone

❖ Patients taking paliperidone should be advised to take the drug orally once daily, preferably in the morning, without regard to meals. Patients should be advised that this drug is contained within a nonabsorbable shell designed to release the drug at a controlled rate. It must be swallowed whole with the aid of liquids and must not be chewed, divided, or crushed.

❖ Patients should be informed that the tablet shell, along with insoluble core components, is eliminated from the body. They should not be concerned if they find a tablet in their stool.

POINTS TO REMEMBER

❖ Psychosis is a major emotional disorder that impairs mental function. A person suffering from psychosis cannot participate in everyday life and shows the hallmark symptom of loss of contact with reality.

❖ Affective disorders are emotional disorders characterized by changes in mood and range from mania (abnormally elevated emotions) to depression (abnormally reduced emotions). Anxiety, a normal physiological emotion, may be a healthy reaction but becomes pathological when it becomes "life altering."

❖ Situational anxiety arises with specific life events and nursing assessment is key to identifying "at-risk" patients.

❖ Benzodiazepines remain the drugs of choice for treatment of anxiety, are most often prescribed, are considered to be fairly safe, and do not interact with many other drugs.

❖ SSRIs are often prescribed because of their superiority to TCAs and MAOIs in terms of adverse-effect and safety profiles.

❖ Nurses need to understand terms used in everyday treatment regimens for mental health disorders. In the past, antipsychotics were called tranquilizers because they produce a state of tranquility. Neuroleptics are thus named because they work on abnormally functioning nerves. Antipsychotics and *neuroleptics* are terms used to refer to the drugs commonly used to treat serious mental health illnesses. They are used to treat BPD, psychoses, schizophrenia, and autism.

❖ Nursing considerations related to psychotherapeutic drugs include astute assessment of medication and drug history and medical history.

❖ Nursing actions focus on adequate use of the nursing process with all types of psychotherapeutic medications and on informing patients that their medications must be taken exactly as prescribed and that they need to avoid alcohol and other CNS depressants (as well as many other medications) to maintain patient safety. Frequent blood studies are needed to monitor therapeutic levels of the drugs.

EXAMINATION REVIEW QUESTIONS

1 For a patient who is in alcohol withdrawal, which medication is most likely to be ordered as treatment for this condition?
a. chlordiazepoxide
b. lithium (Carbolith)
c. alprazolam (Xanax)
d. bupropion (Wellbutrin)

2 For a patient receiving an MAOI, which food product should the patient be instructed to avoid?
a. Milk
b. Shrimp
c. Swiss cheese
d. Grapefruit juice

3 After 4 weeks of treatment for depression, the nurse calls the patient to schedule a follow-up visit. Which finding should the nurse know to look for during the conversation with the patient?
a. Weakness
b. Hallucinations
c. Suicidal ideations
d. Difficulty with urination

4 The nurse is caring for a patient who has been taking clozapine (Clozaril) for 2 months. Which lab test should be monitored while the patient is on this medication?
a. Platelet count
b. Decreased WBC count
c. Liver function studies
d. Kidney function studies

5 Which drug, when administered with lithium, increases the risk of toxicity?
a. Thiazides
b. Levofloxacin
c. Calcium citrate
d. Beta blockers

For answers see http://evolve.elsevier.com/Canada/Lilley/pharmacology/.

CRITICAL THINKING ACTIVITIES

1 A 49-year-old patient comes in with a history of depression. He tells you that he used to be treated for it by a doctor in another country, but he "ran out of pills" a few weeks ago and did not know how to get a refill. He could not remember the name of the pill but said it was for "depression." After a psychiatric evaluation, he is given a 2-week prescription for fluoxetine (Prozac). A few days later, his wife calls to describe "a terrible reaction" that he is having. She says that he is shaking, shivering, has a fever, and is somewhat confused and upset. She thinks he has a bad infection. What do you think has happened, and why?

2 Mrs. B. has inadvertently been given too much lorazepam and is experiencing respiratory arrest. The nurse has identified that the use of the benzodiazepine reversal drug flumazenil is indicated. The dose called for is 0.2 mg delivered over 15 seconds, then another 0.2 mg if consciousness does not occur after 45 seconds, then at 60-second intervals as needed up to a total dose of 1 mg. Flumazenil (Anexate) is available as a 0.1 mg/mL vial. What dose should you draw up into the needle to deliver 0.2 mg each time?

3 A 51-year-old patient arrives at the doctor's office for his annual physical. As the intake nurse, you do a brief assessment and take a short drug history. He states that he has started taking St. John's wort for depression and wants to know what the doctor thinks. You document this in his chart and research this information because you are not that familiar with natural health products. What is St. John's wort? Is it safe for patients to use for depressive symptoms? What information is important to remember about this product? What information is really crucial to share with patients in the future if they state that they are taking this supplement?

For answers see http://evolve.elsevier.com/Canada/Lilley/pharmacology/.

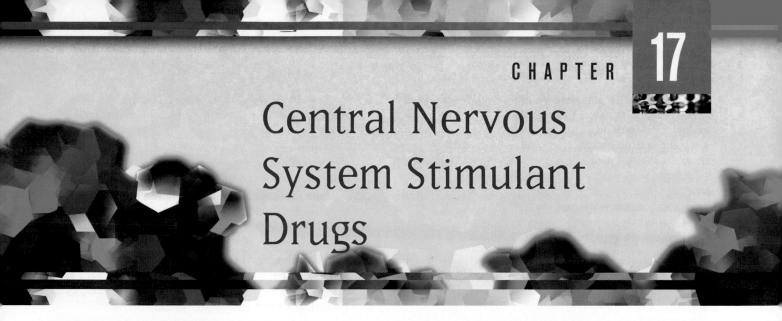

CHAPTER 17

Central Nervous System Stimulant Drugs

Learning Objectives

After reading this chapter, the successful student will be able to do the following:

1 Define the following terms: analeptic, anorexiant, hyperactivity, attention deficit hyperactivity disorder, obesity, and migraine headache.

2 Discuss briefly the prevalence and pathophysiology of attention deficit hyperactivity disorder, narcolepsy, and migraine.

3 Identify the central nervous system (CNS) stimulants with their indications.

4 Discuss the therapeutic effects associated with the use of CNS stimulants.

5 Briefly describe the mechanisms of action, dosage forms, routes of administration, adverse effects, toxic effects, cautions, contraindications, and drug interactions associated with the CNS stimulants.

6 Develop a collaborative plan of care encompassing all phases of the nursing process for a patient taking a CNS stimulant drug.

e-Learning Activities

Web site
(http://evolve.elsevier.com/Canada/Lilley/pharmacology/)

- Animations
- Answers to chapter questions, activities, and case studies
- Calculators and Category Catchers
- Glossary with audio pronunciations
- IV Therapy and Medication Error Checklists
- Multiple-Choice Review Question quizzes
- Nursing Care Plans
- Online Appendices and Supplements
- WebLinks

Drug Profiles

▸▸ **amphetamines**, p. 329
 atomoxetine (atomoxetine hydrochloride)*, p. 330
▸▸ **caffeine**, p. 337
▸▸ **methylphenidate (methylphenidate hydrochloride)***, p. 329
 modafinil, p. 330
 orlistat, p. 334
▸▸ **sibutramine (sibutramine hydrochloride monohydrate)***, p. 334
 sodium oxybate, p. 330
▸▸ **sumatriptan**, p. 335

▸▸ Key drug.

*Full generic name is given in parentheses. For the purposes of this text, the more common shortened name is used.

Glossary

Amphetamines Central nervous system (CNS) stimulants that produce mood elevation or euphoria, increase mental alertness and capacity to work, decrease fatigue and drowsiness, and prolong wakefulness. (p. 328)

Analeptics CNS stimulants that have generalized effects on the brainstem and spinal cord, which, in turn, produce an increase in responsiveness to external stimuli and stimulate respiration. (p. 326)

Anorexiants Drugs used to control or suppress appetite, that also stimulate the CNS. (p. 326)

Attention deficit hyperactivity disorder (ADHD) Syndrome affecting children, adolescents, and adults that involves difficulty maintaining concentration on a given task, hyperactive behaviour, or both. (p. 326)

Cataplexy A condition characterized by abrupt attacks of muscular weakness and hypotonia triggered by an emotional stimulus such as joy, laughter, anger, fear, or surprise. (p. 327)

CNS stimulants Drugs that stimulate specific areas of the brain or spinal cord. (p. 326)

Migraine A common type of recurring painful headache characterized by a pulsatile or throbbing quality, incapacitating pain, and photophobia. (p. 334)

Narcolepsy Syndrome characterized by sudden sleep attacks, cataplexy, sleep paralysis, and visual or auditory hallucinations at the onset of sleep. (p. 327)

Serotonin receptor agonists A new class of CNS stimulants used to treat migraines that work by stimulating 5-HT$_1$ receptors in the brain and are sometimes referred to as *selective serotonin receptor agonists* or *triptans*. (p. 335)

Sympathomimetic drugs CNS stimulants such as noradrenergic drugs (and, to a lesser degree, dopaminergic drugs) whose actions resemble or mimic those of the sympathetic nervous system. (p. 326)

CENTRAL NERVOUS SYSTEM STIMULANTS

Central nervous system (CNS) activity is regulated by a checks-and-balances system that consists of both excitatory and inhibitory neurotransmitters and their corresponding receptors in the brain and spinal cord tissues. CNS stimulation can result from either excessive stimulation of the excitatory neurons or blockade of the inhibitory neurons. **CNS stimulants** are a broad class of drugs that stimulate specific areas of the brain or spinal cord. Most CNS stimulants act by stimulating the excitatory neurons in the brain, enhancing the activity of one or more of the excitatory neurotransmitters in the brain: dopamine (dopaminergic drugs), norepinephrine (noradrenergic drugs), and serotonin (serotonergic drugs). Dopamine is a metabolic precursor of norepinephrine, which is also a neurotransmitter within the sympathetic nervous system (SNS). The actions of noradrenergic drugs often resemble or mimic the actions of the SNS. For this reason, noradrenergic drugs (and, to a lesser degree, dopaminergic drugs) are also called **sympathomimetic drugs**. Other sympathomimetic drugs are discussed further in Chapter 18.

There are three ways to classify CNS stimulant drugs. The first is on the basis of chemical structural similarities. Major chemical classes of CNS stimulants include amphetamines, serotonin agonists, sympathomimetics, and xanthines (Table 17-1). Second, these drugs can be classified according to their site of therapeutic action in the CNS (Table 17-2). Finally, they can be categorized according to five major therapeutic usage categories for CNS stimulant drugs (Table 17-3). These include anti–attention deficit, antinarcoleptic, anorexiant, antimigraine, and analeptic drugs. **Anorexiants** are drugs used to control obesity by suppression of appetite. **Analeptics** are drugs used by clinicians for specific CNS stimulation in certain clinical situations. Some therapeutic overlap exists among these drug categories.

OVERVIEW OF PATHOPHYSIOLOGY

Attention Deficit Hyperactivity Disorder

Attention deficit hyperactivity disorder (ADHD), formerly known as *attention deficit disorder* (ADD), is the most commonly diagnosed psychiatric disorder in children, affecting 3% to 5% of school-aged children. Boys are estimated to be affected from two to nine times as often as girls, although the disorder may be underdiagnosed in girls. Primary symptoms of ADHD centre on a developmentally inappropriate ability to maintain attention span and the presence of hyperactivity and impulsivity. The disorder may involve predominantly attention deficit, predominantly hyperactivity or impulsivity, or a combination of both. It usually begins before 7 years of age (as early as age 3) and is officially diagnosable when

TABLE	17-1

Structurally Related CNS Stimulants

Chemical Category	CNS Stimulant
Amphetamines and related stimulants	dextroamphetamine, methamphetamine methylphenidate
Serotonin agonists	almotriptan, eletriptan, frovatriptan, naratriptan, rizatriptan, sumatriptan, zolmitriptan
Sympathomimetics	Not available in Canada
Xanthines	caffeine, theophylline, aminophylline
Miscellaneous	modafinil, sodium oxybate (CNS depressant), sibutramine (anorexiant), orlistat (lipase inhibitor)

TABLE 17-2	
CNS Stimulants: Site of Action	
Site of Action	**CNS Stimulant**
Cerebral cortex	Amphetamines, phenidates, modafinil
Cerebrovascular system	Serotonin agonists
Hypothalamic and limbic regions	Anorexiants
Medulla and brainstem	Analeptics

symptoms last at least 6 months and occur in at least two different settings, according to the *Diagnostic and Statistical Manual of Mental Disorders*. Symptoms may persist lifelong for both males and females; hyperactivity is less prominent in adolescence and adulthood. Anxiety or mood disorders often coexist with ADHD as well as learning deficiencies and conduct or oppositional disorders. The presence of multiple concurrent conditions may increase the probability of ADHD chronicity.

ADHD involves multiple heterogeneous causes of both genetic and nongenetic etiologies. Studies in monozygotic twins indicate a 92% concordance rate for ADHD, and a child of a parent with ADHD has an up to 50% chance of developing ADHD. Other risk factors for developing ADHD include fetal alcohol syndrome and lead poisoning, as well as brain injury as a result of obstetrical complications or fetal exposure to drugs.

Although multiple neurotransmitters may be involved, a defective dopamine 4 (D_4) receptor gene that results in a deficiency in translating the dopaminergic signal to the second messenger system may be implicated. Other agonists at this site are epinephrine and norepinephrine. Brain abnormalities may also contribute to the development of ADHD. A deficit in the prefrontal cortex may be involved in the pathophysiology of ADHD. The prefrontal cortex is responsible for executive functions such as initiating and sustaining activities, prioritizing, strategizing, and inhibiting impulses that take place. Finally, structural and functional differences in the frontal lobes and basal ganglia have been noted; typically these areas are smaller.

Drug therapy for both child and adult ADHD is essentially the same. Although there is some social controversy regarding the possible overdiagnosis of, and overmedication for, this disorder, management with drugs that modulate dopamine and norepinephrine improve executive functioning and performance.

Narcolepsy

Narcolepsy is a chronic, incurable neurological disorder of unclear origin, in which patients unexpectedly fall asleep, for a few minutes or up to one hour, in the middle of normal daily activities. These "sleep attacks" are reported to cause car accidents or near-misses in 70% or more of patients. In addition to daytime sleepiness, three other major symptoms frequently characterize narcolepsy: **cataplexy**, an associated symptom in at least 70% of narcolepsy cases, which is the sudden loss of voluntary (skeletal) muscle tone with the exception of respiratory and ocular muscles; vivid hypnogenic auditory or visual hallucinations during sleep onset or upon awakening; and brief episodes of total paralysis at the beginning or end of sleep. Another major symptom of the disease is dysfunctional rapid eye movement (REM) sleep. The condition is often associated with strong emotions (for example, joy, laughter, or anger), and commonly the knees buckle and the individual falls to the floor while still awake.

Men and women are equally affected, with approximately 1 in 2500 people affected in Canada. Narcolepsy tends to begin during adolescence or the early twenties and symptoms tend to be lifelong. Some genetic markers that are associated with sleep regulation and with the sleep–wake cycle have been identified. Approximately one half of patients with narcolepsy experience migraine headaches.

DRUGS FOR ATTENTION DEFICIT HYPERACTIVITY DISORDER AND NARCOLEPSY

CNS stimulants are the first-line drugs of choice for both ADHD and narcolepsy. Although there has been some public controversy regarding their use, these drugs have led to a 65% to 75% improvement in symptoms in treated patients compared with a placebo. In general, CNS

TABLE 17-3	
CNS Stimulants and Related Drugs: Therapeutic Categories	
Category	**Drugs**
Analeptic	caffeine, aminophylline, theophylline, modafinil (antinarcoleptic)
Anorexiant	diethylpropion, sibutramine, orlistat (lipase inhibitor)
Anti-ADHD	dextroamphetamine, methamphetamine, methylphenidate, atomoxetine (norepinephrine reuptake inhibitor)
Antimigraine (serotonin agonists)	almotriptan, eletriptan, frovatriptan, naratriptan, rizatriptan, sumatriptan, zolmitriptan
Antinarcoleptic	dextroamphetamine (adjunct), methamphetamine, methylphenidate, sodium oxybate (CNS depressant used for cataplexy)

ADHD, attention deficit hyperactivity disorder; *CNS*, central nervous system.

stimulants elevate mood, produce a sense of increased energy and alertness, decrease appetite, and enhance task performance impaired by fatigue or boredom. Two of the oldest known stimulants are cocaine and amphetamine, which are prototypical drugs for this class. Cocaine is a natural alkaloid, which was first extracted from the plant *Erythroxylon coca* in the mid-nineteenth century but had been used by natives of the Andes for its stimulant effects for centuries before. Caffeine, contained in coffee and tea, is another plant-derived CNS stimulant. Amphetamine sulfate was first synthesized in the late 1800s. It was subsequently used to treat narcolepsy and then to prolong the alertness of soldiers during World War II. Later variants of the drug, which are still used clinically, include dextroamphetamine sulfate and methamphetamine. The drugs currently used to treat both ADHD and narcolepsy include amphetamines as well as nonamphetamine stimulants. Methylphenidate, a synthetic amphetamine derivative, was first introduced for the treatment of hyperactivity in children in 1958. More recently, mixed amphetamine salts (MAS) have been shown to be more effective than nonstimulant ADHD drugs.

Mechanism of Action and Drug Effects

Amphetamines stimulate areas of the brain associated with mental alertness, such as the cerebral cortex and the thalamus. The pharmacological actions of amphetamines and sympathomimetic CNS stimulants are similar to the actions of the SNS in that the CNS and the respiratory system are the primary body systems affected. CNS effects include mood elevation or euphoria, increased mental alertness and capacity for work, decreased fatigue and drowsiness, and prolonged wakefulness. The respiratory effects most commonly seen are relaxation of bronchial smooth muscle, increased respiration, and dilation of pulmonary arteries. Stringent controls have greatly reduced their medical use in Canada, as CNS stimulants are potent drugs with a strong potential for tolerance and psychological dependence. They are therefore classified as Schedule III drugs under the Controlled Drug and Substances Act (see Legal and Ethical Principles on the proper

handling of prescription drugs). These drugs include amphetamine sulfate, its d-isomer dextroamphetamine sulfate (Dexedrine), and mixed amphetamine salts (Adderall XR), which include salts of both amphetamine and dextroamphetamine. Another stimulant, methylphenidate hydrochloride (Biphentin, Concerta, Ritalin), is structurally and functionally similar to amphetamine. Specialists sometimes recommend periodic "drug holidays" (e.g., 1 day per week) without medication to mitigate the addictive tendencies of these drugs.

Amphetamines increase the effects of both norepinephrine and dopamine in CNS synapses by increasing their release and blocking their reuptake. As a result, both neurotransmitters are in contact with their receptors longer, which lengthens their duration of action. The sole nonamphetamine stimulant available in Canada is modafinil (Alertec). Modafinil is also classified as an analeptic. Like amphetamines, it promotes wakefulness. It lacks sympathomimetic properties, however, and appears to work primarily by reducing gamma-aminobutyric acid (GABA)–mediated neurotransmission in the brain. GABA is the principle inhibitory neurotransmitter in the brain. A newer nonstimulant drug, atomoxetine (Strattera), is also being used to treat ADHD. It works by selective inhibition of norepinephrine reuptake.

Indications

Methylphenidate is currently used to treat ADHD and narcolepsy. Dexmethylphenidate is currently indicated for ADHD alone or in the adjunctive treatment of narcolepsy. The newer nonstimulant drug atomoxetine is also now used to treat ADHD. Amphetamine sulfate was used to treat obesity in the early to mid-twentieth century. However, in Canada, amphetamines are not currently approved for this indication. The nonamphetamine stimulant modafinil is indicated for narcolepsy, obstructive sleep apnea/hyponea syndrome, and shift-work sleep disorder.

Contraindications

Contraindications to the use of amphetamine and nonamphetamine stimulants include known drug allergy,

---

⚖ LEGAL & ETHICAL PRINCIPLES

Handling of Prescription Drugs

It is important for the nurse to understand the provincial standards (Regulated Health Professional Act and the Nursing Act) that apply to the handling of all prescription drugs by the registered nurse. The registered nurse extended class (EC) (also called nurse practitioner) can prescribe medications.

The registered nurse is prohibited from doing the following:
- Compounding or dispensing designated drugs for legal distribution and administration
- Distributing the drugs to any individuals who are not licensed or authorized by federal or provincial law

to receive the drugs (e.g., those individuals outside the physician–patient relationship). The penalties for such actions are generally severe.
- Making, selling, keeping, or concealing any counterfeit drug equipment
- Possessing any type of stimulant or depressant drug unless authorized by a legal prescription (as a patient)

It is important to adhere to these legal guidelines to avoid legal penalties, including possible loss of licensure or other severe penalties.

marked anxiety or agitation, glaucoma, Tourette's syndrome, other tic disorders, and therapy with any monoamine oxidase inhibitor (MAOI) within the preceding 14 days. Contraindications specific to atomoxetine include drug allergy, glaucoma, and recent MAOI use as mentioned previously.

Adverse Effects

Both amphetamine and nonamphetamine stimulants have a wide range of adverse effects that most often arise when these drugs are administered at dosages higher than the therapeutic dosages. These drugs tend to "speed up" body systems. For example, effects on the cardiovascular system include increased heart rate and blood pressure. Other adverse effects include angina, anxiety, insomnia, headache, tremor, blurred vision, increased metabolic rate, gastrointestinal (GI) distress, and dry mouth.

Interactions

The drug interactions associated with CNS stimulants vary greatly from class to class. Table 17-4 summarizes some of the more common interactions for all drug classes in this chapter.

TABLE 17-4

CNS Stimulants: Common Drug Interactions

Drug	Mechanism	Result
AMPHETAMINES AND OTHER STIMULANTS		
β-blockers	Increase α-adrenergic effects	Hypertension, bradycardia, dysrhythmias, heart block
CNS stimulants	Additive toxicities	Cardiovascular adverse effects, nervousness, insomnia, convulsions
Digoxin	Additive toxicity	Increased risk of dysrhythmias
MAOIs	Increase release of catecholamines	Headaches, dysrhythmias, severe hypertension
TCAs	Additive toxicities	Cardiovascular adverse effects (dysrhythmias, tachycardia, hypertension)
ANOREXIANTS AND ANALEPTICS		
CNS stimulants	Additive toxicities	Nervousness, irritability, insomnia, dysrhythmias, seizures
MAOIs	Increase release of catecholamines	Headaches, dysrhythmias, severe hypertension
Quinolones	Interfere with metabolism	Reduce clearance of caffeine and prolong caffeine's effect
SEROTONIN AGONISTS		
Ergot alkaloids, SSRIs, MAOIs	Additive toxicity	Cardiovascular adverse effects, nervousness, insomnia, convulsions
Serotonergic drugs	Additive toxicity	Cardiovascular adverse effects, nervousness, insomnia, convulsions

CNS, central nervous system; *MAOI*, monoamine oxidase inhibitor; *SSRIs*, selective serotonin reuptake inhibitors; *TCA*, tricyclic antidepressants.

 DRUG PROFILES

AMPHETAMINES AND RELATED STIMULANTS

The principal drugs used to treat ADHD and narcolepsy are the amphetamine and nonamphetamine stimulants. Dosages and other information appear in the Dosages table on p. 330.

▶▶ amphetamines

The amphetamine salts are the prototypical CNS stimulants used to treat ADHD and narcolepsy. Amphetamine is available in prescription form only for oral use, both as single-component dextroamphetamine sulfate and as a mixture of dextroamphetamine sulfate, dextroamphetamine saccharate, amphetamine sulfate, and amphetamine aspartate.

PHARMACOKINETICS (dextroamphetamine)

Half-Life	Onset	Peak	Duration
PO: 7–14 hr*	PO: 30–60 min	PO: < 2 hr	PO: 10 hr

*pH less than 6.6.

▶▶ methylphenidate hydrochloride

Methylphenidate hydrochloride (Biphentin, Concerta, Ritalin) is also a major drug of choice for the treatment of ADHD and narcolepsy and is the most widely prescribed drug for treatment of ADHD. There is some controversy regarding its use, especially among apprehensive parents. However, with proper diagnosis of the disorder, proper dosing of the drug, and regular medical monitoring,

Continued

DRUG PROFILES (cont'd)

many children can achieve significant improvement in school performance and social skills. Psychosocial problems within a child's family should be ruled out or addressed if they are contributing to the child's problems, regardless of whether the medication is prescribed.

PHARMACOKINETICS (Immediate Release)

Half-Life	Onset	Peak	Duration
PO: 1–3 hr	PO: 30–60 min	PO: 1–3 hr	PO: 4–6 hr

atomoxetine hydrochloride

Atomoxetine hydrochloride (Strattera) is the newest medication approved for treating ADHD in children older than 6 years of age and in adults. It was approved by the U.S. Food and Drug Administration (FDA) in 2002. Atomoxetine assists in increasing attention and decreasing restlessness and impulsiveness in children and adults. This medication is not a controlled substance because it lacks addictive properties, unlike amphetamines. For this reason, it has rapidly gained popularity as a therapeutic option for treating ADHD and has been used to treat over 2 million patients worldwide to date. However, Health Canada and the drug manufacturer did issue a warning describing cases of suicidal thinking and behaviour in small numbers of adolescent patients receiving this medication, similar to its previous warnings regarding adolescent use of antidepressant medications (Chapter 16). Atomoxetine can also cause severe liver injury in rare cases. Atomoxetine currently remains on the market, but prescribers are advised to work with parents in providing prudent monitoring of any young patients taking this medication and to promptly re-evaluate patients showing any behavioural symptoms of concern.

PHARMACOKINETICS

Half-Life	Onset	Peak	Duration
PO: 5 hr	PO: 60 min	PO: 1–2 hr	PO: 24–120 hr

modafinil

Modafinil (Alertec) is indicated for improvement of wakefulness in patients with excessive daytime sleepiness associated with narcolepsy. It has less misuse potential than that of amphetamines and methylphenidate and is a Schedule F drug.

PHARMACOKINETICS

Half-Life	Onset	Peak	Duration
PO: 1 hr	PO: 1–2 mo*	PO: 3 hr	PO: Unknown

*Therapeutic effects.

MISCELLANEOUS NARCOLEPSY DRUGS
sodium oxybate

Sodium oxybate (Xyrem) is the sodium salt of Υ-hydroxybutyrate, one of the notorious "date rape" drugs. It is currently the sole drug approved by Health Canada for the treatment of cataplexy. Recall that cataplexy is a condition characterized by acute attacks of muscle weakness and is often associated with narcolepsy. Distribution of this drug is carefully controlled because of its abuse potential. Prescribers who wish to use this medication for this restricted population of patients must contact the Xyrem Success Program at 1-877-XYREM-88 (1-877-899-7360). Sodium oxybate is currently legally available only through such restricted dispensing programs. It is classified as a Schedule III controlled substance for this limited medical use and is technically a CNS depressant rather than a stimulant. This drug is contraindicated in cases of sleep apnea, substance misuse, or concurrent use of hypnotic drugs.

PHARMACOKINETICS

Half-Life	Onset	Peak	Duration
PO: 30–60 min	PO: 30 min	PO: 30–75 min	PO: 1–5 hr

DOSAGES   Selected CNS Stimulants and Related Drugs

Drug (Pregnancy Category)	Pharmacological Class	Usual Dosage Range	Indications
almotriptan maleate (Axert) (C)	Serotonin receptor agonist	*Adult* PO: 6.25–12.5 mg 1 dose; may repeat in 2 hr for a max of 12.5 mg/24 hr	Acute migraine with or without aura
▸▸amphetamine salts (Adderall XR) (C)	CNS stimulant	*Children 6–12 yr* PO: 5–10 mg once daily in morning, increased weekly until desired effect to a daily max of 30 mg *Adolescents 13–17 yr/Adult* PO: 10 mg once daily in morning, increased weekly to a daily max of 30 mg	ADHD
atomoxetine hydrochloride (Strattera) (C)	Selective norepinephrine reuptake inhibitor	*Children 6 yr and older,* *Adolescents (less than 70 kg)* PO: 0.5–1.4 mg/kg/day divided once or twice daily *Children/Adolescents/Adult (70 kg or more)* PO: 40–100 mg/day divided once or twice daily	ADHD

Continued

DOSAGES   Selected CNS Stimulants and Related Drugs (cont'd)

Drug (Pregnancy Category)	Pharmacological Class	Usual Dosage Range	Indications
caffeine (Caffeine Lite, Caffeinum, Pep-Back, Water Joe) (B)	Xanthine cerebral stimulant	*Adult* PO: 100–200 mg prn	Aids in staying awake
dextroamphetamine sulfate (Dexedrine) (C)	CNS stimulant (sympathomimetic)	*Children 6 yr and older* PO: 2.5–40 mg once daily or bid *Children 12 yr and older/Adult* PO: 5–60 mg once daily	ADHD Adjunctive treatment for narcolepsy
eletriptan hydrobromide (Relpax) (C)	Serotonin receptor agonist	*Adult, 18–65 yr* PO: 20–40 mg ×1 dose; may repeat in 2 hr for a max of 40 mg/24 hr	Acute migraine with or without aura
frovatriptan succinate (Frova) (C)	Serotonin receptor agonist	*Adult* PO: 2.5 mg ×1 dose; may repeat ×1 at 4–24 hr after first dose	Acute migraine with or without aura
methylphenidate hydrochloride, extended-release (Biphentin) (C) methylphenidate hydrochloride, extended-release (Concerta) (C)	CNS stimulant	*Children 6 yr and older* PO: 10–60 mg/day in a single dose *Adult* PO: 10–80 mg once daily in the morning *Children 6–12/Adolescents 13–18* PO: 18–54 mg/day, single dose *Adult over 18* PO: 18–72 mg/day, single dose	ADHD
▸▸methylphenidate hydrochloride (Ritalin, Ritalin SR)	CNS stimulant	*Children 6 yr and older* PO: 5–10 mg tid, max 60 mg *Adult* PO: 20–60 mg/day divided bid–tid	ADHD ADHD
modafinil (Alertec) (C)	CNS stimulant	*Adult over 18* PO: 200–400 mg/day, divided	Narcolepsy, obstructive sleep apnea/hypopnea syndrome, and shift-work sleep disorder
naratriptan hydrochloride (Amerge) (C)	Serotonin agonist	*Adult* PO: 1–2.5 mg at onset of headache	Acute migraine with or without aura
orlistat (Xenical) (B)	Lipase inhibitor	*Adult* PO: 120 mg tid with each meal containing fat	Obesity
rizatriptan (Maxalt, Maxalt RPD) (C)	Serotonin agonist	*Adult* PO: 5–10 mg at onset of headache; may repeat ×1 after 2 hr, up to 20 mg/day	Acute migraine with or without aura
▸▸sibutramine hydrochloride monohydrate (Meridia) (C)	CNS stimulant (anorexiant)	*Adult* PO: 10–15 mg/day	Obesity
sodium oxybate (Xyrem) (B)	CNS depressant	*Adult only* PO: 2.25 g bid; may titrate upward by 1.5 g; max 9 g/day	Cataplexy (associated with narcolepsy)
▸▸sumatriptan (Imitrex) (C)	Serotonin agonist	*Adult* PO: 25–100 mg, repeat after 2 hr to max 200 mg/day SC: 6 mg, repeat in 1 hr; max 12 /day) Nasal spray: 5–20 mg, repeat after 2 hr; max 40 mg/day	Acute migraine with or without aura
zolmitriptan (Zomig, Zomig Rapimelt) (C)	Serotonin agonist	*Adult* Minimum effective dose: 1 mg PO: 2.5 mg at onset of headache; may repeat after 2 hr; max 10 mg/day Note: orally disintegrating tablets may not be broken in half Nasal spray: 2.5–5 mg spray in one nostril at onset of headache	Acute migraine with or without aura

ADHD, attention deficit hyperactivity disorder; *CNS*, central nervous system.

OBESITY

According to Statistics Canada, roughly 23% of Canadians are obese and 59% of the adult population is considered overweight. The incidence of obesity in Canada occurs almost equally among men and women. Obesity was formerly defined as being 20% or more above one's ideal body weight based on population statistics for height, body frame, and gender. More recent data are based on a measurement known as the body mass index (BMI), defined as weight in kilograms divided by height in metres squared (= weight [kg]/[height in metres]2). Overweight is now defined as a BMI of 25 to 29.9 kg/m^2, whereas obesity is defined as a BMI of 30 kg/m^2 or higher. There are now categories to address those individuals who are severely obese (BMI of 40 kg/m^2 or more) and super obese (BMI of 50 kg/m^2 or more). At any given time, one third of women and one quarter of men are trying to lose weight.

Moreover, the incidence of obesity in young people aged 6 to 19 years has increased significantly since 1980. Obesity increases the risk for hypertension, dyslipidemia, coronary artery disease, stroke, type 2 diabetes mellitus, gallbladder disease, gout, osteoarthritis, sleep apnea, and certain types of cancer, including breast and colon cancer. An estimated 80% of obese individuals will develop diabetes in Canada; 8414 deaths (4% of total deaths) were attributable to obesity in 2004. The total direct health care cost of obesity in 2001 was estimated at more than $1.6 billion, which corresponded to 2.2% of the total health care expenditures for all diseases in Canada.

Tracking body weight and body mass index alone may not be sufficient as an indicator of risk. Since visceral fat is strongly correlated with waist circumference, researchers are now recommending that waist measurement become a routine measure in clinical practice. Emerging evidence also suggests that fat deposition within the liver is another factor of fat distribution independently linked to dyslipidemia and insulin resistance. In fact, one study conducted by researchers at Queen's University, Kingston, Ontario, linked visceral fat (fat around the waist or abdomen) to overall mortality in men. Kuk et al. (2006) used computed tomography (CT) scanners to clearly distinguish two different depots of abdominal fat in 291 men (mean age 56.4): intra-abdominal (visceral) fat (excess fat in the abdominal cavity) from abdominal subcutaneous fat (the fat located just under the skin). Logistic regression was used to determine the independent association between the fat depots and all-cause mortality. They found viseral fat to be an independent predictor for mortality. These findings support the importance of setting abdominal obesity as a primary target for obesity reduction and, consequently, the need to educate health care practitioners on the importance of routine measurement of visceral fat by waist circumference.

Yet many people who attempt weight loss do so for cosmetic reasons, not for health reasons. Obese people are often stigmatized, at times even by the health care professionals treating them. See Evidence-Informed Practice on the diagnosis and treatment of obesity in adults.

ANOREXIANTS

By definition, an *anorexiant* is any substance that suppresses appetite. Anorexiants are CNS stimulant drugs used to promote weight loss in obesity. These drugs include diethylpropion (Tenuate) and sibutramine (Meridia). As noted earlier, amphetamines were developed in the 1920s to treat depression and obesity. Stringent regulations have greatly reduced their medical use in Canada and none are currently approved for treating obesity. Orlistat (Xenical) is a related nonstimulant drug.

Mechanism of Action and Drug Effects

Anorexiants are believed to work by suppressing appetite control centres in the brain. Some evidence suggests that they also increase the body's basal metabolic rate, including mobilization of adipose tissue stores and enhanced cellular glucose uptake, as well as reduce dietary fat absorption.

There are some minor differences between these drugs in terms of their individual actions. Diethylpropion resembles amphetamine sulfate in its chemical structures and CNS effects. Diethylpropion is classified as both an anorexiant and an adrenergic (sympathomimetic) drug. However, it appears to suppress appetite centres in the CNS through dopamine- and norepinephrine-mediated pathways. Sibutramine, the newest anorexiant, enhances dopamine, norepinephrine, and serotonin activity in the brain by inhibiting neuronal reuptake of these neurotransmitters. Its dopamine activity is weaker than its norepinephrine and serotonin activity. This kind of serotonergic activity is associated with enhanced feelings of satiety. Both medications also are believed to work in part by raising the patient's metabolic rate as another consequence of their activities in the brain.

Another relatively new drug is orlistat, which differs from the others in that it is not a CNS stimulant per se but works by irreversibly inhibiting the enzyme lipase. This results in absorption of decreased amounts of dietary fat from the intestinal tract and increased fat excretion in the feces.

Indications

Anorexiants are used for the treatment of obesity. However, their effects are often minimal without accompanying behavioural modifications involving diet and exercise. More specifically, these drugs are often used in obese patients with a BMI of 30 or more, or in patients with a BMI of 27 who are also hypertensive or have high cholesterol or diabetes.

Contraindications

Contraindications to anorexiants include drug allergy, any severe cardiovascular disease, uncontrolled hypertension, hyperthyroidism, glaucoma, mental agitation, history of drug abuse, eating disorders (e.g., anorexia, bulimia), and use of MAOIs (Chapter 16) within the previous 14 days. In addition, sibutramine should not be used concurrently with other serotonergic drugs, including selective serotonin reuptake inhibitors (Chapter 16), meperidine,

EVIDENCE-INFORMED PRACTICE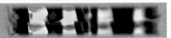

An Applied Evidence-Informed Review of the Diagnosis and Treatment of Obesity in Adults

Background

Because obesity is an epidemic in Canada and leads to substantial morbidity and mortality, a review was conducted to identify effective strategies for managing obesity and to provide a rationale for its diagnosis and treatment. This applied evidence-informed review of research presents information about the diagnostic test characteristics of exact body mass index (BMI) and, for the appropriate and relevant treatment methods identified, reports the number of patients who need to be treated to achieve one positive outcome event. The review integrated support of recommendations from the following scientific bodies known for their work on adult obesity: The National Heart, Lung, and Blood Institute; The World Health Organization; The Canadian Task Force on Preventative Health Care; and The U.S. Preventative Task Force. Data were obtained from pertinent studies identified using MEDLINE, the Database of Abstracts of Reviews of Effectiveness, and the Cochrane Database of Systematic Reviews.

Type of Evidence

This was an applied evidence-informed review of methods for diagnosing and treating adults with obesity. Data in the following areas were summarized: evidence of increased health risk associated with obesity, evidence that reducing weight decreases disease risk, and evidence that reducing weight increases disease risk (e.g., increased risk of hip fracture). The review was based on a compilation and synthesis of the data, focusing on the role of primary care health care providers in the diagnosis and treatment of adult obese patients.

Results of Study

The means of diagnosing obesity in adulthood were identified through the use of BMI rather than the gender-, height-, and age-specific tables used in the past. BMI (weight in kilograms divided by height in metres squared) is easily calculated and seen as a reliable measure for overweight and obese adults. Evidence on treatment modalities was also reviewed and presented. Data on the effectiveness of interventions were reviewed. The weight loss interventions identified as being effective included diet, exercise, behavioural strategies, limited use of pharmacological treatments in combination with strategies that change lifestyle, and surgery for selected morbidly obese patients. Because this chapter concerns central nervous system stimulants, it is relevant to note that serotonin–norepinephrine reuptake inhibitors (e.g., sibutramine) *and* gastrointestinal lipase inhibitors (e.g., orlistat) were the specific drugs mentioned in this review. Surgical interventions discussed in the review were gastric bypass and gastroplasty.

Link of Evidence to Nursing Practice

This review emphasized the importance of using an applied evidence-informed approach to investigating obesity management in adults. Diagnosis and treatment were the focus of the review, and excellent criteria were identified for the health care provider to use in everyday practice. Some of the key points relevant for clinicians to use when treating obese patients are as follows:

- Obesity should be managed as a chronic and relapsing disease.
- BMI should be used as a tool to diagnose obesity in patients and to guide decisions about treatment.
- A reduction of 10% of total body weight (identified as a "modest" reduction) yields results in improving and preventing hypertension, diabetes, and hyperlipidemia.
- Diet combined with exercise proved to be the most effective treatment method; sibutramine should be used with caution pending review by Health Canada.
- Patients should be counselled to set a goal of a 10% decrease in total body weight.
- Patients should be counselled to exercise to increase energy expenditure rather than to attain aerobic fitness.
- Referral to a behavioural program to reinforce the health care provider's counselling should be considered.
- Being an advocate for social policies that promote health, good nutrition, and increased physical activity is important.

This review summarized therapies and lifestyle changes for treating obesity. The importance of viewing obesity management as a lifelong process and applying a "chronic-disease care" model that incorporates collaborative approaches to care was emphasized. Effective methods of diagnosis and treatment of adult obesity were identified. Although the review concentrated on the actions of the primary care provider during the clinical encounter, this was identified as a reactive approach; a more proactive strategy on the part of health care providers is critical to successful therapy. Major changes must occur in the health care of adults and children (because habits start early) to put in place the necessary social policies and good nutrition and exercise habits that are needed to attack this problem. Nurses continue to play an important role in patient care and in the education of the community regarding all types of health care concerns, including the morbidity and mortality associated with obesity.

Based on Orzano, J. A., & Scott, J. G. (2004). Diagnosis and treatment of obesity in adults: An applied evidence-based review. *Journal of the American Board of Family Practice, 17*(5), 359–369. Retrieved May 5, 2009, from http://www.jabfm.org/cgi/content/full/17/5/359

lithium, or dihydroergotamine. Orlistat is contraindicated in cases of chronic malabsorption syndrome or cholestasis.

Adverse Effects

With the exception of diethylpropion, anorexiants may raise blood pressure and cause heart palpitations and even dysrhythmias at higher dosages. Ironically, at therapeutic dosages, they may actually reflexively slow the heart rate. Diethylpropion, however, has little cardiovascular activity. These drugs may also cause anxiety, agitation, dizziness, and headache. In addition to these effects, with sibutramine use, there have been case reports of mania, intestinal obstruction, cardiac arrest, and stroke, among several other serious consequences. However, obese patients commonly have multiple risk factors for such adverse events even when this drug is not taken. The most common adverse effects of orlistat include headache, upper respiratory tract infection (mechanism uncertain), and gastrointestinal distress, including fecal incontinence.

Interactions

Drug interactions for the anorexiants are listed in Table 17-4.

MIGRAINE

A **migraine** is a common type of recurring headache, usually lasting from 4 to 72 hours. Typical features include a pulsatile quality with pain that worsens with each pulse. The pain is most commonly unilateral but may occur bilaterally on both sides of the head. Associated symptoms include nausea, vomiting, *photophobia* (avoidance of light), *phonophobia* (avoidance of sounds), and *osmophobia* (avoidance of odours). In addition, a minority of migraines are accompanied by an aura, which is a predictive set of altered visual or other senses

(formerly termed "classic migraine"). However, most migraines are without an aura (formerly termed "common migraine"). Migraine affects more than 3 million Canadians, or 17% of the population, with a reported incidence in females roughly three times that in males. One Canadian study indicated that people lost an average of 6.5 work days per year because of migraine; 78% of people with migraine felt that it significantly affected their lives, and 62% required bed rest during their attacks, struggling with symptoms. Although migraines can occur at any age, commonly they begin after age 10 and peak between the ages of 25 and 39. They often fade after middle age. Familial inheritance of migraine is also well recognized. There is wide variation in the severity and frequency of attacks among patients and within an individual over time. Precipitating factors include stress, emotionality, hypoglycemia, menses, estrogens (including oral contraceptives), exercise, alcohol, caffeine, cocaine, nitroglycerin, aspartame, and the food additive monosodium glutamate (MSG). Interestingly, over 50% of patients with narcolepsy report nocturnal migraines. Previously, migraines were thought to be caused by compensatory vasodilation when brain circulation was compromised for some unknown reason. According to this "vascular hypothesis," the enhanced intracranial circulation causes headache by displacing tissues within the cranial cavity. A more recent theory can be termed the "neurovascular hypothesis." It focuses on neural structures of the trigeminal nerve itself as well as the vascular structures associated with this nerve, which affect intracranial circulation. This theory is supported by positron emission tomographic (PET) scans of the brain during a migraine attack. These neural structures are believed to have unpredictable episodes of inflammatory dysfunction that results in pain. This inflammatory process, like such processes in general, also causes increased blood flow to the affected area. It is driven by

---

 DRUG PROFILES

ANOREXIANTS

The current major prescription anorexiants is sibutramine. A newer nonstimulant drug included here is the lipase inhibitor orlistat. These two medications offer generally improved safety and adverse effect profiles.

▸▸ sibutramine hydrochloride monohydrate

Sibutramine hydrochloride monohydrate (Meridia) is one of the newest anorexiants and is a prescription medication. Sibutramine works by inhibiting the reuptake primarily of norepinephrine and serotonin (and, to a lesser extent, dopamine), which results in reduced appetite.

PHARMACOKINETICS

Half-Life	Onset	Peak	Duration
PO: 14–16 hr	PO: 8 wk	PO: 6 mo*	PO: 12 mo*

*Therapeutic effects.

orlistat

Orlistat (Xenical), one of the newer anorexiants, is unrelated to other drugs in its category. As noted earlier, it works by binding to gastric and pancreatic enzymes called lipases. Blocking these enzymes reduces fat absorption by roughly 30%. Restricting dietary intake of fat to less than 30% of total calories can help reduce some of the gastrointestinal adverse effects, which include oily spotting, flatulence, and fecal incontinence in 20% to 40% of patients. Decreases in serum concentrations of vitamins A, D, and E and β-carotene are seen as a result of the blocking of fat absorption. Supplementation with fat-soluble vitamins corrects this deficiency.

PHARMACOKINETICS

Half-Life	Onset	Peak	Duration
PO: 1–2 hr	PO: 3 mo*	PO: 6–8 hr	PO: Unknown

*Therapeutic effects.

inflammatory mediator proteins such as the neuropeptides (nerve proteins) *substance P, calcitonin gene–related peptide,* and *neurokinin A,* all of which are potent vasodilators. In particular, falling brain and body serotonin levels are believed to be one major culprit, which is reflected in the design of antimigraine drugs. During a migraine, platelets release serotonin into the circulation where much of it is lost to body metabolism. Two drug classes work against migraine symptoms by enhancing serotonergic transmission in the brain: the ergot alkaloids (Chapter 19) and serotonergic agonists or triptans. These include sumatriptan, almotriptan, eletriptan, naratriptan, rizatriptan, zolmitriptan, and frovatriptan.

ANTIMIGRAINE DRUGS (SEROTONIN AGONISTS)

Serotonin receptor agonists, first introduced in the 1990s, have revolutionized the treatment of migraine headache. Like the ergot alkaloids mentioned in Chapter 19, these drugs work by stimulating serotonin receptors in the brain.

Mechanism of Action and Drug Effects

The chemical name for serotonin is 5-hydroxytryptamine, or 5-HT. Physiologists have further identified two 5-HT receptor subtypes on which these drugs have their greatest effect: 5-HT1B and 5-HT1D. Triptans stimulate these receptors in cerebral arteries, causing vasoconstriction and normally reducing or eliminating headache symptoms. They also reduce the production of inflammatory neuropeptides. This is known as *abortive* drug therapy because it treats a headache that has already started.

Indications

Antimigraine drugs, also referred to as selective serotonin receptor agonists (SSRAs), are indicated for abortive therapy of an acute migraine headache. Although they may be taken during aura symptoms in patients who have auras with their headaches, these drugs are not indicated for *preventive* migraine therapy. Preventive therapy is indicated if migraine attacks occur one or more days per week.

A variety of drugs are used for preventive therapy; most of them are discussed in more detail in other chapters. These include analgesics (e.g., acetaminophen, aspirin, ibuprofen), tricyclic antidepressants (Chapter 16), monoamine oxidase inhibitors (Chapter 16), β-blockers (Chapter 19), calcium channel blockers (Chapters 23 and 25), anticonvulsants (Chapter 14), antiemetics (Chapter 54), sedatives (Chapter 13), and the serotonergic drug cyproheptadine (Chapter 36). The newer serotonin-selective reuptake inhibitor (SSRI) antidepressants (Chapter 16) have not proved effective; in fact, headache is a common adverse effect of this drug class. Among the most commonly used products is a tablet or capsule containing fixed combinations of either acetaminophen or aspirin plus the barbiturate butalbital plus the analeptic caffeine. In addition to potentiating the effects of the analgesics, caffeine can also enhance intestinal absorption of the ergot alkaloids (Chapter 19) and has a vasoconstricting effect, which can reduce cerebral blood flow to ease headache pain. Caffeine also has a diuretic effect, which may ultimately reduce cerebral blood flow through reduced vascular volume secondary to enhanced urinary output. In many cases, preventive drug therapy is sufficient for abortive therapy. When it is not, triptans are now the most commonly prescribed drug class, followed by the ergot alkaloids.

Contraindications

Contraindications to triptans include drug allergy and the presence of serious cardiovascular disease because of the vasoconstrictive potential of these medications.

Adverse Effects

As noted earlier, triptans have potential vasoconstrictor effects, including effects on the coronary circulation. Injectable dosage forms may cause local irritation at the site of injection. Other adverse effects include feelings of tingling, flushing (skin warmth and redness), and a congested feeling in the head or chest.

Interactions

Drug interactions for antimigraine drugs are presented in Table 17-4.

 DRUG PROFILES

SEROTONIN AGONISTS

The serotonin agonists are a new class of CNS stimulants used to treat migraine headache. They can produce relief from moderate to severe migraines within 2 hours in 70% to 80% of patients. They work by stimulating 5-HT$_1$ receptors in the brain and are sometimes referred to as SSRAs or triptans. They are available in a variety of formulations, including oral tablets, sublingual tablets, subcutaneous self-injections, and nasal sprays. A common effect of migraines is nausea and vomiting. Orally administered medications are therefore not tolerated by some patients. For this reason, nonoral (including sublingual) forms are advantageous. They also often have a more rapid onset of

action, producing relief in some patients in 10 to 15 minutes, compared with 1 to 2 hours for tablets. Dosage and other information appears in the Dosages table on p. 331.

▶▶ sumatriptan

Sumatriptan (Imitrex) was the original prototype drug for this class. As noted earlier, there are now seven triptans. Slight pharmacokinetic differences exist between some of these products, but their effects are comparable overall.

PHARMACOKINETICS

Half-Life	Onset	Peak	Duration
PO: 2.5 hr	PO: 0.5–1 hr	PO: 2.5 hr	PO: 4 hr

ANALEPTIC-RESPONSIVE RESPIRATORY DEPRESSION SYNDROMES

Postanaesthetic respiratory depression occurs when a patient's spontaneous respiratory drive does not resume adequately and in a timely manner after general anaesthesia. Analeptic drugs are CNS stimulants used to treat such respiratory depression syndromes. The effects of analeptic drugs are to produce increased response of the brainstem and spinal chord to external stimuli and to stimulate respiration. However, analeptic drugs are now generally used less frequently than in the earlier days of general anaesthesia because of advances in intensive respiratory care, including mechanical ventilation and improved anaesthetic techniques, as well as the availability of newer medications with less toxicity.

Nonetheless, there are several respiratory syndromes for which these medications are sometimes still used. Although these indications are not approved by Health Canada, they are substantiated in the literature. Neonatal apnea, or periodic cessation of breathing in newborn babies, is a common condition seen in neonatal intensive care units. It is especially frequent among premature infants, whose pulmonary structures have not completed their gestational development due to preterm birth. Infants undergoing prolonged mechanical ventilation, especially at high pressures, often develop a chronic lung disease known as bronchopulmonary dysplasia. Respiratory depression may also be secondary to misuse of some drugs. Hypercapnia, or elevated blood levels of carbon dioxide, is often associated with later stages of chronic obstructive pulmonary disease (COPD). Analeptic drugs such as theophylline and aminophylline may be used to treat one or more of these conditions.

ANALEPTICS

Analeptics include the methylxanthines aminophylline, theophylline, and caffeine.

Mechanism of Action and Drug Effects

Analeptics work by stimulating areas of the CNS that control respiration, mainly the medulla and spinal cord. Methylxanthine analeptics (caffeine, aminophylline, and theophylline) also inhibit the enzyme phosphodiesterase. This enzyme breaks down a substance called cyclic adenosine monophosphate (cAMP). When these drugs block this enzyme, cAMP accumulates, resulting in relaxation of smooth muscle in the respiratory tract, dilation of pulmonary arterioles, and stimulation of the CNS in general. Aminophylline is a prodrug (a drug formulated for greater solubility to facilitate administration) that is hydrolyzed (reacts with water molecules) to theophylline in the body; theophylline is metabolized to caffeine. Caffeine has an inherently stronger affinity for CNS stimulation, hence its popularity in coffee, tea, and soft drinks (Table 17-5). As noted previously, it also helps

to potentiate the effects of analgesics used for migraine and has a diuretic effect. The stimulant effects of caffeine are attributed to its antagonism (blocking) of adenosine receptors in the brain. Adenosine is associated with sleep promotion.

Indications

Currently listed indications for analeptics include neonatal apnea, bronchopulmonary dysplasia, hypercapnia associated with COPD, postanaesthetic respiratory depression, and respiratory depression secondary to drugs of misuse (e.g., opioids, alcohol, or barbiturates). However, these latter two conditions are now commonly treated with specific reversal antidote drugs and mechanical ventilation until the overdosed drug wears off. Theophylline and aminophylline are also used for neonatal bradycardia as well as for asthma in older children and adults. Aminophylline is sometimes given intravenously to treat anaphylaxis (Chapter 37).

Contraindications

Contraindications to the use of analeptics include drug allergy, peptic ulcer disease (especially for caffeine), and serious cardiovascular conditions. Concurrent use of other phosphodiesterase-inhibiting drugs such as sildenafil and similar drugs is also not recommended.

Adverse Effects

At higher dosages, analeptics stimulate the vagal, vasomotor, and respiratory centres of the medulla in the

TABLE	17-5

Caffeine-Containing Foods and Drugs

Medications	Amount of Caffeine
NONPRESCRIPTION MEDICATIONS	
Analgesics	
acetaminophen compound caplets/tablets with 8 mg codeine	15–30 mg/caplet/tab
Anacin; Anacin Extra-Strength	32 mg/tab
Atasol, acetylsalicyclic acid compound tablets with 8 mg codeine	15–30 mg/tab
Excedrin Extra-Strength	65 mg/tab
Stimulants	
Alert Aid Caffeine Tablets	200 mg/tab
PRESCRIPTION MEDICATIONS (FOR MIGRAINE)	
Cafergot	100 mg/tab
Fiorinal	40 mg/tab

Beverages	Amount of Caffeine
Cocoa	5–8 mg/237 mL (1 cup)
Coffee (brewed)	3–135 mg/237 mL (1 cup)
Coffee (decaffeinated)	3–5 mg/237 mL (1 cup)
Coffee (instant)	76–106 mg/237 mL (1 cup)
Soft drinks	36–50 mg/355 mL (1 can)
Tea (brewed)	15–50 mg/237 mL

DRUG PROFILES

Analeptic drugs include the methylxanthines aminophylline, theophylline, and caffeine. The profiles for aminophylline and theophylline can be found in Part Six of this book on respiratory system drugs. The antinarcoleptic drug modafinil was discussed in the Narcolepsy section of this chapter. Dosage and other information appears in the Dosages table on p. 331.

▶▶ *caffeine*

Caffeine (Caffeine Lite, Caffeinum, Pep-back, Water Joe) is a CNS stimulant that can be found in over-the-counter (OTC) drugs and combination prescription drugs. It is also contained in many beverages and foods. See Table 17-5 for a few of the many foods and drugs that contain caffeine. Caffeine use is contraindicated in patients with a known hypersensitivity to it and should be used with caution in patients who have a history of peptic ulcers or cardiac dysrhythmias or who have recently suffered a myocardial infarction. In Canada, pure caffeine is only available added to cola-type beverages, and it must be declared in the ingredients list on the product label. Caffeine may not be added to any other food. It is available in oral forms.

PHARMACOKINETICS

Half-Life	Onset	Peak	Duration
PO: 3–4 hr	PO: 15–45 min	PO: 50–75 min	PO: < 6 hr

brainstem, as well as skeletal muscles. Vagal effects include stimulation of gastric secretions, diarrhea, and reflex tachycardia. Vasomotor effects are flushing (warmth, redness) and sweating of the skin. Respiratory effects include elevated respiratory rate (which is normally desired). Skeletal muscle effects are muscular tension and tremors. Neurological effects include reduced deep-tendon reflexes.

Interactions

Drug interactions for the analeptics are presented in Table 17-4.

NURSING PROCESS

Assessment

CNS stimulants are used for a variety of conditions and disorders. They have addictive potential, thus a thorough medical history, physical assessment, and medication history must be obtained before their use. The CNS stimulants used for their anorexiant effect (see discussion in pharmacology section) include drugs that stimulate the release of catecholamines; at higher dosages they suppress appetite, stimulate the respiratory centre, and decrease drug-induced CNS depression (however, seizures may be a consequence of CNS stimulation). Other uses include an improvement in attentiveness and wakefulness. When the patient is about to receive these medications for weight loss, baseline weight and height measurements are needed, as is documentation of vital signs with specific attention to pulse rate and blood pressure. The vital parameters of pulse rate and blood pressure are critical because of the adverse effects associated with these drugs. A nursing history should include questions about lifestyle; exercise; nutritional habits, patterns, and knowledge; family history; self-esteem; stress levels; and mental status, as well as information related to contraindications, cautions, and drug interactions (see Table 17-4). Cardiovascular and cerebrovascular diseases may be exacerbated to life-threatening levels with these drugs. In addition, psychoses may worsen, drug dependence may be exacerbated, and diabetics may need tighter insulin control or a decrease in insulin dosage (mainly because of concurrent dietary changes). Nutritional assessments should be documented and attention given to the levels of fat-soluble vitamins because of their reduction by the medication. The nurse should assess for and document underlying addictive behaviours, hypertension, and other disease states because of the higher risk of exacerbation with these drugs. By contrast, orlistat, the nonstimulant anorexiant, is associated with a lower incidence of systemic adverse effects.

With drugs used for the management of ADHD, cautious and continuous assessment is required. This should include measurement of vital signs and baseline weight and height as well as evaluation of the child's baseline growth and development and complete blood counts as needed. Usual sleep habits and patterns should be noted so that efforts can be made to prevent any sleep disturbances that may occur with these drugs. In addition, it is important to have baseline documentation of difficulties with cognition, attention, and mood so that successful treatment or need for change in therapy is identifiable. Typical behaviour and attention span and history of social problems or problems in school are also important to assess and document before and during therapy. Parental support is important to the success of treatment, so a home assessment is usually performed by staff from supporting organizations such as a public or private school or social services agency. Attention to daily dietary intake before drug therapy is initiated is important because of drug-related weight loss. It is crucial that children not experience too rapid or too much weight loss. Important to the use of these drugs (as with all CNS stimulants) is a thorough heart assessment with attention to heart sounds, any history of chest pain or palpitations, and baseline pulse rate and rhythm and blood pressure. Before administering CNS stimulants, the nurse must carefully gather data from the patient's history that may raise concerns regarding potential contraindications, cautions, and drug interactions (see previous discussion). The nurse should also assess for the use of any natural health products, over-the-counter products, and beverages that may contain ginseng or caffeine (see Natural Health Products: Selected Herbal Compounds Used for Nervous System Stimulation).

The serotonin agonists, commonly used in the treatment of migraines, are not without adverse reactions, contraindications, cautions, and drug interactions. Assessment should include measuring blood pressure, pulse rate and rhythm, and heart sounds, and taking a thorough cardiac history. Because an elevation in blood pressure may occur, even though it is usually only a slight elevation, these drugs should not be used in patients with uncontrolled hypertension. These drugs are not usually prescribed for patients with coronary artery disease unless a thorough heart evaluation has been performed and their use is approved. It is important to reemphasize the significant drug interactions with MAOIs (serotonin agonists should not be administered within 2 weeks of MAOI use). In addition, serotonin agonists should not be taken within 24 hours of use of ergotamine-containing products or even dihydroergotamine or methysergide. Other triptans should not be taken within 24 hours of taking sumatriptan. Because the patient may also take over-the-counter or other prescribed analgesics that contain caffeine, aspirin, or other nonsteroidal anti-inflammatory drugs, allergy to the components should be assessed and any problems with bleeding, gastrointestinal upset, or ulcers should be documented prior to use of these adjunctive therapies.

Nursing Diagnoses

- Anxiety related to the drug's adverse effect of CNS stimulation
- Decreased cardiac output related to the adverse effects of palpitations and tachycardia
- Deficient knowledge related to lack of information about the specific drug regimen
- Disturbed thought processes related to the CNS effects of the drug
- Disturbed sleep pattern (decreased sleep) related to drug effects
- Imbalanced nutrition, more than body requirements, due to presence of obesity
- Imbalanced nutrition, less than body requirements, related to adverse effects of the medication
- Pain related to migraine headaches
- Pain related to adverse effects of the drug such as headache and dry mouth
- Situational low self-esteem related to the impact of obesity, decreased sexual performance, and other adverse effects of the CNS stimulation

Planning

Goals

- Patient will appear less anxious or experiences no anxiety from the medication.
- Patient will be free of heart symptoms and associated complications of drug therapy.
- Patient will remain open to education about related drug and nondrug therapeutic regimens.
- Patient will regain or maintain near-normal body weight and BMI during therapy.

 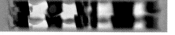 NATURAL HEALTH PRODUCTS

SELECTED HERBAL COMPOUNDS USED FOR NERVOUS SYSTEM STIMULATION*

Common Name(s)	Uses	Possible Drug Interactions (Avoid Concurrent Use)
Ginkgo biloba, ginkgo	To enhance mental alertness; to improve memory or reduce dementia	Warfarin, aspirin
Ginseng	To enhance mental function and concentration	Drugs for diabetes that lower blood sugar (e.g., insulin, oral hypoglycemic drugs), monoamine oxidase inhibitors
Guarana	Nervous system stimulation, appetite suppression	Adenosine, disulfiram, quinolones, oral contraceptives, β-blockers, iron, lithium, phenylephrine (e.g., nasal spray), cimetidine, theophylline, tobacco

Data from Fetrow, C. W., & Avila, J. R. (2000). *The complete guide to herbal remedies*. Springhouse, PA: Springhouse.

*The information in this box does not imply author or publisher endorsement of these products. Though individual consumers often experience satisfying results with natural health products, there is often little, if any, rigorously controlled research to demonstrate their efficacy at treating particular condition(s). Patients should always be advised to communicate regularly with their health care provider(s) about all medications used, including natural health products, to decrease the likelihood of possibly hazardous drug interactions.

- Patient (if a child) will continue to undergo close to normal growth and development while taking medications.
- Patient will experience minimal sleep deprivation.
- Patient will maintain positive self-esteem.
- Patient will appear less anxious.
- Patient will remain adherent to drug therapy and free from complications of treatment.

■ Outcome Criteria

- Patient communicates anxiety, anger, and feelings regarding self-image and self-esteem openly and as needed.
- Patient maintains appropriate weight loss without too rapid losses or gains throughout treatment (if the patient is a child, normal growth and development patterns are continued, with weight and height falling within normal limits on growth chart) while taking CNS stimulants.
- Patient shows improved sensorium and level of consciousness with increased attention span and cognition.
- Patient experiences more restful sleep using non-pharmacological measures.
- Patient's vital signs, especially blood pressure and pulse, remain within normal limits.
- Patient states symptoms (e.g., palpitations, chest pain) to report to the physician immediately.
- Patient reports a decrease in headaches.
- Patient reports that medication is taken as ordered and consistently over the time of the therapeutic protocol.

✎ Implementation

Because anorexiants are generally used for a short period, it is important to emphasize to the patient and all members of the patient's support system that a suitable diet, appropriate independent or supervised exercise program, and behavioural modifications are necessary to support a favourable result and to help the patient cease overeating and experience healthy weight loss. Medications are usually taken first thing in the morning, as ordered, to minimize interference with sleep, and they should not be taken within 4 to 6 hours of sleep. If the patient has been taking these drugs for a prolonged period, there should be a period of weaning upon discontinuation to avoid withdrawal symptoms and any chance of a rebound increase in appetite. Weight should be assessed weekly or as ordered, and often keeping a food diary helps with 24-hour recall of all intake. Caffeine should be avoided, including all caffeine-containing beverages and foods such as coffee, tea, sodas, and chocolate. Other products that contain caffeine include over-the-counter analgesics such as Excedrin, over-the-counter menstrual symptom–related compounds such as Midol, prescription analgesics such as ergotamine with caffeine, butalbital with aspirin and caffeine, and

prescription drugs with an opioid such as butalbital with aspirin, caffeine, and codeine. Dry mouth may be managed with frequent mouth care and the use of sugar-free gum or hard candy. Ice chips may help as well.

Other nursing considerations include emphasis on a holistic approach to treatment of obesity, such as the possible use of hypnosis, biofeedback, and guided imagery as ordered. Keeping a journal to record responses to the drug therapy at home, play, and school is important for charting the effectiveness of the drug for any patient. Counselling is generally a part of the treatment, with the family involved in goal setting for the treatment regimen. The patient should be encouraged to keep follow-up visits with his or her physician. Supplementation with fat-soluble vitamins may be indicated. It is important also to watch for "tolerance" to the anorexiant.

With drugs used for *ADHD*, some children may respond better to certain dosage forms such as immediate release, and dosing should be individualized and based on the patient's needs at different times during their school day (e.g., a noon dose for music lessons later in the afternoon). Scheduling of these medications and close communication with the family and patient are important to successful treatment. It is also important to time medications, as ordered, for periods when symptom control is most needed and sleep not altered. Generally speaking, once-a-day dosing is used with extended-release or long-acting preparations. Adequate and proper dosing will be manifested by good control in behaviour and improvement during school time, and, if extended-release dosage forms work well, the child will not have to take the medication at school. Often a stigma is associated with taking medications at school, thus long-acting preparations or other scheduling may be used to avoid this situation. To help decrease the occurrence of insomnia, the last daily dose should be taken 4 to 6 hours before bedtime. During therapy, the patient should also be monitored for continued physical growth with specific attention to weight. The physician may order times for "medication-free" weekends, holidays, or vacations and the drug may also be discontinued periodically so that the need for the medication can be reassessed.

SSRAs come in a variety of dosage forms. Rizatriptan comes in a disintegrating tablet or wafer that dissolves on the tongue, which leads to rapid absorption even if the patient is experiencing nausea and vomiting; it also comes in oral tablets. Use of the nasal spray or self-injectable forms of the serotonin agonists is desirable, especially in patients experiencing the nausea and vomiting that may occur with migraine headaches. Patient instructions about administration technique are important. Self-injectable forms and nasal sprays also have the benefit of an onset of action of 10 to 15 minutes compared with 1 to 2 hours with tablet forms. Administration of a test dose for all dosage forms is usually recommended. See Patient Education for more information.

Evaluation

Therapeutic responses to drugs used in the management of hyperkinesia include decreased hyperactivity, increased attention span and concentration, and improved behaviour. The therapeutic response to drugs used for the management of narcolepsy is the ability to remain awake. Anorexiants should result in a decrease in the patient's appetite and, therefore, in weight loss. The nurse needs to monitor the patient for the development of adverse effects to these medications; these include changes in mental status, sensorium, mood, affect, and sleep patterns; physical dependency; irritability; and withdrawal symptoms such as headache, nausea, and vomiting.

Therapeutic effects of anorexiants include appetite control and weight loss for the treatment of obesity. Adverse effects of sibutramine include dry mouth, headache, insomnia, and constipation. It is important to monitor for adverse effects of these drugs, including worsening of headache, dry mouth, insomnia, tachycardia, heart irregularities, hypertension, and possible seizures due to excessive CNS stimulation. Therapeutic effects of the anorexiant orlistat include appetite control in obesity. Adverse effects caused mainly by the drug's action of inhibiting lipase include flatulence with an oily discharge, spotting, and fecal urgency. The patient also needs to be closely evaluated for decreases in levels of fat-soluble vitamins (A, D, E, and K) because levels of these vitamins are affected by the decrease in absorption of fats. Therapeutic responses to modafinil include a decrease in sleepiness associated with narcolepsy. Adverse effects for which to monitor with modafinil include headache, nausea, nervousness, and anxiety.

Therapeutic responses to the serotonin agonists include an improvement in the frequency, duration, and severity of migraine headaches with improved daily functioning and performance because of the decrease in headaches. Adverse effects for which to monitor include pain at the injection site (temporary), flushing, chest tightness or pressure, weakness, sedation, dizziness, sweating, increase in blood pressure and pulse rate, and bad taste with the nasal spray formulation, which may precipitate nausea.

PATIENT EDUCATION

CNS Stimulants in General

❖ Patients should be advised to take serotonin agonists at the exact time and frequency as ordered. Generally, medications should be taken exactly as prescribed without skipping, omitting, or adding doses. Sudden withdrawal of medications should be avoided.

❖ Patients should be encouraged to avoid alcohol, over-the-counter cold products, and cough syrups that may contain alcohol, nicotine, and caffeine.

❖ Patients should be encouraged to keep a log of daily activities and record how the drug is working and any adverse effects.

Anorexiants

❖ Patients should be sure to follow all physician instructions regarding medications, diet, and exercise.

❖ Patients should be warned that some of the medications may impair alertness and ability to think. The patient should be cautious in engaging in such activities until these impairments are gone.

❖ Patients should be advised that the unpleasant taste of the drug and dry mouth may be minimized by use of mouth rinses, ice chips, sugarless chewing gum, and hard candies.

Drugs Used to Treat ADHD

❖ Patients should be instructed to take the medication on an empty stomach 30 to 45 minutes before eating, for maximal effects.

❖ Patients should be encouraged to keep scheduled appointments so that the physician can document progress.

❖ Patients should be informed that if the physician thinks use of the medication should be discontinued, a weaning process with careful supervision is usually required.

❖ Patients should be instructed not to crush, chew, or break extended-release or long-acting preparations, and to take these as directed.

❖ Patients should be warned not to increase or decrease dosages because this may lead to complications. If the patient has any questions or concerns, the parents, caregiver, or physician should be contacted.

Antimigraine Drugs

❖ Patients should be instructed to avoid foods containing tyramine, because tyramine is known to precipitate severe headaches. Tyramine-containing foods include beer, wine, aged cheese, food additives, preservatives, artificial sweeteners, chocolate, and caffeine.

❖ Patients should be instructed to gently blow their nose to clear the nasal passages before using a nasal-spray form of an antimigraine drug. With head upright, the patient should close one nostril and insert the nozzle into the open nostril. While a breath is taken through the nose, the spray should be released. The nozzle should be removed, and the

Continued

patient should gently breathe in through the nose and out through the mouth for 10 to 20 seconds. Some distaste may be experienced.

❖ Patients should be warned to avoid doing things that require alertness and rapid, skilled movements while experiencing migraines or taking medications until the patient is feeling normal again.

❖ Patients should be encouraged to keep a journal of all headaches, precipitators, and relievers, and should rate each headache on a scale of 0 to 10, with 0 being no pain and 10 being the worst pain ever. The patient should be sure to record other symptoms such as photophobia, nausea, and vomiting as well as their frequency and duration.

❖ When taking SSRAs, patients should contact the physician immediately if any palpitations, chest pain, or pain or weakness in the extremities occur.

❖ Patients should be informed that injectable forms of sumatriptan should be administered subcutaneously and as ordered. The patient should practise

administering injections (without the medication) with the nurse at the physician's office so that proper technique is used and comfort level achieved.

❖ Patients should be informed that autoinjectors with prefilled syringes may be used. The syringe should be discarded after use.

❖ Patients should be instructed to administer no more than two injections of sumatriptan during a 24-hour period and at least 1 hour should be allowed between injections.

❖ With injections of sumatriptan, patients should be instructed to contact a physician or emergency services immediately if any swelling around the eyes, pain or tightness in the chest or throat, wheezing, or heart throbbing develops.

❖ Patients should be informed of helpful online resources, including http://www.migrainecanada.com, http://www.stresscanada.org, http://www.mindbodycan.com, http://www.aan.com, and http://www.headachenetwork.ca.

POINTS TO REMEMBER

❖ CNS stimulants are drugs that stimulate the brain or spinal cord (e.g., cocaine and caffeine).

❖ Actions of these stimulants mimic those of the SNS neurotransmitters norepinephrine, dopamine, and serotonin.

❖ Sympathomimetic drugs mimic the sympathetic division of the autonomic nervous system.

❖ Included in the family of CNS stimulants are the amphetamines, analeptics, and anorexiants, with therapeutic uses for ADHD, narcolepsy, and appetite control.

❖ Because the analeptics stimulate respiration, they may be used to treat respiratory paralysis caused by overdose of opioids, alcohol, barbiturates, and general anaesthetic drugs.

❖ Anorexiants control or suppress appetite. They may also be used to stimulate the CNS and work by suppressing appetite control centres in the brain.

❖ Contraindications to the use of anorexiants, as well as any CNS stimulant, include hypersensitivity, seizure activity, convulsive disorders, and liver dysfunction.

❖ The serotonin agonists are a newer class of CNS stimulants generally used to treat migraine headaches. Their use should be avoided in patients who have coronary disease.

❖ Amphetamines elevate mood or produce euphoria, increase mental alertness and capacity for work,

decrease fatigue and drowsiness, and prolong wakefulness.

❖ The analeptics have generalized effects on the brainstem and spinal cord, increasing responsiveness to external stimuli and stimulating respiration. Nursing considerations for children who take methylphenidate and other related drugs include recording baseline height and weight before initiating drug therapy and continuing to plot height and weight in a journal during therapy.

❖ Journalling is helpful in evaluating the effects of all drugs used to treat ADHD or migraines as well as in obesity treatment.

❖ Therapeutic responses to drugs used in the treatment of hyperkinesia include decreased hyperactivity, increased attention span and concentration, and improved behaviour patterns.

❖ Adverse effects for which to monitor in individuals taking CNS stimulants include changes in mental status or sensorium, mood, affect, and sleep patterns; physical dependency; and irritability.

❖ Serotonin agonists may be administered subcutaneously, as a nasal spray, or as oral tablets. Any chest pain or tightness, tremors, vomiting, or worsening symptoms should be reported to the physician immediately.

EXAMINATION REVIEW QUESTIONS

1 A patient with narcolepsy will begin treatment with a CNS stimulant. Which of the following adverse effects is this patient likely to encounter?
   a. Bradycardia
   b. Nervousness
   c. Mental clouding
   d. Drowsiness at night

2 At a weight management clinic, a patient who was given a prescription for orlistat (Xenical) calls the clinic hotline because of a "terrible adverse effect." Which of the following adverse affect does the nurse suspect the patient is referring to?
   a. Nausea
   b. Sexual dysfunction
   c. Fecal incontinence
   d. Urinary incontinence

3 If a patient is receiving anorexiants, which of the following nursing diagnoses is the most likely condition being treated for with this drug?
   a. Impaired memory
   b. Deficient fluid volume
   c. Disturbed sleep pattern
   d. Imbalanced nutrition, more than body requirements

4 For a patient with a new prescription for sumatriptan (Imitrex), what teaching topic should he receive before he self-administers this drug?
   a. Proper placement of the transdermal patch
   b. Correct technique for intramuscular injections
   c. Correct technique for subcutaneous injections
   d. The need to dissolve tablets under the tongue completely

5 Which statement is correct to make when reviewing atomoxetine (Strattera) therapy with the parents of an adolescent with ADHD?
   a. "This medication is used only when symptoms of ADHD are severe."
   b. "If adverse effects become severe, stop the medication for 3 to 4 days."
   c. "Be sure to have your child blow his nose before administering the nasal spray."
   d. "Be sure to contact the physician right away if your child expresses of suicidal thoughts."

For answers see http://evolve.elsevier.com/Canada/Lilley/pharmacology/.

CRITICAL THINKING ACTIVITIES

1 The parents of a 10-year-old boy are concerned about the adverse effects of the medication their son is taking for ADHD. What will they need to monitor while he is taking medication for this condition?

2 A patient calls the headache clinic because she is unhappy about her medication. She says, "I've been taking zolmitriptan (Zomig) to prevent headaches, but I am still having them." What does she need to know about the proper use of this drug?

3 Why would you, a nurse practitioner, recommend or not recommend appetite suppressants for an adult who is obese?

For answers see http://evolve.elsevier.com/Canada/Lilley/pharmacology/.

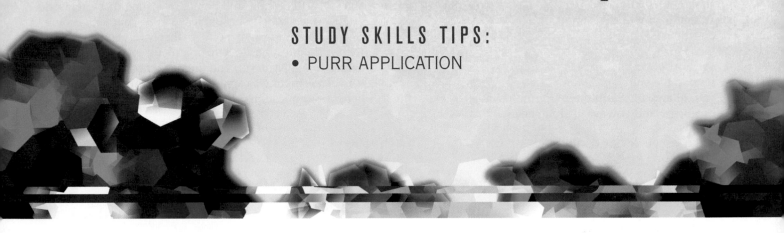

PART THREE
Drugs Affecting the Autonomic Nervous System

STUDY SKILLS TIPS:
- PURR APPLICATION

PURR APPLICATION

Planning for the Part

The PURR model in the Study Skills Tips shows how the process works for individual chapters, but another useful way to use PURR is to take a broader view of the assignment. Chapters have been grouped together into multiple chapter blocks called *parts*, which are meant to put content together in a logical and meaningful way.

Part Title

Begin by looking at the Part Three title, "Drugs Affecting the Autonomic Nervous System." Then look at the part structure. Part Three contains four chapters. All these chapters are concerned with the autonomic nervous system. Before you have done any reading, begin to look for the links that will establish relationships among ideas in individual chapters. You should also look for the broader link that connects the four chapters with each other and with the ideas that have come in earlier parts and will follow in later parts.

Look back at Part Two, "Drugs Affecting the Central Nervous System." Clearly, that part deals with some aspect of the nervous system, as does this part. One learning objective you should establish for yourself is to grasp the relationship between these two parts. You must be able to define and explain *central nervous system* and *autonomic nervous system*. Ask yourself additional questions that will help you establish a connection between these parts: What is the difference in the functions of the central and the autonomic nervous systems? Are there pharmacological drugs that have application in both the central and autonomic nervous systems? Most students focus on the individual chapters, but to fully understand the subject it is essential to grasp the broader scope of chapter and part.

Part Chapters

The next step in applying the Plan step of PURR is to spend a few minutes studying the chapter titles and looking for the relationships that must exist. Part Three has four chapters, and there is a clear pattern in these chapters. Chapters 18 and 19 both contain the term *adrenergic*, so the two chapters are dealing with the same broad topic. However, Chapter 18 covers adrenergic drugs and Chapter 19 covers adrenergic-blocking drugs. Apply questioning strategies at this point: What does "adrenergic" mean? What is an adrenergic drug? These two questions are essential in mastering the content of Chapter 18, and you should ask them almost without thinking. The next step, while easily overlooked, can greatly enhance your understanding when you start to read the material. Note that Chapter 18 deals with drugs and Chapter 19 deals with blocking drugs. There must be a difference between a drug and a blocking drug. Focus now with a few questions that will keep you aware that the content in Chapter 18 has a direct relationship to the content in Chapter 19: What is the difference between a drug and a blocking drug? When is the pharmacological application of a drug appropriate? Under what conditions should a blocking drug be chosen? Then ask a question to help maintain the focus on the concept of the entire part: What aspects of the autonomic nervous system are related to the adrenergic drugs and blocking drugs?

Chapters 20 and 21

Once you begin to focus on the relationship of chapters within a part, certain things will begin to become apparent. Chapters 20 and 21, too, cover drugs and blocking drugs. These two chapters develop the concept as related to cholinergics, rather than adrenergics. But the same questions you used as a focus for Chapters 18 and 19 can be recycled in setting up the study of Chapters 20 and 21. Simply replace the term *adrenergic* with *cholinergic* and you are ready to begin.

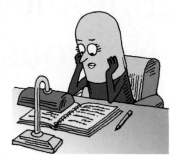

Active Questioning

This is the key concept to master. We have given you a number of sample questions (see Part Title and Part Chapters above) to help you begin the process. These are not the only questions you should ask, but rather samples to help you develop a questioning process.

Some of the questions will prove to be useful when reading the chapters, whereas others will not be applicable. Questions can (and sometimes should) be revised or discarded when the details of the chapter become clearer. The important point is that you begin the part with some questions to help you focus your own reading and learning. Also, you will find that the more you apply active questioning as a part of your learning strategy, the better your questions will become.

CHAPTER 18

Adrenergic Drugs

Learning Objectives

After reading this chapter, the successful student will be able to do the following:

1 Briefly discuss the sympathetic nervous system in relation to drug therapy—specifically, the effects of adrenergic stimulation or sympathomimetic effects.

2 List the drugs classified as adrenergic agonists.

3 Discuss the mechanisms of action, therapeutic effects, indications, adverse and toxic effects, cautions, contraindications, interactions, and available antidotes to overdosage of the adrenergic agonists.

4 Discuss the nursing process as it relates to the administration of adrenergic drugs, including development of a collaborative plan of care for patients and caregivers.

e-Learning Activities

Web site
(http://evolve.elsevier.com/Canada/Lilley/pharmacology/)

- Animations
- Answers to chapter questions, activities, and case studies
- Calculators and Category Catchers
- Glossary with audio pronunciations
- IV Therapy and Medication Error Checklists
- Multiple-Choice Review Question quizzes
- Nursing Care Plans
- Online Appendices and Supplements
- WebLinks

Drug Profiles

▸▸ **dobutamine (dobutamine hydrochloride)***, p. 353
▸▸ **dopamine (dopamine hydrochloride)***, p. 353
▸▸ **epinephrine**, pp. 352, 354
    midodrine, p. 354
▸▸ **norepinephrine (norepinephrine bitartrate)***, p. 354
▸▸ **pseudoephedrine (pseudoephedrine hydrochloride)***, p. 353
▸▸ **salmeterol (salmeterol xinafoate)***, p. 352
▸▸ **salbutamol (salbutamol sulfate)***, p. 352
    tetrahydrozoline, p. 353

▸▸ Key drug.

*Full generic name is given in parentheses. For the purposes of this text, the more common shortened name is used.

Glossary

Adrenergic receptors Receptor sites for the sympathetic neurotransmitters norepinephrine and epinephrine. (p. 346)

α-adrenergic receptors A class of adrenergic receptors that is further subdivided into α_1- and α_2-adrenergic receptors; α_1 and α_2 receptors exist postsynaptically, whereas α_2 receptors also exist presynaptically. Both types are differentiated by their anatomical location in the tissues, muscles, and organs regulated by specific autonomic nerve fibres. (p. 346)

Adrenergics Drugs that stimulate the sympathetic nervous system; also referred to as *adrenergic agonists* or *sympathomimetics* because they mimic the effects of the sympathetic neurotransmitters norepinephrine and epinephrine, and dopamine. (p. 346)

Autonomic functions Bodily functions that are involuntary and result from the physiological activity of the autonomic nervous system. (p. 346)

Autonomic nervous system (ANS) A branch of the peripheral nervous system consisting of the sympathetic nervous system and the parasympathetic nervous system that controls autonomic bodily functions. (p. 346)

β-adrenergic receptors Receptors located on postsynaptic effector cells of cells' tissues, muscles, and organs that are stimulated by specific autonomic nerve fibres; this class of receptors is further subdivided into β_1- and β_2-adrenergic receptors. (p. 346)

Catecholamines Substances that can produce a sympathomimetic response. They are either endogenous catecholamines (such as epinephrine, norepinephrine, and dopamine) or synthetic catecholamines (such as dobutamine). (p. 347)

Dopaminergic receptor A third type of adrenergic receptor located in various tissues and organs and activated by the binding of the neurotransmitter dopamine, which occurs in both endogenous and synthetic (drug) forms. (p. 347)

Mydriasis Pupillary dilation, whether natural (physiological) or drug induced. (p. 350)

Ophthalmics Topically applied eye medications. (p. 350)

Positive chronotropic effect An increase in heart rate. (p. 349)

Positive dromotropic effect An increase in the conduction of cardiac electrical impulses through the atrioventricular node, which results in the transfer of nerve action potentials from the atria to the ventricles, ultimately leading to a systolic heartbeat (ventricular contractions). (p. 349)

Positive inotropic effect An increased force of contraction of the heart muscle (myocardium). (p. 349)

Synaptic cleft The space between either two adjacent nerve cell membranes or the nerve cell membrane and an effector organ cell membrane. (p. 347)

OVERVIEW

Adrenergics are a large group of both exogenous (synthetic) and endogenous (naturally occurring) substances that have a wide variety of therapeutic uses depending on their site of action and their effect on receptors. Adrenergics stimulate the sympathetic nervous system (SNS) and are also called *adrenergic agonists*. They are also known as *sympathomimetics* because they mimic the effects of the SNS neurotransmitters norepinephrine and epinephrine, and dopamine; all three of these are chemically classified as catecholamines. In considering the adrenergic class of medications, it is helpful to understand how the SNS operates in relation to the rest of the nervous system.

SYMPATHETIC NERVOUS SYSTEM

Figure 18-1 depicts the divisions of the nervous system, showing the relationship of the SNS to the entire nervous system. The SNS is the counterpart to the parasympathetic nervous system (PSNS); together they make up the **autonomic nervous system (ANS).** They provide a checks-and-balances system for maintaining the normal homeostasis of the autonomic functions of the human body. **Autonomic functions** are bodily functions that are involuntary and result from physiological activity of the autonomic nervous system. The functions often occur in pairs of opposing actions between the sympathetic and parasympathetic divisions of this nervous system.

Throughout the body there are specific target receptor sites for the catecholamines norepinephrine and epinephrine. These are referred to as **adrenergic receptors,** and it is these sites where adrenergic drugs bind and produce their effects. Adrenergic receptors are located at many anatomic sites. There are two main groups of adrenergic receptors, α-**adrenergic** and β-**adrenergic receptors.**

When these sites are stimulated or blocked, the result is a physiological response. For example, epinephrine reacts with both α- and β-adrenergic receptors, resulting in vasoconstriction and vasodilation, respectively. Both groups of adrenergic receptors have subtypes, designated 1 and 2, providing a further means of checks and balances that control stimulation and blockade, constriction and dilation, and the increased and decreased production of a substance.

The α_1- and α_2-adrenergic receptors are differentiated by their location relative to nerves. The α_1-adrenergic

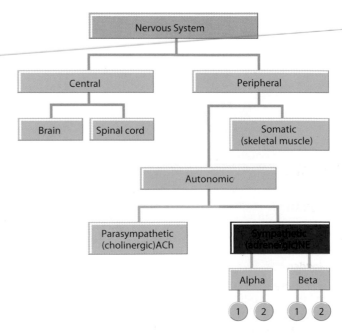

FIG. 18-1 The sympathetic nervous system in relation to the entire nervous system. *ACh*, acetylcholine; *NE*, norepinephrine.

receptors are located on postsynaptic effector cells (the tissue, muscle, or organ that the nerve stimulates). The α_2-adrenergic receptors are located on the presynaptic nerve terminals. They control the release of neurotransmitters. The predominant α-adrenergic agonist response is vasoconstriction and central nervous system (CNS) stimulation.

The β-adrenergic receptors are all located on postsynaptic effector cells. The β_1-adrenergic receptors are located primarily in the heart (Remember: β_1, you have 1 heart); the β_2-adrenergic receptors are located primarily in the smooth muscle of the bronchioles (Remember: β_2, you have 2 lungs), arterioles, and visceral organs. A β-adrenergic agonist response results in bronchial, gastrointestinal (GI), and uterine smooth muscle relaxation; glycogenolysis; and heart stimulation. Table 18-1 contains a more detailed listing of the adrenergic receptors and the responses elicited when they are stimulated by a neurotransmitter or a drug that acts like a neurotransmitter (see also Figure 18-2).

Another type of adrenergic receptor is the **dopaminergic receptor**. When stimulated by dopamine, these receptors cause the vessels of the renal, mesenteric, coronary, and cerebral arteries to dilate, which increases blood flow to these tissues. Dopamine is the only substance that can stimulate these receptors. **Catecholamine** neurotransmitter molecules are produced by the SNS and are stored in vesicles or granules located in the ends of nerves. When the nerve is stimulated, the vesicles move to the nerve

ending and release their contents into the space between the nerve ending and the effector organ, known as the **synaptic cleft.** The released contents of the vesicle (the catecholamines) then have the opportunity to bind to the receptor sites located along the effector organ. Once the neurotransmitter binds to the receptors, the effector organ responds. Depending on the function of the particular organ, this response involves smooth muscle contraction (e.g., skeletal muscles) or relaxation (e.g., gastrointestinal and airway smooth muscles), an increased heart rate, the increased production of one or more substances (e.g., stress hormones), or constriction of a blood vessel. This process is halted by the action of specific enzymes and by reuptake of the neurotransmitter molecules back into the nerve cell (neuron). Catecholamines are specifically metabolized by two enzymes, monoamine oxidase (MAO) and catechol O-methyltransferase (COMT). Each enzyme breaks down catecholamines but is responsible for doing it in a different area. MAO breaks down the catecholamines in the nerve ending, whereas COMT breaks down the catecholamines outside the nerve ending at the synaptic cleft. Neurotransmitter molecules may also be actively taken back up into the nerve ending by the action of protein pumps within the cell membrane, through a phenomenon known as active transport. This restores the catecholamine to the vesicle and provides another means of maintaining an adequate supply of the substance for future sympathetic nerve impulses. This process is illustrated in Figure 18-2. The sympathetic branch of the ANS is often described as having a "fight-or-flight" function because it allows the body to respond in a self-protective manner to dangerous situations.

ADRENERGIC DRUGS

Drugs with effects that are similar to or mimic the effects of the SNS neurotransmitters norepinephrine, epinephrine, and dopamine are referred to as *adrenergics*. Recall that these neurotransmitters are referred to as *catecholamines*. This term also refers specifically to adrenergic drugs that have a basic chemical structure similar to that of norepinephrine, epinephrine, or dopamine. Catecholamines produce a sympathomimetic response and are either endogenous substances such as epinephrine, norepinephrine, and dopamine, or synthetic substances such as dobutamine and phenylephrine.

Catecholamine drugs used therapeutically produce the same result as the endogenous catecholamines. When epinephrine, dobutamine, or any one of the adrenergic drugs is given, it bathes the synaptic cleft. Once there, the drug has the opportunity to induce a response. This can be accomplished in one of three ways: by direct stimulation, by indirect stimulation, or by a combination of the two.

A *direct-acting* sympathomimetic binds directly to the receptor and causes a physiological response (Figure 18-3). Epinephrine is an example of such a drug. An *indirect-acting* sympathomimetic causes the release of the catecholamine from the storage sites (*vesicles*) in the nerve

TABLE 18-1		
Adrenergic Receptor Responses to Stimulation		
Location	**Receptor**	**Response**
CARDIOVASCULAR		
Blood vessels	α_1	Constriction
	β_2	Dilation
Heart muscle	β_1	Increased contractility
Atrioventricular node	β_1	Increased heart rate
Sinoatrial node	β_1	Increased heart rate
ENDOCRINE		
Kidney	β_2	Increased renin secretion
Liver	β_2	Glycogenolysis
Pancreas	α_2	Decreased insulin release
GASTROINTESTINAL		
Muscle	β_2, α_1	Decreased motility
Sphincters	α_1	Constriction
GENITOURINARY		
Bladder sphincter	α_1	Constriction
Penis	α_1	Ejaculation
Uterus	α_1	Contraction
	β_2	Relaxation
RESPIRATORY		
Bronchial muscles	β_2	Dilation
Pupilary muscles of iris	α_1	Mydriasis

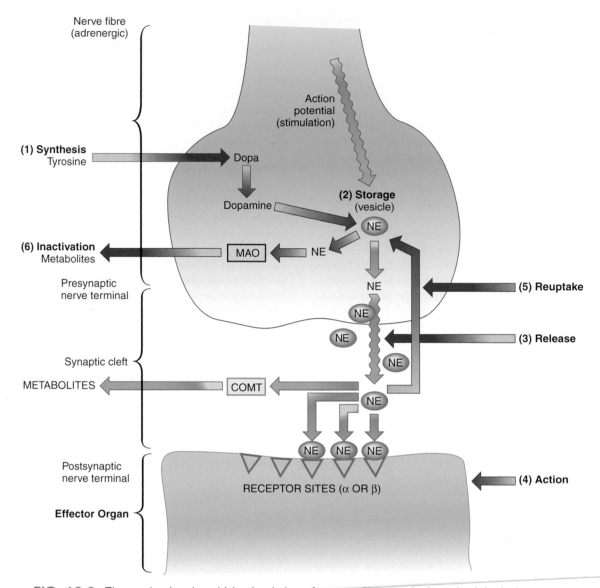

FIG. 18-2 The mechanism by which stimulation of a nerve fibre results in a physiological process; adrenergic drugs mimic this same process. *COMT*, catechol ortho-methytransferase; *MAO*, monoamine oxidase; *NE*, norepinephrine.

endings, which then binds to the receptors and causes a physiological response (Figure 18-4). Amphetamines and other related anorexiants are examples of such drugs. A *mixed-acting* sympathomimetic both directly stimulates the receptor by binding to it and indirectly stimulates the receptor by causing the release of the neurotransmitter stored in vesicles at the nerve endings (Figure 18-5). Ephedrine is an example of a mixed-acting adrenergic drug.

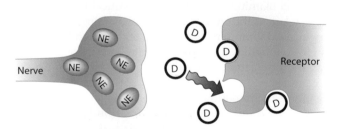

FIG. 18-3 Mechanism of physiological response by direct-acting sympathomimetics. *D*, drug; *NE*, norepinephrine.

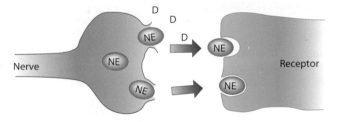

FIG. 18-4 Mechanism of physiological response by indirect-acting sympathomimetics. *D*, drug; *NE*, norepinephrine.

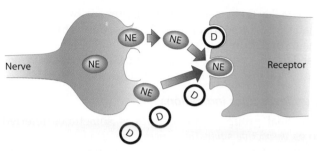

FIG. 18-5 Mechanism of physiological response by mixed-acting sympathomimetics. *D*, drug; *NE*, norepinephrine.

There are also noncatecholamine adrenergic drugs such as phenylephrine, metaproterenol, and salbutamol. These are structurally dissimilar to the endogenous catecholamines and generally have a longer duration of action than either the endogenous or synthetic catecholamines.

Catecholamines and noncatecholamines can act to varying degrees at different types of adrenergic receptors depending on the amount of drug administered. Examples of a few of the catecholamines and the dose-specific selectivity of these drugs for adrenergic receptors are given in Table 18-2. Noncatecholamine drugs show comparable patterns of activity. Although adrenergics work primarily at postganglionic receptors (the receptors that immediately innervate the effector organ, gland, muscle, and so on), they may also work more centrally in the nervous system at the preganglionic sympathetic nerve trunks. The ability to do so depends on the potency of the specific drug and the dose used.

Although adrenergic drugs are classified most technically by their specific receptor activities, they may also be categorized in terms of their clinical effects. For example, phenylephrine is both an α_1-agonist and a vasopressive drug ("pressor"), whereas salbutamol is both a β_2-agonist and a bronchodilator. Both classifications are suitable for most clinical purposes. However, it may sometimes be necessary to carefully choose an adrenergic drug with greater selectivity for a particular receptor type to avoid undesired clinical effects. In this situation, detailed knowledge of the type and degree of receptor selectivity for different drugs may become more important.

Mechanism of Action and Drug Effects

To fully understand the mechanism of action of adrenergics, one must have a working knowledge of normal adrenergic transmission, which takes place at the junction between the nerve (postganglionic sympathetic neuron) and the receptor site of the innervated organ or tissue (effector). The process of SNS stimulation is illustrated in Figure 18-2 and was discussed earlier in this chapter. When adrenergic drugs stimulate α_1-adrenergic receptor sites located on smooth muscles, vasoconstriction most commonly occurs. Many structures of the body are covered by smooth muscles with α-adrenergic receptors on them. The binding of adrenergic drugs to these α_1-adrenergic receptors on the smooth muscle of blood vessels, for example, causes smooth muscle contraction that results in vasoconstriction. However, such drug binding can also cause the relaxation of gastrointestinal smooth muscle, contraction of the uterus and bladder, ejaculation, decreased insulin release, and contraction of the ciliary muscles of the eye, which causes the pupils to dilate (see Table 18-1). Stimulation of α_2-adrenergic receptors, by contrast, actually tends to reverse sympathetic activity, but this action is not of great significance either physiologically or pharmacologically.

There are β_1-adrenergic receptors on the myocardium and in the conduction system of the heart, including the sinoatrial node and the atrioventricular node. When these β_1-adrenergic receptors are stimulated by an adrenergic drug, three effects result: (1) an increased force of contraction **(positive inotropic effect)**, (2) an increase in heart rate **(positive chronotropic effect)**, and (3) an increase in the conduction of cardiac electrical nerve impulses through the atrioventricular node **(positive dromotropic effect)**. Activation of β_2-adrenergic receptors produces relaxation of the bronchi (bronchodilation) and uterus. Stimulation of β_2-adrenergic receptors also causes increased glycogenolysis in the liver and an increase in renin secretion in the kidneys (see Table 18-1).

Indications

Adrenergics, or sympathomimetics, are used in the treatment of a wide variety of illnesses and conditions. Their selectivity for either α- or β-adrenergic receptors and

TABLE 18-2

Catecholamines and Their Dose–Response Relationship

Drug	Dosage	Receptor
dopamine hydrochloride (available premixed only)	Low: 0.5–2 mcg/kg/min Moderate: 2–4 or less than 10 mcg/kg/min High: 20–30 mcg/kg/min	Dopaminergic β_1 α_1
dobutamine hydrochloride	Maintenance: 2–15 mcg/kg/min High: 40 mcg/kg/min	β_1 greater than β_2 greater than α_1
epinephrine hydrochloride (Adrenalin chloride)	Low: 1–4 mcg/min High: 4–40 mcg/min	β_1 greater than β_2, α_1 α_1 greater than or equal to β_1

their affinity for certain tissues or organs determine the settings in which they are most commonly used. Some adrenergics are used as adjuncts to dietary changes in the short-term treatment of obesity. These drugs are discussed in greater detail in Chapter 17.

Respiratory Indications

Certain adrenergic drugs, classified as bronchodilators, have an affinity for the adrenergic receptors located in the respiratory system. Brochodilators tend to preferentially stimulate the β_2-adrenergic receptors rather than the α-adrenergic receptors and result in bronchodilation. Of the two subtypes of β-adrenergic receptors, these adrenergic drugs are predominantly attracted to the β_2-adrenergic receptors on the bronchial, uterine, and vascular smooth muscles and less so to the β_1-adrenergic receptors on the heart. These drugs are helpful in treating conditions such as asthma and bronchitis. Some common bronchodilators that are classified as predominantly β_2-selective adrenergic drugs include ephedrine, epinephrine, fenoterol, formoterol, orciprenaline, salbutamol, salmeterol xinafoate, and terbutaline. These drugs are discussed further in Chapter 37.

Indications for Topical Nasal Decongestants

The intranasal application of certain adrenergics can cause the constriction of dilated arterioles and a reduction in nasal blood flow, thus decreasing congestion. These adrenergic drugs work by stimulating α_1-adrenergic receptors and have little or no effect on β-adrenergic receptors. These nasal decongestants include oxymetazoline and phenylephrine. They are discussed further in Chapter 36.

Ophthalmic Indications

In another topical application, some adrenergics are applied to the surface of the eye. These are called **ophthalmics.** Ophthalmics work much the same way as nasal decongestants except that they affect the vasculature of the eye. When administered, they stimulate α-adrenergic receptors located on small arterioles in the eye and temporarily relieve conjunctival congestion by causing arteriolar vasoconstriction. The ophthalmic adrenergics include brimonidate tartrate, epinephrine, levobunolol hydrochloride, naphazoline, phenylephrine, and tetrahydrozoline.

Adrenergics can also be used to reduce intraocular pressure and dilate the pupils **(mydriasis)**, properties that make them useful in the treatment of open-angle glaucoma. Adrenergics produce these effects by stimulating α- or β_2-adrenergic receptors, or both. The adrenergic used for this purpose is dipivefrin. Opthalmic adrenergic drugs are discussed further in Chapter 58.

Cardiovascular Indications

The final group of adrenergics is sometimes referred to as *vasoactive sympathomimetics*, vasoconstrictive drugs (also known as vasopressive drugs, pressor drugs, or pressors), inotropes, or cardioselective sympathomimetics because they are used to support the cardiovascular system during heart failure or shock. These drugs have a variety of effects on the α- and β-adrenergic receptors, and these effects can also be related to the specific dose of the adrenergic drug. Common vasoactive adrenergic drugs include dobutamine, dopamine, epinephrine, norepinephrine, and phenylephrine.

Contraindications

The usual contraindications to adrenergic drugs are known drug allergy and severe hypertension.

Adverse Effects

Some of the most common unwanted CNS effects of the α-adrenergic drugs are headache, restlessness, excitement, insomnia, and euphoria. Possible cardiovascular adverse effects of the α-adrenergics include chest pain, vasoconstriction, hypertension, tachycardia, and palpitations or dysrhythmias. Effects on other body systems include anorexia or loss of appetite, dry mouth, nausea, vomiting, and, rarely, taste changes.

These drugs can also have unwanted effects on the cardiovascular system, including increased heart rate (positive chronotropy), palpitations (dysrhythmias), and fluctuations in blood pressure. Other significant effects include sweating, nausea, vomiting, and muscle cramps. See Special Populations: Children and Special Populations: The Older Adult for additional information on administration of these drugs in children and the older adult.

The β-adrenergic drugs can adversely stimulate the CNS, causing mild tremors, headache, nervousness, and dizziness. These drugs can also have unwanted effects on the cardiovascular system, including increased heart rate (positive chronotropy), palpitations (dysrhythmias), and fluctuations in blood pressure. Other significant effects include sweating, nausea, vomiting, and muscle cramps.

 SPECIAL POPULATIONS: CHILDREN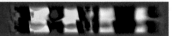

Administration of β-Adrenergic Agonists

- Children are usually more sensitive to most medications; therefore, watch children closely for excessive heart or CNS stimulations with palpitations, tachycardia, irritability, and chest pain.

- Terbutaline is generally not used in children 12 years of age and under.

- Other medications, including over-the-counter medications, should not be used unless a physician has been notified and approves concurrent use.

SPECIAL POPULATIONS: THE OLDER ADULT

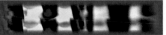

Administration of β-Adrenergic Agonists

- Several physiological changes occur in the cardiovascular system of the older individual. These changes include a decline in the efficiency and contractile ability of the heart muscle and a decrease in cardiac output and stroke volume. In most cases, the older adult adjusts to these changes without too much difficulty; however, if unusual demands are placed on this aging heart, problems and complications may arise. Unusual demands may occur with strenuous activities, excess stress, heat, and medication use. Therefore, when drugs are given that lead to changes in blood pressure, as with the β-adrenergics, the older adult may react negatively with either extremely high or extremely low blood pressure.

- Baroreceptors do not work as effectively in the older adult. Reduced baroreceptor activity may lead to orthostatic hypotension even without medication adverse effects.

- Because of the possible presence of other medical conditions such as hypertension, peripheral vascular disease, and cardiovascular or cerebrovascular disease, the older adult must be monitored carefully before, during, and after administration of adrenergic drugs.

- Vital signs, especially blood pressure and pulse rate, should be monitored frequently and as needed because of the cardiovascular and cerebrovascular effects of adrenergic drugs.

- The older adult (indeed, a patient of any age) should immediately report the occurrence of any chest pain, palpitations, blurred vision, headache, seizures, or hallucinations to the physician or health care provider.

- Cautious use of over-the-counter drugs, natural health products, and other medications is recommended. This caution is advised because of the possibility of polypharmacy, possible drug–drug interactions, and the older adult's increased sensitivity to many drugs and other products.

- The older adult often has decreased motor and cognitive functioning. Therefore, use of additional equipment and certain facilitating aids and provision of special instructions are needed to help ensure proper dosing of medications.

Toxicity and Management of Overdose

The toxic effects of adrenergic drugs are primarily an extension of their common adverse effects (e.g., seizures from excessive CNS stimulation, hypotension or hypertension, dysrhythmias, palpitation, nervousness, dizziness, fatigue, malaise, insomnia, headache, tremor, dry mouth, and nausea). The two most life-threatening toxic effects involve the CNS and the cardiovascular system. In the acute setting, seizures can be effectively managed with diazepam. Intracranial bleeding can also occur, often as the result of an extreme elevation in blood pressure. Such elevated blood pressure increases the risk of hemorrhage not only in the brain but also elsewhere in the body. The best and most effective treatment in this situation is to lower the blood pressure using a rapid-acting sympatholytic (e.g., esmolol; see Chapter 19). This can directly reverse the adrenergic-induced state.

Many adrenergic drugs are either synthetic analogues of the naturally occurring neurotransmitters (norepinephrine, epinephrine, and dopamine) or the actual endogenous adrenergic compounds. The majority of these compounds have very short half-lives, thus their effects are relatively short-lived. Therefore, when these drugs are taken in an overdose or signs and symptoms of toxicity develop, reversing the adverse effects takes a relatively short time. Stopping the drug should quickly cause the toxic symptoms to subside. The recommended treatment for overdose is often managing the symptoms and supporting the patient. If death occurs, it is usually the result of either respiratory failure or cardiac arrest. The treatment of overdose should be aimed at the support of these two body systems.

Interactions

The drug interactions that can occur with adrenergic drugs are significant. Although many of the interactions result only in a diminished adrenergic effect because of direct antagonism at and competition for receptor sites, some reactions can be life threatening. Following are some of the more serious drug–drug interactions involving adrenergic drugs. When α- and β-adrenergic drugs are given with adrenergic antagonists (e.g., some classes of antihypertensive drugs), the drugs directly antagonize each other, which results in reduced therapeutic effects. Administration of adrenergics with anaesthetic drugs or digoxin can cause increased risk of cardiac dysrhythmias. Tricyclic antidepressants, when given with adrenergics, can cause increased vasopressor effects, acute hypertensive crisis, and possibly respiratory depression. Administration of adrenergic drugs with MAO inhibitors can cause a possibly life-threatening hypertensive crisis. Antihistamines and thyroid preparations can increase the effects of adrenergic drugs. Antihypertensives and adrenergics may directly antagonize each other's therapeutic effects.

Laboratory Test Interactions

The α-adrenergic drugs can cause the serum levels of endogenous corticotropin (i.e., adrenocorticotropic hormone), corticosteroids, and glucose to be increased. Therefore, these laboratory test results should be interpreted with caution in patients receiving any of these medications.

Dosages

For the recommended dosages of select adrenergic drugs, see the Dosages tables on pp. 354.

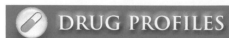
DRUG PROFILES

Adrenergics are used in the treatment of a variety of illnesses, and there are many indications for their use. Their selectivity for either α- or β-adrenergic receptors and their affinity for various tissues or organs define the settings in which they are most commonly used. Four frequently used therapeutic classes of adrenergic drugs are the bronchodilators (Chapter 37), ophthalmic drugs (Chapter 58), nasal decongestants (Chapter 36), and vaso-active drugs, which are emphasized in this chapter and in Chapter 24. It should be noted that receptor selectivity for the α_1, β_1, and β_2 receptor subtypes is relative (as opposed to absolute). Thus, there may be some overlap of drug effects between the different adrenergic classes of drugs, especially at higher dosages.

BRONCHODILATORS

The bronchodilating adrenergic drugs act primarily to stimulate β_2-adrenergic receptors. They are effective as antiasthmatic drugs and are used in the treatment of acute asthma attacks because of their rapid onset of action and efficacy. Ephedrine and epinephrine also possess α-adrenergic activity. Although most of these drugs are prescription-only medications, a few are available over the counter (OTC).

The activation of β_2-adrenergic receptors causes the bronchi to dilate. The selective β_2-adrenergics are the preferred bronchodilators because they produce fewer heart-related adverse effects (e.g., tachycardia) than the nonselective β-adrenergic drugs. These drugs are available primarily in oral, aerosol, and injection forms.

▶▶ epinephrine hydrochloride

Epinephrine hydrochloride (Adrenalin chloride) is a naturally occurring catecholamine produced by the adrenal medulla. It is a potent mixed α- and β-adrenergic drug that produces vasoconstriction, increased blood pressure, heart stimulation, and dilation of the bronchioles. It is the drug of choice for the relief of acute asthma attacks and for the treatment of anaphylaxis. In addition, epinephrine is used to treat open-angle glaucoma, restore heart rhythm in cardiac arrest, and control bleeding in surgical procedures. It is also used as an ophthalmic drug and is administered to prolong the activity of infiltrated local anaesthetics. Its use is contraindicated in several conditions, including hypersensitivity, narrow-angle glaucoma, shock as a result of trauma, general anaesthesia with halogenated drugs, coronary insufficiency, and labour. In addition, its administration with local anaesthetics to the toes or fingers is not recommended because distal circulation may be excessively decreased due to its vasoconstricting properties and the patient may be placed at risk for tissue necrosis (gangrene) and amputation. For those OTC products that contain epinephrine, such as Primatene Mist, cautious (if any) use is recommended because of the potential CNS stimulation and subsequent adverse effects, as well as the potential for drug dependency. See the Dosages table on p. 354 for selected dosage information.

PHARMACOKINETICS

Half-Life	Onset	Peak	Duration
SC: Variable (min)	SC: 5–10 min	SC: 20 min	SC: 4 hr
PO inhaled/IV: Variable (min)	PO inhaled/IV: 1 min	PO inhaled/IV: < 30 min	

▶▶ salbutamol sulfate

Salbutamol sulfate (Airomir, Apo-Salvent, Ventolin) is a selective β_2-adrenergic bronchodilator. Its use is contraindicated in patients with a known hypersensitivity to it. It can be administered orally and by inhalation. The dosage should be individualized. It is available in a metered-dose inhaler and as 2 and 4 mg tablets, oral syrup, inhalation solution, and for intravenous infusion. Salbutamol sulfate is also available for inhalation in combination with ipatropium bromide. See the Dosages table on p. 354 for the most common dosage information.

PHARMACOKINETICS

Half-Life	Onset	Peak	Duration
PO: 4 hr	PO: 30 min	PO: 2.5 hr	PO: 6–8 hr
Inhaled: 4 hr	Inhaled: 5–15 min	Inhaled: 1–1.5 hr	Inhaled: 3–6 hr

▶▶ salmeterol xinafoate

Salmeterol xinafoate (Serevent) is a β_2-agonist indicated for long-term maintenance treatment of asthma, prevention of bronchospasm, and prevention of exercise-induced bronchospasm. It is not indicated for acute exacerbations of asthma or bronchospasms. It is contraindicated in patients with known hypersensitivity to salmeterol. It is available as a 50 mcg/dose blister disk and powder inhalation device. Salmeterol is also available in a combination product with fluticasone propionate (Advair Diskus) (Chapter 37). Recommended dosages are given in the Dosages table on p. 355.

PHARMACOKINETICS

Half-Life	Onset	Peak	Duration
5.5 hr	10–20 min	3 hr	12 hr

NASAL DECONGESTANTS

The sympathomimetic drugs used as nasal decongestants consist of both α- and β-adrenergic drugs. The α-adrenergic activity of these drugs is responsible for causing vasoconstriction in the nasal mucosa. This produces shrinkage of the mucosa, which promotes easier nasal breathing and reduces nasal secretions. However, excessive use of nasal decongestants can lead to greater congestion because of a rebound phenomenon that occurs when use of the product is stopped. This is not seen with the oral drugs. The decongestants are administered topically with nasal drops, which are instilled into each nostril. The ephedrine salts, phenylephrine hydrochloride, and pseudoephedrine can produce nasal decongestion when taken either as single therapy or in multiple therapy such as in combination with allergy, cold, cough, and sinus relief preparations. Phenylephrine

Continued

DRUG PROFILES (cont'd)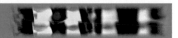

is usually administered via intranasal drops, whereas pseudoephedrine is taken orally. Relative contraindications to the use of the nasal decongestants are the same for all of the drugs and include hypersensitivity, diabetes, hypertension, thyroid disorders, and enlargement of the prostate gland. With routine use, adverse effects due to systemic absorption of nasally administered decongestants are usually minimal. However, all practitioners should be aware of the possibility of systemic adverse effects and educate patients accordingly if they are prescribed these drugs.

▸▸ pseudoephedrine hydrochloride

Pseudoephedrine hydrochloride (Eltor 120, Pseudofrin, Sudafed) is a natural plant alkaloid that is obtained from the ephedra plant. It is a stereoisomer of ephedrine and is a widely used oral decongestant. It is available in oral solution and tablet form. Some dosage forms are available without prescription. It is available in combined form with, for example, acetaminophen, chlorpheniramine maleate, and dextromethorphan as well as in other combinations. Health Canada has recommended that the following products be removed from the market because of severe adverse cardiovascular events: ephedra/ephedrine products containing more than 8 mg of ephedrine or with a label recommending more than 8 mg/dose or 32 mg/day; combination products containing ephedra/ephedrine combined with stimulants (e.g., caffeine or other ingredients that would enhance the activity of ephedra/ephedrine); and ephedra/ephedrine products with labelled or implied claims for appetite suppression, weight loss promotion, metabolic enhancement, increased exercise tolerance, body-building effects, euphoria, increased energy or wakefulness, or other stimulant effects. Some dosage forms are available OTC without prescription. See the Dosages table on p. 355 for recommended dosages.

PHARMACOKINETICS

Half-Life	Onset	Peak	Duration
Variable (min)	15–30 min	30–60 min	4–6 hr
			SR: 8–12 hr

SR, Sustained release.

OPHTHALMIC DECONGESTANTS

Ophthalmic decongestants are adrenergics that are applied topically to the eye. When instilled into the eye, they stimulate α-adrenergic receptors located on the small arterioles in the eye. This results in arteriolar vasoconstriction, which reduces conjunctival congestion and thus decreases redness in the eye. Although epinephrine and phenylephrine can be used as ophthalmic decongestants, naphazoline and tetrahydrozoline are the drugs most widely used.

tetrahydrozoline

Tetrahydrozoline (Visine) is applied topically to the eye to temporarily relieve congestion, itching, and minor irritation in patients with red and irritated eyes. It causes constriction of the blood vessels of the eye and is sometimes also used during some diagnostic eye procedures. It is the active ingredient in such OTC products as Visine and Visine Cool eye drops. Tetrahydrozoline is contraindicated in patients with a hypersensitivity reaction to it and in those with narrow-angle glaucoma. The recommended dosages are given in the Dosages table on p. 355.

PHARMACOKINETICS

Half-Life	Onset	Peak	Duration
Variable (min)	< 3 min	Short (min)	4–8 hr

VASOACTIVE ADRENERGICS

Adrenergics that have primarily cardioselective effects are referred to as *vasoactive adrenergics*. They are used to support a failing heart or to treat shock. They may also be used to treat orthostatic hypotension. These drugs have a wide range of effects on α- and β-adrenergic receptors, depending on the dosage. The vasoactive adrenergics are potent, quick-acting, injectable drugs. Although dosage recommendations are given in the Dosages table, all of these drugs are titrated to the desired physiological response. All of the vasoactive adrenergics (with the exception of midodrine) are rapid in onset, and their effects quickly cease when administration is stopped. Therefore, careful titration and monitoring of vital signs and electrocardiogram (ECG) are required in patients receiving adrenergics.

▸▸ dobutamine hydrochloride

Dobutamine hydrochloride is a β_1-selective vasoactive adrenergic drug that is structurally similar to the naturally occurring catecholamine dopamine. Through stimulation of the β_1 receptors on heart muscle (myocardium), it increases cardiac output by increasing contractility (positive inotropy), which increases the stroke volume, especially in patients with heart failure. Dobutamine is available only in intravenous injectable form. The recommended dosages are listed in the Dosages table on p. 355.

PHARMACOKINETICS

Half-Life	Onset	Peak	Duration
2–5 min	< 2 min	< 10 min	< 10 min

▸▸ dopamine hydrochloride

Dopamine hydrochloride is a naturally occurring catecholamine neurotransmitter in the SNS. It has potent dopaminergic and β_1- and α_1-adrenergic receptor activity, depending on the dosage. When used at low doses, dopamine can dilate blood vessels in the brain, heart, kidneys, and mesentery, which increases blood flow to these areas (dopaminergic receptor activity). At higher infusion rates, dopamine can improve heart contractility and output (β_1-adrenergic receptor activity). Use of the drug is contraindicated in patients who have a catecholamine-secreting tumour of the adrenal gland known as a *pheochromocytoma*. The drug is available in

Continued

DRUG PROFILES (cont'd)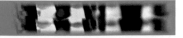

a 5% dextrose solution to be used only as an intravenous injectable drug. The recommended vasoactive dosages are given in the Dosages table on p. 355.

PHARMACOKINETICS

Half-Life	Onset	Peak	Duration
< 2 min	2–5 min	Rapid	10 min

▶▶ epinephrine

Epinephrine (Adrenalin) is also an endogenous vaso-active catecholamine. It acts directly on both the α- and β-adrenergic receptors of tissues innervated by the SNS. It is used in emergency situations and is one of the primary vasoactive drugs used in many advanced cardiac life-support protocols. The physiological response it elicits is dose related. At low dosages, it stimulates primarily β_1-adrenergic receptors, increasing the force of contraction and heart rate. It is also used for anaphylactic shock at these doses because it has significant bronchodilatory effects via the β_2-adrenergic receptors in the lungs. At high dosages (e.g., intravenous drip), epinephrine stimulates primarily α-adrenergic receptors, causing vasoconstriction, which elevates the BP. The dosages recommended for the treatment of various disorders are given in the Dosages table on p. 355.

PHARMACOKINETICS

Half-Life	Onset	Peak	Duration
< 5 min	< 2 min	Rapid	5–30 min

midodrine

Midodrine (Amatine) is a prodrug converted to its active form, desglymidodrine, in the liver. It is this active metabolite that accounts for the primary pharmacological action of midodrine, which is α_1-adrenergic receptor stimulation. This α_1 stimulation causes constriction of both arterioles and veins, resulting in peripheral vasoconstriction. Midodrine is primarily indicated for the treatment of symptomatic orthostatic hypotension. Midodrine is available as 2.5 and 5 mg tablets. Common dosages are given in the Dosages table on p. 355.

PHARMACOKINETICS

Half-Life	Onset	Peak	Duration
3–4 hr	45–90 min	1 hr	6–8 hr

▶▶ norepinephrine bitartrate

Norepinephrine bitartrate (Levophed) acts predominantly by directly stimulating α-adrenergic receptors, which leads to vasoconstriction. It also has some direct-stimulating β-adrenergic effects on the heart (β_1-adrenergic receptors) but none on the lung (β_2-adrenergic receptors). Norepinephrine is directly metabolized to dopamine and is used primarily in the treatment of hypotension and shock. Common dosages are given in the Dosages table on p. 355.

PHARMACOKINETICS

Half-Life	Onset	Peak	Duration
< 5 min	Immediate	1–2 min	1–2 min

DOSAGES   Selected Bronchodilator Drugs

Drug (Pregnancy Class)	Pharmacological Class	Usual Dosage Range	Indications
▶▶epinephrine hydrochloride (Adrenalin chloride) (C)	Adrenergic agonist (α_1, β_1, β_2)	*Children* SC: 0.01 mg/kg (1:1000 solution) to max of 0.5 mg; repeat at 20-min to 4-hr intervals based on response *Adult* IM/SC: 0.2–1 mg (1:1000 solution); repeated at 20-min to 4-hr intervals based on response	
formoterol fumarate (Foradil) (C)	β-adrenergic agonist (β_2-predominant)	*Children 6–16 yr/Adult* Inhalation capsule: 12–24 mcg bid, max 48 mcg	
▶▶salbutamol sulfate (Airomir, Apo-Salvent, Ventolin) (C)	β-adrenergic agonist (β_2-predominant)	*Children over 4 yr* MDI (inhalation aerosol): 1–2 puffs 4 times daily *Adult* MDI (inhalation aerosol): 1–2 puffs 4 times daily *Children 2–6 yr* PO liquid: 0.1 mg/kg tid–qid *Children 6–12 yr* PO liquid: 2 mg tid–qid *Children over 12 yr/Adult* PO liquid: 2–4 mg tid–qid *Adult* IV: 5 mcg/min, increased to 10 mcg/min and 20 mcg/min q15–30 min intervals prn *Adults* Inhalation solution (via nebulizer device): 2.5–5 mg qid diluted in 2.5–5 mL sterile NS *Children 5–12 yr* Inhalation solution (via nebulizer device): 2.5 mg qid diluted in 2–5 mL sterile NS	Bronchodilation

Continued

DOSAGES — Selected Bronchodilator Drugs (cont'd)

Drug (Pregnancy Class)	Pharmacological Class	Usual Dosage Range	Indications
▸▸salmeterol xinofoate (Serevent) (C)	β-adrenergic agonist (β₂-predominant); long-acting	*Children over4 yr/Adult* Inhalation aerosol (Diskus) and(Diskhaler): 1 inhalation (50 mcg) twice daily	Bronchodilation
terbutaline sulfate (Bricanyl) (C)	β-adrenergic agonist (β₂-predominant)	*Children over 6 yr/Adult* MDI inhalation powder: 1–2 inhalation with 5 min between inhalations prn, max 6 inhalations/day	

IM, intramuscular; *IV,* intravenous; *MDI,* metered-dose inhaler; *NS,* normal saline, PO, oral; SC, subcutaneous.

DOSAGES — Selected Nasal and Ophthalmic Decongestant Adrenergics

Drug (Pregnancy Category)	Pharmacological Class	Usual Dosage Range	Indications
▸▸pseudoephedrine hydrochloride (Eltor 120, Pseudofrin, Sudafed) (C)	α-β-adrenergic	**Eltor:** *Children over 12 yr/Adult* PO tabs: 120 mg q12h	Nasal decongestant
tetrahydrozoline (Visine) (C)	α-adrenergic	1–2 drops into eye(s) up to qid	Ophthalmic decongestant

DOSAGES — Selected Vasoactive Adrenergics

Drug (Pregnancy Category)	Pharmacological Class	Usual Dosage Range	Indications
▸▸dopamine hydrochloride (C)	β₁-adrenergic	*Children/Adult* IV infusion: 1–50 mcg/kg/min	Shock syndrome, chronic cardiac decompensatioin
▸▸dobutamine hydrochloride (B)	β₁-adrenergic	*Children/Adult* IV infusion: 2.5–10 mcg/kg/min	Cardiac decompensation
▸▸epinephrine (Adrenalin) (C)	α-β-adrenergic	*Children* SC: 0.01–0.5-mg/kg repeated at 20-min to 4-hr intervals ×2 then q4h prn IV: 0.1 mg over 5–10 min, followed by infusion of 0.1 mcg/kg/min *Adults* SC/IM: 0.2–1 mg, SC repeated at 20-min to 4-hr intervals IV infusion: 0.1–0.25 mg over 5–10 min, repeat q5–15 min *Neonatal* IV: 0.01–0.03 mg q5min as needed *Children* IV: 0.01 mg/kg q5 min as needed over 5–10 min	Bronchial asthma and anaphylaxis
		Adults IV: 0.5 mg q5 min as needed Intracardiac: 0.1–1 mg	Heart resuscitation
midodrine (Amatine) (C)	α₁-adrenergic	*Adults* PO: 2.5–10 mg tid–qid to max 30 mg/day	Chronic orthostatic hypotension
▸▸norepinephrine bitartrate (Levophed) (D)	α-β-adrenergic	*Adults* IV infusion: 8–12 mcg/min titrated to blood pressure	Acute hypotensive states

IM, intramuscular; *IV,* intravenous; *PO,* oral; *SC,* subcutaneous.

NURSING PROCESS

Assessment

Adrenergic drugs have a variety of effects depending on the receptors they stimulate. Stimulation of the α-adrenergic receptors results in vasoconstriction. Stimulation of β_1-adrenergic receptors produces heart stimulation, and stimulation of the β_2-adrenergic receptors results in bronchodilation. Because of these properties, the use of adrenergic agonists requires careful patient assessment and monitoring to maximize therapeutic effects and minimize possible adverse effects. A thorough patient assessment, including a health history and medication history with a listing of the drug allergies, medications routinely used, and over-the counter drugs and natural health products used, should be completed before any drug is administered. Other important assessment questions to pose include the following:

- Are there allergies to any medication, foods, topical products, environmental products, or other substances?
- Does the patient have asthma? If so, how frequent and severe are the attacks, and what factors exacerbate the attacks and help them? Are there any other signs and symptoms besides bronchospasms, wheezing, or dyspnea (shortness of breath)? What previous treatments for asthma have been tried? Are there any successes or failures?
- Is there any history of transient ischemic attacks? Any history of cerebrovascular accident, stroke, hypertension, hypotension, heart irregularities, or other cardiovascular disease?

Assessment of kidney and liver functioning is important before initiating treatment, especially in high-risk patients such as the older adult, because if the drugs cannot be excreted or metabolized properly then adverse effects and toxicity may occur. Assessment of heart functioning is also important because of the heart stimulation associated with these drugs. Adrenergic drugs may cause tachycardia, hypertension, myocardial infarction, or heart failure, so these drugs should be given cautiously or not at all in patients who are at risk for possible worsening of pre-existing disease states or symptoms.

Baseline vital signs should be assessed (e.g., blood pressure, postural blood pressures, pulse rate, temperature, respiratory rate), with further specific attention given to peripheral pulses, skin colour, and capillary refill (and with findings documented). Specific to the use of midodrine is the assessment of postural blood pressures and pulse rates (supine, sitting, and standing, as ordered) before and during drug administration. This should be done for both short- and long-term use of this drug for the management of postural hypotension; the nurse should also watch for other problems such as

dizziness, lightheadedness, and syncope. Assessment of the patient's symptoms and perception of either disease progression or a decrease in symptoms is important for effective and successful treatment.

With other adrenergic drugs, such as those used for bronchodilating effects, the following parameters should be assessed more closely: respiratory status with breath sounds (normal and adventitious); respiratory rate, depth, and pattern; occurrence of difficulty in breathing; activity or exercise tolerance or intolerance; and pulse oximetry readings. Use of a peak flow respiratory meter and measurement of anterior–posterior diameter of the chest wall (increased in chronic lung disorders such as emphysema) may also be part of the assessment process. Physicians may order other respiratory function studies and measurement of arterial blood gas levels, as deemed necessary. Cautions, contraindications, considerations for special populations, and drug interactions should always be assessed prior to use of these and other drugs in this chapter (see the previous discussion on each drug and its related profile and dosage table). In addition, some of these drugs are used only for acute episodes of asthma, whereas other drugs are used year-round as preventative drugs. For example, the drug salmeterol is not used to treat acute attacks. The older adult may react to these drugs with increased sensitivity, which requires close assessment.

Epinephrine and similar drugs are used for their heart, bronchial, antiallergic, ocular, and vasopressor effects. Assessment should focus on vital signs, breath sounds, arterial blood gas levels, and electrocardiogram (ECG) findings. Liver and kidney function test results also need to be assessed and documented. In addition, each system related to the specific action of the drug (e.g., respiratory system and bronchodilation) must be assessed.

Overall, adrenergic drugs work in similar ways, but individual drugs may have some differences in action, indications, and overall considerations. If the overall class of drugs and the way in which they work is known, however, then their related assessment parameters, cautions, contraindications, drug interactions, and considerations for special populations are easy to determine. If the drug is a pure adrenergic agonist, the net effect is stimulation of α-adrenergic receptors with vasoconstriction of blood vessels and subsequent elevation of blood pressure and heart rate. The nurse would then know to expect specific effects from the drug and to anticipate certain adverse effects. The drug may be used for the therapeutic effect of increased blood pressure, but an unwanted adverse effect could be a hypertensive crisis. If the drug is a β-adrenergic agonist, it will stimulate both β_1 and β_2 receptors, which will lead to heart stimulation and bronchodilation. This β_1 action can also result in too much stimulation with severe tachycardia and possibly chest pain if coronary artery disease is present. Thus, by simply knowing the actions of a given drug, the nurse can draw conclusions about, anticipate, and be alert to the drug's therapeutic action, adverse effects, cautions, contraindications, drug interactions, and toxicity.

Nursing Diagnoses

- Decreased cardiac output related to cardiovascular adverse effects of these drugs
- Ineffective tissue perfusion related to intense vasoconstrictive reactions
- Acute pain related to adverse effects of tachycardia and palpitations
- Deficient knowledge regarding therapeutic regimen, adverse effects, drug interactions, and precautions related to use of adrenergic drugs
- Risk for injury related to possible adverse effects (nervousness, vertigo, hypertension, or tremors) or to potential drug interactions
- Disturbed sleep pattern related to CNS stimulation caused by adrenergic drugs
- Nonadherence with drug therapy related to lack of information about the importance of taking the medication as ordered

Planning

Goals

- Patient will experience a reduction in symptoms because of the drug's therapeutic effects.
- Patient will take the drugs as ordered and follow directions explicitly.
- Patient will remain adherent to the drug therapy regimen.
- Patient will demonstrate satisfactory knowledge about the use of the specific medications.

Outcome Criteria

- Patient shows improvement in the disease process or condition for which the medication was given with subsequent decrease in the signs and symptoms of heart and respiratory problems.
- Patient states the importance of pharmacological and nonpharmacological treatment of the respiratory or other conditions that may be present, such as asthma.
- Patient states the importance of adherence to the drug regimen and adherence to the proper dosage of the medication to maximize therapeutic effects and minimize adverse effects.
- Patient experiences minimal adverse effects and complications, such as excessive CNS stimulation, insomnia, tachycardia, chest pain, and tremors.
- Patient states conditions and adverse effects associated with long-term at-home use that should be reported to the physician, such as chest pain, restlessness, and severe insomnia.
- Patient states the importance of scheduling and keeping follow-up appointments with the physician to monitor the effectiveness of drug therapy.

Implementation

There are several nursing interventions that can maximize the therapeutic effects of adrenergic drugs and minimize their adverse effects. The nurse should always check the package inserts concerning dilutional solutions with parenteral dosage forms. For example, subcutaneous administration of the adrenergic agonist epinephrine to patients with asthma requires safe calculations and accurate dosing. A tuberculin syringe used with subcutaneous epinephrine may help with accuracy in both adults and children.

When intravenous infusions of these drugs are administered for shock-related symptoms (hypotension), drugs such as dopamine will be used. Use of epinephrine and some of the other pure α-adrenergics results in vasoconstriction of the renal vessels and subsequent kidney damage or shutdown. Therefore, when any of these drugs are given intravenously, the nurse must be sure to check and be confident that the drug and dosage route are correct. For dopamine and similar drugs, the intravenous site should be checked frequently (e.g., every hour, as needed) for infiltration to be sure that the site remains intact and that the proper rate is being infused. Infiltration of an intravenous solution containing an adrenergic drug may lead to tissue necrosis from excessive vascular vasoconstriction around the intravenous site. Phentolamine is often used for the treatment of infiltration (Chapter 19). Also, with intravenous infusions, the nurse must use only clear solutions and a proper dilutional solution and must always administer the drug with an intravenous infusion pump, with monitoring of the cardiac system. ECG monitoring may also be ordered. All of these drugs should be given per the manufacturer's directions and suggested infusion rates to avoid precipitating dangerously high blood pressure and pulse rate and subsequent complications. (See Legal and Ethical Principles regarding issues that can arise with incorrect infiltrating intravenous infusions.)

When adrenergics are to be administered by an inhaler or nebulizer, patient instruction about correct use, storage, and care of equipment should be complete, thorough, and age-appropriate. The patient also needs to know how to use a spacer correctly because administration with this device is often ordered. Use of a spacer provides more effective delivery of inhaled doses of drug, but patient education must be thorough and easy to understand (see Chapter 6 and Patient Education). With dosing of the adrenergics for bronchodilating effects, often two adrenergics are indicated, but because of different medications and actions, one inhaler may be for use in acute situations and the other may be for long-term and preventive use. This type of treatment

LEGAL & ETHICAL PRINCIPLES

Infiltrating Intravenous (IV) Infusions

Nurses often encounter an infiltrating IV in the routine care of many of their patients. Every action taken is important to the standard of care of the patient and in ensuring that the nurse has acted as any prudent nurse would. The assessment and action taken by the nurse can be important for the patient.

Situation

Ms. Ross was transferred to the critical care unit (CCU) following a four-vessel coronary artery bypass graft surgery. Two hours after admission to the CCU, her BP began to decrease, and she became tachycardic. Postoperative bleeding, tamponade, and myocardial infarction were ruled out as potential etiologies of the cardiogenic shock. On further investigation, it was determined that Ms. Ross was experiencing acute heart failure following damage to the myocardium, which may take hours to days to resolve. A chest X-ray confirmed mild pulmonary edema. In order to improve her BP and cardiac output to increase perfusion to her vital organs, an IV infusion of dopamine was started at 1528 in her right wrist. At midnight, a nurse noted that the intravenous catheter site had a "bruise bluish in colour." The next notation was at 1100 the following day, in which it was recorded that the patient's right arm was swollen and painful with

a large blistered area around the IV catheter site. The same notation was made at 1600. It was not until 1850 that a note indicated that a physician was informed of the infiltration. As a result of the extravasation of dopamine, the patient's lower right arm was permanently scarred.

It was noted that although an infiltration may result from an improper technique, it may also be related to the size of the needle, the status of the patient's veins, or specific intolerance to an intravenous catheter. However, according to the expert nurse's testimony, supported by evidence-informed references, dopamine should be infused into a "large vein," such as in the antecubital fossa, to minimize the risk of extravasation. In addition, dopamine should be monitored continuously for free flow. If extravasation of dopamine occurs, the recommended treatment of the site is infiltration with a saline solution of phentolamine (Rogitine) within 12 hours.

It is essential that nurses are educated about the intravenous administration of dopamine in order to minimize the consequences of extravasation as in this case.

Adapted from McKenry, L. M., Tessier, E., & Hogan, M. (2006). *Mosby's pharmacology in nursing* (22nd ed). St Louis, MO: Mosby.

regimen requires that the patient receive thorough, simple, and complete instructions and explanations about the method of delivery as well as the drugs used. This will help minimize overdosage and risk of severe adverse effects such as hypertension, severe tachycardia, tremors, and CNS overstimulation.

The nurse must emphasize that adrenergic medications are to be used only as prescribed with regard to amount, timing, and spacing of doses. Because of their synergistic effects, for use of adrenergic medications (especially asthmatics) in combination with other types of bronchodilators, the patient must be clear about what to do before, during, and after the dose is delivered. If the patient is taking an inhaled dosage form, an oral or parenteral form of the same or a similar drug may also be prescribed. Through the use of more than one drug of the same drug class and of more than one route of administration, combined therapeutic effects can be achieved. With these regimens, patient education requires particularly close attention in order to prevent exacerbation of adverse effects, minimize drug interactions, and prevent severe vascular and cardiovascular adverse effects. Patients should immediately report any complaints of

chest pain, palpitations, blurred vision, headache, seizures, or hallucinations.

Patients with chronic lung disease who are receiving adrenergic drugs should also avoid anything that may exacerbate their respiratory condition (e.g., food or other allergens, cigarette smoking) and implement measures that may help diminish the risk of respiratory infection. These measures may include avoiding those who are ill with colds and flu, avoiding crowded areas, remaining well nourished and rested, and maintaining fluid intake of up to 3000 mL/day to ensure adequate hydration (unless contraindicated). Keeping a journal of symptoms and any improvement or worsening in their condition while taking the medications may be very helpful.

Salmeterol is not to be used for relief of acute symptoms, and education about its dosing is important. The dosage of salmeterol is usually 2 puffs twice daily 12 hours apart for maintenance effects. For prevention of exercise-induced asthma, it is recommended that patients take 2 puffs $1/_2$ to 1 hour before exercise and no additional doses for 12 hours. Always recheck these orders and directions. If another type of inhalant is used, such as a corticosteroid, the bronchodilator should be used first, with a 5-minute waiting period before taking the second drug. All equipment should be rinsed, and the patient should be encouraged to rinse the mouth thoroughly after the use of any inhalant form of medication.

If ophthalmic forms of these drugs are used, the nurse must make sure that the medication has not expired and is also a clear solution. The eyedropper must not be allowed to touch the eye when the drug is applied, to help prevent contamination of the remaining solution. With ophthalmic administration, drops and ointments should be applied into the conjunctival sac—not directly onto the eye itself.

Oral midodrine should be taken exactly as prescribed. This medication is usually ordered to be given with forcing of fluids before the patient gets out of bed in the morning. Doses of the drug are also often front loaded in their dosing so that most of the doses occur in the morning when patients with orthostatic intolerance are usually more symptomatic. Patients should avoid taking this medication after 1800 to prevent insomnia and possible supine hypertension.

Evaluation

Therapeutic effects of adrenergic drugs include the following. For vasoactive drugs, therapeutic effects include improved cardiac output (with increased urinary output), return to normal vital signs (e.g., blood pressure of 120/80 mm Hg or higher or gradual increases in blood pressure as indicated, pulse rate greater than 60 but less than 120 beats/min), improved skin colour (pallor to pink) and temperature (cool to warm) in extremities, improved peripheral pulses, and increased level of consciousness. Therapeutic effects of drugs given for bronchial indications include a return to a normal respiratory rate (more than 12 but less than 20 breaths/min), improved breath sounds throughout the lung field with fewer adventitious (abnormal) sounds; increased air exchange in all areas of the lungs, including that in the lung bases; decreased to no coughing; decreased dyspnea; improved partial pressure of oxygen and pulse oximeter readings; and tolerance of slowly increasing levels of activity. If the drugs are used for nasal congestion, the patient should report less congestion and improved ability to breathe. Therapeutic effects of midodrine include improved level of functioning and performance of activities of daily living, fewer episodes of postural intolerance (dizziness, lightheadedness, and syncopal episodes), and more energy.

Evaluation for the occurrence of adverse effects with adrenergic drugs includes monitoring for stimulation of the systems that are affected, such as the cardiac system and the CNS. Adverse effects such as heart irregularities, hypertension, and tachycardia may occur. The nurse should be sure to monitor for chest pain as well. With the use of nasal decongestants, adverse effects of rebound nasal congestion, rhinitis, and nasal mucosal ulcerations are possible. See p. 350 for additional information on adverse effects.

PATIENT EDUCATION

- Patients should be educated to always take medications as prescribed; excessive dosing may cause CNS and cardiovascular stimulation, including tachycardia and palpitations.
- Patients should be shown how to self-administer inhaled forms of medication. See Chapter 10 (p. 174) for instructions on using a metered-dose inhaler and a spacer. Patients should be sure to rinse their mouth thoroughly after taking inhaled preparations.
- Patients should report worsening of respiratory symptoms, dyspnea, distress, chest pain, or heart palpitations to the health care provider immediately.
- Patients should not take any other medications (including over-the-counter medications and natural health products) without the physician's approval.

- Patients should be informed that if adrenergic nasal decongestant sprays are used, the phenomenon of rebound nasal congestion may occur with overuse and can be prevented by taking the drug as prescribed.
- Should rebound nasal congestion occur, patients should follow the instructions given by the physician or health care provider and use saline nasal spray for relief.
- Patients should be informed that midodrine use requires careful dosing, as ordered, and patients should use a journal to record adverse effects, improvements in symptoms, or any worsening of symptoms.
- Patients should be advised to rinse their mouth after each inhalation or use of a nebulizer.

POINTS TO REMEMBER

❖ Catecholamines are substances that produce a sympathomimetic response (stimulate the SNS). The naturally occurring or endogenous catecholamines include epinephrine, norepinephrine, and dopamine. An example of an exogenous catecholamine is dobutamine.

❖ Nursing considerations regarding the use of adrenergic agonist drugs to treat respiratory disorders include the following:

• Patients should be taught to avoid respiratory irritants.

• Patients should be instructed to avoid contact with individuals who may have infections to help minimize situations that would exacerbate the original problem.

• Patients should also be told to avoid over-the-counter or prescribed medications because of possible drug interactions with adrenergic agonists.

❖ With nasal preparations, rebound nasal congestion or ulcerations of the nasal mucosa may occur if drugs are overused; therefore, patients need to be educated to use these products only as directed.

❖ Midodrine use requires careful blood pressure monitoring, so education about supine blood pressures and regular documentation of measured blood pressure values is very important to the effective use of the drug.

❖ Inhaled forms of β-agonists are used for their bronchodilating action and must be taken only as prescribed, with caution to avoid any overuse of the drug. Overdosage of these drugs may lead to severe cardiovascular, CNS, and cerebrovascular adverse effects and stimulation.

EXAMINATION REVIEW QUESTIONS

1 When caring for a patient who is receiving β-agonist drug therapy, which of the following effects caused by these drugs does the nurse need to be aware of?
a. Bronchoconstriction
b. Decreased heart rate
c. Increased heart contractility
d. Increased gastrointestinal tract motility

2 During a teaching session for a patient who is receiving inhaled salmeterol, which of the following should the nurse emphasize that the drug is indicated for?
a. Prevention of bronchospasm
b. Reduction of airway inflammation
c. Long-term treatment of sinus congestion
d. Rescue treatment of acute bronchospasms

3 For a patient receiving a vasoactive drug such as intravenous dopamine, which of the following actions by the nurse is most appropriate?
a. Assess the intravenous site hourly to rule out infiltration
b. Monitor the gravity drip infusion closely and adjust as needed
c. Assess the patient's heart function by checking the radial pulse
d. Administer the drug by intravenous boluses according to the patient's blood pressure

4 A patient is receiving dobutamine for worsening of heart failure. Vital signs the day before were as follows: blood pressure, 150/88; pulse rate, 110 beats/min; respiratory rate, 16 breaths/min. Vital signs now are blood pressure, 170/94; pulse rate, 110 beats/min; respiratory rate, 20 breaths/min. The patient is now complaining of "chest tightness." Which statement is most appropriate regarding the patient's symptoms?
a. These changes reflect a need to switch to an oral form of dobutamine.
b. The changes in vital signs are reflective of a therapeutic response to the drug.
c. The patient most likely needs a dose of α-agonist to elevate the heart rate and help treat the heart failure.
d. The presence of chest pain and the changes in vital signs need to be evaluated immediately by the nurse and physician.

5 When a drug is characterized as having a negative chronotropic effect, which of the following should the nurse know to expect?
a. Decreased heart rate
b. Decreased ectopic beats
c. Improved sinoatrial nodal firing
d. Increased force of heart contractions

For answers see http://evolve.elsevier.com/Canada/Lilley/pharmacology/.

CRITICAL THINKING ACTIVITIES

1 Explain why it is important to carefully assess the older adult for the presence of medical conditions before administering any β-adrenergic agonist drugs?

2 Discuss the rationale for careful titration and monitoring of patients receiving vasoactive adrenergic drugs.

3 A patient has had an infiltration of a dopamine infusion. Describe what effects this may have on the patient and the nursing responsibilities when caring for a patient receiving a dopamine infusion.

For answers see http://evolve.elsevier.com/Canada/Lilley/pharmacology/.
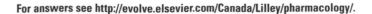

CHAPTER 19

Adrenergic-Blocking Drugs

Learning Objectives

After reading this chapter, the successful student will be able to do the following:

1 Discuss the normal anatomy and physiology of the autonomic nervous system as it pertains to adrenergic-blocking drugs or sympatholytics.

2 List examples of specific drugs categorized as adrenergic antagonists or adrenergic blockers, including α- and β-blockers.

3 Discuss the mechanisms of action, therapeutic effects, indications, adverse and toxic effects, cautions, contraindications, dosages, and routes of administration for the α-blockers, nonselective β-blockers, and β₁- and β₂-blockers.

4 Identify the antidotes used in the treatment of adrenergic-blocking drug overdosage.

5 Develop a collaborative plan of care that includes all phases of the nursing process related to the administration of adrenergic-blocking drugs.

e-Learning Activities

Web site
(http://evolve.elsevier.com/Canada/Lilley/pharmacology/)

- Animations
- Answers to chapter questions, activities, and case studies
- Calculators and Category Catchers
- Glossary with audio pronunciations
- IV Therapy and Medication Error Checklists
- Multiple-Choice Review Question quizzes
- Nursing Care Plans
- Online Appendices and Supplements
- WebLinks

Drug Profiles

    acebutolol (acebutolol hydrochloride)*, p. 369
▸▸ **atenolol**, p. 369
    carvedilol, p. 369
    ergotamine (ergotamine tartrate)*, p. 365
▸▸ **esmolol (esmolol hydrochloride)***, p. 369
    labetalol (labetalol hydrochloride)*, p. 369
▸▸ **metoprolol (metoprolol tartrate)***, p. 369
▸▸ **phentolamine (phentolamine mesylate)***, p. 365
▸▸ **prazosin (prazosin hydrochloride)***, p. 365
▸▸ **propranolol (propranolol hydrochloride)***, p. 370
    sotalol (sotalol hydrochloride)*, p. 370

▸▸ Key drug.

*Full generic name is given in parentheses. For the purposes of this text, the more common shortened name is used.

Glossary

Agonists Drugs with a specific receptor affinity that produce a "mimic" response. (p. 362)

Angina Paroxysmal chest pain caused by myocardial ischemia. (p. 367)

Antagonists Drugs that bind to adrenergic receptors and inhibit or block the action of neurotransmitters, resulting in inhibitory or antagonistic drug effects; also called *inhibitors*. (p. 362)

Cardioprotective Term applied to β-blockers serving to inhibit stimulation of the heart by circulating catecholamines. (p. 367)

Cardioselective β-blockers The β-blocking drugs that are selective for β₁-adrenergic receptors. Also called β₁-blocking drugs. (p. 364)

Dysrhythmias Irregular heart rhythms; almost always called *arrhythmias* in clinical practice. (p. 367)

Extravasation Leaking of fluid from the blood vessel into the surrounding tissues, as in the case of an infiltrated intravenous infusion. (p. 364)

Glycogenolysis The production of glucose from glycogen in the liver, which is reduced by β-blockers. (p. 367)

Intrinsic sympathomimetic activity Paradoxical action of some β-blocking drugs (e.g., acebutolol) that mimics the activity of the sympathetic nervous system. (p. 365)

Lipophilicity The chemical attraction of a substance (e.g., drug molecule) to lipid or fat molecules. (p. 367)

Nonselective β-blockers The β-blocking drugs that block both β₁- and β₂-adrenergic receptors. (p. 364)

Orthostatic hypotension Abnormally low blood pressure that occurs when a person assumes a standing position from a sitting or lying position. (p. 365)

Oxytocics Drugs used to treat postpartum and postabortion bleeding caused by uterine relaxation and enlargement. (p. 363)

Pheochromocytoma Avascular adrenal tumour that is usually benign but secretes epinephrine and norepinephrine and thus often causes central nervous system stimulation and substantial blood pressure elevation. (p. 363)

Sympatholytics Another name for adrenergic antagonists. (p. 362)

Vaughan Williams classification System of classifying antidysrhythmic drugs. (p. 367)

OVERVIEW

The *autonomic nervous system* consists of the *parasympathetic* and *sympathetic* nervous systems. The class of drugs discussed in this chapter works primarily on the sympathetic nervous system (SNS). As discussed in Chapter 18, the adrenergic agonist drugs stimulate the SNS. These drugs are called **agonists** because they bind to receptors and cause a response. The adrenergic blockers have the opposite effect and are therefore referred to as **antagonists.** They also bind to adrenergic receptors but in doing so inhibit or block stimulation of the SNS. They are also referred to as **sympatholytics** because they "lyse," or inhibit, SNS stimulation.

Throughout the body, there are receptor sites for the sympathetic neurotransmitters norepinephrine and epinephrine. These are called the *adrenergic receptors,* and two basic types are found, α and β. There are subtypes of both the α- and β-adrenergic receptors, designated 1 and 2. The α₁- and α₂-adrenergic receptors are differentiated by their location on nerves. The α₁-adrenergic receptors are located on the tissue, muscle, or organ that the nerve is stimulating (postsynaptic effector cells). The α₂-adrenergic receptors are located on the actual nerves that stimulate the presynaptic effector cells. The β₁-adrenergic receptors are located primarily on the heart. The β₂-adrenergic receptors are located primarily on the smooth muscles of the bronchioles and blood vessels. It is at these receptors that adrenergic blockers work, and these drugs are classified by the type of adrenergic receptor they block, α or β or, in a few cases, both. Hence they are called α-*blockers*, β-*blockers*, or α-β–blockers.

α-BLOCKERS

The α-adrenergic–blocking drugs, or α-blockers, interrupt or block the stimulation of the SNS at the α-adrenergic receptor. Various physiological responses occur when the stimulation of the α-adrenergic receptors is inhibited. Adrenergic blockade at the α-adrenergic receptors leads to vasodilation, decreased blood pressure, miosis or constriction of the pupil, or suppressed ejaculation. The ergot alkaloids dihydroergotamine mesylate, ergoloid mesylate, ergotamine tartrate, and ergonovine maleate are α-blockers that are used primarily for their vasoconstrictive properties. The α-blockers doxazosin, prazosin, and terazosin are used as antihypertensive drugs because they cause vasodilation. Both of these two groups of drugs block α-adrenergic receptors, but they also have an affinity for different sites in the body and, therefore, the resultant effects differ. One other α-blocker is phentolamine.

Mechanism of Action and Drug Effects

As mentioned earlier, α-blockers work by blocking or inhibiting the normal stimulation of the SNS. They do this either through direct competition with the SNS neurotransmitter norepinephrine or through a noncompetitive process. Most α-blockers are competitive in their actions. They have a higher affinity for the α-adrenergic receptor than does norepinephrine and can chemically displace norepinephrine molecules from the receptor binding site. Once a competitive α-blocker binds to the receptor, it causes the receptor to be less responsive. This blockade is reversible. Noncompetitive α-blockers work in a different fashion: they also bind to the α-adrenergic receptors, but this type of bond (a *covalent* bond) is irreversible. Regardless of the way in which the blockade is accomplished, the result is a decreased response to stimulation of the SNS. Figure 19-1 illustrates these two mechanisms.

The α-blockers have many effects on the normal physiological functions of the body. The effects of each drug can differ depending on the drug's selectivity for receptors in particular tissues or cells in the body. Ergot alkaloids, for example, can cause peripheral and cerebral vasoconstriction as well as the constriction of dilated arteries. Certain α-blockers can stimulate uterine contractions. Others can block α-adrenergic receptors on both vascular and nonvascular smooth muscle. The vascular smooth muscle receptors for which these α-blockers have

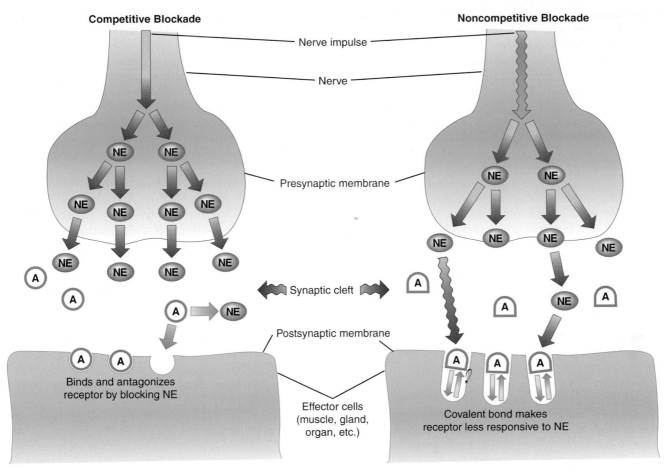

FIG. 19-1 α-Blocker mechanisms for α-adrenergic competitive and noncompetitive blockade. *A*, antagonist; *NE*, norepinephrine.

an affinity are those in the bladder and its sphincters, the gastrointestinal tract and its sphincters, the prostate, and the ureters. The nonvascular smooth muscle receptors for which these drugs have an affinity are in the central nervous system (CNS), liver, and kidneys. Unlike ergot alkaloids, some α-blockers can induce arterial and venous dilation and thus decrease peripheral vascular resistance and blood pressure. Some α-blockers can also influence the concentration of certain neurotransmitters, causing a depletion of catecholamines such as norepinephrine and epinephrine. Others can directly block a neurotransmitter such as serotonin (5-hydroxytryptamine [5-HT]) or indirectly cause it to be depleted.

Indications

The α-blockers have many therapeutic effects, but these effects differ greatly depending on the particular drug. Ergot alkaloids constrict dilated arterioles in the brain that are often responsible for causing vascular headaches, such as migraines. The vasoconstriction that results from the use of the ergot alkaloids helps to relieve the symptoms associated with vascular migraines because of dilated arteries. Ergot alkaloids are also used as **oxytocics,** drugs given to control postpartum and postabortion bleeding caused by uterine relaxation and enlargement. These

drugs stimulate the smooth muscle of the uterus to contract and induce local vasoconstriction.

The α-blockers such as alfuzosin hydrochloride, doxazosin mesylate, prazosin hydrochloride, terazosin hydrochloride, and tamsulosin hydrochloride cause both arterial and venous dilation. This effect reduces peripheral vascular resistance and blood pressure. Consequently, the first three drugs are used to treat hypertension. The α-adrenergic receptors are also present on the vascular smooth muscle of the prostate and the bladder. By blocking the stimulation of α_1 receptors, α-blockers reduce smooth muscle contraction of the bladder neck and the prostatic portion of the urethra. For this reason, α-blockers are used in patients with benign prostatic hyperplasia (BPH) to decrease the resistance to urinary outflow. This reduces urinary obstruction and relieves some of the effects of BPH. Tamsulosin is used exclusively for treating BPH.

Other α-blockers can inhibit excitatory responses to adrenergic stimulation. The α-blockers noncompetitively block α-adrenergic receptors on smooth muscle and various exocrine glands. Because of this action, these particular α-blockers are useful in controlling or preventing hypertension in patients who have a **pheochromocytoma.** A pheochromocytoma is a tumour that forms on the adrenal glands on top of the kidneys and secretes norepinephrine, which causes SNS stimulation. The α-blockers are also useful in the treatment of patients who have increased endogenous α-adrenergic agonist activity, which results in vasoconstriction. Three conditions in which this occurs are Raynaud's disease, acrocyanosis, and frostbite. Phentolamine is an α-blocker useful for the treatment of these syndromes.

Other α-blockers are effective at antagonizing responses caused by injected catecholamines such as epinephrine and norepinephrine. These drugs cause peripheral vasodilation and decrease peripheral resistance by blocking catecholamine-stimulated vasoconstriction. They can also be used to treat pheochromocytomas. Because of their potent vasodilating properties and their fast onset of action, they are used to prevent skin necrosis and sloughing after the **extravasation** of vasopressors such as norepinephrine or epinephrine. When these drugs *extravasate*, or leak out of the blood vessel into the surrounding tissue, they cause vasoconstriction and, ultimately, tissue death, or necrosis. If the vasoconstriction is not reversed quickly, the entire limb can be lost. The α-blocker phentolamine can reverse this potent vasoconstriction and restore blood flow to the ischemic, vasoconstricted area.

Contraindications

Contraindications to the use of α-blocking drugs include known drug allergy and peripheral vascular disease and may also include liver and kidney disease, coronary artery disease, peptic ulcer, and sepsis.

Adverse Effects

The primary adverse effects of α-blockers are those related to their effects on the vasculature. The primary adverse effects of the α-blockers are listed by body system in Table 19-1.

Toxicity and Management of Overdose

In an acute overdose, consultation with a Poison Control Centre is recommended. The patient's stomach should be emptied, usually by gastric lavage. After this, activated charcoal should be administered to bind to the drug and

remove it from the stomach and the circulation. To hasten elimination of the drug bound to the activated charcoal, the first dose should be given with a cathartic such as sorbitol. Symptomatic and supportive measures should be instituted as needed. Blood pressure support with the administration of fluids, volume expanders, and vasopressor drugs and the administration of anticonvulsants such as diazepam for the control of seizures are examples of such measures.

Interactions

The most severe drug interactions with α-blockers are those that potentiate the effects of α-blockers. Generally, the α-blockers are highly protein bound and compete for binding sites with other drugs that are also highly protein bound. Because of the limited sites for binding on proteins and the increased competition for these sites, more free α-blocker molecules circulate in the bloodstream. Drug that is not bound to protein is active, resulting in a more pronounced drug effect. Some of the common drugs that interact with α-blockers and the results of these interactions are listed in Table 19-2.

Dosages

For the recommended dosages of α-blockers, see the Dosages table on p. 366.

β-BLOCKERS

The β-adrenergic–blocking drugs (β-blockers) block SNS stimulation of the β-adrenergic receptors by competing with the endogenous catecholamines norepinephrine and epinephrine. The β-blockers are either selective or nonselective, depending on the type of β-adrenergic receptors they antagonize or block. As mentioned earlier, β_1-adrenergic receptors are located primarily in the heart. The β-blockers selective for these receptors are often referred to as **cardioselective β-blockers,** or β_1-blocking drugs. Other β-blockers block both β_1- and β_2-adrenergic receptors, the latter located primarily on the smooth muscles of the bronchioles and blood vessels. The β-blockers that block both types of β-adrenergic receptors are referred to as **nonselective β-blockers.** The drugs in the β-blocker class can be further categorized

---

TABLE 19-1

α-Blockers: Adverse Effects

Body System	Adverse Effects
Cardiovascular	Palpitations, orthostatic hypotension, tachycardia, edema, dysrhythmias, chest pain
Central nervous	Dizziness, headache, drowsiness, anxiety, depression, vertigo, weakness, numbness, fatigue
Gastrointestinal	Nausea, vomiting, diarrhea, constipation, abdominal pain
Other	Incontinence, nosebleed, tinnitus, dry mouth, pharyngitis, rhinitis

---

TABLE 19-2

α-Blockers: Common Drug Interactions

Drug	Mechanism	Results
β-Blockers Calcium channel blockers Diuretics	Additive effects	Profound hypotension
Protein-bound drugs	Competition for plasma protein-binding sites	Effects of increased free drug levels in plasma

DRUG PROFILES

The α-blockers are prescription-only drugs that are available in oral dosage forms, including tablets and capsules. Most α-blockers are rated as pregnancy category C. Ergot alkaloids, however, are rated as pregnancy category X drugs.

ergotamine tartrate

Ergotamine tartrate is an *ergot alkaloid*. All ergot alkaloids are obtained from the fungus *Claviceps purpurea*, which grows on rye. It causes vasoconstriction of dilated blood vessels in the brain and the carotid arteries. These dilated arteries are responsible for causing vascular headaches such as migraines and cluster headaches. In Canada, ergotamine tartrate is available only in combination with other drugs. The addition of caffeine to ergotamine facilitates the absorption of ergotamine when taken in the oral or suppository form, resulting in a more effective and rapid onset of vasoconstriction. It is contraindicated in patients with peripheral vascular disease, coronary artery disease, severe hypertension, sepsis, shock, or impaired liver or kidney functions, as well as in pregnant women. It is available as a tablet containing 1 mg of ergotamine and 100 mg of caffeine. Several other combination-drug preparations are available in oral tablet form. These combinations vary; some of the other drugs combined with ergotamine in these preparations are belladonna alkaloids, phenobarbital, and dimenhydrinate. Dihydro-ergotamine mesylate is available in an injectable form and as a nasal spray. The five available ergot products should not be taken at the same time as other drugs that strongly inhibit CYP 3A4 liver enzymes. The breakdown of ergotamine in the body is slowed down by these drugs, leading to elevated levels of ergotamine in the body, which can result in serious brain ischemia and thus stroke, or to vasospasm of the extremities, causing gangrene. See the Dosages table on p. 366 for dosing information.

PHARMACOKINETICS

Half-Life	Onset	Peak	Duration
2 hr	30 min–2 hr	4–6 hr	24–48 hr

▶▶ phentolamine mesylate

Phentolamine mesylate (Rogitine) is an α-blocker that reduces peripheral vascular resistance and is used to treat hypertension. It is used to treat the high blood pressure caused by pheochromocytoma as well as in the diagnosis of this catecholamine-secreting tumour. A single intravenous dose of phentolamine is given to the hypertensive patient who is suspected of having the tumour. If the blood pressure declines rapidly, it is highly likely that the patient has a pheochromocytoma. Phentolamine is available only as an intravenous preparation; thus it can then be used to treat the extravasation of vasoconstricting intravenous drugs such as

norepinephrine, epinephrine, and dopamine. When these drugs are given intravenously they can leak out of the vein, especially if the intravenous tube is not correctly positioned. If such a drug is allowed to extravasate into the surrounding tissue, the result is intense vasoconstriction, decreased blood flow, necrosis, and potential loss of the limb. When phentolamine is injected subcutaneously in a circular fashion around the extravasation site, it causes α-adrenergic receptor blockade and vasodilation. This effect increases blood flow to the ischemic tissue and prevents permanent damage. Its use is contraindicated in patients who have shown a hypersensitivity to it, those who have suffered a myocardial infarction, and those with coronary artery disease. The recommended dosages are given in the Dosages table on p. 366.

PHARMACOKINETICS

Half-Life	Onset	Peak	Duration
19 min	Immediate	2 min	15–30 min

▶▶ prazosin hydrochloride

Prazosin hydrochloride (Minipress) is an α_1-adrenergic–blocking drug used primarily to treat hypertension and to reduce urinary obstruction in men with BPH. Other drugs that are chemically and pharmacologically related to prazosin are doxazosin mesylate (Cardura), terazosin hydrochloride (Hytrin), and tamsulosin hydrochloride (Flomax). Its primary antihypertensive effects are related to its selective and competitive inhibition of α_1-adrenergic receptors. In men with BPH, prazosin relieves the impaired urinary flow and urinary frequency by relaxing and dilating the vasculature and smooth muscle in the area surrounding the prostate. It also dramatically lowers blood pressure. A patient's ability to tolerate this drop in blood pressure must be taken into consideration when prescribing α-blockers for the treatment of BPH. Often when patients first start taking α-blockers, they become lightheaded and may faint when standing up after sitting or lying down. This is referred to as **orthostatic hypotension**. Although it is a fairly common problem specific to the α_1-blockers alfuzosin, prazosin, doxazosin, terazosin, and tamsulosin, patients quickly acquire a tolerance to it, usually after the first dose. Often patients taking the first dose are recommended to take it at bedtime and to be careful getting up to circumvent the problem. The use of prazosin is contraindicated in patients who have shown hypersensitivity reactions to it. It is available for oral use in 1, 2, and 5 mg capsules. The normally recommended dosages of prazosin are given in the Dosages table on p. 366.

PHARMACOKINETICS

Half-Life	Onset	Peak	Duration
2–3 hr	2 hr	1–3 hr	10 hr

according to whether they do or do not have **intrinsic sympathomimetic activity**. Drugs with intrinsic sympathomimetic activity (acebutolol, pindolol) not only

block β-adrenergic receptors but also partially stimulate them. This was initially believed to be an advantageous characteristic, but clinical experience has not borne

DOSAGES   Selected α-Adrenergic Blocking Drugs

Drug	Pharmacological Class	Usual Dosage Range	Indications
ergotamine tartrate-caffeine (Cafergot)	α-blocker	*Children 6–12 yr* PO tabs: 1 tab (1 mg ergotamine tartrate); repeat × 2/day; max 3 mg/day or 5 mg/wk Do not exceed 1½/day or 2½ supp/wk	Acute migraine with or without aura
		Adult PO tabs (1 mg ergotamine tartrate): 2 tab; repeat 1 tab at ½-hr intervals; do not exceed 6 mg/attack/day or 10 mg/wk	Migraine
›› phentolamine mesylate (Rogitine)	α-blocker	*Children* IV: 3 mg 1–2 hr preoperatively IM: 1 mg *Adult* IV/IM: 5 mg 1–2 hr preoperatively and repeat if necessary	Hypertension during surgery
		Adult IV: 2.5–5 mg; repeat q5 min until control	Hypertensive episodes with pheochromocytoma
		Children 0.1–0.2 mg/kg up to 10 mg diluted in 10 mL NS into extravasation site *Adult* 5–10 mg diluted in 10 mL NS injected into extravasation site within 12 hr	α-adrenergic drug extravasation
›› prazosin hydrochloride (Minipress)	α₁-blocker	*Adult* PO: 1 mg bid–tid; maintenance range 1–5 mg/day divided bid–qid; max 20 mg/day	Hypertension

IM, intramuscular; *IV*, intravenous; *NS*, normal saline; *PO*, oral.

this out. Some β-blockers also have α receptor–blocking activity, especially at higher doses; examples of these drugs include carvedilol and labetalol. Box 19-1 lists the currently available β-blockers.

Mechanism of Action and Drug Effects

Because β-blockers compete with and block norepinephrine and epinephrine at the β-adrenergic receptors located throughout the body, the β-adrenergic receptor sites can no longer be stimulated by neurotransmitters and SNS stimulation is blocked. Although β-adrenergic receptors are located throughout the body, the most important receptors in terms of the β-blocker drugs are those located on the surface of the heart, the smooth muscle of the bronchi, and the smooth muscle of blood vessels. Cardioselective β₁-blockers block the β₁-adrenergic receptors on the surface of the heart. This effect reduces myocardial stimulation, which, in turn, reduces heart rate, slows conduction through the atrioventricular (AV) node, prolongs sinoatrial (SA) node recovery, and decreases myocardial oxygen demand by decreasing myocardial contractile force (contractility). Nonselective β-blockers also have this effect on the heart, but they block β₂-adrenergic receptors on the smooth muscle of the bronchioles and blood vessels as well.

Smooth muscle also surrounds the airways or *bronchioles* in the lungs. When β₂-adrenergic receptors in the bronchioles are blocked, the smooth muscle contracts, resulting in narrowed airways. This may lead to shortness of breath. In addition, the smooth muscle

BOX 19-1

Currently Available β-Blockers

Nonselective β-Blockers

carvedilol
labetalol (Trandate)*
nadolol (Apo-Nadol)
oxprenolol hydrochloride (Trasicor)
pindolol (Visken)
propranolol hydrochloride (Inderal-LA)
sotalol hydrochloride (Rylosol)
timolol maleate

Cardioselective β-Blockers

acebutolol hydrochloride (Rhotrol, Sectral)
atenolol (Tenormin)
bisoprolol fumarate (Monocor)
esmolol hydrochloride (Brevibloc)
metoprolol tartrate (Betaloc, Lopressor)

*Blocks both α- and β-adrenergic receptors.

that surrounds blood vessels controls the size of the blood vessels and can cause them to dilate or constrict depending on whether the α_1- or β_2-adrenergic receptors are stimulated. When β_2-SNS stimulation at these smooth muscles is blocked by a β-blocker, the muscles are then stimulated by unopposed SNS activity at the α_1-adrenergic receptors, which causes them to contract. This action increases peripheral vascular resistance. Furthermore, catecholamines promote **glycogenolysis,** the production of glucose from glycogen, and mobilize glucose in response to hypoglycemia. Nonselective β-blockers impair this process and impede the secretion of insulin from the pancreas, which causes an elevation of the blood glucose level.

Finally, β-blockers can cause the release of free fatty acids from adipose tissue. This effect may result in moderately elevated blood levels of triglycerides and reduced levels of the "good cholesterol," high-density lipoproteins (HDLs).

Indications

The drug effects vary from β-blocker to β-blocker depending on the specific chemical characteristics of the drug. Some β-blockers are used primarily in the treatment of **angina,** the chest pain that results from cardiac ischemia. These β-blockers work by decreasing demand for myocardial energy and oxygen consumption, which helps shift the supply-and-demand ratio to the supply side and allows more oxygen to get to the heart muscle. This action helps relieve the pain in the heart muscle caused by the lack of oxygen.

Other β-blockers are considered **cardioprotective** because they inhibit stimulation by the circulating catecholamines. Catecholamines are released during myocardial muscle damage such as that caused by a myocardial infarction, or heart attack. When a β-blocker drug occupies myocardial β_1 receptors, circulating catecholamines molecules are prevented from binding to the receptors. Thus, the β-blockers protect the heart from being stimulated by these catecholamines, which would only further increase the heart rate and the contractile force, thereby increasing myocardial oxygen demand. Because of this characteristic, β-blockers are commonly given to patients after they have suffered a myocardial infarction to protect the heart from the stress caused by the compensatory release of catecholamines.

The β-blockers also have a profound effect on the conduction system of the heart. The AV node normally receives impulse stimulation from the SA node and slows it down so that the ventricles have time to fill before they are stimulated to contract. Conduction in the SA node, which spontaneously depolarizes at the most frequent rate, is slowed by β-blockers, which results in a decreased heart rate. The β-blockers also slow conduction through the AV node. The effects of β-blockers on the conduction system of the heart make them useful drugs in the treatment of various types of irregular heartbeats, or **dysrhythmias.** In the **Vaughan Williams classification** of antidysrhythmic drugs (see Chapter 23), all β-blockers are categorized as class II drugs, with the exception of sotalol, which has both class II and class III properties.

The ability of β-blockers to reduce SNS stimulation of the heart, including reducing heart rate and the force of myocardial contraction (systole), renders β-blockers useful in treating hypertension. Traditionally β-blockers were thought to worsen heart failure. However, recent studies have shown benefit to the use of β-blockers. Certain β-blockers, such as carvedilol and metoprolol, have produced the best results to date (see also Evidence-Informed Practice on these two drugs). The form of heart failure that includes a diastolic dysfunction component responds favourably to β-blockers.

Because of their **lipophilicity** (attraction to lipid or fat), other β-blockers (e.g., propranolol) can easily gain entry into the CNS. These β-blockers are used to treat migraine headaches. In addition, the topical application of β-blockers to the eye has been effective in treating ocular disorders such as glaucoma.

Contraindications

Contraindications of β-blockers include known drug allergies and may include uncompensated heart failure, cardiogenic shock, heart block or bradycardia, pregnancy, severe pulmonary disease, and Raynaud's disease.

Adverse Effects

The adverse effects of β-blockers are primarily extensions of their pharmacological activity. Most of these effects are mild and diminish with time. Some of the most serious undesirable effects can be caused by acute withdrawal of the drug. For example, withdrawal of a β-blocker may exacerbate the underlying angina that the drug is being used to treat or it may precipitate a myocardial infarction. The β-blockers may also mask the signs and symptoms of hypoglycemia. Adverse effects induced by β-blockers are listed by body system in Table 19-3.

Toxicity and Management of Overdose

After acute oral overdose of a β-blocker, consultation with a Poison Control Centre is recommended. The stomach should be emptied immediately by induction of emesis or by gastric lavage. Treatment consists primarily of symptomatic and supportive care. Atropine sulfate 1 to 2 mg should be given intravenously for the management of bradycardia. If the bradycardia persists despite atropine treatment, norepinephrine or dopamine may be administered. If the bradycardia still persists, placement of a transvenous heart pacemaker should be considered. For the treatment of severe hypotension, vasopressors should be titrated until the desired blood pressure and heart rate are achieved. Intravenously administered diazepam may be useful for the treatment of seizures.

EVIDENCE-INFORMED PRACTICE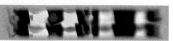

β-Blockers

Background
The β-blockers are used to lower blood pressure and heart rate in patients with heart failure. A recent 5-year longitudinal study of more than 3000 patients was reported in *Lancet* (2003). The study compared clinical outcomes for treatments with carvedilol and metoprolol in patients with chronic heart failure.

Type of Evidence
The β-blockers carvedilol and metoprolol tartrate were compared in a randomized controlled trial known as the Carvedilol or Metoprolol European Trial (COMET).

Results of Study
The median survival time was 1.4 years longer in the group taking carvedilol than in the group taking metoprolol.

Link of Evidence to Nursing Practice
This study had a large sample size of 3000 participants and its result supports the use of β-blockers in the treatment of chronic heart failure. Chronic heart failure presents many challenges for the nursing and medical professions. Four types of drugs have commonly been used to treat heart failure: diuretics, angiotensin-converting enzyme inhibitors, β-blockers, and digitalis glycosides. Most patients with chronic heart failure receive some combination of these drugs. These drugs act to lower blood pressure, and their use in the treatment of chronic heart failure has been targeted at this effect. The lower the blood pressure, the easier it is for blood to be ejected from the left ventricle to the rest of the body. Because the β-blockers lower blood pressure and heart rate, the results found for carvedilol and metoprolol continue to hold promise for patients who have this chronic, debilitating disease. Nurses must look to nursing research to further their knowledge and understanding of diseases and the related pharmacological and nonpharmacological interventions and other treatment regimens. Research findings like these can improve patient care and lead to sound, evidence-informed nursing practice.

Based on Poole-Wilson, P. A., Swedberg, K., Cleland, J., Di Lenarda, A., Hanrath, P., Komajda, M., et al. (2003). Comparison of carvedilol and metoprolol on clinical outcomes in patients with chronic heart failure in the Carvedilol or Metoprolol European Trial (COMET): Randomised controlled trial. *Lancet 362*(9377), 7–13. Riggs, J. M. (2004). New therapies for heart failure. *RN 67*(3), 29–33.

TABLE 19-3

β-Blockers: Common Adverse Effects

Body System	Adverse Effects
Cardiovascular	Atrioventricular block, bradycardia, heart failure, peripheral vascular insufficiency
Central nervous	Dizziness, mental depression, lethargy, hallucinations
Gastrointestinal	Nausea, dry mouth, vomiting, constipation, diarrhea, cramps, ischemic colitis
Hematological	Agranulocytosis, thrombocytopenia
Other	Impotence, rash, alopecia, bronchospasms, dry mouth

Glucagon may be administered for hypoglycemia. Most β-blockers are dialyzable; therefore, hemodialysis may be useful in enhancing elimination in severe overdose.

Interactions

Most of the drug interactions with β-blockers result from either the additive effects of coadministered medications with similar mechanisms of action or the antagonistic effects of drugs. Some of the common drugs that interact with β-blockers and the resulting effects are given in Table 19-4.

Dosages

For information on the recommended dosages for selected β-blockers, see the Dosages table on p. 370.

TABLE 19-4

β-Blockers: Drug Interactions

Drug	Mechanism	Result
Antacids (aluminum hydroxide type)	Decrease absorption	Decreased β-blocker activity
Antimuscarinics/anticholinergics	Antagonism	Reduced β-blocker effects
Diuretics and cardiovascular drugs	Additive effect	Additive hypotensive effects
Neuromuscular-blocking drugs	Additive effect	Prolonged neuromuscular blockade
Oral antihyperglycemic drugs	Antagonism	Decreased hypoglycemic effects

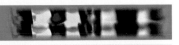

DRUG PROFILES

The β-blockers are prescription-only drugs that are available in oral preparations as tablets and capsules and in parenteral forms as intermittent injections or continuous intravenous infusions. Topically administered forms are also available. Eye drops containing a β-blocker are used in the treatment of glaucoma. Most β-blockers, except acebutolol and sotalol, are rated as pregnancy category C drugs. Acebutolol is a category D drug, and sotalol is a category B drug.

acebutolol hydrochloride

Acebutolol hydrochloride (Rhotrol, Sectral) is a cardioselective β_1-blocker used for the treatment of hypertension and the long-term management of angina pectoris. It is usually used in combination, often with a thiazide diuretic, for the additive antihypertensive effects. However, it may also be used alone as the initial drug in the treatment of hypertension. It may also be used in a multiple drug regimen including a diuretic and a vasodilator for patients with severe hypertension. The regimen has been found to be more effective than acebutolol alone. Acebutolol is one of the few β-blockers that possess intrinsic sympathomimetic activity. Its use is contraindicated in patients who have had a hypersensitivity reaction to it; in those with severe bradycardia, heart block greater than first degree, Raynaud's disease, or malignant hypertension; and in those in cardiogenic shock or heart failure. It is available orally in 100, 200, and 400 mg tablets. The commonly recommended dosages are given in the Dosages table on p. 370.

PHARMACOKINETICS

Half-Life	Onset	Peak	Duration
3–4 hr	1.5–3 hr	2.5–3.5 hr	10–24 hr

▶▶ atenolol

Atenolol (Tenormin) is a cardioselective β-blocker that is commonly used to prevent recurrence of myocardial infarctions in patients who have previously had a myocardial infarction. It is also used in the treatment of hypertension and angina. It is available in 25, 50, and 100 mg tablets for oral use. Atenolol is also available in combination with the diuretic chlorthalidone. See the Dosages table on p. 370 for the recommended dosages.

PHARMACOKINETICS

Half-Life	Onset	Peak	Duration
6–7 hr	PO: 1hr	PO: 2–4 hr	PO: 24 hr

carvedilol

Carvedilol is the newest β-blocker. It has many effects, including acting as a nonselective β-blocker, an α_1-blocker, a calcium channel blocker, and possibly as an antioxidant. Its action on β receptors is 10 times stronger than that on the α_1 receptors. It is used primarily in the treatment of mild, moderate, or severe heart failure of ischemic or nonischemic origin. Carvedilol is also beneficial in hypertension and angina pectoris. It has been shown to slow the progression of heart failure and to decrease the frequency of hospitalization in patients with mild to moderate (class II or III) heart failure. Carvedilol is most commonly added to digoxin, furosemide, and angiotensin-converting enzyme inhibitors when used to treat heart failure. It is contraindicated in patients with class IV decompensated heart failure, asthma, second- or third-degree AV block, cardiogenic shock, or severe bradycardia. It is available as 3.125, 6.25, 12.5, and 25 mg tablets. Recommended dosages are given in the Dosages table on p. 370.

PHARMACOKINETICS

Half-Life	Onset	Peak	Duration
7–10 hr	30 min	1–2.3 hr	24 hr

▶▶ esmolol hydrochloride

Esmolol hydrochloride (Brevibloc) is a potent short-acting β_1-blocker. It is used primarily in acute situations for perioperative management of tachycardia and hypertension in patients in whom there is a concern for compromised myocardial oxygen balance and for rapid control of the ventricular rate in patients with atrial fibrillation or atrial flutter. Because of its short half-life, it is given only as an intravenous infusion, and the serum levels are titrated to control the patient's symptoms. It has a rapid onset and a short duration of action. It is available in a 10 mg/mL vial and a 250 mL premixed solution for intravenous injection. Recommended dosages are given in the Dosages table on p. 370.

PHARMACOKINETICS

Half-Life	Onset	Peak	Duration
9 min	Immediate	5 min	10 min

labetalol hydrochloride

Labetalol hydrochloride (Trandate) is unusual in that it can block both α- and β-adrenergic receptors although the action of labetalol is four times greater on the β-receptors than on the α-receptors. It is used in the treatment of severe hypertension and hypertensive emergencies to quickly lower the blood pressure before permanent damage is done. It is available both for parenteral use as a 5 mg/mL intravenous injection and for oral use as 100, 200, and 300 mg tablets. The normal dosages are given in the Dosages table on p. 371.

PHARMACOKINETICS

Half-Life	Onset	Peak	Duration
6–8 hr	IV: 2–5 min	IV: 5–15 min	IV: 2–4 hr
	PO: 20–120 min	PO: 1–4 hr	PO: 8–24 hr

▶▶ metoprolol tartrate

Metoprolol tartrate (Betaloc Lopressor) is a β_1-blocker that has become popular for use in a patient following myocardial infarction. Recent studies of metoprolol have

Continued

DRUG PROFILES (cont'd)

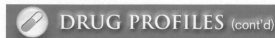

shown increased survival in patients given the drug after they had suffered a myocardial infarction. It is also used in the management of hypertension and angina pectoris. It is available for injection and orally in tablets and extended-release tablets (Lopressor SR). Commonly recommended dosages are given in the Dosages table on p. 371.

PHARMACOKINETICS

Half-Life	Onset	Peak	Duration
IV: 3–4 hr	IV: Immediate	IV: 10 min	IV: 5–8 hr
PO: 3–7 hr	PO: 1 hr	PO: 1.5–5 hr	PO: 24 hr

▶▶ *propranolol hydrochloride*

Propranolol hydrochloride (Inderal-LA) is the prototypical nonselective β_1- and β_2-blocking drug. It was one of the first β-blockers to be used. The lengthy experience using proponolol has revealed many uses for it. In addition to the indications mentioned for acebutolol, propranolol has been used in the treatment of the tachydysrhythmias associated with cardiac glycoside intoxication and for the treatment of hypertrophic subaortic stenosis, pheochromocytoma, thyrotoxicosis (excessive thyroid hormone), migraine headache, and essential tremor, as well as many other conditions. The same contraindications that apply to the cardioselective β-blockers (cited in the discussion on acebutolol) hold for propranolol as well. In addition, its use is contraindicated in patients with

bronchial asthma. It is available as an intravenous injection and orally as long-acting capsules and tablets. The recommended dosages are given in the Dosages table on p. 371.

PHARMACOKINETICS

Half-Life	Onset	Peak	Duration
2–3hr	30 min	1–1.5 hr	6–8 hr

sotalol hydrochloride

Sotalol hydrochloride (Rylosol) is a nonselective β-blocker that has potent antidysrhythmic properties. It is commonly used for the management of difficult-to-treat dysrhythmias. Often these dysrhythmias are life-threatening ventricular dysrhythmias such as sustained ventricular tachycardia. Sotalol has properties characteristic of both a class II and a class III antidysrhythmic drug (see Chapter 23), although many references list it as being one class or the other. Sotalol also has antianginal and antihypertensive properties. Because it is a nonselective β-blocker, it causes some of the adverse effects typical of these drugs, such as hypotension. It is available in oral tablet form. Commonly recommended dosages are given in the Dosages table on p. 371.

PHARMACOKINETICS

Half-Life	Onset	Peak	Duration
7–15 hr	<1 hr	2.5–4 hr	8–12 hr

DOSAGES   Selected β-Adrenergic Antagonists (β-Blockers)

Drug (Pregnancy Class)	Pharmacological Class	Usual Dosage Range	Indications
acebutolol hydrochloride (Rhotrol, Sectral) (D)	β_1-blocker	*Adult* PO: 400–800 mg/day divided bid PO: 200–600 mg/day divided bid	Hypertension Angina pectoris
▶▶ **atenolol (Tenormin) (C)**	β_1-blocker	*Adult* PO: 50–100 mg/day, taken daily PO: 50–200 mg/day divided daily or bid	Hypertension Angina pectoris
bisoprolol fumarate (Monocor) (C)	β_1-blocker	*Adult* PO: 5 mg/day; may be titrated every 2 wks up to max 20 mg/day	Mild to moderate hypertension
carvedilol (C)	α_1- and β-blocker	*Adult* PO: 3.125 mg bid; may double dose every 2 wk to highest tolerated dose, max 50 mg/day	Heart failure
▶▶ **esmolol hydrochloride (Brevibloc) (C)**	β_1-blocker	*Adult* IV: Loading dose, 0.5 mg/kg/min over 1 min, followed by 4 min maintenance of 0.05 mg/kg/min and evaluate	Atrial fibrillation and atrial flutter
		IV: Loading dose, 1.5 mg/kg over 30 sec followed by 0.15–0.3 mg/kg/min infusion	Intraoperative/postoperative tachycardia and hypertension

Continued

DOSAGES   Selected β-Adrenergic Antagonists (β-Blockers)   (cont'd)

Drug (Pregnancy Class)	Pharmacological Class	Usual Dosage Range	Indications
labetalol hydrochloride (Trandate) (C)	α- and β-blocker	**Adult** PO: 200–1200 mg/day divided bid IV: 20 mg over 2 min; additional doses of 40 mg at 10-min intervals until desired effect to max 300 mg; maintenance infusion of 2 mg/min initially and titrated to response	Hypertension Severe hypertension
▸▸metoprolol tartrate (Betaloc, Lopressor) (C)	β₁-blocker	**Adult** PO: 100–400 mg/day divided bid SR tabs: 100–400 mg/day AM IV/PO: 3 bolus injections of 5 mg at 2-min intervals followed in 15 min by 50 mg PO q6h for 48 hr; thereafter 100 mg PO bid	Hypertension angina pectoris, late myocardial infarction Early myocardial infarction
▸▸propranolol hydrochloride (Inderal, Inderal-LA) (C)	β-blocker	**Adult** PO: 80–320 mg/day divided bid–qid PO: 160–320 mg/day PO: 10–30 mg tid–qid 180–240 mg divided tid PO: 20–40 mg tid–qid PO: 40 mg/day PO: 80–160 mg/day divided PO: 60 mg/day divided × 3 days before surgery; give with α-blocker PO: 180–240 mg/day bid–qid IV: 12 mg over 1–2 min, may repeat in 2 min once	Angina pectoris, hypertension Arrhythmias Post–myocardial infarction Hypertrophic subaortic stenosis Essential tremor Migraine prophylaxis Pheochromocytoma surgery Post–myocardial infarction Life-threatening dysrhythmias
sotalol hydrochloride (Rylosol) (B)	β-blocker	**Adult** PO: 160–320 mg/day divided	Life-threatening ventricular dysrhythmias

IV, intravenous; *PO*, oral; *SR*, sustained release.

NURSING PROCESS

 Assessment

Adrenergic-blocking drugs, or sympatholytics, produce a variety of effects on the patient, depending on the type of receptor blocked. Because of the clinical impact of the adrenergic-blocking drugs, primarily on the cardiac and respiratory systems, their use requires careful assessment of the patient to minimize the adverse effects and maximize the therapeutic effects. An understanding of the basic anatomy and physiology of adrenergic receptors and their subsequent actions if stimulated or, in this case, blocked is also critical to carrying out assessment and other aspects of the nursing process and drug therapy. If an adrenergic-blocking drug is nonselective, it blocks both α- and β- (β₁- and β₂-) receptors and has blocking effects on blood vessels (α), heart rate (β₁), and bronchial smooth muscle (β₂). Therefore, if it is a nonselective drug, it will have the following actions:

- α-blocking, causing a block of the sympathetic stimulation of blood vessels (i.e., vasoconstriction); this will result in vasodilation and subsequent decrease in blood pressure.
- β₁-blocking, causing a block of the sympathetic effects on heart rate, contractility, and conduction, with resulting bradycardia, negative inotropic effects (i.e., a decrease in contractility), and a decrease in conduction; this can help in treating several types of dysfunctional irregularities in heart rate.
- β₂-blocking, causing a block of the sympathetic effects on bronchial smooth muscle and of bronchodilating effects from smooth muscle relaxation; this will result in bronchoconstriction in the lungs.

However, if the drug is α, β₁, or β₂ blocking, the resulting effect will be related to the specific receptor or combination thereof. An understanding of these basic physiological concepts helps the nurse to understand critical aspects of the administration of drugs that alter the function of the SNS (in this chapter, drugs that block sympathetic effects).

To begin a thorough assessment, the nurse should gather information about the patient's allergies and past and present medical conditions. Conducting a system overview and taking a thorough medication history should be part of this process. Some questions to pose to the patient follow on the next page:

- Are you allergic to any medications or foods?
- Do you have a history of a chronic obstructive pulmonary disease such as emphysema, asthma, or chronic bronchitis?
- Do you have a history of hypotension, cardiac dysrhythmias, bradycardia, heart failure, or any other cardiovascular disease?

These questions are important because α-blockers may precipitate hypotension, and β-blockers (β_1 and β_2) may precipitate bradycardia, hypotension, heart block, heart failure, bronchoconstriction, or increased airway resistance. Therefore, any pre-existing condition that might be exacerbated by the use of these drugs may become a contraindication or caution. For example, with β_1-blocking drugs, the nurse needs to consider the types of conditions or diseases that would be exacerbated, such as pre-existing bradycardia, decreased heart contractility, and decreased conduction. Another example is with β_2-blocking drugs, with consideration of conditions or diseases involving increased airway resistance because of the β_2-blocking effect of bronchoconstriction. It is critical to remember that these drug classes are used frequently, so adverse effects, cautions, contraindications, and drug interactions must be kept in mind.

Patients should be asked whether they are taking any drugs that could possibly interact with the adrenergic-blocking drug that has been prescribed for them. These interactions include α- and β-agonists (or stimulators). See Tables 19-1 and 19-3 for related adverse effects. See Tables 19-2 and 19-4 for drug interactions.

Nursing Diagnoses

- Ineffective tissue perfusion (cerebral and cardiovascular) related to the adverse effects of the disease of hypertension and the adverse effects of the drug (hypotension)
- Disturbed sensory perception related to the CNS adverse effects of the drug
- Risk for injury related to possible adverse effects of the adrenergic blockers (e.g., postural hypotension, numbness and tingling of the fingers and toes)
- Imbalanced nutrition, less than body requirements, because of nausea and vomiting related to the use of adrenergic blockers
- Ineffective tissue perfusion, cerebral and cardiovascular, related to adverse effects of the disease of hypertension and adverse effects of the drug
- Deficient knowledge related to lack of information about the therapeutic regimen, adverse effects, drug interactions, and precautions to be taken

Planning

Goals

- Patient will maintain and regain adequate tissue perfusion.
- Patient's perception and CNS functioning will remain intact.
- Patient will be free of injury as the result of adverse effects of the medications.
- Patient will take medication exactly as prescribed and with minimal impact on nutrition.
- Patient will experience improvement in hypertension or relief of the symptoms for which the medication was prescribed.
- Patient will remain adherent with the drug therapy regimen.
- Patient will demonstrate an adequate knowledge about the use of the specific medications, their adverse effects, and the appropriate dosing routine to be followed at home.

Outcome Criteria

- Patient states that blood pressure readings are within the normal range and that adverse effects are minimal.
- Patient reports fewer symptoms of hypertension as well as more energy and clearer thinking without profound adverse effects.
- Patient reports no adverse effects of the medications.
- Patient states the importance of both the pharmacological and nonpharmacological treatment of hypertension or other indication for the drug therapy.
- Patient states reasons for adhering to the medication therapy regimen without risking nutritional status.
- Patient reports effective blood pressure lowering or treatment with adrenergic blocker without risks and complications such as syncope, dizziness, and hypotension.
- Patient identifies community resources for monitoring blood pressure (e.g., rescue squads, fire departments).
- Patient demonstrates the correct method of self-measurement of blood pressure using a digital cuff device or using community resources.
- Patient keeps all follow-up appointments with the physician to maintain safe therapy.
- Patient states the possible conditions that the physician should be informed of immediately, such as palpitations, chest pain, insomnia, and excessive agitation.
- Patient follows instructions to avoid sudden withdrawal of hypertensive drugs in order to prevent

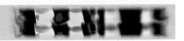

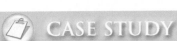 CASE STUDY

Alternative Therapies for Migraine Headaches

A 33-year-old patient has a 15-year history of migraine headaches. She wants to investigate use of natural health products and alternative therapies to prevent and treat her headaches. Her condition has improved over the last 2 years, and she is currently in excellent health. Whenever the headaches are severe, however, she still uses narcotics and antiemetics. Specifically, she takes one capsule of butalbital with aspirin and caffeine (all in one capsule) with 30 mg codeine every 4 to 6 hours as needed for headache along with a 25 mg promethazine hydrochloride oral tablet for associated nausea and prevention of vomiting. You are reviewing information about herbal and alternative therapies with her.

1 Search the Internet. What natural health products are recommended for migraine headaches?
2 In addition to or instead of specific herbal therapies, what other alternative methods may be used to treat migraine headaches?
3 What cautions should you give her about starting herbal therapies?

For answers see http://evolve.elsevier.com/Canada/Lilley/pharmacology/.

rebound hypertensive crises and experiences minimal complications.

Implementation

Several nursing interventions can maximize the therapeutic effects of adrenergic-blocking drugs and minimize their adverse effects. Thorough patient education is required to ensure adherence (see Patient Education). Patients taking α-blockers should be encouraged to change positions slowly to prevent or minimize postural hypotension. When α- or β-blockers are used, apical pulse rate (taken for 1 full minute) and both supine and standing blood pressures should be measured as ordered. Should there be any dizziness, fainting, or lightheadedness, or should blood pressure be lower than 100 mm Hg systolic or pulse rate lower than 60 beats/min, the health care provider should be contacted.

In addition, daily weight measurements are important to monitor the progress of therapy and monitor for edema, one of the adverse effects. A good rule of thumb is that if the patient has an increase of 1 kg or more over a 24-hour period or 2 kg or more within 1 week, the health care provider should be contacted. Other symptoms to be reported include muscle weakness, shortness of breath, and collection of fluid in the lower extremities as noted by difficulty in putting on shoes or socks. The nurse should make sure that the patient is weaned off these medications slowly if indicated because of the rebound hypertension or chest pain that rapid withdrawal can precipitate. The nurse should remember basic anatomy and physiology; this will always help guide nursing actions and considerations related to these drugs.

With any of the adrenergic drugs, the patient's feedback, daily journal-keeping, and adherence to therapy are critical to successful treatment and prevention of adverse effects. In addition, patient education with attention to dietary intake of potassium, fluid intake, daily weight, recording of blood pressure and pulse rates before taking doses, reporting of adverse effects (e.g., postural hypotension and bradycardia), and edema or fluid collection is crucial to patient safety and effective therapy. See Patient Education for more information.

Evaluation

Therapeutic effects for which to monitor in patients receiving adrenergic-blocking drugs include, but are not limited to, the following:

• Decrease in blood pressure, pulse rate, and palpitations in patients with these specific problems before drug therapy
• Alleviation of the symptoms of the disorder for which the drug was indicated
• Return to normal blood pressure and pulse with lowering of the blood pressure toward 120/80 mm Hg and the pulse to within normal limits (60 beats/min) in patients with diagnosed hypertension
• Decrease in chest pain in patients with angina

Patients must also be monitored for occurrence of the adverse effects of these medications, which include bradycardia, depression, fatigue, and hypotension, among others. See Tables 19-1 and 19-3 for other potential adverse effects.

PATIENT EDUCATION

❖ Patients should be educated about the therapeutic effects and adverse effects of their drug therapy.

❖ Patients should be encouraged to always have printed information about their medical conditions and medications (e.g., prescription, over-the-counter drugs, natural health products) on their persons at all times.

❖ Patients should be advised of the importance of always wearing a medical alert bracelet or necklace that identifies the specific medical diagnosis.

❖ Patients should know to update their information frequently with their health care provider, and the changes should be dated. This list could also have a place for the patient to record blood pressures by date and time so that with each visit to the physician, the medication list and blood pressure values are readily available.

❖ Patients should be informed to take medications exactly as prescribed and to never stop taking the drugs abruptly (which can result in rebound hypertension); they should instead contact their health care provider about dosage change or discontinuing any of these medications.

❖ Patients should be encouraged to avoid caffeine and other CNS stimulants while taking adrenergic-blocking drugs, to prevent excessive irritability of the cardiac and central nervous systems.

❖ Patients should be informed to avoid alcohol ingestion because it will lead to vasodilation and a higher risk of hypotension and postural hypotension.

❖ Patients should contact the physician or health care provider if they experience palpitations, chest pain, confusion, weight gain, dyspnea, nausea, or vomiting. Other problems to report include swelling in the feet and ankles, shortness of breath, excessive fatigue, dizziness, and syncope, depression, hallucinations, nightmares, and palpitations.

❖ Patients who are prescribed β-blockers must always take the medication exactly as prescribed, no more and no less, and never try to catch up with their dosing if they have missed more than one dose; in such cases, they should contact the health care provider for further instructions.

❖ Patients should be informed to change positions slowly to avoid dizziness and syncope. Exercise, exposure to heat in the environment or in a sauna, time in a tanning bed (because of greater vasodilation and a greater drop in blood pressure), and use of alcohol may lead to further vasodilation and subsequent syncope.

❖ Patients should report constipation or the development of any urinary hesitancy or bladder distention (discomfort over symphysis pubis) to the health care provider for further directions. Prevention of constipation through diet and fluids should be encouraged.

POINTS TO REMEMBER

❖ Adrenergic-blocking drugs block the stimulation of the α- and β_1- or β_2-adrenergic receptors, with a net result of blocking the effects of either norepinephrine or epinephrine on the receptor. This blocking action leads to a variety of physiological responses depending on which receptors are blocked. Knowing how these receptors work allows the nurse to understand and predict the expected therapeutic effects of the drugs as well as the expected adverse effects.

❖ With α-blockers the predominant response is vasodilation. This response is due to blocking of the α-adrenergic effect of vasoconstriction, which results in blood vessel relaxation.

❖ Vasodilation of blood vessels with the α-blockers results in a drop in blood pressure and a reduction in urinary obstruction that may lead to increased urinary flow rates. These effects need to be monitored in patients taking α-blockers.

❖ β-blockers inhibit the stimulation of β-adrenergic receptors by blocking the effects of the SNS neurotransmitters norepinephrine and epinephrine, and dopamine. Stimulation of β receptors leads to an increase in heart rate, conduction, and contractility. Blocking of β receptors thus results in a decrease in heart rate, conduction, and contractility. Stimulation of β_2-receptors results in bronchial smooth muscle relaxation, or bronchodilation. Blocking of β_2-receptors leads to a decrease in bronchial smooth muscle relaxation, or bronchoconstriction.

❖ β-blockers are classified as either selective or nonselective. Selective β-blockers are also called cardioselective β-blockers and block only the β-adrenergic receptors in the heart that are located on the postsynaptic effector cells (i.e., the cells that nerves stimulate). The beneficial effects of the cardioselective β-blockers include decreased heart rate, reduced cardiac conduction, and decreased myocardial contractility with no bronchoconstriction. These drugs are a good choice for patients with hypertension who also have bronchospastic airway disease or other pulmonary lung disease.

❖ Nonselective β-blockers block both β_1- and β_2-adrenergic receptors and affect the heart and bronchial smooth muscle. These drugs are used to treat patients with hypertension who do not have a problem with bronchospasm or pulmonary airway disease.

❖ Nursing considerations for patients taking β-blockers include teaching patients that they should avoid sudden changes in position because of possible postural hypotension and instructing patients to report rapid weight gain or a decrease in heart rate below 60 beats/min.

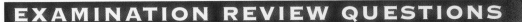

EXAMINATION REVIEW QUESTIONS

1 Which of the following will result when a patient who has experienced infiltration of a peripheral infusion of dopamine is injected with α-blocker phentolamine (Rogitine)?
  a. Local analgesia
  b. Local hypotension
  c. Local vasodilation
  d. Local vasoconstriction

2 Which of the following statements is most correct for a patient taking a β-blocker?
  a. Postural hypotension is not a problem with this drug.
  b. The drug may be discontinued without any time restraints.
  c. Weaning off the medication is necessary to prevent rebound hypertension.
  d. The patient should stop taking the medication at once with a gain of 1 to 2 kg in a week.

3 About which of the following should the nurse provide teaching to a patient who has a new prescription for β-blockers?
  a. Tachycardia
  b. Tachypnea
  c. Bradycardia
  d. Bradypnea

4 For a patient who has had a recent myocardial infarction, which of the following drugs may be prescribed for its cardioprotective effects?
  a. esmolol (Brevibloc)
  b. prazosin (Minipress)
  c. metoprolol (Lopressor)
  d. phentolamine (Rogitine)

5 Which of the following conditions should the nurse assess the patient for before initiating therapy with a nonselective β-blocker?
  a. Pancreatitis
  b. Liver disease
  c. Hypertension
  d. Chronic bronchitis

For answers see http://evolve.elsevier.com/Canada/Lilley/pharmacology/.

CRITICAL THINKING ACTIVITIES

1 Develop patient teaching plans for the use of one of the following medications:
  a. ergotamine tartrate-caffeine
  b. prazosin (Minipress)
  c. atenolol (Tenormin)

2 One of your patients, a 46-year-old mother of two adolescent children, is now taking propranolol (Inderal) for the control of tachycardia and hypertension. What should you tell her if she says, "Well, if it doesn't work after a month or two, I'll just quit taking it!"?

3 A 69-year-old man is given a new prescription for prazosin (Minipress), 1 mg twice a day. The physician asks you to be sure to be "thorough in your teaching" about this drug. What points are important when discussing this drug therapy with your patient?

For answers see http://evolve.elsevier.com/Canada/Lilley/pharmacology/.

CHAPTER 20

Cholinergic Drugs

Learning Objectives

After reading this chapter, the successful student will be able to do the following:

1 Briefly discuss the normal anatomy and physiology of the autonomic nervous system (ANS), including the events that occur during synaptic transmission in the parasympathetic division of the ANS.

2 Briefly discuss the prevalence, etiology, risk factors, and pathophysiology of Alzheimer's disease.

3 List examples of cholinergic drugs, including newer drug therapy for treating Alzheimer's disease and dementia-related conditions.

4 Discuss the mechanisms of action, therapeutic effects, indications, adverse effects, dosage amounts, and routes of administration as well as any antidotes for cholinergic drugs.

5 Develop a collaborative plan of care that includes all phases of the nursing process related to the administration of cholinergic drugs.

e-Learning Activities

Web site
(http://evolve.elsevier.com/Canada/Lilley/pharmacology/)

- Animations
- Answers to chapter questions, activities, and case studies
- Calculators and Category Catchers
- Glossary with audio pronunciations
- IV Therapy and Medication Error Checklists
- Multiple-Choice Review Question quizzes
- Nursing Care Plans
- Online Appendices and Supplements
- WebLinks

Drug Profiles

▸▸ **bethanechol (bethanechol chloride)***, p. 381
▸▸ **donepezil (donepezil hydrochloride)***, p. 382
   galantamine (galantamine hydrobromide)*, p. 382
   memantine (memantine hydrochloride)*, p. 383
▸▸ **physostigmine (physostigmine salicylate)***, p. 382
▸▸ **pyridostigmine (pyridostigmine bromide)***, p. 382
   rivastigmine (rivastigmine hydrogen tartrate)*, p. 382

▸▸ Key drug.

*Full generic name is given in parentheses. For the purposes of this text, the more common shortened name is used.

Glossary

Acetylcholine (ACh) Neurotransmitter responsible for transmission of nerve impulses to effector cells in the parasympathetic nervous system (PSNS). (p. 377)

Acetylcholinesterase (AChE) Enzyme responsible for the breakdown of ACh (also referred to simply as cholinesterase). (p. 378)

Alzheimer's disease A disease characterized by progressive mental deterioration manifested by loss of memory, ability to calculate, and visual–spatial orientations, as well as by confusion and disorientation. (p. 377)

Cholinergic drugs Drugs that stimulate the PSNS by mimicking ACh. (p. 378)

Direct-acting cholinergic agonists Drugs that bind directly to cholinergic receptors to activate them. (p. 378)

Indirect-acting cholinergic agonists Drugs that work indirectly by making more ACh available at the receptor site. (p. 378)

Irreversible cholinesterase inhibitors Drugs that form a permanent covalent bond with cholinesterase. (p. 378)

Miosis Constriction of the pupil. (p. 379)

Muscarinic receptors Effector-organ cholinergic receptors located postsynaptically in the smooth muscle, heart muscle, and glands supplied by parasympathetic fibres; so named because they can be stimulated by the alkaloid muscarine. (p. 377)

Nicotinic receptors Cholinergic receptors located in the ganglia (where presynaptic and postsynaptic nerve fibres meet) of both the PSNS and the sympathetic nervous system; so named because they can be stimulated by the alkaloid nicotine. (p. 377)

Parasympathomimetics Another name for cholinergic drugs that mimic the effects of ACh. (p. 378)

Reversible cholinesterase inhibitors Drugs that bind to cholinesterase for minutes to hours but do not form a permanent bond. (p. 378)

OVERVIEW

Cholinergics, cholinergic agonists, and *parasympathomimetics* are terms referring to the class of drugs that stimulate the parasympathetic nervous system (PSNS). For a better understanding of how these drugs work, it is helpful to know how the PSNS operates in relation to the rest of the nervous system.

PARASYMPATHETIC NERVOUS SYSTEM

The PSNS is the branch of the autonomic nervous system (ANS) with nerve functions generally opposite those of the sympathetic nervous system (SNS) (Figure 20-1). The neurotransmitter responsible for the transmission of nerve impulses to *effector cells* (cells of the target tissues or organs) in the PSNS is **acetylcholine (ACh).** A receptor that binds the ACh and mediates its actions is called a *cholinergic receptor.* There are two types of cholinergic receptors, as determined by their location and their action once stimulated. **Nicotinic receptors** are located in the ganglia of both the PSNS and SNS. They are called *nicotinic* because they can be stimulated by the alkaloid nicotine. The other cholinergic receptors are the **muscarinic receptors.** These receptors are located postsynaptically in the effector organs (i.e., smooth muscle, heart muscle, and glands) supplied by the parasympathetic fibres. They are called *muscarinic* because they are stimulated by the alkaloid muscarine, a substance isolated from mushrooms. Figure 20-2 shows how the nicotinic and muscarinic receptors are arranged in the PSNS.

ALZHEIMER'S DISEASE

Alzheimer's disease (AD) is a progressive, degenerative disease resulting in impairment of memory, judgement, and reasoning as well as language, affective, personality, and behavioural difficulties. AD is the most common form of dementia in Canada, accounting for approximately 47% of all dementias. As the Canadian population ages, the prevalence of AD is expected to rise. By 2041, the

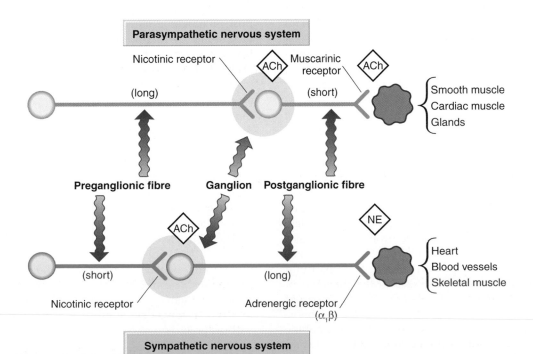

FIG. 20-1 The parasympathetic and sympathetic nervous systems and their relationships to one another. *ACh,* acetylcholine; *NE,* norepinephrine.

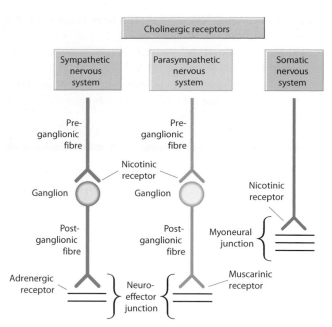

FIG. 20-2 The sympathetic, parasympathetic, and somatic nervous systems. Note the location of the nicotinic and muscarinic receptors within the parasympathetic nervous system.

proportion of the Canadian population over the age of 65 is estimated to be at 23%. Currently, the prevalence of AD among those aged 65 to 74 is 1%, among those aged 75 to 84 is 6.9%, and among those over 85 years is 26%.

The etiology and progression of AD are not well understood. Several factors have been implicated in the disease development; however, a combination of genetic, environmental, and lifestyle triggers seem probable. Four genes have been located that are associated with AD: three different autosomal dominant genes associated with early-onset AD, and the ApoE associated with late-onset AD. The ApoE gene doubles the risk of AD but it occurs in 34% to 65% of individuals with AD; however, 24% to 31% of individuals without AD also have it.

AD is characterized by two abnormalities: amyloid plaques that form between neurons and neurofibrillary tangles found in neurons. β-Amyloid (Aβ) is a general term for protein fragments that the body produces normally. β-Amyloid is a fragment of a protein snipped from another protein called *amyloid precursor protein (APP)*. In a healthy brain, these protein fragments would break down and be eliminated; however, in AD, these fragments accumulate to form hard, insoluble plaques. Neurofibrillary tangles are insoluble twisted fibres found inside brain neurons. They are made up of tau proteins, which form part of a microtubule. The microtubule assists in the transport of nutrients and other important substances from one part of the nerve cell to another. In AD, the tau protein is abnormal and clumps together, and, as a result, the microtubule structures collapse. Neurons do not function properly and eventually die. Choline acetyltransferase, a brain biochemical, is reduced by 90% in the hippocampus and in the cerebral cortex of AD patients. Choline acetyltransferase

is the catalyst for the neurotransmitter ACh, which stimulates higher brain functions of learning and memory. Other neurotransmitters have been implicated in AD; a deficiency in the neurotransmitters norepinephrine, serotonin, and somatostatin may contribute to the behavioural impairments observed in patients with AD.

As AD progresses, brain tissue shrinks. In the early stages of AD, short-term memory begins to decline when the cells in the hippocampus degenerate. As AD spreads through the cerebral cortex, judgement worsens, emotional outbursts may occur, and language is impaired. As AD advances, more nerve cells die, resulting in subsequent changes in behaviour such as wandering and agitation. In the final stages, damage is widespread and brain tissue has shrunk significantly. At this stage, those affected with AD may be unable to feed themselves, speak, recognize people, and control bodily functions. Memory worsens. Constant care is typically necessary. Generally, those with AD live for 8 to 10 years after diagnosis; however, the disease can last for as long as 20 years.

Drugs such as cholinesterase inhibitors are used in the management of AD along with efforts to manage and reduce the severity of the disease through mental stimulation, exercise, and a balanced diet.

CHOLINERGIC DRUGS

Cholinergic drugs mimic the effects of ACh and are therefore sometimes referred to as **parasympathomimetics**. These drugs can stimulate cholinergic receptors directly or indirectly. **Direct-acting cholinergic agonists** bind to cholinergic receptors and activate them. **Indirect-acting cholinergic agonists** act by stimulating postsynaptic nerve cell (neuronal) release of ACh at the receptor site, which allows the ACh to bind to and stimulate the receptor. They do this by inhibiting the action of **acetylcholinesterase (AChE)**, the enzyme responsible for breaking down ACh, which is also referred to simply as cholinesterase. The indirect-acting cholinergic drugs bind to the cholinesterase in one of two ways: reversibly or irreversibly. **Reversible cholinesterase inhibitors** bind to cholinesterase for a period of minutes to hours; **irreversible cholinesterase inhibitors** bind to cholinesterase and form a permanent covalent bond. The body must then generate new enzymes to override the effects of the irreversible drugs. Box 20-1 lists the direct- and indirect-acting cholinergics.

These drugs are used primarily to reduce intraocular pressure (IOP) in patients with glaucoma or in those undergoing ocular surgery (see Chapter 58), to treat gastrointestinal and bladder disorders, to diagnose and treat myasthenia gravis, to treat Alzheimer's disease, and to treat excessive dry mouth (xerostomia) resulting from a disorder known as *Sjögren's syndrome*.

Mechanism of Action and Drug Effects

When ACh directly binds to its receptor, stimulation occurs. Once binding takes place on the membranes of effector cells, the permeability of the cells changes and calcium and sodium are permitted to flow into the cells. This depolarizes the cell membrane and stimulates the effector organ.

The effects of direct- and indirect-acting cholinergics are those generally seen when the PSNS is stimulated. There are many mnemonics to aid in remembering these effects. One way is to think of the PSNS as the "rest-and-digest" system.

Cholinergic drugs stimulate the intestine and bladder, resulting in increased gastric secretions, gastrointestinal motility, and urinary frequency. They also stimulate the pupil to constrict, causing **miosis.** This helps decrease IOP. In addition, parasympathomimetic drugs cause increased salivation and sweating. The cardiovascular effects include decreased heart rate and vasodilation. Cholinergic drugs also cause the bronchi of the lungs to constrict and the airways to narrow.

ACh is needed for normal brain function and is in short supply in patients with Alzheimer's disease. At recommended doses, cholinergics affect primarily the muscarinic receptors, but at high doses the nicotinic receptors can also be stimulated. The desired effects come from muscarinic receptor stimulation; many of the undesirable adverse effects are due to nicotinic receptor stimulation. The effects of the cholinergic drugs are listed in Table 20-1 according to the receptors stimulated.

Indications

The majority of the direct-acting drugs (ACh, carbachol, and pilocarpine) are used topically to reduce IOP in patients with glaucoma or in those undergoing ocular surgery. They are poorly absorbed orally because they have large quaternary amines in their chemical structure. This limits their use to primarily topical application. One exception is the direct-acting cholinergic drug bethanechol chloride, which can be administered

orally. It affects primarily the detrusor muscle of the urinary bladder and the smooth muscle of the gastrointestinal tract. When given, it causes increased bladder and gastrointestinal tract tone and motility, which consequently increases the movement of contents through these areas. It also causes the sphincters in the bladder and the gastrointestinal tract to relax, which allows them to empty. Because of these effects it is used to treat atony of the bladder and gastrointestinal tract, which sometimes occurs after a surgical procedure.

Indirect-acting drugs work by increasing ACh concentrations at the receptor sites, stimulating the effector cells. They cause skeletal muscle contraction and have been shown to improve muscle strength, thus they are used for the diagnosis and treatment of myasthenia gravis. Neostigmine and pyridostigmine are the standard indirect-acting cholinergic drugs used for the symptomatic treatment of myasthenia gravis. Edrophonium is commonly used to diagnose this disorder. Their ability to inhibit cholinesterase also makes them useful for the reversal of neuromuscular blockade produced either by neuromuscular blocking agents (NMBAs) or by anticholinergic poisoning. For this reason, the indirect-acting drug physostigmine is considered the antidote for anticholinergic poisoning and poisoning by irreversible

TABLE 20-1

Cholinergic Drugs: Drug Effects

Body Tissue	Response to Stimulation	
	Muscarinic	**Nicotinic**
PULMONARY		
Bronchi (lung)	Increased secretion, constriction	None
CARDIOVASCULAR		
Blood pressure	Decreased	Increased
Blood vessels	Dilation	Constriction
Heart rate	Slowed	Increased
OCULAR		
Eye	Pupil constriction, decreased accommodation	Pupil constriction, decreased accommodation
GASTROINTESTINAL		
Motility	Increased	Increased
Sphincters	Relaxed	None
Tone	Increased	Increased
GENITOURINARY		
Motility	Increased	Increased
Sphincter	Relaxed	Relaxed
Tone	Increased	Increased
GLANDULAR SECRETIONS	Increased intestinal lacrimal, salivary, and sweat gland secretion	—
SKELETAL MUSCLE	—	Increased contraction

cholinesterase inhibitors such as organophosphates and carbonates, common classes of insecticides. Physostigmine is a restricted drug in Canada and only available through the Special Access Programme.

In the treatment of Alzheimer's disease, cholinergic drugs increase concentrations of ACh in the brain and as a result improve cholinergic function. The ability to increase ACh levels in the brain, by inhibiting cholinesterase and preventing the degradation of endogenously released ACh, increases or maintains memory and learning capabilities. Fortunately, the last two decades have seen the introduction of new medications that are specifically used to arrest or slow the progression of Alzheimer's disease. All are indirect-acting anticholinergic drugs, which means that they are inhibitors of the enzyme cholinesterase. Although their therapeutic efficacy is often limited, indirect-acting anticholinergic drugs can enhance a patient's mental status enough to

make a noticeable, if temporary, improvement in the quality of life for patients and by extension for caregivers and family members. Currently, the most commonly used of these medications is donepezil. It should be kept in mind, however, that patient response to these drugs, as with most other drug classes, is highly variable. For this reason, a failure to respond to maximally titrated doses of one of these drugs should not necessarily rule out an attempt at therapy with another (see Evidence-Informed Practice: Alzheimer's Disease and Galantamine Hydrobromide). Dosage information for all of these drugs appears in the Dosages table on p. 383.

Contraindications

Contraindications to the use of cholinergic drugs include known drug allergy, gastrointestinal or genitourinary tract obstruction (which may require surgical correction), bradycardia, defects in cardiac impulse conduction,

---

EVIDENCE-INFORMED PRACTICE

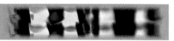

Alzheimer's Disease and Galantamine Hydrobromide

Background

The use of galantamine hydrobromide (Reminyl, Reminyl ER) to treat mild to moderate Alzheimer's disease was investigated in this particular study and found to produce improved cognitive functioning relative to a placebo after 6 months of therapy. This randomized, double-blind, parallel-group, placebo-controlled, flexible-dose study examined the "safety, tolerability, and efficacy" of treatment with Reminyl, using either the non–extended-release or extended-release (ER) dosage form. The study compared cognition and daily living skills of a group of individuals taking Reminyl with those of a group of patients receiving a placebo.

Type of Evidence

This study was conducted over a 6-month period and involved 965 patients. Patients were randomly assigned to receive at least one dose of placebo, Reminyl, or Reminyl ER. The score on the Alzheimer's Disease Cooperative Study–Activities of Daily Living Inventory was used as a secondary outcome measure. Primary outcome measures included scores on the Alzheimer's Disease Assessment Scale–cognitive subscale and the clinician's interview-based impression of change with the use of a caregiver input tool. Observed case analysis at 2, 3, and 6 months was reported.

Results of Study

Results over the 6-month period showed that most patients treated with Reminyl ER experienced "significant improvement in cognition" (including memory, orientation and language) compared with those receiving the placebo. Results of data from the group receiving Reminyl were not shown. However, at 6 months, most patients treated with Reminyl ER also showed no

significant decline from baseline in the performance of activities of daily living (ADLs) and had significantly better ADL scores (e.g., the performance of daily activities such as bathing, dressing, and eating) than those of individuals taking the placebo. It is important to remember that this study involved patients diagnosed with mild to moderate Alzheimer's disease. Treatment with Reminyl ER helped preserve cognitive and related functioning in these patients in home and community settings. This study also found the following to be adverse effects of Reminyl ER: nausea, vomiting, diarrhea, loss of appetite, and weight loss.

Link of Evidence to Nursing Practice

The patients treated with Reminyl ER showed improvement in cognitive functioning. Drug-related adverse events were identified as well. By consulting the findings of drug research and specific clinical trials, nurses remain current and well informed about new and cutting-edge treatments for a variety of diseases, including Alzheimer's disease. The nurse can apply the findings of this study regarding improved cognition and possible adverse effects to the nursing process for individual patients taking the drug to treat Alzheimer's disease. One way to link this evidence to nursing practice is in patient education about the most frequent adverse effects of Reminyl ER use, such as nausea, vomiting, diarrhea, loss of appetite, and weight loss.

Based on: Rockwood, K., Fay, S., Song, X., Macknight, C., and Gorman, M.; Video-Imaging Synthesis of Treating Alzheimer's Disease (VISTA) Investigators. (2006). Attainment of treatment goals by people with Alzheimer's disease receiving galantamine: A randomized controlled trial. *Canadian Medical Association Journal, 174(8)*, 1099–1105.

hyperthyroidism, epilepsy, hypotension, chronic obstructive pulmonary disease, and Parkinson's disease.

Adverse Effects

The primary adverse effects of cholinergic drugs are the consequence of overstimulation of the PSNS. They are extensions of the cholinergic reactions that affect many body functions. The major effects are listed by body system in Table 20-2.

Interactions

The potential drug interactions that can occur with the cholinergics are significant because of their severity. Anticholinergics (such as atropine), antihistamines, and sympathomimetics may antagonize cholinergic drugs and lead to a decreased response to them. Other cholinergic drugs may have additive effects.

TABLE 20-2

Cholinergic Drugs: Adverse Effects

Body System	Adverse Effects
Cardiovascular	Bradycardia, hypotension, conduction abnormalities (atrioventricular block and cardiac arrest)
Central nervous	Headache, dizziness, convulsions
Gastrointestinal	Abdominal cramps, increased secretions, nausea, vomiting
Respiratory	Increased bronchial secretions, bronchospasms
Other	Lacrimation, sweating, salivation, loss of ocular accommodation, miosis

Toxicity and Management of Overdose

There is little systemic absorption of topically administered cholinergic drugs and therefore little systemic toxicity. When administered locally in the eye, the cholinergics can cause temporary ocular changes such as transient blurring and dimming of vision, which can be bothersome to the patient. Systemic toxicity with topically applied cholinergics is seen most commonly when longer-acting drugs are given repeatedly over a long period. This can result in overstimulation of the PSNS and all the previously identified responses. Treatment is generally symptomatic and supportive, and the administration of a reversal drug (e.g., atropine) is rarely required.

The likelihood of toxicity is greater for cholinergics that are given orally or intravenously. The most severe consequence of an overdose is a cholinergic crisis. The symptoms of such a reaction may include circulatory collapse, hypotension, bloody diarrhea, shock, and cardiac arrest. Early signs include abdominal cramps, salivation, flushing of the skin, nausea, and vomiting. Transient syncope, transient complete heart block, dyspnea, and orthostatic hypotension may also occur. These symptoms can be reversed promptly by the administration of atropine, a cholinergic antagonist. Severe cardiovascular reactions or bronchoconstriction may be alleviated by epinephrine, an adrenergic agonist. One way of remembering the effects of cholinergic poisoning is to use the acronym SLUDGE, which stands for **s**alivation, **l**acrimation, **u**rinary incontinence, **d**iarrhea, **g**astrointestinal cramps, and **e**mesis.

Dosages

For recommended dosages of the cholinergic drugs, see the Dosages table on p. 383.

 DRUG PROFILES

As noted earlier, of the direct-acting cholinergic drugs, bethanechol, is the sole drug administered orally. A drug formulation of acetylcholine and the drug carbachol are applied topically to the eye for the treatment of glaucoma or for a reduction in IOP during ocular surgery. These drugs are discussed in greater detail in Chapter 58, as are the indirect-acting cholinergics neostigmine and pyridostigmine, which are used primarily for the treatment of eye disorders or for surgical purposes. The cholinergics are available in oral form as tablets, in topical form as eye drops and gel, and parenterally as intravenous and subcutaneous injections. The cholinergics are all prescription-only drugs.

▶▶ *bethanechol chloride*

Bethanechol chloride (Duvoid, Myotonachol) is a direct-acting cholinergic agonist that stimulates the cholinergic receptors located on the smooth muscle of the bladder. This stimulation results in increased bladder tone, increased motility, and relaxation of the sphincter of the bladder. It is used in the treatment of acute postoperative and postpartum nonobstructive urinary retention and for the management of urinary retention associated with the bladder. It has also been used to prevent and treat the adverse effects of other classes of drugs, such as bladder dysfunction induced by phenothiazine and tricyclic antidepressants. In addition, it is used in the treatment of postoperative gastrointestinal atony and gastric retention, chronic refractory heartburn, and familial dysautonomia, as well as in diagnostic testing for infantile cystic fibrosis. Bethanechol use is contraindicated in patients with hyperthyroidism, peptic ulcer, active bronchial asthma, pronounced bradycardia or hypotension, heart disease or coronary artery disease, epilepsy, and parkinsonism. It should also be avoided in patients with conditions in which the strength or integrity of the gastrointestinal tract

Continued

DRUG PROFILES (cont'd)

or bladder wall is questionable or conditions in which increased muscular activity could prove harmful, such as known or suspected mechanical obstruction. Bethanechol is available in oral-tablet formulations. Commonly recommended dosages are given in the Dosages table on p. 383.

PHARMACOKINETICS

Half-Life	Onset	Peak	Duration
Variable	30–90 min	< 30 min	1–6 hr

▶▶ physostigmine salicylate

Physostigmine salicylate is a synthetic quaternary ammonium compound that is similar in structure to other drugs in this class, including edrophonium, pyridostigmine (see next profile), and neostigmine. In Canada, physostigmine is available only under the Special Access Programme. It is an indirect-acting cholinergic drug that works by inhibiting the action of cholinesterase, the enzyme that breaks down ACh, thus allowing high levels of ACh to remain in the body. It has been shown to improve muscle strength and is therefore used in the symptomatic treatment of myasthenia gravis. It is also useful for reversing the effects of nondepolarizing neuromuscular blocking drugs (NMBAs) after surgery. It may be used in the treatment of severe tricyclic antidepressant overdoses. Its use is contraindicated in patients who have shown a hypersensitivity or had a severe cholinergic reaction to it. It should be used with caution in patients with epilepsy, bronchial asthma, bradycardia, recent coronary artery occlusion, hyperthyroidism, cardiac dysrhythmias, or peptic ulcer. It is available parenterally. Recommended dosages are given in the Dosages table on p. 383.

PHARMACOKINETICS

Half-Life	Onset	Peak	Duration
15–40 min	< 5 min	5 min	30–60 min

▶▶ pyridostigmine bromide

Pyridostigmine bromide (Mestinon, Mestinon-SR) is also a synthetic quaternary ammonium compound and is similar structurally to edrophonium and neostigmine. It is an indirect-acting cholinergic drug and is used in the symptomatic treatment of myasthenia gravis. It is also useful for reversing the effects of nondepolarizing NMBAs after surgery. Its use is contraindicated in patients who have shown a hypersensitivity or had severe cholinergic reaction to it. It should be used with caution in patients with epilepsy, bronchial asthma, bradycardia, recent coronary artery occlusion, vagotonia, hyperthyroidism, cardiac dysrhythmias, or peptic ulcer. It is available in oral form as a regular 60 mg tablet and a 180 mg extended-release tablet. It is classified as pregnancy category B. Recommended dosages are given in the Dosages table on p. 383.

PHARMACOKINETICS

Half-Life	Onset	Peak	Duration
PO: Variable	PO: 20–30 min	PO: 2–5 hr	PO: 6–12 hr

CHOLINERGIC AGONISTS USED SPECIFICALLY FOR ALZHEIMER'S DISEASE

▶▶ donepezil hydrochloride

Donepezil hydrochloride (Aricept) is an indirect-acting anticholinesterase drug that works centrally in the brain to increase levels of ACh by blocking its breakdown. It is used in the treatment of mild to moderate Alzheimer's disease. Drugs with anticholinergic properties should be avoided in patients taking donepezil because these properties may counteract the drug's effects.

Donepezil is taken once a day. It is more specific for cholinesterase in the central nervous system (CNS), which decreases the incidence of drug interactions. Donepezil is available for oral use in regular tablets and rapidly distintegrating tablets. Recommended dosages are given in the Dosages table on p. 383.

PHARMACOKINETICS

Half-Life	Onset	Peak	Duration
PO: 72–80 hr	PO: 3 wk*	PO: 3–4 hr	PO: 2 wk*

*Therapeutic effects.

galantamine hydrobromide

Galantamine hydrobromide (Reminyl) is an indirect-acting cholinergic drug. Its mechanism of action is inhibition of the enzyme cholinesterase. It is indicated for treating patients with mild to moderate dementia associated with Alzheimer's disease. Its only known contraindication is drug allergy. Reduced dosages are recommended for patients with moderate kidney or liver impairment. This drug is *not* recommended for patients with severe kidney or liver impairment. Adverse effects include nausea, vomiting, dizziness, anorexia, and syncope. This drug, along with others in its class, has been shown in some cases to alter cardiac conduction in patients with and without pre-existing cardiovascular disease. Therefore, all patients treated with galantamine, as well as with other cholinergic drugs, should be considered at risk for cardiac conduction effects. Galantamine is available for oral use. It is classified as pregnancy category B. The recommended dosage is given in the Dosages table on p. 384.

PHARMACOKINETICS

Half-Life	Onset	Peak	Duration
PO: 4–10 hr	PO: Variable*	PO: 1 hr	PO: Unknown*

*Onset and duration of drug action for this and other cholinergic drugs used for Alzheimer's dementia are difficult to quantify because both may vary significantly among patients. The practitioner should judge the therapeutic effect of these medications according to the degree of change in the patient's mental status.

rivastigmine hydrogen tartrate

Rivastigmine hydrogen tartrate (Exelon) is an indirect-acting cholinergic drug. Its mechanism of action is

Continued

DRUG PROFILES (cont'd)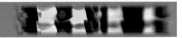

inhibition of the enzyme cholinesterase. It is indicated for the treatment of patients with mild to moderate dementia associated with Alzheimer's disease. Its only known contraindication is drug allergy to rivastigmine or other carbamate compounds. One therapeutic advantage of rivastigmine compared with some similar drugs used to treat Alzheimer's dementia is that dosage adjustments are not needed or recommended for patients with kidney or liver impairment. However, the lowest effective dosage should be used. Common adverse effects include dizziness, headache, nausea, vomiting, diarrhea, and anorexia. Rivastigmine is available in oral form. The recommended dosage is given in the Dosages table below.

PHARMACOKINETICS

Half-Life	Onset	Peak	Duration
1.5 hr	Variable*	1 hr	Unknown*

*Onset and duration of drug action for this and other cholinergic drugs used for Alzheimer dementia are difficult to quantify because both may vary significantly among patients. The practitioner should judge the therapeutic effect of these medications according to the degree of change in the patient's mental status.

MISCELLANEOUS ALZHEIMER'S DISEASE MEDICATION

memantine hydrochloride

In 2004, Health Canada approved a new medication for treating Alzheimer's disease. Memantine hydrochloride (Ebixia) is classified as an *N*-methyl d-aspartate (NMDA) receptor antagonist because of its inhibitory activity at the NMDA receptors in the CNS. Stimulation of these receptors is believed to be part of the Alzheimer disease process. Memantine blocks this stimulation and consequently helps reduce or arrest the patient's degenerative cognitive symptoms. As with all other currently available medications for Alzheimer's disease, the effects of this drug are likely to be temporary but may still provide for some improved quality of life and general functioning for some patients. Its only current contraindication is known drug allergy. No pregnancy category is currently listed. The recommended dosage is given in the Dosages table below.

PHARMACOKINETICS

Half-Life	Onset	Peak	Duration
60–80 hr	Variable	3–8 hr	Unknown

DOSAGES — Selected Cholinergic Agonist Drugs

Drug (Pregnancy Category)	Pharmacological Class	Usual Dosage Range	Indications
▸▸bethanechol chloride (Duvoid, Myotonachol) (C)	Direct-acting muscarinic	*Adult* PO: 10–50 mg tid–qid (usually start with 5–10 mg, repeating hourly until urination, max 50 mg/cycle)	Acute postoperative and postpartum (functional) urinary retention; neurogenic atony
memantine hydrochloride (Ebixia) (C)	NMBA-receptor antagonist	*Adult only* PO: Initial dose is 5 mg/day; may titrate by 5 mg/wk to max 20 mg/day	Moderate to severe Alzheimer's disease
▸▸physostigmine salicylate (C)	Anticholinesterase (indirect acting)	*Children* IM/IV: 0.01–0.03 mg/kg repeated at 5–10 min intervals until desired effect or a dose of 2 mg reached *Adult* IM/IV: 0.5–2 mg repeated q20min if needed	Reversal of anticholinergic drug effects and TCA overdose
▸▸pyridostigmine bromide (Mestinon, Mestinon-SR) (B)	Anticholinesterase (indirect acting)	*Children* PO: 7 mg/kg/day divided into 5–6 doses *Adult* PO: 60–1500 mg/day divided to provide maximum therapeutic effect SR tabs: 180–540 mg once to twice daily	Myasthenia gravis Myasthenia gravis
CURRENTLY AVAILABLE CHOLINERGIC AGONIST DRUGS SPECIFICALLY FOR TREATING ALZHEIMER'S DISEASE			
▸▸donepezil hydrochloride (Aricept) (C)	Cholinesterase inhibitor (indirect acting)	*Adult* PO: 5–10 mg/day as a single dose	Mild, moderate, severe dementia associated with Alzheimer's disease

Continued

DOSAGES	Selected Cholinergic Agonist Drugs (cont'd)		
Drug (Pregnancy Category)	Pharmacological Class	Usual Dosage Range	Indications
galantamine hydrobromide (Reminyl) (B)	Cholinesterase inhibitor (indirect acting)	*Adult* PO: 16–32 mg divided bid ER: 16–32 mg once daily in morning	Mild to moderate dementia associated with Alzheimer's disease
rivastigmine hydrogen tartrate (Exelon) (B)	Cholinesterase inhibitor (indirect acting)	*Adult* PO: 6–12 mg divided bid	Mild to moderate dementia associated with Alzheimer's disease

ER, extended release; *IM*, intramuscular; *IV*, intravenous; *NMBA*, neuromuscular blocking drug; *PO*, oral; *SR*, sustained-release; *TCA*, tricyclic antidepressant.

NURSING PROCESS

Assessment

Cholinergic drugs, or parasympathomimetics, produce a variety of effects stemming from their ability to stimulate the PSNS and mimic the action of ACh. These effects include the following:

- Decreased in heart rate
- Increase in gastrointestinal and genitourinary tone through increased contractility of the smooth muscle
- Increase in the contractility and tone of bronchial smooth muscle
- Increased respiratory secretions
- Miosis (papillary constriction)

For patients taking cholinergic drugs, a thorough head-to-toe physical assessment, nursing history, and medication history should be taken before the drugs are given. Information about patient allergies and past and present medical conditions needs to be assessed and documented prior to administration of the cholinergic drugs. Cautions, contraindications, and drug interactions also need to be identified and documented.

Before a drug for Alzheimer's disease is used, the patient must be assessed for allergies to it, other drugs, or any piperidine derivative. Because galantamine and other related drugs may cause cardiac conduction problems in patients with and without prior heart problems,

it is important to assess heart sounds, any heart problems (e.g., chest pain, irregularities), blood pressure, and pulse rate before and during therapy. Before initiation of drug therapy with donepezil, the nurse should assess and document the patient's vital signs, gastrointestinal and genitourinary history and status, mental status, mood, affect, changes in mental behaviour, depression, and level of consciousness or suicidal tendencies. Once the patient has begun taking the medication, it is critical for the nurse to continue to assess the patient's response to the drug, especially if there is no improvement within a 6-week period. At this point, the health care provider may find it necessary to adjust the dosage. The nurse should assess for the use of natural health products. Ginkgo may be used by some health care providers for organic brain syndrome (see Natural Health Products: Ginkgo). The patient must be assessed for possible medical contraindications and cautions, just as with prescription drugs. See the individual discussions earlier for information regarding other contraindications and drug interactions.

Nursing Diagnoses

- Acute pain related to the adverse effects of abdominal cramping caused by drug therapy
- Deficient knowledge of the therapeutic regimen, adverse effects, drug interactions, and precautions for cholinergic drugs
- Risk for injury related to possible adverse effects of cholinergic drugs (bradycardia and hypotension)

NATURAL HEALTH PRODUCTS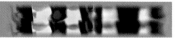

GINKGO *(Ginkgo biloba)*

Overview
The dried leaf of the ginkgo plant contains flavonoids, terpenoids, and organic acids that help ginkgo preparations exert their positive effects as an antioxidant and inhibitor of platelet aggregation.

Common Uses
Organic brain syndrome, peripheral arterial occlusive disease, vertigo, tinnitus

Adverse Effects
Stomach or intestinal upset, headache, bleeding, allergic skin reaction

Potential Drug Interactions
Aspirin, nonsteroidal anti-inflammatory drugs, warfarin, heparin, anticonvulsants, ticlopidine, clopidogrel, dipyridamole, tricyclic antidepressants

Contraindications
None

- Decreased cardiac output related to the cardiovascular adverse effects of dysrhythmias, hypotension, and bradycardia
- Disturbed sensory perception related to the adverse CNS effects of cholinergic drugs

Planning

Goals

- Patient will receive or take medications as prescribed.
- Patient will experience relief of the symptoms for which the medication was prescribed.
- Patient will remain adherent to the drug therapy regimen.
- Patient will demonstrate adequate knowledge concerning the use of the specific medication, its adverse effects, and the appropriate dosing at home.
- Patient will remain free of injury resulting from adverse effects of the medication.

Outcome Criteria

- Patient states the importance of both the pharmacological and nonpharmacological treatment of the gastrointestinal or genitourinary disorder or glaucoma in achieving good health.
- Patient states reasons for adherence to the medication therapy and the risks associated with nonadherence as well as the complications associated with overuse of the medications, such as bronchospasm, increased abdominal cramping, and decreased pulse and blood pressure.
- Patient states conditions under which to contact the physician, such as the occurrence of wheezing, bradycardia, and increased abdominal pain.
- Patient states the importance of scheduling and keeping follow-up appointments with the physician that are related to the management of the disorder for which medication has been prescribed.

Implementation

Several nursing interventions can be implemented to maximize the therapeutic effects of cholinergic drugs and minimize their adverse effects. The nurse should be sure that patients who have undergone surgery ambulate as early as possible as ordered after their procedure to help minimize or prevent gastric and urinary retention and maximize the effects of these medications. For drugs used to treat myasthenia gravis, the oral medication should be given approximately 30 minutes before meals to allow for onset of action and therapeutic effects (e.g., decreased dysphagia). The packaging inserts should always be checked for instructions concerning dilutional drugs and the route of administration. Atropine, the antidote to cholinergic overdose, should be available as necessary and per facility protocol and used only if ordered.

None of the drugs listed in this chapter is used as a "cure" for Alzheimer's disease because there is no cure. The nurse should be honest with the patient, family, significant others, and caregivers about the fact that any of these drugs are given only for symptomatic improvement and not for cure. Of course, the nurse must always adhere to the Canadian Nurses Association's *Code of Ethics*, maintain a high level of professionalism, and respect patients' rights when developing plans of care. Any sharing of information with the patient, family, significant others, and caregivers must be done with the approval of the physician, with good intent, in compliance with any research protocol, and with the goal of being a patient advocate.

When beginning any of these medications, the patient will presumably need continued assistance with activities of daily living and ambulation (because the medication may initially increase dizziness and cause gait imbalances at the initiation of treatment). The patient, family members, and caregivers also need to understand the importance of taking the medication exactly as ordered. In addition, the patient and anyone involved in the patient's daily care should be instructed about how the medication should be taken (such as the importance of taking the drug with food to decrease gastrointestinal upset); should be informed of any possible interactions, concerns, or potential for harm; and should be told the importance of *not* withdrawing the medication abruptly. The patient must be weaned off all drugs over a period of time designated by the physician because of the potential for serious complications if weaning does not occur. Most of the cholinergic agonists have dose-limiting adverse effects that include severe gastrointestinal disturbances (nausea and vomiting). Also, blood pressure readings and corresponding pulse rates should be taken and recorded before, during, and after initiation of therapy. Dizziness with therapy is not unusual and may be an indication of the need for more assistance with care and ambulation. Ataxia may also indicate the need for further assessment and intervention by the nurse and health care provider. In addition, keeping a journal of these parameters as well as information about the patient's mental status, cognition, and ability to perform activities of daily living would be helpful to all involved in the patient's care.

Dosages may be changed by the physician after about 6 weeks if no response to the medication occurs. For patient safety, when galantamine and some of the other newer drugs are used, the nurse must take blood pressure and pulse readings and have electrocardiogram baseline studies available as ordered. The patient should be encouraged to report to the health care provider any new heart distress such as new chest discomfort or palpitations. In summary, because most of the cholinergic drugs are in the group of medications used to treat patients diagnosed with Alzheimer's disease, it is important that the individuals who comprise the support systems for these patients know some of the questions that are helpful to address once a loved one is diagnosed with the disease. These questions follow on the next page:

- What should we expect for our loved one? What will happen to the person emotionally and physically?
- What treatments are available and what drugs are deemed safe? What are the common adverse effects of drug therapy? How can adverse effects be minimized?
- What about diet, fluids, and exercise for our loved one?
- Are there natural health products or over-the-counter drugs that would help with the disease, or should they be avoided in the treatment of the disease?
- What will we need to do for long-term care or other living situations for our loved one?
- What are the expected costs for this person's care now and in the future? What are the costs of drug therapy? What are other costs?
- What kind of help can we all receive emotionally? What about emotional support for our loved one?
- How can this disease affect intimate relationships?
- What type of attorney should we seek out? What about durable power of attorney and living wills? Other types of wills? Are these needed right away if we do not have these legal documents already?
- How do we all go on with our lives when our loved one is changing so drastically?
- Will our lives ever be normal again?
- What about research and clinical trials for treatment regimens? Should we pursue other treatments or do nothing new? What about drugs that are not Health Canada approved?
- How long will this process take? What can we expect over time?

Evaluation

There are several therapeutic effects that must be monitored in patients receiving cholinergic drugs. In patients with myasthenia gravis, the signs and symptoms of the disease should be decreased but may not be completely alleviated. In patients experiencing a decrease in gastrointestinal peristalsis postoperatively, there should be an increase in bowel sounds, the passage of flatus, and the occurrence of bowel movements that indicate increased gastrointestinal peristalsis. In patients who have a hypotonic bladder with urinary retention, micturition (voiding) should occur within approximately 60 minutes of the administration of bethanechol.

The nurse must also be alert to the occurrence of the adverse effects of these medications, including increased respiratory secretions, bronchospasm, nausea, vomiting, diarrhea, hypotension, bradycardia, and conduction abnormalities. For other adverse effects, see Table 20-2.

Therapeutic effects of most of the drugs used to manage Alzheimer's disease–related dementia or cognitive impairment may not occur for up to 6 weeks but include an improvement of the symptoms of the disease. Varying degrees of improvement in mood and a decrease in confusion usually occur. Adverse effects include nausea, vomiting, dizziness, and others. (See individual drug profiles for specific information.) Cardiac conductive disorders and liver dysfunction are the associated adverse effects with galantamine.

PATIENT EDUCATION

- ❖ Family, significant others, and caregivers should be encouraged to participate in the care of patients with Alzheimer's disease.
- ❖ Patients should be encouraged to take medications exactly as ordered and with meals to minimize gastrointestinal upset. They should never double up on medication if a dose has been omitted.
- ❖ Patients should be encouraged to maintain consistent time spacing of doses of medication to optimize therapeutic effects and minimize adverse effects and toxicity.
- ❖ Patients (along with family, significant others, or caregivers) should be encouraged to call the physician or other health care provider if there is any increased muscle weakness, abdominal cramps, diarrhea, dizziness, ataxia, or difficulty breathing.
- ❖ Patients should be informed that if they are taking the medication for the treatment of myasthenia gravis, signs and symptoms associated with the

disease should begin to decrease, and so there should be fewer problems with ptosis (eyelid drooping) and diplopia (double vision), less difficulty swallowing and chewing, and an improvement in muscle weakness.
- ❖ If the medication is being taken for myasthenia gravis, patients should take it 30 minutes before meals so that the drug begins to act before the patient chews and swallows. This will help with strengthening the muscles for chewing and eating.
- ❖ Patients should be taught that if they are taking a sustained-released or extended-release dosage form, it should be taken as is and not crushed, chewed, or broken in any way.
- ❖ Patients should always wear or have on their person an identification bracelet or necklace with medical diagnoses, a list of medications, and any special requirements regarding emergency treatment and allergies.

POINTS TO REMEMBER

❖ *Cholinergics, cholinergic agonists,* and *parasympathomimetics* are all appropriate terms for the class of drugs that stimulate the PSNS (the branch of the ANS that opposes the SNS).

❖ The primary neurotransmitter of the PSNS is ACh. There are two types of cholinergic receptors: nicotinic and muscarinic.

❖ Nicotinic receptors are located on preganglionic nerve fibres in the PSNS, SNS, and adrenal medulla. Muscarinic receptors are located on postsynaptic cells in muscles and glands (*not* on the nerves).

❖ Nursing considerations for the administration of cholinergic drugs include giving the drug as directed and monitoring the patient carefully for the occurrence of bradycardia, hypotension, headache, dizziness, respiratory depression, or bronchospasms.

If these occur in a patient taking cholinergics, the health care provider must be contacted immediately. Nursing considerations for the administration of drugs used to treat Alzheimer's include the following:

❖ It may take about 6 weeks for a therapeutic response to occur.

❖ Heart screening (measurement of blood pressure, postural blood pressures, electrocardiogram) and neurological screening are very important before the initiation of drug therapy.

❖ Any new or different heart adverse effects, such as new chest discomfort or palpitations, should be reported to the physician or health care provider immediately.

❖ Patients taking cholinergics should always be encouraged to change positions slowly to avoid dizziness and fainting resulting from postural hypotension.

EXAMINATION REVIEW QUESTIONS

1 A patient is taking the direct-acting cholinergic drug bethanechol chloride (Duvoid, Myotonachol) before meals. After 3 days, he calls his health care provider's office and complains of nausea and vomiting. Which of the following instructions is appropriate?
a. "If these symptoms continue, take the doses in the evening."
b. "If this continues, you can skip a dose and try it again tomorrow."
c. "Take this medication with meals to reduce gastrointestinal upset."
d. "Continue to take it on an empty stomach to reduce gastrointestinal upset."

2 The family of a patient who has recently been diagnosed with Alzheimer's disease is asking about the new drug prescribed to treat this disease. The patient's wife says, "I'm so excited that there are drugs that can cure this disease! I can't wait for him to start on it." Which of the following replies from the nurse is appropriate?
a. "These effects won't be seen for a few months."
b. "The sooner he starts on the medicine, the sooner it can have this effect."
c. "His response to this drug therapy will depend on how far along he is in the disease process."
d. "These drugs do not cure Alzheimer's disease. Let's talk about what the physician said to expect with this drug therapy."

3 When giving intravenous cholinergic drugs, the nurse must watch for symptoms of a cholinergic crisis. Which of the following is a symptom of this reaction?
a. Tinnitus
b. Hypotension
c. Hypertension
d. Peripheral tingling

4 A patient took an accidental overdose of a cholinergic drug while at home. He goes to the emergency department with severe abdominal cramping and bloody diarrhea. Which drug will the nurse expect to be used to treat this patient?
a. atropine
b. lidocaine
c. physostigmine
d. protamine sulfate

5 A patient with myasthenia gravis has received a prescription for pyridostigmine (Mestinon). Which teaching point is appropriate for this patient?
a. This drug can be given without regard to meals.
b. The drug should be taken 30 minutes after eating meals.
c. The drug should be taken 30 minutes before eating meals.
d. The drug is taken once in the mornings for maximum effect.

For answers see http://evolve.elsevier.com/Canada/Lilley/pharmacology/.

CRITICAL THINKING ACTIVITIES

1 Compare the uses for direct- or an indirect-acting parasympathomimetics and the assessment of the patients who may take these drugs.

2 Describe the symptoms of cholinergic poisoning, or cholinergic crisis, and discuss its treatment.

3 An older adult neighbour wants to take ginkgo (*Ginkgo biloba*) because he is worried about "losing it." He lives alone since being widowed last year and does not have any family members in the area. Review Natural Health Products: Ginkgo in this chapter and other sources, if desired. What would you say to him?

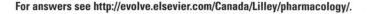

For answers see http://evolve.elsevier.com/Canada/Lilley/pharmacology/.

CHAPTER 21

Cholinergic-Blocking Drugs

Learning Objectives

After reading this chapter, the successful student will be able to do the following:

1 Describe the function of cholinergic receptors contrasting the stimulation of these receptors with the blocking of them.

2 List the drugs that are cholinergic blockers.

3 Discuss the mechanisms of action, therapeutic effects, indications, adverse and toxic effects, routes of administration, contraindications, cautions, and drug interactions of the cholinergic-blocking drugs.

4 Develop a collaborative plan of care that includes all phases of the nursing process related to the administration of the cholinergic-blocking drugs.

e-Learning Activities

Web site
(http://evolve.elsevier.com/Canada/Lilley/pharmacology/)

- Animations
- Answers to chapter questions, activities, and case studies
- Calculators and Category Catchers
- Glossary with audio pronunciations
- IV Therapy and Medication Error Checklists
- Multiple-Choice Review Question quizzes
- Nursing Care Plans
- Online Appendices and Supplements
- WebLinks

Drug Profiles

▸▸ **atropine (atropine sulfate)***, p. 391
▸▸ **benztropine (benztropine mesylate)* (see also Chapter 15)**, p. 392
▸▸ **dicyclomine (dicyclomine hydrochloride)***, p. 392
    glycopyrrolate, p. 392
    scopolamine (scopolamine hydrobromide)*, p. 392
▸▸ **tolterodine (tolterodine L-tartrate)***, p. 392

▸▸ Key drug.

*Full generic name is given in parentheses. For the purposes of this text, the more common shortened name is used.

Glossary

Anticholinergics Another name for cholinergic-blocking or anticholinergic drugs. (p. 389)

Cholinergic-blocking drugs Drugs that block the action of acetylcholine (ACh) and substances similar to ACh at receptor sites in the brain. (p. 389)

Competitive antagonists Drugs or other substances that are antagonists or that resemble an endogenous human substance (metabolite) and interfere with its function in the body, usually by competing for its receptor sites or enzymes; also called *antimetabolites*. (p. 389)

Cycloplegia Paralysis of the ocular lens (p. 389)

Mydriasis Dilation of the pupil of the eye caused by contraction of the dilator muscle of the iris. (p. 389)

OVERVIEW

Cholinergic-blocking drugs (also *cholinergic blockers*), *anticholinergics, parasympatholytics,* and *antimuscarinic drugs* are all terms that refer to the class of drugs that block or inhibit the actions of the neurotransmitter acetylcholine (ACh) at the *muscarinic receptors* in the parasympathetic nervous system (PSNS). Such drugs block the action of cholinergic nerves that transmit impulses through the release of ACh at their synapses. ACh released from a stimulated nerve fibre is then unable to bind to the receptor site and fails to produce a cholinergic effect. This explains why the cholinergic blockers are also referred to as **anticholinergics.** Blocking the parasympathetic nerves allows the sympathetic (adrenergic) nervous system (SNS) to dominate. Because of this ability, cholinergic blockers have many of the same effects as the adrenergics. Figure 21-1 illustrates the site of action of the cholinergic blockers in the PSNS.

Cholinergic blockers have many important therapeutic uses and are one of the oldest groups of therapeutic drugs. Originally they were derived from plant sources, but today these naturally occurring substances are only part of a larger group of cholinergic blockers that include both synthetic and semisynthetic drugs. Box 21-1 lists the currently available cholinergic blockers grouped according to their chemical class.

Mechanism of Action and Drug Effects

Cholinergic blockers are largely **competitive antagonists,** since they compete with ACh for binding at the muscarinic receptors of the PSNS. Once they have bound to the receptor, they inhibit nerve transmission at these receptors. This generally occurs at the neuroeffector junction of smooth muscle, heart muscle, and glands. Cholinergic blockers have little effect at the nicotinic receptors, although at high doses they can have partial blocking effects.

The major sites of action of the anticholinergics are the heart, respiratory tract, gastrointestinal tract, urinary bladder, eye, and exocrine glands. In general, the anticholinergics have effects opposite those of the cholinergics at these sites of action. The blockade of ACh by cholinergic blockers causes the pupils to dilate and

increases intraocular pressure. This can occur because the ciliary muscles and the sphincter muscle of the iris are innervated by cholinergic nerve fibres. Cholinergic blockers can, therefore, keep the sphincter muscle of the iris from contracting and allow unopposed radial muscle stimulation. The result is dilation of the pupil **(mydriasis)** and paralysis of the ocular lens **(cycloplegia)**. This can be detrimental to patients with glaucoma, however, because of the increased intraocular pressure.

In the gastrointestinal tract, cholinergic blockers cause a decrease in gastrointestinal motility, gastrointestinal secretions, and salivation. In the cardiovascular system, cholinergic blockers cause an increase in heart rate. In the genitourinary system, anticholinergics lead to decreased bladder contraction, which can result in urinary retention. In the skin they reduce sweating and in the respiratory system they dry mucous membranes and cause bronchial dilation. These and other effects are listed by body system

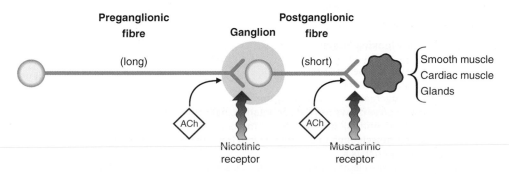

FIG. 21-1 Site of action of cholinergic blockers within the parasympathetic nervous system. *ACh,* acetylcholine.

in Table 21-1. Many of these cholinergic-blocking drugs are available in a variety of forms including intravenous, intramuscular, oral, and subcutaneous preparations.

Indications

At the level of the central nervous system (CNS), cholinergic blockers have the therapeutic effect of decreasing muscle rigidity and diminishing tremors. This is beneficial in the treatment of both Parkinson's disease (see Chapter 15) and drug-induced extrapyramidal reactions. The therapeutic cardiovascular effects of anticholinergics are related to their cholinergic-blocking effects on the heart's conduction system. At low dosages, the anticholinergics may slow the heart rate through their effects on the cardiac centre in the portion of the brain called the *medulla*. At high dosages, cholinergic blockers block the inhibitory vagal (i.e., parasympathetic or cholinergic) effects on the pacemaker cells of the sinoatrial and atrioventricular nodes, which leads to acceleration of the heart rate because of unopposed sympathetic activity. Atropine sulfate is used primarily to treat cardiovascular disorders, such as in the diagnosis of sinus node dysfunction, the treatment of patients with symptomatic second-degree atrioventricular block, and provision of advanced life support in the treatment of sinus bradycardia that is accompanied by hemodynamic compromise.

When the cholinergic stimulation of the PSNS is blocked by cholinergic blockers, the SNS effects go unopposed. In the respiratory tract, this results in decreased secretions from the nose, mouth, pharynx, and bronchi. It also causes relaxation of the smooth muscles in the bronchi and bronchioles, which results in decreased airway resistance and bronchodilation. Because of this effect, the cholinergic blockers have proved beneficial in treating exercise-induced bronchospasms, chronic bronchitis, asthma, and chronic obstructive pulmonary disease.

Gastric secretions and the smooth muscles responsible for producing gastric motility are both controlled by the PSNS, which is primarily under the control of muscarinic receptors. Cholinergic blockers antagonize these receptors, causing decreased secretions, relaxation of smooth muscle, and decreased gastrointestinal motility and peristalsis. For these reasons, cholinergic blockers are commonly used in the treatment of irritable bowel disease and gastrointestinal hypersecretory states.

The effects that anticholinergics have on the bladder make them useful in the treatment of genitourinary tract disorders such as reflex neurogenic bladder and incontinence. They relax the detrusor muscles of the bladder and increase constriction of the internal sphincter. The ability of cholinergic blockers to decrease glandular secretions also makes them potentially useful drugs for reducing gastric and pancreatic secretions in patients with acute pancreatitis. They are also used preoperatively to reduce salivary secretions, which aids in intubation and other procedures (e.g., endoscopy) involving the oral cavity.

Contraindications

Contraindications to the use of anticholinergic drugs include known drug allergy, narrow-angle glaucoma, acute asthma or other cause of respiratory distress, myasthenia gravis, acute cardiovascular instability (some exceptions were listed previously), and gastrointestinal or genitourinary tract obstruction or other acute gastrointestinal or genitourinary illness.

Adverse Effects

Many body systems are affected adversely by cholinergic blockers because of their site of action. The muscarinic receptors are located in a variety of tissues, organs, and glands throughout the body. Therefore, blockade of the muscarinic receptors by the anticholinergics produces a wide range of effects, some desirable, as described in the previous section, and some not so desirable, depending on the clinical situation. The adverse effects of cholinergic blockers are listed by body system in Table 21-2.

Other factors contributing to the wide variety of possible adverse effects of cholinergic blockers are the relative affinity of the muscarinic receptors for specific drugs and the drug dosage. Certain patient populations are also more susceptible to the effects of these drugs.

TABLE 21-1

Cholinergic Blockers: Drug Effects

Body System	Cholinergic-Blocking Effects
Cardiovascular	Small doses: decrease heart rate Large doses: increase heart rate
Central nervous	Small doses: decrease muscle rigidity and tremors Large doses: cause drowsiness, disorientation, hallucinations
Eye	Dilate pupils (mydriasis), decrease accommodation by paralyzing ciliary muscles (cycloplegia)
Gastrointestinal	Relax smooth muscle tone of gastrointestinal tract, decrease intestinal and gastric secretions, decrease motility and peristalsis
Genitourinary	Relax detrusor muscle of bladder, increase constriction of internal sphincter; these two effects may result in urinary retention
Glandular	Decrease bronchial secretions, salivation, sweating
Respiratory	Decrease bronchial secretions, dilate bronchial airways

TABLE 21-2

Cholinergic Blockers: Adverse Effects

Body System	Cholinergic-Blocking Effects
Cardiovascular	Increased heart rate, dysrhythmias
Central nervous	Central nervous system excitation, restlessness, irritability, disorientation, hallucinations, delirium
Eye	Dilated pupils, decreased visual accommodation, increased intraocular pressure
Gastrointestinal	Decreased salivation, gastric secretions, motility
Genitourinary	Urinary retention
Glandular	Decreased sweating
Respiratory	Decreased bronchial secretions

These groups include infants, older adults, fair-skinned children with Down syndrome, and children with spastic paralysis or brain damage.

Interactions

The potential drug interactions that can occur with cholinergic blockers are significant and often involve additive or synergistic drug effects. Knowledge of the broad categories of drugs that should not be coadministered with cholinergic blockers can help prevent potentially serious consequences. Additive cholinergic effects occur when antihistamines, phenothiazines, tricyclic antidepressants (TCAs), and monoamine oxidase inhibitors (MAOIs) are given with cholinergic blockers.

Toxicity and Management of Overdose

The dosage of cholinergic blockers is particularly important because there is a relatively small difference between therapeutic and toxic doses. Drugs with this characteristic are commonly referred to as having a narrow therapeutic index. The treatment of cholinergic blocker overdose consists of symptomatic and supportive therapy. Consultation with a Poison Control Centre is recommended. The patient should be hospitalized and close, continuous monitoring, including continuous electrocardiogram (ECG) monitoring, should be initiated. The stomach should be emptied by whichever means is most appropriate, usually through lavage. Activated charcoal has proven to be effective in removing unabsorbed drug from the gastrointestinal tract.

Fluid therapy and other standard measures used for the treatment of shock should be instituted as needed. Delirium, hallucinations, coma, and cardiac dysrhythmias respond favourably to physostigmine treatment. Its routine use as an antidote for cholinergic blocker overdose is controversial, however, and it is available in Canada only under the Special Access Programme. It has the potential to produce severe adverse effects such as seizures and cardiac asystole and should therefore be reserved for the treatment of patients who show extreme delirium or agitation or who could inflict injury on themselves.

Dosages

For the recommended dosages of selected cholinergic blockers, see the Dosages table on p. 393.

DRUG PROFILES

Among the oldest and best known naturally occurring cholinergic blockers are the belladonna alkaloids. It is the belladonna alkaloid contained in the anticholinergic drugs that is responsible for their therapeutic effects. Of these, atropine is the prototypical drug; it has been in use for hundreds of years and continues to be widely administered because of its effectiveness. Besides atropine, scopolamine is the other major naturally occurring drug. These drugs come from a variety of plants within the potato family *(Solanaceae)*. Some examples are *Atropa belladonna* (deadly nightshade), *Hyoscyamus niger* (henbane), and *Datura stramonium* (jimsonweed or thorn apple).

Many of the semisynthetic and synthetic cholinergic blockers are therapeutically useful drugs. They are used in the treatment of a variety of illnesses and conditions ranging from irritable bowel syndrome to the symptoms of the common cold and are also administered preoperatively to dry up secretions. The cholinergic blockers are the synthetic derivatives of the plant-derived belladonna alkaloids and are generally more specific in binding predominantly with muscarinic receptors. They may also be associated with fewer adverse effects.

▸▸ atropine sulfate

Atropine sulfate is a naturally occurring antimuscarinic. It may be prepared synthetically but is usually obtained by extraction from members of the *Solanaceae* family of plants (which includes deadly nightshade or jimsonweed, as noted earlier). In general, atropine is more potent than scopolamine in its cholinergic-blocking effects on the heart and in its effects on the smooth muscles of the bronchi and intestines. Atropine is effective in the treatment of many of the conditions listed in the Indications section. It is also used preoperatively to reduce salivation and gastrointestinal secretions, as is glycopyrrolate. Its use is contraindicated in patients with angle-closure glaucoma, adhesions between the iris and lens, certain types of asthma (not cholinergic associated), advanced liver or kidney dysfunction, hiatal hernia associated with reflux esophagitis, intestinal atony, obstructive gastrointestinal or genitourinary conditions, and severe ulcerative colitis and toxic megacolon. It is available as a parenteral injection in several concentrations, as well as ophthalmic preparations (Chapter 58). The recommended dosages are given in the Dosages table on p. 393.

Continued

DRUG PROFILES (cont'd)

PHARMACOKINETICS

Half-Life	Onset	Peak	Duration
IV: 2.5 hr	IV: Immediate	IV: 2–4 min	IV: 4–6 hr

‣ *benztropine mesylate*

For a discussion of benztropine mesylate, see the Drug Profiles section on p. 279 in Chapter 15.

‣ *dicyclomine hydrochloride*

Dicyclomine hydrochloride (Bentylol) is a synthetic antispasmodic cholinergic blocker used primarily in the treatment of functional disturbances of gastrointestinal motility such as irritable bowel syndrome and spastic constipation. It has also been used for the treatment of colic and enterocolitis in infants. It is most commonly administered in oral form as either a 10 or 20 mg tablet. It is also available as orally administered syrup at a strength of 10 mg/5 mL. As a parenteral preparation, it is available as a 10 mg/mL intramuscular injection. Intravenous administration is not recommended. Use of the drug is contraindicated in infants less than 6 months of age, patients who have a known hypersensitivity to anticholinergics, and those with obstructive uropathy, gastrointestinal tract obstruction, myasthenia gravis, paralytic ileus and intestinal atony, severe ulcerative colitis, reflux esophagitis, glaucoma, or unstable cardiovascular status. The recommended dosages can be found in the Dosages table on p. 393.

PHARMACOKINETICS

Half-Life	Onset	Peak	Duration
9–10 hr	1–2 hr	1–1.5 hr	3–4 hr

glycopyrrolate

Glycopyrrolate is a synthetic antimuscarinic drug that blocks receptor sites in the autonomic nervous system that controls the production of secretions and the concentration of free acids in the stomach. It is most commonly used as a preoperative medication to reduce salivation and excessive secretions in the respiratory and gastrointestinal tracts. It is also used in the management of gastrointestinal disorders when oral medication is not tolerated or rapid cholinergic effect is required. Its use is contraindicated in patients who are hypersensitive to it and in those with glaucoma, myasthenia gravis, gastrointestinal or genitourinary obstruction, paralytic ileus, or intestinal atony as well as in the older adult or in debilitated patients with chronic lung disease, severe ulcerative colitis, liver or kidney disease, toxic megacolon, tachycardia, or unstable cardiovascular status in acute hemorrhage. Glycopyrrolate is available parenterally as a 0.2 mg/mL intramuscular or intravenous injection. The normal recommended dosages are given in the Dosages table on p. 393.

PHARMACOKINETICS

Half-Life	Onset	Peak	Duration
Variable	IV: 1 min	IV: 10–15 min	IV: 4 hr
	IM: 20–40 min	IM: 30–45 min	IM: 4–6 hr

scopolamine hydrobromide

Scopolamine hydrobromide (Transderm-V) is another naturally occurring cholinergic blocker and one of the principal belladonna alkaloids. It appears to be the most potent antimuscarinic for the prevention of motion sickness. Although its mechanism of action in the CNS is not well understood, it is believed to prevent motion-induced nausea by correcting the imbalance between ACh and norepinephrine in the higher centres in the brain, particularly in the vomiting centre, that is responsible for the symptoms of motion sickness. Ipratropium, a derivative of scopolamine, has potent effects on the lungs and is discussed in Chapters 36 and 37. Scopolamine is available in several different delivery systems that make it useful for various indications. For the prevention of motion sickness, it is available in a convenient transdermal delivery system, a patch that can be applied just behind the ear 12 hours before the antiemetic effect is required. The patch provides protection for 3 days. It is also available in two parenteral formulations for injection by various routes: intravenous, intramuscular, and subcutaneous. The transdermal patch (Transderm-V) is available by prescription. The contraindications that apply to atropine apply to scopolamine as well. The recommended dosages for various indications can be found in the Dosages table on p. 393.

PHARMACOKINETICS

Half-Life	Onset	Peak	Duration
Variable	IV: 30–60 min	IV: 30–45 min	IV: 4 hr
	Patch: 4–5 hr	Patch: 12 hr	Patch: 72 hr

‣ *tolterodine L-tartrate*

Tolterodine L-tartrate (Detrol, Detrol LA) is a relatively new muscarinic receptor blocker now being widely promoted for treatment of urinary frequency, urgency, and urge incontinence caused by bladder (detrusor) overactivity. Another, much older drug that is commonly used to treat these conditions is oxybutynin, which is also one of the most commonly prescribed. Other drugs used include hyoscine butylbromide (Buscopan), flavoxate hydrochloride, and the tricyclic antidepressant imipramine. The newest drug for this purpose is solifenacin (Vesicare). These drugs are less commonly used than tolterodine because of their antimuscarinic adverse effects, particularly dry mouth. Tolterodine appears to be associated with a much lower incidence of dry mouth, in part because of its pharmacological specificity for the bladder instead of the salivary glands.

Tolterodine should not be used in patients with narrow-angle glaucoma or urinary retention. Patients with markedly decreased liver function or poor metabolizers taking drugs that inhibit cytochrome P450 enzyme 3A4 (CYP3A4), such as erythromycin or ketoconazole, should begin with 1 mg twice a day rather than the recommended dose of 2 mg twice a day. It is available as 1 and 2 mg tablets. Recommended dosages are given in the Dosages table on p. 393.

PHARMACOKINETICS

Half-Life	Onset	Peak	Duration
2–4 hr	1 hr	1–2 hr	5 hr

DOSAGES   Selected Cholinergic Blocking (Anticholinergic) Drugs

Drug (Pregnancy Category)	Pharmacological Class	Usual Dosage Range	Indications
▸▸atropine sulfate (C)	Anticholinergic	*Infants and Children* IM/SC: 0.01–0.02 mg/kg/dose 30–60 min preoperative (minimum, 0.1 mg/dose; maximum 0.6 mg/dose) IV/endotracheal tube: 0.01–0.02 mg/kg/dose; max 5 mg IV: 0.02–0.05 mg/kg initial dose q10–20 min until effect, then q1–4hr × 24 hr Inhalation: 0.03–0.05 mg/kg/dose in 3–5 mL NS tid–qid; max 2.5 mg/dose	Preoperative (for secretion control), therapeutic anticholinergic effect Treatment of bradycardia Antidote to organophosphate poisoning (e.g., insecticides) Bronchospasm
		Adult IM: 1 mg IV: 0.5–1 mg every 3–5 min to 0.03–0.04 mg/kg IM/IV: 1–2 mg/dose, repeat q 5–60 min until disappearance of muscarinic symptoms; continue until definite improvement Inhalation: 0.025 mg/kg/dose in 3–5 mL NS tid–qid; max 2.5 mg/dose	Hypotonic gastrointestinal radiography Treatment of bradycardia Antidote to organophosphate poisoning (e.g., insecticides) Bronchospasm
▸▸dicyclomine hydrochloride (Bentylol) (B)		*Children* PO: 5–10 mg tid–qid *Adult* PO: 80–160 mg/day divided tid–qid	Irritable bowel syndrome
glycopyrrolate (B)		*Children* IV: 0.005 mg/kg, may repeat q 2–3 min prn; max 0.1 mg/dose IM: 0.005 mg/kg *Adult* IV: 0.1 mg; may repeat q 2–3 min prn IM: 0.005 mg/kg 30–60 min preoperative *Adult and children* IM/IV: 0.2 mg for each 1 mg of neostigmine or 5 mg of pyridostigmine IM/IV: 0.1–0.2 mg tid–qid	Intraoperative control of secretions Preoperative for control of secretions Intraoperative control of secretions Preoperative control of secretions Reversal of neuromuscular blockade Gastrointestinal disorders
oxybutynin chloride (Ditropan, Ditropan XL) (C)		*Adult* PO: 5 mg bid–qid *Adult only* PO ER tab: 5–30 mg/day as single or divided doses *Children over 5 yr* PO: 5 mg bid–tid	Antispasmodic for neurogenic bladder (e.g., following spinal cord injury), overactive bladder
oxybutynin (Oxytrol) (C)		*Adult* Transdermal: 3.9 mg/day applied twice weekly	Treatment of overactive bladder; urgency; frequency
scopolamine hydrobromide (Transderm-V) (C)		*Children* IM/IV/SC: 0.006 mg/kg/dose *Adult* IM/IV/SC: 0.3–0.6 mg; may repeat 3–4/day Transdermal patch: 1.5 mg patch behind ear q3days (delivers approx 1 mg scopolamine over 3 days); apply at least 12 hr before transportation	Preoperative control of secretions Preoperative control of secretions Motion sickness
solifenacin succinate (Vesicare) (C)		*Adult* PO: 5–10 mg daily	Treatment of overactive bladder
▸▸tolterodine L-tartrate (Detrol, Detrol LA) (C)		*Adult* PO: 1–2 mg bid PO ER cap: 2–4 mg daily	Treatment of overactive bladder

ER, extended release; *IM*, intramuscular; *IV*, intravenous; *NS*, normal saline; *PO*, oral; *SC*, subcutaneous.

NURSING PROCESS

Assessment

Anticholinergic drugs (parasympatholytics or cholinergic antagonists or blockers) produce a number of effects that result from the blocking of cholinergic receptors. Because of the variety of effects at different body sites (e.g., smooth muscle relaxation, decreased glandular secretion, mydriasis), the nurse must take a complete medical and medication history and perform a thorough head-to-toe assessment to help identify these contraindications or cautions to the use of the drugs. Drug interactions should also be noted. The head-to-toe assessment will also help in documenting baseline findings and providing data for evaluating drug effectiveness. Cautions, contra-indications, and drug interactions have been presented in the pharmacology section. Lifespan considerations for the older adult include increased susceptibility to the adverse effects of confusion, delirium, constipation, blurred vision, and tachycardia; thus the older adult requires more careful assessment and monitoring. See Special Populations: The Older Adult for the care of the older adult with an overactive bladder.

Nursing Diagnoses

- Ineffective tissue perfusion (cardiopulmonary) related to drug-induced tachycardia

- Risk for injury related to possible excessive CNS stimulation and adverse effects resulting in tremors, confusion, sedation, and amnesia
- Constipation related to adverse effects of anticholinergic (cholinergic-blocking) drugs
- Impaired gas exchange related to thickened respiratory secretions from adverse effects of the drug
- Urinary retention related to loss of bladder tone from adverse effects of the drug.
- Risk for injury related to decreased sweating and loss of normal heat-regulating mechanisms (especially in the older adult and in those who engage in excessive exercise or who are in high environmental temperatures) and possible heat stroke due to effects of the drug on the temperature-regulating mechanisms
- Risk for falls related to changes in vision related to the mydriatic (pupil dilating) effects of the medication
- Deficient knowledge related to the lack of information about the therapeutic regimen, adverse effects, drug interactions, and precautions for the use of anticholinergic drugs.

Planning

Goals

- Patient will self-administer medications as prescribed.
- Patient will experience relief of symptoms for which the medication was prescribed.
- Patient will remain adherent to the drug therapy regimen.

SPECIAL POPULATIONS: THE OLDER ADULT

Overactive Bladder

Overactive bladder is estimated to affect approximately 1 in 5 Canadians over the age of 35, and the incidence increases with age.

Some questions to pose to the older adult about this condition include the following:
- Do you suddenly experience a strong urge to urinate?
- Do you urinate more than eight times within a 24-hour period?
- Do you have to get up more than two times during the night to urinate?
- Do you have "wetting" accidents?
- Are these "wetting" accidents related to the uncontrollable urge to urinate?

If the patient answers "yes" to some of these questions, the patient should be encouraged to contact the patient's primary health care provider. A referral to a urologist may or may not be necessary.

Various treatments are available in Canada. Some of these drug treatments have been presented in this chapter; one other drug (released in 2006) is a different option for men and women experiencing the symptoms

of overactive bladder. Solifenacin succinate (Vesicare) is taken once daily and treats all of the major symptoms of overactive bladder, including urgency, frequency, and urge-related incontinence.

Solifenacin succinate was found to reduce the number of incontinence episodes over 12 weeks in studies of the drug involving more than 3000 patients with overactive bladder symptoms; 5 to 10 mg dosing of the drug produced alleviation of all of the major symptoms. Use of this drug is contraindicated in patients with glaucoma, certain gastrointestinal or genitourinary tract problems, severe constipation, or urinary retention. Adverse effects include dry mouth, constipation, and blurred vision. If a patient experiences severe abdominal pain or is constipated for 3 or more days, the patient should contact his or her health care provider immediately.

Modified from http://myWebMD.com/content/tools/1/quiz/_over-active_bladder.htm, http://www.astellas.com/ca/en/urology_vesi-care_info.html; and Kosier, J. H., Combest, W., & Newton, M. (2006). Medication minute. Solifenacin succinate (VESIcare): Overactive bladder therapy. *Urologic Nursing, 26*(6), 496–497.

- Patient will demonstrate adequate knowledge about the use of the specific medications, adverse effects, and appropriate dosing at home.
- Patient will be injury-free from adverse effects from the medication.

■ Outcome Criteria

- Patient states the rationale for the use of cholinergic blockers in preoperative preparation, such as decreasing the risk of complications associated with anesthesia.
- Patient states the importance of adherence to the medication regimen, such as avoiding complications of Parkinson's disease.
- Patient states the importance of taking the medication as prescribed and not suddenly withdrawing the medication because of the risk of increasing adverse effects.
- Patient states the adverse effects that the physician should be notified of immediately if they occur (e.g., palpitations, dysrhythmias, chest pain).
- Patient keeps follow-up appointments with the physician to avoid the adverse effects of complications from treatment or nonadherence to the drug regimen.

▨ Implementation

A preventive focus for nursing care is important to the effective use of cholinergic-blocking drugs, especially with regard to patient teaching about how to possibly decrease the need for cholinergic-blocking drugs. There are several nursing interventions that may also maximize the therapeutic effects of anticholinergics and minimize the adverse effects, such as giving the drug on time and according to the physician's order. For example, solifenacin (Vesicare) should be taken exactly as directed, and patients should be encouraged to contact their health care provider if symptoms do not improve. See Patient Education for more information.

Because drugs such as atropine and glycopyrrolate are compatible with some of the commonly used preoperative medications such as meperidine and morphine, they may be used in combination with these drugs and mixed in the same syringe for parenteral, preanesthetic medication. Whenever several medications are mixed together in one syringe, doses must always be calculated carefully and compatibilities always double-checked carefully. When administering an anticholinergic ophthalmic solution, the nurse must always check the concentration of medication and apply pressure (i.e., for 15 to 30 seconds) with a tissue to the inner canthus of the eye. This helps minimize the possibility of systemic absorption of the drug. Atropine may be combined with other cholinergic-blocking drugs (e.g., hyoscyamine) for treatment of lower urinary tract discomfort. This combination decreases genitourinary spasms and genitourinary hypermotility.

When a cholinergic-blocking drug is used to treat urinary tract disorders or dysfunction, the patient needs to be aware of the importance of taking the drug exactly as ordered, which may be up to four times a day, depending on the drug. In addition, in patients with altered kidney or liver function, the dose or frequency of dosing of oxybutynin may need to be decreased because of the potential for toxicity. If anticholinergic drugs are taken at the same time as a CYP3A4 inhibitor (e.g., erythromycin), the possibility of complications exists. Oxybutynin should be taken as directed with fluids 1 hour before or 2 hours after meals, if tolerated. Tolterodine should be taken as directed and with food. Also associated with the cholinergic-blocking drugs are the adverse effects of constipation and inability to sweat or perspire. See Patient Education for more information on these specific drugs.

▨ Evaluation

Monitoring goals and outcome criteria should be a starting place for effective evaluation of therapy with these medications. In particular, therapeutic effects for cholinergic-blocking drugs include the following:

- For Parkinson's disease, patients experience improved ability to carry out the activities of daily living and fewer problems with tremors, salivation, and drooling.
- For relief of gastrointestinal symptoms such as hyperacidity, patients report improved comfort and a decrease in symptoms of abdominal pain, nausea, vomiting, and heartburn.
- For urological problems, patients show an improvement in urinary patterns with less hypermotility and increased time between voiding.
- In preoperative situations, patients experience fewer bronchospasms with induction of anesthesia and fewer problems with secretions because the cholinergic blockers (anticholinergic drugs) dry out secretions, making them viscous.

The nurse must also monitor the patient for the occurrence of adverse effects such as constipation, tachycardia, tremors, confusion, hallucinations, CNS depression (which occurs with large dosages of atropine), sedation, urinary retention, hot and dry skin, and fever. Toxicity associated with cholinergic-blocking drugs includes possible CNS depression, with confusion and hallucinations, and cardiovascular stimulation, with severe tachycardia and palpitations.

PATIENT EDUCATION

- Patients should be encouraged to take the drug exactly as prescribed and to take the exact amount to prevent overdosage, which could cause life-threatening problems, especially in the cardiovascular and central nervous systems.
- Patients should be taught to practise regular oral hygiene with brushing of teeth twice daily and flossing. They can minimize the adverse effect of dry mouth through maintaining a high fluid intake (if not contraindicated), using artificial saliva drops or gum, and sucking on sugar-free hard candy as needed. Regularly scheduled dental visits should be encouraged because of the association between dry mouth and dental caries or gum disease.
- Patients should be encouraged to exercise care when first taking the medications and to be cautious when engaging in activities such as driving a car or operating machinery because of the blurred vision that commonly occurs with cholinergic-blocking drugs.
- Patients should be informed of the adverse effect of increased sensitivity to light. Wearing dark or tinted glasses or sunglasses is encouraged.
- Patients should be encouraged to consult their health care provider before taking any other medications, including prescription drugs, over-the-counter medications, or natural health products.

- The older adult or patients taking higher dosages of these medications should be informed that the risk of experiencing heat stroke or hyperthermia is increased because of the drug's interference with the normal heat-regulating mechanisms. The older adult should be educated on how to prevent these problems (e.g., stay in a cool or shaded environment if outside in warm temperatures, wear protective clothing and hats or caps, take fluids regularly, avoid excessive heat and strenuous exercise in warm environments, and avoid saunas or hot tubs). In addition, fans, air conditioners, and adequate ventilation may help prevent overheating.
- Patients should be encouraged to contact the health care provider if they experience urinary hesitancy or retention, constipation, palpitations, tremors, confusion, sedation, amnesia, excessive dry mouth (especially if the patient has a chronic lung infection or other chronic lung disease), fever, alterations in gait, excessive dizziness, or difficulty urinating.
- Patients should be informed that anticholinergic-related constipation may be managed with increased bulk and fibre by dietary intake or the use of over-the-counter fibre-containing supplements (as ordered) and fluids.

POINTS TO REMEMBER

- *Cholinergic blockers, anticholinergics, parasympatholytics,* and *antimuscarinics* are all terms that refer to the drugs that block or inhibit the actions of acetylcholine (ACh) in the PSNS.
- The use of the cholinergic blockers allows the SNS to dominate. They are classified chemically as natural, semisynthetic, and synthetic anticholinergics. Anticholinergics may be competitive antagonists (blockers) and compete with ACh at the muscarinic

receptors. In high dosages, they result in partial blocking actions at nicotinic receptors. Anticholinergics bind to and block ACh at muscarinic receptors located on the cells stimulated by the parasympathetic nerve.
- The nurse should assess for possible contraindications such as benign prostatic hypertrophy, glaucoma, tachycardia, myocardial infarction, heart failure, and hiatal hernia.

EXAMINATION REVIEW QUESTIONS

1 Which of the following points should the nurse remind the older adult of when taking anticholinergics?
a. Avoid exposure to high temperatures.
b. Limit liquid intake to avoid fluid overload.
c. Begin an exercise program to avoid adverse effects.
d. Stop the medication if excessive dryness of the mouth occurs.

2 Which of the following are contraindications to the use of anticholinergics?
a. Chronic bronchitis
b. Peptic ulcer disease
c. Irritable bowel syndrome
d. Benign prostatic hypertrophy (BPH)

3 Which of the following are adverse effects associated with the use of cholinergic blockers?
a. Diarrhea
b. Dry mouth
c. Diaphoresis
d. Decreased sensorium

4 Which of the following effects will the nurse administering a cholinergic-blocking drug expect to see?
a. Miosis
b. Increased muscle rigidity
c. Increased bronchial secretions
d. Decreased gastrointestinal motility and peristalsis

5 During the assessment of a patient about to receive a cholinergic-blocking drug, the nurse should determine whether the patient is taking any drugs that may potentially interact with the anticholinergic. Which of the following drugs might these include?
a. Antibiotics, such as penicillin
b. Narcotics, such as morphine sulfate
c. Tricyclic antidepressants, such as amitriptyline
d. Anticonvulsants, such as phenobarbital

For answers see http://evolve.elsevier.com/Canada/Lilley/pharmacology/.

CRITICAL THINKING ACTIVITIES

1 The nurse is preparing to administer preoperative medications to a 75-year-old woman who is undergoing minor surgery. She has a history of smoking, heart failure, and glaucoma. Why should the nurse not administer the ordered atropine preoperatively to this patient? Explain the rationale for contacting the physician about this drug interaction and your subsequent action.

2 The nurse is caring for a patient who has just experienced a cardiac arrest while in the intensive care unit. The patient has a second-degree heart block and sinus bradycardia with a heart rate of 30 beats/min and has lost consciousness. The nurse determines that the cholinergic blocker _____ should be given to _____ the heart rate. (*Choose two responses*)
a. dicyclomine
b. tolterodine
c. atropine
d. increase
e. decrease

3 You are on a deep-sea fishing trip with friends. One of the participants shows you the patch she is wearing because she gets "terribly seasick." She tells you that she has never used this patch before but that her friends recommended that she try it. After 3 hours, you notice that she is very restless and irritable. What drug do you think is contained in this patch? Are these expected adverse effects or a worse problem? Explain.

4 In preparation for emergency surgery, the preoperative order was to give 0.5 mg of atropine to your patient intravenously. The vial concentration is 1 mg/mL. In the haste of this emergency situation, 5 mL of the atropine solution is given. How many milligrams of atropine were given to your patient? What effects can you expect to see? What treatment will you expect to be ordered for this problem?

5 What are the advantages of the synthetic derivatives over the natural belladonna alkaloids?

For answers see http://evolve.elsevier.com/Canada/Lilley/pharmacology/.

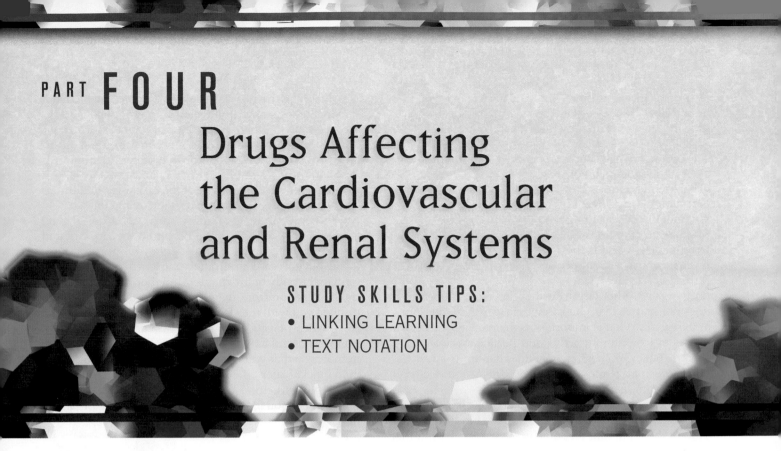

Drugs Affecting the Cardiovascular and Renal Systems

STUDY SKILLS TIPS:
- LINKING LEARNING
- TEXT NOTATION

LINKING LEARNING

The Part Three Study Skills Tips stressed the importance of planning for the part as a whole. With that in mind, what is the focus of Part Four? The part title is "Drugs Affecting the Cardiovascular and Renal Systems." What is the first question you think you should ask about this part? You might begin by asking, "What are cardiovascular and renal systems?" This is an obvious question and might seem to be so basic that it need not be asked, but the next eight chapters will all develop around this part title. Asking the obvious question is sometimes the best way to get started.

Chapter Structure

Just as there is a structure to each part in the text, there is also a structure in the chapters. This structure is a repeating model created to organize the material and present it in the clearest way possible.

Chapter Objectives

Each chapter begins with a set of objectives. It is tempting to ignore the objectives and get right on with the task of reading the chapter, but it is helpful to spend a little time to read the objectives and think about what they reveal about the content of the chapter.

Example Based on Chapter 22 Objectives

Objective 1. Differentiate between the following terms: *inotropic, chronotropic,* and *dromotropic.*

What can you learn from this objective? First, there is the vocabulary. This objective makes it clear that you have some terms to learn, and it may be helpful to have some blank note cards available to start setting up vocabulary cards for this chapter. Write each of the terms on a separate card and complete the card as the terms are introduced and explained in the chapter.

The next thing that stands out is that the three terms contain a common element, *tropic.* This should bring active questioning into play. What does the suffix *tropic* mean? Asking this question now is a way of noting that these three terms do have some common meaning.

Objective 2: Briefly discuss the effect of cardiac glycosides and other positive inotropic drugs on the failing or diseased heart.

From this statement comes the potential for a new question relating to the first objective. What do *inotropic, chronotropic,* and *dromotropic* have to do with the heart? Just as it is essential to see the relationship between parts and chapters, it is also essential to see relationships within the chapters. These two objectives should cause you to consider those relationships and make your own learning much more active.

Chapter Headings

The next chapter structure to consider in this process is the chapter headings. Chapter 22 has the major sections Overview, Heart Failure and Cardiac Dysrhythmias, Cardiac Glycosides, Phosphodiesterase Inhibitors, Miscellaneous Heart Failure Drugs, and Nursing Process. What is the importance of this heading structure? It tells you that the authors will focus on the pharmacological aspects first and then explain how these relate to nursing.

The section Cardiac Glycosides is broken down into subsections in this chapter. Spend several minutes considering the organization of these subsections. The first subtopic to be treated is under the heading Mechanism of Action and Drug Effects. What is the mechanism of action of cardiac glycosides? How 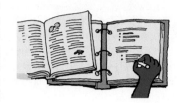 do they act? What effect do they have on the heart? It does not matter that you cannot answer these questions at this point. What is important is that you ask them as a means of fostering an active and participatory learning attitude when you begin to read the chapter. Think, question, anticipate, and then read. This sequence will enhance your learning.

Continue this process of looking at the subtopics and thinking ahead to what will be explained in the chapter. These subsections are the same in every chapter, and this thinking process should quickly become automatic.

Glossary

This chapter structure has already been stressed in previous Study Skills Tips, and it is essential to learning. The glossary is a mini-dictionary for each chapter. Words that have not been introduced earlier in the text and that are central to the content of this chapter are presented here. The listing is in alphabetical order, which means that the glossary terms will not necessarily occur in the same order in the body of the chapter.

As you read the terms in the glossary, be aware of the nature of the definition. A glossary definition is specific and brief. It is a useful place to begin to learn the new terms in the chapter, but the definition presented may not be enough for full understanding. You will find that full understanding will come after reading the chapter and encountering the term within the fuller context of sentences and paragraphs of text that explain not only the term but also how it applies in the particular situation.

Glossary and Text Relationship

The term *inotropic agent* is defined in the Chapter 22 glossary. As you read it, you understand that inotropic has to do with force or energy of muscle contractions. The glossary states that a positive inotropic agent is a drug that increases myocardial contractility. Some of this information is clear, and some of it is still somewhat hazy. It should become clearer when connected with the chapter text. The first paragraph of the chapter introduces inotropic agents: "Drugs that increase the force of myocardial contraction are called positive **inotropic drugs**—drugs that have a beneficial role in the treatment of a failing heart muscle."

With this sentence you should have a much clearer understanding of what is meant by inotropic agents, as well as knowing that there are positive inotropic drugs. You see the core definition as presented in the glossary and you read to determine how that core definition is expanded and exemplified in the body of the text. It would be useful to make note of the expanded definitions on the vocabulary note cards previously mentioned.

When preparing vocabulary cards, it is not a good idea to simply copy the definition from the glossary and assume that this definition will serve your purpose. Wait to fill out the card until after you encounter the same term in the body of the chapter, and then pick and choose the information from the glossary and the text that will provide you with the clearest understanding of the term. Also, when placing information on vocabulary cards, it is always useful to include the chapter number and page numbers so that you can locate the source of your definition quickly later.

Chapter structures can provide you with a clear picture of what you are expected to learn and the organizational pattern in which the material will be presented. Being aware of the structures and making use of them in this way will improve your concentration when you begin to read the chapter for understanding 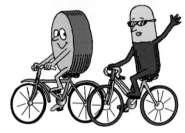 and memory. The time spent working with chapter structure is not wasted and does not significantly increase the study time of the chapter. In fact, the time you spend working with the objectives, headings, and glossary will generally save time when you are doing intensive reading and study.

TEXT NOTATION

Highlighting or underlining text materials can be helpful when rehearsing and reviewing materials after the study reading. The problem, as discussed in the *Study Guide*, is that it is often difficult to limit the quantity of material that is marked. Although a good general guideline is to try to limit yourself to marking no more than 20% to 25% of the total, this guideline applies to large blocks of material. However, some paragraphs contain essential information and must be marked extensively, whereas other paragraphs may need only one or two sentences marked. In this Study Skills Tips section, the object is to look at how the author's structure and language can help you select what should be marked.

Text Notation Application

Reproduced below are the first two paragraphs from Chapter 27 with model underlining completed, followed by a discussion of the reasons for these particular choices.

You should not view the underlining shown here as a "perfect" model. The decision as to what to mark is an individual choice based on a number of factors, including prior experience with the subject matter and awareness of personal learning objectives and needs. This example is intended to provide you with a basic model to adapt to your own learning style and needs.

Chapter 27, 1st Paragraphs Under "Overview" and "Physiology of Fluid Balance"

"Fluid and electrolyte management is one of the cornerstones of patient care. Most disease processes, tissue injuries, and surgical procedures greatly influence the physiological status of fluids and electrolytes in the body. A prerequisite to understanding fluid and electrolyte management is knowledge of the extent and composition of the various body fluid compartments."

"Approximately 60% of the adult human body is water or the *total body water* (TBW). Total body water is distributed among the three main compartments in the following proportions: **intracellular fluid (ICF)**, 67%; **interstitial fluid (ISF)**, 25%; and plasma volume (PV), 8%. This distribution is illustrated in Figure 27-1. The actual volume of fluid that would normally be distributed in each compartment in an average 70 kg man with a TBW content of 60% of his total body weight is shown in Table 27-1."

Discussion. The first thing you should notice is that the underlining here exceeds the 20% to 25% guideline. These are the first paragraphs in the chapter. First paragraphs are usually introductions to the topic and may vary a great deal in the quantity of important information. This selection seemed to contain a number of key points that must be considered. Because the content seems important, more is underlined.

Sentence 1 was chosen because of the word "cornerstones." This word suggests that fluid management is extremely important in patient care—the reader must be sure to keep that focus throughout the chapter. Paying careful attention to the author's word choices plays a major role in selecting materials for text notation.

Paying attention to language led to the third sentence, which begins, "A prerequisite to understanding. . . " That phrase should immediately capture your attention. The phrase says that there is something that must be understood before anything else that follows will make complete sense. The phrase should also serve as an instant cue to generate a question for reading: "What is the prerequisite to understanding fluid and electrolyte management?" This question is answered directly by the sentence containing the phrase. The phrase serves as a language cue that there is something important. This, in turn, suggests that you probably will want to underline or highlight some information. The question helps you select what should be marked. Everything you do at this point serves as a guide to help you establish clear learning objectives and makes the process of selecting the best information for marking easier.

The next segment was chosen because it stands out from the body of the paragraph. *"Total body water"* is italicized. This is a print convention used as a means of putting emphasis on something that the author believes to be of special importance. The decision to underline words and phrases that are already emphasized is a personal one. You may feel that since the author has already marked it, you have no need to add your own marks. Some students find that their own marking, even of italicized or bold print material, serves as a double reminder of the importance of the information. Remember, text notation is highly personal. Whether you choose to add your own marking or not, there is one aspect of this phrase that is essential. "Total body water" is part of the vocabulary of fluids and electrolytes. That means it is time to add to your vocabulary cards.

This term served as a lead-in to the next key point marked. The next statement is "Total body water is distributed among the three main compartments. . . " Whenever you see a phrase with a number and a word such as "main," you should be aware that this is potentially important material. This phrase should generate a new question that will aid in your selection of material to mark: "What are the three main compartments?" You see immediately that the rest of this sentence answers that question and therefore identifies what needs to be marked. This marking also identifies three additional vocabulary items to be added to your cards for this chapter. As you set up your cards, be careful. One fluid is "intra-," and the second is "inter-." It would be easy to confuse the two, but they have different meanings. If you are not sure what the difference is between *intra-* and *inter-*, consult a dictionary.

Chapter 27, Paragraph Two of "Physiology of Fluid Balance"

". . .The TBW can be described as being inside or outside of the blood vessels, or vasculature. If this terminology is used, then the term **intravascular fluid (IVF)** describes fluid inside the blood vessels, and the term **extravascular fluid (EVF)** describes the fluid outside the blood vessels. Examples of EVF include lymph and cerebrospinal fluid. As you learn these concepts, recall the difference between the prefixes intra- (inside), inter- (between), and extra- (outside). The term **plasma** is used to describe the fluid that flows through the blood vessels that is intravascular. . . ISF is the fluid that is in the space between cells, tissues, and organs. Both plasma and ISF make up extracellular volume. Both ISF and ICF make up extravascular volume. These terms are often confused and misused. Table 27-1 lists these definitions for further clarity and understanding."

Discussion. The language conventions and the print conventions **bold** and *italics* are the same that were used to help in the previous paragraph. This paragraph also makes a point about the possibility of confusing or misusing the terms introduced. Being told that there is confusing material suggests that it is crucial that you be able to identify, define, and explain each of the terms used, and that it will take some careful thnking to do so. There is one additional point in this paragraph that is important. The last sentence points you to a table, Table 27-1. There are many tables in this text. Tables are often used to simplify complex material and to clarify the relationships between the items presented. In these opening paragraphs, with the repeated reference to the confusing nature of the descriptions, Table 27-1 will almost certainly be important to your learning.

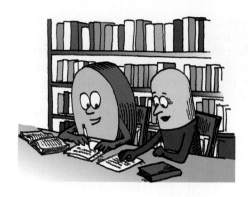

CHAPTER 22

Positive Inotropic Drugs

Learning Objectives

After reading this chapter, the successful student will be able to do the following:

1 Differentiate between the following terms: *inotropic*, *chronotropic*, and *dromotropic*.

2 Briefly discuss the pathophysiology of heart failure and dysthrythmias.

3 Briefly discuss the effect of cardiac glycosides and other positive inotropic drugs on the failing or diseased heart.

4 Compare the mechanisms of action, pharmacokinetics, indications, dosages, dosage forms, routes of administration, cautions, contraindications, adverse effects, and toxicity of the cardiac glycosides and other positive inotropic drugs.

5 Briefly discuss rapid versus slow digitalization, including nursing considerations.

6 Identify significant drugs, laboratory tests, and food interactions associated with cardiac glycosides and other positive inotropic drugs.

7 Develop a collaborative plan of care that includes all phases of the nursing process for patients undergoing treatment with cardiac glycosides or other positive inotropic drugs.

e-Learning Activities

Web site
(http://evolve.elsevier.com/Canada/
Lilley/pharmacology/)

- Animations
- Answers to chapter questions, activities, and case studies
- Calculators and Category Catchers
- Glossary with audio pronunciations
- IV Therapy and Medication Error Checklists
- Multiple-Choice Review Question quizzes
- Nursing Care Plans
- Online Appendices and Supplements
- WebLinks

Drug Profiles

▸▸ **digoxin**, p. 410
   digoxin immune Fab, p. 410
   milrinone (milrinone lactate)*, p. 411

▸▸ Key drug.

*Full generic name is given in parentheses. For the purposes of this text, the more common shortened name is used.

Glossary

Atrial fibrillation   A common cardiac dysrhythmia involving atrial contractions that are so rapid that they prevent full repolarization of myocardial fibres between heartbeats. (p. 404)

Automaticity   A property of specialized excitable tissue that allows self-activation through the spontaneous development of an action potential, as in the pacemaker cells of the heart. (p. 405)

Cardiac glycosides   Glycosides (carbohydrates that yield a sugar and a nonsugar upon hydrolysis) that are derived from the plant species *Digitalis purpurea* and are used in the treatment of heart disease. (p. 405)

Chronotropic drugs   Drugs that influence the rate of the heartbeat. (p. 404)

Dromotropic drugs   Drugs that influence the conduction of electrical impulses. (p. 404)

Ejection fraction   The proportion of blood that is ejected during each ventricular contraction compared with the total ventricular filling volume. (p. 404)

Heart failure   An abnormal condition in which cardiac pumping is impaired as the result of myocardial infarction, ischemic heart disease, or cardiomyopathy. (p. 404)

Inotropic drugs   Drugs that affect the force or energy of muscular contractions, particularly contraction of the heart muscle. (p. 404)

Left ventricular end-diastolic volume (LVEDV)   The total amount of blood in the ventricle before it contracts, or the preload. (p. 404)

Phosphodiesterase inhibitors   A group of inotropic drugs that work by inhibiting the enzyme *phosphodiesterase*. (p. 408)

Refractory period   The period during which a pulse generator (e.g., the sinoatrial node of the heart) is unresponsive to an input signal of specified amplitude and it is impossible for the myocardium to respond. (p. 405)

Therapeutic window   The range of drug levels in the blood that is considered beneficial as opposed to toxic or ineffective. (p. 407)

OVERVIEW

It is estimated that heart failure affects 1% to 2% of the general population, or approximately 450,000 Canadians, and over 50,000 new cases are diagnosed each year. Twenty percent of these Canadians are 65 years of age or older. Estimates are that there are 106,130 admissions of 85,679 patients with heart failure to Canadian hospitals. Of these, 32.7% were re-admissions within 1 year, and in-hospital mortality was 15.8%. These statistics mirror trends reported in Europe and the United States. It is estimated that by 2050, the number of patients hospitalized for heart failure will triple. The burden to the Canadian health care system is estimated at between 1.4 and 2.3 billion dollars. Therefore, any drug that can lengthen survival in affected patients or help the failing heart perform its essential functions is extremely valuable. Drugs that increase the force of myocardial contraction are called positive **inotropic drugs**—drugs that have a beneficial role in the treatment of a failing heart muscle. Drugs that increase the rate at which the heart beats are called positive **chronotropic drugs.** Drugs may also affect how quickly electrical impulses travel through the conduction system of the heart (the sinoatrial [SA] node, atrioventricular [AV] node, bundle of His, and Purkinje fibres). Drugs that accelerate conduction are referred to as positive **dromotropic drugs.** The focus of this chapter is on two of the main classes of positive inotropic drugs: *cardiac glycosides* and *phosphodiesterase inhibitors*.

HEART FAILURE AND CARDIAC DYSRHYTHMIAS

Heart failure is a pathological state in which the heart is unable to pump blood in sufficient amounts from the ventricles (i.e., cardiac output is insufficient) to meet the body's metabolic needs. The signs and symptoms typically associated with heart failure constitute the syndrome of heart failure. This syndrome can be limited to the left ventricle (producing pulmonary edema and symptoms of dyspnea or cough) or to the right ventricle (producing symptoms such as pedal edema, jugular venous distention, ascites, and liver congestion), or it may affect both ventricles.

In patients with heart failure, the overworked, failing heart cannot meet the demands placed on it and blood is not ejected efficiently from the ventricles. This occurs because the **ejection fraction** (the amount of blood ejected with each contraction) compared with the total amount of blood in the ventricle just before contraction (**left ventricular end-diastolic volume**) is decreased. (Normally, the ejection fraction is approximately 65% [0.65] of the total volume in the ventricle.) As more blood accumulates in the right and left ventricles, more pressure builds up in the blood vessels leading to the heart. The retrograde transmission of this increased hydrostatic pressure from the left ventricle leads to pulmonary congestion, whereas elevated right ventricular pressure causes systemic venous congestion and peripheral edema.

Because the heart cannot then meet the increased demands placed on it, the blood supply to certain organs is reduced. The organs most dependent on blood supply, the brain and heart, are the last to be deprived of blood. As an organ that is relatively less dependent on blood supply, the kidney has its blood supply shunted away. Therefore, the filtration of fluids and removal of waste products is impaired. When these fluids and waste products accumulate, the patient experiences symptoms such as pulmonary edema and shortness of breath, and peripheral edema resulting from kidney failure.

The physical defects producing heart failure are of two types: (1) a heart defect (myocardial deficiency such as myocardial infarction or valve insufficiency), which leads to inadequate cardiac contractility and ventricular filling; and (2) a defect outside the heart (e.g., systemic defects such as coronary artery disease, pulmonary hypertension, or diabetes), which results in an overload on an otherwise normal heart. Either or both of these defects may be present in a given patient. Common causes of myocardial deficiency and systemic defects are listed in Box 22-1.

A dysfunctional heart rhythm is technically termed a cardiac dysrhythmia. In practice, however, the term arrhythmia is also used, even though it literally means "no rhythm," or absence of heartbeat. In patients with supraventricular dysrhythmias, **atrial fibrillation**, or atrial flutter, the atria (the upper chambers of the heart) are contracting several hundred times a minute. Not only are the atria contracting too frequently, but several areas in the atria besides the SA node are then acting as the pacemaker of the heart. Normally, the AV node controls how slowly or quickly impulses arrive in the ventricles. The AV node also has the ability to receive all of these depolarizations and to allow only a certain number to

Myocardial Deficiency and Increased Workload: Common Causes

Myocardial Deficiency

Inadequate Contractility
Cardiomyopathy
Coronary artery disease
Infection
Myocardial infarction

Inadequate Filling
Atrial fibrillation
Infection
Ischemia
Tamponade

Increased Workload

Pressure Overload
Hypertension
Outflow obstruction

Volume Overload
Anemia
Congenital abnormalities
Hypervolemia
Thyroid disease

pass through to the ventricles. This keeps the patient from going into ventricular fibrillation, which can be fatal. It also allows the ventricles time to fill with blood, which is essential for normal perfusion. During atrial fibrillation or flutter, patients may show symptoms of heart failure.

All cells in the heart can depolarize spontaneously, a property called **automaticity.** The **refractory period** occurs when the cardiac cells are re-adjusting their sodium and potassium levels following depolarization. During this time, the cardiac cells cannot depolarize again. The sodium–potassium adenosine triphosphatase (ATPase) pump is responsible for the movement of potassium ions in and sodium ions out of the cardiac cells after they have depolarized, an action potential has been generated, and the electrical impulse has been promulgated through the myocardium. In patients with supraventricular tachy-dysrhythmias such as atrial fibrillation or flutter, the AV node may be circumvented and a greater number of electrical impulses than normal may arrive in the ventricle before the refractory period is over. This can potentially cause ventricular tachydysrhythmias (e.g., ventricular tachycardia or fibrillation), which are potentially more serious than the supraventricular tachydysrhythmias mentioned earlier. Figure 22-1 illustrates the conduction system of the heart. The heart conduction system and the abnormalities responsible for causing dysrhythmias are described in greater detail in Chapter 23.

CARDIAC GLYCOSIDES

Cardiac glycosides are one of the oldest and most effective groups of heart drugs. Not only do they have beneficial effects on the failing heart but they also help control the ventricular response to atrial fibrillation or flutter. They were originally obtained from either the *Digitalis purpurea* or the *Digitalis lanata* plant, both commonly referred to as *foxglove.* For this reason, cardiac glycosides are sometimes referred to as digitalis glycosides. Digoxin is the most frequently prescribed cardiac glycoside and the only one currently available in Canada. Another drug with a similar-sounding name, *digitoxin,* is no longer on the Canadian market. Cardiac glycosides have been the mainstay of therapy for heart failure for more than 200 years, and they continue to be one of the most commonly used positive inotropic drugs. The widespread and enduring popularity of digitalis is the result of many years of clinical use. Critically ill patients can be restored to near-normal states within hours after initiating digoxin therapy, a process known as *digitalization.*

See Special Populations: Children for information on the use of cardiac glycosides in children with heart failure.

Data questioning the use of cardiac glycosides were recently released, however. Digoxin therapy as a first-line treatment for heart failure did not improve mortality rates. Angiotensin-converting enzyme (ACE) inhibitors and diuretics were recommended as the key drugs to offer therapeutic benefit; nevertheless, digoxin may still offer benefit in some patients (see Evidence-Informed Practice: The DIG Trial).

While the emphasis in this chapter regarding heart failure is on systolic dysfunction or inadequate ventricular

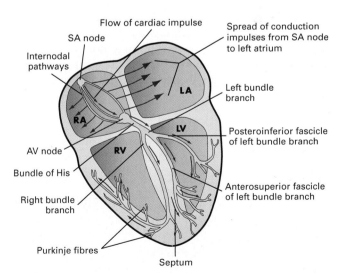

FIG. 22-1 Conduction system of the heart. *AV,* atrioventricular; *LA,* left atrium; *LV,* left ventricle; *RA,* right atrium; *RV,* right ventricle; *SA,* sinoatrial. (Lewis, S. M., Heitkemper, M. M., & Dirksen, S. R. (2009). *Medical-surgical nursing: Assessment and management of clinical problems* (2nd Canadian ed., Goldsworthy, S., & Barry, M. A., eds.). St. Louis, MO: Mosby.)

SPECIAL POPULATIONS: CHILDREN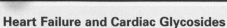

Heart Failure and Cardiac Glycosides

- The cause, symptoms, treatment, and prognosis of heart failure in children vary depending on age. In infants, the cause of heart failure is generally congenital heart defects or other structural problems. In older children, the structure of the heart may be normal but the heart muscle may be weakened. Symptoms of heart failure differ depending on age and become worse with age because the heart must keep up with increased oxygen demands and energy demands.

- Symptoms may include poor growth, difficulty in feeding, and tachypnea; in older children, inability to tolerate exercise and other activities, the need to rest more often, and dyspnea with minimal exertion occur more frequently.

- Treatment is generally age and cause specific. For septal defects, surgery or medication may be indicated. For more complex problems, surgery may be needed within the first few weeks of life.

- Medications used include furosemide (a loop diuretic), angiotensin-converting enzyme inhibitors, β-blockers, and sometimes digoxin to help with heart-pumping efficiency.

- Digoxin should be given on a regular time schedule 1 hour before or 2 hours after feeding. Dosing of the drug must be accompanied by close monitoring and individualized nursing care.

- Correct calculation of dosages is important to safe and cautious nursing care. A one-decimal-point placement error will result in a 10-fold dosage error, which could be fatal.

- All medication calculations should be double-checked by a second registered nurse or by a pharmacist or physician because of the narrow margin for error. Toxicity manifests in children as nausea, vomiting, bradycardia, anorexia, and dysrhythmias.

- The physician should be notified immediately should the following symptoms indicative of heart failure develop: increased fatigue, sudden weight gain (1 kg or more in 24 hours), or respiratory distress.

Source: The Hospital for Sick Children Web site information on congestive heart failure. Available at http://www.aboutkidshealth.ca/HeartConditions/

---

contractions (systole) during the pumping of the heart, it is also important to note the less common condition of diastolic dysfunction, or inadequate ventricular filling, during ventricular relaxation (diastole). This condition is most commonly associated with left ventricular hypertrophy secondary to chronic hypertension. However, it may also result from cardiomyopathy (e.g., virus-induced), pericardial disease, and diabetes. Unlike with systolic heart failure, inotropic drugs (including digoxin) and vasodilators (see Chapter 25) may not be the drugs of choice for diastolic failure. Diuretic drugs (see Chapter 26), on the other hand, are often used as part of therapy for both conditions.

Mechanism of Action and Drug Effects

The primary beneficial effect of a cardiac glycoside (e.g., digoxin) is thought to be an increase in myocardial contractility. This occurs secondary to the inhibition of the sodium-potassium ATPase pump. When the action of this enzyme complex is inhibited, the cellular sodium concentration and, subsequently, the calcium concentration increase. The overall result is enhanced myocardial contraction. Digoxin also augments (cholinergic or parasympathetic) vagal tone, resulting in increased diastolic filling between heartbeats secondary to reduced heart rate. This further enhances cardiac efficiency and output.

Cardiac glycosides also change the electrical conduction properties of the heart, markedly affecting the conduction system and cardiac automaticity. Cardiac glycosides decrease the velocity (rate) of electrical conduction and prolong the refractory period in the conduction system. The particular area of the conduction system where this occurs is between the atria and the ventricles (SA node to AV node). The cardiac cells remain in a state of depolarization for a longer period and are unable to start another electrical impulse, which also reduces heart rate and improves cardiac efficiency.

The cardiac glycoside digoxin produces the following dramatic inotropic, chronotropic, dromotropic, and other heart effects:

- A positive inotropic effect, resulting in an increase in the force and velocity of myocardial contraction without a corresponding increase in oxygen consumption
- A negative chronotropic effect, producing a reduced heart rate
- A negative dromotropic effect that decreases automaticity at the SA node, decreases AV nodal conduction, reduces conductivity at the bundle of His, and prolongs the atrial and ventricular refractory periods
- An increase in stroke volume
- A reduction in heart size during diastole
- A decrease in venous blood pressure and vein engorgement
- An increase in coronary circulation
- Promotion of diuresis as the result of improved blood circulation
- Palliation of exertional and paroxysmal nocturnal dyspnea, cough, and cyanosis

Indications

Cardiac glycosides are used primarily in the treatment of heart failure and supraventricular dysrhythmias.

EVIDENCE-INFORMED PRACTICE

 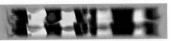

The DIG Trial

Background

Congestive heart failure is a major public health problem in Canada and other developed countries. The Digitalis Investigation Group (DIG) trial was a multicentre random-ized, double-blind, placebo-controlled trial conducted in Canada and the United States that evaluated the effects of digoxin on all-cause mortality and on hospitalization for heart failure in patients with heart failure.

Type of Evidence

In the main trial, 3397 patients with left ventricular ejec-tion fractions of 0.45 or less were randomly assigned to digoxin and 3403 to placebo in addition to diuret-ics and angiotensin-converting enzyme (ACE) inhibit-ors. All patients were followed up for a minimum of 28 months. The ancillary DIG trial followed up an addi-tional 988 patients with heart failure, but with a left ven-tricular ejection fraction greater than 0.45.

Results of Study

After a mean follow-up of 37 months, patients in the first trial who received digoxin had lower risks of death and hospital admission for worsening heart failure. The results of the ancillary trial (after a mean follow-up of 37 months) demonstrated no overall effect. Post-hoc analyses from the DIG trial had correlated digoxin lev-els less than 1.0 nmol/L with decreased mortality and digoxin levels greater than 1.5 nmol/L with increased mortality (Ahmed et al., 2006). These results have been confirmed by large prospective, randomized trials.

Link of Evidence to Nursing Practice

Congestive heart failure (CHF) is the most common cause of cardiovascular hospital admission. Digoxin has been available for over 200 years and is widely used. The implementation of evidence-informed therapy for heart failure management is clinically efficacious. However, there is still uncertainty surrounding the appropriateness of its role and value in treating patients with heart failure. Critics of the DIG trial cite that the trial participants were primarily White and male, with an average of 64 years of age, whereas the more typical population of patients with heart failure are in their late seventies and early eighties, have substantial comorbidity, and include a greater pro-portion of women and non-White people. Nurses should be informed of current evidence to support management of heart failure but also be familiar with potential pitfalls.

Based on Ahmed, A., Rich, M. W., Love, T. E., Lloyd-Jones, D. M., Aban, I. B., Colucci, W. S., et al. (2006). Digoxin and reduction in mortality and hospitalization in heart failure: A comprehensive *post hoc* analysis of the DIG trial. *European Heart Journal, 27,* 178–186; The Digitalis Investigation Group. (1997). The effect of digoxin on mortality and morbidity in patients with heart failure. *New England Journal of Medicine, 336*(8), 525–533.

In heart failure, the therapeutic effects of digoxin are sec-ondary to its ability to increase the force of contraction, its positive inotropic action. This has many therapeutic benefits. Increasing the force of contraction increases the volume of blood ejected as a percentage of the left ventricular end-diastolic volume or preload (i.e., the ejection fraction). Because more blood is ejected with each contraction of the heart, less blood remains in the ventricle and thus less pressure builds up. Consequently, the symptoms of pulmonary edema, pulmonary hyper-tension, and right-sided ventricular failure subside and tissue perfusion improves.

Another benefit of this positive inotropic action is that it promotes diuresis by ensuring that adequate blood is supplied to the kidneys. As a result, fluids are more completely filtered and waste products removed, which relieves shortness of breath and pulmonary edema.

Cardiac glycosides are also effective in the treatment of supraventricular dysrhythmias such as atrial fibrillation and atrial flutter because of their negative chronotropic and negative dromotropic actions. Automaticity, conduc-tion velocity, and the refractory period are all affected. Digoxin can slow the depolarization of the SA node and other areas of the atria that may be acting as pacemakers. Thus, the cardiac glycosides, such as digoxin, directly slow conduction through the AV node (decreasing the ventricular rate) and increase the vagal action on the heart.

In addition, the cardiac glycosides lengthen the refractory period, which allows the correct levels of sodium and potassium ions to be reached before depolarization.

Contraindications

Contraindications to the use of cardiac glycosides include known drug allergy and may include second- or third-degree heart block, atrial fibrillation (also an indication, so this is a clinical judgement call), ventricular tachycar-dia or fibrillation, heart failure resulting from diastolic dysfunction, and subaortic stenosis (obstruction in the left ventricle below the aortic valve). However, these drugs may be used to treat some of these conditions, if recommended by a competent cardiologist, depending on the given clinical situation

Adverse Effects

The adverse effects associated with cardiac glycoside use can be serious. The primary cardiac glycoside in use today is digoxin, and close monitoring of the patient's clinical response and observation for the possible development of toxic symptoms are essential. Digoxin has a narrow **therapeutic window;** the range of drug levels in the blood that is considered therapeutic is small (1–2.5 nmol/L). Monitoring of digoxin levels after the drug reaches steady state is necessary only if there is sus-picion of toxicity, nonadherence, or deteriorating kidney function. The digoxin target range is 0.64–1.54 nmol/L in patients with heart failure. A retrospective analysis of the Digitalis Investigation Group (DIG) Trial suggests that a decrease in mortality is associated with serum digoxin concentrations of 0.64–1.15 nmol/L, a neutral effect on mortality with 1.28–1.49 nmol, and a potential adverse effect on survival at concentrations greater than 1.54 nmol/L (see Evidence-Informed Practice: The DIG Trial). Low potassium levels can increase the potential for toxicity, known specifically for this drug as digitoxicity. Therefore, it is important to frequently check serum electrolyte levels. Estimates are that as many as 20% of patients taking digoxin exhibit symptoms of toxicity. Older adult patients with heart failure are at increased risk for adverse effects from digoxin, which are often nonspecific and can occur at serum digoxin concentrations generally considered therapeutic. The common undesirable effects associated with cardiac glycoside use are listed in Table 22-1.

Toxicity and Management of Overdose

The treatment strategies for digoxin toxicity depend on the severity of the symptoms. These strategies can range from simply withholding the next dose to instituting aggressive therapies. Consultation with a Poison Control Centre is recommended. The steps usually taken in the management of cardiac glycoside toxicity are listed in Table 22-2.

When significant toxicity develops as a result of cardiac glycoside therapy, the administration of digoxin immune Fab may be indicated. *Digoxin immune Fab* is an antibody that recognizes digoxin as an antigen and forms an antibody–antigen complex, thus inactivating the free digoxin. Digoxin immune Fab therapy is not indicated for every patient who is showing signs of digoxin toxicity. The following are the clinical settings in which its use may be indicated:

- Hyperkalemia (a serum potassium level over 5 mmol/L) in a patient with digitoxicity
- Life-threatening cardiac dysrhythmias, sustained ventricular tachycardia or fibrillation, and severe sinus bradycardia or heart block unresponsive to atropine treatment or cardiac pacing
- Life-threatening digoxin overdose: more than 10 mg of digoxin in adults; more than 4 mg of digoxin in children

Interactions

A number of significant drug interactions are possible with cardiac glycosides. The common ones are listed in Table 22-3. Bran, taken in large amounts, may decrease the absorption of oral digitalis drugs. The herbal supplement hawthorne can reduce the effectiveness of cardiac glycosides. Hawthorne is used for hypertension and angina. Other specific drug interactions are mentioned in Table 22-3.

Use of a digoxin preparation can also interfere with the results of several laboratory tests. It can cause the plasma levels of estrone to be raised and the levels of lactate dehydrogenase and testosterone to be lowered. It can also cause the erythrocyte sodium concentration to be increased and the erythrocyte potassium concentration to be reduced.

In addition to interacting with other drugs and laboratory tests, digoxin can interact with certain foods and natural health products. The consumption of excessive amounts of potassium-rich foods can decrease its therapeutic effect, whereas the consumption of excessive amounts of licorice can increase digoxin toxicity as the result of the hypokalemia produced. St. John's wort (*Hypericum perforatum*) may interfere with intestinal digoxin absorption, resulting in low serum concentrations of digoxin.

Dosages

For dosage information on the cardiac glycosides, see the Dosages table on p. 411. Because of the fine line between therapeutic and toxic dosage levels for many patients, also see Preventing Medication Errors: The Importance of Decimal Points.

PHOSPHODIESTERASE INHIBITORS

As the name implies, **phosphodiesterase inhibitors** (PDIs) are a group of inotropic drugs that work by inhibiting an enzyme called *phosphodiesterase*. The inhibition of this enzyme results in two beneficial effects in an individual with heart failure: a positive inotropic response and vasodilation. For this reason, this class of drugs is also referred to as *inodilators* (inotropes and dilators). These

TABLE 22-1

Cardiac Glycosides: Common Adverse Effects

Body System	Adverse Effect
Cardiovascular	Any type of dysrhythmia including bradycardia or tachycardia
Central nervous	Headache, fatigue, malaise, confusion, convulsions
Ocular	Coloured vision (i.e., green, yellow, or purple), halo vision, or flickering lights
Gastrointestinal	Anorexia, nausea, vomiting, diarrhea

TABLE 22-2

Digoxin Toxicity: Step-by-Step Management

Step	Instructions
1	Discontinue administration of the drug.
2	Begin continuous electrocardiographic monitoring for cardiac dysrhythmias; administer any appropriate antidysrhythmic drugs as ordered.
3	Determine serum digoxin and electrolyte levels.
4	Administer potassium supplements for hypokalemia if indicated, as ordered.
5	Institute supportive therapy for gastrointestinal symptoms (nausea, vomiting, or diarrhea).
6	Administer digoxin antidote (i.e., digoxin immune Fab) if indicated, as ordered.

TABLE 22-3

Cardiac Glycosides: Drug Interactions

Interacting Drug	Mechanism	Result
Antidysrhythmics calcium (parenteral) reserpine	Increase cardiac irritability	Increased digoxin toxicity
amphotericin B chlorthalidone Laxatives Loop diuretics Steroids (kidney) Sympathomimetics Thiazide diuretics	Produce hypokalemia	Increased digoxin toxicity
Antacids Antidiarrheals cholestyramine colestipol sucralfate	Decrease oral absorption	Reduced therapeutic effect
Anticholinergics	Increase oral absorption	Increased therapeutic effect
Barbiturates	Induce enzyme	Reduced therapeutic effect
β-blockers	Block β_1 receptors in heart	Enhanced bradycardic effect of digoxin
Calcium channel blockers	Block calcium channels in myocardium	Enhanced bradycardic and negative inotropic effects of digoxin
amiodarone quinidine verapamil	Decrease clearance	Increased digoxin levels (2×); digoxin dose should be reduced 50%

drugs were discovered during the quest for positive inotropic drugs with a better therapeutic window than that of digoxin. Milrinone is the sole phosphodiesterase inhibitor available in Canada. Milrinone shares a similar pharmacological action with methylxanthines such as theophylline. They both inhibit phosphodiesterase, which results in an increase in intracellular cyclic adenosine monophosphate (cAMP). However, milrinone is more specific for phosphodiesterase type III, found in high concentrations in the heart and vascular smooth muscle.

Mechanism of Action and Drug Effects

The mechanism of action of PDIs differs from that of other inotropic drugs such as cardiac glycosides and catecholamines. The beneficial effects of a PDI come from the intracellular increase in cAMP; normally, the phosphodiesterase enzyme prevents the buildup of cAMP. Milrinone works by selectively inhibiting phosphodiesterase type III, which results in more calcium for the heart to use in muscle contraction. The increased calcium in heart muscle is also taken back up into its storage sites

 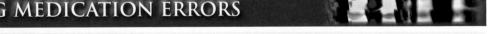

PREVENTING MEDICATION ERRORS

The Importance of Decimal Points

Incorrect decimal placement can be lethal when calculating digoxin dosages. According to the Institute for Safe Medication Practices Canada (ISMP-Canada), trailing zeros should NOT be used after decimal points. In the case of digoxin, if a "1 mg" dose is ordered, and written as "1.0 mg," the order could be misread as "10 mg," and the patient would receive 10 times the ordered dose.

The ISMP also recommends that leading zeroes be used if a dose is less than a whole number. For example, ".25 mg" can look like "25 mg," resulting in a dose that is 100 times the ordered dose. Instead, the order should be written as "0.25 mg" to avoid any errors.

Of course, such an error would likely be caught when the nurse realizes how many 250 mcg digoxin tablets it would take to give a "25 mg" dose, or how many millilitres would be needed for an intravenous dose. However, such errors have occurred. Consider what would happen if a digoxin overdose leads to digoxin toxicity and the serious effects this would have on the patient.

For more information, visit http://www.ismp-canada.org/download/ISMPCSB2006-04Abbr.pdf

DRUG PROFILES

Cardiac glycosides get their name from their chemical structures. Glycosides are complex, steroid-like structures linked to sugar molecules. Because the particular drugs derived from the digitalis plant have potent actions on the heart, they are referred to as *cardiac glycosides,* with digoxin being, by far, the most commonly prescribed digitalis preparation. Digoxin is currently the only prescribed digitalis preparation. Digoxin should be used with a diuretic and angiotensin-converting enzyme (ACE) inhibitor for optimum therapeutic effect.

▶▶ *digoxin*

Digoxin (Lanoxin) is an effective drug for the treatment of both heart failure and atrial fibrillation and flutter. It may also be used clinically to improve myocardial contractility and thus reverse cardiogenic shock or other low cardiac output states. Digoxin use is contraindicated in patients who have shown a hypersensitivity to it and in those with ventricular tachycardia and fibrillation, heart disease associated with beriberi, or hypersensitive carotid sinus syndrome. Normal therapeutic drug levels of digoxin should be between 0.8 and 2 ng/mL. Levels higher than 2 ng/mL are typically desirable for the treatment of atrial fibrillation. Digoxin effectiveness in systolic heart failure is thought to be linked more with its neurohormonal effects and less with its positive inotropic effects. The neurohormonal effects of digoxin (decreased norepinephrine, decreased vagal tone) are evident only at lower digoxin serum levels (0.9–1.5 nmol/L).

Digoxin is available in oral and injectable forms. Because of the narrow therapeutic index and potential for errors in administration, digoxin is available in parenteral formulations of 0.05 mg/mL for children and 0.25 mg/mL for adults. In addition, as digoxin has a long duration of action and half-life (see Pharmacokinetics below), a loading, or "digitalizing," dose is often given to bring serum levels of the drug up to a desirable therapeutic level more quickly. See the Dosages table on p. 411 for the recommended digitalizing doses and the daily oral and intravenous dosages for adults and children.

PHARMACOKINETICS

Half-Life	Onset	Peak	Duration
33–44 hr	30–120 min	2–6 hr	2–4 days

digoxin immune Fab

Digoxin immune Fab (Digibind) is the antidote for severe digoxin overdose and is indicated for the reversal of life-threatening cardiotoxic effects such as severe sinus bradycardia, second- or third-degree heart block, severe ventricular tachycardia or fibrillation, and severe hyperkalemia. It has a unique mechanism of action. Digoxin immune Fab binds to free (unbound) digoxin, which reverses the drug effects and symptoms of toxicity. Use of digoxin immune Fab is contraindicated in patients who have known hypersensitivity to it. It is available only in parenteral form (38 mg vial).

The dosage of digoxin immune Fab varies according to the amount of digoxin to neutralize. It most often is calculated by the number of vials. It is commonly dosed on the basis of the patient's serum digoxin level in conjunction with the patient's weight. Each vial containing 38 mg of purified digoxin-specific Fab fragments will bind approximately 0.05 mg of digoxin. For recommended dosages, the nurse should consult the manufacturer's latest dosage recommendations.

It is important to know that after digoxin immune Fab is given, all subsequent digoxin serum levels will be elevated for days to weeks because of the presence of both the free (unbound) digoxin (toxic digoxin) and the digoxin that has been bound by the digoxin immune Fab (nontoxic digoxin). Therefore, after its administration, the clinical signs and symptoms of digoxin toxicity, rather than the digoxin serum levels, should be used to monitor the effectiveness of reversal therapy.

PHARMACOKINETICS

Half-Life	Onset	Peak	Duration
15–20 hr	Immediate	Immediate	Days to weeks

---

in the sarcoplasmic reticulum at a much faster rate than normal. As a result, the heart muscle relaxes and is more compliant. The smooth muscle that surrounds blood vessels also relaxes, causing dilation of the systemic or pulmonary blood vessels, which, in turn, decreases the workload of the heart. The effects on heart muscle result in an increase in the force of contraction (i.e., positive inotropic action). In summary, phosphodiesterase inhibitors have positive inotropic and lusitropic (relaxing blood vessels) and vasodilatory effects. They may also increase the heart rate in some instances and, consequently, have positive chronotropic effects.

Indications

Milrinone is primarily used as an *inodilator* for the short-term management of heart failure. In the treatment of heart failure, the therapeutic benefits of this inodilator are its inotropic and vasodilatory effects. This inodilator has 10 to 100 times greater affinity for smooth muscle surrounding blood vessels than it does for heart muscle. Thus the primary beneficial effects of the inodilator may come from its ability to dilate blood vessels. This dilation causes a reduction in afterload, or the force against which the heart has to pump to eject its volume of blood.

Traditionally, a PDI is administered to patients who can be closely monitored and who have not responded adequately to digoxin, diuretics, or vasodilators. A PDI such as milrinone does not require a receptor-mediated action to increase contraction. In contrast to other positive inotropic drugs, such as β-agonists (e.g., dobutamine, dopamine), stimulation of a receptor is required to increase contraction. The repetitive stimulation of these receptors can cause the body to become less sensitive to the drug over time. In patients with end-stage heart failure who require positive inotropic support, a continual dosage increase is often needed to maintain positive results. As the dosage of the positive inotropic drug is increased, however, it produces more adverse heart effects. Because milrinone does not use receptors to increase the force of contraction, the drug does not pose this problem. Many hospitals that treat large numbers of patients with heart failure now treat those experiencing end-stage heart failure with weekly 6-hour infusions of milrinone. This has been shown to increase patients' quality of life and decrease the number of re-admissions to the hospital for exacerbations of heart failure.

Contraindications

Contraindications to the use of a PDI include known drug allergy and may include the presence of severe aortic or pulmonary valvular disease and heart failure resulting from diastolic dysfunction.

Adverse Effects

The primary adverse effect seen with milrinone therapy is ventricular dysrhythmia, occurring in approximately 12% of patients treated with this drug. Some other adverse effects are hypotension (3.1%), headache (2.4%), angina pectoris and chest pain (1.4%), hypokalemia (0.7%), tremor (0.5%), and thrombocytopenia (0.5%).

Toxicity and Management of Overdose

No specific antidote exists for an overdose of milrinone. Hypotension secondary to vasodilation is the primary effect seen with excessive doses of this drug. The recommendation is to reduce the dose or temporarily discontinue the PDI if excessive hypotension occurs. This should be done until the patient's condition is stabilized. Consultation with a Poison Control Centre and general measures for circulatory support are also recommended.

Interactions

Concurrent administration of diuretics (see Chapter 26) may cause significant hypovolemia and reduced cardiac filling pressure. The patient should be appropriately monitored in a critical care setting to detect and respond to these problems. Also, additive inotropic effects may be seen with coadministration of digoxin. Furosemide must not be injected into intravenous lines of milrinone because it will precipitate immediately.

Dosages

For dosage information on milrinone, see the Dosages table on p. 412.

 DRUG PROFILES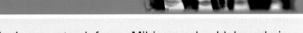

milrinone lactate

Milrinone lactate is the only available phosphodiesterase inhibitor in Canada. Milrinone is referred to as an inodilator because it exerts both positive inotropic and vasodilatory effects. This drug is contraindicated in patients who have shown hypersensitivity to it. Milrinone is available only in parenteral form. Milrinone should be administered with a loading dose followed by a continuous infusion (maintenance dose).

PHARMACOKINETICS

Half-Life	Onset	Peak	Duration
2.3 hr	5–15 min	6–12 hr	8–10 hr

DOSAGES   Drugs for Heart Failure

Drug (Pregnancy Category)	Pharmacological Class	Usual Dosage Range	Indications
▸▸ digoxin (Lanoxin) (C)	Digitalis cardiac (cardiotonic) glycoside	*Children* Digitalizing dose IV: Premature: 0.015–0.025 mg/kg Full term: 0.020–0.030 mg/kg 1–24 mo: 0.030–0.050 mg/kg 2–5 yr: 0.025–0.035 mg/kg 5–10 yr: 0.015–0.030 mg/kg Over10 yr: 0.008–0.012 mg/kg PO: Premature: 0.020–0.030 mg/kg Full term: 0.025–0.035 mg/kg 1–24 mo: 0.035–0.060 mg/kg 2–5 yr: 0.030–0.040 mg/kg 5–10 yr: 0.020–0.035 mg/kg Under10 yr: 0.010–0.015 mg/kg Usual maintenance dose: 25%–35% of digitalizing dose *Adult* PO/IV: Usual digitalizing dose: 1–1.5 mg/day; usual maintenance dose: 0.125–0.5 mg/day	Heart failure, atrial fibrillation

Continued

DOSAGES Drugs for Heart Failure (cont'd)			
Drug (Pregnancy Category)	**Pharmacological Class**	**Usual Dosage Range**	**Indications**
milrinone lactate (C)	Phosphodiesterase inhibitor	*Adult* PO/IV: Usual digitalizing dose: 1–1.5 mg/day; usual maintenance dose: 0.125–0.5 mg/day IV loading dose: 50 mcg/kg over 10 min IV continuous infusion dose: 0.375–0.75 mcg/kg/min	Heart failure Heart failure
nesiritide (Natrecor) (C)	Recombinant human type-B natriuretic peptide	*Adult only* (use in children not yet established) IV: Initial bolus of 2 mcg/kg, followed by continuous infusion of 0.01 mcg/kg/min	Acutely decompensated heart failure in patients with dyspnea at rest or with minimal activity

MISCELLANEOUS HEART FAILURE DRUGS

The newest class of medications for heart failure currently includes only one drug: nesiritide (Natrecor). This drug is classified as a synthetic *recombinant* version of human B-type natriuretic peptide (BNP), a synthetic hormone that has vasodilating effects on both arteries and veins. BNP is secreted by the ventricles of the heart in response to pressure or volume overload in the ventricles. BNP levels are elevated in patients with left ventricular dysfunction and are thought to balance the effects of the renin–angiotension–aldosterone (RAA) system by causing sodium and water excretion, vasodilation, reduced aldosterone secretion, decreased hypertrophy, and inhibition of the sympathetic nervous system and the RAA system. BNP levels correlate with both the severity of symptoms and the prognosis in congestive heart failure. A "recombinant" drug is one manufactured using recombinant DNA technology. This method is described further in later chapters, including Chapter 51.

The vasodilating effect of nesiritide takes place not only in the heart but also throughout the body. A related hormone that occurs naturally in the body is atrial natriuretic peptide (ANP). ANP is released primarily from myocytes in the right atrium in response to high blood pressure. ANP affects vascular permeability by reducing water, sodium, and adipose loads on the circulatory system, thereby reducing blood pressure. *Vascular permeability* is the ability of plasma to flow between blood vessels and their surrounding tissues, which serves as one way for the body to regulate blood pressure. The effects of nesiritide on vascular permeability have yet to be studied.

At this time, nesiritide is generally used in the critical care setting as a final effort to treat severe, life-threatening acute heart failure, often along with several other cardiostimulatory medications. The manufacturer recommends that nesiritide not be used as a first-line drug for this purpose. Its only current contraindication is drug allergy, although it is not recommended for use in patients with low cardiac filling pressures, as typically measured in the critical care unit. The drug received a Notice of Compliance by Health Canada in 2008 on the basis of promising evidence of clinical effectiveness for the treatment of a serious, life-threatening, or severely debilitating illness. Currently identified drug interactions include additive hypotensive effects with coadministration of ACE inhibitors (Chapter 25) and diuretics (Chapter 26). Recommended dosages are given in the Dosages table above.

NURSING PROCESS

Assessment

Before a cardiac glycoside or other positive inotropic drug is administered, a thorough assessment of the patient is required so that the drug can be used in the safest manner possible. An assessment of the patient's past and present medical histories (especially in the presence of heart, hypertensive, or kidney diseases) and complete medication history may yield findings that either dictate cautious use of the drug or even contraindicate its use (Table 22-4). Before the nurse initiates therapy with digoxin or another positive inotropic drug, a number of clinical parameters and other data need to be assessed. These include the following:

- Blood pressure, pulse rate (both apical and radial for 1 full minute), and heart sounds (see also text below on heart assessment)
- Peripheral pulse location and grading
- Capillary refill
- Presence of edema

- Breath sounds
- Weight
- Intake and output amounts
- Serum laboratory values such as potassium, sodium, magnesium, and calcium
- Electrocardiogram
- Kidney function laboratory test values (blood urea nitrogen and creatinine levels)
- Liver function test results (levels of aspartate aminotransferase, alanine aminotransferase, creatine phosphokinase, lactate dehydrogenase, and alkaline phosphatase)
- Medication history and profile regarding prescription drugs, over-the-counter drugs, and natural health products—for example, herbal products (e.g., Siberian ginseng) may increase digitalis drug levels; consuming large amounts of bran with digoxin will decrease the drug's absorption
- Dietary habits and a recall of meals and snacks for the previous 24 hours
- Inquiries about the intake of moderate to large amounts of bran or taking bran at the same time as the digitalis drug (which decreases the drug's absorption)
- Smoking history
- Alcohol intake

Other assessment data include thorough monitoring of electrolytes because of the narrow therapeutic range with digoxin. With a narrow therapeutic range, there is but a small difference between a therapeutic serum level of digoxin and a toxic level. Because low levels of certain electrolytes (e.g., hypokalemia) may precipitate this drug's toxicity, close assessment is critical to preventing complications and further problems. Other laboratory tests include those for serum calcium, magnesium, and sodium levels before and during drug therapy. In addition, the occurrence of any edema (weight gain of 1 kg a day or 2 kg or more in 1 week) needs to be reported to the health care provider. The following systems should also be included in the assessment:

- Neurological assessment, noting headache, depression, weakness, changes in level of consciousness, alertness and orientation versus confusion, presence of restlessness, fatigue, lethargy, or occurrence of nightmares
- Gastrointestinal assessment, with attention to changes in appetite, diarrhea versus constipation, nausea, and vomiting
- Heart assessment, with documentation of any irregularities, pulse rate of less than 60 beats/min or more than 100 beats/min, abnormal heart sounds, and abnormal ECG findings (if ordered)
- Vision and sensory assessment, with notation of any changes such as green–yellow halos surrounding the peripheral field of vision.

Also assess for complaints of anorexia, nausea, and vomiting, which indicate cardiac glycoside toxicity. See Table 22-1 for more information related to adverse effects. Cautions, contraindications, and drug interactions should also be assessed (see Tables 22-1, 22-2, and 22-3).

In summary, a head-to-toe physical assessment with thorough medical and medication history taking will help prevent adverse and toxic reactions by identifying them early in the therapy. These drugs, although helpful in the management of heart failure, are not without risk of toxicity. It is also important to assess support systems at home because safe and effective therapy depends on close observation, monitoring of parameters such as daily weight, attention to complaints by the patient, and evaluation of how the patient is feeling.

TABLE 22-4

Conditions Predisposing to Digitalis Toxicity

Condition or Disease	Significance
Advanced age	Because of decreased kidney function and the resultant diminished drug excretion along with decreased body mass in this patient population, a lower dose than usual is needed to prevent toxicity. Polypharmacy may also lead to toxicity.
Atrioventricular block	Heart block may worsen with increasing levels of digitalis.
Dysrhythmias	Dysrhythmias may occur that did not exist before digitalis use and could be related to digitalis toxicity.
Hypercalcemia	The patient is at higher risk of sinus bradycardia, dysrhythmias, and heart block.
Hypokalemia	The patient's risk of serious dysrhythmias is increased and the patient is more susceptible to digitalis toxicity.
Hypothyroid, respiratory, or kidney disease	Patients with these disorders require lower doses because they cause delayed kidney drug excretion.
Liver dysfunction	Hepatic elimination of digitoxin is decreased, which necessitates a reduction in doasge.
Use of cardiac pacemaker	A patient with this device may exhibit digitalis toxicity at lower doses than normal.
Ventricular fibrillation	Ventricular rate may actually increase with digitalis use.

Nursing Diagnoses

- Ineffective tissue perfusion, cardiopulmonary, related to the pathophysiological influence of heart failure
- Deficient knowledge related to the first-time use of a cardiac glycoside or positive inotropic drug and subsequent lack of information on heart failure and its treatment
- Risk for injury related to limited information on the pathological impact of heart failure and the potential adverse effects of drug therapy
- Imbalanced nutrition less than body requirements, related to gastrointestinal adverse effects from digoxin toxicity
- Nonadherence to therapy related to lack of information about the drug's effects and adverse effects

Planning

Goals

- Patient will exhibit improved cardiac output once therapy is initiated.
- Patient will state use, action, adverse effects, and toxic effects of therapy.
- Patient will be free from injury related to medication therapy.
- Patient will have an improved appetite, or patient will be free of anorexia while taking positive inotropic drugs.

In planning for the administration of these preparations, the nurse must check the dosage and always double-check calculations as well as the patient's laboratory values. Administration of parenteral dosage forms needs preplanning so that all necessary equipment is gathered before giving the drug.

Outcome Criteria

- Patient has improved to strong peripheral pulses, increased endurance for activity, decreased fatigue, and pink, warm extremities.
- Patient has increased urinary output resulting from therapeutic effects of the drug.
- Patient has improved heart and lung sounds with decreased dysrhythmias and crackles.
- Patient loses appropriate weight and has less edema from the therapeutic effects of the drug (increased urinary output because of increased cardiac output).
- Patient's skin and mucous membranes (colour and temperature) are improved to pink and warm.
- Patient maintains appetite while on therapy and reports anorexia, nausea, or vomiting immediately to the health care provider.

- Patient is free of toxicity as evidenced by absence of bradycardia and no complaints of anorexia, nausea, or vomiting.
- Patient demonstrates proper technique for measuring radial pulse for 1 full minute before taking medication.
- Patient is able to state drug-related problems that must be reported to the health care provider, such as palpitations, dysrhythmias, chest pain, and pulse less than 60 beats/min or greater than 120 beats/min.

Implementation

Before administering any cardiac glycoside, all electrolyte and drug levels should be checked to be sure they are within normal limits. The nurse should *always* count the patient's apical pulse rate (auscultate the apical heart rate—found at the point of maximal impulse at the fifth left midclavicular intercostal space—*for 1 full minute*). If the pulse is 60 beats/min or less or greater than 120 beats/min, the dose should be withheld and the health care provider notified of the problem. Withholding of the dose is usually indicated; however, health care facilities and health care providers have their own protocols that apply to individual patients. In addition, the health care provider should be contacted if the patient experiences any of the following signs and symptoms (which may indicate digitalis toxicity): anorexia, nausea, vomiting, diarrhea, or visual disturbances such as blurred vision or the perception of green or yellow halos around objects. Remember that most institutions and nursing units follow a protocol or policy on digitalis and its administration.

Other nursing interventions include checking the dosage form and prescribed amounts and the physician's order carefully to make sure that the correct drug dosage ordered has been dispensed (e.g., 0.125 or 0.25 mg). Oral digoxin may be administered with meals but not with foods high in fibre, such as bran, because the fibre, will bind to the digitalis and lead to altered absorption and bioavailability of the drug. If the medication is to be given intravenously, it is critical to patient safety to infuse undiluted intravenous forms at approximately 0.25 mg/min or over longer than a 5-minute period, or per hospital protocol. The administration of intramuscular forms of cardiac glycosides is extremely painful and is not indicated or recommended because tissue necrosis and erratic absorption are often the outcome. Digoxin is incompatible with many other medications in solution or syringe, and compatibility must be double-checked before parenteral administration. The nursing interventions for patients undergoing digitalization must be considered separately. Although not commonly used in contemporary practice, digitalization may still be performed in some areas of practice for the management of heart failure. Rapid digitalization (to achieve faster onset of action) is generally reserved for patients with heart failure and in acute distress. Such patients are hospitalized because digitalis toxicities can appear quickly in this setting and are directly correlated with the high drug concentrations used. Should the patient undergoing rapid digitalization exhibit any of the manifestations of toxicity, the health care provider should be contacted immediately. These patients should be observed constantly and serum drug and potassium levels measured frequently.

Slow digitalization is generally performed on an outpatient basis in patients with heart failure who are not in such acute distress. In this situation, it takes longer for toxic effects to appear (depending on the specific drug's half-life) than with rapid digitalization. The main advantages of slow digitalization are that it can be performed on an outpatient basis, oral dosage forms can be used, and it is safer than rapid digitalization. The disadvantages are that it takes longer for the therapeutic effects to occur and the symptoms of toxicity are more gradual in onset and, therefore, more insidious.

Should toxicity occur and digoxin rise to a life-threatening level, the antidote, digoxin immune Fab, should be administered as ordered. It is given parenterally over 30 minutes and in some scenarios given as an intravenous bolus (or IV push) (e.g., if cardiac arrest is imminent). All vials of the drug should be refrigerated. The drug, stable for 4 hours after being mixed, should be used immediately and, if not used within this time frame, be discarded. Compatible solutions for dilution should be checked prior to infusion of the antidote. Blood pressure, apical pulse rate/rhythm, electrocardiogram, and serum potassium levels must be closely monitored and documented. The nurse must always watch for changes from patient baseline assessment values in the following: muscle strength; tremor; muscle cramping; mental health status; heart irregular rhythms (from hypokalemia); and confusion, thirst, and cold clammy skin (from hyponatremia). If toxicity improves, these signs and symptoms will improve (from baseline).

Intake and output, heart rate, blood pressure, daily weight, respiration rate, heart sounds, and breath sounds should be recorded. Any evidence of hypokalemia should be noted and reported to the physician immediately. When giving these drugs (e.g., digoxin, milrinone, digoxin immune Fab) parenterally, an infusion pump must be used unless the order is to give them IV push.

Evaluation

Monitoring patients after the administration of positive inotropic drugs is critical for identifying therapeutic effects and adverse effects. Because positive inotropic drugs increase the force of myocardial contractility (positive inotropic effect), alter electrophysiological properties (decrease rate, negative chronotropic effect), and decrease AV node conduction (negative dromotropic effect), the therapeutic effects include the following:

- Increased urinary output
- Decreased edema
- Decreased shortness of breath, dyspnea, and crackles
- Decreased fatigue
- Resolution of paroxysmal nocturnal dyspnea
- Improved peripheral pulses, skin colour, and temperature

While monitoring for therapeutic effects, it is essential (because of the low therapeutic index of digitalis preparations) that the nurse assess the patient for the development of toxic effects described earlier. Monitoring laboratory values such as serum creatinine, potassium, calcium, sodium, and chloride levels, as well as monitoring the serum levels of digoxin (0.8–2.0 ng/mL), is important to ensure safe and efficacious treatment.

Therapeutic effects of milrinone include an improvement in heart function with a corresponding alleviation of the patient's heart failure. Adverse effects to monitor include hypotension, dysrhythmias, headache, ventricular fibrillation, chest pain, and hypokalemia. Patients taking milrinone should be evaluated for significant hypotension; should this occur, the drug should be discontinued or the infusion rate decreased per the physician's orders.

PATIENT EDUCATION

- Patients should be instructed to measure the radial pulse rate before each dose of digoxin. For the older adult or physically or mentally challenged patients, it is important that home health care personnel supervise the medication regimen or that a hospital-based or cardiologist-managed heart failure clinic supervise therapy. This is important because these individuals are at risk for drug interactions, adverse effects, and toxicity.
- Patients should keep a journal at home in which they record the following: date, time of dose, amount of medication taken, dietary intake, weight, any unusual adverse effects or changes in condition, pulse rate, and any other miscellaneous comments.
- Patients should be encouraged to contact the physician or health care provider if they have any unusual complaints, if the pulse rate is below 60 beats/min or is erratic, if the pulse rate is 120 beats/min or greater, or if they are experiencing anorexia, nausea, or vomiting.
- Patients should be encouraged to report any of the following: palpitations or a feeling that the heart is racing, a change in heart rate, dizziness, fainting or blackout spells, or weight gain (1 kg or more in 24 hours or 2 kg or more in 1 week).
- Patients should be encouraged to immediately report any changes in visual acuity to the health care provider or home health care nurse.
- Patients should be informed to wear a medical alert bracelet or necklace or otherwise make sure their medical and medication histories and information are with them at all times. They must make sure that all information is updated frequently or with each visit to the physician.
- Patients should be encouraged to measure their weight daily, at the same time each day and with the same amount of clothing on because weight is an important indicator of fluid volume overload or exacerbation of heart failure. Be emphatic about the importance of adherence to medications, reducing the stress on the heart, rest and relaxation, watching the weight daily, and keeping follow-up appointments with the physician, heart failure clinic, nurse practitioner, or other health care provider.
- Digoxin is usually taken once a day, and patients should be encouraged to take it at the same time every morning. If a dose is missed, the patient may take the omitted dose if no more than 12 hours have passed from the time the drug was to have been taken.
- If more than 12 hours have passed, patients should know to not skip that dose, not double up on the next digoxin dose, and to contact the health care provider immediately for further instructions.
- Patients should never abruptly stop their digoxin (or other positive inotropics) because this could precipitate more heart problems and complications.
- Patients should be encouraged to consume foods high in potassium, especially if they are also taking a potassium-depleting diuretic. Encourage them to report any weakness, fatigue, or lethargy immediately to the health care provider.
- Patients should be encouraged to report any worsening of dizziness or dyspnea or the occurrence of any unusual problems.
- Patients should avoid using antacids or eating ice cream, milk products, yogourt, or cheese for 2 hours before or after taking medication to avoid interference with the drug.

POINTS TO REMEMBER

- *Inotropic* drugs affect the force of myocardial contraction: *positive inotropics* (e.g., digoxin) increase the force of contractions and *negative inotropics* (e.g., β-blockers, calcium channel blockers) decrease the force of myocardial contractility.
- *Chronotropic* drugs affect the rate at which the heart beats (beats/min): *positive chronotropic* drugs (e.g., epinephrine, atropine) increase the heart rate and *negative chronotropic* drugs decrease the heart rate.
- *Dromotropic* drugs affect the conduction of electrical impulses through the heart: *positive dromotropic* drugs increase the speed of electrical impulses through the heart, whereas *negative dromotropic* drugs have the opposite effect.
- Nurses need to be aware of important physiological concepts such as ejection fraction. A patient's *ejection fraction* reflects the contractility of the heart and is approximately 65% (0.65) in a normal heart. This value decreases as heart failure progresses; therefore, patients with heart failure have low ejection fractions because their hearts are failing to pump effectively.
- Nurses should be knowledgeable regarding contraindications to the use of digoxin, which include the following: a history of allergy to the digitalis medications, ventricular tachycardia and fibrillations, and AV block.
- Patients need to be aware of conditions that predispose to digitalis toxicity, including hypokalemia, hypercalcemia, hypothyroid states, kidney dysfunction, and advanced age.
- Patients should be educated to measure pulse rate and daily weight and to record these daily.
- Nurses should always measure the apical pulse rate for 1 full minute when digoxin is administered, and patients should be instructed on measuring radial pulse rates when at home.
- Patients should be encouraged to notify the health care provider immediately at the first signs of anorexia, nausea, or vomiting, or bradycardia with a pulse rate below 60 beats/min if taking digoxin.
- Nurses must be aware that hypotension, dysrhythmias, and thrombocytopenia are major adverse effects of milrinone use.

EXAMINATION REVIEW QUESTIONS

1 Which of the following signs and symptoms of cardiac glycoside toxicity should the nurse teach the patient to be aware of?
   a. Increased urine output
   b. Dizziness when standing up
   c. Visual changes such as photophobia
   d. Flickering lights or halos around lights

2 During assessment of a patient who is receiving digoxin, which finding would indicate an increased possibility of toxicity?
   a. Digoxin level of 1.5 ng/mL
   b. Apical pulse rate of 62 beats/min
   c. Serum potassium level of 2 mmol/L
   d. Serum potassium level of 4.8 mmol/L

3 When monitoring a patient receiving an intravenous infusion of milrinone, which adverse effect must the nurse be alert for?
   a. Anemia
   b. Proteinuria
   c. Thrombocytopenia
   d. Decreased blood urea nitrogen and creatinine levels

4 When a patient is experiencing digitalis toxicity, in which of the following situations would it be appropriate to treat with digoxin immune Fab (Digibind)?
   a. Supraventricular dysrhythmias
   b. Apical heart rate of 60 beats/min
   c. Hypokalemia (serum potassium level lower than 3.5 mmol/L)
   d. Hyperkalemia (serum potassium level higher than 5 mmol/L)

5 Before beginning oral digoxin therapy, the nurse would note that some drugs would cause a decrease in the absorption of the digoxin if the two are taken together. Which of the following would cause this effect?
   a. Potassium
   b. Loop diuretics
   c. Antidiarrheals
   d. Antidepressants

For answers see http://evolve.elsevier.com/Canada/Lilley/pharmacology/.

CRITICAL THINKING ACTIVITIES

1 A nurse intravenously administered 125 mg of digoxin instead of 0.125 mg. The patient has developed a severe heart block dysrhythmia, and the slow heart rate has not responded to administration of atropine and other measures. The patient will be receiving digoxin immune Fab. Explain how this medication works in this situation. How could this situation have been prevented?

2 Your patient, a 78-year-old-man, has a potassium level of 3.0 mmol/L. He states that he has been nauseous and without an appetite and has experienced some diarrhea. He has been taking digoxin for the past few weeks for the treatment of recently diagnosed heart failure. Discuss the implication of hypokalemia in a patient who is on digoxin and any negative consequences.

3 Explain why an older patient with hypothyroid disease is at increased risk for digitalis toxicity.

For answers see http://evolve.elsevier.com/Canada/Lilley/pharmacology/.

CHAPTER 23

Antidysrhythmic Drugs

Learning Objectives

After reading this chapter, the successful student will be able to do the following:

1 Describe the anatomy and physiology of a normal heart, including conduction, rate, and rhythm, and compare them with those of a heart with abnormal conduction and rhythm.

2 Define the term *dysrhythmia* and explain its causes and consequences for the patient.

3 Identify the most commonly encountered dysrhythmias.

4 Compare the dysrhythmias with regard to their basic characteristics, their impact on the structures of the heart, and related symptoms.

5 Contrast the classes of antidysrhythmic drugs, citing prototypes in each class and describing their mechanisms of action, indications, routes of administration, dosing, any related drug protocols, adverse effects, cautions, contraindications, drug interactions, and any toxic reactions.

6 Develop a collaborative plan of care that includes all phases of the nursing process for patients receiving each class of antidysrhythmics.

e-Learning Activities

Web site
(http://evolve.elsevier.com/Canada/Lilley/pharmacology/)

- Animations
- Answers to chapter questions, activities, and case studies
- Calculators and Category Catchers
- Glossary with audio pronunciations
- IV Therapy and Medication Error Checklists
- Multiple-Choice Review Question quizzes
- Nursing Care Plans
- Online Appendices and Supplements
- WebLinks

Drug Profiles

adenosine, p. 435
▸▸ amiodarone (amiodarone hydrochloride)*, p. 434
▸▸ atenolol, p. 433
▸▸ diltiazem (diltiazem hydrochloride)*, p. 435
esmolol (esmolol hydrochloride)*, p. 433
flecainide (flecainide acetate)*, p. 432
ibutilide (ibutilide fumarate)*, p. 434
▸▸ lidocaine (lidocaine hydrochloride)*, p. 431
▸▸ metoprolol (metoprolol tartrate)*, p. 433
mexiletine (mexiletine hydrochloride)*, p. 432
procainamide (procainamide hydrochloride)*, p. 431
propafenone (propafenone hydrochloride)*, p. 432
▸▸ propranolol (propranolol hydrochloride)*, p. 433
quinidine (quinidine sulfate)*, p. 431
▸▸ sotalol (sotalol hydrochloride)*, p. 434
▸▸ verapamil (verapamil hydrochloride)*, p. 435

▸▸ Key drug.

*Full generic name is given in parentheses. For the purposes of this text, the more common shortened name is used.

Glossary

Action potential Electrical activity consisting of a self-propagating series of polarizations and depolarizations that travel across the cell membrane of a nerve fibre during the transmission of a nerve impulse and across the cell membrane of a muscle cell during contraction or other activity of the cell. (p. 419)

Action potential duration (APD) For a cell membrane, the interval beginning with baseline (resting) membrane potential followed by depolarization and ending with repolarization to baseline membrane potential. (p. 421)

Arrhythmia Literally "no rhythm," meaning absence of a heartbeat rhythm (i.e., no heartbeat at all). More commonly used in clinical practice to refer to any variation from the normal rhythm of the heartbeat. (p. 419)

Cardiac Arrhythmia Suppression Trial (CAST) The name of the major research study conducted by the National Heart, Lung, and Blood Institute to investigate the possibility of eliminating sudden cardiac death in patients with asymptomatic, non–life-threatening ectopy that has arisen after a myocardial infarction. (p. 432)

Depolarization The movement of positive and negative ions on either side of a cell membrane across the membrane in a direction that tends to bring the net charge to zero. (p. 420)

Dysrhythmia Any disturbance or abnormality in the rhythm of the heartbeat. (p. 419)

Effective refractory period (ERP) The period after the firing of an impulse during which a cell may respond to a stimulus but the response will not be passed along or continued as another impulse. (p. 421)

Internodal pathways (Bachmann's bundle) Special pathways in the atria that carry electrical impulses spontaneously generated by the sinoatrial node. These impulses cause the heart to beat. (p. 422)

Relative refractory period (RRP) The time after generation of an action potential during which a nerve fibre will show a (reduced) response only to a strong stimulus. (p. 421)

Resting membrane potential (RMP) The transmembrane voltage that exists when cell membranes of heart muscle (or other muscle or nerve cells) are at rest. (p. 419)

Sodium–potassium adenosine triphosphatase (ATPase) pump A mechanism for transporting sodium and potassium ions across the cell membrane against an opposing concentration gradient. (p. 419)

Sudden cardiac death Unexpected, fatal cardiac arrest. (p. 432)

Threshold potential (TP) The critical state of electrical tension required for spontaneous depolarization of a cell membrane. (p. 422)

Vaughan Williams classification The system most commonly used to classify antidysrhythmic drugs. (p. 425; see also Table 23-3, p. 425)

DYSRHYTHMIAS AND NORMAL CARDIAC ELECTROPHYSIOLOGY

A **dysrhythmia** is any deviation from the normal rhythm of the heart. The term **arrhythmia** (literally "no rhythm") implies asystole, or no heartbeat at all because a patient who has no heart rhythm is in asystole, or dead. A synonymous term is dysrhythmia, which is the primary term used in this chapter and book. Dysrhythmias can develop in association with many conditions. Some of the more common ones arise after a myocardial infarction (MI) or heart surgery or as the result of coronary artery disease. These dysrhythmias are usually serious and may require treatment with an antidysrhythmic drug or nonpharmacological therapies (discussed later in this chapter), although not all require medical treatment. A cardiologist is usually consulted to make the judgement.

Disturbances in heart rhythm are the result of abnormally functioning cardiac cells. Therefore, an understanding of the pathological mechanism responsible for dysrhythmias first requires review of the electrical properties of cardiac cells. Figure 22-1 on p. 405 illustrates the overall anatomy of the conduction system of the heart. Figure 23-1 illustrates some of the properties of this system with reference to a single cardiac cell. Within a resting cardiac cell there is a net negative charge relative to the outside of the cell. This difference in the electronegative charge exists in all types of cardiac cells and is referred to as the **resting membrane potential (RMP).** The

RMP results from an uneven distribution of ions (sodium, potassium, and calcium) across the cell membrane. This is known as polarization. Each ion moves primarily through its own specific channel, which is a specialized protein molecule that sits across the cell membrane. These proteins work continuously to restore the specific intracellular and extracellular concentrations of each ion. At RMP, the ionic concentration gradient (distribution) for the different ions is such that potassium ions are more highly concentrated intracellularly, whereas sodium and calcium ions are both more highly concentrated extracellularly. For this reason, potassium is generally thought of as an intracellular ion, whereas sodium and calcium are generally thought of as extracellular ions. Negatively charged intracellular and extracellular ions such as chloride (Cl^-) and bicarbonate ($HCO3^-$) also contribute to this uneven distribution of ions, which is known as a polarized state. This polarized distribution of ions is maintained by the **sodium–potassium adenosine triphosphatase (ATPase) pump,** an energy-requiring ionic pump. The energy that drives this pump comes from molecules of adenosine triphosphate (ATP), which are a major source of energy in cellular metabolism. Cardiac cells become excited when there is a change in this distribution of ions across their membranes (RMP) that leads to the propagation of an electrical impulse. This change is known as an **action potential.** Action potentials normally occur in a continuous and regular manner in the cells of the heart conduction system, such as the sinoatrial (SA) node, atrioventricular (AV) node, and the His–Purkinje system, because all of these tissues have the property of spontaneous electrical excitability known as automaticity. This excited state creates action potentials, which, in turn, generate electrical impulses that travel through the myocardium ultimately to create the heartbeat via contraction of heart muscle fibres.

An action potential has five phases. *Phase 0* is also called the upstroke because it appears as an upward line on the graph of an action potential, as shown in Figures 23-2*A* and *B*. Both of these figures graphically illustrate the cycle of electrical changes that create an action potential. Note the variation in the shape of the curve of the graph, depending on the relative conduction speed of the specific tissue involved (SA node versus Purkinje fibre). A faster rate of conduction corresponds to a steeper slope on the graph. During phase 0, the resting cardiac cell membrane suddenly becomes highly permeable to sodium ions, which rush from outside of the cell membrane to inside (influx) through what are known as the fast channels or sodium channels. This disruption of the earlier polarized state of the membrane is known as **depolarization**. Depolarization can be thought of as a temporary equalization of positive and negative charges across the cell membrane. This releases spurts of electrochemical energy that drive the resulting electrical impulses through adjacent cells.

Phase 1 of the action potential begins a rapid period of *repolarization* that continues through *phases 2* and *3* to *phase 4*, which is the RMP. In phase 1, the sodium channels close and the concentrations of each ion begin to move back toward their ion-specific RMP levels. During phase 2, calcium ion influx occurs through the *slow channels* or calcium channels. They are called slow channels because the calcium influx occurs relatively more slowly than the earlier sodium influx. Potassium ions then flow from inside of the cell to outside (efflux) through specific potassium channels to offset the elevated positive charge caused by the influx of sodium and calcium ions. In the case of the Purkinje fibres, this causes a partial plateau (flattening on the graph) during which the overall membrane potential changes only slightly, as seen in Figure 23-2*B*.

In phase 3, the ionic flow patterns of phases 0 to 2 are changed by the sodium–potassium ATPase pump (or, more simply, the sodium pump), which re-establishes the baseline polarized state by restoring both intracellular and extracellular concentrations of sodium, potassium, and calcium (see Figure 23-1). As a result, the cell membrane is ultimately repolarized to its baseline level or RMP (phase 4). Note that this entire process occurs over roughly 400 milliseconds—that is, four hundred thousandths (less than half) of 1 second.

However, there is some variation in this period between different parts of the conduction system. As an example, Figure 23-3 illustrates the pattern of movement of sodium, potassium, and calcium ions into and out of a Purkinje cell during the phases of the action potential. Note that there are several important differences in the action potentials of SA nodal cells and Purkinje cells. The RMP in the Purkinje cell is approximately −80 to −90 mV, compared with −50 to −60 mV in the SA nodal cell (which is also comparable with that in AV nodal cells). The level of the RMP for a given type of cell is an important determinant of the *rate* of its impulse conduction to other cells. The less negative (i.e., the closer to zero) the RMP at the onset of phase 0 of the action potential, the slower is the upstroke *velocity* of phase 0. The *slope* of phase 0 is directly related to the impulse velocity. An upstroke with a steeper slope indicates faster conduction velocity. Thus, in the Purkinje cells, electrical conduction is relatively fast, and electrical impulses are conducted quickly. Many antidysrhythmic drugs affect the RMP and sodium channels; this effect, in turn, influences the rate of impulse conduction. These cells are referred to as *fast-response cells*, or *fast-channel cells*, and Purkinje fibres can therefore be thought of as fast-channel tissue. Many antidysrhythmic drugs affect the RMP and sodium channels, which, in turn, influences the rate of impulse conduction.

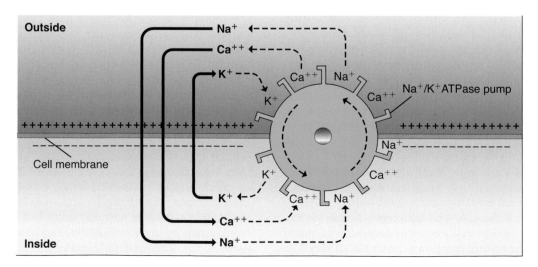

FIG. 23-1 Resting membrane potential of a cardiac cell. *ATPase*, adenosine triphosphatase

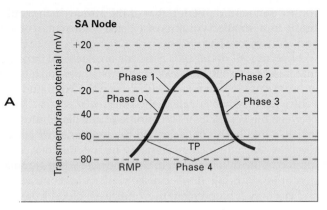 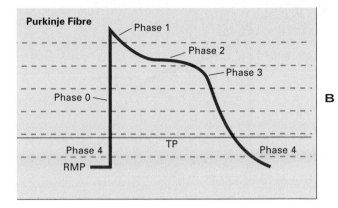

FIG. 23-2   Action potentials. *RMP*, resting membrane potential; *SA*, sinoatrial; *TP*, threshold potential.

In contrast to Purkinje fibres, the cells of the SA node, which have RMPs of –50 to –60 mV (i.e., less negative and closer to zero than those of Purkinje cells), have a slower upstroke velocity, or a slower phase 0. This is illustrated in Figure 23-2*A* as an upstroke curve that is less steep, indicating a relatively slower rate of electrical conduction in these cells.

Again, AV nodal cells are comparable to SA nodal cells in this regard. This slower upstroke in the SA and AV nodes is primarily dependent on the entry of calcium ions through the slow channels or calcium channels mentioned previously in the discussion of phase 3 in both nodal and Purkinje cells. This means that nodal action potentials are affected by calcium influx as early as phase 0, an effect that is less pronounced in the Purkinje action potentials, where calcium influx is more predominantly a phase 3 phenomenon. The nodes are therefore called slow-channel tissue, and conduction in these cells is slower than that in other parts of the conduction system. Drugs that affect calcium ion movement into or out of these cells (e.g., calcium channel blockers) tend to have significant effects on the SA and AV nodal conduction rates.

The interval between phase 0 and phase 4 is called the **action potential duration (APD)** (Figure 23-4). The period between phase 0 and midway through phase 3 is called the *absolute* or **effective refractory period (ERP).** During the ERP, the cardiac cell cannot be stimulated to depolarize and generate another action potential. During the remainder of phase 3 until the return to the RMP (phase 4), the cardiac cell can be depolarized again if it receives a powerful enough impulse (such as one induced by drug therapy or supplied by an electrical pacemaker). This period is referred to as the **relative refractory period (RRP).** If a cardiac cell receives a strong enough stimulus during the RRP, it will be when the cell is at a relatively less negative membrane potential (i.e., closer to zero than when at RMP), which will result in a slower upstroke (phase 0) and slower impulse conduction than if it were stimulated while at RMP. Figure 23-4 illustrates these aspects of an action potential. Again, the actual shape of the action potential curve varies in different parts of the conduction system.

The RMP of certain cardiac cells gradually decreases (becomes less negative) over time in ongoing cycles, and this is probably secondary to small changes in the flux of

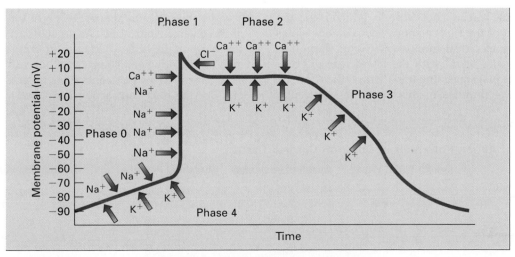

FIG. 23-3   Purkinje fibre action potential.

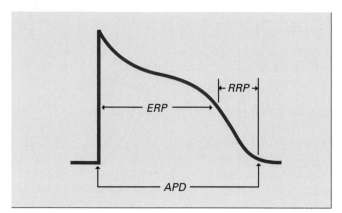

FIG. 23-4 Aspects of an action potential. *APD*, action potential duration; *ERP*, effective refractory period; *RRP*, relative refractory period.

sodium and potassium ions. Depolarization eventually occurs when a certain critical voltage is reached **(threshold potential [TP])**. This process of spontaneous depolarization is referred to as *automaticity*, or *pacemaker activity*, as mentioned earlier in this section. It is normal when it occurs in the SA node (see Figure 22-1, p. 405). When spontaneous depolarizations occur elsewhere, however, dysrhythmias often result.

Although the SA node, AV node, and His–Purkinje cells all possess the property of automaticity, only the SA node is the pacemaker of the heart because it spontaneously depolarizes the most frequently. The SA node has an intrinsic rate of 60 to 100 depolarizations or beats per minute; that of the AV node is 40 to 60 beats/min; and that of the ventricular Purkinje fibres is 40 or fewer beats/min. The action potentials and other properties in different areas of the heart are compared in Table 23-1.

As the pacemaker of the heart, the SA node, which is located near the top of the right atrium, generates the electrical impulse that ultimately produces the heartbeat. First, however, this impulse travels through the atria via specialized pathways called the **internodal pathways (Bachmann's bundle).** This causes contraction of atrial myocardial fibres, which creates the first heart sound. Next, the impulse reaches the AV node, which is located near the bottom of the right atrium. The AV node slows this fast-moving electrical impulse just long enough to allow the ventricles to fill with the blood that the contracting atria are just squeezing into them. If the AV node did not slow the impulse in this way, the ventricular

contraction would overlap that of the atria, which would result in a smaller volume of ejected ventricular blood and reduced cardiac output.

Next, the AV nodal cells generate an electrical impulse that passes into the *bundle of His* (or His bundle), a band of heart muscle fibres located between the right and left ventricles in what is called the *ventricular septum* (wall between the ventricles). The bundle of His distributes the impulse into both ventricles via the *right* and *left bundle branches*. Each branch terminates in the *Purkinje fibres* located in the myocardium of the ventricles. The stimulation of the Purkinje fibres causes ventricular contraction and ejection of blood from the ventricles. Blood from the right ventricle is pumped into the pulmonary circulation, whereas blood from the left ventricle is pumped into the systemic circulation to supply the rest of the body. The His bundle and Purkinje fibres are so named for the medical scientists who first identified them. Together, they are often referred to in the literature as the His–Purkinje system. Any abnormality in cardiac automaticity or impulse conduction often results in some type of dysrhythmia.

Electrocardiography

The electrophysiological heart events described in detail earlier correspond more simply to the tracings of an electrocardiogram, abbreviated as ECG or EKG. *EKG,* which originates from a German spelling, is used more commonly in the United States. Figure 23-5 illustrates the basic elements of a normal ECG tracing. The P wave corresponds to spontaneous impulse generation in the SA node followed immediately by depolarization of atrial myocardial fibres and their muscular contraction. This normally determines the heart rate and is affected by the balance between sympathetic and parasympathetic nervous system tone, the intrinsic automaticity of the SA nodal tissue, the mechanical stretch of atrial fibres due to incoming blood volume, and heart drugs. The QRS complex (or QRS interval) corresponds to depolarization and contraction of ventricular fibres. The J point marks the start of the ST segment, which corresponds to the beginning of ventricular repolarization. The T wave corresponds to completion of the repolarization of these ventricular fibres. As an analogy, depolarization can be thought of as discharge or contraction of heart muscle fibres, whereas repolarization can be thought of as a relaxation of just-contracted muscle fibres to prepare for the next contraction (heartbeat). Note that the

---

TABLE 23-1

Comparison of Action Potentials in Different Cardiac Tissues

Tissue	Action Potential Wave	Speed of Response	Threshold Potential (mV)	Conduction Velocity (m/sec)
SA node		Slow	−60	Less than 0.05
Atrium		Fast	−90	1
AV node		Slow	−60	Less than 0.05
His–Purkinje system		Fast	−95	3
Ventricle		Fast	−90	1

AV, atrioventricular; *SA,* sinoatrial.

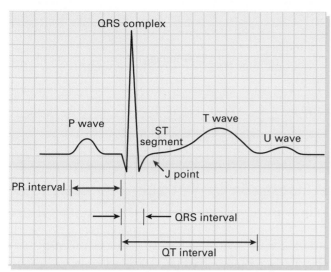

FIG. 23-5 The waves and intervals of a normal electrocardiogram. (From Goldberger A. L. (2006). Clinical electrocardiography: A simplified approach (*7th* ed.). St. Louis, MO: Mosby.)

repolarization of the atrial fibres is obscured on the ECG tracing by the QRS complex and thus has no corresponding deflection in the tracing.

The U wave is not always present, and its physiological basis is uncertain. When it does occur, it is believed to arise from repolarization of Purkinje fibres or delayed repolarization of the ventricular cells that are among the last to depolarize earlier in the cycle of the heartbeat. The PR and QT intervals and the ST segment

are parts of the ECG tracing that are often altered in recognizable ways by disease or by the adverse effects of certain types of drug therapy or drug interactions, as discussed in later sections of this chapter.

Common Dysrhythmias

A variety of cardiac dysrhythmias are recognized. Some are easier to treat than others using drug therapy and interventional cardiology procedures such as pacemakers, catheter ablation, cardioversion, and implantable cardioverters–defibrillators. These nonpharmacological techniques are described in a later section of this chapter. Dysrhythmias are subdivided into several broad categories depending on their anatomical site of origin in the heart. Supraventricular dysrhythmias originate above the ventricles in the SA or AV node or atrial myocardium. Ventricular dysrhythmias originate below the AV node in the His–Purkinje system or ventricular myocardium. Dysrhythmias that originate outside the conduction system (i.e., in atrial or ventricular cells) are known as ectopic, and their specific points of origin are called ectopic foci (foci is the plural of the Latin word focus). Conduction blocks are dysrhythmias that involve disruption of impulse conduction between the atria and ventricles through the AV node and may also originate in the His–Purkinje system, directly affecting ventricular function. Less commonly, impulse conduction between the SA and AV node is affected. Several of the most common dysrhythmias are described in Table 23-2, and corresponding ECG tracings are provided. They are also described further in the following text.

TABLE	23-2

Common Types of Dysrythmias

Dysrhythmia	Description	ECG Tracing
SUPRAVENTRICULAR DYSRHYTHMIAS		
Atrial fibrillation (AF)	Rapid, ineffective atrial contractions	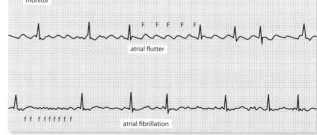
Atrial flutter	Milder form of AF, but often progresses to AF	
Paroxysmal supraventricular tachycardia (PSVT)	Heart rate of 180–200 beats/min or higher	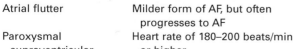
CONDUCTION BLOCKS		
First-degree AV block	Mildest degree, often asymptomatic	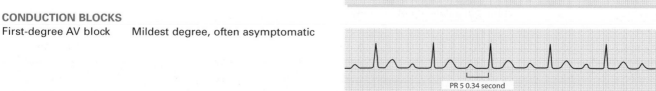

Continued

TABLE 23-2

Common Types of Dysrhythmias (cont'd)

Dysrhythmia	Description	ECG Tracing
Second-degree AV block (Mobitz type I)	Progressive lengthening of PR interval with each beat until impulse is not conducted	
Second-degree AV block (Mobitz type II)	Similar to Mobitz type I, but more consistent in terms of number of failed impulses per unit of time	
Third-degree AV block (complete heart block)	No SA nodal impulses reach ventricles (but heartbeat often still occurs from ventricles' own automaticity—i.e., ectopic ventricular beats)	
VENTRICULAR DYSRHYTHMIAS		
Premature ventricular contractions (PVCs)	Contractions generated by impulses arising from ectopic foci within ventricular myocardium	
Nonsustained ventricular tachycardia (NSVT)	Relatively brief period (20 sec or less) in which ventricles contract rapidly on their own as well as in response to AV impulses	
Sustained ventricular tachycardia (SVT)	Same as above but more prolonged	
Torsades de pointes (TdP)	Rapid ventricular tachycardia preceded by QT interval prolongation (often progresses to ventricular fibrillation)	
Ventricular fibrillation (VF)	Rapid, ineffective ventricular contractions (fatal if not reversed)	

APB, atrial premature beat; *AV*, atrioventricular; *ECG*, electrocardiogram; *SA*, sinoatrial; *VF*, ventricular fibrillation; *VPB*, ventricular premature beat.

Among the supraventricular dysrhythmias, atrial fibrillation is a particularly common condition. It is characterized by rapid atrial contractions that only incompletely pump blood into the ventricles. Atrial fibrillation is notable in that it predisposes the patient to stroke because the blood tends to stagnate in the incompletely emptied atria and is therefore more likely to clot. If such blood clots manage to make their way into the left ventricle, they may be embolized to the brain and cause a stroke. Although theoretically there would be a similar risk for pulmonary embolism, this seems to be less of a clinical concern with atrial fibrillation than the risk of stroke. Patients with ongoing atrial fibrillation are often given anticoagulant therapy with warfarin to reduce the likelihood of stroke.

AV nodal re-entrant tachycardia (AVNRT) is a conduction disorder that often gives rise to a dysrhythmia known as paroxysmal supraventricular tachycardia (PSVT). (The word paroxysmal means "sudden.") AVNRT occurs when electrical impulse transmission from the AV node into the His–Purkinje system of the ventricles is disrupted. As a result, some of the impulses circle backward (retrograde impulses) and re-enter the atrial tissues to produce a tachycardic response. In Wolff–Parkinson–White (WPW) syndrome, ectopic impulses that begin near the AV node actually bypass the AV node and reach the His–Purkinje system before the normal AV-generated impulses. This is one cause of ventricular tachycardia, although it is technically supraventricular in origin.

Varying degrees of AV block (often called heart block) involve varying levels of disrupted conduction of impulses from the AV node and His–Purkinje system to the ventricles. Although first-degree AV block is often asymptomatic, third-degree block, or complete heart block, often requires use of a heart pacemaker to ensure adequate ventricular function. There can also be blocks within the His–Purkinje system of the ventricles known as bundle branch blocks.

Premature ventricular contractions (PVCs) occur when impulses originate from ectopic foci within the ventricles (His–Purkinje system). PVCs probably occur period ally in many people; they become problematic when they occur frequently enough to compromise systolic blood volume. Ventricular tachycardia refers to a rapid heartbeat from impulses originating in the ventricles. It can be nonsustained (brief) or sustained, requiring definitive treatment. Worsening ventricular tachycardia can deteriorate into torsades de pointes, an intermediate dysrhythmia that often further deteriorates into ventricular fibrillation. Ventricular fibrillation is fatal if not reversed, which most often requires electrical defibrillation. Interestingly, torsades de pointes often responds preferentially to intravenous magnesium sulfate.

ANTIDYSRHYTHMIC DRUGS

Numerous drugs are available to treat dysrhythmias. These drugs are categorized according to where and how they affect cardiac cells. Although other classifications are described in the literature, the most commonly used system is the **Vaughan Williams classification.** This system is based on the electrophysiological effect produced by the particular drugs on the action potential. This approach identifies four major classes of drugs. Class I antidysrhythmics are considered membrane-stabilizing drugs, but they are further divided into Ia, Ib, and Ic drugs, depending on the magnitude of their effects on phase 0, the APD, and the ERP. Class II drugs are β-blockers that depress phase 4 depolarization. Class III drugs primarily prolong repolarization during phase 3. Class IV drugs depress phase 4 depolarization and prolong repolarization during phases 1 and 2. Calcium channel blockers (CCBs) (slow channel blockers) such as verapamil belong to class IV. The drugs in these four classes are listed in Table 23-3.

There is a gradual current trend away from the use of class Ia drugs. The formerly available class Ic drug encainide was removed from the market after research indicated that its risk of inducing fatal cardiac dysrhythmias overshadowed its dysrhythmia suppression

TABLE   23-3

Vaughan Williams Classification of Antidysrhythmic Drugs

Functional Class	Drugs
Class I: Membrane-stabilizing drugs; fast sodium channel blockers	
Ia: ↑ blockade of sodium channel, delay repolarization, ↑ APD	disopyramide, procainamide, quinidine,
Ib: ↑ blockade of sodium channel, accelerate repolarization, ± APD	lidocaine, mexiletine, phenytoin
Ic: ↑↑↑ blockade of sodium channel ± on repolarization; also suppress re-entry	flecainide, propafenone
Class II: β-blocking drugs	All β-blockers
Class III: Drugs whose principal effect on cardiac tissue is to ↑ APD	amiodarone, ibutilide sotalol*
Class IV: Calcium channel blockers	diltiazem, verapamil
Other: Antidysrhythmic drugs that have the properties of several classes and therefore cannot be placed in one particular class	adenosine, digoxin

APD, action potential duration; ↑, increase; ↓, decrease; ±, increase or decrease.

*Sotalol also has class II properties.

easons, the other two class Ic drugs, ...fenone, are generally used only in ... other drugs. Nonetheless, several ...pes remain available in Canada as ...d are included in this discussion. ...... drugs have emerged as among the most widely used antidysrhythmics at this time. The class IV drugs (calcium channel blockers), unlike most of the other classes, have limited usefulness in tachydysrhythmias (dysrhythmias involving tachycardia), unlike most of the other classes. The role of class II drugs (β-blockers) continues to grow in the field of cardiology, including in dysrhythmia management. Digoxin, the cardiac glycoside discussed in Chapter 22, still has a place in dysrhythmia management, especially in the prevention of dangerous ventricular tachydysrhythmias secondary to atrial fibrillation.

Mechanism of Action and Drug Effects

Antidysrhythmic drugs work by correcting, to varying degrees and by various mechanisms, abnormal heart electrophysiological function. As membrane-stabilizing drugs, class I drugs exert their actions on the sodium (fast) channels. However, as already noted, there are some slight differences in the actions of the drugs in this class; consequently, they are divided into three additional subclasses. These subclasses are Class Ia, Ib, and Ic drugs, and they depend on the magnitude of the effects of each drug on phase 0, the APD, and the ERP. Class Ia drugs (quinidine, procainamide, and disopyramide) block the sodium channels; more specifically, they delay repolarization and increase the APD. Class Ib drugs (mexiletine, phenytoin, and lidocaine) also block the sodium channels, but unlike class Ia drugs, they accelerate repolarization and decrease the APD. Phenytoin (Dilantin) is more commonly used as an anticonvulsant (Chapter 14) than as an antidysrhythmic drug. Class Ic drugs (flecainide and propafenone) have a more pronounced effect on the blockade of sodium channels but have little effect on repolarization or the APD.

Class II drugs (acebutolol, esmolol, propranolol) are β-adrenergic blockers (β-blockers). They are commonly used as antianginal drugs (Chapter 24) and as antihypertensives (Chapters 19 and 25). They work by reducing or blocking sympathetic nervous system stimulation to the heart and, consequently, the transmission of impulses in the heart's conduction system. This results in depression of phase 4 depolarization. These drugs mostly affect slower-conducting cardiac tissue.

Class III drugs (amiodarone ibutilide, dofetilide, and sotalol) increase the APD by prolonging repolarization in phase 3. They affect fast tissue and are most commonly used to manage dysrhythmias that are difficult to treat. Sotalol actually has properties of both class II and class III and is often listed as a member of one or the other class, depending on the specific reference used.

Class IV drugs are the calcium channel blockers, which, similar to β-blockers, are also used as both antianginal drugs (Chapter 24) and antihypertensives (Chapter 25). As their name implies, they act specifically by inhibiting the channel pathways, reducing the influx of calcium ions during action potentials. This results in depression of phase 4 depolarization. Diltiazem and verapamil are the calcium channel blockers most commonly used to treat cardiac dysrhythmias.

The mechanisms of action of the major classes of antidysrhythmics are summarized in Table 23-4. The effects for the various classes of drugs are summarized in Box 23-1.

Indications

Antidysrhythmic drugs are effective in treating a variety of cardiac dysrhythmias. The antidysrhythmic drugs and the most common indications for their use are listed in Table 23-5.

Contraindications

Contraindications to the use of antidysrhythmic drugs include known drug allergy to a specific product and may include second- or third-degree AV block, bundle branch block, cardiogenic shock, sick sinus syndrome, or any other major ECG changes, depending on the clinical judgement of a cardiologist. The reason for these concerns is that all antidysrhythmic drugs are potentially dysrhythmogenic and can therefore worsen existing dysrhythmias. The risk of such an effect is greater in

TABLE 23-4

Antidysrhythmic Drugs: Mechanisms of Action

Vaughan Williams class	I	II	III	IV
Action	Blocks sodium channels, affects phase 0	Decreases spontaneous depolarization, affects phase 4	Prolongs APD	Blocks slow calcium channels
Tissue	Fast	Slow	Fast	Slow
Effect on action potential				

APD, action potential duration.

BOX 23-1

Effects of Antidysrhythmic Drugs

Class Ia (disopyramide, quinidine, procainamide)

- Depress myocardial excitability
- Prolong the ERP
- Eliminate or reduce ectopic foci stimulation
- Decrease inotropic effect
- Have anticholinergic (vagolytic) activity

Class Ib (lidocaine, mexiletine, phenytoin)

- Decrease myocardial excitability in the ventricles
- Eliminate or reduce ectopic foci stimulation in the ventricles
- Have minimal effect on the SA node and automaticity
- Have minimal effect on the AV node and conduction
- Have minimal anticholinergic (vagolytic) activity

Class Ic (flecainide, propafenone)

- Produce dose-related depression of cardiac conduction, especially in the bundle of His–Purkinje system
- Have minimal effect on atrial conduction
- Eliminate or reduce ectopic foci stimulation in the ventricles
- Have minimal anticholinergic (vagolytic) activity
- Flecainide use now reserved for the most serious dysrhythmias

Class II (acebutolol, esmolol, propranolol)

- Block β-adrenergic heart stimulation
- Reduce SA nodal activity
- Eliminate or reduce atrial ectopic foci stimulation
- Reduce ventricular contraction rate
- Reduce cardiac output and blood pressure

Class III (amiodarone, ibutilide, dofetilide, sotalol*)

- Prolong the ERP
- Prolong the myocardial action potential
- Block both α- and β-adrenergic heart stimulation

Class IV (diltiazem, verapamil)

- Prolong AV nodal ERP
- Reduce AV nodal conduction
- Reduce rapid ventricular conduction caused by atrial flutter

---

AV, atrioventricular; *ECG,* electrocardiogram; *ERP,* effective refractory period; *SA,* sinoatrial.

*Sotalol also has class II properties.

TABLE 23-5

Antidysrhythmic Drugs: Indications

Drug	Indications
CLASS IA	
disopyramide procainamide quinidine	Atrial fibrillation, premature atrial contractions, premature ventricular contractions, ventricular tachycardia, Wolff–Parkinson–White syndrome
CLASS IB	
lidocaine mexiletine phenytoin	Ventricular dysrhythmias only (premature ventricular contractions, ventricular tachycardia, ventricular fibrillation)
CLASS IC	
flecainide propafenone	Severe ventricular dysrhythmias and supraventricular tachycardia dysrhythmias, atrial fibrillation and flutter
CLASS II	
β-blockers atenolol esmolol metoprolol propranolol	Both supraventricular and ventricular dysrhythmias (act as general myocardial depressants)
CLASS III	
amiodarone	Life-threatening ventricular tachycardia or fibrillation
dofetilide	Atrial fibrillation or flutter resistant to other drugs
sotalol*	Same as amiodarone
CLASS IV	
calcium channel blockers diltiazem verapamil	Paroxysmal supraventricular tachycardia; rate control for atrial fibrillation and flutter

*Sotalol also has class II properties.

already existing AV conduction delays. The safe prescribing of antidysrhythmic drugs is an area that requires strong clinical expertise and careful judgement on a case-by-case basis.

Adverse Effects

Adverse effects common to most antidysrhythmics include hypersensitivity reactions, nausea, vomiting, and diarrhea. Other common effects include dizziness, headache, and blurred vision. In addition, many antidysrhythmic are capable of producing new dysrhythmias (prodysrhythmic effect). As with any drug class, there are also cases of unpredictable or idiosyncratic adverse effects that are not related to drug concentration in the body. The belief is that such effects will eventually be explained by genetic variations. Table 23-6 summarizes the most commonly reported adverse effects by specific drug. Effects that pertain specifically to the ECG tracing are summarized in Table 23-7.

patients with structural heart damage (e.g., after myocardial infarction). In particular, with AV block and bundle branch block, there is a danger of drug-induced ventricular failure if a given drug should further compromise

TABLE   23-6

Common Adverse Effects of Antidysrhythmic Drugs

Drug	Adverse Effects
adenosine, amiodarone	Flushing
adenosine, amiodarone, β-blockers, disopyramide, flecainide, lidocaine, mexiletine,	Dyspnea
adenosine, β-blockers, flecainide, mexiletine	Chest pressure or pain
amiodarone	Photosensitivity, skin discoloration (blue–grey skin), hypothyroidism, hyperthyroidism, liver enzyme elevations
amiodarone	Pulmonary toxicity (hypersensitivity pneumonitis, pulmonary fibrosis)
amiodarone, β-blockers	Heart failure
amiodarone, β-blockers, disopyramide, procainamide, verapamil	Hypotension
amiodarone, β-blockers, quinidine (secondary to antibodies to drug-platelet complexes)	Thrombocytopenia or other coagulation abnormalities
amiodarone, digoxin, disopyramide, dofetilide, flecainide, ibutilide, lidocaine, mexiletine, phenytoin, procainamide, propafenone, quinidine	Central nervous system effects, including one or more of the following (specific adverse effects may vary with drug): tinnitus, hearing loss, visual disturbances, confusion, delirium, psychosis, giddiness, hallucinations, depression, dizziness, paresthesias, stupor, coma, seizures, fatigue, headache, tremor, anxiety, gait disturbance, somnolence (sleepiness), insomnia
amiodarone, diltiazem	Edema
amiodarone, diltiazem, disopyramide, dofetilide, flecainide, ibutilide, lidocaine, mexiletine, propafenone, quinidine (note that almost any drug can cause gastrointestinal adverse effects)	Gastrointestinal effects, including one or more of the following (specific adverse effects may vary with drug): nausea, vomiting, diarrhea, abdominal pain, anorexia, constipation, weight gain, flatulence, bloating, taste disturbance
amiodarone, dofetilide, flecainide, ibutilide, moricizine, phenytoin, propafenone, sotalol, verapamil	Prodysrhythmic effects (see also Table 23-7)
amiodarone, moricizine	Decreased libido
amiodarone, phenytoin	Venous irritation, thrombophlebitis
β-blockers	Hyperkalemia, hypoglycemia, hyperglycemia
β-blockers	Urticaria and other more serious dermatological reactions (e.g., Stevens–Johnson syndrome, toxic epidermal necrolysis)
β-blockers, disopyramide	Elevated cholesterol, triglyceride levels
β-blockers, disopyramide, flecainide, lidocaine, mexiletine, procainamide, propafenone, quinidine	Rash, pruritus (itching)
β-blockers, disopyramide, flecainide, mexiletine, procainamide, propafenone	Muscular pain or weakness
β-blockers, procainamide	Agranulocytosis
disopyramide	Hypokalemia
lidocaine	Arterial spasms
lidocaine, procainamide	Elevated defibrillatory threshold
procainamide	Raynaud's disease (idiopathic peripheral vascular compromise)
procainamide (especially in slow acetylators) and quinidine	Drug-induced lupus-like syndrome (idiosyncratic): arthralgia, fever, pleuropericarditis, hepatomegaly, positive result on antinuclear antibody test
quinidine	Fever
quinidine	Hemolytic anemia
quinidine (especially when taken with anticoagulants)	Bleeding

Toxicity and Management of Overdose

The main toxic effects of the antidysrhythmics involve the heart, circulation, and central nervous system (CNS). Specific antidotes are not available, and the management of an overdose involves maintaining adequate circulation and respiration using general support measures and any required symptomatic treatment (Table 23-8).

Interactions

Antidysrhythmics can interact with many different categories of drugs. The most serious drug interactions are those that result in dysrhythmias, hypotension or hypertension, respiratory distress, or any excessive therapeutic or toxic drug effects. Drug interactions occur when the presence of one drug strengthens or weakens

TABLE 23-7

Common Electrocardiographic Effects of Antidysrhythmic Drugs

Drug	Effect
adenosine, propafenone	Atrial fibrillation
amiodarone, β-blockers, digoxin, diltiazem, lidocaine, phenytoin, propafenone, verapamil	Bradycardia
amiodarone, β-blockers, diltiazem, disopyramide, lidocaine, propafenone, quinidine, verapamil	AV nodal disturbance or block
amiodarone, β-blockers, disopyramide, lidocaine, quinidine, verapamil	SA nodal disturbance or depression
amiodarone, β-blockers, lidocaine, propafenone	His–Purkinje block (bundle branch block)
amiodarone, digoxin, disopyramide, dofetilide, ibutilide, lidocaine, procainamide, propafenone, quinidine, sotalol	Ventricular tachycardia (with lidocaine, often occurs in association with supraventricular tachycardia; with sotalol, often occurs secondary to torsades de pointes)
digoxin	Supraventricular (atrial) tachycardia
digoxin, verapamil	Asystole
disopyramide, dofetilide, ibutilide, procainamide, propafenone, quinidine	Prolonged QRS or QT interval
disopyramide, dofetilide, ibutilide, quinidine, procainamide, sotalol	Torsades de pointes
mexiletine, propafenone	Premature ventricular contractions

AV, atrioventricular; *SA* sinoatrial.

TABLE 23-8

Selected Antidysrhythmic Drugs: Management of Overdose

Drug	Toxic Effect	Management
acebutolol	Bradycardia	1–3 mg IV atropine divided
	Bronchospasm	β$_2$-adrenergic or theophylline
	Cardiac failure	Digitalization
	Hypotension	Vasopressor
		Glucagon
adenosine	Usually self-limiting because of a short half-life	Competitive antagonists: caffeine or theophylline
amiodarone	Bradycardia	β-adrenergic drug
	Hypotension	Positive inotropic drug or vasopressor
digoxin	Decrease clearance because of drug interactions with other antidysrhythmic drugs (e.g., quinidine, verapamil, amiodarone)	See Chapter 22 for more information
disopyramide	Loss of consciousness, cardiac and respiratory arrest	Neostigmine for anticholinergic effects, activated charcoal, and hemodialysis
esmolol	Same as for acebutolol	Same as for acebutolol
flecainide	Reduced heart rate	Dopamine or dobutamine; acidify alkaline urine
lidocaine	Convulsions	Diazepam or thiopental
mexiletine	Bradycardia, hypotension	Atropine; acidify urine to promote excretion
phenytoin	Circulatory and respiratory arrest, convulsions	Life support measures when required
procainamide	Cardiac depression	IV pressor drugs and supportive measures
	Convulsions	Diazepam and mechanically assisted respiration
propafenone	Same as for acetbutolol	Same as for acetbutolol
propranolol	Cardiac dysrhythmias	Sodium lactate (reduces toxicity except in alkalosis); lidocaine
quinidine	Same as acebutolol	Same as acebutolol
sotalol	Convulsions	Diazepam or short-acting barbiturate
verapamil	Heart failure	Dopamine or dobutamine
	Conduction problems	Isoproterenol
	Hypotension	Cardiac pacing
		Vasopressors, 10% calcium gluconate solution

IV, intravenous.

the pharmacological effects of another. This is most commonly seen when the first drug affects the activity of the enzymes that metabolize the second drug, either speeding or slowing its elimination. One particular interaction common to many antidysrhythmics is the potentiation of anticoagulant activity with warfarin (Coumadin). Because many patients receiving antidysrhythmic therapy also need warfarin, prothrombin time and international normalized ratio (INR) should be monitored appropriately and necessary adjustments made to the warfarin dosage. Other common interactions are summarized in Table 23-9. To explain the mechanism for each interaction is beyond the scope of this text. Readers needing more detailed information are encouraged to consult the *Compendium of Pharmaceuticals and Specialties (CPS)* or other appropriate references.

TABLE   23-9

Common Drug Interactions for Selected Antidysrhythmic Drugs

Antidysrhythmic Drug	Interacting Drugs	Effects
amiodarone	Other antidysrhythmics, cimetidine, quinolone antibiotics, selective serotonin reuptake inhibitors, ritonavir	Enhanced amiodarone activity
amiodarone	phenytoin, cholestyramine, rifampin	Reduced amiodarone activity
amiodarone	cyclosporine, digoxin, fentanyl, phenytoin, methotrexate, theophylline	Possible toxicity of these drugs
β-blockers	Other antidysrhythmics, cimetidine, clonidine, epinephrine, ergot alkaloids, oral contraceptives, diphenhydramine, haloperidol, hydralazine, hydroxychloroquine, loop diuretics	Enhanced β-blocker activity
β-blockers	Antacids, cholestyramine, ampicillin, rifampin, nonsteroidal antiinflammatory drugs (e.g., ibuprofen), phenothiazines (e.g., promethazine, quinolone antibiotics, salicylates, thyroid hormones	Reduced β-blocker activity
β-blockers	haloperidol, benzodiazepines, ergot alkaloids, gabapentin	Possible toxicity of these drugs
β-blockers	Sulfonylureas	Reduced hypoglycemic effect of these drugs
calcium channel blockers (ver-apamil or diltiazem)	Other antidysrhythmics, cimetidine, ranitidine	Enhanced calcium channel blocker activity
calcium channel blockers (verap-amil or diltiazem)	phenytoin, rifampin	Reduced calcium channel blocker activity
calcium channel blockers (ver-apamil or diltiazem)	Anaesthetics, doxorubicin, benzodiazepines, buspirone, carbamazepine, digoxin, statins, steroids, tacrolimus, sirolimus, theophylline, vincristine	Possible toxicity of these drugs
disopyramide	Other antidysrhythmics, digoxin (possibly beneficial), macrolide antibiotics, quinolone antibiotics, antipsychotics	Enhanced disopyramide activity
disopyramide	phenytoin, rifampin	Reduced disopyramide activity
dofetilide, ibutilide	Other antidysrhythmics, cimetidine, amiloride, ketoconazole, tri-methoprim–sulfamethoxazole, metformin, megestrol, prochlorperazine, triamterene, verapamil	Enhanced dofetilide or ibutilide activity
dofetilide, ibutilide	Potassium-wasting diuretics (i.e., thiazides, loop diuretics)	Hypokalemia, hypomagnesemia
flecainide	Other antidysrhythmics	Enhanced flecainide activity
lidocaine	Other antidysrhythmics, cimetidine	Enhanced lidocaine activity
procainamide	Other antidysrhythmics, anticholinergics, quinidine, cimetidine, ranitidine, quinolone antibiotics, antipsychotics, trimethoprim	Enhanced procainamide activity
propafenone	Other antidysrhythmics, cimetidine, quinidine, selective serotonin reuptake inhibitors (e.g., fluoxetine)	Enhanced propafenone activity
propafenone	rifampin	Reduced propafenone activity
propafenone	cyclosporine, digoxin, theophylline	Possible toxicity of these drugs
quinidine	Barbiturates, cholinergics, rifampin, disopyramide, phenytoin, nifedipine	Reduced quinidine activity
quinidine	Other antidysrhythmics, antacids, cimetidine, verapamil, anticholinergics, digoxin, anticoagulants, β-blockers, tricyclic antidepressants	Enhanced quinidine activity*

*Note that enhanced activity of any antidysrhythmic drug may reach the level of drug toxicity, including potentially fatal cardiac dysrhythmias.

DRUG PROFILES

Because the four classes of antidysrhythmics produce a variety of effects on the action potential of the cardiac cell, they exert a major effect on cardiac electrophysiological function. The diversity of therapeutic effects and the attendant adverse effects pose a special challenge to the nurse, who is responsible for ensuring the safe and efficacious use of these drugs. Because the aspects of the nursing process that relate to the administration of antidysrhymiacs differs for each of the four classes of drug, each group is discussed separately. Dosage and other information appears in the Dosages table on p. 436.

CLASS IA DRUGS

Class Ia drugs are considered membrane-stabilizing drugs because they possess local anaesthetic properties. They stabilize the membrane and have depressant effects on phase 0 of the action potential. These drugs include disopyramide, procainamide, and quinidine.

procainamide hydrochloride

The electrophysiological effect of procainamide hydrochloride (Procan SR) is similar to that of quinidine, but it differs from quinidine in that its indirect effect (anticholinergic action) is weaker. Procainamide is useful in the management of atrial and ventricular tachydysrhythmias. It is reported to be more effective in the treatment of ventricular disturbances, especially in suppressing premature ventricular contractions (PVCs) and preventing the recurrence of ventricular tachycardia. The intravenous form of procainamide is generally preferred over the intravenous form of quinidine. Procainamide is chemically related to the local anaesthetic procaine.

Significant adverse effects of the drug include ventricular dysrhythmias and blood disorders. It can cause a lupus erythematosus–like syndrome, which occurs in approximately 30% of patients on long-term therapy. It can also cause gastrointestinal effects such as nausea, vomiting, and diarrhea, but these are less intense than those of quinidine. Other adverse effects include fever, thrombocytopenia, maculopapular rash, urticaria, pruritus, flushing, and torsades de pointes resulting from prolongation of the QT interval. Use of procainamide is contraindicated in patients who have shown hypersensitivity reactions to it and in those with complete heart block, lupus erythematosus, and second- or third-degree heart block. It is available in both oral and injectable forms.

PHARMACOKINETICS

Half-Life	Onset	Peak	Duration
IV/IM: 3 hr	IV/IM: 10–30 min	IV/IM: 10–60 min	IV/IM: 3 hr
PO: 3 hr	PO: 0.5–1 hr	PO: 1–2 hr	PO: 3 hr (8 hr for extended-release dosage form)

quinidine sulfate

Quinidine sulfate has both a direct action on the electrical activity of the heart and an indirect (anticholinergic) effect. Its anticholinergic action results in inhibition of the parasympathetic nervous system and allows sympathetic nervous system activity to go unopposed. This accelerates the rate of electrical impulse formation and conduction. Significant adverse effects of quinidine include cardiac asystole and ventricular ectopic beats. Like other cinchona alkaloids and the salicylates, quinidine can cause cinchonism. Symptoms of mild cinchonism include tinnitus, vertigo, headache, dizziness, loss of hearing, slight blurring of vision, and gastrointestinal upset. Contraindications to use of the drug include hypersensitivity to it, thrombocytopenic purpura resulting from previous therapy, AV block, intraventricular conduction defects, and abnormal rhythms (proarrhythmic effects such as torsades de pointes). Quinidine is available in parenteral form.

PHARMACOKINETICS

Half-Life	Onset	Peak	Duration
PO: 6–7 hr	PO: 1–3 hr	PO: 0.5–6 hr	PO: 6–8 hr (12 hr for sustained-release dosage form)

CLASS IB DRUGS

Class Ib drugs share many characteristics with class Ia drugs but are grouped together because they act preferentially on ischemic myocardial tissue. They have little effect on conduction velocity in normal tissue. Class Ib drugs have a weak depressive effect on phase 0 depolarization, the APD, and the ERP. They include lidocaine, mexiletine, and phenytoin.

▶▶ lidocaine hydrochloride

Lidocaine hydrochloride (Xylocaine) is the prototypical Ib drug. It is one of the most effective drugs for the treatment of ventricular dysrhythmias, but it can only be administered intravenously because it has an extensive first-pass effect (i.e., when taken orally, the liver metabolizes most of it to inactive metabolites). Because of its extensive liver metabolism, dosage reduction by 50% is recommended for patients in frank liver failure or cirrhosis. Dosage reductions may also be necessary in patients with kidney impairment because of extensive excretion of the drug and its metabolites by the kidney.

Lidocaine exerts its effects on the conduction system of the heart by making it difficult for the ventricles to develop a dysrhythmia, an action known as *raising the ventricular fibrillation threshold*. It accomplishes this by decreasing the sensitivity of the cardiac cell membrane to impulses and decreasing the cell's ability to depolarize on its own (decreasing automaticity). Many of these effects are accomplished by blockade of fast sodium channels.

Lidocaine is the drug of choice for treating the acute ventricular dysrhythmias associated with myocardial infarction (MI). Significant adverse effects include central nervous system (CNS) toxicities such as twitching, convulsions, and confusion; respiratory depression or arrest; and the cardiovascular effects of hypotension, bradycardia, and dysrhythmias. Use of lidocaine is contraindicated

Continued

in patients who are hypersensitive to its use, who have severe SA or AV intraventricular block, or who have Stokes–Adams or Wolff–Parkinson–White syndrome. Lidocaine is available only in parenteral form for intramuscular injection or intravenous administration. Intramuscular administration is recommended only in extenuating circumstances, such as when the patient is symptomatic and no intravenous or ECG equipment is available.

PHARMACOKINETICS

Half-Life	Onset	Peak	Duration
IV/IM: 8 min, 1–2 hr (terminal)	IV/IM: 45–90 sec	IV/IM: 5–10 min	IV/IM: 20 min to 1.5 hr

mexiletine hydrochloride

Mexiletine hydrochloride is structurally and pharmacologically similar to lidocaine, and its effects on the conduction system of the heart are also similar. A response to parenteral lidocaine does not predict a response to mexiletine. Mexiletine effectively suppresses PVCs in patients experiencing an acute MI, chronic coronary artery disease, or digitalis toxicity and in those undergoing heart surgery. It has proved particularly useful when taken in combination with selected class Ia or Ic drugs or with β-blockers.

The most frequent adverse effects are nausea, vomiting, dizziness, and tremor. These reactions are usually not serious, however, and are dose related and minimized by taking the drug with food or an antacid. Contraindications to its use include hypersensitivity, cardiogenic shock, and second- or third-degree AV block. Mexiletine is available only for oral use.

PHARMACOKINETICS

Half-Life	Onset	Peak	Duration
PO: 6.7 – 17.2 hr	PO: 0.5–2 hr	PO: 1.5–4 hr	Unknown

CLASS IC DRUGS

Class Ic drugs (flecainide, propafenone) have a more pronounced effect on sodium channel blockade than the Ia and Ib drugs but have little effect on repolarization or the APD. These drugs significantly slow conduction in the atria, AV node, and ventricles. Because of their marked effect on conduction, these drugs strongly suppress PVCs, reducing or eliminating them in a large number of patients.

flecainide acetate

Flecainide acetate (Tambocor) is a chemical analogue of procainamide. A large, multicentre, double-blind, placebo-controlled study called the **Cardiac Arrhythmia Suppression Trial** (**CAST**) was conducted by the National Heart, Lung, and Blood Institute to determine whether the incidence of **sudden cardiac death** could be reduced in post-MI patients with asymptomatic non–life-threatening ectopy through the use of flecainide. The findings showed that the excessive mortality and nonfatal cardiac arrest rates in patients treated with this drug were actually comparable with or higher than those seen in patients who received

the placebo. Because of these findings, Health Canada required that the labelling of flecainide be revised to indicate that its use be limited to the treatment of documented life-threatening ventricular dysrhythmias such as sustained ventricular tachycardia. Treatment with this drug should be initiated in the hospital. This drug is not indicated for the management of less severe dysrhythmias such as nonsustained ventricular tachycardia or frequent PVCs.

Although flecainide is better tolerated than quinidine or procainamide and is more effective than mexiletine, it is more proarrhythmic. It is this proarrhythmic potential that limits its use to the management of life-threatening dysrhythmias. Flecainide has a negative inotropic effect and depresses left ventricular function. Less serious but more common noncardiac adverse effects include dizziness, visual disturbances, and dyspnea. Contraindications to its use include hypersensitivity, cardiogenic shock, second- or third-degree AV block, and non–life-threatening dysrhythmias. Flecainide is available only for oral use.

PHARMACOKINETICS

Half-Life	Onset	Peak	Duration
12–27 hr	30 min	3 hr	3–5 days*

*Therapeutic levels.

propafenone hydrochloride

Propafenone hydrochloride (Rythmol) is similar in action to flecainide. It reduces the fast inward sodium current in Purkinje fibres and, to a lesser extent, in myocardial fibres. Unlike other class I drugs, propafenone has mild β-blocking effects. This may contribute to its overall effects on the conduction system. It is also believed to have calcium channel blocking effects, which may contribute to its mild negative inotropic effects.

Until recently, propafenone's use has been limited to the treatment of documented life-threatening ventricular dysrhythmias such as sustained ventricular tachycardia. Recent findings suggest that at low dosages it has benefit in the treatment of atrial fibrillation as well, although it is not officially approved for this use in Canada. Treatment should also be started while the patient is in the hospital. Unlike flecainide, however, propafenone can be given to patients with depressed left ventricular function. It may be a better antidysrhythmic drug than disopyramide, procainamide, and quinidine in these patients. However, it should be used with caution in patients with heart failure, because of the β-blocking properties and dose-dependent negative inotropic effects.

Propafenone is generally well tolerated. The most commonly reported adverse reaction is dizziness. Patients may also complain of a metallic taste, constipation, and headache, along with nausea and vomiting. These gastrointestinal adverse effects may be reduced by taking propafenone with food. Propafenone is contraindicated in patients with a known hypersensitivity to it and in those with bradycardia, bronchial asthma, significant hypotension, uncontrolled heart failure, cardiogenic shock, or conduction disorders. It is available only for oral use.

Continued

DRUG PROFILES (cont'd)

PHARMACOKINETICS

Half-Life	Onset	Peak	Duration
2–17 hr	Unknown	3 hr	3–4 days*

*Steady state.

CLASS II DRUGS

Class II antidysrhythmics are also known as β-*blockers*. These drugs work by reducing or blocking sympathetic nervous system (SNS) stimulation to the heart and the heart's conduction system. By doing this, β-blockers prevent catecholamine-mediated actions on the heart. This action is known as a cardioprotective quality of β-blockers. The resulting cardiovascular effects include a reduced heart rate, delayed AV node conduction, reduced myocardial contractility, and decreased myocardial automaticity. The pharmacologically induced effects of the β-blockers are especially beneficial after an MI because of the many catecholamines released at this time, making the heart hyper-irritable and predisposed to many types of dysrhythmias. The β-blockers offer protection from these potentially dangerous complications. Several studies have demonstrated a significant reduction (averaging 25%) in the incidence of sudden cardiac death after MI in patients treated with β-blockers on an ongoing basis.

Although there are several β-blockers, only a few are used as antidysrhythmic drugs. The β-blocker drugs currently approved by Health Canada for this purpose are acebutolol, esmolol, propranolol, and sotalol (which has class II and III properties). Selected drugs are described here. The class II drugs are classified as pregnancy category C drugs except acebutolol, pindolol, and sotalol, which are all category B drugs.

▶▶ atenolol

Atenolol (Tenormin) is a cardioselective β-blocker, which means that it preferentially blocks the $β_1$-adrenergic receptors that are located primarily in the heart. Non-cardioselective β-blockers block not only the $β_1$-adrenergic receptors on the heart but also the $β_2$-adrenergic receptors in the lungs and, therefore, could exacerbate a pre-existing asthma or chronic obstructive pulmonary disease. In addition to having class II antidysrhythmic properties, atenolol is useful in the treatment of hypertension and angina. Its use is contraindicated in patients with severe bradycardia, second- or third-degree heart block, heart failure, cardiogenic shock, or a known hypersensitivity. Atenolol is available in oral form.

PHARMACOKINETICS

Half-Life	Onset	Peak	Duration
PO: 6–7 hr	PO: 1 hr	PO: 2–4 hr	PO: 24 hr

esmolol hydrochloride

Esmolol hydrocloride (Brevibloc) is a short-acting β-blocker with pharmacological and electrophysiological effects on the heart's conduction system that are similar to those of atenolol. Esmolol is also a cardioselective β-blocker that primarily and preferentially blocks the $β_1$-adrenergic receptors in the heart. It is used in the acute treatment of supraventricular tachyarrhythmias or dysrhythmias that originate above the ventricles and are fast instead of slow. It is also used to control hypertension and tachyarrhythmias that develop after an acute MI. Use of esmolol is contraindicated in patients with a known hypersensitivity to it or in those with hypotension, severe bradycardia, second- or third-degree heart block, heart failure, cardiogenic shock, or severe asthma. Esmolol is available only in injectable form.

PHARMACOKINETICS

Half-Life	Onset	Peak	Duration
IV: 9 min	IV: Rapid	IV: Rapid	IV: Short

▶▶ metoprolol tartrate

Metoprolol tartrate (Lopresor) is another cardioselective β-blocker commonly given after an MI to reduce the risk of sudden cardiac death. It is also used in the treatment of hypertension and angina. The contraindications to metoprolol use are the same as those to atenolol and esmolol. It is available in both oral and injectable forms.

PHARMACOKINETICS

Half-Life	Onset	Peak	Duration
PO: 3.5 hr	PO: 1 hr	PO: 1.5–2 hr	PO: 24 hr

▶▶ propranolol hydrochloride

Propranolol hydrochloride (Inderal) was one of the first β-blockers introduced into clinical practice, in 1968. It was then primarily used in the treatment of dysrhythmias. Propranolol is a nonspecific β-blocker that blocks both $β_1$- and $β_2$-adrenergic receptors in the heart and lungs. Its primary effect on the conduction system of the heart is the blockade of cardiac $β_1$-adrenergic receptors, which prevents catecholamine-mediated stimulation of the heart. The resulting cardiovascular effects are a reduced heart rate, delayed AV node conduction, reduced myocardial contractility, and decreased myocardial automaticity. Propranolol is also believed to have membrane-stabilizing properties that may play a small role in its overall antidysrhythmic effect.

Because propranolol is the oldest of this class of drugs, there are now numerous indications for its use. Hypertension, angina, supraventricular dysrhythmias, ventricular tachycardia, the tachyarrhythmias associated with cardiac glycoside toxicity, hypertrophic subaortic stenosis, pheochromocytoma, thyrotoxicosis, migraines, post-MI, and essential tremor are just some of its many uses. The contraindications to propranolol use are the same as those for atenolol. It is available in both oral and parenteral forms.

PHARMACOKINETICS

Half-Life	Onset	Peak	Duration
IV: 3–5 hr	IV: 2 min	IV: 15 min	IV: 3–6 hr
PO: 3–5 hr	PO: 30 min	PO: 1–1.5 hr	PO: 8–11 hr

Continued

▶▶ *sotalol hydrochloride*

Sotalol hydrochloride (Rhylosol) is another nonselective β-blocker used to treat dysrhythmias. It is unique in that it possesses antidysrhythmic properties similar to those of the class III drugs (such as amiodarone) while simultaneously exerting β-blocker or class II effects on the conduction system of the heart. In addition, sotalol has prodysrhythmic properties similar to those of the class Ic drugs. This means that while patients are taking sotalol, it can cause serious dysrhythmias such as torsades de pointes or a new ventricular tachycardia or fibrillation. For this reason, sotalol is usually reserved for the treatment of documented life-threatening ventricular dysrhythmias such as sustained ventricular tachycardia. Contraindications to sotalol use include hypersensitivity to it, bronchial asthma, cardiogenic shock, and sinus bradycardia. Sotalol is available only in the oral form.

PHARMACOKINETICS

Half-Life	Onset	Peak	Duration
PO: 10–20 hr	PO: 1–2 hr	PO: 2.5–4 hr	PO: 12–24 hr

CLASS III DRUGS

Class III drugs include amiodarone, sotalol (which also has class II properties), ibutilide, and dofetilide. Amiodarone controls dysrhythmias by inhibiting repolarization and markedly prolonging refractoriness and the APD. Ibutilide and dofetilide are both indicated for conversion of atrial fibrillation or flutter to a normal sinus rhythm. Amiodarone is indicated for the management of life-threatening ventricular tachycardia or ventricular fibrillation that is resistant to other drug therapy. Amiodarone has also been effective in the treatment of sustained ventricular tachycardias. Amiodarone has recently been used more frequently to treat atrial dysrhythmias.

▶▶ *amiodarone hydrochloride*

Amiodarone hydrochloride markedly prolongs the APD and the ERP in all cardiac tissues. Besides exerting these dramatic effects, it is also known to block both the α- and β-adrenergic receptors of the SNS. Clinically, it is one of the most effective antidysrhythmic drugs for controlling supraventricular and ventricular dysrhythmias. It is indicated for the management of sustained ventricular tachycardia, ventricular fibrillation, and nonsustained ventricular tachycardia.

Amiodarone has many undesired adverse effects that are attributable to its chemical properties. Amiodarone is lipophilic, or fat loving. Therefore, it can penetrate and concentrate in the adipose tissue of any organ in the body, where it may cause unwanted effects. It also has iodine in its chemical structure. One organ that sequesters iodine from the diet is the thyroid gland. As a result, amiodarone can cause either hypothyroidism or hyperthyroidism. Adverse reactions occur in approximately 75% of patients treated with this drug, but the incidence is higher and the severity greater with higher dosages (those exceeding 400 mg/day) and prolonged therapy. The most common adverse effect is corneal microdeposits, which may cause visual halos, photophobia, and dry eyes. This occurs in virtually all adults who take the drug for longer than 6 months.

The most serious adverse effect is pulmonary toxicity, which is fatal in about 10% of patients. Pulmonary toxicity involves a clinical syndrome of progressive dyspnea and cough accompanied by damage to the alveoli that can result in pulmonary fibrosis. Another serious complication of amiodarone therapy is that it may not only treat dysrhythmias but also provoke them. Amiodarone has an exceptionally long half-life, approaching many days. As a result, the therapeutic effects as well as any adverse effects of amiodarone may linger long after the drug has been discontinued. In fact, it may take as long as 2 to 3 months after the drug has been discontinued for some adverse effects to subside.

For all these reasons, although it is effective, amiodarone is typically considered a drug of last resort. Therapy is usually started in the hospital and is closely monitored until the patient's serum levels are within a therapeutic range. Use of amiodarone is contraindicated in patients who have a known hypersensitivity to it and in those with severe sinus bradycardia, or second- or third-degree heart block. For patients on long-term oral amiodarone therapy after intravenous amiodarone administration is discontinued, recommended conversions are available (Table 23-10). This drug is marketed in both oral and injectable forms.

PHARMACOKINETICS

Half-Life	Onset	Peak	Duration
PO: 26–107 days	PO: 1–3 wk	PO: 3–12 hr	PO: 10–150 days

ibutilide fumarate

Ibutilide fumarate (Corvert) is a class III antidysrhythmic drug. Dofetilide (Tikosyn) is a similar drug with similar indications. Unlike the other two drugs in the class III group of antidysrhythmics, ibutilide is indicated for atrial dysrhythmias. Atrial fibrillation and atrial flutter cause irregular contractions of the heart and can lead to serious conditions such as decreased cardiac output, heart failure, low blood pressure, and stroke. Although other pharmacological therapies are used to treat atrial fibrillation and flutter, ibutilide and dofetilide are the only drugs available for rapid conversion of these two conditions to normal sinus rhythm. The only other treatment that can produce rapid conversion is electrical cardioversion. Although it is effective, electrical cardioversion carries the risk, expense, and inconvenience of both the procedure itself and the anaesthesia it requires.

Ibutilide is dosed on the basis of patient weight. Use of ibutilide is contraindicated in patients who have previously demonstrated hypersensitivity to it. As with other antidysrhythmic drugs, ibutilide should be used with caution because it can also produce fatal dysrhythmias, most significantly ventricular tachycardia and torsades de pointes. Class Ia antidysrhythmic drugs (e.g., disopyramide, quinidine, and procainamide) and other class III drugs (e.g., amiodarone and sotalol) should not

Continued

DRUG PROFILES (cont'd)

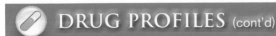

be administered concomitantly with ibutilide, nor should they be given within 4 hours after infusion of ibutilide because of their potential to prolong refractoriness. Ibutilide is available only in the injectable form.

PHARMACOKINETICS

Half-Life	Onset	Peak	Duration
6 hr	10 min	30 min	4 hr

CLASS IV DRUGS

Class IV antidysrhythmic drugs are calcium channel blockers. Although more than nine such drugs are currently available, only a few are commonly used as antidysrhythmics. Besides being effective antidysrhythmics, calcium channel blockers are useful in the treatment of hypertension (Chapter 25) and angina. Verapamil and diltiazem are the most commonly used calcium channel blockers for the following:

- Treating dysrhythmias, specifically those that arise above the ventricles (paroxysmal supraventricular tachycardia [PSVT])
- Controlling the ventricular response to atrial fibrillation and flutter by slowing conduction and prolonging refractoriness of the AV node (i.e., preventing the ventricles from beating as fast as the atria)

These drugs block the slow inward flow of calcium ions into the slow (calcium) channels in cardiac conduction tissue. The conduction effects of these drugs are limited to the atria and the AV node, where conduction is prolonged and the tissues are made more refractory to stimulation. These drugs have little effect on ventricular tissues.

▶▶ diltiazem hydrochloride

Diltiazem hydrochloride (Apo-DiltiazTZ, Cardizem) is primarily indicated for the temporary control of a rapid ventricular response in a patient with atrial fibrillation or flutter and PSVT. Its use is contraindicated in patients with hypersensitivity, acute MI, pulmonary congestion, Wolff–Parkinson–White syndrome, severe hypotension, cardiogenic shock, sick sinus syndrome, or second- or third-degree AV block. Diltiazem is available in both oral and parenteral forms.

PHARMACOKINETICS

Half-Life	Onset	Peak	Duration
PO: 3.5–6 hr	PO: 0.5–1 hr	PO:2–4 hr	PO: 4–8 hr
			PO: 12 hr*

*For extended-release product.

▶▶ verapamil hydrochloride

Verapamil hydrochloride (Apo-Verap, Covera-HS, Isoptin SR) has actions similar to those of diltiazem in that it also inhibits calcium ion influx across the slow calcium channels in cardiac conduction tissue. This results in dramatic effects on the AV node. Verapamil is used to prevent and convert recurrent PSVT and to control ventricular response in atrial flutter or fibrillation. It can also temporarily control a rapid ventricular response to these frequent atrial stimulations, usually decreasing the heart rate by at least 20%. Not only is verapamil used for the management of dysrhythmias, but it is also used to treat angina, hypertension, and hypertrophic cardiomyopathy. The contraindications that apply to diltiazem apply to verapamil as well. It is also available in both oral and parenteral forms.

PHARMACOKINETICS

Half-Life	Onset	Peak	Duration
PO: 2.8–7.4 hr	PO: 30 min	PO: 1–2 hr	PO: 6–8 hr
IV: 2–5 hr	IV: 1–2 min	IV: 3–5 min	IV: 10–60 min

UNCLASSIFIED ANTIDYSRHYTHMICS
adenosine

Adenosine (Adenocard) is an unclassified antidysrhythmic drug. It is a naturally occurring nucleoside that slows the electrical conduction time through the AV node and is indicated for the conversion of PSVT to sinus rhythm. It is particularly useful when the PSVT has failed to respond to verapamil or when a patient has a coexisting condition such as heart failure, hypotension, or left ventricular dysfunction that limits the use of verapamil. Its use is contraindicated in patients with second- or third-degree heart block, sick sinus syndrome, atrial flutter or fibrillation, or ventricular tachycardia, as well as in those with a known hypersensitivity to it. It has an extremely short half-life of less than 10 seconds. For this reason, it is administered only intravenously as a fast intravenous push. It commonly causes asystole for a period of seconds. All other adverse effects are minimal because of its short duration of action. Adenosine is available only in parenteral form.

PHARMACOKINETICS

Half-Life	Onset	Peak	Duration
< 10 sec	1 min	Immediate	1–2 min

TABLE 23-10

Recommended Conversions Between Oral and Intravenous Amiodarone Therapies

Duration of Amiodarone IV Infusion	Initial Daily Dose of Oral Amiodarone
Less than 1 wk	800–1600 mg
1–3 wk	600–800 mg
More than 3 wk	400 mg

IV, intravenous.

DOSAGES — Selected Antidysrhythmic Drugs

Drug (Pregnancy Category)	Pharmacological Class	Usual Dosage Range	Indications
adenosine (Adenocard) (C)	Unclassified antidysrhythmic	*Children less than 50 kg* IV: 0.05–0.1 mg/kg rapid bolus; may be repeated *Adult* IV: 6 mg bolus over 1–2 sec; a second rapid bolus of 12 mg as needed (prn), which may be repeated a second time as needed	Supraventricular tachycardia, conversion to normal sinus rhythm
▸▸amiodarone hydrochloride (D)	Class III antidysrhythmic	*Adult* IV: 150 mg over 10 min, then 60 mg/hr for 6 hr, then 30 mg/hr as maintenance dose PO: 800–1600 mg/day for 1–3 wk, reduced to 600–800 mg/day for 5 wk; usual maintenance dose 400 mg/day PO: 200–400 mg/day	Ventricular dysrhythmias Atrial dysrhythmias
▸▸atenolol (Tenormin)(B)	β₁-blocker (class II antidysrhythmic)	*Adult* PO: 25–100 mg/day	Post-MI
▸▸diltiazem hydrochloride (Apo-Diltiaz TZ, Cardizem)	Calcium channel blocker	*Adult* IV: Bolus dose 0.25 mg/kg over 2 min, second dose 0.35 mg/kg over 2 min after 15 min as needed, then 5–10 mg/hr or higher by continuous infusion	Supraventricular dysrhythmias
disopyramide (Apo-Diltiaz TZ, Cardizem)	Class Ia antidysrhythmic	*Adult* PO: 400–800 divided daily; LA: 250 mg bid	Ventricular dysrhythmias
esmolol hydrochloride (Brevibloc) (C)	β₁-blocker (class II antidysrhythmic)	*Adult* IV: Bolus dose of 0.5 mg/kg/min followed by 4 min of 0.05 mg/kg/min and evaluate	Supraventricular tachyarrhythmias
flecainide acetate (Tambocor) (C)	Class Ic antidysrhythmic	*Adult* PO: 50 mg q12h; increase 50 mg bid q4d until desired effect; max 300 mg/day 100 mg q12h; increase 50 mg bid q4d as needed; usual dose 150 mg q12h; max 400 mg/day	Paroxysmal supraventricular tachycardia Sustained ventricular tachycardia
ibutilide fumarate (Corvert) (C)	Class III antidysrhythmic	*Adult* IV: 0.5 mg infusion over 10 min (if less than 60 kg, then 0.005 mL/kg)	Atrial fibrillation or flutter
▸▸lidocaine hydrochloride (Xylocaine) (B)	Class Ib antidysrhythmic	*Children* IV: Suggested bolus dose, 1 mg/kg; usual maintenance infusion rate, 20–50 mcg/kg/min *Adult* IV: Bolus dose 50–100 mg; may be repeated in 10 min; do not exceed 200–300 mg over 1 hr; usual maintenance infusion rate 1–2 mg/min	Ventricular dysrhythmias Ventricular dysrhythmias
▸▸metoprolol tartrate (Lopresor) (C)	β₁-blocker	*Adult* PO: 100 mg bid	Early MI Late MI
mexiletine hydrochloride (C)	Class Ib antidysrhythmic	*Adult* PO: Loading dose 400 mg; then 400–800 mg in 2–6 hr; maintenance is 400–800 mg divided bid–tid	Ventricular dysrhythmia

Continued

DOSAGES Selected Antidysrhythmic Drugs (cont'd)

Drug (Pregnancy Category)	Pharmacological Class	Usual Dosage Range	Indications
procainamide hydrochloride (Procan SR) (C)	Class Ia antidysrhythmic	*Adult* PO: initial dose, 1.25 g; 0.75 g in 1 hr; 0.05–1 g q2h until results or tolerance PO: initial dose 1 g; 50 mg/kg divided q3h until results or tolerance SR (maintenance): 50 mg/kg divided q6h doses IV: 20 mg/min (total 17 mg/kg), then maintenance infusion of 1–4 mg/min	Atrial fibrillation, paroxysmal atrial tachycardia Ventricular tachycardia Rapid dysrhythmia control
propafenone hydrochloride (Rhythmol) (C)	Class Ic antidysrhythmic	*Adult* PO:150 mg q8h; increase at 3-4 day intervals to 300 mg q12h; max 300 mg q8h	Sustained ventricular dysrhythmias
▸▸propranolol hydrochloride (Inderal) (D)	β-blocker (class II antidysrhythmic)	*Adult* IV: 1–3 mg; if needed, repeated in 2 min and additional doses as needed q4h; begin PO as soon as possible PO: 60–320 mg/day divided bid–qid	Serious dysrhythmias
quinidine sulfate	Class Ia antidysrhythmic	*Adult* IV: 200–300 mg q6–8h or loading dose 12 mg/kg with maintenance dose of 6 mg/kg q4–6h	Ventricular and supraventrical dysrhythmias Atrial fibrillation or flutter Conversion of atrial fibrillation Premature atrial and ventrical contractions Paroxysmal supraventrical tachycardia
▸▸sotalol hydrochloride (Rhylosol) (C)	Class II antidysrhythmic	*Adult* PO: 160–320 mg/day divided into 2 doses	Life-threatening dysrhythmias
▸▸verapamil hydrochloride (Apo-Verap, Covera-HS, Isoptin SR) (C)	Calcium channel blocker (class IV antidysrhythmic)	*Children* IV: 0–1 yr: 0.1–0.2 mg/kg bolus over 2 min; repeat dose after 30 min IV: 1–15 yr: 0.1–0.3 mg/kg bolus over 2 min; do not exceed 5 mg dose; repeat dose not exceeding 10 mg may be given after 30 min *Adult* PO: Start with 80 mg tid–qid; daily range 240–480 mg IV: 5–10 mg bolus over 2 min; repeat dose of 10 mg after 30 min	Supraventricular tachyarrhythmias Supraventricular tachyarrhythmias

IV, intravenous; *LA,* extended release, *MI,* myocardial infarction; *PO,* oral; *SR,* sustained release.

NURSING PROCESS

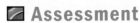

▨ Assessment

Before administering any class I antidysrhythmics to a patient, the nurse must perform a thorough physical assessment and nursing assessment and obtain a complete medical history. Contraindications, cautions, and drug interactions for all of the antidysrhythmic drugs have been presented in the pharmacology section of the chapter as well as in various tables in the text. Other focuses of assessment include a baseline ECG with interpretation of the results and vital signs with attention to heart rate, rhythm, and character. Heart sounds and blood pressure, including postural blood pressures, should also be noted. Other signs and symptoms for which to assess include apical-radial pulse deficits, jugular vein distention, edema, prolonged capillary refill (longer than 5 seconds), decreased urinary output, activity intolerance, chest pain or pressure, dyspnea, syncope or dizziness, fatigue, nausea, changes in alertness, anxiety, and abnormal serum electrolyte levels. Kidney and liver function studies are usually ordered to determine if dosages need to be adjusted because of age and altered excretion or metabolism of drugs. Altering of dosages is necessary in these situations to help prevent excessive accumulation and toxicity. (See also Evidence-Informed Practice: Antidysrhythmics and the Older Adult.)

Blood counts should be assessed for problems with clotting (e.g., thrombocytopenia). Baseline neurological functioning and identification of any neuromuscular deficits, such as muscle weakness, should be documented. These problems may be exacerbated by some of the antidysrhythmics (e.g., amiodarone, procainamide). Other concerns associated with antidysrhythmics require close inspection of the skin for bruising and bleeding, as well as notation of bleeding gums, black tarry stools, hematuria, or hematemesis. All cautions, contraindications, and drug interactions should be assessed prior to use of these drugs as well as other classes of antidysrhythmics (see previous discussion).

One important drug interaction to re-emphasize is that of grapefruit juice, which inhibits metabolism by cytochrome P450 3A4 liver enzymes (review *metabolism* in Chapter 2). This interaction with quinidine leads to increased blood levels and further risk of cinchonism.

Use of lidocaine requires assessment of the central nervous and cardiovascular systems, with attention to heart rate and blood pressure. Further assessment of respiratory, thyroid, liver, and hypertensive conditions is needed with use of amiodarone. Use of this drug with fentanyl (an opioid) and St. John's wort (a natural health product) should be avoided because of subsequent hypotension and bradycardia.

Pharmacokinetic Bridge to Nursing Practice

◼ Amiodarone

A study of long-term oral amiodarone therapy for the treatment of dysrhythmias provides a different perspective on

---

📄 EVIDENCE INFORMED PRACTICE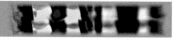

Antidysrhythmics and the Older Adult

Background
A review article presented a thorough examination of research studies and clinical trials investigating the management of dysrhythmia in the older adult. As noted in the article, the most interesting and recent application of pacemaker implantation has been for cardiac resynchronization in patients with advanced heart failure. Chronic heart failure is increasing in prevalence. Because the older adult is more susceptible to atrial fibrillation, life-threatening ventricular dysrhythmias, and symptomatic bradycardia, it is very important for the clinician to be able to identify abnormal rhythms and initiate appropriate therapies to help prevent stroke and improve quality of life and survival. Data are reviewed in this article, but it is the summary of the treatment modalities that is noteworthy.

Type of Evidence
This article provided a review of clinical trials and management of irregularities in heart rate in the older adult. It also presented a review of treatment regimens.

Results of Study
Older adults are at increased risk for both atrial and ventricular irregularities even though they may be clinically healthy, and irregularity occurrence increases the risk of other problems in these patients. The options of a new generation of oral anticoagulants and percutaneously implanted devices that may soon play a more expanded role in the management of atrial fibrillation were discussed in this study. Data from large clinical trials have shown that the use of automatic implanted cardioverter defibrillators (AICDs) to treat ventricular tachydysrhythmias

improves the survival of these patients, in the appropriate setting. Biventricular pacing is also a treatment modality with an identifiable role in reducing morbidity in patients with heart failure. Other studies and trials evaluating the role of treatment modalities in the management of heart irregularities in the older adult were also reviewed in this article. The treatment methods examined have provided the older adult with the possibility of improved quality of life, decreased morbidity, and longer survival.

Link of Evidence to Nursing Practice
Older adults are subject to a variety of insults to their physiological and psychological status, and even if they are in normal health for their age, the risk for abnormal heart conditions and rhythms is high. The studies reviewed in this article provide evidence of improved quality of life and reduced morbidity and mortality with the use of these treatment modalities. It is important for the nurse to be aware of reliable, valid clinical trial data such as those examined in the article so that the nurse can support the patient and family throughout implementation of new treatment plans, including use of antidysrhythmics, anticoagulants, implanted pacemakers, cardioverters and defibrillators, and biventricular pacing. Research findings, such as the trial data reviewed in this article, may continue to improve patient care and lead to sound, evidence-informed medical and nursing practice.

Based on Wenger, N. K., Helmy, T., Patel, A. D., & Hanna, I. R. (2005). Approaching cardiac arrhythmias in the elderly patient, *Medscape General Medicine*, 7(4). Retrieved November 14, 2008, from http://www.medscape.com/viewarticle/514471

pharmacokinetics. To aid in evaluating the complex pharmacokinetic properties of amiodarone and developing an optimal dosing schedule for the drug in long-term oral drug therapy, serum concentrations of the drug and its metabolite, desethylamiodarone, were monitored in 345 Japanese patients receiving amiodarone (Kashima et al., 2005). Serum concentrations of the drug and its metabolite were determined by a test called chromatography. In 245 participants who took fixed maintenance dosages of the drug for 6 months, there were small variations in the ratio of serum level of the actual drug and the serum level of its metabolite. (Review *metabolism* and related concepts in Chapter 2.) Other pharmacokinetic properties of amiodarone included an average clearance that was found to be slightly higher in women than in men, even though there was no difference between men and women with regard to age, dosage, or duration of action of the dose. Japanese patients had little variation in pharmacokinetics. From this study, one can see how important it is to fully understand basic pharmacokinetic principles (e.g., dosing, clearance, drug metabolism, serum concentrations) and appreciate their value as a critical component of drug therapy and the nursing process. It is also important to note that ethnoculture, gender, age, and racial or ethnic group have an impact on the way each person responds to a drug and how each drug may vary in its action.

Nursing Diagnoses

- Decreased cardiac output related to the pathology of the dysrhythmia
- Ineffective tissue perfusion related to the physiological impact of dysrhythmias
- Risk for injury related to the drug adverse effects of hypotension, dizziness
- Deficient knowledge related to lack of experience with drug therapy
- Impaired gas exchange (decreased) related to adverse reaction to the medications
- Disturbed body image related to changes in lifestyle and sexual functioning caused by the disease process as well as by the adverse effects of the drugs
- Nonadherence to the medication regimen due to unpleasant adverse effects and lack of knowledge

Planning

Goals

- Patient will be free of injury throughout duration of drug therapy.
- Patient will demonstrate adequate knowledge about drug therapy and related instruction.
- Patient will regain normal respiratory patterns and experience minimal respiratory-related adverse effects during drug therapy.
- Patient will regain normal or near-normal cardiac output and tissue perfusion.

- Patient will experience improved tolerance to activity and improved general sense of well-being.
- Patient will be free of complications associated with the drug therapy.
- Patient will maintain intact self-esteem and body image during drug therapy.
- Patient will report any increase in the symptoms of the dysrhythmia.
- Patient will demonstrate adequate knowledge of drug therapy and its adverse effects.

Outcome Criteria

- Patient's symptoms of dysrhythmia, such as shortness of breath and chest pain, are decreased or alleviated by drug or nondrug therapy or a combination of both.
- Patient has normal breathing patterns (rate and rhythm) and no shortness of breath, cough, or chest pain.
- Patient exhibits signs and symptoms of improved cardiac output and tissue perfusion as evidenced by regular apical and radial pulses; vital signs within normal limits; and a decrease in weight, edema, crackles, and shortness of breath, attributable to adherence to therapy.
- Patient states the common adverse effects of the drug being taken, such as constipation, dry mouth, and dizziness.
- Patient experiences an increase in energy and stamina and is able to carry out activities of daily living without symptoms.
- Patient states the importance of adhering to the medication regimen and of scheduling and attending follow-up visits with the physician or health care provider.
- Patient openly discusses feelings of inadequacy and low self-esteem, fears, and negative feelings about self.

Implementation

When being given class I antidysrhythmics, patients should continue to have their pulse rates (and other vital signs) monitored; if pulse rate is lower than 60 beats/min, the physician should be notified. Initially, the ECG and vital signs must be monitored closely because of possible prolongation of the QT interval by more than 50%. The end result may be the occurrence of a variety of conduction disturbances. Oral dosage forms should be taken as ordered and with food and fluids to help minimize gastrointestinal upset. Intravenous dosing of any of the antidysrhythmic classes of drugs should be through use of an infusion pump. The quinidine salts have ingredients that are specific to the given drugs and so the forms are not interchangeable.

Any chest pain, hypotension, gastrointestinal distress, dizziness or syncope, blurred vision, change in respiratory status, or edema should be reported to the physician immediately. Weight gain of 1 kg or more in 24 hours or 2 kg or more in 1 week should also be reported.

Hypersensitivity to some of these drugs may occur 3 to 20 days into the therapy and is manifested by fever.

Vials of lidocaine are usually identified as for cardiac or not for cardiac use, and it is important to remember this distinction when reading the vial's label. Lidocaine solutions need to be used with extreme caution, and the nurse should be aware that the *plain* solution is used in various cardiac situations. Lidocaine is also used as an anaesthetic; the different concentrations of the drug are crucial to remember, as are their corresponding indications. It is also important to know that lidocaine comes in a solution with epinephrine, a potent vasoconstrictor. This combined solution comes in handy when suturing or repairing wounds or lacerations to help anaesthetize (from the lidocaine) the area and control bleeding of the area (epinephrine vasoconstricts and decreases bleeding). The solution with epinephrine must never be used intravenously and never used except as a topical anaesthetic with vasoconstrictor properties. Thus careful reading of a label is important when using lidocaine or any of these drugs.

Parenteral solutions are usually stable for 24 hours. If the patient is also taking β-blockers, be sure to report any shortness of breath, edema, or skin rash. If the parenteral solution of any of these drugs appears discoloured, it should be discarded and not used. Gastrointestinal upset occurs with amiodarone during administration of loading doses and may be prevented by taking oral doses with food. Provision of a high-fibre diet along with forcing fluids is also recommended to minimize constipation. If anorexia occurs, specific dietary changes should be made to improve appetite. See Patient Education for more information.

🖎 Evaluation

The monitoring of patients receiving all classes of antidysrhythmics is important to confirm the therapeutic effects as well as identify the adverse and toxic effects.

- *Class I:* Therapeutic effects include improved cardiac output; decreased chest discomfort; decreased fatigue; improved vital signs, skin colour, and urinary output; and conversion of irregularities to normal rhythm. Adverse effects include bradycardia, dizziness, headache, cinchonism, chest pain, heart failure, and peripheral edema. Toxic effects range from heart failure and bradycardia to CNS-related effects such as confusion or convulsions.

- *Class II:* Therapeutic effects include improved cardiac output; decreased chest discomfort; decreased fatigue; regular pulse rate or improvement in irregularities; and improved vital signs, skin colour, and urinary output. Adverse effects include bradycardia, dizziness, headache, and peripheral edema. Toxic effects consist of heart failure, bradycardia, bronchospasms, hypotension, and conduction problems.

- *Class III:* Therapeutic effects include improved cardiac output; greater regularity in rhythm; decreased chest discomfort; decreased fatigue; and improved vital signs, skin colour, and urinary output. Adverse effects include peripheral neuropathies, extrapyramidal symptoms, headache, fatigue, lethargy, bradycardia, hypotension, dysrhythmias, severe orthostatic hypotension (bretylium use only), microdeposits on the cornea with visual disturbances, hypothyroidism or hyperthyroidism, nausea, vomiting, constipation, liver dysfunction with abnormal liver enzyme activity, electrolyte imbalances, photosensitivity, blue–grey skin colour changes, severe pulmonary changes with development of pneumonitis, alveolitis at high dosages, pulmonary fibrosis, and pulmonary muscle weakness. The patient's thyroid function should be monitored carefully during therapy so that abnormal function can be identified before any further adverse effects appear. Toxic effects include hypotension or hypertension and bradycardia.

- *Class IV:* Therapeutic effects include improved cardiac output; decreased chest discomfort; decreased fatigue; and improved vital signs, skin colour, and urinary output. Adverse effects include bradycardia, heart failure, hypotension, AV conduction disorders, ventricular asystole, peripheral edema, and constipation. Toxic effects include hypotension, bradycardia, heart failure, and conduction disorders.

PATIENT EDUCATION

- Patients should be warned not to crush or chew any of the oral sustained-release preparations. If portions of a tablet or capsule are noted in the patient's stool, the patient should know it is from the wax matrix of the drug dosage form. This means the drug matrix has not been absorbed and the physician should be contacted.
- If the use of an oral preparation is associated with gastrointestinal distress, the patient should be informed to take the drug with food.
- Patients should be informed that if they need to use an antacid, it should be taken either 2 hours before or after taking the drug.
- Patients should be informed that a well-balanced diet without an excess of alkaline ash foods, which include citrus fruits, vegetables, and milk, is recommended and that fluid intake should be increased up to 3 L/day (unless contraindicated).
- Patients should be encouraged to limit and/or avoid the intake of caffeine (see Table 17-5 in Chapter 17 for a listing of foods and beverages containing caffeine).
- Patients should be instructed to take medications exactly as prescribed without doubling up or omitting doses. If the patient forgets a dose or is ill and cannot take a dose, the patient should know to contact the health care provider for further instructions.
- Patients should be instructed to not abruptly discontinue their drug but to continue taking it as prescribed. They should be cautioned that sudden withdrawal of the drug or stopping it on their own may be life threatening or lead to severe complications.
- Patients should be instructed on how to take their pulse and blood pressure or to use community resources such as the local fire station, pharmacy, or physician's office for a pulse and blood pressure check.
- Patients should be informed that a daily or weekly journal of symptoms, adverse effects, daily weights, a rating of how they feel, activity tolerance, blood pressure, and pulse rates will help with therapy. Also encourage them to weigh themselves at the same time every day and while wearing the same amount of clothing.

- Patients should be instructed to call the physician immediately if there is a weight gain of 1 kg or more in 24 hours or 2 kg or more in 1 week.
- Patients should be cautioned to change positions slowly because postural hypotension can be an adverse effect of these drugs. Moving too quickly may lead to dizziness, syncope, and subsequent injury or falls.
- At the beginning of therapy or with any dosage increase, patients should be encouraged to avoid driving and other hazardous activities until sedating adverse effects are resolved.
- Patients should be instructed on ways to manage dry mouth, such as use of sugarless gum or candy, eating ice chips, or rinsing the mouth frequently with water. Frequent dental visits are also encouraged.
- Patients should be cautioned to avoid exertion, hot weather, and saunas or hot tubs because of the possibility of fainting due to further blood vessel dilation from the heat and a subsequent drop in blood pressure (combined with adverse effects of hypotension with some of these drugs).
- Patients should know to report any dizziness, shortness of breath, or chest pain to their physician.
- Patients should be made to fully understand the need for carrying medical identification at all times, including an identification bracelet that lists disorders, medications, and allergies.
- With amiodarone, photosensitivity is an adverse effect, so patients should be advised to avoid sun exposure and should wear sun-protective clothing and dark glasses when going outside. Sunscreens are ineffective because they do not block ultraviolet B light. Barrier sun blocks such as zinc or titanium chloride are needed.
- With amiodarone, patients should be instructed on the need to report any blue–grey discoloration of the skin (often after 1 year, and especially on the face, neck, and arms) immediately to the health care provider. Patients should also report any jaundice, fever, numbness or tingling of extremities, blurred vision, or increased sensitivity to light.

POINTS TO REMEMBER

❖ The SA node, AV node, and bundle of His–Purkinje cells are all areas in which there is automaticity (cells can depolarize spontaneously). The SA node is the pacemaker because it can spontaneously depolarize easier and faster than the other areas.

❖ Any disturbance or abnormality in the pattern of the heartbeat/pulse rate is termed a *dysrhythmia.* Antidysrhythmic drugs are used to correct dysrhythmias; however, they may also cause dysrhythmias and for this reason are said to be *prodysrhythmic.* The Vaughan Williams classification system is most commonly used to classify antidysrhythmic drugs. It classifies groups of drugs according to where and how they affect cardiac cells and according to their mechanisms of action, as follows:

• *Class I:* membrane-stabilizing drugs (e.g., examples are class Ia: quinidine; class Ib: lidocaine; class Ic: flecainide)

• *Class II:* β-adrenergic blockers that depress phase 4 depolarization (e.g., propranolol)
• *Class III:* drugs that prolong repolarization in phase 3 (e.g., amiodarone)
• *Class IV:* calcium channel blockers that depress phase 4 depolarization (e.g., verapamil)

❖ Nursing actions for the antidysrhythmics include astute nursing assessment and close monitoring of the heart rate, blood pressure, heart rhythms, general well-being, skin colour, temperature, and heart and breath sounds. The therapeutic responses to antidysrhythmics include a decrease in blood pressure in hypertensive patients, a decrease in edema, and restoration of a regular pulse rate without major irregularities or with improved regularity compared to the irregularity that existed before therapy.

❖ Patient education about the dosage schedule and the adverse effects that the patient should report to the physician is important for safe and effective therapy.

EXAMINATION REVIEW QUESTIONS

1 A patient with a rapid, irregular heart rhythm is being treated in the emergency department with adenosine. During administration of this drug, which adverse effect should the nurse be prepared to monitor the patient for?
 a. Hypertension
 b. Muscle tetany
 c. Transitory asystole
 d. Nausea and vomiting

2 When assessing a patient who has been taking amiodarone for 6 months, which adverse reaction might the nurse identify?
 a. Urticaria
 b. Dysphagia
 c. Glycosuria
 d. Photophobia

3 The nurse is assessing a patient who has been taking quinidine and asks about adverse effects. Which of the following adverse effects is associated with the use of quinidine?
 a. Tinnitus
 b. Chest pain
 c. Muscle pain
 d. Excessive thirst

4 A patient calls the family practice office to report that he saw his pills in his stools when he had a bowel movement. What should be the nurse's response?
 a. "The pills are not being digested properly. You should be taking them with food."
 b. "The pills are not being digested properly. You should be taking them on an empty stomach."
 c. "What you are seeing is the waxy matrix that contained the medication, but the drug has been absorbed."
 d. "This indicates that you are not tolerating this medication and will need to switch to a different form."

5 Which condition would be a caution for the use of a class I antidysrhythmic?
 a. Tachycardia
 b. Hypertension
 c. Kidney dysfunction
 d. Ventricular dysrhythmias

For answers see http://evolve.elsevier.com/Canada/Lilley/pharmacology/.

CRITICAL THINKING ACTIVITIES

1 What special nursing considerations are important when administering adenosine to a patient who is experiencing PSVT that has not responded to treatment with calcium channel blockers?

2 Mrs. L. is about to be discharged home and will be taking quinidine for the treatment of ventricular ectopy. What instructions are important for her to understand before her discharge?

3 Many precautions are associated with the use of amiodarone (Cordarone). Discuss problems that you would warn a patient about when taking this drug, especially in the summer in hot climates. What serious adverse effect may occur?

For answers see http://evolve.elsevier.com/Canada/Lilley/pharmacology/.

CHAPTER 24

Antianginal Drugs

Learning Objectives

After reading this chapter, the successful student will be able to do the following:

1 Explain the pathophysiology related to myocardial ischemia and the subsequent experience of angina.

2 Describe the factors that may precipitate angina as well as measures that decrease its occurrence.

3 Compare the major classes of antianginal drugs (nitrates, calcium channel blockers, and β-blockers) with regard to their mechanisms of action, dosage forms, routes of administration, cautions, contraindications, drug interactions, adverse effects, patient tolerance, toxicity, and patient education.

4 Develop a collaborative plan of care incorporating all phases of the nursing process related to the administration of antianginal drugs.

e-Learning Activities

Web site
(http://evolve.elsevier.com/Canada/Lilley/pharmacology/)

- Animations
- Answers to chapter questions, activities, and case studies
- Calculators and Category Catchers
- Glossary with audio pronunciations
- IV Therapy and Medication Error Checklists
- Multiple-Choice Review Question quizzes
- Nursing Care Plans
- Online Appendices and Supplements
- WebLinks

Drug Profiles

amlodipine (amlodipine besylate)*, p. 452
▸▸ atenolol, p. 450
▸▸ diltiazem (diltiazem hydrochloride)*, p. 452
▸▸ isosorbide (isosorbide dinitrate)*, p. 447
▸▸ metoprolol (metoprolol tartrate)*, p. 450
▸▸ nitroglycerin, p. 447

▸▸ Key drug.

*Full generic name is given in parentheses. For the purposes of this text, the more common shortened name is used.

Glossary

Acute coronary syndrome (ACS) A group of clinical symptoms compatible with acute myocardial ischemia. (p. 444)

Angina pectoris Chest pain occurring when the heart's supply of blood carrying oxygen and energy-rich nutrients is insufficient to meet the demands of the heart. (p. 444)

Atherosclerosis A common form of arteriosclerosis involving deposits of fatty, cholesterol-containing material (plaques) within arterial walls. (p. 444)

Chronic stable angina Chest pain that occurs from atherosclerosis that results in long-term but relatively stable level of obstruction in one or more coronary arteries. (p. 444)

Coronary arteries Arteries that deliver oxygen to the heart muscle. (p. 444)

Coronary artery disease (CAD) Any one of the abnormal conditions that can affect the arteries of the heart and produce pathological effects, especially a reduced supply of oxygen and nutrients to the myocardium. (p. 444)

Ischemia Inadequate blood supply to an organ. (p. 444)

Ischemic heart disease Inadequate blood supply to the heart via the coronary arteries. (p. 444)

Myocardial infarction (MI) Gross necrosis of the myocardium following interruption of blood supply; it is almost always caused by atherosclerosis of the coronary arteries and is commonly called heart attack. (p. 444)

Reflex tachycardia A rapid heartbeat caused by a variety of autonomic nervous system effects, such as blood pressure changes, fever, or emotional stress. (p. 447)

Unstable angina Early stage of progressive coronary artery disease. (p. 444)

Vasospastic angina Ischemia-induced myocardial chest pain caused by spasms of the coronary arteries. (p. 444)

ANGINA PECTORIS AND CORONARY ARTERY DISEASE

Acute coronary syndrome (ACS) is a group of clinical symptoms compatible with acute myocardial ischemia. This can occur as a result of insufficient blood and oxygen supply to the myocardium that is due to *coronary artery disease*. The heart is an efficient organ that requires a large supply of oxygen to meet the extraordinary demands placed on it. The heart's much-needed oxygen supply is delivered to the myocardium through the **coronary arteries**. The inability to provide an adequate supply of oxygen to an organ is **ischemia**. When the organ involved is the heart, the condition is called **ischemic heart disease**. Ischemic pain results when the supply of oxygen and energy-rich nutrients in the blood is insufficient to meet the demands of the heart. This condition is called **angina pectoris**, or chest pain.

Ischemic heart disease is the leading cause of death in Canada (see Special Populations: Women on the differences between men and women concerning heart disease). The primary cause is obstruction of the coronary arteries resulting from **atherosclerosis**. When atherosclerotic plaques project from the walls into the lumens of the coronary vessels, they become narrow. The supply of oxygen and energy-rich nutrients required for the heart to meet the demands placed on it is then decreased. This disorder is called **coronary artery disease (CAD).** An acute result of CAD and of ischemic heart disease is **myocardial infarction (MI)**, or heart attack. It occurs when blood flow through the coronary arteries to the myocardium is completely obstructed such that part of the myocardium cannot receive any of the blood-borne nutrients (especially oxygen) necessary for normal function. If this process is not reversed immediately, that area of the heart will die and become *necrotic* (dead or nonfunctioning). Damage to a large enough area of the myocardium can be disabling or fatal.

The rate at which the heart pumps and the strength of each heartbeat (contractility) also influence oxygen demands on the heart. There are numerous influences that can increase heart rate and contractility and thus increase oxygen demand. These include caffeine, exercise, and stress. These influences result in stimulation of the sympathetic nervous system, which results in increased heart rate and contractility. In an already overburdened heart, such as in a person with CAD, this can worsen the balance between myocardial oxygen supply and demand and result in angina. Some drugs used to treat angina are aimed at correcting this imbalance between myocardial oxygen supply and demand by decreasing heart rate and contractility; nitrates, β-blockers, and calcium channel blockers are examples.

The pain of angina is a result of the following process. Under ischemic conditions when the myocardium is deprived of oxygen, the heart shifts to anaerobic metabolism to meet its energy needs. One of the byproducts of anaerobic metabolism is lactic acid. The accumulation of lactic acid and other metabolic byproducts stimulates chemosensitive and mechanoreceptive receptors of nerve cells found within heart muscle fibres and around the coronary vessel, producing the heart pain known as *angina*. It is the same pathophysiological mechanism responsible for causing the soreness in skeletal muscles after vigorous exercise.

There are three classic types of chest pain, or angina pectoris. **Chronic stable angina**, also referred to as *classic angina* and *effort angina*, occurs as a result of atherosclerosis. Chronic stable angina is triggered by either exertion or stress (cold, fear, or emotions). The nicotine in tobacco, as well as alcohol, coffee, and other drugs that stimulate the sympathetic nervous system, can also exacerbate angina. The pain of chronic stable angina is commonly intense but subsides within 15 minutes of either rest or appropriate antianginal drug therapy. **Unstable angina** is usually the early stage of progressive CAD. It often culminates in MI in subsequent years. For this reason, unstable angina is also called preinfarction angina. Another term for this type of angina is crescendo angina because the pain increases in severity, as does the frequency of attacks. In the later stages, pain may even occur while the patient is at rest. **Vasospastic angina** results from spasm of the layer of smooth muscle that surrounds the atherosclerotic coronary arteries. In contrast to chronic stable angina, this type of pain often occurs at rest and without any precipitating cause. It does seem to follow a regular pattern, however, usually occurring at the same time of day. This type of angina is also called *Prinzmetal's angina* or variant angina. Dysrhythmias and electrocardiogram (ECG) changes often accompany these different types of anginal attacks.

ANTIANGINAL DRUGS

The three main classes of drugs used to treat angina pectoris are the nitrates and nitrites, the β-blockers, and the calcium channel blockers. Their therapeutic effects

SPECIAL POPULATIONS: WOMEN

Heart Disease in Women

- Women's lifetime risk of developing coronary artery disease by the age of 40 years is one in three.
- Socioeconomic status is a risk factor for women; women with low incomes have a 61% increase in risk of cardiovascular disease mortality over that for high-income women.
- Women are more likely than men to have unstable angina.
- Women experience more atypical symptoms of acute coronary syndrome than do men, such as chest pain other than substernal or left-sided or no chest pain, fatigue, and shoulder pain.
- 45% of women die within 5 years of onset of heart failure because of coronary artery disease.
- Women delay seeking emergency care for chest pain longer than men, which can be critical for treatment to be effective.
- Women are less likely than men to receive aggressive testing or to receive angioplasty or emergency bypass.
- Women should maintain a body mass index (BMI) of between 18.5 and 24.9.
- Women should exercise daily for 30 minutes of moderate intensity (e.g., brisk walking) and for 60 to 90 minutes if weight loss is necessary.
- Alcohol should be limited to no more than one drink per day.
- Sodium intake should be less than 2.3 g per day.
- Aspirin therapy and heart disease risk reduction: 81–325 mg should be used in high-risk women; in healthy and lower-risk women 65 years or older; and in lower-risk women under 65 when the benefit for ischemic stroke prevention outweighs the adverse effects of aspirin. Aspirin is not used as risk reduction for myocardial infarction in healthy women under age 65.
- Avoid supplements of vitamin E, vitamin C, beta carotene, and folic acid (except during childbearing years) with or without B_6 and B_{12}.
- There is a critical period in young adulthood to middle-age when women should avoid risk factors; by doing so, they can diminish risk of heart disease in later life.
- Fasting lipid levels including triglycerides, low-density lipoprotein-cholesterol (LDL-C), and high-density lipoprotein-cholesterol (HDL-C) should be measured every 1 to 3 years in postmenopausal women or at 50 years or over; more frequent testing is recommended for those with abnormal values.
- Elevated triglyceride levels and low levels of HDL-C are more prominent and significant independent risk factors in women.

Source: Herrmann, C. (2008). Raising awareness of women and heart disease—Women's hearts are different. *Critical Care Nursing Clinics of North America, 20*(3), 251–263; Quinn, J. R. (2008). Update on women and heart disease. *Nursing Management, 39*(8), 22–28; Pilote, L., Dasgupta, K., Guru, V., Humphries, K. H., McGrath, J., Norris, C., et al. (2007). A comprehensive view of sex-specific issues related to cardiovascular disease. *Canadian Medical Association Journal, 176*(6 Suppl.), S1–S44.

are summarized and compared in Table 24-1. There are three main therapeutic objectives of antianginal drug therapy. It must (1) minimize the frequency of attacks and decrease the duration and intensity of the anginal pain; (2) improve the patient's functional capacity with as few adverse effects as possible; and (3) prevent or delay the worst possible outcome, MI. The overall goal of antianginal drug therapy is to increase blood flow to the ischemic myocardium, decrease myocardial oxygen demand, or both. Figure 24-1 illustrates how drug therapy works to alleviate angina. Existing evidence suggests that drug therapy may be at least as effective as angioplasty in treating this condition.

NITRATES/NITRITES

Nitrates have long been the mainstay of both the prophylaxis and treatment for angina and other heart problems. This class of antianginal drugs was first discovered by Sir Thomas Lauder Brunton in England, who noted that amyl nitrite was just as effective as venesection (venipuncture with drainage of blood volume) in the management of angina. A few years later, a chemically related substance, glyceryl trinitrate (nitroglycerin), was successfully isolated and used for this purpose. Today, there are several chemical derivatives of these early precursors, all of which are organic nitrate esters. They are available in a wide variety of preparations, including sublingual, chewable, and oral tablets; capsules; ointments; patches; a translingual spray; and intravenous solutions. The following nitrates are the rapid- and long-acting nitrates available for clinical use:

- amyl nitrite (rapid acting), nitroglycerin (both rapid and long acting)
- isosorbide dinitrate (both rapid and long acting)
- isosorbide mononitrate (primarily long acting)

Mechanism of Action and Drug Effects

Medicinal nitrates and nitrites, more commonly referred to as simply *nitrates*, dilate all blood vessels. They predominantly affect venous vascular beds; however, they also have a dose-dependent arterial vasodilator effect.

TABLE 24-1					
Antianginal Drugs: Therapeutic Effects					
Therapeutic Effect	**Nitrates**	**β-Blockers***	**Nifedipine**	**Verapamil**	**Diltiazem**
SUPPLY					
Blood flow	↑↑	↑	↑↑↑	↑↑↑	↑↑↑
Duration of diastole	0	↑↑↑	0/↑	↑↑↑	↑↑
DEMAND					
Preload	↓↓	↑	↓/0	0	0/↓
Afterload	↓	0/↓	↓↓↓	↓↓	↓↓
Contractility	0	↓↓↓	↓	↓↓↓	↓↓
Heart rate	0/↑	↓↓↓	0/↑	↓↓	↓↓

↓, Decrease; ↑, increase; 0, little or no effect.

*In particular those that are cardioselective and do not have intrinsic sympathomimetic activity.

†*Preload* is pressure in the heart caused by blood volume. The nitrates effectively move part of this blood out of the heart and into blood vessels, thereby decreasing preload or filling pressure.

These vasodilatory effects are the result of relaxation of the smooth muscle cells that are part of the wall structure of veins and arteries. Particularly notable, however, is the potent dilating effect of nitrates on the coronary arteries, both large and small. This effect causes redistribution of blood and therefore oxygen to previously ischemic myocardial tissue and reduction of anginal symptoms. By causing venous dilation, the nitrates reduce venous return

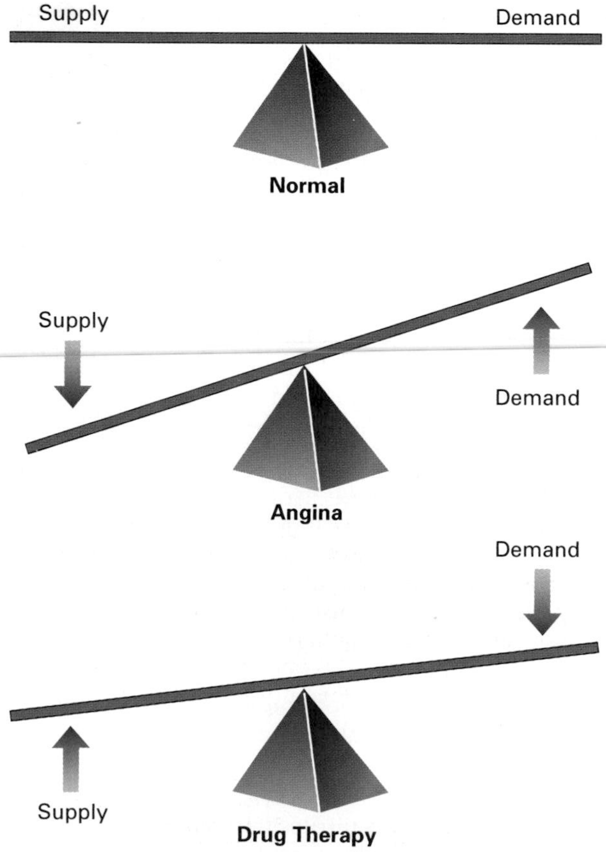

FIG. 24-1 Benefit of drug therapy for angina through increasing oxygen supply and decreasing oxygen demands.

and, in turn, reduce the left ventricular end-diastolic volume (or preload), which results in a lower left ventricular pressure. Left ventricular systolic wall tension is thus reduced, as is myocardial oxygen demand. These and other nitrate drug effects are summarized in Table 24-1.

Coronary arteries that are diseased and have been narrowed by atherosclerosis can still be dilated as long as there remains smooth muscle surrounding the coronary artery and the atherosclerotic plaque does not completely obstruct the arterial lumen. Exercise-induced spasms of atherosclerotic coronary arteries can also be reversed or even prevented by administration of nitrates, thus enabling patients to carry out healthy physical activity.

Indications

The nitrates are used for stable, unstable, and vasospastic (Prinzmetal's) angina. Long-acting dosage forms are used more for prevention of anginal episodes. Rapid-acting dosage forms, most often sublingual nitroglycerin tablets or spray, or an intravenous drip in the hospital setting, are used to treat acute anginal attacks.

Contraindications

Contraindications to the use of nitrates include known drug allergy, severe anemia, closed-angle glaucoma, hypotension, or severe head injury. This is because the vasodilation effects of nitrates can worsen these latter conditions. In anemia, a drug-induced hypotensive episode can further compromise already reduced tissue oxygenation.

Adverse Effects

Nitrates are well tolerated, and most adverse effects are usually transient and involve the cardiovascular system. The most common undesirable effect is headache, which generally diminishes in intensity and frequency soon after the start of therapy. Other cardiovascular effects include tachycardia and postural hypotension. If nitrate-induced vasodilation occurs too rapidly, the cardiovascular system overcompensates and increases the heart rate, a condition referred to as **reflex tachycardia**. This may occur when significant vasodilation occurs that involves the systemic veins. When this happens, there is a large shift in blood volume toward the systemic venous circulation and away from the heart. Baroreceptors (blood pressure receptors) in the heart then falsely sense that there has been a dramatic loss of blood volume. At this point, the heart begins beating more rapidly to move the apparently smaller volume of blood more quickly throughout the body, especially toward the vital organs (including the heart itself). However, the same baroreceptors soon sense that there has not been a loss of blood volume but that the volume of blood missing in the heart is now in the periphery (e.g., venous system), and the heart rate slows back to normal.

Methemoglobinemia is an extremely rare adverse effect and usually occurs in patients with an inherited genetic propensity for the condition. Topical nitrate dosage forms can produce various types of contact dermatitis (skin inflammations), but these are actually reactions to the dosage delivery system and not to the nitroglycerin contained within it.

Tolerance to the antianginal effects of nitrates can occur surprisingly quickly in some patients, especially in those taking long-acting formulations or taking nitrates continuously. In addition, cross-tolerance can arise when a patient receives more than one nitrate dosage form. To prevent this, a regular nitrate-free period allows certain enzymatic pathways to replenish themselves. A common regimen with transdermal patches is to remove them at night for 8 hours and apply a new patch in the morning. This practice has been shown to prevent tolerance to the beneficial effects of nitrates.

Interactions

Nitrate antianginal drugs can produce additive hypotensive effects when taken in combination with alcohol, β-blockers, calcium channel blockers, phenothiazines, and erectile-dysfunction drugs such as sildenafil (Viagra).

Dosages

The organic nitrates are available in an array of forms and dosages. See the Dosages table on p. 448 for more information.

 DRUG PROFILES

▶▶ *isosorbide dinitrate*

Isosorbide dinitrate (Apo-ISDN, Cedocard SR) is an organic nitrate and thus a powerful explosive. It exerts the same effects as the other nitrates. When isosorbide dinitrate is metabolized in the liver, it is broken down into two active metabolites, both of which have the same therapeutic actions as isosorbide dinitrate. Isosorbide dinitrate is available as rapid-acting sublingual tablets, immediate-release tablets, and long-acting oral dosage forms.

PHARMACOKINETICS

Half-Life	Onset	Peak	Duration
>PO: Variable	PO: 20–40 min	PO: Unknown	PO: 4–6 hr
SL: Variable	SL: 2–5 min	SL: Unknown	SL: 1–3 hr
SR: Variable	SR: Up to 4 hr	SR: Unknown	SR: 6–8 hr

PO, oral; *SL*, sublingual; *SR*, sustained-release

▶▶ *nitroglycerin*

Nitroglycerin is the prototypical nitrate and is made by many pharmaceutical companies; therefore, it has many different trade names (e.g., Nitro-Dur, Nitrostat). It has traditionally been the most important drug used in the symptomatic treatment of ischemic heart conditions such as angina. When given orally, nitroglycerin goes to the liver to be metabolized before it can be active in the body. During this process, a large amount of the nitroglycerin is removed from the circulation. This is called a large first-pass effect (discussed in Chapter 2). For this reason, nitroglycerin is administered by many other routes to

bypass the first-pass effect. It also is available in many formulations and has proved useful for the treatment of a variety of cardiovascular conditions. Tablets or the aerosol spray administered by the sublingual and buccal routes are used for the treatment of chest pain or angina of acute onset and for the prevention of angina when patients have known angina predictors. Use of these routes is advantageous for alleviating these acute conditions because the area under the tongue and inside the cheek is highly vascular. This means that the nitroglycerin is absorbed quickly and directly into the bloodstream, hence its therapeutic effects occur rapidly.

Nitroglycerin is also available as a metered-dose aerosol that is sprayed onto or under the tongue. Nitroglycerin is available in an intravenous form that is used for blood pressure control in hypertensive patients perioperatively; for the treatment of ischemic pain, heart failure, and pulmonary edema associated with acute MI; and in hypertensive emergency situations. Topical dosage formulations are used for the long-term prophylactic management of angina pectoris. Topical formulations offer the same advantages as sublingual and buccal formulations in that they also bypass the liver and the first-pass effect. They also allow for the continuous slow delivery of nitroglycerin so that a steady dose of nitroglycerin is supplied to the patient. See Preventing Medication Errors: Rate versus Dose.

PHARMACOKINETICS

Half-Life	Onset	Peak	Duration
SL: 1–4 min	SL: 2–3 min	SL: Unknown	SL: 0.5–1 hr

DOSAGES   Selected Antianginal Nitrate Coronary Vasodilators

Drug (Pregnancy Category)	Pharmacological Class	Usual Dosage Range	Indications
▸▸isosorbide dinitrate (Apo-ISDN, Cedocard SR) (C)	Antianginal nitrate coronary vasodilator	*Adult* SL: 5–10 mg × 3 PO: 10–30 mg tid SR: 20–40 mg bid, 7 hr apart	Angina
▸▸nitroglycerin (Nitro-Dur, Nitrostat) (C)	Antianginal nitrate coronary vasodilator	*Adult* IV (continuous infusion by pump): 5–20 mcg q3–5 min Ointment: 2.5–5 cm ribbon q6–8h, up to 10–12.5 cm ribbon q4h Spray: 0.4–0.8 mg (1–2 sprays) onto or under the tongue prn SL: 0.3–0.6 mg q5 min, 3 times Transdermal: daily in A.M., leave on 12–14 hr (0.2–0.8 mg/hr)	Angina

IV, intravenous; *PO*, oral; *SL*, sublingual; *SR*, sustained-release.

PREVENTING MEDICATION ERRORS

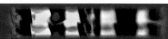

Rate versus Dose

The Institute of Safe Medication Practice (ISMP) reported an incident in which a nitroglycerin intravenous drip was set to infuse at 60 mL/hour rather than 60 mcg/min. With the medication concentration used (50 mg/250 mL) the patient actually received 200 mcg/minute instead of the ordered 60 mcg/min. Investigation of this incident revealed that the nurses were using a handwritten, non-standard dosing table rather than one that corresponded to the available concentrations of premixed solutions in the hospital. According to the report, the patient became hypotensive but recovered.

Several preparations of nitroglycerin for injection, which differ in concentration, vial volume, or both, are available. It is crucial that the nurse understands the difference between "mL/hr" and "mcg/min" when programming infusion pumps; rates are not interchangeable with ordered doses. In addition, use of standardized dosing charts that correspond to available concentrations of solutions is important. Some facilities also require double-checking of infusion pump settings before beginning drug therapy. However, because there is no fixed optimum dose of nitroglycerin, each patient must be titrated to response.

For more information, see http://www.ismp.org/Newsletters/nursing/Issues/NurseAdviseERR200506.pdf

β-BLOCKERS

The β-adrenergic blockers, more commonly referred to as β-blockers, have become the mainstay in the treatment of several cardiovascular diseases. These include angina, MI, dysrhythmias (Chapter 23), and hypertension (Chapter 25). Most available β-blockers demonstrate antianginal efficacy, although not all have been approved for this use. β-Blockers approved as antianginal drugs are atenolol, metoprolol, nadolol, and propranolol (see also Chapter 19).

Mechanism of Action and Drug Effects

The primary drug effects of the β-blockers are related to the cardiovascular system. As discussed in Chapters 18 and 19, the β_1-adrenergic receptors, located in the heart's conduction system and throughout the myocardium, are the predominant β-adrenergic receptors in the heart. The β-adrenergic receptors are normally stimulated by the binding of the neurotransmitters epinephrine and norepinephrine. These catecholamines are released in greater quantities during times of exercise or other stress to stimulate the heart muscle to contract more strongly. At the normal heart rate of 60 to 80 beats/min, the heart spends 60% to 70% of its time in diastole. As the heart rate increases during stress or exercise, the heart spends more and more time in systole and less and less time in diastole. The physiological consequence is that the coronary arteries receive increasingly less blood, and eventually the myocardium becomes ischemic. In an ischemic heart, the increased oxygen demand from increasing contractility (systole) also leads to increasing degrees of ischemia and chest pain. The physiological act of systole requires energy in the form of adenosine triphosphate and oxygen. Therefore, any decrease in the energy demands on the heart is beneficial for alleviating conditions such as angina, in which the supply of these vital substances is already deficient because of the ischemia. When β-receptors are blocked by β-blockers, the rate at which the pacemaker (sinoatrial node) fires decreases, and the time it takes for the node to recover increases. The β-blockers also slow conduction through the atrioventricular node and reduce myocardial contractility (negative inotropic effect). Both of these effects serve to slow the heart rate (negative chronotropic effect). These effects reduce myocardial oxygen demand, which aids in the treatment of angina by reducing the workload of the heart. Slowing the heart rate is also beneficial in patients with ischemic heart disease because the coronary arteries have more diastolic time to fill with oxygen- and nutrient-rich blood and deliver these substances to the myocardial tissues.

The β-blockers also have many therapeutic effects after an MI. After a patient has a MI, there is a high level of circulating catecholamines (norepinephrine and epinephrine), the release of which has been triggered by the myocardial damage resulting from the infarction. These catecholamines will produce several harmful consequences if their actions go unopposed. They essentially irritate the heart. They cause the heart rate to increase, causing a further imbalance in the supply-and-demand ratio, and they irritate the conduction system of the heart, which can result in dysrhythmias that can be fatal. The β-blockers block all of these harmful effects, and their use has been shown to improve the chances for survival in such patients. Unless strongly contraindicated, they are given to all patients in the acute stages after an MI.

The β-blockers also suppress the activity of the hormone renin, which is the first step in the renin–aldosterone–angiotensin system. Renin is a potent vasoconstrictor released by the kidneys when they sense that they are not being adequately perfused. When β-blockers inhibit the release of renin, the blood vessels to and in the kidney dilate, which reduces blood pressure (Chapter 25).

Indications

As mentioned earlier, indications for the use of β-blockers include angina and MI. They are also commonly used in hypertension (see Chapter 25), cardiac dysrhythmias (as described in Chapter 23), and essential tremor. Some non–Health Canada–approved but common uses include migraine headache and, in low doses, even the tachycardia associated with "stage fright."

The β-blockers are most effective in the treatment of typical exertional angina (i.e., that caused by exercise) because the usual physiological increase in the heart rate and systolic blood pressure that occurs during exercise or stress is blunted, thereby decreasing the myocardial oxygen demand. For an individual (often the older adult) with significant angina, "exercise" may simply be carrying out the activities of daily living (ADLs) (bathing, dressing, cooking, housekeeping, etc.), which can become a major stressor for such patients.

Contraindications

There are a number of contraindications associated with the use of β-blockers, including systolic heart failure and serious conduction disturbances, because of the effects of β-receptor blockade on heart rate and myocardial contractility. They should be used with caution in patients with bronchial asthma because any level of blockade of β2 receptors can promote bronchoconstriction through unopposed parasympathetic (vagal) tone (see Adverse Effects). These contraindications are relative rather than absolute and depend on patient-specific risks and expected benefits of this drug therapy. Other relative contraindications include diabetes mellitus (because of masking of hypoglycemia-induced tachycardia) and peripheral vascular disease (the drug may further compromise cerebral or peripheral blood flow).

Adverse Effects

The adverse effects of β-blockers result from the ability of the drug to block β-adrenergic receptors (β_1 and β_2) in various areas of the body. Therefore, blocking of β_1 receptors may lead to a decrease in heart rate, cardiac output, and cardiac contractility, whereas blocking of β_2 receptors may result in bronchoconstriction and increased airway resistance in patients with asthma or chronic obstructive pulmonary disease. β-Blockers may lead to heart rhythm problems, decreased sinoatrial (SA) and atrioventricular (AV) nodal conduction, a decrease in systolic and diastolic blood pressures, and possible peripheral receptor blockade and decreased renin release from the kidneys. β-Blockers are associated with masking tachycardia associated with hypoglycemia. Fatigue, insomnia, and weakness may be related to negative effects on the heart and the central nervous system. The β-blockers can also cause both hypoglycemia and hyperglycemia, which is of particular concern in diabetic patients. Other common β-blocker–related adverse effects are listed in Table 24-2.

Interactions

There are many important drug interactions that involve the β-blockers. The more common and important of these interactions are listed in Table 24-3.

Dosages

For information on the dosages of selected β-blockers, see the Dosages table on p. 450.

TABLE 24-2

β-Blockers: Adverse Effects

Body System	Adverse Effects
Cardiovascular	Bradycardia, hypotension, second- or third-degree heart block, heart failure
Central nervous	Dizziness, fatigue, mental depression, lethargy, drowsiness, unusual dreams
Metabolic	Altered glucose and lipid metabolism
Other	Wheezing, dyspnea, erectile dysfunction

TABLE	24-3

β-Blockers: Common Drug Interactions

Drug	Mechanism	Result
Anticholinergics	Antagonistic effects	Decreased level of β-blocker
Cimetidine	Decreases metabolism	Increased levels and pharmacodynamic effects of propranolol and metoprolol
Diuretics and antihypertensives	Additive effects	Hypotension
Insulin and oral antihyperglycemic drugs	Additive hypoglycemic effects	Hypoglycemia; possibly requiring dosage adjustment of β-blocker or antihyperglycemic drugs
Phenothiazine	Additive hypotensive effects	Hypotension and cardiac arrest
Phosphodiesterase type 5 inhibitors (e.g., sildenafil [Viagra])	Additive hypotensive effects	Potentially life-threatening hypotension

DRUG PROFILES

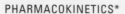

As pointed out earlier, β-blockers are the mainstay in the treatment of a wide range of cardiovascular diseases, including hypertension, angina, and the acute stages of MI. The three most commonly used β-blockers are carvedilol, metoprolol, and atenolol. Carvedilol is not indicated for angina but is instead indicated for congestive heart failure, essential hypertension, and left ventricular dysfunction. As noted previously, atenolol, metoprolol, nadolol, and propranolol all are indicated for angina. The drug profile for carvedilol is given in Chapter 19 on p. 369.

▶▶ atenolol

Atenolol (Tenorim) is a cardioselective β₁-adrenergic receptor blocker and is indicated for the prophylactic treatment of angina pectoris. Use of atenolol after MI has been shown to decrease mortality. It is available in oral form.

PHARMACOKINETICS*

Half-Life	Onset	Peak	Duration
6–7 hr	1 hr	2–4 hr	24 hr

▶▶ metoprolol tartrate

Metoprolol tartrate (Lopresor, Lopresor SR) is another cardioselective β₁-adrenergic receptor blocker, with many of the same characteristics as atenolol. Metoprolol tartrate is used for the prophylactic treatment of angina. It has shown similar efficacy in reducing mortality in patients who have had an MI and in treating angina. It is available in both oral and parenteral forms.

PHARMACOKINETICS

Half-Life	Onset	Peak	Duration
3.5 hr	1 hr	1.5–2 hr	13–19 hr

DOSAGES	Selected β-Adrenergic Drugs

Drug (Pregnancy Category)	Pharmacological Class	Usual Dosage Range	Indication
▶▶ atenolol (Tenormin) (C)	β₁-blocker	**Adult** PO: 50–200 mg/day as a single dose	Angina
▶▶ metoprolol tartrate (Lopresor, Lopresor SR) (C)	β₁-blocker	**Adult** PO: 100–400 mg/day divided bid SR: 100–200 mg taken in the morning	Angina

CALCIUM CHANNEL BLOCKERS

There are three chemical classes of calcium channel blockers (CCBs). The most common smooth muscle–selective class is the *dihydropyridines,* represented by amlodipine. Note that dihydropyridines are easy to recognize because the drug name ends in *-pine. Nondihydropyridines,* of which there are only two currently used clinically, comprise the other two classes of CCBs: *phenylalkylamines* (e.g., verapamil) and *benzothiazepines* (e.g., diltiazem) (Table 24-4). Although they all block calcium channels, their chemical structures and, thus, mechanisms of action differ slightly. Many CCBs are available, with more being developed. Those that are used for the treatment of chronic stable angina are amlodipine, diltiazem, nifedipine, and verapamil.

Mechanism of Action and Drug Effects

Calcium plays an important role in the excitation–contraction coupling process that occurs in the heart and vascular smooth muscle cells, as well as in skeletal muscle. Preventing calcium from entering into this process thus prevents muscle contraction and promotes relaxation. Relaxation of the smooth muscles that surround the coronary arteries causes them to dilate. This dilation increases blood flow to the ischemic heart, which, in turn, increases the oxygen supply and helps shift the supply

TABLE 24-4

Classification of Calcium Channel Blockers

Generic Name	Trade Name	Available Routes
BENZOTHIAZEPINES		
diltiazem hydrochloride	(Apo-Diltiaz TZ, Cardizem CD)	PO/IV
DIHYDROPYRIDINES		
amlodipine besylate	Norvasc	PO
felodipine	Plendil	PO
nifedipine	Adalat	PO
nimodipine	Nimotop	PO
PHENYLALKYLAMINES		
verapamil hydrochloride	Covera-HS, Isoptin	PO/IV

IV, intravenous; *PO*, oral.

and demand back to normal. This dilation also occurs in the arteries throughout the body, which results in a decrease in the force (systemic vascular resistance) against which the heart has to exert when delivering blood to the body (afterload). Decreasing the afterload reduces the workload of the heart and thus reduces myocardial oxygen demand. This is the primary beneficial antianginal effect of the dihydropyridine CCBs such as amlodipine and nifedipine, but these drugs have a smaller negative inotropic effect than that of verapamil and diltiazem.

Other cardiovascular effects of the CCBs include depression of the automaticity of and conduction through the sinoatrial and atrioventricular nodes because of their effects on the calcium channels (slow channels) within these tissues. For this reason, they are useful in treating cardiac dysrhythmias (Chapter 23). Finally, the CCBs reduce myocardial contractility and peripheral and coronary artery tone. Verapamil and diltiazem also decrease heart rate. Their strongest antianginal properties are secondary to their effects on myocardial contractility and the smooth muscle tone of peripheral and coronary arteries.

Indications

The therapeutic benefits of the CCBs are numerous. Because of their acceptable adverse-effect and safety profiles, they are considered first-line drugs for the treatment of such conditions as angina, hypertension, and supraventricular tachycardia. The CCBs are often particularly effective for the treatment of coronary artery spasms (vasospastic or Prinzmetal's angina). However, they may not be as effective as β-blockers in blunting exercise-induced elevations in heart rate and blood pressure. The CCBs are also used for the short-term management of atrial fibrillation and flutter (Chapter 23), migraine headaches (Chapter 17), and Raynaud's disease (a type of peripheral vascular disease). Interestingly, the dihydropyridine CCB nimodipine is indicated solely as an adjunct for cerebral artery spasms associated with intracranial aneurysm rupture.

Contraindications

Contraindications to the use of CCBs include known drug allergy, acute MI, second- or third-degree atrioventricular block (unless the patient has a pacemaker), and hypotension.

Adverse Effects

The adverse effects of the CCBs are limited and primarily relate to overexpression of their therapeutic effects. The most common of the CCB-related adverse effects are listed in Table 24-5.

Interactions

The drug interactions that can occur with CCBs vary with the particular drug, although there are not actually many such interactions. One of particular note, because of its beneficial effect, is the interaction that occurs between cyclosporin and diltiazem. Because diltiazem interferes with the metabolism and elimination of cyclosporin (thus cyclosporin is not broken down as quickly), smaller doses of cyclosporin are needed. This smaller dosage is advantageous because one of cyclosporin's most common and devastating effects is that it can destroy the kidney and cause kidney failure. One particular food interaction is that with grapefruit juice, which can reduce the metabolism of calcium channel blockers. Other important drug interactions that involve CCBs are listed in Table 24-6.

Dosages

For information on the dosages of selected CCBs, see the Dosages table on p. 452.

TABLE 24-5

Calcium Channel Blockers: Adverse Effects

Body System	Adverse Effects
Cardiovascular	Hypotension, palpitations, tachycardia or bradycardia, heart failure
Gastrointestinal	Constipation, nausea
Other	Dermatitis, dyspnea, rash, flushing, peripheral edema, wheezing

TABLE 24-6

Calcium Channel Blockers: Common Drug Interactions

Drug	Mechanism	Result
β-blockers	Additive effects	Bradycardia and atrioventricular block
digoxin	Interference with elimination	Possible increased digoxin levels
H₂ blockers	Decreased clearance	Elevated levels of CCBs

DRUG PROFILES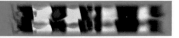

▶▶ *diltiazem hydrochloride*

Diltiazem hydrochloride (Apo-Diltiaz TZ, Cardizem) has both cardiac-depressant and vasodilator actions and is thus able to reduce arterial pressure without producing the same degree of reflex cardiac stimulation caused by dihydropyridines. It has a particular affinity for the cardiac conduction system and is effective for the oral treatment of angina pectoris resulting from coronary insufficiency, for coronary artery spasm, and for hypertension. It is one of the few CCBs that are also available in parenteral form, which is used for the treatment of atrial fibrillation and flutter along with paroxysmal supraventricular tachycardia. Verapamil is another CCB with similar indications. Two sustained-delivery formulations of diltiazem are available: a controlled-delivery-release capsule, which is taken once a day, and a sustained-release capsule, taken two to three times daily. In addition to numerous brands of these two dosage forms, the drug is also available in several strengths of immediate-release capsule and intravenous forms.

PHARMACOKINETICS

Half-Life	Onset	Peak	Duration
5–7 hr	30 min	7–11 hr	Up to 24 hr*

*With extended-release dosage forms.

amlodipine besylate

Amlodipine besylate (Norvasc) is currently the most popular CCB of the dihydropyridine subclass. It is indicated for both angina and hypertension and is available only for oral use.

PHARMACOKINETICS

Half-Life	Onset	Peak	Duration
30–50 hr	30–50 min	6–12 hr	24 hr

DOSAGES   Selected Calcium Channel–Blocking Drugs

Drug (Pregnancy Category)	Pharmacological Class	Usual Dosage Range	Indications
amlodipine besylate (Norvasc) (C)	Calcium channel blocker	*Adult* PO: 5–10 mg/day	Angina
▶▶ diltiazem hydrochloride (Apo-Diltiaz TZ, Cardizem) (C)	Calcium channel blocker	*Adult* PO: Initial dose 30 mg qid ac and at bedtime; range of 240–360 mg divided in 3–4 doses Sustained-released capsule: 120–360 mg, divided bid–tid Controlled-delivery capsule: 120–360 mg once daily	Angina
verapamil hydrochloride (Apo-Verap, Covera-HS, Isoptin SR) (C)	Calcium channel blocker	*Adult* PO: 120 mg tid–qid PO HS (extended release): 180–360 daily each evening; max 480 mg/day	Angina

SUMMARY OF ANTIANGINAL PHARMACOLOGY

In patients with CAD, the clinical symptoms result from a lack of or inadequate delivery of blood carrying oxygen and nutrients to the heart, which results in ischemic heart disease. Antianginal drugs such as nitrates, nitrites, β-blockers, and CCBs are used to reduce ischemia by increasing the delivery of oxygen- and nutrient-rich blood to cardiac tissues or by reducing oxygen consumption by the coronary vessels. Either of these mechanisms can reduce ischemia and lead to a decrease in anginal pain. Nitrates and nitrites work primarily by decreasing venous return to the heart (preload) and decreasing systemic vascular resistance (afterload). The CCBs decrease calcium influx into the smooth muscle, causing vascular relaxation. This either reverses or prevents the spasms of coronary vessels that cause the anginal pain associated with Prinzmetal's or chronic angina. The β-blockers slow the heart rate and decreasing contractility, thereby decreasing oxygen demands. Although these groups of drugs have similar clinical effects, the nursing process required for each is somewhat specific in terms of the characteristics and effects of the drugs and the indications for and contraindications to their use.

PHARMACOKINETIC BRIDGE TO NURSING PRACTICE

Not only are the pharmacokinetic properties of nitrates interesting, but their specific properties are critical to safe and accurate nursing care. Moreover, the patient's understanding of nitrate pharmacokinetics is also important because the level of the patient's knowledge may strongly influence adherence with the drug regimen and effectiveness of treatment for angina. The pharmacokinetics differ for the various dosage forms of nitroglycerin and are as follows:

- Intravenous infusion: onset within 1–2 minutes (fastest of all dosage forms), peak time not applicable, duration of action 3–5 minutes
- Sublingual tablet: onset of action 2–3 minutes, peak action unknown, duration of action 0.5–1 hour
- Transmucosal tablet: onset 2–5 minutes, peak within 4–10 minutes, and duration of 3–5 hours
- Extended-release tablet: onset in 20–45 minutes, peak action varies, and duration of action between 3-8 hours
- Topical ointment: onset 15–60 minutes, peak within $\frac{1}{2}$ to 2 hours, and duration of 3–8 hours
- Transdermal patch: onset 30–60 minutes, peak 1–3 hours, and duration of action 8–12 hours.

If the goal of treatment is to abort or treat a sudden attack of angina, then rapid onset of action is needed, so the clinical decision (by the physician) would be to prescribe either intravenous infusion, sublingual tablet (and/or lingual spray, which has a similar onset time), or transmucosal tablet. These dosage forms have pharmacokinetics that allow quick access of the drug to the bloodstream and lead to more rapid vasodilation. This action provides more oxygenated blood to the myocardium and aborts acute attacks. If symptoms persist, more drastic medical management would be indicated. The quick-onset nitroglycerin dosage forms may also be used by the patient before engaging in activities known to provoke angina, such as increased physical activity, sexual intercourse, or other forms of physical exertion. If the purpose of treatment is maintenance therapy, the nitrate form must have other pharmacokinetic properties, such as a longer onset of action (because stopping an attack is not needed in this situation) and, more importantly, a longer duration of action to provide protection against angina. Use of ointments, transdermal patches, or extended-release preparations would be appropriate in such cases. If there is an acute episode of angina while on maintenance therapy, rapid onset of action would be indicated (as ordered). Thorough knowledge about a drug and its pharmacokinetics will allow the nurse to make safe and sound decisions about drug therapy for patients with angina.

NURSING PROCESS

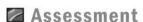

Assessment

Before administering antianginal drugs, health and medication history (e.g., listing of all prescription drugs, over-the-counter products, and natural health products) should be completed and documented. Weight, height, and vital signs, with attention to supine, sitting, and standing blood pressures, should also be noted. A systolic blood pressure reading of less than 90 mm Hg should be reported to the

physician before a dose of any of these drugs is given. Apical pulse rates are preferred with drugs impacting blood pressure or heart rate and should be taken for 1 full minute with attention to rhythm and character. If the pulse rate is 60 beats/min or below, the physician should be contacted for further instructions. The nurse should also assess for any contraindications, cautions, and drug interactions (see the previous discussion in the pharmacology section). The patient's chest pain should also be thoroughly assessed, with documentation about onset, type, character (e.g., sharp, dull, piercing, squeezing, radiating), intensity, location, duration, precipitating factors (e.g., physical exertion, exercise, eating, stress, sexual intercourse), alleviating factors, and presence of nausea or vomiting. The physician may order an ECG, and the results should be reported and documented.

The significant drug interaction with sildenafil, tadalafil, or vardenafil (used for erectile dysfunction) and nitrates is important to note because of potential worsening of hypotensive responses, paradoxical bradycardia, and increased angina with risk of heart or cerebrovascular complications (from decreased perfusion). The older adult often has difficulty with blood pressure control because of normal age-related periods of hypotension, and use of antianginals may lead to worsening of hypotensive responses, paradoxical bradycardia, and increased angina. If patients are taking nitrates on a long-term basis, it is important to assess continued therapeutic responses because patients may develop tolerance to the drug's effects. The physician should be notified if the patient begins to have more angina; another antianginal or vasodilating drug may be ordered.

Nonselective β-blockers or $β_2$-blockers are contraindicated in patients with bronchospastic disease because of the drug-related effects of bronchoconstriction and increased airway resistance. If asthma or other respiratory problems are present, β-blockers should not be used. In addition, there are also concerns about the use of β-blockers in patients with hyperthyroidism, impaired kidney or liver function, peripheral vascular disease, or diabetes. Hypoglycemia may occur in patients with previously controlled diabetes and nonselective β-blockers may also exacerbate pre-existing heart failure. Assessment for edema is important because of drug-related edema. Weight gain of 1 kg or more over 24 hours or 2 kg or more in 1 week should be reported.

Nursing Diagnoses

- Decreased cardiac output related to the pathology of CAD
- Ineffective tissue perfusion related to the physiological impact of CAD
- Risk for injury related to the drug adverse effects of hypotension with subsequent dizziness and/or syncope
- Acute pain related to the pathological impact of tissue ischemia on the heart

- Impaired physical mobility related to the impact of cellular ischemia
- Deficient knowledge related to first-time use of these drugs and a new diagnosis

Planning

Goals

- Patient will experience fewer episodes of chest pain because of appropriate use of antianginal medication.
- Patient will be able to perform activities of daily living and increase mobility with greater comfort, less chest pain, and increased stamina and energy.
- Patient will tolerate moderate, supervised exercise while taking antianginals.
- Patient will remain free of injury while on drug therapy.
- Patient will state the actions to take when chest pain is unrelieved.
- Patient will state rationale for medication therapy as well as the adverse effects to report.

Outcome Criteria

- Patient states that there are more frequent periods of comfort while carrying out activities of daily living, engaging in supervised exercise, and performing moderate activity without recurring angina and without major adverse effects on follow-up with the physician.
- Patient states measures to decrease risk of injury, such as changing positions slowly, keeping legs moving when in a still position, increasing fluid intake with medication regimen, and removing rugs or carpets that can cause tripping or slipping.
- Patient states symptoms that should be reported to the physician, such as syncope, excessive dizziness, severe headache, or increase in episodes of chest pain or its severity.

Implementation

It is crucial for the nurse to always review and record the patient's vital signs and description of chest pain for the duration of therapy. Various dosage forms and routes of administration are used with the following nursing considerations:

- For any dosage form: The drug should always be administered while the patient is seated to avoid falls or injury from drug-induced hypotension, which may last for up to 30 minutes after dosing of the drug. When administering nitrates, the patient's chest pain should be monitored, with rating of the pain on a scale of 1 to 10, before, during, and after therapy. The

patient's response to drug therapy should be monitored through assessment of the patient's blood pressure, pulse rate, and presence of headache, dizziness, or lightheadedness. With the patient in a supine position, an appropriate dose of a nitrate should produce a clinical response of a fall in blood pressure of about 10 mm Hg, a rise in heart rate of 10 beats/min, or both. Should the patient's systolic blood pressure fall to less than 90 mm Hg or pulse rate to less than 60 beats/min, the physician should be contacted.

- For oral dosage forms: These should be taken as ordered before meals and with 180 mL of water. Extended-release preparations should not be crushed, chewed, or altered in any way. Acetaminophen may be given if there is a drug-related headache.
- For sublingual or buccal forms: Tablets are to be placed under the tongue (sublingual) or between the inner cheek mucosa and gum (buccal) as directed and not swallowed until the drug is completely dissolved. Remember that nitrates should be kept in its original packaging or container (e.g., sublingual or buccal tablets come in a small amber-coloured glass container with a metal lid). Avoid exposure to light, plastic, cotton filler, and moisture.
- *For spray:* Upon initiating treatment with nitroglycerin pump spray, especially when changing from another form of nitroglycerin, the patient should be monitored by the physician to determine the minimum effective dose. Each metered dose contains 0.4 mg of nitroglycerin. The patient is instructed to spray one to two metered doses onto or under the tongue without inhaling. The container should be held in a vertical position with the nozzle head up. The opening in the nozzle head should be held as closely as possible to the mouth.
- For ointment: The proper dosing paper supplied by the drug company should be used to apply a thin layer on clean, dry, hairless skin of the upper arms or body. Areas below the knees and elbows should be avoided. The ointment should not be applied with the fingers unless using a gloved finger, to avoid contact with the skin and subsequent absorption. A tongue depressor may also be used, but in most situations the ointment may be squeezed directly from the tube onto the proper dosing paper. Once the ointment is in place, it should not be rubbed into the skin, and the area should be covered with an occlusive dressing if not provided (e.g., plastic wrap). Application sites should be rotated, and all residue from the previous dose of ointment (or transdermal patch) should be gently removed with soap and water and the area patted dry.
- For transdermal forms: The patch should be applied to a clean, residue-free, hairless area, and sites should be rotated. If cardioversion or use of an automated

electrical defibrillator is required, the patch should be removed to avoid burning of the skin and damage to the defibrillator paddles. Be sure to locate and remove the old patch and any residual drug.

- For intravenous forms: Intravenous dosing is for use in emergency situations only and in settings with close automatic monitoring of the blood pressure and pulse and constant ECG monitoring. Intravenous administration of nitrates may lead to sudden and severe hypotension, cardiovascular collapse, and shock. Always check for incompatibilities, use the proper diluent, and give intravenous solutions only through an infusion pump and as ordered. Intravenous dosage forms are available as ready-to-use injectable doses and are administered using specific nonpolyvinylchloride (non-PVC) plastic intravenous bags and tubing. The non-PVC infusion kits are used to avoid absorption or uptake of the nitrate by the intravenous tubing and bag. This packaging prevents decomposition of the nitrate (with breakdown) into cyanide when the drug is exposed to light. Intravenous forms of nitroglycerin are stable for about 96 hours after preparation. If parenteral solutions are not clear and are discoloured, the solution should be discarded.

With isosorbide, tablets are best taken on an empty stomach; however, if the patient complains of headache or gastrointestinal upset, the medicine should be taken with meals. Oral tablets of isosorbide can be crushed; however, the sublingual and extended-release forms should not be crushed or chewed. In addition, if a "chewable" form is to be given, it should not be crushed, even though it is chewable. As with sublingual nitroglycerin, the patient should not swallow the medication until it is completely dissolved. If dizziness or lightheadedness occurs, assist and encourage the patient to change positions slowly. The nurse should monitor the patient's blood pressure, including orthostatic blood pressures, as well as anginal episodes with documentation of their severity and frequency.

CCBs should be given as ordered, and the patient should take them as ordered without sudden or abrupt withdrawal. Weight should be measured daily (see the discussion of β-blockers), and the patient should be constantly monitored for edema and shortness of breath. The patient should be instructed to move and change positions slowly and with caution to prevent syncope. The nurse should also advise the patient on how to prevent constipation. Should the patient experience heart irregularities, pronounced dizziness, nausea, or dyspnea, the physician should be contacted immediately. Intravenous administration of either CCBs or β-blockers requires use of an infusion pump and careful monitoring. See Patient Education for more information.

The β-blockers should be given as ordered and taken with or without food and without abrupt withdrawal. The patient's weight should be assessed every day at the same time, and if there is a gain of 1 kg or more in 24 hours or 2 kg or more in 1 week, the physician should be contacted immediately. With the use of these drugs, measures should be taken to reduce the incidence of orthostatic hypotension, such as having the patient dangle the legs before standing. Any dizziness, lightheadedness, mental depression, confusion, rash, or unusual bleeding or bruising should be reported to the physician. The patient should be informed that alcohol, saunas, hot tubs, hot showers, and hot weather or a hot environment will exacerbate vasodilation and increase the occurrence of orthostatic hypotension and raise the risk for dizziness, syncope, and falls (as with all antianginals). With β-blockers, constipation may be a problem, which can be prevented by a high-fibre diet and increased water intake. Should the patient report that parts of any sustained-release forms of medication are appearing in the stool, the medication is possibly moving too rapidly through the gastrointestinal tract and the patient may need to be switched to another dosage form. The patient should be taught to monitor blood pressure correctly and to keep a journal in which the patient records all blood pressure readings, weights, and response to the medication regimen. Also, remember that the therapeutic effects of the β-blockers may take up to 1 to 2 weeks to appear. See Patient Education for more information on antianginals.

Evaluation

Patients taking antianginals must be monitored carefully for the occurrence of an allergic reaction, which may be manifested by dyspnea, swelling of the face, or hives. Evaluation of therapeutic effects includes assessing how goals and outcomes have been met, such as appropriate decrease in blood pressure, increase in cardiac output and tissue perfusion with decrease in angina, and a gradual increase in activity level and performance of activities in daily living without exacerbation of anginal episodes. In addition, the patient should be monitored for adverse reactions such as headache, lightheadedness, dizziness, and decreased blood pressure, which may indicate the need to decrease the dosage. If the patient is receiving intravenous nitroglycerin, the nurse should evaluate for the development of pedal edema, abnormal skin turgor, nausea, vomiting, crackles, dyspnea, and orthopnea. If the patient experiences blurred vision, dry mouth, an excessive drop in blood pressure and pulse rate, excessive facial or neck flushing, or worsening of angina, the physician should be notified immediately.

PATIENT EDUCATION

Nitroglycerin

❖ Patients should be instructed that keeping a journal is a good way of documenting how he or she feels, including how many anginal episodes occur, what happens, the character and intensity of the pain, frequency, and precipitating and relieving factors. Encourage the patient to also make notes about how the medication is tolerated.

❖ Patients taking capsules or extended-release dosage forms should be encouraged to not chew, crush, or alter the dosage form.

❖ Aerosol and sublingual forms: Patients taking aerosol dosage forms should be taught to not shake the canister before lingual spraying and to avoid inhaling or swallowing the lingual aerosol until the drug is dispersed. With sublingual forms, instruct the patient to take the medication at the first sign of chest pain and repeat every 5 minutes for up to a total of 3 doses. New recommendations are that if the patient is still having chest pain after 1 dose of sublingual nitroglycerin, he or she should immediately call 911. The sublingual dose should be placed under the tongue and the patient should avoid swallowing until the tablet is dissolved, with no eating or drinking until the drug has completely dissolved.

❖ Patients should be taught about the best place to keep the medication away from moisture, light, heat, and cotton filler and to keep the medication in its original packaging (e.g., nitroglycerin in amber-coloured glass container). Inform the patient to expect burning or stinging once the medication is placed under the tongue; if it does not burn, then the drug may have lost its potency and a new prescription must be obtained.

❖ It is important to emphasize that the medication is only potent for 3 to 6 months. Patients should be reminded to always have a fresh supply of the drug on hand, to plan ahead if travelling, and (irrespective of the dosage form) to be seated or lying down when taking the medication to avoid falls secondary to a drop in blood pressure.

❖ *Transmucosal* tablets should be placed under the upper lip in the buccal pouch, which is located between the cheek and gum. Patients should be cautioned to avoid chewing or swallowing transmucosal dosage forms.

❖ With all forms of nitrates, patients should be educated on adverse effects such as flushing of the face, dizziness, fainting, brief throbbing headache, increase in heart rate, and lightheadedness. Inform them that headaches associated with nitrates last approximately 20 minutes (with sublingual forms) and may be easily managed with acetaminophen. If headaches are bothersome with the dosing of oral forms, the drug should be taken with meals, and patients should contact their physician if adverse effects continue.

Educate patients that blurred vision, dry mouth, or severe headaches may indicate drug overdose which requires immediate medical attention.

❖ Patients should be taught that while taking antianginals, they should avoid alcohol, hot environmental temperatures, saunas, hot tubs, and excessive exertion because these will lead to worsening of vasodilation with hypotension, possible fainting, or other heart events.

❖ If the physician prescribes it, the patient should be taught to take the nitroglycerin before stressful activities or events such as emotional situations, consumption of large meals, smoking, or sudden increase in activity (e.g., sexual intercourse). The patient should be instructed to follow the physician's directions very closely.

❖ With ointment forms, patients should be told to use the appropriate dosage paper for application of ointment and not to use the fingers to apply the medicine. The medication can be pressed evenly directly from the tube onto the paper and to its dosing line. The patient should squeeze a thin line of ointment onto the paper and follow instructions regarding its application and the use of an occlusive dressing.

❖ With transdermal nitrate use, patients should be taught to apply the patch at the same time each day and to be sure to have only one patch in place at a time, with all residue cleansed off the skin before a new patch (or ointment) is applied. Educate about avoiding skin folds, hairy areas, and any area distal to the knees or elbows. Other instructions are as follows: A patch should never be placed on irritated or open skin. If the transdermal patch becomes loose, the patient should take it off, gently remove the residue with soap and water, pat the area dry, and place another patch in another area. Rotation of sites is helpful in prevention of irritation with this form and with ointments. Sometimes the physician may order the patient to remove the patch for 8 hours at a specified time to prevent tolerance to the drug, because resistance does develop over time. Provide clear instructions about this type of regimen.

Isosorbide Dinitrate

❖ Patients should be educated about oral nitrates (e.g., dinitrate form is poorly absorbed, but its metabolite, isosorbide mononitrate, is active and well absorbed).

❖ Patients should be taught to take the medication exactly as prescribed and while lying down, to avoid injury from sudden drop in blood pressure with subsequent dizziness, lightheadedness, and fainting.

❖ Patients should be clearly informed that dosing may be scheduled for three times a day with a 12-hour drug-free interval, such as dosing at 0700, 1300, and 1900. The 12-hour drug-free interval will help prevent tolerance.

- Patients should be educated about not altering the dosage form; for example, no oral dosage form should be crushed. Oral tablet forms, as with all oral medications, should be taken with at least 180 to 240 mL of water.
- Patients should be instructed to keep a journal of episodes of angina along with blood pressure and pulse readings.
- Patients should be taught that while taking these

drugs, they should always move cautiously and slowly, change positions gradually, and move their legs about or dangle them while sitting for a few moments before standing to prevent dizziness and fainting.
- Patients should be taught that brands of these drugs should never be changed from one to the other and to avoid alcohol, heat, and saunas (see the previous tips for nitroglycerin).

POINTS TO REMEMBER

- Angina pectoris (chest pain) occurs because of a mismatch between the oxygen supply and oxygen demand, with either too high a demand for oxygen or too little oxygen delivery.
- The heart is an aerobic (oxygen-requiring) muscle, and when it does not receive enough oxygen, pain (angina) occurs. When the coronary arteries that deliver oxygen to the heart muscle become blocked, a heart attack (MI) occurs. CAD is an abnormal condition of the arteries (blood vessels) that deliver oxygen to the heart muscle. These arteries may become narrowed, which results in reduced flow of oxygen and nutrients to the myocardium.
- Nitrates, CCBs, and β-blockers may be used to treat the symptoms of angina.
- Nitroglycerine is the prototypical nitrate. Nitrates dilate constricted coronary arteries, helping to increase the supply of oxygen and nutrients to the heart muscle. Nitrates also dilate all other blood vessels, which leads to the following effects: venous dilation results in a decrease of blood return to the heart (decreased preload), whereas arterial dilation results in a decrease of peripheral resistance (decreased afterload—that is, the pressure or force against which the left ventricle must pump). Isosorbide dinitrates were the first group of oral drugs used to treat angina. Nitroglycerin is the main intravenous nitrate used to treat angina and hypertensive crises.

- The β-blockers are also used to relieve angina by decreasing the heart rate, which helps reduce the workload of the heart and decreases the oxygen demand of the heart.

Nursing considerations for the use of all antianginals include the following:
- Dosage forms for nitrates include conventional tablets, sublingual and buccal tablets, controlled-release and sustained release capsules, transdermal patch, topical ointment, and intravenous injection. Specific nursing interventions are associated with each dosage form. Hypotension is the most common adverse effect for all dosage forms. Extended-release tablets or transdermal patches are generally used for long-term angina prophylaxis, whereas lingual sprays and sublingual tablets are used for acute treatment.
- Quick-onset nitrates should be used to treat acute anginal attacks.
- CCBs and β-blockers may be associated with the adverse effects of postural hypotension, dizziness, headache, and edema.
- The nonselective β-blockers may exacerbate congestive heart failure, respiratory bronchospastic problems, and hypoglycemia.
- If the patient's pulse rate is 60 beats/min or lower, the physician should be contacted for further instructions.
- The patient should be sure to keep a fresh supply of sublingual nitroglycerin because the drug is only stable for 3 to 6 months.

EXAMINATION REVIEW QUESTIONS

1 A patient has a new prescription for transdermal nitroglycerin patches. Which of the following are these patches most appropriately used for?
a. To prevent palpitations
b. To relieve exertional angina
c. To prevent the occurrence of angina
d. To reduce the severity of anginal episodes

2 Which of the following statements will a nurse with adequate knowledge about the administration of intravenous nitroglycerin recognize as being correct?
a. The intravenous form is given by bolus injection.
b. Intravenous nitroglycerin can be given via gravity drip infusions.
c. Because the intravenous forms are short-lived, the dosing must be every 2 hours.
d. Intravenous nitroglycerine must be protected from exposure to light through use of special tubing.

3 Which statement by the patient reflects the need for additional patient education about the CCB diltiazem (Cardiazem)?
a. "I can take this drug to stop acute anginal attacks."
b. "When the long-acting forms are taken, the drug cannot be crushed."
c. "I understand that food and antacids alter this drug's absorption orally."
d. "This drug may cause my blood pressure to drop, so I should be careful when getting up."

4 A nurse is assessing a patient with angina who is to start β-blocker therapy. Which of the following assessed conditions may be a problem if these drugs are used?
a. Asthma
b. Hypertension
c. Essential tremors
d. Exertional angina

5 A 68-year-old man has been taking the nitrate isosorbide dinitrate for 2 years for angina. He recently has been experiencing erectile dysfunction and wants a prescription for sildenafil (Viagra). Which response would the nurse most likely hear from the prescriber?
a. "These drugs are compatible with each other, and so I'll write a prescription."
b. "He will have to take a lower dose of the isosorbide if he wants to take sildenafil."
c. "Taking sildenafil with the nitrate may result in severe hypotension, so a contraindication exists."
d. "I'll write a prescription, but if he uses it, he needs to stop taking the isosorbide for one dose."

For answers see http://evolve.elsevier.com/Canada/Lilley/pharmacology/.

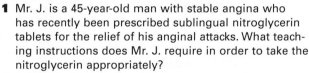

CRITICAL THINKING ACTIVITIES

1 Mr. J. is a 45-year-old man with stable angina who has recently been prescribed sublingual nitroglycerin tablets for the relief of his anginal attacks. What teaching instructions does Mr. J. require in order to take the nitroglycerin appropriately?

2 Mrs. A. has been shovelling snow all morning. You are also shovelling the snow in your yard, and you see her suddenly sit down in her driveway. When you go over to check on her, she says that she took a nitroglycerin pill at the first sign of chest pain, just like the doctor told her to. The chest pain is gone at this time. What, if anything, should she have done differently?

3 Your patient has been switched from sublingual nitroglycerin to a transdermal form. What instructions do you need to give him regarding the difference in his therapeutic regimen?

For answers see http://evolve.elsevier.com/Canada/Lilley/pharmacology/.

CHAPTER 25

Antihypertensive Drugs

Learning Objectives

After reading this chapter, the successful student will be able to do the following:

1. Briefly discuss the normal anatomy and physiology of the autonomic nervous system, including the events that take place within the sympathetic and parasympathetic divisions and how they relate to long-term and short-term control of blood pressure.

2. Define hypertension with comparison of primary and secondary hypertension and their related manifestations.

3. Describe the protocol for treating hypertension as detailed in the Canadian Hypertension Education Program Guidelines, including the rationale for its use.

4. List the criterion pressure values (in millimetres of mercury) for the new hypertension categories of normal pressure, prehypertension, hypertension stage 1, and hypertension stage 2 as defined in the Canadian Hypertension Education Program Guidelines.

5. Using the most recent guidelines, compare the drugs used in the pharmacological management of hypertension with regard to mechanism of action, specific indications, adverse effects, toxic effects, cautions, contraindications, dosages, and routes of administration.

6. Discuss the rationale for the nonpharmacological management of hypertension.

7. Develop a collaborative plan of care that includes all phases of the nursing process for patients receiving antihypertensive drugs.

e-Learning Activities

Web site
(http://evolve.elsevier.com/Canada/
Lilley/pharmacology/)

- Animations
- Answers to chapter questions, activities, and case studies
- Calculators and Category Catchers
- Glossary with audio pronunciations
- IV Therapy and Medication Error Checklists
- Multiple-Choice Review Question quizzes
- Nursing Care Plans
- Online Appendices and Supplements
- WebLinks

Drug Profiles

aliskiren (aliskiren fumarate)*, p. 477
bosentan (bosentan monohydrate)*, p. 478
▸▸ captopril, p. 473
carvedilol, p. 470
▸▸ clonidine (clonidine hydrochloride)*, p. 470
enalapril (enalapril sodium)*, p. 473
epoprostenol (epoprostenol sodium)*, p. 478
▸▸ hydralazine (hydralazine hydrochloride)*, p. 477
▸▸ losartan (losartan potassium)*, p. 475
prazosin (prazosin hydrochloride)*, p. 470
sodium nitroprusside, p. 477
treprostinil (treprostinil sodium)*, p. 479

▸▸ Key drug.

*Full generic name is given in parentheses. For the purposes of this text, the more common shortened name is used.

Glossary

α₁-blockers Drugs that primarily cause arterial and venous dilation through their action on peripheral sympathetic neurons. (p. 466)

Antihypertensive drugs Drugs used to treat hypertension. (p. 460)

Cardiac output The amount of blood ejected from the left ventricle, measured in litres per minute. (p. 464)

Centrally acting adrenergic drugs Drugs that modify the function of the sympathetic nervous system in the brain by stimulating α₂-receptors, which has a reverse sympathetic effect causing a decrease in blood pressure. (p. 466)

Essential hypertension An elevated systemic arterial pressure for which no cause can be found and which is often the only significant clinical finding; also called *primary* or *idiopathic hypertension.* (p. 464)

Ganglionic blocking drugs Drugs that prevent nerves from responding to the action of acetylcholine by occupying the receptor sites for acetylcholine (i.e., nicotinic receptors) on sympathetic and parasympathetic nerve endings. (p. 460)

Hypertension A common, often asymptomatic disorder in which blood pressure persistently exceeds 140/90 mm Hg. (p. 460)

Idiopathic hypertension Hypertension with no known primary cause; also called *primary hypertension.* (p. 464)

Nicotinic receptor The receptor and site of action for acetylcholine in both the parasympathetic and sympathetic nervous systems. (p. 466)

Orthostatic hypotension A common adverse effect of adrenergic drugs involving a sudden drop in blood pressure when patients change position, especially when rising from a seated or horizontal position. (p. 468)

Prodrug A drug that is inactive in its administered form and must be biotransformed in the liver to its active form. (p. 471)

Secondary hypertension High blood pressure known to be associated with a primary disease, such as kidney, pulmonary, endocrine, or vascular disease. (p. 464)

OVERVIEW

Significant advancements have been made in the detection, evaluation, and treatment of high blood pressure, or **hypertension**. Over the past 40 years, the development of new antihypertensive medications has had an enormous impact on the quality of life of affected persons by reducing the incidence of complications associated with hypertension and decreasing the adverse effects associated with these drugs. Drug therapy for hypertension first became available in the early 1950s with the introduction of **ganglionic blocking drugs**. However, unpleasant adverse effects and inconsistent therapeutic effects were common problems with these **antihypertensive drugs.** In 1953 the vasodilator hydralazine was introduced and in 1958 the thiazide diuretics became available. These drugs offered important advantages over the previous antihypertensive drug therapies. In addition, with the discovery of these newer drugs came a better understanding of the disease process itself.

Since that time, several additional drug categories have emerged, including loop diuretics (also called potassium-wasting diuretics), potassium-sparing diuretics, β-blockers (β-receptor antagonists), angiotensin-converting enzyme (ACE) inhibitors, $α_1$-antagonists, $α_2$-agonists, angiotensin II receptor blockers (ARBs), calcium channel blockers (CCBs), and vasodilators. Although some of the medications mentioned in this chapter represent older classes of drugs, all are current therapeutic options listed in the treatment guidelines for hypertension published by the Canadian Hypertension Education Program (CHEP). For this reason, these selected older drugs are discussed in this chapter along with the newer drug classes.

HYPERTENSION

As the current population ages, by the year 2025 it is expected that 1.56 billion adults over 18 years of age worldwide will have hypertension. In Canada, over five million people have some form of hypertension. Fifty percent of Canadian adults over the age of 65 have hypertension, and of those who have a normal blood pressure at age 65, more than 90% will develop hypertension. In Canada, it is estimated that 46% of women and 38% of men aged 60 and over are taking antihypertensive medications. The incidence of hypertension is also higher among some ethnic groups—Blacks, Aboriginal peoples, and the Asian population, for example. (See Ethnocultural Implications: Antihypertensive Drug Therapy in Black Patients, and Hypertension in Aboriginal Peoples as well as Special Populations: The Older Adult, Children and the Adolescent, and Women: Hypertension for a discussion of hypertension in different ethnocultural groups and special populations.) Not only does hypertension affect a large portion of our society, but it also has many severe consequences if left untreated. Hypertension is a major risk factor for coronary artery disease, cardiovascular disease, and death resulting from cardiovascular causes. It is the most important risk factor for stroke and heart failure, and it is a major risk factor for kidney failure and peripheral vascular disease. Blacks and Aboriginal peoples are at higher risk than Whites of developing stroke, heart disease, and end-stage kidney disease.

The diagnosis and management of hypertension have varied considerably over the years, resulting in a great deal of misunderstanding in how to treat this disorder. Since 2000, the Canadian Hypertension Education Program (CHEP) and the Heart and Stroke Foundation of Canada have produced and updated yearly evidence-informed recommendations for the detection, assessment, and treatment of hypertension, assembled by the 43 members of the CHEP Evidence-Based Recommendations Task Force. Each year, the recommendations focus on a change from previous guidelines or an important initiative (Boxes 25-1 and 25-2). CHEP's intent is to educate health care professionals and the general public about the consequences of hypertension and the importance of adequate prevention and treatment in order to reduce the burden of cardiovascular disease. Nurses have a key role to play in the primary prevention, detection, and treatment of hypertension.

Hypertension prevention efforts at the provinvial level include a recent population blood pressure survey conducted in Ontario, which found markedly improved

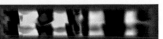

ETHNOCULTURAL IMPLICATIONS

Antihypertensive Drug Therapy in Black Patients

The following are some important generalizations about demographics and the drugs used to treat hypertension:

- β-Blockers and angiotensin-converting enzyme (ACE) inhibitors have been found in Canada to be more effective in lowering blood pressure in Whites than in Blacks.
- Calcium channel blockers and diuretics have been shown to be more effective in Black patients than in White patients in Canada.
- Captopril used as monotherapy to treat hypertension has been found in the United States to elicit a lesser response in Black patients, who are considered to be low-renin hypertensives, than in the general treatment population.
- Losartan used as monotherapy for hypertension has been found to be less effective in Black patients than in other racial groups in Canada because Black patients are low-renin hypertensives.

These findings are important to remember in the care of patients, whether they are in an inpatient setting, are being seen by a physician or a nurse practitioner, or are being screened by a nurse in the community. The significance of these ethnocultural factors is that they allow a better understanding of the dynamics of pharmacological treatment in hypertensive patients of different ethnic groups and also underscore the importance of a thorough nursing assessment that includes attention to ethnocultural influences. They also allow an appreciation of individual responses to drug therapy and aid in achieving more successful treatment of the disease. These responses are often considered by health care providers in selecting first-line therapy.

Results of many studies in Canada have supported a difference between Blacks and Whites in response to antihypertensive drugs; however, conflicting findings have been found in this area. Although researchers have reported that, on average, Blacks and Whites differ slightly in their responses to antihypertensive drugs, a meta-analysis published in the March 2004 issue of *Hypertension* found that the majority of American Blacks and Whites in the studies analyzed had similar responses to some of the more commonly used antihypertensives such as diuretics, β-blockers, calcium channel blockers, and ACE inhibitors. In this analysis, which pooled data on the use of common antihypertensives in some 9300 Whites and 2900 Blacks in America, 81% to 95% of Blacks and Whites were found to experience similar changes in blood pressure in response to each of the four groups of commonly used drugs. This analysis concluded that race, as examined in this context, had little value in predicting response to these drugs and that the responses of the two groups were overlapping. Clinical decisions may thus be more efficient and of greater therapeutic value if drug treatment is based on considerations relevant to the given individual, such as indications and medical history, rather than solely on race. In summary, it is important for nurses to fully understand all the ethnocultural and multifactor influences on pharmacological therapies so that the nursing process can be implemented thoroughly and effectively.

Based on Rakel, R. E., & Bope, E. T. (2008). *Conn's current therapy 2008,* Philadelphia: Saunders; Sehgal, A. (2004). Overlap between Whites and Blacks in response to antihypertensive drugs. *Hypertension* 4, 566–572.

ETHNOCULTURAL IMPLICATIONS

Hypertension in Aboriginal Peoples

Hypertension among the Aboriginal peoples exceeds that of all Canadians in all major age and gender groups. Challenges to treatment exist because of limited access to ambulatory care and the reluctance to receive medical treatments. To address this challenge, in June 2008, the Aboriginal Hypertension Management Program (AHMP)

was launched. This program has adapted educational tools to make hypertension treatment more ethnoculturally sensitive and appropriate. The program is being piloted over 18 months in two First Nations communities in Ontario: Manitoulin Island–Aundeck Omni Kaning and Whitefish River First Nation communities.

rates of awareness of treatment and control of hypertension. The results of the survey suggest that Ontario has the highest rate of treatment and control of hypertension in the world. Currently, a national blood pressure survey is under way.

To identify those with hypertension, all adults require ongoing regular assessment of blood pressure. More recent CHEP guidelines include the classification of prehypertension. Those individuals who have prehypertension or

high normal blood pressure (130–139/85–89 mm Hg) are considered at higher risk of developing hypertension. It is estimated that of those who have high normal blood pressure and are overweight, 40% will develop hypertension within 2 years while an additional 20% will develop hypertension within 4 years.

Whereas previous guidelines recommended a stepped-care pharmacological approach to treating the illness, many practitioners believe that this approach

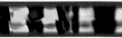

SPECIAL POPULATIONS: THE OLDER ADULT

Hypertension

Hypertension often presents as elevation of systolic blood pressure in the older adult population. Diastolic pressures plateau or decrease in the mid-fifties while systolic pressures increase. Cardiovascular morbidity and mortality are closely correlated to elevations in systolic blood pressure, and control of systolic pressures in the older adult remains a challenge. In 2008, the Hypertension in the Very Elderly Trial (HYVET), a randomized, double-blind, placebo-controlled trial, assessed the benefit-to-risk ratio of treating hypertensive patients aged 80 years and older.

The landmark results showed that treatment with indapamide, a nonthiazide diuretic, with or without perindopril, an angiotensin-converting enzyme (ACE) inhibitor, to achieve a target blood pressure of 150/80 mm Hg was associated with significant reductions in stroke and a 30% reduction in the rate of fatal or nonfatal stroke and heart failure. This study refutes previous claims that aggressive treatment of hypertension in patients over the age of 80 would produce more risks than benefits.

 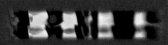

SPECIAL POPULATIONS: CHILDREN AND THE ADOLESCENT

Hypertension

The prevalence of hypertension in children and adolescents is estimated at between 2% and 14% and is increasing because of rising obesity rates. Hypertension in obese children is estimated to be between 11% and 30%. Hypertension in children and adolescents is often secondary to underlying disease or may be an early onset of primary hypertension. The measurement of blood pressure is based on age- and gender-determined parameters. *Hypertension* is defined as blood pressure equal to or greater than the 95th percentile for age, gender, and height on three separate occasions. Blood pressure between the 90th and 95th percentile is considered *prehypertensive*. Secondary causes of hypertension require a full evaluative diagnostic workup. Management with nonpharmacological treatment for primary hypertension

as recommended by the Canadian Hypertension Education Program includes a healthy diet with a decreased intake of dietary salt, saturated fat, and cholesterol, as well as increased consumption of fresh fruits and vegetables, low-fat dairy products, dietary fibre, whole grains, and proteins from plant sources. Regular physical activity should be encouraged to prevent childhood obesity. Non-pharmacological interventions in childhood should be emphasized because of emerging evidence for an early programming effect in the development of hypertension later in life (Koshy, Grisaru, & Midgley, 2008). The use of diuretics, β-blockers, the angiotensin-converting enzyme (ACE) inhibitors, and angiotensin II receptor blockers (ARBs) are effective as pharmacological treatment.

SPECIAL POPULATIONS: WOMEN

Hypertension

Younger women generally have lower systolic blood pressures than do men, whereas after age 50, the rate of blood pressure increases significantly to surpass that of men. The risk of developing hypertension over a woman's lifetime is 86% to 90% compared with 81% to 83% for men. Menopause may contribute to the rise in blood pressure as women get older, based on a number of factors, although the use of estrogen-replacement

therapy appears to have little overall effect on the elevation of blood pressure. Women benefit from the same drug classifications as those used for men in the treatment of hypertension. Because of their teratogenic effect, angiotensin-converting enzyme (ACE) inhibitors and angiotensin II receptor blockers (ARBs) are not used in women intending to become pregnant.

no longer adequately reflects the current range of pharmacological alternatives available or furnishes the type of care dictated by the level of scientific understanding of the disorder. Individualized therapy was proposed as a more appropriate treatment strategy than stepped care because it allows specific patient circumstances to be addressed and pharmacological alternatives to be

considered. In this individualized approach, there is the recognition that some patients may require two or more medications, even as initial therapy, depending on their individual cardiovascular risk factors such as obesity, diabetes, and family history. Health care providers are encouraged to adopt an individualized approach to the planning of drug therapy that takes into consideration

BOX 25-1 2008 CHEP Hypertension Guidelines

The main theme of the 2008 Canadian Hypertension Education Program (CHEP) evidence-informed guidelines, introduced for the accurate measurement of and treatment of hypertension, was the endorsement of home blood pressure monitoring. Detailed patient guidelines include which monitors to purchase as well as advice on how to measure blood pressure accurately. The guidelines continued to emphasize an individualized approach to therapy as a means of addressing specific patient characteristics and needs and identifying pharmacological alternatives. Some of the major points can be summarized as follows:

- Encourage hypertensive patients to use an approved blood pressure–measuring device and to use proper technique to assess blood pressure at home. Blood pressure measured at home is a stronger predictor of cardiovascular events than office-based readings. Home measurement can help confirm the diagnosis of hypertension, improve blood pressure control, reduce the need for medications, help to identify white-coat and masked hypertension, and improve medication adherence in nonadherent patients. An Internet-based toolbox to assist patients in managing hypertension through home blood pressure measurement and lifestyle change can be found at http://www.heartandstroke.ca/bp.
- Adults with high normal blood pressure require annual blood pressure assessment. One in five adult Canadians has high normal blood pressure (130–139/85–89 mm Hg) and up to 60% of them will develop hypertension within 4 years.
- All Canadian adults need to have their blood pressure assessed at all appropriate clinical visits. One in five adult Canadians has hypertension, and for those aged 55 with normal blood pressure, 90% will develop hypertension if they live an average age. All adults require ongoing assessment of blood pressure throughout their lives.
- Optimal management of blood pressure requires assessment of overall cardiovascular risk. Over 90% of hypertensive Canadians have other cardiovascular risks. Identifying and managing these other risks (e.g., unhealthy diet, inactivity, abdominal obesity, dyslipidemia, diabetes) can reduce cardiovascular disease by over 60% in hypertensive patients.

- Lifestyle modifications such as a healthy diet, regular physical activity, moderation in alcohol, reductions in dietary sodium, and, in some patients, stress reduction are effective in reducing blood pressure and cardiovascular risk. Routine simple and brief interventions introduced by the health care provider markedly increase the probability of a patient adhering to lifestyle changes.
- Treat to target. In general, blood pressure should be lowered to less than 140/90 mm Hg and in those with diabetes or chronic kidney disease, to less than 130/80 mm Hg.
- Combinations of therapies (both drug and lifestyle) are generally necessary to achieve target blood pressures. Most patients require more than one antihypertensive drug as well as lifestyle changes to achieve recommended blood pressure targets.
- Monitor patients whose blood pressure is above target regularly and increase the intensity of treatment until the targets are achieved. Regular follow-up along with titration of therapy is required to achieve blood pressure targets.
- Focus on adherence. Nonadherence to therapy is an important cause of poor blood pressure control. Patient adherence to therapy should be assessed on each visit, and interventions to improve adherence should be a part of clinical routine.

The key message of the 2007 CHEP guidelines was the importance of assessing blood pressure in all Canadian adults and to regularly assess blood pressure in those with high normal values. In addition, the 2007 recommendations supported increasing evidence that hypertension can be prevented through education to reduce the intake of dietary sodium. In 2008, CHEP emphasized the necessity for all appropriate adult Canadians with hypertension to practise home blood pressure monitoring. In this theme it was recognized that greater patient involvement in care potentially improves treatment and control.

Source: Canadian Hypertension Education Program. (2008). *2008 key messages.* Retrieved November 22, 2008, from http://hypertension.ca/chep/recommendations/summaries/key-messages/. Reproduced by permission of Canadian Hypertension Education Program (2008).

BOX 25-2 2009 CHEP Hypertension Guidelines

In 2009, CHEP marks its 10th anniversary in updating recommendations for the management of hypertension. Recommendations include treating blood pressure to less than 140/90 mm Hg in most patients. One of the primary themes for 2009 is managing hypertension in the patient with diabetes, with the focus "on reducing death and cardiovascular disease in people with diabetes by encouraging health care professionals to ensure their patients' blood pressure is maintained less than 130/80 mm Hg" (CHEP, 2009). Lifestyle modification combined with three, four, or more drugs may be necessary for blood pressure control in individuals with diabetes. Management gaps include suboptimal use of pharmacotherapy in younger

hypertensive people with multiple cardiovascular risk factors and a low rate of useful lifestyle changes after a hypertension diagnosis. In 2009, CHEP specifically recommended not to combine an ACE inhibitor with an angiotensin receptor blocker in people with uncomplicated hypertension, diabetes (without micro- or overt albuminuria), chronic kidney disease (without proteinuria), or ischemic heart disease (without heart failure).

Source: Canadian Hypertension Education Program. (2009). *2009 Canadian hypertension education program recommendations: The short clinical summary—an annual update.* Retrieved September 21, 2009, from http://hypertension.ca/chep/wp-content/uploads/2009/07/2009-short-clinical-summary-final-2.pdf

the demographic concerns for the patient, the presence of concomitant diseases, the use of concurrent therapies, and the patient's quality of life.

The classification scheme used to categorize individual cases of hypertension has been simplified to the following four stages based on blood pressure measurements: normal, prehypertension, stage 1 hypertension, and stage 2 hypertension. This revised classification scheme is presented in detail in Table 25-1.

Hypertension can also be defined by its cause. When the specific cause of hypertension is unknown, it may be called **essential, idiopathic**, or *primary* **hypertension.** About 90% of the cases of hypertension are of this type. Secondary hypertension makes up the other 10%. **Secondary hypertension** is most commonly the result of another disease such as pheochromocytoma (adrenal tumour), pre-eclampsia (a pregnancy complication involving acute hypertension, among other symptoms), or renal artery disease. It may also result from the use of certain medications. If the cause of secondary hypertension can be eliminated, the blood pressure usually returns to normal.

Blood pressure is determined by the product of cardiac output and systemic vascular resistance (SVR). **Cardiac output** is the amount of blood that is ejected from the left ventricle and is measured in litres per minute. Normal cardiac output is 4 to 8 L/min. SVR is the force (resistance) the left ventricle has to overcome to eject its volume of blood. Numerous factors interact to regulate these two major variables and keep the blood pressure within normal limits. These are illustrated in Figure 25-1. These are the same factors that can cause high blood pressure and are the targets of action of many of the antihypertensive drugs.

Another form of hypertension is referred to as *masked hypertension*. This occurs when a patient's office blood pressure is less than 140/90 mm Hg but the ambulatory or home blood pressure readings are in the hypertensive range. According to several recent studies, cardiovascular risk is similar between those with masked hypertension and those with sustained hypertension. The prevalence of masked hypertension in Canada may be approximately 8%. *White-coat hypertension* is defined as high blood pressure occurring in a medical setting despite normal ambulatory pressure and is associated with anxiety and nervousness.

ANTIHYPERTENSIVE DRUGS

As previously mentioned, the drug therapy for hypertension should be individualized to accommodate or complement the specific needs or concerns of the patient. Important considerations in planning drug therapy are

TABLE 25-1

Classification and Management of Blood Pressure

Blood Pressure Measurements and Classification				Initial Drug Therapy	
BP Classification	Target SBP* (mm Hg)	Target DBP* (mm Hg)	Lifestyle Modification	Without Compelling Indications[†]	With Compelling Indications[†]
Optimum	Less than 120	and less than 80	Awareness		
Normal	120–129	80–89	Awareness		
High normal or prehypertension	130–139	or 85–89	Yes	No antihypertensive drug indicated; annual follow-up	Drug(s) for compelling indications[‡]
Stage 1 hypertension	140–159	or 90–99	Yes	Thiazide-type diuretics for most; may consider ACE inhibitor, ARB, BB, CCB, or combination	Drug(s) for compelling indications; other antihypertensive drugs (diuretic, ACE inhibitor, ARB, BB, CCB) prn
Stage 2 hypertension	160 or higher	or 100 or higher	Yes	Two-drug combination for most[§] (usually thiazide-type diuretic and ACE inhibitor, ARB, BB, or CCB).	

ACE, angiotensin-converting enzyme; *ARB*, angiotensin II receptor blocker; *BB*, β-adrenergic blocker; *BP*, blood pressure; *CCB*, calcium channel blocker; *DBP*, diastolic blood pressure; *SBP*, systolic blood pressure.

*Treatment determined by highest BP category.

[†]Compelling indications include heart failure, previous myocardial infarction, high cardiovascular risk, diabetes mellitus, chronic kidney disease, and previous stroke.

[‡]Treat patients with chronic kidney disease or diabetes to BP goal of less than 130/80 mm Hg.

[§]Initial combined therapy should be used cautiously in those at risk for orthostatic hypotension.

Source: Canadian Hypertension Education Program. (2007). *2007 CHEP recommendations for the management of hypertension.* Retrieved September 17, 2009, from http://www.hypertension.ca/chep/wp-content/uploads/2007/10/chep-2007-spiral-mar16.pdf; U.S. Department of Health and Human Services. (2003). *Seventh report of the Joint National Committee on prevention, detection, evaluation, and treatment of high blood pressure (JNC-7).* Washington, DC: National Institutes of Health.

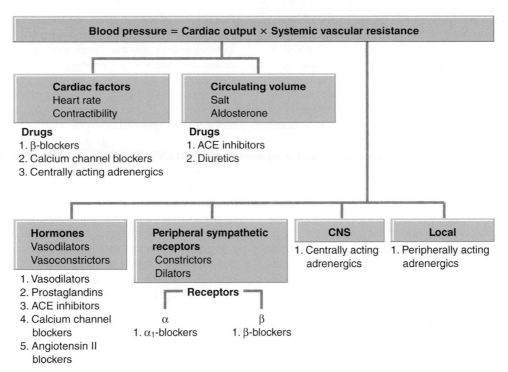

FIG. 25-1 Normal regulation of blood pressure and corresponding mechanisms. *ACE*, angiotensin-converting enzyme; *CNS*, central nervous system.

whether the patient has concomitant medical problems and what the impact of drug therapy on the patient's quality of life will be. For example, one very common adverse effect of almost any antihypertensive drug is sexual dysfunction in male patients, which is the most common reason for nonadherence to drug therapy. Demographic factors, ethnocultural implications, the ease of medication administration, (e.g., a once-a-day dosing schedule or transdermal administration), and cost are other important considerations.

There are seven main categories of pharmacological drugs: diuretics, adrenergic drugs, vasodilators, angiotensin-converting enzyme (ACE) inhibitors, angiotensin II receptor blockers (ARBs), calcium channel blockers (CCBs), and vasodilators. Because all antihypertensive drugs (with the exception of diuretics) have some vasodilatory action, those in the last category are also called *direct vasodilators* to differentiate them. Drugs in these classes are used either alone or in combination. The categories and subcategories of antihypertensive drugs are listed in Box 25-3. The diuretics are discussed in detail in Chapter 26.

REVIEW OF AUTONOMIC NEUROTRANSMISSION

The stimulation of the two divisions of the autonomic nervous system (ANS), the parasympathetic (PSNS) and sympathetic (SNS) nervous systems, is controlled by the neurotransmitters acetylcholine (ACh) and norepinephrine. The receptors for both divisions of the ANS are located throughout the body in a variety of tissues.

BOX 25-3

Categories and Subcategories of Antihypertensive Drugs

Adrenergic Drugs
- Centrally and peripherally acting adrenergic neuron blockers
- Centrally acting α_2-receptor agonists
- Peripherally acting α_1-receptor blockers
- Peripherally acting β-receptor blockers (β-blockers)
- Cardioselective (β_1-receptor blockers)
- Nonselective (β_1- and β_2-receptor blockers)
- Peripherally acting dual α_1- and β-receptor blockers

Angiotensin-Converting Enzyme Inhibitors

Angiotensin II Receptor Blockers

Calcium Channel Blockers
- Benzothiazepines
- Dihydropyridines
- Phenylalkylamines

Diuretics
- Loop diuretics
- Potassium-sparing diuretics
- Thiazides and thiazide-like diuretics

Renin Inhibitors

Vasodilators
- Act directly on vascular smooth muscle cells, *not* through α- or β-receptors

ANS physiology can be reviewed in greater detail in the introductory sections of Chapters 18 through 21. The preganglionic receptor for ACh in both the SNS and PSNS is the **nicotinic receptor**. It gets its name from the fact that the administration of the ganglionic stimulant nicotine first revealed its existence. In both systems, this receptor is located between the preganglionic and postganglionic fibres. The receptor located between the postganglionic fibre and the effector cells (i.e., the postganglionic receptor) is called the muscarinic or cholinergic receptor in the PSNS and the adrenergic or noradrenergic receptor (i.e., α- or β-receptor) in the SNS. Physiological activity at muscarinic receptors is stimulated by ACh and cholinergic agonist drugs (Chapter 20) and is inhibited by cholinergic antagonists (anticholinergic drugs, Chapter 21). Similarly, physiological activity at adrenergic receptors is stimulated by norepinephrine and epinephrine and adrenergic agonist drugs (Chapter 18) and inhibited by antiadrenergic drugs (adrenergic blockers, i.e., α- or β-receptor blockers; Chapter 19). Figure 25-2 shows how these receptors are arranged in both the PSNS and SNS and indicates their corresponding neurotransmitters.

ADRENERGIC DRUGS

Adrenergic drugs are a large group of antihypertensive drugs, as listed in Box 25-3. The β-blockers and combined α-β-blockers have been discussed in detail in Chapter 19. The adrenergic drugs discussed here exert their antihypertensive action at different sites.

Mechanism of Action and Drug Effects

Five specific drug subcategories are included in the adrenergic antihypertensive drugs, as indicated in Box 25-3. Each of these subcategories of drugs can be described as having central action (in the brain) or peripheral action (at the heart and blood vessels). These drugs include the adrenergic neuron blockers (central and peripheral), the α₂-receptor agonists (central), the α₁-receptor blockers (peripheral), the β-receptor blockers (peripheral), and the combination α₁- and β-receptor blockers (peripheral).

The centrally acting α₂-adrenergic drugs clonidine and methyldopa act by modifying the function of the SNS. Because SNS stimulation leads to an increased heart rate and force of contraction, the constriction of blood vessels, and the release of renin from the kidney, the result is hypertension. The **centrally acting adrenergic drugs** act by stimulating the α₂-adrenergic receptors in the brain. The α₂-adrenergic receptors are unique in that receptor stimulation actually reduces sympathetic outflow, in this case from the central nervous system (CNS). The resulting lack of norepinephrine production reduces blood pressure. This stimulation of the α₂-adrenergic receptors also affects the kidneys, reducing the activity of renin. Renin is the hormone and enzyme that converts the protein precursor angiotensinogen to the protein angiotensin I (AI), the precursor of angiotensin II (AII), a potent vasoconstrictor that raises blood pressure.

In the periphery, the **α₁-blockers** doxazosin, prazosin, and terazosin also modify the function of the SNS. However, they do so by blocking the α₁-adrenergic receptors, which, when stimulated by circulating norepinephrine, produce increased blood pressure. Consequently, when these receptors are blocked, blood pressure is decreased. The drug effects of the α₁-blockers are primarily related to their ability to dilate arteries and veins, which reduces peripheral vascular resistance and subsequently decreases

TARGET <140 mm Hg systolic and <90 mm Hg diastolic

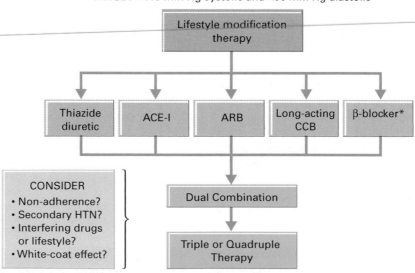

*Not indicated as first-line therapy for patients over 60

FIG. 25-2 Hypertension treatment algorithm.

blood pressure. This produces a marked decrease in the systemic and pulmonary venous pressures and an increase in cardiac output. The α_1-blockers also increase urinary flow rates and decrease outflow obstruction by preventing smooth muscle contractions in the bladder neck and urethra. This can be beneficial in cases of benign prostatic hypertrophy (BPH; discussed later in this chapter).

The β-blockers also act in the periphery and include propranolol and atenolol as well as several other drugs. These drugs are discussed in more detail in Chapter 23 because they also have antidysrhythmic properties. Their antihypertensive effects are related to their reduction of the heart rate through β_1-receptor blockade. Furthermore,

β-blockers cause a reduction in the secretion of the hormone *renin* (see ACE inhibitors section), which, in turn, reduces both AII-mediated vasoconstriction and aldosterone-mediated volume expansion. Long-term use of β-blockers reduces peripheral vascular resistance.

Two dual-action α_1- and β-receptor blockers, which also act in the periphery at the heart and blood vessels, are currently available. These two drugs are labetalol and the newer drug carvedilol. These drugs have the dual antihypertensive effects of reduction in heart rate (β_1-receptor blockade) and vasodilation (α_1-receptor blockade). Figure 25-3 illustrates the site and mechanism of action for the antihypertensive drugs.

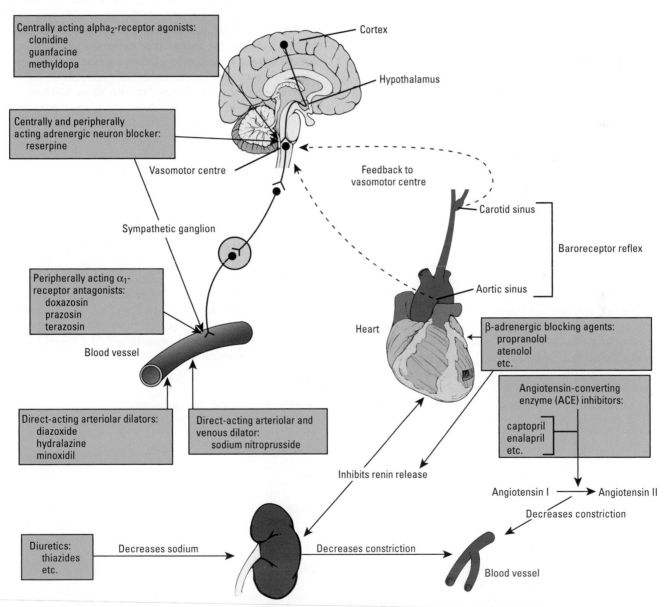

FIG. 25-3 Site and mechanism of action for the antihypertensive drugs. Note: Reserpine is not available in Canada. (Source: U.S. Department of Health and Human Services. (1997). The sixth report of the Joint National Committee on detection, evaluation, and treatment of high blood pressure (JNC-VI). Washington, DC: National Institutes of Health. In S. M. Lewis, M. M. Heitkemper, & S. R. Dirksen (Eds.). (2003). *Medical-surgical nursing: Assessment and management of clinical problems* (6th ed.). St. Louis, MO: Mosby.)

Indications

All of the drugs mentioned are used primarily for the treatment of hypertension, either alone or in combination with other antihypertensive drugs. Various forms of glaucoma may also respond to treatment with some of these drugs. Clonidine has several unlabelled uses (that is, uses not approved by Health Canada but still common), including prophylaxis for migraine headaches and the treatment of severe dysmenorrhea or menopausal flushing. It is also useful in managing withdrawal symptoms in persons with opioid, nicotine, or alcohol dependency. The α_1-blockers doxazosin, prazosin, and terazosin have been used to relieve the symptoms associated with BPH. They have also proven to be effective in the management of severe heart failure when used with cardiac glycosides (Chapter 22) and diuretics (Chapter 26).

Contraindications

Contraindications to the use of the adrenergic antihypertensive drugs include known drug allergy and may also include acute heart failure, concurrent use of monoamine oxidase inhibitors (Chapter 16), severe depression, peptic ulcer, colitis, and severe liver or kidney disease. Asthma may also be a contraindication to the use of any non-cardioselective β-blocker (e.g., carvedilol). As mentioned in Chapter 22, vasodilating drugs may also be contraindicated in cases of heart failure that occur secondary to diastolic dysfunction.

Adverse Effects

As with all drug classes, adrenergic drugs can cause adverse effects. The most common adverse effects of adrenergic drugs include postural and postexercise hypotension, dry mouth, drowsiness, sedation, dizziness, edema, constipation, and sexual dysfunction (e.g., erectile dysfunction). Other effects include headaches, sleep disturbances, nausea, rash, peripheral pooling of blood, and heart disturbances such as palpitations. There is also a high incidence of **orthostatic hypotension** (a sudden drop in blood pressure during changes in position) in patients taking adrenergic drugs. This sudden drop in blood pressure can lead to a situation known as *first-dose syncope,* in which the hypotensive effect is severe enough to cause the patient to lose consciousness with the first dose of medication.

In addition, the abrupt discontinuation of the centrally acting α_2-receptor blockers can result in rebound hypertension. This effect may occur with other antihypertensive drug classes as well. Nonselective drugs are more commonly associated with bronchoconstriction (because of unrestrained parasympathetic tone) as well as metabolic inhibition of glycogenolysis in the liver, which can lead to hypoglycemia. However, hyperglycemic episodes are also among the adverse effects reported for this drug class.

Any change in the dosing regimen for cardiovascular medications should be undertaken gradually and with appropriate patient monitoring and follow-up. Although the same is true for most other classes of medications, abrupt dosage changes of cardiovascular medications, either up or down, can be especially hazardous for the patient. Some of these drugs can also cause disruptions in blood count as well as in serum electrolyte levels and kidney function. Periodic monitoring of white blood cell count, serum potassium and sodium levels (see also Evidence-Informed Practice), and urinary protein levels is recommended.

Interactions

Adrenergic drugs interact primarily with CNS depressants such as alcohol, benzodiazepines, and opioids. The additive effects of these combinations of drugs increase CNS depression. Terazosin can produce a reduced hematocrit reading. Other drug interactions that can occur with selected adrenergic drugs are summarized in Table 25-2. This list is merely representative and is not exhaustive. The nurse should always keep a drug information handbook available to check in cases in which a specific drug interaction is suspected.

Dosages

For information on the dosages of selected adrenergic antihypertensive drugs, see the Dosages table on p. 470.

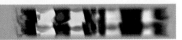

EVIDENCE-INFORMED PRACTICE

Benefits of Reduced Dietary Sodium Additives in Hypertension Management

Background
Based on data from clinical trials, this Canadian study investigated the significance of excess consumption of dietary sodium (salt) to the development of hypertension in Canadians.

Type of Evidence
The researchers used data from the 2004 Canadian Community Health Survey.

Results of Study
More dietary sodium than daily recommendations was consumed by 85% of Canadian men and 60% of Canadian women aged 19 to 70. Salt added to food was not included in these estimations. The researchers estimated that one million Canadians have hypertension because of an excessive intake of dietary sodium, resulting in direct health care costs of over 430 million dollars per year. Reducing sodium intake by 1840 mg/day would lead to a decrease in systolic blood pressure by 5.06 mm Hg and in diastolic blood pressure by 2.7 mm Hg.

Link of Evidence to Nursing Practice
Hypertension is the leading risk factor for mortality in Canada and worldwide. Health Canada recommends a daily intake of 1200 to 1500 mg of sodium for a healthy adult. According to Statistics Canada, the average Canadian has a daily sodium intake of over 3100 mg (equivalent to $1\frac{1}{2}$ teaspoons), 77% of which is found primarily in processed foods. Foods that make up 19% of the sodium in individuals' diets are pizzas, hamburgers, hotdogs, and sandwiches, with soups accounting for 7%, and pasta, 6%. Estimates are that one quarter of Canadian adults (approximately five million) have hypertension, with more than 9 in 10 Canadians expected to develop high blood pressure if they have an average lifespan of about 80 years. While Health Canada's new Eating Well with Canada's Food Guide recommends that Canadians reduce their sodium intake, the World Health Organization (WHO) advocates a regulated approach. The WHO suggests that governmental policies restricting the amount of sodium added to food by food industries is more effective. Nurses can play a significant role in educating their patients about hypertension and how to reduce sodium intake. Reducing dietary sodium intake within the context of a healthy diet can substantially reduce the incidence of hypertension among Canadians who have normal blood pressure. Therefore, a population health approach to reducing dietary sodium is an appropriate strategy.

The 2008 and 2009 CHEP recommendations for lifestyle modifications to prevent and treat hypertension include the following:
- Restrict dietary sodium intake to less than 100 mmol/day (and 65 mmol/day to 100 mmol/day in hypertensive patients). NOTE: The sodium and salt content terminology is confusing. Conversion: 2300 mg sodium is approximately one teaspoon of salt (sodium chloride), 100 mmol of sodium or salt, or 5.8 g (5800 mg) of salt (NaCl).
- Perform 30 to 60 minutes of aerobic exercise, 4 to 7 days per week.
- Maintain a healthy body weight (body mass index [BMI] 18.5 kg/m^2 to 24.9 kg/m^2) and waist circumference (smaller than 102 cm for men and smaller than 88 cm for women).
- Limit alcohol consumption to no more than 14 units per week in men or nine units per week in women.
- Follow a diet that is reduced in saturated fat and cholesterol, and one that emphasizes fruits, vegetables, and low-fat dairy products, dietary and soluble fibre, whole grains, and protein from plant sources.
- Consider stress management in selected individuals with hypertension.

Based on Canadian Hypertension Education Program. (2008). *2008 key messages.* Retrieved November 22, 2008, from http://hypertension.ca/chep/recommendations/summaries/key-messages/; Joffres, M. R., Campbell, N. R. C., Manns, B., &Tu, K. (2007). Estimate of the benefits of a population-based reduction in dietary sodium additives on hypertension and its related health care costs in Canada. *Canadian Journal of Cardiology, 23*(6), 437–443.

TABLE 25-2

Adrenergic Drugs: Drug Interactions

Drug	Interacts With	Mechanism	Result
clonidine	Opioids, sedatives, hypnotics, anaesthetics, alcohol	Additive	Increased CNS depression
	TCAs, MAOIs, appetite suppressants, amphetamines	Opposing actions	Decreased hypotensive effects
	Diuretics, nitrates, other antihypertensive drugs	Additive	Increased hypotensive effects
	β-blockers, cardiac glycosides	Additive	May potentiate bradycardia and increase the rebound hypertension in clonidine withdrawal
prazosin	Diuretics, other hypotensive drugs	Additive	Increased hypotension
	indomethacin	Opposing effects	Decreased hypotensive effect
	verapamil	Increased serum prazosin levels	Increased hypotension

CNS, central nervous system; *MAOIs,* monoamine oxidase inhibitors; *TCAs,* tricyclic antidepressants.

DRUG PROFILES

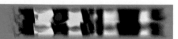

α_2-ADRENERGIC RECEPTOR STIMULATORS (AGONISTS)

Of the available α_2-receptor agonists, clonidine and methyldopa, clonidine is by far the most commonly used and the prototype drug for this drug class. Methyldopa is also used in the treatment of hypertension and is the drug of choice for treating hypertension in pregnancy. However, these drugs are not typically prescribed as first-line antihypertensive drugs because their use is associated with a high incidence of adverse effects such as orthostatic hypotension, fatigue, and dizziness. They may be used as adjunct drugs in the treatment of hypertension after other drugs have failed or may be used in conjunction with other antihypertensives such as diuretics.

▶▶ clonidine hydrochloride

Clonidine hydrochloride (Catapres, Dixarit) is used primarily for its ability to decrease blood pressure. It is used alone or in combination with thiazide diuretics. Clonidine is used in patients in whom treatment with a diuretic or β-blocker was ineffective or had unacceptable adverse effects. Clonidine has a better safety profile than the other centrally acting adrenergics and has the advantage of being available in several dosage formulations, including both topical and oral preparations. Clonidine should not be discontinued abruptly because of severe rebound hypertension. Its use is contraindicated in patients who have shown hypersensitivity reactions to it. See the Dosages table below for recommended dosages.

PHARMACOKINETICS

Half-Life	Onset	Peak	Duration
12–16 hr	30–60 min	3–5 hr	8 hr

α_1-BLOCKERS

The α_1-blockers include doxazosin mesylate (Cardura), prazosin hydrochloride (Minipress), tamsulosin hydrochloride (Flomax), and terazosin hydrochloride (Hytrin). They are the newest of the adrenergics and have the best safety and efficacy profiles, but they are not without adverse effects. Their use is contraindicated in patients who have shown a hypersensitivity to them. They are available only as oral preparations. Tamsulosin is not used to manage blood pressure but is indicated solely for symptomatic management of BPH. This use is described further in Chapter 35 on men's health drugs.

prazosin hydrochloride

Prazosin hydrochloride (Minipress) is the oldest of the α_1-blockers and the prototype for this drug class. Prazosin reduces both peripheral vascular resistance and blood pressure through dilation of both arterial and venous blood vessels. It is beneficial in the treatment of hypertension, the relief of symptoms of obstructive BPH, and as an adjunct to cardiac glycosides and diuretics in the treatment of severe heart failure. Recommended dosages are given in the Dosages table below.

PHARMACOKINETICS

Half-Life	Onset	Peak	Duration
2–3 hr	2 hr	3 hr	10 hr

DUAL-ACTION α_1-AND β-RECEPTOR BLOCKERS

carvedilol

Carvedilol, a newer drug, was approved by Health Canada in 1996. Its use in the ambulatory care setting is growing, and it seems to be well tolerated by most patients. In addition to hypertension, it is also indicated for mild, moderate, or severe heart failure in conjunction with digoxin, diuretics, and ACE inhibitors. Its contraindications include known drug allergy, cardiogenic shock, severe bradycardia or decompensated heart failure, primary obstructive valve disease, liver impairment, bronchospastic conditions such as asthma, and heart problems involving the conduction system. Dosage information appears in the Dosages table below.

PHARMACOKINETICS

Half-Life	Onset	Peak	Duration
7–10 hr	1–2 hr	2–3 hr	Unknown

DOSAGES   Selected Antihypertensive Drugs: Adrenergic Agonists and Antagonists

Drug (Pregnancy Category)	Pharmacological Class	Usual Dosage Range	Indications
carvedilol (C)	Peripherally acting α_1-, β_1-, and b_2-receptor antagonist (blocker)	*Adult* PO: 3.125 to 25 mg bid	Hypertension (primary indication is heart failure)
▶▶clonidine hydrochloride (Catapres, Dixarit) (C)	Centrally acting α_2-receptor agonist	*Adult* PO: Initial dose 0.1 mg/day bid; may titrate up to a maximum of 0.6 mg/day, divided bid	Hypertension (may have other unlabelled uses including psychiatric, cardiovascular, and gastrointestinal problems)
prazosin hydrochloride (Minipress) (C)	Peripherally acting α_1-receptor antagonist	*Adult* PO: Initial dose 0.5 mg at bedtime; then 0.5 mg bid–tid; titrate up to maximum of 20 mg/day	Hypertension

ANGIOTENSIN-CONVERTING ENZYME INHIBITORS

The ACE inhibitors are a large group of antihypertensive drugs. There are currently 10 ACE inhibitors available for clinical use, in addition to various combination drug products in which a thiazide diuretic or a CCB is combined with an ACE inhibitor. The available ACE inhibitors are captopril (Capoten), benazepril hydrochloride (Lotensin), cilazapril (Inhibace), enalapril sodium (Vasotec), fosinopril sodium (Monopril), lisinopril (Prinvil, Zestril), perindopril erbumine (Coversyl), quinapril hydrochloride (Accupril), ramipril (Altace), and trandolapril (Mavik). These drugs are safe and effective and are often used as the first-line drugs in the treatment of both heart failure and hypertension. Some of the distinguishing characteristics of the drugs that make up this large class of antihypertensives are summarized in Table 25-3. The ACE inhibitors as a class are similar and differ in only a few of their chemical properties, but there are some significant differences among them in their clinical properties. Knowing these differences can help the practitioner select the proper drug for a particular patient.

Captopril has the shortest half-life and therefore must be dosed more frequently than any of the other ACE inhibitors. This may be an important drawback to its use in a patient who has a history of nonadherence with medication therapy. On the other hand, it may be best to start with a drug that has a short half-life in a patient who is still critically ill and may not tolerate medications well, so that if problems arise they will be short-lived. Both captopril and enalapril can be dosed multiple times a day.

Captopril and lisinopril are the only two ACE inhibitors that are not prodrugs. A **prodrug** is a drug that is inactive in its administered form and must be biotransformed in the liver to its active form in order to be effective. This characteristic of captopril and lisinopril is an important advantage in treating a patient with liver dysfunction; because all of the other ACE inhibitors are prodrugs, their transformation to active form in such patients tends to be hindered.

Enalapril is the only ACE inhibitor available in a parenteral preparation. All other drugs are available only in oral formulations. All of the newer ACE inhibitors, such as benazepril, fosinopril, lisinopril, quinapril, and ramipril, have long half-lives and long durations of action, which allows them to be given once a day. This is particularly beneficial for a patient who is taking many other medications and may have difficulty keeping track of the dosing schedules for each one. A once-a-day medication regimen promotes better patient adherence.

All ACE inhibitors have detrimental effects on the unborn fetus and neonate. They are classified as pregnancy category C drugs for women in their first trimester and as pregnancy category D drugs for women in their second or third trimester. ACE inhibitors should be used in pregnant women only if there are no safer alternatives. Fetal and neonatal morbidity and mortality have been reported in at least 50 women who were receiving ACE inhibitors during their pregnancies.

Many of the ACE inhibitors are combined with either a diuretic or a CCB. The advantages of such combination products are convenience and improved patient adherence. Often an individual with hypertension or heart failure must take many medications, including an ACE inhibitor, to control hypertension. Use of combination products leads to greater patient adherence because fewer medications need to be taken. Examples of combination ACE inhibitor–CCB products available currently in Canada are perinopril and indapamide (Coversyl Plus LD) and trandolapril and verapamil (Tarka).

Mechanism of Action and Drug Effects

As is often the case with pharmaceutical innovations, the development of the ACE inhibitors was spurred by the discovery of an animal substance found to have beneficial effects in humans. This particular animal substance was the venom of the South American viper, which was found to inhibit kininase activity. Kininase is an enzyme that normally breaks down bradykinin, a potent vasodilator in the human body.

TABLE 25-3

ACE Inhibitors: Distinguishing Characteristics

Generic Name	Trade Name	Combination With Hydrochlorothiazide	Interval	Route	Prodrug
benazepril hydrochloride	Lotensin	None	Once a day	PO	Yes
captopril	Capoten	None	Multiple	PO	No
cilazapril	Inhibace	Inhibace Plus	Once a day	PO	Yes
enalapril sodium	Vasotec	Vaseretic	Multiple	PO/IV	Yes
fosinopril sodium	Monopril	None	Once a day	PO	Yes
lisinopril	Prinvil,	Prinzide 12.5 and 25	Once a day	PO	No
	Zestril	Zestoretic 12.5 and 25	Once a day	PO	No
perindopril erbumine	Coversyl	None	Once a day	PO	Yes
quinapril hydrochloride	Accupril	Accuretic	Once a day	PO	Yes
ramipril	Altace	None	Once to twice daily	PO	Yes
trandolapril	Mavik	None	Once a day	PO	Yes

ACE, angiotensin-converting enzyme; *IV*, intravenous; *PO*, oral.

The ACE inhibitors have several beneficial cardiovascular effects. As their name implies, they inhibit the angiotensin-converting enzyme, which is responsible for converting angiotensin I (AI) to angiotensin II (AII). AII is a potent vasoconstrictor and induces aldosterone secretion by the adrenal glands. Aldosterone stimulates sodium and water resorption, which can raise blood pressure. Together, these processes are referred to as the renin–angiotensin–aldosterone system.

The primary effects of the ACE inhibitors are cardiovascular and renal. Their cardiovascular effects are due to their ability to reduce blood pressure by decreasing systemic vascular resistance (SVR); they prevent the breakdown of the vasodilating substance bradykinin and substance P (another potent vasodilator), thus preventing the formation of AII. These combined effects decrease afterload, or the resistance against which the left ventricle must pump to eject its volume of blood during contraction. The ACE inhibitors are beneficial in the treatment of heart failure because they prevent sodium and water resorption by inhibiting aldosterone secretion. This causes diuresis, which decreases blood volume and return to the heart. This process, in turn, decreases preload, or the left ventricular end-diastolic volume, and consequently the work required of the heart.

Indications

The therapeutic effects of the ACE inhibitors are related to their potent cardiovascular effects. They are excellent antihypertensives and adjunctive drugs for the treatment of heart failure. They may be used alone or in combination with other drugs such as diuretics in the treatment of hypertension or heart failure.

The beneficial hemodynamic effects of the ACE inhibitors have been studied extensively. Because of their ability to decrease SVR (a measure of afterload) and preload, ACE inhibitors can stop the progression of left ventricular hypertrophy, which is sometimes seen after a myocardial infarction (MI), a pathological process known as ventricular remodelling. The ability of ACE inhibitors to prevent ventricular remodelling is termed a cardioprotective effect. ACE inhibitors have been shown to decrease morbidity and mortality rates in patients with heart failure. They should be considered the drugs of choice for hypertensive patients with heart failure. ACE inhibitors have also been shown to have a protective effect on the kidneys because they reduce glomerular filtration pressure. This is one reason why they are among the cardiovascular drugs of choice for diabetic patients.

The therapeutic effects of the ACE inhibitors are listed in Table 25-4, which lists the body substances on which ACE inhibitors act and the resulting beneficial hemodynamic effects.

Contraindications

Contraindications to the use of ACE inhibitors include known drug allergy, especially a previous reaction of angioedema (laryngeal swelling; see description under Adverse Effects) to an ACE inhibitor. Patients with a baseline potassium of 5.0 mmol/L or higher may not be suitable candidates for ACE inhibitor therapy because these drugs can promote hyperkalemia. All ACE inhibitors are contraindicated in lactating women, in children, and in patients with bilateral renal artery stenosis.

Adverse Effects

Major CNS effects of the ACE inhibitors include fatigue, dizziness, mood changes, and headaches. A characteristic dry, nonproductive cough is reversible with discontinuation of the therapy. A first-dose hypotensive effect can cause a significant decline in blood pressure. Other adverse effects include loss of taste, proteinuria, hyperkalemia, rash, pruritus, anemia, neutropenia, thrombocytosis, and agranulocytosis. In patients with severe heart failure whose kidney function may depend on the activity of the renin–angiotensin–aldosterone system, treatment with ACE inhibitors may cause acute kidney failure. ACE inhibitors tend to promote potassium resorption in the kidney, even though they also promote sodium excretion because of their reduction of aldosterone secretion. For this reason, serum potassium levels should be monitored regularly. This is particularly important when there is concurrent therapy with potassium-sparing diuretics, although many patients tolerate both types of drug therapy with no major problems. One rare, but potentially fatal, adverse effect is *angioedema*, a strong vascular reaction involving inflammation of submucosal tissues, which can progress to anaphylaxis.

Toxicity and Management of Overdose

The most pronounced symptom of an overdose of an ACE inhibitor is hypotension. Treatment is symptomatic

TABLE 25-4			
ACE Inhibitors: Therapeutic Effects			
Body Substance	**Effect in Body**	**ACE Inhibitor Action**	**Resulting Hemodynamic Effect**
Aldosterone	Causes sodium and water retention	Prevents its secretion	Diuresis = ↓ plasma volume = ↓ filling pressures or ↓ preload
Angiotensin II	Potent vasoconstrictor	Prevents its formation	↓ SVR = ↓ afterload
Bradykinin	Potent vasodilator	Prevents its breakdown	↓ SVR = ↓ afterload

ACE, angiotensin-converting enzyme; ↓, decreased; *SVR*, systemic vascular resistance.

and supportive and includes the administration of intravenous fluids to expand the blood volume. Hemodialysis is effective for the removal of captopril, enalapril, lisinopril, and perindopril.

Interactions

Nonsteroidal anti-inflammatory drugs can reduce the antihypertensive effect of ACE inhibitors. Concurrent use of ACE inhibitors and other antihypertensives or diuretics can have hypotensive effects. Giving lithium and ACE inhibitors together can result in lithium toxicity. Potassium supplements and potassium-sparing diuretics, when administered with ACE inhibitors, may result in hyperkalemia. As noted earlier, monitoring of serum potassium becomes especially important in these cases. Acetone may be falsely detected in the urine of patients taking captopril.

Dosages

For information on the dosages for selected ACE inhibitors, see the Dosages table below.

 DRUG PROFILES

ACE INHIBITORS

▸▸ **captopril**

Captopril (Capoten) was the first ACE inhibitor to become available and is considered the prototypical drug for the class. Several large multicentre studies have shown its clinical efficacy in minimizing or preventing the left ventricular dilation and dysfunction (also called ventricular remodelling) that can arise in the acute period after an MI and consequently improving the patient's chances of survival. It can also reduce the risk of heart failure in these patients and thus the need for subsequent hospitalizations for the treatment of heart failure. Because it has the shortest half-life of all of the currently available ACE inhibitors, captopril is an excellent drug for hospitalized patients who are in a fragile condition but require afterload and preload reduction to decrease the workload of a failing heart. A long-acting drug may reduce these hemodynamic variables significantly and have lingering effects for which it may be difficult to compensate acutely. Recommended dosages are given in the Dosages table below.

PHARMACOKINETICS

Half-Life	Onset	Peak	Duration
< 2 hr	15 min	1–2 hr	2–6 hr

enalapril sodium

Enalapril sodium (Vasotec) is the only currently available ACE inhibitor available in both oral and parenteral preparations. The parenteral formulation (enalaprilat) is an active drug. It offers the hemodynamic benefit of inhibiting ACE activity in an acutely ill patient who cannot tolerate oral medications. Although its half-life is slightly longer than that of captopril, it may in some instances still have to be given twice a day. The oral form of enalapril differs from captopril in that it is a prodrug and the patient must have a functioning liver for the drug to be converted into its active form. As with captopril, it has been shown in many large studies to improve a patient's chances of survival after an MI and to reduce the incidence of heart failure and thus the need for subsequent hospitalizations for the treatment of heart failure. Recommended dosages are given in the Dosages table below.

PHARMACOKINETICS*

Half-Life	Onset	Peak	Duration
PO: < 2 hr	PO: 1 hr	PO: 4–6 hr	PO: 12–24 hr

*For oral enalapril.

DOSAGES Selected Antihypertensive Drugs: ACE Inhibitors and Angiotensin II Receptor Blockers

Drug (Pregnancy Category)	Pharmacological Class	Usual Dosage Range	Indications
▸▸ captopril (Capoten) (C, first trimester; D, second and third trimesters)	ACE inhibitor	*Adult* PO: 25–150 mg bid–tid	Hypertension, heart failure
enalapril sodium (Vasotec, Vaseretic*) (C, first trimester; D, second and third trimesters)	ACE inhibitor	*Children (less than 16 years)* PO: 0.08 mg/kg (up to 5 mg) once daily	Hypertension
		Adult PO: 10–40 mg/day as a single dose or in 2 divided doses	Hypertension
		PO: 5–20 mg/day as a single or divided dose with digoxin and diuretic; max 40 mg/day	Heart failure
		IV: 1.25 mg q6h over a 5-min period *PO: Usual dose 1–2 tabs/day	Hypertension

Continued

DOSAGES	Selected Antihypertensive Drugs: ACE Inhibitors and Angiotensin II Receptor Blockers (cont'd)			
Drug (Pregnancy Category)	**Pharmacological Class**	**Usual Dosage Range**		**Indications**
▶▶**losartan potassium (Cozaar, *Hyzaar)** (C, first trimester; D, second and third trimesters)	Angiotensin II receptor blocker	*Adult* PO: 50–100 mg once daily *PO: 1 tab once daily		Hypertension
valsartan (Diovan, Diovan-HCT*) (C, first trimester; D, second and third trimesters)		*Adult* PO: 80–320 mg in a single dose *PO: maximum recommended dose is 320 mg valsartan and 25 mg hydrochlorothiazide		

ACE, angiotensin-converting enzyme; *IV,* intravenous; *PO,* oral.

*Fixed-combination tablet with hydrochlorothiazide.

ANGIOTENSIN II RECEPTOR BLOCKERS

The ARBs are one of the newest classes of antihypertensives and include losartan potassium (Cozaar), eprosartan mesylate (Teveten), valsartan (Diovan), irbesartan (Avapro), candesartan cilexetil (Atacand), and telmisartan (Micardis).

Mechanism of Action and Drug Effects

ARBs block the binding of AII to type 1 AII receptors (AT1 receptors). ACE inhibitors such as enalapril block conversion of AI to AII, but AII may also be formed by other enzymes that are not blocked by ACE inhibitors. For comparison, recall that ACE inhibitors block the breakdown of bradykinins and substance P, which accumulate and may cause adverse effects such as cough but might also contribute to the drugs' antihypertensive and heart and nephroprotective effects. Bradykinins are potent vasodilators and help to reduce blood pressure by dilating arteries and decreasing SVR.

In contrast to ACE inhibitors, the ARBs affect primarily vascular smooth muscle and the adrenal gland. By selectively blocking the binding of AII to the type 1 AII receptors in these tissues, ARBs block vasoconstriction and the secretion of aldosterone. AII receptors have been found in other tissues throughout the body, but the effects of ARB blocking of these receptors is unknown.

Clinically, ACE inhibitors and ARBs appear to be equally effective for the treatment of hypertension. Both are well tolerated, but ARBs do not cause cough. There is evidence that ARBs are better tolerated and have lower mortality (after MI) than ACE inhibitors. It is not yet clear whether ARBs are as effective as ACE inhibitors in treating heart failure (cardioprotective effects) or in protecting the kidneys, as in diabetes. Both classes of drugs are contraindicated for use in the second or third trimester of pregnancy. Whether one or more of these drugs, particularly the newer drugs, could prove to have unique adverse effects with long-term use is unknown.

Indications

The therapeutic effects of ARBs are related to their potent vasodilating properties. They are excellent antihypertensives and adjunctive drugs for the treatment of heart failure. They may be used alone or in combination with other drugs such as diuretics in the treatment of hypertension or heart failure. The beneficial hemodynamic effects of ARBs are their ability to decrease SVR (a measure of afterload). Their use is rapidly growing, and many more studies are verifying their beneficial effects. Currently these drugs are used primarily in patients who have been intolerant of ACE inhibitors.

Contraindications

The only usual contraindications to the use of ARBs are known drug allergy, pregnancy, and lactation. ARBs such as losartan should be used cautiously in the older adult and in patients with kidney dysfunction because of increased sensitivity to its effects and risk for more adverse effects in the older adult. As with other antihypertensives, blood pressure and apical pulse rate should be assessed before and during drug therapy.

Adverse Effects

The most common adverse effects of ARBs are upper respiratory infections and headache. Occasionally, dizziness, inability to sleep, diarrhea, dyspnea, heartburn, nasal congestion, back pain, and fatigue can occur. Rarely, anxiety, muscle pain, sinusitis, cough, and insomnia can also occur. Hyperkalemia is much less likely to occur than with the ACE inhibitors.

Toxicity and Management of Overdose

Overdose may manifest as hypotension and tachycardia; bradycardia occurs less often. Treatment is symptomatic and supportive and includes the administration of intravenous fluids to expand the blood volume.

Interactions

ARBs can interact with cimetidine, phenobarbital, and rifampin. The drugs that interact with ARBs, the mechanism responsible, and the result of the interaction are summarized in Table 25-5. In addition, as is the case with ACE inhibitors, ARBs can promote hyperkalemia, especially when taken concurrently with potassium supplements (although this occurs much less frequently than with ACE inhibitors). However, patients' individual chemistry varies widely and so monitoring of the serum potassium level is necessary for each patient. Potassium supplements may still be indicated for those patients with a tendency toward hypokalemia (whether acute or chronic).

Dosages

For information on the dosages for selected ARBs, see the Dosages table on p. 474.

TABLE	25-5
Angiotensin II Receptor Blockers: Drug Interactions	

Drug	Mechanism	Result
cimetidine	Competes for metabolism	Increased ARB effect
lithium	Inhibits lithium elimination	Increased lithium concentrations
phenobarbital, rifampin	Increases metabolism	Decreased ARB effect

---

DRUG PROFILES

▶▶ losartan potassium

Losartan potassium (Cozaar) has been shown to be beneficial in patients with hypertension and heart failure. Numerous studies are showing the beneficial effects of ARBs, including losartan, in the treatment of heart failure. These studies indicate that ARBs are better tolerated and produce a marginally lower mortality rate (after MI) than treatment with ACE inhibitors.

The use of losartan is contraindicated in patients who are hypersensitive to any component of the product. It should be used with caution in patients with kidney or liver dysfunction and in patients with renal artery stenosis. Breastfeeding women should not take losartan because it can cause serious adverse effects to the nursing infant. Losartan is available in combination with the thiazide diuretic, hydrochlorothiazide (Hyzaar). Recommended dosages are given in the Dosages table on p. 474.

PHARMACOKINETICS

Half-Life	Onset	Peak	Duration
6–9 hr	Unknown	3–4 hr	24 hr

CALCIUM CHANNEL BLOCKERS

CCBs have already been discussed in some detail in the two previous chapters on antidysrhythmic drugs (Chapter 23) and antianginal drugs (Chapter 24). As a class of medications, they are used for several indications and have many beneficial effects and relatively few adverse effects. CCBs are primarily used for the treatment of hypertension and angina. Their effectiveness in treating hypertension is related to their ability to cause smooth muscle relaxation by blocking the binding of calcium to its receptors, preventing contraction of the smooth muscle. Because of their effectiveness and safety, they have been added to the list of first-line drugs for the treatment of hypertension. CCBs are used for many other indications as well. They are effective antidysrhythmics and they can prevent the cerebral artery spasms that can occur after a subarachnoid hemorrhage (nimodipine). They are also sometimes used in the treatment of Raynaud's disease and migraine headache.

DIURETICS

The diuretics are a highly effective class of antihypertensive drugs. They are currently listed as the first-line antihypertensives in the CHEP guidelines for the treatment of hypertension. They may be used as monotherapy or in combination with drugs of other antihypertensive classes. Their primary therapeutic effect is decreasing the plasma and extracellular fluid volumes, which results in decreased preload. This leads to a decrease in cardiac output and total peripheral resistance, all of which decrease the workload of the heart. This large group of antihypertensives is discussed in detail in Chapter 26. The thiazide diuretics (e.g., hydrochlorothiazide) are the most commonly used diuretics for hypertension.

VASODILATORS

Vasodilators act directly on arteriolar and venous smooth muscle to cause relaxation. They do not work through adrenergic receptors. Sodium nitroprusside is useful in the management of hypertensive emergencies when the blood pressure is severely or moderately elevated. However, there is a potential consequence of impending end-organ damage, particularly in the brain, heart, or eyes.

Mechanism of Action and Drug Effects

The mechanism of action of the direct-acting vasodilators that makes them useful as antihypertensive drugs is their ability to directly elicit peripheral vasodilation. This effect results in a reduction in SVR. More recently, minoxidil (in its topical form) has received attention because of its effectiveness in restoring hair growth, described further in Chapter 57. Hydralazine and minoxidil act primarily through arteriolar vasodilation, whereas nitroprusside has both arteriolar and venous effects.

Indications

All of the vasodilators can be used to treat hypertension, either alone or in combination with other antihypertensives. Sodium nitroprusside is reserved for the management of hypertensive emergencies. Minoxidil in its topical form is used to restore hair growth.

Contraindications

Contraindications include known drug allergy and may also include hypotension, cerebral edema, head injury, acute MI, or coronary artery disease.

As mentioned in Chapter 22, vasodilating drugs may also be contraindicated in cases of heart failure secondary to diastolic dysfunction.

Adverse Effects

The adverse effects of hydralazine include dizziness, headache, anxiety, tachycardia, edema, nasal congestion, dyspnea, anorexia, nausea, vomiting, diarrhea, anemia, agranulocytosis, hepatitis, peripheral neuritis, systemic lupus erythematosus (SLE), and rash. Minoxidil adverse effects include T-wave electrocardiogram changes, pericardial effusion or tamponade, angina, breast tenderness, rash, and thrombocytopenia. Sodium nitroprusside adverse effects include bradycardia, decreased platelet aggregation, rash, hypothyroidism, hypotension, methemoglobinemia, and, rarely, cyanide toxicity. Cyanide ions are a byproduct of nitroprusside metabolism. However, most drug dosages do not produce a large enough number of these ions to cause any serious effects.

Toxicity and Management of Overdose

Hydralazine toxicity or overdose produces hypotension, tachycardia, headache, and generalized skin flushing. Treatment is supportive and symptomatic and includes the administration of intravenous fluids, digitalization if needed, and the administration of β-blockers for the control of tachycardia.

Minoxidil overdose or toxicity can precipitate excessive hypotension. Treatment is supportive and symptomatic and includes the administration of intravenous fluids. Norepinephrine and epinephrine should not be used to reverse the hypotension because of the possibility of excessive cardiac stimulation.

The main symptom of sodium nitroprusside overdose or toxicity is excessive hypotension. This drug is normally administered only to patients receiving intensive care. Under these conditions, the infusion rate is usually carefully titrated to immediately visible results on a cardiovascular monitor that provides constant measurements of blood pressure from centrally placed venous or arterial catheters. For this reason, excessive hypotension is usually avoidable. When it does occur, discontinuation of the infusion has an immediate effect because the drug is metabolized rapidly (nitroprusside has a half-life

of 10 minutes). Treatment for the hypotension is supportive and symptomatic; if necessary, pressor drugs can be infused to quickly raise blood pressure. The chemical structure of nitroprusside contains cyanide groups, which are released upon its metabolism in the body and can theoretically result in cyanide toxicity, although this is extremely rare. Should this unlikely event occur, treatment can be administered using a standard cyanide antidote kit that includes sodium nitrite and sodium thiosulfate for injection and amyl nitrite for inhalation. However, the usual release of cyanide ions accompanying therapy with this drug rarely, if ever, reaches sufficient concentration to paralyze respirations, as can be the case with concentrated occupational or wartime exposure to cyanide.

Interactions

Although the incidence of drug interactions with the direct-acting vasodilators (especially sodium nitroprusside) is low, as a class of drugs they are associated with a variety of drug interactions. These are summarized in Table 25-6.

Dosages

For dosage information for selected vasodilator drugs, see the Dosages table on p. 477.

TABLE	25-6

Direct-Acting Vasodilators: Drug Interactions

Drug	Mechanism	Result
HYDRALAZINE		
Adrenergics	Antagonism	Decreased hypotensive effect
Antihypertensives	Additive effects	Increased hypotensive effect
Monoamine oxidase inhibitors	Altered biotransformation	Increased hypotensive effect
MINOXIDIL		
Antihypertensives/ thiazides	Additive effects	Increased hypotensive effect
guanethidine	Additive effects	Significant hypotensive effect
SODIUM NITROPRUSSIDE		
Ganglionic-blocking drugs	Additive effects	Increased hypotensive effect

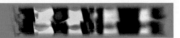

 ## DRUG PROFILES

▸▸ hydralazine hydrochloride

Hydralazine hydrochloride (Apresoline, Novo-Hylazin) is less commonly used now than when it first became available, but it is still effective for selected patients. It can be taken orally for routine cases of **essential hypertension** and it is also available in injectable form for hypertensive emergencies. However, in addition to drug allergy, its currently listed contraindications include coronary artery disease and mitral valve dysfunction, such as that related to childhood rheumatic fever. Available tablet strengths are 10 mg, 25 mg, and 50 mg, and the injectable form is 20 mg/mL. It is classified as pregnancy category C. See the Dosages table below for dosage information.

PHARMACOKINETICS

Half-Life	Onset	Peak	Duration
IV: 1–3 hr	IV: 5–20 min	IV: 30–45 min	IV: 2–4 hr
PO: 3–7 hr	PO: 20–30 min	PO: 1–2 hr	PO: 6–12 hr

sodium nitroprusside

Sodium nitroprusside (Nipride) is normally used in the critical care setting for severe hypertensive emergencies and is titrated to effect by intravenous infusion. Its use is contraindicated in patients with a known hypersensitivity to it and in those with the compensatory hypertension associated with coarctation or arteriovenous shunt, congenital Leber's optic atrophy, or tobacco amblyopia (both of which may predispose the patient to cyanide toxicity), severe heart failure, and known inadequate cerebral perfusion (especially during neurosurgical procedures). Because of the risk for cyanide toxicity at maximal doses (up to 10 mcg/kg/min) for extended periods, its use at such dosages is limited to no longer than 10 minutes. See the Dosages table on p. 477 for dosage information.

PHARMACOKINETICS

Half-Life	Onset	Peak	Duration
2 min	< 2 min	2–5 min	1–10 min

DOSAGES **Selected Antihypertensive Drugs: Vasodilators**

Drug (Pregnancy Category)	Pharmacological Class	Usual Dosage Range	Indications
▸▸hydralazine hydrochloride (Apresoline, Novo-Hylazin) (C)	Direct-acting peripheral vasodilator	*Adult* PO: 10 mg qid for 2–4 days, followed by 25 mg qid for balance of week; second and subsequent weeks 50 mg qid, then adjust to lowest effective dose for maintenance IV: 5–40 mg prn	Hypertension
minoxidil (Loniten) (C)		*Children less than 12 yr* PO: 0.25–1 mg/kg/day divided; max 50 mg/day *Children over 12 yr/Adult* PO: 10–40 mg/day divided; max 100 mg/day	
sodium nitroprusside (Nipride) (C)		*Children/Adult* IV: 0.58 mcg/kg/min	

IV, intravenous; *PO,* oral.

 ## DRUG PROFILES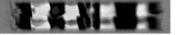

RENIN INHIBITORS

Direct renin-inhibitors are the most recent classification of drugs to be used in the treatment of primary hypertension. The sole drug in this class is aliskiren.

▸▸ aliskiren fumarate

Aliskiren fumarate (Rasilez) is the first in the new class of low–molecular weight renin inhibitors, indicated for the treatment of mild to moderate hypertension. Its use

is currently recommended as monotherapy or in combination with other antihypertensive drugs such as thiazide diuretics, ACE inhibitors, or dihydropyridine CCBs because of its synergistic effects.

The renin–angiotensin system plays a key role in blood pressure regulation. Renin, stored and released by the juxtaglomerular cells of the afferent arteriole of the kidney, is the first enzyme in the renin–angiotensin–aldosterone system. This system plays a role in blood pressure control. The release of renin is triggered by low blood volume, reduced kidney perfusion, or increased sympathetic

Continued

DRUG PROFILES (cont'd)

nervous system activity. Renin splits angiotensinogen to angiotensin I (AI), which is converted by the angiotensin-converting enzyme to angiotensin II (AII), a potent vasoconstrictor. Renin also stimulates the release of catecholamines from the adrenal medulla. AII directly causes arterial smooth muscle to contract, leading to vasoconstriction and consequently an increase in blood pressure. In addition, AII stimulates the production of aldosterone, which causes the tubules of the kidneys to increase reuptake of sodium and water, increasing plasma volume and blood pressure. Chronic increases in AII promote inflammation and fibrosis that are associated with end-organ damage.

Aliskiren has a unique mechanism of action: it binds directly to the renin enzyme and blocks the conversion of angiotensinogen to AI and AII. This action suppresses the entire system, resulting in a reduction in plasma renin activity as well as in AI, AII, and aldosterone. Other antihypertensive drugs that work on the renin–angiotensin–aldosterone system, such as the ACE inhibitors and ARBs, result in a compensatory rise in the plasma renin levels because of their suppression of the negative feedback loop. Because of aliskiren's extended half-life, this compensatory rise in plasma renin does not occur. The antihypertensive effect occurs within 2 weeks after initiating therapy with 150 mg per day and a maximum effect is reached after 4 weeks.

Its use is contraindicated in those who are hypersensitive to it. Aliskiren is generally well tolerated. The most common adverse effects include headache, dizziness, fatigue, and dose-related gastrointestinal effects such as diarrhea. The concomitant use of aliskiren with cyclosporine is not recommended.

Aliskiren is available in oral formulations. The common adult dosage for this drug is 150–300 mg PO, once daily. It is classified as pregnancy category C during the first trimester and category D during the second or third trimesters.

PHARMACOKINETICS

Half-Life	Onset	Peak	Duration
24 hr	30 min	1–3 hr	7–8 days*

*Steady state.

DRUG PROFILES

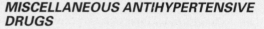

MISCELLANEOUS ANTIHYPERTENSIVE DRUGS

Three newer medications, bosentan, epoprostenol, and trepostinil, exemplify some of the most recent antihypertensive drugs to be made available in Canada.

bosentan monohydrate

Bosentan monohydrate (Tracleer), currently the single novel drug in a new drug class, acts by blocking the receptors of the hormone endothelin. Normally this hormone acts to stimulate the narrowing of blood vessels by binding to endothelin receptors (ET_A and ET_B) in the endothelial (innermost) lining of blood vessels and in vascular smooth muscle. Bosentan reduces blood pressure by blocking this action. However, currently its use is specifically indicated only for pulmonary artery hypertension in patients with moderate to severe heart failure. Its use is contraindicated in patients with known drug allergy, pregnancy, or significant liver impairment, and in patients receiving concurrent drug therapy with cyclosporine or glyburide. Recommended dosages are given in the Dosages table on p. 479.

PHARMACOKINETICS

Half-Life	Onset	Peak	Duration
5.4 hr	Variable	3–5 hr	Unknown

epoprostenol sodium

Epoprostenol sodium (Flolan), also known as prostacyclin, a metabolite of arachidonic acid, is a naturally occurring prostaglandin that lowers blood pressure through a combined mechanism of action by direct dilation of both pulmonary and systemic arterial blood vessels and by inhibiting platelet aggregation. The vasodilatory effects of epoprostenol reduce right and left ventricular afterload and increase cardiac output and stroke volume. Epoprostenol is indicated specifically for the long-term treatment of primary pulmonary artery hypertension and secondary pulmonary hypertension due to scleroderma in patients with moderate to severe heart failure who do not respond to traditional therapy. Its use is contraindicated in patients with known drug hypersensitivity and in patients with heart failure associated with severe left ventricular systolic function.

Epoprostenol is administered using a portable pump through a central venous catheter via the subclavian or jugular vein. Intense patient education and access to medical care is required because of potential problems with the drug delivery system.

Because epoprostenol is a potent inhibitor of platelet aggregation, risk for bleeding is an important consideration in its use. The most common adverse effects noted are dizziness, headache, nausea and vomiting, diarrhea, jaw pain, flushing, flulike symptoms, and anxiety and nervousness. Thrombocytopenia has also been reported. This drug is unique in that it is diluted to the nanogram level for administration. Recommended dosages are given in the Dosages table on p. 479.

PHARMACOKINETICS

Half-Life	Onset	Peak	Duration
IV: 10 min	2.7 min	Unknown	min*

*Steady state

Continued

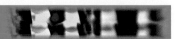

treprostinil sodium

Treprostinil sodium (Remodulin) lowers blood pressure through a combined mechanism of action by dilating both pulmonary and systemic blood vessels and by inhibiting platelet aggregation. As with bosentan, treprostinil is indicated specifically for long-term management of pulmonary artery hypertension in patients with moderate to severe heart failure. Its only current contraindication is

known drug allergy. Like epoprostenol, it is diluted to the nanogram level for administration. Recommended dosages are given in the Dosages table below.

PHARMACOKINETICS

Half-Life	Onset	Peak	Duration
SC: 4 hr	Unknown	Unknown	hr*

*Steady state

DOSAGES   Miscellaneous Antihypertensive Drugs

Drug	Pharmacological Class	Usual Dosage Range	Indications
bosentan monohydrate (tracleer) (X)	Endothelin-receptor antagonist	*Adult only* PO: Initial dose of 62.5 mg bid 4 wk, then increase as tolerated to maintenance dose of 125 mg bid	Pulmonary artery hypertension in moderate to severe heart failure
epoprostenol sodium (Flolan) (B)	Vasodilator and platelet aggregation inhibitor	*Adult only* IV: 2 ng/kg/min continuous infusion, may increase by 1–2 ng/kg/min until effect	Pulmonary artery hypertension in severe heart failure
treprostinil sodium (Remodulin) (B)	Vasodilator and platelet aggregation inhibitor	*Adult only* Continuous subcutaneous infusion: 0.625– 1.25 ng/kg/min	Pulmonary artery hypertension in severe heart failure

NURSING PROCESS

A variety of drugs are used to treat hypertension. Although much of the nursing process related to their use is similar for all these drug classes of antihypertensives, there are some considerations specific to the use of each particular drug class. Therefore, both general and specific information on these drugs and drug groups is presented.

It is important for the nurse to understand the hypertension guidelines regarding evaluation, classification, and diagnosis of hypertension, risk factors, and identifiable causes of hypertension. These guidelines enable earlier identification and management and aid in teaching patients the blood pressure measurement techniques that apply to adults aged 18 years and older. One of the major changes in the newer reports is the creation of a "prehypertension" category of hypertension, defined as a systolic blood pressure of 120 to 139 mm Hg or diastolic blood pressure of 80 to 89 mm Hg, or both. These guidelines were developed and implemented to encourage the management, both pharmacological and nonpharmacological, of hypertension early in the disease process instead of later when multiple-organ damage may be present.

Assessment

Before administering any antihypertensive drug to a patient, the nurse should obtain a thorough health history and perform a head-to-toe physical examination, which

are crucial for ensuring safe drug therapy. Parameters to measure and document include blood pressure, pulse, respirations, and pulse oximetry readings. Results of laboratory tests, especially those indicative of fluid and electrolyte imbalances, heart function and heart tissue damage, kidney function, and liver function should be monitored. These laboratory tests may include the following:

- Serum sodium, potassium, chloride, magnesium, and calcium
- Serum levels of troponin, which is usually elevated within 4 to 6 hours after onset of a heart attack and may be a reliable indicator up to 14 days after a heart attack
- Kidney function studies, including blood urea nitrogen and serum and urinary creatinine
- Liver function studies, including serum transaminase alanine aminotransferase (formerly called serum glutamic pyruvic transaminase) and aspartate aminotransferase

Because hypertension may lead to heart, vascular, kidney, liver, and retinal damage, assessment to determine how much organ damage has occurred is necessary. Laboratory tests will most likely be complemented by more sophisticated scans and imaging studies. Noninvasive ophthalmoscopic examination of the eye structures (e.g., optic nerve, optic disc, vasculature) by a professionally trained health care practitioner (e.g., nurse practitioner, physician, ophthalmologist, optometrist) allows easy visualization of the structures impacted by hypertension. If hypertensive retinopathy is present, the exam will reveal narrowing of blood vessels in the eye, oozing of fluid from these blood vessels, spots on the retina, swelling of the macula and optic nerve, or bleeding in the back of the eye. These problems may be prevented by controlling the blood pressure or treating hypertension with appropriate follow-up once it is diagnosed.

The nurse must also assess for conditions, factors, or variables that may be underlying causes for a patient's hypertension, such as the following:

- Addison's disease
- Coarctation of the aorta
- Coronary heart disease
- Ethnoculture and race or ethnicity
- Cushing's disease
- Family history of hypertension
- Nicotine use
- Obesity
- Peripheral vascular disease
- Pheochromocytoma
- Renal artery stenosis
- Kidney or liver dysfunction
- Stressful lifestyle

With many of these factors, antihypertensive drugs must be used with caution, as discussed earlier in the pharmacology section; contraindications to their use must be given particular attention. The older adult and those with chronic illnesses are of special concern because these patients are at high risk for further compromise of their physical condition if they suffer from uncontrolled or untreated hypertension or the adverse effects of antihypertensives (e.g., fluid loss, dehydration, electrolyte imbalances, hypotension). For complete drug interactions associated with antihypertensives, see the pharmacology section in this chapter.

Use of α-*adrenergic agonists* requires close assessment of the patient's blood pressure, pulse rate, and weight before and during treatment because of their strong vasodilating properties and hypotensive adverse effects. These drugs may also be associated with fluid retention and edema, so assessment of heart and breath sounds, monitoring of intake and output, and assessment for dependent and peripheral edema are necessary. The α-adrenergic drugs should always be used carefully because of associated hypotension-induced dizziness and syncope and should be used especially cautiously in the older adult or other patients with pre-existing dizziness and syncope. First-dose syncope generally occurs within 30 to 90 minutes of taking this drug and is often preceded by an increase in heart rate (120 to 160 beats/min). Careful assessment of blood pressures (supine and standing) and corresponding pulse rates is required before each dose of the drug and 30 to 60 minutes after the drug is given, especially for the first dose or two of the medication.

Blood pressures and pulse rates (supine and standing) should always be assessed with any of the antihypertensive drugs, as should cautions, contraindications, and drug interactions. *Centrally acting* α-*blockers* require assessment of white blood cell counts, serum potassium and sodium, and protein in the urine. The route of administration for the given drug order should also be noted because of different concerns related to a specific route (e.g., assessment of skin sites for readiness for transdermal application [e.g., with clonidine]).

The β-*blockers* and their mechanisms of action are important to remember prior to giving these drugs to a patient because of the risk of complications in certain patient populations. If a drug is a nonselective β-blocker, it blocks both β_1- and β_2-receptors and will block both heart and respiratory effects, whereas if a drug is only a β_1-blocking drug, the cardiac system will be affected (pulse rate and blood pressure will decrease), but there will be no β_2-effects, thus limiting any concern for respiratory problems (e.g., bronchoconstriction). If a patient needs a β-blocker but has a restrictive airway problem, nonselective β-blockers should not be used in order to avoid bronchoconstriction; a β_1-specific blocker would be used to avoid a negative impact on the lungs. However, if there is no history of respiratory illnesses or concerns, these drugs may be very effective as antihypertensives. In addition, for patients with congestive heart failure, it is important to understand that β-blockers also have a negative inotropic effect on the heart (decrease contractility); their use would lead to worsening of heart failure, creating the need for a completely different type of antihypertensive.

With use of β-blockers, assessment should include measurement of blood pressure and apical pulse rate immediately before each dose; if the systolic blood pressure is less than 90 mm Hg or the pulse rate is less than 60 beats/min, the physician should be notified because of the risk of adverse effects (e.g., hypotension, bradycardia). The drug would usually be withheld as ordered or per protocol. These blood pressure and pulse rate parameters are also applicable to the use of other antihypertensives. Breath sounds and heart sounds should be assessed before and during drug therapy.

Use of *ACE inhibitors* requires assessment of blood pressure, apical pulse rate, and respiratory status (because of the adverse effect of a dry, hacking, persistent cough). It is important to take blood pressure immediately before initial and subsequent doses of the drug so that extreme fluctuations may be identified early. Serum potassium, sodium, and chloride levels should also be assessed. Baseline heart functioning will most likely be ordered prior to initiation of therapy. Proteinuria is simple to assess through use of the dipstick method on the patient's first voided urine sample of the morning. Because of adverse effects of neutropenia and other blood disorders, a complete blood count should be performed before and during therapy, as ordered.

ARBs should be used very cautiously in the older adult and in patients with kidney dysfunction because of increased sensitivity to the drug's effects and risk for more adverse effects.

Vasodilators require baseline neurological assessment with noting of level of consciousness and cognitive ability. These should be used with extreme caution in the older adult because they are more sensitive to the drug's effect on lowering of blood pressure and subsequent problems with hypotension, dizziness, and syncope. See Chapters 23, 24, and 26 for further discussion of other antihypertensives.

In summary, many assessment parameters are similar for the various groups of antihypertensives. The difference in the level of assessment depends on the drug's impact on blood pressure as well as the individual's response to the medication and any pre-existing illness or condition. Other aspects to be assessed in any patient receiving these drugs, as well as most other drugs, include the patient's ethnocultural background, racial or ethnic group, reading level, learning needs, developmental and cognitive status, financial status, mental health status, support systems, and overall physical health. Always encourage patients to learn how to assess and monitor themselves and their individual responses to drug therapy.

Nursing Diagnoses

- Deficient knowledge related to a new prescribed drug regimen and lack of familiarity with medications and lifestyle changes
- Nonadherence to drug therapy related to lack of familiarity with or acceptance of the disease process
- Sexual dysfunction related to adverse effects of some antihypertensive drugs
- Risk for injury (e.g., possible falls) related to adverse effects of the antihypertensive drug, such as dizziness, orthostatic hypotension, and syncope
- Acute pain related to headache as an adverse effect of drug therapy
- Ineffective tissue perfusion (renal, cardiac, cerebral) related to the impact of the disease process or possible severe hypotensive adverse effects of drug therapy
- Excess fluid volume related to adverse effects of edema
- Imbalanced nutrition, less than body requirements, related to the drug's adverse effects (e.g., impaired taste or loss of appetite)
- Constipation related to adverse effects of antihypertensive drugs
- Risk for injury (e.g., possible falls) related to possible CNS adverse effects such as paresthesia, sedation, tremors, weakness, and seizures
- Risk for injury to mucous membranes related to the adverse effects of the medication and decreased saliva (dry mouth)
- Disturbed body image related to the adverse effects of antihypertensives (e.g., erectile dysfunction, sexual dysfunction, weight gain, fatigue)

Planning

Nursing goals for antihypertensive therapy should focus on educating the patient and the patient's family on the need for adequate management to prevent end-organ damage. These goals include making sure the patient understands the nature of the disease, its symptoms, and treatment, and the importance of adhering to the treatment regimen. The patient must also come to terms with the diagnosis and with the fact that there is no cure for the disease, thus treatment will be lifelong. The influence of chronic illness and the importance of nonpharmacological therapy, stress reduction, and follow-up care must also be emphasized. The nurse needs to plan for ongoing assessment of blood pressure, weight, diet, exercise, smoking habits, alcohol intake, adherence to therapy, and sexual function in the patient receiving therapy for hypertension.

Goals

- Patient will take the drug exactly as prescribed.
- Patient will experience relief of symptoms for which the medication was prescribed (e.g., a decrease in blood pressure).
- Patient will demonstrate adequate knowledge about the use of the specific medication, its adverse effects, and the appropriate dosing at home.
- Patient will be free of injury resulting from adverse effects of the medication.
- Patient will state the rationale and importance of antihypertensive therapy.
- Patient will describe measures to implement in order to decrease the impact of the adverse effects of antihypertensive therapy.
- Patient will report any change in sexual patterns and function, bowel pattern changes, or activity intolerance.
- Patient will remain adherent to the therapy regimen.

Outcome Criteria

- Patient states the risks and complications of potent antihypertensive drugs, such as tremors, decreased sweating, tachycardia, and hypotension.
- Patient states conditions to report to the physician, such as syncope or chest pain.
- Patient states the importance of lifelong adherence to drug therapy for hypertension to decrease end-organ damage and complications.
- Patient follows instructions to change position slowly, monitor blood pressure, keep follow-up appointments with the physician, and keep a journal to help monitor the effects of therapy.
- Patient communicates openly with nurses and other members of the health care team regarding the disease, its treatment, and any concerns related to changes in body image.
- Patient reports to the physician immediately any pitting edema of the feet, hands, or sacral area or weight gain of 1 kg or more within 24 hours or 2 kg or more in 1 week.
- Patient maintains normal nutritional status through adherence to a prescribed diet high in fibre and fluids and avoidance of alcohol.

Implementation

Nursing interventions generally can help patients achieve stable blood pressure while minimizing adverse effects. Many patients have problems adhering to treatment because the disease itself is silent or without symptoms.

Patients are thus unaware of their blood pressure or think that if they do not feel ill there is nothing wrong with them, which poses many problems for treatment. Also, the antihypertensives are associated with multiple adverse effects that may impact patients' self-concept and sexual function. Often these adverse effects lead patients to abruptly stop taking the medication. It is important to inform patients that with *all* antihypertensives any abrupt withdrawal is a serious concern because of the risk of developing rebound hypertension, characterized by a sudden and extremely high elevation of blood pressure. This places the patient at risk for a stroke or other cerebral or heart adverse event. Prevention of this through patient education is critical to patient safety. Other interventions related to each major group of drugs are discussed subsequently. See Patient Education for more information.

Patients taking α-adrenergic *agonists*, such as methyldopa, will need to monitor their blood pressure and pulse rate at home or have these taken for them by a family member who has received instructions or by other qualified medical personnel. The blood pressure machines found in pharmacies do not provide as accurate readings as the devices designed for home use (see Box 25-1). The α-adrenergic agonists are also associated with severe hypotension and first-dose syncope. To avoid injury, be sure patients are supine with the first dose of this drug. More than likely, these drugs will be prescribed to be given at bedtime to allow the patient to sleep through the drug's first-dose syncope. It may take 4 to 6 weeks for the drug to achieve its full therapeutic effects, so education about delayed onset of action and bedtime dosing is important to prevent injury. The patient must also be continually monitored for dizziness, syncope, edema, and other adverse effects (e.g., shortness of breath, exacerbation of pre-existing heart disorders). Diuretics may be ordered as adjunctive therapy to minimize the adverse effects of edema, but they may lead to more dizziness and electrolyte problems. Serum creatinine, blood urea nitrogen, potassium, and sodium should be measured during the initiation and titration of antihypertensives.

Centrally acting α-*blockers* require the same type of nursing interventions as other α-blockers; however, as their name indicates, the mechanism of action of these drugs is central, so adverse effects are often more pronounced (e.g., hypotension, sedation, bradycardia, edema). See Patient Education for more information.

The β-*blockers* are either nonselective (block both β$_1$- and β$_2$-receptors; e.g., propranolol) or cardioselective (block mainly β$_1$-receptors; e.g., atenolol). With any β-blocker, careful adherence to the drug regimen is crucial to patient safety. Patients taking β-blockers may experience an exacerbation of respiratory diseases such as asthma, bronchospasm, and chronic obstructive pulmonary disease (increased bronchoconstriction due to β$_2$-blocking), or an exacerbation of heart failure because of the drug's negative inotropic effects (decreased contractility due to β$_1$-blocking). Proper instructions about reporting adverse effects and for taking blood pressure and pulse rates must

be clear and concise. In addition, if a β$_1$-blocker causes shortness of breath, it is most likely because of edema or exacerbation of congestive heart failure. Any dizziness, depression, confusion, or unusual bleeding or bruising should be reported to the health care provider immediately. See Patient Education for more information.

ACE inhibitors must also be taken exactly as prescribed. If angioedema occurs, the physician should be contacted immediately. Should the drug need to be discontinued, weaning is recommended (as with all antihypertensives) to avoid rebound hypertension. Serum sodium and potassium levels should be monitored during therapy. Serum potassium levels increase as an adverse effect with these drugs and may lead to hyperkalemia with more complications. Urine samples may be checked for proteinuria and, because anorexia may also be an adverse effect, dietary and fluid intake should be monitored closely. Impaired taste may occur as an adverse effect and last up to 2 to 3 months after the drug has been discontinued. It is also important to educate the patient that it takes several weeks to see the full therapeutic effects and that potassium supplements should not be used with these drugs (because of the adverse effect of hyperkalemia).

ARBs must also be taken exactly as prescribed. They are often tolerated best with meals, as with many antihypertensives. The dosage should not be changed nor the medication discontinued unless prescribed by the physician. With ARBs, if the patient has hypovolemia or liver dysfunction the dosage may need to be reduced. A diuretic such as hydrochlorothiazide may be ordered in combination with an ARB for patients who have hypertension with left ventricular hypertrophy. Losartan is also an option for patients at risk for stroke and for those who are hypertensive and have left ventricular hypertrophy. Most importantly, with ARBs, any unusual shortness of breath, dyspnea, weight gain, chest pain, or palpitations should be reported to the health care provider immediately.

Some nursing considerations for *vasodilators* are similar to those for other antihypertensives; however, their impact on blood pressure may be more drastic depending on the specific drug and dosage. Hydralazine given by injection may result in reduced blood pressure within 10 to 80 minutes after administration and requires close monitoring of the patient. With hydralazine, systemic lupus erythematosus (SLE) may be an adverse effect if the patient is taking more than 200 mg orally per day. If signs and symptoms of SLE occur, the drug should be discontinued, the physician should be contacted immediately, and the patient should be closely monitored. Electrocardiographic changes, cardiovascular inadequacies, and hypotension may have pronounced effects on the patient's heart status, thus the drug should *never* to be given without adequate monitoring and frequent assessment. Pyridoxine may help to diminish the adverse effect of peripheral neuritis.

Sodium nitroprusside must always be diluted per manufacturer guidelines. Because sodium nitroprusside is a potent vasodilator, there may be extreme decreases in the patient's blood pressure. Close monitoring is therefore important for preventing further complications. Severe drops in blood pressure may lead to irreversible ischemic injuries and even death. The nurse must remember that sodium nitroprusside should never be infused at the maximum dose rate for more than 10 minutes. If this drug does not control a patient's blood pressure after 10 minutes, it will most likely be ordered to be discontinued. To help prevent complications of cyanide and thiocyanate toxicity, the nurse should do the following: (1) Dilute the medication properly and avoid use of any solution that has turned blue, green, or red; (2) infuse only using a volumetric infusion pump, not through ordinary intravenous sets; (3) continuously monitor blood pressure during the infusion (often by invasive measures), and (4) when more than 500 mcg/kg of sodium nitroprusside is administered at a rate faster than 2 mcg/kg/min, be aware that this may result in production of cyanide at a more rapid rate than the patient can eliminate unaided. (See Lab Values Related to Drug Therapy for more information.)

CCBs and related nursing interventions are discussed only briefly here because these drugs are covered in Chapters 23 and 24. Drugs like enalapril and verapamil are to be taken exactly as prescribed with the warning to the patient not to puncture, open, or crush the extended-release or sustained-release tablets and capsules. The nurse must be aware that CCBs are negative inotropic drugs (used to decrease cardiac contractility) because this action may induce more signs of heart failure if CCBs are given with drugs that are used to increase heart contractility, such as digitalis glycosides. Monitoring of blood pressure and pulse rate before and during therapy will aid in prevention or early detection of any problems related to the negative inotropic effects (decreased contractility), negative chronotropic effects (decreased heart rate), and negative dromotropic effects (decreased conduction.)

The nurse must remember always to base nursing interventions on a thorough assessment and plan of care that includes consideration of the patient's ethnocultural group. This is particularly important with antihypertensives because research studies have documented differences in responses to antihypertensives among different racial and ethnic groups. Some ethnic groups respond less favourably to certain drugs than to others. As with any disease, patients must be treated with respect and with an appreciation for a holistic approach to health care in which all physical, psychosocial, and spiritual needs are taken into consideration (see Ethnocultural Implications: Hypertension in Aboriginal Peoples on p. 461).

In summary, some educational information on the particular group of drugs or specific drugs prescribed for the patient must be conveyed to the patient. The nurse must remember that patient education is of critical importance and plays an important part in ensuring adherence to the drug regimen and in decreasing the incidence of problems related to these medications.

 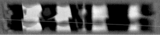

LAB VALUES RELATED TO DRUG THERAPY

Related to Drug Therapy for Sodium Nitroprusside

Laboratory Test	Normal Ranges	Rationale for Assessment
Serum methemoglobin and serum cyanide	Normally there are no values with appropriate drug levels of sodium nitroprusside	Use of sodium nitroprusside may be associated with sequestration of hemoglobin (Hgb) as methemoglobin. The appearance of this clinically significant adverse effect of methemoglobinemia is rare (less than 10%). Patients receiving this drug at the maximum rate of 10 mcg/kg/min would take 16 or more hours to reach a total accumulated dose of 10 mg/kg, so serum laboratory testing is used to measure the amount of methemoglobin. Significant clinical signs of this adverse effect include impaired oxygen delivery despite adequate cardiac output. When the sequestration is diagnosed, the treatment of choice is 1 to 2 mg/kg of methylene blue given intravenously over several minutes to allow binding of the metabolic byproduct of cyanide to methemoglobin as cyanmethemoglobin, but this should only be given as ordered and with extreme caution. In addition, sodium nitroprusside may lead to toxic reactions, even with doses that are within recommended dosage ranges; toxic reactions are evident by extreme hypotension, cyanide toxicity, or thiocyanate toxicity. Cyanide level assays are performed to detect if cyanide levels are in body fluids, but this is a difficult test to interpret and so not the most reliable method of monitoring. Other laboratory tests that may prove to be helpful in diagnosing cyanide toxicity include alterations of acid–base balance and venous oxygen concentrations. Actual cyanide levels in the blood may lag behind peak cyanide levels by an hour or more. Signs of thiocyanate toxicity include ringing of the ears (tinnitus), miosis, and hyperreflexia as well as methemoglobinemia.

Evaluation

Because patients with hypertension are at high risk for cardiovascular injury, it is critical that they adhere to both their pharmacological and nonpharmacological treatment regimens. Monitoring patients for the adverse effects (e.g., orthostatic hypotension, dizziness, fatigue) and toxic effects of the various types of antihypertensive drugs helps the nurse to identify potentially life-threatening complications. The most important aspect of the evaluation process is collecting data and monitoring patients for evidence of controlled blood pressure. Blood pressure should be maintained at less than 140/90 mm Hg. If compelling indications, such as diabetes mellitus or kidney disease, are present, then the blood pressure goal is lower than 130/80 mm Hg. Blood pressure should be monitored at periodic intervals, and patient education about self-monitoring is important to the safe use of antihypertensives. In addition, the physician needs to examine the fundus of the patient's eyes because this is a more reliable indicator of the long-term effectiveness of treatment than blood pressure readings.

The patient must constantly be monitored for the development of end-organ damage and for specific problems that the medication can cause. Male patients receiving antihypertensives should be counselled and constantly monitored for any sexual dysfunction. This is important to do because if the patient experiences the dysfunction and is not expecting it, he may not report the problem and decide to stop taking the medication abruptly. Such action places the patient at high risk for rebound hypertension and possible stroke or other complications. Communication is critical in such situations. Follow-up visits to the physician are important for monitoring these and other adverse effects and checking patient adherence.

Therapeutic effects of antihypertensives in general include an improvement in blood pressure and in the disease process. Patients should report a return to a normal baseline of blood pressure with improved energy levels and improved signs and symptoms of hypertension, such as less edema, improved breath sounds, no abnormal heart sounds, capillary refill in less than 5 seconds, and less shortness of breath (dyspnea). Adverse effects for which to monitor include all of the specific adverse effects discussed in the pharmacology section of the chapter as well as those described for each group of drugs earlier in the Nursing Process section.

 CASE STUDY

Hypertension

Hypertension was diagnosed in G.S. when she was 33 years old. Both her mother and sister have hypertension, and both were also in their thirties when it was diagnosed. G.S.'s most current blood pressure reading is 150/96 mm Hg, and for this reason the nurse practitioner has recommended that she see her primary care provider. After examining her, the physician prescribes atenolol (Tenormin) and relaxation therapy. After 14 days of this therapy, G.S.'s blood pressure is 145/86 mm Hg. Stress reduction has been the biggest obstacle in her treatment because she is a lawyer in a prominent law firm and has found that her blood pressure is consistently elevated (160/100 mm Hg) whenever she measures it at work.

1. What should G.S. know about the expected therapeutic effects and adverse effects of atenolol?
2. Discuss the differences between a drug such as atenolol and the drug propranolol (Inderal).
3. What lifestyle changes would you, as her nurse, recommend that G.S. make and, even more important, what information would you give to help her change her lifestyle and more effectively reduce the stress in her life?

For answers, see http://evolve.elsevier.com/Canada/Lilley/pharmacology/.

 IN MY FAMILY

West African Health Beliefs and Taboos, and Cures for Hypertension

(as told by P.B., from the Dan Tribe, Monrovia, Liberia; and O.I., from Ile-Ife, Oshun, Nigeria)

[P.B.] "In Liberia it is believed that illnesses are from evil spirits and the herbs counteract the work of the evil spirits. As well, that sickness is the result of being evil throughout life and the illness is the outcome of being evil. They also believe that some illnesses cannot be cured. . . . A bread fruit tree is [used] to heal hypertension. The leaves are boiled and the ill person drinks the liquid. It keeps the blood pressure on a minimal level."

[O.I.] "There are some taboos for every family in the town and you must not disobey the taboo of your family. [For example], 'you must not walk in the sun if you're pregnant,' 'you must not eat certain meat,' etc. So if someone has a disease or sickness, it might be because of the disobedience to those taboos...[For hypertension] there is a leaf that grows naturally near every house called 'Erin'; this leaf will be squeezed with water and liquid will be sieved from the leaf and the affected individual will drink the liquid obtained."

PATIENT EDUCATION

Antihypertensives in General

- Patients should be taught to take medications exactly as prescribed by the physician, to never double or omit doses, and to contact their physician if these instructions are not followed.
- Patients should be informed that successful therapy requires adherence to medications as well as any dietary restrictions (e.g., decreasing fatty foods or those high in cholesterol).
- Patients should always monitor stress levels and use biofeedback, imagery, or relaxation techniques or massage, as needed. Exercise, if approved by the physician, may also help in the management of hypertension. It serves to relieve stress and is usually inclusive of supervised, prescribed exercise.
- Patients should be encouraged to avoid smoking and excessive alcohol intake as well as excessive exercise, hot climates, saunas, hot tubs, and hot environments. Heat may precipitate vasodilation and lead to worsening of hypotension with risk of fainting and injury.
- Patients should be reminded of the importance of follow-up appointments because laboratory tests may be needed for the duration of therapy.
- Patients should be taught to keep medications out of the reach of children.
- Patients should be encouraged to always wear a medical alert bracelet or necklace and carry a medical identification card specifying the patient's diagnosis, noting allergies, and listing all medications taken (e.g., prescribed drugs, over-the-counter [OTC] medications, and natural health products). The same information should be kept in a visible location in the patient's car and in the patient's home on the refrigerator for emergency medical personnel.
- Patients should weigh themselves daily at the same time every day and with the same amount of clothing, and record the weight in a journal.
- Patients should be instructed to record blood pressure frequently, including postural blood pressures. Patients should feel comfortable in taking their blood pressure and pulse rate. Patients should practise as needed and should never hesitate to ask for assistance.
- Patients should be encouraged to inform all health care providers (e.g., dentist, surgeon) that he or she is taking an antihypertensive drug.
- Patients should be sure to move purposefully and cautiously and to change positions slowly because of the possible adverse effect of postural hypotension and associated risk for dizziness, light-headedness, and possible fainting and falls. Patients should be educated that a strategy to manage or minimize the lightheadness and dizziness associated with antihypertensive drugs is to stagger the drugs (e.g., take the β-blocker at 0800 and the ACE inhibitor at 1000).
- Patients should be informed to always keep an adequate supply of hypertensive medications on hand, especially while travelling.

- Patients should be reminded of the importance of scheduling periodic eye examinations (e.g., every 6 months) because of the need to evaluate treatment effectiveness and the impact of hypertension on the vasculature of the eyes.
- Patients should be cautioned not to stop taking the medication just because of feeling better. With successful therapy, the patient's condition will improve, but lifelong therapy is usually required.
- Patients should be encouraged to use saliva substitutes, sugar-free hard candy, or frequent fluids for management of dry mouth.
- Patients should be informed about measures to help with constipation, such as forcing fluids, increasing fibre and roughage, and contacting the physician for consultation if there is no relief of this adverse effect. Use of over-the-counter agents, natural health products, or a prescription drug may be indicated.
- Sexual dysfunction may occur with antihypertensives, so patients should be encouraged to be open with reporting and discussing any problems or concerns. Emphasize to the patient that should this adverse effect occur, there are options to help alleviate the problem, such as combination therapy that allows lower dosages of drugs to be used, as well as use of other types of antihypertensives. The patient should always report any problems to the physician, because solutions are usually available.
- Patients should know to never abruptly stop taking the medication for any reason, including sexual problems, because of the risk of severe rebound hypertension. Avoiding abrupt withdrawal of *any* of the antihypertensives is critical to patient safety.
- Patients should be aware that antihypertensives may lead to depression, so any change in emotional status should be reported to the health care provider.

α-Adrenergic Agonists

- Patients should be informed about avoiding alcohol and heat because of exacerbation of vasodilation and subsequent worsening of hypotension, leading to dizziness and possible fainting (syncope). This is appropriate for any of the antihypertensives.
- Patients should be careful at first with activities such as driving or activities requiring alertness. The patient may have to postpone driving and other activities until the drowsiness stops.
- Patients should report any jaundice, unexplained fever, or flulike symptoms to the physician immediately.
- Patients should be encouraged to take daily weight measurements each morning before breakfast, at the same time and wearing the same amount of clothing each day. Information should be recorded in a daily journal along with blood pressure readings. The patient should be instructed to report an increase in weight by 1 kg or more over a 24-hour period or 2 kg or more in 1 week.

Continued

❖ Patients should be informed that centrally acting blockers may affect sexual functioning (e.g., causing erectile dysfunction or decreased libido) and to contact their health care provider if this adverse effect becomes problematic. Other treatment options may be indicated.

β-Blockers

❖ Patients should be cautioned to move and change positions slowly to avoid possible dizziness, fainting, and falls and should be instructed to report a pulse rate of less than 60 beats/min, any peripheral numbness, dizziness, weight gain (see earlier), or systolic blood pressure of 90 mm Hg or lower to the physician.

❖ Patient should be encouraged to avoid prolonged sitting or standing and excessive physical exercise, as these may lead to exacerbation of hypotensive effects; patients can counteract these activities with healthier alternatives such as pumping the feet up and down while sitting.

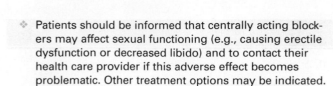

POINTS TO REMEMBER

❖ All antihypertensives in some way affect cardiac output and SVR.

❖ Cardiac output is the amount of blood ejected from the left ventricle measured in litres per minute.

❖ SVR is the force the left ventricle must overcome to eject its end-diastolic volume.

❖ The major classes of antihypertensives are the diuretics (see Chapter 26), α-blockers, centrally active α-blockers, β-blockers, ACE inhibitors, vasodilators, CCBs, and ARBs. One new class of drugs, the renin inhibitors, was also introduced in 2008.

❖ ACE inhibitors act by blocking a critical enzyme system responsible for the production of angiotensin II (a potent vasoconstrictor). They prevent (1) vasoconstriction caused by angiotensin II, (2) aldosterone secretion and therefore sodium and water resorption, and (3) the breakdown of bradykinin (a potent vasodilator) by angiotensin II.

❖ ARBs act by blocking the binding of angiotensin at the receptors; the result is a decrease in blood pressure.

❖ CCBs may be used to treat angina, dysrhythmias, and hypertension and help to reduce blood pressure by causing smooth-muscle relaxation and dilation of blood vessels. If calcium is not present, then the smooth muscle of the blood vessels cannot contract.

Aspects of the nursing process related to the use of antihypertensives include the following:

❖ A thorough nursing assessment should include assessment for any underlying causes of hypertension, such as kidney or liver dysfunction, a stressful lifestyle, Cushing's disease, Addison's disease, renal artery stenosis, peripheral vascular disease, or pheochromocytoma.

❖ The nurse should always assess for the presence of contraindications, cautions, and potential drug interactions before administering any of the antihypertensive drugs. Contraindications include a history of MI or chronic kidney disease. Cautious use is recommended in patients with renal insufficiency and glaucoma. Drugs that interact with antihypertensive drugs include other antihypertensive drugs, anaesthetics, and diuretics.

❖ Patients should be managed using both pharmacological and nonpharmacological strategies. They should be encouraged to consume a diet low in fat, reduce their salt intake, and make any other necessary modifications in their diet (such as an increase in fibre), engage in regular supervised exercise, and reduce the amount of stress in their lives.

❖ Therapeutic effects include fewer hypertension-related symptoms, such as chest pain and severe headaches, and decreased blood pressure readings.

❖ Adverse effects for which to constantly monitor include tachycardia, confusion, CNS depression, and constipation.

EXAMINATION REVIEW QUESTIONS

1 Which of the following adverse effects is of most concern for the older adult patient taking antihypertensive drugs?
   a. Dry mouth
   b. Hypotension
   c. Restlessness
   d. Constipation

2 When giving antihypertensive drugs, for which of the following classes of drugs must the nurse consider giving the first dose at bedtime?
   a. β-Blockers such as prazosin (Minipress)
   b. Diuretics such as furosemide (Lasix)
   c. ACE inhibitors such as captopril (Capoten)
   d. Vasodilators such as hydralazine (Apresoline)

3 A 56-year-old man started antihypertensive drug therapy 3 months ago and is in the office for a follow-up visit. While the nurse is taking his blood pressure, he informs the nurse that he has had some problems with sexual intercourse. Which of the following would be the most appropriate response by the nurse?
   a. "Not to worry. Tolerance will develop."
   b. "The physician can work with you on changing the dosage or drugs."
   c. "Sexual dysfunction happens with this therapy, and you must learn to accept it."
   d. "This is an unusual occurrence, but it is important to stay on your medications."

4 When a patient is being taught about the potential adverse effects of an ACE inhibitor, which of the following should be mentioned as possibly occurring when this drug is taken to treat hypertension?
   a. Nausea
   b. Sedation
   c. Hypokalemia
   d. Dry, nonproductive cough

5 A patient has a new prescription for an adrenergic drug. During a review of the patient's list of current medications, which would cause concern about a possible interaction with this new prescription?
   a. An oral anticoagulant taken daily
   b. A multivitamin with iron taken daily
   c. A benzodiazepine taken as needed for allergies
   d. A nonsteroidal anti-inflammatory drug taken as needed for joint pain

For answers see http://evolve.elsevier.com/Canada/Lilley/pharmacology/.

CRITICAL THINKING ACTIVITIES

1 Primary hypertension has been diagnosed in a 53-year-old woman, and the β-blocker carvedilol has been prescribed. Before initiating therapy, what past medical conditions should the nurse inquire about during the nursing assessment?

2 A 78-year-old woman has been admitted to the emergency department for the treatment of a possible acute MI and and has another diagnosis of acute hypertensive crisis. One of the physician's orders is to start a sodium nitroprusside infusion. What is the purpose of using sodium nitroprusside?

3 A 63-year-old Black man has a new diagnosis of stage 2 hypertension. He has been treated for type 2 diabetes for 2 years but admits that he does not follow his diet as he should. His urinalysis shows traces of protein, but his retinal examination shows no defects. What drug therapy would you expect to see ordered for this patient? What is the treatment goal for this patient? Explain.

For answers see http://evolve.elsevier.com/Canada/Lilley/pharmacology/.

CHAPTER 26

Diuretic Drugs

Learning Objectives

After reading this chapter, the successful student will be able to do the following:

1 Describe the normal anatomy and physiology of the kidney.

2 Briefly discuss the impact of the kidney on blood pressure regulation.

3 Describe how diuretics work in the kidney.

4 Distinguish among the different classes of diuretics with regard to mechanisms of action, indications, dosages, routes of administration, adverse effects, toxicity, cautions, contraindications, and drug interactions.

5 Develop a collaborative plan of care that includes all phases of the nursing process for patients receiving diuretics.

e-Learning Activities

Web site
(http://evolve.elsevier.com/Canada/Lilley/pharmacology/)

- Animations
- Answers to chapter questions, activities, and case studies
- Calculators and Category Catchers
- Glossary with audio pronunciations
- IV Therapy and Medication Error Checklists
- Multiple-Choice Review Question quizzes
- Nursing Care Plans
- Online Appendices and Supplements
- WebLinks

Drug Profiles

acetazolamide, p. 492
amiloride (amiloride hydrochloride)*, p. 497
▸▸ **furosemide,** p. 494
▸▸ **hydrochlorothiazide,** p. 499
▸▸ **mannitol,** p. 495
metolazone, p. 499
▸▸ **spironolactone,** p. 497
triamterene, p. 497

▸▸ Key drug.

*Full generic name is given in parentheses. For the purposes of this text, the more common shortened name is used.

Glossary

Afferent arterioles The small blood vessels branching from the renal artery approaching the glomerulus (proximal part of the nephron). (p. 490)

Aldosterone A mineralocorticoid steroid hormone produced by the adrenal cortex that mediates the actions of the renal tubule in the regulation of sodium and potassium balance in the blood. (p. 490)

Ascites An abnormal intraperitoneal accumulation of fluid (defined as a volume of 500 mL or greater) containing large amounts of protein and electrolytes. (p. 494)

Collecting duct The most distal part of the nephron between the distal convoluted tubule and the ureters, which lead to the urinary bladder. (p. 490)

Distal convoluted tubule The part of the nephron immediately distal to the ascending loop of Henle and proximal to the collecting duct. (p. 490)

Diuretics Drugs or other substances that tend to promote the formation and excretion of urine. (p. 489)

Efferent arterioles The small blood vessels exiting the glomerulus. At this point, blood has completed its filtration in the glomerulus. (p. 490)

Filtrate   The material that passes through a filter. In the kidney, the filter is the glomerulus, and the filtrate is the extracted material from the blood (normally liquid) that ultimately becomes urine. (p. 490)

Glomerular capsule   The open, rounded, and most proximal part of the proximal convoluted tubule that surrounds the glomerulus and receives the filtrate from the blood. (p. 490)

Glomerular filtration rate (GFR)   The volume of ultrafiltrate extracted per unit of time from the plasma flowing through the glomeruli of the kidney. (p. 490)

Glomerulus   The cluster of kidney capillaries that marks the beginning of the nephron and is immediately proximal to the proximal convoluted tubule. (p. 490)

Loop of Henle   The part of the nephron that is immediately distal to the proximal convoluted tubule. (p. 490)

Nephron   The microscopic functional filtration unit of the kidney, consisting of (in anatomical order from proximal to distal) the glomerulus, proximal convoluted tubule, loop of Henle, distal convoluted tubule, and the collecting duct, which empties urine into the ureters. There are approximately one million nephrons in each kidney. (p. 490)

Open-angle glaucoma   Elevated pressure in an eye because of obstruction of the outflow of aqueous humor, but access to the trabecular meshwork remains open. (p. 491)

Proximal convoluted tubule   The part of the nephron that is immediately distal to the glomerulus and proximal to the loop of Henle. (p. 490)

Ultrafiltration   Filtration at a microscopic level; the term is often used to describe the filtration function of the kidneys, with the filtrate referred to more specifically as ultrafiltrate. (p. 490)

OVERVIEW

Each kidney has approximately one million *glomeruli*: these are the sites at which the blood is filtered. Within each glomerulus is a small tuft of capillaries. Blood enters through a tiny vessel called the *afferent arteriole* and leaves through the *efferent arteriole*. These two vessels thus regulate the inflow and outflow resistance of the intervening glomerular capillaries, thereby controlling the filtration pressure.

Diuretics are the drugs that accelerate the rate of urine formation through a variety of mechanisms. The result is the removal of sodium and water from the body. Diuretics were discovered accidentally when a mercury-based antibiotic was noted to have a potent diuretic effect. Thus began the early developmental stages of diuretic drugs. All the major classes of diuretic drugs in use today were developed between 1950 and 1970, and they remain among the most commonly prescribed

drugs in the world. Diuretics, preferably a thiazide, play a key role as first-line drugs in the treatment of hypertension. The ALLHAT study provides the best evidence justifying a diuretic as first-line management (see Research: The ALLHAT Study). The hypotensive activity of diuretics occurs as a result of many different mechanisms. Diuretics cause direct arteriolar dilation, which decreases peripheral vascular resistance. They also reduce extracellular fluid volume, plasma volume, and cardiac output, which may account for the decrease in blood pressure. Diuretics have long been the mainstay of therapy for not only hypertension but also heart failure. Two of their advantages are their relatively low cost and their favourable safety profile compared with that of many other drug classes. The primary disadvantage with their use is the metabolic adverse effects that can result from excessive fluid and electrolyte loss. Such effects are usually dose related and are therefore controllable with dosage *titration* (careful adjustment).

RESEARCH

The ALLHAT study

Results from the Antihypertensive and Lipid-Lowering Treatment to Prevent Heart Attack Trial (ALLHAT), one of the largest hypertension clinical trials conducted in North America, revealed that the less expensive thiazide diuretics are more effective than the more expensive newer antihypertensives on the market. The ALLHAT, a double-blind trial, involved 42,418 participants from Canada and the United States in a 5-year study to compare the impact of four antihypertensive drugs: chlorthalidone (a thiazide diuretic), amlodipine (a calcium channel blocker), lisinopril (an angiotensin-converting enzyme inhibitor), and doxazosin (an α-blocker). Forty-seven percent of the participants were women. Early on, the study involving doxazosin was terminated because of adverse

cardiovascular events. Although the benefits of the three remaining drugs turned out to be quite similar, overall, chlorthalidone had fewer adverse cardiovascular events and lowered systolic blood pressure better than the other two drugs. The pragmatic message is that the diuretic chlorthalidone should be the first-line drug used in the management of hypertension.

Source: ALLHAT Officers and Coordinators for the ALLHAT Collaborative Research Group. (2002). Major outcomes in high-risk hypertensive patients randomized to angiotensin-converting enzyme inhibitor or calcium channel blocker vs. diuretic: The Antihypertensive and Lipid-Lowering Treatment to Prevent Heart Attack Trial (ALLHAT). *Journal of the American Medical Association, 288*, 2981–2997.

Within this chapter, the essential properties and actions of some important classes of diuretic drugs—carbonic anhydrase inhibitors, loop diuretics, osmotic diuretics, potassium-sparing diuretics, and thiazide and thiazide-like diuretics—are reviewed. Following an overview of kidney function, the diuretic drug classes will be discussed.

KIDNEY PHYSIOLOGY

The kidney plays an important role in the day-to-day functioning of the body. It filters toxic waste products from the blood while also conserving essential substances. This delicate balance between elimination of toxins and retention of essential chemicals is maintained by the **nephron.** The nephron is the primary structural unit in the kidney, and each kidney contains approximately one million nephrons. It is in the nephron that diuretic drugs exert their effect. The initial filtering of the blood takes place in the **glomerulus,** a cluster of capillaries surrounded by the **glomerular capsule**. The rate at which blood flows into and out of the glomerulus and filtering occurs is the **glomerular filtration rate (GFR),** which is used to gauge how well the kidneys are functioning. Normally about 180 L of blood is filtered through the nephrons per day. The GFR is regulated by **afferent arterioles,** small blood vessels entering the glomerulus, and **efferent arterioles,** small blood vessels exiting the glomerulus. A mnemonic, or memory aid, that may be helpful to remember which arteriole is which is "A for *approach* and *afferent*" and "E for *exit* and *efferent*." Alterations in blood flow such as those that occur in a patient in shock can thus have a dramatic effect on kidney function. In situations of low blood flow, the kidney receives less blood; therefore, less diuretic arrives to its site of action. For this reason, diuretics may have diminished effects, although they are often used to restore or enhance kidney blood flow and glomerular filtration in such situations. This is particularly true of the loop diuretics.

The **proximal convoluted tubule,** or simply the *proximal tubule,* anatomically follows the glomerulus and reabsorbs 60% to 70% of the sodium and water from the filtered fluid (*ultrafiltrate,* resulting from the process of **ultrafiltration**) back into the bloodstream. Blood vessels surround the nephrons and allow substances to be directly reabsorbed from or secreted into the bloodstream. This process is one of active transport that requires energy in the form of adenosine triphosphate molecules. The active transport of sodium and potassium ions back into the blood causes the passive reabsorption of chloride and water. The chloride ions (Cl^-) and water passively follow the sodium ions (Na^+) and, to a lesser extent, potassium ions (K^+) by osmosis. Another 20% to 25% of sodium is reabsorbed into the bloodstream in the ascending **loop of Henle**. In the loop of Henle, the chloride is actively reabsorbed and the sodium passively follows. The remaining 5% to 10% of sodium reabsorption takes place in the **distal convoluted tubule**, or the *distal tubule,* which anatomically follows the ascending loop of Henle. In the distal tubule, sodium is actively filtered in exchange for potassium or hydrogen ions, a process regulated by the hormone **aldosterone**. The **collecting duct** is the final common pathway for the **filtrate** (material extracted from the blood) that started in the glomerulus. It is in the glomerulus that antidiuretic hormone acts to increase the absorption of water back into the bloodstream, thereby preventing it from being lost in the urine. The nephron and the sites of action of the different classes of diuretics are shown in Figure 26-1.

DIURETIC DRUGS

Diuretics are classified according to their sites of action within the nephron, their chemical structure, and their diuretic potency. The sites of action of diuretics are determined by the way in which they affect the solute (electrolyte) and water transport systems located along the nephron (see Figure 26-1). The commonly used classes of drugs and individual drugs in these classes are listed in Table 26-1. The most potent diuretics are the loop diuretics, followed by mannitol, metolazone (a thiazide-like diuretic), the thiazides, and the potassium-sparing diuretics. The potency of these diuretics is a function of where they act in the nephron to inhibit sodium and water reabsorption. The more sodium and water prevented from reabsorption, the greater the diuresis and, consequently, the greater the potency.

CARBONIC ANHYDRASE INHIBITORS

Carbonic anhydrase inhibitors (CAIs) are chemical derivatives of sulfonamide antibiotics. As their name implies, CAIs inhibit the activity of the enzyme carbonic anhydrase, which is found in the kidneys, eyes, and other parts of the body. The site of action of the CAIs is the location of the carbonic anhydrase enzyme system along the nephron, primarily in the proximal tubule. For example, acetazolamide acts principally in the proximal tubule, which is directly distal to the glomerulus.

Mechanism of Action and Drug Effects

The carbonic anhydrase system in the kidney is located distal to the glomerulus in the proximal tubules, where approximately two thirds of all sodium and water are reabsorbed into the blood. A specific active transport system, located in the proximal tubules, operates the exchanges of sodium for hydrogen ions. For sodium and water to be reabsorbed back into the blood, hydrogen must be exchanged for it. Carbonic anhydrase facilitates hydrogen ions for this exchange. When its actions are inhibited by a CAI such as acetazolamide, little sodium and water can be reabsorbed into the blood, and they are eliminated with the urine. The CAIs reduce the formation of hydrogen (H^+) and bicarbonate (HCO_3^-) ions from carbon dioxide and water by the noncompetitive, reversible inhibition of carbonic anhydrase activity. This results in a reduction in the availability of these ions, primarily hydrogen, for use by active electrolyte transport systems.

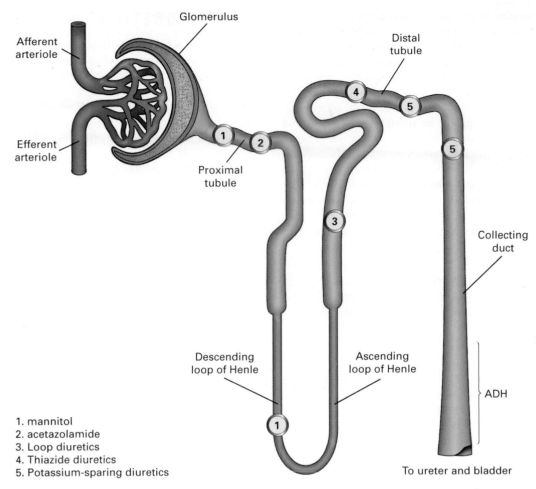

1. mannitol
2. acetazolamide
3. Loop diuretics
4. Thiazide diuretics
5. Potassium-sparing diuretics

FIG. 26-1   The nephron and diuretic sites of action. *ADH*, antidiuretic hormone.

The reduction of the formation of bicarbonate and hydrogen ions by CAIs can have many effects on other parts of the body. Metabolic acidosis induced by CAIs is beneficial in preventing certain seizure conditions. In addition, both the respiratory and metabolic acidosis induced by CAIs may increase oxygenation during hypoxia by increasing ventilation, cerebral blood flow, and the dissociation of oxygen from oxyhemoglobin, all of which is usually beneficial to the patient. An undesirable effect of CAIs is elevation of the blood glucose level, which causes glycosuria in patients with diabetes. This action may result in part from CAI-enhanced potassium loss in the urine.

Indications

The therapeutic applications of CAIs are wide and varied. They are commonly used in the treatment of glaucoma, edema, epilepsy, and high-altitude sickness.

CAIs are used principally as adjunct drugs in the long-term management of **open-angle glaucoma** that cannot be controlled by topical miotic drugs or epinephrine derivatives alone. Administration of CAIs together can increase the outflow of the aqueous humor; its obstruction is responsible for the glaucoma. They are also used short term in conjunction with miotics to lower intraocular pressure in preparation for ocular surgery in patients with acute ocular disorders or narrow-angle glaucoma and as an adjunct in the treatment of secondary glaucoma.

TABLE	26-1

Classification of Diuretics

Class	Drugs
Carbonic anhydrase inhibitors	acetazolamide, methazolamide
Loop diuretics	bumetanide, ethacrynic acid, furosemide
Osmotic diuretics	mannitol
Potassium-sparing diuretics	amiloride, spironolactone, triamterene
Thiazide and thiazide-like diuretics	chlorthalidone, chlorothiazide, hydrochlorothiazide, indapamide, metolazone, trichlormethiazide

Note: The drug classes in this table are presented in alphabetical order, not in the order of preferred use (e.g., thiazide diuretics are often the first drug of choice, followed by loop diuretics).

CAIs, particularly acetazolamide, are used to manage edema secondary to heart failure that has become resistant to other diuretics. However, as a class, CAIs are much less potent diuretics than loop diuretics or thiazides, and the metabolic acidosis they induce diminishes their diuretic effect in 2 to 4 days.

Acetazolamide may be a useful adjunct to other anticonvulsants in the prophylactic management of various forms of epilepsy. Tolerance to the anticonvulsant effects of CAIs develops quickly, however, and CAIs may be ineffective for prolonged therapy. Acetazolamide is also effective in both the prevention and treatment of the symptoms of high-altitude sickness. These symptoms include headache, nausea, shortness of breath, dizziness, drowsiness, and fatigue.

Contraindications

Contraindications to the use of CAIs include known drug allergy as well as hyponatremia, hypokalemia, severe kidney or liver dysfunction, adrenal gland insufficiency, and cirrhosis.

Adverse Effects

The more common undesirable effects of CAIs are metabolic abnormalities such as acidosis and hypokalemia. The CAIs may also produce drowsiness, anorexia, paraesthesias, hematuria, urticaria, photosensitivity, and melena.

Interactions

Significant drug interactions that occur with CAIs include an increase in digitalis toxicity when CAIs and digitalis are given together, as a result of the hypokalemia that CAIs may induce. The concomitant use of CAIs and corticosteroids may also cause hypokalemia. Use of CAIs with oral hypoglycemic drugs and quinidine may induce greater activity or toxicity of the latter drugs.

Dosages

For information on the dosages of acetazolamide, see its profile in the Drug Profiles section.

LOOP DIURETICS

Loop diuretics (bumetanide, ethacrynic acid, and furosemide) are potent diuretics. Bumetanide and furosemide are chemically related to the sulfonamide antibiotics.

Mechanism of Action and Drug Effects

Loop diuretics have kidney, cardiovascular, and metabolic effects. Their kidney effects are their major mechanism of action. Loop diuretics act primarily along the thick ascending limb of the loop of Henle, blocking chloride and, secondarily, sodium reabsorption. Loop diuretics increase urinary calcium excretion and cause a significant increase in magnesium excretion. They are also believed to activate kidney prostaglandins, which results in dilation of the blood vessels of the kidneys, the lungs, and the rest of the body (i.e., reduction in kidney, pulmonary, and systemic vascular resistance). The beneficial hemodynamic effects of loop diuretics are a reduction in both the preload and central venous pressures, the filling pressures of the ventricles. These actions make them useful in the treatment of edema associated with heart failure, liver cirrhosis, and kidney disease.

Loop diuretics are particularly useful when rapid diuresis is needed because of their rapid onset of action. In addition, the diuretic effect lasts at least 2 hours. Loop diuretics possess a distinct advantage over thiazide diuretics in that their diuretic action continues even when the creatinine clearance decreases to below 25 mL/min. This means that despite diminishing kidney function, loop diuretics can still act. Because of their potent diuretic effect and the duration of this effect, loop diuretics are effective in a single daily dose. This allows the kidney tubule time to partially compensate for the potassium depletion and other electrolyte disturbances that often accompany round-the-clock diuretic therapy. Despite this, the major adverse effect of loop diuretics is electrolyte disturbances. Prolonged administration of high doses can result in hearing loss stemming from ototoxicity, although this is rare.

To summarize, loop diuretics produce a potent diuresis and subsequent loss of fluid. The resulting decreased fluid volume leads to a decreased return of blood to the

---

 DRUG PROFILES

Although there are two CAIs (see Table 26-1), by far the most widely prescribed is acetazolamide, and thus it is the only CAI profiled.

acetazolamide

Use of acetazolamide (Acetazolam) is contraindicated in patients who have a known hypersensitivity to it and to sulfonamides, as well as in those with significant liver or kidney dysfunction, low serum potassium or sodium levels, acidosis, and adrenal gland failure. Acetazolamide is available in oral and parenteral forms. The parenteral

form is available through the Special Access Programme, Health Canada. The extended-release capsule is recommended for use in glaucoma and high-altitude sickness. A recommended dosage for children is oral administration of 8 to 30 mg/kg/day in 3 divided doses. A common oral dosage for adults is 250 mg to 1 g daily in divided doses. Acetazolamide is classified as pregnancy category C.

PHARMACOKINETICS

Half-Life	Onset	Peak	Duration
PO: 10–15 hr	PO: 1 hr	PO: 2–4 hr	PO: 8–12 hr

heart, or decreased filling pressures. This sequence of events has the following cardiovascular effects:

- Reduces blood pressure
- Reduces pulmonary vascular resistance
- Reduces systemic vascular resistance
- Reduces central venous pressure
- Reduces left ventricular end-diastolic pressure

The metabolic effects of loop diuretics are secondary to the electrolyte losses resulting from potent diuresis. Major electrolyte losses include loss of sodium and potassium and, to a lesser extent, calcium. Changes in the plasma levels of insulin, glucagon, and growth hormone levels have been associated with loop diuretic therapy.

Indications

Loop diuretics are used to manage edema associated with heart failure and liver or kidney disease, manage hypertension, and increase the kidney excretion of calcium in patients with hypercalcemia. As with certain other classes of diuretics, they may also be indicated in cases of heart failure resulting from diastolic dysfunction.

Contraindications

Contraindications to the use of loop diuretics include known drug allergy and may include allergy to sulfonamide antibiotics, hepatic coma, or severe electrolyte loss.

Adverse Effects

Common undesirable effects of loop diuretics are listed in Table 26-2. Other less common effects associated with bumetanide therapy are muscle cramps, dry mouth, arthritic pain, and encephalopathy. These are more likely to occur in patients with pre-existing liver disease, which may require selection of a different drug. Ethacrynic acid may cause neutropenia and, rarely, episodes of Henoch–Schönlein purpura. Furosemide can produce erythema multiforme, exfoliative dermatitis, photosensitivity, and, in rare cases, aplastic anemia.

Because of the increased urinary calcium secretion, loop diuretics can lead to bone loss if used long term. Several studies have implicated loop diuretics in bone loss and resultant osteoporotic hip and other fractures in older adult men.

Toxicity and Management of Overdose

Electrolyte loss and dehydration, which can result in circulatory failure, are the main toxic effects of loop diuretics that require attention. Treatment involves electrolyte and fluid replacement.

Interactions

Loop diuretics exhibit both neurotoxic and nephrotoxic properties, and they produce additive effects when given in combination with drugs that have similar toxicities. The drug interactions are summarized in Table 26-3.

Loop diuretics also affect certain laboratory results. They cause increases in the serum levels of uric acid, glucose, alanine aminotransferase, and aspartate aminotransferase. Their combined use with a thiazide (particularly metolazone) results in the blockade of sodium and water reabsorption at multiple sites in the nephron, a property referred to as *sequential nephron blockade*, which increases their effects. The reduction of vascular resistance induced by loop diuretics may be impeded when taken concurrently with nonsteroidal anti-inflammatory drugs (NSAIDs) because these two drug classes have opposite effects on prostaglandin activity.

Dosages

For the recommended dosages of loop diuretics, see the Dosages table on p. 495.

TABLE 26-2

Loop Diuretics: Common Adverse Effects

Body System	Adverse Effects
Central nervous	Dizziness, headache, tinnitus, blurred vision
Gastrointestinal	Nausea, vomiting, diarrhea
Hematological	Agranulocytosis, thrombocytopenia, neutropenia
Metabolic	Hypokalemia, hyperglycemia, hyperuricemia, hypomagnesemia, increased urinary calcium excretion

TABLE 26-3

Loop Diuretics: Common Drug Interactions

Drug	Mechanism	Results
Aminoglycosides chloroquine vancomycin	Additive effect	Increased neurotoxicity, notably ototoxicity
Corticosteroids digoxin	Hypokalemia	Additive hypokalemia Increased digoxin toxicity
lithium	Decrease in kidney excretion	Increased lithium toxicity
NSAIDs	Inhibition of kidney prostaglandins	Decreased diuretic activity
Sulfonylureas	Decrease in glucose tolerance	Hyperglycemia

NSAIDs, nonsteroidal anti-inflammatory drugs.

DRUG PROFILES

The currently available loop diuretics are bumetanide, ethacrynic acid, and furosemide. As a class they are potent diuretics, but potency varies for the different drugs. The equipotent doses for the drugs are as follows:

PHARMACOKINETICS

bumetanide	ethacrynic acid	furosemide
1 mg	50 mg	40 mg

▸▸ furosemide

Furosemide (Lasix, Lasix Special, Novo-Semide) is by far the most commonly used loop diuretic in clinical practice and the prototypical drug in this class. Structurally it is related to the sulfonamide antibiotics (Chapter 38). It has all of the therapeutic and adverse characteristics of the loop diuretics mentioned earlier. It is primarily used in the management of pulmonary edema and the edema associated with heart failure, liver disease, nephrotic syndrome, and **ascites** (the accumulation of fluid in the peritoneal area). It has also been used in the treatment of hypertension, usually that caused by heart failure.

Furosemide is contraindicated in patients who have shown a hypersensitivity to sulfonamides; in infants and lactating women; and in patients suffering from anuria, hypovolemia, and electrolyte depletion. It is available in oral form as 40 mg/5 mL and 10 mg/mL solutions. It is also available as 20, 40, and 80 mg tablets and as a special 500 mg high-dosage formulation intended exclusively for patients with severely impaired kidney function who do not respond to traditional doses of furosemide. In parenteral form, it is available as a 10 mg/mL injection. Recommended dosages are given in the Dosages table on p. 495.

PHARMACOKINETICS

Half-Life	Onset	Peak	Duration
PO: 1–2 hr	PO: 1 hr	PO: 1–2 hr	PO: 4–8 hr
IV: 1 hr	IV: 30 min	IV: 1 hr	IV: 2 hr

OSMOTIC DIURETICS

The osmotic diuretics include mannitol, urea, organic acids, and glucose. Mannitol, a nonabsorbable solute, is the most commonly used.

Mechanism of Action and Drug Effects

Mannitol works along the entire nephron. Its major site of action, however, is the proximal tubule and descending limb of the loop of Henle. Because it is nonabsorbable, it produces osmotic pressure in the glomerular filtrate, which, in turn, pulls fluid, primarily water, into the renal tubules from the surrounding tissues. This process also inhibits the tubular reabsorption of water and solutes, which produces a rapid diuresis. Ultimately, this reduces cellular edema and increases urine production, causing diuresis. However, it produces only a slight loss of electrolytes, especially sodium. Therefore, mannitol is not indicated for patients with peripheral edema because it does not promote sufficient sodium excretion.

Mannitol may induce vasodilation and in doing so increases both glomerular filtration and kidney plasma flow. This makes it an excellent drug for preventing kidney damage during acute kidney failure. It is also often used to reduce intracranial pressure and cerebral edema resulting from head trauma. In addition, mannitol treatment may be tried when elevated intraocular pressure is unresponsive to other drug therapies.

Indications

Mannitol is the osmotic diuretic of choice. It is commonly used in the treatment of patients in the early, oliguric phase of acute kidney failure. For it to be effective in this setting, however, enough kidney blood flow and glomerular filtration must still remain to enable the drug to reach the kidney tubules. Increased kidney blood flow resulting from the dilation of blood vessels supplying blood to the kidneys is another therapeutic benefit of mannitol therapy in such patients. It can also be used to promote the excretion of toxic substances, reduce intracranial pressure, and treat cerebral edema. In addition, it can be used as a genitourinary irrigant in the preparation of patients for transurethral surgical procedures and as supportive treatment in patients with edema induced by other conditions.

Contraindications

Contraindications to the use of mannitol include known drug allergy, severe kidney disease, pulmonary edema (loop diuretics are used instead), and active intracranial bleeding.

Adverse Effects

The significant undesirable effects of mannitol include convulsions, thrombophlebitis, and pulmonary congestion. Other less significant effects are headaches, chest pains, tachycardia, blurred vision, chills, and fever.

Interactions

There are no drugs that interact significantly with mannitol.

Dosages

For the recommended dosages of mannitol, see the Dosages table on p. 495.

DRUG PROFILES

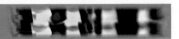

▸▸ *mannitol*

Mannitol (Osmitrol, Resectisol) is the prototypical osmotic diuretic. Its use is contraindicated in patients with a hypersensitivity to it as well as in those suffering from anuria, severe dehydration, pulmonary congestion, or cerebral hemorrhage. Treatment should be terminated if severe heart or kidney impairment develops after the initiation of therapy. It is available only in parenteral form as 5%, 10%, 20%, and 25% solutions for intravenous injection. It is also available with sorbital for irrigations. Mannitol

may crystallize when exposed to low temperatures. This is more likely to occur when concentrations exceed 15%. For this reason, mannitol should always be administered intravenously through a filter, and vials of the drug are often stored in a warmer in the pharmacy. Recommended dosages are given in the Dosages table on p. 495.

PHARMACOKINETICS

Half-Life	Onset	Peak	Duration
IV: 1.5 hr	IV: 0.5–1 hr	IV: 0.25–2 hr	IV: 6–8 hr

DOSAGES   Selected Loop Diuretics and Osmotic Diuretics

Drug (Pregnancy Category)	Pharmacological Class	Usual Dosage Range	Indications
bumetanide (Burinex) (C)	Loop diuretic	*Adult* PO: 0.5–2 mg/day as a single dose; max 10 mg/day; intermittent dose schedule recommended	Edema
ethacrynic acid (Edecrin)	Loop diuretic	*Children* PO: Initial dose 25 mg/day; careful titration 25 mg increases to effect *Adult* PO: 50–100 mg/day; max 200 mg/day IV: 0.5–1 mg/kg	Heart failure, hypertension, kidney failure, pulmonary edema, cirrhosis
▸▸furosemide (Lasix, Lasix Special, Novo-Semide) (C)	Loop diuretic	*Children* IM/IV: 0.5–1 mg/kg; do not exceed 1 mg/kg/day PO: 0.5–1 mg/kg q4h; max 2 mg/kg/day divided *Adult* IM/IV: 20–40 mg/dose; max 100 mg/day; PO: 20–80 mg/day as a single dose; max 200 mg/day	Heart failure, hypertension, kidney failure, pulmonary edema, cirrhosis
▸▸mannitol (Osmitrol, Resectisol) (C)	Osmotic diuretic	*Adult* IV infusion: 50–200 g/day, 1.5–2 g/kg over 30–60 min Suggested loading dose of 25 g, followed by an infusion rate to produce a urine flow of at least 100 mL/hr	Renal failure; abnormally high intraocular and intracranial pressure

IM, intramuscular; *IV,* intravenous; *PO,* oral.

POTASSIUM-SPARING DIURETICS

The currently available potassium-sparing diuretics are amiloride, spironolactone, and triamterene (in Canada triamterene is available only in combination with hydrochlorothiazide). These diuretics are also referred to as aldosterone-inhibiting diuretics because they block the aldosterone receptors. In fact, spironolactone is a competitive antagonist of aldosterone and for this reason causes sodium and water to be excreted and potassium to be retained. It is the most commonly used of the three drugs.

Mechanism of Action and Drug Effects

Potassium-sparing diuretics act in the collecting ducts and distal convoluted tubules, where they interfere with sodium–potassium exchange. Spironolactone competitively binds to aldosterone receptors and therefore blocks the reabsorption of sodium and water that is induced by aldosterone secretion. These receptors are found primarily in the distal tubule. Amiloride and triamterene do not bind to aldosterone receptors; however, they inhibit both aldosterone-induced and basal sodium reabsorption, working in both the distal tubule and collecting ducts.

SPECIAL POPULATIONS: CHILDREN

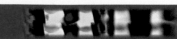

Use of Diuretics

- Dosages of diuretic medications for children should be calculated carefully, regardless of whether the patient is in the hospital or in the home setting. Weight should be measured daily at the same time every day so that therapeutic effects and adverse effects of diuretics can be assessed. Because children are at greater risk for adverse effects and toxicity, they require closer and more cautious daily assessment to avoid excess fluid volume and electrolyte loss, hypotension, and shock.

- The half-life of furosemide is increased in neonates, so the interval between doses may need to be lengthened, as ordered by the physician.

- Oral forms of diuretics may be taken with food or milk and should be taken early in the day and at the same time every day.

- Lengthy exposure to either heat or sun should be avoided because it may precipitate heat stroke,

exhaustion, and fluid volume loss in children taking diuretics.

- Thiazide diuretics cross the placenta and to the fetus and small amounts are distributed in breast milk. Thus breastfeeding is not advised for mothers who are taking these drugs. For children, oral solutions of thiazide diuretics are available.

- Laboratory tests that may be altered by diuretics include increased serum levels of calcium, bilirubin, creatinine, glucose, and uric acid. Adverse effects, including potassium depletion and loss of volume, may be worse in children because of age and increased sensitivity to these drugs.

- Loop diuretics may also interfere with laboratory findings in children. Blood urea nitrogen, uric acid, and serum glucose levels may be increased, whereas calcium, chloride, magnesium, potassium, and sodium levels may be decreased.

They are often prescribed for children with heart failure because their heart problems are often accompanied by an excess secretion of aldosterone, and the loop and thiazide diuretics are often ineffective in their management (see also Special Populations: Children, on use of diuretics in children).

Because approximately 3% of the total filtered urine volume reaches the collecting ducts, the potassium-sparing diuretics are relatively weak compared with the thiazide and loop diuretics. When diuresis is needed, they are generally used as adjuncts to thiazide treatment. This combination is beneficial in two respects. First, the drugs have synergistic diuretic effects; second, the two drugs counteract the adverse metabolic effects of each other. The thiazide diuretics cause potassium, magnesium, and chloride to be lost in the urine, and the potassium-sparing diuretics counteract this effect by elevating the potassium and chloride levels.

Indications

The therapeutic applications of the potassium-sparing diuretics vary depending on the particular drug. Spironolactone and triamterene are used in the treatment of hyperaldosteronism and hypertension and to reverse the potassium loss caused by the potassium-wasting (e.g., loop, thiazide) diuretics. One common feature of heart failure is a hyperactive renin–angiotensin–aldosterone system. Research has identified this hyperactivity as a causative factor in permanent ventricular myocardial wall damage, known as remodelling, following myocardial infarction. Clinical drug trials are increasingly demonstrating a cardioprotective benefit of spironolactone, because of its aldosterone-inhibiting activity, in preventing this remodelling process. The uses for amiloride are similar to those for spironolactone and triamterene, but amiloride

is less effective in the long term. It maybe more effective than spironolactone or triamterene in the treatment of metabolic alkalosis, however. It is primarily used in the management of heart failure. As with certain other classes of diuretics, potassium-sparing diuretics may also be indicated in cases of heart failure due to diastolic dysfunction.

Contraindications

Contraindications to the use of potassium-sparing diuretics include known drug allergy, hyperkalemia (e.g., serum potassium level greater than 5.5 mmol/L), and severe kidney failure or anuria. Triamterene may also be contraindicated in cases of severe liver failure.

Adverse Effects

Potassium-sparing diuretics have several common undesirable effects, which are listed in Table 26-4. There are also some significant adverse effects specific to individual drugs. Spironolactone can cause gynecomastia, amenorrhea, irregular menses, and postmenopausal bleeding. Triamterene may reduce folic acid levels and cause the formation of kidney stones and urinary casts. It may also precipitate megaloblastic anemia. Hyperkalemia also may occur when potassium-sparing

TABLE 26-4

Potassium-Sparing Diuretics: Common Adverse Effects

Body System	Adverse Effects
Central nervous	Dizziness, headache
Gastrointestinal	Cramps, nausea, vomiting, diarrhea
Other	Urinary frequency, weakness, hyperkalemia

diuretics are used in combination with each other or with other potassium-sparing drugs such as angiotensin-converting enzyme (ACE) inhibitors (see Chapter 25, as well as the Interactions section that follows). However, adverse effects from triamterene use are rare.

Interactions

The concomitant use of potassium-sparing diuretics and lithium, ACE inhibitors, or potassium supplements can result in significant drug interactions. The administration of ACE inhibitors or potassium supplements in combination with potassium-sparing diuretics can result in hyperkalemia. When lithium and potassium-sparing diuretics are given together, lithium toxicity can result. NSAIDs can inhibit kidney prostaglandins, decreasing blood flow to the kidneys and thus decreasing the delivery of diuretic drugs to this site of action. This, in turn, can lead to a diminished diuretic response.

Dosages

For the recommended dosages of potassium-sparing diuretics, see the Dosages table below.

 DRUG PROFILES

amiloride hydrochloride

Amiloride hydrochloride (Midamor) is generally used in combination with a thiazide or loop diuretic in the tretament of heart failure. Hyperkalemia may occur in approximately 10% of the patients who take amiloride alone. It should be used with caution in patients with kidney impairment or diabetes mellitus and in the older adult. It has only weak antihypertensive properties. Amiloride is available only in oral form. It is also available in combination with hydrochlorothiazide (Moduret, Novamilor). Recommended dosages are given in the Dosages table below.

PHARMACOKINETICS

Half-Life	Onset	Peak	Duration
6–9 hr	2 hr	6–10 hr	24 hr

▸▸ spironolactone

Structurally, spironolactone (Aldactone) is a synthetic steroid that blocks aldosterone receptors. It is used in high dosages for the treatment of ascites, a condition commonly associated with cirrhosis of the liver. The serum potassium level should be monitored frequently in patients who have impaired kidney function or who are currently taking potassium supplements because hyperkalemia is a common complication of spironolactone therapy. It is the potassium-sparing diuretic most commonly prescribed for children who have heart failure because heart failure in children often causes excess aldosterone to be secreted, which, in turn, results in increased sodium and water reabsorption. Recently, spironolactone has been shown to reduce morbidity and mortality rates in patients with severe heart failure when added to standard therapy (see Research: The Randomized Aldactone Evaluation Study). This is believed to be primarily due to its reduction of ventricular remodelling after myocardial infarction. Of the three commonly used potassium-sparing diuretics, spironolactone has the greatest antihypertensive activity. It is available only in oral form. It is also available in combination with hydrochlorothiazide (Aldactazide, Apo-Spirazide). Recommended dosages are given in the Dosages table below.

PHARMACOKINETICS

Half-Life	Onset	Peak	Duration
13–24 hr	1–3 days	2–3 days	2–3 days

triamterene

The pharmacological properties of triamterene are similar to those of amiloride. Like amiloride, triamterene acts directly on the distal renal tubule of the nephron to depress the reabsorption of sodium and the excretion of potassium and hydrogen, processes otherwise stimulated at that site by aldosterone. It has little or no antihypertensive effect. It is available only in combination with hydrochlorothiazide (Riva-Zide). Recommended dosages are given in the Dosages table below.

PHARMACOKINETICS

Half-Life	Onset	Peak	Duration
2–3 hr	2–4 hr	6–8 hr	12–16 hr

DOSAGES   Selected Potassium-Sparing Diuretic Drugs

Drug (Pregnancy Category)	Pharmacological Class	Usual Dosage Range	Indications
amiloride hydrochloride (Midamor) (B)	Potassium-sparing diuretics	*Adult* PO: 5–20 mg/day	Edema, heart failure (as an adjunct to potassium-sparing diuretics)
▸▸ spironolactone (Aldactone) (D)	Potassium-sparing diuretics	*Children* PO: 3 mg/kg/day single or divided; 1–2 mg/kg maintenance *Adult* PO: 25–200 mg/day	Edema, hypertension, heart failure, ascites
triamterene 50 mg/ hydrochlorothiazide 25 mg (Riva-Zide) (D)	Potassium-sparing diuretics	*Adult* PO: 1–4 tablets daily after meals	Diuretic–antihypertensive

RESEARCH

The Randomized Aldactone Evaluation Study (RALES)

The landmark RALES was a randomized, blinded placebo-controlled trial involving 1663 patients (822 received spironolactone, 841 placebo) with a mean age of 65 years. Participants were primarily White men with severe (class III and IV) heart failure and a left ventricular ejection fraction (LVEF) less than 35%. Subjects received 25 mg of spironolactone in addition to existing therapy (digoxin, β-blockers, and ACE inhibitors). Subjects were closely monitored over a 2-year period. Those receiving spironolactone had a 30% reduced mortality. As a result, spironolactone has become a standard treatment in patients with severe heart failure. Guidelines suggest the use of spironolactone for patients with an LVEF less than 30% and either severe symptomatic chronic heart failure or acute heart failure following acute myocardial infarction, unless there is renal dysfunction or hyperkalemia. A rise in potassium may occur following treatment with spironolactone and may be severe. Potassium should be monitored three times per week when initiated or with dose adjustment and once monthly when stabilized. Generally, a potassium level of 4.4–5.4 mmol/L is desirable when using diuretics.

Source: Pitt, B., Zannad, F., Remme, W. J., Cody, R., Castaigne, A., Perez, A., et al. for The Randomized Aldactone Evaluation Study Investigators. (1999). The effect of spironolactone on morbidity and mortality in patients with severe heart failure. *New England Journal of Medicine, 341*(10), 709–717.

THIAZIDES AND THIAZIDE-LIKE DIURETICS

Thiazide and thiazide-like diuretics are generally considered equivalent in their effects. Thiazide diuretics, as with several of the loop diuretics, are chemical derivatives (benzothiadiazines) of sulfonamide antibiotics. Chlorthalidone is distinguished by its prolonged half-life of up to 72 hours. Metolazone may be more effective than other drugs in this class in the treatment of patients with kidney dysfunction. Hydrochlorothiazide is undoubtedly the most commonly prescribed and the least expensive of the generic preparations. Thiazide diuretics include chlorothiazide, hydrochlorothiazide, and trichlormethiazide. Thiazide-like diuretics are similar in action to the thiazides and include chlorthalidone, indapamide, and metolazone. Of all of these drugs, hydrochlorothiazide and metolazone are by far the most commonly prescribed in practice, although the others currently remain on the Canadian market.

Mechanism of Action and Drug Effects

Thiazides are used as adjunct drugs in the management of heart failure, liver cirrhosis, and edema of various origins. The primary site of action of thiazides and thiazide-like diuretics is the distal convoluted tubule, where they inhibit the reabsorption of sodium, potassium, and chloride. This results in osmotic water loss. Thiazides also cause direct relaxation of the arterioles, which reduces afterload. Decreased preload and decreased afterload are the beneficial hemodynamic effects. This makes them effective for the treatment of both heart failure and hypertension.

As kidney function decreases, the efficacy of thiazides diminishes, probably because delivery of the drug to the site of activity is impaired. Thiazides generally should not be used if the creatinine clearance is less than 30 to 50 mL/min. Normal creatinine clearance is 125 mL/min. The only exception is metolazone, which remains effective to a creatinine clearance of 10 mL/min. The major adverse effects of the drugs stem from the electrolyte disturbances they produce. They are noted for precipitating hypokalemia and hypercalcemia, as well as metabolic disturbances such as hyperlipidemia, hyperglycemia, and hyperuricemia.

Indications

Thiazide and thiazide-like diuretics are also approved by Health Canada for the treatment of hypertension and edematous states. Any of these drugs can be used either as monotherapy or in combination with other drugs. This group of diuretics may also be useful as adjunct drugs in the treatment of edema related to heart failure, liver cirrhosis, and corticosteroid or estrogen therapy. As with certain other classes of diuretics, they may be indicated in cases of heart failure due to diastolic dysfunction.

Contraindications

Contraindications to the use of thiazides and thiazide-like diuretics include known drug allergy, hepatic coma (metolazone), anuria, and severe kidney failure.

Adverse Effects

Major adverse effects of thiazide and thiazide-like diuretics relate to the electrolyte disturbances they cause. These are mainly reduced potassium levels and elevated levels of calcium, lipids, glucose, and uric acid. Other effects, such as gastrointestinal disturbances, skin rashes, photosensitivity, thrombocytopenia, pancreatitis, and cholecystitis, are less common. Dizziness and vertigo are common adverse effects of metolazone therapy and are attributed to sudden shifts in the plasma volume brought about by the drug. Headache, impotence, and reduced libido are other important adverse effects of these drugs. Many of these adverse effects are dose related and are seen at higher doses, especially those above 25 mg. The more common adverse effects of thiazide and thiazide-like diuretics are listed in Table 26-5.

TABLE 26-5

Thiazide and Thiazide-Like Diuretics: Potential Adverse Effects

Body System/Process	Adverse Effects
Central nervous	Dizziness, headache, blurred vision, paraesthesia, decreased libido
Gastrointestinal	Anorexia, nausea, vomiting, diarrhea, pancreatitis, cholecystitis
Genitourinary	Erectile dysfunction
Hematological	Jaundice, leukopenia, purpura, agranulocytosis, aplastic anemia, thrombocytopenia
Integumentary	Urticaria, photosensitivity
Metabolic	Hypokalemia, glycosuria, hyperglycemia, hyperuricemia, hypochloremic alkalosis

Toxicity and Management of Overdose

An overdose of these drugs can lead to an electrolyte imbalance resulting from hypokalemia. Symptoms include anorexia, nausea, lethargy, muscle weakness, mental confusion, and hypotension. Treatment involves electrolyte replacement.

Interactions

Thiazides and related drugs interact with corticosteroids, diazoxide, digitalis, and oral hypoglycemic. The mechanisms and results of these interactions are summarized in Table 26-6. Excessive consumption of licorice can lead to an additive hypokalemia in patients taking thiazides.

Dosages

For information on the dosages for thiazide and thiazide-like diuretics, see the Dosages table on p. 500.

TABLE 26-6

Thiazide and Thiazide-Like Diuretics: Common Drug Interactions

Drug	Mechanism	Result
Corticosteroids	Additive effect	Hypokalemia
diazoxide	Additive effect	Hyperkalemia
digoxin	Hypokalemia	Increased digoxin toxicity
lithium	Decreased clearance	Increased lithium toxicity
NSAIDs	Inhibition of kidney prostaglandins	Decreased diuretic activity
Oral antidiabetic drugs	Antagonism	Reduced therapeutic hypoglycemic effect

 # DRUG PROFILES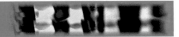

▶▶ hydrochlorothiazide

Hydrochlorothiazide, which is considered the prototypical thiazide diuretic, is a commonly prescribed and inexpensive thiazide diuretic. It is also a safe and effective diuretic. Hydrochlorothiazide is used in combination with many other drugs: amiloride, angiotensin II receptor antagonists, methyldopa, propranolol, spironolactone, triamterene, hydralazine, ACE inhibitors, β-blockers, and labetalol. Dosages exceeding 50 mg/day rarely produce additional clinical results and may only increase drug toxicity. This property is known as the *ceiling effect.* Hydrochlorothiazide use is contraindicated in patients with a known hypersensitivity to thiazides or sulfonamides and in those suffering from anuria, kidney decompensation, or hypomagnesemia. It is available only in oral form. Recommended dosages are given in the Dosages table on p. 500.

PHARMACOKINETICS

Half-Life	Onset	Peak	Duration
2.5–14.8 hr	2 hr	4–6 hr	6–12 hr

metolazone

Metolazone (Zaroxolyn) is a thiazide-like diuretic that appears to be more potent than thiazide diuretics. This greater potency is most visible in patients with kidney dysfunction. One striking advantage of metolazone is that it remains effective to a creatinine clearance as low as 10 mL/min. It may also be given in combination with loop diuretics to obtain a potent diuresis in patients with severe symptoms of heart failure. Metolazone is contraindicated in patients with a known hypersensitivity to thiazides or sulfonamides, in those with anuria, and in pregnant or lactating women. It is available only in oral form. Recommended dosages are given in the Dosages table on p. 500.

PHARMACOKINETICS

Half-Life	Onset	Peak	Duration
6–20 hr	1 hr	2 hr	12–24 hr

DOSAGES	Thiazide and Selected Thiazide-Like Diuretic Drugs		
Drug (Pregnancy Category)	Pharmacological Class	Usual Dosage Range	Indications
hydrochlorothiazide (B)	Thiazide diuretic	*Neonates and Infants under 6 mo* PO: 2.5–3.5 mg/kg/day divided bid *Infants over 6 mo and Children under 12 yr* PO: 2.5 mg/kg/day divided bid *Adult* PO: 25–200 mg/day, usually divided PO: 12.5–100 mg/day *Older Adult* PO: 12.5–25 mg/day	Edema, hypertension, heart failure, nephrotic syndrome
metolazone (Zaroxolyn) (B)	Thiazide-like diuretic	*Children* PO: 0.2–0.4 mg/kg/day *Adult* PO: 2.5–20 mg/day	Edema, hypertension, heart failure, nephrotic syndrome

IN MY FAMILY

Wax Gourd Soup for Nephritis
(as told by L.Z, of Chinese descent)

"One of my family members has had nephritis; some traditional Chinese physicians have recommended that he drink wax gourd soup. The ingredients of the soup include 500 g of wax gourd and 30 g of red adzuki bean; add a tiny bit of salt, then boil all the ingredients with about 2–3 litres of water for 30 minutes. Chinese people believe that wax gourd helps increase urine output and decrease edema and has a hydrating effect."

NURSING PROCESS

Assessment

Before giving a patient any type of diuretic, the nurse should obtain a complete history, including medication history and nursing history. A thorough physical assessment should be completed and all findings documented. Because fluid volume levels and electrolyte concentrations are affected by diuretics, the patient's baseline fluid volume status (as indicated by vital signs, weight, and intake and output measurements) should be assessed and documented. Postural blood pressures (lying, sitting, standing) should be assessed before and during drug therapy because of diuretic-induced fluid volume loss. This volume loss may lead to postural hypotension or a drop in blood pressure (e.g., of 20 mm Hg or more) upon standing. Skin turgor, status of moisture levels of mucous membranes, and capillary refill are also important to assess with diuretic therapy.

Serum potassium, sodium, chloride, magnesium, calcium, uric acid, and creatinine levels should also be measured and documented as ordered. Other laboratory studies may include arterial blood gases and blood pH. Cautious use of diuretics, with close monitoring of fluid volume status, electrolytes, and vital signs, is recommended in patients with the following disorders or conditions: hypokalemia, hypovolemia, kidney disease, liver disease, lupus erythematosus, diabetes, chronic obstructive pulmonary disease, and gout. Loop diuretics are more potent than thiazides, combination products, and potassium-sparing diuretics, so these drugs may pose more problems for patients of any age. Patients with altered kidney or liver functioning may react more sensitively to diuretics and subsequent fluid volume loss. Cautions, contraindications, and drug interactions associated with all of the diuretics need to be considered in the nursing assessment for any of these drugs. Potassium-sparing diuretics may lead to hyperkalemia, and the patient's blood levels of potassium need to be closely monitored. In addition, a significant concern that must be part of the nursing assessment for loop diuretics is that they adversely react with other medications that are ototoxic or nephrotoxic (e.g., sulfonamide antibiotics).

Nursing Diagnoses

- Decreased cardiac output related to adverse effects of diuretics
- Deficient fluid volume related to drug effects of diuretics
- Risk for injury related to postural hypotension and dizziness

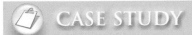

Diuretic Therapy

Primary hypertension has been diagnosed in Ms. G., a 47-year-old woman. Blood pressure readings have been ranging between 158 and 172 mm Hg systolic and 94 and 110 mm Hg diastolic. Average blood pressure over the past month has been 156/98 mm Hg. There is a strong family history of hypertension. Ms. G. is a single parent of two adolescents. She is also trying to keep up with her responsibilities as a full-time assistant professor of education at a local urban university and works more than 40 hours a week. There is no evidence of kidney insufficiency or heart damage at this time, nor is there evidence of retinopathy or other signs and symptoms of end-organ disease. No other problems are reported. Ms. G. is started on 50 mg of hydrochlorothiazide daily with a small dose of the β-blocker atenolol.

1. Discuss the antihypertensive effects of hydrochlorothiazide.

2. What information must you share with this patient to increase adherence and decrease adverse effects? What should she be educated about concerning her disease process and the impact of adherence to the drug therapy regimen?

3. What should be included in her daily regimen (e.g., exercise, diet, journalling)?

4. What other nonpharmacological measures should you tell the patient about that can better help her control her blood pressure?

For answers see http://evolve.elsevier.com/Canada/Lilley/pharmacology/.

• Deficient knowledge related to lack of experience with newly prescribed diuretic therapy
• Acute pain related to occurrence of headache from adverse effects of diuretics
• Nonadherence to the treatment regimen because of lack of information about the adverse effects of medications

Planning

Goals

• Patient will regain fluid and electrolyte balance.
• Patient will remain free of the complications associated with diuretic use.
• Patient will remain free of injury while on diuretics.
• Patient will remain adherent to the therapy regimen.

Outcome Criteria

• Patient maintains normal levels of electrolytes (sodium, potassium, and chloride values) while taking diuretics.
• Patient continues to show or regains normal cardiac output while on diuretic therapy as evidenced by vital signs, adequate intake, and output within normal limits (pulse less than 100 and higher than 60 beats/min; blood pressure 120/80 mm Hg; urine output less than or equal to 30 mL/hr).
• Patient's skin is pliable and without edema or dryness.
• Patient rises slowly and changes positions slowly and cautiously while receiving diuretics.
• Patient states the importance of and rationale for follow-up visits with the physician, such as monitoring for adverse effects, dehydration, and fluid and electrolyte imbalances.

• Patient reports dizziness, fainting, palpitations, tingling, confusion, or disorientation to the physician immediately.

Implementation

Blood pressure, pulse rate, intake and output, and daily weight should continue to be measured and recorded during diuretic therapy. Changes from the initial assessment data that would alert the nurse to possible problems with the drug therapy include complaints of weakness, fatigue, tremor, or muscle cramping, changes in mental health status, and cold clammy skin. Diuretic therapy may also precipitate heart irregularities, thus heart rate and rhythm are important parameters to continue to watch and document. Fluid loss may lead to constipation, requiring measures to prevent this through dietary changes or use of naturally occurring bulk formers (e.g., Metamucil-type drugs). Diuretics should always be given exactly as directed but with consideration of the patient's age and related needs. Dosing and timing of the drugs are often very important to enhance therapeutic effects and minimize adverse effects. Because diuretics taken late in the afternoon or evening may lead to nocturia, the patient may experience sleep deficit, so these medications should be scheduled for morning dosing. Safety concerns exist with nocturia, especially with the older adult because getting up in the middle of the night with possible confusion and dizziness may create the potential for falls and injury (see also Special Populations: The Older Adult: Diuretic Therapy).

Loop diuretics (if taken at high doses as ordered) may put patients at greater risk for volume and electrolyte depletion (e.g., hypokalemia, hyponatremia, dehydration). Monitoring of therapy should include frequent blood pressure and pulse rate, hydration status, capillary refill, and daily weights. Acute hypotensive episodes may also occur with higher doses of loop diuretics and precipitate syncope and falls, so safety measures should be implemented. Most oral diuretics should be taken with food to help minimize gastric upset. If giving intravenous dosage forms, it is crucial to check for diluents as well as drug incompatibilities. Rates of infusion should be confirmed and an infusion pump used. With potassium-sparing diuretics, potassium is reabsorbed and not excreted , so hyperkalemia, rather than hypokalemia, may become problematic. Signs and symptoms of hyperkalemia include nausea, vomiting, diarrhea, and abdominal cramping (Chapter 27) and should be reported immediately. See Patient Education for more information.

Evaluation

The therapeutic effects of diuretics include the resolution of or reduction in edema, fluid volume overload, heart failure, or hypertension or a return to normal intraocular pressures (if used for that purpose). The patient must also be monitored for the occurrence of adverse reactions to the diuretics, such as metabolic acidosis (arterial blood gas values should be monitored), drowsiness, lethargy, hypokalemia, tachycardia, hypotension, leg cramps, restlessness, and a decrease in mental alertness. With potassium-sparing diuretics, hyperkalemia may be the adverse effect to monitor for with the therapeutic regimen. All goals and outcome criteria should be used in the evaluation process.

SPECIAL POPULATIONS: THE OLDER ADULT

Diuretic Therapy

- Measurements of the patient's height, weight, intake and output, blood pressure, pulse rate, respiratory rate, temperature; assessment of breath and heart sounds and edematous areas; and monitoring of serum sodium, potassium, and chloride levels should occur before and during diuretic drug therapy so that adverse effects and complications can be minimized or identified early.

- It should be emphasized to the older adult that diuretics should be taken at the same time every day. They are generally ordered to be taken in the morning to help prevent nocturia (voiding at night), which can result in lack of sleep. More importantly, nocturia can lead to injury if the individual needs to get out of bed to void, becomes dizzy or confused, and falls. A bedside commode may be used to decrease the risk of injury. If the older adult patient is living alone and has minimal or no assistance with the medication regimen, visits from a home health or other health professional may help ensure the safety, efficacy, and adherence not only in taking the medication but also in following all aspects of the therapeutic regimen.

- Caution should be exercised in the administration of diuretics to older adults because they are more sensitive to the therapeutic effects and adverse effects of these drugs (often reacting to smaller dosages of

medication than are required by other patients), such as dehydration, electrolyte loss, dizziness, and syncope.

- Patients should be encouraged to change positions slowly because of the risk of orthostatic hypotension and subsequent falls and injury. Daily weights, blood pressures, and overall well-being should be recorded daily.

- Carrying a card outlining medical history, blood pressure readings, names and telephone numbers for contact persons, and a list of medications is important to ensure safety and minimize potential complications. The card should be formatted such that it can fit in a wallet, with a copy placed on the refrigerator door or in another visible location so that it will be easily available to emergency personnel. Copies of the card should be given to the caregiver(s), family members, significant others, physicians, dentist, and relevant health care personnel. The card should be updated at regular intervals by the patient or another adult or by a physician involved in the patient's care. A card like this can be made easily using standard card stock or an index card. It can be placed in a wallet sleeve or be laminated, and information can be entered using an erasable pen or pencil. A sample showing the headings and content for such a card is provided on the next page:

Continued

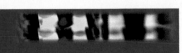

SPECIAL POPULATIONS: THE OLDER ADULT (cont'd)

1. Name: _____

2. Age: _____   3. Blood type: _____

4. Drug/food allergies: _____

5. Medical history (circle all that apply, and write in any not listed):

Anemia	Depression	Nerve problems
Asthma	Diabetes	Pacemaker or defibrillator device
Bleeding problems	Difficulty swallowing	Recent weight gain
Blood clots	Heart problems	Recent weight loss
Breathing problems	High blood pressure	Stroke
Cancer	Low blood pressure	Thyroid problems

   Others: _____

6. Current medications:

    Prescription drugs

    Name of drug: _____

    Dose amount: _____

    Frequency of doses: _____

    Condition for which drug is taken: _____

    Over-the-counter drugs

    Name of drug: _____

    Dose amount: _____

    Frequency of doses: _____

    Condition for which drug is taken: _____

    Herbals, vitamins, and other preparations

    Name of drug: _____

    Dose amount: _____

    Frequency of doses: _____

    Condition for which substance is taken: _____

7. Surgery (list all):

    Date: _____ Type and purpose: _____

    Any complications: _____

8. Prosthetics used: _____

9. Dental problems or concerns: _____

10. Wear glasses _____ Use hearing aid(s) _____ Need help with mobility _____

11. Other important information that should be known in case of emergency: _____

    _____

12. Contact names and telephone numbers: _____

PATIENT EDUCATION

Patients taking diuretics should be informed about the following:

- They should maintain proper nutritional intake and fluid volume status with attention to eating potassium-rich foods, except when contraindicated or when taking potassium-sparing diuretics.
- Foods high in potassium include bananas, oranges, dates, raisins, plums, fresh vegetables, potatoes (white and sweet), meat, fish, apricots, whole-grain cereals, and legumes.
- Potassium supplementation may be recommended by a physician when a patient's potassium level is below 3 mmol/L (Chapter 27).
- Frequent laboratory tests may be indicated at the beginning of therapy and during the use of diuretics.
- They need to change positions slowly and to rise slowly after sitting or lying to prevent dizziness and possible fainting (syncope).
- Forcing fluids may be needed, if not contraindicated, to maintain adequate hydration.
- They should report any unusual adverse effects or problems to their health care provider immediately.
- Keeping a daily journal noting weight, how the patient feels each day, and any other important information relative to their diagnosis and medical treatment is important.
- They can prevent constipation with an increase in fibre, bulk, roughage, and fluids if not contraindicated.
- Patients should be informed about the signs and symptoms of hypokalemia, such as weakness, leg cramps, and other cramping. In addition, encourage patients to avoid hot climates, excessive sweating, fever, and the use of saunas or hot tubs. Heat raises core body temperature and causes further loss of potassium and sodium through sweat. Should the patient experience excessive sweating, vomiting, or other fluid loss, hypovolemia may be exacerbated.
- Patients taking a diuretic along with a digitalis preparation should be instructed on how to monitor pulse rate; education should be extended to the patient's family members and caregivers. Emphasize the warning signs and symptoms of digitalis toxicity, such as anorexia, nausea, vomiting, and bradycardia (a pulse rate of less than 60 beats/min).
- Patients with diabetes mellitus who are also taking thiazide, loop diuretics, or both should be educated about close monitoring of blood glucose levels. These diuretics may cause elevation of blood glucose.

POINTS TO REMEMBER

- The five main types of diuretics are CAIs and loop, osmotic, potassium-sparing, thiazide, and thiazide-like diuretics.
- The loop, potassium-sparing, thiazide, and thiazide-like diuretics are most commonly used.
- The nurse must remember that the loop diuretics are more potent than the thiazides, combination diuretics, and potassium-sparing diuretics. The two most commonly prescribed loop diuretics are furosemide and bumetanide.
- Thiazide diuretics are the most commonly used diuretics and the least expensive because several generic preparations are available.
- Hydrochlorothiazide is considered the prototypical thiazide diuretic and is used as adjunctive therapy to manage liver cirrhosis, edema, and heart failure. Related adverse metabolic effects for which the nurse needs to monitor include hypokalemia, hypercalcemia, hyperlipidemia, hyperglycemia, and hyperuricemia.
- Adverse effects for which the nurse should monitor patients taking loop or thiazide diuretics include metabolic alkalosis, drowsiness, lethargy, hypokalemia, tachycardia, hypotension, leg cramps, restlessness, and decreased mental alertness. When potassium-sparing diuretics are used, hyperkalemia with nausea, vomiting, and diarrhea may occur.
- Nurses must have a thorough knowledge of kidney anatomy and physiology and how it relates to the action of the diuretics; for example, if a loop diuretic is given, its site of action is the loop of Henle, and it causes the excretion of sodium, potassium, and chloride into the urine.
- Methods for monitoring for excess and deficit fluid volume states include assessment of skin and mucous membranes, pulse rate, intake and output, and daily weights. The nurse should always be concerned about the more vulnerable patient populations, such as older adults, those with a chronic illness, and patients with altered kidney or liver function.

EXAMINATION REVIEW QUESTIONS

1 The nurse is reviewing the medications that have been ordered for a patient who has received a new prescription for a loop diuretic. Which of the following may have a possible interaction with the loop diuretic?
a. NSAIDs
b. warfarin
c. penicillins
d. vitamin C

2 When monitoring laboratory test results for patients receiving loop and thiazide diuretics, which of the following must the nurse look for?
a. Decreased serum glucose levels
b. Increased serum levels of sodium
c. Decreased serum levels of potassium
d. Increased serum levels of potassium

3 When the nurse is checking the laboratory data for a patient taking spironolactone (Aldactone), which result would be a potential concern?
a. Serum sodium level of 140 mmol/L
b. Serum potassium level of 3.6 mmol/L
c. Serum potassium level of 5.8 mmol/L
d. Serum magnesium level of 0.8 mmol/L

4 Which of the following statements should be included in patient education for an 81-year-old female with heart failure who is taking daily doses of spironolactone (Aldactone)?
a. "Avoid foods that are high in potassium."
b. "Be sure to eat foods that are high in potassium."
c. "A weight gain of 1–1.25 kg in 24 hours is normal."
d. "Change positions slowly because this drug causes severe hypertension-induced syncope."

5 A patient with diabetes has a new prescription for a thiazide diuretic. Which statement should the nurse include when teaching the patient about the thiazide drug?
a. "There is nothing for you to be concerned about when you are taking the thiazide."
b. "You should take the thiazide at night to avoid interactions with the diabetes medicine."
c. "Monitor your blood glucose closely because the thiazide may cause the levels to decrease."
d. "Monitor your blood glucose closely because the thiazide may cause the levels to increase."

For answers see http://evolve.elsevier.com/Canada/Lilley/pharmacology/.

CRITICAL THINKING ACTIVITIES

1 Mr. G. is a 64-year-old man who has been admitted to the coronary care unit because he is experiencing heart failure. He has been given 80 mg of furosemide q6h but has experienced no relief of the pulmonary and peripheral edema. The physician would like to change his diuretic to bumetanide. What is the equivalent daily dose of bumetanide?

2 What type of teaching would be appropriate for a patient who is beginning treatment with a potassium-sparing diuretic?

3 Describe the antihypertensive effects of loop diuretics in the treatment of hypertension.

For answers see http://evolve.elsevier.com/Canada/Lilley/pharmacology/.

CHAPTER **27**

Fluids and Electrolytes

Learning Objectives

After reading this chapter, the successful student will be able to do the following:

1   Identify the fluid and electrolyte solutions commonly used in the management of fluid and electrolyte disorders.

2   Discuss the mechanisms of action, indications, dosages, routes of administration, contraindications, cautions, adverse effects, toxicity, and drug interactions of fluid and electrolyte solutions.

3   Compare the solutions used to expand or decrease a patient's fluid volume and electrolytes; consider how they work and why they are used and specific antidotes to any toxic effects.

4   Develop a collaborative plan of care that includes all phases of the nursing process for patients receiving fluid and electrolyte solutions.

e-Learning Activities

Web site
(http://evolve.elsevier.com/Canada/Lilley/pharmacology/)

- Animations
- Answers to chapter questions, activities, and case studies
- Calculators and Category Catchers
- Glossary with audio pronunciations
- IV Therapy and Medication Error Checklists
- Multiple-Choice Review Question quizzes
- Nursing Care Plans
- Online Appendices and Supplements
- WebLinks

Drug Profiles

albumin, p. 512
dextran, p. 512
potassium supplements, p. 516
sodium chloride, p. 510, 517
sodium polystyrene sulfonate, p. 516

Glossary

Blood   The fluid that circulates through the heart, arteries, capillaries, and veins, carrying nutriment and oxygen to the body cells. Blood consists of *plasma*, its liquid component, and three major solid components in the form of *erythrocytes* (red blood cells, or RBCs), *leukocytes* (white blood cells, or WBCs), and *platelets*. (p. 507)

Colloidal   Describes a state of matter in which large molecules or aggregates of molecules that do not precipitate and that measure between 1 and 100 nm are dispersed in another medium. (p. 508)

Colloid oncotic pressure (COP)   The osmotic pressure exerted by a colloid in solution such as that produced when the concentration of protein in the plasma on one side of a blood vessel cell wall membrane is higher than that in the neighbouring *interstitial fluid* (ISF). (p. 508)

Crystalloids   A substance in a solution that diffuses through a semipermeable membrane. (p. 508)

Dehydration   Excessive loss of water from the body tissues that is accompanied by an imbalance in the essential electrolyte concentrations. (p. 508)

Edema   The abnormal accumulation of fluid in interstitial spaces. (p. 508)

Extracellular fluid (ECF)   That portion of the body fluid comprising the ISF and blood plasma. (p. 507)

Extravascular fluid (EVF)   Fluids in the body that are outside the blood vessels. (p. 507)

Gradient   A difference in the concentration of a substance on two sides of a permeable barrier. (p. 508)

Hydrostatic pressure (HP)   The pressure exerted by a liquid. (p. 508)

Hyperkalemia Abnormally high potassium concentration in the blood, most often because of defective kidney excretion, but it can also be due to excessive dietary potassium. (p. 514)

Hypernatremia Abnormally high sodium concentration in the blood; may be due to defective kidney excretion, but more commonly it results from excessive dietary sodium or aggressive therapy. (p. 517)

Hypokalemia Abnormally low potassium concentration in the blood, the major intracellular cation in the bloodstream. (p. 514)

Hyponatremia Abnormally low sodium concentration in the blood, caused by either inadequate excretion of water or excessive water in the bloodstream. (p. 517)

Interstitial fluid (ISF) ECF that fills in the spaces between most of the cells of the body; an *interstice* is a small space within a tissue. (p. 507)

Intracellular fluid (ICF) Fluid located within cell membranes throughout most of the body; contains dissolved solutes that are essential to maintaining electrolyte balance and healthy metabolism. (p. 507)

Intravascular fluid (IVF) The fluid inside the blood vessels. (p. 507)

Isotonic Having the same concentration of a solute as another solution, thereby exerting the same osmotic pressure as that solution, such as an isotonic saline solution that contains an amount of salt equal to that found in the ICF and ECF. (p. 508)

Osmotic pressure The pressure exerted on a semipermeable membrane separating a solution from a solvent, the membrane being impermeable to the solutes in the solution and permeable only to the solvent. (p. 508)

Plasma The watery, straw-coloured fluid component of lymph and blood in which the leukocytes, erythrocytes, and platelets are suspended. (p. 507)

Serum The clear, cell-free portion of the blood from which fibrinogen has also been separated during the clotting process, as typically carried out with a laboratory sample. (p. 507)

OVERVIEW

Fluid and electrolyte management is one of the cornerstones of patient care. Most disease processes, tissue injuries, and surgical procedures greatly influence the physiological status of fluids and electrolytes in the body. A prerequisite to understanding fluid and electrolyte management is knowledge of the span and composition of the body fluid compartments.

PHYSIOLOGY OF FLUID BALANCE

Approximately 60% of the adult human body is water, or the *total body water* (TBW). Total body water is distributed among the three main compartments in the following proportions: **intracellular fluid (ICF)**, 67%; **interstitial fluid (ISF)**, 25%; and plasma volume (PV), 8%. This distribution is illustrated in Figure 27-1. The actual volume of fluid that would normally be distributed in each compartment in an average 70 kg man with a TBW content of 60% of his total body weight is shown in Table 27-1.

The terms used to identify the spaces within which the TBW is distributed can be quite confusing. There are two basic approaches to distinguishing the locations of the fluid. The TBW can be described as being inside or outside of the blood vessels, or vasculature. If this terminology is used, then the term **intravascular fluid (IVF)** describes fluid inside the blood vessels and the term **extravascular fluid (EVF)** describes the fluid outside the blood vessels. Examples of EVF include lymph and cerebrospinal fluid. As you learn these concepts, recall the difference between the prefixes intra- (inside), inter- (between), and extra- (outside). The term **plasma** is used to describe the intravascular fluid that flows through the blood vessels. **Serum**, a closely related term, is the cell-free portion of the **blood** that fibrinogen is separated from during the clotting process. Fluid can also be described as being within the cells or outside the cells. ISF is the fluid that is in the space between cells, tissues, and organs. Both plasma and ISF make up extracellular volume. Both ISF and ICF make up extravascular volume. These terms are often confused and misused. Table 27-1 lists these definitions for further clarity and understanding.

What, then, keeps fluid inside the blood vessels? All the fluid outside the cells, the **extracellular fluid (ECF)**, which is composed of both the plasma and the ISF, has approximately the same concentration of electrolytes. However, there is one big difference between the plasma and the ISF. The plasma has a protein concentration four times greater than that of the ISF. These proteins are primarily albumin but also include globulin and fibrinogen. The reason for this higher intravascular concentration of

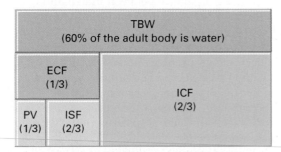

FIG. 27-1 Distribution of total body water (TBW). *ECF*, extracellular fluid; *ICF*, intracellular fluid; *ISF*, interstitial fluid; *PV*, plasma volume.

TABLE 27-1		
Fluid Location: Descriptive Terms and Actual Volumes*		
Name	**Location**	**Actual Volumes**
IF THE POINT OF REFERENCE IS THE CELLS, THEN THESE TERMS ARE USED:		
Intracellular fluid (ICF)	Inside the cells	28,000 mL
Extracellular fluid (ECF)	Outside the cells	14,000 mL (composed of both intravascular plasma and ISF)
IF THE POINT OF REFERENCE IS THE BLOOD VESSELS, THEN THESE TERMS ARE USED:		
Intravascular fluid or plasma volume (PV)	Inside blood vessels	3500 mL
Extravascular fluid (EVF)	Outside blood vessels	38,500 mL
IF THE POINT OF REFERENCE IS THE TISSUES, THEN THESE TERMS ARE USED:		
Interstitial fluid (ISF)	In the spaces between cells, tissues, and organs but not in the plasma or the cells	10,500 mL

*Values given are for a 70 kg man with a total body water of 60% of his total body weight.

protein is that these solutes (proteins) have a molecular mass that exceeds 69,000 daltons, making them too large to pass through the walls of the blood vessels. Because of the difference in concentration of plasma proteins, fluid flows from the area of low protein concentration in the interstitial compartment to the area of high concentration inside the blood vessel to try to create an **isotonic** environment on either side of the blood vessel wall. (*Isotonic* means an equal concentration of solutes across a membrane.) The protein in the blood vessels exerts a constant **osmotic pressure** that prevents the leakage of too much plasma through the capillaries into the tissues. Because proteins suspended in plasma constitute a **colloidal** state (i.e., a state of dispersion of molecules or aggregates of molecules within a medium), this particular pressure is called **colloid oncotic pressure (COP)**; normally it is 24 mm Hg. The opposing pressure, exerted by the ISF, is called **hydrostatic pressure (HP)**. Normally it is 17 mm Hg, which is less than the COP. The phenomenon of COP is illustrated in Figure 27-2.

This regulation of the volume and composition of body water is essential for life because it is the medium in which all metabolic reactions occur. The body maintains the volume and composition remarkably constant by maintaining a balance between intake and excretion. The amount of water gained each day is kept roughly equal to the amount of water lost. When, for some reason, the body cannot maintain this equilibrium, therapy with select agents becomes necessary. If the amount of water gained exceeds the amount of water lost, a water excess, or overhydration, occurs. Such fluid excesses often accumulate in interstitial spaces, such as in the pericardial sac, intrapleural space, peritoneal cavity, joint capsules, and lower extremities. This accumulation is referred to as **edema**. If the quantity of water lost exceeds that gained, a water deficit, or **dehydration**, occurs. Death often occurs when 20% to 25% of the TBW is lost.

Dehydration leads to a disturbance in the balance between the amount of fluid in the extracellular compartment and that in the intracellular compartment.

Sodium is the principal extracellular electrolyte and plays a primary role in maintaining water concentration in the body because of its highly osmotic chemistry. In the initial stages of dehydration, water is lost first from the extracellular compartments. The nature of further fluid losses, COP changes, or both depends on the type of clinical dehydration (Table 27-2). Clinical conditions that can result in dehydration and fluid loss, as well as the symptoms of dehydration and fluid loss, are listed in Table 27-3.

When fluid that has been lost must be replaced, there are three categories of agents that can be used to accomplish this: crystalloids, colloids, and blood products. The clinical situation dictates which category of agent is most appropriate.

CRYSTALLOIDS

Crystalloids are fluids given by intravenous (IV) injection that supply water and sodium to maintain the osmotic **gradient** (i.e., difference in salt concentrations) between the extravascular and intravascular compartments.

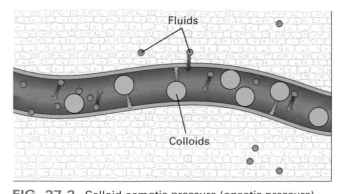

FIG. 27-2 Colloid osmotic pressure (oncotic pressure). As shown, the colloids inside the blood vessel are too large to pass through the vessel wall. The resulting oncotic pressure exerted by the colloids draws fluid from the surrounding tissues and other extravascular spaces into the blood vessels and keeps fluid inside the blood vessel.

TABLE 27-2

Types of Dehydration

Type of Dehydration	Characteristics
Hypertonic	Occurs when water loss is greater than sodium loss, resulting in a concentration of solutes outside the cells and causing the fluid inside the cells to move to the extracellular space, thus dehydrating the cells. Example: Elevated temperature resulting in perspiration
Hypotonic	Occurs when sodium loss is greater than water loss, resulting in higher concentrations of solute inside the cells, thus pulling fluid from outside the cells (plasma and interstitial spaces) into the cells. Examples: Kidney insufficiency and inadequate aldosterone secretion
Isotonic	Occurs with a loss of sodium and water from the body, resulting in a decrease in the volume of extracellular fluid. Examples: Diarrhea and vomiting

TABLE 27-3

Conditions Leading to Fluid Loss and Associated Symptoms*

Condition	Associated Symptoms
Bleeding	Tachycardia and hypotension
Bowel obstruction	Reduced perspiration and mucous secretions
Diarrhea	Reduced urine output (oliguria)
Fever	Dry skin and mucous membranes
Vomiting	Reduced lacrimal (tears) and salivary secretions

*Note: There may be overlap involving more than one of the symptoms depending on the patient's specific condition.

Their plasma volume-expanding capacity is related to the sodium concentration. The different crystalloids are listed in Table 27-4.

Mechanism of Action and Drug Effects

Because crystalloids work by osmosis, hypertonic saline (3% sodium chloride) is more efficient than normal saline (NS) (0.9% sodium chloride) for expanding the PV.

Crystalloid solutions contain fluids and electrolytes that are normally found in the body. They do not contain proteins (colloids), which are necessary to maintain the COP and prevent water from leaving the plasma compartment. In fact, the administration of large quantities of crystalloid solutions for fluid resuscitation decreases the COP, attributable to a dilutional effect. Compared with the distribution of colloids, crystalloids are distributed faster into the interstitial and intracellular compartments, making crystalloids better for treating dehydration than for expanding the PV alone, such as in hypovolemic shock. That is, crystalloids cannot expand the PV on a longer-term basis, nor can colloids; even in the short term, much larger fluid volumes are required.

Indications

They are used to compensate for insensible fluid losses, replace fluids when there are body fluid deficits, and manage specific fluid and electrolyte disturbances. Crystalloids also promote urinary flow. They are much less expensive than colloids and blood products. In addition, there is no risk of viral transmission or anaphylaxis and no alteration in the coagulation profile associated with their use, unlike blood products. The choice of whether to use a crystalloid or colloid depends on the severity of the condition. Following are the common indications for either crystalloid or colloid replacement therapy:
- Acute liver failure
- Acute nephrosis
- Adult respiratory distress syndrome
- Burns
- Cardiopulmonary bypass
- Hypoproteinemia
- Reduction of the risk of deep vein thrombosis (DVT)
- Kidney dialysis
- Shock

TABLE 27-4

Crystalloids

Product	Composition (mmol/L)						Volume (mL)	Cost*
	Na	Cl	K	Ca	Mg	Lactate		
NS	154	154	0	0	0	0	1000	1
Hypertonic saline	513	513	0	0	0	0	500	1
Lactated Ringer's	130	109	4	3	0	28	1000	2.5×
D5W	0	0	1	0	0	0	1000	2×
Plasma-Lyte	140	103	10	5	3	8	1000	5×

Ca, calcium; *Cl*, chloride; *D5W*, 5% dextrose in water; *K*, potassium; *Mg*, magnesium; *Na*, sodium; *NS*, normal saline.

*Relative cost; example: D5W is two times the cost of hypertonic saline.

Contraindications

Contraindications to the use of crystalloids include known drug allergy to a specific product and hypervolemia and may include severe electrolyte disturbance, depending on the type of crystalloid used.

Adverse Effects

Crystalloids are a safe and effective means of replacing needed fluid. They do, however, have some unwanted effects. Because they contain no large particles, such as proteins, they do not stay within the blood vessels and can leak out of the plasma into the tissues and cells. This leakage may result in edema anywhere in the body because of osmosis from the crystalloid; peripheral edema and pulmonary edema are two common examples. Crystalloids also dilute the proteins that are in the plasma, further reducing the COP. Because crystalloids cannot carry oxygen, their use may result in decreased oxygen tension as a result of a dilutional effect on erythrocyte concentration. Typically, large volumes (litres of fluid) are required for crystalloids to be effective. As a result, large or prolonged infusions may worsen acidosis or alkalosis or adversely affect central nervous system (CNS) function from fluid overload. Another disadvantage of crystalloids is that their effects are relatively short-lived.

Interactions

Interactions with crystalloid solutions are rare because they are similar if not identical to normal physiological substances. Certain electrolytes contained in lactated Ringer's solution may be incompatible with other electrolytes, forming a chemical precipitate.

Dosages

For the recommended dosages of crystalloids, see Table 27-5.

TABLE 27-5

Crystalloids and Colloids: Dosing Guidelines

	Crystalloids and Colloids			
	0.9% NS	3% NS	5% Colloid*	25% Colloid†
TO RAISE PLASMA VOLUME BY 1 L, ADMINISTER:				
	5–6 L	1.5–2 L	1 L	0.5 L
FLUID COMPARTMENT DISTRIBUTED TO:				
Plasma	25%	25%	100%	200%–300%
Interstitial space	75%	75%	0	Decreased fluid levels
Intracellular space	0	0	0	Decreased fluid levels

NS, normal saline.

*Iso-oncotic solutions such as 5% albumin, dextran 70, and hetastarch.
†Hyperoncotic solutions such as 25% albumin.

 DRUG PROFILES

The most commonly used crystalloid solutions are normal saline (NS or 0.9% sodium chloride) and lactated Ringer's solution. The available crystalloid solutions and their compositions are summarized in Table 27-4. Sodium chloride is also discussed briefly in relation to electrolytes, in the section Physiology of Electrolyte Function (p. 514) and in the Nursing Process section.

sodium chloride

Sodium chloride (salt, NaCl) is available in several concentrations. The most common concentration is 0.9%. This is the physiologically normal concentration of sodium chloride, and for this reason it is referred to as *normal saline* (NS). Other available concentrations are 0.45% (half-normal) and 3% (hypertonic saline). These solutions have different indications and are used in different situations, depending on how urgently fluid volume restoration is needed and the extent of the sodium loss.

Because sodium chloride is a physiological fluid that is present throughout the body's water, there are no hypersensitivity reactions to it. It is safe to administer during any stage of pregnancy, but it is contraindicated in patients with hypernatremia, hyperchloremia, or both. Hypertonic saline injections (3%) are contraindicated in the presence of increased, normal, or only slightly decreased serum electrolyte concentrations. Aside from the 0.45%, 0.9%, and 3% solutions, sodium chloride is also available as a 650 mg tablet. The dose of sodium chloride administered depends on the clinical situation. The volume of crystalloid or colloid needed to expand the plasma volume by 1 litre (1000 mL), given in Table 27-5, can be used as a general guide to dosing.

PHARMACODYNAMICS

Plasma Volume Expansion	Colloid Oncotic Pressure	Duration of Expansion
60–70 mL*	30 mm Hg	Few hours

*500 mL of NS will expand the plasma volume by 60 to 70 mL.

COLLOIDS

Colloids are protein substances that increase the colloid oncotic pressure (COP) and effectively move fluid from the interstitial compartment to the plasma compartment by pulling the fluid into the blood vessels. Normally, this task is performed by the three blood proteins: albumin, globulin, and fibrinogen. However, for them to be effective, the total protein level must be within the range of 74 g/L. If the protein level drops below 53 g/L, the COP then drops below the HP and fluid shifts into the tissues. When this happens, colloid replacement therapy is required to reverse this process by increasing the COP. The COP decreases with age and also with hypotension and malnutrition. The commonly used colloids are listed in Table 27-6.

Mechanism of Action and Drug Effects

The mechanism of action of colloids is related to their ability to increase the COP. Recall that because the colloids cannot pass into the extravascular space, ordinarily there is a higher concentration of solutes (solid particles) inside the blood vessels (intravascular space) than outside the blood vessels. Fluid thus moves toward this hypertonic area from the extravascular space in an attempt to make it isotonic. Because colloids increase the blood volume, they are sometimes called *plasma expanders.* They also make up part of the total plasma volume.

Colloids increase the COP and move fluid from outside the blood vessels to inside the blood vessels. They can maintain the COP for several hours. Colloids are naturally occurring products and consist of proteins (albumin), carbohydrates (dextrans or starches), and animal collagen (gelatin). Usually they contain a combination of both small and large particles. The small particles are eliminated quickly and promote diuresis and perfusion of the kidneys; the larger particles maintain the plasma volume. Albumin is the exception, as it contains particles that are all the same size.

Indications

Colloids are used to treat a wide variety of conditions (see list on p. 509). Clinically, colloids are superior to crystalloids in their ability to expand the plasma volume. However, crystalloids are less expensive and are less likely to promote bleeding. On the other hand, crystalloids are more likely to cause edema because of the larger

TABLE	27-6

Commonly Used Colloids

Product	Composition (mmol/L)		Volume (mL)	Cost[†]
	Na	Cl		
5% Albumin	145	145	500	10×
25% Albumin	145	145	100	10×
Dextran 70*	154	154	500	1
Dextran 40*	154	154	500	2×
Hetastarch	154	154	500	5×

Na, sodium; *Cl,* chloride.

[†]Using the cost of dextran 70 as the means of comparison.
*Dextran is available in NaCl, which has 154 mmol/L of both Na and Cl. It is also available in 5% dextrose in water (D5W), which contains no Na or Cl.

volumes needed to achieve the desired clinical effect, yet they are still superior to colloids for emergency short-term plasma volume expansion.

Contraindications

Contraindications to the use of colloids include known drug allergy to a specific product and hypervolemia and may include severe electrolyte disturbance.

Adverse Effects

Colloids are relatively safe agents, although there are some disadvantages to their use. They have no oxygen-carrying ability and contain no clotting factors, unlike blood products. Because of this, they can alter the coagulation system through a dilutional effect, resulting in impaired coagulation and, possibly, bleeding. They may also dilute the plasma protein concentration, which, in turn, may impair the function of platelets. Rarely, dextran therapy causes anaphylaxis or kidney failure.

Interactions

Because colloid solutions are so compatible with many drugs, they are sometimes used as the medium for delivering them. The anaesthetic drug propofol (Diprivan) (Chapter 12) is an example. It is delivered in a 10% lipid emulsion.

Dosages

For the recommended dosages of colloids, see Table 27-5.

 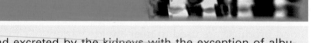

DRUG PROFILES

The specific colloid used for replacement therapy varies from institution to institution. The three most commonly used are 5% albumin, dextran 40, and hetastarch. They have a fast onset and a long duration of action. With the exception of albumin, they are metabolized in the liver and excreted by the kidneys with the exception of albumin. Albumin is metabolized by the reticuloendothelial system and excreted by the kidneys and the intestines. Hetastarch is a synthetic colloid with properties similar to albumin and dextran.

Continued

DRUG PROFILES (cont'd)

albumin

Albumin (Alburex, Albutein, Butimate, Plasbumin) is a natural protein that is normally produced by the liver. It is responsible for generating about 70% of the COP. Human albumin is a sterile solution of serum albumin that is prepared from pooled blood, plasma serum, or placentas obtained from healthy human donors. It is pasteurized (heated at 60°C for 10 hours) to destroy any contaminants.

Albumin is contraindicated in patients with a known hypersensitivity to it and in those with heart failure, severe anemia, or kidney insufficiency. Albumin is available only in parenteral form in 5% and 25% concentrations. It is classified as pregnancy category C. See Table 27-5 for the dosing guidelines.

PHARMACOKINETICS

Half-Life	Onset	Peak	Duration
16 hr	< 15 min	Unknown	< 24 hr

dextran

Dextran is a solution of glucose. It is available in two concentrations—dextran 40 and the more concentrated dextran 70, which has a molecular weight similar to that of albumin. Dextran 40 is more commonly used and is a low-molecular-weight polymer of glucose. It is a derivative of sugar that has actions similar to those of human albumin in that it expands the plasma volume by drawing fluid from the interstitial space to the intravascular space.

Dextran is contraindicated in patients with hypersensitivity to it and in those with heart failure, kidney insufficiency, and extreme dehydration. It is available only in parenteral form in either a 5% dextrose solution or a 0.9% sodium chloride solution. It is classified as pregnancy category C. See Table 27-5 for the dosing guidelines.

PHARMACOKINETICS

Half-Life	Onset	Peak	Duration
2–6 hr (D-40)	< 5 min	Unknown	4–6 hr
12 hr (D-70)	1 hr	Unknown	12 hr

BLOOD PRODUCTS

Blood products are biological drugs. All of them can augment the plasma volume. Red blood cell (RBC)-containing products can improve tissue oxygenation as well and also augment plasma volume. Blood products are also the most expensive and are less available than crystalloids and colloids because they are natural products and require human donors. The available blood products are listed in Table 27-7. They are most often indicated when a patient has lost 25% or more blood volume.

Mechanism of Action and Drug Effects

The mechanism of action of blood products is related to their ability to increase the COP and, hence, the plasma volume. They do so in the same manner as colloids and crystalloids, by pulling fluid from the extravascular space to the intravascular space. Because of this property they are also considered plasma expanders. Red blood cell products also have the ability to carry oxygen. They can maintain the COP for several hours to days, and because they come from human donors, they have all the benefits (and hazards) that human blood products have. They are administered when a person's body is deficient in these products.

Indications

Blood products are used to treat a wide variety of clinical conditions; the blood product used depends on the specific indication. The available blood products and specific conditions they are used to treat are listed in Table 27-8.

Contraindications

There are no absolute contraindications to the use of blood products. However, because of the risk for transfer of infectious disease, although remote, their use should be based on careful clinical evaluation of the patient's condition.

Adverse Effects

Blood products can produce undesirable effects, some potentially serious. Because blood products have a human source, they can be incompatible with the recipient's immune system. These incompatibilities are screened prior to the administration of the particular blood product by determining the respective blood types of the donor and recipient and by cross-matching to determine compatibility between selected blood proteins. This helps to reduce the likelihood of the recipient rejecting the blood products, which would, in turn, precipitate transfusion reactions and anaphylaxis. Blood products can also transmit pathogens,

TABLE 27-7

Blood Products

Product	Dosage	Cost*
Cryoprecipitate	1 unit	1
Fresh frozen plasma	1 unit	1.7×
Packed red blood cells	1 unit	2.2×
Plasma protein fractions	1 unit	1
Whole blood	1 unit	3.3×

*Using the cost of cryoprecipitate as the means of comparison.

TABLE   27-8

Blood Products: Indications

Blood Product	Indication
Cryoprecipitate and plasma protein fraction	To manage acute bleeding (greater than 50% blood loss slowly or 20% acutely)
Fresh frozen plasma	To increase clotting factor levels in patients with a demonstrated deficiency
Packed red blood cells	To increase oxygen-carrying capacity in patients with anemia, in patients with substantial hemoglobin deficits, and in patients who have lost up to 25% of their total blood volume
Whole blood	Same as for packed red blood cells, except that whole blood is more beneficial in cases of extreme (greater than 25%) loss of blood volume, since whole blood also contains plasma, the chief fluid volume of the blood; it also contains plasma proteins, the chief osmotic component, which help draw fluid back into blood vessels from surrounding tissues

such as hepatitis and human immunodeficiency virus (HIV), from the donor to the recipient. Various preparation techniques are now used to reduce the risk of pathogen transmission, resulting in a drastic reduction in the incidence of blood-transferred infections.

therefore, they interact with few substances. Calcium and drugs such as aspirin, which normally affect coagulation, may interact with these substances when infused in the body in much the same way they interact with the body's blood products.

Interactions

As with crystalloids and colloids, blood products are similar if not identical to normal physiological substances;

Dosages

For the dosage guidelines pertaining to blood products, see Table 27-9.

TABLE   27-9

Suggested Guidelines for Blood Products: Management of Bleeding

Amount of Blood Loss	Fluid of Choice
Less than or equal to 20% (slow loss)	Crystalloids
20%–50% (slow loss)	Nonprotein plasma expanders (dextran and hetastarch)
Greater than 50% (slow loss) or 20% (acutely)	Whole blood or packed red blood cells and/or fresh frozen plasma and plasma protein fraction PPF and FFP
Greater than or equal to 80% lost	As above, but for every 5 units of blood given, administer 1–2 units of fresh frozen plasma and 1–2 units of platelets to prevent hemodilution of clotting factors and bleeding

 DRUG PROFILES

Packed red blood cells and fresh frozen plasma are among the most commonly used blood products. All blood products are derived from pooled human blood donors. Other less commonly used, but still important, blood products include whole blood, plasma protein fraction, cryoprecipitate, and platelets.

PACKED RED BLOOD CELLS

Packed red blood cells are obtained by centrifugation of whole blood and their separation from plasma and the other cellular elements. The advantage to packed red blood cell use is that their oxygen-carrying capacity is better than that of the other blood products, and they are less likely to cause cardiac fluid overload. Their disadvantages include high cost, limited shelf life, fluctuating availability, and their risk for virus transmission, allergic

reactions, and bleeding abnormalities. The suggested guidelines are given in Table 27-9.

FRESH FROZEN PLASMA

Fresh frozen plasma is obtained by centrifugation of whole blood and removing the cellular elements. The resulting plasma is then frozen at −18°C. Fresh frozen plasma is not recommended for routine fluid resuscitation, but it may be used as an adjunct to massive blood transfusion in the treatment of patients with underlying coagulation disorders. The plasma-expanding capability of fresh frozen plasma is similar to that of dextran but slightly less than that of hetastarch. The disadvantage of fresh frozen plasma is that it can transmit pathogens. The suggested guidelines are given in Table 27-9.

PHYSIOLOGY OF ELECTROLYTE BALANCE

Recall that the chemical composition of the fluid compartments varies from compartment to compartment. The principal electrolytes in the extracellular fluid are sodium cations (Na^+) and chloride anions (Cl^-); the major electrolyte of the intracellular fluid is the potassium cation (K^+).

Other important electrolytes are calcium (see Lab Values Related to Drug Therapy), magnesium, and phosphorus. These different chemical components are vital to the normal function of all body systems. They are controlled by the renin–angiotensin–aldosterone system, antidiuretic hormone system, and sympathetic nervous system. When these neuroendocrine systems are out of balance, adverse electrolyte imbalances commonly result.

 LAB VALUES RELATED TO DRUG THERAPY

Calcium

Laboratory Test	Normal Ranges	Rationale for Assessment
Serum calcium	2.18–2.58 mmol/L or 1.05–1.30 mmol/L (ionized level)	Calcium supplementation may be deemed necessary whenever the level of calcium drops below normal ranges. In addition to reporting normal levels of serum calcium, ionized calcium levels need to be reported. Serum ionized calcium is the amount of calcium not bound to protein. Clinical signs and symptoms of hypocalcemia include abnormal neuromuscular contractions and tremors. Other assessment tests for the presence of abnormal neuromuscular contractions are the Chvostek's and Trousseau's signs, two classic tests. Chvostek's sign is elicited by gently tapping the face at a point just anterior to the ear and below the zygomatic bone with the blunt end of a reflex hammer. A positive response for hypocalcemia includes twitching of the ipsilateral facial muscles and is suggestive of neuromuscular excitability secondary to hypocalcemia. Trousseau's sign is elicited by inflating a sphygmomanometer cuff (blood pressure cuff) for several minutes. A positive response includes muscular contraction with flexion of the wrist and metacarpophalangeal joints, hyperextension of the fingers, and flexion of the thumb on the palm. This muscle contraction is indicative of neuromuscular excitability secondary to hypocalcemia. These tests, in addition to serum calcium testing, may be helpful in confirming the presence of hypocalcemia.

Modified from Urbano, F. L. (2000). Signs of hypocalcemia: Chvostek's and Trousseau's signs. *Hospital Physician, 36*(3), 43–45.

POTASSIUM

Potassium cations (with a positive charge) are the most abundant electrolytes inside cells (the intracellular space), where the normal concentration is approximately 150 mmol/L. Approximately 95% of potassium in the body is intracellular. In contrast, the potassium content outside the cells in the plasma ranges from 3.5 to 5.0 mmol/L. These plasma levels are critical to normal body function.

Potassium is obtained from a variety of foods, the most common being fruits and juices, fish, vegetables, poultry, meats, and dairy products. It is estimated that for normal body functions to be maintained, a person must consume 5 to 10 mmol of potassium per day. Fortunately, the average adult daily diet usually provides 35 to 80 mmol of potassium, which is well above the required daily amount. Excess dietary potassium is usually excreted in urine. However, if the kidneys lose their ability to filter and secrete waste products, potassium can accumulate, leading to toxic levels. These, in turn, can precipitate ventricular fibrillation and cardiac arrest. Hyperaldosteronism and potassium-sparing diuretics can alter

normal potassium balance as well. **Hyperkalemia** refers to an excessive serum potassium level, defined as a serum potassium level exceeding 5.5 mmol/L. There are several causes of hyperkalemia. As identified, kidney failure can result in hyperkalemia; other causes are as follows:
- Angiotensin-converting enzyme (ACE) inhibitors
- Burns
- Excessive loss from cells
- Infections
- Metabolic acidosis
- Potassium supplements
- Potassium-sparing diuretics
- Trauma

Hypokalemia is a deficiency of potassium; it is more a result of excessive potassium loss than of poor dietary intake. As with hyperkalemia, there are multitudes of clinical conditions that can cause hypokalemia, including the following:
- Alkalosis
- Burns*

*Burn patients can exhibit either hyperkalemia or hypokalemia.

- Corticosteroids
- Diarrhea
- Hyperaldosteronism
- Increased secretion of mineralocorticoids (hormones of the adrenal cortex)
- Ketoacidosis
- Large amounts of licorice
- Loop diuretics
- Malabsorption
- Prolonged laxative misuse
- Starvation diets
- Thiazide diuretics
- Thiazide-like diuretics
- Vomiting

Too little serum potassium can also greatly increase the toxicity associated with digitalis preparations, and this can precipitate serious ventricular dysrhythmias.

The early detection of hypokalemia is important in the prevention of serious, life-threatening consequences of this metabolic disturbance if left undetected. The key to early detection is recognizing its early symptoms, which are generally mild and can easily be missed in assessment. Both the early (mild) symptoms and late (severe) symptoms of hypokalemia are listed in Box 27-1. The treatment of hypokalemia involves identification and treatment of the cause and restoring the serum potassium levels to normal (greater than 3.5 mmol/L). The consumption of potassium-rich foods can usually correct mild hypokalemia, but clinically significant hypokalemia requires the oral or parenteral administration of a potassium supplement, which usually contains potassium chloride.

Mechanism of Action and Drug Effects

The importance of potassium as the primary intracellular electrolyte is evidenced by the enormous number of life-sustaining reactions and everyday physiological functions that require it—functions that are taken for granted and that would not be possible without it. Muscle contraction, the transmission of nerve impulses, and the regulation of heartbeats (the pacemaker function of the heart) are some of the functions that would not be possible without potassium.

Potassium is also essential for the maintenance of acid–base balance, isotonicity, and the electrodynamic characteristics of the cell. It plays a role in many enzymatic reactions, and it is an essential component of gastric secretion, kidney function, tissue synthesis, and carbohydrate metabolism.

Indications

Potassium replacement therapy is called for in the treatment or prevention of potassium depletion in patients whenever dietary measures prove inadequate. Potassium salts used for this purpose include potassium chloride, potassium phosphate, and potassium acetate. The chloride is necessary to correct the hypochloremia (low chloride) that commonly accompanies potassium deficiency, and phosphate is used to correct hypophosphatemia.

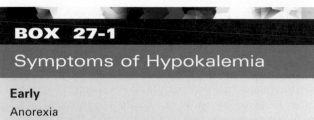

BOX 27-1

Symptoms of Hypokalemia

Early

Anorexia
Hypotension
Lethargy
Mental confusion
Muscle weakness
Nausea

Late

Cardiac dysrhythmias
Neuropathy
Paralytic ileus
Secondary alkalosis

The acetate salt may be used to raise the blood pH in acidotic conditions.

Other therapeutic effects of potassium are related to its role in the contraction of muscles and the maintenance of the electrical characteristics of cells. Potassium salts may be used to stop irregular heartbeats (dysrhythmias) and to manage the tachyarrhythmias that can occur after heart surgery. Potassium may also be used to treat thallium poisoning and to help increase muscular strength in some patients with myasthenia gravis.

Contraindications

Contraindications to potassium replacement products include known drug allergy to a specific drug product, hyperkalemia from any cause, severe kidney disease, acute dehydration, untreated Addison's disease, severe hemolytic disease, and conditions involving extensive tissue breakdown (e.g., multiple trauma, severe burns).

Adverse Effects

The adverse effects of oral potassium therapy are primarily limited to the gastrointestinal tract and occur with the oral administration of potassium preparations. These gastrointestinal effects include diarrhea, nausea, and vomiting. More significant ones include gastrointestinal bleeding and ulceration. The parenteral administration of potassium usually produces pain at the injection site. Cases of phlebitis have been associated with intravenous administration, and the excessive administration of potassium salts can lead to hyperkalemia and toxic effects.

Toxicity and Management of Overdose

The toxic effects of potassium are the result of hyperkalemia. Symptoms include muscle weakness, paraesthesia, paralysis, convulsions, cardiac rhythm irregularities that can result in ventricular fibrillation, and cardiac arrest. The treatment instituted depends on the degree of the hyperkalemia and ranges from regimens for reversing life-threatening problems to simple dietary restrictions. In the event of severe hyperkalemia, the intravenous administration of sodium bicarbonate, calcium gluconate or chloride, or dextrose solution with insulin is often required. These drugs correct severe hyperkalemia by causing a rapid intracellular shift of potassium ions, thus reducing the serum potassium concentration. Such interventions are often followed by orally or rectally administered sodium polystyrene sulfonate (e.g., Kayexalate) or hemodialysis to eliminate the extra potassium from the body. Less critical levels can be reduced with dietary restrictions.

Interactions

Concurrent use of potassium-sparing diuretics and angiotensin-converting enzyme (ACE) inhibitors can produce a hyperkalemic state. Concurrent use of diuretics, amphotericin B, and mineralocorticosteroids can produce a hypokalemic state.

Dosages

Fluid and electrolyte therapy involves replacing any deficit losses and providing maintenance levels for specific patient requirements. Accordingly, specific dosage amounts of fluids or electrolytes depend on several clinical factors, including the following:
- Specific patient losses
- Efficacy of patient physiological systems involved in fluid and electrolyte metabolism, especially adrenal, cardiovascular, and kidney functions
- Current drug therapy for pathological conditions that complicate the amount and duration of replacement
- Selection of oral or parenteral replacement formulations

Suggested dosage guidelines with subsequent adjustments for potassium are 10 to 20 mmol administered orally several times a day or parenteral administration of 30 to 60 mmol every 24 hours.

DRUG PROFILES

potassium supplements

Potassium supplements are administered to prevent or treat potassium depletion. The acetate, bicarbonate, chloride, citrate, and gluconate salts of potassium are available for oral administration. The parenteral salt forms of potassium for intravenous administration are acetate, chloride, and phosphate.

The dosage of potassium supplements is usually expressed in millimoles (mmol; equal to milliequivalents [mEq]) of potassium and depends on the requirements of the individual patient. These salt forms of potassium and the number of grams of each needed to yield 40 mmol or mEq are given in Table 27-10.

Potassium is contraindicated in patients with severe kidney disease, severe hemolytic disease, or Addison's disease and in those suffering from hyperkalemia, acute dehydration, or extensive tissue breakdown stemming from multiple traumas. Potassium is available in many different oral and intravenous formulations. It is available in oral form as a tablet and powder for solution, as an extended-release capsule and tablet, and as an elixir and solution. It is also available as an injection for intravenous use. Potassium is calssified as pregnancy category A.

PHARMACOKINETICS

Half-Life	Onset	Peak	Duration
IV: Variable	IV: Immediate	IV: Rapid	IV: Variable
PO: Variable	PO: 30 min	PO: 30 min	PO: Variable

sodium polystyrene sulfonate (potassium exchange resin)

Sodium polystyrene sulfonate (Kayexalate, K-Exit Poudre) is known as a *cation exchange resin* that is used to treat hyperkalemia. For this purpose, it is usually administered orally via a nasogastric tube or as an enema. Its action is in the intestine, where potassium ions from the body are exchanged for sodium ions in the resin. Although the drug effects in each case are unpredictable, approximately 1 mmol of potassium is lost from the body per gram of resin administered. It has no listed contraindications, but it can cause disturbances in electrolytes other than potassium, such as calcium and magnesium. For this reason, patients' electrolytes should be closely monitored during treatment with sodium polystyrene sulfonate. It is typically dosed in multiples of 15 to 30 g until desired effect on serum potassium. It is available in a powder for reconstitution and as an oral suspension. It is classified as pregnancy category C.

TABLE 27-10

Potassium: Salt Forms

Salt Form	Amount (g) Needed to Yield 40 mmol of Potassium
Acetate	3.9
Chloride	3.0
Citrate	4.3
Dibasic phosphate	3.5
Gluconate	9.4
Monobasic phosphate	5.4

SODIUM

Although sodium was discussed under colloids earlier in this chapter, it is also presented here in the electrolyte section because it is most commonly given for replenishing purposes. Sodium is the counterpart to potassium in that potassium is the principal cation (positively charged substance) inside cells, and sodium is the principal cation outside cells. The normal concentration of sodium outside cells is 135 to 145 mmol/L, and it is maintained through the dietary intake of sodium in the form of sodium chloride, which is obtained directly from salt; fish; meats; and other foods flavoured, seasoned, or preserved with salt.

Hyponatremia is the condition of sodium loss or deficiency and occurs when the serum levels decrease below 135 mmol/L. It is manifested by lethargy, hypotension, stomach cramps, vomiting, diarrhea, and seizures. Some of the same conditions that cause hypokalemia can also cause hyponatremia; these are listed on p. 514. Other causes of hyponatremia are excessive perspiration, occurring during hot weather or physical work; prolonged diarrhea or vomiting, especially in young children; kidney disorders; and adrenocortical impairment.

Hypernatremia is the condition of sodium excess and occurs when the serum levels of sodium exceed 145 mmol/L. Some of the symptoms are water retention (edema) and hypertension. The most common cause is poor kidney excretion stemming from kidney malfunction. Inadequate water consumption and dehydration are other causes. Symptoms of hypernatremia include red, flushed skin; dry, sticky mucous membranes; increased thirst; temperature elevation; and decreased or absent urination.

Mechanism of Action and Drug Effects

As one of the body's electrolytes, sodium performs many physiological roles necessary for the normal functions of the body. It is the major cation in extracellular fluid and is principally involved in the control of water distribution, fluid and electrolyte balance, and osmotic pressure of body fluids. Sodium also participates along with both chloride and bicarbonate in the regulation of acid–base balance. Chloride, the major extracellular anion (negatively charged substance), closely complements the physiological action of sodium. Sodium is also capable of causing diuresis.

Indications

Sodium is primarily administered in the treatment or prevention of sodium depletion when dietary measures have proved inadequate. Sodium chloride is the primary salt used for this purpose. Mild hyponatremia is usually treated with the oral administration of sodium chloride tablets, fluid restriction, or both. Pronounced sodium depletion is treated with NS or lactated Ringer's solution administered intravenously. (These drugs are discussed earlier in this chapter.)

Contraindications

The only usual contraindications to the use of sodium replacement products are known drug allergy to a specific product and hypernatremia.

Adverse Effects

The oral administration of sodium chloride can cause gastric upset consisting of nausea, vomiting, and cramps. Venous phlebitis can be a consequence of its parenteral administration.

Toxicity and Management of Overdose

Hypernatremia leads to hypertension, edema, thirst, tachycardia, weakness, convulsions, and possibly coma. Treatment consists of increased fluid intake and dietary restrictions. In more serious cases, diuretics may be required to enhance urinary sodium excretion. Intravenous administration of dextrose in water solution (e.g., D5W, D10W) may also be helpful, by both intravascular sodium dilution and enhanced urine volume output.

Interactions

Sodium is not known to interact significantly with any drugs.

Dosages

Fluid and electrolyte therapy involves replacing any deficit losses and providing maintenance levels for specific patient requirements. Accordingly, specific dosage amounts of fluids or electrolytes depend on several clinical factors, as follows:
- Specific patient losses
- Efficacy of patient physiological systems involved in fluid and electrolyte metabolism, especially adrenal, cardiovascular, and kidney functions
- Current drug therapy for pathological conditions that complicate the amount and duration of replacement
- Selection of oral or parenteral replacement formulations
  Suggested dosage guidelines with subsequent adjustments for sodium chloride are 1 to 2 g administered orally several times a day or parenteral administration of 1 L of sodium chloride injection (NS).

 DRUG PROFILES

sodium chloride

Sodium chloride (salt, NaCl) is used primarily as a replacement electrolyte for either the prevention or treatment of sodium loss. It is also used as a diluent for the infusion of compatible drugs and in the assessment of kidney function after a fluid challenge. Sodium chloride is contraindicated in patients who are hypersensitive to it. It is available in many intravenous preparations and in oral form. It is classified as pregnancy category C.

PHARMACOKINETICS

Half-Life	Onset	Peak	Duration
Unknown	Immediate	Rapid	Variable

NURSING PROCESS

Assessment

For fluid replacement, patients' needs vary, and any medications or solutions ordered should be given exactly as ordered and without substitution. However, it is also important to always confirm the order against authoritative resources. The nurse is responsible for making sure that whatever is given or done to the patient is accurate and safe and meets standards of care. As a brief review, parenterally administered hydrating solutions (e.g., 5% dextrose in water [D5W]) are used primarily to prevent dehydration. Isotonic solutions (e.g., 0.9% normal saline) are customarily used to augment extracellular volume in patients experiencing blood loss, severe vomiting, or any condition that leads to a chloride loss equal to or greater than the sodium loss. Isotonic normal saline (0.9% NS) is also used as diluting fluid for blood transfusions because D5W results in hemolysis of red blood cells (in transfusions). Hypertonic solutions (3%) are used to treat hypotonic expansion, such as that resulting from water intoxication.

As soon as physician orders have been verified and checked for accuracy and completeness, assessment of the medication/solution, the patient, and the intravenous site (if applicable) should be done. The nurse must also assess the following areas related to intravenous infusions of fluids and electrolytes: solution to be infused, infusion equipment, infusion rate of solution/medication per minute, concentration of parenteral solution, related mathematical calculations, laboratory values (e.g., sodium, chloride, potassium), and parenteral compatibilities. More specific assessment of the patient who is to receive a parenteral replacement solution should focus on gathering information on the patient's medical history, including diseases of the gastrointestinal tract, kidney, heart, or liver. A medication history should focus on a listing of prescription drugs, over-the-counter (OTC) medications, and natural health products. A dietary history is also important and should include specific dietary habits and a dietary recall of the last 24 hours. Fluid volume and electrolyte status (through laboratory testing, urinary specific gravity, vital signs, and intake and output) should be assessed and documented. Because the skin and mucous membranes also reflect a patient's hydration status, they are important to assess, including skin turgor and rebound elasticity of skin over the top of the hand and other areas over the body. The findings should be documented as "immediate" turgor or "delayed" turgor. Count the number of seconds that the patient's skin stays in the pinched-up position; normal return is immediate or within 3 to 5 seconds.

To begin assessment of potassium levels, it is important to know that the normal range is 3.5 to 5 mmol/L; levels below 3.5 mmol/L (hypokalemia) may result in a variety of problems such as heart irregularities and muscle weakness. Tartrazine sensitivity, noted mostly in patients with aspirin allergies, should be assessed carefully if a patient is taking potassium chloride because of a risk of cross-sensitivity. Potassium supplementation should be avoided or used with extreme caution in patients taking ACE inhibitors and with potassium-sparing diuretics (such as spironolactone). These drugs are associated with adverse effects of hyperkalemia and could worsen hyperkalemia and possibly result in severe cardiac compromise and even cardiac arrest if given with potassium supplementation. Oral potassium supplements are irritants and can be ulcerogenic. If a patient has a history of ulcers or gastrointestinal bleeding, the supplementation should not be given orally and the physician should be contacted for further instructions.

Normal ranges of serum potassium often vary depending on the institution and physician. In order to identify and treat hyperkalemia, the normal range of potassium must be established. In some labs, potassium levels of 5.3 mmol/L may be identified as abnormally high, whereas other labs may identify 5.0 mmol/L as being abnormally high. High (and low) serum potassium levels should be reported. A serum level exceeding 5.5 mmol/L is considered by most sources as being toxic and dangerous to the patient and should be reported immediately to the physician. With close monitoring of patients, the dangerous effects of hyperkalemia may be prevented if it is identified early and treated appropriately, thus avoiding potentially life-threatening complications (see previous discussion of hyperkalemia).

Vein access remains an issue with parenteral potassium supplementation because of irritation to the veins with infiltration or if the concentration has not been mixed thoroughly. Some important factors to consider for peripheral venous access include the following (for potassium, sodium, fluid, and any other sort of medication given per the intravenous route):

- Attempt use of distal veins first.
- Know the purpose of using potassium and other electrolytes.
- Set the rate as ordered and recalculated for infusion.
- Know the anticipated duration of therapy.
- Assess the overall condition of the veins.
- Know the restrictions imposed by the patient's history (e.g., affected arm of a patient who has had a mastectomy and lymph node dissection).

For the patient who has had a mastectomy or stroke, these situations may be associated with inadequate circulation and lead to edema and other complications.

Sodium is another electrolyte used in some intravenous replacement solutions. Hyponatremia, or serum sodium below 135 mmol/L, if not resolved with dietary or oral intake, may need to be treated with parenteral infusions. Venous access sites should be carefully chosen because of possible irritation of the vein and subsequent phlebitis. If there is overzealous replacement, hyponatremic states may lead to hypernatremia and fluid overload, edema, worsening of heart failure, dyspnea, and rales. Continual monitoring of vital signs, hydration status of skin and mucus membrane, and level of consciousness is important for safe intravenous replacement and for prevention of further complications.

Hypernatremia also requires careful assessment. Identification of any precipitating events, medical concerns, and at-risk patient situations is important to finding early solutions for treatment. The at-risk population for hypernatremia includes the older adult, patients with renal and cardiovascular diseases, patients receiving sodium supplements or with increased sodium intake, and those with decreased fluid intake. Recent evidence suggests that reducing dietary salt intake will help reduce the risk for developing heart disease, the recommendation being limiting salt intake to 1000 to 1500 mg per day. All electrolytes require assessment of cautions, contraindications, and drug interactions.

Albumin and other colloids are associated with cautions, contraindications, and drug interactions that need to be assessed. It is also important to assess the patient's hematocrit (Hct), hemoglobin (Hgb) levels, and serum protein levels. Monitoring of the patient's blood pressure, pulse rate, respiratory status, and intake and output amounts should be documented. Assessment for dyspnea or hypoxia should also be noted and reported prior to use of these drugs. Laboratory interference is seen with alkaline phosphatase, which is increased when albumin is given.

When giving blood or blood components, the nurse should obtain a thorough history regarding transfusions received and the patient's response. Any history of adverse reactions to transfusions should be reported to the physician and the nature of these reactions documented. It is also important to assess the status of venous access areas and to check the patient's laboratory values (e.g., Hct, Hgb, white blood cells [WBCs], red blood cells [RBCs], platelets, and clotting factors). Baseline vital signs should be noted before infusing blood or blood products. Even the general appearance of the patient, energy level, ability to carry out activities of daily living, and colour of extremities are important to note. During the infusion of blood components, be alert to the occurrence of fever and of blood in the urine, which are indicative of an adverse reaction.

In summary, safety and caution are top priorities in treating patients receiving any drug, including fluid and electrolyte replacements. Because excess levels of fluid and electrolytes and deficits may pose tremendous risks to patients, the nurse must assess these thoroughly. In addition, with so many patients receiving therapies in the home setting, the nurse has even more responsibility for astute and thorough assessment before, during, and after therapy.

Nursing Diagnoses

- Risk for falls related to fluid and electrolyte imbalances
- Risk for imbalanced fluid volume related to drug-induced fluid excesses or deficits and electrolyte excesses or deficits
- Risk for injury related to complications of the transfusion or infusion of blood products, blood components, or related agents
- Deficient knowledge about treatment regimen related to lack of patient education about electrolyte disturbances and influence of treatment

Planning

Goals

- Patient will experience minimal problems with volume overload related to the transfusion or infusion.
- Patient will begin minimal exercise and will show increased tolerance daily.
- Patient will participate in activities as tolerated.
- Patient will state measures to implement to minimize injury related to altered blood component levels or altered fluid and electrolyte levels.
- Patient will state the rationale for treatment and the adverse effects of replacement agents.
- Patient will state symptoms and problems to report to the physician.

Outcome Criteria

- Patient remains free of injury as the result of adverse reactions (dizziness, volume overload, hypersensitivity) to the transfusion or infusion or as the result of an allergic reaction.
- Patient regains the ability to engage in normal or near-normal exercise, showing increased tolerance daily as evidenced by walking small distances and increasing to regular supervised exercise.
- Patient participates in activities according to ability to tolerate them without dyspnea or chest pain.
- Patient demonstrates a return to normal or near-normal values of blood components or fluid and electrolyte levels.
- Patient sees the physician for follow-up, as ordered, to monitor laboratory values pertinent to treatment.

Implementation

Continued monitoring of the patient during fluid or electrolyte therapy is crucial to ensure safe and effective treatment. It is also important to continue monitoring to identify adverse effects early and to help prevent complications of overzealous treatment or undertreatment. All serum electrolyte levels should not exceed normal ranges (see the pharmacology section).

With parenteral dosing, the nurse must monitor infusion rates as well as appearance of the fluid or solution (i.e., potassium and saline solutions are clear, whereas albumin is brown, clear, and viscous). The intravenous site must also be monitored frequently per facility policy and nursing standards of care for evidence of infiltration (e.g., swelling, skin cool to the touch around intravenous site, absent or decreased flow rate and no blood return from the intravenous catheter) or thrombophlebitis (e.g., swelling, redness, heat and pain at site). Volume overload, drug toxicity, fever, infection, and emboli are other complications of intravenous therapy.

With the administration of any fluid and electrolyte solution, a steady and even flow rate must be maintained to prevent complications. Infusion rates must follow physician's orders, and calculations must be rechecked for accuracy. The intravenous site, tubing, bag, fluids, and solutions as well as expiration dates should all be checked, in case of infusion of replacement fluids or electrolytes. Always act in a cautious, safe, and thorough manner when administering fluids and electrolyte solutions, and remember that older adults and children have increased sensitivity to these solutions and fluids (as well as to most medications). Patients at risk for deficits in volume, especially older adults, should be informed of the impact of a hot, humid environment on physiological functioning and of exacerbation by excess perspiration. Water is central to every metabolic reaction that occurs within the body, and when there are deficits, physiological reactions are negatively affected and composition of fluids and electrolytes altered. For any age group, staying hydrated at all times is a preventive measure.

Oral preparations of potassium should be prescribed whenever possible, instead of parenteral dosage forms. The oral dosage forms should be prepared per manufacturer inserts or per policy and standard of care. Generally, oral forms of potassium must not be taken with food, to minimize gastric distress or irritation. Powder or effervescent forms should be prepared according to the package guidelines and mixed thoroughly with at least 120 to 180 mL of fluids prior to actual administration of the medication. Enteric-coated and sustained-released forms may still result in gastric upset and lead to ulcer development (ulcerogenic). Although the risk for gastrointestinal adverse effects may be minimized with these dosage forms, the medicine should still be taken with food or a snack. The safest and most effective intervention includes frequent and close monitoring for complaints of nausea, vomiting, abdominal pain, or bleeding (such as blood in the stool or the occurrence of hematemesis, or blood in vomitus). Should abnormalities be noted, continue to monitor the vital signs and other parameters, and report the findings to the physician immediately. Serum levels of potassium should be monitored during therapy as well.

With the patient who is at risk for hypokalemia, provide educational materials and patient teaching to encourage the patient to eat certain foods high in potassium. The minimal daily requirement for potassium is between 40 and 50 mmol for adults and 2 to 3 mmol/kg of body weight for infants. Information on foods containing potassium should be shared with the patient; these foods include some of the following: two medium-sized bananas or a 240 mL glass of orange juice contains 45 mmol; 20 large dried apricots contain 40 mmol; and a level teaspoon of salt substitute (KCl) contains 60 mmol of potassium. Conversely, if the patient is already hyperkalemic, these food items should be avoided. See previous discussion on the use of Kayexylate to treat hyperkalemia. See Patient Education for more information.

Potassium chloride is the salt customarily used for intravenous infusions. Potassium chloride comes with the concern and caution of avoiding overdosage because of the possibility of causing cardiac arrest. It is always important to remember that intravenous dosage forms of potassium MUST always be given in a DILUTED form. There is NO use or place for UNDILUTED potassium because undiluted potassium is associated with cardiac arrest. Therefore, parenteral forms of potassium should be diluted properly. Most pharmacies now "premix" the infusion; however, it is still imperative to double-check the concentration and amount of diluent. Never assume that whatever was premixed is 100% correct. Diluted potassium should also be given only in situations where there is adequate urine output of at least 30 mL/hour. Manufacturer instructions and policy protocols generally recommend that intravenous solutions be given at concentrations less than 40 mmol/L of potassium and a rate not exceeding 20 mmol/hr. Another precautionary measure that must be followed is to avoid adding KCl to an already existing intravenous solution because the exact concentration would not be accurately calculated, thus risking complications, overdosage, or toxicity. Make sure that all intravenous fluids are labelled appropriately and documented, as with any medication. If there is need for very close monitoring of the intravenous fluid rate, an infusion pump may be used. There is no place for intravenous push or intravenous bolus potassium replacement.

Replacement of sodium carries the same concern for dosing and route of administration. In situations where the patient is only mildly depleted, an increase in oral intake of sodium should be tried. Food items high in sodium include ketchup, mustard, cured meats, cheeses, potato chips, peanut butter, popcorn, and table salt. In some situations, salt tablets may be necessary. If the patient is given salt tablets, it is important that the patient also take plenty of fluids of up to 3000 mL/24 hr, unless contraindicated. If the sodium deficit requires intravenous replacement, venous-access issues and drip rate are as important to consider as with volume and potassium infusions (see previous discussion regarding intravenous infusion and intravenous sites).

The intravenous infusion of albumin and other colloids should always be done slowly and cautiously and with careful monitoring to prevent fluid overload and possible heart failure, especially in those patients who are at particular risk for heart failure. Fluid overload is evidenced by shortness of breath, crackles in the bases of lungs, decreased pulse oximeter readings, edema of dependent areas, and increase in weight. Serum hematocrit and hemoglobin values should also be determined before, during, and after therapy so that any dilutional factors can be determined. For example, if a patient has received albumin and other colloids too quickly and hypervolemia results, the patient's hemoglobin and hematocrit may actually be decreased. This decrease would be due to a dilutional factor from too much volume as related to concentration of solutes. Clinically, the patient would appear to be anemic, but, in fact, the deficit would be attributed to the increase in volume. It is also important to remember that albumin should be given at room temperature.

For infusion of blood, it is essential to always check the expiration date of blood and blood components to make sure that the blood is not outdated. Under NO circumstances should outdated blood be used! Policies at most hospitals and other health care agencies require that blood and blood products be double-checked by another registered nurse BEFORE the blood is infused. This is important in preventing confusion of blood types. Blood types should always be a major concern because of the possible complications that can occur—some life threatening—if the wrong blood type is given or if the blood is given to the wrong person. The "Ten Rights" of drug administration are critical in all that nurses do with medications, and administering blood is no exception.

When infusing blood and blood products, all vital signs and related parameters should be documented before, during, and after administration of a blood product, component (e.g., plasma protein fraction, platelets, and fresh frozen plasma), or solution. The patient should then be assessed and the findings documented. Vital signs should also be checked and recorded. Immediate effects of a transfusion reaction develop within a few minutes or hours after the start of transfusion and may include apprehension, restlessness, flushed skin, increased pulse and respirations, dyspnea, rash, joint or lower back pain, swelling, fever and chills (a febrile reaction beginning 1 hour after the start of administration and possibly lasting up to 10 hours), nausea, weakness, and jaundice. These signs and symptoms should be reported to the physician immediately. Regardless of when the reaction occurs, the blood or product should be stopped and intravenous line kept patent with isotonic NS solution infusing at a low drip. Always follow the facility's protocol for transfusion reactions.

In summary, patients taking any type of fluid or electrolyte substance, colloid, or blood component should be encouraged to immediately report unusual adverse effects to their physician. Such complaints include chest pain, dizziness, weakness, and shortness of breath.

Evaluation

The therapeutic response to fluid, electrolyte, and blood or blood component therapy includes normalization of fluid volume and laboratory values, including red blood cells, white blood cells, hemoglobin, hematocrit, sodium, potassium, and calcium. In addition to these laboratory values, evaluation of the patient's heart, respiratory, musculoskeletal, and gastrointestinal functioning is also important. Energy levels and tolerance to activities of daily living should return to normal. There should be improved skin colour and minimal to no dyspnea, chest pain, weakness, or fatigue. Blood volume that has been correctly treated will be evidenced by a return to normal for laboratory values, improved vital signs, an increase in energy, and near-normal O_2 saturation levels. The therapeutic response to albumin therapy includes an elevation of blood pressure, decreased edema, and increased serum albumin levels. Monitoring for the adverse effects of any of these drugs and solutions should occur frequently and include monitoring for distended neck veins, shortness of breath, anxiety, insomnia, expiratory crackles, frothy, blood-tinged sputum, and cyanosis.

PATIENT EDUCATION
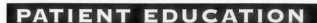

- As needed, patients should be educated about the difference in signs and symptoms of hyponatremia and hypernatremia. Hyponatremia manifests as lethargy, hypotension, stomach cramps, vomiting, diarrhea, and possibly seizures. Hypernatremia manifests as red, flushed skin; dry, sticky mucous membranes; increased thirst; temperature elevation; and a decrease in or absence of urination.
- Patients should inform all personal health care professionals about all medications they are taking, including OTC drugs, natural health products, and prescription drugs.
- Patients should be educated about how to take oral potassium chloride. Include directions about mixing any powdered or liquid solutions in at least 120 to 240 mL of cold water or juice, drinking the entire mixture slowly, and taking the dose with food.
- Patients taking potassium supplements should inform their health care provider if they experience gastrointestinal upset, abdominal pain, muscle cramps or weakness, fatigue, or irregular heartbeat. Inform the patient about the many drug interactions, including those with antacids, diuretics, and digitalis drugs.
- Patients should be educated about foods high in potassium such as bananas, oranges, leafy green vegetables, spinach, potatoes, lentils, fish, chicken, turkey, ham, beef, and milk.
- Patients should be informed that sustained-release capsules and tablets must be swallowed whole and should not be crushed, chewed, or allowed to dissolve in the mouth by sucking. This would increase adverse effects.
- Patients should be encouraged to report any difficulty in swallowing, painful swallowing, or feeling as if the capsule or tablet is stuck in their throat. Other serious adverse effects that need to be reported include vomiting of coffee ground–like material, stomach or abdominal pain, swelling, and black or tarry stools.
- Patients should be informed that extended-release dosage forms should be taken in full. If difficulty in swallowing occurs with the whole tablet, and if approved by their health care provider, patients could break the tablet in half and take each half separately, drinking one half a glass of water (120 mL) with each and taking the entire dose within a few minutes. Dissuade the patient from saving a half for later. If the tablet must be dissolved as prescribed, the patient should know to allow 2 minutes for the tablet to dissolve in 120 mL of water, stir for 30 seconds, and then drink immediately. Adding 30 mL of water to the glass with swirling and then drinking the residual will enable adequate dosing. Water is recommended as the solution for mixing the extended dosage.
- Patients should be instructed to dissolve effervescent tablets as directed, with emphasis on taking at least 90 mL of cold water per tablet. The dose should be taken as soon as fully dissolved, sipping the mixture over 5 to 10 minutes and taking the dose after food to minimize gastrointestinal upset.
- Patients should be informed that salt substitutes contain potassium, so another alternative should be recommended if patients are hyperkalemic.
- Patients should be informed to report any feelings of irritation (e.g., burning) at the intravenous site at any time.
- Patients should be informed to take salt tablets as prescribed, with caution, and with adequate fluid intake.

POINTS TO REMEMBER

- Total body water is divided into intracellular (inside the cell) and extracellular (outside the cell) compartments. Fluid volume outside cells is either in the plasma (intravascular volume) or between the tissues, cells, or organs (intracellular volume).
- Colloids are large protein particles that cannot leak out of the blood vessels because their size prevents them from passing through the vessel wall. Examples of colloids include albumin, hetastarch, and dextran. Albumin must be administered with caution because of the high risk for hypervolemia and possibly heart failure. The nurse needs to monitor intake and output, weights, and heart and breath sounds, as well as laboratory values appropriate to the situation and for albumin.
- Blood products are also known as *oxygen-carrying resuscitation fluids*. They are the only class of fluids that are able to carry oxygen because they are the only fluids that contain hemoglobin. Patients should show improved energy and increasing tolerance for activities of daily living. The nurse should also monitor pulse oximeter readings.
- Dehydration may be hypotonic, resulting from the loss of salt; hypertonic, resulting from fever with perspiration; or isotonic, resulting from diarrhea or vomiting. Each form of dehydration is treated differently. The nurse should carefully assess intake and output as well as skin turgor, urine specific gravity, and blood values of potassium, sodium, and chloride.
- Hypertonic solutions should be given slowly (less than 100 mL/hr) because of the risk for hypervolemia due to overzealous replacement.
- Symptoms of hypokalemia include lethargy, weakness, fatigue, respiratory difficulty, paralysis, and possible paralytic ileus. CAUTION: When replacing potassium via intravenous infusions, the nurse should never give undiluted potassium chloride because it can result in ventricular fibrillation and cardiac arrest as a result of hyperkalemia. Nursing units should only use diluted potassium (e.g., 1000 mL of

intravenous fluids premixed by the manufacturer of the drug and intravenous fluids). The nurse should never exceed recommended dosages of potassium (e.g., usual dose per 1000 mL of intravenous fluids is 40 mmol). Treatment of hyperkalemia is with the use of Kayexylate. Adverse effects that the nurse needs to be aware of include nausea, stomach pain, loss of appetite, and constipation, or diarrhea may occur. If these effects persist or worsen, notify the physician immediately. Unlikely to occur are swelling, muscle cramps, dizziness, and mental or mood changes. If they do occur, they should be reported promptly.

❖ Blood products may cause hemolysis of red blood cells; therefore, adverse reactions such as fever, chills, and back pain should be watched for continually. Hematuria may occur if the hemolysis reaction is present. If noted, the nurse should notify the physician immediately, the intravenous infusion discontinued, and the nature of the reactions and all actions taken documented. Vital signs and frequent monitoring of the patient before, during, and after infusions are critical to patient safety. Blood products should be given only with NS 0.9% because D5W will also cause hemolysis of the blood product.

EXAMINATION REVIEW QUESTIONS

1 While setting up a transfusion of packed red blood cells, which principle must the nurse remember to follow?
  a. Check the patient's vital signs after the infusion is completed.
  b. Flushed skin and fever are expected reactions to a blood transfusion.
  c. The intravenous line should be flushed with NS before the blood is added to the infusion.
  d. The intravenous line should be flushed with dextrose before the blood is added to the infusion.

2 When preparing an intravenous solution that contains potassium, which of the following must the nurse know is a contraindication to the potassium infusion?
  a. Diarrhea
  b. Dehydration
  c. Serum potassium of 2.8 mmol/L
  d. Serum potassium of 5.6 mmol/L

3 Which of the following is a contraindication for albumin when assessing a patient who has an order for albumin administration?
  a. Heart failure
  b. Severe burns
  c. Acute liver failure
  d. Fluid-volume deficit

4 The nurse is preparing an infusion for a patient who has deficient clotting due to hemophilia. Which type of infusion will this patient receive?
  a. Albumin 5%
  b. Packed red blood cells
  c. Whole blood
  d. Fresh frozen plasma

5 While monitoring a patient who is receiving an infusion of 3% NS, which of the following should the nurse look for?
  a. Bradycardia
  b. Hypotension
  c. Fluid overload
  d. Decreased skin turgor

For answers see http://evolve.elsevier.com/Canada/Lilley/pharmacology/.

CRITICAL THINKING ACTIVITIES

1 Contrast the three types of dehydration. List an example of each type.
2 Discuss the importance of crystalloids and their therapeutic effectiveness. Provide examples of crystalloids and the conditions for which they would be ordered.
3 Compare the use of crystalloids with that of colloids.

For answers see http://evolve.elsevier.com/Canada/Lilley/pharmacology/.

CHAPTER 28

Coagulation Modifier Drugs

Learning Objectives

After reading this chapter, the successful student will be able to do the following:

1 Briefly review hemostasis, coagulation, and platelet physiology.

2 Discuss the mechanisms of action of coagulation modifiers such as anticoagulants, antiplatelet drugs, antifibrinolytics, and thrombolytics.

3 Compare the indications, cautions, contraindications, adverse effects, routes of administration, and dosages of coagulation modifiers.

4 Discuss the administration procedures for coagulation modifiers.

5 Identify drug interactions associated with the use of coagulation modifiers, specific observations related to their use, and available antidotes.

6 Develop a collaborative plan of care that includes all phases of the nursing process for patients receiving anticoagulants, antiplatelet drugs, antifibrinolytics, and thrombolytics.

e-Learning Activities

Web site
(http://evolve.elsevier.com/Canada/Lilley/pharmacology/)

- Animations
- Answers to chapter questions, activities, and case studies
- Calculators and Category Catchers
- Glossary with audio pronunciations
- IV Therapy and Medication Error Checklists
- Multiple-Choice Review Question quizzes
- Nursing Care Plans
- Online Appendices and Supplements
- WebLinks

Drug Profiles

▸▸ **alteplase**, p. 540
   argatroban, p. 531
▸▸ **aspirin**, p. 536
▸▸ **clopidogrel (clopidogrel bisulfate)***, p. 536
   desmopressin (desmopressin acetate)*, p. 538
▸▸ **enoxaparin (enoxaparin sodium)***, p. 531
▸▸ **eptifibatide** p. 536
▸▸ **heparin (heparin sodium)***, p. 532
   lepirudin, p. 532
▸▸ **streptokinase**, p. 540
▸▸ **warfarin (warfarin sodium)***, p. 532

▸▸ Key drug.

*Full generic name is given in parentheses. For the purposes of this text, the more common shortened name is used.

Glossary

Anticoagulant A substance that prevents or delays coagulation of the blood. (p. 526)

Antifibrinolytic drug A drug that promotes the formation of clots through prevention of the lysis of fibrin. (p. 526)

Antiplatelet drug A drug that prevents platelet plugs from forming; this effect can help prevent cardiovascular disease such as myocardial infarctions and strokes. (p. 526)

Antithrombin III (AT-III) A substance that inactivates three major activating factors of the clotting cascade: activated II (thrombin), activated X, and activated IX. (p. 529)

β-Hemolytic streptococci (group A) The pyogenic streptococci of group A that cause hemolysis of red blood cells in blood agar in the laboratory setting. (p. 538)

Clot Insoluble solid elements of blood (cells, fibrin threads, etc.) that have chemically separated from the liquid (plasma) component of the blood. (p. 525)

Coagulation   The sequential process by which the multiple coagulation factors of the blood interact in the coagulation cascade, ultimately forming an insoluble fibrin clot. (p. 525)

Coagulation cascade   The series of steps beginning with the *intrinsic* or *extrinsic* pathways of coagulation and proceeding through the formation of a *fibrin clot*. (p. 525)

Deep vein thrombosis (DVT)   The formation of a thrombus in one of the deep veins of the body, most commonly the iliac and femoral veins. (p. 528)

Embolus   A blood clot (thrombus) that has been dislodged from the wall of a blood vessel and is travelling throughout the bloodstream. (p. 525)

Fibrin   A stringy, insoluble protein produced by the action of thrombin on fibrinogen during the clotting process; a major component of blood *clots* or *thrombi* (see Thrombus). (p. 525)

Fibrinogen   A plasma protein that is converted into fibrin by thrombin in the presence of calcium ions. (p. 535)

Fibrinolysis   The continual process of fibrin decomposition produced by the actions of the enzymatic protein fibrinolysin. (p. 526)

Fibrinolytic system   An area of the circulatory system undergoing fibrinolysis. (p. 526)

Fibrin-specificity   Property of newer thrombolytic drugs to activate plasminogen to plasmin in the presence of established clots having fibrin threads. (p. 539)

Hemorheological drug   A drug that alters the function of platelets without compromising their blood-clotting properties. (p. 526)

Hemostasis   Arrest of bleeding, either by the physiological properties of vasoconstriction and coagulation or by mechanical, surgical, or pharmacological means. (p. 525)

Hemostatic   A procedure, device, or substance that arrests the flow of blood. (p. 532)

Plasmin   The enzymatic protein that breaks down fibrin into fibrin degradation products; it is derived from plasminogen. (p. 526)

Plasminogen   A plasma protein that is converted to plasmin. (p. 526)

Pulmonary embolus (PE)   The blockage of a pulmonary artery by foreign matter such as fat, air, tumour, or a thrombus that usually arises from a peripheral vein. (p. 528)

Stroke   Occlusion of the blood vessels of the brain by an embolus, thrombus, or cerebrovascular hemorrhage, resulting in ischemia of the brain tissue. (p. 526)

Thromboembolic event   An event in which a blood vessel is blocked by an embolus carried in the bloodstream from the site of its formation. (p. 528)

Thrombolytic drug   A drug that dissolves thrombi by functioning similarly to *tissue plasminogen activator*. (p. 526)

Thrombus   Technical term for a blood clot (plural: *thrombi*); an aggregation of platelets, fibrin, clotting factors, and the cellular elements of the blood that is attached to the interior wall of a vein or artery, sometimes occluding the lumen of the vessel. (p. 525)

Tissue plasminogen activator   A naturally occurring plasminogen activator secreted by vascular endothelial cells in the walls of the blood vessels. Thrombolytic drugs are based on this blood component. (p. 525)

HEMOSTASIS AND COAGULATION

Hemostasis is a process that stops bleeding from an injured blood vessel, requiring the combined activity of vascular, platelet, and plasma factors. Hemostasis can be accomplished by mechanical means (e.g., compression to the bleeding site) or by surgical means (e.g., surgical clamping or cauterization of a blood vessel). When hemostasis occurs because of physiological clotting of blood, it is called **coagulation**, or the process of blood-clot formation. A **clot** is the insoluble solid elements of blood (cells, fibrin threads, etc.) that have chemically separated from the liquid (plasma) component of the blood. The technical term for a blood clot is **thrombus**, and a thrombus that is not stationary but moves through blood vessels from its point of origin is called an **embolus**. Normal hemostasis involves the complex interaction of substances that promote clot formation and substances that either inhibit coagulation or dissolve the formed clot. Substances that promote coagulation include *platelets, von Willebrand factor, activated clotting factors*, and *tissue thromboplastin*. Substances that inhibit coagulation include *prostacyclin, antithrombin III*, and *proteins C and S*.

Additionally, **tissue plasminogen activator** is a natural substance that dissolves clots that are already formed.

The coagulation system is illustrated in Figures 28-1 and 28-2. It is a cascade (or **coagulation cascade**) because each activated clotting factor serves as a catalyst that amplifies the next reaction. The result is a large concentration of a clot-forming substance called **fibrin**. The coagulation cascade is typically divided into the intrinsic and extrinsic pathways, and these pathways are activated by different types of injury. When blood vessels are damaged by penetration from the outside (e.g., a knife or bullet wound), thromboplastin, a substance contained in the walls of blood vessels, is released. This initiates the *extrinsic pathway* by activating factors VII and X (see Figure 28-1). All of the components of this *intrinsic pathway* are present in the blood in their inactive forms (see Figure 28-2). This pathway is activated when factor XII comes in contact with exposed collagen on the *inside* of damaged blood vessels. Figures 28-1 and 28-2 illustrate the steps that occur in the extrinsic and intrinsic pathways, respectively, and the factors involved. They also illustrate the site of action of two commonly used anticoagulant drugs: warfarin and heparin.

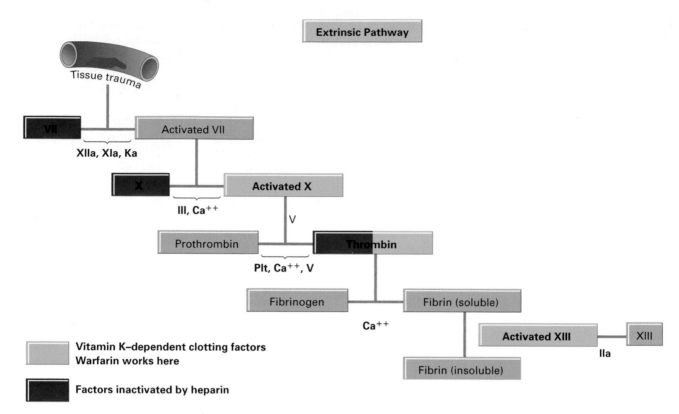

FIG. 28-1 Coagulation pathway and factors: extrinsic pathway. *Plt*, platelets.

Once a clot is formed and fibrin is present, the **fibrinolytic system** is activated. This system initiates the breakdown of clots and serves to balance the clotting process. **Fibrinolysis** is the reversal of the clotting process; it is the mechanism by which formed thrombi are *lysed* (broken down) to prevent excessive clot formation and blood vessel blockage. The fibrin in the clot binds to a circulating protein known as **plasminogen**. Through this process, plasminogen is converted to **plasmin**, the enzymatic protein that eventually breaks down the fibrin thrombus into *fibrin degradation products*. In this way, the thrombus is kept localized, which prevents it from becoming an embolus that can travel to obstruct a major blood vessel in the lung, heart, or brain. Figure 28-3 illustrates the fibrinolytic system.

COAGULATION-MODIFYING DRUGS

Coagulation-modifying drugs aid the body in reversing or achieving hemostasis, and they can be broken down into several main categories based on their actions. **Anticoagulants** inhibit the action or formation of clotting factors and, therefore, prevent clots from forming. **Antiplatelet drugs** prevent platelet plugs from forming by inhibiting platelet aggregation; this inhibition can

be beneficial in preventing heart attacks and strokes. A **stroke** is ischemia of brain tissue arising from occlusion of the blood vessels of the brain by an embolus, thrombus, or cerebrovascular hemorrhage. Other drugs, by contrast, alter platelet function without preventing platelets from working. These drugs are sometimes referred to as **hemorheological drugs**. Sometimes clots form and totally block a blood vessel. When this happens in one of the coronary arteries, a heart attack occurs, and the clot blocking the blood vessel must be lysed to prevent or minimize damage to the myocardial muscle. **Antifibrinolytic drugs**, also known as hemostatic drugs, have the opposite effect of these other classes of drugs; they actually *promote* blood coagulation and are helpful in managing conditions in which excessive bleeding would be harmful.

The **thrombolytic drugs** lyse (break down) clots, or *thrombi*, that have already formed. This action differentiates thrombolytics from the anticoagulants, which can only prevent the formation of a clot. The drugs in each category of coagulation modifiers are listed in Table 28-1. Understanding the individual coagulation modifiers and their mechanisms of action requires a basic working knowledge of the coagulation pathway and coagulation factors, which is provided in the next section.

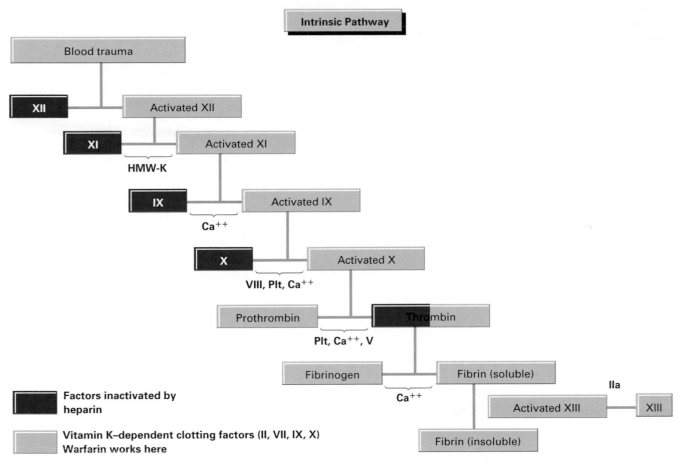

FIG. 28-2 Coagulation pathway and factors: intrinsic pathway. *HMW-K*, high-molecular-weight kininogen; *Plt*, platelets.

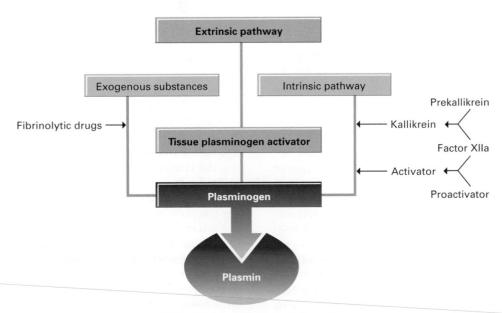

FIG. 28-3 The fibrinolytic system.

TABLE 28-1

Coagulation Modifiers: Comparison of Drug Subclasses

Type of Coagulation Modifier and Mechanism of Action	Drug Class	Individual Drugs
PREVENT CLOT FORMATION: ANTICOAGULANTS		
Inhibits clotting factors (thrombin) and Xa	Heparins	Unfractionated heparin (heparin sodium) and low-molecular-weight heparins (dalteparin sodium [Fragmin], enoxaparin sodium [Lovenox], nadroparin calcium [Fraxiparine], tinzaparin sodium [Innohep])
Inhibits vitamin K–dependent clotting factors II, VII, IX, and X	Coumadins	warfarin sodium (Coumadin)
Inhibits clotting factors IIa and Xa	Glycosaminoglycans	danaparoid sodium (Orgaran)
Inhibits thrombin (factor IIa)	Direct thrombin inhibitors	antithrombin III (human) (Thrombate), lepirudin (Refludan), argatroban (Argatroban), bivalirudin (Angiomax)
Inhibits factor Xa	Selective factor Xa inhibitor	fondaparinux (Arixtra)
THROMBOLYTICS		
Lyse a preformed clot	Thrombolytic enzymes	streptokinase (Streptase)
	Tissue plasminogen activators alteplase (Activase, Cathflo), reteplase (Retavase), tenecteplase (TNKase)	
	Recombinant human activated protein C	drotrecogin alfa (Xigris)
ANTIPLATELET DRUGS		
Interfere with platelet function	Aggregation inhibitors	clopidogrel (Plavix)
	Aggregation inhibitors/ vasodilators	treprostinil (Remodulin)
	Glycoprotein IIb/IIIa inhibitors	abciximab (Reopro), eptifibatide (Integrilin), tirofiban (Aggrastat)
	Miscellaneous	anagrelide (Agrylin), dipyridamole (Aggrenox)
PROMOTE CLOT FORMATION: ANTIFIBRINOLYTICS		
Prevent lysis of fibrin	Systemic hemostats	aminocaproic acid (Amicar),tranexamic acid (Cyklokapron), aprotinin (Trasylol)
Reduce blood viscosity	Hemorrheologics	pentoxyfilline (Trental)
REVERSAL DRUGS	Heparin antagonist	protamine sulfate
	warfarin sodium antagonist	vitamin K

ANTICOAGULANTS

Anticoagulants are drugs that prevent the formation of a clot by inhibiting certain clotting factors. They are only used prophylactically because they have no direct effect on a blood clot that has already formed or on ischemic tissue injured as the result of an inadequate blood supply caused by the clot. By decreasing blood coagulability, anticoagulants prevent intravascular thrombosis. Their uses vary from preventing clot formation to preventing the extension of a preformed clot, or a thrombus. Coagulation studies should be monitored when patients are receiving anticoagulants. These are discussed in the appropriate sections throughout this chapter. The *D-dimer* (*D* stands for domain), also known as *fibrin degradation fragment*, is a small protein fragment produced during the degradation of a blood clot by fibrinolysis. D-dimer is used to diagnose thrombotic states.

Once a clot forms on the wall of a blood vessel, it may dislodge and travel through the bloodstream. This travelling clot is referred to as an embolus. If an embolus travels and lodges in a coronary artery, it results in a myocardial infarction (MI); if it travels to the brain, it causes a stroke; if it travels to the lungs, it is a **pulmonary embolus (PE)**; and if it travels to the veins in the legs, it causes **deep vein thrombosis (DVT)**. Collectively, these complications are called **thromboembolic events** because they involve a thrombus becoming an embolus and causing an adverse cardiovascular event. Anticoagulants can prevent all of these from occurring if used in the correct manner. There are both orally and parenterally administered anticoagulants. Each drug has a slightly different mechanism of action and indications. Each class of anticoagulants has risks, primarily that of bleeding. The mechanisms of action of the anticoagulants vary depending on the drug. Drug classes of anticoagulants include older drugs, such as unfractionated heparin and warfarin. There are also several newer drug classes, including low-molecular-weight heparins (LMWHs), glycosaminoglycans, antithrombin drugs, and a selective factor Xa inhibitor. Dosages, indications, and other relevant information appear in the corresponding Dosages table on p. 533.

Mechanism of Action and Drug Effects

Anticoagulants are also called *antithrombotic* drugs because they all work to prevent the formation of a clot or thrombus, also called thrombosis. All anticoagulants work in the clotting cascade but do so at different points. As shown in Figures 28-1 and 28-2, heparin works by binding to a substance called **antithrombin III** (AT-III), which shuts off three main activating factors: activated II (also called thrombin), activated X, and activated IX. (Factors XI and XII are also inactivated but do not play as important a role as the other three factors.) Of these, the thrombin is the most sensitive to the actions of heparin. AT-III is the major natural inhibitor of thrombin in the blood. The overall effect of heparin is that it turns off the coagulation pathway and prevents clots from forming. As previously noted, however, it cannot lyse a clot. The drug name "heparin" usually refers to *unfractionated* heparin, which is a relatively large molecule, and is derived from animal sources. In contrast, LMWHs are synthetic and have a smaller molecular structure. They include enoxaparin (Lovenox), dalteparin (Fragmin), and tinzaparin (Innohep), and all three work similarly to heparin. Unlike heparin, however, which primarily binds to activated factors II, X, and IX, LMWHs are much more specific for activated factor X (Xa) than for activated factor II (IIa thrombin), giving LMWHs a much more predictable anticoagulant response. As a result, frequent laboratory monitoring of bleeding times such as activated partial thromboplastin times (aPTTs), which is imperative with unfractionated heparin, is not required with LMWHs.

Warfarin sodium (Coumadin) also acts by inhibiting vitamin K synthesis by bacteria in the gastrointestinal tract. This, in turn, inhibits production of clotting factors II, VII, IX, and X. These four factors are normally synthesized in the liver and are known as *vitamin K–dependent clotting factors.* As with heparin, the final effect is the prevention of clot formation. Figures 28-1 and 28-2 show where in the clotting cascade this occurs.

The *glycosaminoglycan* class currently includes one drug, danaparoid. This drug prevents fibrin formation by inhibiting clotting factors Xa (in conjunction with AT-III) and IIa (in conjunction with both AT-III and *heparin cofactor II [HC II]*). In contrast, fondaparinux (Arixtra) inhibits thrombosis through its molecular specificity against factor Xa alone. There are also currently four antithrombin drugs, one natural and three synthetic, which inhibit the thrombin molecules directly. The natural drug is human antithrombin III (Thrombate), which is isolated from the plasma of human donors. The three synthetic drugs include lepirudin (Refludan), argatroban (Argatroban), and bivalirudin (Angiomax). All of these drugs work similarly to inhibit thrombus formation.

Indications

The ability of anticoagulants to prevent clot formation is of benefit in certain settings where there is a high likelihood of clot formation. These include myocardial infarction, unstable angina, atrial fibrillation, indwelling devices such as mechanical heart valves, and conditions in which blood flow may be slowed and blood may pool, such as major orthopedic surgery. The ultimate consequence of a clot can be a stroke or a heart attack, a DVT, or a pulmonary embolism; therefore, the prevention of these serious consequences is the ultimate benefit of anticoagulants. Warfarin is indicated for *prevention* of any of these events, whereas both unfractionated heparins and LMWHs are used for both prevention and treatment. LMWHs, especially enoxaparin, are also routinely used as anticoagulant bridge therapy in situations in which a patient must stop warfarin for surgery or other invasive medical procedures. The remainder of the antithrombotic drugs have similar but more restricted indications, which are listed in the corresponding Dosages table on p. 533.

Contraindications

Contraindications to the use of anticoagulants are generally similar for the different drugs and include known drug allergy to a specific product and usually include any acute bleeding process of high risk for such an occurrence, as well as thrombocytopenia. Some examples include leukemia or other major blood dyscrasias, pregnancy, gastrointestinal obstruction, serious inflammation (e.g., colitis), infection, and recent surgery or other invasive medical procedure. Warfarin is strongly contraindicated in pregnancy, whereas the other anticoagulants are rated in lower pregnancy categories (B or C).

Adverse Effects

Bleeding is the main complication of anticoagulation therapy, and the risk increases with increasing dosages. Such bleeding may be localized (e.g., hematoma at site of injection) or systemic. It also depends on the nature of the patient's underlying clinical disorder and is increased in patients who are also taking high doses of aspirin or other drugs that impair platelet function. One particularly notable common adverse effect of heparin is *heparin-induced thrombocytopenia* (HIT), also called *heparin-associated thrombocytopenia* (HAT). Thrombocytopenia is is an independent marker of risk for death and life-threatening events. It is an allergic reaction mediated by the production of immunoglobulin (Ig)G antibodies. Immune complexes bind to circulating platelets, resulting in platelet activation, which triggers increased platelet activation and thrombin generation. The greatest risk to the patient with HIT is this paradoxical occurrence of thrombosis, something that heparin normally prevents or alleviates. The incidence of this disorder ranges from 5% to 15% of patients and is higher with *bovine* (cow-derived) than with *porcine* (pig-derived) heparins. As listed in the Dosages table (p. 533), the direct thrombin inhibitors lepirudin and argatroban are both specifically indicated for treating HIT. Other adverse effects are listed in Table 28-2.

TABLE 28-2

Anticoagulants: Common Adverse Effects

Drug Subclass	Adverse Effects
Direct thrombin inhibitors	Bleeding, dizziness, chest discomfort, nausea, constipation, chills, shortness of breath, fever, urticaria, heart and kidney failure (lepirudin, argatroban), cardiac dysrhythmias (argatroban), hypotension (argatroban and bivalirudin)
Glycosaminoglycans	Bleeding, insomnia, headache, dizziness, rash, pruritus, nausea, constipation, vomiting, fever, injection site pain, edema, joint pain, asthenia, anemia, urinary retention, urinary tract infection
Heparins	Bleeding, hematoma, nausea, anemia, thrombocytopenia, fever, edema
Selective factor Xa inhibitors	Bleeding, hematoma, dizziness, confusion, rash, gastrointestinal distress, urinary tract infection, urinary retention, anemia

Interactions

The drug interactions involving the oral anticoagulants are profound and complicated; the drugs and the result of an interaction are given in Table 28-3. The main interaction mechanisms responsible for increasing anticoagulant activity include the following:

- Enzyme inhibition of biotransformation (metabolism)
- Displacement of the drug from inactive protein-binding sites
- Decrease in vitamin K absorption or synthesis by the bacterial flora of the large intestine
- Alteration in the platelet count or activity

TABLE 28-3

Anticoagulants: Drug Interactions

Drug	Mechanism	Result
WARFARIN SODIUM		
acetaminophen (high doses)		
amiodarone	Displaces from inactive protein-binding sites	
bumetanide		
furosemide		Increased anticoagulant effect
aspirin/other NSAIDs		
Broad-spectrum antibiotics	Decreases platelet activity	
cephalosporin		
Mineral oil	Interferes with vitamin K	
vitamin E		
Barbiturates		Decreased anticoagulant effect
carbamazepine	Enzyme inducer	
rifampin		
amiodarone		
cimetidine		
ciprofloxacin		
erythromycin		
ketoconazole	Enzyme inhibitor	Increased anticoagulant effect
metronidazole		
omeprazole		
Sulfonamides		
cholestyramine	Impairs absorption of warfarin	Decreased anticoagulant effect
sucralfate		
HEPARIN		
aspirin/other NSAIDs	Decrease platelet activity	
Cephalosporins		
ethacrynic acid		
Oral anticoagulants	Additive	Increased anticoagulant effect
Penicillins		
Thrombolytics		
Glycosaminoglycans, direct thrombin inhibitors, selective factor Xa inhibitors	Additive	Increased bleeding risk
Any other anticoagulant, antiplatelet, or thrombolytic drugs		

NSAID, nonsteroidal anti-inflammatory drug.

Drugs that can increase the activity of heparin include aspirin, intravenous (IV) ethacrynic acid, and oral anticoagulants. Antihistamines, digitalis, and tetracyclines may partially antagonize the anticoagulant effects of heparin by inducing (promoting activity of) enzymes that metabolize heparin. The drugs that cause this are listed in Table 28-3. As for laboratory test interactions, heparin can alter the serum levels of lipids, glucose, thyroxine, aspartate aminotransferase (AST), and alanine aminotransferase (ALT) and can affect triiodothyronine (T$_3$) uptake.

Toxicity and Management of Overdose

Treatment of the toxic effects of anticoagulants is aimed at reversing the underlying cause. Although the toxic effects of heparin, LMWHs, and warfarin are hemorrhagic in nature, the management for each is different. Symptoms that may be attributed to toxicity or an overdose of anticoagulants are hematuria, melena (blood in stools), petechiae, ecchymoses, and gum or mucous membrane bleeding. Should either heparin or warfarin toxicity occur, the anticoagulant should be discontinued. This strategy may be sufficient to reverse the toxic effects of heparin because of its short half-life (approximately 90 minutes). In severe cases or when large doses have been given intentionally (i.e., during cardiopulmonary bypass for heart surgery), IV injection of protamine sulfate is indicated. Protamine sulfate is a specific heparin antidote and forms a complex with heparin, completely reversing its anticoagulant properties. This occurs in as few as 5 minutes. In general, 1 mg of protamine can reverse the effects of 100 units of heparin. Heparin comes from three different sources, and each source has a different anticoagulant potency.

In theory, however, the protamine dosing should vary depending on the type of heparin given (1 mg of protamine for 90 units of heparin sodium from bovine lung tissue, 100 units of heparin calcium from porcine intestinal mucosa, and 115 units of heparin sodium from porcine intestinal mucosa). Protamine may also be used to reverse the effects of LMWHs. A 1 mg dose of protamine equal to that of the LMWH should be used (e.g., 1 mg protamine/1 mg enoxaparin). If the heparin overdose has resulted in a large blood loss, replacement with packed red blood cells (PRBCs) may be necessary.

If warfarin sodium toxicity or overdose occurs, again, the first step is to discontinue the warfarin. Similar to heparin, the toxicity associated with warfarin use is an extension of its therapeutic effects on the clotting cascade. However, because warfarin functionally inactivates the vitamin K–dependent clotting factors and because these clotting factors are synthesized in the liver, it may take 36 to 42 hours before the liver can resynthesize enough clotting factors to reverse the warfarin effects. IV injection of vitamin K (phytonadione) can hasten the return to normal coagulation. The dose and route of administration of vitamin K depend on the clinical situation and its acuity (i.e., how quickly the warfarin-induced effects must be reversed). High doses of vitamin K (10 to 15 mg) given intravenously should reverse the anticoagulation within 6 hours. If warfarin therapy needs to be resumed, warfarin resistance is likely to occur because a large dose of vitamin K will maintain its wafarin reversal effects for up to 1 week. The use of low doses of vitamin K, if clinically feasible, may minimize this effect. In acute situations in which bleeding is severe and the time it would take for the vitamin K to take effect is too great, it may be necessary to administer transfusions of human plasma or clotting factor concentrates.

Dosages

For the dosage information of anticoagulants, see the Dosages table on p. 533.

 DRUG PROFILES

Of all the anticoagulants, only warfarin is available for oral use. The rest are by IV or subcutaneous (SC) injection only. Intramuscular (IM) injection of these drugs is contraindicated because of their propensity to cause anticoagulation with large ecchymoses at the site of injection.

argatroban

Argatroban, which has the same trade name, is a synthetic direct thrombin inhibitor derived from the amino acid L-arginine. Argatroban exerts its anticoagulant effects by inhibiting thrombin catalyzed or induced reactions, including fibrin formation; activation of coagulation factor XIII, factor V, factor VIII, and protein C; and platelet aggregation. It is indicated both for active HIT and for percutaneous coronary intervention (PCI) procedures in patients at risk for HIT (i.e., those with history). It is only given intravenously.

PHARMACOKINETICS

Half-Life	Onset	Peak	Duration
30–50 min	Immediate	1–3 hr	Dependent on length of infusion

▶▶ enoxaparin sodium

Enoxaparin sodium (Lovenox) is the prototype LMWH and is obtained by enzymatically cleaving large unfractionated heparin molecules into small fragments. These smaller fragments of heparin have a greater affinity for factor Xa than for factor IIa and have a higher degree of bioavailability and a longer elimination half-life than unfractionated heparin. Laboratory monitoring, as done for heparin, is not necessary with enoxaparin because of its high bioavailability and greater affinity for factor Xa. Enoxaparin is available only in injectable form.

Continued

DRUG PROFILES (cont'd)

Other anticoagulants with comparable pharmacology and indications include danaparoid sodium (Oragaran) and fondaparinux sodium (Arixtra).

PHARMACOKINETICS

Half-Life	Onset	Peak	Duration
4.5 hr	3–5 hr	3 hr	12 hr

▸▸ *heparin sodium*

Heparin sodium (Hepalean, Heparin LEO) is a natural mucopolysaccharide anticoagulant obtained from porcine intestinal mucosa or from beef lung. One brand name for some of the commonly used heparin products is Hepalean-Lok, often called Hep-Lok. This brand name, however, refers only to small vials of aqueous heparin IV flush solutions used to maintain patency of heparin lock IV insertion sites. This use for heparin is fundamentally different from the systemic use of heparin for its anticoagulant cardiovascular effects as discussed in this chapter. Heparin solutions used for heparin lock flushes are usually in a lower concentration than heparin used for systemic cardiovascular purposes. Some institutions routinely use normal saline (0.9%) as a flush for heparin lock IV ports and have moved away from using heparin flush solutions for this purpose. Heparin is only available in injectable form in multiple strengths ranging from 10 to 40,000 units per mL.

PHARMACOKINETICS

Half-Life	Onset	Peak	Duration
1–2 hr	SC: 20–60 min IV: Immediate	SC: 2–4 hr	Dose-dependent

lepirudin

Lepirudin (Refludan) is a recombinant, yeast-derived inhibitor of thrombin. It is used specifically for heparin-induced thrombocytopenia (HIT). It is also indicated for anticoagulation in adult patients with acute coronary syndromes (unstable angina/acute myocardial infarction without ST elevation) combined with aspirin. As with heparin, lepirudin is monitored using the *aPTT*. Argatroban is another drug in this class with the same indication. Other drugs in this class with more variable indications include human antithrombin III (for hereditary deficiency), desirudin (for DVT prophylaxis), and bivalirudin (for unstable angina).

PHARMACOKINETICS

Half-Life	Onset	Peak	Duration
1 hr	Not listed	Not listed	Dependent on length of infusion

▸▸ *warfarin sodium*

Warfarin sodium (Coumadin) is a pharmaceutical derivative of the natural plant anticoagulant known as *coumarin*. Warfarin is the most commonly prescribed oral (PO) anticoagulant and is only available for oral use. Use of this drug requires careful monitoring of the prothrombin time/International Normalized Ratio (PT/INR), which is a standardized measure of the degree to which a patient's blood coagulability has been reduced by the drug. The INR measures the intrinsic pathway. A normal INR (without warfarin) is 1.0, whereas a therapeutic INR (with warfarin) ranges from 2 to 3.5, depending on the indication for use of the drug (e.g., a range of 2 to 3 is recommended for prophylaxis for DVT and treatment and prevention of pulmonary embolus, whereas a range of 2.5 to 3.5 is recommended for mechanical heart valves). A patient older than 65 years may have a lower INR threshold for bleeding complications and should be monitored accordingly.

PHARMACOKINETICS

Half-Life	Onset	Peak	Duration
0.5–3 days	12–24 hr	3–4 days	2–5 days

PLATELET PHYSIOLOGY

Another class of coagulation modifiers that prevent clot formation comprises antiplatelet drugs. The anticoagulants exert their effect in the clotting cascade. In contrast, antiplatelet drugs act to prevent platelet adhesion to the site of blood vessel injury, which occurs before the clotting cascade. An understanding of the role of platelets in the clotting process is essential to understanding how antiplatelet drugs work.

Platelets normally flow through blood vessels without adhering to their surfaces. Blood vessels can be injured by a disruption of blood flow, trauma, or the rupture of plaque from a vessel wall. When such events occur, substances such as collagen and fibronectin, which are present in the walls of blood vessels, become exposed. Collagen is a potent stimulator of platelet adhesion, as is a prevalent component of the platelet membranes, glycoprotein IIb/IIIa (GP IIb/IIIa). Once platelet adhesion occurs, stimulators (compounds such as adenosine diphosphate [ADP], thrombin, thromboxane A_2 [TXA_2], and prostaglandin H_2) are released from the activated platelets. These stimulators cause platelets to aggregate (accumulate) at the site of injury. Once at the site of vessel injury, platelets change shape and release contents, which include ADP, serotonin, and platelet factor 4 (PF4). The hemostatic function of these substances is twofold: first, they function as platelet recruiters, attracting additional platelets to the site of injury; second, they are potent *vasoconstrictors*. Vasoconstriction limits blood flow to the damaged blood vessel to reduce blood loss.

A platelet plug that has formed at a site of vessel injury is not stable and can be dislodged. The clotting cascade is therefore stimulated to form a more permanent *fibrin* plug (blood clot). The role of platelets and their relationship to the clotting cascade are illustrated in Figure 28-4.

DOSAGES   Selected Anticoagulant Drugs

Drug (Pregnancy Category)	Pharmacological Class	Usual Dosage Range	Indications
argatroban (Argatroban) (B)	Synthetic thrombin inhibitor	*Adult* IV: 2–10 mcg/kg/min until aPTT in desired range	Thromboprevention and treatment in HIT, and in PCI in patients at risk for HIT
antithrombin III (Human; Thrombate III) (B)	Human antithrombin	*Adult* IV: calculated by weight on the basis of desired AT-III level	Hereditary AT-III deficiency in surgical, obstetrical, or thrombosis settings
bivalirudin (Angiomax) (B)	Synthetic thrombin inhibitor	*Adult* IV: 0.75 mg/kg bolus, then 1.785 mg/kg/hr (with aspirin, 325 mg daily)	Thromboprevention in unstable angina
dalteparin sodium (Fragmin) (B)	LMWH	*Adult* SC: 2500–5000 units once daily	DVT prophylaxis
▸▸enoxaparin sodium (Lovenox) (B)	LMWH	*Adult* SC: 30–100 mg every 12 hours	Prevention and treatment of thromboembolic and ischemic processes in postoperative, unstable angina and in post-MI situations
heparin (Hepalean, Heparin LEO) (C)	Natural anticoagulant	*Children* IV: Initial 50 units/kg, then 12–25 units/kg/hr, increased by 2–4 units/kg/hr q6–8h prn *Adult* SC: 10,000–20,000 units followed by 8000–10,000 units tid IV: 10,000 units followed by 5000–10,000 units 4–6 ×/day IV infusion: 20,000–40,000 units/day ACT or aPTT determines maintenance dose	Thrombosis/embolism, coagulopathies (e.g., DIC), DVT, and PE prophylaxis, clotting prevention (e.g., open heart surgery, dialysis)
lepirudin (Refludan) (B)	Synthetic thrombin inhibitor	*Adult* IV: 0.4 mg/kg bolus, then 0.15 mg/kg continuous infusion × 2–10 days	Thromboprevention in patients with HIT
tinzaparin (Innohep) (B)	LMWH	*Adult* SC: 175 units/kg once daily	DVT prophylaxis only
▸▸warfarin sodium (Coumadin) (X)	Coumarin anticoagulant	*Adult* PT or INR determines maintenance dose, usually 2–10 mg/day	Thromboprevention and treatment in DVT, PE, atrial fibrillation, post-MI

ACT, activated clotting time; *aPTT*, activated partial thromboplastin time; *AT-III*, antithrombin-III; *DIC*, disseminated intravascular coagulation; *DVT*, deep vein thrombosis; *HIT*, heparin-induced thrombocytopenia; *INR*, International Normalized Ratio; *IV*, intravenous; *LMWH*, low-molecular-weight heparin; *MI*, myocardial infarction; *PCI*, percutaneous coronary intervention; *PE*, pulmonary embolus; *PT*, prothrombin time; *SC*, subcutaneous.

ANTIPLATELET DRUGS

The mechanisms of action of the antiplatelet drugs vary depending on the drug. Aspirin, clopidogrel, dipyridamole, pentoxifylline, anagrelide, abciximab, tirofiban, and eptifibatide all affect the normal function of platelets. Dosage, indications, and other information appear in the Dosages table on p. 536.

Mechanism of Action and Drug Effects

Many of the antiplatelet drugs affect the *cyclooxygenase* pathway, one of the common final enzymatic pathways in the complex arachidonic acid pathway that operates within platelets and on blood vessel walls. This pathway,

as it functions in both platelets and blood vessel walls, is illustrated in Figure 28-5.

Aspirin (acetylsalicylic acid) is also widely used for its analgesic, anti-inflammatory, and antipyretic (antifever) properties (Chapter 45). As for aspirin's anticoagulant effects, it acetylates and inhibits cyclooxygenase in the platelet irreversibly such that the platelet cannot regenerate this enzyme. Therefore, the effects of aspirin last the lifespan of a platelet, or 7 days. This irreversible inhibition of cyclooxygenase within the platelet prevents the formation of TXA_2, a substance that causes blood vessels to constrict and platelets to aggregate. Consequently, by preventing TXA_2 formation, aspirin prevents these actions, resulting in dilation of the blood vessels and

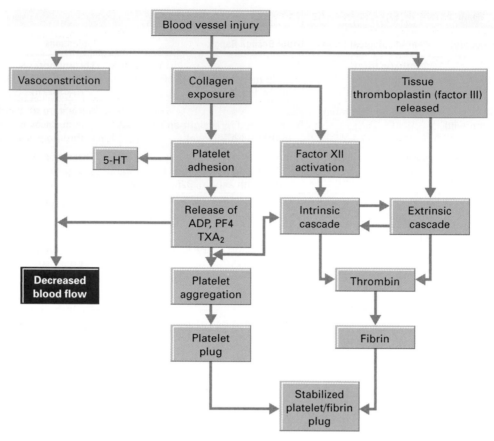

FIG. 28-4 Relationship between platelets and the clotting cascade. *ADP*, adenosine diphosphate; *5-HT*, serotonin; *PF4*, platelet factor 4; *TXA$_2$*, thromboxane A$_2$.

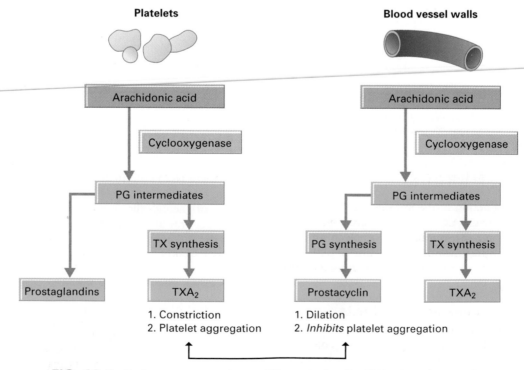

FIG. 28-5 Cyclooxygenase pathway. *PG*, prostaglandin; *TXA$_2$*, thromboxane A$_2$.

prevention of platelets from aggregating or forming a clot. In addition, aspirin may also affect vitamin K–dependent clotting factors VII, IX, and X, by interfering with the action of vitamin K, in a manner similar to warfarin. Ironically, aspirin has the additional limitation of preventing the formation of prostacyclin, a beneficial anticoagulant substance released by healthy endothelial cells from prostaglandin H_2 that causes blood vessel dilation and inhibits platelet aggregation. However, this procoagulant effect of aspirin is not as pronounced as its anticoagulant effects.

Dipyridamole, another antiplatelet drug, also acts to inhibit platelet aggregation by preventing the release of ADP, PF4, and TXA_2, substances that stimulate platelets to aggregate or form a clot. Figure 28-4 explains how these substances function to accomplish platelet aggregation. Dipyridamole may also directly stimulate the release of prostacyclin and inhibit the formation of TXA_2 (see Figure 28-5).

Clopidogrel belongs to one of the newest classes of antiplatelet drugs called the *ADP inhibitors*. Its use has largely superseded that of the original ADP inhibitor ticlopidine. Clopidogrel's mechanism of action is entirely different from that of aspirin, as it inhibits platelet aggregation by altering the platelet membrane so that it can no longer receive the signal to aggregate and form a clot. This signal is in the form of **fibrinogen** molecules (plasma proteins converted into fibrin by thrombin in the presence of calcium ions), which attach to glycoprotein receptors (GP IIb/IIIa) on the surface of the platelet. Clopidogrel inhibits the activation of this receptor. Clopidogrel has been shown to be somewhat better than aspirin at reducing the number of heart attacks, strokes, and vascular deaths in at-risk patients.

Pentoxifylline, another antiplatelet drug, is a methylxanthine derivative with properties similar to those of other methylxanthines, such as caffeine and theophylline (Chapter 37). It was one of the earliest antiplatelet drugs, but is now much less commonly used. It reduces the viscosity of blood by increasing the flexibility of red blood cells (RBCs) and reduces the aggregation of platelets. It is sometimes referred to as a *hemorrheological drug*, or a drug that alters the fluid dynamics of the blood. The antiplatelet effects of pentoxifylline are attributed to its inhibition of ADP, serotonin, and PF4 (see Figure 28-4). Pentoxifylline also stimulates the synthesis and release of prostacyclin from blood vessels (see Figure 28-5). In addition, it may have effects on the fibrinolytic system by raising the plasma concentrations of the tissue plasminogen activator (see Figure 28-3).

The newest available antiplatelet class of drugs is the GP IIb/IIIa inhibitors. They act by blocking the receptor protein by the same name that occurs in the platelet wall membranes. This protein plays a role in promoting the aggregation of platelets in preparation for fibrin clot formation. Currently available drugs in this class are tirofiban (Aggrastat), eptifibatide (Integrilin), and abciximab (ReoPro).

Indications

The therapeutic effects of antiplatelet drugs depend on the particular drug. Aspirin has multiple therapeutic effects, although many of the effects vary depending on the dose. Aspirin is recommended for stroke prevention in daily doses of 50 to 325 mg. Clopidogrel is also used for reducing the risk for fatal and nonfatal thrombotic stroke and is used for prophylaxis against transient ischemic attacks (TIAs) as well for post-MI *thromboprevention* (i.e., prevention of the formation of thrombi). Dipyridamole is used as an adjunct to warfarin in the prevention of postoperative thromboembolic complications. It is also used to decrease platelet aggregation in other thromboembolic disorders.

GP IIb/IIIa inhibitors are used to treat acute unstable angina, MI, and during PCI such as angioplasty. Their purpose is mainly for thromboprevention. This treatment approach is based on the fact that prevention of thrombus formation is easier and less risky overall than lysing a formed thrombus. Pentoxifylline is indicated for peripheral vascular disease.

Contraindications

Contraindications to the use of antiplatelet drugs include known drug allergy to a specific product, thrombocytopenia, active bleeding, leukemia, traumatic injury, gastrointestinal ulcer, vitamin K deficiency, and recent stroke.

Adverse Effects

The potential adverse effects of the antiplatelet drugs can be serious, and they all pose a risk for inducing a serious bleeding episode. The most common adverse effects are listed in Table 28-4.

TABLE	28-4

Antiplatelet Drugs: Adverse Effects

Body System	Adverse Effects
ASPIRIN	
Central nervous	Stimulation, drowsiness, dizziness, confusion, flushing
Gastrointestinal	Nausea, vomiting, gastrointestinal bleeding, diarrhea, heartburn
Hematological	Thrombocytopenia, agranulocytosis, leukopenia, neutropenia, hemolytic anemia, bleeding
CLOPIDOGREL	
Cardiovascular	Chest pain, hypertension, edema
Central nervous	Flulike symptoms, headache, dizziness, fatigue
Gastrointestinal	Abdominal pain, dyspepsia, diarrhea, nausea
Miscellaneous	Epistaxis and integumentary disorders, including rash and pruritus
GP IIB/IIIA INHIBITORS	Bleeding, bradycardia, dizziness, edema, leg pain, pelvic pain, chills

Interactions

There are some potentially dangerous drug interactions that can occur with antiplatelet drugs. The concurrent use of dipyridamole with aspirin, clopidogrel, or nonsteroidal anti-inflammatory drugs (NSAIDs) produces additive antiplatelet activity and increased bleeding potential. There may also be allergic cross-reactivity between aspirin and NSAIDs. Large doses of aspirin have a hypoglycemic effect and may enhance the effect of oral hypoglycemic drugs. The combined use of steroids or NSAIDs with aspirin can increase the risk of ulcers and gastrointestinal bleeding because of a synergistic effect. The combined use of aspirin and heparin with GP IIb/IIIa inhibitors also further enhances antiplatelet activity and increases the likelihood of a serious bleeding episode. In spite of all of these potentially harmful interactions, it is not uncommon to see patients on daily maintenance doses of aspirin for thrombopreventive purposes. The most commonly used dose in this situation is the "baby aspirin" dose of 81 mg instead of the standard adult dose of 325 mg.

Dosages

For information on the dosages of selected antiplatelet drugs, see the Dosages table below.

 DRUG PROFILES

Antiplatelet drugs are effective in the management of thromboembolic disorders. Each has unique pharmacological properties, and, therefore, they all are somewhat different from one another.

▶▶ *aspirin*

Aspirin is available in many combinations with other prescription and nonprescription drugs and has numerous product names. One unique contraindication for aspirin is its use in children and teenagers with flulike symptoms. This situation is associated with cases of Reye's syndrome, a rare, acute, and sometimes fatal condition involving liver and central nervous system (CNS) damage (Chapter 45). Aspirin is available in both oral and rectal forms.

PHARMACOKINETICS

Half-Life	Onset	Peak	Duration
PO: 3.5–4.5 hr	PO: 15–30 min	PO: 1–2 hr	PO: 4–6 hr

▶▶ *clopidogrel bisulfate*

Clopidogrel bisulfate (Plavix) is currently the most widely used ADP inhibitor. It has superseded ticlopidine (Ticlid) because of the associated serious adverse reactions with ticlopidine, including life-threatening neutropenia and agranulocytosis. It was initially believed that clopidogrel might be free from such adverse effects. However, there are some emerging case reports of clopidogrel-associated hematological adverse effects of comparable severity. This drug is available only in oral form.

PHARMACOKINETICS

Half-Life	Onset	Peak	Duration
PO: 8 hr	PO: 1–2 hr*	PO: 1 hr*	PO: 7–10 days

*Onset and peak values can be reduced by giving a loading dose of 300–375 mg.

▶▶ *eptifibatide*

Eptifibatide (Integrilin) is a GP IIb/IIIa inhibitor, along with tirofiban (Aggrastat) and abciximab (ReoPro). They are usually administered in critical care or heart catheterization lab settings, where continuous cardiovascular monitoring is the norm. All are available only for intravenous use.

PHARMACOKINETICS

Half-Life	Onset	Peak	Duration
IV: 2–2.5 hr	IV: 1 hr	IV: Unknown	IV: 4 hr

DOSAGES Selected Antiplatelet Drugs

Drug (Pregnancy Category)	Pharmacological Class	Usual Dosage Range	Indications
▶▶ aspirin (C/D)	Salicylate antiplatelet	*Adult* PO: 81–325 mg/day	MI prophylaxis TIA prophylaxis
▶▶ clopidogrel bisulfate (Plavix) (B)	ADP inhibitor	*Adult* PO: 75 mg daily; 300–375 mg may be given as a one-time loading dose for patients with unstable angina, non-ST-segment elevation	Reduction of atherosclerotic events; acute coronary syndrome without ST-segment elevation
▶▶ eptifibatide (Integrilin) (B)	GP IIb/IIIa inhibitor	*Adult Only* IV: Single bolus followed by continuous infusion; specific doses are based on patient weight from 37 to 121 kg*	Unstable angina/non–ST-segment elevation MI

ADP, adenosine diphosphate; *GP*, glycoprotein; *IV*, intravenous; *MI*, myocardial infarction; *PO*, oral; *TIA*, transient ischemic attack.

*See manufacturer's directions for specific dose.

ANTIFIBRINOLYTIC DRUGS

The individual antifibrinolytic drugs have varying mechanisms of action, but all prevent the lysis of fibrin, the substance that helps make the platelet plug insoluble and anchors the clot to the damaged blood vessel (see Figures 28-1 and 28-2). The term *antifibrinolytic* means to prevent the lysis of fibrin; in doing so, these drugs promote clot formation. For this reason, they are also called hemostatic drugs. They have the opposite effects of anticoagulant and antiplatelet drugs, which prevent clot formation. There are two synthetic antifibrinolytics, tranexamic acid and desmopressin, and one natural antifibrinolytic drug, aprotinin. Dosages, indications, and other information for desmopessin appear in the designated Dosages table on p. 538. There are also hemostatic drugs that are used *topically* (on the skin or tissue surface) in surgical settings to stop excessive bleeding. These include topical thrombin, microfibrillar collagen, absorbable gelatin, and oxidized cellulose.

Mechanism of Action and Drug Effects

Antifibrinolytics vary in several ways, depending on the particular drug. The antifibrinolytic drugs and their proposed mechanisms of action are described in Table 28-5.

The drug effects of the antifibrinolytics are specific and limited. They do not have many effects beyond their hematological ones. Tranexamic acid and aprotinin prevent the breakdown of fibrin, which prevents the destruction of the formed platelet clot. Desmopressin causes a dose-dependent increase in the concentration of plasma factor VIII (von Willebrand factor) and an increase in the plasma concentration of tissue plasminogen activator. The overall effect is increased platelet aggregation and clot formation. This drug is also an analogue of antidiuretic hormone (ADH) and is discussed further in Chapter 30.

Indications

Antifibrinolytics are useful in both the prevention and treatment of excessive bleeding resulting from systemic hyperfibrinolysis or surgical complications. They have also proved successful in arresting excessive oozing from surgical sites such as chest tubes and in reducing the total blood loss and duration of bleeding in the postoperative period. Desmopressin may also be used in patients who have hemophilia A or type I von Willebrand's disease.

Contraindications

Contraindications to the use of antifibrinolytic drugs include known drug allergy to a specific product and disseminated intravascular coagulation (DIC), which could be worsened by these drugs.

Adverse Effects

The adverse effects of antifibrinolytic drugs are uncommon and mild. However, there have been rare reports of antifibrinolytic drugs causing thrombotic events, such as acute cerebrovascular thrombosis and acute MI. The common adverse effects of antifibrinolytics are listed in Table 28-6.

Interactions

The concurrent use of drugs such as estrogens or oral contraceptives with tranexamic acid and aprotinin may have an additive effect, resulting in increased coagulation. Few specific interactions have been reported for desmopressin, although it should be given cautiously in patients receiving lithium, large doses of epinephrine, demeclocycline, heparin, or alcohol because these combinations may lead to a reduced antidiuretic response to desmopressin. Drugs such as chlorpropamide and fludrocortisone may potentiate the antidiuretic response, resulting in edema.

Dosages

For information on the dosages for desmopressin, see the Dosages table on p. 538.

TABLE 28-5

Antifibrinolytics: Mechanisms of Action

Antifibrinolytic Drug	Mechanism of Action
Synthetic drug: tranexamic acid	Forms a reversible complex with plasminogen and plasmin. By binding to the lysine-binding site of plasminogen, tranexamic acid displaces plasminogen from the surface of fibrin. This prevents plasmin from lysing the fibrin clot. Therefore, the drug can only work if a clot has formed.
Natural drug: aprotinin	Inhibits the proteolytic enzymes trypsin, plasmin, and kallikrein, which lyse proteins that destroy fibrin clots. By inhibiting these enzymes, aprotinin prevents the degradation of the fibrin clot. It is also thought to inhibit the action of the complement system.
Other: desmopressin (DDAVP)	Works by increasing von Willebrand factor, which anchors platelets to damaged vessels via the GP IIb platelet receptor. It appears that desmopressin acts as a general endothelial stimulant, stimulating factor VIII, prostaglandin I_2, and plasminogen-activated release.

GP, glycoprotein.

TABLE 28-6

Antifibrinolytics: Adverse Effects

Body System	Adverse Effects
Cardiovascular	Dysrhythmias, orthostatic hypotension, bradycardia
Central nervous	Headache, dizziness, fatigue, hallucinations, psychosis, convulsions
Gastrointestinal	Nausea, vomiting, abdominal cramps, diarrhea

DRUG PROFILES

desmopressin acetate

Desmopressin acetate (DDAVP, Minirin, Octostim) is a synthetic polypeptide. It is structurally similar to vasopressin, or antidiuretic hormone (ADH), the natural human posterior pituitary hormone. Because of these physical characteristics, it is often used to increase the reabsorption of water by the collecting ducts in the kidneys. This action prevents or controls polydipsia, polyuria, and dehydration in patients with diabetes insipidus caused by a deficiency of endogenous posterior pituitary vasopressin or in patients with polyuria and polydipsia resulting from trauma or surgery in the pituitary region.

Desmopressin also causes a dose-dependent increase in plasma factor VIII (von Willebrand factor), along with an increase in tissue plasminogen activator, resulting in increased platelet aggregation and clot formation. Desmopressin is contraindicated in patients with a known hypersensitivity to it and in those with nephrogenic diabetes insipidus. It is available in both injectable and intranasal dosage forms as well as oral disintegrating tablets. Desmopressin nasal spray and tablets are used for primary nocturnal enuresis.

PHARMACOKINETICS

Half-Life	Onset	Peak	Duration
< 2 hr	15–30 min	1.1–2 hr	8–12 hr

DOSAGES   Desmopressin

Drug (Pregnancy Category)	Pharmacological Class	Usual Dosage Range	Indications
desmopressin acetate (DDAVP, Minirin, Octostim) (B)	Synthetic posterior pituitary hormone	*Children* IV: 0.3 mcg/kg infused over 20–30 min; preoperative use: drug is administered 30 min before surgery IV: 10 mcg/m² infused over 20–30 min; preoperative use: drug is administered 30 min before surgery	Surgical and postoperative hemostasis and management of bleeding in patients with hemophilia A or type I von Willebrand's disease

THROMBOLYTIC DRUGS

Thrombolytics are coagulation modifiers that lyse thrombi in the coronary arteries. This action re-establishes blood flow to the blood-starved heart muscle. If the blood flow is re-established early, the heart muscle and left ventricular function can be preserved. If blood flow is not re-established early, the affected area of the heart muscle becomes ischemic and eventually necrotic and nonfunctional.

Thrombolytic therapy was first introduced in 1933 when a substance that would break down fibrin clots was isolated from a patient's blood. This substance was determined to be produced by a bacterium, β-**hemolytic streptococci (group A)**, growing in the patient's blood. The substance was eventually called streptokinase (SK).

Although SK was first used in a patient in 1947 to dissolve a clotted hemothorax, it was not until 1958 that the first patient with an acute MI received SK. In 1960, a naturally occurring human plasminogen activator called urokinase became available, which was found to exert fibrinolytic effects on pulmonary emboli. However, the results of early thrombolytic trials, conducted during the 1960s and 1970s and consisting of patients who had had

an acute MI, were not taken seriously by the medical community. It was not until the 1980s that DeWood and colleagues demonstrated that the underlying cause of acute MIs was a coronary artery occlusion. This marked the start of rapid growth in the use of thrombolytic drugs for the early treatment of acute MI.

Since that time, several new thrombolytics have become available for this and other clinical uses. Tissue plasminogen activator (t-PA) and anisoylated plasminogen streptokinase activator complex (APSAC) are two such drugs. With the arrival of these new thrombolytics came several large landmark thrombolytic research studies (GUSTO Investigators, 1993; Baigent et al., 1998). These studies demonstrated that early thrombolytic therapy could result in a 50% reduction in mortality, a reduction in infarct size, an improvement in left ventricular function, and a reduction in the incidence and severity of congestive heart failure. These findings and developments, along with a better understanding of the pathogenesis of acute MIs, have led the way in the advancements made in the treatment of acute MIs. Currently available thrombolytic drug classes include thrombolytic enzymes (streptokinase [Streptase]), tissue plasminogen activators (anistreplase [Eminase], alteplase [t-PA, Activase], reteplase [Retavase], and tenecteplase [TNKase]), and a recombinant human activated protein C (drotrecogin alfa [Xigris]). Dosages, indications, and other information appear in the designated Dosages table on p. 540.

Mechanism of Action and Drug Effects

A fine balance exists between the formation and dissolution of a clot. Recall that the coagulation system is responsible for forming clots, whereas the fibrinolytic system is responsible for dissolving clots. The natural fibrinolytic system within blood takes days to break down a clot or thrombus. This is of little value, however, in the case of a clotted blood vessel supplying blood to the heart muscle. While necrosis of the myocardium would not be prevented by these natural means, thrombolytic therapy activates the fibrinolytic system to break down the thrombus in the blood vessel quickly so that delivery of blood to the heart muscle via the coronary arteries is quickly re-established. This action prevents myocardial muscle and heart function from being destroyed. Thrombolytics accomplish this by activating the conversion of plasminogen to plasmin, which breaks down, or lyses, the thrombus (see Figure 28-3). Plasmin is a *proteolytic* enzyme, meaning it breaks down proteins. Plasmin is a relatively nonspecific serine protease that is capable of degrading such proteins as fibrin, fibrinogen, and other procoagulant proteins such as factors V, VIII, and XII. In other words, the substances that form clots are destroyed by plasmin. Essentially, thrombolytic drugs work by mimicking the body's own process of clot destruction. Although the individual thrombolytic drugs are somewhat diverse in their actions, they all have this common result.

Streptokinase (SK), the original thrombolytic enzyme, binds with plasminogen to form an SK–plasminogen complex, which then acts on other plasminogen molecules to form plasmin. The plasmin formed then lyses the clots. SK is not clot specific, however. SK activates fibrinolysis throughout the body; it breaks down not only the thrombus in the coronary artery but also clots anywhere in the body. This effect can be helpful with clots in the leg, for example. The APSAC is an SK–plasminogen complex that has been chemically modified by acylation, allowing a prolonged half-life. In contrast to the newer thrombolytic drugs, the thrombolytic enzymes are not clot specific, which increases the risk for bleeding complications. The newer thrombolytics have chemical specificity for fibrin threads (**fibrin-specificity**) and work primarily at the site of a clot. They still carry some bleeding risk, but much less than that of the thrombolytic enzymes.

Tissue plasminogen activator (t-PA) is a naturally occurring plasminogen activator secreted by vascular endothelial cells (the walls of blood vessels). However, the amount secreted naturally is not sufficient to dissolve a coronary thrombus quickly enough to restore circulation to the heart and preserve heart muscle. t-PA is now manufactured through recombinant DNA techniques and thus can be administered in sufficient quantities to dissolve a coronary thrombus quickly. It is fibrin specific (clot specific), so only the fibrin clot stimulates t-PA to convert plasminogen to plasmin. Therefore, it has as great a propensity to induce a systemic thrombolytic state, compared with thrombolytic enzymes.

Indications

The purpose of all thrombolytic drugs is to activate the conversion of plasminogen to plasmin, the enzyme that breaks down a thrombus. The presence of a thrombus that interferes significantly with normal blood flow on either the venous or the arterial side of the circulation is an indication for the use of thrombolytic therapy. An exception to this may be a thrombus that has formed in blood vessels that directly connect with the central nervous system (CNS). The indications for thrombolytic therapy include acute MI, arterial thrombosis, DVT, occlusion of shunts or catheters, pulmonary embolus, and acute ischemic stroke.

Contraindications

Contraindications to the use of thrombolytic drugs include known drug allergy to the specific product and to any preservatives and concurrent use with other drugs that alter clotting.

Adverse Effects

The most common undesirable effect of thrombolytic therapy is internal, intracranial, and superficial bleeding. Other problems include hypersensitivity, anaphylactoid reactions, nausea, vomiting, and hypotension. These drugs can also induce cardiac dysrhythmias.

Toxicity and Management of Overdose

Acute toxicity primarily causes an extension of the adverse effects of the thrombolytic drug. Treatment is symptomatic and supportive, as thrombolytic drugs have a relatively short half-life and no specific antidotes.

Interactions

The most common effect of drug interactions is an increased bleeding tendency resulting from the concurrent use of anticoagulant, antiplatelet, or other drugs that affect platelet function.

One laboratory test interaction that can occur with thrombolytic drugs is a reduction in the plasminogen and fibrinogen levels.

Dosages

For information on the dosages for SK and alteplase, see the Dosages table on p. 540.

DRUG PROFILES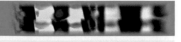

All thrombolytic drugs exert their effects by activating plasminogen and converting it to plasmin, which is capable of digesting fibrin, a major component of clots. In Canada, tenecteplase is the preferred thrombolytic drug in many areas.

▸ alteplase

Alteplase (Activase, Cathflo) is a naturally occurring t-PA secreted by vascular endothelial cells. The pharmaceutically available t-PA is made through recombinant DNA techniques, and modified hamster ovary cells produce the substance. It is clot (fibrin)-specific and, therefore, does not produce a systemic lytic state. In addition, because it is present in the human body in a natural state, its administration for therapeutic use does not induce an antigen–antibody reaction. Therefore, it can be readministered immediately in the event of reinfarction. The t-PA has a very short half-life of 5 minutes. It is believed to open the clogged artery faster, but its action is short-lived. Therefore, it is given concomitantly with heparin to prevent reocclusion of the infarcted blood vessel. Alteplase is also available only in parenteral form. There is a smaller dosage form known as Cathflo Activase that is used to flush clogged IV or arterial lines.

PHARMACOKINETICS

Half-Life	Onset	Peak	Duration
5 min	Unknown	Varies with dose	Unknown

▸ streptokinase

Streptokinase (SK, Streptase) is the oldest thrombolytic drug, produced from β-hemolytic streptococci. It binds with plasminogen, and this SK–plasminogen complex then acts on other plasminogen molecules to form plasmin. SK is not clot specific. Because it is made from a nonhuman source, it is antigenic and may provoke allergic reactions. This occurs when the body's immune system recognizes it as a foreign antigen and launches an antibody against it, resulting in an antigen–antibody reaction. These antibodies develop approximately 5 days after SK therapy and persist for 6 months to 1 year. It is recommended that patients not be retreated with SK or APSAC during this period.

Hypotension secondary to vasodilation occurs in approximately 10% to 15% of patients given SK. SK is contraindicated in patients with known hypersensitivity to it, in patients who have recently undergone surgery, and those with active internal bleeding, aneurysm, uncontrolled hypotension, intracranial or intraspinal neoplasm, and trauma. It is available only in parenteral form.

PHARMACOKINETICS

Half-Life	Onset	Peak	Duration
18 min, then 83 min	1 hr	Varies with dose	24–36 hr

DOSAGES   Selected Thrombolytic Drugs

Drug (Pregnancy Category)	Pharmacological Class	Usual Dosage Range	Indications
▸ alteplase (Activase, Cathflo) (C)	Thrombolytic enzyme	**Adult** IV: 100 mg over 90 min given as a 15 mg IV bolus, then 50 mg over 30 min, then 35 mg over 60 min	Acute MI
▸ streptokinase (SK, Streptase) (C)	Thrombolytic enzyme	**Adult** IV: 1.5 million units infused within 60 min or intracoronary infusion initiated with a bolus of 20,000 units followed by 2000 units/min for 1 hr	Acute MI
		IV: Loading dose of 250,000 units over 30 min followed by a maintenance infusion of 100,000 units/hr for 24–72 hr	DVT, arterial thrombosis and embolism, PE
		IV: 250 000 units into each occluded limb of the cannula over 25–35 min and clamped for 2 hr followed by aspiration of the infusion cannula with saline and reconnection of the cannula	Arteriovenous cannula occlusion

DVT, deep vein thrombosis; *IV,* intravenous; *MI,* myocardial infarction; *PE,* pulmonary embolism.

NURSING PROCESS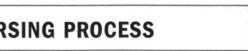

A variety of conditions warrant the use of coagulation modifiers, including the clotting of a peripheral inserted catheter (PIC) line or a central venous catheter; clot prevention in coronary artery bypass grafting, major vessel injury, and thrombophlebitis; and treatment of venous or arterial thromboembolism. The drugs used to treat these different conditions are varied in their mechanisms of action and have general as well as specific nursing process–related issues.

▨ Assessment

The nursing process related to these drugs will be discussed by drug class with specific drugs mentioned, as deemed appropriate. Nursing assessment associated with *all coagulation-modifying* drugs should begin with a thorough nursing history, medication history, and brief physical assessment, including the following: medical history, family history, dietary habits, changes in body weight over time, activities of daily living, exercise habits, employment activities, success with previous medication and treatment regimens, blood pressure, pulse rate, respirations, body weight, and height. Laboratory tests usually ordered include baseline complete blood counts, hemoglobin, hematocrit, lipoprotein fractionation, triglyceride and cholesterol levels, and clotting studies. The appropriate serum laboratory tests that should be performed for baseline and maintenance levels are presented in Lab Values Related to Drug Therapy.

Assessment of the skin and of areas identified as potential SC injection sites for heparin and LWMHs is important for carrying out safe administration techniques. For these specific drugs, *avoid* any area within 5 cm of the umbilicus as well as open wounds, scars, open or abraded areas, incisions, drainage tubes, stomas, and areas of bruising or oozing because these sites are at higher risk for further tissue trauma with injection of anticoagulant. The area being referenced here is the subcutaneous fatty area across the lower abdomen and between the iliac crests.

There should be a thorough assessment of the following at-risk factors as related to the patient's clotting disorder: immobility; history of limited activity or prolonged bed rest (e.g., generally for more than 5 days); dehydration; obesity; smoking; congestive heart failure;

LAB VALUES RELATED TO DRUG THERAPY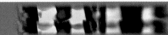

Anticoagulants and Antiplatelets

Laboratory Test	Normal Ranges	Rationale for Assessment
Partial thromboplastin time (PTT)	Normal control values are between 21 and 35 seconds, with therapeutic ranges aimed at 1.5 to 2.5 times the normal control value. Some laboratory testing centres use values between 2 to 2.5 times the normal control value.	This blood test detects defects in the intrinsic thromboplastin system and is used to monitor anticoagulant/heparin therapy. If patient values are more than 2.5 times the control value, the patient may be receiving too much anticoagulant, and the dosage will need adjustment by the physician. If patient values are less than 1.5, then the patient may not be receiving enough anticoagulant and is at risk for clotting.
aPTT (activated partial thromboplastin time)	With heparin therapy, aPTT values should fall between 1.5 and 2.5 times the control or baseline value. Normal control values are 25 to 35 seconds, so therapeutic values should then be approximately 45 to 70 seconds.	Therapeutic levels of aPTT indicate decreased levels of clotting factors and subsequent clotting activity. aPTT is a more sensitive part of PTT and often replaces it. It is used to see if there are deficiencies in the patient's intrinsic coagulation pathway and monitor heparin therapy. aPTT is sensitive to changes in blood clotting factors, except for factor VII. Therefore, it is used to reflect normal blood coagulation. With continuous IV infusions of heparin, aPTT levels can be drawn at any time, but with intermittent infusions the aPTT should be drawn approximately 1 hour before a dose of heparin is scheduled to be given.
Prothrombin time (PT)	The normal control PT value ranges from 11 to 13 seconds, with therapeutic levels of anticoagulation aimed at 1.5 times the control or about 18 seconds.	Prothrombin is a vitamin K–dependent protein, a major component of the clotting process. It reflects the activity of clotting and is used to monitor effectiveness of warfarin therapy. PT values vary with each laboratory centre and are based on the specifics of the testing procedure.
International Normalized Ratio (INR)	Target levels of INR range from 2 to 3 or average 2.5. For individuals taking warfarin for treatment of recurring systemic clots or emboli or having mechanical heart valves, the goal of INR may be 2.5 to 3.5, with a middle value of 3.	This is a routine test to evaluate coagulation while patients are on warfarin. When the therapy is initiated, the INR and PT should be done daily until a "stable" daily dose is reached or when a dose maintains the PT and INR within therapeutic ranges and does not cause bleeding. INR results actually reflect a dose of warfarin given 36 to 72 hours prior to the actual testing. Advantages of INR testing include the fact that there is more consistency among laboratories and a more consistent warfarin dosage. Some laboratories will report both INR and PT together.

mitral or aortic stenosis; coronary heart disease with documented athero- or arteriosclerosis; peripheral vascular disease; pelvic, gynecological/genitourinary, abdominal, orthopedic, or major vascular surgery; history of thrombophlebitis, deep vein thrombosis, thromboembolism, including pulmonary embolism, myocardial infarct, or atrial fibrillation; edema of the periphery; trauma to the lower extremities; use of oral contraceptives; and current extended air travel time. If the patient has a positive history of clotting disorders, thromboembolism, or both, be sure to assess and document the following:

- For thrombophlebitis of the leg: presenting signs and symptoms such as calf edema, pain, warmth, or redness directly over the vessel (more indicative of a superficial clot); increased diameter measurement of the calf of the affected leg; pain in the calf with dorsiflexion (often called Homan's sign; however, this is a very controversial method of assessment) or pain upon gentle compression of the calf muscle against the tibial bone
- For pulmonary embolism: chest pain, cough, dyspnea, tachypnea, drop in O_2 saturation (by oximetry or blood gasses), hemoptysis, tachycardia, drop in blood pressure, and possible shock

With use of the *parenteral anticoagulant* heparin, assessment of the patient is essential to quality nursing care and should include allergies, contraindications, cautions, and drug interactions. It is also necessary to assess conditions that pose an at-risk situation for a patient, such as severe hypertension, ulcer disease, ulcerative colitis, aneurysms, malignant hypertension, alcoholism, and head injuries. An important caution for heparin use is with pregnancy or lactation; however, should there be a need for an anticoagulant in pregnancy, heparin is the drug of choice, not warfarin. Other relevant information is presented in Table 28-1. (See also the Case Study for a typical example of heparin therapy.) For patient safety, nurses must remember that heparin is NOT interchangeable unit for unit with another class of anticoagulants, *the low-weight-molecular heparins (LWMHs)*. Heparin sodium contains benzyl alcohol, thus allergy to this additional

component needs to be assessed. The nurse should also note if the natural health products ginkgo and ginseng are being used because they may affect blood coagulation.

Although the use of LMWHs leads to fewer adverse reactions in some patients, LWMHs are still associated with the contraindications, cautions, and drug interactions previously discussed. The same parameters discussed earlier with heparin use are also appropriate with the use of LWMHs. In addition, LWMHs contain sulfites and benzyl alcohol, so allergies to these substances should be assessed. As noted earlier, the LWMHs differ from standard heparin as well as among themselves, so they are not interchangeable. Indications for LWMHs may include outpatient anticoagulant therapy, which is a trend for the use of these drugs because they are given subcutaneously. They also require less frequent and less close monitoring than that with heparin use. Clotting studies should also be assessed prior to therapy.

For use of warfarin, the nurse needs to know its related contraindications, cautions, and drug interactions, discussed previously in this chapter. All of the parameters and laboratory studies listed earlier for use of coagulation-modifying drugs are applicable to warfarin. Because of the drug's action, warfarin should be withdrawn—as ordered—prior to dental procedures or in the event of any evidence of tissue necrosis, gangrene, diarrhea, intestinal flora imbalances, and steatorrhea, all of which require close assessment. Because warfarin is indicated for prophylaxis and long-term treatment of a variety of thromboembolic disorders (see the pharmacaology section for specifics), it requires constant and astute assessment of the patient and of clotting activities or lack thereof. Most health care providers use standard protocols of warfarin to assist in the dosing of the drug based on INR values. The most common starting dose for warfarin is 5 mg daily. However, the dose can range from 1 to 10 mg and occasionally even higher (e.g., 12 mg), depending on individual patient response. In most situations, dosage for adults is between 1 and 5 mg orally every day. In addition, warfarin's pharmacokinetics are important to assess and understand because it takes

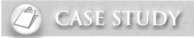 **CASE STUDY**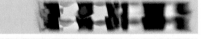

Heparin Therapy

In the past 2 years, Mr. L., a 56-year-old attorney, has had three episodes of DVT. All occurred without complications, and all were treated successfully with anticoagulant therapy and bed rest. He has now arrived at the emergency department because of increased pain and swelling that has lasted for the past 3 days in his left calf. Initially he is given 5000 units of heparin. On admission to the hospital for anticoagulant therapy, he is started on a continuous infusion of 25,000 units of heparin in 1000 mL of 0.9% sodium chloride.

1. What nursing actions should be implemented to ensure the accuracy and safety of the continuous heparin infusion?

2. What patient findings would indicate a therapeutic response to the heparin therapy?
3. Mr. L. suddenly complains of numbness and tingling in his lower extremities with accompanying changes in muscle strength and sensation 12 hours after the initiation and continuation of heparin therapy. What would be the most appropriate nursing actions to implement?

DVT, deep vein thrombosis.
For answers, see http://evolve.elsevier.com/Canada/Lilley/pharmacology/.

about 3 days for the drug to reach a steady state. Patients on heparin may receive warfarin prior to discontinuation of heparin for anticoagulation.

With *antiplatelet* drugs, a thorough nursing history, medication history, and physical assessment should be performed. Although possible drug interactions, cautions, and contraindications need to be watched for, close assessment of any bleeding is most important to patient safety. Because aspirin, NSAIDs, and other antiplatelets alter bleeding times, these drugs should be withheld for 5 to 7 days prior to surgical procedures. Specific guidelines are generally given by the physician to avoid the concurrent use of other anticoagulants, antiplatelets, and fibrinolytics. With aspirin and its related ototoxicity, it is important to not give drugs that have the same adverse effect (e.g., ototoxicity), such as with aminoglycosides (e.g., vancomycin).

Baseline cardiovascular assessment is needed with documentation of general history, history of chest pain, complete blood count, hemoglobin, hematocrit, platelet counts, prothrombin time, and INR values. Baseline documentation provides values against which therapy values can be compared. Along with these parameters, if platelet counts are at or fall below 150×10^9/L, the physician should be notified, and antiplatelet therapy will most likely not be initiated (or will be discontinued).

It is important to patient safety to re-emphasize that aspirin should not be used in children and adolescents, in any patient with any bleeding disorder, in children with flulike symptoms, in pregnant or lactating women, or in patients with a vitamin K deficiency or peptic ulcer disease. In these situations there would be major consequences if aspirin were used; for example, there is a high risk for Reye's syndrome with aspirin use in children and teenagers, as well as for teratogenic effects, ulcers, or bleeding tendencies. The nurse must know how each of the drugs acts in the body so that there is a sound knowledge base for critical thinking–based decision— for example, to call the physician and to not administer two antiplatelets at the same time or give a thrombolytic with heparin, warfarin, aspirin, or NSAIDs. This type of critical drug information is important in ensuring that the patient receives the safest and most appropriate care during all phases of the nursing process.

The *glycoprotein IIb/IIIa inhibitors,* for example, eptifibatide (Integrilin), tirofiban (Aggrastat), and abciximab (ReoPro), are associated with the same baseline assessment information (e.g., vital signs, medical history, history of chest pain and heart disease, complete blood cell counts, hemoglobin, hematocrit, kidney function tests, platelet counts). Prior to and during therapy, should platelet counts fall below 150×10^9/L or be at that level to begin with, the physician should be contacted for further orders.

Antifibrinolytics require the same astute assessment of baseline parameters and laboratory testing; however, there are additional concerns for patients with altered heart, kidney, or liver functioning. In these situations, the physician may need to decrease the dosage of medication.

Serum potassium levels should be noted prior to therapy because of the potential for drug-induced hyperkalemia.

Thrombolytics also require similar assessment parameters, baseline complete blood cell counts, and clotting studies. There is always major concern and contraindications for the use of alteplase (Activase, t-PA) and other thrombolytics (e.g., active internal bleeding, history of stroke, cerebral neoplasms, arteriovenous malformation, aneurysms, known bleeding disorders, severe uncontrolled hypertension, intracranial or intraspinal surgery or trauma within, for example, the past 2 months). Any arterial puncture, venous cut-down sites, PIC line sites, and central-infusion ports or sites should be constantly assessed for bleeding. Intramuscular injections may pose problems with bleeding, thus other dosage forms may be indicated. As with any drugs that alter clotting and platelet activity, the thrombolytics are associated with risk for bleeding from wounds or the gastrointestinal, genitourinary, or respiratory tracts, so any drainage, urine, stool, emesis, sputum, and secretions should be assessed for presence of blood.

Nursing Diagnoses

- Ineffective tissue perfusion related to the clotting disorder or thrombus formation
- Impaired physical mobility related to tissue injury or decreased tissue perfusion from coagulation disorders
- Risk for injury related to possible adverse reactions to any of the drugs that alter blood clotting
- Deficient knowledge related to medication treatment regimen because of lack of information
- Acute pain related to symptoms of underlying clotting disorder or ischemia
- Activity intolerance related to underlying tissue disorder or ischemia

Planning

Goals

- Patient will experience increased comfort and relief of pain.
- Patient will exhibit improved blood flow as the result of the therapeutic effects of the anticoagulants.
- Patient will remain free from injury stemming from either the disease or the medication being taken.
- Patient will be adherent to the lifestyle changes required and to the medication therapy.
- Patient will demonstrate adequate knowledge regarding medication therapy and its potential adverse effects.

Outcome Criteria

- Patient experiences relief of symptoms such as decreased pain, swelling, and edema once tissue perfusion is regained as the result of medication therapy.
- Patient shows improved circulation with warm extremities or strong pedal pulses or experiences a return to predisease state of tissue perfusion.

- Patient is free of bruising, bleeding problems, or any other adverse reaction to the medication.
- Patient states the rationale for the use of the medication regimen, such as decreased clotting or clot formation.
- Patient states the nature of and rationale for the lifestyle changes needed, such as improved diet, exercise, and smoking cessation.
- Patient states the adverse effects, how to monitor for complications of the anticoagulants, the importance of coming in for follow-up appointments with the physician and of frequent laboratory studies, and when to contact the physician to prevent complications such as hemorrhage.

■ Implementation

Vital signs, heart sounds, peripheral pulses, and neurological checks are routinely monitored in all patients during and immediately after anticoagulant therapy. The laboratory values to be monitored are presented in Lab Values Related to Drug Therapy on p. 541. If there is any change in pulse rate or rhythm, blood pressure, or level of consciousness, or unexplained restlessness occurs, contact the physician immediately, as it may indicate bleeding or hemorrhage.

Knowledge of the proper techniques of administration is crucial for safe and effective use of any clotting-altering drug (Box 28-1). The anticoagulant is given via the subcutaneous (SC) or intravenous (IV) routes and not intramuscularly. Inadvertent intramuscular injection can be easily avoided if the nurse uses only SC syringes that include a 1.5 cm, 25- to 28-gauge needle. No major harm would result from a subcutaneous dose inadvertently given intravenously. If rapid anticoagulation is needed, the physician generally orders IV heparin, either by continuous or intermittent infusion. During continuous IV infusion or SC injection, monitoring of daily clotting studies may be ordered. The effects are reversed with the IV administration of protamine sulfate. With SC heparin, several doses of protamine sulfate may be needed to reverse the anticoagulant effect because of the variable rates of absorption of this dosage form. See Box 28-1 for the procedure for the intermittent or continuous IV administration of heparin.

LMWHs are given by subcutaneous injection in the abdominal area using the same techniques as those used for administering heparin, with a few differences. Solutions may be clear to pale yellow in colour. Usual length of therapy is approximately 5 to 10 days, and it is important to constantly be aware of any bleeding problems while the patient is taking this and other clot-altering drugs. Complete blood counts, platelet counts, and stool for occult blood are all tests that will most likely be done during therapy for monitoring purposes. Tests for occult blood in the stool can be done if the occult stool test paper with its developer is available. It simply helps to identify hidden blood in the stool, which may occur as an adverse effect with LMWHs as well as with any clotting-altering drugs.

When the oral anticoagulant warfarin is prescribed, therapy is often initiated while the patient is still on heparin so that when the heparin is eventually discontinued, the blood levels of warfarin have been allowed for and therapeutic anticoagulation levels are achieved. Because the full therapeutic effect of warfarin does not occur until 4 to 5 days after the first dose, the patient who has been on heparin for anticoagulation and is switched to warfarin must have this overlap of activity to maintain the prevention of clotting. The administration procedures for warfarin are outlined in Box 28-1.

Monitoring the clotting studies is still of utmost priority, as is watching for any clotting or bleeding problems. For conversion from heparin to an oral anticoagulant such as warfarin, the dose of the oral drug should be the usual initial amount, with PT-INR levels used to help the physician determine the next appropriate dosage of warfarin. Once there is continuous therapeutic anticoagulation coverage and warfarin is established, the heparin or LWMH may then be discontinued without tapering. Should uncontrolled bleeding occur with any of these medications, the nurse must take action to control the bleeding and institute emergency measures to stabilize the patient's condition. The physician should also be contacted immediately.

Of benefit with the use of anticoagulants is the use of antidotes. The antidote to hemorrhage or uncontrolled bleeding resulting from heparin or LMWH therapy is protamine sulfate. This antidote is given intravenously and may be given in an undiluted form over a 10-minute time frame, *not exceeding* 5 mg/min or 50 mg in any 10-minute period. The benchmark dose is based on the fact that 1 mg of protamine sulfate neutralizes 90 to 115 units of heparin. Too-rapid infusion may lead to acute hypotensive episodes, bradycardia, dyspnea, and transient feelings of warmth and flushing. aPTT ranges and hematocrit levels are generally used at this point to monitor bleeding, clotting, and risk for bleeding. Any changes in blood pressure and pulse rate must also be watched for. The antidote to oral anticoagulant (warfarin sodium) therapy is vitamin K, given preferably via the SC route, although oral, IV, and IM dosage forms are also available. This drug may lead to rare occurrences of severe reactions such as dyspnea, dizziness, rapid or weak pulse, chest pain, and hypotension that may progress to shock and cardiac arrest. The nurse needs to continually monitor the patient's vital signs, heart parameters, and bleeding times and clotting studies.

The patient being treated with *antiplatelets* (or any clot-altering drug) should be constantly monitored for signs and symptoms of bleeding during and after their use. These symptoms include epistaxis, hematuria, hematemesis, easy or excessive bruising, blood in the stools, and bleeding gums. If the patient undergoes invasive procedures or receives injections, appropriate pressure should be applied to bleeding sites, and all areas of venous or arterial catheter insertion should be closely watched for bleeding.

BOX 28-1 — Heparin Administration

Subcutaneous Heparin Administration

- After thoroughly checking the physician's order, assess the patient for the existence of any allergies, contraindications, or cautions, or drug interactions.
- Wash hands thoroughly. A tuberculin syringe is used because it is the correct gauge and needle length. For a 25- to 28-gauge needle, the length of the needle is 1.5 to 2 cm.
- See Chapter 10 for specific information on technique for giving heparin or LWMH injections and for a review on safe medication administration.
- Check the injection site for bleeding or bruising and document any pertinent information. Technique is important with subcutaneous injections of heparin (Chapter 10). Do not massage or rub the site before or after the injection. Do not aspirate before injecting, to prevent hematoma formation.
- Make sure the patient is comfortable, then remove your gloves and wash your hands. Document your intervention and any other pertinent data.

Intravenous Heparin Administration

- Always double-check the specific physician's order for dosage, rate of infusion, and time and route before beginning therapy and always practise the "Rights" of medication administration to prevent overdosing or erroneous dosing. Make sure the proper diluent is used and the compatibility of solutions or other drugs is checked before beginning the infusion.
- For the continuous IV administration of heparin, an IV pump must be used to ensure a precise rate of infusion.
- Continuous dosing is preferred over intermittent dosing because continuous dosing helps with blood levels of the drug, whereas intermittent IV dosing is associated with higher risks for bleeding abnormalities.
- The use of continuous IV infusions generally begins with a loading dose and is followed by a maintenance dose. Be aware that dosage adjustments are made exactly as ordered. The patient's aPTT level and other related clotting studies are used as parameters for dosing of heparin or LWMHs.
- For intermittent infusions, a heparin lock was formerly used. Heparin locks are now referred to as intermittent infusion locks or saline locks (because the locks are flushed with isotonic saline and not heparin).
- Intermittent infusions of heparin are usually ordered to be given every 4 to 6 hours because of heparin's short half-life. Intermittent infusions and all other types of IV infusions include use of needle-less systems.
- Regardless of the type of IV infusion (e.g., intermittent or continuous IV infusion), it is crucial to check the site to determine whether infiltration has occurred so that hematoma formation may be prevented. If infiltration is suspected, the lock should be removed and replaced in a new site before the next scheduled infusion. Document your actions in the nurse's notes.
- Therapeutic dosage of heparin is guided by aPTT with a targeted level of 1.5 to 2.5 times the control or normal. aPTTs are drawn within 24 hours of beginning therapy, 24 to 48 hours after therapy starts, and 1 to 2 times weekly for about 3 to 4 weeks on an average. With long-term therapy, aPTTs are monitored 1 to 2 times per month.

Oral Anticoagulant Administration

- It is important to recheck the physician's orders and the patient's medication and medical history before administering the drug. Always check to make sure the patient has no known hypersensitivity to the drug.
- Scored tablets may be crushed and may be given with or without food.
- There are many more drugs that can interact with oral anticoagulants than with heparin, especially those that are highly protein bound (such as the ones listed in Table 28-3). Always check the patient's medication list before initiating therapy with warfarin.
- Dosages of warfarin are calculated on the basis of INR blood values. INRs are also used to monitor the effectiveness of therapy. Remember, however, dosing is highly individualized.
- Oral anticoagulants should be administered at the same time every day to maintain steady blood levels.
- Document the dose, time of administration, and any other pertinent facts.

aPTT, activated partial thromboplastin time; *INR,* International Normalized Ratio; *LMWH,* low-molecular-weight heparin.

Extended-release dosage forms should be taken in their entire dosage form and without chewing or crushing. It is recommended that enteric-coated aspirin be taken with 180 to 240 mL of water and with food to help prevent gastrointestinal upset. To avoid irritation to the esophagus, make sure the patient knows to remain upright and to not lie down for up to 30 minutes after the dose of aspirin. If the aspirin has a strong, vinegar-like odour, discard the drug. With clopidogrel therapy, interventions are similar to that of aspirin. The patient should report any of the following: aches in the joints, back pain, dizziness, severe headache, dyspepsia, flulike signs and symptoms, and epigastric pain.

Antiplatelet drugs are often discontinued, as ordered, for 7 days prior to surgery. However, some surgical procedures (e.g., cardiovascular surgery) may warrant that patient remain in an anticoagulated state intraoperatively. Oral forms of dipyridamole should be taken on an empty stomach; however, if it is not tolerated, it may be taken with food. If nausea occurs, cola, unsalted crackers, or dry toast may help alleviate this adverse effect. In addition, it may take up to 2 to 3 months of continuous therapy for the drug to reach therapeutic levels. Encourage patients to change positions slowly and to take their time going from lying to sitting to standing because of dizziness and postural hypotension that are adverse effects of antiplatelets and all other drugs in this chapter.

Nursing considerations associated with *glycoprotein (GP) IIb/IIIa inhibitors* such as abciximab, eptifibatide, and tirofiban include close monitoring of all vital signs, electrocardiogram (ECG) readings, peripheral pulses, heart sounds, skin colour, and temperature. These measures are all important parts of nursing care during and after the use of these drugs. Because these drugs are used in combination with heparin to treat individuals suspected of having acute coronary syndrome or with percutaneous transluminal coronary angioplasty (PTCA), there is always concern for the stability of the patient as well as a high risk for serious bleeding and extension of an acute myocardial infarct. The patient in this situation is at risk for other medical complications, and this risk may be intensified by the drug. Avoidance of further invasive procedures while the patient is on this type of drug is important to help prevent risks for bleeding. If invasive procedures are required, it is crucial to constantly monitor for bleeding and observe all vital parameters before, during, and after the procedure.

Intravenous tirofiban should be protected from light, and any unused solutions should be discarded 24 hours after an infusion has been started. No other drugs should be used with this drug infusion, except for heparin, which may be given through the same IV line. Abciximab, in particular, can be given by bolus or by continuous infusions with infusion rates monitored closely (PTCA). Manufacturer guidelines identify the need for a sterile, nonpyrogenic, low protein–binding 0.2- or 0.22-micron filter. While the vascular shield is in position, the patient should be on complete bed rest with the head of the bed elevated at 30 degrees. The affected extremity should be maintained in a straight position; peripheral pulses, colour, and temperature of distal extremities should be constantly monitored. Once the sheath is removed, application of pressure to the femoral artery is required for at least 30 minutes, either by manual or mechanical pressure. A pressure dressing should be applied once bleeding has stopped. The site should be closely monitored for any oozing or bleeding.

If there is serious bleeding, the GP IIb/IIIa receptor inhibitor and heparin (the usual protocol for PTCA) should be discontinued immediately, the patient should be monitored closely, and the physician should be notified immediately for emergency treatment. Always move and handle these patients with caution, and avoid unnecessary trauma or injury because of the risk for hematoma formation or bleeding. DO NOT take blood pressures in the lower extremities, but keep a close and constant watch on the patient's blood pressure (for hypotension) and pulse rate (for tachycardia), as well as for any complaints of abdominal or back pain, severe headache, and any other signs and symptoms of hemorrhage. When removing adhesive or sticky tape, always be careful to not tear or rip the skin, which would lead to tissue trauma and further risk for bleeding. aPTT levels should

be monitored after the procedure, along with very close monitoring for bleeding with attention to intramuscular injection sites, arterial or venous puncture sites, and bleeding from nasogastric tubes and urinary catheters. These procedures should be avoided, if at all possible, during or immediately after the angioplasty.

With *antifibrinolytics*, it is important to have an understanding of the rationale for the use of these drugs, such as to stop bleeding from overdoses of thrombolytic drugs or to control bleeding during heart surgery. Aminocaproic acid and tranexamic acid are usually given intravenously until bleeding is controlled. Antifibrolytics require close patient monitoring, and if there is any change in motor strength or level of consciousness, the physician should be notified. Nurses need to apply their knowledge of certain adverse effects of drugs (like these) so that nursing care may be focused on prevention of complications, maintenance of safety, and a return to a healthier state. Because of drug-induced skeletal myopathies, creatine kinase and other liver function studies should be monitored. It is also important to monitor heart rate and blood pressure with attention to quality and strength of peripheral pulses. For the patient with hemophilia, tranexamic acid may be used to help decrease bleeding from dental extractions. Close monitoring of patients for any oral bleeding is important with postdental care at home.

Nursing considerations related to *thrombolytics* are very similar to those for drugs previously discussed in this chapter. Specifically, their IV administration should be prepared per manufacturer guidelines and per protocol. Invasive procedures should be avoided during the use of these drugs, as should simultaneous use of anticoagulants or antiplatelets. IV infusion sites should be monitored frequently for bleeding, redness, and pain. Intramuscular injections of other drugs are contraindicated to prevent tissue damage and bleeding. Any bleeding from gums or mucous membranes or the occurrence of epistaxis and increased pulse (greater than 100 beats/min) should be reported to the physician immediately, and all vital signs should be monitored frequently. Other nursing considerations include monitoring for hypotension, restlessness, and a decrease in hemoglobin and hematocrit, which should be reported to the physician immediately. Patients should be instructed to report pink, red, or cloudy urine; black, tarry stools or frank red blood in the stools; abdominal or chest pain; dizziness; or severe headache.

Reconstitution for IV dosing should be done with NaCl or D5W. Solutions should be rolled gently and not shaken to maintain a stable solution. Continual monitoring of INR, aPTT, platelets, and fibrinogen levels should occur and within 2 to 3 hours after the use of thrombolytics. The patient's fibrinogen level may be measured to check for actual fibrinolysis. With the breakdown of fibrin (or fibrinolysis), INR or aPTT levels will increase or be prolonged. Should bleeding occur, the physician will most likely discontinue the drug and replace fibrinogen with infusions of whole blood plasma or with cryo-precipitate. Antifibrinolytics (e.g., aminocaproic acid/tranexamic acid) may also be given. Important features that patients need to know for several of the clot-altering drugs are listed in Patient Education.

◼ Evaluation

Monitoring for the therapeutic and adverse effects of clot-altering drugs is crucial for their safe use. Because these drugs are used for a variety of purposes, therapeutic responses vary. Some of the therapeutic effects include decreased chest pain and a decrease in dizziness, as well as other neurological symptoms. Adverse effects may include a fall in blood pressure, headache, hematoma formation, irritation and pain at the injection site, hemorrhage, thrombocytopenia, shortness of breath, chills, and fever. Early signs of drug overdose for any of the clot-altering drugs include bleeding of the gums while brushing teeth, unexplained nosebleeds or bruising, and heavier-than-usual menstrual bleeding. Abdominal pain, back pain, bloody or tarry stools, bloody urine, constipation, blood in the sputum, severe or continuous headaches, and the vomiting of frank red blood or a coffee ground–like substance indicating old blood are all possible indications of internal bleeding.

The adverse effects of aspirin use include gastrointestinal upset or bleeding, heartburn, headache, hepatitis, thrombocytopenia, agranulocytosis, leukopenia, neutropenia, hemolytic anemia, prolonged PT, tinnitus, hearing loss, rapid pulse, wheezing, hypoglycemia, hyponatremia, and hypokalemia. Adverse effects of anti-platelets include postural hypotension, headache, weakness, syncope, gastrointestinal upset, rash, flushing of the face, and dizziness. It is necessary to continually monitor liver, kidney, and clotting function in patients on long-term aspirin and other anti-clotting therapy.

Therapeutic effects of clopidogrel and similar drugs include a decrease in the occurrence of clotting events such as transient ischemic attacks (TIAs) and strokes. Adverse effects for which to monitor with these drugs include increased bleeding tendencies, flulike symptoms, headache, fatigue, chest pain, and epistaxis.

Therapeutic levels of anticoagulants and other clot-altering drugs are monitored by laboratory tests such as aPTT, PT, and INR and are presented in Lab Values Related to Drug Therapy on p. 541. Remember, however, that aPTT levels are used with heparin, and PT and INR with warfarin. To determine the effects of heparin therapy, the aPTT should have a therapeutic value of 1.5 to 2.5 times the control value. Once the level of the particular drug stabilizes and maintenance therapy is ongoing, clotting studies may be drawn at 1- to 4-week intervals, depending on the specific drug, patients' responses, and their overall physical condition. In case of the need for reversal of the anticoagulation effects, there are antidotes available, for example, heparin with an antidote of protamine sulfate and warfarin with the antidote of vitamin K (see Implementation section).

Therapeutic effects of antifibrinolytics include the arrest of oozing of blood from a surgical site or a decrease in blood loss.

The continuous monitoring of the patient for the signs and symptoms of internal or external bleeding is crucial during both the initiation and maintenance of therapy. Because of the complexity and life-threatening nature of the conditions for which these drugs are used, the nurse must continually monitor and re-evaluate the patient's response to the treatment, document responses accordingly, and always keep goals and outcome criteria within the plan of care to serve as a benchmark. From the evaluation phase, the goal is that the patient will emerge with full therapeutic effects and minimal adverse and toxic effects as related to drug therapy.

PATIENT EDUCATION

❖ Patients should be taught that these drugs are given for specific purposes (e.g., prevention of serious complications related to clotting, such as with strokes, heart attacks, heart valve replacements, mini-strokes [TIAs, or transient ischemic attacks], deep vein thrombosis in the legs). It is important to understand that a healthy lifestyle is an important part of therapy and will most likely include a healthy diet with the right foods, weight reduction if needed, smoking cessation, blood pressure management, and stress reduction.

❖ Patients should be informed that medications must be taken exactly as prescribed because too little may lead to a clot and too much may lead to bleeding. Regular follow-up appointments are an important part of patient care, with frequent blood tests to monitor therapeutic effects versus adverse effects of the

medication. The results of the blood tests will assist health care providers to determine proper dosage.

❖ Patients should be encouraged to inform all their health care providers, including dentists, about their medications.

❖ Patients should be encouraged to carry an identification card at all times and wear a medical alert necklace or bracelet that states the medical diagnosis and drugs being taken. Including the physician's name and phone number and any allergies is also recommended.

❖ Home heparin therapy may require that patients receive injections for a certain period. The LWMHs are usually used in these situations. Patients need to understand that if they are switched to warfarin (Coumadin) from heparin, there may be an overlap of

Continued

taking the warfarin and heparin for approximately 3 to 5 days to allow therapeutic levels of the oral warfarin to occur before discontinuing heparin. This process may occur in the hospital or at home. Enoxaparin (LWMH) is usually given for up to 3 months. Complete and thorough instructions and return demonstrations are an important part of patient education (Chapter 9).

❖ Patients should be taught the importance of reporting any unusual bleeding from anywhere on the body, onset of a severe headache, blurred vision, vomiting of blood, dizziness, fainting, fever, muscular or limb weakness, rash, nose bleeds, or any excessive vaginal or menstrual bleeding.

❖ Patients should be educated about applying direct pressure for 3 to 5 minutes or longer as needed for any superficial bleeding.

❖ Patients should be encouraged to keep a journal on how they are feeling daily as well as how they are tolerating their medication. They should also include any adverse effects or problems.

❖ To help prevent clot formation in the arteries, the physician may prescribe other interventions to help reduce risk factors for cardiovascular disease, such as a low-fat, low-cholesterol diet; medication to lower cholesterol if deemed necessary; weight reduction if ordered; controlling blood pressure if hypertensive; avoidance and cessation of smoking; stress management; and regular exercise.

❖ Patients should be educated on how to help prevent clot formation in their leg veins. If they are prone to blood clots in the legs or deep vein thrombosis, there are measures they can take to help minimize situations that may make the blood flow slow or sluggish, such as not wearing tight-fitting clothing, minimizing sitting for prolonged periods of time, not crossing their legs at the knees, not wearing tight-fitting socks, avoiding periods of prolonged bed rest, making sure to stop and walk around every 1 to 2 hours when on long trips, staying well hydrated, and doing leg and foot exercises.

❖ With any of the anticoagulants (oral, heparin, LWMHs) or clot-altering drugs, patients should be encouraged to avoid brushing their teeth with a hard-bristled toothbrush, shaving with a straight razor, and engaging in any activity that would increase the risk for tissue injury. They should understand why they need to be very careful when shaving, trimming their nails, gardening, or participating in rough or contact sports, and they should take every precaution to protect themselves from injury.

❖ Patients should be educated that while on anticoagulants they should avoid eating large amounts of foods high in vitamin K, such as broccoli, brussels sprouts, collard greens, kale, lettuce, mustard greens, and tomatoes. These foods will interact with the drug and decrease its effectiveness.

❖ Capsicum pepper, feverfew, garlic, ginger, ginkgo, and ginseng are some natural health products that have potential interactions, especially to warfarin, and patients should receive a list of commonly encountered drug interactions. Patients should know to report any of the following to their physician immediately: decrease in urine output; constant ringing in the ears; swelling of the feet, ankles, or legs; dark urine; clay-coloured stools; abdominal pain; rash (discontinue use if rash occurs); and blurred vision or the perception of halos around objects.

❖ Patients should be educated to never make up for any missed doses and to not double-up on doses. If in doubt about what to do, they should contact their physician for further instructions.

❖ Patients should be instructed to take aspirin or aspirin–like products with at least 240 mL of water and with food to help avoid stomach upset. Taking oral warfarin with food may help prevent gastrointestinal upset.

❖ Patients should be informed that use of any of these medications requires that containers be kept out of the reach of children and medications be kept in a container with a childproof top or lid. All equipment, syringes, and needles should be kept out of reach of children and other individuals.

POINTS TO REMEMBER

❖ Coagulation modifiers act by (1) preventing clot formation, (2) promoting clot formation, (3) lysing a preformed clot, or (4) reversing the action of anticoagulants.

❖ Anticoagulants, antiplatelet drugs, antifibrinolytics, thrombolytics, and reversal drugs are all examples of coagulation modifiers. The coagulation system is as follows: Clot formation takes place concurrently as clot destruction; clot destruction is governed by the fibrinolytic system; clot formation is accomplished by the coagulation pathway, of which there is an extrinsic and an intrinsic pathway.

❖ Warfarin prevents clot formation by inhibiting vitamin K–dependent clotting factors (II, VII, IX, and X) and is used prophylactically to prevent clots from forming; it cannot lyse preformed clots.

❖ The degree of anticoagulation (for any of the medications) is monitored by the prothrombin time (PT).

❖ Heparin prevents clot formation by binding to antithrombin III. By doing so, it blocks certain activating factors. The overall effect is to shut down the coagulation pathway and prevent clots from forming. Heparin does not lyse (break down) a clot. Nurses should remember that heparin is given intravenously or subcutaneously.

❖ Antiplatelet drugs prevent clot formation by preventing platelet involvement in clot formation. All antiplatelets affect normal platelet function and should be given to patients only after thorough assessment of the patient with a medical history and medication profile.

Continued

❖ Antifibrinolytics prevent lysis of fibrin, thus promoting clot formation; they have the opposite effects of anticoagulants. Thrombolytics are able to lyse preformed clots in blood vessels that supply the heart with oxygenated blood. Examples of drugs include streptokinase (SK) and anisoylated plasminogen streptokinase activator complex (APSAC). SK is derived from group A β-hemolytic streptococci and converts plasminogen to plasmin, which breaks down thrombi. Therapeutic effects that the nurse should monitor for include improved tissue perfusion, decreased chest pain, and prevention of further myocardial damage. Adverse effects include nausea, vomiting, hypotension, and bleeding.

❖ The therapeutic effects of most coagulation modifier drugs include improved circulation, tissue perfusion, decreased pain, and prevention of further tissue damage. Before using any of these drugs, it is important for the nurse to perform a thorough physical assessment and record findings, as well as monitor any pertinent laboratory values such as INR, aPTT, and PT.

❖ Nursing care is individualized according to the patient, thorough assessment data, existing medical conditions, and the specific drug. It is the nurse's responsibility to know everything about the patient and the drug for safe administration and for quality nursing care.

EXAMINATION REVIEW QUESTIONS

1 The nurse is monitoring a patient who is receiving antithrombolytic therapy in the emergency room for a possible myocardial infarction. Which of the following adverse effects would be the highest concern at this time?
a. Dizziness
b. Irregular heart rhythm
c. BP 130/98 mm Hg
d. Slight bloody oozing from the IV insertion site

2 A patient is receiving instructions for warfarin therapy, and asks the nurse about what medications she can take for headaches. Which type of medication should the nurse tell her to avoid?
a. Opioids
b. NSAIDs
c. Acetaminophen (Tylenol)
d. There are no restrictions while on warfarin.

3 The nurse is teaching a patient about self-administration of the LMWH enoxaparin (Lovenox). Which statement should be included in this teaching session?
a. "Be sure to massage the injection site thoroughly after receiving the drug."
b. "We will need to teach a family member how to give this drug in your arm."
c. "This drug needs to be taken at the same time every day with a full glass of water."
d. "This drug is given in the folds of your abdomen, but at least 5 cm away from your navel."

4 A patient is receiving warfarin (Coumadin) therapy as part of the treatment for a pulmonary embolism. Which laboratory test results should the nurse monitor to check the drug's effectiveness?
a. aPTT levels
b. PT-INR levels
c. Platelet counts
d. Vitamin K levels

5 A patient has received a double dose of heparin during surgery and is bleeding through his incision site. While the surgeons are working to stop the bleeding at the incision site, what action will the nurse prepare to do at this time?
a. Obtain an order for packed red blood cells.
b. Prepare to give intravenous vitamin K as an antidote.
c. Call the blood bank for an immediate platelet transfusion.
d. Prepare to give intravenous protamine sulfate as an antidote.

For answers see http://evolve.elsevier.com/Canada/Lilley/pharmacology/.

CRITICAL THINKING ACTIVITIES

1 Mrs. F.W., age 63, has had hip replacement surgery and will be receiving enoxaparin (Lovenox) 30 mg SC every 12 hours. Explain the rationale behind this medication order.

2 If a patient decides to take garlic tablets to reduce his cholesterol level, is there a concern if he is taking warfarin? Explain.

3 Explain the rationale for a patient to receive warfarin and heparin together.

For answers see http://evolve.elsevier.com/Canada/Lilley/pharmacology/.

CHAPTER **29**

Antilipemic Drugs

Learning Objectives

After reading this chapter, the successful student will be able to do the following:

1 Explain the pathophysiology of primary and secondary hyperlipidemia, including causes and risk factors.

2 Discuss the different types of lipoproteins and their role in cardiovascular diseases and in hyperlipidemia.

3 List the drug classes with specific drugs that are used to treat hyperlipidemia.

4 Compare the drugs used to treat hyperlipidemia, including the rationale for treatment, indications, mechanisms of action, dosages, routes of administration, adverse effects, toxicity, cautions, contraindications, and associated drug interactions.

5 Develop a collaborative plan of care that includes all phases of the nursing process for the patient receiving an antilipemic drug.

e-Learning Activities

Web site
(http://evolve.elsevier.com/Canada/Lilley/pharmacology/)

- Animations
- Answers to chapter questions, activities, and case studies
- Calculators and Category Catchers
- Glossary with audio pronunciations
- IV Therapy and Medication Error Checklists
- Multiple-Choice Review Question quizzes
- Nursing Care Plans
- Online Appendices and Supplements
- WebLinks

Drug Profiles

▸▸ **atorvastatin (atorvastatin calcium)***, p. 558
▸▸ **cholestyramine**, p. 559
 ezetimibe, p. 561
 gemfibrozil, p. 561
▸▸ **nicotinic acid**, p. 560

▸▸ Key drug.

*Full generic name is given in parentheses. For the purposes of this text, the more common shortened name is used.

Glossary

Antilipemic A drug that reduces lipid levels. (p. 551)

Apolipoprotein The protein component of a lipoprotein. (p. 551)

Cholesterol A fat-soluble crystalline steroid alcohol that is found in animal fats and oils and egg yolk and widely distributed in the body, especially in bile, blood, brain tissue, liver, kidneys, adrenal glands, and myelin sheaths of nerve fibres. (p. 551)

Chylomicrons Minute droplets of lipoproteins; the forms in which dietary fats are absorbed from the small intestine. (p. 551)

Exogenous lipids Lipids originating outside the body or an organ (e.g., dietary fats) or produced as the result of external causes, such as a disease caused by a bacterial or viral drug foreign to the body. (p. 552)

Foam cells The characteristic initial lesion of atherosclerosis, also known as the *fatty streak*. (p. 553)

HMG–CoA reductase inhibitors A class of cholesterol-lowering drugs that act by inhibiting the rate-limiting step in cholesterol synthesis; also commonly referred to as *statins* (see *statins*). (p. 555)

Hypercholesterolemia A condition in which greater-than-normal amounts of cholesterol are present in the blood. (p. 552)

Lipoprotein Conjugated protein in which lipids form an integral part of the molecule. (p. 551)

Statins A class of cholesterol-lowering drugs more formally known as *HMG–CoA reductase inhibitors.* (p. 555)

Triglycerides A compound consisting of a fatty acid (oleic, palmitic, or stearic) and a type of alcohol known as *glycerol.* (p. 551)

OVERVIEW

An understanding of **antilipemic** drugs begins with an understanding of how **cholesterol** and **triglycerides** are transported and used in the human body and how lipoproteins, apolipoproteins, receptors, and enzyme systems are involved in these processes. Also essential is an understanding of the basic mechanisms underlying lipid abnormalities and the link between hyperlipidemia and coronary heart disease (CHD). Armed with this knowledge, the clinician can develop and implement a rational approach to treatment using both nonpharmacological and pharmacological interventions. Some patients also use dietary supplements for control of hyperlipidemia (see Natural Health Products).

LIPIDS AND LIPID ABNORMALITIES

Primary Forms of Lipids

Triglycerides and cholesterol are the two primary forms of lipids in the blood. Triglycerides function as an energy source and are stored in adipose tissue. Cholesterol is primarily used to make steroid hormones, cell membranes, and bile acids. Triglycerides and cholesterol are both water-insoluble fats that must be bound to specialized lipid-carrying proteins called **apolipoproteins**. This combination of triglycerides and cholesterol with an apolipoprotein is referred to as a **lipoprotein**. Lipoproteins transport lipids via the blood. They are made up of a lipid core of triglycerides or cholesterol esters, or both, which is surrounded by a thin layer of phospholipids, apolipoproteins, and cholesterol. There are various types of lipoproteins, and they are classified according to their density and the type of apolipoproteins they contain. These types of lipoproteins and their classification are listed in Table 29-1.

Cholesterol Homeostasis

There is a complex range of biochemical factors and reactions that are all part of physiological (normal) cholesterol homeostasis. Figure 29-1 summarizes the major concepts that are described. Fats are taken into the body through the diet and are broken down in the small intestine to form triglycerides. These triglycerides are, in turn, incorporated into **chylomicrons** in the cells of the

 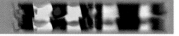

NATURAL HEALTH PRODUCTS

GARLIC *(allium sativum)*

Overview
Garlic obtains its pharmacological effects from the active ingredient allinin.

Common Uses
Antispasmodic, antiseptic, antibacterial and antiviral, antihypertensive, antiplatelet, lipid-lowering activity

Adverse Effects
Dermatitis, vomiting, diarrhea, anorexia, flatulence, antiplatelet activity

Potential Drug Interactions
May inhibit iodine uptake, warfarin, diazepam, protease inhibitors

Contraindications
Contraindicated in patients about to undergo surgery within 2 weeks and in patients with human immunodeficiency virus (HIV) or diabetes
Follow manufacturer directions on container for use of specific preparations.

FLAX

Overview
Flax is a flowering annual found in the Europe, Canada, and the United States. Both the seed and the oil of the plant are used medicinally.

Common Uses
Atherosclerosis, hypercholesterolemia, hypertriglyceridemia; gastrointestinal distress (especially constipation); menopausal symptoms; and bladder inflammation, among other uses

Adverse Effects
Diarrhea, allergic reactions

Potential Drug Interactions
Antidiabetic drugs: Theoretically can potentiate hypoglycemic effects
Anticoagulant drugs: Theoretically can potentiate anticoagulant effects by reducing platelet aggregation and prolonging bleeding time

Contraindications
Pregnancy, bowel obstruction; use with caution in diabetes and cardiovascular disease
Follow manufacturer directions on container for use of specific preparations.

TABLE 29-1

Lipoprotein Classification

Lipid Content	Lipoprotein Classification	Protein Content
Most ↑ Least	Chylomicron VLDL LDL IDL HDL	Least ↓ Most

HDL, high-density lipoprotein; *IDL,* intermediate-density lipoprotein; *LDL,* low-density lipoprotein; *VLDL,* very-low-density lipoprotein.

intestinal wall, which are then absorbed into the lymphatic system. The primary purpose of chylomicrons is to transport lipids obtained from dietary sources **(exogenous lipids)** from the intestines to the liver to be used to make steroid hormones, lipid structural components for peripheral body cells, and bile acids.

The liver is the major organ where lipid metabolism occurs. The liver produces *very-low-density lipoprotein (VLDL)* from both endogenous and exogenous sources. The major role of VLDL is the transport of endogenous lipids to peripheral cells. Once VLDL is circulating, it is enzymatically cleaved by lipoprotein lipase and loses triglycerides, thus creating *intermediate-density lipoprotein (IDL)*. IDL is soon also cleaved by lipoprotein

lipase, creating *low-density lipoprotein (LDL)*. Cholesterol is almost all that is left in LDL after this process. Any tissues that require LDL, such as endocrine cells, possess LDL receptors. LDL and about half of IDL are reabsorbed from the circulation into the liver by means of LDL receptors on the liver.

HDL is produced in the liver and intestines and is also formed when chylomicrons are broken down. Lipids that are not used by peripheral cells are transferred as cholesterol esters to HDL. HDL then transfers the cholesterol esters to IDL to be returned to the liver. HDL is responsible for the "recycling" of cholesterol. HDL is sometimes referred to as the good lipid (or "good cholesterol") because it is believed to be cardioprotective.

If the liver has an excess amount of cholesterol, the number of LDL receptors on the liver decreases, resulting in an accumulation of LDL in the blood. One explanation for **hypercholesterolemia** (cholesterol in the blood), therefore, is this down-regulation (reduced production) of liver LDL receptors. A major function of the liver is to manufacture cholesterol, a process that requires acetyl coenzyme A (CoA) reductase. Inhibition of this enzyme thus results in decreased cholesterol production by the liver.

Atherosclerotic Plaque Formation

Fundamental to the study of hyperlipidemia is an understanding of the processes by which lipids and lipoproteins participate in the formation of atherosclerotic

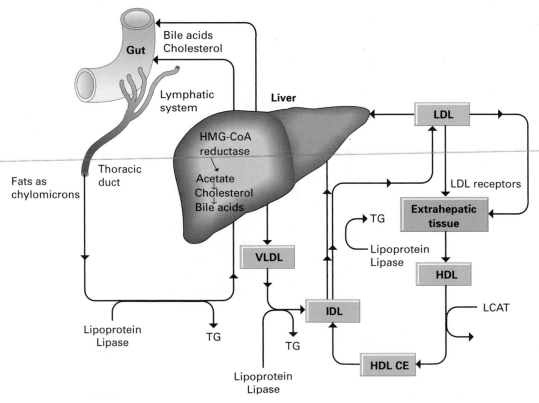

FIG. 29-1 Cholesterol homeostasis. *CE,* cholesterol ester; *HDL,* high-density lipoprotein; *HMG–CoA,* hydroxymethylglutaryl-coenzyme A; *IDL,* intermediate-density lipoprotein; *LCAT,* lecithin cholesterol acetyltransferase; *LDL,* low-density lipoprotein; *TG,* triglyceride; *VLDL,* very-low-density lipoprotein.

plaque and, subsequently, the development of coronary heart disease. The primary event that causes atherosclerosis appears to be repeated, subtle injury to the artery's wall through various mechanisms, including smoking, elevated blood pressure, diabetes mellitus, and elevated cholesterol. An ongoing inflammatory response plays a central role in all stages of atherogenesis. When serum cholesterol levels are elevated, LDLs are oxidized by reactive oxygen free radicals produced by endothelial cells. In response to the injury, circulating monocytes adhere to the smooth endothelial surface of the coronary vasculature. These monocytes burrow into the next layer of the blood vessel (subendothelial tissue) and differentiate into macrophage cells, which then absorb the oxidized LDLs and slowly become large **foam cells**, the characteristic precursor lesion of atherosclerosis, also known as the *fatty streak*. Once this process is established, it is usually present throughout the coronary and systemic circulation. There is also smooth muscle proliferation and migration from the tunica media to the intima in response to cytokines secreted by damaged endothelial cells. This process eventually forms a fibrous capsule covering the fatty streak.

Link Between Cholesterol and Coronary Artery Disease

Numerous epidemiological trials, such as the Framingham Study and the Lipid Research Clinics Prevalence Cohort, have shown that as blood cholesterol levels increase in a population, the incidence of death and disability related to coronary artery disease (CAD) also increases. The risk for CAD in patients with cholesterol levels of 5.2 mmol/L is three to four times greater than that for patients with levels lower than 4.0 mmol/L. The absolute incidence of CAD in premenopausal women and women on estrogen replacement therapy is approximately 25% less than that of men. This lower risk is thought to be secondary to the effects of estrogen because the risk of CAD rises considerably in postmenopausal women. There has been emerging controversy, however, regarding this long-standing belief because two recent estrogen replacement therapy (ERT) trials (Women's Health Initiative and Heart and Estrogen/progestin Replacement Study) did not demonstrate prevention of cardiovascular events in women receiving ERT. Other experimental studies that looked for any benefits of low-dose estrogen therapy in *male* patients also did not demonstrate significant cardioprotective efficacy (The Coronary Drug Project, 1973).

Approximately 75,000 heart attacks occur in Canada each year. It is the leading cause of death among both men and women. Thus, the thrust of treatment is two-pronged: primary prevention of cardiac events in patients with risk factors and secondary prevention of subsequent cardiac events in individuals who have previously suffered a heart event (e.g., myocardial infarction [MI]). The benefits of primary prevention as it refers to cholesterol reduction have been illustrated in a variety of recent trials. Some of the larger and more recent trials are the Lipid Research Clinics Coronary Primary Prevention Trial (LRC-CPPT), the Helsinki Heart Study, and the West of Scotland Coronary Prevention Study (WOS). The LRC trial used the drug cholestyramine, the Helsinki study used the drug gemfibrozil, and the WOS used the hydroxymethylglutaryl (HMG)–CoA reductase inhibitor pravastatin. These studies help reinforce the belief that in patients with known risk factors for coronary heart disease, drug therapy with an antilipemic drug can reduce the occurrence of such disease. First-time heart attack as well as death caused by heart disease can be reduced with drug therapy.

Data from new clinical trials have emerged that support a more vigorous approach to lipid lowering in specific patient groups. Several of these recent studies, such as the Treatment to New Targets (TNT), Incremental Decrease in Endpoints through Aggressive Lipid lowering (IDEAL), and PRavastatin Orator Vastatin Evaluation and Infection Therapy (PROVE-IT) studies, indicate that a lower low-density lipoprotein cholesterol (LDL-C) target is appropriate for high-risk individuals. Others, such as the Anglo-Scandinavian Cardiac Outcome Trial (ASCOT), demonstrate treatment benefit for intermediate-risk groups, even in the absence of overt dyslipidemia.

The benefits of cholesterol reduction as secondary prevention have been illustrated in a number of recent trials as well. Some of the larger trials are the Cholesterol-Lowering Atherosclerosis Study (CLAS), the Familial Atherosclerosis Treatment Study, the Scandinavian Simvastatin Survival Study (4S trial), and the Treating to New Targets (TNT) trial. CLAS used the drugs colestipol and niacin, the Familial Atherosclerosis Treatment Study used the drugs niacin/colestipol and lovastatin/colestipol, and the 4S trial used the drug simvastatin. At the completion of the TNT trial, evidence showed that the aggressive reduction of LDL levels to less than 2.2 mmol/L reduced the risk of cardiovascular events by 22%. These secondary prevention trials demonstrated that in patients with documented CAD, treatment with a cholesterol-lowering drug has many positive outcomes, including decreased coronary events, regression of coronary atherosclerotic lesions, and prolonged survival.

Preventive measures taken early in a person's life to reduce and maintain cholesterol levels in a desirable range should have a dramatic effect in terms of preventing CAD and the resulting death and disability. These measures include lifestyle modifications such as in diet, weight, and activity level. Diets lower in saturated fat and higher in fibre and plant chemicals known as sterols and stanols, as well as perhaps the substitution of soy-based proteins for animal proteins, appear to promote healthier lipid profiles. These are among the latest dietary recommendations by the third National Cholesterol Education Program Adult Treatment Panel III (NCEP ATP III) from the National Institutes of Health. Consuming fatty fish or dietary supplements containing omega-3 fatty acids appears to have beneficial effects on triglyceride and HDL levels and is currently recommended by the Heart and Stroke Foundation of Canada (2008). The Heart and Stroke Foundation also strongly emphasizes the substantial therapeutic benefits of even modest weight reduction and of exercise in both the improvement of lipid profiles and reduction of the likelihood of heart disease. The Canadian Clinical Practice Guidelines for the Management of Dyslipidemia and the Prevention of Cardiovascular Disease stress that therapeutic lifestyle measures such as diet, exercise, smoking cessation, and weight loss along with targeted medications are necessary to achieve target cholesterol-level goals (McPherson, Frohlich, Fodor, & Genest, 2006).

Hyperlipidemias and Treatment Guidelines

The decision to prescribe hyperlipemic drugs as an adjunct to diet therapy in patients with an elevated cholesterol level should be based on the patient's clinical profile. This includes the patient's age, sex, menopausal status, family history, and response to dietary treatment, as well as the presence of risk factors (other than hyperlipidemia) for premature CAD and the cause, duration, and phenotypic pattern of the patient's hyperlipidemia.

Major sources of guidance for antilipemic treatment at the disposal of health care professionals in Canada and the United States have been the *Clinical Practice Guidelines for the Management of Dyslipidemia and the Prevention of Cardiovascular Disease* and the *United States National Cholesterol Education Program* (NCEP). These programs have two main thrusts, both aimed at reducing the total risk of CAD in the North American population. One is focused on the entire population and consists of general guidelines for the prevention of CAD, including appropriate dietary intake of total cholesterol and saturated fat, weight control, physical activity, and the control of other lifestyle risk factors. The other aspect is focused on the management of individual patients who are at increased risk for CAD. In these guidelines, the selection of diet and drug therapy options is determined by the presence of certain risk factors. In an effort to standardize risk assessment across North America, the most recent Canadian guidelines are the first to include CAD risk equivalents. Three levels of risk—high, intermediate, and low—have been statistically calculated to equate one's 10-year risk for a major coronary event (e.g., MI) for those patients who do not currently have CAD. These risk factors and risk equivalents are listed in Box 29-1.

When the decision to institute drug therapy has been made, the choice of drug should then be determined by the specific lipid profile of the patient. There are five identified patterns or phenotypes of hyperlipidemia, and these are determined by the nature of the plasma concentrations of total cholesterol, triglycerides, and lipoprotein fractions (HDL, LDL, IDL, VLDL). The categories of hyperlipidemia are listed in Table 29-2. The process of characterizing a patient's specific lipid profile in this way is referred to as *phenotyping*.

One of the basic principles of the Canadian and NCEP guidelines is that all reasonable nonpharmaceutical means of controlling the blood cholesterol level (e.g.

BOX 29-1

Coronary Heart Disease: Risk Factors

Positive Risk Factors

- Age
- Male: over 45 years
- Female: over 55 years, or women with premature menopause not on estrogen replacement therapy
- Family history: History of premature CAD (e.g., MI or sudden death before 55 years of age in father or other male first-degree relative, or before 65 years of age in mother or other female first-degree relative)
- Current cigarette smoker
- Hypertension: greater than 140/90 mm Hg, or on antihypertensive medication
- Low-density lipoprotein/high-density lipoprotein levels greater than 5.0 mmol/L
- Diabetes mellitus

Negative Risk Factors

- High HDL cholesterol: **greater than or equal to 1.6 mmol/L**—if the HDL cholesterol is **greater than or equal to 1.6 mmol/L**, subtract one risk factor

CAD, coronary artery disease; *HDL*, high-density lipoprotein; *MI*, myocardial infarction.

---

diet, exercise) should be tried for at least 6 months and found to fail before drug therapy is considered. Because drug therapy for hyperlipidemias entails a long-term commitment to the therapy, factors that should be considered before initiation of therapy are the type and severity of dyslipidemia, the age and lifestyle of the patient, the relative indications and contraindications of different drugs and drug categories for the patient, potential drug interactions, adverse effects, and the overall cost of therapy. Major changes in updated 2006 Canadian dyslipidemia guidelines include a lower low-density lipoprotein cholesterol (LDL-C) treatment target (lower than 2.0 mmol/L) for high-risk patients and a slightly higher intervention point for the initiation of drug therapy in most low-risk individuals (LDL-C of 5.0 mmol/L or a total cholesterol to high-density lipoprotein cholesterol ratio of 6.0).

New information on the impact of abdominal obesity, family history of premature CAD, chronic kidney disease, and presence of subclinical atherosclerosis on cardiovascular risk has been added to the updated Canadian and NCEP guidelines. The value of nontraditional risk factors such as apolipoprotein (apo) B, high-sensitivity C-reactive protein (hsCRP), lipoprotein(a) (Lp[a]), and glycosylated hemoglobin in the prediction of cardiovascular risk and the current status of homocysteine measurement or treatment have also been discussed. The treatment decisions that should be made on the

TABLE 29-2

Types of Hyperlipidemias

Phenotype	Lipoprotein Elevated	Lipid Composition	
		Cholesterol (mmol/L)	Triglyceride
I	Chylomicrons	Greater than 7.8	Greater than 34.2
IIa	LDL	Greater than 7.8	Normal equal to or about 1.7
IIb	LDL, VLDL	Greater than 7.8	Normal equal to or about 1.7
III	IDL	Greater than 10.6	Greater than 6.8 (1–3 × higher than cholesterol)
IV	VLDL	Normal or mildly elevated Greater than 6.5	Greater than 4.6
V	VLDL, chylomicrons	Greater than 7.8	Greater than 22.8

IDL, intermediate-density lipoprotein; *LDL,* low-density lipoprotein; *VLDL,* very-low-density lipoprotein.

basis of LDL cholesterol levels are listed in Table 29-3. The updated guidelines even recommend optional use of drug therapy to reduce LDL to less than 70 mg/dL in very high–risk patients and to less than 100 mg/dL in moderately high–risk patients. "Very high–risk" patients include those with active cardiovascular disease as well as other major risk factors such as diabetes, continued smoking, or *metabolic syndrome. Metabolic syndrome* is a set of risk factors associated with obesity, including hyper-triglyceridemia and low HDL. Features of metabolic syndrome are listed in Box 29-2. "Moderately high–risk" patients include those who have no cardiovascular disease but have two or more risk factors.

There are currently four established classes of drugs used to treat dyslipidemia: HMG–CoA reductase inhibitors **(statins)**, bile acid sequestrants, the B-vitamin niacin (vitamin B₃, also known as *nicotinic acid*), and the fibric acid derivatives (fibrates). In addition to all of these drugs, the newest drug, *ezetimibe (Ezetrol),* is a cholesterol absorption inhibitor. In many cases, patient outcomes are improved with combinations of these drugs. One of the newest examples of this is the combination tablet Vytorin, which contains both the statin drug atorvastatin and ezetimibe (not yet available in Canada).

HMG–CoA REDUCTASE INHIBITORS

The rate-limiting enzyme in cholesterol synthesis is known as HMG–CoA reductase. The class of medications that competitively inhibit this enzyme, the **HMG–CoA reductase inhibitors**, are the most potent of the drugs available for reducing plasma concentrations of LDL cholesterol and are the most prescribed drug class in Canada. Lovastatin was the first drug in this class to be approved for use. Five additional rHMG–CoA reductase inhibitors have become available on the Canadian market: pravastatin, simvastatin (see Research: Statin Drugs Have Positive Effects on Cardiovascular System and Hypertension), atorvastatin, rosuvastatin, and flu-vastatin. Because of the shared suffix of their generic names, these drugs are often collectively referred to as *statins.* The maximum extent to which lipid levels are lowered may not occur until 6 to 8 weeks after the start of therapy. Few direct comparisons of the statins have been published. However, the authors of the published account of one such study concluded that the following doses of drugs would yield the same reduction in the LDL cholesterol level: simvastatin, 10 mg; pravastatin, 20 mg; and lovastatin, 20 mg. This particular study did not assess fluvastatin, rosuvastatin, or atorvastatin.

TABLE 29-3

Target Lipid Levels

Risk Categories and Target Lipid Levels			
		Target Level	
Risk Category	10-Year Risk	LDL-C (mmol/L)	Total Cholesterol: HDL–C ratio
High	Equal to or greater than or 20% or history of diabetes mellitus or any atherosclerotic disease	Less than 2.0 *and*	Less than 4.0
Moderate	10%–19%	Less than 3.5 *and*	Less than 5.0
Low	Less 10%	Less than 5 *and*	Less than 6.0

C, cholesterol; *HDL,* high-density lipoprotein; *LDL,* low-density lipoprotein.

Note: Although specific targets for triglyceride levels are no longer recommended, the guidelines emphasize that a plasma triglyceride concentration of less than 1.7 mmol/L is optimal. Canada's target lipid levels are based on LDL-C levels. In addition, the total-cholesterol to HDL ratio is considered to be of greater importance than HDL levels alone.

BOX 29-2

Identifying Features of Metabolic Syndrome

- Abdominal obesity
- Men: Waist circumference over 102 cm, European male over 94 cm, Asian male over 90 cm
- Women: Waist circumference over 88 cm, European and Asian females over 80 cm
- Serum triglycerides equal to or greater than 1.7 mmol/L
- HDL-C:
  - Men: less than 1 mmol/L
  - Women: less than 1.3 mmol/L
- Blood pressure greater than 130/85 mm Hg
- Fasting blood glucose 5.7 –7 mmol/L

HDL-C, high-density lipoprotein cholesterol.

Mechanism of Action and Drug Effects

Statins lower the blood cholesterol level by decreasing the rate of cholesterol production. The liver requires HMG–CoA reductase to produce cholesterol. It is the rate-limiting enzyme in the reactions needed to make cholesterol. The statins inhibit this enzyme and consequently decrease cholesterol production. When less cholesterol is produced, the liver increases the number of LDL receptors to augment the recycling of LDL from the circulation back into the liver, where it is needed for the synthesis of other needed substances such as steroids, bile acids, and cell membranes. Lovastatin and simvastatin are administered as inactive drugs or prodrugs that must be biotransformed into their active metabolites in the liver. In contrast, pravastatin is administered in its active form.

Indications

The statins are recommended by the 2006 Canadian dyslipidemia guidelines as first-line drug therapy for hypercholesterolemia (elevated LDL cholesterol, or LDL-C), the most common and dangerous form of dyslipidemia. More specifically, they are indicated for the treatment of type IIa and IIb hyperlipidemia and have been shown to reduce the plasma concentrations of LDL cholesterol by 30% to 40%. Their cholesterol-lowering properties are dose dependent in that the larger the dose that is given, the greater are the cholesterol-lowering effects achieved. A 10% to 30% decrease in the concentrations of plasma triglycerides has also been observed in patients receiving any of these drugs. Another important therapeutic effect of the statins is an overall tendency for the HDL cholesterol level to increase by 2% to 15%, a known beneficial risk factor (i.e., a negative risk factor) against cardiovascular disease.

These drugs appear to be equally effective in their ability to reduce LDL cholesterol concentrations. However, simvastatin and atorvastatin are more potent on a milligram basis. Atorvastatin appears to be more effective at lowering triglycerides than other HMG–CoA reductase inhibitors. Combined drug therapy with more than one class of antilipemic drugs may be necessary for desired results; the statins are often combined with niacin or fibrates for this purpose, despite the risk for increased adverse drug effects (see Adverse Effects).

Contraindications

Contraindications to the use of HMG–CoA reductase inhibitors (statins) include known drug allergy and pregnancy. Other contraindications may include liver disease or elevation of liver enzymes.

Adverse Effects

Generally, the HMG–CoA reductase inhibitors available for clinical use have proved to be well tolerated, with significant adverse effects being fairly uncommon. Mild, transient gastrointestinal disturbances, rash, and

 RESEARCH

Statin Drugs Have Positive Effects on Cardiovascular System and Hypertension

The Heart Protection Study was a multicentre, randomized, double-blind, placebo-controlled study of some 20,000 patients ages 40 to 80 years who had nonfasting total blood cholesterol concentrations of at least 3.5 mmol/L. Trial participants had heart disease or were likely to develop heart disease because of a pre-existing disease such as diabetes or history of stroke. A dose of 40 mg of simvastatin or placebo was administered for an average of 5 years. Outcomes showed major benefits of simvastatin in reducing the risks of fatal and nonfatal heart attacks and strokes as well as in reducing the need for bypass surgery and angioplasty. The likelihood of stroke was reduced by 2.5%, and the likelihood of death from coronary heart disease was reduced by 18%. Benefits of statin therapy were demonstrated for a range of individuals, including patients with cardiovascular disease, diabetes, and peripheral vascular disease.

These effects were found 2 years after initiation of medication and continued for as long as drug therapy was given.

Source: Heart Protection Collaborative Study Group. (2002). MRC/BHF heart protection study of cholesterol lowering with simvastatin in 20, 536 individuals: A randomized placebo-controlled trial. *Lancet, 360,* 7–22.

headache have been the most common problems. These and other less common adverse effects are listed in Table 29-4. Elevations in liver enzymes may also occur, and the patient should be monitored for excessive elevations, which may indicate the need for alternative drug therapy. Dose-dependent elevations in liver enzyme activity to values greater than three times the upper limit of normal have been noted in approximately 0.4% to 1.9% of patients taking HMG–CoA reductase inhibitors. The serum creatine phosphokinase (CPK) concentrations may be increased by more than 10 times the normal level in patients receiving these drugs. Most of these patients have remained asymptomatic, however. In August 2001, Bayer Corporation voluntarily recalled from the market its drug cerivastatin (Baycol) because of increasing numbers of serious adverse effects.

A less common but still clinically important adverse effect is myopathy (muscle pain), which may progress to a serious condition known as *rhabdomyolysis*. Rhabdomyolysis involves the breakdown of muscle protein leading to *myoglobinuria*, which is the urinary elimination of the muscle protein myoglobin, the oxygen-carrying pigment of muscle tissue that is similar to a single subunit of hemoglobin (Hgb). This abnormal urinary excretion of protein can place a severe strain on the kidneys, possibly leading to acute kidney failure and possibly death. This myopathy is uncommon (less than 0.1%) during monotherapy for dyslipidemia with statins alone, and it appears to be dose dependent (40 mg) and more common in patients receiving a statin in combination with cyclosporine, niacin, gemfibrozil (a fibrate), or erythromycin. Patients receiving statin therapy should be advised to immediately report any unexplained muscular pain or discomfort to their health care provider. When recognized reasonably early, rhabdomyolysis is usually reversible with discontinuation of the statin drug. In March 2005, Health Canada issued a Public Health Advisory summarizing the adverse events of myopathy and rhabdomyolysis cases associated with use of rosuvastatin (Crestor), one of the newer statin drugs. AstraZeneca Canada Pharmaceuticals, the manufacturer of this drug, altered the drug labelling, listing risk factors for myopathy symptoms. These include hypothyroidism, personal or family history of hereditary muscular disorders, previous history of muscular toxicity with another statin or fibrate, alcohol misuse, situations in which an increase in plasma levels may occur, concurrent use of fibrates, and patients with serious kidney problems. Asian patients (those of Filipino, Chinese, Japanese, Korean, Vietnamese, or South Asian origin) may be at greater risk of developing rhabdomyolysis.

Although these adverse effects are relatively uncommon and although much benefit is often derived from statins use, prescribers are advised to use minimal effective doses, with regular laboratory blood monitoring of liver and kidney function (every 3 to 6 months). Patients should also be educated about these serious, although

TABLE 29-4

HMG–CoA Reductase Inhibitors: Adverse Effects

Body System	Adverse Effects
Central nervous	Headache, dizziness, blurred vision, ophthalmoplegia, fatigue, nightmares, insomnia
Gastrointestinal	Constipation, cramps, diarrhea, nausea,
Miscellaneous	Myalgias, skin rashes

uncommon, adverse drug effects, and instructed to immediately report signs of toxicity, including muscle soreness, changes in urine colour, fever, malaise, nausea, or vomiting.

Toxicity and Management of Overdose

Limited data are available on the nature of toxicity and overdose in patients taking HMG–CoA reductase inhibitors. Treatment, if needed, is supportive and based on the presenting symptoms.

Interactions

HMG–CoA reductase inhibitors should be used cautiously in patients taking oral anticoagulants. In addition, the coadministration of HMG–CoA reductase inhibitors with other classes of antilipemics, oral anticoagulants, oral antidiabetic drugs, erythromycin, gemfibrozil, insulin, niacin, and even grapefruit juice has been observed to lead to the development of rhabdomyolysis, although this occurs rarely. Patients are advised to limit grapefruit juice to less than 1 litre daily, which is probably more than most people drink anyway. The mechanism of this interaction is as follows: Components in grapefruit juice inactivate one of the cytochrome P450 enzymes, specifically CYP3A4, in both the liver and the intestines. This enzyme plays a key role in statin metabolism. The presence of grapefruit juice in the body may, therefore, result in sustained levels of unmetabolized statin drug, increasing the risk for major drug toxicity (e.g., rhabdomyolysis).

Dosages

For dosage information on atorvastatin, see Drug Profiles.

Other Antilipemic Drugs

BILE ACID SEQUESTRANTS

Bile acid sequestrants, also referred to as *bile acid–binding resins* and *ion-exchange resins,* include cholestyramine and colestipol. Both drugs have been used widely for more than 20 years and have been evaluated extensively in well-controlled clinical trials. They were actually the original prescription anticholesterol drugs. They have proven efficacy, but their powdered forms are somewhat messy to use. Colestipol is also available in tablet form. Bile acid sequestrants are generally considered

DRUG PROFILES

HMG–COA REDUCTASE INHIBITORS (STATINS)

The HMG–CoA reductase inhibitors (statins) are all potent inhibitors of the enzyme that catalyzes the rate-limiting step in the synthesis of cholesterol. There are currently six statins available in Canada: atorvastatin calcium (Lipitor), fluvastatin sodium (Lescol), lovastatin (Advicor, Mevacor), pravastatin sodium (Pravasa), rosuvastatin calcium (Crestor), and simvastatin (Zocor). There are minor differences between the drugs in this class of antilipemics; the most dramatic difference is potency. All six drugs are prescription only and are contraindicated in pregnant or lactating women (category X) and in those suffering from active liver dysfunction or with elevated serum transaminase levels of unknown cause. There is little evidence to recommend one drug over another, with the exception of fluvastatin, which may be somewhat less effective than the others.

▶▶ atorvastatin calcium

Atorvastatin calcium (Lipitor) is the most commonly used drug in this class of cholesterol-lowering drugs. It is used to lower total and LDL cholesterol as well as triglycerides. It is indicated for the treatment of type IIa

and IIb hyperlipidemias, type III dysbetalipoproteinemia, and type IV hypertriglyceridemia. Atorvastatin has also been shown to raise the HDL component. All statins are generally administered once daily, in the evening, which is thought to be the time when cholesterol synthesis occurs, when the activity of HMG–CoA reductase is at its highest. Cholesterol synthesis is thought to peak in the early morning hours. The other statins can be taken without regard to meals, with the exception of lovastatin, which is absorbed better with meals. Atorvastatin is the sole statin approved for use in children. It is particularly effective for the treatment of heterozygous familial hypercholesterolemia in boys and postmenarchal girls aged 10 to 17 years. The recommended dosage for atorvastatin is 10 to 80 mg daily. It is available only in tablet form. Atorvastin is also available in a combination with the calcium channel blocker, amlodipine besylate (Caduet), indicated for patients at cardiovascular risk.

PHARMACOKINETICS

Half-Life	Onset	Peak	Duration
13–16 hr	1–2 hr	2 wk*	Unknown

*Maximum therapeutic effect.

second-line drugs in most cases in place of the more potent statins. However, they are still a suitable alternative in patients intolerant of the statins. Generally, bile acid sequestrants lower the plasma concentrations of LDL cholesterol by 15% to 30%. They also increase the HDL cholesterol level by 3% to 8% and increase liver triglyceride and VLDL production, which may result in a 10% to 50% increase in the triglyceride level.

Mechanism of Action and Drug Effects

Bile acid resins bind bile, preventing the reabsorption of bile acids from the small intestine. Instead, an insoluble bile acid–resin (drug) complex is excreted in the bowel movement. Bile acids are necessary for the absorption of cholesterol from the small intestine and yet are also synthesized from cholesterol by the liver. This is one natural way that the liver excretes cholesterol from the body. The more that bile acids are excreted in feces, the more the liver converts cholesterol to bile acids. This action reduces the level of cholesterol in the liver and, thus, in the circulation. The liver then attempts to compensate for the loss of cholesterol by increasing the number of high-affinity LDL receptors on the liver's surface. Circulating LDL molecules bind to these receptors to be taken up into the liver, which also has the benefit of reducing circulating LDL in the bloodstream.

Indications

Bile acid sequestrants may be used as primary or adjunct drug therapy in the management of type II

hyperlipoproteinemia. One common strategy is to use them along with statins for an additive drug effect in reducing LDL cholesterol. Cholestyramine is also used to relieve the pruritus associated with partial biliary obstruction.

Contraindications

Contraindications to the use of bile acid sequestrants include known drug allergy and biliary or bowel obstruction.

Adverse Effects

The adverse effects of colestipol and cholestyramine are similar. Constipation is a common problem and may be accompanied by heartburn, nausea, belching, and bloating. These adverse effects tend to disappear over time, however. Many patients require additional education and support to help them manage the gastrointestinal effects and adhere to the medication regimen. It is important that therapy be initiated with low doses and patients instructed to take the drugs with meals to reduce the adverse effects. By increasing dietary fibre intake or taking a fibre supplement such as psyllium (Metamucil and others), as well as increasing fluid intake, patients may relieve constipation and bloating. Mild increases in the triglyceride levels may also occur from the use of bile acid sequestrants. The most common adverse effects of the bile acid sequestrants are bleeding, headache, tinnitus, and a burnt odour of the urine. Common gastrointestinal adverse effects are constipation, heartburn, nausea, belching, and bloating. These drugs may also cause mild increases in the triglyceride levels.

DRUG PROFILES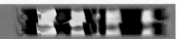

BILE ACID SEQUESTRANTS

The bile acid sequestrants cholestyramine and colestipol are indicated for the treatment of type IIa and IIb hyperlipidemia. They lower the cholesterol level, particularly the LDL cholesterol level, by increasing the destruction of LDL. However, their use may result in increases in the VLDL cholesterol level. Because of the high incidence of gastrointestinal adverse effects in patients taking these drugs, adherence to the prescribed dosage schedules is often poor. However, educating patients about the purpose and expected adverse effects of therapy can help improve adherence. Patients must be warned not to take bile acid sequestrants concurrently with other drugs, because the drug interactions can be pronounced. Thus other drugs must be taken at other times of the day—this cannot be overemphasized.

▶▶ **cholestyramine**

Cholestyramine (Novo-Cholamine) is a prescription-only drug that is contraindicated in patients with a known hypersensitivity to it and in those with complete biliary obstruction. It may interfere with the distribution of fat-soluble vitamins to the fetus or nursing infant of pregnant or nursing women taking the drug.

Toxicity and Management of Overdose

Because the bile acid sequestrants are not absorbed, an overdose could cause obstruction of the gastrointestinal tract. Therefore, treatment of an overdose involves restoring gut motility.

Interactions

The significant drug interactions associated with the use of bile acid sequestrants are limited to the absorption of concurrently administered drugs. All drugs should be taken at least 1 hour before or 4 to 6 hours after the administration of ion-exchange resins. In addition, high doses of a bile acid sequestrant will decrease the absorption of fat-soluble vitamins (A, D, E, and K).

Dosages

For dosage information on cholestyramine and colestipol hydrochloride, see the Dosages table on p. 562.

NICOTINIC ACID

Nicotinic acid (Niacin, Niaspan) is not only a unique lipid-lowering drug, it is also a vitamin. For its lipid-lowering properties to be realized, much larger doses of nicotinic acid are required than when it is used as a vitamin. Nicotinic acid is a B vitamin, specifically vitamin B_3 (also known as *niacin*). It is an effective and inexpensive medication that exerts favourable effects on the plasma concentrations of all lipoproteins. Nicotinic acid is often given in combination with other antilipemic drugs to enhance the lipid-lowering effects.

Mechanism of Action and Drug Effects

Although the exact mechanism of action of niacin is unknown, the beneficial effects are thought to be related to its ability to inhibit lipolysis in adipose tissue, decrease esterification of triglycerides in the liver, and increase the activity of lipoprotein lipase. The drug effects of nicotinic acid are primarily limited to its ability to reduce the metabolism or catabolism of cholesterol and triglycerides. Nicotinic acid decreases LDL levels moderately (10% to 20%), decreases the triglyceride levels (30% to 70%), and increases the HDL levels moderately (20% to 35%). Nicotinic acid is also a vitamin needed for many bodily processes. In large doses, it may produce vasodilation that is limited to the cutaneous vessels. This effect seems to be induced by prostaglandins. Nicotinic acid also causes the release of histamine, resulting in an increase in gastric motility and acid secretion. Nicotinic acid may also stimulate the fibrinolytic system to break down fibrin clots.

Indications

Nicotinic acid has been shown to be effective in lowering triglyceride, total serum cholesterol, and LDL cholesterol levels. It also increases HDL cholesterol levels. Nicotinic acid may also lower the lipoprotein (a) level, except in patients with severe hypertriglyceridemia. It has been shown to be effective in the treatment of types IIa, IIb, III, IV, and V hyperlipidemia.

Nicotinic acid's effects on triglyceride levels begin to be noticed after 1 to 4 days of therapy, with the decrease in the levels ranging from 20% to 80%. The decline in LDL levels is less, with the maximum decrease ranging from 10% to 15%. The maximum effects of niacin are seen after 3 to 5 weeks of continuous therapy.

Contraindications

Contraindications to the use of nicotinic acid include known drug allergy and may include liver disease, hypertension, peptic ulcer, and any active hemorrhagic process.

Adverse Effects

Nicotinic acid can cause flushing, pruritus, and gastrointestinal distress. Small doses of aspirin or nonsteroidal anti-inflammatory drugs may be taken 30 minutes before niacin to minimize the cutaneous flushing. These undesirable effects can also be minimized by starting patients on a low initial dosage and increasing it gradually and by having patients take the drug with meals. The most common adverse effects and those associated with niacin therapy are listed in Table 29-5.

TABLE **29-5**

Nicotinic Acid: Potential Adverse Effects

Body System	Adverse Effects
Gastrointestinal	Abdominal discomfort, gastrointestinal distress
Integumentary	Cutaneous flushing, pruritus, hyperpigmentation
Other	Blurred vision, glucose intolerance, hyperuricemia, dry eyes (rare), hepatotoxicity

Interactions

The major drug interactions associated with nicotinic acid are minimal. One interaction to note, however, is that when nicotinic acid is taken concomitantly with an HMG–CoA reductase inhibitor, the likelihood of myopathy development is greatly increased.

Dosages

For dosage information on niacin, see the Dosages table on p. 562.

 DRUG PROFILES

▶▶ *nicotinic acid*

Used alone or in combination with other lipid-lowering drugs, nicotinic acid (niacin, vitamin B₃) (Nio-dan, Niaspan) is an effective, inexpensive medication that has beneficial effects on LDL cholesterol, triglyceride, and HDL cholesterol levels. Extended-release Advicor is currently the only available combined formulation of niacin and lovastatin. Drug therapy with nicotinic acid is usually initiated at a small daily dose taken with or after meals to minimize the adverse effects. Liver dysfunction has been observed in individuals taking sustained-release forms of niacin, not immediate-release forms. However, newer extended-release dosage forms, which dissolve more slowly than the immediate-release forms, appear to have even better adverse-effect profiles, including less hepatotoxicity and flushing of the skin. Niacin is contraindicated in patients who have shown a hypersensitivity to it; in those with peptic ulcer, liver disease, hemorrhage, or severe hypotension; and in lactating women. It is also not recommended for patients with gout. Niacin is available over the counter and by prescription.

PHARMACOKINETICS

Half-Life	Onset	Peak	Duration
20–60 min	Unknown	30–70 min	Unknown

FIBRIC ACID DERIVATIVES

Current fibric acid derivatives include bezafibrate, gemfibrozil and gemfibrozil. These drugs primarily affect triglyceride levels but may also lower total cholesterol and LDL cholesterol levels and raise HDL cholesterol levels. Collectively, they are referred to as *fibrates*.

Mechanism of Action and Drug Effects

Fibric acid drugs are believed to work by activating lipoprotein lipase, the enzyme responsible for the breakdown of cholesterol. This enzyme usually cleaves a triglyceride molecule from VLDL or LDL, leaving behind a lipoprotein. Fibric acid derivatives can also suppress the release of free fatty acid from adipose tissue, inhibit the synthesis of triglycerides in the liver, and increase the secretion of cholesterol into bile. Fibric acid derivatives have been shown to reduce triglyceride levels and serum VLDL and LDL concentrations. Independent of their lipid-lowering actions, fibric acid derivatives can also induce changes in blood coagulation. This involves a tendency for them to decrease platelet adhesiveness. They can also increase plasma fibrinolysis, the process that causes fibrin and, therefore, clots to be broken down.

Indications

The fibric acid derivatives bezafibrate, gemfibrozil, and fenofibrate decrease triglyceride levels and increase HDL cholesterol levels approximately 25%. They decrease LDL concentrations in patients with type IIa and IIb hyperlipidemias and increase LDL levels in patients with type IV and V hyperlipidemias. They are indicated for the treatment of type III, IV, and V hyperlipidemias and, in some cases, the type IIb form, although other classes of antilipemics are usually attempted first.

Contraindications

Contraindications to the use of fibrates include known drug allergy and may include severe liver or kidney disease, cirrhosis, or gallbladder disease.

Adverse Effects

As a class, the most common adverse effects of fibric acid derivatives are abdominal discomfort, diarrhea, nausea, headache, blurred vision, increased risk for gallstones, and prolonged prothrombin time. Liver function tests may also show increased enzyme levels. The more common adverse effects are listed in Table 29-6.

TABLE 29-6

Fibric Acid Derivatives: Potential Adverse Effects

Body System	Adverse Effects
Gastrointestinal	Nausea, vomiting, diarrhea, gallstones, acute appendicitis
Genitourinary	Erectile dysfunction, decreased urine output, hematuria, increased risk for urinary hematuria, increased risk for urinary tract infections and viral infections
Other	Drowsiness, dizziness, rash, pruritus, alopecia, vertigo, headache

Toxicity and Management of Overdose

The management of fibrate overdose, which is uncommon, is supportive care based on presenting symptoms. Gastrointestinal decontamination or use of gastric lavage may be indicated for large overdoses.

Interactions

Gemfibrozil can enhance the action of oral anticoagulants, thus necessitating careful dose adjustments of these latter drugs. The risk for myositis, myalgia, and rhabdomyolysis is increased when fibrates are given with a statin. Fenofibrate may also raise the blood level of ezetimibe if taken concurrently.

Laboratory test interactions that can occur in patients taking gemfibrozil include a decrease in the hemoglobin (Hgb) level, hematocrit (Hct) value, and white blood cell count. In addition, the aspartate aminotransferase (AST), activated clotting time (ACT), lactate dehydrogenase, and bilirubin levels can be increased.

Dosages

For dosage information on bezafibrate, gemfibrozil and fenofibrate, see the Dosages table on p. 562.

 DRUG PROFILES

FIBRIC ACID DERIVATIVES (FIBRATES)

The fibric acid derivatives bezafibrate, gemfibrozil, and fenofibrate are prescription-only drugs. They are contraindicated in patients with hypersensitivity, pre-existing gallbladder disease, significant liver or kidney dysfunction, and primary biliary cirrhosis. Fibrates decrease triglyceride and increase HDL levels by approximately 25%. They are effective for the treatment of mixed hyperlipidemia.

gemfibrozil

Gemfibrozil (Lopid) is a fibric acid derivative that decreases the synthesis of apolipoprotein B (Apo B) and lowers the VLDL level. It can also increase the HDL level. In addition, it is highly effective for lowering plasma triglyceride levels. In a large trial, the Helsinki study, the triglyceride levels of the group receiving gemfibrozil were reduced by as much as 43% compared with the control group. The total cholesterol and LDL levels were reduced by 11% and 10%, respectively, and the HDL level was increased by 10%. Gemfibrozil is indicated for the treatment of type IV and V hyperlipidemias and, in some cases, type IIb. The specific dosing recommendations are given in the Dosages table on p. 562.

PHARMACOKINETICS

Half-Life	Onset	Peak	Duration
1.3–1.5 hr	Unknown	1–2 hr	Unknown

CHOLESTEROL ABSORPTION INHIBITORS
ezetimibe

Ezetimibe (Ezetrol) is currently the sole cholesterol absorption inhibitor, approved by Health Canada in 2003. Ezetimibe has a novel mechanism of action. It selectively inhibits absorption of cholesterol and related sterols in the small intestine. The result is a reduction in several blood lipid parameters: total cholesterol, LDL cholesterol (LDL-C), Apo B, and triglycerides. However, serum levels of HDL cholesterol (HDL-C) have been shown to actually increase with the use of ezetimibe. These beneficial effects appear to be further enhanced when ezetimibe is taken with a statin drug, rather than either type of drug taken alone, although ezetimibe may be used as monotherapy.

In several small studies, ezetimibe was not shown to interact significantly with cimetidine, warfarin, digoxin, oral contraceptives, glipizide, or antacids. However, fibric acid derivatives (fibrates) have been shown to significantly increase the serum levels of ezetimibe. It is not yet known whether this is harmful; currently, concurrent use of ezetimibe and fibrates is not recommended. The use of ezetimibe with bile acid sequestrants has been shown to reduce the serum level of ezetimibe by 55% and 80% in two small studies. Concurrent use of these two types of drugs is not yet contraindicated, but it should be recognized that the extent of LDL reduction normally promoted by ezetimibe is likely to be reduced with this drug combination. When used with a statin, there is a synergistic reduction in LDLs.

Ezetimibe is contraindicated in cases of demonstrated allergy to the drug or active liver disease or unexplained elevations in serum liver enzymes. The drug is currently available only as a 10 mg tablet for once-daily dosing. It may be taken with or without food, and for patient convenience, may be dosed at the same time as a statin drug, if prescribed.

PHARMACOKINETICS

Half-Life	Onset	Peak	Duration
22 hr	Unknown	4–12 hr	Unknown

DOSAGES Selected Antilipemic Drugs

Drug (Pregnancy Category)	Pharmacological Class	Usual Dosage Range	Indications
▶▶atorvastatin calcium (Lipitor) (X)	HMG–CoA reductase inhibitor	*Adult* PO: 10–80 mg/day	Hyperlipidemia
bezafibrate (PMS-Bezafibrate, Bezalip SR) (C)	Fibric acid derivative	*Adult* PO: 200 bid–tid mg/day SR: 400 daily	Hyperlipidemia
▶▶cholestyramine (Novo-Cholamine) (C)	Antilipemic ion-exchange resin	*Adult* PO: Powder, 4–8 g daily to bid	Hyperlipidemia
colestipol hydrochloride (Colestid) (C)	Antilipemic ion-exchange resin	*Adult* PO: Granules: 5–30 g/day once or in divided doses; tabs: 2–16 g/day	Hyperlipidemia
ezetimibe (Ezetrol) (C)	Cholesterol absorption inhibitor	*Adult* PO: 10 mg 1 ×/day	Hyperlipidemia
fenofibrate (Lipidil) (C)	Fibric acid derivative	*Adult* PO: 67 mg/day initial dose; max 200 mg/day	Hyperlipidemia
gemfibrozil (Lopid) (C)	Fibric acid derivative	*Adult* PO: 600 mg bid 30 min before meals in A.M. and P.M.	Hyperlipidemia
▶▶nicotinic acid (Niacin, Niaspan) (A; C if dose exceeds RDA)	B vitamin	*Adult* PO: initial dose 50 mg tid; double q5 days to 1.5–2 g/day; max 4 g/day	Hyperlipidemia
simvastatin (Zocor) (X)	HMG–CoA reductase inhibitor	*Adult* PO: 10–40 mg/day; max 80 mg/day	Hyperlipidemia

PO, oral; *RDA,* recommended daily allowance; *SR,* sustained release.

NURSING PROCESS

 ## Assessment

Before initiating antilipemic therapy in a patient, the nurse should obtain thorough health and medication histories, including any over-the-counter drugs, natural health products, and prescription drugs. Hypersensitivity to any of these drugs is also important to document. The nurse must assess the patient's dietary patterns, exercise program and frequency, weight, height, and vital signs, and documentation over time, such as weeks of data, particularly food intake. Use of tobacco, alcohol, and social drugs, with information about frequency, amount, and duration of use, should be documented. Some of the lipid disorders are hereditary and require a thorough assessment of the family history. Positive risk factors for coronary artery disease (CAD) include some of the following:

- Age (male 45 years or older; female 55 years or older)
- Smoking
- HDL levels of 0.9 mmol/L or less
- Diabetes mellitus
- Family history of premature CAD

Cautions, contraindications, and drug interactions should be assessed prior to the use of any of the antilipemics. Serum lipid values and lipoprotein levels also need to be assessed and include the following normal ranges: (1) lipids—cholesterol levels 3.6 to 5.2 mmol/L; (2) triglycerides 0.45 to 1.69 mmol/L; and (3) lipoproteins—LDL less than 3.4 mmol/L and HDL greater than 1.2 mmol/L (men) and greater than 1.4 mmol/L (female). With use of cholestyramine, which contains aspartame, it is of particular interest to know if there is a history of phenylketonuria (PKU). Patients with PKU cannot properly process the amino acid phenylalanine, a component of protein. High levels of phenylalanine lead to behavioural, cognitive, and learning dysfunction as early as 3 weeks of age. Dietary restrictions must continue throughout the lifespan, with adult patients requiring monthly testing of phenylalanine. Because aspartame is a dipeptide comprising aspartic acid and phenylalanine, its intake would lead to an increase in the source of phenylalanine. Therefore, another class of antilipemics other than cholestyramine would be indicated to prevent further complications from this disorder.

HMG–CoA reductase inhibitors (the statins) must not be used in patients younger than 10 years of age. In those patients who do qualify for taking HMG–CoA reductase inhibitors, the nurse must assess for all contraindications, cautions, and drug interactions (discussed in the pharmacology section of this chapter). The patient's intake of alcohol is important to assess in terms of the amount consumed and over what period because of the potential of liver dysfunction associated with most lipid-lowering drugs. If the liver is already damaged, these drugs adversely affect it further. Assessment of liver enzymes indicative of liver function should also be performed, including aspartate aminotransferase (AST), creatine phosphokinase (CPK), and alanine aminotransferase (ALT). Lipid/lipoprotein levels need to be assessed before, during, and after drug therapy with the statins and with other antilipemic drugs. Myopathies and rhabdomyolysis should also be assessed for during and after drug therapy. Should blood levels of transaminases increase and myopathy or rhabdomyolysis occur, the drug will most likely be discontinued by the physician.

With these drugs as well as others in this class, cultural influences need to be assessed in relation to the individual's belief on how to control diet and cholesterol levels. Cultural practices need to be considered also because of possible herbal and homeopathic therapies.

In patients taking bile acid sequestrants, niacin, and fibric acid derivatives, the nurse needs to assess for these drugs' related contraindications and cautions and to always check for the numerous drug interactions.

Nursing Diagnoses

- Imbalanced nutrition, more than body requirements, related to poor dietary habits of high fat intake
- Deficient knowledge related to a lack of knowledge about the disease and related complications
- Deficient knowledge related to a lack of understanding of drug therapy and need for lifestyle changes
- Impaired home maintenance related to lack of experience with lifestyle changes and unfamiliar medication therapy
- Imbalanced nutrition, less than body requirements, related to vitamin A, D, E, and K deficits from adverse effects of antilipemics

Planning

Goals

- Patient will remain adherent to both nonpharmacological and pharmacological therapy.
- Patient will remain free of the complications associated with antilipemics because of appropriate use of the drug.
- Patient will visit physician regularly and as indicated for the treatment of hyperlipidemia and to repeat laboratory studies until normal values return.
- Patient will maintain homeostasis and nutritional well-being while taking the antilipemic drug.

Outcome Criteria

- Patient states the importance of pharmacological and nonpharmacological therapy to overall health and safety, such as decreasing the risk for CAD.
- Patient states the rationale of therapy as well as its adverse effects and expected therapeutic effects (i.e., decreasing lipid levels, gastrointestinal adverse effects, and therapeutic response of improved lipid profile).
- Patient states those conditions that the physician should be notified of, such as jaundice and abdominal pain.
- Patient states that cholesterol levels should return to less than 5.2 mmol/L within approximately 6 to 8 weeks.
- Patient states the importance of follow-up care with the physician to monitor for changes in liver function studies as well as lipid levels.
- Patient states measures to adequately maintain levels of fat-soluble vitamins.

Implementation

Patients who are taking antilipemics for a long period may have altered levels of fat-soluble vitamins and thus require supplementation of vitamins A, D, and K. Antilipemics may also affect the liver and biliary systems, and they may have gastrointestinal effects such as constipation. Appropriate actions need to be taken to avoid or minimize constipation, such as increasing intake of fibre and fluids. Monitoring of blood levels according to the health care provider's instructions often includes serum transaminase and other liver function studies.

With HMG–CoA reductase inhibitors, serum levels of ALT, AST and CPK are often measured every 6 to 8 weeks for the first 6 months of statin therapy and then usually every 3 to 6 months thereafter. If a lipid profile is ordered, emphasize to the patient that they should fast for 12 to 14 hours and that the following levels are desired: cholesterol less than 5.2 mmol/L; triglycerides less than 1.69 mmol/L; LDL less than 3.4 mmol/L; and HDL more than 1.2 mmol/L (men) and more than 1.4 mmol/L (women). (See also Lab Values Related to Drug Therapy.) Because severe cardiovascular diseases and strokes are associated with cholesterol levels of 6.2 mmol/L, LDLs more than 4.14 mmol/L, and HDLs less than 0.9 mmol/L, it is critical to the maintenance of health and prevention of complications to continue with any prescribed nonpharmacological and pharmacological therapies (regardless of the specific antilipemic used). These drugs should never be discontinued abruptly.

Bile acid sequestrants often come in powder form and should be mixed thoroughly with fruit (e.g., crushed pineapple) or other food or fluids (at least 120 to 180 mL of fluid). Another option is to mix with Metamucil and orange juice or lemonade the night before, refrigerate,

LAB VALUES RELATED TO DRUG THERAPY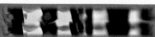

Coronary Heart Disease

Laboratory Test	Normal Ranges	Rationale for Assessment
Lipid panel with serum cholesterol, triglycerides, and lipids	Serum cholesterol levels less than 5.2 mmol/L Triglyceride levels less than 1.69 mmol/L Low-density lipoprotein (LDL) cholesterol level less than 2.6 mmol/L) High-density lipoprotein (HDL) cholesterol level 1.56 mmol/L or greater Very low–density lipoprotein (VLDL) less than 3.4 mmol/L	A lipid panel is a serum test that measures lipids, fats, and fatty substances used as a source of energy in the body. Lipids include cholesterol, triglycerides, HDL, and LDL. When a lipid panel is ordered, the levels include all of the following: total cholesterol, triglycerides, HDL, LDL, VLDL, ratio of total cholesterol to HDL, and ratio of LDL to HDL. Lipid levels are important to health status and are indicators of health; if there are abnormalities (e.g., high cholesterol, triglycerides, HDL, VLDL and LDL levels), the individual is at increased risk for heart disease and stroke. Dietary and other lifestyle changes may be implemented to help decrease the bad cholesterol levels (LDL and VLDL) and elevate the good cholesterol levels (HDL). Medical treatment protocols may also be implemented to help prevent heart attack and stroke.

Based on McPherson, R., Frohlich, J., Fodor, G., & Genest, J. (2006). Canadian Cardiovascular Society position statement—Recommendations for the diagnosis and treatment of dyslipidemia and prevention of cardiovascular disease. *Canadian Journal of Cardiology, 22*(11), 913–927.

and drink the mixture the next day after shaking it well. The powder may not mix completely at first, but patients should be sure to mix the dose as much as possible and then dilute any undissolved portion with additional fluid. The powder should be dissolved for at least 1 full minute without stirring. Stirring is not recommended with most powders because it causes them to clump. Powder and granule dosage forms are *never* to be taken in dry form.

It is important that colestipol be taken 1 hour before or 4 to 6 hours after any other oral medication or meals because of the high risk for drug–drug or drug–food interactions. Cholestyramine should be taken just before or with meals and never given to a patient with PKU because it contains aspartame. To prevent injuries from falls, patients should be encouraged to change positions slowly and to lie down should they get dizzy (from orthostatic hypotension).

With niacin, flushing of the face may occur, so the patient should be made aware of this adverse effect. Postural hypotensive adverse effects require that the patient change positions slowly and with caution and to lie down should further dizziness occur. To avoid gastrointestinal upset, patients should take these medications with fluids or food. With niacin, aspirin and careful drug titration after a doctor's order may help prevent some of the adverse effects, including flushing of the skin and hyperuricemia.

Evaluation

Evaluation of goals and outcome criteria is the best place to begin when trying to evaluate the therapeutic versus adverse effects of these medications. Cholesterol and triglyceride levels are used to monitor the patient's response to the medication regimen; specific levels should be mentioned in the nursing assessment. While on antilipemics and as a part of a change in lifestyle, patients should remain on a low-fat, low-cholesterol diet. Patients receiving an antilipemic drug need to be monitored for therapeutic and adverse effects during therapy. The therapeutic effects of both nonpharmacological and pharmacological measures are evidenced by a decrease in cholesterol and triglyceride levels to within normal levels (see Lab Values Related to Drug Therapy). Another commonly monitored marker, as a risk factor for atherosclerotic heart disease, is highly sensitive C-reactive protein. Any elevation of this protein is associated with greater risk for major ischemic heart disease (e.g., myocardial infarction). Nonpharmacological measures include following a low-fat, low-cholesterol diet; supervised, moderate exercise; weight loss; cessation of smoking and drinking; and relaxation therapy.

If there is no response to pharmacological therapy after about 3 months, the medication is generally withdrawn. Fenofibrate may be increased at 4- to 8-week intervals depending on the triglyceride levels. Adverse effects to monitor for include gastrointestinal upset, increased liver enzyme levels, hepatomegaly, myalgias, and other effects mentioned earlier in the chapter. Patients should be closely monitored for baseline kidney and liver function throughout the treatment regimen as well as for the development of liver or kidney dysfunction.

PATIENT EDUCATION

- Patients should be encouraged to notify their health care providers should there be any new or troublesome symptoms or if there is persistent gastrointestinal upset, constipation, gas, bloating, heartburn, nausea, vomiting, abnormal or unusual bleeding, or yellow discoloration of the skin. Other symptoms to report include muscle pain, decreased sex drive, impotence, and difficulty urinating.
- Patients should be encouraged to keep all medications, including antilipemics, out of the reach of children and protected with childproof lids or tops.
- Patients should be educated about the need for eating plentiful amounts of raw vegetables, fruit, and bran and at least 2000 mL of fluids a day to prevent the constipation that is commonly associated with antilipemics.
- Patients should be encouraged to inform all health care providers about all medications they are taking, including over-the-counter medications, natural health products, and antilipemics. Antilipemics are highly protein-bound, and thus they are associated with many drug interactions, including drugs that a dentist may prescribe. In addition, antilipemics may alter clotting if taken on a long-term basis, so bleeding may occur during dental work.
- Patients should be educated about early signs of a peptic ulcer, including nausea and abdominal discomfort followed by abdominal pain and distention, and that these should be reported immediately to their physician.
- Patients should be taught to engage in moderate daily exercise as ordered by their physician and with supervision at first, especially if they are not used to exercising, and to change positions slowly because of possible dizziness and the risk for falls.
- Patients should be instructed that if a once-a-day dosage scheme is chosen, the medications should be taken with the evening meal.
- Patients should be encouraged to store these medications away from heat and moisture to avoid alteration in the drug and its components.
- With the HMG–CoA reductase inhibitors, or "statin" drugs, patients should be educated about the following measures:
  - Take the medication with at least 6 oz of water or with meals to help minimize gastric upset.
  - It may take several weeks before therapeutic results are seen, and frequent laboratory testing will occur at about every 3 to 6 months.
  - If taking one of the statin drugs, an ophthalmic examination is needed prior to and during therapy because of the problems reported with visual acuity.
  - Other adverse effects may include a decrease in libido. If there are any severe muscle aches or pain, chest pain, or other unexplained pain, patients should contact their physician immediately.
- Patients taking a bile acid sequestrant should make sure that they contact their health care provider immediately if stools appear black and tarry.
- Patients should receive nutritional consultation and assistance with menu planning for a low-fat diet.
- Patients should be encouraged to never abruptly discontinue their medication.

POINTS TO REMEMBER

- There are two primary forms of lipids: triglycerides and cholesterol.
- Triglycerides function as an energy source and are stored in adipose tissue.
- Cholesterol is primarily used to make steroid hormones, cell membranes, and bile acids.
- Lipids and lipoproteins participate in the formation of atherosclerotic plaque, which leads to coronary artery disease, and nurses need to understand the pathology involved in this disease process so that they can provide appropriate patient education.
- Nurses need to understand that when plaque forms in the blood vessels that supply the heart with needed oxygen and nutrients, there will be an eventual decrease in the lumen size of blood vessels and a reduction in the amount of oxygen and nutrients that can reach the heart.
- Antilipemic drugs are used to lower the high levels of lipids within the blood (triglycerides and cholesterol). The major classes of antilipemics are as follows:
  - HMG–CoA reductase inhibitors
  - Bile acid sequestrants
  - Nicotinic acid
  - Fibric acid derivatives
  - Cholesterol absorption inhibitor (Ezetrol)
  - The mechanisms of action vary with each class and each drug.
- Nurses need to thoroughly understand the effects of the HMG–CoA reductase inhibitors and that they lower blood cholesterol levels by decreasing the rate of cholesterol production and inhibit the enzyme necessary for the liver to produce cholesterol. While taking nursing history, it is important for the nurse to assess the patient for any possible drug interactions and for a history of PKU (as related to use of cholestyramine).
- Fat-soluble vitamins may need to be prescribed for patients taking these medications long term because of the effects of antilipemics on the liver's production of fat-soluble vitamins.
- When using the powder or granule oral-based forms of these drugs, they must be mixed with noncarbonated liquids and *never* taken dry.
- Monitoring for adverse effects with the antilipemics includes monitoring liver and kidney function studies.
- The statins have gained much attention for their adverse effects of muscle aches and pain from the breakdown of muscle tissue. Some patients suffer irreversible kidney damage and severe pain with use of statins and may have to alter dosages or drugs as ordered by their health care provider.

EXAMINATION REVIEW QUESTIONS

1 The nurse is administering a bile acid sequestrant drug. Which action should the nurse recommend that the patient use to reduce the adverse effects?
  a. Increase dietary fibre intake.
  b. Take the medication with grapefruit juice.
  c. Take the medication dry without mixing it.
  d. Take a small dose of aspirin or an NSAID 30 minutes before the dose.

2 When administering nicotinic acid, which adverse effect does the nurse need to monitor for?
  a. Headache
  b. Constipation
  c. Low back pain
  d. Cutaneous flushing

3 Which point is important to emphasize to a patient taking an antilipemic drug?
  a. Take it on an empty stomach before meals.
  b. A low-fat diet is not necessary while on these medications.
  c. It is important to report muscle pain as soon as possible.
  d. Improved cholesterol levels should be evident within 2 weeks.

4 When assessing a patient before giving a new order for an antilipemic medication, which condition would be a potential contraindication?
  a. Hyperlipidemia
  b. Diabetes insipidus
  c. Pulmonary fibrosis
  d. Elevated levels in liver studies

5 Which of the following products, if taken concurrently with a statin, would increase a patient's risk of developing rhabdomyolysis?
  a. NSAIDs
  b. Gemfibrozil
  c. Orange juice
  d. Fat-soluble vitamins

For answers see http://evolve.elsevier.com/Canada/Lilley/pharmacology/.

CRITICAL THINKING ACTIVITIES

1 Flushing of the face and neck may occur with the administration of nicotinic acid. What would you suggest to a patient to help decrease these reactions and their unpleasantness?

2 Is the statement that follows true or false? Explain your answer.

Antilipemics may be safely taken without concern for other medications, especially prescribed medications, and may be discontinued abruptly.

3 Your patient has just informed you that he was told that it was okay to take his colestipol powder without fluids. Are you concerned about this? Explain your answer.

For answers see http://evolve.elsevier.com/Canada/Lilley/pharmacology/.

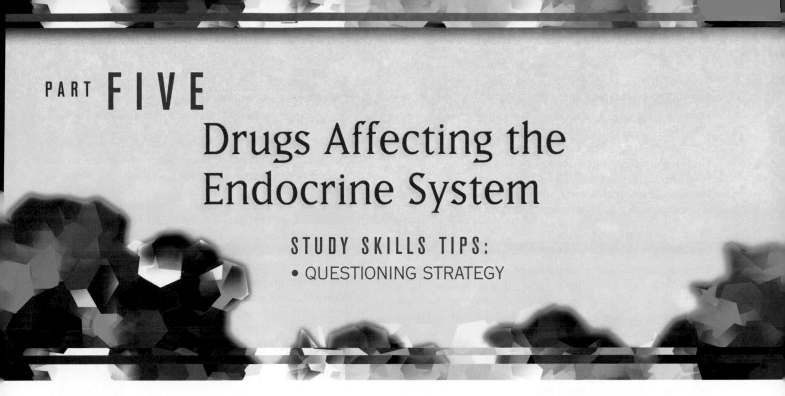

PART FIVE

Drugs Affecting the Endocrine System

STUDY SKILLS TIPS:
- QUESTIONING STRATEGY

QUESTIONING STRATEGY

One of the best ways to learn is to become actively involved with the text. The best way to get involved is to ask questions.

Part Title

As you begin each new part, ask a question to focus your attention. In Part Five, this question is: "What is the endocrine system?" This same question could be asked of Parts Two through Nine by simply replacing "endocrine" with the appropriate system for the specific part. Looking at the chapter titles in the part tells us that the endocrine system has to do with pituitary drugs, thyroid and antithyroid drugs, antidiabetic drugs, adrenal drugs, women's health drugs, and men's health drugs. Although this answer is general, it is a beginning and helps keep you aware of what you need to learn from each chapter.

Chapter Titles

Chapter titles provide the first mechanism to generate questions. The first question to ask is: "What is this chapter about?" That question is also answered immediately. "What is Chapter 30 about?" It is about pituitary agents.

The question to ask next is: "What do pituitary (Chapter 30), thyroid and antithyroid (Chapter 31), antidiabetic and hypoglycemic (Chapter 32), adrenal (Chapter 33), women's health (Chapter 34), and men's health (Chapter 35) refer to?" Take the chapter title and state it as a question. What do you know about these subjects?

Chapter Objectives

To enhance your study, turn each chapter objective into one or more questions. Here are some possible questions using the objectives from Chapter 32.

Objective 1
Discuss the normal actions and functions of the pancreas.
- What are the normal actions and functions of the pancreas?

Objective 2
Compare type 1 and type 2 diabetes mellitus with reference to age of onset, signs and symptoms, pharmacological and nonpharmacological treatment, incidence, and etiology.
- What is type 1 diabetes mellitus?
- What is type 2 diabetes mellitus?
- How do types 1 and 2 diabetes mellitus differ?

Since the objectives tell you what the authors expect you to know at the end of the chapter, starting out with questions based on the objectives will improve your learning and probably save you time.

Chapter Headings

The same principle can be applied to each of the topic headings set out in the chapter. Continuing to use Chapter 32 as a model, here are some samples of questions that might be useful as preparation for reading.

Type 1 Diabetes Mellitus
- What is type 1 diabetes?
- What is mellitus?

As you start to process the chapter headings, you will also notice that they begin to answer some of the questions from the chapter objectives. This is a good time to begin setting up vocabulary cards.

Mechanism of Action and Drug Effects

- What is the mechanism of action of insulin?
- Is there more than one mechanism?
- What are the most important drug effects of insulin?
- Where do these effects take place?
- What is the evidence of these effects?

The idea is to focus on the major content of the chapter and establish a guide for learning as you read.

Print Conventions Within the Body of the Chapter

Print conventions are useful in this study skills strategy. The use of *italics*, **bold**, <u>underlining</u>, and multiple colours of ink are examples of print conventions. They are designed to catch your attention. Use them as a basis for questions.

Chapter 32

In the first paragraph of this chapter, the first obvious print convention is the word **glucose**. It is printed in bold. If you let your eyes float down the page and do not read anything, this word stands out. It must be important.

- What is glucose?
- What is the relationship between glucose and type 1 diabetes mellitus?

There are more words on the first page of the chapter text that are in the same print style. Apply the same procedure to these terms. Also, note that two of the terms, *glycogen* and *glycogenolysis*, must have some direct relationship, since the second term contains the first word. The basic question in each case is, "What does the term mean?" However, there should be more to your questions than just the basics. Glycogenolysis seems to mean that there is some operation or activity taking place. Ask yourself the following:

- What happens in glycogenolysis?
- Where does glycogenolysis occur?
- When does glycogenolysis occur?
- How does it relate to type 1 diabetes mellitus?

Chapter Tables

Tables give a summary of information discussed in the chapter. You can learn a great deal from tables if you take the time.

Look at Table 32-1. The table summarizes characteristics of type 1 and type 2 diabetes. There are two obvious questions for each type.

- What is type 1 (type 2) diabetes?
- What are its characteristics?

Use these questions to study Table 32-1, and you will find that all the information you need in order to respond to these questions is found here. It may be useful to make a first pass throughout the chapter focusing only on the tables before you begin to read. You will learn a great deal about some of the topics, and you will have established background information that will help you ask better questions and read with better understanding.

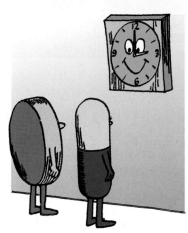

The time you spend asking questions makes the reading and learning go more quickly. Another benefit is that some of the questions you ask will appear on tests. These questions will be easy for you to answer, which will give you test-taking confidence and, in the end, better grades. After you use the strategy for two or three chapters, you will find that the benefits far outweigh the time it takes.

CHAPTER 30

Pituitary Drugs

Learning Objectives

After reading this chapter, the successful student will be able to do the following:

1 Describe the normal function of the anterior and posterior aspects of the pituitary gland and the impact of the pituitary gland on the human body.

2 Compare the indications, mechanisms of action, dosages, routes of administration, adverse effects, cautions, contraindications, and drug interactions of the pituitary drugs.

3 Develop a collaborative plan of care that includes all phases of the nursing process for patients receiving pituitary drugs, such as corticotrophin, desmopressin, octreotide, somatropin, and vasopressin.

e-Learning Activities

Web site
(http://evolve.elsevier.com/Canada/Lilley/pharmacology/)

- Animations
- Answers to chapter questions, activities, and case studies
- Calculators and Category Catchers
- Glossary with audio pronunciations
- IV Therapy and Medication Error Checklists
- Multiple-Choice Review Question quizzes
- Nursing Care Plans
- Online Appendices and Supplements
- WebLinks

Drug Profile

▶▶ **cosyntropin**, p. 573

▶▶ Key drug.

Glossary

Hypothalamus The gland that lies below the thalamus and directly above the pituitary gland. The hypothalamus–pituitary unit is the most dominant portion of the entire endocrine system; secretion of hormones from the anterior pituitary is under strict control by hypothalamic hormones. (p. 570)

Negative feedback loop In endocrinology, when the production of one hormone by its source gland is controlled by the levels of a second hormone, which is produced by a second gland after being stimulated by the hormone from the first gland. (p. 571)

Neuroendocrine system The system that regulates the reactions of the organism to both internal and external stimuli and involves the integrated activities of the endocrine glands and the nervous system. (p. 570)

Pituitary gland An endocrine gland suspended in a pocket of bone beneath the hypothalamus, to which it is connected by a stalk containing nerve fibres and blood vessels. The pituitary gland supplies numerous hormones that control many vital processes. (p. 570)

ENDOCRINE SYSTEM

The maintenance of physiological stability is the primary goal of the endocrine system. It must accomplish this task despite constant changes in the internal and external environments. Every cell and, thus, every organ in the body come under its influence. The endocrine system communicates with the approximately 50 million target cells in the body via hormones. *Hormones* are a large group of natural substances with chemical structures that are highly specific for causing physiological effects in the cells of their target tissues.

They are secreted into the bloodstream in response to the body's needs and travel through the blood to their site of action, the target cell.

For decades the pituitary gland was believed to be the master gland that regulated and controlled the other endocrine glands in this diverse system. However, the discovery of strong evidence that the central nervous system (CNS), specifically, the **hypothalamus** (a gland above and behind the pituitary gland), controls the pituitary has led to the abandonment of this older belief. The hypothalamus and pituitary are now viewed as functioning together as an integrated unit, the most dominant portion of the entire endocrine system, with primary direction coming from the hypothalamus. For this reason, the system is now commonly referred to as the **neuroendocrine system**. In fact, the endocrine system can be considered in much the same way as the CNS, each being a system for signalling and each operating in a stimulus-and-response manner. Together these two systems essentially govern all bodily functions.

The **pituitary gland** is made up of two distinct glands—the *anterior pituitary (adenohypophysis)* and the *posterior pituitary (neurohypophysis).* They are individually linked to and communicate with the hypothalamus, and each gland secretes its own set of hormones. These hormones are listed in Box 30-1 and shown in Figure 30-1.

BOX 30-1

Hormones of the Anterior and Posterior Pituitary

Anterior Pituitary (Adenohypophysis)

Adrenocorticotropic hormone (ACTH)
Follicle-stimulating hormone (FSH)
Growth hormone (GH)
Luteinizing hormone (LH)
Prolactin (PH)
Thyroid-stimulating hormone (TSH)

Posterior Pituitary (Neurohypophysis)

Antidiuretic hormone (ADH)
Oxytocin

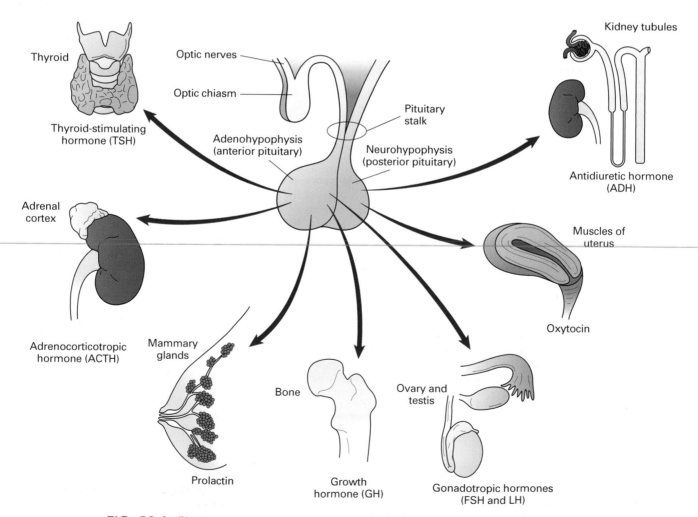

FIG. 30-1 Pituitary hormones. (From McKenry, L. M., Tessier, E., & Hogan, M. A. (2006). *Mosby's pharmacology in nursing.* (22nd ed.). St. Louis, MO: Mosby.)

Hormones are either water or lipid soluble. The water-soluble hormones are protein-based substances such as the catecholamines norepinephrine and epinephrine. The receptors for these hormones are usually located on cell membranes. These hormones bind to their receptors on the cell surface, from where they either directly activate the cell to perform a function or cause a chemical signal to be sent by means of a second messenger to generate an appropriate cellular response. The lipid-soluble hormones consist of the steroid and thyroid hormones. They are capable of crossing the plasma membrane through the process of simple diffusion and of binding with receptors within the cell nucleus, where they stimulate a specific cellular response.

The activity of the endocrine system is regulated by a system of surveillance and signalling that is usually dictated by the body's ongoing needs. Hormone secretion is commonly regulated by the **negative feedback loop**, illustrated as follows: when gland X releases hormone X, this stimulates target cells to release hormone Y. When there is an excess of hormone Y, gland X "senses" this and inhibits its release of hormone X.

PITUITARY DRUGS

There are a variety of drugs that affect the pituitary gland. They are used as replacement therapy to balance a hormone deficiency and as diagnostic aids to determine whether there is hypofunction or hyperfunction of a patient's hormonal functions. The currently identified anterior and posterior pituitary hormones and the drugs that mimic or antagonize their actions are listed in Table 30-1. Many of these hormones have been synthesized commercially; some of them have already been discussed in other chapters.

The anterior pituitary drugs discussed in this chapter include cosyntropin, somatropin, and octreotide; the posterior pituitary drugs discussed here are vasopressin and desmopressin.

Mechanism of Action and Drug Effects

The mechanisms of action of the pituitary drugs differ according to the drug, but overall, they either augment or antagonize the natural effects of the pituitary hormones. Exogenously administered cosyntropin (synthetic corticotropin) elicits all of the same pharmacological responses as those elicited by the endogenous *adrenocorticotropic hormone* (ACTH). Regardless of whether it is exogenous or endogenous in origin, cosyntropin travels to the adrenal cortex located just above the kidneys and stimulates the secretion of the mineralocorticoid cortisol (the drug form is hydrocortisone sodium succinate [Solu-Cortef]). Cortisol has many anti-inflammatory effects,

TABLE 30-1

Anterior and Posterior Pituitary Hormones and Drugs

Hormone	Function and Mimicking Drug
ANTERIOR PITUITARY	
Adrenocorticotropic hormone (ACTH)	Targets adrenal gland; mediates adaptation to physical and emotional stress and starvation; redistributes body nutrients; promotes synthesis of adrenocortical hormone (glucocorticoids, mineralocorticoids, androgens); involved in skin pigmentation
	Cosyntropin (synthetic corticotropin): Diagnosis of adrenocortical insufficiency
Follicle-stimulating hormone (FSH)	Stimulates oogenesis and follicular growth in females and spermatogenesis in males
	Menotropins: Same pharmacological effects as FSH; many of the other gonadotropins also stimulate FSH (Chapter 34).
Growth hormone (GH)	Regulates anabolic processes related to growth and adaptation to stressors; promotes skeletal and muscle growth; increases protein synthesis; increases liver glycogenolysis; increases fat mobilization
	Somatropin, somatrem: Human GH for hypopituitary dwarfism
	Octreotide: A synthetic polypeptide structurally and pharmacologically similar to GH release–inhibiting factor; it inhibits GH
Luteinizing hormone (LH)	Stimulates ovulation and estrogen release by ovaries in females; stimulates interstitial cells in males to promote spermatogenesis and testosterone secretion
	Gonadotropins: Many of the drugs discussed in Chapter 34 stimulate LH
Prolactin (PH)	Targets mammary glands; stimulates lactogenesis and breast growth
	Bromocriptine: Inhibits action of PH and therefore inhibits lactogenesis (Chapter 34)
Thyroid-stimulating hormone (TSH)	Stimulates secretion of thyroid hormones T_3 and T_4 by the thyroid
	Thyrotropin: Increases the production and secretion of thyroid hormones (Chapter 31)
POSTERIOR PITUITARY	
Antidiuretic hormone (ADH)	Increases water reabsorption in distal tubules and collecting duct of nephron; concentrates urine; causes potent vasoconstriction
	Vasopressin: ADH; performs all the physiological functions of ADH
	Desmopressin: A synthetic vasopressin
Oxytocin	Targets mammary glands; stimulates ejection of milk and contraction of uterine smooth muscle
	Pitocin: Has all the physiological actions of oxytocin (see Chapter 34)

T_3 triiodothyronine; T_4 thyroxine.

including reduction of inflammatory leukocyte functions, edema, and scar tissue formation. Cortisol also promotes kidney retention of sodium, which can result in edema and hypertension.

The drug that mimics growth hormone (GH) is somatropin. This drug promotes growth by stimulating anabolic (tissue-building) processes, including nitrogen retention and increased cellular protein synthesis; liver glycogenolysis (to raise blood sugar levels); lipid mobilization from body fat stores; and retention of sodium, potassium, and phosphorus. Somatropin promotes linear growth in children who lack normal amounts of the endogenous hormone.

A drug that antagonizes the effects of the natural GH, by inhibiting GH release, is octreotide. It is a synthetic polypeptide that is structurally and pharmacologically similar to GH release–inhibiting factor, also called somatostatin. It also reduces plasma concentrations of vasoactive intestinal polypeptide (VIP), a protein secreted by a type of tumour known as VIPoma that causes profuse watery diarrhea.

The drugs that affect the posterior pituitary, such as vasopressin and desmopressin, mimic the actions of the naturally occurring antidiuretic hormone (ADH). They increase water reabsorption in the distal tubules and collecting ducts of the nephrons, resulting in concentrated urine and, thus, reduced water excretion by up to 90%. Vasopression is also a potent vasoconstrictor (hence, its name) in larger doses and is thus used in certain hypotensive emergencies. Desmopressin causes a dose-dependent increase in the plasma levels of factor VIII (antihemophilic factor), von Willebrand's factor (acts closely with factor VIII), and tissue plasminogen activator. These properties make it useful in treating certain blood disorders. The drug form of oxytocin mimics the endogenous hormone, promoting uterine contractions (Chapter 34).

Indications

Cosyntropin is used in the diagnosis, but not usually the treatment, of adrenocortical insufficiency. Upon diagnosis, the actual drug therapy for adrenocortical insufficiency generally involves replacement hormonal therapy using drug forms of the deficient corticosteroid hormones. These drugs are discussed in more detail in Chapter 33. Cosyntropin is also used for the treatment of multiple sclerosis and corticotropin insufficiency caused by long-term corticosteroid use (e.g., prednisone therapy in asthma patients). Its anti-inflammatory and immunosuppressant properties may be useful in patients with normal adrenocortical function.

Somatropin is a recombinantly made human GH. It is effective in stimulating skeletal growth in patients with an inadequate secretion of normal endogenous GH, such as those with hypopituitary dwarfism.

Octreotide is of benefit in alleviating certain symptoms of carcinoid tumours stemming from the secretion of VIP, including severe diarrhea and flushing, and potentially life-threatening hypotension associated with a carcinoid crisis.

Vasopressin and desmopressin are also occasionally used after cranial surgery that may involve the pituitary gland. Because of their vasoconstrictor properties, they are useful in the treatment of various types of bleeding, particularly gastrointestinal hemorrhage. Because of its effects on blood-clotting factors, desmopressin is useful in the treatment of hemophilia A and type I von Willebrand's disease.

Contraindications

Contraindications for the use of pituitary drugs vary with each individual drug and are listed in each of the drug profiles included in this chapter. Because even small amounts of these drugs can initiate major physiological changes, they should all be used with extreme caution in patients with acute or chronic illnesses such as migraine headaches, epilepsy, and asthma.

Adverse Effects

Most of the adverse effects of the pituitary drugs are specific to the individual drug. Drugs possessing similar hormonal effects generally have similar adverse effects. The most common adverse effects of the pituitary drugs described here are listed in Tables 30-2 to 30-4.

Interactions

Selected interactions involving pituitary drugs are summarized in Table 30-5.

Dosages

For the recommended dosages of these select pituitary drugs, see the Dosages table on p. 574.

TABLE 30-2	
Cosyntropin–Zinc Hydroxide (Synacthen Depot): Common Adverse Effects	
Body System	**Adverse Effects**
Central nervous	Convulsions, dizziness, euphoria, insomnia, headache, depression, psychosis
Gastrointestinal	Nausea, vomiting, peptic ulcer perforation, pancreatitis, abdominal distension, ulcerative esophagitis
Genitourinary	Water and sodium retention, hypokalemia, alkalosis, calcium loss
Musculoskeletal	Hypocalcemia with possible pathological bone fractures
Ocular	Cataracts
Other	Sweating, acne, hyperpigmentation, weakness, muscle atrophy, myalgia, arthralgia

TABLE 30-3

Desmopressin and Vasopressin: Common Adverse Effects

Body System	Adverse Effects
Cardiovascular	Increased blood pressure
Central nervous	Drowsiness, headache, lethargy, flushing
Gastrointestinal	Nausea, heartburn, cramps
Genitourinary	Uterine cramping
Other	Nasal irritation and congestion, tremor, sweating, vertigo

TABLE 30-4

Growth Hormone Analogues: Common Adverse Effects

Body System	Adverse Effects
Central nervous	Headache
Endocrine	Hyperglycemia, ketosis, hypothyroidism
Genitourinary	Hypercalciuria
Other	Rash, urticaria, antibodies to GH, inflammation at injection site

GH, growth hormone.

TABLE 30-5

Selected Drug Interactions Involving Pituitary Drugs

Pituitary Drug	Interacting Drug	Potential Result
desmopressin	carbamazepine, chlorpropamide, clofibrate	Enhanced desmopressin effects
	lithium, alcohol, demeclocycline, heparin	Reduced desmopressin effects
octreotide	cyclosporine	Case report of transplant rejection
	vitamin B_{12}	Reduced vitamin B_{12} levels (monitor B_{12} levels with chronic therapy)
somatropin	Glucocorticoids	Reduction of growth effects
vasopressin	carbamazepine, fludrocortisone, tricyclic antidepressants	Enhanced antidiuretic effect
	norepinephrine, lithium, heparin, alcohol	Reduced antidiuretic effect

 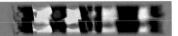
DRUG PROFILES

▸▸ *cosyntropin*

Cosyntropin (Cortrosyn, Synacthen Depot) is intended for short-term use only. It is available in two parenteral forms: a regular form (Cortrosyn) that may be given by intravenous (IV), intramuscular (IM), or subcutaneous (SC) injection; and a repository (depot) form (Synacthen, cosytropin with a zinc hydroxide complex) that is administered intramuscularly and has a more prolonged effect. The longer-acting depot form is contraindicated in those with Cushing's syndrome, osteoporosis, heart failure, peptic ulcer disease, hypertension or primary adrenocortical insufficiency or hyperfunction, untreated infections, acute psychosis, and those who have undergone recent surgery.

Both Cortrosyn and Synacthen Depot may be used as diagnostic agents in screening patients who may have adrenocortical insufficiency; however, Cortrosyn has a rapid effect; a 30-minute test of adrenal function can be preformed as an outpatient procedure. Synacthen Depot has been used in collagen diseases, panhypopituitarism, acquired hemolytic jaundice, and other disorders. Common dosages are listed in the Dosages table on p. 574.

PHARMACOKINETICS

Half-Life	Onset	Peak	Duration
Unknown	Rapid	1 hr	3 days*

*For repository form.

DOSAGES Selected Pituitary Drugs

Drug (Pregnancy Category)	Pharmacological Class	Usual Dosage Range	Indications
▸▸cosyntropin (Cortrosyn, Synacthen Depot) (C)	Adrenal cortex–stimulating hormone	*Children** 3–6 yr: 0.25–0.5 mg every 2–8 days 6–15 yr: IM depot: 0.25–1 mg every 2–8 days *Adult* IV: 250 mcg in 500 mL of D5W over 6 hr IM: 250 mcg IM depot: 0.5–1 mg q48–72h	Diagnosis of adrenocortical insufficiency Exacerbation of multiple sclerosis, others
desmopressin (DDAVP melt, Minirin, Octostim) (C)	ADH, antihemophilic hormone	*Children 6 yr and over/Adult* Intranasal spray: 150–300 mcg PO: 0.1 mg at bedtime, titrated upward as needed to max 0.4 mg/day based on diurnal response *Children 3 mo–12 yr* Intranasal spray: 5–30 mcg divided daily, bid–tid *Adult* Intranasal spray: 10–40 mcg divided daily–tid IV/SC: 0.3 mcg/kg; max IV 20 mcg *Children/Adult* IV infusion: 0.3 mcg/kg, diluted in 50 mL of NS (use 10 mL of saline diluent in patients weighing less than 10 kg)	Primary nocturnal enuresis Central diabetes insipidus Hemophilia A and type 1 von Willebrand's disease
octreotide acetate (Sandostatin, Sandostatin LAR) (c)	Somatostatin (GH inhibitor) analogue	*Adult†* IV/SC: Initial dose of 100–300 mcg bid–tid; may titrate up to 1500 mcg tid Depot IM: 20–30 mg q4 wk IV/SC: 100–600 mcg/day divided bid–qid Depot IM: 200–300 mcg q4 wk	Acromegaly Metastatic carcinoid tumours (to control flushing and diarrhea symptoms) VIPomas
somatropin (Humatrope, Nutropin, Saizen, Serostim) (C)	GH analogue	*Children/Adult* Dosages are individualized and vary widely among the many available products; a typical dosage regimen is 0.18–0.24 mg/kg/wk daily SC injections; consult product insert. Serostim: SC once daily at bedtime; dosage calculated by weight	Growth failure; AIDS-related wasting syndrome (Serostim only)
vasopressin (Pressyn, Pressyn AR) (C)	Natural or synthetic ADH	*Children/Adult* IM/SC 0.25–0.5 mL q3–4 hr Intranasal: individually determined	Diabetes insipidus; prevention or treatment of postoperative abdominal distension; dispersal of abdominal gas to improve imaging in abdominal X-ray studies

ADH, antidiuretic hormone; *D5W,* 5% dextrose in water; *GH,* growth hormone; *NS,* normal saline.

*Children's dosage must be carefully individualized and should be monitored by a pediatric endocrinologist.

†Normally used only in adults.

NURSING PROCESS

☑ Assessment

Before administering any of the pituitary drugs, the nurse should perform a thorough nursing assessment, obtain a complete medication history, and document findings. Questions about hypersensitivity should be posed to the patient and documented. Baseline weight, blood pressure, serum glucose levels, cholesterol, and electrolytes should be assessed and documented.

Contraindications, cautions, and drug interactions for the use of pituitary drugs vary with each individual drug and are listed in Box 30-2. Small doses of these drugs may initiate major physiological changes, so they should be used with special caution in patients with acute or chronic illnesses such as migraine headache, epilepsy, asthma, and other chronic disease processes. Other growth hormones should be avoided when using other drugs that antagonize their effects.

BOX 30-2   Pituitary Drugs: Assessment Data

Assessment Parameters	Cautions and Drug Interactions	Contraindications
COSYNTROPIN	*Cautions:*	
Allergy to pork because of cross-sensitivity	Clotting disorders	Adrenocortical hypo- and hyperfunction (primary)
Baseline vital signs	Gout	Allergy
Blood glucose levels	History of tuberculosis (possible re-emergence of the disease)	Fungal infections
CBC, intake and output, weight	Hypothyroidism	Heart failure
Chest X-ray study	Kidney dysfunction	No long-term therapy in children
Cortisol levels	Lactation	Osteoporosis
Electrolyte values	Latent tuberculosis	Recent surgery
	Liver disease	Scleroderma
	Mental health disorders	Ulcer disease
	Myasthenia gravis	
	Pregnancy	
	Seizures	
	Drug Interactions:	
	Alcohol	
	amphotericin B (increases hypokalemia)	
	aspirin	
	Digoxin (increased risk for toxicity)	
	Diuretics	
	Hypocalcemia	
	Insulin	
	Live virus vaccines (may lead to viral replication)	
	Liver enzyme inducers (may decrease drug's effect)	
	Oral hypoglycemics	
	Potassium supplements	
	Steroids	
DESMOPRESSIN	*Cautions:*	
CBC: leukocytes	Asthma	Allergy to drug or to TCAs
ECG	Children under 12 yr	BPH
Heart enzymes	Chronic migraines	Children under 12 yr
Vital signs with BP lying and standing q4h	Depression or suicidal tendencies	Glaucoma
Weight every wk	Increased intraocular pressure	MI (recovery phase)
	Narrow-angle glaucoma	Seizure disorder
	Seizure disorder	
	Drug Interactions:	
	Alcohol	
	carbamazepine	
	chlorpropamide	
	clofibrate (result in additive effects of the desmopressin)	
	Heparin (may result in decreased therapeutic effects of the desmopressin)	
	lithium	
OCTREOTIDE	*Cautions:*	
	Chronic kidney failure	Allergy
	Insulin, oral hypoglycemics, glucagons, and growth hormone (alters blood glucose)	
	Insulin-dependent diabetes	

Continued

BOX 30-2 — Pituitary Drugs: Assessment Data (cont'd)

Assessment Parameters	Cautions and Drug Interactions	Contraindications
SOMATROPIN AND SOMATREM GH antibodies Thyroid function studies	*Cautions:* Cancer Diabetes mellitus Hypothyroidism Pregnancy *Drug interactions:* Corticosteroids (impaired growth) Glucocorticoids Thyroid hormones	Closed epiphyseal plates Drug allergy Intracerebral lesions

VASOPRESSIN
Edema
Intake and output
Pulse and vital signs, especially
  with IM/IV dosage forms
Weight
	Cautions:
	Asthma
	Coronary artery disease
	Kidney and heart diseases
	Migraines
	Nephritis
	Pregnancy
	Seizures
	Vascular disease
	
	Drug interactions:
	Alcohol
	carbamazepine
	chlorpropamide
	clofibrate
	Drugs for water loss (e.g., furosemide, mannitol,
	  ethacrynic acid)
	epinephrine
	fludrocortisone
	Ganglionic blocking drugs (e.g., mecamylamine)
	Heparin
	lithium
	norepinephrine
	TCAs (e.g., amitriptyline, nortriptyline)
	Urea
		Allergy
		Chronic kidney disease

BP, blood pressure; *BPH*, benign prostatic hypertrophy; *CBC*, complete blood count; *ECG*, electrocardiogram; *GH*, growth hormone; *IM*, intramuscular; *IV*, intravenous; *MI*, myocardial infarction; *TCA*, tricyclic antidepressant.

Nursing Diagnoses

- Disturbed body image related to specific disease processes or drug adverse effects and their influence on physical characteristics
- Excess fluid volume related to adverse effects of pituitary drugs
- Fatigue related to adverse effects of the pituitary drugs
- Acute pain related to gastrointestinal adverse effects of the pituitary drugs
- Deficient knowledge related to new treatment with pituitary drugs

Planning

Goals

- Patient will maintain positive body image.
- Patient will maintain normal fluid volume and electrolyte status while on pituitary drugs.
- Patient will return to normal or pretherapy levels of activity.
- Patient will experience little to no pain related to drug-induced gastrointestinal upset or epigastric distress.
- Patient will remain adherent to medication therapy.
- Patient with be free of injury related to adverse effects of medications.

Outcome Criteria

- Patient openly expresses fears, anxieties, and concerns to health care professionals about body image changes related to disease process and drug therapy.
- Patient's sodium level is within normal limits while on drug therapy.
- Patient states ways to decrease edema caused by drug, such as dietary precautions.
- Patient experiences only minimal gastrointestinal upset and gastric distress by taking drug with food or at mealtimes.
- Patient states measures to employ to diminish the risk for falls related to the musculoskeletal and neurological (seizures) adverse effects of drug.
- Patient performs activities of daily living and other normal activities without difficulty.
- Patient states the importance of follow-up visits to the physician for monitoring of adherence, therapeutic effects, and adverse reactions.

Implementation

Cosyntropin is available in intramuscular, subcutaneous, and intravenous forms and in a repository form. Intramuscular injections should be administered using a 21-gauge needle. Intravenous injections should be given over 2 minutes, or as designated in the packaging insert, and should be diluted with the recommended amounts of normal saline solution. This drug should never be stopped or doses changed without a physician's order. Patients on long-term therapy will need to be weaned off the drug with medical supervision. Dentists and other physicians involved in the patient's care should be aware of cosyntropin therapy up to the previous 12 months. Patients receiving cosyntropin should avoid vaccinations during drug therapy.

Patients who are receiving synthetic corticotropin and corticotropin-like drugs should be encouraged to maintain adequate hydration of up to 2000 mL per day, unless this is contraindicated. Fluids should be low in sodium content, especially if the patient has heart disorders. In addition, doses should not be changed or stopped without a physician's order. It is also very important for the patient to be aware of adverse effects that need to be reported to their physician. These include muscle twitching (positive Trousseau's sign or Chvostek's signs) from possible hypocalcemia, muscle weakness, numbness, tingling and cramping (from hypokalemia), nausea, vomiting, ECG changes, and irritability. Emotional status, mood, and ability to sleep may be affected by cosnytropin; these adverse effects or problems need to be monitored and documented throughout the treatment regimen.

Desmopressin should be administered according to physician's orders because it may vary for each indication (i.e., diabetes insipidus versus other forms of pituitary dysfunction). Injection sites for somatropin should be rotated; injections are usually given subcutaneously (somatrem may be given intramuscularly as well).

Vasopressin is administered intravenously, into the ventral gluteal muscle, or in the subcutaneous tissue but only as prescribed by the physician. To minimize adverse effects, drink one or two glasses of water when receiving this medication or as directed by a doctor. Always check the clarity of the parenteral solutions before using the medication. If there are visible particles or any fluid discoloration, the solution should not be used. Be alert to the adverse effects of nausea, diarrhea, pallor, abdominal pain, and flatus (gas). If these worsen or persist, the physician or health care provider should be notified immediately. Severe headache, sweating, chest pain, tremors, heart irregularities, unexplained weight gain, blood in the stool, black tarry stools, or seizure activity should be reported to the physician.

Evaluation

Once goals and outcome criteria have been evaluated, therapeutic responses to these drugs should be evaluated. For cosyntropin, there should be less inflammation and improved symptoms as related to the indication. For desmopressin and vasopressin, severe thirst should be reduced and urinary output improved. With somatropin, increased growth should occur in patients in whom this is indicated.

For cosyntropin and somatropin, expected adverse effects include dependent edema, moon face, pulmonary edema, infection, and mental health status changes such as increased aggressive behaviour and irritability. Somatropin may increase serum calcium levels. Desmopressin and vasopressin may cause adverse effects similar to those of cosyntropin and somatropin but with additional adverse effects of hypertension, nausea, gastrointestinal upset, tremors, respiratory distress, and drowsiness. Allergic reactions to these drugs may include rash, urticaria, fever, and dyspnea. If these problems occur, the drug should be discontinued and the physician notified.

PATIENT EDUCATION

❖ Patients should be encouraged to avoid alcohol while taking these medications.

❖ Patients should be encouraged to avoid abrupt discontinuation of these drugs because of the negative impact on pituitary hormones and the impact on blood levels of the hormones.

❖ Patients should be counselled that the drug does not lead to a cure but does help alleviate the symptoms of the disease.

❖ Patients and anyone else involved in their care should be properly educated on the routes and techniques of drug administration. With children, demonstration of the technique of administration should be done with the family or caregiver before discharge and re-evaluated with repeat demonstrations. Written instructions should always be used with patients of any age.

❖ Patients should be encouraged to keep a journal about the drug therapy and how the drugs are being tolerated.

❖ As with any medication or illness, patients should be encouraged to keep a medical alert bracelet, necklace, or card (in the wallet) on the individual at all times.

❖ Patients should be encouraged to notify their physician if they experience fever, sore throat, joint pain, or muscular pain.

POINTS TO REMEMBER

❖ The pituitary gland is composed of two distinct glands: anterior and posterior. Each distinct gland has its own set of hormones: *anterior:* thyroid-stimulating hormone (TSH), growth hormone (GH), adrenocorticotropic hormone (ACTH), prolactin (PH), follicle-stimulating hormone (FSH), luteinizing hormone (LH); *posterior:* antidiuretic hormone (ADH), oxytocin.

❖ Pituitary drugs are used to either mimic or antagonize the action of endogenous pituitary hormones.

❖ Drugs that mimic the action of endogenous pituitary hormones include cosyntropin, somatropin, vasopressin, and desmopressin.

❖ Drugs that antagonize the actions of endogenous pituitary hormones include octreotide, which suppresses or inhibits certain symptoms related to carcinoid tumours.

❖ Nursing assessment for patients receiving cosyntropin should include baseline vital signs, electrolyte values (sodium, potassium, chloride), blood glucose levels, chest X-ray studies, weight, and cortisol levels. Patients taking desmopressin should be assessed with documentation of vital signs, including both supine and standing blood pressures and pulse rates. Other assessment data should include complete blood count heart and liver enzyme activity, electrocardiogram, and weight.

❖ Patients receiving somatropin should have thyroid function and growth hormone levels assessed and documented. Assessment should include vital signs, intake and output amounts, weight, and presence and status of edema.

EXAMINATION REVIEW QUESTIONS

1 During a teaching session for a patient who will be taking cosyntropin, which statement should the nurse include?
 a. "Restrict fluids to avoid fluid volume excess."
 b. "Vaccinations should be avoided while on this medication."
 c. "Stop taking the medication if you experience adverse effects."
 d. "Be sure to increase your sodium and potassium intake while on this drug."

2 During an assessment of a patient who has been taking cosyntropin for 4 weeks, which assessment finding should the nurse recognize as being a possible indication of hypocalcemia?
 a. Joint pain
 b. Muscle twitching
 c. Decreased reflexes
 d. Visual disturbances

3 The nurse is reviewing the medication list for a patient who will be starting therapy with somatropin. Which drug has effects that need to be addressed before the patient starts this new drug?

 a. Penicillin
 b. Thyroid hormones
 c. Antidepressant therapy
 d. NSAID therapy for arthritis

4 A patient who is about to be given cosyntropin is also taking a diuretic, intravenous heparin, penicillin, and an opioid as needed for pain. What possible interaction should the nurse should observe for?
 a. Decreased effectiveness of the penicillin
 b. Increased sedation if the opioid is given
 c. Hypokalemia because of interaction with the diuretic
 d. Decreased anticoagulation because of interaction with the heparin

5 When monitoring the therapeutic effects of intranasal desmopressin in a patient who has diabetes insipidus, which assessment would the nurse look for as an indication that the medication therapy is successful?
 a. Decreased thirst
 b. Decreased diarrhea
 c. Improved nasal patency
 d. Increased insulin levels

For answers see http://evolve.elsevier.com/Canada/Lilley/pharmacology/.

CRITICAL THINKING ACTIVITIES

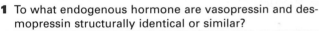

1 To what endogenous hormone are vasopressin and desmopressin structurally identical or similar?

2 Discuss the purpose of octreotide therapy for a patient who has a cancerous tumour.

3 Your patient is excited that he is beginning therapy with pituitary drugs and is positive about a cure. What would be your most appropriate response, and why?

For answers see http://evolve.elsevier.com/Canada/Lilley/pharmacology/.

Thyroid and Antithyroid Drugs

Learning Objectives

After reading this chapter, the successful student will be able to do the following:

1 Briefly describe the normal anatomy and physiology of the thyroid gland.

2 Discuss the functions of the thyroid gland and related hormones.

3 Describe the differences in the diseases resulting from hyposecretion and hypersecretion of the thyroid gland.

4 Identify the drugs used to treat hyposecretion and hypersecretion disorders of the thyroid gland.

5 Discuss the mechanisms of action, indications, dosages, routes of administration, contraindications, cautions, drug interactions, and adverse effects of the drugs used to treat hypothyroidism and hyperthyroidism.

6 Develop a collaborative plan of care that includes all phases of the nursing process for patients receiving thyroid replacement and for patients receiving antithyroid drugs.

e-Learning Activities

Web site
(http://evolve.elsevier.com/Canada/Lilley/pharmacology/)

- Animations
- Answers to chapter questions, activities, and case studies
- Calculators and Category Catchers
- Glossary with audio pronunciations
- IV Therapy and Medication Error Checklists
- Multiple-Choice Review Question quizzes
- Nursing Care Plans
- Online Appendices and Supplements
- WebLinks

Drug Profiles

▸▸ **levothyroxine (levothyroxine sodium)***, p. 583
▸▸ **propylthiouracil**, p. 585

▸▸ Key drug.

*Full generic name is given in parentheses. For the purposes of this text, the more common shortened name is used.

Glossary

Hyperthyroidism A condition characterized by excessive production of the thyroid hormones. Also called *thyrotoxicosis*. (p. 582)

Hypothyroidism A condition characterized by diminished production of the thyroid hormones. (p. 581)

Thyroid-stimulating hormone (TSH) An endogenous substance (also called *thyrotropin*) secreted by the pituitary gland that controls the release of thyroid gland hormones and is necessary for the growth and function of the thyroid gland. (p. 581)

Thyroxine (T$_4$) The principle thyroid hormone that influences the metabolic rate. (p. 580)

Triiodothyronine (T$_3$) A secondary thyroid hormone that also affects body metabolism. (p. 580)

THYROID FUNCTION

The thyroid gland lies across the larynx in front of the thyroid cartilage commonly known as the "Adam's apple." Its lobes extend laterally on both sides of the front of the neck. The thyroid gland is responsible for the secretion of three hormones essential for the proper regulation of metabolism: **thyroxine (T$_4$)**, **triiodothyronine (T$_3$)**, and calcitonin (Chapter 34). It is also close to and communicates with the parathyroid gland, which lies just above and behind it. The parathyroid gland consists of two pairs of bean-shaped glands. These glands are made up of encapsulated cells, which are responsible for maintaining adequate levels of calcium in the extracellular fluid, primarily by mobilizing calcium from bone.

T_4 and T_3 are produced in the thyroid gland through the iodination and coupling of the amino acid tyrosine. The iodide (I–, the ionized form of iodine) required for this process is acquired from the diet, and approximately 1 mg of iodide is needed per week. This iodide is sequestered by the thyroid gland, where it is absorbed from the blood and concentrated to 20 times its blood level. In the blood it is also converted to iodine (I_2), which is combined with tyrosine to make diiodotyrosine. The combination of two molecules of diiodotyrosine results in the formation of thyroxine, which has four iodine molecules in its structure (T_4). Triiodothyronine is formed by the coupling of one molecule of diiodotyrosine with one molecule of monoiodotyrosine, making three iodine molecules in its structure (T_3). The biological potency of T_3 is almost four times greater than that of T_4, but T_4 is present in much greater quantities. After the synthesis of these two thyroid hormones, they are stored in a complex with thyroglobulin (a protein that contains tyrosine and an amino acid) in the follicles in the thyroid gland called the *colloid*. When the thyroid gland is signalled to do so, the thyroglobulin–thyroid hormone complex is then enzymatically broken down to release T_3 and T_4 into the circulation. This entire process is triggered by **thyroid-stimulating hormone (TSH)**, also called *thyrotropin*. Its release from the anterior pituitary is stimulated when the blood levels of T_3 and T_4 are low.

The thyroid hormones are involved in a wide variety of bodily processes. They regulate lipid and carbohydrate metabolism; are essential for normal growth and development; control the heat-regulating system (thermoregulatory centre); and have several effects on the cardiovascular, endocrine, and neuromuscular systems. Therefore, hyperfunction or hypofunction of the thyroid gland can lead to a wide range of serious consequences.

HYPOTHYROIDISM

There are three types of **hypothyroidism,** or reduced production of the thyroid hormones. *Primary hypothyroidism* stems from an abnormality in the thyroid gland and occurs when the thyroid gland is not able to perform one of its many functions, such as releasing the thyroid hormones from their storage sites, coupling iodine with tyrosine, trapping iodide, or converting iodide to iodine, or any combination of these functions. It is the most common of the three forms of hypothyroidism. *Secondary hypothyroidism* begins at the level of the pituitary gland and results from reduced secretion of the TSH needed to trigger the release of the T_3 and T_4 stored in the thyroid gland. *Tertiary hypothyroidism* is caused by a reduced level of the thyrotropin-releasing hormone (TRH) from the hypothalamus. This, in turn, reduces TSH and thyroid

hormone levels. Knowledge of the underlying cause of hypothyroidism allows one to treat the cause and thus eliminate the deficiency.

Hypothyroidism can also be classified by when it occurs in life. Hyposecretion of thyroid hormone during youth may lead to *cretinism,* a condition characterized by low metabolic rate, retarded growth and sexual development, and possibly intellectual disabilities. Hyposecretion of thyroid hormone in adults may lead to *myxedema,* a condition characterized by decreased metabolic rate. It also involves loss of mental and physical stamina, gain in weight, loss of hair, firm edema, and yellowish dullness of the skin.

Some forms of hypothyroidism may result in the formation of a goitre, an enlargement of the thyroid gland resulting from its overstimulation by elevated levels of TSH. The TSH level is elevated because there is little or no thyroid hormone in the circulation.

THYROID-AUGMENTATION DRUGS

All three types of hypothyroidism are amenable to thyroid hormone replacement using thyroid preparations. These drugs can be either natural or synthetic in origin. The natural thyroid preparations are derived from the thyroids of animals such as cattle and hogs. There is currently only one such preparation available in Canada, which is called, simply, thyroid, or desiccated thyroid. *Desiccation* is the term for the drying process used to prepare this drug form, which basically consists of pulverized animal thyroid gland. All of the natural preparations are standardized according to their iodine content.

The synthetic thyroid preparations are levothyroxine (T_4), liothyronine (T_3), and liotrix, the latter drug containing a combination of T_4 and T_3 in a 4:1 ratio. The approximate clinically equivalent doses of the drugs are given in Table 31-1. This information is useful for guiding dosage adjustments when switching a patient from one thyroid hormone to another.

Mechanism of Action and Drug Effects

Thyroid drugs function in the same manner as endogenous thyroid hormones, affecting many body systems. At the cellular level they act to induce changes in the metabolic rate, including protein, carbohydrate, and lipid metabolism, and increase oxygen consumption, body temperature, blood volume, and overall cellular

TABLE 31-1

Thyroid Drugs: Clinically Equivalent Doses

Thyroid Drug	Approximate Equivalent Dose
NATURAL THYROID PREPARATION	
Desiccated thyroid	60–65 mg
SYNTHETIC THYROID PREPARATIONS	
levothyroxine	Equal to or greater than 100 mcg
liothyronine	25 mcg

growth and differentiation. Thyroid drugs also stimulate the cardiovascular system by increasing the number of myocardial β-adrenergic receptors. This increase in receptors, in turn, increases the sensitivity of the heart to catecholamines and ultimately increases cardiac output. Additionally, thyroid hormones increase kidney blood flow and the glomerular filtration rate, which results in a diuretic effect.

Indications

The thyroid preparations are given to replace what the thyroid gland cannot produce to achieve normal thyroid levels (euthyroid). The thyroid preparations are used in the treatment of all three forms of hypothyroidism, although levothyroxine is generally the preferred drug because its hormonal content is standardized and its effect is, therefore, predictable. Thyroid drugs can also be used for the diagnosis of suspected hyperthyroidism (as a TSH-suppression test) and in the prevention or treatment of various types of goitres. They are also used for replacement hormonal therapy in patients whose thyroid glands have been surgically removed or destroyed by radioactive iodine in the treatment of thyroid cancer or hyperthyroidism.

Hypothyroidism should also be treated during pregnancy, with the dose of prescribed thyroid hormones adjusted every 4 weeks to maintain the TSH at the lower end of the normal range. Fetal growth may be retarded if maternal hypothroidism is untreated during pregnancy.

Contraindications

Contraindications to thyroid preparations include known drug allergy to a given drug product, recent myocardial infarction (MI), adrenal insufficiency, or hyperthyroidism.

Adverse Effects

The adverse effects of thyroid medications are usually the result of overdose. The most significant adverse effect is cardiac dysrhythmia with the risk for life-threatening or fatal irregularities. Other more common undesirable effects are listed in Table 31-2.

Interactions

The metabolism of many drugs is affected by the altered body metabolism of hypothyroid and states. For example, many drugs administered to a patient with hypothyroidism will have an extended effect because of delayed metabolism of the drug in the liver and decreased kidney glomerular filtration rate. In addition, drug absorption via the intestine and parenterally injected drugs may be slowed. Consequently, dosages of many drugs may need to be reduced. Thyroid drugs increase the degradation of vitamin K–dependent clotting factors and enhance the activity of warfarin, which may require reduced doses. Cholestyramine, calcium supplements, and aluminum-containing antacids bind to thyroid hormone in the gastrointestinal tract, possibly decreasing the absorption of both drugs.

Levothyroxine can increase requirements for insulin and digoxin; consequently, dosages may need to be increased when patients are changing from a hypothyroid to a euthyroid state. In addition, the use of thyroid hormones increases cardiac responsiveness to epinephrine, dopamine, or dobutamine and may increase the risk of dysrhythmias. Drugs that increase the metabolism of levothyroxine are phenytoin, carbamazepine, rifampin, sertraline, and phenobarbital; the dosage of levothyroxine may need to be increased to maintain optimum levothyroxine levels.

Dosages

For the recommended dosages of the thyroid drugs, see the Dosages table on p. 583.

HYPERTHYROIDISM

The excessive secretion of thyroid hormones, or **hyperthyroidism**, may be caused by several different diseases and drugs. Some of the more common diseases are Graves' disease, which is the most common cause; Plummer's disease, which is also known as *toxic nodular disease* and is the least common cause; multinodular disease; and thyroid storm, which is usually induced by stress or infection.

Hyperthyroidism can affect multiple body systems, resulting in an overall increase in metabolism. Commonly reported symptoms are diarrhea, flushing, increased appetite, muscle weakness, fatigue, palpitations, irritability, nervousness, sleep disorders, heat intolerance, and altered menstrual flow.

ANTITHYROID DRUGS

The treatment of hyperthyroidism may be aimed at treating either the primary cause or the symptoms of the disease. Antithyroid drugs, iodides, ionic inhibitors, and radioactive isotopes of iodine are used to treat the underlying cause, and drugs such as β-blockers are used to treat the symptoms. The focus of this discussion is the antithyroid drugs, the *thioamide* derivatives, methimazole and propylthiouracil. In addition to the thioamides, radioactive iodine may be used to treat hyperthyroidism. Radioactive iodine (^{131}I) destroys the thyroid gland, in a process known as ablation. It does this by emitting

TABLE 31-2

Thyroid Drugs: Common Adverse Effects

Body System	Adverse Effects
Cardiovascular	Tachycardia, palpitations, angina, dysrhythmias, hypertension, cardiac arrest
Central nervous	Insomnia, tremors, headache, anxiety
Gastrointestinal	Nausea, diarrhea, increased or decreased appetite, cramps
Other	Menstrual irregularities, weight loss, sweating, heat intolerance, fever

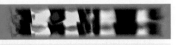

DRUG PROFILES

There are several drugs that may be used for hypo-thyroidism. The most commonly used are the synthetic drugs, although some patients get better results with the animal-derived products. Many factors must be considered before the initiation of drug therapy with a thyroid drug, including the desired ratio of T_3 to T_4, the cost, and the desired duration of effect. All thyroid drugs are contraindicated in patients who have had a hypersensitivity reaction to them in the past and in those suffering from adrenal insufficiency, MI, or hyperthyroidism.

There is a wide range of replacement doses for hypo-thyroidism, requiring individualized therapy and monitoring to ensure an adequate dose. When a euthyroid state is established, the daily maintenance dose of levothyroxine does not vary to a great extent. However, as the patient ages, dosages may need to be lowered. Once treatment is initiated, plasma TSH levels begin to decrease within hours and are usually normal within 2 weeks. It may take up to 6 weeks for full effect in some patients. Once a euthyroid state is achieved, the dosage of most of the other drugs that the patient may be taking can be adjusted to reflect a return to a normal rate of metabolism.

▶▶ levothyroxine sodium

Levothyroxine sodium (Eltroxin, Euthyrox, Synthroid), or T_4, is the most commonly prescribed synthetic thyroid

hormone and is generally considered the drug of choice. One advantage it has over the natural thyroid preparations is that it is chemically pure, being 100% T_4 (thyroxine). Thus its drug effects are more predictable than those of both natural thyroid products, which contain T_3 and T_4 in varying ratios (depending on the animal source), and synthetic T_3/T_4 combination drugs. Levothyroxine's half-life is long enough that it needs to be administered only once a day. It is available in oral (PO) form and in parenteral form. Liothyronine (Cytomel) and desiccated thyroid (Thyroid) are other drug examples.

Switching between different brands of levothyroxine during treatment can destabilize the course of treatment and should be minimized. Thyroid function tests should be monitored more carefully when switching is necessary. Limited drug supply or cost concerns may be reasons for switching, as when the patient's insurance provider's drug formulary requirements limit the patient's coverage.

Common dosages are given in the Dosages table below.

PHARMACOKINETICS

Half-Life	Onset	Peak*	Duration*
9–10 days	2 days	3–4 wk	1–3 wk

*Therapeutic effects.

DOSAGES Selected Thyroid Drugs

Drug (Pregnancy Category)	Pharmacological Class	Usual Dosage Range	Indications
desiccated thyroid (Thyroid) (A)	Desiccated (dried) animal thyroid gland	*Children 0–12 yr* PO: 15–90 mg/day *Adult* PO: 15–120 mg/day	Congenital hypothyroidism Hypothyroidism
▶▶levothyroxine sodium (Eltroxin, Euthyrox, Synthroid) (A)	Synthetic levothyroxine (thyroid hormone T_4)	*Children 0–12 yr* PO: 3–15 mcg/kg/day *Adult* PO: 1 – 1.7 mcg/kg/day IM/IV: 50% of oral dose IV: 300–500 mcg in a single dose; repeat next day 75–100 mcg if necessary	Congenital hypothyroidism Hypothyroidism Myxedema coma
liothyronine (Cytomel)*(A)	Synthetic liothyronine (thyroid hormone T_3)	*Adult* PO: 25–75mcg/day PO: 50–100 mcg daily PO: 20–50 mcg daily	Hypothyroidism Myxedema Cretinism

*Liothyronine is synonymous with triiodothyronine (T_3).

destructive β-rays once it is taken up into the follicles of the thyroid gland. Radioactive iodine is a commonly used treatment for both hyperthyroidism and thyroid cancer. Surgery is a nonpharmacological way of treating hyperthyroidism that involves removal of part of the thyroid gland. It is usually an effective way to treat hyperthyroidism, but lifelong hormone replacement therapy is normally required.

Mechanism of Action and Drug Effects

Methimazole and propylthiouracil act by inhibiting the incorporation of iodine molecules into the amino acid tyrosine, a process required to make both monoiodotyrosine and diiodotyrosine, the precursors of T_3 and T_4. This inhibition of iodine impedes the formation of thyroid hormone. Propylthiouracil has the added ability to inhibit the conversion of T_4 to T_3 in the peripheral circulation. Neither drug can inactivate already existing thyroid hormone.

The drug effects of methimazole and propylthiouracil are limited primarily to the thyroid gland; their overall effect is a decrease in the thyroid hormone level. The administration of these drugs to patients with hyperthyroidism lowers the high levels of thyroid hormone, thereby normalizing the overall metabolic rate. A euthyroid state is usually reached in 6 to 8 weeks. Individuals with severe hyperthyroidism may require larger initial doses (large doses may be divided for better therapeutic effect). Symptoms of hyperthyroidism will usually subside with 4 to 8 weeks of initiating therapy. When circulating thyroid hormones are normalizing, tapering of the drug dose can be started, with monthly dosage changes. Therapy continues for 12 to 24 months.

Indications

Antithyroid drugs are used to palliate hyperthyroidism and to prevent the surge in thyroid hormones that occurs after the surgical treatment of or during radioactive iodine therapy for hyperthyroidism or thyroid cancer. In some types of hyperthyroidism, such as that seen in Graves' disease, long-term administration of antithyroid drugs (several years) may induce a spontaneous remission. Surgical resection of the thyroid (thyroidectomy) is often used in patients who are intolerant of antithyroid drug therapy and in pregnant women, in whom both antithyroid drugs and radioactive iodine therapy are usually contraindicated.

Contraindications

The only usual contraindication to the use of the two antithyroid drugs is known drug allergy. These drugs should be avoided in pregnancy whenever possible. However, they are sometimes used in the lowest effective dose to treat hyperthyroidism that is exacerbated by the metabolic demands of pregnancy.

Adverse Effects

The most damaging or serious adverse effects of the antithyroid medications are liver and bone marrow toxicity. These and the more common adverse effects of methimazole and propylthiouracil are listed in Table 31-3. During the time a patient is in a hyperthyroid state, the rate of metabolism of many drugs may be elevated, so drug dosages may need to be higher to achieve therapeutic effects.

Interactions

Drug interactions that occur with antithyroid drugs include additive leukopenic effects when they are taken in conjunction with other bone marrow depressants and an increase in the activity of oral anticoagulants.

Dosages

See the Dosages table on p. 585 for the recommended dosages of methimazole and propylthiouracil.

PHARMACOKINETIC BRIDGE TO NURSING PRACTICE

Thyroid replacements possess specific characteristics, as with many drugs, based on their pharmacokinetics. Nurses must understand the pharmacokinetics to think critically through a clinical situation with patients who are taking the specific drug. Understanding the specifics of what occurs to the drugs once they have been administered will enable the nurse to be more competent in decision making with the patient and will lead to a more quality, efficient, and knowledge-based collaborative plan of care.

For the drug levothyroxine sodium (Eltroxin, Euthyrox, Synthroid), the pharmacokinetic characteristics include a half-life of 9 to 10 days, onset of action of 2 days, peak effects within 3 to 4 weeks, and duration of action of 1 to 3 weeks. It takes 4 to 5 days for the drug to be decreased in the body by 50% or to have it eliminated by this amount. Peak effects occur in up to 4 weeks, and the drug will stay in the blood for up to 3 weeks after it has been discontinued. Because of this prolonged half-life, the risk for toxicity is of concern. Toxicity is manifested by weight loss, tachycardia, nervousness, tremors, hypertension, headache, insomnia, menstrual irregularities, and heart irregularities. Another important pharmacokinetic property is that the drug is more than 99% protein bound. A highly protein-bound drug acts like a "biological" sustained-release drug and remains in the body longer and so is more likely to be in the serum to react with other drugs (therefore, more drug interactions occur with highly protein-bound drugs). In addition, the protein-binding characteristic may lead to toxicity from the drug remaining in the blood for prolonged periods of time.

Knowing the pharmacokinetics of levothyroxine is critical to the safe and efficient administration of the drug. Given the drug's pharmacokinetics, the effects of

TABLE 31-3	
Antithyroid Drugs: Common Adverse Effects	
Body System	**Adverse Effects**
Central nervous	Drowsiness, headache, vertigo, fever, paraesthesia
Gastrointestinal	Nausea, vomiting, diarrhea, jaundice, hepatitis, loss of taste
Genitourinary	Smoky-coloured urine, decreased urine output
Hematological	Agranulocytosis, leukopenia, thrombocytopenia, hypothrombinemia, lymphadenopathy, bleeding
Integumentary	Rash, pruritus, hyperpigmentation
Musculoskeletal	Myalgia, arthralgia, nocturnal muscle cramps
Renal	Increased blood urea nitrogen and serum creatinine
Other	Enlarged thyroid, nephritis

DRUG PROFILES

▸▸ *propylthiouracil*

Propylthiouracil is a thioamide antithyroid drug. Approximately 2 weeks of therapy with propylthiouracil may be necessary before symptoms improve. It is available only in oral form as 50 and 100 mg tablets. Common dosages are given in the Dosages table below. Methimazole is the only alternative drug in this class.

PHARMACOKINETICS

Half-Life	Onset	Peak*	Duration
1–1.5 hr	3–4 wk†	6–10 wk	2–3 hr

*Therapeutic effects.
†Effects on serum thyroid hormone concentration may occur within 60 min of a single dose.

DOSAGES Selected Antithyroid Drugs

Drug (Pregnancy Category)	Pharmacological Class	Usual Dosage Range	Indications
methimazole (Tapazole) (D)	Antithyroid	*Children* PO: 0.4 mg/kg/day divided tid *Adult* PO: 15–60 mg/day divided tid	Hyperthyroidism
▸▸propylthiouracil (generic only) (D)	Antithyroid	*Neonate* PO: 5–10 mg/kg divided tid *Children 6–10 yr* PO: 50–150 mg/day divided tid *Children over 10 yr* PO: 150–300 mg/day divided tid *Adult* PO: 100–150 mg/day divided bid–tid	Hyperthyroidism

levothyroxine are long acting and pose more risks. In summary, it is important to understand the significance of pharmacokinetics as it applies to this specific drug as a hormone replacement.

NURSING PROCESS

▨ Assessment

Assessment of the patient taking thyroid supplements for hypothyroidism includes monitoring of vital signs to compare them with future vital signs. T_3 and T_4 levels should also be assessed before and during drug therapy. Thyroid-stimulating hormone (TSH) levels will need to be assessed as well. It is important to take a medical history and a medication history to be aware of the prescription, nonprescription, and over-the-counter drugs as well any natural health products. Cautions, contraindications, and drug interactions associated with the use of thyroid hormone (discussed previously in the pharmacology section) should be assessed prior to the initiation of these drugs. Menstruation may be affected by changes in hormone levels, so a baseline reproductive and gynecological history should be taken. It is also important to remember that certain thyroid hormones may work faster than others (see the Pharmacokinetic Bridge to Nursing Practice section). Lifespan considerations include those related to older adults because of their increased sensitivity to thyroid effects (see Special

Populations: The Older Adult: Thyroid Hormones). Individualization of dosage is recommended because no two patients are ever identical in their responses.

For antithyroid drugs, such as propylthiouracil and methimazole, it is important to first assess vital signs as well as signs and symptoms of thyroid crisis, or what is often called "thyroid storm." These include tachycardia, heart irregularities, fever, heart failure, flushed skin, confusion, apathetic attitude, behavioural changes, possible hypotension, and vascular collapse. Baseline weight and intake/output measurements should also be assessed in patients receiving antithyroid and thyroid preparations. Assessing for thyroid storm also means assessing for potential causes, including thyroidectomy or abrupt withdrawal of antithyroid drugs. Other causes include excess thyroid replacement or failure to give antithyroid medications before thyroid surgery. Related cautions, contraindications, and drug interactions of antithyroid drugs must also be assessed prior to use.

▨ Nursing Diagnoses

- Risk for injury related to the adverse effects of the medication
- Risk for infection related to the bone marrow depression caused by antithyroid drug
- Acute pain related to the adverse effects of the drug
- Decreased cardiac output related to the adverse effects of the thyroid drugs
- Deficient knowledge related to lack of experience with self-administration of the drug

SPECIAL POPULATIONS: THE OLDER ADULT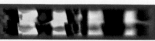

Thyroid Hormones

- The older adult is much more sensitive to thyroid hormone replacement therapy (as they are more sensitive to most drugs). They are also more likely to suffer more adverse reactions to thyroid hormones than patients in any other age group.
- They have more adverse consequences because their liver and kidney functions are decreased and the drug is highly protein bound.

- If the older adult begins to experience stumbling, falling, depression, incontinence, cold intolerance, and weight gain, he or she should contact the physician.
- With the older adult, it is also important to note that drug therapy should be individualized and initiated with caution. If higher doses are necessary, increases should be with the doctor's guidance and done gradually.

Planning

Goals

- Patient will remain free from injury as the result of the adverse effects of the drug.
- Patient will be monitored closely (e.g., for thyroid levels) while taking the drug.
- Patient will remain free of infection while receiving antithyroid drugs.
- Patient will maintain normal energy levels while on thyroid drugs.
- Patient will experience minimal adverse effects resulting from the drug.
- Patient will state the rationale of the use of the thyroid drug and its adverse effects and the need for adherence by stating such information.

Outcome Criteria

- Patient states the measures to implement to decrease the likelihood of injury related to the drug's adverse effects, such as frequent laboratory checks and monitoring of vital signs.
- Patient states the importance of follow-up appointments with the physician for frequent blood studies and monitoring of therapeutic effects.
- Patient states ways to decrease the risk of infection while receiving an antithyroid drug, such as avoiding persons with infections, eating a proper diet, and getting adequate rest.
- Patient uses relaxation techniques to deal with the nervousness and irritability caused by the drugs or the diseases.

Implementation

When administering thyroid drugs, it is important for the nurse to give the drug at the same time each day to maintain consistent blood levels of the drug. If possible, it is best to administer thyroid drugs once daily in the morning to decrease the likelihood of insomnia that may result from evening dosing. If needed, tablets may be crushed.

It is also important to avoid interchanging brands, as there can be problems with bioequivalence between different manufacturers. If the patient is scheduled to undergo any radioactive isotope studies, the thyroid drug is usually discontinued about 4 weeks before the test, but only on a physician's order.

Evaluation

A therapeutic response to thyroid drugs is reflected by disappearance of the symptoms of hypothyroidism, including depression, constipation, loss of appetite, weight gain, cold intolerance, syncope, and dry and brittle hair. Increased nervousness, irritability, mood changes, angina, and palpitations are adverse effects that need to be reported to the physician immediately. Signs that a patient is receiving inadequate doses include a return of the symptoms of hypothyroidism (see Hypothyroidism section).

A therapeutic response to antithyroid drugs is characterized by weight gain, decreased pulse, a return to a normal blood pressure, and decreased serum levels of T_4. Symptoms of overdose include cold intolerance, depression, and edema. The patient should be encouraged to report the development of any swelling, sore throat, lesions, or other signs of inflammation. Signs that a patient is not receiving adequate doses include tachycardia, insomnia, irritability, fever, and diarrhea.

PATIENT EDUCATION

- Patients should be informed to never discontinue the drug abruptly and that drug therapy is lifelong.
- Patients should be taught the importance of keeping follow-up visits, because thyroid function tests are essential for assessing the patient's health, and of documenting therapeutic and adverse effects.
- Patients should be encouraged not to interchange brands and to be sure that the pharmacy is refilling their drug with the correct brand.
- Patients should be told the importance of reporting chest pain, weight loss, tremors, and insomnia.
- Parents and caregivers should be informed that children may suffer from hair loss at the beginning of therapy but that it is reversible.
- Because children may exhibit increased aggressiveness during the first few months of therapy, parents should be educated about this possible behavioural change.
- Patients should be encouraged to keep a journal of daily energy levels and appetite during the initiation of drug therapy.
- Patients should be informed that it may take up to 3 weeks to see the full therapeutic effects of thyroid drugs.
- Patients should be informed that antithyroid medications are better tolerated when taken with meals or a snack. These drugs should be taken at the same time every day to maintain consistent blood levels of the drug, and they should never be withdrawn abruptly.
- Patients taking antithyroid (or thyroid) drugs should be encouraged to not take any over-the-counter (OTC) medications without physician approval.
- Patients taking antithyroid medications should be encouraged to avoid eating foods high in iodine, such as soy, tofu, turnip, seafood, and some breads.
- Patients should avoid using iodized salt or should decrease its intake, as prescribed.
- Patients or caregivers should be educated on how to take a pulse rate and record it.
- Patients should be encouraged to report illnesses, weight gain, cold intolerance, and depression to the physician immediately.

POINTS TO REMEMBER

- Thyroxine (T_4) and triiodothyronine (T_3) are the two hormones produced by the thyroid gland; thyroid hormone is made by iodination and coupling with the amino acid tyrosine.
- Thyroid replacement is generally done carefully by a health care provider, with frequent monitoring of serum levels until there appears to be stabilization. Nurses must monitor and review laboratory values to be sure that serum levels are within normal limits to avoid possible toxicity.
- Hyperthyroidism is caused by excessive secretion of thyroid hormone from the thyroid gland and may be attributed to different diseases (Graves' disease, Plummer's disease, and multinodular disease) or drugs. Important information about the patient's medical history should always be assessed and documented appropriately.
- Patients should report the occurrence of excitability, irritability, or anxiety to their health care provider because these symptoms may indicate levothyroxine toxicity.
- With antithyroid medications, the nurse should be aware of possible toxic reactions such as agranulocytosis, pancytopenia, and life-threatening hepatitis.

EXAMINATION REVIEW QUESTIONS

1 When monitoring the lab values of a patient who is taking antithyroid drugs, which of the following should the nurse know to watch for?
a. Decreased blood urea nitrogen
b. Increased platelet counts
c. Increased blood glucose levels
d. Decreased white blood cell counts

2 The pharmacy has called a patient to notify her that the current brand of thyroid replacement hormone is on back order. The patient calls the clinic to ask what she should do. What is the best response by the nurse?
a. "You should stop the medication until your current brand is available."
b. "Go ahead and take the other brand that the pharmacy has available for now."
c. "You can split the thyroid pills that you have left so that they will last longer."
d. "Let me ask your physician what should be done; we will need to watch how you do if you switch brands."

3 When assessing the older adult patient, which of the following nonspecific symptoms of hypothyroidism should the nurse look for?
a. Leukopenia, anemia
b. Weight loss, dry cough
c. Loss of appetite, polyuria
d. Cold intolerance, depression

4 To help with the insomnia associated with thyroid hormone replacement therapy, which of the following should the nurse encourage the patient to do?
a. Take the dose first thing in the morning.
b. Use a sedative to assist with falling asleep.
c. Reduce the dosage as needed if sleep is impaired.
d. Take one half the dose at lunch time and the other half 2 hours later.

5 The nurse is teaching a patient who has a new prescription for thyroid hormone. Which adverse effect should the patient notify the physician of?
a. Anxiety
b. Headache
c. Palpitations
d. Appetite changes

For answers see http://evolve.elsevier.com/Canada/Lilley/pharmacology/.

CRITICAL THINKING ACTIVITIES

1 Your patient has been taking thyroid drugs for about 16 months and has recently noted palpitations and some heat intolerance. Should you be concerned about this, or is this a fairly benign reaction to thyroid replacement? Explain your answer.

2 Explain "thyroid storm" and potential causes.

3 A 33-year-old man, a new admission from the medical-surgical unit to the step-down critical care unit, underwent a thyroidectomy 2 days ago. While reviewing the orders, you note that the patient is to be started on a thyroid drug upon transfer to your unit. The written orders specify that 25 mcg of levothyroxine should be given once daily. However, the pharmacy has sent 25 mcg of liothyronine, another thyroid replacement product. Because the dose of each is the same, is it safe to administer the liothyronine? Explain your answer.

For answers see http://evolve.elsevier.com/Canada/Lilley/pharmacology/.

CHAPTER 32

Antidiabetic Drugs

Learning Objectives

After reading this chapter, the successful student will be able to do the following:

1 Discuss the normal actions and functions of the pancreas.

2 Compare type 1 and type 2 diabetes mellitus with reference to age of onset, signs and symptoms, pharmacological and nonpharmacological treatment, incidence, and etiology.

3 Discuss the factors influencing blood glucose level in individuals without diabetes and in patients with type 1 and type 2 diabetes mellitus.

4 Identify the drugs used to manage type 1 and type 2 diabetes mellitus.

5 Discuss the mechanisms of action, indications, contraindications, cautions, drug interactions, and adverse effects associated with the various categories of insulin and the oral antihyperglycemic drugs.

6 Compare rapid-, regular-, intermediate-, and long-acting insulins with reference to their onset of action, peak effects, duration of action, indications, adverse effects, cautions, contraindications, drug interactions, dosages, and routes.

7 Compare the signs and symptoms and related treatment of hypoglycemia and hyperglycemia.

8 Develop collaborative plans of care that include all phases of the nursing process for patients with type 1 or type 2 diabetes, focusing on drug regimens.

e-Learning Activities

Web site
(http://evolve.elsevier.com/Canada/Lilley/pharmacology/)

- Animations
- Answers to chapter questions, activities, and case studies
- Calculators and Category Catchers
- Glossary with audio pronunciations
- IV Therapy and Medication Error Checklists
- Multiple-Choice Review Question quizzes
- Nursing Care Plans
- Online Appendices and Supplements
- WebLinks

Drug Profiles

acarbose, p. 604
▸▸ gliclazide, p. 605
glimepiride, p. 605
▸▸ glyburide, p. 605
▸▸ insulin aspart, insulin glulisine, insulin lispro, p. 598
▸▸ insulin detemir, insulin glargine, p. 599
▸▸ insulin isophane, p. 599
▸▸ metformin (metformin hydrochloride)*, p. 605
premixed insulins, p. 599
▸▸ regular insulin, p. 598
repaglinide, p. 605
▸▸ rosiglitazone (rosiglitazone maleate)*, p. 605

▸▸ Key drug.

*Full generic name is given in parentheses. For the purposes of this text, the more common shortened name is used.

Glossary

Diabetes mellitus A complex disorder of carbohydrate, fat, and protein metabolism resulting primarily from the lack of insulin secretion by the β-cells of the pancreas or from defects in the insulin receptors; it is commonly referred to simply as *diabetes*. There are two major types of diabetes: *type 1* and *type 2* (see Glossary entries below). (p. 591)

Diabetic ketoacidosis (DKA) Severe metabolic complication of uncontrolled diabetes, which, if untreated, leads to diabetic coma and death. (p. 594)

Gestational diabetes Diabetes that develops during pregnancy. It may resolve after pregnancy but may also be a precursor of type 2 diabetes. (p. 595)

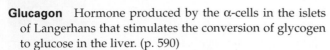
Glucagon   Hormone produced by the α-cells in the islets of Langerhans that stimulates the conversion of glycogen to glucose in the liver. (p. 590)

Glucose   A simple sugar that serves as a major source of energy. (p. 590)

Glycogen   A polysaccharide that is the major carbohydrate stored in animal cells. (p. 590)

Glycogenolysis   The breakdown of glycogen to glucose. (p. 590)

Hemoglobin A₁c (HbA₁c)   Hemoglobin molecules to which glucose molecules are bound; blood levels of hemoglobin A_{1c} are used as a diagnostic measurement of average daily blood glucose in the monitoring of diabetes; it is also called *glycosylated hemoglobin* or *glycated hemoglobin.* (p. 606)

Hyperglycemia   A fasting blood glucose level of 7 mmol/L or higher or a nonfasting blood glucose level of 11.1 mmol/L or higher. (p. 591)

Hyperosmolar nonketotic syndrome (HNKS)   A metabolic complication of uncontrolled diabetes, similar in severity to DKA but without ketosis and acidosis. (p. 594)

Hypoglycemia   A blood glucose level of less than 2.8 mmol/L. (p. 607)

Impaired fasting glucose level   A prediabetic state defined as a fasting glucose level of at least 6.1 mmol/L but lower than 6.9 mmol/L; it is sometimes called *prediabetes.* (p. 592)

Insulin   A naturally occurring hormone secreted by the β-cells of the islets of Langerhans in the pancreas in response to increased levels of glucose in the blood. (p. 590)

Ketones   Organic chemical compounds produced through the oxidation of secondary alcohols (e.g., fat molecules), including dietary carbohydrates. (p. 590)

Polydipsia   Chronic excessive intake of water; it is a common symptom of diabetes. (p. 590)

Polyphagia   Excessive eating; it is a common symptom of diabetes. (p. 590)

Polyuria   Increased frequency or volume of urinary output; it is a common symptom of diabetes. (p. 590)

Type 1 diabetes mellitus   Diabetes mellitus that is a genetically determined autoimmune disorder involving a complete or nearly complete lack of insulin production; it most commonly develops in children or adolescents. (p. 592)

Type 2 diabetes mellitus   A type of diabetes that most commonly presents in middle age. The disease may be controlled by lifestyle modifications, oral drug therapy, insulin, or a combination of these measures, but patients are not necessarily dependent on insulin. (p. 593)

PANCREAS

The pancreas is a large, elongated organ located behind the stomach. It is both an exocrine gland (secreting digestive enzymes through the pancreatic duct) and a ductless endocrine gland (secreting hormones directly into the bloodstream). The endocrine functions of the pancreas are the focus of this chapter. Two main hormones are produced by the pancreas: *insulin* and *glucagon.* Both hormones play an important role in the regulation of the endocrine system, specifically the use, mobilization, and storage of glucose by the body. **Glucose** is one of the primary sources of energy for the cells of the body. It is also the simplest form of carbohydrate (sugar) found in the body and is often referred to by the name of its D-isomer form, *dextrose.* There is a normal amount of glucose that circulates in the blood to meet body requirements for quick energy. However, not all of the glucose consumed is needed. When the quantity of glucose in the blood is sufficient, the excess is stored as **glycogen** in the liver and, to a lesser extent, in skeletal muscle tissue, where it remains until the body needs it. Glucose is also stored in adipose tissue as triglyceride body fat. **Insulin** is the hormone responsible for initiating storage of excess glucose as glycogen in the various tissues.

Insulin serves several important metabolic functions in the body. It stimulates carbohydrate metabolism in skeletal and heart muscles and in adipose tissue by facilitating the transport of glucose into these cells. In the liver, insulin facilitates the phosphorylation of glucose to glucose-6-phosphate, which is then converted to glycogen for storage. By facilitating glucose storage in the liver as glycogen, insulin keeps the glomerular filtrate of the kidney free of glucose. Without insulin, the kidneys are unable to absorb the excess glucose in the glomerular filtrate and lose large amounts of glucose (a critical body nutrient and energy source), **ketones**, and other solutes into the urine. This loss of nutrient energy sources eventually leads to **polyphagia**, weight loss, and malnutrition. The presence of these solutes in the distal kidney tubules and collecting ducts also draws large volumes of water into the urine through *osmotic diuresis*, which leads to **polyuria**, dehydration, and **polydipsia**. Polydipsia results from increased *serum osmolality* (i.e., relatively greater concentrations of solutes in the body caused by excessive urinary water loss).

When more circulating glucose is needed, glycogen, primarily that stored in the liver, is converted to glucose through a process called **glycogenolysis.** The hormone responsible for initiating this process is **glucagon,** a protein hormone consisting of a single chain of amino acids (polypeptide chain). Its molecules are approximately one half the size of those of insulin. Glucagon is released from the α-cells of the islets of Langerhans in the pancreas. The β-cells of these same islets secrete insulin, a protein hormone composed of two amino acid chains (acidic A chain and basic B chain) joined by a disulfide linkage. Glucagon has only minimal effects on muscle glycogen and adipose tissue triglyceride stores.

There is a continuous homeostatic balance in the body between the actions of insulin and those of glucagon. This natural balance serves to maintain physiologically optimal blood glucose levels, which normally range between 4 and 6 mmol/L. In diabetes, glucose levels are in excess of this range. Because of the critical role of the pancreas in producing and maintaining insulin and glycogen, *pancreatic transplantation* is now sometimes undertaken to treat diabetes that has not been successfully controlled by other means. Another treatment involves continuous insulin administration via a mechanized *insulin pump.*

Other substances that function as glucose regulators include *cortisol, epinephrine,* and *growth hormone.* These work synergistically with glucagon to counter the effects of insulin and cause increases in the blood glucose level. Insulin also has a direct effect on fat metabolism. It stimulates lipogenesis and inhibits lipolysis and the release of fatty acids from adipose cells. In addition, insulin stimulates protein synthesis and promotes the intracellular shift of potassium and magnesium, thereby decreasing elevated blood concentrations of these electrolytes. The actions of insulin are also antagonized by the following body substances: somatropin (growth hormone); the adrenomedullary hormones epinephrine and norepinephrine; the adrenocortical hormones cortisol and aldosterone; thyroid hormones; and estrogens.

DIABETES MELLITUS

Diabetes mellitus, more commonly referred to simply as *diabetes*, is primarily a disorder of carbohydrate metabolism that involves either a deficiency of insulin, a tissue (e.g., muscle, liver) resistance to insulin, or both. Whatever the cause of the diabetes, the result is hyperglycemia. **Hyperglycemia** is a state involving excessive concentrations of glucose in the blood and results when the normal counterbalancing actions of glucagon and insulin fail to maintain normal glucose homeostasis (i.e., serum levels of 4 to 6 mmol/L). Complications in protein and fat metabolism (*dyslipidemia;* Chapter 29) are also involved. Currently, the key diagnostic criterion for diabetes mellitus is hyperglycemia indicated by a fasting plasma glucose (FPG) of more than 7 mmol/L. Diagnostic indicators are described in more detail in Box 32-1.

Uncontrolled hyperglycemia correlates strongly with serious long-term adverse health effects related to both *macroangiopathy* and *microangiopathy. Macroangiopathy* involves large vessel damage that is usually related to deposition of atherosclerotic plaque. This damage compromises central as well as peripheral circulation. In contrast, *microangiopathy* involves damage to the capillary vessels, which impairs peripheral circulation. In addition, both autonomic and somatic nerve damage occur, caused primarily by the metabolic changes themselves and, to a lesser degree, by the compromised circulation. Box 32-2 lists common long-term complications of diabetes.

Diabetes mellitus is, in fact, not a single disease but rather a group of diseases. For this reason, it is often regarded as a syndrome rather than a disease. In some cases, diabetes is caused by a relative or absolute lack of insulin that is believed to result from the destruction of β-cells in the pancreas. As a result, insulin cannot be produced. Hyperglycemia can also be caused by defects in insulin receptors. The proteins that serve as insulin receptors normally occur in several tissues, including liver, muscle, and adipose tissue. These proteins customarily function in coordination with insulin molecules to remove glucose molecules from the blood. When these proteins become defective, they no longer respond normally to insulin molecules. The result is that glucose molecules remain in the blood, rather than being stored in the tissues.

Two major types of diabetes mellitus are currently recognized and designated by the Canadian Diabetes Association (CDA): type 1 and type 2. Type 1 diabetes was previously also called *insulin-dependent diabetes mellitus (IDDM)* or *juvenile-onset diabetes.* Type 2 diabetes was previously also called *non–insulin-dependent diabetes mellitus (NIDDM)* or *adult-onset diabetes.* The numerical designations for both conditions were adopted by the CDA as the preferred terms in 1995.

The previous designations were abandoned for several reasons. One reason is that many patients with type 2 diabetes *do* eventually become dependent on insulin therapy for control of their illness. A second reason is that the current epidemic of child and adult obesity in Canada is resulting in an increasing incidence of type 2 diabetes in children and adolescents (see Special Populations: Children and the Adolescent: Diabetes Mellitus). This condition is now called *maturity-onset diabetes of youth (MODY)* and refers in general to hyperglycemia in persons younger than 25 years of age. Obesity is one of the major risk factors for the development of type 2 diabetes. Non-White ethnic groups, including Blacks,

BOX 32-1

Criteria for Diagnosis of Diabetes

Symptoms of diabetes plus casual plasma glucose concentration equal to or higher than 11.1 mmol/L. "Casual" means measured at any time of the day without regard to time since the last meal. The classic symptoms of diabetes include polyuria, polydipsia, and unexplained weight loss.
OR
Fasting plasma glucose level equal to or higher than 7 mmol/L. "Fasting" is defined as no caloric intake for at least 8 hours.
OR
Two-hour postload glucose level equal to or higher than 11.1 mmol/L *(impaired glucose tolerance)* during an *oral glucose tolerance test (OGTT)*. Note that the OGTT is not recommended for routine clinical use.
Any positive result of the above assessments should be confirmed by repeat testing at a later date.

BOX 32-2 Major Long-Term Consequences of Diabetes (Type 1 and Type 2)

Pathology	Possible Consequences
MACROVASCULAR (ATHEROSCLEROTIC PLAQUE)	
Cerebral arteries	Stroke
Coronary arteries	Myocardial infarction
Peripheral vessels	Peripheral vascular disease (e.g., neuropathies [see below], foot ulcers, possible amputations)
MICROVASCULAR (CAPILLARY DAMAGE)	
Nephropathy (kidney damage)	Proteinuria (microalbuminuria), chronic kidney failure (may require dialysis or kidney transplantation)
Neuropathy (autonomic and somatic nerve damage, due to both metabolic alterations and compromised circulation)	Autonomic nerve damage—for example, diabetic gastroparesis, bladder dysfunction, lack of awareness of hypoglycemia Somatic nerve damage—for example, diabetic foot ulcer, leg or foot amputation (resulting from undetected injuries due to loss of sensation and from compromised circulation)
Retinopathy (retinal damage)	Partial or complete blindness

Source: Canadian Diabetes Association Clinical Practice Guidelines Expert Committee. (2008). Canadian Diabetes Association 2008 clinical practice guidelines for the prevention and management of diabetes in Canada. *Canadian Journal of Diabetes, 32*(Suppl. 1), S1–S201.

Asians, Hispanics, and Aboriginal peoples, are at higher risk for developing type 2 diabetes than are Whites. The usual differences between type 1 and type 2 diabetes mellitus are listed in Table 32-1.

Interestingly, approximately 10% of patients with type 2 diabetes have circulating antibodies, which suggests an autoimmune origin for the disease. This condition is known as *latent autoimmune diabetes in adults (LADA)* and is basically a more slowly progressing form of type 1 diabetes. The most common signs and symptoms of any type of diabetes are elevated blood glucose level (higher than 7 mmol/L) or **impaired fasting glucose level** (6.1 mmol/L or higher but less than 6.9 mmol/L)

and polyuria, polydipsia, polyphagia, glucosuria, weight loss, and fatigue.

Type 1 Diabetes Mellitus

Type 1 diabetes mellitus is characterized by a lack of insulin production or by the production of defective insulin, which results in acute hyperglycemia. Affected patients require exogenous insulin to lower the blood glucose level and prevent diabetic complications. It is believed that a genetically determined autoimmune reaction gradually destroys the insulin-producing β-cells of the pancreatic islets of Langerhans (Figure 32-1). The *preclinical* phase of β-cell destruction may be prolonged,

 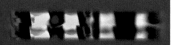
SPECIAL POPULATIONS: CHILDREN AND THE ADOLESCENT

Diabetes Mellitus

- Diabetes mellitus is the most common endocrine disease in children.
- Type 2 diabetes and other types of diabetes such as genetic defects in β-cell function and maturity-onset diabetes of the young (MODY) are more prevalent.
- Glycemic targets should be graduated with age; cognitive impairment has been associated with severe hypoglycemia in children under the age of 6.
- Children with new-onset diabetes require control with two daily injections of short-acting or rapid-acting insulin analogues combined with an intermediate- or long-acting insulin.

- Fasting blood glucose screening for type 2 diabetes should be done every 2 years for children 10 years of age or younger (if puberty has occurred) with the following risk factors: obesity; high-risk ethnic group (Aboriginal peoples, Hispanics, South Asians, Asians, or Blacks) or first- or second-degree family member with type 2 diabetes or diabetes in utero exposure; manifestations of insulin resistance (acanthosis nigricans, polycystic ovary disease, hypertension, dyslipidemia, nonalcoholic fatty liver disease); impaired glucose tolerance; or use of antipsychotic medications.

TABLE 32-1

Type 1 and Type 2 Diabetes Mellitus: Characteristics

Characteristic	Type 1	Type 2
Etiology	Autoimmune destruction of β-cells in the pancreas	Multifactorial genetic defects; strong association with obesity and insulin resistance resulting from a reduction in the number or activity of insulin receptors
Incidence	10% of cases	90% of cases
Onset	Juvenile onset, age younger than 20 yr	Previously maturity onset, age older than 40 yr; now increasingly seen in younger adults and children and adolescents, attributed to obesity epidemic
Endogenous insulin	Little or none	Normal levels
Insulin receptors	Normal	Decreased or defective
Body weight	Usually nonobese	Obese (80% of cases)
Treatment	Insulin	Weight loss, diet and exercise, oral hypoglycemics if necessary; only about one third of all patients need insulin

possibly lasting several years. At some critical point, a rapid transition from preclinical to clinical type 1 diabetes occurs. This transition may be triggered by a specific event such as an acute illness or major emotional stress. An unidentified viral infection is also strongly suspected as an environmental trigger. The stressor(s) triggers the release of the counter-regulatory hormones cortisol and epinephrine. These hormones then mobilize glucagon to release glucose from the storage sites in the liver. This only further increases the already rising levels of glucose in the blood secondary to islet cell damage. At some point during this cascade of events an autoimmune reaction may be initiated that destroys the insulin-producing β-cells of the pancreatic islets of Langerhans. The result is essentially a complete lack of endogenous insulin production by the pancreas, which necessitates chronic replacement insulin therapy.

Historically, oral antidiabetic drugs (discussed later in this chapter) have not been effective in treating type 1 diabetes, although this is being investigated by a small number of researchers.

Type 2 Diabetes Mellitus

Type 2 diabetes mellitus, once thought to be a mild form of type 1 diabetes mellitus, is an important disorder that is often poorly treated. Of all the forms of diabetes mellitus, it is by far the most common, accounting for at least 90% of all cases of diabetes mellitus and affecting as much as 20% of the population over 70 years of age. Over 1.7 million people in Canada have type 2 diabetes. In part because this form of diabetes does not always require insulin therapy, many common and dangerous misconceptions about type 2 diabetes mellitus exist: that it is a mild form of diabetes; that it is easy to treat; and that tight metabolic control is unnecessary because these patients, who are mostly older adults, will die before diabetic complications develop. The clinical realities of this disease demonstrate otherwise, however.

Type 2 diabetes mellitus is caused by both insulin resistance and insulin deficiency, but an absolute lack of insulin does not exist as in type 1 diabetes. As previously noted, one of the normal roles of insulin is to facilitate

the uptake of circulating glucose molecules and into tissues to be used as energy. In type 2 diabetes, all of the main target tissues of insulin (muscle, liver, and adipose tissue) are hyporesponsive or resistant to the effects of insulin. Not only is the absolute number of insulin

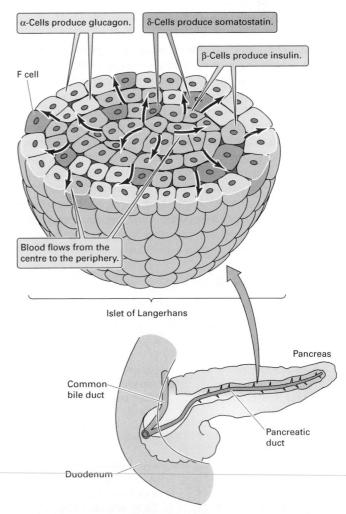

FIG. 32-1 Islet of Langerhans. (From Boron, W. F., & Boulapaep, E. L. (2003). *Medical physiology*. Philadelphia: Saunders.)

receptors in the target tissues reduced, but their individual sensitivity and responsiveness to insulin is decreased as well. Therefore, it is possible for a patient with type 2 diabetes mellitus to have normal or elevated levels of insulin and still have high blood glucose levels. Another reason for this paradoxical situation is that the altered insulin receptor dynamics cause the liver to overproduce glucose, which exacerbates the existing hyperglycemic condition. All of these processes result in impaired *postprandial glucose metabolism,* another problematic feature of type 2 diabetes that contributes to the dangerous hyperglycemic state.

In addition to the reduction in the number and sensitivity of insulin receptors in type 2 diabetes, there is often reduced insulin secretion by the pancreas. This insulin deficiency results from a loss of the normal responsiveness of the β-cells in the pancreas to elevated blood glucose levels. When the β-cells do not recognize glucose they do not secrete insulin, and the normal insulin-facilitated transport of glucose into cells of muscle, liver, and adipose tissue does not occur. This situation is analogous to the loss of responsiveness of insulin receptors to insulin described earlier. Both insulin resistance and insulin deficiency may induce or aggravate one another.

Type 2 diabetes is a multifaceted disorder. Although loss of blood glucose control is its primary sign, several other significant conditions are strongly associated with the disease. These include obesity, coronary heart disease, dyslipidemia, hypertension (Chapter 25), microalbuminuria (spilling of protein into the urine), and changes in the blood that increase the risk for thrombotic events. For patients with type 2 diabetes, the Canadian Diabetes Association recommends the regular use of aspirin for prevention of coronary artery heart disease and antilipemic drug therapy (Chapter 29), when applicable, in addition to any necessary antidiabetic drug therapy. These comorbidities are strongly associated with the development of type 2 diabetes and are collectively referred to as *metabolic syndrome* (also known as *insulin-resistance syndrome*).

Approximately 90% of patients with diabetes are obese at the time of initial diagnosis. Obesity worsens insulin resistance because adipose tissue is often the site of a large proportion of the body's defective insulin receptors. These precipitating factors of type 2 diabetes, and the disease itself, are highly inherited (hereditary). However, the current obesity epidemic, driven by both widespread lack of exercise and a high-fat, high-carbohydrate diet, is increasingly leading to the occurrence of this disease even in adolescents.

Acute Diabetic Complications: Diabetic Ketoacidosis and Hyperosmolar Nonketotic Syndrome

When blood glucose levels are high but no insulin is present to allow glucose to be used for energy production, the body may break down fatty acids for fuel, producing ketones as a metabolic byproduct. If this production occurs to a sufficient degree, **diabetic ketoacidosis (DKA)** may result. DKA is a complex, multisystem complication of uncontrolled diabetes. Without treatment, DKA will lead to coma and death. DKA is characterized by extreme hyperglycemia, the presence of ketones in the serum, acidosis, dehydration, and electrolyte imbalances. Approximately 25% to 30% of patients with newly diagnosed type 1 diabetes mellitus present with DKA. Another complication of comparable severity that is triggered by extreme hyperglycemia is **hyperosmolar nonketotic syndrome (HNKS).** The most common precipitator of DKA and HNKS is some type of physical or emotional stress. It was formerly believed that DKA occurred only in type 1 diabetes and HNKS occurred only in type 2 diabetes. However, it is now recognized that both disorders can occur with diabetes of either type. This overlap is increasingly common with the rapidly decreasing age of type 2 diabetic patients.

Table 32-2 describes the subtle differences between these two acute diabetic complications. Treatment for either involves fluid and electrolyte replacement as well as intravenous insulin therapy (more common for DKA).

TABLE 32-2

Comparison of Some Salient Features of Diabetic Ketoacidosis and Hyperosmolar Nonketotic Syndrome

	Condition	
Feature	**Diabetic Ketoacidosis**	**Hyperosmolar Nonketotic Syndrome**
Age of patient	Usually younger than 40 yr	Usually older than 40 yr
Duration of symptoms	Usually less than 2 days	Usually longer than 5 days
Cerebral edema	Often subclinical; occasionally clinical	Not evaluated if subclinical; rarely clinical
Ketone bodies	At least 4+ in 1:1 dilution	Less than 2+ in 1:1 dilution
pH	Low	Normal
Serum glucose level	Usually less than 44 mmol/L	Usually higher than 44 mmol/L
Serum HCO_3 level	Low	Normal
Serum K level	High, normal, or low	High, normal, or low
Serum Na level	More likely to be normal or low	More likely to be normal or high
Serum osmolality	Usually less than 350 mOsm/kg	Usually more than 350 mOsm/kg
Prognosis	3% to 10% mortality	10% to 20% mortality
Subsequent course	Insulin therapy required in virtually all cases	Insulin therapy not required in many cases

From Harmel, A. P., & Mathur, R. (2004). *Davidson's diabetes mellitus: Diagnosis and treatment (5th ed.).* Philadelphia: Saunders.

Gestational Diabetes

Gestational diabetes is a type of hyperglycemia that develops during pregnancy. Relatively uncommon, it occurs in approximately 4% of pregnancies. The use of insulin is necessary to decrease the risk of birth defects. In most cases, gestational diabetes resolves after delivery. However, as many as 30% of patients are estimated to develop type 2 diabetes within 10 to 15 years. This percentage is higher among Aboriginal women.

All pregnant women should have blood glucose screenings at regular prenatal visits. Women who develop gestational diabetes should be screened for lingering diabetes 6 to 8 weeks post partum. They should also be advised of their increased risk for recurrent diabetes and of the importance of regular medical checkups. Women who are known to be diabetic before pregnancy should ideally have detailed prepregnancy counselling (and, therefore, a planned pregnancy) and prenatal care from a physician experienced in managing pregnancies in diabetic women. Specific drug-therapy issues pertaining to gestational diabetes are discussed further in the Insulins section.

Prevention and Screening

Both macrovascular and microvascular problems are now recognized at fasting plasma glucose (FPG) levels as low as 7 mmol/L, with *fasting* being defined loosely as an overnight fast (no food from midnight until after the blood sample is taken in the morning). *Impaired fasting glucose level* is defined as an FPG level higher than or equal to 6.1 mmol/L but less than 6.9 mmol/L. This condition often proves to be a precursor to diabetes and thus is sometimes referred to as *prediabetes*. Another recognized prediabetic condition is *impaired glucose tolerance,* which is identified using an oral glucose challenge test (see Box 32-1). The Canadian Diabetes Association recommends that all adults 40 years of age and older be screened for elevated FPG levels every 3 years. Several preventive measures are also recommended. Reducing alcohol consumption is helpful because alcohol is broken down in the body to simple carbohydrates, which leads to increases in blood glucose level. Regular exercise also lowers blood glucose levels by increasing insulin receptor sensitivity; the loss of this is a primary problem in type 2 diabetes. Exercise also reduces body fat and tends to reduce high blood pressure.

Nonpharmacological Treatment Interventions

Patients diagnosed with type 1 diabetes almost always require insulin therapy. However, the initial treatment of type 2 diabetes should consist of weight loss and lifestyle changes. In some cases, these interventions may be sufficient to arrest the disease and avoid the need for drug therapy. Even a modest weight loss of 5% of the initial body weight can reduce the risk of disease progression from impaired glucose tolerance to type 2 diabetes by 60%. The benefits of weight loss are that it not only lowers the blood glucose and lipid levels of these patients but also reduces another common comorbidity, hypertension.

Other recommended lifestyle changes include improved dietary habits (e.g., consumption of a diet higher in protein and lower in fat and carbohydrates), smoking cessation, reduced alcohol consumption, and regular physical exercise. Cigarette smoking doubles the risk of cardiovascular disease in patients with diabetes, largely because of its effects on peripheral vascular circulation and respiratory function. In fact, smoking cessation would probably save far more lives than antihypertensive, antilipemic, and antidiabetic drug treatments combined. Alcohol consumption in diabetics can result in either hyperglycemia or hypoglycemia, depending on the patient's nutritional status. Alcohol metabolism in the liver reduces gluconeogenesis and contributes to a further drop in blood sugar levels when an individual with diabetes has not eaten for a while and his or her glucose resources are exhausted. This response is particularly critical in people with diabetes taking medications that can cause hypoglycemia. Chronic alcohol consumption in well-nourished persons with diabetes can lead to hyperglycemia. The Canadian Diabetes Association's recommendation of alcohol intake for individuals with diabetes is the same as that for the general population (e.g., no more than two standard drinks/day, no more than 14 standard drinks/wk for men, and no more than 9 standard drinks for women/wk). Moderate amounts of alcohol consumed with food do not cause acute hyperglycemia or hypoglycemia.

Antidiabetic Drugs

The two major classes of drugs used to treat diabetes mellitus are insulins and oral hypoglycemic drugs. These drugs are more broadly referred to as *antidiabetic drugs,* and they are aimed at producing a normoglycemic or euglycemic (normal blood sugar) state. These drugs are discussed in detail in the following sections.

INSULINS

The primary treatment for type 1 diabetes mellitus is insulin therapy. Patients with type 2 diabetes are not generally prescribed insulin until lifestyle changes and oral drug therapy no longer provide adequate glycemic control. Two main sources of insulin are currently available: extracted from domesticated animals or synthesized in laboratories using recombinant deoxyribonucleic acid (DNA) technology. Insulin was originally isolated from cattle; however, beef-derived insulin is no longer available on the Canadian market. Insulin isolated from pigs, known as *porcine insulin,* has a chemical structure that differs from human insulin by only one amino acid. Porcine insulin has also been supplanted by human-derived insulin products. Beef insulin can be imported from the United Kingdom through Health Canada's Special Access Programme (SAP).

The development of recombinant DNA technologies has led to widespread use of recombinant insulins that follow the natural chemical structure of the human insulin molecule. Recombinant insulin is produced with bacteria or yeast that have been altered to contain the genetic information necessary for them to reproduce an insulin that is exactly like human insulin. The pharmacokinetic properties of insulin (onset of action, peak effect, and duration of action) can also be altered by making minor modifications to either the insulin molecule or the final drug formulation. This practice has led to the development of several different insulin preparations, including combination insulin products that contain more than one type of insulin in the same solution. Chemical manipulation of insulin activity helps to meet the often individualized time-oriented metabolic demands for insulin of patients with diabetes. Table 32-3 compares the pharmacokinetic parameters of commonly prescribed insulin products.

Further modifications can be accomplished by mixing compatible insulin preparations in the syringe before administration. There are many premixed insulins containing a combination of two insulins, each with a different duration of action. This is usually a mix of fast-acting and longer-acting insulin in fixed proportions. These products eliminate the difficulty that some individuals encounter while mixing insulin. Patients should be thoroughly educated about how, when, and whether they should (or should not) mix different types of insulin. Some combinations are chemically incompatible and can result in undesirable alteration of glycemic effects.

Mechanism of Action and Drug Effects

Exogenously administered insulin functions as a substitute for the endogenous hormone. It serves to replace the insulin that is either not made at all or is made defectively in the body of a patient with diabetes. The drug effects of exogenously administered insulin are many and may involve many body systems. They are the same as those of normal endogenous insulin. That is, exogenously administered insulin restores the patient's ability to metabolize carbohydrates, fats, and proteins; to store glucose in the liver; and to convert glycogen to fat stores.

Indications

All insulin preparations can be used to treat both type 1 and type 2 diabetes, but each patient requires careful customization of the dosing regimen for optimal glycemic control. Additional therapeutic approaches such as lifestyle modifications (e.g., improved dietary and exercise habits) are also indicated; type 2 diabetes requires oral drug therapy as well. The use of intensive insulin therapy and tight glucose control is described in Box 32-3.

Contraindications

Contraindications to the use of all insulin products include known drug allergy to a specific product. Insulin should never be administered to an already hypoglycemic patient.

Adverse Effects

Hypoglycemia resulting from an insulin overdose can result in shock and possibly death. This is the most immediate and serious adverse effect of insulin. Other more common adverse effects of insulin therapy are listed in Table 32-4. Some of the effects listed (e.g., tachycardia, delirium, sweating) can be associated with *either* hypoglycemia or hyperglycemia. The *clinical* symptoms of these two conditions can overlap, thus underscoring the need to teach patients and their caregivers to measure and track their blood glucose levels when any acute symptoms arise.

Interactions

Drug interactions that can occur with the insulins are significant. The β-blockers, chlorthalidone, corticosteroids, diazoxide, epinephrine, ethacrynic acid, furosemide, isoniazid, niacin, phenytoin, thiazides, sympathomimetic drugs, and thyroid hormones (both endogenous and

TABLE 32-3

Human Insulins and Analogues: Comparison of Pharmacokinetic Properties

Insulin Preparation	Brand Name	Onset of Action	Peak Action	Duration of Action
aspart* glulisine* lispro*	NovoRapid Apidra Humalog	10–15 min	60–90 min	3–5 hr
Human regular	Humulin R	30 min	2–3 hr	6.5 hr
Human NPH	Humulin N Novolin ge NPH	1–3 hr	5–8 hr	Up to 18 hr
detemir*	Levemir	3–4 hr 90 min	None	22–26 hr 16–24 hr
glargine*	Lantus	90 min	None	24 hr

Source: Canadian Diabetes Association Clinical Practice Guidelines Expert Committee. (2008). Canadian Diabetes Association 2008 clinical practice guidelines for the prevention and management of diabetes in Canada. *Canadian Journal of Diabetes, 32*(Suppl. 1), S1–S201.

*Insulin analogue.

BOX 32-3 Intensive Insulin Therapy and Tight Glucose Control

The importance of tight glucose control in patients with type 1 and type 2 diabetes appears obvious. In fact, the value of patients' maintaining especially careful control of their blood glucose levels was demonstrated in three large research studies in the 1990s: the Diabetes Control and Complications Trial (DCCT; 1993) sponsored by the National Institutes of Health, the Kumamoto study in Japan (1995), and the United Kingdom Prospective Diabetes Study (UKPDS; 1998). The DCCT focused on patients with type 1 diabetes only and demonstrated improved outcomes with intensive insulin therapy. Intensive therapy was defined as either three insulin injections daily or administration of a rapid-acting insulin (regular, lispro, or aspart) by continuous subcutaneous insulin infusion (CSII). External CSII pumps are now being used in clinical practice. They are normally preprogrammed to deliver a basal dose of insulin round the clock, with premeal boluses delivered via the pump as needed. The patient can adjust these bolus doses on the basis of premeal blood glucose measurements. The Kumamoto study and UKPDS both focused on patients with type 2 diabetes and included the use of both insulin and oral antidiabetic drugs.

All three studies showed that patients who optimize, or even merely improve, their blood glucose control have a reduced incidence of long-term complications associated with the disease. These complications include both microvascular effects (retinopathy, nephropathy, neuropathy) and macrovascular effects (myocardial infarction, stroke, and peripheral vascular disease). The reductions in microvascular and neuropathic complications were especially dramatic, whereas the reductions in macrovascular complications were observable but not statistically significant. Nonetheless, such studies underscore the importance of helping each patient maintain the best possible glycemic control through an individualized treatment regimen.

Shichiri, M., Kishikawa, H., Ohkubo, Y., & Wake, N. (2000). Long-term results of the Kumamoto Study on Optimal Diabetes Control in type 2 diabetic patients. *Diabetes Care, 23*(Suppl. 2), B21–B29.

The Diabetes Control and Complications Trial Research Group. (1993). The effect of intensive treatment of diabetes on the development and progression of long-term complications in insulin-dependent diabetes. *New England Journal of Medicine, 329*(14), 977–986.

United Kingdom Prospective Diabetes Study Group. (1998). United Kingdom Prospective Diabetes Study 24: A 6-year, randomized, controlled trial comparing sulfonylurea, insulin, and metformin therapy in patients with newly diagnosed type 2 diabetes that could not be controlled with diet therapy. *Annals of Internal Medicine, 128*(3), 165–175.

TABLE 32-4

Insulin: Common Adverse Effects

Body System	Adverse Effect
Cardiovascular	Tachycardia, palpitations
Central nervous	Headache, lethargy, tremors, weakness, fatigue, delirium, sweating
Metabolic	Hypoglycemia
Other	Blurred vision, dry mouth, hunger, nausea, flushing, rash, urticaria, anaphylaxis

exogenous) can antagonize the hypoglycemic effects of insulin (which results in elevated blood glucose levels). Alcohol, anabolic steroids, sulfa drugs, angiotensin-converting enzyme (ACE) inhibitors, guanethidine, monoamine oxidase inhibitors (MAOIs), propranolol, and salicylates can increase insulin's hypoglycemic effects, which leads to lower blood glucose levels.

Dosages

See the Dosages table on p. 600 for the recommended dosages of the insulin drugs.

 ## DRUG PROFILES

INSULINS

The primary treatment for both type 1 diabetes and gestational diabetes is insulin therapy. There are currently four major classes of insulin, as determined by their pharmacokinetic properties: rapid-acting, short-acting, intermediate-acting, and long-acting insulin (Table 32-5). As previously mentioned, insulin is usually a therapy of last resort for type 2 diabetes. However, some clinicians elect to prescribe insulin earlier than previously done for patients who achieve less than desirable glycemic control with oral antihyperglycemic drugs or experience adverse reactions to them.

The insulin dosage regimen for all patients with diabetes is highly individualized and may consist of one or more types of insulin administered at either fixed doses or variable doses in response to self-measurements of blood glucose. Because porcine (pork-derived) insulin products are derived from a different animal species, they are more likely to be allergenic. For this reason, they are seldom used today in developed countries, except in the unusual case of a patient who has intolerance for other insulins or achieves better glycemic control with a porcine product.

Colour and appearance of insulins is important to understand for patient safety and for the prevention of adverse effects and complications. Several insulins appear

Continued

DRUG PROFILES (cont'd)

as clear, colourless solutions. These include regular insulin, insulin glulisine (Apidra), insulin lispro (Humalog), and insulin glargine (Lantus). Other insulins, such as NPH insulin (Humulin N, Novolin ge NPH) are white, opaque (cloudy) solutions. The importance of the insulin's colour and appearance to nursing care is discussed further in the Implementation subsection under Nursing Process. If an insulin is rapid or short acting, then the nurse knows to expect that the insulin will be clear, whereas intermediate-acting insulin is cloudy. Comparative pharmacokinetic parameters for several commonly used insulin products appear in Table 32-3.

Two special patient populations that require careful attention during insulin therapy are children and pregnant women. Insulin dosages for both groups are calculated by weight, as they are for the general adult population. The usual dosage range is 0.5 to 1 units/kg/day as a total daily dose. However, the nurse must be aware of a few important differences regarding the use of some of the more unusual insulin products in children. The rapid-acting insulin lispro is approved for use in children older than 3 years of age and is often used concurrently with oral sulfonylurea therapy (discussed later in the chapter). However, the combination lispro product Humalog 25 that contains 75% insulin lispro protamine (an intermediate-acting insulin) and 25% insulin lispro (a rapid-acting insulin) is *not* currently approved for use in children younger than 18 years of age. The other rapid-acting product, insulin aspart (NovoRapid), also is *not* currently approved for children. Any insulin therapy for children that falls outside of standard dosing guidelines should be prescribed by a trained pediatric endocrinologist, who must also provide careful monitoring of the patient. Children need age-appropriate education and supervision from health care professionals and parents. This includes a safe and gradual transfer of responsibility for self-management of their illness.

Pregnant women also require special care for diabetes management. Gestational diabetes reportedly occurs in approximately 3.5% of non-Aboriginal and up to 18% of Aboriginal pregnancies. Although many of these mothers will return to a normal glycemic state after pregnancy, they also have a 30% to 60% risk of developing diabetes again in later life. Although all currently available oral and injectable antidiabetic drugs are classified as pregnancy category B or C, oral medications are generally not recommended for pregnant patients because of a lack of firm safety data. In contrast, insulin use in pregnant women is much better studied and understood. For this reason, insulin therapy is the only currently recommended drug therapy for pregnant women with diabetes. Approximately 15% of women who develop gestational diabetes require insulin therapy during pregnancy. All insulin products are classified as pregnancy category B drugs except for the glargine and aspart products, which are pregnancy category C drugs.

Insulins, both endogenous and exogenous, do not normally cross the placenta. However, insulin is normally excreted into human milk. Because this is a natural process, nursing mothers may still receive insulin therapy.

Nevertheless, it is currently unknown whether insulin glargine is excreted in breast milk, and so it should not be used in women while they are breastfeeding. Optimization of insulin therapy and diet are especially important for a nursing mother because inadequate or excessive glycemic control may reduce milk production. Effective glycemic control during pregnancy is also essential because infants born to women with gestational diabetes have a twofold to threefold greater risk of congenital anomalies. The incidence of stillbirth is directly related to the degree of maternal hyperglycemia. Weight reduction is generally *not* advised for these women, however, because it can jeopardize fetal nutritional status.

RAPID–ACTING INSULINS

▶▶ insulin aspart, insulin glulisine, and insulin lispro

Currently three insulin analogues are classified as rapid acting. They have a rapid onset of action of 10 to 15 minutes but also a shorter duration of action than that of other insulin categories. These products include insulin lispro (Humalog), insulin aspart (NovoRapid), and, most recently, insulin glulisine (Apidra). Their effects are most like those of the endogenous insulin produced from the pancreas in response to a meal. After a meal, the glucose that is ingested stimulates the pancreas to secrete insulin. This insulin then chemically facilitates uptake of the excess glucose at hepatic insulin receptor sites for storage in the liver as glycogen. In individuals with diabetes mellitus, the insulin response to a glucose load at meals is deficient; therefore, a rapid-acting insulin product is often used within 15 minutes of mealtime. This corresponds to the time required for the onset of action of these products.

Insulin lispro was approved by Health Canada in 1998, becoming the first new insulin product to appear on the market in many years. Produced using recombinant DNA technology, the rapid-acting insulins are able to more closely mimic the body's natural rapid insulin output after consumption of a meal than are previous insulin products. For this reason, they are usually given within 15 minutes before beginning or within 20 minutes after starting a meal. Both insulin lispro and insulin glulisine are approved for use in subcutaneous (not intravenous) continuous infusion pumps, which are now more frequently used in children and patients with severe diabetes. The successful use of this device, as with diabetes treatment in general, requires a motivated and attentive patient.

SHORT-ACTING INSULIN

▶▶ regular insulin

Regular insulin (Humulin R, Novolin ge Toronto) is currently the only insulin classified as short acting. Some references still classify it as a rapid-acting insulin. However, the rapid-acting insulins, aspart, glulisine, and lispro, are human insulin analogues. They are insulin molecules with synthetic alterations to their chemical structures that alter their onset or duration of action.

Continued

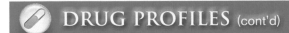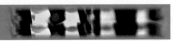

Such alteration gives the rapid-acting insulins a faster onset of action and a shorter time to peak plasma level but also a shorter duration of action than that of regular insulin, hence the newer designation for regular insulin as a short-acting product. Regular insulin is the only insulin product that can be administered via intravenous bolus, intravenous infusion, or even intramuscularly. These routes, especially the intravenous infusion route, are often used in cases of DKA or coma associated with uncontrolled type 1 diabetes.

Regular insulin solution was the first medicinal insulin product developed and was originally isolated from bovine (cow) and porcine (pig) sources. It is now primarily made from human insulin sources using recombinant DNA technology.

INTERMEDIATE-ACTING INSULINS

▶▶ insulin isophane

Currently available intermediate-acting insulin products include two basic isophane types (also known as NPH): (1) (Humulin N) and (2) Novolin ge NPH. NPH is an acronym for *neutral protamine Hagedorn* insulin, the original name of this type of insulin. Novolin ge NPH insulin is a sterile suspension of zinc insulin crystals and protamine sulfate in buffered water for injection; it is produced by recombinant DNA technology in *Saccharomyces cerevisiae*. Humulin N is a human biosynthetic NPH polypeptide hormone of rDNA origin; it is produced by a genetically altered *Escherichia coli* strain. These insulins appear as a cloudy or opaque suspension. Because of their intermediate onset of action, the effects of these insulins are slower to occur and more prolonged than those of endogenous insulin.

LONG-ACTING INSULINS

▶▶ insulin detemir and insulin glargine

Two long-acting basal insulin products are now available: insulin detemir (Levemir) and insulin glargine (Lantus). Insulin detemir and insulin glargine are normally clear, colourless solutions. They are recombinant DNA–produced insulin analogues. These two insulin products are unique in that they provide a constant level of insulin in the body, which enhances their safety because the effects do not rise and fall as with other insulins. Therapy is often initiated with once-daily dosing, although glargine may be dosed every 12 hours, depending on the patient's glycemic response. Both these long-acting insulin products have longer onsets and durations of action than those of endogenous (regular) insulin. Because they help provide a more prolonged, consistent blood glucose level, they are sometimes referred to as basal insulins. Often for those patients being switched from twice-daily NPH to glargine, the initial daily glargine dose is reduced to 80% of the previous total NPH dose, with a range of 2 to 100 units.

PREMIXED INSULINS

Currently available premixed combination insulin products contain a fixed ratio of insulin—a percentage of a rapid-acting or short-acting insulin to a percentage of intermediate-acting insulin—that works together in the body to optimize glycemic control. The numerical designations indicate the relative percentages of each of the two components in the product. In each case, the numbers add to up 100%. These insulins include biosynthetic Humulin 30/70, Novolin ge (30/70, 40/60, and 50/50; mixtures containing Novolin ge Toronto and Novolin ge NPH, respectively, in the proportions indicated by the ratio in the product name), and NovoMix 30, biphasic insulin aspart (dual-release human insulin analogue suspension containing 30% soluble insulin aspart and 70% insulin aspart protamine crystals). These products were developed to more closely simulate the varying levels of endogenous insulin that occur normally in the general population.

To maintain constant blood glucose levels both after and between meals, insulin must be present. In most insulin regimens, patients take a combination of a rapid-acting insulin to manage the surges in glucose that occur after meals and an intermediate- or long-acting insulin for the period between meals when glucose levels are lower. However, this requires the mixing and administration of different types of insulins. Fixed-combination products were developed in an attempt to simplify the dosage process. Premixed insulin preparations are usually given once or twice daily when a rapid initial effect together with a more prolonged effect is desired. The effect of Novolin ge mixtures begins after approximately 30 minutes, is maximal between 2 and about 12 hours, and terminates after approximately 24 hours. The percentage of rapid- and short-acting with the intermediate-acting components in each of the available fixed insulin products is specified in the Dosages table on p. 601.

SLIDING-SCALE INSULIN DOSING

Another strategy for dosing insulin is the *sliding-scale method*. In this method, subcutaneous doses of short-acting (regular) or rapid-acting (lispro or aspart) insulin are adjusted according to blood glucose test results. This method is typically used in hospitalized patients whose insulin requirements may vary dramatically because of stress (e.g., infections, surgery, acute illness), inactivity, or variable caloric intake including receipt of *total parenteral nutrition (TPN)*. Sliding-scale insulin administration may also be used in patients with type 1 diabetes on intensive insulin therapy. When an individual is on a sliding-scale insulin regimen, blood glucose concentrations are determined several times a day (e.g., before meals and at bedtime for patients on normal meal schedules, or every 4 to 6 hours around the clock for patients on TPN or enteral tube feedings). This enables the patient to obtain fasting blood glucose values and values before meals. Subcutaneously administered regular insulin is then ordered in an amount that increases with the increase in blood glucose. The use of sliding-scale insulin has been the subject of some controversy, however, because of perceived lack of effectiveness in achieving optimal glycemic control in hospitalized patients.

TABLE 32-5

Available Insulin Products

Activity Classification	Human Recombinant Insulins
RAPID ACTING	
insulin aspart	NovoRapid
insulin glulisine	Apidra
insulin lispro	Humalog
SHORT ACTING	
regular	Humulin R, Novolin ge Toronto
INTERMEDIATE ACTING	
isophane insulin suspension (NPH)	Humulin N, Novolin ge NPH
LONG ACTING	
insulin detemir	Levemir
insulin glargine	Lantus
MIXED HUMAN INSULINS	
Percentage regular/NPH insulin (30/70), biosynthetic insulin (40/60), biosynthetic insulin (50/50), biosynthetic	
MIXED HUMAN ANALOGUES	
insulin lispro, insulin protamine (30/70)	NovoMix 30

ORAL ANTIHYPERGLYCEMIC DRUGS

As previously described, type 2 diabetes is usually a heterogeneous illness. Effective treatment involves several elements, including lifestyle modifications (e.g., diet, exercise, smoking cessation), careful monitoring of blood glucose, and possible therapy with one or more drugs. In addition, the treatment of associated comorbid conditions can further complicate the entire process. Type 2 diabetes is characterized by insulin resistance and an ongoing reduction in β-cell function. Thus glucose levels will worsen over time and necessitate ever-changing treatment.

If normal blood glucose levels are not achieved after 2 to 3 months of lifestyle modifications, treatment with an oral antihyperglycemic drug is often prescribed. However, the patient should be clearly advised that the ability of any drug therapy to improve the health of any patient with diabetes is aided by appropriate changes in diet and activity level. Such drug therapy may fail or become inadequate without an effort by the patient to make behavioural changes. Once-daily dosage forms of oral drugs are increasingly popular, as is the case with insulins (e.g., glargine). With drug therapy in general, reduced frequency of dosing is associated with increased patient adherence to the drug regimen and improved therapeutic outcomes.

The *Canadian Diabetes Association 2008 Clinical Practice Guidelines for the Prevention and Management of Diabetes in Canada* maps out strategies for managing type 2 diabetes,

DOSAGES   Human-Based Insulin Products

Drug (Pregnancy Category)	Pharmacological Class	Usual Dosage Range	Indications
RAPID ACTING			
⇒ insulin aspart (NovoRapid) (C) insulin glulisine (Apidra) (C) insulin lispro (Humalog) (B)	Human recombinant rapid-acting insulin analogues	*Children/Adult* SC: 0.5–1 unit/kg/day; doses are highly individualized to desired glycemic control; rapid-acting insulins are best given 15 min before a meal All three drugs may be given per sliding scale; they may also be given via continuous SC infusion pump (but not IV)	Diabetes mellitus, type 1 and type 2
SHORT ACTING			
⇒ regular insulin (Humulin R, Novolin ge Toronto) (B)	Human recombinant short-acting insulin	SC only: Same dosage as insulin aspart, insulin glulisine, and insulin lispro; SC doses of regular insulin are best given 30 to 60 min before a meal. Regular insulin may also be given per sliding scale and is the only insulin that can be given IV as a continuous infusion	Diabetes mellitus, type 1 and type 2
INTERMEDIATE ACTING			
⇒ isophane insulin suspension (NPH, Humulin N, Novolin ge NPH) (B)	Human recombinant intermediate-acting insulin analogues	SC only: Same dosage as insulin aspart, insulin lispro, insulin glulisine, and regular insulin	Diabetes mellitus, type 1 and type 2

Continued

DOSAGES   Human-Based Insulin Products (cont'd)

Drug (Pregnancy Category)	Pharmacological Class	Usual Dosage Range	Indications
LONG ACTING			
▸▸**insulin detemir (Levemir) (C) insulin glargine (Lantus) (C)**	Human recombinant long-acting insulin analogues	SC only: Same dosage as others but is approved only for once- or twice-daily dosage (basal dosing)	Diabetes mellitus, type 1 and type 2
PREMIXED INSULIN PRODUCTS			
biphasic insulin aspart (NovoMix 30) insulin lispro protamine suspension 75% (50%) and insulin lispro 25% (50%) (Humalog Mix 25; Humalog Mix 50) (B)	Human recombinant intermediate-acting and rapid-acting premixed insulin product	SC only: Same dosage as others	Diabetes mellitus, type 1 and type 2
regular insulin 30% and NPH 70% (Humulin 30/70; Novolin ge 30/70) (B) regular insulin 40% and NPH 60% (B) regular insulin 50% and NPH 50% (B)	Human recombinant intermediate-acting and short-acting premixed insulin products		

IV, intravenous; *SC,* subcutaneous.

including early treatment with medication. Figure 32-2 shows the target organs for orally administered anti-hyperglycemic drugs. New research recommends that the sooner glycosylated hemoglobin (A_{1c}) level targets are achieved (A_{1c} of less than 7% is considered normal), the better the long-term outcomes are (see Table 32-6 for correlations of A_{1c} levels with mean serum glucose levels). The A_{1c} measures the average blood glucose level over the previous 3 months and can be used to predict the risk for diabetes complications. One of the recommended

guidelines is starting combination therapy using two drugs from two different classes of oral hypoglycemic drugs if the A_{1c} exceeds 9%. The use of submaximal doses of the drugs results in a more rapid and better glycemic control and fewer adverse effects than with monotherapy at maximal dosages. There is debate over which drugs should be used initially and which drugs should be added later. Nevertheless, the patient should be clearly advised that the ability of any drug therapy to improve health depends on appropriate changes in diet and activity level.

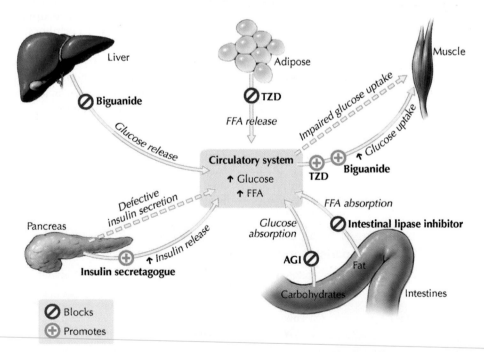

FIG. 32-2 Major target organs and actions of orally antihyperglycemic therapy for type 2 diabetes mellitus. *AGI,* α-glucosidase inhibitor; *FFA,* free fatty acid; *TZD,* thiazolidenedione. (Source: Cheng, A.Y.Y. and Fantus, G.I. (2005). Oral antihyperglycemic therapy for type 2 diabetes mellitus. *Canadian Medical Association Journal, 172*(2), 213-226. Reprinted from *CMAJ* by permission of the publisher. © 2005 CMA Media Inc. This work is protected by copyright and the making of this copy was with the permission of Access Copyright. Any alteration of its content or further copying in any form whatsoever is strictly prohibited unless otherwise permitted by law.)

PART FIVE   Drugs Affecting the Endocrine System

TABLE 32-6

Diabetes Care: Correlation of Glycosylated Hemoglobin Levels with Mean Serum Glucose Levels

Hemoglobin A$_{1c}$ (%)	Mean Serum Glucose Levels (mmol/L)
6	7.5
7	9.5
8	11.5
9	13.5
10	15.5
11	17.5
12	19.5

Mechanism of Action and Drug Effects

Sulfonylureas

The sulfonylureas are a group of oral antidiabetic drugs that are able to stimulate insulin secretion from the β-cells of the pancreas. This increased insulin then helps transport the glucose out of the blood and into the tissues, cells, and organs in which it is needed. Because of these actions, the sulfonylureas may be broadly considered oral hypoglycemic drugs. The sulfonylureas have many other beneficial effects besides their ability to stimulate insulin release from the pancreas. They may also enhance the actions of insulin in muscle, liver, and adipose tissue, enabling these tissues to take up and store glucose more easily as a later source of energy. They may increase the availability of insulin by preventing the liver from breaking insulin down as fast as it ordinarily would (reduced liver clearance). In summary, the overall effect of the sulfonylureas is that they improve both insulin secretion and the sensitivity to insulin in tissues.

The sulfonylureas have been the anchor of oral pharmacological therapy for type 2 diabetes mellitus for more than 30 years. Their primary beneficial effect in patients with type 2 diabetes mellitus is to stimulate insulin secretion from β-cells in the pancreas. These drugs work best during the early stages of the disease when the patient still has β-cell function.

Selected sulfonylurea drugs and their comparative durations of action are listed in Table 32-7. Although the first-generation drugs listed are less commonly used now than they were earlier, they are still available and preferred by some patients and prescribers. The action of these drugs forces the extra glucose out of the blood (the site of its harmful effects) and into cells, tissues, and organs (where it can be used as energy or stored as fuel). The sulfonylurea compounds also increase the sensitivity of the insulin receptor proteins in the cells of the muscles, liver, and fat to the effects of insulin.

Meglitinides

Repaglinide and nateglinide are currently the only two drugs in the meglitinide class. They are structurally different from the sulfonylureas but have a similar mechanism of action in that they also increase insulin secretion from the pancreas.

Biguanide

Metformin, a drug that had been used for over 30 years in Canada, is currently the only drug classified as a *biguanide*. Like the sulfonylureas, it is now among the most commonly used oral drugs for treating type 2 diabetes. Metformin differs significantly from the sulfonylureas in that it does not increase insulin secretion from the pancreas and thus does not cause hypoglycemia.

Metformin is believed to exert its beneficial effects in type 2 diabetes mellitus via three mechanisms: (1) it decreases glucose production by the liver by reducing gluconeogenesis; (2) it decreases intestinal absorption of glucose; and (3) it improves insulin receptor sensitivity in the liver, skeletal muscle, and adipose tissue, resulting in increased glucose uptake by these organs. This results in increased peripheral glucose uptake and use and decreased liver production of triglycerides and cholesterol. The use of metformin in individuals with prediabetes can reduce the risk of progression to type 2 diabetes by 30%. Metformin is available in combination with rosiglitazone (Avandamet).

Thiazolidinediones

The third major drug category to emerge for the oral treatment of type 2 diabetes mellitus is the thiazolidinediones. Thiazolidinediones are also referred to as *insulin-sensitizing drugs*, as well as *glitazones*. The first

TABLE 32-7

Sulfonylurea Drugs: Qualitative Comparison of Pharmacokinetic Properties

Drug	Potency	Onset of Action	Duration of Action	Active Metabolite?
FIRST GENERATION				
chlorpropamide* (Novo-Propamide)	Low	Fast	Very long	Yes
tolbutamide*	Low	Fast	Short	No
SECOND GENERATION				
glimepiride (Amaryl)	High	Intermediate	Long	Yes
gliclazide (Diamicron, Diamicron MR, generic)	High	Fast	Long	No
glyburide (Diaβeta, Euglucon, generic)	High	Slow	Long	Yes

*Still available in Canada, but rarely used.

drug in this class to be used in the United States, Japan, and the United Kingdom was troglitazone (Rezulin). In 2000, it was removed from the market because of concerns about liver toxicity; it was never introduced in Canada. The two newer thiazolidinediones currently available in Canada are pioglitazone and rosiglitazone. They offer efficacy similar to that of troglitazone with less risk of toxicity. Thiazolidinediones act to decrease insulin resistance by enhancing the sensitivity of insulin receptors in the liver, skeletal muscle, and adipose tissue. These drugs are also known to directly stimulate peripheral glucose uptake and storage, as well as inhibit glucose and triglyceride production in the liver. Thiazolidinediones have no known effect on insulin secretion. The use of a thiazolidinedione in individuals with prediabetes can reduce the risk of progression to type 2 diabetes by 60%.

α-Glucosidase Inhibitor

Less commonly used than the oral drug classes described previously is the α-glucosidase inhibitor acarbose. This α-glucosidase inhibitor acts by reversibly inhibiting the enzyme α-glucosidase. This enzyme is found in the brush border (villi) of the small intestine and is responsible for the hydrolysis of oligosaccharides and disaccharides to glucose and other monosaccharides. When α-glucosidase is blocked, glucose absorption is delayed. The timing of administration of the α-glucosidase inhibitor is important. When an α-glucosidase inhibitor is taken with the first mouthful of a meal, excessive postprandial blood glucose elevation (a glucose "spike") can be prevented or reduced. The use of acarbose in individuals with prediabetes can reduce the risk of progression to type 2 diabetes by 30%.

Indications

Sulfonylurea drugs are used to lower the blood glucose levels in patients when diet and lifestyle changes have failed to do so, although β-cell function must be preserved for the drugs to have this action. The biguanide metformin is indicated as monotherapy in patients with type 2 diabetes mellitus. It is used as an adjunct to dietary measures to lower blood glucose levels when hyperglycemia cannot be satisfactorily managed through diet alone. Metformin may be used concomitantly with a sulfonylurea when dietary measures and metformin or a sulfonylurea drug alone does not result in adequate glycemic control. The thiazolidinediones (or glitazones) are most commonly used alone or with a sulfonylurea, metformin, or insulin in patients with type 2 diabetes mellitus.

Contraindications

Contraindications to the use of all antihyperglycemic drugs generally include known drug allergy and active hypoglycemia. They may also include severe liver or kidney disease, depending on the required metabolic pathways of the drug in question. These oral drugs are generally not used during pregnancy; insulin therapy is safer for the fetus and provides for the more careful glycemic control that is critical during pregnancy.

Adverse Effects

Sulfonylureas

The most serious adverse effects of sulfonylureas involve the hematological system and include agranulocytosis, hemolytic anemia, thrombocytopenia, and cholestatic jaundice. Effects on the gastrointestinal system include nausea, epigastric fullness, and heartburn. Erythema, photosensitivity, hypoglycemia, and morbilliform and maculopapular eruptions are other undesirable effects.

Meglitinides

The most commonly reported adverse effects of the meglitinides include headache, hypoglycemia, dizziness, weight gain, joint pain, and upper respiratory infection or flulike symptoms.

Biguanide

The biguanide metformin primarily affects the gastrointestinal tract. The most common adverse effects of therapy with metformin are abdominal bloating, nausea, cramping, a feeling of fullness, and diarrhea. These effects are usually self-limiting and transient and can be lessened by starting with low dosages, titrating up slowly, and taking the medication with food. Less common adverse effects with metformin are a metallic taste and reduction in vitamin B_{12} levels. Lactic acidosis is rare with metformin and is lethal in 50% of cases. Unlike sulfonylureas, metformin does not cause hypoglycemia.

Thiazolidinediones

Rosiglitazone and pioglitazone both may cause moderate weight gain, edema, and mild anemia, possibly as a result of fluid retention. The safety of thiazolidinedione use in pregnant women, in children, and in patients with heart failure has not been established. There is concern that liver toxicity may be an effect of the entire class of thiazolidinediones. Laboratory measurement of liver alanine aminotransferase (ALT) levels is recommended, before treatment is begun, to assess baseline liver function, and ALT levels should be measured periodically thereafter per clinical judgement. If the ALT level rises above 2.5 to 3 times the normal upper limit, ALT monitoring should be done more frequently, and the drug should be discontinued if ALT levels do not return to normal values.

α-Glucosidase Inhibitor

The α-glucosidase inhibitor acarbose also has adverse effects that primarily involve the gastrointestinal tract. Its use can cause flatulence, diarrhea, and abdominal pain. At high dosages, it may also elevate liver enzymes (transaminases). Unlike sulfonylureas, acarbose does not cause hypoglycemia, hyperinsulinemia, or weight gain.

Interactions

Sulfonylureas

The potential drug interactions that can occur with sulfonylureas are significant. Their hypoglycemic effect is increased when they are taken concurrently with alcohol, anabolic steroids, β-blockers, chloramphenicol, guanethidine, MAOIs, oral anticoagulants, phenylbutazone, or sulfonamides. Natural health products reported to increase the likelihood of hypoglycemia when given with sulfonylureas include garlic and ginseng.

Drugs capable of reducing the hypoglycemic effect of sulfonylureas include adrenergics, corticosteroids, thiazides, and thyroid preparations. In addition, the drugs in some drug classes have sufficient chemical similarity to the sulfonylureas that *allergic cross-reactivity* may be seen. These drug classes include loop diuretics (e.g., furosemide) and sulfonamide antibiotics (e.g., sulfamethoxazole). Sulfonylureas may also interact with alcohol in a way similar to disulfiram (Antabuse), which is used to deter alcohol ingestion in individuals with chronic alcoholism. This *disulfiram-type reaction* includes acute discomforts such as vomiting and hypertensive episodes.

Meglitinides

The hypoglycemic effects of the meglitinides may be increased if they are given with drugs such as fluconazole, gemfibrozil, nonsteroidal anti-inflammatory drugs, pioglitazone, and sulfonamides. Reduced hypoglycemic effects have been reported with drugs such as phenobarbital, phenytoin, carbamazepine, nafcillin, and thiazide diuretics.

Biguanide

Metformin concentrations can be increased when the drug is given concomitantly with furosemide and nifedipine. When it is given with cationic drugs such as cimetidine or digoxin, competition for kidney tubular secretion occurs, which results in increased metformin concentrations. In addition, the concurrent use of metformin with iodinated (iodine-containing) radiological contrast medium has been associated with both acute kidney failure and lactic acidosis. For these reasons, metformin therapy should be discontinued at least 48 hours before the patient undergoes any radiological study that requires such contrast medium and should be withheld for at least 48 hours after the procedure. The integrity of the patient's kidney function should also be confirmed via blood sampling following the procedure before the patient is allowed to resume metformin therapy.

Thiazolidinediones

Clinically important interactions between rosiglitazone and other drugs have not been reported. Levels of low-density lipoprotein and high-density lipoprotein cholesterol increase between 12% and 19% in individuals taking rosiglitazone, but triglyceride levels may actually decrease. Pioglitazone, by contast, is partly metabolized by cytochrome P450 3A4 (CYP3A4). Serum concentrations of pioglitazone may be increased if the drug is taken concurrently with a CYP3A4 inhibitor such as ketoconazole. However, pioglitazone raises low-density lipoprotein cholesterol only slightly and lowers serum triglyceride concentrations.

α-Glucosidase Inhibitor

Other potential drug interactions include medications that can cause hyperglycemia as an adverse effect, including loop and other types of diuretics, corticosteroids, estrogens, phenothiazines, thyroid replacement hormones, antiepileptic drugs, the antilipemic drug niacin, sympathomimetics (often found in over-the-counter cold products), digoxin, and intestinal adsorbents.

Dosages

For the recommended dosages of oral antihyperglycemic drugs, see the Dosages table on p. 606.

 DRUG PROFILES

Sulfonylurea drugs are the oldest class of oral drugs used for diabetes. There are two categories, or generations, of sulfonylurea drugs. The first-generation sulfonylureas are the older low-potency drugs tolbutamide and chlorpropamide. These drugs are still available in Canada but are now used much less frequently than newer drugs. The second-generation sulfonylureas are the newer high-potency drugs gliclazide, glyburide, and glimepiride.

The newer drug categories include the biguanides, α-glucosidase inhibitors, meglitinides, and thiazolidinediones. Currently, the only biguanide used in Canada is metformin. Acarbose is the only available α-glucosidase inhibitor in Canada. The meglitinides include repaglinide and nateglinide. The newest class of drugs used to treat patients with type 2 diabetes mellitus is the thiazolidinediones. Pioglitazone and rosiglitazone belong to this class and are currently the only thiazolidinediones available.

acarbose

Acarbose (Glucobay) is currently the sole available α-glucosidase inhibitor. Acarbose works by blunting elevated blood sugar levels after a meal. To act optimally, it is taken with the first mouthful of each meal. It may also be taken concomitantly with sulfonylurea drugs or with metformin. Acarbose is contraindicated in patients with a hypersensitivity to α-glucosidase inhibitors, diabetic ketoacidosis, cirrhosis, inflammatory bowel disease, colonic ulceration, partial intestinal obstruction, or chronic intestinal disease.

PHARMACOKINETICS

Half-Life	Onset	Peak	Duration
2–3 hr	1–1.5 hr	14–24 hr	9–15 hr

Continued

DRUG PROFILES (cont'd)

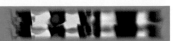

gliclazide

Gliclazide (Diamicron, Diamicron MR, generic) is a second-generation sulfonylurea drug with a potency much greater than that of the first-generation drugs. For this reason, the common doses of gliclazide are smaller compared with the higer dosages of 100 to 500 mg for the first-generation drugs. In contrast to the other second-generation drug glyburide, gliclazide has a rapid onset and short duration of action, with no active metabolites. This combination of features confers many benefits. The rapid onset of action allows it to function much like the body normally does in response to meals when greater levels of insulin are required rapidly to deal with the increased glucose in the blood. When a patient with type 2 diabetes mellitus takes gliclazide, it rapidly stimulates the pancreas to release insulin. This, in turn, facilitates the transport of extra glucose from the blood into the cells of the muscles, liver, and adipose tissues.

Its short duration of action, compared with that of glyburide, prevents long-term stimulation of the β-cells in the pancreas, which may otherwise cause the β-cells to become resistant to the effects of the sulfonylurea drugs. Long-term β-cell stimulation may also cause the pancreas to make too much insulin, thereby inducing hyperinsulinemia, which can cause the muscle, liver, and fat tissues to become resistant to the effects of insulin.

Gliclazide use is contraindicated in cases of known drug allergy as well as in type 1 or brittle diabetes. Unlike most other oral antihyperglycemic drugs, it is not contraindicated in patients with severe kidney failure. It works best if given 30 minutes before meals. This allows the timing of the insulin secretion induced by the gliclazide to correspond to the elevation in the blood glucose level induced by the meal in much the same way as endogenous insulin levels are raised in a person without diabetes.

PHARMACOKINETICS

Half-Life	Onset	Peak	Duration
10.4 hr	1–1.5 hr	4–6 hr	10–24 hr

glimepiride

Glimepiride (Amaryl) is the newest of the sulfonylurea drugs. It has properties comparable with those of glyburide and gliclazide, except that it has an onset of action that is intermediate between that of gliclazide and glyburide, as indicated in Table 32-7. Common dosages are listed in the Dosages table on p. 606.

PHARMACOKINETICS

Half-Life	Onset	Peak	Duration
5–9 hr	2–3 hr	2–3 hr	24 hr

glyburide

Glyburide (Diaβeta, Eugulon, Med Glybe) is another second-generation sulfonylurea drug. It differs from the first-generation oral hypoglycemic drugs in its greater potency and from gliclazide in its slower onset and longer duration of action and the fact that it has active metabolites. These differences can have significant consequences. Because of its relatively slow onset of action, glyburide is less desirable for the treatment of the short-term elevations in the blood glucose levels that occur after meals. However, its longer duration of action is more suitable for the long-term, constant stimulation of the pancreas, resulting in the release of a constant amount of insulin. This may be beneficial in controlling blood glucose levels during the night and throughout the day. It has similar contraindications to gliclazide.

PHARMACOKINETICS

Half-Life	Onset	Peak	Duration
10 hr	1–1.5 hr	4 hr	24 hr

metformin hydrochloride

Metformin hydrochloride (Glucophage) is currently the sole biguanide oral antihyperglycemic drug. It acts primarily by inhibiting liver glucose production and increasing the sensitivity of peripheral tissue to insulin. Because its mechanism of action differs from that of sulfonylurea drugs, it may be given concomitantly with these drugs.

Metformin's use is contraindicated in patients with a hypersensitivity to biguanides, liver or kidney disease, alcoholism, or cardiopulmonary disease.

PHARMACOKINETICS

Half-Life	Onset	Peak	Duration
1.7–3 hr	< 1 hr	1–3 hr	24 hr

repaglinide

Repaglinide (GlucoNorm) is one of two antihyperglycemic drugs classed as meglitinides. The other is nateglinide (Starlix). Meglitinides have a mechanism of action similar to that of the sulfonylureas, as they also stimulate the release of insulin from pancreatic β-cells. They are often particularly helpful in the treatment of patients who have erratic eating habits, because the drug dose is skipped when a meal is missed. Contraindications include known drug allergy.

PHARMACOKINETICS

Half-Life	Onset	Peak	Duration
2–3 hr	15–60 min	1 hr	4–6 hr

rosiglitazone maleate

Rosiglitazone maleate (Avandia) is classified as a glitazone or thiazolidinedione derivative. It is marketed for the treatment of patients with type 2 diabetes. Rosiglitazone and pioglitazone (Actos) can be used alone or with a sulfonylurea, metformin, or insulin. Thiazolidinedione antihyperglycemic drugs act by decreasing insulin resistance. As noted earlier, the safety of these drugs for use in pregnant women, children, and individuals with heart failure has not been established.

PHARMACOKINETICS

Half-Life	Onset	Peak	Duration
3–4 hr	Unknown	1 hr	Unknown

DOSAGES Selected Oral Antihyperglycemic Drugs

Drug (Pregnancy Category)	Pharmacological Class	Usual Dosage Range	Indications
acarbose (Glucobay) (B)	α-glucosidase inhibitor	*Adult* PO: 50–100 mg tid, taken with first bite of meal	Type 2 diabetes mellitus
chlorpropamide (Novo-Propamide) (C)	First-generation sulfonylurea	*Adult* PO: 100–500 mg daily	Type 2 diabetes mellitus
▸▸ gliclazide (Diamicron, Diamicron MR) (C)	Second-generation sulfonylurea	*Adult* PO: 80–320 mg daily (doses above 160 mg divided, bid) MR: 30–120 mg once daily	Type 2 diabetes mellitus
glimepiride (Amaryl) (C)	Second-generation sulfonylurea	*Adult* PO: 1–8 mg daily	Type 2 diabetes mellitus
▸▸ glyburide (Diaβeta, Eugulon, Med Glybe) (C)	Second-generation sulfonylurea	*Adult* PO: 2.5–20 mg/day with first meal	Type 2 diabetes mellitus
▸▸ metformin hydrochloride (Glucophage) (B)	Biguanide	*Children/Adult* PO: 500 mg tid–qid or 850 mg bid–tid daily; max daily dose 2550 mg for adults and 2000 mg for children 10–16 yr	Type 2 diabetes mellitus
repaglinide (GlucoNorm) (C)	Meglitinide	*Adult* PO: 0.5–4 mg tid taken with meals	Type 2 diabetes mellitus
▸▸ rosiglitazone maleate (Avandia) (C)	Thiazolidinedione	*Adult* PO: 4–8 mg divided once to twice daily	Type 2 diabetes mellitus
COMBINATION ORAL DRUGS rosiglitazone/glimepiride (Avandryl) (C)	Combination thiazolidinedione/ sulfonylurea	*Adult* PO: 4 mg/1 mg; 4 mg/2 mg; 4 mg/4 mg (1 tab) daily	Type 2 diabetes mellitus
rosiglitazone/ metformin (Avandemet) (C)	Combination thiazolidinedione/ biguanide	*Adult* PO: 4 mg /500 mg–8 mg/2000 mg bid	Type 2 diabetes mellitus

MR, modified release; *PO*, oral.

MISCELLANEOUS ANTIDIABETIC DRUGS

Amylin Mimetic

Pramlintide (Symlin; pregnancy category C), an *amylin mimetic* not yet available in Canada, is in clinical trials, being investigated as a potential antidiabetic drug. *Amylin* is a natural hormone protein in the body that is stored and secreted with insulin from the pancreas in response to food intake. It affects the postprandial blood levels of glucose in the following three ways:

1. It slows gastric emptying.
2. It suppresses glucagon secretion, which reduces liver glucose output.
3. It centrally modulates appetite and satiety (sense of having eaten enough).

Pramlintide acts by mimicking the action of amylin, thus enhancing the effects caused by the natural hormone. The drug is indicated for use in patients with type 1 or type 2 diabetes receiving mealtime insulin who have failed to achieve optimal glucose control with insulin and oral antidiabetic drugs. Its use is contraindicated in patients with known drug allergy (including allergy to its *metacresol* component), gastroparesis or other impaired gastrointestinal motility, hypoglycemia, or **hemoglobin A_{1c} (HbA$_{1c}$)** level of more than 9%; in patients who are poorly adherent to insulin therapy or self-monitoring of blood glucose level; and in children.

Adverse effects include self-limiting nausea, vomiting, and dizziness, especially in overdose. The drug itself does not cause hypoglycemia, but if the patient is taking a pre-prandial rapid- or short-acting insulin product, the insulin dose usually needs to be reduced by 50%. Pramlintide can delay the oral absorption of any drug and should be given at least 1 hour before any concentration-dependent oral medication (including oral contraceptives and anti-biotics). It can also alter insulin pharmacokinetics in the body and should not be mixed with any insulin products.

Recommended dosage ranges are from 15 to 60 mcg for type 1 diabetes and 60 to 120 mcg for type 2 diabetes, given before any major meal (defined as more than 250 kcal or more than 30 g of carbohydrates). The drug is given only by subcutaneous injection.

Incretin Mimetic

Another group of potential antidiabetic drugs comprises the *incretin mimetics*. *Incretins* are hormones that regulate the rate through which nutrients transit the gastrointestinal tract and thereby regulate the rate of delivery of nutrients such as glucose into the circulation. These actions occur because incretins have a powerful effect on gastrointestinal motility, particularly gastric emptying. In addition, they stimulate production of insulin from the pancreas and have other hormonal actions. The result is reduction of both fasting and postprandial glucose concentrations in patients with type 2 diabetes. There are two major *incretins* that have been studied: glucagon-like peptide-1 (GLP-1) and glucose-dependent insulinotropic peptide (GIP).

Exenatide is currently being investigated in Canada. Exenatide (Byetta; pregnancy category C) is a GLP-1 receptor agonist that acts by *mimicking incretin and thereby binding to and positively enhancing the GLP-1 receptor activity*. Exenatide is indicated only for patients with type 2 diabetes and is contraindicated in those with drug allergy or type 1 diabetes. Possible adverse effects include hypoglycemia, dizziness, and nausea. Like pramlintide, this drug can delay absorption of other orally administered drugs because of its slowing of gastric emptying. In patients who also receive metformin, the metformin dose does not need to be changed because metformin does not cause hypoglycemia. However, in patients taking sulfonylurea drugs the dose may need to be reduced if hypoglycemia appears on initiation of exenatide therapy. The usual starting dosage is 5 mcg within 1 hour of both the morning and evening meals. If needed, the dosage may be increased to 10 mcg twice daily before meals after 1 month on the 5 mcg dose. Factors influencing exenatide's implementation are cost and the lack of information about its effect on diabetic complications, as well as the use of other antidiabetic medications.

Inhaled Insulin

The drug Exubera, an inhaled insulin product, was withdrawn from the market by the manufacturer Pfizer because it was not shown to be more effective than injected insulin, dosages could not be adjusted as easily as injected insulin, and it had the potential risk of lung problems.

Dipeptidyl Peptidase-4 Inhibitors

A new class of drugs aimed at controlling incretin levels in the body is the dipeptidyl peptidase-4 (DPP-4) inhibitors. Sitagliptin (Januvia) is the only drug of this class available in Canada. DPP-4 is an enzyme found in many tissues of the body. This enzyme rapidly breaks down the incretin hormones. A DPP-4 inhibitor such as stialiptin slows the breakdown of incretins, thus increasing their elimination half-life (keeping them active for a longer period of time), and assists in regulating blood glucose levels. Stiagliptin is highly specific for the DPP-4 receptor and lowers blood glucose. Combination therapy with metformin provides dramatic improvements in blood glucose levels. The usual dosage is a daily dosage of 100 mg. Adverse effects include sore throat, headache, and diarrhea.

HYPOGLYCEMIA

Hypoglycemia is an abnormally low blood glucose level (generally below 2.8 mmol/L). When the cause is organic and the effects are mild, treatment usually consists of dietary modifications, primarily a higher intake of protein and lower intake of carbohydrates, to prevent a rebound postprandial hypoglycemic effect. Hypoglycemia is also a common adverse effect of many antidiabetic drugs when their pharmacological effects are greater than expected. Because the brain needs a constant amount of glucose to function, early symptoms of hypoglycemia include the central nervous system (CNS) manifestations of confusion, irritability, tremor, and sweating. Later symptoms include hypothermia and seizures. Without adequate restoration of normal blood and CNS glucose levels, coma and death will occur.

GLUCOSE-ELEVATING DRUGS

Oral forms of concentrated glucose are available for patients to use in the event of a hypoglycemic crisis. Dosage forms of these include rapidly dissolving buccal tablets and semisolid gel forms designed for oral use and rapid mucosal absorption. Table sugar, which is sucrose, will not produce as rapid an effect as the glucose products intended for use by patients with diabetes because sucrose is a *disaccharide* (two-molecule) sugar that must first be digested in the body to yield glucose as a *monosaccharide* (one-molecule) byproduct. In the hospital setting, intravenous glucose is an obvious option. Concentrations of up to 50% dextrose in water (D50W) are most often used for this purpose. Although solutions with glucose concentrations of up to 70% are also available, these are usually used for total parenteral nutrition (TPN) preparations rather than acute treatment of hypoglycemia.

In addition to oral and intravenous glucose, two other drugs are specifically used for the treatment of hypoglycemia. Glucagon, a natural hormone secreted by the pancreas, has been synthesized in the laboratory and is now available as an injection to be given when a quick response to hypoglycemia is needed. Diazoxide is another drug that may be given to correct abnormally low blood glucose levels. It works by inhibiting the release of insulin from the pancreas and is most commonly given to patients with long-term illnesses that are causing hypoglycemia. An example of such an illness is pancreatic cancer, which causes the pancreas to oversecrete insulin, resulting in too much insulin in the blood, or hyperinsulinemia. The oral form of diazoxide is used for these purposes. There is also an intravenous form used for the treatment of hypertensive emergencies (very high blood pressure) in critical care unit settings.

PHARMACOKINETIC BRIDGE TO NURSING PRACTICE

Provision of insulin therapy by continuous subcutaneous insulin infusion (CSII) is becoming an option for selected patients with diabetes to minimize the risks and complications of the disease. Other treatment options used to achieve tight control are multiple daily injections of insulin (MDI), but the onset, peak, and duration of action of the drug will depend on the specific insulin used. With CSII, normal serum glucose levels are maintained by the continuous delivery of basal insulin with food intake, primarily carbohydrate consumption, being covered by bolus doses of insulin. Insulin pumps (e.g., CSII) lead to a more rapid, consistent absorption of the drug, and hypoglycemia is reduced. Research has also shown that use of an insulin pump helps to decrease the occurrence of elevated prebreakfast serum glucose levels, or what is often called the *dawn phenomenon* (referring to the dawn of the day). Because the insulin pump delivers insulin through the subcutaneous route and the infusion is a continuous one, fewer problems occur that were previously associated with once- or twice-daily injections. Patients using CSII achieve mean serum glucose and HbA_{1c} levels that remain somewhat lower than those associated with MDI, thus creating less risk for hypoglycemia. With a thorough understanding of new and different drugs (with their associated pharmacokinetic properties), the nurse can help patients achieve a higher quality of life, minimize risks, and maximize wellness.

NURSING PROCESS

◩ Assessment

Before administering any type of antidiabetic drug, the nurse must assess the patient's knowledge about the disease and recommended treatments. Head-to-toe physical assessment, medication history, and nursing assessment need to be completed and documented. A medication history should include a list of current medications, including over-the-counter (OTC) drugs and natural health products. Assessment of appropriate laboratory test results (e.g., fasting blood glucose level, HbA_{1c} level) should include any abnormalities compared with baseline levels. The physician's order for insulin must also be assessed so that the correct route, type of insulin (e.g., clear [rapid- or short-acting] or cloudy [intermediate-acting or NPH]), and dosage are implemented correctly. With assessment, it is important to note that allergic reactions are less likely to occur with recombinant human insulins than with porcine insulins because of the former's similarity with endogenous insulin. Contraindications, cautions, and drug interactions associated with the various forms of insulin (discussed in the pharmacology section)

should be thoroughly assessed prior to giving any insulin. Oral antihyperglycemic drugs also require close assessment of contraindications, cautions, and drug interactions. Other drugs that have chemical–structural similarity with sulfonylureas (e.g., furosemide, sulfamethoxazole) need to be noted because of the increased risk for cross-sensitivity. See Table 32-8 on special considerations for use of the different antidiabetic medications.

Diabetes in people over the age of 60 is metabolically distinct and the management should differ from that in individuals under the age of 60. Lifestyle interventions are effective in preventing diabetes in the older adult at high risk for developing diabetes. Rosiglitazone and acarbose are effective in preventing diabetes in the high-risk older adult, whereas metformin is not. As the risk for hypoglycemia increases with age, sulfonylureas should be used cautiously. The initial dose is one half of the dose used for younger individuals. Gliclazide and gliclaside MR and glimepiride are preferred because of reduced hypoglycemia. The use of premixed insulins and insulin pens minimizes dosage errors and improves glycemic control.

The nurse must also be aware that malnourished older adults may react adversely to the biguanide metformin. Contraindications, cautions, and drug interactions for this drug class (discussed previously in the pharmacology section), as well as the interaction between metformin and the radiopaque dyes used for certain diagnostic purposes (e.g., computed tomography [CT] scan with contrast), must be considered. This interaction is associated with an increased risk for kidney dysfunction. With thiazolidinediones, one important caution is their use in patients with elevated ALT levels. Baseline ALT levels should thus be measured before drug therapy is begun and periodically thereafter (e.g., every 3 months or as ordered).

Unstable serum glucose levels require immediate attention, so any signs and symptoms of hypoglycemia (e.g., acute onset of nervousness, sweating, lethargy, weakness, cold and clammy skin, change in sensorium) or symptoms of hyperglycemia (e.g., tachycardia, blood glucose levels that exceed 8 mmol/L, changes in respiration [Kussmaul's respiration]) must be assessed. Assessment is even more critical for a patient with diabetes who is under stress, has an infection or is ill, is pregnant or lactating, or is experiencing trauma or any change in health status. When receiving treatment, patients with diabetes are at risk of hypoglycemia, with the potential danger of losing consciousness; constant assessment of serum glucose levels and neurological status is thus required.

Ethnocultural factors must also be considered in relation to adherence to a therapeutic regimen. See Ethnocultural Implications: Type 2 Diabetes Among the Canadian Aboriginal Population as an example.

◩ Nursing Diagnoses

- Risk for injury related to neurological deficits (e.g., neuropathies) associated with diabetes mellitus

TABLE 32-8

Considerations for the Use of Antihyperglycemic Drugs and Insulin

Drug	Children Considerations	Pregnancy and Lactation Considerations	Older Adult Considerations
gliclazide glimepiride	Safety and efficacy not established	Not recommended in pregnancy; unknown if this drug crosses into breast milk	Hypoglycemia is more difficult to identify in the older adult. Age-related kidney dysfunction may increase sensitivity to the glucose-lowering action.
glyburide	Safety and efficacy not established	Crosses the placenta and is found in breast milk; not recommended for pregnant or lactating women	Age-related kidney dysfunction may lead to toxic effects and significant risk of hypoglycemic responses.
insulin	No age-related precautions in children; use of insulin lispro contraindicated in children younger than 18 years of age	Drug of choice for treatment during pregnancy; not secreted into breast milk, but lactation may decrease actual insulin requirements	The older adult with altered visual, cognitive, or motor abilities may have difficulty maintaining safe adherence to the drug regimen.
metformin	Safety and efficacy not established	Distributed into breast milk in animals	The older adult may require dosage adjustment if kidney dysfunction occurs. Negligible risk of hypoglycemia as monotherapy
nateglinide repaglinide	Safety and efficacy not established	Unknown if these drugs are distributed into breast milk	No age-related precautions, but the older adult is more prone to hypoglycemia (negligible if used as monotherapy)
pioglitazone rosiglitazone	Safety and efficacy not established	Unknown if these drugs cross the placenta or if they are distributed into breast milk; not recommended for pregnant or lactating women	No age-related concerns

 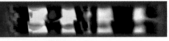

ETHNOCULTURAL IMPLICATIONS

Type 2 Diabetes Among the Canadian Aboriginal Population

- The prevalence of type 2 diabetes in Canadian Aboriginal children aged 5 to 18 years is approximately 1%; the Plains Cree in Central Canada have the highest prevalence.
- Aboriginal people are diagnosed with type 2 diabetes at a younger age.
- Aboriginal women have greater than two times the risk of developing gestational diabetes compared with that for non-Aboriginal women; they also have a higher prevalence of pre-existing type 2 diabetes during pregnancy. An increased prevalence of prediabetes and metabolic syndrome exists among them as well.
- Cardiovascular disease, peripheral artery disease, neuropathy, and kidney disease are more common complications in the Aboriginal population.

- Genetic susceptibility and local genetic mutations combined with social stressors, high rates of physical inactivity, and diets composed of refined sugars contribute to the high rates of diabetes in the Aboriginal population.
- Screening for diabetes in individuals with risk factors should be done every 1 to 2 years.
- Primary prevention programs must be ethnoculturally sensitive and initiated by Aboriginal communities to empower individuals and promote change.
- Various communities in the provinces/territories are taking action to identify and manage diabetes, such as the Aboriginal Diabetes Wellness Program in northern Alberta and the Ontario Aboriginal Diabetes Strategy.

- Risk for infection related to the pathological impact of diabetes associated with altered immune system function
- Imbalanced nutrition, more than body requirements, leading to weight gain associated with diabetes mellitus

- Deficient knowledge related to lack of information about diabetes mellitus, its management, and the prevention of disease-related complications
- Ineffective therapeutic regimen management related to lack of experience with a significant daily treatment regimen

☑ Planning

■ Goals

- Patient will remain free from injury and complications of diabetes.
- Patient will remain free of infection.
- Patient will maintain adequate weight control and dietary habits in the overall management of diabetes.
- Patient will state the effects of diabetes on body function.
- Patient will remain adherent to the medical regimen and adhere to treatment protocols.
- Patient will state the importance of adherence to drug regimens, lifestyle changes, dietary restrictions, and high-risk behaviours.
- Patient will state the action and adverse effects of insulin or the oral antihyperglycemic drugs.

■ Outcome Criteria

- Patient performs self-assessment and foot care as directed and as needed to maintain healthy skin.
- Patient immediately reports elevated temperature, lesions or sores that do not heal well, and any unusual redness of any area to the health care provider.
- Patient observes the diet recommended by the Canadian Diabetes Association or other dietary advisor according to the physician's orders or nutritional consult.
- Patient eats a healthy diet, gets sufficient rest and relaxation, and notifies the physician should any unusual problems occur with changes in customary activity (e.g., nausea and vomiting).
- Patient keeps all scheduled appointments with health care providers to monitor therapeutic effectiveness and assess for complications of therapy.
- Patient takes medication as scheduled, monitors blood glucose levels, and watches for any signs and symptoms of hyperglycemia or hypoglycemia.

☑ Implementation

With any patient who is to receive insulin or oral anti-hyperglycemic drugs, the nurse must always check the blood glucose levels (and other related laboratory values) before administering the drug so that accurate baseline glucose levels are obtained and available if the prepared dosage should be carried out with another registered nurse. Insulin should be rolled between the hands before the prescribed dosage is withdrawn to avoid air getting in the syringe and prevent inaccurate dosage administration. Insulin may be stored at room temperature if it is to be used within 1 month; otherwise, it must be refrigerated. Refrigeration is also recommended in warm or hot climates or temperatures. If insulin is discoloured or past the expiry date, it should not be used. For information about the handling, mixing, storage, and administration of insulin see Box 32-4.

Insulin should be administered subcutaneously at a 90-degree angle unless the patient is emaciated, in which case it is administered at a 45-degree angle. Only regular insulin may be administered intravenously; however, this route is controversial because of absorption of the insulin into the intravenous bag and tubing. Only insulin syringes should be used; they are easy to identify because they have orange caps and are calibrated in units, not millilitres (mL). The syringe has an ultrafine preattached needle that is 29 gauge (and 12.7 mm [½ inch] in length). When mixing insulins (if ordered), the regular or rapid-acting insulin (unmodified and *clear*) should be withdrawn first, followed by withdrawal of the intermediate-acting or NPH (modified and cloudy) insulin, but only after the appropriate amount of air has been injected (which is equal to the prescribed number of units) into the vials. Air should be injected into the intermediate insulin vial, followed by injection of air into the regular or rapid- or short-acting insulin vial. This helps prevent contamination of the rapid-acting insulin by the intermediate-acting insulin (see Table 32-3 and Chapter 10). Some fixed combinations of insulin products come premixed.

Understanding the action of the insulin and its related pharmacokinetics (e.g., onset, peak, duration) is critical to safe care and for patient education. For example, it is important to know that lispro insulin is more rapidly absorbed than regular insulin, with an onset of action of 15 minutes and peak effect of 1 to 2 hours, so lispro must be given 15 minutes before meals, compared with 30 minutes before meals with regular insulin. Lispro insulin mixed with NPH should be given immediately after the insulins are mixed and also 15 minutes before meals. The physician's orders should be checked for any dietary changes (e.g., possible increase in carbohydrates and decrease in fat intake to avoid postprandial hypoglycemia).

Regardless of whether porcine or recombinant human insulin is used, understanding the peak, onset, and duration of action of the specific insulin will help the nurse determine when the drug should be taken. The intermediate-acting insulins, such as NPH and the many combination products of regular and intermediate insulin, have onsets of action ranging from 30 minutes to 1 to 2 hours; therefore, the nurse must work with this time interval to ensure that the patient eats at the correct time (i.e., immediately before or at the time of onset of action). In the hospital setting, meal trays must arrive on the unit before giving insulin to avoid time lapses and subsequent hypoglycemic episodes. The nurse must also be sure that other forms of allowed foods are available to the patient in case meals are delayed and insulin has already been administered.

Patients may require dosing by a sliding-scale method, which includes subcutaneous regular insulin doses adjusted according to serum glucose test results. Sliding scale may be used for hospitalized diabetic patients experiencing drastic changes in serum glucose levels due to physical or emotional stress, infections, surgery, acute

BOX 32-4   Administration, Handling, and Storage of Insulin

Dosages, Storage, Handling, and Mixing

1. Individualize insulin dosages (e.g., use sliding scales as ordered) and monitor closely for adequate control of hypoglycemia and hyperglycemia.

2. Adjust dosages, as ordered, to achieve premeal and bedtime serum glucose levels of 5 mmol/L to 7 mmol/L in adults.

3. Store insulin for current use at room temperature. Avoid extreme temperatures and exposure to sunlight because the insulin's protein structure will be permanently denatured. Extra vials not in use should be stored in the refrigerator. Vials being used in high environmental temperatures should also be stored in the refrigerator, but insulin should *never* be given cold. Never freeze insulin. To maintain drug stability, insulin should be stored for up to 1 month at room temperature and for up to 3 months in the refrigerator.

4. Discard unused vials if they have not been used for several weeks (or follow hospital policy). Do not use any insulin that does not have the proper clarity or colour (e.g., clear for regular, cloudy for NPH).

5. Store prefilled insulin syringes in the refrigerator for up to 1 week. Store the syringe with the needle pointing upward to avoid clogging within the hub of the needle.

Administration

1. Administer insulin subcutaneously (see Chapter 10); however, regular insulin may be given intravenously in special situations (e.g., drip in patient with diabetic ketoacidosis; in postoperative patients) if ordered.

2. Roll the drug vial gently between the hands without shaking to avoid bubble formation in the vial, which may lead to inaccurate dosage withdrawal (regular insulin does not need to be rolled). Give mixed insulins within 5 minutes of mixing to avoid binding of the solution and subsequent altered activity of the drugs. Premixed insulin suspensions should not be used if the precipitate has become lumpy or granular in appearance or has formed a deposit of solid particles on the wall of the vial or cartridge. These insulin suspensions should also not be used if the contents remain clear after the vial or cartridge has been shaken carefully.

3. Administer insulin at the recommended times, but always with meals or meal trays ready. Give insulin lispro approximately 15 minutes before meals (it has a quicker onset of action) and only after monitoring the patient's fasting serum glucose level (as with all insulin administration). Give regular and rapid-acting insulin 30 minutes before a meal, and give NPH insulin 30 to 45 minutes before mealtime.

4. When giving regular and NPH insulin at the same time (if ordered), mix the two appropriately (see discussion of mixing insulins in the Implementation subsection under Nursing Process). This mixture is usually given at least 30 minutes before mealtime.

5. Administer insulin subcutaneously at a 90-degree angle in most cases. If the patient is emaciated, a 45-degree angle may be more effective. Insulin syringes should always be used (see previous discussion and Chapter 10).

6. The abdomen provides the most consistent and rapid site for injection of insulin. Instruct patients taking insulin injections to rotate sites within the same general location for about 1 week before moving to a new location (e.g., all injections for a week in the upper right thigh before moving a little lower on the right thigh). This technique allows for better insulin absorption. Each injection site should be at least 0.5 to 1 inch away from the previous injection site. If this practice is followed, it will be approximately 6 weeks before the patient will have to rotate to a totally new area of the body. Note the following sites for subcutaneous insulin injections: thigh areas (front and back) and outer areas of the upper arm (middle third of the upper arm between the shoulder and the elbow).

7. Continuous subcutaneous insulin injections, multiple daily injections, or both may be ordered for tight glucose control.

---

illness, inactivity, or variable caloric intake, as well as in patients needing intensive insulin therapy. When this insulin regimen is used, blood glucose levels are measured several times a day (e.g., every 4 hours, every 6 hours, or at specified times such as 0700, 1100, 1600 hours, and midnight) to obtain fasting and premeal blood glucose values.

Oral antihyperglycemic drugs are usually administered at least 30 minutes before meals. Some sulfonylureas are to be taken with breakfast, α-glucosidase inhibitors are always to be taken with the first mouthful of each main meal, and the thiazolidinediones are to be given once daily or in two divided doses. Exact timing of the dose should always be checked against the physician's order and with consideration of the drug's onset of action. With any antihyperglycemic drug or insulin, it is important for the nurse and patient to know what to do if symptoms of hypoglycemia occur; for example, the patient should take glucagon; eat glucose tablets or gel, corn syrup, or honey; drink fruit juice or a nondiet soft drink; or eat a small snack such as crackers or half a sandwich. It is critical to the safe and efficient use of oral antidiabetics that food will be or is being tolerated before the dose is given. If the oral drug or insulin is taken and no meal is consumed or it is consumed at a later time than usual, the hypoglycemia may be problematic and result in negative health consequences and possible unconsciousness.

If the patient receiving metformin is to undergo diagnostic studies with contrast dye, the physician will need to discontinue the drug prior to the procedure and restart it after the tests, only after re-evaluation of the patient's kidney status. Because rosiglitazone and pioglitazone may both cause moderate weight gain and edema, it is important to weigh the patient daily at the same time every day and with the same amount of clothing. Several combination drug products are also available, including rosiglitazone plus metformin as well as rosiglitazone plus glimepiride, which should be given exactly as prescribed.

In special situations (e.g., the patient is NPO and is taking either an oral antihyperglycemic drug or insulin), it is crucial for the nurse to follow the physician's orders regarding drug administration. If there are no written orders about this situation, make sure to contact the physician for further instructions. If a patient is on NPO status but is receiving an intravenous solution of dextrose, the physician may still order insulin, but this should always be clarified. The physician should also be contacted if a patient becomes ill and unable to take the usual dosage of an oral antidiabetic drug (or insulin). Patients should always wear a medical alert bracelet, necklace, or tag with the diagnosis, list of medications, and emergency contact information.

It is also important that the nurse stay informed and up-to-date about the latest research on diabetes. For example, there is a strong correlation between diabetes and heart disease, and microvascular problems are recognized as occurring at FPG levels of 7 mmol/L. As noted earlier, the Canadian Diabetes Association recommends that all adults 40 years of age and older be tested for elevated FPG levels every 3 years. Lifestyle changes for patients with high FPG levels may include decreased alcohol consumption, regular exercise to help lower blood glucose levels by increasing insulin sensitivity, and periodic medical follow-up. See Evidence-Informed Practice: Optimal Glycemic Control for more information on specific nursing research related to diabetes and its application to nursing practice. The Case Study gives an example of nursing implementation.

In summary, there are many nursing considerations related to drug therapy in patients with diabetes mellitus. Patient education is very important and should begin the moment the patient has entered the health care system or upon diagnosis. Instruction tailored to the patient's educational level and given with the use of appropriate teaching–learning concepts and teaching aids can be crucial to patient adherence. The nurse should be sure that all resources are made available to patients (e.g., financial assistance, visual assistance, dietary plans, daily menus, CDA information, transportation assistance, and Meals on Wheels and other community resources). See Patient Education for more specific information.

Evaluation

It is important for the nurse to understand current therapeutic guidelines. The prevailing key diagnostic criterion for diabetes mellitus is hyperglycemia with an FPG of higher than 7 mmol/L; however, the therapeutic response to insulin and any of the oral antidiabetic drugs is a decrease in blood glucose to the level prescribed by the physician or to near-normal levels. Most often, fasting blood glucose levels (not less than 4 mmol/L or greater than 5.5 mmol/L, or a level designated by the physician) are used to measure the degree of glycemic control. To measure the patient's adherence to the therapy regimen for several months previously, the level of HbA_{1c} is measured. This value reflects how well the patient has been managing diet and drug therapy.

Patients with diabetes need to be monitored frequently by health care providers (as well as at home) to make sure that they are adhering to the therapy regimen as evidenced by normalization of blood test results. Monitor the patient for indications of hypoglycemia or hyperglycemia and insulin allergy. With insulin lispro, because the onset of action is more rapid than with regular insulin and the duration of action is shorter, it is crucial for the nurse and the patient to monitor blood glucose levels very closely until the dosage is regulated and blood glucose is at the level the physician desires. Should a patient be changed from one insulin or oral antidiabetic drug to another, glucose levels must be monitored very closely at home or by the health care professional. Always evaluate whether identified goals and outcome criteria are being met, and plan nursing care accordingly.

EVIDENCE-INFORMED PRACTICE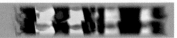

Optimal Glycemic Control

Background
Research has confirmed that optimal glycemic control often achieved through intensive insulin therapy, though it carries many challenges, can help some patients with diabetes reduce complications and experience a better quality of life. More than 1.8 million Canadians, or 5.5% of the population, have diabetes mellitus, and serious complications and organ damage can result from the pathological process. Heart disease, kidney disease, vascular disease, blindness, and amputations are the most common of the severely debilitating and fatal complications. One possible regimen that can minimize risks and major complications and allow a more normal lifestyle is intensive insulin therapy, given by means of continuous subcutaneous insulin infusions (CSII) via a pump or through multiple daily injections (MDI). Research has shown that tight insulin control through intensive therapy may well be the way to reduce morbidity and mortality.

Type of Evidence
The Diabetes Control and Complications Trial (DCCT) compared intensive therapy with conventional therapy in a population of 1441 teenagers and young adults with type 1 diabetes. Intensive therapy involved hospitalization for stabilization of the disease and for patient education, frequent dosing of insulin guided by the results of at least four serum glucose tests a day, four daily insulin injections or use of insulin pump, monthly office visits, frequent telephone calls between the patients and nurse educators, dietary consultation, and exercise. Follow-up investigations occurred 4 years later.

Results of Study
The study found a 39% to 76% reduction in the incidence of complications associated with diabetes in those receiving intensive therapy. Specifically, the findings of the DCCT showed that lowering blood glucose levels reduced the risk of eye disease by 75%, of kidney disease by 50%, and of nerve disease by 60%. DCCT participants were not expected to have many heart-related problems because their average age was 27 years when the study was initiated; however, electrocardiography, blood pressure tests, and serum laboratory tests of lipid levels were performed for all participants to look for signs of cardiovascular disease. The study showed that the participants who received intensive therapy had significantly lower risks of developing hyperlipidemia and subsequent cardiovascular and coronary heart disease. The risks of intensive therapy identified in the DCCT included hypoglycemia severe enough to require the assistance of another individual. Because of this risk, DCCT researchers did not recommend intensive therapy for patients younger than 13 years of age, patients with heart disease or advanced complications, older adults, or patients with a history of frequent severe hypoglycemia.

A follow-up investigation 4 years later (in 1997), the Epidemiology of Diabetes Interventions and Complications study, found that the original intensive-therapy group continued to have a lower risk of eye, nerve, and kidney disease, even though control had become less intensive. In 2003, some 6 years later, the patients still had reduced rates of nerve damage. Because of the long-term nature of the study and the moderately sized research sample, the results hold promise for the treatment of diabetics in those individuals willing to invest the required time, energy, and lifestyle changes.

Link of Evidence to Nursing Practice
Patients who are the best candidates for CSII are those who are diligent and committed to self-management of their diabetes, are willing to spend the time it takes to record serum glucose levels and insulin values in a journal four or more times a day, will make monthly or more frequent visits to their health care providers, and are able to monitor carbohydrate intake closely. Individuals who have motor or cognitive impairments and those who are not committed to the intensive therapy may be unable to adhere to the strict regimen. The evidence strongly indicates the value of tight control of glucose levels in reducing long-term complications associated with diabetes. Not all patients are willing to spend the time and effort required to achieve tight glucose control, and the regimen is very stressful; however, every patient has the right to be informed of this option and its associated benefits and risks.

This study produced ground-breaking results and has made an impact on the care of diabetic patients today. Many of the 1441 participants have been involved in the research for more than 20 years. To obtain more information for patients, see the Canadian Diabetes Association Web site (http://www.diabetes.ca). In practising evidence-informed nursing, nurses look at new treatment approaches and their potential for improving patient care, as with the new therapy examined in this study. Although the costs of intensive therapy are high, they are offset by the decrease in other medical expenses related to the complications of diabetes and by the improved quality of life.

Based on National Institute of Diabetes and Digestive and Kidney Diseases (2004). *National diabetes statistics, 2004.* Available at http:/diabetes.niddk.nih.gov/dm/pubs/statistics/index.htm; Dow N (2005). Tight insulin control: Making it work. *RN 68*(7):44–52; National Institute of Diabetes and Digestive and Kidney Diseases (2001). *Diabetes Control and Complications Trial (DCCT).* Available at http://diabetes.niddk.nih.gov/dm/pubs/control; American Diabetes Association (2004). *Intensive diabetes control yields less nerve damage years later.* Available at www.diabetes.org/for-media/2004-press-releases/neuropathy.jsp.

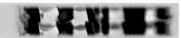

CASE STUDY

Diabetes Mellitus

B.G. is a 58-year-old man who received a diagnosis of type 2 adult-onset diabetes mellitus 10 years ago; he has needed to take insulin for the last 2 years. He has been recovering, without complications, from a laparoscopic cholecystectomy; however, his blood glucose levels have shown significant fluctuations over the last 24 hours. The physician has changed his insulin to lispro (Humalog) to evaluate whether there is any better control of his blood glucose levels.

1. What is the rationale for the use of oral antihyperglycemic drugs in a patient with type 2 diabetes? Why do some patients with type 2 diabetes need to begin taking insulin? What can be done to measure the control of the patient's diabetes over the short term and long term?

2. What are the pharmacokinetics related to lispro?

3. What special instructions, if any, should be given to B.G. about lispro before he is discharged home from the hospital?

For answers see http://evolve.elsevier.com/Canada/Lilley/pharmacology/.

IN MY FAMILY

Fenugreek Seeds

(as told by M.P., of Indian (Hindu) descent)

"To help lower their blood sugar, my grandparents [and M.P.'s father] incorporate the use of fenugreek as an adjunct to their prescribed medication [of Metformin 2× 500 mg]. . . . The fenugreek seeds are soaked in water overnight and then consumed with milk first thing in the morning. . . . After he [M.P.'s father] started consuming the fenugreek seeds, he noticed that his blood sugar levels had decreased significantly. According to my father and grandparents, they have not experienced any side effects from using fenugreek along with Metformin, although my grandmother says that pregnant women are not advised to consume this mixture because it relaxes the uterus."

PATIENT EDUCATION

- ❖ Patients should always be encouraged to wear a medical alert bracelet or necklace and to carry a medical alert card.

- ❖ Patients should be instructed on drawing up insulin, its storage, the equipment needed, mixing (if ordered) insulins, and the technique for insulin injections. Demonstrate how to draw up the prescribed dose of insulin, how to inject the drug properly, how to rotate insulin injection sites, and how to keep notes in a journal.

- ❖ Patients should be instructed on how to monitor blood (serum) glucose levels at the prescribed intervals, and the specific glucometer machine's instructions should be emphasized. Thorough instructions about the importance of exercise, hygiene, foot care, the prescribed dietary plan, and weight control should also be given.

- ❖ Patients should be encouraged to avoid smoking and alcohol, follow all dietary instructions, and never skip meals or skip insulin.

- ❖ Patients should be instructed on the difference between hypoglycemia and hyperglycemia (see Hypoglycemia and Hyperglycemia sections for specific signs and symptoms), and emphasize the treatment of each—for example, having quick sources of glucose on hand (such as candy, sugar packets, OTC glucose tablets, sugar cubes, honey, corn syrup, orange juice, and nondiet soda beverages) for hypoglycemia, and having more insulin on hand for hyperglycemia. Encourage patients to have quick dosage forms of glucose available at all times!

- ❖ Patients should be informed about situations or conditions that lead to altered serum glucose (e.g., fever, illness, stress, increased activity or exercise, surgery, emotional distress). Encourage the patient to contact their health care provider if any of these occur.

- ❖ Patients should be educated about the importance of knowing premeal blood glucose levels prior to taking insulin and that insulin is given in relation to meal times, specifically breakfast.

- ❖ Patients should be instructed to store insulin at room temperature, unless the patient is travelling or is in a hot climate, because heat will alter insulin.

- ❖ Patients should be taught the importance of having adequate supplies of insulin and equipment and making sure to store them safely and away from children. If needed, magnifying-glass attachments are available for syringes and vials.

Continued

- Patients should be given a demonstration of mixing of insulins (see Chapter 10 and previous discussion in this chapter) and rotation of injection sites.
- Patients should be informed to notify the physician if the patient notes any yellow discoloration of the skin, dark urine, fever, sore throat, weakness, or unusual bleeding or easy bruising (with any antidiabetic drug regimen).
- Patients should be encouraged to review Canadian Diabetes Association (CDA) recommendations for fasting blood glucose level measurement. For adults, the CDA recommends maintaining preprandial glucose levels of 4 to 7 mmol/L, peak postprandial levels of 10 mmol/L, and a glycosylated hemoglobin (HbA_{1c}) level below 7%.
- Patients should be taught the importance of HbA_{1c} monitoring (e.g., at least two times a year for those with good glycemic control; quarterly for patients not at goal, having changed their therapy, or not being adherent to the therapy). These recommendations apply to patients taking oral antidiabetic drugs as well.
- Patients should be encouraged to review lifestyle modifications, including weight control and glucose level maintenance with diet and exercise, drug therapy, or a combination of these strategies. Patients with type 2 diabetes will have a greater therapeutic response to diet and exercise and glucose level control than will those with type 1 diabetes. Follow CDA recommendations for fasting serum glucose level measurement. Educate patients about the importance of supervised exercise until their condition stabilizes. A nutritional consult may be needed, with specific menu planning to help the patient with changes in intake (e.g., low-fat diet with 160 to 300 g of carbohydrates).
- Patients should be taught the importance of CDA recommendations for control of diabetes—for example, 150 minutes of moderate- to vigorous-intensity aerobics each week, spread over at least 3 days of the week as well as resistance exercise three times per week. For patients with any neurological changes in

the extremities due to diabetes, exercise will most likely include use of a treadmill, prolonged walking, swimming or aquatic aerobics, bicycling, rowing, chair exercises, arm exercises, and non–weight-bearing exercises.
- Patients with any form of diabetes should be advised that lifelong treatment and control, with strict management of drug therapy and glucose monitoring, are critical to reducing complications.
- Patients should be instructed to perform strict foot care, beginning with assessment of feet and toes every day. Other actions to prevent infections of the foot and possible gangrene (from diabetes-induced decreased circulation) include the following:
  • Soaking feet daily or as ordered in lukewarm water (a thermometer may be needed to check water), with adequate drying and application of moisturizing lotion afterward
  • Checking feet and legs for colour, temperature, edema, and the appearance of any open sores or reddened areas
  • Contacting the health care provider for further instructions if there is suspicion of any type of wound or alteration in skin intactness
  • Having frequent pedicures and trimming of nails done by a podiatrist or a licensed, certified individual
  • Reporting any unusual changes in the skin and intactness of the feet or nails or nail beds
- Patients should be educated about not skipping meals or medications; if problems with either occur, patients should contact their health care provider.
- Some of the oral antihyperglycemic drugs cause sensitivity to light, thus patients should always wear protective eyewear and sunscreen and avoid unprotected sun exposure (including use of tanning beds).
- Patients should be advised that some oral antihyperglycemic drugs interact negatively with alcohol and cause a disulfiram-type reaction characterized by acute illness with vomiting and hypertension.

POINTS TO REMEMBER

- Insulin normally facilitates removal of glucose from the blood and its storage as glycogen in the liver.
- Type 1 diabetes mellitus was formerly known as insulin-dependent diabetes (IDDM) or juvenile-onset diabetes. Little or no endogenous insulin is produced by individuals with type 1 diabetes. It is much less common than type 2 diabetes and affects only about 10% of all patients. Patients with type 1 diabetes usually are not obese.
- The primary treatment for type 1 diabetes mellitus is insulin therapy. Patients with type 2 diabetes are not generally prescribed insulin until other measures—lifestyle changes and oral drug therapy—no longer provide adequate glycemic control.
- There are currently two main sources of insulin. It can be extracted from domesticated animals or synthesized in laboratories using recombinant deoxyribonucleic acid (DNA) technology. Insulin was originally isolated

from cattle, but beef-derived insulin is no longer available because of the risk of "mad cow" disease.
- For those with type 2 diabetes, effective treatment involves several elements, including lifestyle modifications (e.g., diet, exercise, smoking cessation), careful monitoring of blood glucose levels, and possibly therapy with one or more drugs. If normal blood glucose levels are not achieved after 2 to 3 months of lifestyle modifications, treatment with an oral antihyperglycemic drug is often prescribed.
- Complications associated with diabetes include retinopathy, neuropathy, nephropathy, hypertension, cardiovascular disease, and coronary artery disease.
- The nurse should always check for allergies to specific medications and to pork before giving insulin.
- Patients need to learn the signs and symptoms of hypoglycemia and hyperglycemia and the methods of treating them at home. They also need to know when to contact the physician.

Continued

❖ A quick form of glucose should be kept available for patients taking arcabose because of the hypoglycemic reactions associated with this type of oral hypoglycemic. The nurse should make sure that patients know to keep such forms of glucose accessible for management at home.

❖ Review CDA recommendations for fasting serum glucose levels (e.g., maintenance of preprandial glucose levels of 4 to 7 mmol/L, peak postprandial levels of 10 mmol/L, and a glycosylated hemoglobin [HbA_{1c}] level below 7%).

❖ Exact timing of the dose of insulin or oral antidiabetic drug should always be carefully checked against the physician's order and with consideration of the drug's pharmacokinetics, including onset of action, peak, and duration of action.

❖ Information on foot care and the prevention of infection should be part of the patient education given to individuals with diabetes.

❖ The techniques of continuous subcutaneous insulin infusions (CSII) and multiple daily injections (MDI) hold promise for patients by giving them tight control of serum glucose levels, which can help decrease the complications of diabetes.

❖ The nurse must remember that oral antidiabetic drugs are not to be used in pregnant women.

EXAMINATION REVIEW QUESTIONS

1 Which of the following is most appropriate regarding the nurse's administration of lispro to a hospitalized patient?
a. It should be given half an hour before a meal.
b. It should be given half an hour after a meal.
c. It should given 15 minutes before the patient begins a meal.
d. The timing of the insulin injection does not matter with lispro.

2 Which of the following statements would be appropriate to include in the patient teaching for type 2 diabetics?
a. "Insulin injections are never used with type 2 diabetes."
b. "Because you are not taking insulin injections, it is not necessary to measure your blood glucose levels."
c. "Alcohol should be avoided because it can cause your blood glucose to fall to lower-than-normal levels."
d. "Patients with type 2 diabetes usually have better control over their diabetes than those with type 1 diabetes."

3 Which of the following is a therapeutic response to oral antihyperglycemic drugs?
a. Weight gain of 5 kg
b. Fewer episodes of DKA
c. Hemoglobin A_{1c} levels of 6%
d. Glucose levels of 9.5 mmol/L

4 When teaching the patient about drugs that interact with insulin, which of the following over-the-counter products should the nurse instruct the patient to avoid, unless otherwise instructed by the physician?
a. Vitamin C
b. Cough syrups
c. Iron supplements
d. Acetaminophen products

5 A patient with type 2 diabetes has a new prescription for repaglinide (GlucoNorm). After a week, she calls the office to ask what to do because she keeps missing meals. "I work right through lunch sometimes, and I'm not sure if I should take it or not. What should I do?" What is the nurse's best response?
a. "Go ahead and take the pill when you first remember that you missed it."
b. "You should try not to skip meals, but if that happens, you should also skip that dose of repaglinide."
c. "Take both pills with the next meal and try to eat a little extra to make up for what you missed at lunchtime."
d. "We will probably need to change your prescription to insulin injections because you can't eat meals on a regular basis."

For answers see http://evolve.elsevier.com/Canada/Lilley/pharmacology/.

CRITICAL THINKING ACTIVITIES

1 Type 1 diabetes mellitus has recently been diagnosed in a 109 kg, 25-year-old woman. When she is admitted to your unit for additional testing and control of her diabetes, she is placed on a 1500 calorie diet for diabetes control and prescribed 30 units of NPH insulin to be given every day at 0730. At 1600 on the first day of therapy she becomes diaphoretic, weak, and pale. What should you do, and how would you explain these symptoms to this patient?

2 Compare the action of metformin (Glucophage) with that of regular insulin, glyburide (Diaβeta), and acarbose (Glucobay). What other oral antidiabetic drug(s) have an action similar to that of metformin?

3 What actions would be necessary in the nursing care of the patient with type 1 diabetes mellitus who is on NPO status for surgery but has orders for the usual morning dose of Humulin N insulin? Explain your answer.

For answers see http://evolve.elsevier.com/Canada/Lilley/pharmacology/.

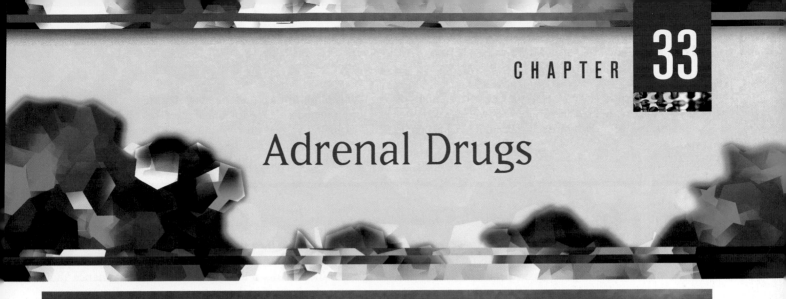

CHAPTER 33

Adrenal Drugs

Learning Objectives

After reading this chapter, the successful student will be able to do the following:

1 Discuss the normal anatomy, physiology, and related functions of the adrenal glands, including specific hormones released from the glands.

2 Briefly compare the hormones secreted by the adrenal medulla with those secreted by the adrenal cortex.

3 Contrast Cushing's syndrome and Addison's disease.

4 Compare the actions and functions of glucocorticoids and mineralocorticoids, including their effect in the body, which diseases alter them, and how they are used in pharmacotherapy.

5 Contrast the mechanisms of action, indications, dosages, routes of administration, cautions, contraindications, drug interactions, and adverse effects for glucocorticoids and mineralocorticoids.

6 Develop a collaborative plan of care that includes all phases of the nursing process for patients taking adrenal drugs.

e-Learning Activities

Web site
(http://evolve.elsevier.com/Canada/
Lilley/pharmacology/)

- Animations
- Answers to chapter questions, activities, and case studies
- Calculators and Category Catchers
- Glossary with audio pronunciations
- IV Therapy and Medication Error Checklists
- Multiple-Choice Review Question quizzes
- Nursing Care Plans
- Online Appendices and Supplements
- WebLinks

Drug Profiles

▸▸ **fludrocortisone (fludrocortisone acetatel*,** p. 622
▸▸ **prednisone,** p. 622

▸▸ Key drug.

*Full generic name is given in parentheses. For the purposes of this text, the more common shortened name is used.

Glossary

Addison's disease A life-threatening condition caused by failure of adrenocortical function. (p. 619)

Adrenal cortex The outer portion of the adrenal gland. (p. 618)

Adrenal medulla The inner portion of the adrenal gland. (p. 618)

Aldosterone A mineralocorticoid hormone produced by the adrenal cortex that acts on the kidney tubule to regulate sodium and potassium balance in the blood. (p. 618)

Cortex General anatomical term for the outer layers of a body organ or other structure. (p. 618)

Corticosteroids Any of the natural or synthetic adrenocortical hormones. (p. 618)

Cushing's syndrome A metabolic disorder characterized by abnormally increased secretion of the adrenocortical steroids. (p. 619)

Epinephrine An endogenous hormone secreted into the bloodstream by the adrenal medulla; also a synthetic drug that is an adrenergic vasoconstrictor and increases cardiac output. (p. 618)

Glucocorticoids A major group of corticosteroid hormones that regulate carbohydrate, protein, and lipid metabolism and inhibit the release of corticotropin. (p. 618)

Medulla General anatomical term for the most interior portions of an organ or structure. (p. 618)

Mineralocorticoids A major group of corticosteroid hormones that regulate electrolyte and water balance; in humans the primary mineralocorticoid is aldosterone. (p. 618)

Norepinephrine An adrenergic hormone, also secreted by the adrenal medulla, that increases blood pressure by causing vasoconstriction but does not appreciably affect cardiac output; it is the immediate metabolic precursor to epinephrine. (p. 618)

ADRENAL SYSTEM

The adrenal gland is an endocrine organ that sits on top of the kidneys like a cap. It is composed of two distinct parts called the **adrenal cortex** and the **adrenal medulla**, which structurally and functionally are different from one another. The term **cortex** refers to the outer layers of various organs (e.g., cerebral cortex), while the term **medulla** refers to the most internal layers. The adrenal cortex comprises approximately 80% to 90% of the adrenal gland; the remainder is the medulla. The adrenal cortex is made up of regular endocrine tissue (hormone driven), and the adrenal medulla is made up of neurosecretory tissue (driven by both hormones and peripheral autonomic nerve impulses). Therefore, the adrenal gland actually functions as two different endocrine glands, each secreting different hormones.

The adrenal medulla secretes two important hormones, both of which are catecholamines: **epinephrine,** or adrenaline, which accounts for about 80% of the secretion, and **norepinephrine,** or noradrenaline, which accounts for the other 20%. (Both these hormones are discussed in Chapter 18 and are not described further in this chapter in any detail.) Some characteristics of the adrenal cortex and the adrenal medulla and the hormones secreted by each are presented in Table 33-1.

The hormones secreted by the adrenal cortex, which are the focus of this chapter, are broadly referred to as **corticosteroids** because they arise from the cortex and are made from the steroid cholesterol. There are two types of corticosteroids: **glucocorticoids** and **mineralocorticoids**. The corticosteroids are secreted by two different layers, or zones, of the cortex. The *zona glomerulosa*, the outer layer, secretes the mineralocorticoids, and the *zona fasciculata*, which lies under the zona glomerulosa, secretes glucocorticoids. A third, inner layer, the zona reticularis, secretes small amounts of sex hormones. All the hormones secreted by the adrenal cortex are steroid hormones; that is, they have the steroid chemical structure.

Mineralocorticoids play an important role in regulating mineral salts (electrolytes) in the body, hence their name. In humans, the only physiologically important mineralocorticoid is **aldosterone**. Its primary role is to maintain normal levels of sodium in the blood (sodium homeostasis) by causing sodium to be reabsorbed from the urine back into the blood in exchange for potassium and hydrogen ions. In this way, aldosterone not only regulates blood sodium levels but also influences potassium levels of the blood and blood pH.

Overall, corticosteroids are necessary for many vital bodily functions. Some of the significant functions are listed in Box 33-1. Without these hormones, life-threatening consequences may arise.

Adrenal corticosteroids are synthesized as needed; the body does not store them as it does other hormones. The body levels of these hormones are regulated by the hypothalamic–pituitary–adrenal (HPA) axis in much the same way as the levels of hormones secreted by the organs discussed in Chapters 30, 31, and 32 (pituitary, thyroid, and pancreas) are regulated. As the name implies, this axis consists of a highly organized system of communication between the adrenal gland, the pituitary gland, and the hypothalamus. As is the case for the other endocrine glands, it uses hormones as the messengers and a negative feedback mechanism as the controller and maintainer of the process (Figure 33-1). This feedback mechanism operates as follows: When the level of a particular corticosteroid is low, corticotropin-releasing hormone is released from the hypothalamus into the bloodstream and travels to the anterior pituitary, where it triggers the release of adrenocorticotropic hormone (ACTH; also called corticotropin). ACTH is then transported in the blood to the adrenal cortex, where it stimulates the production of corticosteroids. Corticosteroids

TABLE 33-1

Adrenal Gland: Characteristics

Type of Tissue	Type of Hormone	Specific Drugs/Hormones
ADRENAL CORTEX		
Endocrine	Glucocorticoids	adrenocorticotropic hormone (ACTH), betamethasone, cortisone, dexamethasone, hydrocortisone, methylprednisolone, prednisolone, triamcinolone
	Mineralocorticoids	aldosterone, desoxycorticosterone, fludrocortisone
ADRENAL MEDULLA		
Neuroendocrine	Catecholamines	epinephrine, norepinephrine

BOX 33-1

Adrenal Cortex Hormones: Biological Functions

Glucocorticoids

Anti-inflammatory actions
Carbohydrate and protein metabolism
Fat metabolism
Maintenance of normal blood pressure
Stress effects

Mineralocorticoids

Blood pressure control
Maintenance of pH levels in blood
Maintenance of serum potassium levels
Sodium and water reabsorption

are then released into the bloodstream. When they reach peak levels, a signal (negative feedback) is sent to the hypothalamus, and the HPA axis is inhibited until the level of corticosteroid again falls below physiological threshold, at which point the axis is stimulated once again (see Figure 33-1).

Oversecretion (hypersecretion) of adrenocortical hormones can lead to a group of signs and symptoms called **Cushing's syndrome**. Hypersecretion of glucocorticoids results in the redistribution of body fat from the arms and legs to the face, shoulders, trunk, and abdomen, which leads to the characteristic "moon face." This glucocorticoid excess can be due to any one of several causes, including ACTH-dependent adrenocortical hyperplasia or tumour, ectopic ACTH-secreting tumour, or excessive administration of steroids. The hypersecretion of aldosterone, or primary aldosteronism, leads to increased water retention and muscle weakness resulting from the potassium loss.

Undersecretion (hyposecretion) of adrenocortical hormones causes the condition **Addison's disease**. Addison's disease is associated with decreased blood sodium and glucose levels, increased potassium levels, dehydration, and weight loss. The combination of a mineralocorticoid (fludrocortisone) and a glucocorticoid (prednisone or some other suitable drug) is used for treatment.

ADRENAL DRUGS

All the naturally occurring corticosteroids are available as exogenous drugs. Higher-potency synthetic analogues are also available. Adrenal glucocorticoids, an extremely large group of steroids, are categorized in various ways. They can be classified by whether they are a natural or synthetic cortiosteroid, by the method of administration (e.g., systemic, topical), by their salt and water retention potential (mineralocorticoid activity), by their duration of action (i.e., short, intermediate, or long acting), or by

some combination of these methods. The only corticosteroid drug with exclusive mineralocorticoid activity is fludrocortisone. Its uses are much more specific than those of the glucocortocoids and are discussed in the designated drug profile for fludrocortisone. The currently available synthetic adrenal hormones and adrenal steroid inhibitors are listed in Table 33-2.

Mechanism of Action and Drug Effects

The action of corticosteroids is related to their involvement in the synthesis of specific proteins. There are several steps to this process. Initially, the steroid hormone binds to a receptor on the surface of a target cell to form a steroid–receptor complex, which is then transported through the cytoplasm to the nucleus of that target cell. Once inside the nucleus of the target cell, the complex stimulates the cell's deoxyribonucleic acid (DNA) to produce messenger ribonucleic acid (mRNA), which is then used as a template for the synthesis of a specific protein. It is these proteins that exert specific effects.

Most of the corticosteroids exert their effects by modifying enzyme activity; therefore, their role is more intermediary than direct. Recall that the naturally occurring mineralocorticoid aldosterone affects electrolyte and fluid balance by acting on the distal kidney tubule to promote sodium reabsorption from the nephron into the blood, which pulls water and fluid along with it. Fluid and water retention occurs, which leads to edema and hypertension. Aldosterone also promotes potassium and hydrogen excretion.

The glucocorticoid drugs hydrocortisone (called *cortisol* in its naturally occurring form) and cortisone have

Hypothalamic–Pituitary–Adrenal (HPA) Axis

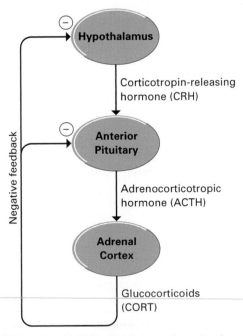

FIG. 33-1   Negative feedback control mechanism of adrenocortical hormones. *CORT*, glucocorticoids; *HPA*, hypothalamic–pituitary–adrenal.

TABLE 33-2

Available Synthetic Corticosteroids

Hormone Type	Method of Administration	Individual Drugs
Adrenal steroid inhibitor	Systemic	ketoconazole, mitotane
Glucocorticoid	Topical	amcinonide, betamethasone benzoate, betamethasone dipropionate, betamethasone valerate, clobetasol propionate, desoximetasone, dexamethasone, diflucortolone valerate, flumethasone pivalate, fluocinolone acetonide, fluocinonide, fluticasone propionate, halcinonide, halobetasol propionate, hydrocortisone acetate, hydrocortisone valerate, methylprednisolone acetate, mometasone furoate, prednicarbate, triamcinolone acetonide
	Systemic	beclomethasone, cortisone, dexamethasone, fludrocortisone, hydrocortisone, methylprednisolone, prednisolone, prednisone, triamcinolone
	Inhaled	beclomethasone, budesonide, flunisolide, fluticasone
	Nasal	beclomethasone dipropionate, budesonide, flunisolide, fluticasone, mometasone, triamcinolone acetonide
Mineralocorticoid	Systemic	fludrocortisone acetate

some mineralocorticoid activity and, therefore, have some of the same effects as aldosterone (i.e., fluid and water retention). Their other main effect is inhibition of inflammatory and immune responses. Glucocorticoids primarily inhibit or assist in controlling the inflammatory response by stabilizing the cell membranes of inflammatory cells, *lysosomes;* decreasing the permeability of capillaries to the inflammatory cells; and decreasing the migration of white blood cells into already inflamed areas. They may lower fever by reducing the release of interleukin-1 from white blood cells. They also stimulate erythroid cells that eventually become red blood cells. Glucocorticoids also promote the breakdown (catabolism) of protein, the production of glycogen in the liver (glycogenesis), and the redistribution of fat from the peripheral areas to the central areas of the body.

Indications

All systemically administered glucocorticoids have a similar clinical efficacy but differ in their potency and duration of action and in the extent to which they cause

salt and fluid retention (Table 33-3). Glucocorticoids have broad indications, including the following:

- Adrenocortical deficiency
- Adrenogenital syndrome
- Bacterial meningitis (particularly in infants)
- Cerebral edema
- Collagen diseases (e.g., systemic lupus erythematosus)
- Dermatological diseases (e.g., exfoliative dermatitis, pemphigus)
- Endocrine disorders (thyroiditis)
- Gastrointestinal diseases (e.g., ulcerative colitis, regional enteritis)
- Exacerbations of chronic respiratory illnesses such as asthma and chronic obstructive pulmonary disease
- Hematological disorders (reduce bleeding tendencies)
- Ocular disorders (nonpyogenic inflammations)
- Organ transplantation (decrease immune response to prevent organ rejection)
- Leukemias and lymphomas (palliative management)
- Nephrotic syndrome (remission of proteinuria)
- Spinal cord injury

TABLE 33-3

Systemic Glucocorticoids: A Comparison

Drug	Origin	Duration of Action	Equivalent Dose (mg)*	Salt and Water Retention Potential
betamethasone	Synthetic	Long	0.60	Minimal
cortisone	Natural	Short	25	High
dexamethasone	Synthetic	Long	0.75	Minimal
hydrocortisone	Natural	Short	20	High
methylprednisolone	Synthetic	Intermediate	4	Low
prednisone	Synthetic	Intermediate	5	Low
prednisolone	Synthetic	Intermediate	5	Low
triamcinolone	Synthetic	Intermediate	4	Minimal

*Drugs with higher potency require smaller milligram doses than those with lower potency. This column illustrates the approximate dose equivalency between different drugs that is expected to achieve a comparable therapeutic effect.

Glucocorticoids are also administered by inhalation for the control of steroid-responsive bronchospastic states. Nasally administered glucocorticoids are used to manage allergic rhinitis and to prevent the recurrence of polyps after surgical removal (Chapter 37). Topical steroids are used in the management of inflammations in the eye, ear, and skin.

Contraindications

Contraindications to the administration of glucocorticoids include drug allergy, cataracts, glaucoma, peptic ulcer disease, psychiatric and mental health problems, and diabetes mellitus, as adrenal drugs may intensify these diseases. Because of their immunosuppressant properties, glucocorticoids are often avoided in the presence of any serious infection, including septicemia, systemic fungal infections, and varicella. One exception to this rule is tuberculous meningitis, for which glucocorticoids may be used to prevent inflammatory central nervous system damage. Caution is required when using glucocorticoids in any patient with gastritis, reflux disease, ulcer disease, or diabetes, as well as with heart, kidney, or liver dysfunction.

Adverse Effects

The potent metabolic, physiological, and pharmacological effects of the corticosteroids can influence every body system, so they can produce a wide variety of significant undesirable effects. The more common of these adverse effects are summarized in Table 33-4.

Interactions

Systemically administered corticosteroids can interact with many drugs:

- Their use with non–potassium-sparing diuretics (e.g., thiazides, loop diuretics) can lead to severe hypocalcemia and hypokalemia.
- Their use with aspirin, other nonsteroidal anti-inflammatory drugs, and other ulcerogenic drugs produces additive gastrointestinal effects.

- Their use with anticholinesterase drugs produces weakness in patients with myasthenia gravis.
- Their use with immunizing biologicals inhibits the immune response to the biological agent.
- Their use with oral antihyperglycemic drugs may reduce the hypoglycemic effects of the antihyperglycemic.

There are many other drugs that can interact with glucocorticoids. These drugs include the following: thyroid hormones, antifungal drugs (such as fluconazole), barbiturates, hydantoins, oral anticoagulants, oral contraceptives, potassium-depleting diuretics, and theophylline. Concerns about these specific drugs and interactions include the following:

- Antifungals decrease kidney clearance of adrenal drugs.
- Barbiturates increase the metabolism of prednisone and similar drugs.
- Oral contraceptives can increase the half-life of adrenal drugs.

Other drug interactions may be possible between adrenal drugs and over-the-counter (OTC) drugs and natural health products. The nurse should educate the patient to read package labelling and consult with a pharmacist when in doubt.

Dosages

For information on the recommended dosages of adrenal drugs, see the Dosages table on p. 623.

NURSING PROCESS

Assessment

Before administering any of the adrenal drugs, the nurse should perform a thorough physical assessment to determine the patient's nutritional and hydration status, baseline weight, intake and output, vital signs

TABLE 33-4

Corticosteroids: Common Adverse Effects

Body System	Adverse Effects
Cardiovascular	Heart failure, cardiac edema, hypertension, because of electrolyte imbalances (e.g., hypokalemia, hypernatremia)
Central nervous	Convulsions, headache, vertigo, mood swings, psychic impairment, nervousness, insomnia
Endocrine	Growth suppression, Cushing's syndrome, menstrual irregularities, carbohydrate intolerance, hyperglycemia, hypothalamic–pituitary–adrenal axis suppression
Gastrointestinal	Peptic ulcers with possible perforation, pancreatitis, ulcerative esophagitis, abdominal distension
Integumentary	Fragile skin, petechiae, ecchymoses, facial erythema, increased risk of infection and delayed wound healing, hirsutism, urticaria
Musculoskeletal	Muscle weakness, loss of muscle mass, osteoporosis
Ocular	Increased intraocular pressure, glaucoma, exophthalmos, cataracts
Other	Weight gain

DRUG PROFILES

CORTICOSTEROIDS

The systemic corticosteroids consist of 13 chemically different but pharmacologically similar hormones. They all exert varying degrees of glucocorticoid and mineralocorticoid effects. Their differences are due to slight changes in their chemical structures.

Corticosteroids can cross the placenta and produce fetal abnormalities. They may also be secreted in breast milk and cause abnormalities in the nursing infant. Their use is contraindicated in patients who have exhibited hypersensitivity reactions to them in the past and in patients with fungal or bacterial infections. Short- or long-term use can lead to a condition known as *steroid psychosis*. In addition, the cessation of long-term treatment with these drugs requires a tapering of the daily dose because the administration of the exogenous hormones causes the endogenous production of the hormones to stop. Tapering of daily doses allows the hypothalamic–pituitary–adrenal axis the time to recover and to start stimulating the normal production of the endogenous hormones.

▶▶ *fludrocortisone acetate*

Fludrocortisone acetate (Florinef) is contraindicated in cases of systemic fungal infection. Adverse effects generally pertain to water retention and include congestive heart failure, hypertension, and elevated intracerebral pressure (e.g., leading to seizures). Other potential adverse effects involve several body systems and include skin rash, menstrual irregularities, peptic ulcer, hyperglycemia, potassium loss, hypokalemic alkalosis, muscle pain and weakness, compression bone fractures, glaucoma, and thrombophlebitis, among others. Drug interactions include anabolic steroids (increased edema), barbiturates, hydantoins, rifamycins (increased fludrocortisone clearance), estrogens (reduced fludrocortisone clearance), amphotericin B and thiazide and loop diuretics (hypokalemia), anticoagulants (enhanced or reduced anticoagulant activity), antidiabetic drugs (reduced activity leading to hyperglycemia), digoxin (increased risk for dysrhythmias due to fludrocortisone-induced hypokalemia), salicylates (reduced efficacy), and vaccines (increased risk of neurological complications). Fortunately, adverse effects and serious drug interactions secondary to fludrocortisone therapy are uncommon because of the relatively small doses of the drug that are normally prescribed. This drug is available only in oral form. Recommended dosages are given in the Dosages table on p. 623.

PHARMACOKINETICS

Half-Life	Onset	Peak	Duration
18–36 hr	10–20 min	PO: 1.7 hr	Unknown

▶▶ *prednisone*

Prednisone (Winpred, generic) is one of the four intermediate-acting glucocorticoids; others are methylprednisolone, prednisolone, and triamcinolone. The glucocorticoids drugs have half-lives that are more than double those of the short-acting corticosteroids (2 to 5 hours), thus they have much longer durations of action. Prednisone is the preferred oral glucocorticoid for anti-inflammatory or immunosuppressant purposes. Along with methylprednisolone and prednisolone, it is also used for exacerbations of chronic respiratory illnesses such as asthma and chronic bronchitis. This drug has only minimal mineralocorticoid properties and thus by itself is inadequate for the management of adrenocortical insufficiency (Addison's disease). Prednisone is available in oral tablets. Prednisolone, a prednisone metabolite, is the liquid drug form of prednisone. Recommended dosages are given in the Dosages table on p. 623.

PHARMACOKINETICS

Half-Life	Onset	Peak	Duration
18–36 hr	Unknown	1–2 hr	36 hr

(notably blood pressure ranges), skin condition, and immune status. Important baseline laboratory values include serum sodium, serum potassium, blood urea nitrogen, serum glucose, and serum hemoglobin and hematocrit. The serum tests are important because of the adverse effects that are expected with adrenal drugs. For example, serum potassium levels usually decrease and blood glucose levels increase when a glucocorticoid such as prednisone is given. In addition, the patient's muscle strength and body stature should be assessed and documented. Liver functioning may also be assessed through liver enzyme testing. All of these parameters must be assessed and documented before, during, and after therapy so that baseline comparisons will be available to evaluate therapeutic effectiveness and adverse effects.

Specific contraindications, cautions, and drug interactions (including prescription drugs, over-the-counter drugs, and natural health products) associated with adrenal drugs should be assessed thoroughly (discussed in the pharmacology section of this chapter). Assessment of variables associated with lifespan includes concerns related to use of these medications during pregnancy and lactation. Growth suppression may occur in children receiving long-term adrenal drug therapy (e.g., glucocorticoids) if the epiphyseal plates of the long bones have not closed; however, there are often situations in which the benefits outweigh the risks of the drug's adverse effects. The older adult is more prone to adrenal suppression with prolonged adrenal therapy and may require dosage alterations by the physician to minimize the impact of the drug on muscle mass, plasma volume, kidney and liver functions, blood pressure, and serum glucose and electrolyte levels. These drugs may exacerbate muscle weakness and fatigue as well as osteoporosis. Because the adrenal drugs are associated with sodium retention, patients with edema and

DOSAGES   Selected Antiadrenal and Corticosteroid Drugs

Drug (Pregnancy Category)	Pharmacological Class	Usual Dosage Range	Indications
dexamethasone (Dexasone, generic) (C)	Synthetic long-acting glucocorticoid	*Children* PO/IV: 0.5–2 mg/kg/day divided q6h *Adult* PO/IV/IM: 0.75–9 mg/day divided bid–qid	Wide variety of endocrine (including adrenocortical insufficiency), rheumatic, collagen, dermatological, allergic, ocular, respiratory, hematological, neoplastic, gastrointestinal, and nervous system disorders; edematous states
dexamethasone sodium phosphate (Dexamethasone-Omega) (C)	Synthetic long-acting repository glucocorticoid	*Adult* IM: 8–16 mg q1–3 wk Intralesional: 0.8–1.6 mg Intra-articular and soft tissue: 4–16 mg q1–3 wk	Same as dexamethasone Inflammation Inflammation
▸▸fludrocortisone acetate (Florinef) (C)	Synthetic mineralocorticoid	*Children (including infants)/Adult* PO: 0.1–0.2 mg daily	Addison's disease; salt-losing adrenogenital syndrome
hydrocortisone (Cortef) (C)	Natural short-acting glucocorticoid	*Children* PO: 2.5–10 mg/kg/day divided q6–8h *Adult* PO: 20–240 mg/day	Adrenocortical insufficiency; many inflammatory conditions
hydrocortisone sodium succinate (C)	Natural, water-soluble, short-acting glucocorticoid	*Children* IV/IM: 1.5 mg/kg/day divided daily–bid *Adult* IV/IM: 100–500 mg q2–6h, depending on condition and patient response	Adrenocortical insufficiency
▸▸prednisone (Winpred, generic) (C)	Synthetic intermediate-acting glucocorticoid	*Children* PO: 0.05–2 mg/kg/day divided daily–qid *Adult* PO: 0.55–30 mg/kg/day	Wide variety of endocrine (including adrenocortical insufficiency) and rheumatic, collagen, dermatological, allergic, ocular, respiratory, hematological, neoplastic, gastrointestinal, and nervous system disorders; edematous states

IM, intramuscular; *IV*, intravenous; *PO*, oral.

heart disease must be closely assessed for exacerbation of these conditions.

Nursing Diagnoses

- Imbalanced nutrition, more than body requirements, related to increased appetite resulting from adrenal drug therapy
- Disturbed body image related to the physiological effects of diseases of the adrenal gland on the body or the cushingoid appearance due to drug therapy (with prednisone)
- Excess fluid volume related to fluid retention associated with glucocorticoid and mineralocorticoid use
- Risk for infection related to anti-inflammatory, immunosuppressive, metabolic, and dermatological effects of long-term glucocorticoid therapy
- Impaired skin integrity related to the adverse effects of glucocorticoids
- Risk for injury related to adverse effects of adrenal drug therapy, such as changes in sensorium and confusion

Planning

Goals

- Patient will describe the healthy diet to follow during treatment.
- Patient will experience minimal body image disturbances.
- Patient will exhibit minimal complications resulting from the fluid retention caused by mineralocorticoid therapy.
- Patient will be free of infection during adrenal drug therapy.
- Patient's skin and mucous membranes will remain intact during treatment.
- Patient will maintain normal fluid and electrolyte levels.
- Patient will remain free of changes in sensorium and possible confusion or dizziness from adrenal drug therapy.
- Patient will state adverse symptoms to report immediately to the physician.

Outcome Criteria

- Patient eats adequate food according to the food guide pyramid and, with adequate menu planning, maintains weight within normal range.
- Patient conveys anxiety about body image disturbances to health care providers.
- Patient experiences minimal problems with fluid volume excess and weight does not increase more than 1 kg/wk.
- Patient notifies the physician if fever (over 38°C) occurs.
- Patient performs frequent mouth and skin care to prevent infections and maintain intact skin.
- Patient implements measures to minimize major electrolyte imbalances during adrenal drug therapy.
- Patient changes positions slowly and walks carefully to prevent injuries resulting from dizziness or syncope (occurring as a result of postural hypotension).
- Patient identifies symptoms to report to the physician, such as weight gain of more than 1 kg/wk, shortness of breath, edema, dizziness, and syncope.
- Patient experiences minimal effects when weaned from adrenal drugs such as prednisone.

Implementation

The nurse must understand how glucocorticoids function so that education reflecting the fundamental concepts can be provided to the patient. Such education can help maximize therapeutic effects and minimize adverse effects. Points to remember when giving glucocorticoids include the following:

- Hormone production by the adrenal gland is influenced by time of day and follows a diurnal (daily or 24-hour) pattern with peak levels occurring early in the morning between 0600 and 0800, a decrease occurring during the day, and a lower peak occurring in the late afternoon between 1600 and 1800.
- Cortisol levels increase in response to both emotional and physiological stress.
- Cortisol levels also increase when endogenous levels decrease because of a physiological negative feedback system.
- When exogenous glucocorticoids are given, endogenous levels decrease; for endogenous production to resume, exogenous levels must be decreased gradually so that hormone levels respond to the negative feedback system.
- The best time to give exogenous glucocorticoids is early in the morning (0600 to 0900) because this leads to the least amount of adrenal suppression.

Some of the systemic forms of adrenal drugs (e.g., prednisone) may be given by the oral, intramuscular, intravenous, or rectal route. Parenteral forms should be diluted according to manufacturer guidelines and intravenous dosages administered over the recommended time span. Intramuscular forms should always be administered into a large muscle, such as the ventral gluteal site, with rotation of sites (if giving frequent injections) to prevent tissue trauma and irritation.

Oral dosage forms should be given with milk, food, or nonsystemic antacids (such as A_1, Ca^2, or Mg), unless contraindicated, to minimize gastrointestinal upset. Another option is for the physician to order an H_2-receptor antagonist or a proton pump inhibitor to prevent ulcer formation (glucocorticoids are often ulcerogenic). Patients should be encouraged to avoid alcohol, aspirin, and nonsteroidal anti-inflammatory drugs to minimize gastric irritation and gastric bleeding. In long-term therapy, alternate-day dosing of glucocorticoids will help minimize adrenal suppression. With oral and all other forms of glucocorticoids that are given short or long term, abrupt withdrawal must be avoided. Abrupt withdrawal of adrenal drugs (e.g., prednisone) may lead to Addisonian crisis, which may be life threatening. Signs and symptoms of Addison's disease or adrenal insufficiency include fatigue, nausea, vomiting, and hypotension.

Other adrenal drug dosage forms include intra-articular, intrabursal, intradermal, intralesional, and intrasynovial routes. Intra-articular injections should not be overused; should a joint be injected with medication, the patient should rest that area for up to 48 hours after the injection. Topical dosage forms are also available and may be applied to the skin or eye or administered by inhalation as ordered. These drug dosage forms should be used as ordered and only according to the instructions in the package insert, which may specify the use of an occlusive dressing. The skin should be clean and dry before application of a topical drug. Gloves should be worn and the medication applied with either a sterile tongue depressor or a cotton-tipped applicator. Sterile technique should be used if the skin is not intact.

Nasally administered glucocorticoids (e.g., beclomethasone) should be used exactly as ordered. Any written instructions that come with the product should be read and followed carefully. Patients should be instructed that before using the nasal spray, they should first clear the nasal passages and then use the spray per instructions. After the nasal passages are cleared, the container is placed gently inside the nasal passage and the medication is released at the same time that the patient breathes in through the nose. Glucocorticoid inhalers should be used specifically as ordered, and negative consequences of overuse should be explained to the patient. Inhalers containing adrenal drugs (e.g., corticosteroids) may lead to oral mucosal, oral-cavity, laryngeal, or pharyngeal fungal (candidiasis) infections. After inhalers with these medications are used, the patient should always rinse the mouth with lukewarm water to prevent fungal overgrowth and further complications. Hoarseness, fungal infections (candidiasis), throat irritation, and dry mouth are possible adverse effects associated with the use of inhaled corticosteroids and should be reported to the health care provider immediately. See Chapter 10 and Patient Education for more information.

If a patient is receiving long-term maintenance glucocorticoid therapy and requires surgery, the nurse should be sure that the patient's medical records are reviewed carefully. In addition, all nursing documentation and notes should be reviewed. If the preoperative orders do not include the maintenance dosage, the nurse should contact the surgeon or other physician and ensure that they are aware of the situation and the possible need for a rapid-acting corticosteroid. After surgery, the dosage of steroid may well be increased, with a gradual decrease in dosage over several days until the patient returns to baseline. The nurse should keep in mind that healing may be decreased if the patient has been on long-term therapy.

Because of their suppressed immune systems, patients taking corticosteroids should avoid contact with people with infections and should report any fever, increased weakness and lethargy, or sore throat. Monitoring nutritional status, weight, fluid volume, electrolyte status, skin turgor, and glucose levels during therapy is important to ensure safe and effective therapy. Administration in one daily morning dose is recommended to minimize adrenal suppression. Physicians or health care providers should be notified if there is any weakness, joint pain, dyspnea, fever, dysrhythmias, depression, edema, or other unusual symptoms.

Evaluation

A therapeutic response to corticosteroids includes a resolution of the underlying manifestations of the disease, such as a decrease in inflammation, increased feeling of well-being, less pain and discomfort in the joints, decrease in lymphocytes, or other improvement in the condition for which the medication was ordered. Adverse effects include weight gain; increased blood pressure; pulse irregularities; sodium increase and potassium loss; mental health status changes such as aggression, depression, or psychosis; electrolyte disturbances; elevated glucose levels; decreased healing; gastrointestinal upset; and ulcer-related symptoms. Systemic drugs may cause potassium depletion, which manifests as fatigue, nausea, vomiting, muscle weakness, and dysrhythmias. Cushing's syndrome is characterized by moon face, truncal obesity, increase in blood glucose and sodium levels and a loss of potassium, wasting of muscle mass, buffalo hump, and other features presented in the Adrenal System section of this chapter. Cataract formation and osteoporosis may also occur. Addisonian crisis occurs with a rapid drop of cortisol level (e.g., abrupt withdrawal of medication) and is manifested by hypotension, weight loss, dehydration, and decreased blood glucose level.

PATIENT EDUCATION

❖ Patients should be instructed on the importance of drug therapy and its method of administration, to follow exact instructions, and to never stop the medication abruptly. Abrupt withdrawal from adrenal drugs is not recommended because this may precipitate an adrenal crisis.

❖ Patients should be encouraged to contact the physician if there are situations that prevent proper dosing. If a once-a-day dose is missed, the patient should take the dose as soon as possible after remembering that the dose was missed. If the dose is not remembered until close to the time for the next dose, then the patient should skip the dose and resume the dosing on the next day without doubling up. Inform the patient of what to expect with long-term glucocorticoid therapy, including changes in body appearance with acne, buffalo hump, truncal obesity, moon face, thinning of the extremities, and cataract formation.

❖ Patients should be educated about the importance of bone health and prevention of falls because long-term therapy may lead to osteoporosis. The physician may suggest a daily supplement of oral calcium and vitamin D.

❖ Patients should be informed to report to the physician any signs and symptoms of acute adrenal insufficiency, such as anorexia, hypotension, hypoglycemia, weakness, nausea, psychological changes, and restlessness. The patient should also report vomiting and diarrhea or other acute illnesses. Other problems to report include weight gain, lower extremity edema, muscle weakness, and severe or continual headache.

❖ Patients should be instructed to take fludrocortisone with food or milk to minimize gastrointestinal upset. Weight gain of >1 kg/24 hr or >2 kg/wk with any adrenal drug should be reported to the physician as soon as possible.

❖ Patients should be encouraged to use a journal to document responses to treatment, blood pressure readings, daily weight measurements, and any adverse effects experienced.

❖ Patients should keep return appointments with the physician so that electrolyte levels can be monitored. Also, emphasize the importance of maintaining a low-sodium and high-potassium diet as ordered.

❖ Patients should be encouraged to wear a medical identification bracelet or necklace with the diagnosis and list of medications and allergies. A medical card with important relevant information should be kept on the person at all times and updated frequently.

POINTS TO REMEMBER

❖ The adrenal gland is an endocrine organ located on top of the kidneys and is composed of two distinct tissues: the adrenal cortex and the adrenal medulla. The adrenal medulla secretes two important hormones: epinephrine (80%) and norepinephrine (20%); the adrenal cortex secretes the two classes of *corticosteroids:* glucocorticoids and mineralocorticoids.

❖ Biological functions of glucocorticoids include anti-inflammatory actions; maintenance of normal blood pressure; carbohydrate, protein, and fat metabolism; and stress effects.

❖ Biological functions of mineralcorticoids include sodium and water reabsorption, blood pressure control, and maintaining of potassium levels and pH levels of blood.

❖ Patients taking adrenal drugs may receive them by various routes, such as orally, intramuscularly, intravenously, intranasally, intra-articularly, and by inhalation; some are also administered by means of a rectal enema.

❖ Nurses should follow the manufacturer's guidelines for dilution and administration. Intramuscular forms of adrenal drugs should be administered deep into a large muscle, such as the ventral gluteal site. Steroid inhalers should be used as ordered and only after adequate patient education; patients should rinse the mouth after their use to avoid oral fungal infections (oral candidiasis) and oral–pharyngeal irritation.

❖ Parenteral forms should be diluted and administered according to the manufacturer's guidelines.

❖ Adverse effects to monitor for include weight gain, increase in blood pressure, pulse irregularities, mental health status alterations such as aggression or depression, electrolyte disturbances, elevated blood glucose levels, changes in nutrition status, decreased healing, gastrointestinal tract upset, and ulcer-related symptoms.

❖ With once-a-day dosing of corticosteroids, adrenal suppression may be minimized if the dose is given between 0600 and 0900, but they should only be given as ordered.

EXAMINATION REVIEW QUESTIONS

1 Which of the following statements is correct regarding corticosteroids?
   a. They have few adverse effects.
   b. They are often used for their anti-inflammatory effects.
   c. They may be administered only by inhalant dosage forms.
   d. They may be used long term without major complications.

2 Which statement of the patient shows a poor understanding of the teaching about oral corticosteroid therapy that the patient has received?
   a. "I should take this drug with food or milk."
   b. "I will report any fever or sore throat symptoms."
   c. "I will stay away from anyone who has a cold or infection."
   d. "I can stop this medication if I have severe adverse effects."

3 During long-term corticosteroid therapy, the nurse should monitor the patient for Cushing's syndrome. Which of the following characteristics is usually manifested by this syndrome?

   a. Weight loss
   b. Truncal obesity
   c. Muscle thickening
   d. Thickened hair growth

4 A patient has been prescribed a daily dose of prednisone. At what time of day should the patient take the medication to help reduce adrenal suppression?
   a. In the morning
   b. At lunchtime
   c. At dinnertime
   d. At bedtime

5 Which teaching is appropriate for a patient who is taking an inhaled glucocorticoid for asthma?
   a. "Blow your nose after taking the medication."
   b. "Do not rinse the mouth after taking the medication."
   c. "Exhale while pushing in on the canister of the inhaler."
   d. "Rinse the mouth thoroughly after taking the medication."

For answers see http://evolve.elsevier.com/Canada/Lilley/pharmacology/.

CRITICAL THINKING ACTIVITIES

1 A 19-year-old man is admitted through the emergency department after a motorcycle accident. He is conscious upon admission, has stable vital signs, and has minimal cuts and abrasions on the left side of his body. You perform a thorough neurological examination and find absence of sensation to light touch and pinprick and lower extremity paralysis. Reflexes are absent below the groin area. The physician orders high-dose intravenous methylprednisolone. What is the purpose of this medication, and what should you, as the nurse, watch for while the patient is receiving this medication?

2 You are caring for a patient who is taking 100 mg of hydrocortisone orally. The physician decides that he is more familiar with prednisone and wants to change the patient's medication to the equivalent oral dose of prednisone. What will be the equivalent dose of prednisone?

3 Discuss how drug therapy benefits patients with Addison's disease.

For answers see http://evolve.elsevier.com/Canada/Lilley/pharmacology/.

CHAPTER 34

Women's Health Drugs

Learning Objectives

After reading this chapter, the successful student will be able to do the following:

1 Discuss the normal anatomy and physiology of the female reproductive system and the variety of related disorders that are treated with estrogens and progestins.

2 Discuss the hormonally mediated feedback system and how it regulates the female reproductive system.

3 Describe the disorders affecting women's health and the drugs used to treat these disorders.

4 Describe the rationale for the treatments involving estrogen, progesterone, uterine motility–altering drugs, alendronate, and other drugs related to women's health, with indications, adverse effects, cautions, contraindications, drug interactions, dosages, and routes of administration.

5 Develop a collaborative plan of care that includes all phases of the nursing process for patients receiving any drug related to women's health (e.g., estrogens, progestins, oral contraceptives, uterine mobility–altering drugs, alendronate, and related drugs).

e-Learning Activities

Web site
(http://evolve.elsevier.com/Canada/Lilley/pharmacology/)

- Animations
- Answers to chapter questions, activities, and case studies
- Calculators and Category Catchers
- Glossary with audio pronunciations
- IV Therapy and Medication Error Checklists
- Multiple-Choice Review Question quizzes
- Nursing Care Plans
- Online Appendices and Supplements
- WebLinks

Drug Profiles

▸▸ **alendronate (alendronate sodium)***, p. 639
   calcitonin, p. 640
   choriogonadotropin alfa, p. 642
   clomiphene (clomiphene citrate)*, p. 642
▸▸ **dinoprostone**, p. 644
▸▸ **ergonovine (ergonovine maleate)***, p. 644
▸▸ **estrogen**, p. 632
▸▸ **medroxyprogesterone (medroxyprogesterone acetate)***, p. 635
   megestrol (megestrol acetate)*, p. 635
▸▸ **menotropins**, p. 642
▸▸ **oxytocin**, p. 644
   raloxifene (raloxifene hydrochloride)*, p. 640
   teriparatide, p. 640

▸▸ Key drug.

*Full generic name is given in parentheses. For the purposes of this text, the more common shortened name is used.

Glossary

Chloasma Hyperpigmentation from the hormone melanin in the skin, involving brownish macules on the cheeks, forehead, lips, and neck. (p. 632)

Corpus luteum The structure that forms on the surface of the ovary after every ovulation and acts as a short-lived endocrine organ that secretes progesterone. (p. 628)

Endocrine glands Glands that secrete one or more hormones directly into the blood. (p. 628)

Estrogens The collective term for one of two major classes of female sex steroid hormones (the other class is *progestins*); of the estrogens, estradiol is responsible for most estrogenic physiological activity. (p. 628)

Fallopian tubes The passages through which ova are carried from the ovaries to the uterus. (p. 628)

Gonadotropin The hormone that stimulates the testes and ovaries. (p. 628)

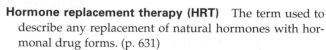

Hormone replacement therapy (HRT) The term used to describe any replacement of natural hormones with hormonal drug forms. (p. 631)

Implantation The attachment to, penetration of, and embedding of the fertilized ovum in the lining of the uterine wall. (p. 628)

Menarche The first menses in a young woman's life, and the beginning of cyclic menstrual function. (p. 629)

Menopause The cessation of menses that marks the end of a woman's childbearing capability. (p. 629)

Menses The normal flow of blood that occurs during menstruation. (p. 628)

Menstrual cycle The recurring cycle of changes in the endometrium in which the decidual layer is shed, regrows, proliferates, is maintained for several days, and is shed again at menstruation unless a pregnancy begins. (p. 628)

Nucleic acids Compounds involved in energy storage and release as well as in the determination and transmission of genetic characteristics. (p. 631)

Osteoporosis A condition characterized by the progressive loss of bone density and thinning of bone tissue; it is associated with an increased risk of fractures. (p. 638)

Ova Female reproductive or germ cells (singular: *ovum*; also called *eggs*). (p. 628)

Ovarian follicles The location of egg production and ovulation in the ovary; the follicle is the precursor to the corpus luteum. (p. 628)

Ovaries The pair of female gonads located on each side of the lower abdomen beside the uterus. They store the ova and release an ovum during the ovulation stage of the menstrual cycle. (p. 628)

Ovulation The rupture of the ovarian follicle, which results in the release of an unfertilized ovum into the peritoneal cavity, where it then normally enters the fallopian tube. (p. 628)

Progestins The collective term for one of the two major classes of female hormones (the other class is *estrogens*). (p. 628)

Puberty The period of life when the ability to reproduce begins. (p. 628)

Uterus The hollow, pear-shaped female organ in which the fertilized ovum is implanted (see *implantation*) and the fetus develops. (p. 628)

Vagina Part of the female genitalia that forms a canal from its external orifice through its vestibule to the uterine cervix. (p. 628)

OVERVIEW OF FEMALE REPRODUCTIVE FUNCTIONS

The female reproductive system consists of the **ovaries, fallopian tubes, uterus,** and **vagina** and the external structure known as the *vulva*. The development of these primary sex structures, the initiation of their subsequent reproductive functions (starting at **puberty**), and their maintenance are controlled by pituitary **gonadotropin** hormones and the female sex steroid hormones, the **estrogens** and **progestins.** Pituitary gonadotropins include follicle-stimulating hormone (FSH) and luteinizing hormone (LH). Both play a primary role in hormonal communication between the pituitary gland (Chapter 30) and the ovaries in the continuous regulation of the **menstrual cycle.**

Estrogens are also responsible for stimulating the development of secondary female sex characteristics, including breast, skin, and bone development and distribution of body fat and hair. Progestins help create optimal conditions for pregnancy in the endometrium after **ovulation** and also promote **menses** in the absence of a fertilized ovum.

The ovaries (female gonads) are paired glands located on each side of the uterus. They function both as **endocrine glands** and as reproductive glands. As reproductive glands, they produce within the **ovarian follicles** mature **ova,** which are then ovulated or released into the space in the peritoneal cavity between the ovary and the fallopian tube. Fingerlike projections known as *fimbriae* lie adjacent to each ovary and serve to "catch" the released ovum and guide it into the fallopian tube. Once inside the fallopian tube the ovum is moved through its lumen to the uterus.

This movement is accomplished through the muscular contractions of the tube walls and the actions of ciliated cells inside the lumen of the tube, which "beat" in the direction of the uterus. Fertilization of the ovum, when it occurs, often takes place in the fallopian tube.

As endocrine glands, the ovaries are responsible for producing the two major classes of sex steroid hormones, estrogens and progestins. Chemically, each of the two major classes includes several distinct hormones. However, only two of the hormones occur in significant amounts and have the greatest physiological activity—the estrogen *estradiol* and the progestin *progesterone*. Estradiol is the principal secretory product of the ovary and has several estrogenic effects. One effect is the regulation of gonadotropin (FSH, LH) secretion via negative feedback to the pituitary gland (Figure 34-1). Other effects include promotion of the development of women's secondary sex characteristics, monthly endometrial growth, thickening of vaginal mucosa, thinning of cervical mucus, and growth of the ductal system of the breasts. Progesterone is the principal secretory product of the **corpus luteum** and has progestational effects, including promotion of tissue growth and secretory activity in the endometrium following the estrogen-driven *proliferative phase* of the menstrual cycle. This important secretory process is required for endometrial egg **implantation** and maintenance of pregnancy. Other effects of progesterone include induction of menstruation when fertilization has not occurred, and, during pregnancy, inhibition of uterine contractions, increased viscosity of cervical mucus (which protects the fetus from external contamination), and growth of the alveolar glands of the breasts.

Female Reproductive Axis

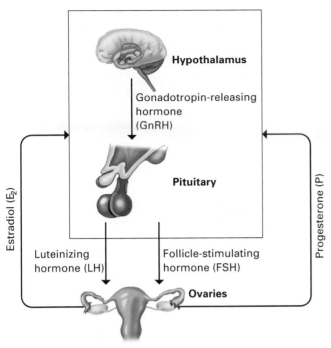

FIG. 34-1 Regulation of gonadotropin (FSH, LH) secretion by estradiol. *E₂*, estradiol; *FSH*, follicle-stimulating hormone; *GnRH*, gonadotropin-releasing hormone; *LH*, luteinizing hormone; *P*, progesterone.

The uterus consists of three layers: the outer protective *perimetrium*, the muscular *myometrium*, and the inner mucosal layer, the *endometrium*. The myometrium provides the powerful smooth muscle contractions needed for childbirth. The endometrium is the site of the following:

- Implantation of a fertilized ovum and subsequent development of the fetus
- Initiation of labour and birthing of the infant
- Menstruation

The vagina provides a common passageway for birthing and menstrual flow. In addition, it is a receptacle for the penis during sexual intercourse and the sperm after ejaculation.

The menstrual cycle usually takes approximately 1 month. Menstrual cycles begin during puberty with the first menses **(menarche)** and cease at **menopause**, which, in most women, occurs between 45 and 55 years of age. The hormonally controlled menstrual cycle consists of four distinct but interrelated phases that occur in overlapping sequence. Phase names correspond to activity in either the ovarian follicle or the endometrium (Table 34-1).

- **Phase 1:** The *menstruation phase*, which initiates the cycle and lasts from 5 to 7 days.
- **Phase 2:** The *follicular phase*, during which a mature ovum develops from an ovarian follicle. This phase is also called the *proliferative* or *preovulatory phase* and is characterized by rising estrogen secretion from the ovary and LH secretion from the pituitary gland. It terminates on or about day 14 of the cycle.

- **Phase 3:** The *ovulation phase* involves release of the unfertilized ovum from the ovary. This process occurs over approximately 24 to 48 hours, beginning around day 14. Both estrogen and LH levels peak near this time.
- **Phase 4:** The final phase of the cycle is the *luteal* or *postovulatory phase*. It is also known as the *secretory phase*. It occurs when the corpus luteum forms from the ruptured ovarian follicle. The corpus luteum is a mass of secretory cells on the surface of the ovary. Its primary function is to produce progesterone, which helps optimize the endometrial mucosa for implantation of a fertilized ovum. The corpus luteum also serves as an initial source of progesterone needed during early pregnancy. This function is later assumed by the developing placenta. If fertilization does not occur, the rising progesterone levels in the blood initiate menstruation. The corpus luteum then degenerates, and the menstrual cycle begins again on or about day 28.

Figure 34-2 illustrates the sequence of hormone secretions and related events that take place during the menstrual cycle.

Female Sex Hormones

ESTROGENS

There are three major endogenous estrogens: estradiol, estrone, and estriol. All are synthesized from cholesterol in the ovarian follicles and have the basic chemical structure of a steroid, known as the *steroid nucleus*. For this reason, they are sometimes referred to as *steroid hormones*. Estradiol is the principal and most active of the three estrogens and represents the end product of estrogen synthesis.

The exogenous estrogenic drugs, those used as drug therapy, were developed because most of the endogenous estrogens are inactive when taken orally. The synthetic drugs fall into two categories, steroidal and nonsteroidal, as follows:

Steroidal:
- Conjugated estrogens (Premarin)
- Synthetic conjugated estrogens (Estrace)
- Esterified estrogens (Neo-Estrone)
- Estradiol cypionate (Estinate)

TABLE	34-1

Phases of the Menstrual Cycle

Phase	Ovarian Follicle Activity	Endometrium Activity
Phase 1	Menstruation	Menstruation
Phase 2	Follicular phase (preovulatory)	Proliferative phase
Phase 3	Ovulation	Ovulation
Phase 4	Luteal phase (postovulatory)	Secretory phase

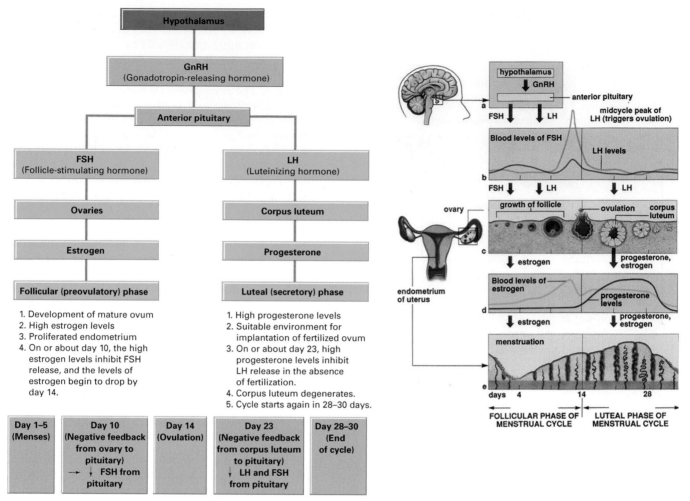

FIG. 34-2 Hormonal activity during the monthly menstrual cycle. Gonadotropin-releasing hormone (GnRH) from the hypothalamus stimulates the pituitary gland, causing it to secrete follicle-stimulating hormone (FSH) early in the cycle (coinciding with menses) and later luteinizing hormone (LH). FSH stimulates the ovaries to produce estrogen (primarily estradiol). Later in the cycle, the combined surges in the levels of estrogen, GnRH, FSH, and LH stimulate ovulation. The corpus luteum then secretes estrogen and progesterone, providing negative feedback to the hypothalamus and pituitary gland to reduce GnRH, FSH, and LH secretions. If the ovum (egg) is not fertilized by a spermatozoon, levels of estrogen and progesterone then fall to their monthly lows, GnRH and FSH rise again, and the onset of menses begins a new cycle. (Artwork reproduced with permission from University of California Santa Barbara, UCSB SexinfoOnline. Available at http://www.soc.ucsb.edu/sexinfo/article/the-menstrual-cycle. All rights reserved.)

- Estradiol transdermal (Climara, Estracomb, Estraderm, Estradot, Oesclim, others)
- Estradiol vaginal (Estring, Premarin, Vagifem)
- Estradiol valerate
- Estrone (Folliculum)
- Estropipate (Ogen)
- Ethinyl estradiol and norethindrone (Alesse, Minestrin 1/20, many others)

Nonsteroidal:
- Diethylstilbestrol (Stilbestrol)

The most popular estrogen product in use today is the conjugated estrogen. *Conjugated estrogens* are a combination of natural estrogen compounds equivalent to the average estrogen composition of the urine of pregnant mares, hence its brand name of Premarin. There is also a nonanimal source for this conjugated estrogen product. The product Estrace is composed of one estrogen,

17β-estradiol, which is structurally identical to estradiol produced by the female ovary but is obtained from soybeans. This product was developed in response to consumer demand from women who wanted an alternative to an animal-derived product. Some women obtain other natural estrogen products from naturopathic prescribers or natural health products such as black cohosh and evening primrose oil and prefer these to standard prescription drugs such as Premarin. Patients report varying degrees of satisfaction with the numerous products available, and it can take both time and patience to find the best choice for a given individual (see Natural Health Products). Ethinyl estradiol is one of the more potent estrogens and is most commonly found in oral contraceptive drugs.

Nonsteroidal estrogen products are no longer available for use in Canada for obstetric use because of major

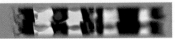

 NATURAL HEALTH PRODUCTS

POSTMENOPAUSE

BLACK COHOSH (Actaea racemosa and Cimicifuga racemosa)
- Preparations of black cohosh are made from its roots and rhizomes of bugpane
- Onset of action is 2 to 4 weeks
- Thought to reduce frequency and intensity of hot flashes and other menopausal symptoms
- Action: may have estrogenic effects

CHASTEBERRY (Vitex agnus-castus)
- Berry from the Chaste tree, a small shrub-like tree native to Central Asia and the Mediterranean region

- Thought to reduce libido, vaginal dryness, difficult or painful coitus
- Action: may have effects on FSH, LH, dopamine

EVENING PRIMROSE OIL (Oenothera biennis)
- Used for its action on vasomotor symptoms
- Thought to contain essential fatty acid, γ-linoleic acid

SOY
- Contains isoflavins with weak estrogenic effects

VALERIAN (Valerian officinalis)
- Root used by women to reduce menstrual cramps

adverse effects with the use of diethylstilbestrol (DES). Box 34-1 describes this important episode in medical history. Diethylstilbestrol (Stilbestrol), however, is Health Canada approved for palliative treatment of inoperable prostate cancer.

Mechanism of Action and Drug Effects

The binding of estrogen to estrogen receptors stimulates the synthesis of **nucleic acids** (deoxyribonucleic acid [DNA] and ribonucleic acid [RNA]) and proteins, which are the building blocks for all living tissue. Estrogens are also required at puberty for *feminization,* the development and maintenance of the female reproductive system and the development of female secondary sex characteristics.

Estrogens produce their effects in estrogen-responsive tissues, which have a large number of estrogen receptors. These tissues include the female genital organs, the breasts, the pituitary gland, and the hypothalamus. At the time of puberty, the production of estrogen increases greatly. This causes the initiation of menses, breast development, redistribution of body fat, softening of the skin, and other feminizing changes. Estrogens play a role in the shaping of body contours and development of the

skeleton. For instance, long bones are usually inhibited from growing, with the result that females are usually shorter than males.

Indications

Estrogens are used in the treatment or prevention of a variety of disorders that primarily result from estrogen deficiency. These conditions are listed in Box 34-2. **Hormone replacement therapy (HRT)** to counter such estrogen deficiency is most commonly known for its benefits in treating menopausal symptoms (e.g., hot flashes).

Contraindications

Contraindications for estrogen administration include known drug allergy, any estrogen-dependent cancer, undiagnosed abnormal vaginal bleeding, pregnancy, active thromboembolic disorder (e.g., stroke, thrombophlebitis), or a history of such a disorder.

Adverse Effects

The most serious adverse effects of the estrogens are thromboembolic events. Infrequently, estrogens cause erythema multiforme, a rare skin disorder characterized

BOX 34-1   Diethylstilbestrol

Between 1940 and 1971, an estimated six million mothers and their fetuses were exposed to diethylstilbestrol (DES). The drug was used to prevent reproductive problems such as miscarriage, premature delivery, intrauterine fetal death, and toxemia. This use resulted in significant complications of the reproductive systems of both female and male offspring. In 2003, the Marketed Health Products Directorate and the Therapeutic Products Directorate of Health Canada issued a health professional advisory in a letter advising of the risk of genital and obstetrical complications in those

exposed in utero, with recommended screening guidelines. Complications suspected to result from DES exposure are to be reported to the Canadian Adverse Drug Reaction Monitoring Program (CADRMP). D.E.S. Action Canada is a consumer organization that provides information and advocates on behalf of those exposed to DES. In addition, two large groups have been established to monitor DES complications: the International Registry for Research on Hormonal Transplacental Carcinogenesis and the National Cooperative Diethylstilbestrol Adenosis (DESAD) Project.

BOX 34-2

Indications for Estrogen Therapy

- Atrophic vaginitis (shrinkage of the vagina or urethra)
- Dysmenorrhea (painful or difficult menstruation)
- Hypogonadism
- Kraurosis vulvae (atrophy and shrinkage of the skin of the vulva)
- Oral contraception (in combination with a progestin)
- Osteoporosis treatment and prophylaxis
- Ovarian failure or castration
- Prevention of postpartum lactation
- Prostate cancer (palliative treatment of advanced inoperable cases)
- Uterine bleeding
- Vasomotor symptoms of menopause (e.g., hot flashes)

TABLE 34-2

Estrogens: Common Adverse Effects

Body System	Adverse Effects
Cardiovascular	Hypertension, thrombophlebitis, edema
Dermatological	Chloasma (facial skin discoloration; also called melasma) hirsutism, alopecia
Gastrointestinal	Nausea, vomiting, diarrhea, constipation, abdominal pain
Genitourinary	Amenorrhea, breakthrough uterine bleeding, enlarged uterine fibromyomas
Other	Tender breasts, fluid retention, decreased carbohydrate tolerance, headaches

by macules, papules, or subdermal vesicles with a multiform appearance on the hands and forearms. It can be recurrent or may run a severe course and terminate fatally in Stevens–Johnson syndrome, one of the most severe dermatological drug reactions. The most common undesirable effect of estrogen use is nausea. Often, photosensitivity may occur with estrogen therapy. One common dermatological effect of note is known as **chloasma**. This may be distressing to the patient in terms of her body image as it consists of brownish, macular spots that often occur on the forehead, cheeks, lips, and neck. This and other undesirable effects are listed in Table 34-2.

Interactions

Several drugs and drug classes that can potentially reduce the effectiveness of oral contraceptives can possibly result in an unintended pregnancy. These include the following:

- Antibiotics
- Barbiturates
- griseofulvin
- isoniazid
- rifampin

The effectiveness of other drugs may be reduced when they are taken with oral contraceptives. These include the following:

- Anticonvulsants
- Antihyperglycemic drugs
- β-blockers
- guanethidine
- Hypnotics
- Oral anticoagulants
- theophylline
- Tricyclic antidepressants
- Vitamins

Dosages

For the recommended dosages of oral contraceptives, see the Dosages table on p. 633.

DRUG PROFILES

▶▶ *estrogen*

Estrogen is indicated for the treatment of many clinical conditions, primarily those resulting from estrogen deficiency (see Box 34-2). Many of these conditions occur around menopause, when the endogenous estradiol level is declining. Any estrogen capable of binding to the estrogen receptors in target organs can alleviate menopausal symptoms. As a general rule, the smallest dosage of estrogen that relieves the symptoms or prevents the condition is used. Although many women receive estrogen or estrogen-progestin therapy for many months or years, some clinicians (and patients) may prefer that the patient be weaned from estrogen therapy in light of known adverse effects.

Two recent studies performed as part of the Women's Health Initiative (WHI), a large research program consisting of a set of clinical trials and an observational study sponsored by the National Institute of Health (NIH), demonstrated the detrimental effects of estrogen and combined estrogen/progestin therapy. Both studies attempted to determine the value of hormone replacement therapy (HRT), if any, in preventing diseases and conditions commonly affecting older women, including breast

Continued

DRUG PROFILES (cont'd)

cancer, heart disease, stroke, and hip fracture. The WHI was launched in 1991 under the direction of the National Heart, Lung, and Blood Institute (NHLBI). In one of the WHI studies of HRT, research subjects who took a certain estrogen/progestin were found to have an increased risk of breast cancer, heart disease, stroke, and blood clots, although their risks for hip fractures and colon cancer were reduced (Manson et al., 2003). These preliminary results were so alarming that this study of combined estrogen/progestin therapy was prematurely discontinued in 2002. A part of the WHI study focusing on cognitive function, the WHI Memory Study, also identified adverse cognitive effects in women receiving combination estrogen/progestin therapy (Schumaker et al., 2003). These patients showed an increased risk of developing dementia and demonstrated reduced performance on tests of cognitive function.

A second HRT study was begun, in which women who had undergone hysterectomy received estrogen alone without progestin. In March 2004, however, these participants were advised to stop taking the assigned drug because the estrogen-only therapy appeared to be associated with an increased risk of stroke. The data also indicated that estrogen therapy had no effect on the rates of coronary heart disease or breast cancer but was associated with a reduced rate of hip fracture (Cauley et al., 2003). Given these results, the view of the NHLBI is that the increased risk of stroke does not justify the use of preventive therapy in healthy women, especially since no beneficial effect on heart disease (risk reduction) was demonstrated. Follow-up of the WHI study subjects is expected to continue until 2010.

At this time, the NHLBI recommends that estrogen *not* be used for the prevention of cardiovascular disease.

However, HRT, given in the lowest effective dosages and for the shortest possible duration of treatment, is still recommended for alleviation of menopausal symptoms, according to the needs of each patient. Also recommended is the use of topical hormonal products if treatment is required only for vulvovaginal atrophy. In addition, although estrogen therapy is still endorsed for the prevention of postmenopausal osteoporosis, the recommendation is that they only be considered for women judged to be at especially high risk for osteoporosis. The nonestrogen osteoporosis drugs should also be strongly considered as an alternative or supplementary therapy.

The principal pharmacological effects of all estrogens are similar because there are only slight differences in their chemical structure. These differences yield drugs of different potencies, which, in turn, make them useful for a variety of indications. They also allow the drugs to be given by different routes of administration and often at highly customized doses.

Many fixed estrogen/progestin combination products have emerged over the years. Their use is commonly referred to as *continuous-combined hormone replacement therapy*. The rationale for the development of these drugs is that the use of estrogen therapy alone has been associated with an increased risk of endometrial hyperplasia, a possible precursor of endometrial cancer. The addition of continuously administered progestin to an estrogen regimen reduces the incidence of endometrial hyperplasia associated with unopposed estrogen therapy. Examples of these fixed combinations are conjugated estrogens with medroxyprogesterone acetate, norethindrone acetate with ethinyl estradiol, and estradiol with norethindrone acetate.

DOSAGES   Selected Estrogenic Drugs

Drug (Pregnancy Category)	Pharmacological Class	Usual Dosage Range	Indications
▸▸conjugated estrogens (Premarin) (X)	Estrogenic hormones	PO: 0.3–1.25 mg daily PO: 0.625 mg/day PO: 1.25 mg/day cyclically, 3 wk on, 1 wk off or continuously	Atrophic vaginitis, vulvular atrophy Menopausal symptoms, osteoporosis Female castration, primary ovarian failure
estradiol (Climara, Estrace) (X)	Estrogenic hormone	PO: 1 mg daily, adjusted to needs of patient PO: 0.5 mg daily cyclically, can be titrated up or down	Menopausal symptoms Osteoporosis prophylaxis
estradiol (Estring, Estraderm, Estrogel) (X)	Estrogenic hormone	Transdermal patch: 2.5 g patch twice weekly for 50 mcg/day, adapted to patient needs Metered dose pump: 2 actuations applied with hands over large area of skin in a uniform manner Estring: Inserted as deeply as possible into upper 1/3 of vaginal vault, left for 3 mo	Menopausal symptoms Menopausal urogenital symptoms

PROGESTINS

Available progestational drugs, or progestins, include both natural and synthetic drugs. Progesterone is the most active natural progestational hormone and is the primary progestin component in most drug formulations. It is produced by the corpus luteum after each ovulation and during pregnancy by the placenta. In addition, there are two other major natural progestins. The first is 17-hydroxyprogesterone, an inactive metabolite of progesterone. The second is pregnenolone, a chemical precursor to all steroid hormones that is synthesized from cholesterol in the ovary as was described for the estrogens. Because orally administered progesterone is relatively inactive and parenterally administered progesterone causes local reactions and pain, chemical derivatives were developed that are effective orally and also more potent. Their actions are also more specific and of longer duration. The following are some of the most commonly used progestins:

- medroxyprogesterone acetate (Depo-Provera, Medroxy, Premplus, Provera)
- megestrol (Megace)
- norethindrone acetate (Mestranol)
- norgestrel (Ovral)
- progesterone (Crinone, Prometrium)

Mechanism of Action and Drug Effects

All of the progestin products produce the same physiological responses as those produced by progesterone. These responses include induction of secretory changes in the endometrium, including diminished endometrial tissue proliferation; an increase in the basal body temperature; thickening of the vaginal mucosa; relaxation of uterine smooth muscle; stimulation of mammary alveolar tissue growth; feedback inhibition (negative feedback) of the release of pituitary gonadotropins (FSH and LH); and alterations in menstrual blood flow, especially in the presence of estrogen.

Indications

Progestins are useful in the treatment of functional uterine bleeding caused by a hormonal imbalance, fibroids, or uterine cancer; the treatment of primary and secondary amenorrhea; in the adjunctive and palliative treatment of some cancers and endometriosis; and alone or in combination with estrogens in the prevention of conception. They may also be helpful in preventing a threatened miscarriage and alleviating the symptoms of premenstrual syndrome. Specifically, medroxyprogesterone and

progesterone have been used to treat hormone imbalance, primary or secondary amenorrhea, and functional bleeding of the uterus, although medroxyprogesterone is the one most commonly used. Norethindrone and norgestrol may be used to treat female hormone imbalance and endometriosis but are more commonly used alone or in combination with estrogens as contraceptives. Megestrol is commonly used as adjunct therapy in the treatment of breast and endometrial cancers. When estrogen replacement therapy is initiated after menopause, progestins are often included to decrease endometrial proliferation that can be caused by unopposed estrogen. Formulations of progesterone itself are also used to treat female infertility (see Dosages table on p. 635).

Contraindications

Contraindications to use of progestins are similar to those for estrogens, as listed earlier.

Adverse Effects

The most serious undesirable effects of progestin use include liver dysfunction, commonly manifested as cholestatic jaundice; thrombophlebitis; and thromboembolic disorders such as pulmonary embolism. The more common adverse effects are listed in Table 34-3.

Interactions

There are reports of possible decreases in glucose tolerance when progestins are taken with antidiabetic drugs, and the dosage of the antidiabetic drug may need to be adjusted. The concurrent use of medroxyprogesterone or norethindrone or rifampin induces increased metabolism of the progestin.

Dosages

For recommended dosages of the progestins, see the Dosages table on p. 635.

TABLE 34-3

Progestins: Common Adverse Effects

Body System	Adverse Effects
Gastrointestinal	Nausea, vomiting
Genitourinary	Amenorrhea, spotting, changes in menstrual flow, changes in cervical erosion and secretions
Other	Edema, weight gain or loss, allergic rash, pyrexia, somnolence or insomnia, depression

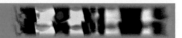

DRUG PROFILES

▶▶ medroxyprogesterone acetate

Medroxyprogesterone acetate (Depo-Provera, Medroxy, Premplus, Provera-Pak) inhibits the secretion of pituitary gonadotropins, which prevents follicular maturation and ovulation. It also stimulates the growth of mammary tissue and has an antineoplastic action against endometrial cancer. Medroxyprogesterone is used to treat uterine bleeding, secondary amenorrhea, endometrial cancer, and endometriosis and is also used as a contraceptive. Its most common use is to prevent endometrial cancer caused by estrogen replacement therapy. It is sometimes used as adjunct therapy in certain types of cancer (Chapter 49). Medroxyprogesterone is available in oral and parenteral preparations.

PHARMACOKINETICS

Half-Life	Onset	Peak	Duration
14.5 hr	Unknown	IM: 2–7 hr	IM: 3 mo

▶▶ megestrol acetate

Megestrol acetate (Megace) is a synthetic progestin that differs structurally from progesterone-only in the addition of a methyl group on the steroid nucleus and a double bond. Although megestrol shares the actions of the progestins, it is primarily used in the palliative management of recurrent, inoperable, or metastatic endometrial or breast cancer. It is used in the management of anorexia, cachexia, or unexplained substantial weight loss in patients with acquired immune deficiency syndrome (AIDS). In addition, it may be used to stimulate appetite and promote weight gain in patients with cancer. It is available only for oral use.

PHARMACOKINETICS

Half-Life	Onset	Peak	Duration
34 hr	6–8 wk	1–3 hr	4–10 mo

DOSAGES | Selected Progestational Drugs

Drug (Pregnancy Category)	Pharmacological Class	Usual Dosage Range	Indications
▶▶medroxyprogesterone acetate (Depo-Provera, Medroxy, Premplus, Provera-Pak) (X)	Progestin	PO: 5–10 mg/day for set number of days or cyclically (smaller doses may be given on a continuous daily basis)	Amenorrhea, uterine bleeding
		PO: 2.5–10 mg daily on last 10–13 days of each month to accompany estrogen dosing	Vasomotor symptoms of menopause
		PO: 200–400 mg/day	Endometrial cancer
		PO: 400–800 mg/day divided	Breast cancer
		IM: 50 mg/wk or 100 mg q2 wk × 6 mo	Endometriosis
megestrol acetate (Megace, Megace OS) (X)	Progestogen	PO (Megace Os): 400–800 mg/day	Anorexia, cachexia, or significant weight loss in patients with HIV/AIDS or in patients with cancer
		PO: 160 mg/day	Palliative or adjunctive breast carcinoma
		PO: 80–320 mg/day divided	Endometrial carcincoma
		PO: 120 mg/day, single dose	Advanced hormone-responsive carcinoma of prostate
progesterone (Crinone*, Prometrium) (X)	Progestin	Intravaginal gel: 90 mg once to twice daily for up to 12 wk	Reproduction failure and in vitro fertilization therapy
		PO: 200 mg at bedtime or 300 mg bid for set number of days or cyclically†	Hormone replacement therapy
		IM: 5–10 mg daily for 6–8 days	Amenorrhea or functional uterine bleeding

IM, intramuscular; *PO*, oral.

*These products are sometimes used to promote or maintain pregnancy as part of an assisted reproductive technology regimen.
†Formulation contains peanut oil and is contraindicated in patients with peanut allergy.

CONTRACEPTIVE DRUGS

Contraceptive drugs are medications used to prevent pregnancy. *Contraceptive devices* are nondrug methods of pregnancy prevention such as intrauterine devices (IUDs), male and female condoms, and cervical diaphragms. For their own safety, patients must be informed that contraceptive drug therapy, including spermicidal drugs, serves only to prevent pregnancy and does not protect them from the transmission of sexually transmitted infections, including HIV/AIDS. Spermicidal drugs, such as the over-the-counter foams for intravaginal use, most often contain the spermicide nonoxynol-9, which kills sperm cells to prevent pregnancy but does not necessarily kill microbes that cause sexually transmitted infections, including HIV infection.

Aside from sexual abstinence, oral contraceptives are the most effective form of birth control currently available. Estrogen/progestin combinations, often referred to as "the pill," are oral contraceptives that contain both estrogenic and progestational steroids. The most common estrogenic component is ethinyl estradiol, a semisynthetic steroidal estrogen. The most common progestin component is norethindrone.

Currently available oral contraceptives may be biphasic, triphasic, or monophasic, in terms of the doses taken at different times of the menstrual cycle. The monophasic and triphasic oral contraceptives are the most numerous on the market and the most widely prescribed. Some patients (e.g., those with menstrual irregularities) may require special assistance in selecting drug products with their prescribers. Three other important contraceptive medications are a long-acting injectable form of medroxyprogesterone, a transdermal contraceptive patch, and, most recently, an intravaginal contraceptive ring (NuvaRing). The etonogestrel-ethinyl estradiol slow-release vaginal ring is a soft, flexible, clear plastic ring that measures 54 mm in diameter. It can be inserted by the user into the vagina, where it is held in place and slowly releases the hormones for 3 weeks. It is removed for a 1-week ring-free interval. During the ring-free period, the user usually menstruates within a few days. A new ring is inserted to begin a new cycle. The ring's method of action is similar to that of the combined oral contraceptive pill. The ring does not provide a physical barrier to sperm and it does not prevent sexually transmitted infections.

Biphasic drugs contain a fixed estrogen dose but a low progestin dose for the first 10 days and a higher dose for the rest of the cycle and are available in 21- or 28-day dosage packages. Triphasic oral contraceptives contain three different estrogen–progestin dose ratios that are administered sequentially during the cycle and are provided in 21- or 28-day dosage packages. Triphasic products closely duplicate the normal hormonal levels of the female cycle. These contraceptives also come in monophasic forms, in which the estrogen and progestin doses are the same throughout the cycle. Oral contraceptives

that are progestin-only drugs are also available. Another new approach is extended dosing of oral contraceptives.

Mechanism of Action and Drug Effects

Contraceptive drugs prevent ovulation by inhibiting the release of gonadotropins and by increasing uterine mucous viscosity, which results in (1) decreased sperm movement and fertilization of the ovum, and (2) possible inhibition of implantation (nidation) of a fertilized egg (zygote) into the endometrial lining.

Oral contraceptives have many of the same hormonal effects as those normally produced by the endogenous estrogens and progesterone. The contraceptive effect results mainly from suppression of the hypothalamic–pituitary system that they induce, which, in turn, prevents ovulation. Other incidental benefits to their use are that they improve menstrual cycle regularity and decrease blood loss during menstruation. A decreased incidence of functional ovarian cysts and ectopic pregnancies has also been associated with their use.

Indications

Oral contraceptives are used primarily to prevent pregnancy. In addition, they are used to treat endometriosis and hypermenorrhea and to produce cyclic withdrawal bleeding in patients with amenorrhea. Occasionally, combination oral contraceptives are used to provide postcoital emergency contraception. Emergency contraception pills are not effective if the woman is already pregnant (i.e., egg implantation has occurred). They should be taken within 72 hours of unprotected intercourse with a follow-up dose 12 hours after the first dose. They are intended to prevent pregnancy after known or suspected contraceptive failure or unprotected intercourse. Triphasil, Min-Ovral, and Alesse are three ethinyl estradiol/levonorgestrel combination drugs that are commonly used for this indication. One new oral contraceptive of note is Seasonale, which includes both estrogen and progestin components. It is sold in packages containing 3 months' worth of medication, including 1 week's worth of nonhormonal tablets, because Seasonale reduces a woman's menstrual cycles to once every 3 months.

The Dosages table on p. 637 provides selected examples of the many contraceptive drugs available. All act in a similar fashion to prevent pregnancy. If they are used during pregnancy, however, they can cause termination of pregnancy. Drugs that are intended for termination of pregnancy are known as abortifacients and are discussed later in this chapter.

Contraindications

Contraindications to the use of oral contraceptives include known drug allergy to a specific product, pregnancy, and known high risk for or history of thromboembolic events such as myocardial infarction, venous thrombosis, pulmonary embolism, or stroke.

Adverse Effects

Common adverse effects associated with the use of oral contraceptives are listed in Table 34-4. These effects include hypertension, thromboembolism, alterations in carbohydrate and lipid metabolism, increases in serum hormone concentrations, and alterations in serum metal and plasma protein levels. The estrogen component appears to be the source of most of these metabolic effects.

TABLE   34-4

Oral Contraceptives: Common Adverse Effects

Body System	Adverse Effects
Cardiovascular	Hypertension, thrombophlebitis, edema, thromboembolism, pulmonary embolism, myocardial infarction
Central nervous	Dizziness, headache, migraines, depression, stroke
Gastrointestinal	Nausea, vomiting, diarrhea, anorexia, pancreatitis, cramps, constipation, increased appetite, increased weight, cholestatic jaundice
Genitourinary	Amenorrhea, cervical erosion, breakthrough bleeding, dysmenorrhea, breast changes

Interactions

Several drugs and drug classes can potentially reduce the effectiveness of oral contraceptives, which can possibly result in an unintended pregnancy. These include the following:

- Antibiotics
- griseofulvin
- isoniazid
- rifampin

The effectiveness of other drugs may be reduced when they are taken with oral contraceptives. These include the following:

- Anticonvulsants
- Antihyperglycemic drugs
- β-Blockers
- guanethidine
- Hypnotics
- Oral anticoagulants
- theophylline
- Tricyclic antidepressants
- Vitamins

Dosages

For the recommended dosages of oral contraceptives, see the Dosages table below.

DOSAGES   Selected Contraceptive Medications

Drug (Pregnancy Category)	Pharmacological Class	Usual Dosage Range	Indications
ORAL CONTRACEPTIVES			
levonorgestrel/ethinyl estradiol (Ortho 7/7/7, Tri-Cyclen, Triquilar, Triphasil) (X)	Triphasic	3 or 4 monthly phases of variable estrogen and progestin combinations; 21- or 28-day products; 28-day products contain 7 inert tabs	Prevention of pregnancy
norethindrone and ethinyl estradiol (Symphasic) (X)	Biphasic	Fixed estrogen–variable progestin 21- or 28-day products. For the most reliable contraceptive action, patient should take all preparations according to instructions from the prescriber or patient information product insert, at intervals not to exceed 24 h	Prevention of pregnancy
norethindrone and ethinyl estradiol	Monophasic	Fixed estrogen/progestin combinations; 21- or 28-day products; 28-day products contain 7 inert tabs	Prevention of pregnancy
INJECTABLE CONTRACEPTIVES (DEPOT)			
▸▸**medroxyprogesterone acetate (Depo-Provera) (X)**	Progestin-only injectable contraceptive	IM: 150 mg q3 mo	Prevention of pregnancy
TRANSDERMAL CONTRACEPTIVES			
norelgestromin and ethinyl estradiol (X)	Fixed-combination estrogen/progestin transdermal contraceptive	Transdermal patch: 1 patch applied weekly × 3 each month, scheduled around menses in week 4	Prevention of pregnancy
INTRAVAGINAL CONTRACEPTIVES			
etonogestrel/ethinyl estradiol vaginal ring (NuvaRing) (X)	Fixed-combination estrogen/progestin intravaginal contraceptive	One ring inserted into vagina by patient and left in place for 3 weeks, followed by 1-week removal. A new ring is then inserted 1 week later.	Prevention of pregnancy

IM, intramuscular.

CURRENT DRUG THERAPY FOR OSTEOPOROSIS

Bone homeostasis is a dynamic process, maintained through a balanced coordination between bone reabsorption by osteoclasts and bone formation by osteoblasts. *Osteoblasts,* which are found on the outer surfaces of the bones and in the bone cavities, synthesize bone matrix. They secrete collagen which strands together to form osteoids, the spiral fibres of bone matrix. Calcium salts and phosphorus, retrieved from the blood, precipitate and bond with osteoids. Through this process the bone matrix is mineralized and strengthened. Estrogen receptors are also found on osteoblast surfaces; estrogens increase the number of osteoblasts, which increases collagen production. *Osteoclasts,* by contrast, continually reabsorb bone matrix and reabsorption is followed by new bone formation, thus achieving a balance of bone mass.

A variety of factors influence bone development: nutrition, exposure to sunlight, hormonal secretions, and physical exercise. Vitamin D is necessary for calcium absorption in the small intestine. When vitamin D is lacking, as in those with limited sun exposure, calcium may be poorly absorbed. Consequently, bone matrix is deficient in calcium, resulting in weak bones. Vitamins A and C also are needed for normal bone growth and development.

Approximately 1 in 4 Canadian women and 1 in 8 men aged 50 years or over currently are affected by **osteoporosis**, a condition characterized by the progressive loss of bone density and thinning of bone tissue; an additional 60% have decreased bone mineral density, or *osteopenia.* The prevalence of osteoporosis increases with age from approximately 6% at 50 years of age to over 50% above 80 years of age. Menopause is a critical period during which bone mineral density (BMD) decreases. There is an average BMD decrease of 6.8% over 5 years in the hip. The Canadian Multicentre Osteoporosis Study (CaMos; Berger et al., 2008) also found that significant BMD loss occurs after age 70, mainly in the hip bone. In men, BMD decreases more gradually, although it starts earlier, around the age of 40. Canadian White women over 50 years of age have a 40% lifetime risk of developing an osteoporotic fragility fracture, a 17.5% lifetime risk of sustaining a hip fracture, and a 16% lifetime risk of a wrist fracture.

The annual Canadian cost for treating osteoporosis and fractures is $1.9 billion each year and is expected to reach $32.5 billion by 2018 as the population ages. Seventy percent of approximately 25,000 hip fractures in Canada are osteoporosis related. Death results in approximately 20% of cases and disability in 50% of those who survive. Risk factors for postmenopausal osteoporosis include White or Asian descent, slender body build, early estrogen deficiency, smoking, alcohol consumption, low-calcium diet, sedentary lifestyle, and family history of osteoporosis. Although osteoporosis is a disorder that affects mostly women, up to 20% of people with this condition are men.

Supplementation with calcium and vitamin D is recommended for all women and men considered at risk for osteoporosis (e.g., those with a family history of the disorder). The recommended calcium intake usually ranges from 1000 to 1500 mg daily depending on age, frame, and hormone status. The Society of Obstetricians and Gynecologists, in their 2006 practice guidelines, recommend routine supplementation of 1000 mg of calcium and 400 units of vitamin D as mandatory adjunct therapy to the main pharmacological interventions. In February 2006, the National Heart, Lung, and Blood Institute (NHLBI) announced the results of the calcium–vitamin D trial of the Women's Health Initiative, which monitored patients for 7 years to examine the preventive effects of calcium and vitamin D supplementation. The conclusion was that such supplements led to a more modest than expected reduction in hip and other fractures, had no preventive effects with regard to colon polyps or cancer as previously believed, and increased the risk of kidney stones (Jackson et al., 2006). More current studies have found that vitamin D may provide cancer preventive effects (Huncharek, Muscat, & Kupelnick, 2009; IARC Working Group on Vitamin D, 2008; Lappe et al., 2007; McCullough et al., 2003), the evidence of potential benefit is limited and inconsistent. Thus more research is being conducted to clarify the available evidence.

Three major drug classes are currently the foundation of treating existing osteoporosis and osteopenia: the bisphosphonates, the selective estrogen receptor modulators (SERMs), and the hormones calcitonin and teriparatide. Available bisphosphonates used for osteoporosis prevention and treatment include etidronate, alendronate, and risedronate. Zoledronic acid (Aclasta), classed as a bone metabolism regulator by Health Canada, is a once-yearly intravenous infusion for the treatment of osteoporosis in postmenopausal women to reduce the incidence of hip, vertebral, and nonvertebral fractures. It is considered a biphosphonate. Currently, raloxifene and tamoxifen are the available SERMs. Tamoxifen is used primarily in oncology settings and is discussed further in Chapter 49. Raloxifene has been investigated mainly for use in the prevention of osteoporosis, although many studies suggest that it may be beneficial in the treatment of osteoporosis as well. A drug form of the hormone calcitonin is also commonly used.

Mechanism of Action and Drug Effects

Bisphosphonates work by inhibiting osteoclast-mediated bone reabsorption, which, in turn, indirectly enhances bone mineral density. Osteoclasts are bone cells that break down bone, causing calcium to be reabsorbed into the circulation; this reabsorption eventually leads to osteoporosis if not controlled or countered by adequate new bone formation. These drugs have become the primary drugs of choice for this condition because their use is backed by the strongest clinical evidence indicating reversal of lost bone mass and reduction of fracture risk.

Raloxifene acts to prevent osteoporosis by stimulating estrogen receptors on bone and increasing bone density in a manner similar to the estrogens themselves. Like the natural thyroid hormone, calcitonin directly inhibits osteoclastic bone reabsorption.

In contrast to the other therapies described thus far, which inhibit bone reabsorption, teriparatide is the first and currently the only drug available that acts by stimulating bone formation. It is a derivative of parathyroid hormone and acts to treat osteoporosis by modulating the body's metabolism of calcium and phosphorus in a manner similar to natural parathyroid hormone.

Indications

Raloxifene is used primarily for the prevention of postmenopausal osteoporosis. The bisphosphonates and calcitonin are used in both the prevention and treatment of osteoporosis. Teriparatide is used mainly for the subset of osteoporosis patients at highest risk of fracture (e.g., those with prior fracture).

Contraindications

Contraindications to bisphosphonate use include drug allergy, hypocalcemia, esophageal dysfunction, and the inability to sit or stand upright for at least 30 minutes after taking the medication. Zoledronic acid should not be used in individuals with severe kidney impairment

Use of SERMs is contraindicated in women with a known allergy to these drugs, in women who are or may become pregnant, and in women with a venous thromboembolic disorder, including deep vein thrombosis, pulmonary embolism, and retinal vein thrombosis, or with a history of such a disorder.

Contraindications to calcitonin use include drug allergy or allergy to salmon (the drug is salmon derived). Contraindications to the use of teriparatide include drug allergy.

Adverse Effects

The primary adverse effects of SERMs are hot flashes and leg cramps. Like estrogens, SERMS can increase the risk of venous thromboembolism, and they are teratogenic. Leukopenia may also occur and predispose the patient to infections. Postmenopausal women taking raloxifene are no more likely to develop breast, uterine, or ovarian cancer than women taking a placebo. The most common adverse effects of bisphosphonates include headache, gastrointestinal upset, and joint pain. However, the bisphosphonates are usually well tolerated. There is a risk of esophageal burns with biphosphonate medications if they become lodged in the esophagus before reaching the stomach. For this reason, the patient should take biphosphonates with a full glass of water and remain sitting upright or standing for at least 30 minutes. Common adverse effects of calcitonin include flushing of the face, nausea, diarrhea, and reduced appetite. Common adverse effects of teriparatide include chest pain, dizziness, hypercalcemia, nausea, and arthralgia.

Interactions

Cholestyramine and ampicillin decrease the absorption of raloxifene, and raloxifene can decrease the effects of warfarin. Calcium supplements and antacids can interfere with the absorption of the bisphosphonates, thus these drugs should be spaced 1 to 2 hours apart to avoid this interaction. Calcium supplements, although often needed by patients with osteoporosis, are also more likely to cause hypercalcemia in patients receiving calcitonin. There have been case reports of teriparatide-associated hypercalcemia that has been implicated in digitalis toxicity.

Dosages

For the recommended dosages of osteoporosis drugs, see the Dosages table on p. 640.

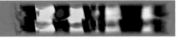

DRUG PROFILES

▶▶ alendronate sodium

Alendronate sodium (Fosamax) is an oral bisphosphonate and the first nonestrogen–nonhormonal option for preventing bone loss. This drug acts by inhibiting or reversing osteoclast-mediated born reabsorption. Recall that osteoclasts are the bone cells that cause breakdown or reabsorption of bone tissue as part of their normal physiology. Unchecked osteoclastic activity often leads to osteoporosis if not managed, so this drug class represents a major breakthrough in the treatment of osteoporosis. It is indicated for the prevention and treatment of osteoporosis in men and in postmenopausal women. It is also indicated for the treatment of glucocorticoid-induced osteoporosis in men and for the treatment of Paget's disease in women.

Data show that alendronate may reduce the risk of hip fracture by 51%, spinal fracture by 47%, and wrist fracture by 48%. Precaution should be taken in patients with dysphagia, esophagitis, esophageal ulcer, or gastric ulcer because the drug can be irritating. Case reports of esophageal erosions have been published. It is recommended that alendronate be taken immediately upon rising in the morning with 240 mL of water and that the patient not lie down for at least 30 minutes after taking it. When patients whose condition has been stabilized on alendronate are hospitalized and cannot adhere to these recommendations, the medication is often withheld. Alendronate has an extremely long-term half-life,

Continued

DRUG PROFILES (cont'd)

and missing several days without taking a dose will do little to reduce the therapeutic efficacy of the drug.

Both alendronate and a similar drug, risedronate, are available only in tablet form for daily or weekly oral use. Alendronate/cholecalciferol (Fosavance) is also available for once-weekly administration. Risendronate with calcium (Actonel Plus Calcium) is available for a monthly administration course. Risendronate is also available in a 75 mg tablet, for monthly duet administration (on two consecutive days per month on the same calendar days each month), or a 150 mg tablet for once-a-month administration on the same calendar day per month.

PHARMACOKINETICS

Half-Life	Onset*	Peak*	Duration
> 10 yr because of storage of drug in bone tissue	3 wk	Unknown	Unknown

*Therapeutic effect.

calcitonin

Calcitonin (Miacalin NS), in its drug forms, is derived from salmon (fish) sources. It is available as a nasal spray.

PHARMACOKINETICS (NASAL SPRAY)

Half-Life	Onset	Peak	Duration
43 min	Unknown	30–40 min	Unknown

raloxifene hydrochloride

Raloxifene hydrochloride (Evista) is an SERM. It is used primarily for the prevention of postmenopausal osteoporosis. Interestingly, raloxifene has positive effects on cholesterol levels, but it is not normally used specifically for this purpose. It may not be the best choice for women near menopause because the use of this drug is associated with hot flashes. It is available only for oral use.

PHARMACOKINETICS

Half-Life	Onset	Peak	Duration
27 hr	Unknown	Unknown	Unknown

teriparatide

Teriparatide (Forteo) is currently the only drug in the newest class of medications used in the treatment of osteoporosis. It is a derivative of parathyroid hormone and works to treat osteoporosis by modulating the body's metabolism of calcium and phosphorus in a manner similar to natural parathyroid hormone. It is currently available only in injectable form in a 3 mL cartridge for pen use in a strength of 250 mcg/mL.

PHARMACOKINETICS

Half-Life	Onset	Peak	Duration
Unknown	2 hr	4–6 hr	16–24 hr

DOSAGES   Selected Drugs Used Specifically for Osteoporosis

Drug (Pregnancy Category)	Pharmacological Class	Usual Dosage Range	Indications
▸▸alendronate sodium (Fosamax) (C)	Bisphosphonate	PO: 5 mg daily PO: 10 mg daily or 70 mg once per week	Prevention and treatment of postmenopausal osteoporosis
calcitonin salmon (Miacalin NS) (C)	Bone metabolism regulator	Nasal spray: 200 units (1 spray) alternating nostrils daily	Osteoporosis treatment
etidronate disodium (Didronel) (C)	Biphosphonate	PO: 90-day cycle: etidronate 400 mg daily × 14 days, then calcium carbonate 1250 mg daily × 76 days	Prevention and treatment of postmenopausal osteoporosis
raloxifene hydrochloride (Evista) (X)	Selective estrogen receptor modulator	PO: 60 mg daily	Osteoporosis prevention and treatment
teriparatide (Forteo) (C)	Parathyroid hormone derivative	SC: 250 mcg once daily in thigh or abdomen × 18 mo	Osteoporosis treatment
zoledronic acid (Aclasta, Zometa) (C)	Biphosphonate	IV: 5 mg (in 100 mg ready-to-use solution) over 15 min	Osteoporosis treatment

IM, intramuscular; *PO*, oral; *SC*, subcutaneous.

Drug Therapy Related to Pregnancy, Labour, Delivery, and the Postpartum Period

FERTILITY DRUGS

Infertility in women generally results from the absence of ovulation (anovulation), which normally is caused by imbalances of female reproductive hormones. Such imbalances can occur at the level of the hypothalamus, the pituitary gland, the ovary, or any combination of these. Supplements of estrogens or progestins may be used to fortify the blood levels of these hormones when ovarian output is inadequate. The use of the drug forms of these hormones was described in the Estrogens and Progestins sections earlier in this chapter.

Hormone deficiencies at the hypothalamic and pituitary levels are often treated with gonadotropin ovarian stimulants. These drugs stimulate increased secretion of gonadotropin-releasing hormone (GnRH) from the hypothalamus, which then results in increased secretion of FSH and LH from the pituitary gland. These hormones, in turn, stimulate the development of ovarian follicles and ovulation. They also stimulate ovarian secretion of estrogens and progestins that are part of the normal ovulatory cycle.

Proper selection and dosage adjustment of fertility drugs often requires the expertise of a fertility specialist. The medical techniques used in the treatment of infertility, including drug therapy, are collectively referred to as *assistive reproductive technology*. One common specific technique is *in vitro fertilization*, in which a woman's ovum is fertilized with her partner's sperm in a laboratory setting and the fertilized ovum is then medically implanted into the woman's uterus. Infants born from the use of this technique are often referred to as "test tube babies." The success of such fertilization techniques may be further aided by the use of ovulation-stimulant drugs such as clomiphene, menotropins, and choriogonadotropin alfa.

Mechanism of Action and Drug Effects

Clomiphene is a nonsteroidal ovulation stimulant that works by blocking estrogen receptors in the uterus and brain. This results in a false signal of low estrogen levels to the brain. The hypothalamus and pituitary gland then increase their production of GnRH (from the hypothalamus) and FSH and LH (from the pituitary), which stimulates the maturation of ovarian follicles. Ideally, this leads to ovulation and increases the likelihood of conception in a previously infertile woman.

Menotropins is a standardized mixture of FSH and LH derived from the urine of postmenopausal women. The FSH component stimulates the development of ovarian follicles, which leads to ovulation. The LH component stimulates the development of the corpus luteum, which supplies female sex hormones (estrogens and progestins) during the first trimester of pregnancy. Choriogonadotropin alfa is a recombinant form (i.e., developed with recombinant DNA technology) of the hormone human chorionic gonadotropin (hCG). This hormone is naturally produced by the placenta during pregnancy and can be isolated from the urine of pregnant women. It is an analogue of LH and can provide a substitute for the natural LH surge that promotes ovulation. It does this by binding to LH receptors in the ovary and stimulating the rupture of mature ovarian follicles and subsequent development of the corpus luteum. Human chorionic gonadotropin also maintains the viability of the corpus luteum during early pregnancy. This is critical because the corpus luteum provides the supply of estrogens and progestins necessary to support the first trimester of pregnancy until the placenta assumes this role. Choriogonadotropin alfa is often given in a carefully timed fashion following FSH-active therapy such as with menotropins or clomiphene, when patient monitoring indicates sufficient maturation of ovarian follicles.

Indications

Fertility drugs are used primarily for the promotion of ovulation in anovulatory female patients. They may also be used to promote spermatogenesis in infertile men. Progesterone formulations are also used to treat female infertility.

Contraindications

Contraindications to the use of ovarian stimulants include known drug allergy to any specific product and may also include primary ovarian failure, uncontrolled thyroid or adrenal dysfunction, liver disease, pituitary tumour, abnormal uterine bleeding, ovarian enlargement of uncertain cause, sex hormone–dependent tumours, and pregnancy.

Adverse Effects

The most common adverse effects of the ovulation stimulants are listed in Table 34-5.

TABLE	34-5

Fertility Drugs: Most Common Adverse Effects

Body System	Adverse Effects
Cardiovascular	Tachycardia, phlebitis, deep vein thrombosis, hypovolemia
Central nervous	Dizziness, headache, flushing, depression, restlessness, anxiety, nervousness, fatigue
Gastrointestinal	Nausea, bloating, constipation, abdominal pain, vomiting, anorexia
Other	Urticaria, ovarian hyperstimulation, multiple pregnancies, blurred vision, diplopia, photophobia, breast pain, fever

Interactions

Few drug interactions occur with fertility drugs. The most notable are tricyclic antidepressants, the butyrophenones (e.g., haloperidol), the phenothiazines (e.g., promethazine), and the antihypertensive drugs methyldopa and reserpine. When any of these drugs are taken with fertility drugs, prolactin concentrations may be increased, which may impair fertility.

Dosages

For recommended dosages of the fertility drugs, see the Dosages table below.

DRUG PROFILES

choriogonadotropin alfa

Choriogonadotropin alfa (Ovidrel) is a synthetic recombinant analogue of natural hCG and has effects similar to those of this hormone. These effects include the rupture of mature ovarian follicles (and ovulation) and maintenance of the corpus luteum. Choriogonadotropin alfa is currently available only in injectable form.

PHARMACOKINETICS

Half-Life	Onset	Peak	Duration
5.6 hr	2 hr	6 hr	36 hr

clomiphene citrate

Clomiphene citrate (Clomid, Serophene) is primarily used to stimulate the production of pituitary gonadotropins, which, in turn, induce the maturation of the ovarian follicle and, eventually, ovulation. It is currently available only for oral use.

PHARMACOKINETICS

Half-Life	Onset	Peak	Duration
5 days	4–12 days	Unknown	1 mo

▶▶ menotropins

Menotropins (Menopur, Pergonal) is a purified preparation of the gonadotropins FSH and LH that is extracted from the urine of postmenopausal women. Other available medications with similar composition and functions include urofollitropin (Bravelle), follitropin alfa (Gonal-f), and follitropin beta (Puregon). Contraindications for all of these drugs are listed in the Fertility Drugs section. Menotropins is available only as a parenteral injection.

PHARMACOKINETICS

Half-Life	Onset	Peak	Duration
Unknown	Unknown	Unknown	Unknown

DOSAGES Selected Fertility Drugs

Drug (Pregnancy Category)	Pharmacological Class	Usual Dosage Range	Indications
choriogonadotropin alfa (Ovidrel) (X)	Ovulation stimulant, recombinant	SC/IM: 250 mcg given 1 day after last dose of follicle stimulant (e.g., menotropins)	Female infertility
clomiphene citrate (Clomid, Serophene) (X)	Ovulation stimulant	PO: 50–100 mg daily for 5 days; cycle repeatable depending on response	Female infertility in selected patients
▶▶ **menotropins (Menopur, Pergonal) (X)**	Gonadotropins (FSH/LH) ovulation stimulant	SC: 225–450 units daily for 20 days (max) adjusted according to response, followed by chorionic gonadotropin	Female infertility, male infertility

IM, intramuscular; *PO*, oral; *SC*, subcutaneous.

Uterine-Active Drugs

A variety of medications are used to alter the dynamics of uterine contractions to either promote or prevent the start or progression of labour. In the immediate postpartum period, medications may also be used to promote rapid shrinkage of the uterus in order to reduce the risk of postpartum hemorrhage.

UTERINE STIMULANTS

The uterus is a highly muscular organ that has a complex network of smooth muscle fibres and a large blood supply. The uterus undergoes several changes during normal gestation and childbirth that at different times make it either resistant or susceptible to hormones and drugs. Three types of drugs are used to stimulate uterine contractions: ergot derivatives, prostaglandins, and the hormone oxytocin. These drugs are often collectively referred to as oxytocics, after the naturally occurring hormone oxytocin, whose action they mimic. Oxytocin is one of the two hormones secreted by the posterior lobe of the pituitary gland. The other is vasopressin, which is also known as antidiuretic hormone. Prostaglandin, the other class of oxytocic drugs, is a natural hormone involved in regulating the network of smooth muscle fibres of the uterus. This network is known as the *myometrium*. The third major class of oxytocic drugs, the ergot alkaloids, consists also of potent simulators of uterine muscle.

Mechanism of Action and Drug Effects

The uterus of a woman who is not pregnant is relatively insensitive to oxytocin. During pregnancy, the uterus becomes more sensitive to oxytocin and is most sensitive at term (the end of pregnancy).

During childbirth, oxytocin stimulates uterine contraction, whereas during lactation it promotes the movement of milk from the mammary glands to the nipples.

Prostaglandins cause potent contractions of the myometrium and may also play a role in the natural induction of labour. When prostaglandin concentrations increase during the final few weeks of pregnancy, mild myometrial contractions, commonly known as Braxton–Hicks contractions, are stimulated.

Indications

Oxytocin is available in a synthetic injectable form (e.g., Pitocin). This drug is used to induce labour at or near full-term gestation and to enhance labour when uterine contractions are weak and ineffective. Oxytocic drugs are also used to prevent or control uterine bleeding after delivery, to induce completion of an incomplete abortion (including miscarriages), and to promote milk expression during lactation.

The prostaglandins may be used therapeutically to induce labour by softening the cervix (cervical ripening) and enhancing uterine muscle tone. They may also be used to stimulate the myometrium to induce abortion during the second trimester when the uterus is resistant to oxytocin. Examples of these drugs are dinoprostone and misoprostol.

Ergot alkaloids are used after delivery of the infant and placenta to prevent postpartum uterine atony (lack of muscle tone) and hemorrhage.

Contraindications

Contraindications to the use of labour-inducing uterine stimulants include known drug allergy to a specific product and may include pelvic inflammatory disease, cervical stenosis, uterine fibrosis, high-risk intrauterine fetal positions before delivery, placenta previa, hypertonic uterus, uterine prolapse, or any condition in which vaginal delivery is contraindicated (e.g., increased bleeding risk). Contraindications to the use of abortifacients include known drug allergy, the presence of an IUD, ectopic pregnancy, concurrent anticoagulant therapy or bleeding disorder, inadequate access to emergency health care, or the inability to understand or adhere to follow-up instructions.

Adverse Effects

The most common undesirable effects of oxytocic drugs are listed in Table 34-6.

Interactions

Few clinically significant drug interactions occur with oxytocic drugs. The most common and important of these involve sympathomimetic drugs. Combining drugs that produce vasoconstriction, such as sympathomimetics, with the oxytocic drugs can result in severe hypertension.

Dosages

For the recommended dosages of selected oxytocic drugs, see the Dosages table on p. 644.

TABLE	34-6

Oxytocic Drugs: Most Common Adverse Effects

Body System	Adverse Effects
Cardiovascular	Hypotension or hypertension, chest pain
Central nervous	Headache, dizziness, fainting
Gastrointestinal	Nausea, vomiting, diarrhea
Genitourinary	Vaginitis, vaginal pain, cramping
Other	Leg cramps, joint swelling, chills, fever, weakness, blurred vision

DRUG PROFILES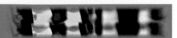

▶▶ dinoprostone

Dinoprostone (Prostin E_2, Cervidil, Prepidil) is a synthetic derivative of the naturally occurring hormone prostaglandin E_2. It is used for ripening of an unfavourable cervix in pregnant women at or near term with a medical or obstetric need for labour induction. It is available for vaginal use in various dosage forms and for oral use.

PHARMACOKINETICS

Half-Life	Onset	Peak	Duration
Gel: N/A	Gel: Rapid	Gel: 30–45 min	Gel: Unavailable
PO: 1 min	PO: 10 min	PO: Unavailable	PO: 2–3 hr

▶▶ ergonovine maleate

The ergot alkaloid ergonovine maleate is used primarily in the immediate postpartum period to enhance myometrial tone and reduce the likelihood of postpartum uterine hemorrhage. Its use is contraindicated in patients with a known hypersensitivity to ergot medications and in those with pelvic inflammatory disease. It should also not be used for augmentation of labour, before delivery of the placenta, or during a spontaneous abortion. Ergonovine is available in oral injectable forms.

PHARMACOKINETICS

Half-Life	Onset	Peak	Duration
PO: < 2 hr	PO: 5–15 min	PO: 30 min	PO: 3 hr
IM: N/A	IM: < 5 min	IM: Not listed	IM: Not listed

▶▶ oxytocin

The drug oxytocin is the synthetic form of the endogenous hormone oxytocin and has all of its pharmacological properties.

PHARMACOKINETICS

Half-Life	Onset	Peak	Duration
IV: 3–5 min	IV: Immediate	IV: Immediate	IV: 2–3 hr
IM: 3–5 min	IM: < 5 min	IM: Immediate	IM: 2–3 hr

DOSAGES   Selected Uterine Stimulants

Drug (Pregnancy Category)	Pharmacological Class	Usual Dosage Range	Indications
▶▶dinoprostone (Prostin E_2, Cervidil, Prepidil) (X)	Prostaglandin E_2 abortifacient and cervical ripening drug	Vaginal insert (Cervidil) 10 mg placed transversely into posterior vaginal fornix (the space behind cervix)	Cervical ripening for induction of labour
		Cervical gel (Prostin E_2 gel): 1 mg in posterior fornix of vaginal canal; 1–2 mg repeated once in 6 hr	Cervical ripening for induction of labour
		Tablets (Prostin E_2): 0.5 mg followed by 0.5 mg each hour, not to exceed 1.5 mg	Elective and indicated induction of labour
		Vaginal gel (Prepidil): 0.5 mg into internal cervical os	Cervical ripening for induction of labour
▶▶ergonovine maleate (X)	Oxytocic ergot alkaloid	IM: 200 mcg after delivery of placenta, repeatable at 2- to 4-hr intervals, up to 5 doses	Postpartum uterine atony and hemorrhage
		IV: 200 mcg in 5 mL NS over 1 min	Emergency situations of excessive uterine bleeding
misoprostol (X)	Prostaglandin	PO: 400 mcg 12 hr before procedure	Termination of pregnancy (off-label use)
		Intravaginally: 400 mcg 4 hr before suction curettage	
▶▶oxytocin (X)	Oxytocic hypothalamic hormone	IV infusion: 1–20 microunits/min, titrated to effect	Labour induction
		IV: 5–10 units by slow injection	Postpartum uterine atony and hemorrhage
		IM: 5–10 units in a single dose after delivery of placenta	

IM, intramuscular; *IV*, intravenous; *NS*, normal saline; *PO*, oral.

UTERINE RELAXANTS

When contractions of the uterus begin before term, it may be desirable to stop labour because premature birth increases the risk of neonate death. Postponing delivery by relaxing the uterine smooth muscles and helping prevent contractions and the induction of labour increases the likelihood of the infant's survival. However, this measure is generally employed only after the 20 weeks of gestation because spontaneous labour occurring before then is commonly associated with a nonviable fetus and thus is usually not interrupted. Only uterine contractions occurring between about 20 and 37 weeks of gestation are considered premature labour.

The nonpharmacological treatment of premature labour includes bed rest, sedation, and hydration. Drugs given to inhibit labour and maintain the pregnancy are called *tocolytics*. Tocolytics have generally been found useful only in the short term to delay labour to allow for the administration of corticosteroids to accelerate the maturity of fetal lung development. Generally, tocolytics can delay labour for approximately 48 hours. Clear evidence that tocolytics reduce neonatal mortality or serious neonatal morbidity is limited. Currently available tocolytics such as indomethacin, calcium antagonists, and magnesium sulfate have not been shown to improve outcomes. There is currently a Canadian-led nitroglycerin trial under way, funded by the Canadian Institute of Health Research, to determine if nitroglycerin is an effective tocolytic. Because of the lack of evidence on the use of tocolytics in Canada, further discussion on this class of drugs is not warranted here.

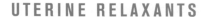

NURSING PROCESS

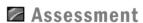 Assessment

In this section, estrogen and progesterone drugs are discussed first, and then medroxyprogesterone, megestrol, menotropins, the gonadotropins, and clomiphene are covered. Information on uterine motility–altering drugs is then provided, followed by a discussion of dinoprostone and, finally, consideration of the bisphosphonates, selective estrogen receptor modulators, teriparatide, and calcitonin.

Before initiating therapy with any of the hormonal drugs (e.g., estrogens, progestins) or other women's health–related drugs, the patient's blood pressure, weight, blood glucose levels, and results of liver and kidney function tests should be documented. Drug allergies, contraindications, cautions, and drug interactions should also be assessed and documented. Patient assessment should include thorough medication history, medical history, and menstrual history, as well as documentation of vital signs,

weight, any underlying heart disease and malignant diseases, and hormonal levels, if appropriate. Assessment of emotional stability is also important because of possible therapy-related depression. Results of the patient's last physical exam, clinician-performed breast exam, and gynecological exam should be noted as well.

Estrogen-only hormones should be given only after the following disorders and conditions have been ruled out: abnormal uterine bleeding, thromboembolic disorders, pregnancy, incomplete long-bone growth, photosensitivity (a more common adverse effect with conjugated estrogens), estrogen receptor–positive breast cancer, personal history or family history of breast cancer, early menstruation, pregnancies late in life, endocrine disorders, kidney or liver dysfunction, fluid retention disorders, and seizure activity. Assessment should include questions about breast examination and breast self-examination practices and dates of when the patient had her last complete physical examination and Papanicolaou (Pap) smear. The nurse must also assess the patient's baseline level of knowledge about estrogens and use of hormones, whether for contraception or replacement therapy. The patient's readiness to learn, educational level, and degree of adherence to other medication regimens must also be assessed. The success of treatment with oral contraceptives, hormonal replacement medication, and other therapies depends heavily on the patient understanding the instructions.

With oral contraceptive drugs (e.g., combination estrogen/progestin drugs), in addition to the assessment described above for estrogen-only hormones, patients should be assessed for cerebral and coronary vascular disease, jaundice, thromboembolic disorders and malignancies of the reproductive tract, or abnormal vaginal bleeding. Patients should be closely monitored if they have any of the following disorders: uncontrolled hypertension, migraine headaches, visual disturbances, hyperlipidemia, asthma, blood dyscrasias, diabetes mellitus, congestive heart failure, depression, and seizures. The concern is for exacerbation of any of these problems or disorders and subsequent complications. Patients who smoke should also be closely monitored because of the increased risk of complications in smokers, especially those older than 35 years. Smoking history should include documentation of number of packs per day and number of years the patient has smoked. When combination oral contraceptives are used in emergency situations for postcoital conception, the same contraindications, cautions, and drug interactions apply even if for one-time use.

With hormones that are progestin/progesterone only, much of the information described earlier for estrogens is applicable. Although medroxyprogesterone and megestrol have similar actions, their indications are varied. Medroxyprogesterone is used for amenorrhea and abnormal uterine bleeding, whereas megestrol is indicated in the palliative treatment of breast and endometrial cancers and promotion of increased appetite in patients with AIDS. Assessment of the appropriate parameters related to these drugs and their actions should be noted as well.

An understanding of menotropins is critical to patient safety, and assessment of the patient's knowledge about the drug and its use is important. Human chorionic gonadotropin is usually administered only after laboratory tests have determined the sufficiency of follicular development. A complete physical assessment is needed with attention to the menstrual–reproductive history and heart, kidney, and liver functioning. Abdominal assessment is important, with pre-existing diseases and abdominal pain noted. If the ovary is overstimulated, moderate ovarian enlargement with or without abdominal pain and distention may occur. If overstimulation is severe, the patient may experience nausea, vomiting, diarrhea, oliguria, ascites, electrolyte disturbances, and thromboembolic events.

Use of clomiphene requires assessment of the patient's medical and medication histories as well as a thorough review of the menstrual history. It is particularly important to assess reproductive status and uterine status because use of the drug may result in multiple births. Family stability and economic status must be assessed because of the risk of multiple births; everyone concerned needs as healthy a home as possible. Heart, liver, and kidney status must also be assessed, as ordered.

Before administering uterine stimulants (e.g., oxytocin or prostaglandins), the nurse should measure and document the patient's blood pressure, pulse, and respiration. Fetal heart rate and contraction-related fetal heart rates should also be determined and recorded. Because oxytocin therapy is associated with vasopressive and antidiuretic effects, it especially important to know fluid volume status. The nurse should know that when these drugs are administered, maternal blood pressure will decrease initially but will then rise (occasionally by up to 30%), and cardiac output and stroke volume will subsequently increase. Assessment for complications associated with the use of these drugs should include measurement of all vital signs, monitoring of intake and output, and observation for signs and symptoms of water intoxication (e.g., headache, fatigue,

nausea, anorexia, lethargy, disorientation, seizures or coma, tachycardia, hypotension, and muscular cramps and weakness), which may even be fatal if not appropriately identified. Fetal distress and uterine contractions for either hypertonic or hypotonic patterns should be assessed frequently and documented.

For labour and delivery, the patient's cervix should be ready for induction or be rated at a Bishop score of 5 or higher. The *Bishop scale* is a scoring system based on station, dilation, effacement, position, and consistency to assist in predicting whether induction of labour will be required. Constant monitoring of maternal blood pressure, pulse, contractions, and fluid status, as well as fetal heart rate is needed.

Oxytocin is not used during the first trimester except in some cases of spontaneous or induced abortion. The same considerations apply to the ergot alkaloids (e.g., ergonovine), and the patient's vital signs and fetal heart rate should be assessed. A baseline neurological assessment is important with attention to seizures. The nurse should continually assess for the signs of acute overdose, including nausea, vomiting, abdominal pain, numbness and tingling of the extremities, and hypertension. Contraindications, cautions, and drug interactions (previously discussed in the pharmacy section) also need to be considered.

The use of dinoprostone or other prostaglandin E_2 drugs is indicated in specific situations requiring termination of pregnancy. The presence of fibroids, pelvic inflammatory disease, pelvic stenosis, respiratory disease, and recent or past pelvic surgery should be asked about and documented.

For bisphosphonates, such as alendronate, there are many contraindications, cautions, and drug interactions. Assessment of the following is thus important to patient safety: occurrence of thromboembolisms, perimenopausal state, deep vein thrombosis, pulmonary embolism, concurrent estrogen therapy, anticipated immobility or bed rest (the drug should be discontinued 72 hours before the patient becomes immobile), aspiration risk, kidney or liver dysfunction, high levels of calcium, the use of other drugs considered to be gastrointestinal irritants, the presence of esophageal abnormalities, delayed esophageal emptying, and the inability to remain upright in either a sitting or standing position. (Remaining

⊕ IN MY FAMILY

The Yogourt Tampon

(as told by S.T., fifth-generation Canadian of British descent)

"For a yeast infection, my mother had two suggestions. One is applying a thin layer of cornstarch on the external genitalia to pull out extra moisture. More important, though, is the yogurt-covered tampon. From a fresh, unopened container of plain yogurt, put a small portion of yogurt in a clean bowl. Cover a clean tampon with the yogurt, and insert the tampon as you normally would. Leave it in for a couple of hours or until the next time you urinate. My mom swears by the yogourt tampon."

upright helps prevent esophageal erosion and ulcers from reflux of the drug back into the esophagus.) Drug interactions discussed earlier in the chapter need to be considered, and any drugs associated with gastrointestinal distress or ulcers (e.g., aspirin, nonsteroidal anti-inflammatory drugs) should be avoided. Other drugs in this category require similar assessment. Concerns about prolonged immobility should be addressed as well.

Nursing Diagnoses

- Disturbed body image related to the effects of abnormal hormonal estrogen or progestin levels, problems with pregnancy, osteoporosis, or other female diseases or disorders
- Anxiety related to female disorders and possible complications of associated therapy
- Deficient knowledge related to lack of information about first-time drug therapy
- Acute pain resulting from a disorder of the female reproductive tract and related drug therapy
- Ineffective sexuality patterns related to abnormal levels of estrogen
- Decisional conflict related to the risks versus benefits of postmenopausal estrogen replacement therapy
- Risk for injury to the mother in relation to the adverse effects of uterine mobility–altering drugs
- Risk for injury to the infant in realtion to premature labour or the adverse effects of tocolytics.
- Risk for infection related to possible drop in white blood cell count because of the effects of SERMs

Planning

Goals

- Patient will be free of body image disturbances.
- Patient will state the rationale for hormonal replacement, combination oral contraceptives, osteoporosis drugs, uterine relaxants, or fertility drugs.
- Patient will state the adverse effects of specific medications.
- Patient will state the importance of adherence to hormonal therapy and other recommended pharmacological and nonpharmacological measures for the treatment of premature labour, pre-eclampsia, or fertility disorders.
- Patient will openly state the need for improved sexual functioning and image before and during treatment.
- Patient will state fears and concerns about the use of hormonal therapy.
- Patient will state fears and concerns about pregnancy and its outcome.

Outcome Criteria

- Patient openly expresses concerns, fears, and anxieties about body image changes and the need for medication.

- Patient is adherent to pharmacological and non-pharmacological therapy regimens and achieves successful management of osteoporosis, breast cancer, infertility, pre-eclampsia, or premature labour, or experiences effective birth control.
- Patient is free of complications and disturbing adverse effects associated with each group of drugs, such as chest pain, leg pain, blurred vision, thrombophlebitis, and leukopenia.
- Patient returns for regular follow-up visits with the physician to monitor the therapeutic and adverse effects of treatment.
- Patient engages in positive sexual patterns and habits while receiving hormonal therapy.
- Patient is free of complications associated with uterine mobility–altering drugs.

Implementation

Both estrogens and progestins should be administered as ordered in the lowest dosages possible and the doses titrated as needed. Intramuscular doses should be given deep in large muscle masses and the injection sites rotated. Oral forms should be taken with food or milk to minimize gastrointestinal upset. Progestin-only oral contraceptive pills are taken daily. It is important for the patient to take this oral contraceptive at the same time every day so that effective hormonal serum levels are maintained. Because use of the progestin-only pill leads to a higher incidence of ovulatory cycles, there is an associated increased rate of failure. The nurse should remember that this type of pill is usually prescribed for those women who are unable to tolerate estrogens or for whom estrogens are contraindicated. The progestin-only contraceptive is often more effective in women who are over 35 years of age. Combination estrogen/progestin pills contain low doses of drug. Low-dose monophasic and multiphasic types are provided as 21 days of pills followed by 7 days of placebo pills, and the patient needs to understand how this treatment regimen functions. The nurse should emphasize to the patient that the reduction of estrogen has been associated with a decrease in adverse effects and a decrease in the risk for liver tumours, hypertension, and cardiovascular changes; however, more breakthrough bleeding will occur.

Medroxyprogesterone should be given as ordered. Megestrol is given orally and the patient should know whether the drug is being given to improve appetite so that appropriate dietary measures can be implemented. Menotropins should be given as ordered and requires frequent monitoring for the duration of therapy. Nausea, vomiting, dizziness, shortness of breath, severe headache, blurred vision, or swelling of the feet should be reported. Gonadotropin hormones are usually given intramuscularly, and if they are given in conjunction with menotropins, the dose is usually given 1 day after the last menotropin dose.

Fertility drugs such as clomiphene are often self-administered. The provision of specific instructions on how to administer the drug at home and how to monitor drug effectiveness is very important to improve the success of treatment. Journal tracking of the medication regimen is helpful to those involved in the care of the infertile patient or couple. See Patient Education for more information.

Oxytocin should be administered only as ordered, and any instructions or protocol should be strictly followed. The cervix must be ripe (see earlier discussion in the pharmacology section). Prostaglandin E_2 may be instilled vaginally to help accomplish this if the mother's cervix is not ripe or at a Bishop score of 5 or higher. Because oxytocin has vasopressive and antidiuretic properties, the patient is at risk for hypertensive episodes as well as fluid retention; constant monitoring of maternal blood pressure and pulse rate as well as fetal monitoring is therefore required. Patients should report any of the following: strong contractions, edema, symptoms of water intoxication, palpitations, chest pain, and any changes in fetal movement.

Intravenous infusions (use of infusion pumps) of oxytocin should be administered with the proper dilutional fluid and rate. To minimize the adverse effects of the drug, intravenous piggyback dosing is often ordered so that the diluted oxytocin solution can be discontinued immediately if maternal or fetal decline occurs while an intravenous line with hydration is maintained. Doses are generally titrated as ordered and are based on the progress of labour and degree of fetal tolerance to the drug. Should the labour progress at 1 cm/hr dilation, oxytocin may no longer be needed. The decision is made by the physician and on an individual basis. Generally speaking, with oxytocin therapy, if there are hypertensive responses or major changes in the maternal vital signs or if the fetal heart rate decreases or if fetal movement stops, the physician should be contacted immediately. Hyperstimulation may also occur. If contractions are more frequent than every 2 minutes and last longer than 1 minute later (and are accompanied by changes in other parameters), the infusion should be stopped and the physician contacted immediately. If this does occur, it is critical to place the patient on the left side, maintain administration of intravenous fluids, and give oxygen as ordered (generally via tight face mask at 10 to 12 L/min). If there is concern about overstimulation, discuss concerns with the physician and document actions thoroughly.

Dinoprostone is given by vaginal suppository to those who are 12 to 20 weeks pregnant and are seeking termination and to patients in whom evacuation of the uterus is needed for the management of incomplete spontaneous abortion or intrauterine fetal death (up to 28 weeks). The drug should be given exactly as ordered, and the patient should be monitored closely.

The success of therapy with drugs such as alendronate depends on providing thorough patient teaching and ensuring that the patient understands all aspects of the drug regimen. With alendronate, the nurse must emphasize the need to take the medication upon rising in the morning, and with a full glass (180 to 240 mL) of water at least 30 minutes before taking any food, other fluids, or other medications. In addition, the nurse must emphasize that the patient should remain upright, in either a standing or sitting position, for approximately 30 minutes after taking the drug to help prevent esophageal erosion or irritation. The patient taking raloxifene should be informed that the drug should be discontinued 72 hours before and during prolonged immobility. Therapy may be resumed once the patient becomes fully ambulatory and as ordered. See Patient Education for more teaching tips for the patient.

☒ Evaluation

Therapeutic responses to the drugs discussed in this chapter should be measured by evaluating whether goals and outcome criteria have been met. Many drugs have been discussed here, often with several indications for their use; thus the therapeutic response would be occurrence of the indicated therapeutic effect. With any of the indicated effects, the nurse needs to monitor for the associated adverse effects and toxicity. Therapeutic effects of estrogens may range from prevention of pregnancy to a decrease in menopausal symptoms to reduction in the size of a tumour. Adverse effects of estrogens may include thromboembolism, edema, jaundice, abnormal vaginal bleeding, hyperglycemia, nausea, vomiting, increased appetite, and weight gain. Therapeutic responses to progestins include a decrease in abnormal uterine bleeding and the disappearance of menstrual disorders (i.e., amenorrhea). The adverse effects of progestins include edema, hypertension, heart symptoms, changes in mood and affect, and jaundice.

Therapeutic effects of oxytocin and other uterine stimulants include stimulation of labour and control of postpartum bleeding, and adverse reactions may include drop in pulse rate, dysrhythmias, severe abdominal pain, and shock-like symptoms (e.g., decrease in blood pressure, increase in pulse rate). These adverse effects may indicate a dangerous complication and medical emergency.

Therapeutic effects of fertility drugs include successful fertilization. Adverse reactions include hot flashes, abdominal discomfort, blurred vision, gastrointestinal upset, nervousness, depression, weight gain, and hair loss. Multiple births and birth defects are other possible consequences of therapy. The therapeutic effects of *dinoprostone* include therapeutic termination of pregnancy; adverse effects are severe cramping and bleeding. Therapeutic effects of *alendronate* and related drugs include increased bone density and prevention or management of osteoporosis; adverse effects include leukopenia, decreased platelet levels, thrombophlebitis, hot flashes, and leg cramps.

PATIENT EDUCATION

- Patients should be informed that hormonal drugs are usually tolerated better if taken with food or milk to minimize gastrointestinal upset.
- With use of oral contraceptives and any form of hormone replacement therapy with estrogens or progestins, patients should be encouraged to openly discuss concerns about the medications. The patient should be assured that although risks may be associated with hormone replacement therapy, the physician will weigh each case individually and make the decision in each situation on the basis of benefits versus risks, but with the ultimate decision lies with the patient.
- With estrogens and progestins, patients should be encouraged to report the following to the health care provider immediately: chest pain, leg pain, blurred vision, headache, neck stiffness, neck pain, loss of vision, numbness of extremities, severe headache, edema, yellow discoloration of the skin or sclera, clay-coloured stools, and abnormal vaginal bleeding.
- Patients should be advised to report any weight gain of more than 2 kg in 1 week or 1 kg or greater within a 24-hour period to the health care provider. The patient should also report any breakthrough bleeding, change in menstrual flow, and breast tenderness.
- Patients should be instructed to take oral contraceptives exactly as ordered and get follow-up annual examinations, including a pelvic examination, Pap smear, and practitioner-performed breast examination. Patients should be instructed, with return demonstration, in performing monthly breast self-examinations and about the ideal time to perform a breast self-examination (e.g., 7 to 10 days after the menses). Follow-up appointments and annual examinations by a health care provider must be emphasized.
- Patients should be instructed to avoid sunlight or be sure to apply sunscreen because of increased sensitivity to sunlight and the ultraviolet light from tanning beds.
- With the use of progesterone-only intravaginal gel with other gels, patients should be sure to insert the other gels at least 6 hours before or after the progesterone-based product.
- Progesterone-filled intrauterine inserts are placed in the uterine cavity by a physician. Patients should receive thorough education regarding their use, which is for 1 year after insertion; the inserts need to be replaced after that time. Patients should report abnormal uterine bleeding, cramping, abdominal pain, and amenorrhea to the physician.
- Patients using an estrogen/progestin vaginal ring for contraception should be informed about what to expect with its insertion and that it should be removed 3 weeks later and a new ring inserted 1 week after that. Use of this contraceptive device calls for thorough teaching and follow-up, including insertion and removal techniques and a return demonstration, before the patient leaves the physician's office. Inform patients that menstruation will follow in about 2 to 3 days after the ring is removed. They should replace the used ring in its foil pouch, discard it in the trash, and not flush it down the toilet.
- With emergency oral contraception, patients should take the first dose of this drug as soon as possible after intercourse because it is more effective when taken early, but it may be taken up to 72 hours after the event. A second dose is taken 12 hours later. One product contains only progestin, and one is a combination of progestin and estrogen; the two are equally effective when prescribed appropriately.
- Patients should be instructed to take the dose of oral contraceptives at the same time every day. If one dose is missed, the patient should take the dose as soon as it is remembered and use a backup form of contraception. More specific instructions should be provided for the omission of more than one pill or 1 day's dosage and should be specific to the prescribed oral contraceptive drug. For patient safety and adherence, provide patients with contact information for getting answers for questions about dosing and missed doses.
- Patient should be instructed about the fact that oral contraceptives may prevent pregnancy, but sexual intercourse is only considered safe if the contraceptive is combined with the use of condoms to prevent sexually transmitted infections.
- Patients should be informed about the significant interactions between oral contraceptives and certain antibiotics (Chapters 38 and 39) and the need for backup contraception. Encourage patients to always inquire about this interaction when taking antibiotics and to use a backup form of contraception. St. John's wort may also diminish the effectiveness of the oral contraceptive, so provide additional information about this potential drug interaction.
- Patients taking bisphosphonates (e.g., alendronate) should be instructed to take the drug exactly as prescribed and to take it at least 30 minutes before the first morning beverage, food, or other medication. It must be taken with at least 180 to 240 mL of water. Patients must understand the importance of remaining upright for at least 30 minutes after taking the medication to prevent esophageal and gastrointestinal adverse effects. Esophageal irritation, dysphagia, severe heartburn, and retrosternal pain must be reported to the physician immediately to prevent severe reactions.
- Patients should be encouraged to inquire about taking supplemental calcium and vitamin D if taking bisphosphonates and to inquire about the best timing of their dosing.
- Patients should be encouraged to make lifestyle changes as recommended, such as doing weight-bearing exercises (e.g., walking), stopping smoking, and limiting or eliminating alcohol intake.

POINTS TO REMEMBER

❖ Three major estrogens are synthesized in the ovaries: estradiol (the principal estrogen), estrone, and estriol. Exogenous estrogens can be classified into two main groups: steroidal estrogens (e.g., conjugated estrogens, esterified estrogens, estradiol) and the nonsteroidal estrogen diethylstilbestrol.

❖ Progestins have a variety of uses, including treatment of uterine bleeding and amenorrhea and adjunctive and palliative treatment of some cancers.

❖ Oral contraceptives containing a combination of estrogens and progestins are the most effective form of birth control currently available.

❖ Uterine stimulants (sometimes called *oxytocic drugs*) include ergot derivatives, prostaglandins, and oxytocin.

❖ Uterine relaxants (often called tocolytic drugs) are used to stop preterm labour and maintain pregnancy by halting uterine contractions.

❖ A thorough nursing assessment is necessary to ensure the safe and effective use of female reproductive drugs. Information should be obtained on the patient's past medical problems, history of menses and difficulties with menstrual cycle, medications taken (prescribed and over-the-counter), number of pregnancies and miscarriages, last menstrual period, and any related surgical or medical treatments.

❖ The nurse is responsible for determining the response of the mother and fetus to drugs such as oxytocin through monitoring of the frequency of contractions, the progress of labour, and fetal tolerance. The dose should be titrated per the physician's order.

❖ Drugs that alter uterine motility are potentially dangerous to the mother and the fetus. The nurse should watch the infusion carefully while closely monitoring the patients (mother and fetus). Intravenous infusions should be given only with intravenous pumps.

EXAMINATION REVIEW QUESTIONS

1 The nurse is assessing a patient who is to receive dinoprostone. Which of the following would be a contraindication to the use of this drug?
 a. Ectopic pregnancy
 b. Incomplete abortion
 c. Pregnancy at 15 weeks
 d. Gastrointestinal upset or ulcer disease

2 When teaching a patient who is taking oral contraceptive therapy for the first time, which of the following adverse effects should the nurse tell the patient about?
 a. Polyuria
 b. Dizziness
 c. Nausea and vomiting
 d. Tingling in the extremities

3 Which of the following situations is an indication for an oxytocin infusion?
 a. Hypertonic uterus
 b. Induction of labour at full term
 c. Termination of a pregnancy at 12 weeks
 d. Cervical stenosis in a patient who is in labour

4 After a patient has been taught about drug therapy with the SERM raloxifene, which statement from the patient reflects a good understanding of the instruction?
 a. "After I take this drug I must sit upright for at least 30 minutes."
 b. "One advantage of this drug is that it will reduce my hot flashes."
 c. "I will need to stop taking this drug at least 3 days before I travel to Europe."
 d. "I can continue this drug even when travelling as long as I take it with 240 mL of water each time."

5 A patient calls the clinic because she has realized that she has missed one dose of an oral contraceptive. Select all the statements that are appropriate responses from the nurse.
 a. "Wait 7 days, then start a new pack of pills."
 b. "Don't worry, you are still protected from pregnancy."
 c. "Please come in to the clinic for a re-evaluation of your therapy."
 d. "Go ahead and take the missed dose now, along with today's dose."
 e. "You will need to use a backup form of contraception until the next cycle."

For answers see http://evolve.elsevier.com/Canada/Lilley/pharmacology/.

CRITICAL THINKING ACTIVITIES

1 K.T. has spent 14 hours in labour and has made little progress. This is her first pregnancy, and she is exhausted, and the uterine contractions have decreased in strength. She is now receiving an oxytocin infusion. What will you monitor while she is receiving this drug?

2 Why are oxytocics such as oxytocin and ergonovine used to treat postpartum and postabortion bleeding caused by uterine relaxation and enlargement?

3 Explain the primary mechanism by which oral contraceptives prevent pregnancy.

For answers see http://evolve.elsevier.com/Canada/Lilley/pharmacology/.

CHAPTER 35

Men's Health Drugs

Learning Objectives

After reading this chapter, the successful student will be able to do the following:

1 Discuss the normal anatomy, physiology, and functions of the male reproductive system.

2 Compare the male reproductive drugs in terms of their rationale for use, dosages, and dosage forms.

3 Describe the mechanisms of action, dosages, adverse effects, cautions, contraindications, drug interactions, and routes of administration for men's health drugs.

4 Develop a collaborative plan of care that includes all phases of the nursing process for patients receiving men's health drugs for the treatment of benign prostatic hypertrophy, sexual dysfunction, hormone deficiency, or prostate cancer.

e-Learning Activities

Web site
(http://evolve.elsevier.com/Canada/Lilley/pharmacology/)

- Animations
- Answers to chapter questions, activities, and case studies
- Calculators and Category Catchers
- Glossary with audio pronunciations
- IV Therapy and Medication Error Checklists
- Multiple-Choice Review Question quizzes
- Nursing Care Plans
- Online Appendices and Supplements
- WebLinks

Drug Profiles

finasteride, p. 656
▶▶ **sildenafil (sildenafil citrate)***, p. 656
▶▶ **testosterone**, p. 656

▶▶ Key drug.

*Full generic name is given in parentheses. For the purposes of this text, the more common shortened name is used.

Glossary

Anabolic activity Any metabolic activity that promotes growth of body tissues, such as the activity produced by testosterone that results in the development of bone and muscle tissue; also called *anabolism*. (p. 652)

Androgenic activity The activity produced by testosterone that promotes the development and maintenance of the male reproductive system and other male secondary sex characteristics. (p. 652)

Androgens Male sex hormones responsible for mediating the development and maintenance of male sex characteristics. (p. 652)

Benign prostatic hypertrophy (BPH) Nonmalignant enlargement of the prostate gland. (p. 653)

Catabolism The opposite of anabolic activity; any metabolic activity that results in the breakdown of body tissues. (p. 652)

Erythropoietic effect The effect of stimulating the production of red blood cells (*erythropoiesis*). (p. 652)

Prostate cancer A malignant tumour within the prostate gland. (p. 654)

Prostate-specific antigen Protein produced in the epithelial cells of the prostate and absorbed into the bloodstream. (p. 655)

Testosterone The main androgenic hormone. (p. 652)

OVERVIEW OF THE MALE REPRODUCTIVE SYSTEM

The male reproductive system consists of several structures, the testes and seminiferous tubules being the most important to the discussion within this chapter because they produce the primary male hormones. The *testes,* a pair of oval glands located in the scrotal sac, are the male gonads. The testes produce male sex hormones. The *seminiferous tubules,* channels in the testes, are the site of spermatogenesis, the process by which mature sperm cells are produced.

Androgens are the group of male sex hormones (primarily testosterone) that mediate the normal development and maintenance of the primary male sex characteristics (normal male genital anatomy), as well as the secondary sex characteristics (Figure 35-1). Secondary male sex characteristics include advanced development of the prostate, seminal vesicles (two glands adjacent to the prostate), penis, and scrotum, as well as male hair distribution, laryngeal enlargement and thickening of the vocal cords, and male body musculature and fat distribution. Androgens must be secreted in adequate amounts for these characteristics to appear. The most important androgen is **testosterone**, which is produced from clusters of interstitial cells embedded between the seminiferous tubules. As well as possessing **androgenic activity**, testosterone also promotes the development of bone and muscle tissue, inhibits protein **catabolism**, and promotes retention of nitrogen, phosphorus, potassium, and sodium. These functions contribute to its **anabolic activity**. Testosterone initiates the synthesis of specific proteins needed for androgenic and anabolic activity by binding to chromatin, strands of deoxyribonucleic acid (DNA), in the nuclei of interstitial cells. In addition, testosterone appears to have an **erythropoietic effect** in that it stimulates the production of red blood cells (Chapter 56).

ANDROGENS AND OTHER DRUGS PERTAINING TO MEN'S HEALTH

There are several synthetic derivatives of testosterone, developed with the intention of improving on the pharmacokinetic and pharmacodynamic characteristics of the naturally occurring hormone. One way that this was accomplished was by combining esters with testosterone, which prolonged the duration of action of the hormone. For example, testosterone propionate is formulated as an oily solution and its hormonal effects last for 2 to 3 days. The effects of testosterone cypionate and testosterone enanthate in oil last much longer and they can be administered once every 2 to 4 weeks. Orally administered testosterone has poor pharmacokinetic and pharmacodynamic characteristics because most of the dose is metabolized and destroyed by the liver before it can reach the circulation (first-pass effect). To circumvent this

problem, researchers developed methyltestosterone and fluoxymesterone (both are controlled substances in Canada). Newer transdermal dosage forms for testosterone, including skin patches and a gel, have provided another way to circumvent the first-pass effect.

There are other chemical derivatives of the naturally occurring testosterone known as *anabolic steroids.* These are synthetic drugs that closely resemble the natural hormone but possess high anabolic activity. One anabolic steroid drug product, nandrolone decanoate (Deca-Durabolin), is currently commercially available in Canada by prescription, as adjuvant treatment for senile and postmenopausal osteoporosis, for certain types of anemia such as aplastic and sickle cell, and for metastatic breast cancer. Nandrolone is also used in conditions in which tissue building or protein-sparing action is required, such as in acquired immune deficiency syndrome (AIDS) wasting syndrome (debilitation related to disease-induced nutritional malabsorption). Anabolic steroids have a great potential for misuse by athletes, particularly body builders and weight lifters, who may take doses up to 100 times greater than those used to treat medical conditions, because of the muscle-building properties. Most steroids used by athletes are smuggled, stolen, or made in clandestine laboratories. Veterinary drugs are often used. Steroidal "supplements," such as dehydroepiandrosterone (DHEA), are converted into testosterone or a similar compound in the body that if taken in large amounts can have similar effects as anabolic steroids. These substances are not available in Canada but are found in health food stores and sold over the Internet. Improper use of these substances can have many serious consequences, such as sterility, cardiovascular disease, and liver cancer. For this reason, anabolic steroids are regulated under the Controlled Drugs and Substances Act Schedule IV. The trafficking, possession for the purpose of trafficking, possession for the purpose of exporting, and production, import, and export of anabolic steroids are all illegal. This classification implies that misuse of the drug can lead to psychological or physical dependence, or both. Steroids can produce a variety of psychological effects that range from euphoria to hostility. Another synthetic androgen is danazol. Its labelled uses include endometriosis and fibrocystic breast disease in women.

Mechanism of Action and Drug Effects

The drug forms of the natural and synthetic androgens and the synthetic anabolic steroids have effects similar to those of the endogenous androgens. These include stimulation of the normal growth and development of the male sex organs (primary sex characteristics) and development and maintenance of the secondary sex characteristics. One reason for the growth-promoting effects of androgens is that they stimulate the synthesis of ribonucleic acid (RNA) at the cellular level, thereby promoting cellular growth and reproduction. They also slow the breakdown of amino acids. These properties

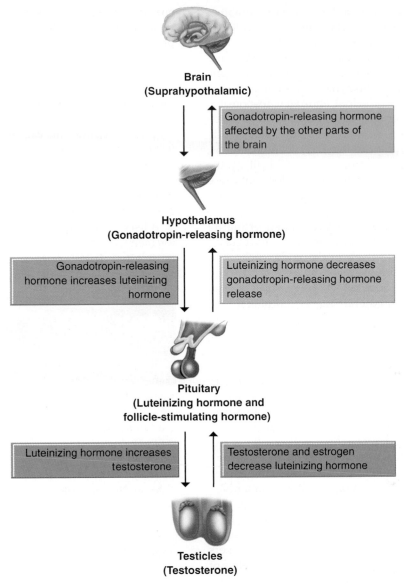

Brain
(Suprahypothalamic)

Gonadotropin-releasing hormone
affected by the other parts of
the brain

Hypothalamus
(Gonadotropin-releasing hormone)

Gonadotropin-releasing
hormone increases luteinizing
hormone

Luteinizing hormone decreases
gonadotropin-releasing hormone
release

Pituitary
(Luteinizing hormone and
follicle-stimulating hormone)

Luteinizing hormone increases
testosterone

Testosterone and estrogen
decrease luteinizing hormone

Testicles
(Testosterone)

FIG. 35-1 Regulation of male characteristics by testosterone.

contribute to an increased synthesis of body proteins, which aids in the formation and maintenance of muscle tissue. Another potent anabolic effect of androgens is the retention of nitrogen, also essential for protein synthesis. Nitrogen promotes the storage in the body of inorganic phosphorus, sulfate, sodium, and potassium, all of which have important metabolic roles, including protein synthesis, nerve impulse conduction, and muscle contractions. All of these effects result in weight gain and an increase in muscular strength. Finally, androgens also stimulate the production of erythropoietin by the kidney, resulting in enhanced erythropoiesis (red blood cell synthesis). However, the administration of exogenous androgens causes the release of endogenous testosterone to be inhibited as the result of feedback inhibition of the pituitary luteinizing hormone. Large doses of exogenous androgens may also suppress sperm production as the result of feedback

inhibition of pituitary follicle-stimulating hormone, leading to infertility.

Androgen inhibitors are drugs that block the effects of naturally occurring (endogenous) androgens in the body. Because this is accomplished via inhibition of a specific enzyme, 5α-reductase, these drugs are also called 5α-reductase inhibitors. As previously mentioned, androgens maintain secondary sex characteristics, one of which is the growth and maintenance of the prostate. For unknown reasons, normal male physiology results in a common enlargement of the prostate known as **benign prostatic hypertrophy (BPH)**. This process begins as early as 30 years old and is present in at least 85% of men by the age of 80 years. The most troubling symptom is usually varying degrees of obstructed urinary outflow. Although surgical treatment by transurethral resection of the prostate (TURP) is a common strategy, BPH is also amenable to treatment with a 5α-reductase inhibitor. There are currently two 5α-reductase inhibitors available, finasteride and dutasteride. Finasteride, the prototype drug for this class, inhibits 5α-reductase, the enzyme that normally converts testosterone to 5α-dihydrotestosterone (DHT). DHT is actually a somewhat more potent type of testosterone and is the principal androgen responsible for stimulating prostatic growth, as well as other male primary and secondary sex characteristics. Finasteride can dramatically lower prostatic DHT concentrations, which eases the passage of urine made difficult by the enlarged prostate. Fortunately, finasteride does not cause the antiandrogen adverse effects that might be expected, such as loss of muscle strength and fertility.

The drug effects of finasteride are limited primarily to the prostate, but it may also affect 5α-reductase–dependent processes elsewhere in the body, such as in the hair follicles, skin, and liver. For example, it has been noted that men taking finasteride experience increased hair growth. Therefore, finasteride is also indicated for the treatment of male-pattern baldness. Research has demonstrated that the inhibition of 5α-reductase prevents the thinning of hair caused by increased levels of DHT. Finasteride is indicated for treating baldness only in men, not in women, even though testosterone and DHT serve to promote normal male hair growth (e.g., facial hair), as well as hair loss (baldness or alopecia), in both sexes. Finasteride can be teratogenic in pregnant women and its use in women of any age (pregnant or not) is still not recommended by its manufacturer. Another medication, minoxidil, can be used topically to treat baldness in both men and women. It is discussed in more detail in Chapter 57.

Another class of drugs that may be used to help alleviate the symptoms of obstruction due to BPH is the α₁-adrenergic blockers. These drugs are discussed in greater detail in Chapter 19. The α₁-adrenergic blockers that are most commonly used for symptomatic relief of obstruction secondary to BPH are terazosin (Hytrin), doxazosin (Cardura), and tamsulosin (Flomax). Tamsulosin appears to have greater specificity for the α₁-receptors in the prostate and thus may cause less hypotension.

There are also two other classes of androgen inhibitors. The first class includes the androgen receptor blockers flutamide (Euflex), nilutamide (Anadron), and bicalutamide (Casodex). They block the activity of androgen hormones at the level of the receptors in target tissues (e.g., prostate). For this reason, androgen receptor blockers are used in the treatment of **prostate cancer.** The second class is the gonadotropin-releasing hormone (GnRH) analogues leuprolide (Eligard, Lupron), goserelin (Zoladex), and triptorelin (Trelstar). They inhibit the secretion of pituitary gonadotropin, which eventually leads to a decrease in testosterone production. Both androgen receptor blockers and GnRH analogues are used most commonly to treat prostate cancer and are discussed in further detail in Chapter 49.

Sildenafil (Viagra), a phosphodiesterase type 5 (PDE5) inhibitor, is the first oral drug approved for the treatment of erectile dysfunction (ED). Sildenafil inhibits the enzyme phosphodiesterase, which, in turn, allows the buildup of the chemical cyclic guanosine monophosphate (cGMP) in the penis. The cGMP causes relaxation of the smooth muscle in the corpora cavernosa (erectile tubes) of the penis and permits the inflow of blood. Nitric oxide is also released inside the corpora cavernosa during sexual stimulation and contributes to the erectile effect. Two drugs that are similar but have a longer duration of action are vardenafil (Levitra) and tadalafil (Cialis). A second type of drug used to treat erectile dysfunction is the prostaglandin alprostadil (Calverject, Muse). This drug must be given by injecting it directly into the erectile tissue of the penis or pushing a suppository form of the drug into the urethra.

A list of all of the drugs mentioned in the chapter used for men's health appears in Box 35-1. More information on selected drugs appears in the Drug Profiles section.

BOX 35-1

Currently Available Men's Health Drugs

α₁-Adrenergic Blockers

alfuzosin hydrochloride
doxazosin mesylate
tamsulosin
terazosin

Anabolic Steroids

nandrolone

Other Androgens

danazol
testosterone

Antiandrogens

bicalutamide
flutamide
nilutamide

5α-Reductase Inhibitors

dutasteride
finasteride

Gonadotropin-Releasing Hormone Analogues

goserelin acetate
leuprolide acetate
triptorelin pamoate

Peripheral Vasodilator

minoxidil

Phosphodiesterase Type 5 Inhibitors for Erectile Dysfunction

sildenafil citrate
tadalafil
vardenafil hydrochloride

Antiandrogens and gonadotropin-releasing hormone analogues are discussed in the antineoplastic drug chapters (Chapters 48 and 49).

Indications

The primary use for androgens is in hormone replacement therapy. Indications for other types of drugs discussed in this chapter are listed in Table 35-1.

Contraindications

Contraindications to the use of androgenic drugs include known androgen-responsive tumours. Use of sildenafil, tadalafil, and vardenafil is also contraindicated in men with major cardiovascular disorders, particularly if they use nitrate medications such as nitroglycerin. Finasteride is contraindicated in women (especially pregnant women) and children.

Adverse Effects

Although adverse effects are rare, some of the most devastating effects of androgenic steroids occur in the liver, where they cause the formation of blood-filled cavities, a

condition known as *peliosis of the liver.* This condition is a potential consequence of the long-term administration of androgenic anabolic steroids and can be life threatening. Other serious liver effects are liver cancer, cholestatic hepatitis, jaundice, and abnormal liver function. Fluid retention is another undesirable effect of androgens and may account for some of the weight gain seen in persons taking them. The serious adverse effects that can be caused by androgens far outweigh the advantages gained from their use in those seeking improved athletic ability. Other less serious adverse effects of androgens are listed in Table 35-2.

The PDE5 inhibitors sildenafil, tadalafil, and vardenafil appear to have relatively favourable adverse-effect profiles. In patients with pre-existing cardiovascular disease, especially those taking nitrates (e.g., nitroglycerin, isosorbide mononitrate, dinitrate), these drugs can lower blood pressure substantially, potentially leading to more serious adverse events. Headache, flushing, and dyspepsia are the most common adverse effects reported. *Priapism,* or abnormally prolonged penile erection, is another relatively uncommon, but possible, adverse effect of both the erectile dysfunction drugs and the androgens. This condition is a medical emergency and warrants urgent medical attention. It is simply due to an excessive therapeutic drug response. The PDE5 inhibitors have also been recognized to cause temporary, minor visual changes known as nonarteritic ischemic optic neuropathy in a small number of users. In 2006, Health Canada issued a safety warning that the condition had been reported in a small number of users of the PDE5 inhibitors.

Finasteride has been reported to cause loss of libido, loss of erection, ejaculatory dysfunction, hypersensitivity reactions, gynecomastia, and severe myopathy. The drug has also caused a 50% decrease in **prostate-specific antigen (PSA)** concentrations (proteins produced in the epithelial cells of the prostate and absorbed into the bloodstream). Pregnant women should not handle crushed or broken tablets on a regular basis because of

TABLE 35-1

Men's Health Drugs: Indications

Drug	Indication(s)
danazol	Endometriosis
	Fibrocystic breast disease
finasteride	Benign prostatic hyperplasia (BPH)
	Male androgenetic alopecia
minoxidil	Hypertension
	Male androgenetic alopecia
nandrolone	Senile and postmenopausal osteoporosis
	Metastatic breast cancer
sildenafil, tadalafil, vardenafil	Erectile dysfunction
testosterone	Primary or secondary hypogonadism

TABLE 35-2

Men's Health Drugs: Selected Adverse Effects

Drug Class	Adverse Effects
α_1-Adrenergic blockers	Tachycardia, hypotension, chest pain, syncope, depression, dizziness, drowsiness, asthenia, rash, pruritus, erectile dysfunction, urinary frequency, upper body muscular pain, dyspnea, flulike symptoms, visual changes, headache
Androgens (including anabolic steroids)	Headache, increased or reduced libido, anxiety, depression, acne, male-pattern baldness, hirsutism, nausea, abnormal liver function tests, liver neoplasms, priapism, polycythemia, elevated cholesterol, anaphylaxis (injection)
5α-Reductase inhibitors	Reduced libido, reduced semen volume, hypotension, dizziness, drowsiness
Peripheral vasodilator (topical minoxidil)	Topical route usually limited to localized dermatological reactions, including erythema, dermatitis, eczema, pruritus; possible systemic reactions theoretically include edema, chest pain, hyper- or hypotension, headache, dizziness, nausea, vomiting, diarrhea, sexual dysfunction, anemia, thrombocytopenia, and muscular pain
Phosphodiesterase type 5 inhibitors	Dizziness, headache, dyspepsia, nasal congestion, muscular pain, chest pain, hyper- or hypotension, rash, dermatitis, abnormal liver function tests, dry mouth, nausea, vomiting, diarrhea, gingivitis, priapism

the possibility of topical absorption, which can lead to teratogenic effects.

Interactions

When used with oral anticoagulants, all androgens can significantly increase or decrease anticoagulant activity. They can also enhance the hypoglycemic effects of oral antihyperglycemic drugs. Concurrent use with cyclosporine increases the risk of cyclosporine toxicity and is not recommended.

Dosages

For recommended dosages of the men's health drugs, see the Dosages table on p. 657.

DRUG PROFILES

finasteride

Finasteride (Propecia, Proscar) use is contraindicated in patients who have shown a hypersensitivity to it and in pregnant women. It is considered potentially dangerous for a pregnant woman even to handle crushed or broken tablets. The drug is currently available in two tablet strengths. The lower strength of 1 mg is indicated for androgenic alopecia in men. The higher strength of 5 mg is indicated for BPH. A similar but newer drug, dutasteride, is also indicated for BPH and is currently available in 0.5 mg capsule form. Both drugs are contraindicated in women and children. Refer to the Dosages table on p. 657 for dosage information.

PHARMACOKINETICS

Half-Life	Onset	Peak	Duration
4–15 hr*	3–12 mo†	8 hr‡	Unknown

*Varies with age.
†To reduce prostate size.
‡To lower DHT concentrations.

▶▶ sildenafil citrate

Sildenafil citrate (Viagra) is the first oral drug approved by Health Canada for the treatment of erectile dysfunction. Another currently available drug for the treatment of erectile dysfunction is an injectable form of the prostaglandin alprostadil. Sildenafil potentiates the physiological sexual response, causing penile erection after sexual arousal by relaxing smooth muscle and increasing blood flow into the penis.

Sildenafil is contraindicated in patients with a known hypersensitivity to it. Sildenafil can potentiate the hypotensive effects of nitrates, thus its administration to patients who are using organic nitrates in any form, either regularly or intermittently, is contraindicated. Dosage information for sildenafil and vardenafil appears in the Dosages table on p. 657. Another drug added to this class of phosphodiesterase type 5 inhibitors is tadalafil.

PHARMACOKINETICS

Half-Life	Onset	Peak	Duration
4 hr	0.5–1 hr	1 hr	4 hr

▶▶ testosterone

Testosterone (Andriol, Androderm, AndroGel, Delatestryl, Depo-Testosterone, Testim) is a naturally occurring anabolic steroid. It is used for primary and secondary hypogonadism but may also be used to treat oligospermia (low sperm count) and inoperable breast cancer in women, where its purpose is to counteract tumour-enhancing estrogen activity. When it is used as hormone replacement therapy, a transdermal product is desirable. There are presently two transdermal patch formulations available, which are designed to mimic the normal circadian variation in testosterone concentration seen in young healthy men; the maximum testosterone levels occur in the early morning hours and the minimum concentrations occur in the evening. The transdermal delivery product Androderm is always applied to the skin surface of the back, abdomen, upper arms, or thighs. The area should not be oily, damaged, hairy, or irritated. The patch should never be applied to the scrotal skin or bony prominences because of the risk of burn-like blisters. Androderm has a central drug delivery reservoir surrounded by a peripheral adhesive area.

Testosterone is contraindicated for use in patients with severe kidney, heart, or liver disease, hypersensitivity or genital bleeding, and in pregnant or lactating women. Testosterone is a Schedule IV controlled substance under the Controlled Drugs and Substances Act. It is available as intramuscular injections, transdermal patches, and a capsule. Common dosages are listed in the Dosages table on p. 657.

PHARMACOKINETICS

Half-Life	Onset	Peak	Duration
10–100 min	1–2 hr	2–4 hr	2 hr–4 wk depending on dosage form

PHARMACOKINETIC BRIDGE TO NURSING PRACTICE

Drugs used to manage erectile dysfunction (e.g., sildenafil) essentially work in the same way as does the body to assist the patient in achieving an erection. The related pharmacokinetics must be understood so that the drug is given safely and effectively. Sildenafil is a rapidly absorbed drug with maximal plasma concentrations within 30 to 120 minutes after oral dosing and if taken on an empty stomach. Peak time is at an average of 60 minutes. If the drug is taken with a high-fat meal, absorption will be delayed, and it may take an additional 60 minutes for the drug to reach peak levels. This is yet another example of how specific drug pharmacokinetics can be affected by variables in a patient's everyday life and habits. Another pharmacokinetic property is that patients who are 65 years of age or older have reduced clearance

DOSAGES   Selected Men's Health Drugs

Drug (Pregnancy Category)	Pharmacological Class	Usual Dosage Range	Indications
danazol (Cyclomen) (X)	Pituitary gonadotropin inhibitor	PO: 200–800 mg/day divided bid or qid for 3–6 mo	Endometriosis
		PO: 100–400 mg/day divided bid for up to 4–6 mo or regression of symptoms	Fibrocystic breast disease
dutasteride (Adovart) (X)	5α-reductase inhibitor	PO: 0.5 mg daily	Benign prostatic hypertrophy
finasteride (Propecia, Proscar)	5α-reductase inhibitor	PO: 1 mg daily (Propecia)	Male androgenic alopecia (baldness)—males only
		PO: 5 mg daily (Proscar)	Benign prostatic hypertrophy
sildenafil citrate (Viagra) (B)	Phosphodiesterase 5 inhibitor	PO: 25–100 mg 1 hr before sexual activity; no more than once daily	Erectile dysfunction
testosterone cypionate (Depo-Testosterone) (X)	Androgen	IM: 200–400 mg q3–4 wk	Erectile dysfunction due to testicular deficiency, male climacteric
			Eunuchism, eunuchoidism (failure of the testes to develop)
		IM: 100–200 mg q3–6 wk	Oligospermia (low sperm count)
		IM: 200–400 mg q3–4 wk	Anabolic effect, osteoporosis
testosterone enanthate (Delatestryl) (X)	Androgen	IM: 100–400 mg q4 wk	Hypogonadism
testosterone, transdermal (Androderm, Androgel, Testim 1%) (X)	Androgenic hormone	**Over 18** Androderm patch (applied to skin of back, abdomen, upper arms, or thighs): 2.5–5 mg/day	Male hypogonadism
		AndroGel (applied to shoulders, arms, or abdominal skin): 5–10 g daily (delivers 50–100 mg of testosterone)	Male hypogonadism
testosterone undeconate (Andriol) (X)	Androgen	PO: 120–160 mg, divided bid for 2–3 wks	Male hypogonadism
vardenafil hydrochloride (Levitra) (X)	Phosphodiesterase 5 inhibitor	PO: 5–20 mg 25–60 min before sexual activity; no more than once daily	Erectile dysfunction

of sildenafil and may experience increased plasma concentrations of free (or pharmacologically active) drug. This could possibly lead to drug accumulation and possible toxicity. (See Special Populations: The Older Adult on sildenfil use in older men.)

NURSING PROCESS

Assessment

Before any drug is given to a patient for the treatment of benign or malignant diseases of the male reproductive tract, presenting symptoms should be thoroughly assessed and a complete history of past and present medical diseases or conditions should be obtained. In addition, assessment of the patient's urinary elimination patterns should be documented. The physician usually performs a rectal examination for BPH or other pathology and documents findings and will order a serum PSA test before initiating

therapy. Special handling precautions should be followed for some of these drugs because of potential teratogenic effects (e.g., finasteride should not be handled by pregnant nurses or caregivers). The patient should also be assessed for liver impairment. For patients with prostate cancer, PSA levels should be assessed before therapy and as needed because levels should decrease with successful treatment. (See also Ethnocultural Implications: Men's Health Concerns and Screening regarding prostate cancer.)

Drugs for erectile dysfunction should be given only after a medical–physical examination, a thorough nursing assessment, and a medication history have been completed. Serum phosphorus levels also need to be documented. Bowel sounds and bowel patterns should be assessed, noting any dysphagia or gastrointestinal motility disorders (which may occur with sildenafil). Contraindications, cautions, and drug interactions (previously discussed in the pharmacology section) should be assessed prior to the use of this drug (and all drugs in this class).

With testosterone and related drugs, the patient should be assessed for diabetes and heart disease

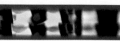

SPECIAL POPULATIONS: THE OLDER ADULT

Sildenafil: Use and Concerns

- Over 10 million men experience erectile dysfunction in North America. The incidence of erectile dysfunction increases as age increases. About 2% of affected men are in their forties and 23% are 65 years of age or older.

- Sildenafil (Viagra) is a prescription medication that is commonly ordered to treat erectile dysfunction, but it is not without concerns and cautions for the patient. This is especially true for the older adult, who generally has other medical conditions (e.g., kidney disorders, hypertension, diabetes) and is usually taking more than one other prescribed medication.

- Liver function declines with age; therefore, drugs may not be metabolized as effectively in older adults as they are in younger adults. In addition, sildenafil is highly protein bound, which causes it to stay in the body longer and thus create more drug interactions.

- A decreased dosage of sildenafil is generally indicated for patients over 65 years of age and for those with liver or kidney impairment.

- Adverse effects to be concerned about in all patients, particularly older patients, include headache, flushing, urinary tract infection, diarrhea, rash, and dizziness.

- Sildenafil should be used cautiously in patients who have heart disease and angina because these patients are at greater risk for complications, especially if they are taking nitrates for their cardiovascular disease. Sildenafil produces an 8 to 10 mm decrease in systolic blood pressure and a 5 to 6 mm decrease in diastolic blood pressure that begin 1 hour after taking a dose. The effect can last for approximately 4 hours.

- Discussing topics of a sexual nature may be comfortable for some patients but may produce anxiety in others. It is important for nurses to be aware of ethnocultural and gender differences in how individuals perceive their own sexuality and how they generally deal with sexual-performance issues.

- Nurses must be respectful of each individual's beliefs and feelings about not only sexuality but also other parts of the patient's being. This requires knowledge, sensitivity, and objectivity.

Source: Lacy, C. F., Armstrong, L. L., Goldman, M. P., & Lance, L. L. (2008). *Drug information handbook* (17th ed.). Hudson, OH: Lexi-Comp.

because of possible edema and subsequent added stress on the heart. Because androgenic anabolic steroids (e.g., testosterone) may increase weight, have a negative impact on bone growth, and elevate serum levels of potassium, chloride, nitrogen, phosphorus, and cholesterol, the nurse should assess for obesity, recent weight gain, bone disorders, and electrolyte imbalances before, during, and after therapy. Height, vital signs, and intake and output should be assessed and results of the following laboratory tests analyzed: kidney function tests (blood urea nitrogen and creatinine levels), heart enzyme assay, liver function tests (lactate dehydrogenase, creatine phosphokinase, and bilirubin levels), and PSA levels. A history of male breast cancer, prostate cancer, or gynecomastia should also be ruled out prior to drug therapy.

 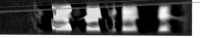

ETHNOCULTURAL IMPLICATIONS

Men's Health Concerns and Screening

Prostate cancer is the leading cancer diagnosed among men in Canada. Black men in North America have the highest rate of prostate cancer in the world. Of all racial and ethnic groups, Black men have the highest risk of being diagnosed with prostate cancer and have a greater chance of dying from it than White men. The risk of developing prostate cancer is less common among Asian and Aboriginal men. The causes of the higher rates of prostate cancer in Black men are largely unknown; however, higher mortality rates are associated with late detection. Another factor is that dark skin absorbs less sunlight than does light skin, which may contribute to the higher incidence of prostate cancer among men of African or Caribbean descent.

Researchers have studied the impact of ethnoculture on health-seeking behaviours among many of the racial and ethnic groups (e.g., Asians, Native Americans, Hispanics) in an attempt to gain greater understanding about the role of ethnoculture in health-related behaviours. Despite this research, however, little is known about the impact of ethnoculture on health-seeking behaviours among Black men. A goal of Healthy People 2010 is to eliminate disparities among racial and ethnic groups. For example, compared with other groups, Black men suffer a higher burden of disease because of health, social, political, and psychological factors, to the degree that they have been labelled an endangered species. More studies need to focus on the relationship between ethnoculture and communication with health care providers as it affects the Black male's knowledge, health belief systems, and health practices regarding prostate cancer screening.

From Braithwaite, R. L. (2001). The health status of black men. In R. L. Braithwaite and S. E. Taylor (Eds.), *Health issues in the black community (2nd ed.)*. San Francisco: Jossey-Bass Publishers; Woods, D. V., Montgomery, S. B., Belliard, J. C., Ramírez-Johnson, J., & Wilson, C. M. (2005). Culture, black men, and prostate cancer: What is reality? *Cancer Control, Journal of the Moffitt Cancer Centre*. Available at http://www.medscape.com/viewarticle/497924

Nursing Diagnoses

- Disturbed body image related to sexual dysfunction or diseases of the male reproductive tract
- Fatigue related to the adverse effects of medications
- Excess fluid volume related to possible adverse effects (sodium retention)
- Impaired urinary elimination related to BPH
- Ineffective sexuality patterns related to the effects of treatment with testosterone and drugs used for erectile dysfunction
- Sexual dysfunction (male) related to inability to perform sexually due to erectile dysfunction
- Risk for injury related to the adverse effects of therapy with drugs used for erectile dysfunction
- Risk for situational low self-esteem related to sexual dysfunction secondary to medications or disease states
- Deficient knowledge related to misinterpretation of information about self-medication

Planning

Goals

- Patient will maintain positive body image.
- Patient will maintain normal activity levels during drug therapy with testosterone.
- Patient will maintain normal sodium and fluid volume levels during drug therapy.
- Patient will retain near-normal urinary elimination patterns.
- Patient will experience minimal alterations in sexual integrity and function during testosterone therapy.
- Patient will remain adherent to drug therapy regimen.
- Patient will state feelings and concerns about actual or perceived changes in sexual patterns and functioning.

Outcome Criteria

- Patient expresses feelings, fears, and anxieties concerning potential for alteration in body image related to disease process or the adverse effects of treatment with testosterone and related men's health drugs.
- Patient maintains healthy activity level during drug therapy and suffers minimal fatigue with gradual increase in activities of daily living.
- Patient states measures to be taken (such as dietary changes) to minimize edema related to sodium retention from the use of large dosages of testosterone.
- Patient verbalizes feelings, anxieties, and fears of alteration in sexual patterns or functioning during drug therapy.
- Patient takes medications as prescribed and with appropriate follow-up.

Implementation

Finasteride may be given orally without regard to meals; the medication should be protected from exposure to light and heat. When used for treatment of the urinary symptoms of BPH, finasteride and related drugs should be administered orally for approximately 6 months, at the end of which time the condition should be re-evaluated. Patients taking drugs for erectile dysfunction should be warned about potential adverse effects, such as flushing of the face, headache, nasal congestion, heartburn, diarrhea, urinary tract infections, blue-tinged vision, blurred vision and light sensitivity, and dizziness. There have been concerns in the media about heart-related deaths associated with this drug, so patient education is crucial to patient safety. Additionally, the patient has the right to accurate and appropriate education about risk factors and concerns about level of activity and physical exertion. See Patient Education for more information.

The therapeutic effects of testosterone are maximized when the drug is taken as ordered and at regular intervals so that steady levels are maintained. If the drug is being used for hypogonadism or induction of puberty, dosages may be managed differently, so that at the end of the growth spurt the patient is placed on maintenance dosages. Androderm patches should be placed on clean, dry skin on the back, abdomen, upper arms, or thighs; the scrotum and bony areas (shoulder, hip) should be avoided. Often these patches are to be changed every 7 days. Because various types of transdermal patches are available, the nurse should be sure that the patient understands which type of patch is to be used and where and how it is to be applied. If the drug is given intramuscularly, the vial of medication should be mixed thoroughly by agitating it before withdrawing the prescribed amount of medication. See Natural Health Products for a description of saw palmetto, a natural health product often taken to relieve symptoms of enlarged prostate.

Evaluation

The therapeutic effects of drugs related to the male reproductive tract include improvement of the condition and signs and symptoms for which the patient is being treated, such as hypogonadism, sexual dysfunction, erectile dysfunction, and urinary elimination problems caused by BPH. The therapeutic effects may not be seen for 6 to 12 months, so it is important for the nurse to observe and monitor the patient for the intended effects of the drugs. In addition, the nurse should evaluate for the adverse effects of these medications (see the pharmacology section for specific adverse effects). Goals and outcome criteria should always be evaluated to see if the patient's needs have been met.

NATURAL HEALTH PRODUCTS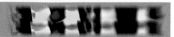

SAW PALMETTO *(Serenoa repens, Sabul serrulata)*

Overview
Saw palmetto is derived from a tree that is also known as the American dwarf palm. The therapeutically active part of the tree is its ripe fruit. Saw palmetto is believed to inhibit dihydrotestosterone and 5α-reductase.

Common Uses
Diuretic, urinary antiseptic, treatment of benign prostatic hypertrophy, treatment of alopecia

Adverse Effects
Gastrointestinal upset, headache, back pain, dysuria

Potential Drug Interactions
Anti-inflammatory drugs, hormones such as estrogen replacement therapy and oral contraceptives, immunostimulants

Contraindications
None

PATIENT EDUCATION

❖ With finasteride, patients should be instructed, at their educational level, about the drug's therapeutic effects and adverse effects. Adverse effects include erectile dysfunction, decrease in the amount of ejaculate, and decreased libido; however, the nurse should emphasize that these adverse effects may be transient and that sexual functioning is not otherwise altered. The nurse should also inform the patient of the special handling precautions for female family members, significant others, or caregivers who are pregnant or of childbearing age. This includes not handling any broken or crushed tablets, which could result in exposure to the drug and the risk of teratogenic effects.

❖ With sildenafil, patients should be informed that the drug should be taken about 1 hour before sexual activity and that patients should not be taking this medication if they are also taking nitrates.

❖ Patients should be warned that sildenfil causes blurred vision, sensitivity to light, and loss of blue–green colour discrimination in approximately 3 to 10% of patients. This occurs as a result of the drug's inhibition of the photoreceptor cells in the retina (and occurs more frequently at higher dosages). This effect is mild and lasts for a brief time; however, airplane pilots need to be cautioned because they rely on green and blue lights for landing the planes.

❖ Patients should be informed that drug therapy for erectile dysfunction is not effective without sexual stimulation and arousal.

❖ With testosterone, patients should be educated about the therapeutic and adverse effects with use of age-appropriate education strategies. Follow-up appointments should be emphasized as an important aspect of effective therapy.

❖ Patients should be educated about the transdermal dosage form and how it should be discarded in a trash can once the drug has been unwrapped and applied, so that accidental application or ingestion by children (or anyone else) may be prevented.

❖ Patients taking testosterone capsules should be informed that the drug should be taken with a meal and swallowed without chewing. The blister package should be protected from light and moisture and not refrigerated.

❖ Patients should be encouraged to report any of the following adverse effects in order to receive further instructions: for male patients, swelling of the extremities, jaundice, or prolonged painful erections; for female patients, hoarseness, deepening of the voice, menstrual irregularities, acne, or facial hair growth. Dosage amounts may be changed or the drug may be discontinued by the physician should these effects occur.

❖ Patients should be educated about avoiding abrupt withdrawal of testosterone.

POINTS TO REMEMBER

❖ The most commonly used drugs related to male health and the male reproductive tract are finasteride, sildenafil, and testosterone. The nurse needs to know how these drugs work and what their adverse effects, contraindications, cautions, and drug interactions are for their safe and effective use.

❖ Testosterone is responsible for the development and maintenance of the male reproductive system and secondary sex characteristics. Oral testosterone has poor pharmacokinetic and pharmacodynamic characteristics, thus it is usually recommended that testosterone be administered via injection (parenteral route) or a transdermal patch.

❖ Patients taking testosterone should be told to avoid abrupt withdrawal of the medication. Weaning off the drug, if ordered, is generally done over several weeks.

❖ Finasteride is usually indicated to stop growth of the prostate in men with BPH and to treat men with androgenic alopecia. Finasteride may be given orally without regard to meals but should be protected from exposure to light and heat.

❖ Patients taking drugs for erectile dysfunction (e.g., sildenafil) should be warned about potential adverse effects, such as flushing of the face, headache, nasal congestion, heartburn, diarrhea, urinary tract infections, blue-tinged vision, blurred vision and light sensitivity, and dizziness.

❖ Because there are major concerns about heart-related deaths associated with nitrates and drugs used for erectile dysfunction, patient education should focus on prevention of drug interactions and related adverse effects and complications.

❖ The therapeutic effects of drugs related to the male reproductive tract include improvement of the condition and signs and symptoms for which the patient is being treated, such as hypogonadism, sexual dysfunction, erectile dysfunction, and urinary elimination problems caused by BPH. It is important to note that the therapeutic effects of most of the drugs do not occur immediately and may take 6 to 12 months.

EXAMINATION REVIEW QUESTIONS

1 Which is important to monitor when a patient is taking finasteride (Proscar)?
a. PSA levels
b. Blood pressure
c. Fluid retention
d. Complete blood count

2 The nurse is performing an assessment of a patient who is asking for a prescription for sildenafil (Viagra). Which of the following findings would be a contraindication to its use?
a. Age 65 years
b. History of hypertension
c. Medication list that includes nitrates
d. Medication list that includes saw palmetto

3 During a counselling session for a group of teenage athletes, the use of androgenic steroids is discussed. Which of the following is a rare but devastating effect of androgenic steroid use that the nurse should discuss?
a. Bradycardia
b. Kidney failure
c. Peliosis of the liver
d. Tachydysrhythmias

4 The nurse is teaching a patient about the possible adverse effects of erectile dysfunction drugs. If the patient experiences priapism, or an erection that lasts longer than 4 hours, which of the following should he know to do?
a. Seek medical attention
b. Turn on his left side and rest
c. Apply an ice pack for 30 minutes
d. Stay in bed until the erection ceases

5 A patient is asking about the use of saw palmetto for prostate health. Which of the following drugs interact with saw palmetto?
a. Nitrates
b. Antihypertensive drugs
c. Acetaminophen (Tylenol)
d. Nonsteroidal anti-inflammatory drugs

For answers see http://evolve.elsevier.com/Canada/Lilley/pharmacology/.

CRITICAL THINKING ACTIVITIES

1 How do finasteride and testosterone differ in their mechanisms of action?

2 Why might an androgen be prescribed to a patient who has anemia?

3 Develop a teaching plan about the risks of anabolic steroids for an 18-year-old male football player and weight lifter.

For answers see http://evolve.elsevier.com/Canada/Lilley/pharmacology/.
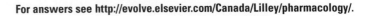

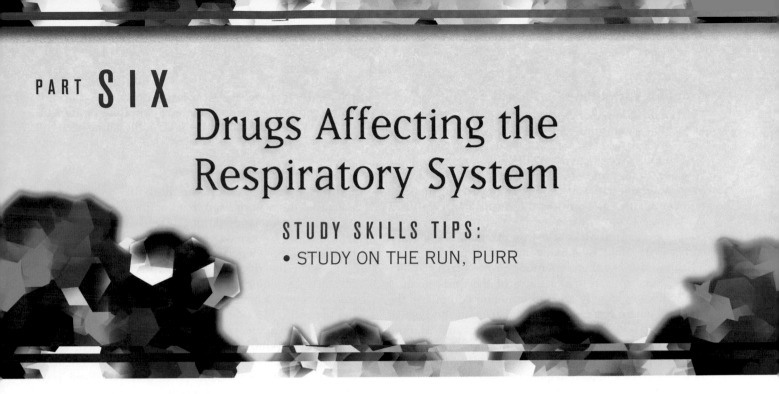

PART SIX

Drugs Affecting the Respiratory System

STUDY SKILLS TIPS:

- STUDY ON THE RUN, PURR

STUDY ON THE RUN, PURR

Study on the Run (SOTR) is about making use of small blocks of time that pop up in your day. The steps Plan, Rehearse, and Review do not require that the entire chapter be covered in one study session. These steps benefit learning through repetition of material. The more you repeat something, the better you will recall it on a test.

Where Is the Time?

Small blocks of time are everywhere in your day; it is just a matter of becoming aware of them. Finishing an exam early, standing in the checkout line, or even waiting for the washing machine to finish the last spin before you change loads can be time used for 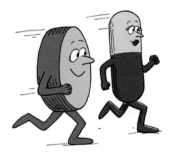 SOTR. Remember, every minute of time you use this way is a minute of time you will not have to find later.

SOTR and Plan

These study skills sections have repeatedly stressed the importance of questioning as an essential component of the Plan step. Look at the chapter objectives for Chapter 36. There are three objectives presented for this chapter. Work on the questions for as many of these objectives as you can in the time that you have. If you complete questions for only two objectives, do not think that you are failing to complete something. Instead, learn to view what you have done as that much less to do later. The time you spend now frees up

that much more time during your large blocks of study time for intense study reading.

Will you forget the questions you generated before you have the opportunity to read the chapter? If you make it a habit to ask questions, you will find that you remember the focus questions well. If you have trouble remembering your questions, use a pencil. Write questions in the margins of the text. Gradually, you will find that questioning has become such an automatic procedure that you will not need to write down the questions; you will remember them.

SOTR and Vocabulary

One of the most challenging aspects of a course like this is the almost overwhelming vocabulary load. As if the new vocabulary were not enough, you also need to keep reviewing previous parts and chapters because a term that was introduced three chapters ago has reappeared and you do not remember it clearly. Creating your own vocabulary cards is a perfect SOTR activity.

The basic card model is simple. The word, common form, prefix, or suffix appears on the card front. The back of the card may have just a little information, the minimum being a definition of what is on the front, or the back of the card may contain considerable information. By including part, chapter, and page number on the back you can locate the term quickly if the need arises. In addition, you may want to add a specific example from the text or one of your own creation to help clarify the term. Put as much information on the back as you find useful. It might also be helpful to colour code your cards. For example, all cards having to do with the cardiac system could be pink and all cards relating to the respiratory system, blue.

Creating Vocabulary Cards with SOTR

Use the time between classes to create personal vocabulary cards. Grab your text and your blank note cards. Open to the next chapter you will be studying. Flip over to the glossary pages. Write the first word from the glossary on the front of a blank note card. Flip the card over. Write the part and chapter numbers and the page number for the glossary on the card. Pick a standard location for this. Put these numbers in a top corner or a bottom corner, but make sure you put them in the same corner every time. Eventually, this practice will become a habit and make the preparation process faster. It also helps when you are making use of the cards because you will know exactly what information you put on the card and where you put it. Put this card aside and repeat the process with the next term in the glossary. In those few minutes before you go to class, you can complete the basic preparation for a full set of cards covering the 17 terms in the Chapter 36 glossary.

Note that the paragraph above did not suggest copying the definition in the glossary at this time. The term may be much easier to understand when used in the context of a sentence and a paragraph. If, as you read the chapter, you feel that the glossary definition is also useful to have on this card, you can always flip back, using the location information you put on the card.

SOTR and Vocabulary Review

Your vocabulary cards are ideal for SOTR action. Carry a deck of cards with you at all times. Whenever you have even a minute or two, you can pull out a stack of cards—cards from previous chapters or the current chapter. Use the oral ask-and-answer method discussed in the *Study Guide*. For instance, the first term in the glossary for Chapter 36 is *adrenergic*. Ask yourself aloud, "What is an *adrenergic*?" Then try to answer the question aloud. Answer: "An adrenergic is a drug that stimulates the sympathetic nerve fibres of the autonomic nervous system." It is not necessary to recall the exact answer presented in the glossary or chapter. What is important is that you respond with a clear and meaningful answer. The answer given above is not exactly the same as that stated in the glossary, but the general concept is the same. Once you have stated your answer, turn the card over and check to

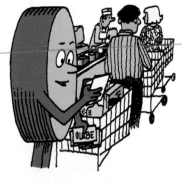

make sure that you were correct. Each time you do this with a term, you are strengthening your long-term memory and will find that it takes less and less time to recall the terms you need.

SOTR and Chapter Review

It can be overwhelming if you think that review means rereading the material and that you therefore need large blocks of uninterrupted time. There is a much more efficient way to review, and it works well in short time blocks, making it a perfect technique for SOTR.

Look at the first page of Chapter 36. You should instantly see a number of visible structures that make it easy to review key terms and concepts without rereading the entire block of material. First, there is the chapter title: *Antihistamines, Decongestants, Antitussives, and Expectorants*. What are antihistamines? This is a question you would have generated when you were engaged in the Plan step of PURR. Now that you have read the chapter, repeat the question and answer it aloud. Answer aloud because you will hear what you say—you will either know the material or need to mark it to come back and reread. Now ask a more complex question: "What is the role of antihistamines? What do they do?" Now try to answer these questions. If you can, then you do not need to reread to find out what antihistamines are. Next, you will notice some words are in **bold print**. Apply the same process. Using the bold face words and phrases as stimulus, ask questions and try to answer them to your own satisfaction. If you cannot develop a satisfactory answer, then you know that some rereading is needed. But it is very focused. You are not trying to reread everything on the page, only the material right there associated with the term.

Looking under the first major heading, Antihistamines, you will see a list. Look at the previous sentence: "This explains why the release of excessive amounts of histamine can lead to anaphylaxis and severe allergic symptoms and result in any or all of the following physiological changes." Ask questions. If you can answer them, no reading is necessary. If you cannot answer them, you know that the answers are found immediately after this sentence in the indented list. Use the structures in the chapter to accomplish focused review. Comprehension is improved, long-term memory is strengthened, and your test grades will reflect this.

The benefits of SOTR are enormous. There is no drawback. You are using time that otherwise would be "wasted." This time now becomes productive study time. The more active you become in looking for SOTR opportunities, the more you will find.

CHAPTER 36

Antihistamines, Decongestants, Antitussives, and Expectorants

Learning Objectives

After reading this chapter, the successful student will be able to do the following:

1 Provide specific examples of the drugs categorized as antihistamines, decongestants, antitussives, and expectorants.

2 Discuss the mechanisms of action, indications, contraindications, cautions, drug interactions, adverse effects, dosages, and routes of administration for antihistamines, decongestants, antitussives, and expectorants.

3 Develop a collaborative plan of care that includes all phases of the nursing process for patients taking antihistamines, decongestants, antitussives, and expectorants.

e-Learning Activities

Web site
(http://evolve.elsevier.com/Canada/Lilley/pharmacology/)

- Animations
- Answers to chapter questions, activities, and case studies
- Calculators and Category Catchers
- Glossary with audio pronunciations
- IV Therapy and Medication Error Checklists
- Multiple-Choice Review Question quizzes
- Nursing Care Plans
- Online Appendices and Supplements
- WebLinks

Drug Profiles

codeine (codeine phosphate)*, p. 678
▸▸ **dextromethorphan (dextromethorphan hydrobromide)***, p. 678
▸▸ **diphenhydramine (diphenhydramine hydrochloride)***, p. 673
▸▸ **guaifenesin**, p. 678
▸▸ **loratadine**, p. 673
oxymetazoline (oxymetazoline hydrochloride)*, p. 678

▸▸ Key drug.

*Full generic name is given in parentheses. For the purposes of this text, the more common shortened name is used.

Glossary

Adrenergics (sympathomimetics) Drugs that stimulate the sympathetic nerve fibres of the autonomic nervous system that use epinephrine or epinephrine-like substances as neurotransmitters. (p. 672)

Anticholinergics (parasympatholytics) Drugs that block the action of acetylcholine and similar substances at acetylcholine receptors, resulting in the inhibition of the transmission of parasympathetic nerve impulses. (p. 672)

Antigens Substances that, upon entering the body, can induce specific immune responses and, in turn, react with the specific products of this response, such as antibodies and specifically sensitized T lymphocytes. (p. 669)

Antihistamines Substances capable of reducing the physiological and pharmacological effects of histamine, including a wide variety of drugs that block histamine receptors. (p. 666)

Antitussive A drug that reduces coughing, often by inhibiting neural activity in the cough centre of the central nervous system (CNS). (p. 666)

Corticosteroids Any of the hormones produced by the adrenal cortex, either in natural or synthetic form. (p. 672)

Decongestants Drugs that reduce congestion or swelling, especially of the upper or lower respiratory tract. (p. 666)

Empirical therapy A method of treating disease on the basis of observations and experience, without an understanding of the precise cause of or mechanism responsible for the disorder or the way in which the therapeutic drug or procedure produces improvement or cure. (p. 666)

Expectorants Drugs that increase the flow of fluid in the respiratory tract, usually by reducing the viscosity of bronchial and tracheal secretions and facilitating their removal by the cough reflex and ciliary action. (p. 666)

Histamine antagonists Drugs that compete with histamine for binding sites on histamine receptors. (p. 667)

Influenza A highly contagious infection of the respiratory tract caused by a myxovirus and transmitted by airborne droplets. (p. 666)

Nonsedating antihistamines Newer medications that work peripherally to block the actions of histamine and therefore do not have the CNS effects of many of the older antihistamines; also called *second-generation antihistamines* or peripherally acting antihistamines. (p. 671)

Reflex stimulation An irritation of the respiratory tract occurring in response to an irritation of the gastrointestinal tract. (p. 676)

Rhinovirus Any of aproximately 100 serologically distinct ribonucleic acid (RNA) viruses that cause approximately 40% of acute respiratory illnesses. (p. 666)

Sympathomimetic drugs A class of drugs whose effects mimic those resulting from the stimulation of organs and structures by the sympathetic nervous system. (p. 673)

Upper respiratory tract infection (URI) Any infectious disease of the upper respiratory tract, including the common cold, laryngitis, pharyngitis, rhinitis, sinusitis, and tonsillitis. (p. 666)

COLD MEDICATIONS

Most common colds result from a viral infection, most often a **rhinovirus** or an **influenza** virus. These viruses typically invade the tissues (mucosa) of the upper respiratory tract (nose, pharynx, and larynx) to cause an **upper respiratory tract infection (URI)**. The inflammatory response elicited by these invading viruses stimulates excessive mucus production. This fluid drips behind the nose, down the pharynx, and into the esophagus and lower respiratory tract, resulting in symptoms typical of a cold: sore throat, coughing, and upset stomach. The irritation of the nasal mucosa often triggers the sneeze reflex and causes the release of several inflammatory and vasoactive substances. Consequently, the small blood vessels in the nasal sinuses dilate, leading to nasal congestion.

The treatment of the common symptoms of URI involves the combined use of **antihistamines** (to reduce the effects of histamine), nasal **decongestants** (to reduce congestion or swelling in the respiratory tract), **antitussives** (to reduce coughs), and **expectorants** (to reduce the viscosity of bronchial and tracheal secretions). Many of these drugs are available over the counter. However, they can only relieve the symptoms of a URI; they are ineffective in eliminating the causative pathogen. Antivirals are currently the only drugs that can do this, but treatment with antivirals is often hampered because the viral cause cannot be readily identified. Thus the treatment rendered can only be based on what is believed to be the most likely cause, given the presenting clinical symptoms. Such treatment is called **empirical therapy**. Some patients seem to gain benefit from the use of natural health products and other supplements, such as vitamin C, in preventing the onset of cold signs and

symptoms or in decreasing their severity. One product commonly used for colds is echinacea (see Natural Health Products). The practitioner should recognize, however, that controlled research data on the efficacy of natural health products are limited. Also, some natural health products can have significant drug–drug or drug–disease interactions (see Evidence-Informed Practice).

ANTIHISTAMINES

Histamine is a biological compound synthesized in the mast cells in the body, where it is released in response to a stimulus such as injury or an allergen. Upon release from mast cells, histamine causes dilation of capillaries, contraction of smooth muscle, stimulation of gastric acid secretion, and acceleration of the heart rate. Histamine contracts many smooth muscles, such as those of the bronchi and gut, but powerfully relaxes others, including those of fine blood vessels. It is a potent stimulus to gastric acid production. Histamine is also a neurotransmitter in the CNS. There are two types of cellular receptors for histamine. Histamine$_1$ (H$_1$) receptors mediate smooth muscle contraction and dilation of capillaries, and histamine$_2$ (H$_2$) receptors mediate the acceleration of the heart rate and gastric acid secretion. Thus the release of excessive amounts of histamine can lead to anaphylaxis and severe allergic symptoms and result in any or all of the following physiological changes:

- Constriction of smooth muscle, especially in the stomach and lungs
- Increase in body secretions
- Vasodilation, lowering blood pressure and increasing permeability of the vessel walls, so that fluids escape into the surrounding tissues, resulting in edema

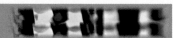

NATURAL HEALTH PRODUCTS

ECHINACEA *(Echinacea)*

Overview
The three species of echinacea are *Echinacea angustifolia, Echinacea pallida,* and *Echinacea purpurea.* Echinacea has been shown in clinical trials to reduce cold symptoms and recovery time when taken early in the illness. This result is probably due to its immunostimulant effects. Currently, there is no strong research evidence to warrant recommending echinacea for urinary tract infections, wound healing, or prevention of colds; further study is needed to show evidence of its therapeutic effects and indications.

Common Uses
Stimulation of the immune system, antisepsis, treatment of antiviral infections and influenza-like respiratory infections, promotion of healing of wounds, and treatment of chronic ulcerations

Adverse Effects
Dermatitis, upset stomach or vomiting, dizziness, headache, unpleasant taste

Potential Drug Interactions
Amiodarone, cyclosporine, phenytoin, methotrexate, ketoconazole, barbiturates; tolerance likely to develop if used for more than 8 weeks. Because some preparations have a high alcohol content, they may cause acetaldehyde syndrome in patients taking disulfiram (Antabuse) to prevent alcohol misuse (Chapter 9).

Contraindications
Contraindicated in patients with acquired immune deficiency syndrome (AIDS), tuberculosis, connective tissue diseases, multiple sclerosis

GOLDENSEAL *(Hydrastis canadensis)*

Overview
Goldenseal is native to wooded areas in Canada and the eastern United States. The dried root of the perennial plant is most commonly used for its biologically active alkaloids. These components have been shown to have antibacterial, antifungal, and antiprotozoal activity. The alkaloid berberine has both anticholinergic and antihistaminic activity.

Common Uses
Treatment of upper respiratory tract infections, allergies, nasal congestion, and numerous genitourinary, skin, ophthalmic, and otic conditions. It is often combined with echinacea in cold remedy products.

Adverse Effects
Gastrointestinal distress, emotional instability, mucosal ulceration (e.g., when used as a vaginal douche).

Potential Drug Interactions
Gastric acid suppressors (including antacids, histamine H_2 blockers [e.g., ranitidine], proton pump inhibitors [e.g., omeprazole]): theoretically reduced effectiveness because of acid-promoting effect of herb

   Antihypertensives: theoretically reduced effectiveness because of vasoconstrictive activity of herb

Contraindications
Acute or chronic gastrointestinal disorders; pregnancy (has uterine-stimulant properties); should be used with caution by those with cardiovascular disease

Source: Basch, E. M., & Ulbricht, C. E. (2005). *Natural standard herb and supplement book.* St. Louis, MO: Elsevier Mosby; Skidmore-Roth L. (2004). *Mosby's handbook of herbs and natural supplements* (2nd ed.). St. Louis, MO: Mosby.

Antihistamines are drugs that directly compete with histamine for specific receptor sites. For this reason, they are also called **histamine antagonists**. Antihistamines that compete with histamine for the H_2 receptors are called *histamine$_2$ (H_2) antagonists* or *H_2 blockers* and include such drugs as cimetidine, ranitidine, famotidine, and nizatidine. Because they act on the gastrointestinal system, they are discussed in detail in Part Nine, which focuses on the drugs that affect this system. The focus of this chapter is on the H_1 antagonists (also called *H_1 blockers*); these drugs are more commonly known as *antihistamines*. All antihistamines compete with histamine for the H_1 receptors in areas such as the smooth muscle surrounding blood vessels and bronchioles. They also affect secretions of the lacrimal, salivary, and respiratory mucosal glands, which are the primary anticholinergic actions of antihistamines. Antihistamines are useful drugs because approximately 10% to 20% of the general population is sensitive to environmental allergens. Histamine is a major inflammatory mediator of many allergic disorders, such as allergic rhinitis (e.g., hay fever and mould, dust allergies), anaphylaxis, angioedema, drug fevers, insect bite reactions, and urticaria (itching).

H_1 antagonists include drugs such as diphenhydramine, chlorpheniramine, and fexofenadine. Because of their antihistaminic properties, they are of greatest value in the treatment of nasal allergies, particularly seasonal hay fever. They are also given to relieve the symptoms of the common cold, such as sneezing and runny nose. When used in this way, the effect of antihistamines is purely palliative, not curative, as they can suppress the symptoms of a cold but can do nothing to destroy the virus causing it. The antihistaminic, anticholinergic, and sedative properties of H_1 antagonists also make them useful for the treatment of problems such as vertigo, motion sickness, insomnia, and cough. The clinical efficacy of the different antihistamines is extremely similar, although they all have varying degrees of antihistaminic, anticholinergic, and sedating properties (Figure 36-1). The particular actions of, and hence indications for, a particular antihistamine are determined by its specific chemical makeup. These drugs also differ from each other in their potency and their adverse effects, especially in the degree of drowsiness they produce. Several classes of antihistamines are listed in Table 36-1, along with their anticholinergic and sedative effects.

EVIDENCE-INFORMED PRACTICE

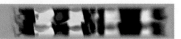

The Natural Health Product COLD-fX

Background
There is growing interest in the role of ginseng as an effective upper respiratory prophylaxis. COLD-fX, derived from the roots of the North American ginseng *Panax quinquefolius*, is an expensive complementary over-the-counter natural health remedy. Recently, it received Health Canada approval to be marketed by the manufacturer with the health claim that COLD-fX boosts the immune system and consequently reduces cold and flu symptoms. It is the number one natural health product sold in Canada. This Canadian study examined the efficacy of ginseng in preventing upper respiratory tract infections.

Type of Evidence
This randomized, double-blind, placebo-controlled study consisted of 323 subjects between the ages of 18 and 65 (average of 42 years old and over 60% female) who had experienced two or more colds in the year before the study. Participants were excluded if they had received influenza immunization in the previous 6 months. Participants took either two capsules of COLD-fX per day or a placebo for 4 months after the onset of the influenza season. Subjects maintained a daily log of cold-related symptoms and adverse effects.

Results of Study
There were 149 patients in the placebo arm and 130 patients in the COLD-fX arm that completed the study. To measure symptoms, the Jackson index was used, which assesses eight cold symptoms (sneezing, nasal obstruction, nasal discharge, sore throat, cough, headache, chilliness, and malaise) by use of a three- or four-point response range. This study used a modified Jackson scale and concluded that patients receiving COLD-fX experienced fewer colds per person over the 4-month period. Adverse effects were similar in both groups.

Link of Evidence to Nursing Practice
In order to knowledgeably inform patients, it is important for nurses to be familiar with the evidence of natural health product claims. This study indicated that when taken for 4 months to prevent colds and flu, COLD-fX could decrease the number of colds by 0.25 colds in adults who had more than two colds in the previous year. Health Canada's recommendations are that COLD-fX "helps reduce the frequency, severity and duration of cold and influenza symptoms by boosting the immune system." There are no published trials to date that support COLD-fX as treatment of colds and flu. The routine use of COLD-fX is not recommended. Frequent hand washing may be just as effective in reducing the incidence of colds and influenza.

Based on Predy, G. N., Goel, V., Lovlin, R., Donner, A., Stitt, L., & Basu, T. K. (2005). Efficacy of an abstract of North American ginseng containing poly-furanosyl-saccharides for preventing upper respiratory tract infections: A randomized controlled trial. *Canadian Medical Association Journal, 173*(9), 1043–1048.

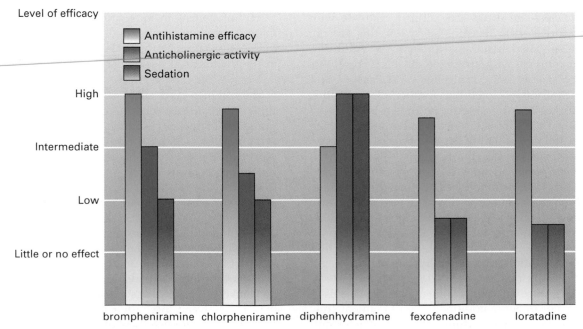

FIG. 36-1 Comparison of efficacy and adverse effects of selected antihistamines.

TABLE 36-1

Effects of Selected Antihistamines

Chemical Class	Anticholinergic Effects	Sedative Effects	Comments
ALKYLAMINES			
brompheniramine	Moderate	Low	Cause less drowsiness and more CNS stimulation; suitable for
chlorpheniramine	Moderate	Low	daytime use
ETHANOLAMINES			
clemastine	High	Moderate	Substantial anticholinergic effects; commonly cause sedation;
dimenhydrinate	High	High	at usual dosages, drowsiness occurs in about 50% of patients;
diphenhydramine	High	High	diphenhydramine and dimenhydrinate also used as antiemetics
ETHYLENEDIAMINES			
pyrilamine	Low to none	Low	Weak sedative effects, but adverse gastrointestinal effects are
tripelennamine	Low to none	Moderate	common
PHENOTHIAZINE			
promethazine	High	High	Drugs in this class are principally used as antipsychotics; some are useful as antihistamines, antipruritics, and antiemetics
PIPERIDINES			
azatadine	Moderate	Moderate	Commonly used in the treatment of motion sickness; hydroxyzine
cyproheptadine	Moderate	Low	is used as a tranquilizer, sedative, antipruritic, and antiemetic
hydroxyzine	Moderate	Moderate	
MISCELLANEOUS			
fexofenadine	Low to none	Low to none	Few adverse anticholinergic or sedative effects; almost exclusively
loratadine	Low to none	Low to none	antihistaminic effects, can be taken during the day because no sedative effects occur; in general, they are longer acting and have fewer adverse effects

Mechanism of Action and Drug Effects

During an allergic reaction, histamine and other substances are released from mast cells, basophils, and other cells in response to **antigens** circulating in the blood. Histamine molecules then bind to and activate other cells in the nose, eyes, respiratory tract, gastrointestinal tract, and skin, producing characteristic allergic signs and symptoms (Figure 32-2). For example, in the respiratory tract, histamine causes extravascular smooth muscle (e.g., in the bronchial tree) to contract, whereas antihistamines cause it to relax. Also, histamine causes pruritus by stimulating nerve endings. Antihistamines can prevent or alleviate this itching.

The circulating histamine molecules normally bind to histamine receptors on basophils and mast cells, stimulating further release of histamine stored within these cells. Antihistamine drugs compete with histamine for unoccupied histamine receptors on the surfaces of basophils and mast cells. This action blocks the circulating histamine from binding to the receptor and prevents the further release and actions of histamine stored within these cells. Therefore, antihistamines are most effective when given early in a histamine-mediated reaction before all of the free histamine molecules bind to cell membrane receptors. This binding of H_1 blockers to the receptors prevents the adverse consequences of histamine binding: vasodilation; increased gastrointestinal, respiratory, salivary, and lacrimal secretions; and increased capillary permeability with resulting edema. The drug effects of antihistamines are listed in Table 36-2.

Indications

Antihistamines are most beneficial in the management of nasal allergies, seasonal or perennial allergic rhinitis (e.g., hay fever), and some of the typical symptoms of the common cold. They are also useful in the treatment of allergic reactions, motion sickness, Parkinson's disease (because of their anticholinergic effects), and vertigo. They are sometimes used as a sleep aid because of the CNS drowsiness effect.

Contraindications

Use of antihistamines is generally contraindicated in cases of known drug allergy. They should also not be used as the sole drug therapy during acute asthmatic attacks. In such cases, a rapid-acting bronchodilator such as salbutamol or, in extreme cases, epinephrine is usually the most urgently needed medication. Other contraindications may include narrow-angle glaucoma, heart disease, kidney disease, hypertension, bronchial asthma, chronic obstructive pulmonary disease, peptic ulcer disease, seizure disorders, benign prostatic hypertrophy, and pregnancy. Fexofenadine is not recommended for children under 6 years of age or those with kidney impairment. Desloratadine is not recommended for children. Loratadine is not recommended for children under

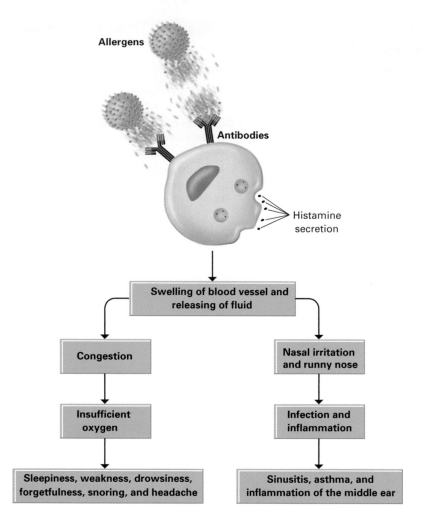

FIG. 36-2 Mediation of the allergic response by histamine.

2 years of age. Antihistamines should generally be used with caution in patients with impaired liver function or kidney insufficiency, as well as in lactating mothers.

Adverse Effects

Drowsiness is usually the chief complaint of people who take antihistamines, but the sedative effects vary among drug class (see Table 36-1). Fortunately, sedative effects are much less common, although still possible, with newer "nonsedating" drugs. Anticholinergic (drying) effects of antihistamines can cause adverse effects such as dry mouth, changes in vision, difficulty urinating, and constipation. Reported adverse effects of antihistamines are listed in Table 36-3.

TABLE 36-2		
Antihistamines: Drug Effects		
Body System	**Histamine Effects**	**Antihistamine Effects**
Cardiovascular (small blood vessels)	Dilates blood vessels, increases blood vessel permeability (allows substances to leak into tissues)	Reduces dilation of blood vessels and increased permeability
Immune (release of substances commonly associated with allergic reactions)	Released from mast cells along with several other substances, which results in allergic reactions	Does not stabilize mast cells or prevent the release of histamine and other substances, but does bind to histamine receptors and prevents the actions of histamine
Smooth muscle (on exocrine glands)	Stimulates salivary, gastric, lacrimal, and bronchial secretions	Reduces salivary, gastric, lacrimal, and bronchial secretions

TABLE 36-3	
Antihistamines: Reported Adverse Effects	
Body System	**Adverse Effects**
Cardiovascular	Local anaesthetic (quinidine-like) effect on the cardiac conduction system, which can result in dysrhythmias, arrest, hypotension, palpitations, syncope, dizziness, death (see Interactions section)
Central nervous	Sedation (mild drowsiness to deep sleep), dizziness, muscular weakness, paradoxical excitement, restlessness, insomnia, nervousness, seizures
Gastrointestinal	Anorexia, nausea, vomiting, diarrhea or constipation, hepatitis, jaundice
Other	Dryness of mouth, nose, and throat; urinary retention; erectile dysfunction; vertigo; visual disturbances; blurred vision; tinnitus; headache; rarely agranulocytosis, hemolytic anemia, leukopenia, thrombocytopenia, pancytopenia

Interactions

When fexofenadine is administered with erythromycin or ketoconazole, increased fexofenadine concentrations can result. Rifampin reduces the absorption of fexofenadine. Ketoconazole, cimetidine, and erythromycin may increase concentrations of loratadine. Alcohol, monoamine oxidase inhibitors (MAOIs), and CNS depressants may increase the CNS depressant effects of diphenhydramine and cetirizine. Concurrent use of anticholinergic drugs and MAOIs may also lead to more anticholinergic adverse effects such as dry mouth and constipation. Antihistamine effects may be potentiated excessively by interactions with apple, grapefruit, and orange juice as well as St. John's wort. An allergist will usually recommend discontinuation of antihistamine drug therapy at least 4 days prior to allergy testing.

Dosages

For the recommended dosages for selected antihistamines, see the Dosages table on p. 673.

 DRUG PROFILES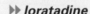

Although some antihistamines are prescription drugs, most are available over the counter. Antihistamines are available in many dosage forms to be administered orally, intramuscularly, intravenously, or topically.

NONSEDATING ANTIHISTAMINES

A major advance in antihistamine therapy occurred with the development of the **nonsedating antihistamines** loratadine, cetirizine, and fexofenadine. These drugs were developed partly to eliminate many of the unwanted adverse effects (mainly sedation) of the older antihistamines. These drugs act peripherally to block the actions of histamine and therefore do not have the CNS effects that many older antihistamines have. For this reason, these drugs are also called *peripherally acting antihistamines;* they tend not to cross the blood–brain barrier, unlike their traditional counterparts. Another advantage of these drugs over the older antihistamines is that they have longer durations of action, which allows some to be taken only once a day. This dosage further increases adherence. The three drugs replace the two original nonsedating antihistamines terfenadine and astemizole, which were withdrawn from the Canadian market following several cases of fatal drug-induced cardiac dysrhythmias. Fexofenadine is actually the active metabolite of terfenadine but is not associated with severe heart effects. Loratadine and cetirizine are also not associated with adverse heart effects.

▶▶ loratadine

Loratadine (Claritin) is a nonsedating antihistamine that is taken only once a day. Structurally, it is similar to cyproheptadine and azatadine, but unlike these drugs it does not cross the blood–brain barrier to cause sedation effects. Loratadine is used to relieve the symptoms of seasonal allergic rhinitis (e.g., hay fever) as well as chronic urticaria. Loratadine and its primary active metabolite, desloratidine (Aerius), are both available as over-the-counter drugs.

Drug allergy is the only contraindication to the use of loratadine. The drug is available in oral form as a 10 mg tablet, as a 1 mg/mL syrup, as a 10 mg rapidly disintegrating tablet, and in a combination tablet with the decongestant pseudoephedrine. See the Dosages table on p. 673 for dosage information.

PHARMACOKINETICS

Half-Life	Onset	Peak	Duration
19–24 hr	1–3 hr	8–12 hr	24 hr

TRADITIONAL ANTIHISTAMINES

The traditional antihistamines are the first-generation drugs that work both peripherally and centrally. They also have anticholinergic effects, which, in some cases, make them more effective than nonsedating antihistamines. Some of the commonly used older drugs are diphenhydramine,

Continued

DRUG PROFILES (cont'd)

brompheniramine, chlorpheniramine, dimenhydrinate, meclizine, and promethazine. They are used either alone or in combination with other drugs for the symptomatic relief of many disorders ranging from insomnia to motion sickness. Many patients respond to and tolerate the older drugs, and because many are available as generic preparations, they are much less expensive. These drugs are available both over the counter and by prescription.

▸▸ *diphenhydramine hydrochloride*

Diphenhydramine hydrochloride (Allerdryl, Allernix, Benadryl, others) is an older, traditional antihistamine that acts both peripherally and centrally. It is still often used as a hypnotic drug because of its sedating effects. This use is not generally advised in the older adult, however, because of the "hangover" effect and increased potential for falls. Diphenhydramine is one of the most commonly used antihistamines, in part because of its excellent safety profile and efficacy. It has the greatest range of therapeutic indications of any antihistamine available. It is used for the relief or prevention of histamine-mediated allergies and motion sickness, for postoperative nausea and vomiting, for the treatment of Parkinson's disease (because of its anticholinergic effects), and the promotion of sleep. It is also used in conjunction with epinephrine in the management of anaphylaxis and in the treatment of acute dystonia reactions.

Diphenhydramine use is contraindicated in patients with a known hypersensitivity to it, nursing mothers, neonates, and patients with lower respiratory tract symptoms. It is available in oral, parenteral, and topical preparations. In oral form, diphenhydramine is available as caplets and capsules, chewable tablets, liquid, and in several combination products that contain other cough and cold medications. In parenteral form, diphenhydramine is available as an injection. In topical form, diphenhydramine is available as a cream. It is also available in combination with several other drugs that are commonly given topically as creams and lotions, such as calamine, camphor, and zinc oxide. The recommended dosages for the oral and injectable forms are given in the Dosages table on p. 673.

PHARMACOKINETICS

Half-Life	Onset	Peak	Duration
2–7 hr	15–30 min	1–2 hr	4 hr

DECONGESTANTS

Nasal congestion occurs as a result of excessive nasal secretions and inflamed and swollen nasal mucosa. The primary causes of nasal congestion are allergies and URIs, especially the common cold. During a cold, the blood vessels that surround the nasal sinus are usually dilated, swollen, and engorged with plasma, white blood cells, mast cells, histamines, and many other blood components that are involved in fighting infections of the respiratory tract. This swelling, or dilation, blocks the nasal passages, resulting in nasal congestion. There are three separate groups of nasal decongestants: **adrenergics (sympathomimetics)**, which are the largest group; **anticholinergics (parasympatholytics)**, which are less commonly used; and selected topical **corticosteroids** (intranasal steroids).

Nasal decongestants can be taken orally to produce a systemic effect, can be inhaled, or can be administered topically into the nose. Each method of administration has advantages and disadvantages. Decongestants administered by the oral route include pseudoephedrine, which is available over the counter. A commonly used nasal decongestant spray is phenylephrine, also available over the counter.

Drugs administered by the oral route produce prolonged decongestant effects, but the onset of activity is more delayed and the effect less potent than that of decongestants applied topically. However, the clinical problem of rebound congestion associated with topically administered drugs is almost nonexistent with oral dosage forms. *Rebound congestion* occurs because of the rapid absorption of the drug through mucous membranes and delivery to adrenergic receptors within respiratory tissues, followed by a more rapid decline in therapeutic activity. Oral dosage forms, by contrast, provide a more gradual increase and decline in pharmacological activity because of the time required for gastrointestinal absorption. Inhalation decongestants used orally include desoxyephedrine and propylhexedrine, neither of which is available on the Canadian market. The inhaler available in Canada contains oxymetazoline hydrochloride, a sympathomimetic associated with rebound congestion.

Topical administration of adrenergics into the nasal passages produces a potent decongestant effect with a prompt onset of action. However, sustained use of topical adrenergics for several days can cause rebound congestion, which only exacerbates the condition. Decongestants suitable for nasal inhalation include the following:
- oxymetazoline hydrochloride (Afrin, Claritin, Dristan, Drixoral, Vicks, others)
- phenylephrine hydrochloride (Mydfrin)
- xylometazoline hydrochloride (Balminil, Otrivin)

Inhaled intranasal steroids and anticholinergic drugs are not generally associated with rebound congestion and are often used prophylactically to prevent nasal congestion in patients with chronic upper respiratory symptoms. Commonly used intranasal steroids include the following:
- beclomethasone dipropionate (Qvar, Rivanase)
- budesonide (Pulmicort, Pulmicort Turbuhaler, Rhinocort, Rhinocort Turbuhaler, Symbicort Turbuhaler)
- flunisolide (Rhinalar)
- fluticasone propionate (Flonase)
- mometasone furoate (Nasonex)
- triamcinolone acetonide (Nasacort)

DOSAGES   Selected Antihistamines

Drug (Pregnancy Category)	Pharmacological Class	Usual Dosage Range	Indications
NONSEDATING ANTIHISTAMINES			
cetirizine hydrochloride (Reactine) (B)	H₁ antihistamine	*Children 2–6 yr* 5 mg once daily or divided bid *Children 6–12 yr* 10 mL once daily or divided bid *Children 12 yr and older/Adult* 5–10 mg once daily, max 20 mg/day	Allergic rhinitis, chronic urticaria
desloratadine (Aerius) (B)	H₁ antihistamine	*Children 2–5 yr* 1.25 mg once daily *Children 6–11 yr* 2.5 mg once daily *Children 12 yr and older/Adult* Tab: 5 mg once daily Syrup: 10 mg once daily	Allergic rhinitis, chronic urticaria
fexofenadine hydrochloride (Allegra) (B)	H₁ antihistamine	*Children over 12 yr/Adult* 60 mg bid or 120 mg once daily	Allergic rhinitis, chronic urticaria
▸▸loratadine (Claritin) (B)	H₁ antihistamine	*Children 2–9 yr* 5 mg once daily *Children 12 yr and older/Adult* 10 mg once daily	Allergic rhinitis, chronic urticaria
TRADITIONAL ANTIHISTAMINES (MORE COMMONLY ASSOCIATED WITH SEDATION)			
chlorpheniramine maleate (Chlor-Tripilon; less sedating) (B)	H₁ antihistamine	*Children 2–5 yr* 1 mg (¼ of a 4-mg tab) q4–6h, max 6 mg/24 hr *Children 6–11 yr* 2 mg q4–6h, max 12 mg/24 hr *Children 12 and over/Adult* 4 mg q4–6h, max 24 mg/24 hr	Allergic rhinitis
▸▸diphenhydramine hydrochloride (Allerdryl, Allernix, Benadryl; more sedating) (B)	H₁ antihistamine	*Children equal to or over 10 kg* IM/IV: 12.5–25 mg tid–qid *Adult* IM/IV: 25–50 mg tid–qid *Children under 2 yr* Liquid: 2.5 mL q4–6h *Children 2–5 yr* Liquid: 5 mL q4–6h *Children 6–under 12 yr* Elixir: 5–10 mL q4–6h, max 4 doses/day; liquid: 10–20 mL q4–6h, max 4 doses/day Allergic disorders, PD, night-time insomnia, motion sickness *Children 12 yr and older/Adult* PO: 50 mg at bedtime	Night-time insomnia

IM, intramuscular; *IV*, intravenous; *PD*, Parkinson's disease; *PO*, oral.

Currently, the only commonly used intranasal anticholinergic is the ipratropium bromide (Atrovent) nasal spray.

Mechanism of Action and Drug Effects

Nasal decongestants are most commonly used for their ability to shrink engorged nasal mucous membranes and relieve nasal stuffiness. Adrenergic drugs (e.g., oxymetazoline) accomplish this by constricting the small arterioles that supply the structures of the upper respiratory tract, primarily the blood vessels surrounding the nasal sinuses. When these blood vessels are stimulated by α-adrenergic drugs they constrict. Because sympathetic nervous system (SNS) stimulation produces the same effect, these drugs are sometimes referred to as **sympathomimetic drugs,** or *sympathomimetics.* Once these blood vessels shrink, the nasal secretions in the swollen mucous membranes are better able to drain, either externally through the nostrils or internally through reabsorption into the bloodstream or lymphatic circulation.

Nasal steroids target the inflammatory response elicited by the invading organisms (viruses and bacteria) or other antigens (e.g., allergens). The body responds to antigens by producing inflammation in an effort to isolate or wall off the area and by attracting cells of the immune system to consume and destroy the offending antigens. Steroids exert their anti-inflammatory effect by causing the cells to be turned off or rendered unresponsive. It should be kept in mind, however, that the goal is not complete immunosuppression of the respiratory tract but rather the modulation of inflammatory symptoms to improve patient comfort and air exchange. Intranasal steroids are also discussed in Chapter 37.

Indications

Nasal decongestants reduce nasal congestion associated with acute or chronic rhinitis, the common cold, sinusitis, and hay fever or other allergies. They may also be used to reduce swelling of the nasal passages and to facilitate visualization of the nasal and pharyngeal membranes before surgery or diagnostic procedures.

Contraindications

Contraindications to the use of decongestants include drug allergy and, in the case of adrenergic drugs, narrow-angle glaucoma, uncontrolled cardiovascular disease, hypertension, diabetes, hyperthyroidism, and prostatitis. Other contraindications may include situations in which patients are unable to close their eyes (such as after a stroke) and patients with a history of stroke or transient ischemic attacks, cerebral arteriosclerosis and long-standing asthma, benign prostatic hyperplasia, or diabetes.

Adverse Effects

Adrenergic drugs are usually well tolerated. Possible adverse effects include nervousness, insomnia, palpitations, and tremor. The most common adverse effects of intranasal steroids are localized and include mucosal irritation and dryness as well as the possibility of nose bleeds because of the thinning of the nasal mucosa with long-term use.

Although a topically applied adrenergic nasal decongestant can be absorbed into the bloodstream, the amount is usually not significant enough to cause systemic effects in normal doses. Excessive doses of these drugs are more likely to cause systemic effects elsewhere in the body. These may include cardiovascular effects such as hypertension and palpitations and CNS effects such as headache, nervousness, and dizziness. The systemic effects are the result of α-adrenergic stimulation of the heart, blood vessels, and CNS.

Interactions

There are few significant drug interactions with nasal decongestants. Systemic sympathomimetic drugs and sympathomimetic nasal decongestants are more likely to cause drug toxicity when given together. MAOIs may result in additive pressor (e.g., increase in blood pressure) effects when given with sympathomimetic nasal decongestants.

Other drugs that interact with nasal decongestants include guanethidine, MAOIs, methyldopa, and urinary acidifiers and alkalinizers.

Dosages

For the recommended dosages of oxymetazoline, the only nasal decongestant profiled, see the Dosages table on p. 678.

DRUG PROFILES

Many of the decongestants are available over the counter; the more potent drugs that can cause serious adverse effects are available only by prescription. Use of adrenergic drugs is usually contraindicated in patients with diabetes, hypertension, heart disease, thyroid dysfunction, prostatitis, or known hypersensitivity. Although nasal steroids are relatively safe, they too are contraindicated in some circumstances, including nasal mucosal infections (because of their ability to depress the body's immune response as part of their anti-inflammatory effect) or known drug allergy.

Many inhaled corticosteroids (e.g., beclomethasone, dexamethasone, and flunisolide) are discussed in greater detail in Chapter 37. The adrenergic drug oxymetazoline is discussed here. Both these drug categories are generally first-line drugs for the treatment of chronic nasal congestion.

oxymetazoline hydrochloride

Oxymetazoline hydrochloride (Afrin, Claritin, Dristan, Drixoral, Vicks) is chemically and pharmacologically similar to the other sympathomimetic drug, xylometazoline. When these drugs are administered intranasally, they cause dilated arterioles to constrict, thereby reducing nasal blood flow and congestion. Oxymetazoline and its chemically related cousins have the same contraindications as the other nasal decongestants. Common dosages for this drug are given in the Dosages table on p. 678.

PHARMACOKINETICS

Half-Life	Onset	Peak	Duration
Unknown	5–10 min	Unknown	2–6 hr

ANTITUSSIVES

Coughing is a normal physiological function that serves the purpose of removing potentially harmful foreign substances and excessive secretions from the respiratory tract. The cough reflex is stimulated when receptors in the bronchi, alveoli, and pleura (lining of the lungs) are stretched. This causes a signal to be sent to the cough centre in the medulla of the brain, which, in turn, stimulates the cough. Although coughing is primarily a beneficial response, there are times when it is not useful and may even be harmful (e.g., after a surgery such as hernia repair, or in cases of nonproductive cough or "dry cough"). In such situations, it may enhance patient comfort and reduce respiratory distress to inhibit this otherwise normal response through the use of an antitussive drug. There are two main categories of antitussives: opioid and nonopioid. Although all opioid drugs have antitussive effects, only codeine and its semisynthetic derivative hydrocodone are used as antitussives. Both drugs are effective in suppressing the cough reflex and, if used in the prescribed manner, their use should not lead to dependency. Codeine and hydromorphone are usually incorporated into combination formulations with other respiratory drugs and are rarely used alone for the purpose of cough suppression.

Nonopioid antitussive drugs are less effective than opioid drugs. They are available either alone or in combination with other drugs in an array of over-the-counter cold and cough preparations. Dextromethorphan is the most widely used of these antitussive drugs and is a derivative of the synthetic opioid levorphanol.

Mechanism of Action and Drug Effects

The opioid antitussives codeine and hydrocodone suppress the cough reflex through direct action on the cough centre in the CNS (medulla). Opioid antitussives also provide analgesia and have a drying effect on the mucosa of the respiratory tract, which also increases the viscosity of respiratory secretions. This helps reduce symptoms such as runny nose and postnasal drip. The nonopioid cough suppressant dextromethorphan acts in the same way. Because it is not an opioid, however, it does not have analgesic properties, nor does it cause addiction or CNS depression.

Indications

Although they have other properties, such as the analgesic effect of the opioid drugs, antitussives are used primarily to arrest the cough reflex when the cough is nonproductive or harmful.

Contraindications

The only absolute contraindication to the antitussives is drug allergy. Relative contraindications include opioid dependency (for opioid antitussives) and high risk for respiratory depression (e.g., in frail older adults). Patients with these conditions are often able to tolerate lower drug dosages and still experience some symptom relief.

Additional contraindications and cautions include the following:
- *codeine* (see hydrocodone)
- *dextromethorphan:* contraindications of hyperthyroidism, advanced heart and vessel disease, hypertension, glaucoma, and having taken MAOIs within the past 14 days
- *diphenhydramine* (see Antihistamines section)
- *hydrocodone:* contraindication with alcohol and extreme caution with CNS depression, anoxia, high serum levels of carbon dioxide (hypercapnia), and respiratory depression, and cautions of increased intracranial pressure, impaired kidney function, and liver diseases, as well as benign prostatic hyperplasia, Addison's disease, and chronic obstructive pulmonary disease.

Adverse Effects

Following are the common adverse effects of selected antitussive drugs:
- *codeine:* sedation, nausea, vomiting, lightheadedness, and constipation
- *dextromethorphan:* dizziness, drowsiness, and nausea
- *diphenhydramine:* sedation, dry mouth, and other anticholinergic effects
- *hydrocodone:* sedation, nausea, vomiting, lightheadedness, and constipation

Interactions

Few drug interactions occur with the use of opioid antitussives and dextromethorphan. Opioid antitussives (codeine and hydrocodone) may potentiate the effects of other opioids, general anaesthetics, tranquilizers, sedatives and hypnotics, tricyclic antidepressants (TCAs), MAOIs, alcohol, and other CNS depressants. Dextromethorphan may also potentiate the serotonergic effects of MAOIs, thus concurrent administration is contraindicated.

Dosages

For the recommended dosages of selected antitussive drugs, see the Dosages table on p. 678.

DRUG PROFILES

Antitussives come in many oral dosage forms and are available both with and without a prescription. Most of the narcotic antitussives are available only by prescription because of the associated misuse potential. Dextromethorphan is the most popular non-narcotic antitussive available over the counter.

codeine phosphate

Codeine phosphate (Dimetane-Expectorant-C, Dimetapp-C, CoActifed, Robitussin AC, others) is a popular opioid antitussive drug. It is used in combination with many other respiratory medications to control coughs. Because it is an opioid, it is potentially addictive and can depress respirations as part of its CNS-depressant effects. For this reason, codeine-containing cough suppressants are more tightly controlled (Controlled Drugs and Substances, Schedule I) but commonly available by prescription. Cough suppressants containing codeine are also available behind the counter in the pharmacy.

Cough suppressants are available in many oral dosage forms: solutions, tablets, capsules, and suspensions. Their use is contraindicated in patients with a known hypersensitivity to opiates and in those suffering from respiratory depression, increased intracranial pressure, seizure disorders, or severe respiratory disorders.

Common dosages are listed in the Dosages table on p. 678.

PHARMACOKINETICS

Half-Life	Onset	Peak	Duration
2.9 hr (plasma)	30–60 min	1–2 hr	4–6 hr

▸▸ dextromethorphan hydrobromide

Dextromethorphan hydrobromide (Benylin DM-E, Buckley's, Dimetapp-DM, Robitussin-DM, Vicks) is a nonopioid antitussive that is available alone or in combination with many other cough and cold preparations. It is widely used because it is safe and nonaddictive and does not cause respiratory or CNS depression. Its use is contraindicated in cases of drug allergy, asthma or emphysema, or persistent headache. Dextromethorphan is available as lozenges, solution, liquid-filled capsules, granules, caplets, tablets (chewable, extended-release, and film-coated), and an extended-release syrup. It is classified as pregnancy category C. Common dosages are listed in the Dosages table on p. 678.

PHARMACOKINETICS

Half-Life	Onset	Peak	Duration
Unknown	15–30 min	Unknown	3–6 hr

EXPECTORANTS

Expectorants aid in the expectoration (i.e., coughing up and spitting out) of excessive mucus that has accumulated in the respiratory tract, by breaking down and thinning out the secretions. Expectorants are administered orally either as single drugs or in combination with other drugs to facilitate the flow of respiratory secretions by reducing the viscosity of tenacious secretions. The actual clinical effectiveness of expectorants is highly questionable, however. Placebo-controlled clinical evaluations have failed to strongly confirm that expectorants reduce the viscosity of sputum. More recently, Health Canada has warned against their use in children under the age of 6 (see Special Populations: Children). Despite this, expectorants are popular drugs and are contained in many over-the-counter cold and cough preparations. They provide symptom relief for many users. The most common expectorant used in over-the-counter products is guaifenesin (formerly known as glyceryl guaiacolate).

Mechanism of Action and Drug Effects

Expectorants' mechanism of action is through **reflex stimulation.** Loosening and thinning of the respiratory tract secretions occurs in response to an irritation of the gastrointestinal tract produced by the drug. Guaifenesin is the only such drug currently available in Canada. In the past, there were several iodine-containing expectorants on the Canadian market; however, they are no longer available.

Indications

Expectorants are used for the relief of productive cough associated with the common cold, bronchitis, laryngitis, pharyngitis, pertussis, influenza, and measles. They may also be used for the suppression of coughs caused by chronic paranasal sinusitis. By loosening and thinning sputum and the bronchial secretions, they may also indirectly diminish the tendency to cough.

Contraindications

Contraindications include drug allergy and possibly hyperkalemia (for potassium-containing expectorants).

Adverse Effects

The adverse effects of the expectorant guaifenesin are minimal and include nausea, vomiting, and gastric irritation.

Interactions

The drug interactions most commonly associated with expectorant use are minimal.

Dosages

The recommended dosages of guaifenesin, the only expectorant profiled, are given in the Dosages table on p. 678.

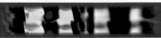

SPECIAL POPULATIONS: CHILDREN

Over-the-Counter Cough and Cold Medication Use in Young Children

On the basis of an increased number of adverse events, in December 2008, Health Canada issued new mandates requiring manufacturers to label cough and cold drugs with the recommendation that children under 6 years should not be given the drugs. The new labelling has been in place since fall 2009. No comprehensive studies have investigated the therapeutic effects of cough and cold medication in children. Furthermore, from January 1995 to 2008, Health Canada received 164 reports of adverse events related to over-the-counter cough and cold medications in children under 12. Of these, 105 were considered serious. Of 124 adverse reactions in children under the age of 6 years, 80 were considered serious. Five children under the age of 2 who were given cough and medications died; however, it is unclear whether misuse or overdose of the medications was the reason for the deaths. Some of the reported adverse effects included decreased level of consciousness, abnormal or rapid heart rhythm, convulsions, and hallucinations.

Children under the age of 6 years generally have more frequent colds than do older children and thus are likely to be exposed more frequently to these medications. The following are recommendations that the nurse can provide parents, legal guardians, and caregivers regarding cold and cough medications for young children:

- Do not use over-the-counter cough and cold medicines in children under 6 years of age. Younger children are less likely to be able to communicate a potential adverse effect from a cough and cold medicine and are less likely to ask their parents or caregivers for help in the same way a child over 6 years of age.

- Do not give children medications labelled as only for adults.
- Talk to your health care provider if you have questions about the proper use of over-the-counter cough and cold medicines.
- Instead of giving medication, parents should make sure their children receive plenty of fluids, get lots of rest, and remain in a comfortable environment when they come down with a cold.
- If symptoms worsen, last for more than a week, or are accompanied by a fever higher than 38°C or the production of thick phlegm, see a health care provider.
- To prevent overdoses, do not give more than one kind of cough and cold medicine to a child.
- For children older than 6 years, always follow all the instructions carefully, including the dosing and length-of-use directions, and use the dosing device if one is included.
- For babies and young children, it is important to rule out serious illnesses that have cold-like signs and symptoms (for example, pneumonia, earache, or other infections). This is especially important if symptoms do not improve or if the child's condition worsens.
- The common cold is a viral infection for which there is no cure. Cough and cold medicines offer only temporary relief of symptoms.
- There is no evidence that over-the-counter cough and cold drugs benefit children. Cold symptoms usually are self-limiting.

 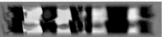

DRUG PROFILES

▶▶ *guaifenesin*

Guaifenesin (Balminil, Robitussin, others) is a commonly used expectorant. It is used in the symptomatic management of coughs of varying origins. It is beneficial for the treatment of nonproductive coughs because it thins the mucus in the respiratory tract that is difficult to cough up. There is little published pharmacokinetic data on guaifenesin; its half-life is estimated to be approximately 1 hour.

This short half-life helps explain why it is usually dosed several times throughout the day. However, although guaifenesin remains popular, there is some evidence to suggest that it has no greater therapeutic activity than water in terms of loosening respiratory tract secretions. See the Dosages table on p. 678 for the common dosages.

NURSING PROCESS

☑ Assessment

When the patient is to be given drugs to treat symptoms related to the respiratory tract, the nurse should begin the assessment by gathering data about the condition and determining whether the symptoms are caused by an allergic reaction. The patient's medical history and medication profile, a thorough head-to-toe physical assessment, and a nursing history are all critical to understanding possible causes, risks, or links to diseases or conditions such as allergy, a cold, or influenza. For example, if an allergic reaction to a drug, food, or substance has occurred, the patient

DOSAGES   Selected Decongestant, Expectorant, and Antitussive Drugs

Drug	Pharmacological Class	Usual Dosage Range	Indication
codeine phosphate (as part of a combination product such as Dimetane-Expectorant-C, Dimetapp-C, CoActifed, Robitussin AC, others) (C)	Opioid antitussive	*Children 2–6 yr* 2.5 mL q4–6h *Children 6 yr to under 12 yr* 5 mL q4–6h *Children over 12 yr/Adult* 10 mL q4–6h	Cough suppression
▸▸dextromethorphan hydrobromide (as part of a combination product such as Benylin DM-E, Buckley's, Dimetapp-DM, Robitussin-DM, Vicks, others)	Nonopioid antitussive	*Children 2–5 yr* 2.5 mL q6h *Children 6–11 yr* 5 mL q6h *Children over 12 yr/Adult* 10 mL q6h	Cough suppression
▸▸guaifenesin (100 mg/mL) (Balminil, Robitussin, others)	Expectorant	*Children 2 yr to under 6 yr* 2.5 mL q6h *Children 6 yr to under 12 yr* 5 mL q6h 10–20 mL q6h	Relief of respiratory congestion, cough suppression
oxymetazoline hydrochloride (Afrin, Claritin, Dristan, Drixoral, Vicks) (C)	α-Adrenergic vasoconstrictor	*Children over 6 yr/Adult* 0.05%, 2 or 3 sprays in each nostril q12h prn, usually for no more than 3–5 days; children 6–12: max 2 doses/24 h	Relief of nasal congestion

may be experiencing signs and symptoms such as hives, wheezing or bronchospasm, tachycardia, or hypotension, whereas if the cause is a cold or influenza, the symptoms will be different and should be treated completely differently in most cases. The drug of choice is then selected on the basis of severity of the symptoms and their cause.

Before administering the traditional antihistamines such as diphenhydramine, chlorpheniramine, or brompheniramine, the nurse must ensure that the patient has no allergies to this group of medications, even though these drugs are used for allergic reaction. Contraindications, cautions, and drug interactions need to be assessed with this and all other drugs. Use of the antihistamines is of concern in patients who are having an acute asthma attack and those with lower respiratory tract disease or who are at risk for pneumonia. The rationale for not using these drugs in these situations is that antihistamines dry up secretions; if the patient cannot expectorate the secretions, the secretions may become viscous (thick), occlude airways, and lead to atelectasis or further infection or occlusion of the bronchioles. It is also important to know that these drugs may lead to paradoxical reactions in the older adult, with subsequent irritability as well as dizziness, confusion, sedation, and hypotension.

Most nonsedating antihistamines (e.g., fexofenadine, loratadine, desloratadine, cetirizine) are not to be used in patients younger than 6 years of age. Allergies and other contraindications, cautions, and drug interactions should be assessed prior to use. With the traditional and nontraditional antihistamines, it is important to remember that if allergy testing is to be performed, these medications should be discontinued at least 4 days before the testing, but only with a physician's order.

With antitussive therapy, assessment is tailored to the patient and the specific drug. Most of these drugs result in sedation, dizziness, and drowsiness, so assessment of the patient's safety is important. A history of allergies, contraindications, cautions, and drug interactions should be completed and documented. Respiratory assessment (as with all of the drugs in this chapter) should include rate, rhythm and depth, breath sounds, presence of cough, and description of cough and sputum if present. For individuals with chronic respiratory disease, the physician may order serum levels of carbon dioxide, PaO_2, and other blood gas information (e.g., blood pH).

Use of decongestants requires assessment of contraindications, cautions, and drug interactions. Because decongestants are available in oral, nasal drops and sprays, and eye drop dosage forms, any condition that could affect the functional structures of the eye or nose may be a possible caution or contraindication. Decongestants may increase blood pressure and heart rate, so the patient's blood pressure, pulse, and other vital parameters should be assessed and documented.

Inhaled intranasal steroids and anticholinergic drugs are not generally associated with rebound congestion but may be used prophylactically to prevent nasal congestion in patients with chronic upper respiratory tract symptoms. Contraindications, cautions, and drug interactions, as with all the drugs in this chapter, need to be thoroughly assessed prior to use. For patients who have a cough and need to mobilize secretions more easily, expectorants are often recommended or prescribed. Assessment of cough and sputum, if present, should be noted in addition to all of the previously identified parameters.

Nursing Diagnoses

- Impaired gas exchange related to the disorder, condition, or disease affecting the respiratory system and respiratory-related signs and symptoms
- Deficient knowledge related to the effective use of cold medications and other related products due to lack of information and patient teaching
- Ineffective airway clearance related to diminished ability to cough or a suppressed cough reflex (with antitussives)
- Risk for injury related to sensory-perceptual alterations from drug-induced drowsiness or the sedating effects of many of these drugs

Planning

Goals

- Patient will state the rationale for the use of an antihistamine, expectorant, antitussive, or decongestant.
- Patient will state the adverse effects of the medication.
- Patient will state the importance of adherence to the therapy regimen.
- Patient will identify symptoms to report to the physician.
- Patient will state the importance of follow-up appointments with the physician.
- Patient will convey relief of symptoms with treatment.
- Patient will regain near-normal or normal (baseline) respiratory patterns and function.
- Patient will remain free of excessive drowsiness or sedation.

Outcome Criteria

- Patient remains adherent to the antihistamine, antitussive, decongestant, or expectorant medication regimen until symptoms are resolved or the physician orders discontinuation.
- Patient takes medications exactly as prescribed to avoid complications of therapy, experience maximal effectiveness, and minimize adverse effects.
- Patient reports any of the following symptoms to the physician immediately: increase in cough, congestion, shortness of breath, chest pain, fever (a temperature above 38°C), or any change in sputum production or colour (i.e., if not clear or if a change from baseline).
- Patient identifies specific safety precautions to help prevent injury related to drug-induced CNS-depressant adverse effects, such as moving purposefully and slowly, asking for assistance as needed, minimizing the use of other CNS-depressant drugs, and, if an older adult or at high risk for injury, obtaining assistance with activities of daily living and with mobility.
- Patient reports resolution of symptoms and an improved health status, such as return of temperature to baseline, return of secretions or sputum to clear colour and normal consistency, return to normal breathing rate and patterns, and clearing of breath sounds.

Implementation

Patients taking traditional antihistamines (e.g., diphenhydramine) should take the medications as prescribed. Most of these medications, including the over-the-counter antihistamines, are best tolerated when taken with meals. Although food taking may slightly decrease absorption of antihistamines, it has the benefit of minimizing the gastrointestinal upset that the drugs may cause. Patients who experience dry mouth should be encouraged to chew or suck on candy (sugar-free if needed) or over-the-counter throat, cough, or cold lozenges, or to chew gum. Patients should also perform frequent mouth care to ease the dryness and related discomfort. Because of the potential for serious drug interactions, other over-the-counter or prescribed cold or cough medications should not be taken with antihistamines unless they were previously approved or ordered by the physician. Dosage amounts and routes may vary depending on whether the patient is an older adult, young adult, or child under the age of 12 years, so proper dosing and usage should be encouraged. Blood pressure and other vital signs should be monitored as needed. Older adults and children should be monitored for any paradoxical reactions, which are common with these drugs.

If patients are receiving any of the newer second-generation nonsedating antihistamines, the drugs should be taken carefully and as directed. Reduced dosages may be needed for patients who are older adults or have decreased kidney functioning. These newer H_1 receptor antagonist drugs do not cross the blood–brain barrier as readily as do older antihistamines and are therefore less likely to cause sedation. They are generally well tolerated with minimal adverse effects.

With antitussives, chewable or lozenge forms of the drugs should be used exactly as ordered. Drowsiness or dizziness may occur with the use of antitussives; therefore, patients should be cautioned about driving a car or engaging in other activities that require mental alertness until they feel normal again. If the antitussive contains codeine, the CNS-depressant effects of the narcotic opiate may further depress breathing and respiratory effort. Other antitussives, such as dextromethorphan, as well as the codeine-containing drugs should be given at evenly spaced intervals so that the drug reaches a steady state.

Patients taking decongestants, such as pseudoephedrine or phenylephrine, are generally using the drugs for nasal decongestion. These drugs come in oral dosage forms, including sustained-release and chewable forms. With the use of any of the drugs discussed in this chapter and with the respective disorders or diseases they are intended for, it is also important to encourage fluid intake of up to 3000 mL a day, unless contraindicated. The fluid helps liquefy secretions, assists in

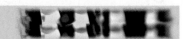

CASE STUDY

Decongestants

A 22-year-old college student has had allergy symptoms since moving into his dormitory. When he calls the student health centre, he is told to try an over-the-counter nasal decongestant. He tries this and is excited about the relief he experiences until 2 weeks later, when his symptoms return. He calls the student health centre again, upset because his symptoms are now worse.

1. What explanation do you have for the worsening symptoms?

2. What patient education should he have received about this type of drug?

3. What other over-the-counter drugs and nonpharmacological measures could be suggested for this situation?

_____

For answers see http://evolve.elsevier.com/Canada/Lilley/pharmacology/.

breaking up thick secretions, and makes it easier to cough up secretions. See Patient Education for teaching tips on these drugs.

Evaluation

A therapeutic response to drugs given to treat respiratory conditions, such as antihistamines, antitussives, decongestants, and expectorants, includes resolution of the symptoms of the condition for which the drugs were originally prescribed or taken. These symptoms may include cough; nasal, sinus, or chest congestion; nasal, salivary, and lacrimal gland hypersecretion; sneezing; watery, red, or itchy eyes; itchy nose; allergic rhinitis; motion sickness; and allergic symptoms. Some of the antihistamines, such as diphenhydramine, are also helpful as sleep aids, and a therapeutic response when taken for this purpose would be the successful induction of sleep. Adverse effects for which to monitor in patients using any of these drugs include excessively dry mouth, drowsiness, oversedation, dizziness (lightheadedness), paradoxical excitement, nervousness, dysrhythmias, palpitations, gastrointestinal upset, urinary retention, fever, dyspnea, chest pain, palpitations, headache, or insomnia, depending on the drug prescribed. (See Table 36-3 for other common adverse effects.)

IN MY FAMILY

Cough Cures

(as told by M.F., of Filipino descent)

Ampalaya (bittermelon): "My parents would often grind the leaves until the juice comes out. My brother and I used to drink it when we were kids whenever we had cough. Ampalaya loosens the mucus. Since it is very bitter in taste, it also helps us cough out the phlegm easier and [makes us] feel better or less stuffy on the chest. We never drank it with other medications. Ampalaya is really bitter, and it would only make us vomit and waste the medicine. We drank it twice a day for cough."

Oregano: "My mom grinds the oregano leaves to get the juice out of it. We drink it [in] a small cup, two to three times a day when we have cough. It is less bitter than ampalaya, so I preferred drinking this when I was small. Oregano also helps loosen the mucus, making it easier to cough out the phlegm."

PATIENT EDUCATION

❖ Patients should be educated about the possibility of tolerance to the sedating effects of traditional antihistamines. Patients should be informed to avoid activities that require alertness until tolerance to sedation occurs or until a patient accurately judges that the drug has no impact on motor skills or responses to motor activities. Other areas for patient education include a list of drugs for the patient to avoid, including alcohol and CNS depressants.

❖ Patients should be encouraged to take fluids unless contraindicated. With traditional and nonsedating antihistamines, patients may require use of a humidifier to help liquefy sections, making expectoration of sputum easier.

❖ Patients with upper or lower respiratory symptoms or disease processes should know to avoid dry air, smoke-filled environments, and allergens.

❖ Patients should be encouraged to always check possible drug interactions because of the many over-the-counter and prescription drugs that could lead to adverse effects if taken concurrently.

❖ Patients should be educated about taking the medication with food to help avoid gastrointestinal upset.

❖ Patients should be informed to report to the health care provider any difficulty breathing, palpitations, hallucinations, or tremors.

❖ Patients taking antitussives should be advised to take these with caution and to be fully aware of the importance of reporting fever, chest tightness, change in sputum from clear to coloured, difficult or noisy breathing, activity intolerance, and weakness.

❖ Patients should be instructed to use decongestants only as ordered and to adhere to dose and frequency instructions. Emphasize the fact that frequent, long-term, or excessive use of decongestants (whether oral forms or nasal inhaled forms) may lead to rebound congestion in which the nasal passages become more congested as the effects of the drug wear off; when this occurs, the patient generally uses more of the drug, precipitating a vicious cycle with more congestion. Patients should be encouraged to report excessive dizziness, heart palpitations, weakness, sedation, or excessive irritability to the physician.

❖ Patients taking expectorants should avoid alcohol or use of products containing alcohol, and they should not use these medications for longer than 1 week. If cough or symptoms continue, they should know to contact their physician. Fluids should be encouraged (unless contraindicated) to help thin secretions for easier expectoration.

POINTS TO REMEMBER

❖ There are two types of histamine blockers: H_1 blockers and H_2 blockers. H_1 blockers are the drugs that most people are referring to when they use the term *antihistamine*. H_1 blockers prevent the harmful effects of histamine and are used to treat seasonal allergic rhinitis, anaphylaxis, and reactions to insect bites, for example. H_2 blockers are used to treat gastric acid disorders, such as hyperacidity or ulcer disease.

❖ Patients should be educated thoroughly about the purposes of their medications, the expected adverse effects, and the drugs that possibly lead to negative interactions. Patients should be informed about the availability of newer, nonsedating antihistamines. Patients taking a nonsedating antihistamine or, for that matter, any drug should know to inform their physicians and other health care providers (e.g., dentists) that they are taking this medication. The nurse should be sure to educate patients about measures to avoid dry mouth associated with nonsedating antihistamines. Decongestants consist of adrenergics and corticosteroids. Decongestants act by causing constriction of the engorged and swollen blood vessels in the sinuses, thus decreasing pressure and allowing the mucus to drain. Nurses must understand the

action of these drugs and know relevant important information such as significant adverse effects, including heart- and CNS-stimulating effects that may result in palpitations, insomnia, restlessness, and nervousness.

❖ Nonopioid antitussive drugs may also cause sedation, drowsiness, or dizziness. Patients should not drive a car or engage in other activities that require mental alertness if these adverse effects occur. Codeine-containing antitussives may lead to CNS depression; they should be used cautiously and should not be mixed with anything containing alcohol.

❖ Any of the drugs presented in this chapter may interact with many over-the-counter preparations, especially other over-the-counter cold products; therefore, patients should always check the package insert to determine drug interactions.

❖ Decongestants and expectorants are recommended to treat cold symptoms, but patients should be encouraged to report to the physician a fever of over 38°C, cough, or other symptoms lasting longer than 4 days with decongestants or any other of the drugs presented in this chapter.

EXAMINATION REVIEW QUESTIONS

1 When assessing a patient who is to receive a decongestant, which of the following should the nurse recognize as being a potential contraindication to this drug?
a. Fever
b. Glaucoma
c. Ulcer disease
d. Allergic rhinitis

2 When giving decongestants, which can have α-stimulating effects, which of the following adverse effects should the nurse assess for?
a. Fever
b. Bradycardia
c. Hypertension
d. CNS depression

3 The nurse is reviewing a patient's medication orders for prn (as necessary) medications that can be given to a patient who has pneumonia with a productive cough. Which drug should the nurse choose?
a. An antitussive
b. An expectorant
c. An antihistamine
d. A decongestant

4 Which of the following patients would benefit most from antitussive cough medication?
a. A patient who has influenza
b. A patient with a productive cough
c. A patient with chronic paranasal sinusitis
d. A patient who has had recent abdominal surgery

5 A patient is taking a decongestant to help reduce symptoms of a cold. Which possible symptom should the nurse instruct the patient to observe for that may indicate an adverse effect of this drug?
a. Dry mouth
b. Increased cough
c. Slower heart rate
d. Heart palpitations

For answers see http://evolve.elsevier.com/Canada/Lilley/pharmacology/.

CRITICAL THINKING ACTIVITIES

1 Why should antihistamines be used with caution in asthmatic patients?

2 Discuss the problem of rebound congestion when nasal spray decongestants are used. Does this phenomenon also occur with oral decongestants? Explain your answer.

3 What additional nursing interventions would be helpful to an older adult without major medical problems who is taking guaifenesin?

For answers see http://evolve.elsevier.com/Canada/Lilley/pharmacology/.

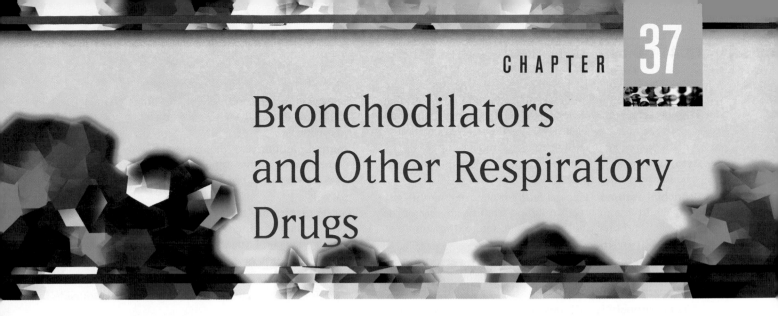

CHAPTER 37

Bronchodilators and Other Respiratory Drugs

Learning Objectives

After reading this chapter, the successful student will be able to do the following:

1 Describe the anatomy and physiology of the respiratory system.

2 Briefly review the pathophysiology of the common disorders of the lower respiratory tract: asthma, chronic bronchitis, and emphysema.

3 Discuss the impact of respiratory drugs on lower and upper respiratory tract diseases and conditions.

4 List the classifications of drugs, with specific examples of each class. Discuss the mechanisms of action, indications, contraindications, cautions, drug interactions, dosages, routes of administration, adverse effects, and toxic effects of bronchodilators and other respiratory drugs.

5 Develop a collaborative plan of care that includes all phases of the nursing process for patients who use bronchodilators or other respiratory drugs.

e-Learning Activities

Web site
(http://evolve.elsevier.com/Canada/Lilley/pharmacology/)

- Animations
- Answers to chapter questions, activities, and case studies
- Calculators and Category Catchers
- Glossary with audio pronunciations
- IV Therapy and Medication Error Checklists
- Multiple-Choice Review Question quizzes
- Nursing Care Plans
- Online Appendices and Supplements
- WebLinks

Drug Profiles

fluticasone (fluticasone propionate)*, p. 696
ipratropium (ipratropium bromide)*, p. 691
methylprednisolone, p. 696
▸▸ **montelukast (montelukast sodium)***, p. 694
▸▸ **salbutamol (salbutamol sulfate)***, p. 689
▸▸ **theophylline**, p. 692

▸▸ Key drug.

*Full generic name is given in parentheses. For the purposes of this text, the more common shortened name is used.

Glossary

Allergen Any substance that evokes an allergic response. (p. 685)

Allergic asthma Bronchial asthma caused by hypersensitivity to an allergen or allergens. (p. 685)

Alveoli Microscopic sacs in the lungs where oxygen is exchanged for carbon dioxide; also called *air sacs*. (p. 684)

Antibodies Immunoglobulins produced by lymphocytes in response to bacteria, viruses, or other antigenic substances. (p. 685)

Antigen A substance (usually a protein) that, upon entering the body, causes the formation of an antibody and reacts specifically with that antibody. (p. 685)

683

Asthma Recurrent and reversible shortness of breath that occurs when the airways of the lung (bronchi and bronchioles) become narrow as a result of bronchospasm, inflammation, and edema of the bronchial mucosa. (p. 684)

Asthma attack The onset of wheezing together with difficulty breathing. (p. 685)

Bronchial asthma General term for recurrent and reversible shortness of breath resulting from narrowing of the bronchi and bronchioles; it is often referred to simply as asthma. (p. 684)

Bronchodilators Medications that improve airflow by relaxing bronchial smooth muscle cells (e.g., xanthines, adrenergic agonists). (p. 688)

Chronic bronchitis Chronic inflammation of the bronchi. (p. 686)

Emphysema A condition of the lungs characterized by enlargement of the air spaces distal to the bronchioles. (p. 686)

Immunoglobulins Proteins belonging to any of five structurally and antigenically distinct classes of antibodies present in the serum and external secretions of the body. (p. 685)

Lower respiratory tract (LRT) The division of the respiratory system composed of organs located almost entirely within the chest. (p. 684)

Status asthmaticus A prolonged asthma attack. (p. 685)

Upper respiratory tract (URT) The division of the respiratory system composed of organs located outside the chest cavity (thorax). (p. 684)

OVERVIEW

The main function of the respiratory system is to deliver oxygen to, and remove carbon dioxide from, the cells of the body. To perform this deceptively simple task, an intricate system of tissues, muscles, and organs—the *respiratory system*—is required. It consists of two divisions, or tracts: the upper and lower respiratory tracts. The **upper respiratory tract (URT)** is composed of the structures that are located outside the chest cavity, or *thorax*. These are the nose, nasopharynx, oropharynx, laryngopharynx, and larynx. The **lower respiratory tract (LRT)** is located almost entirely within the chest and is composed of the trachea, all segments of the bronchial tree, and the lungs. The URT and LRT have four main accessory structures that aid in their overall function. These are the oral cavity (mouth), the rib cage, the muscles of the rib cage (intercostal muscles), and the diaphragm. The URT and LRT together with the accessory structures make up the respiratory system, and the elements of this system are in constant communication with each other as they perform the vital function of respiration and the exchange of oxygen for carbon dioxide.

Air is a mixture of many gases. During inhalation, oxygen molecules from the air diffuse across the semipermeable membranes of the **alveoli** (*air sacs*), where they are exchanged for carbon dioxide molecules, which are exhaled. The lungs also filter, warm, and humidify the air. The oxygen is then delivered to the cells by the blood vessels of the circulatory system. The respiratory system transfers the oxygen it has extracted from inhaled air to the hemoglobin protein molecules contained within red blood cells. It is also here that the cellular metabolic waste product carbon dioxide is collected from the tissues by the red blood cells. This waste is then transported back to the lungs via the circulatory system, where it diffuses back across the alveolar membranes and is then exhaled into the air. The respiratory system also plays a central role in speech, smell, and regulation of pH (acid–base balance).

DISEASES OF THE RESPIRATORY SYSTEM

Several diseases impair the function of the respiratory system. Those that affect the URT include colds, rhinitis, and hay fever. These conditions and the drugs used to manage them are discussed in Chapter 36. *Chronic obstructive pulmonary disease (COPD)* is an umbrella term used to describe chronic lung diseases that cause limitations in lung airflow. The more familiar terms *chronic bronchitis* and *emphysema* are no longer used but are now included within the COPD diagnosis. In 1997, the Global Initiative for Chronic Obstructive Lung Disease (GOLD) was launched in collaboration with the National Heart, Lung, and Blood Institute, National Institutes of Health (NIH), USA, and the World Health Organization (WHO). The GOLD provides guidelines on a disease state characterized by airflow limitation that is not fully reversible. The airflow limitation is usually both progressive and associated with an abnormal inflammatory response of the lungs to noxious particles or gases. **Asthma** that is persistent and present most of the time despite treatment is also considered a COPD. Cystic fibrosis and infant respiratory distress syndrome are other disorders that affect the LRT, but because their treatment places more emphasis on nonpharmacological than on pharmacological measures, they are not a focus of the discussion in this chapter.

ASTHMA

Bronchial asthma is defined as a recurrent and reversible shortness of breath and occurs when the airways of the lung (bronchi and bronchioles) become narrow as a result of bronchospasm, inflammation and edema of the bronchial mucosa, and the production of viscid (sticky) mucus. The alveolar ducts and alveoli distal to the bronchioles remain open, but the obstruction to the airflow in the airways prevents carbon dioxide from getting out of the air spaces and oxygen from getting into them. Wheezing and difficulty breathing are the symptoms.

When an episode has a sudden and dramatic onset, it is referred to as an **asthma attack**. Most asthma attacks are short, and normal breathing is subsequently recovered. However, an asthma attack may be prolonged for several minutes to hours and may not respond to typical drug therapy. This condition, known as **status asthmaticus,** often requires hospitalization. The onset of asthma occurs before 10 years of age in 50% of patients and before 40 years of age in approximately 80% of patients.

Asthma is not considered a disease but a symptom complex with many different etiologies and a number of predisposing, causal, and contributing risk factors. Asthma tends to run in families. Environmental triggers such as a viral infection, allergens, and pollutants are thought to interact with a hereditary predisposition to produce disease. It is estimated that approximately 3 million Canadians have asthma; approximately 10% are children, and 12.5% of the population older than 12 years of age has asthma. Generally, it is thought that asthma prevalence is increasing, particularly among adult women. However, some new research contradicts these statistics. Researchers in Ottawa, Ontario, studied approximately 500 adults in eight different cities across Canada, all diagnosed with asthma. The researchers found that 30% did not have asthma. Based on further testing, 150 of 496 did not have asthma. When treatments were stopped, there was no sign of asthma. The researchers suggested that asthma is often assumed to be the problem when a patient complains of wheezing or difficulty breathing.

Allergic asthma is caused by hypersensitivity to an allergen(s) in the environment. An **allergen** is any substance that elicits an allergic reaction. The offending allergens are substances such as dust, mould, pollen, and animal dander, which are present in the environment throughout the year. Cigarette smoke, including secondhand smoke, is another common allergen. Exposure to the offending allergen causes an immediate reaction called the *early-phase response.* This is mediated by hypersensitive antibodies already present in the patient's body that sense the allergen to be a foreign substance, or **antigen**. The **antibody** in asthma sufferers is usually **immunoglobulin** E (IgE), which is one of the five types of antibodies in the body (the others are IgG, IgA, IgM, and IgD). On exposure to the allergen, the patient's body responds by mounting an immediate and potent antigen–antibody reaction. This reaction occurs on the surface of cells such as mast cells, which are rich in histamines, leukotrienes (LTs), and other mediators, and stimulates the release of inflammatory mediators. This reaction, in turn, triggers the mucosal swelling and bronchoconstriction that are characteristic of an allergic asthma attack. The early-phase response lasts approximately 1 hour. The sequence of events in early-phase response is listed in Box 37-1.

Approximately 50% of patients with asthma experience a *late-phase response,* 4 to 6 hours after the initial response. It is thought that the mediators produced in the early-phase response attract additional inflammatory mediators, especially leukotrienes, which create a self-sustaining cycle of inflammation and obstruction. The clinical symptoms are the same as during the early phase. As a result of the inflammation, airways become sensitized or hyper-responsive such that subsequent episodes of asthma may be triggered not only by allergens but also by respiratory stimuli such as strong odours, cold weather, and strenuous work or exercise. The risk factors that contribute to the etiology of asthma and their most likely causes are summarized in Table 37-1.

The National Asthma Task Force and the Canadian Asthma Consensus Group have established guidelines for the diagnosis and management of asthma, published in 2000 and 1999, respectively. The Global Initiative

TABLE 37-1

Etiology of Asthma

Factors	Most Likely Cause
Predisposing	Atopy (inherited allergic reaction), gender, genetics
Causal	Indoor allergens: dust, dander, cockroach, mould; outdoor allergens: pollens, fungi; occupational sensitizers
Contributing	Respiratory infections, air pollution, smoking, low income

BOX 37-1   Sequence of Events in Early-Phase Response of Asthma

- The offending allergen provokes the production of hypersensitive antibodies (most commonly IgE) that are specific to the allergen. This immunological response initiates patient sensitivity.
- The IgE antibodies are homocytotrophic (that is, they have an affinity for similar cells) and collect on the surface of mast cells and basophils, thus sensitizing the patient to the allergen.
- Subsequent allergen contact provokes the antigen–antibody reaction on the surface of mast cells.
- Mast cell integrity is then violated, and these cells release chemical mediators. They also synthesize and then release other chemical mediators. These mediators include bradykinin, eosinophil chemotactic factor of anaphylaxis (ECF-A), histamine, prostaglandins, and slow-reacting substance of anaphylaxis (SRS-A).
- The released chemical mediators, especially histamine and SRS-A, trigger the bronchial constriction and the asthma attack.

for Asthma (GINA) is an initiative between the U.S. National Heart, Lung, and Blood Institute, the NIH, and the WHO to reduce world asthma prevalence, morbidity, and mortality. On the basis of these guidelines, drugs are no longer classified as either anti-inflammatory or bronchodilator medications but as long-term control and quick-relief medications. The specific drugs in each classification are listed in Box 37-2. The guidelines advocate a stepwise treatment approach (see Table 37-2 and Figure 37-1) and an individualized action plan.

According to new WHO estimates, COPD is expected to become the third leading cause of death by 2030. "Much of the increase in COPD is associated with projected increases in tobacco use and the exposure to smoke from the combustion of solid fuels indoors, for heating and cooking," says Dr. Cruz, Medical officer for the Chronic Respiratory Diseases group in WHO. "Tobacco use is highly prevalent in many countries, especially in low- and middle-income countries. Smoking cigarettes from adolescence to adulthood costs on average 10 years of life" (WHO, 2008).

When pulmonary tissues are exposed to noxious gases and particles, the physiological response is inflammation. When the exposure is chronic, the inflammatory response is also chronic. The inflammation associated with COPD occurs throughout the pulmonary tissue, including the parenchyma and vasculature. The inflammatory cells secrete numerous mediators including tumour necrosis factor (TNF), interleukin 8 (IL-8), and leukotriene B4 (LT-B4). The mediators are believed to contribute to the damage of lung structures. The larger airways (i.e., trachea, bronchi, and bronchioles larger than 2–4 mm) respond by increasing mucus-secreting glands, increasing the number of goblet cells, and decreasing mucociliary function. These changes lead to hypersecretion of mucus, chronic cough, and increased susceptibility to bacterial infection. The small bronchi and bronchioles (smaller than 2 mm) also go through repeating cycles of injury and repair to the airway walls. This results in remodelling and eventually permanent scaring, thickening, and consolidation.

It is the hypersecretion and decreased mucociliary function that define patients *at risk* for COPD. The destruction, scaring, thickening, and subsequent remodelling of the smaller airways is what leads to the decreased pulmonary function that characterizes *mild, moderate,* and *severe* COPD. Damage to the pulmonary vasculature leads to pulmonary hypertension, cor pulmonale, and the hypoxia/hypercapnia seen in patients with *severe* COPD.

CHRONIC BRONCHITIS

Chronic bronchitis is a continuous inflammation of the bronchi, although it is actually inflammation of the bronchioles that obstructs airflow. Manifestations must continue for at least 3 months of the year for 2 consecutive years to be defined as chronic bronchitis. Chronic bronchitis involves the excessive secretion of mucus and

---

BOX 37-2

Classifications of Drugs Used to Treat Asthma

Long-Term Control

Inhaled or oral glucocorticosteroids
Ipratropium

Rapid-Relief

Inhaled short-acting β₂-agonists

Adjunct Therapy

Antiallergic, nonsteroidal drugs (e.g., sodium
cromoglycate, nedocromil)
Leukotrine-receptor agonists
Long-acting β₂-agonists

---

certain pathological changes in the bronchial structure. The disease can arise as the result of repeated episodes of acute bronchitis or in the context of chronic generalized diseases. It is usually precipitated by prolonged exposure to bronchial irritants. One of the most common irritants is cigarette smoke. Some patients acquire the disease by other predisposing factors such as viral or bacterial pulmonary infections during childhood. Others may have mild impairment of the ability to inactivate proteolytic enzymes, which then damage the airway mucosal tissues. Unknown genetic characteristics may be responsible as well.

EMPHYSEMA

In **emphysema**, alveolar walls are destroyed and air spaces enlarged. This appears to stem from the effect of

---

TABLE 37-2

Stepwise Approach to the Management of Asthma

Step	Drug Classification
Step 1: Mild intermittent	Short-acting inhaled β₂-agonists prn
Step 2: Mild persistent	Sodium cromoglycate or nedocromil (particularly in children) and low-dose inhaled corticosteroids (preferred) plus short-acting inhaled β₂-agonists prn Theophylline and antileukotriene drugs considered second line
Step 3: Moderate persistent	Medium-dose inhaled corticosteroids Long-acting bronchodilator (salmeterol preferred) Short-acting inhaled β₂-agonists prn
Step 4: Severe persistent	High-dose inhaled corticosteroids Long-acting bronchodilators Systemic corticosteroids Short-acting inhaled β₂-agonists prn

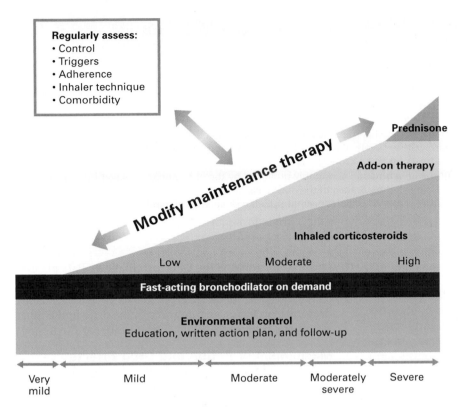

Regularly assess:
• Control
• Triggers
• Adherence
• Inhaler technique
• Comorbidity

Prednisone

Add-on therapy

Inhaled corticosteroids

Low   Moderate   High

Fast-acting bronchodilator on demand

Environmental control
Education, written action plan, and follow-up

Very mild   Mild   Moderate   Moderately severe   Severe

FIG. 37-1 Continuum of treatments for asthma management. (Reprinted with permission from Becker, A., Watson, W., Ferguson, A., Dimich-Ward, H., & Chan-Yeung, M. (2004). The Canadian asthma primary prevention study: Outcomes at 2 years of age. *Journal of Allergy and Clinical Immunology, 113,* 650–656.)

proteolytic enzymes released from leukocytes in the setting of alveolar inflammation. The partial destruction of alveolar walls reduces the surface area where oxygen and carbon dioxide are exchanged, thus impairing effective respiration. As with chronic bronchitis, smoking appears to be the primary precipitant of the underlying inflammation. There is also an associated genetic component in some people known as *alpha-antitrypsin deficiency*.

TREATMENT OF DISEASES OF THE LOWER RESPIRATORY TRACT

Given a greater understanding of the pathophysiology of asthma and COPD, the emphasis of research has shifted to the role played by inflammatory cells and their mediators. This is also reflected in the medication classes used to treat COPD, although bronchodilators still play an important role. A synopsis of the mechanisms of action of the classes of antiasthmatic drugs is provided in Table 37-3.

The GOLD guidelines updated in 2008 identify four stages of disease severity for COPD.

Stage I: Mild COPD

Spirometry shows mild airflow limitations due to chronic cough, mucus production, and the beginning of damage to the lungs. Patients may not be aware of the symptoms. Some characteristics of this stage include the following:
• Ratio of forced expiratory volume over 1 second to forced vital capacity (FEV_1/FVC) less than 70%
• FEV_1 equal to or greater than 80% predicted
• Presence of chronic symptoms such as cough and sputum production

Stage II: Moderate COPD

At this stage, airflow is getting worse. Symptoms become noticeable, and dyspnea occurs with everyday exertion. This is when most people go to their doctor for the first time. Characteristics include the following:
• FEV_1/FVC less than 70%
• FEV_1 greater than or equal to 50% but less than 80% predicted
• Chronic symptoms (cough, sputum production)

Stage III: Severe COPD

At this stage, there is very limited airflow. Dyspnea occurs after minimal exertion, to the point where even small tasks like leaving the house or going upstairs are a major issue. Characteristics include the following:
• FEV_1/FVC less than 70%
• FEV_1 greater than or equal to 30% but less than 50% predicted
• Chronic symptoms (cough, sputum production)

Stage IV: Very Severe COPD

At this stage, complications such as respiratory failure and heart failure begin to develop. Quality of life is extremely impaired and the symptoms become life threatening. Characteristics include the following:
• FEV_1/FVC less than 70%
• FEV_1/FVC less than 30% predicted or FEV_1 less than 50% predicted plus chronic respiratory failure
• Classification based on postbronchodilator FEV_1
• Respiratory failure: arterial partial pressure of oxygen (PaO_2) less than 60 mm Hg with or without $PaCO_2$ greater than 50 mm Hg while breathing at sea level

TABLE 37-3

Mechanisms of Antiasthmatic Drug Action

Antiasthmatic	Mechanism in Asthma Relief
Anticholinergics	Block cholinergic receptors, thus preventing the binding of cholinergic substances that cause constriction and increase secretions
Antileukotriene drugs	Modify or inhibit the activity of leukotrienes, which decreases arachidonic acid–induced inflammation and allergen-induced bronchoconstriction
β-agonists and xanthine derivatives	Raise intracellular levels of cAMP, which, in turn, produces smooth muscle relaxation and dilates the constricted bronchi and bronchioles
Corticosteroids	Prevent the inflammation commonly provoked by the substances released from mast cells
Mast cell stabilizers (sodium cromoglycate and nedocromil)	Stabilize the cell membranes of the mast cells in which the antigen–antibody reactions take place, preventing the release of substances such as histamine

cAMP, cyclic adenosine monophosphate.

BRONCHODILATORS

Bronchodilators are an important part of the pharmacotherapy for all COPDs. Bronchodilators relax bronchial smooth muscle bands to dilate the bronchi and bronchioles that are narrowed as a result of the disease process. There are three classes of such drugs: β-agonists, anticholinergics, and methylxanthine derivatives.

β-ADRENERGIC AGONISTS

The β-agonists are a large classification of drugs commonly used during the acute phase of an asthmatic attack to quickly reduce airway constriction and restore airflow to normal. They are agonists or stimulators of the adrenergic receptors in the sympathetic nervous system. The β- and α-adrenergic receptors are discussed in Chapters 18 and 19. The β-agonists imitate the effects of norepinephrine on these receptors. For this reason, they are also called *sympathomimetic bronchodilators*. Available asthma-related drugs in this class include salbutamol (e.g., Airomir, Ventolin), isoproterenol, epinephrine, and ephedrine. Under the Montreal Protocol treaty of 1996, Canada agreed to discontinue the use of ozone-layer depleting chlorofluorocarbons (CFCs) as a propellant in metered-dose inhalers and introduced the use of hydrofluoroalkane (HFA) propellants as environmentally friendly alternatives. The formulations using HFAs are equally bioavailable, effective,

safe, and tolerable as the CFC formulations. Patients may experience a different taste and a softer, warmer spray than with CFC inhalers. HFA products deliver smaller droplets than CFCs, and delivery of the drug to the lungs is improved; consequently, a spacer is not required.

Mechanism of Action and Drug Effects

The β-agonists dilate airways by stimulating the β_2-adrenergic receptors located throughout the lungs. There are three subcategories of β-agonists, based on their selectivity for β_2-receptors:

1. Nonselective adrenergic drugs, which stimulate the α-, β_1-(cardiac), and β_2-(respiratory) receptors. Example: epinephrine
2. Nonselective β-adrenergic drugs, which stimulate both β_1- and β_2-receptors. Example: isoproterenol
3. Selective β_2-drugs, which primarily stimulate the β_2-receptors. Example: salbutamol

These drugs can also be categorized according to their routes of administration as oral, injectable, or inhalational drugs. The β-agonist bronchodilators are listed in Table 37-4.

The bronchioles are surrounded by smooth muscle. If this smooth muscle contracts, the airways are narrowed and the amount of oxygen and carbon dioxide exchanged is reduced. The action of β-agonist bronchodilators begins at the specific receptor stimulated and ends with the dilation of the airways, but many reactions

TABLE 37-4

β-Agonist Bronchodilators

Drug	Type	Brand Names	Route of Administration
ephedrine	α-βs	None (various generic)	PO, IM, IV, SC
epinephrine	α-β	(Adrenalin)	SC, IM, inhalation
fenoterol	β_2	Duovent UDV (combined with ipratropium)	Inhalation
formoterol	β_2	Foradil, Oxeze	Inhalation
isoproterenol	β_1-β_2	None	IV, inhalation
salbutamol	β_2	Airomir, Ventolin	PO, inhalation
salmeterol	β_2	Serevent	Inhalation
terbutaline	β_2	Bricanyl	Inhalation

IM, intramuscular; *IV*, intravenous; *PO*, oral; *SC*, subcutaneous.

must take place at the cellular level for bronchodilation to occur. When a β_2-adrenergic receptor is stimulated by a β-agonist, adenylate cyclase, an enzyme needed to make cyclic adenosine monophosphate (cAMP), is activated. The increased levels of cAMP made available by adenylate cyclase cause bronchial smooth muscles to relax, which results in bronchial dilation and increased airflow into and out of the lungs.

Nonselective adrenergic agonist drugs such as epinephrine also stimulate α-adrenergic receptors, causing constriction within the blood vessels. This vasoconstriction reduces the amount of edema or swelling in the mucous membranes and limits the quantity of secretions normally produced by these membranes. In addition, such drugs also stimulate β_1-receptors, resulting in cardiovascular adverse effects such as an increase in heart rate, force of contraction, and blood pressure as well as central nervous system (CNS) effects such as nervousness and tremor.

Drugs such as salbutamol that predominantly stimulate the β_2 receptors have more specific drug effects. By stimulating specifically the β_2-adrenergic receptors of the bronchial and vascular smooth muscles, they cause bronchodilation and may also have a dilating effect on the peripheral vasculature, resulting in a decrease in diastolic blood pressure. In addition, the β_2-agonists are thought to stimulate the sodium–potassium adenosine triphosphatase ion pump in cell membranes. This action facilitates a temporary shift of potassium ions from the bloodstream into the cells, resulting in a temporary decrease in serum potassium levels. For this reason, β_2-agonists are also useful in treating patients with acute hyperkalemia. Finally, stimulation of β_2-receptors in uterine smooth muscle can cause beneficial uterine relaxation (see Indications).

Indications

The primary respiratory therapeutic effect of the β-agonists is the relief of severe bronchospasm associated with acute exacerbations of bronchial asthma and chronic bronchitis. They are also used for beneficial therapeutic effects outside the respiratory system. Because some of these drugs have the ability to stimulate both β_1- and α-adrenergic receptors, they may be used to treat hypotension and shock. They can also stimulate a shift of potassium out of the blood and into cells. For this reason, as noted earlier, β_2-agonists can be used to treat hyperkalemia (e.g., that associated with kidney failure).

Contraindications

Contraindications include drug allergy, uncontrolled cardiac dysrhythmias, and high risk of stroke (because of the vasoconstrictive drug actions).

Adverse Effects

Mixed α-β agonists produce the greatest array of undesirable effects, including insomnia, restlessness, anorexia, heart stimulation, hyperglycemia, tremor, and vascular headache. The adverse effects of the nonselective β-agonists are limited to β-adrenergic effects, including heart stimulation, tremor, anginal pain, and vascular headache. The β_2-drugs can cause both hypertension and hypotension, as well as vascular headaches and tremor. Overdose management may include careful administration of a β-blocker while the patient is under close observation. Because the half-life of most adrenergic agonists is often relatively short, however, the patient may just be observed while the body eliminates the medication.

Interactions

The use of a nonselective β-blocker with β-agonist bronchodilators antagonizes the bronchodilation. The use of β-agonists with monoamine oxidase inhibitors and other sympathomimetics is best avoided because of the enhanced risk for hypertension. Concurrent use with xanthines and digoxin increases the risk of cardiac toxicity and may also reduce digoxin serum levels. Hypokalemia and electrocardiographic changes are more likely to occur with concurrent use of diuretics. Patients with diabetes may require an adjustment in the dose of their antihyperglycemic drugs, particularly patients receiving epinephrine, because of the increased blood glucose levels that can occur.

Dosages

For recommended dosages of selected β-agonists, see the Dosages table on p. 690.

 DRUG PROFILES

▸▸ *salbutamol sulfate*

Salbutamol sulfate (Airomir, Ventolin) is one of four β_2-specific bronchodilating β-agonists. Other similar drugs are formoterol (Oxeze), salmeterol (Serevent), and terbutaline (Bricanyl). Although salbutamol is the most commonly used drug in this class, salmeterol has a unique 12-hour duration of action, which makes it an attractive alternative. If salbutamol is used too frequently, dose-related adverse effects may be seen because salbutamol loses its β_2-specific actions, especially at larger doses. As a consequence, the β_1-receptors are stimulated,

which causes nausea, increased anxiety, palpitations, tremors, and an increased heart rate.

Salbutamol is available for oral, parenteral, and inhalational use. Inhalation dosage forms include metered-dose inhalers (MDI) as well as solutions for inhalation. It is also available combined with ipratropium (Combivent) for inhalations.

PHARMACOKINETICS

Half-Life	Onset	Peak	Duration
Inhaled:	Inhaled:	Inhaled:	Inhaled:
3–4 hr	5–15 min	60–90 min	3–6 hr

DOSAGES Bronchodilators

Drug (Pregnancy Category)	Pharmacological Class	Usual Dosage Range	Indications
epinephrine (Adrenalin) (C)	α-β–agonist	*Children* SC: 0.01–0.03 mg/kg q5 min prn IV: 0.1 mg over 5–10 min followed by continuous infusion 0.1–1.5 mcg/kg/min *Adult* SC/IM: 0.2–1.0 mg q10–15 min–q4h IV: 0.1–0.25 mg	Relief of bronchospasm and allergic manifestations
ipratropium bromide (Atrovent HFA) (B)	Anticholinergic	*Children over 18/Adult* MDI: 2 puffs tid–qid Nasal spray, 0.03%: 2 sprays bid–tid Nasal spray, 0.06%: 2 sprays bid–tid–qid *Children 5–12 yr* Inhalation solution: 125–250 mcg tid–qid *Adult* Inhalation solution: 250–500 mcg tid–qid	COPD Rhinorrhea Acute asthma exacerbation COPD
▸ salbutamol sulfate (Airomir, Ventolin) (C)	β₂-agonist	*Children 2–6 yr* PO: 0.1 mg/kg tid–qid *Children 6–12 yr* PO: 2 mg tid–qid *Children 12 and over/Adult* PO: 2–4 mg tid–qid *Children 5–12 yr* Inhalation: 1.25–2.5 mg qid *Adult* Inhalation: 2.5–5 mg qid *Children 4 yr and over* MDI: 1 puff q3–4/day *Adult* MDI: 1–2 puffs qid *Adult* IV: 5 mcg/min–20 mcg/min diluted, continuous infusion	Prevention or relief of bronchospasm Severe bronchospasm, status asthmaticus

COPD, chronic obstructive pulmonary disease; *IM,* intramuscular; *IV,* intravenous; *MDI,* metered-dose inhaler; *PO,* oral; *SC,* subcutaneous.

ANTICHOLINERGICS

Currently, two anticholinergic drugs are used in the treatment of COPD: ipratropium bromide and tiotropium bromide monohydrate.

Mechanism of Action and Drug Effects

On the surface of the bronchial tree are receptors for acetylcholine (ACh), the neurotransmitter for the parasympathetic nervous system. When the parasympathetic nervous system releases ACh from its nerve endings, the neurotransmitter binds to the ACh receptors on the surface of the bronchial tree, which results in bronchial constriction and narrowing of the airways. Anticholinergic drugs block these ACh receptors to prevent bronchoconstriction. This action indirectly causes airway dilation.

Indications

Because their actions are slow and prolonged, anticholinergics are used for prevention of the bronchospasm associated with chronic bronchitis or emphysema and not for the management of acute symptoms.

Contraindications

The only usual contraindication to the use of the bronchial anticholinergic drugs is drug allergy, including allergy to atropine. Previously, soy lecithin was used as a suspension agent in some of the inhalational formulations; however, this ingredient is not used because of possible allergies to peanut oils, peanuts, soybeans, and other legumes (beans).

Adverse Effects

The most commonly reported adverse effects of ipratropium and tiotropium therapy are related to the drugs' anticholinergic effects and include dry mouth or throat, nasal congestion, heart palpitations, gastrointestinal distress, headache, coughing, and anxiety. Its use is contraindicated in patients with a known hypersensitivity to it or to atropine or any of its derivatives.

Drug Interactions

Possible additive toxicity may occur when anticholinergic bronchodilators are taken with other anticholinergic drugs.

Dosages

See the Dosages table on p. 690.

 ## DRUG PROFILES

ipratropium bromide

Ipratropium bromide (Atrovent) is the oldest and most commonly used anticholinergic bronchodilator. It is pharmacologically similar to atropine (Chapter 21). It is available as a liquid aerosol for inhalation and as an MDI (Atrovent HFA). A newer but similar drug is tiotropium (Spiriva), which is formulated for once-daily dosing. When used in combination with a β-agonist such as fenoterol hydrobromide (Duovent UDV) or salbutamol (Combivent), ipratropium is indicated for acute asthmatic attacks. Both combinations are available as inhalation solutions.

PHARMACOKINETICS

Half-Life	Onset	Peak	Duration
1.6 hr	5–15 min	1–2 hr	4–5 hr

XANTHINE DERIVATIVES (ALSO CALLED XANTHINES)

The natural xanthines consist of the plant alkaloids caffeine, theobromine, and theophylline, but only theophylline and caffeine are currently used clinically. Synthetic xanthines include aminophylline and oxtriphylline. Caffeine, which is actually a metabolite of theophylline, has other uses described later.

Mechanism of Action and Drug Effects

The mechanisms of action of the different xanthine drugs are similar. They cause bronchodilation by increasing the levels of the energy-producing substance cAMP. They do this by competitively inhibiting phosphodiesterase, the enzyme responsible for breaking down cAMP. In patients with COPD, cAMP plays an integral role in the maintenance of open airways. Higher intracellular levels of cAMP contribute to smooth muscle relaxation and inhibit IgE-induced release of the chemical mediators that drive allergic reactions (histamine, slow-reacting substance of anaphylaxis [SRS-A], and others).

Xanthine derivatives have other beneficial drug effects besides those involving respiratory function. Theophylline is metabolized to caffeine in the body, whereas aminophylline is metabolized to theophylline. Theophylline and other xanthines also stimulate the CNS, but to a lesser degree than caffeine. This stimulation of the CNS has the beneficial effect of acting directly on the medullary respiratory centre to enhance respiratory drive. In large doses, theophylline and its derivatives may stimulate the cardiovascular system, which results in both an increased force of contraction (positive inotropy) and an increased heart rate (positive chronotropy). The increased force of contraction raises cardiac output and, consequently, blood flow to the kidneys. This action, in combination with the ability of the xanthines to dilate blood vessels in and around the kidney, increases the glomerular filtration rate, producing a diuretic effect.

Indications

Xanthines are used to dilate the airways in patients with asthma, chronic bronchitis, or emphysema. They may be used in mild to moderate cases of acute asthma and as an adjunct drug in the management of COPD. However, xanthines are now de-emphasized as treatment for milder asthma because of their greater potential for drug interactions and the greater interpatient variability in therapeutic drug levels in the blood. Because of their relatively slow onset of action, xanthines are more often used for the prevention of asthmatic symptoms than for the relief of acute asthma attacks. However, they are often preferred as adjunct bronchodilators for patients with chronic bronchitis or emphysema.

Caffeine is primarily used without prescription as a CNS stimulant, or analeptic (Chapter 17), to promote alertness (e.g., for long-duration driving or studying). It is also used as a heart stimulant in infants with bradycardia and to enhance respiratory drive in infants in neonatal critical care units. It is not normally used clinically in adults for these purposes, although theoretically it would have similar effects.

Contraindications

Contraindications to therapy with xanthine derivatives include drug allergy, uncontrolled cardiac dysrhythmias, seizure disorders, hyperthyroidism, and peptic ulcers. Caffeine, a metabolite of theophylline, is known as a secretagogue. Such compounds stimulate gastric secretions, hence the contraindication of peptic ulcer.

Adverse Effects

The common adverse effects of the xanthine derivatives include nausea, vomiting, and anorexia. In addition, gastroesophageal reflux has been observed to occur during sleep in patients taking these drugs. Heart adverse effects include sinus tachycardia, extrasystole, palpitations, and ventricular dysrhythmias. Transient increased urination and hyperglycemia are other possible adverse effects. Overdose and other toxicity of xanthine derivatives are usually treated by the administration of repeat doses of activated charcoal. Theophylline has a narrow therapeutic index requiring individual patient dosage calculation.

Interactions

The use of xanthine derivatives with any of the following drugs causes the serum level of the xanthine derivative to be increased: allopurinol, cimetidine, macrolide antibiotics (e.g., erythromycin), quinolones (e.g., ciprofloxacin), influenza vaccine, rifampin, and oral contraceptives. Their use with sympathomimetics, or even caffeine, can produce additive heart and CNS stimulation. A reported natural health product interaction is the tendency of St. John's wort (Hypericum perforatum) to enhance the rate of xanthine drug metabolism, presumably by enhancing the activity of the enzymes in the liver that normally metabolize the xanthine. Thus, higher dosages of theophylline and other xanthine derivatives may be needed in patients using this popular natural health product. Cigarette smoking has a similar effect because of the enzyme-inducing effect of nicotine. Food interactions include charcoal broiling and high-protein and low-carbohydrate foods. These substances may reduce serum levels of xanthines through various metabolic mechanisms.

Dosages

For the recommended dosages of selected theophylline salts, see the Dosages table below.

 DRUG PROFILES

▶▶ theophylline

Theophylline (Theolair, Uniphyl) is the most commonly used xanthine derivative. It is available in oral, rectal, injectable (as aminophylline), and topical dosage forms. Besides theophylline, which occurs in various salt forms, the other xanthine bronchodilators used clinically for the treatment of bronchoconstriction are aminophylline and oxtriphylline. Both of these drugs are theophylline prodrugs that are metabolized to theophylline in the body. Aminophylline is the most commonly used of these prodrugs and is sometimes given intravenously to patients with status asthmaticus who have not responded to fast-acting β-agonists such as epinephrine.

The beneficial effects of theophylline can be maximized by maintaining levels in the blood within a certain target range. If these levels become too high, many unwanted adverse effects can occur. If the levels become too low, the patient receives little therapeutic benefit. Although the optimal level may vary from patient to patient, a common target therapeutic range for theophylline in the blood is usually 55 to 110 mmol/L. The Canadian Asthma Consensus guidelines recommend that a serum concentration of 28 to 55 mmol/L will reduce adverse effects without loss of therapeutic benefit. Laboratory monitoring of drug blood levels is common to ensure adequate dosage, especially in the hospital setting.

PHARMACOKINETICS

Half-Life	Onset	Peak	Duration
PO: 7–9 hr*	PO: Unknown	PO: 1–2 hr	PO: Varies with dosage form

*Depending on pulmonary, heart, and liver functions; smoking history; and dosage form.

DOSAGES Theophylline Salts

Drug (Pregnancy Category)	Pharmacological Class	Usual Dosage Range	Indications
aminophylline (Phyllocontin) (C)	Xanthine-derived bronchodilator	*Children 6 mo–16 yr* IV: 0.2–0.9 mg/kg/h continuous infusion	Asthma, COPD
		Adult PO: 225–350 mg bid IV: 0.7 mg/kg/h continuous infusion	Asthma, COPD
▶▶theophylline (Theolair, Uniphyl) (C)	Xanthine-derived bronchodilator	*Children over 1 yr*/Adult* 16 mg/kg/day to max 400 mg/day in 3–4 divided doses	Asthma, COPD

*The dosage schedules and dosage forms used vary widely with age and clinical status.

NONBRONCHODILATING RESPIRATORY DRUGS

Bronchodilators are just one type of drug used to treat asthma, chronic bronchitis, and emphysema; these drugs include β-adrenergic agonists and xanthines. There are also other drugs that are effective in suppressing underlying causes of some of these respiratory illnesses. These include antileukotriene drugs (montelukast and zafirlukast), and corticosteroids (beclomethasone, budesonide, dexamethasone, flunisolide, fluticasone, and triamcinolone). Another drug class known as mast cell stabilizers is now rarely used. However, these drugs are still listed in the Canadian Consensus guidelines as alternative therapy and include cromolyn, ketotifen and nedocromil. As their class name implies, they work by stabilizing the cell membranes of mast cells to prevent the release of inflammatory mediators such as histamine. Based on a Cochrane review, ketotifen used alone or in combination with other interventions seems to improve the control of asthma and wheezing in children with mild and moderate asthma. The two adverse effects of ketotifen are sedation and weight gain.

ANTILEUKOTRIENE DRUGS

A newer class of asthma medications called *leukotriene-receptor antagonists (LTRAs)*, or antileukotriene drugs, is available. Antileukotriene drugs became the first new class of asthma medications to be introduced in Canada in more than 20 years, when the first of these was made available in the 1990s.

Before the development of antileukotriene drugs, most asthma treatments focused on relaxing the contraction of bronchial muscles with bronchodilators. In the last decade, researchers have begun to understand how asthma symptoms are caused by the immune system at the cellular level. A chain reaction starts when a trigger allergen, such as cat hair or dust, initiates a series of chemical reactions in the body. Several substances are produced, including a family of molecules known as *leukotrienes*. In people with asthma, leukotrienes cause inflammation, bronchoconstriction, and mucus production. This, in turn, leads to coughing, wheezing, and shortness of breath. Antileukotriene drugs prevent leukotrienes from attaching to receptors located on circulating immune cells (e.g., lymphocytes in the blood) and immune cells within the lungs (e.g., alveolar macrophages). This alleviates asthma symptoms in the lungs by reducing inflammation.

Mechanism of Action and Drug Effects

The antileukotriene drugs montelukast (Singulair) and zafirlukast (Accolate) act directly by binding to the D4 leukotriene-receptor subtype (LTD4) in respiratory tract tissues and organs. The drug effects of antileukotriene drugs are primarily limited to the lungs. Through their reduction of leukotriene synthesis or action, they prevent smooth muscle contraction of the bronchial airways, decrease mucus secretion, and reduce vascular permeability (which reduces edema). Other antileukotriene effects of antileukotriene drugs include prevention of the mobilization and migration of such cells as neutrophils and leukocytes into the lungs. This effect also serves to reduce airway inflammation.

Indications

The antileukotriene drugs montelukast and zafirlukast are used for the prophylaxis and long-term treatment of asthma in adults and children. Montelukast is considered safe in children 2 years of age and older and zafirlukast in children 12 years of age and older. Montelukast is the most widely used of these drugs and has also been approved for treatment of allergic rhinitis, a condition discussed in Chapter 36. These drugs are not intended for the management of acute asthmatic attacks. Improvement with their use is typically seen in about 1 week.

Contraindications

Drug allergy or other previous adverse drug reaction is the primary contraindication to use of antileukotriene drugs. Allergy to povidone, lactose, titanium dioxide, or cellulose derivatives is also important to note because these are inactive ingredients in these drugs.

Adverse Effects

The adverse effects of antileukotriene drugs differ depending on the specific drug. Zafirlukast can cause headaches, nausea, and diarrhea. This drug may also lead to liver dysfunction. For this reason, liver enzyme levels should be monitored regularly in patients taking these drugs, especially early in the course of therapy.

There have been some case reports of Churg–Strauss syndrome in patients receiving montelukast. This syndrome is characterized by systemic necrotizing vasculitis (destruction of blood vessels) and is often manifested by tender subcutaneous nodules, large skin plaques, and markedly elevated eosinophil count in the blood (eosinophilia). It is usually treated with systemic (intravenous or oral) corticosteroid therapy.

Interactions

Montelukast has fewer drug interactions than does zafirlukast. It does not interact with theophylline, warfarin, digoxin, prednisone, or either the estrogen or progestin components of combination oral contraceptives. Phenobarbital decreases montelukast concentrations. For information on the drugs that interact with zafirlukast, see Table 37-5.

Dosages

For recommended dosages of selected antileukotriene drugs, see the Dosages table on p. 694.

Drug Interactions: Antileukotriene Drugs

Drug	Mechanism	Result
MONTELUKAST (SINGULAIR)		
phenobarbital, rifampin	Increased metabolism	Decreased montelukast levels
ZAFIRLUKAST (ACCOLATE)		
Aspirin	Decreased clearance	Increased zafirlukast levels
erythromycin	Decreased bioavailability	Decreased zafirlukast levels
theophylline	Decreased bioavailability	Decreased zafirlukast levels
tolbutamide, phenytoin, carbamazepine	Inhibited metabolism	Increased tolbutamide, phenytoin, and carbamazepine levels
warfarin	Decreased clearance	Increased warfarin levels

DRUG PROFILES

Antileukotriene drugs are a new class of asthma medications. As noted earlier, there are two antileukotriene drugs currently available: zafirlukast and montelukast. They are used primarily for oral prophylaxis and long-term treatment of asthma. These drugs are not recommended for treatment of acute asthma attacks.

▶▶ montelukast sodium

Montelukast sodium (Singulair) is the latest drug to become available in the antileukotriene class. It belongs to the same subcategory of antileukotriene drugs as zafirlukast. Montelukast and zafirlukast block LTD4 receptors

to augment the inflammatory response. Montelukast offers the advantage of being Health Canada approved for use in children 2 years of age and older. It also has fewer adverse effects and drug interactions than zafirlukast. Use of montelukast is contraindicated in patients with a known hypersensitivity to it. It is availableonly for oral use. Common dosages are given in the Dosages table below.

PHARMACOKINETICS

Half-Life	Onset	Peak	Duration
2.7–5.5 hr	30 min	3–4 hr	24 hr
		Chewable tablet: 2.5 hr	

DOSAGES **Selected Antileukotriene Drugs**

Drug (Pregnancy Category)	Pharmacological Class	Usual Dosage Range	Indications
▶▶ montelukast sodium (Singulair) (B)	Leukotriene-receptor antagonist	*Children 2–5 yr* PO (chewable tablet, oral granules): 4 mg daily, evening *Children 6–14 yr* PO (chewable tablet): 5 mg daily, evening	Prophylaxis and maintenance treatment of asthma
		Adult over 15 yr PO: 10 mg daily, evening	Asthma and seasonal allergic rhinitis
zafirlukast (Accolate) (B)	Leukotriene-receptor antagonist	*Children 12 yr and over/Adult* PO: 20 mg bid	Prophylaxis and long-term treatment of asthma

CORTICOSTEROIDS

Corticosteroids, also known as glucocorticoids, are either naturally occurring or synthetic drugs used in the treatment of asthma and COPD because of their anti-inflammatory effects. All have actions similar to those of the natural steroid hormone cortisol, which is chemically the same as the drug hydrocortisone. Synthetic steroids are now more commonly used in drug therapy. They can be administered by inhalation, orally, and intravenously in severe cases of asthma when the drug cannot transfer to the airways because of airway obstruction. Corticosteroids administered by inhalation have an advantage over orally administered corticosteroids in that their action is limited to the topical site

in the lungs. This generally prevents systemic effects. The chemical structures of the corticosteroids given by inhalation have also been slightly altered to limit their systemic absorption from the respiratory tract. The corticosteroids administered by inhalation include the following:

- beclomethasone dipropionate (Gen-Beclo AQ, Qvar, Rivanase AQ)
- budesonide (Pulmicort Nebuamp, Pulmicort Turbuhaler, Rhinocort Aqua, Rhinocort Turbuhaler)
- fluticasone furoate (Avamys)
- fluticasone propionate (Flonase, Flovent Diskus, Flovent HFA)
- mometasone furoate monohydrate (Nasonex)
- triamcinolone acetonide (Nasacort AQ)

The systemic use of corticosteroids is described in Chapter 33. The most commonly used systemic corticosteroids for respiratory illness include the following:

- prednisone (oral)
- methylprednisolone (Solu-Medrol) (intravenous)

Mechanism of Action and Drug Effects

Although the exact mechanism of action of the corticosteroids has not been determined, it is conjectured that they have the dual effect of both reducing inflammation and enhancing the activity of β-agonists. The corticosteroids previously mentioned produce their anti-inflammatory effects through a complex sequence of actions. The overall effect is to prevent nonspecific inflammatory processes. These include the accumulation of inflammatory mediators as well as altered vascular permeability (which causes edema).

Essentially, corticosteroids act by stabilizing the membranes of cells that normally release harmful bronchoconstricting substances (e.g., histamine, slow-reacting substance of anaphylaxis [SRS-A]). These cells include leukocytes *or* white blood cells (WBCs). There are five types of WBCs, each with its own specific characteristics. The five types of WBCs, their role in the inflammatory process, and the way in which corticosteroids inhibit their normal action, combat inflammation, and produce bronchodilation are summarized in Table 37-6. In particular, inflammatory mediators are primarily released by lymphocytes in the circulation as well as by mast cells and alveolar macrophages. These latter two cell types are stationary (noncirculating) inflammatory cells that remain localized in the tissues and organs of the respiratory tract.

Corticosteroids have also been shown to restore or increase the responsiveness of bronchial smooth muscle to β-adrenergic receptor stimulation, which results in more pronounced stimulation of the β$_2$-receptors by

β-agonist drugs such as salbutamol. It may take several weeks of continuous therapy before the full therapeutic effects of the corticosteroids are realized.

Indications

Inhaled corticosteroids are used for the primary treatment of bronchospastic disorders to control the inflammatory responses believed to be the underlying cause of asthma and COPD. They are often used concurrently with bronchodilators, primarily β-adrenergic agonists. The systemic (versus inhaled) use of corticosteroids for a variety of illnesses is described in Chapter 33. In respiratory illnesses, systemic corticosteroids are generally used only for acute exacerbations. Their long-term use is avoided because of the associated long-term adverse effects (discussed below). The *National Asthma Education and Prevention Program* (NAEPP) recommends long-term use only in cases of truly disabling illness in which the benefits of the drug therapy arguably outweigh the adverse effects. When a more pronounced anti-inflammatory effect is needed, however, as in an acute exacerbation of asthma or other COPD, intravenous corticosteroids (e.g., methylprednisolone) are often used.

Contraindications

Drug allergy is the primary contraindication. Corticosteroids are not intended as sole therapy for acute asthma attacks.

Inhaled corticosteroids are contraindicated in patients who are hypersensitive in response to glucocorticoids, in patients whose sputum tests positive for Candida organisms, and in patients with systemic fungal infection.

Adverse Effects

The main undesirable local effects of typical doses of inhaled corticosteroids include pharyngeal irritation,

TABLE 37-6

White Blood Cells (Leukocytes)

Specific WBC*	Role in Inflammation	Corticosteroid Effect
GRANULOCYTES		
Basophils (0.5%–1%)	Contain histamine, an inflammation-causing substance, and heparin, an anticoagulant	Stabilize cell membranes so that histamine is not released
Eosinophils (2%–5%)	Function primarily in allergic reactions and in protecting against parasitic infections; ingest inflammatory chemicals and antigen–antibody complexes	Little, if any, effect
Neutrophils (65%)	Contain powerful lysosomes (small bodies that hold cellular digestive enzymes); release chemicals that destroy invading organisms and also attack other WBCs	Stabilize cell membranes so that inflammation-causing substances are not released
AGRANULOCYTES		
Lymphocytes (25%)	Two types: T lymphocytes and B lymphocytes; T cells attack infecting microbial or cancerous cells; B cells produce antibodies against specific antigens	Decrease activity of lymphocytes
Monocytes (3%–5%)	Produce macrophages, which can migrate out of the bloodstream to such places as mucous membranes, where they are capable of engulfing large bacteria or virus-infected cells	Inhibit macrophage accumulation in already inflamed areas, thus preventing more inflammation

*Value in parentheses is the percentage of all leukocytes by the given type.

coughing, dry mouth, and oral fungal infections. Most of the drug effects of inhaled corticosteroids are limited to their topical sites of action in the lungs. Because of the chemical structure of the inhaled dosage forms, there is relatively little systemic absorption of the drugs when they are administered by inhalation at normal therapeutic doses. However, the degree of systemic absorption is more likely to be increased in patients who require higher inhaled doses. When there is significant systemic absorption, which is most likely with high-dose intravenous or oral administration, corticosteroids can affect any of the organ systems in the body. Some of these systemic drug effects include adrenocortical insufficiency, increased susceptibility to infection, fluid and electrolyte disturbances, endocrine effects, CNS effects (insomnia, nervousness, seizures), and dermatological and connective tissue effects, including brittle skin, bone loss, and osteoporosis.

One significant point pertains to patients who are switched from inhaled corticosteroids after receiving systemic corticosteroids, especially at high dosages for an extended period. Patient deaths from adrenal gland failure have been reported in cases when the switch to inhaled corticosteroids was made quickly and the dosage of systemic corticosteroids was not reduced gradually. Prevention of this requires careful clinical monitoring with slow tapering of drug dosages. The patient dependent on systemic corticosteroids may need up to 1 year of recovery time after discontinuation of systemic therapy.

There is also evidence that bone growth is suppressed in children and adolescents taking corticosteroids. This suppression is more apparent in children receiving larger systemic (versus inhaled) dosages over longer treatment durations. Growth should be tracked (e.g., with standardized charts) and medications reevaluated should growth suppression become evident. In some cases, supplemental growth hormone may be prescribed.

Interactions

Drug interactions are more likely to occur with systemic (versus inhaled) corticosteroids. Corticosteroids may increase serum glucose levels, possibly requiring adjustments in dosages of antidiabetic drugs. Because of interactions related to metabolizing enzymes, they may also raise the blood levels of the immunosuppressants cyclosporine and tacrolimus. Likewise, the antifungal drug itraconazole may reduce clearance of the steroids, whereas phenytoin, phenobarbital, and rifampin may enhance it. There is also greater risk for hypokalemia with concurrent use of potassium-depleting diuretics such as hydrochlorothiazide and furosemide.

Dosages

For recommended dosages of selected corticosteroids, see the Dosages table on p. 697.

MONOCLONAL ANTIBODIES

The newest asthma drug is the breakthrough recombinant humanized IgG$_1$ monoclonal anti-IgE antibody omalizumab (Xolair). Omalizumab is used for the management of allergy-specific asthma. A Chinese hamster ovary cell suspension culture in a medium containing gentamicin is used to produce omalizumab.

Mechanism of Action and Drug Effects

Omalizumab acts by selectively binding with and forming complexes with unbound IgE. Omalizumab also blocks the high-affinity receptors on the surfaces of the mast cells and basophils to which antibodies attach. This action reduces the amount of IgE available to trigger the allergic–inflammatory cascade. In addition, histamine release from basophils is reduced by approximately 90% following stimulations with an allergen compared with pretreatment values. Omalizumab also reduces both early- and late-phase asthmatic responses and decreases eosinophil numbers in sputum.

 DRUG PROFILES

fluticasone propionate

Fluticasone propionate is administered intranasally (Flonase)—(one inhalation in each nostril daily) and by oral inhalation (Flovent Diskus, Flovent HFA)—(usually one inhalation by mouth twice daily). Recently fluticasone became available in combination with the long-acting bronchodilator salmeterol xinaforte (Advair Diskus, Advait Inhalation Aerosol).

PHARMACOKINETICS

Half-Life	Onset	Peak	Duration
Inhaled: 3 hr	Inhaled: Unknown	Inhaled: Unknown	Inhaled: Up to 1 day

methylprednisolone

Methylprednisolone is a systemic corticosteroid available in an injectable (Solu-Medrol) form.

PHARMACOKINETICS

Half-Life	Onset	Peak	Duration
IV: 3–4 hr	IV: 1–2 hr	IV: Unknown	IV: 24–36 hr

DOSAGES   Selected Corticosteroids

Drug (Pregnancy Category)	Pharmacological Class	Usual Dosage Range	Indications
budesonide (Pulmicort Nebuamp, Pulmicort Turbuhaler, Rhinocort Aqua, Rhinocort Turbuhaler) (C)	Synthetic glucocorticoid	*Children over 6 yr/Adult* MDI: 200–400 mcg daily, divided bid *Children and Adult* Nasal spray: 2 sprays in each nostril bid or 4 sprays in each nostril once daily *Children 3 mo–12 yr* Inhalation solution: 0.25–1 mg, daily, bid *Adult* Inhalation solution: 1–2 mg daily, bid	Asthma prophylaxis and maintenance treatment Allergic rhinitis Asthma prophylaxis and maintenance treatment
fluticasone propionate (Flonase, Flovent Diskus, Flovent HFA) (C)	Synthetic glucocorticoid	*Children 12 mo–4 yr* Flovent HFA, Diskus: 100 mcg daily, bid, using a Babyhaler spacer device with a face mask *Children 4–16 yr* Flovent HFA, Diskus: 50–200 mcg bid *Adolescents 16 yr and older/Adult* Flovent HFA, Diskus: 100–500 mcg daily bid Flovent HFA, 3 strengths available: 50, 125, 250 mcg/actuation Flovent Diskus, inhalation powder, 4 strengths available: 50, 100, 250, 500 mcg/actuation *Children 4–11 yr* Flonase metered-dose nasal spray: 1–2 sprays (50 mcg/each metered dose) in each nostril bid (max 200 mcg daily) *Children 12 yr and older/Adult* Flonase metered-dose nasal spray: 2 sprays (50 mcg/each metered dose) in each nostril bid (max 400 mcg/day)	Asthma prophylaxis and maintenance treatment Seasonal allergic rhinitis including hay fever, and perennial rhinitis poorly responsive to conventional treatment; management of associated sinus pain and pressure
methylprednisolone sodium succinate (Solu-Medrol) (C)	Synthetic glucocorticoid	Dose varies as above, but usually 30 mg/kg IV over 30 min, q4–6h × 48 hr, usually tapered down Oral taper: usually from 24 to 2 mg daily	Exacerbations of asthma or other COPD
prednisone (Winpred, others) (C)	Synthetic glucocorticoid	Dose varies widely, depending on severity of disease; usual oral dose 1-100 mg daily, usually tapered down	Exacerbations of asthma or other COPD

COPD, chronic obstructive pulmonary disease; *IV*, intravenous; *MDI*, metered-dose inhaler.

Indications

Omalizumab is indicated for adults and adolescents, 12 years of age and older, diagnosed with moderate to severe persistent allergic asthma who are poorly controlled on conventional therapy, experience adverse effects secondary to high-dose or prolonged corticosteroid treatment, or who have frequent exacerbations because of poor medication adherence.

Contraindications

Omalizumab's use is contraindicated in patients with known hypersensitivity to either omalizumab or any component of the formulation.

Adverse Effects

In clinical trials, adverse events seen with omalizumab included injection-site reactions such as bruising, itching, pain, redness, stinging, swelling, or rash; diarrhea; epistaxis; headache; hematoma; menorrhagia; and nausea and vomiting.

NURSING PROCESS

Assessment

The net drug effect of β-agonists, xanthine derivatives, anticholinergics, leukotriene-receptor antagonists (or antileukotrienes), and corticosteroids is improved airflow in airway passages and increased oxygen supply. Cautions, contraindications, and drug interactions (discussed previously in the pharmacology section) should be assessed before any of these drugs is administered. In a thorough assessment of patients receiving any of the respiratory drugs, the patient's skin colour, temperature, respiration rate (which should be more than 12 but less than 24 breaths/min), depth and rhythm, breath sounds, blood pressure, and pulse should be monitored as needed. The nurse should also determine if the patient is having problems with cough, dyspnea, orthopnea, or hypoxia, or has other signs or symptoms of respiratory distress. The patient should also be assessed for the presence of any of the following: sternal retractions, cyanosis, restlessness, activity intolerance, heart irregularities, palpitations, hypertension, tachycardia, or use of accessory muscles to breathe. The anterior–posterior diameter of the thorax should be determined, and pulse oximetry should be assessed to determine oxygen saturation levels. Assess for history of allergies and specific allergens (e.g., dust mites, pollen, mould, mildew, and nuts or other foods). If a cough is present, its character, frequency, and presence of sputum should be noted. The colour of sputum should also be noted.

A complete medication history, noting prescription drugs, over-the-counter drugs, natural health products, alternative therapies, use of nebulizers and humidifiers, use of a home air conditioner, and intactness of heating and air conditioning system should be documented. Note the characteristics of any respiratory symptoms (e.g., seasonally induced, exercise- or stress-induced) and if there is a family history of respiratory diseases. Identify any environmental exposures and precipitating or alleviating factors for any respiratory symptoms and disease processes. An excellent resource for asthma may be found online at http://www.asthmacontrol.com/. Assessment of smoking habits should also be done because of potential exacerbation of respiratory symptoms and problems. Also, nicotine interacts with many respiratory drugs.

Heart status may be compromised because of respiratory distress; thus blood pressure, pulse rate, heart sounds, and electrocardiogram (ECG), if ordered, need to be assessed. The physician may order blood gases with attention to pH, oxygen, carbon dioxide levels, and serum bicarbonate levels. The patient's nail beds should be assessed for abnormalities (e.g., clubbing, cyanosis), as well as the area around the lips. Restlessness may be due to hypoxia, so this symptom should be further evaluated. If chest X-ray, CT, or magnetic resonance imaging (MRI) have been ordered, the findings need to be reviewed. Along with a physical assessment, the nurse needs to assess the patient's emotional state because anxiety, stress, and fear may only further compromise the patient's respiratory status and oxygen levels. The patient's age should also be noted because of increased sensitivity to drugs in older adults and children.

While the cautions, contraindications, drug interactions, and general overview of respiratory assessment associated with the β-agonists (discussed in the pharmacology section) need to be considered, it is particularly important that assessment of allergies to the fluorocarbon propellant (in inhaled dosage forms) also be noted. Assess the patient's intake of caffeine (e.g., chocolate, tea, coffee, candy, and sodas) and the patient's use of over-the-counter medications containing caffeine (e.g., appetite suppressants, pain relievers). The intake of caffeine is important to determine because caffeine has sympathomimetic effects and causes an increase in adverse effects

that are similar to those associated with salbutamol and other β-agonists (e.g., tachycardia, hypertension, headache, nervousness, tremors). Educational level and readiness to learn should also be assessed in preparation of patient education (e.g., instructions about the use of dosage forms such as MDIs).

With respiratory anticholinergic drugs, their cautions, contraindications, and drug interactions should be noted. Assessments for patients taking these drugs should include those mentioned earlier for respiratory drugs as well as assessment for any history of benign prostatic hypertrophy (because of drug-induced urinary retention) or glaucoma (because of drug-induced increase in intraocular pressure). Ipratropium and its aerosol forms have been associated with bronchospasms, so the patient should be assessed for pre-existing problems with the use of MDIs.

Assessment with the use of xanthine derivatives (e.g., theophylline) should include identification of any contraindications, cautions, and drug interactions. Cardiovascular and CNS stimulation may occur with these drugs, thus requiring astute heart and neurological assessment. Gastrointestinal upset may occur with the xanthenes as well, so assessment of bowel patterns and pre-existing disease (e.g., ulcers) is also important. Results of a renal panel and liver function tests should be assessed if these are ordered. As with anticholinergics, xanthines may cause urinary retention, so baseline assessment of urinary patterns and benign prostatic hypertrophy is important. A dietary assessment should include questions about consumption of a low-carbohydrate, high-protein diet and intake of charcoal-broiled meat. These dietary practices may lead to increased theophylline elimination and possibly decreased therapeutic levels; a high-carbohydrate, low-protein diet may decrease excretion of the drug and lead to theophylline toxicity. Effects of the xanthines may be increased by other xanthine-containing foods (e.g., those containing caffeine). Other concerns include prescription drugs and use of over-the-counter drugs containing caffeine (e.g., some antimigraine drugs). See Special Populations: The Older Adult for assessment precautions regarding use of xanthines in older adults.

With corticosteroids, baseline assessment of vital signs, breath sounds, and heart sounds should be done. Age should be noted because corticosteroids are not recommended in children in whom growth is still occurring. As with the other drugs in this chapter, awareness of basic information about these drugs, in particular their action, is important for safe use and prevention of medication errors. For example, glucocorticoids are used for their anti-inflammatory effects, β-agonists and xanthines for their bronchodilating effects, and anticholinergics for their blockage of cholinergic receptors. Knowing what the drugs do and why they are used helps prevent or decrease medication errors and adverse effects. (See Chapter 33 for more information on these anti-inflammatory and adrenal drugs.)

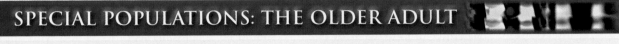

SPECIAL POPULATIONS: THE OLDER ADULT

- Xanthine derivatives should be administered cautiously along with careful monitoring in older adults; sensitivity to xanthines is increased in this patient population because of decreased drug metabolism.

- The older adult should be assessed for signs and symptoms of xanthine toxicity, which include nausea, vomiting, restlessness, insomnia, irritability, and tremors. The nurse should be cautious in assessing restlessness and concluding that it is drug related because it may be caused by hypoxia secondary to respiratory difficulties and not by the medication itself.

- The older adult should be told never to chew or crush sustained-released dosage forms; to be careful of drug interactions, especially with other asthma-related drugs or bronchodilators; and to take the medication at the same time every day.

- The older adult should be advised never to omit or double up on doses. If a dose is missed, the patient should contact the physician or health care provider for further instructions.

- Monitoring of serum levels of the drug should be initiated to avoid possible toxicity and to make sure blood levels are therapeutic. Assistance with transportation and expenses may be needed and can be obtained from community resources.

- Lower dosages may be necessary initially in the older adult because of not only their increased sensitivity to the drug but also the possibility of decreased liver and kidney functioning. Close monitoring for adverse effects and toxicity should be part of daily therapy, and palpitations and increased blood pressure (from cardiovascular and central nervous system stimulation) should be noted and reported.

With antileukotrienes, it is important to assess for contraindications, cautions, and drug interactions. Liver functioning should be determined because of specific concerns about the use of these drugs in patients with altered liver function. As with other medications, the older adult is more sensitive to these drugs.

Nursing Diagnoses

- Impaired gas exchange related to pathophysiological changes caused by respiratory disease
- Fatigue related to the disease process
- Risk for injury related to bronchospasms of the disease and to the adverse effects of respiratory medications
- Anxiety related to the "unknown" associated with respiratory disease and to the adverse effects of drug therapy
- Disturbed sensory perception related to CNS stimulation caused by bronchodilators
- Deficient knowledge related to unfamiliarity with drug treatment regimen and the disease process
- Ineffective tissue perfusion related to the adverse effects of salbutamol and other β-agonist drugs
- Nonadherence to the drug regimen related to undesirable adverse effects of drug therapy

Planning

Goals

- Patient will experience minimal exacerbations of the disease while adherent to the drug regimen.
- Patient will state the importance of rest for recovery.
- Patient will be free of injury related to the disease or the adverse effects of the drug.

- Patient will remain adherent to the drug regimen and to the nonpharmacological therapies.
- Patient will follow up with health care providers as instructed by the physician.
- Patient will not increase or decrease the dosage or stop taking the medication without the approval of the physician.
- Patient's respiratory status will improve because of adherence to the drug therapy.
- Patient's circulation will remain intact and strong during therapy.

Outcome Criteria

- Patient briefly describes the disease process, its signs and symptoms, and the precipitating factors.
- Patient states measures to take to prevent injury resulting from the disease or the adverse effects of the drug, such as taking drugs as prescribed.
- Patient is well rested, with plans to rest during periods of exacerbation.
- Patient states the expected adverse effects of the drug being taken, such as palpitations, nervousness, mood changes, and insomnia.
- Patient contacts the physician if increased dyspnea, shortness of breath, increased cough, or fever occurs.
- Patient states the importance of taking the drug as prescribed, the reasons for not increasing or decreasing the dosage of the drug, and the importance of not stopping the drug therapy, to prevent complications and exacerbations related to the disease or to the adverse effects of medications.
- Patient states situations to report to the physician that are indicative of poor circulation, such as swelling of the feet, bluish discoloration of nail beds or lips, coolness of the extremities, and heart palpitations.

Implementation

Nursing interventions that apply to patients with respiratory disease processes (e.g., COPD, asthma, other upper and lower respiratory tract disorders) include patient education and an emphasis on adherence and prevention, in addition to the specific actions related to the prescribed drug therapy. Measures to implement in order to prevent, relieve, or decrease the manifestations of the disease should be emphasized to the patient at all times, and the patient's awareness of specific precipitating factors should be increased. Bronchodilators and other respiratory drugs should be given exactly as prescribed and by the prescribed route (e.g., parenterally, orally, by intermittent positive pressure breathing, or by inhalation). The proper method for administering the inhaled forms of these drugs should be demonstrated to the patient, who should provide a return demonstration. The patient should also be strongly discouraged from taking more than the prescribed dose of β-agonists, xanthenes, and other respiratory drugs because of their excessive demands on the heart and the cardiac and CNS stimulations (hypertension and tachycardia) that may occur.

The use of MDIs requires coordination to inhale the medication correctly and to ensure approximately 10% of the drug delivered to the lungs. One minute should be allowed between puffs, and the use of a spacer may be indicated to increase the amount of drug delivered. During the 1-minute interval, some bronchodilation occurs, which facilitates penetration of the second puff. Dry powder inhalers are small, hand-held devices that deliver a specific amount of dry micronized powder with each inhaled breath. Their use does not require the same coordination as that for MDIs, they deliver about 20% of the drug to the lung, and they have no propellants and thus pose no problems for the environment. One minute should be allowed between each puff. A nebulizer dosage form delivers small amounts of misted droplets of the drug to the lungs through a small mouthpiece or mask. Although a nebulizer may take a longer time to deliver the drug to the lungs than do the inhalers, the nebulizer dosage form may be more effective for some patients. See Chapter 10 for more information.

β-agonists should be taken exactly as prescribed, and recommended dosage and frequency should be adhered to, as overdosage may be life threatening. Oral sustained-released tablets should not be crushed or chewed and should be taken with food to avoid gastrointestinal upset. Inhaled forms and their instructions are presented in Patient Education. Before, during, and after therapy with these drugs, it is important to reassess the respiratory status and breath sounds. Anticholinergic drugs used for respiratory diseases (e.g., ipratropium) should be taken daily as ordered and with appropriate use of the MDI. See Patient Education for further information on the administration of this drug. Exact instructions should be included in the physician's order for the medication and may vary. Rinsing the mouth with water immediately after use of any inhaled or nebulized drug may help prevent mucosal irritation and dryness.

Xanthine derivatives should also be given exactly as prescribed. If they are to be administered parenterally, the nurse should determine the correct diluent and rate of administration. IV infusion pumps should be used to ensure dosage accuracy and help prevent toxicity. Too rapid an infusion may lead to profound hypotension, with possible syncope, tachycardia, seizures, and even cardiac arrest. To prevent a sudden increase in drug release and the irritating effects on the gastric mucosa, timed-release preparations should not be crushed or chewed. Oral forms should be taken with food to avoid gastrointestinal upset. Suppository forms of the drug should be refrigerated, and patients should notify the physician if rectal burning, itching, or irritation occurs. The patient should continue to be monitored for respiratory status and improvement in baseline condition during drug therapy.

Inhaled glucocorticoids should also be used exactly as prescribed, with cautions about overuse. The medication should be taken every day as ordered, regardless of whether the patient is feeling better or not. Often these drugs (e.g., flunisolide) are used as maintenance drugs and are taken twice daily for maximal response. An inhaled β$_2$-agonist may be used before the inhaled glucocorticoid to provide bronchodilation before administration of the anti-inflammatory drug. The bronchodilator inhaled drug is generally taken several minutes before the glucocorticoid or corticosteroid aerosol. All equipment (inhalers or nebulizers) should be kept clean, with filters cleaned and changed (nebulizers) and in good working condition. Use of a spacer may be indicated, especially if success with inhalation is limited. Rinsing of the mouth immediately after use of the inhaler or nebulizer dosage forms of corticosteroids and glucocorticoids is recommended to help prevent overgrowth of oral fungi and oral candidiasis (thrush).

Children may need a physician's order to have these medications on hand at school and during athletic events or physical education. Peak flow meter use is also encouraged among patients of all ages to better regulate their disease. Journalling may help in recording peak flow levels, signs and symptoms of the disease, any improvement, and any adverse effects associated with therapy. Systemic forms of glucocorticoids should be used with caution in children because use of these drugs may lead to suppression of the hypothalamic–pituitary–adrenal axis and to subsequent growth stunting. However, the benefits of these drugs are considerable and outweigh the risks. Inhaled forms and use of short-term systemic therapy are often combined in children. The nurse should continue to monitor the patient's condition during therapy with a focus on the respiratory, cardiac, and central nervous systems.

The antileukotrienes montelukast and zafirlukast are given orally. Of most concern are the montelukast chewable tablets, which contain aspartame and approximately 0.842 mg of phenylamine per 5 mg tablet. Patient education for the leukotriene-receptor antagonists should stress that they are indicated for long-term management of asthma but not of acute asthma. Montelukast granules are taken either directly into the mouth or mixed with 1 teaspoon of apple sauce or other cold or room-temperature soft food. The granules are not to be dissolved in liquid for administration. Once the granule packet is opened, the granules should be taken within 15 minutes. The drugs should be taken every night on a continuous schedule, even after symptoms improve. Fluid intake should increase, as with all the respiratory drugs, to help decrease the viscosity of secretions.

 Evaluation

The therapeutic effects of any of the drugs used to improve the control of acute or chronic respiratory symptoms and diseases and treat or help prevent respiratory diseases include the following: a decrease in dyspnea, wheezing, restlessness, and anxiety; improved respiratory patterns with return to normal rate and quality; improved activity tolerance and arterial blood gas levels; improved quality of life; and decreased severity and incidence of respiratory symptoms. The therapeutic effects of bronchodilators (e.g., xanthines, β-agonists) include decreased symptoms and increased ease of breathing. Blood levels of theophylline should be between 55 and 110 mmol/L (10 to 20 mg/L) and should be frequently monitored. Peak flow meters are easy to use and help reveal early decreases in peak flow caused by bronchospasms. They also serve to monitor treatment effectiveness. Other respiratory drugs should produce the therapeutic effects related to the specific drug. Adverse effects for which to monitor in all drugs in this chapter are presented in the respective drug profiles and drug tables. Therapeutic effects include an improvement in control of the acute or chronic respiratory disease process. Achievement of goals and outcomes should also be evaluated.

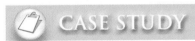 CASE STUDY

Chronic Obstructive Pulmonary Disease

Ms. B. is a 73-year-old woman who had worked in the local traffic tunnel for about 25 years and has had chronic obstructive pulmonary disease (COPD) for approximately 10 years, caused by exposure to workplace environmental pollutants and by cigarette smoking. She is now retired and is frequently admitted to the hospital for treatment of her condition. She quit smoking 8 years ago. She is now in the hospital for treatment of an acute exacerbation of the COPD and an upper respiratory tract infection. The physician has ordered the following: aminophylline intravenously per respiratory therapy protocol, intravenous continuous infusion at a rate of 0.8 mg/kg/hr; chest physiotherapy bid and prn; cephalothin sodium antibiotic therapy, 1 g intravenously in 30 mL normal saline q8h; measurement of intake and output; daily weight measurement; assessment of vital signs, with breath sounds

q2h and prn until stable; and salbutamol inhaler, 2 puffs q4h per respiratory therapy protocol.

1. What nursing interventions would be most appropriate for helping this patient conserve energy while enhancing O_2 and CO_2 gas exchange?
2. What is the rationale for the continuous intravenous infusion of aminophylline?
3. What are the reasons for prescribing the salbutamol inhaler and the antibiotic? Be specific about the rationale for each.
4. What would be the most important patient education guidelines to discuss with Ms. B. concerning the use of an oral xanthine drug (theophylline) and the salbutamol inhaler at home?

For answers see http://evolve.elsevier.com/Canada/Lilley/pharmacology/.

PATIENT EDUCATION

β-Agonists

- Patients should be sure to maintain healthy living habits, such as undergoing regular health checkups, drinking adequate fluids, eating three balanced meals daily, and engaging in consistent exercise as tolerated and as ordered.
- Patients with asthma, bronchitis, or COPD should be encouraged to avoid exposure to conditions or situations that may lead to bronchoconstriction and worsening of the disorder (e.g., allergens, stress, smoking, and air pollutants).
- Patients should be educated about precipitating events for their respiratory problems or symptoms, as well as measures to help alleviate them. Patients should receive adequate information about their medications, over-the-counter drugs, and natural health products as well as about all actions that will help prevent or control the their illnesses.
- Patients should be instructed in the proper use and care of MDIs, dry powder inhalers, and other such devices, as described in Patient Education for corticosteroids. (Also see Chapter 10 and Figures 10-90 through 10-93 for more specific information.)

Xanthines

- Patients should be educated about interactions between nicotine and xanthines. Smoking decreases the blood concentrations of aminophylline and theophylline. Other interactions associated with xanthines include charcoal-broiled foods that may decrease serum levels of the drug.
- Patient should be made aware of food and beverage items that contain caffeine (e.g., chocolate, coffee, cola, cocoa, tea) because of exacerbation of CNS stimulation.
- Patients should be encouraged to keep follow-up appointments because of the importance of monitoring therapeutic levels of medications.
- Patients should be instructed to take the medication round the clock to maintain steady-state drug levels and to never chew or crush extended-release preparations. Educate the patient to take granules directly into the mouth or mix with apple sauce. Any problems such as headaches, insomnia, restlessness, muscle twitching, nausea, vomiting, gastrointestinal pain, palpitations, and seizures should be reported immediately to the health care provider.

Anticholinergics

- Patients should be informed that ipratropium is used prophylactically to decrease the frequency and severity of asthma and has to be taken as ordered and generally year-round for therapeutic effectiveness.
- Patients should be encouraged to drink fluids with use of anticholinergics and with all other respiratory drugs, unless contraindicated. Fluids decrease the thickness of secretions and help with expectoration of sputum.

- Patients taking any respiratory drugs (including anticholinergics) should be instructed to take the prescribed number of puffs from an inhaler and no more than two puffs with one dosing or as ordered. Educate patients about the proper use of the MDI with or without a spacer (which applies to inhaled drugs in this chapter), how to use a dry powder inhaler, and how to properly clean and store the equipment. One to two minutes should be allowed between each puff from the inhaler.

Corticosteroids

- Patients should be instructed that in addition to adhering to the dosing and frequency of these drugs, if inhaled forms are used, good oral hygiene (e.g., rinsing of the mouth) should be practised after the last inhalation. Rinsing the mouth with water is appropriate and necessary to prevent oral fungal infections.
- Patients should be instructed about keeping inhalers clean, including (once a week) removing the medication canister from the plastic casing and washing the casing in warm, soapy water. Once the casing is dry, the patient can replace the canister and cap the mouthpiece.
- Patients should be taught to keep track of the doses left in the MDI as follows: The number of doses in the canister should be noted, and the number of days the doses will last should be calculated. For example, assume that two puffs are taken four times a day, and the inhaler has a capacity of 200 inhalations. Two puffs four times a day equals eight inhalations per day. Eight dividing 200 yields 25; that is, the inhaler will last approximately 25 days. The MDI should be marked with the date it will be empty and a refill obtained a few days before that date. Note that using extra doses will alter the refill date.
- Each patient should be encouraged to always check the expiration dates of all medications.
- Patients should be encouraged to keep an asthma action plan, which is a personalized program developed by the physician and the patient for managing the asthma. Generally, those individuals who use individualized plans have better asthma control.
- Patients should be encouraged to keep a journal of the medications being taken, how the medications work, what progress is being made in alleviating the asthma or illness, and how they are feeling every day. Any adverse effects should also be recorded.
- Patients should be instructed to wear a medical alert bracelet or necklace and to carry a medical card with their diagnoses and list of medications and allergies. Emergency contact persons and phone numbers should also be listed.
- Patients using an intranasal dosage form should be instructed on how to clear the nasal passage before drug administration. The patient should tilt the head slightly forward and insert the spray tip into one

Continued

nasal passage, pointing the tip toward the inflamed nasal turbinates. The medication should be pumped into the nasal passage as the patient sniffs inward while holding the other nostril closed; the procedure is then repeated in the other nasal passage. Any unused portion should be discarded after 3 months.

❖ Patients need to be aware that excess levels of systemic corticosteroids may lead to cushingoid symptoms; even though an inhaler minimizes this problem, education about it is very important to patient safety. Signs and symptoms of cushingoid syndrome include moon face, acne, an increase in fat pads, and swelling. These signs and symptoms are at a higher risk of occurrence if these drugs are given systemically, either orally or parenterally.

❖ In addition, patients should be informed that Addison's crisis can occur if a systemic corticosteroid is abruptly discontinued, so any dosage forms of these drugs should be weaned prior to withdrawal of the medication. The problems that the patient may

experience include nausea, shortness of breath, joint pain, weakness, and fatigue. If these occur, the patient should know to contact the physician immediately.

❖ Patients should be instructed to always check for drug interactions with any type of medication.

❖ Patients should be encouraged to report to the physician any weight gain of 1 kg or more in 24 hours or 2 kg or more in 1 week.

Leukotriene Antagonists

❖ Patients should be instructed on the action and purpose of leukotriene antagonists (e.g., used for maintenance therapy and not for treatment of an acute attack of bronchospasms).

❖ Patients should be told to report worsening of the underlying asthma or any adverse effects of drug therapy that are not tolerable.

❖ Patients should be instructed to report any abdominal pain, jaundice, nausea, or vomiting to the physician.

POINTS TO REMEMBER

❖ The β-agonists may stimulate α- and β-receptors, β$_1$- and β$_2$-receptors, or just β$_2$-receptors. The β$_2$-stimulants are the most specific for the lungs and have the fewest adverse effects.

❖ Xanthines include drugs such as caffeine and theophylline and work by inhibiting phosphodiesterase. Phosphodiesterase breaks down cAMP, which is needed to relax smooth muscles.

❖ Theophylline is the most common xanthine; aminophylline is the parenteral form of theophylline.

❖ A major anticholinergic, ipratropium bromide, is the only anticholinergic drug used for the treatment of COPD.

❖ Anticholinergic drugs are used for maintenance effects and not for relief of acute bronchospasms; their action is to block the bronchoconstrictive effects of ACh.

❖ Corticosteroids are also used for the treatment of respiratory disorders and have many indications. The most commonly used ones are beclomethasone, dexamethasone, flunisolide, and triamcinolone.

Corticosteroids exert their action by stabilizing the membranes of cells that release harmful bronchoconstricting substances.

❖ Contraindications to β-agonist use include heart disease and seizure disorders. Use of anticholinergics is contraindicated in patients with benign prostatic hypertrophy or glaucoma.

❖ Use of xanthine derivatives is contraindicated in patients with a history of gastrointestinal tract disorders or peptic ulcer disease.

❖ The antileukotriene drugs montelukast and zafirlukast are given orally. Adverse effects include headache, dizziness, insomnia, and dyspepsia.

❖ The nurse should be sure to give the patient proper instructions on the use of MDIs, dry powder inhalers, and other inhalant equipment. Keeping equipment clean and in a good state of repair is important, so adequate instructions should be provided not only for their use but also for their cleaning and storage.

EXAMINATION REVIEW QUESTIONS

1 A patient who has a history of asthma is experiencing an acute episode of shortness of breath and needs to take a medication for immediate relief. Which medication will the nurse choose for this situation?
a. A β-agonist, such as salbutamol
b. A corticosteroid, such as fluticasone
c. An anticholinergic, such as ipatropium
d. An antileukotriene, such as montelukast

2 After a nebulizer treatment with the β-agonist salbutamol, the patient complains of feeling a little "shaky," with slight tremors of the hands. His heart rate is 98 beats/min, increased from the pretreatment rate of 88 beats/min. Which of the following is causing this reaction?
a. An allergic reaction to the medication
b. An idiosyncratic reaction to the medication
c. An expected adverse effect of the medication
d. An indication that he has received an overdose of the medication

3 A patient has been receiving an aminophylline (xanthine derivative) infusion for 24 hours. When monitoring for adverse effects, which of the following should the nurse know to expect?
a. CNS depression
b. Sinus tachycardia
c. Increased appetite
d. Temporary urinary retention

4 A patient will be receiving a new prescription for the antileukotriene montelukast (Singulair). Which of the following does the drug do?
a. Improve the respiratory drive
b. Reduce inflammation in the airway
c. Stimulate immediate bronchodilation
d. Loosen and remove thickened secretions

5 After taking a dose of an inhaled corticosteroid, such as fluticasone, what is the most important action the patient should perform next?
a. Rinse out the mouth with water
b. Hold the breath for 60 seconds
c. Repeat the dose in 15 minutes if feeling short of breath
d. Follow the corticosteroid with a bronchodilator inhaler, if ordered

For answers see http://evolve.elsevier.com/Canada/Lilley/pharmacology/.

CRITICAL THINKING ACTIVITIES

1 Your patient is taking a xanthine derivative and should not ingest xanthine-containing beverages. What are some examples of these beverages, and why is it important to avoid consuming them while taking a xanthine derivative?

2 Discuss the necessary patient education regarding the use of leukotriene modifiers, especially the rationale for the emphasis on taking the medication daily as ordered.

For answers see http://evolve.elsevier.com/Canada/Lilley/pharmacology/.

PART SEVEN
Anti-infective and Anti-inflammatory Drugs

STUDY SKILLS TIPS:

- NURSING PROCESS
- ASSESSMENT
- NURSING DIAGNOSES
- EVALUATION

NURSING PROCESS

This study section focuses on the Nursing Process sections, using Chapter 38 as an example. Consider the following statement:

"The discussion of the nursing process will <u>focus</u> on each <u>major classification of antibiotics</u> to convey <u>general and specific information</u> about the various antibiotics."

The underlining in this paragraph points out the important information. The Nursing Process section focuses on major classifications, and you need to see both *general* and *specific* information about the classifications. Although the paragraph is only one sentence long, it clearly defines what you need to keep in mind as you study this section.

ASSESSMENT

When you read the Nursing Process section of a chapter, ask yourself. What do I need to learn? What do I need to know? What do I need to be able to do? Consider the following sentence from Chapter 38.

"To ensure <u>effective treatment</u>, in general, <u>before the administration</u> of any antibiotic, it is <u>crucial to assess for a history of or symptoms indicative of hypersensitivity or allergic reactions (mild reactions with rash, pruritus, or hives to severe reactions with laryngeal edema, bronchospasms, hypotension, and possible cardiac arrest). Further assessment</u> should include the <u>patient's age, weight, and baseline vital signs with body temperature as well as examination of the results of any laboratory studies that have been ordered, including liver function studies (aspartate aminotransferase [AST] level and alanine aminotransferase [ALT] level), kidney function studies (usually blood urea nitrogen and creatinine levels), heart function studies and tests (pertinent laboratory tests, electrocardiogram, or ultrasonography if indicated), culture and sensitivity tests, and complete blood count (CBC) with hemoglobin/hematocrit (Hgb/Hct) levels and platelet/clotting values.</u>"

In Chapter 38, you are assessing patients in relation to the pharmacological interventions discussed. Some underlining has been done to bring focus to the things you need to be aware of as you study.

The word *crucial* tells you this is something that cannot be ignored. Ask yourself, what is crucial? The answer is found in the sentence. You need to have data collected on the patient. The sentence goes on to identify the kind of data that should be available, and the sentence makes it clear that it has to be done "before the administration of any antibotic."

The first item is "hypersensitivities." Some individuals are allergic to certain antibiotics; it would be dangerous and possibly fatal to administer an antibiotic to a patient who is hypersensitive to it. Assessment for this also connects with effective treatment. As you consider each of the underlined elements in this sentence, keep in mind its relationship to effectiveness and appropriateness.

The patient's age should be known. Chapter 3 deals with concerns related to the older adult and of children. Children and older adult patients respond to drugs differently from young adults. This response would directly affect dosage and possibly even the choice of antibiotics to be administered. Again, this factor is directly related to the "effective treatment" referred to in this sentence.

Another piece specifies liver, kidney, and heart functioning. Try to recall information that related the specific antibiotics to these functions.

One more aspect of this sentence is the use of standard medical abbreviations. In earlier Study Skills Tips, it was suggested that you prepare vocabulary cards for these abbreviations. You need to know what CBC, Hgb, and Hct mean, what they measure, and how they relate to the appropriate administration of antibiotics. If these letters are not meaningful to you, then you will not be able to link what you know about the antibiotics with what you must know about administering them. Many test 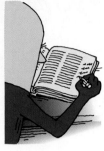 questions on nursing examinations use the standard abbreviations, and you must know them instantly and be able to relate them to the situation covered.

NURSING DIAGNOSES

Again start with the question, "What am I supposed to learn?" The focus is on administration of antibiotics. What should you look for in working with patients that affects the administration of antibiotics?

This same procedure should be applied to the sections on Planning, Outcome Criteria, and Implementation. Consider what each of these headings suggests about the nursing process, and read and evaluate the information, relating it to what you have already learned. Also, consider the implications of the information as possible test questions that may ask you to do more than recall specific facts. As an example, consider the following case:

Patient A, age 23 years, has a fever of 38.2°C. She was admitted yesterday and delivered a healthy infant 8 hours ago. She is breastfeeding the newborn. What antibiotics might be administered for the fever? What specific antibiotics should be used with caution or eliminated from consideration?

This case demonstrates the need to read and think critically. You need to remember the specific facts from the chapter and be able to take a case study example and apply those facts to that specific situation.

EVALUATION

This is the final section under Nursing Process. What are you supposed to evaluate? Consider the second sentence under this section in Chapter 38.

"The therapeutic effects of antibiotics include a decrease in the signs and symptoms of the infection; a return to normal vital signs, including temperature and negative results on culture and sensitivity tests; normal results for CBC; and improved appetite, energy level, and sense of well-being." This sentence makes it clear that you are evaluating the patient and the response to the antibiotics being administered. In evaluating the patient, what should you look for? Given the focus in the nursing process on contraindications, cautions, hypersensitivity, and reactions related to the administration of antibiotics, you should be evaluating two aspects of the patient.

First, you should look for the positive responses indicating that the patient is responding well to treatment. When you read the next sentence in this section, you see: "Evaluation for adverse effects includes monitoring for. . . ." This says that your role in evaluation is to monitor the patient for negative responses and to be prepared to educate the patient about these effects and possible steps to alleviate them.

The Nursing Process section in each chapter should be read carefully and thoughtfully, because it is in this section that you begin to see how the complex pharmacological material presented earlier in the chapter applies to your role as a nurse. This material should be read with the same concern and care that you have given to the earlier part of the chapter; this is the section in which you think about *applying* all you have learned. Apply the 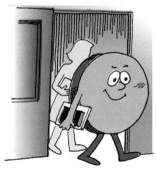 PURR model, and be an active questioner and reader, and you will be successful in working with the Nursing Process in each chapter.

Antibiotics Part 1: Sulfonamides, Penicillins, Cephalosporins, Macrolides, and Tetracyclines

Learning Objectives

After reading this chapter, the successful student will be able to do the following:

1 Discuss the general principles of antibiotic therapy.

2 Explain how antibiotics work to eradicate infections from the body.

3 Discuss the pros and cons of antibiotics with attention to the overuse or misuse of antibiotics and the development of drug resistance.

4 Classify the antibiotics by general category, including sulfonamides, penicillins, cephalosporins, macrolides, and tetracyclines.

5 Discuss the mechanisms of action, indications, cautions, contraindications, routes of administration, and drug interactions for the sulfonamides, penicillins, cephalosporins, macrolides, and tetracyclines.

6 Identify drug-specific adverse effects and toxic effects of each of the antibiotic classes listed earlier and cite measures to decrease their occurrence.

7 Discuss the concept of superinfection, including how it occurs and how to prevent it.

8 Develop a collaborative plan of care that includes all phases of the nursing process for patients receiving drugs in each of the following classes of antibiotics: sulfonamides, penicillins, cephalosporins, macrolides, and tetracyclines.

e-Learning Activities

Web site
(http://evolve.elsevier.com/Canada/Lilley/pharmacology/)

- Animations
- Answers to chapter questions, activities, and case studies
- Calculators and Category Catchers
- Glossary with audio pronunciations
- IV Therapy and Medication Error Checklists
- Multiple-Choice Review Question quizzes
- Nursing Care Plans
- Online Appendices and Supplements
- WebLinks

Drug Profiles

▸▸ **amoxicillin**, p. 717
ampicillin, p. 718
▸▸ **azithromycin, clarithromycin**, p. 725
▸▸ **cefazolin (cefazolin sodium)***, p. 720
cefepime (cefepime hydrochloride)*, p. 721
▸▸ **cefoxitin (cefoxitin sodium)***, p. 720
ceftazidime (ceftazidime pentahydrate)*, p. 720
▸▸ **ceftriaxone (ceftriaxone sodium)***, p. 721
cefuroxime (cerfuroxime sodium)*, p. 720

▸▸ **cephalexin**, p. 720
cloxacillin (cloxacillin sodium)*, p. 717
▸▸ **doxycycline hyclate**, p. 728
▸▸ **erythromycin**, p. 724
▸▸ **imipenem-cilastatin**, p. 721
meropenem, ertapenem, p. 721
▸▸ **penicillin G, penicillin V potassium**, p. 717
pivmecillinam (pivmecillinam hydrochloride)*, piperacillin (piperacillin sodium)*, p. 718
sulfamethoxazole-trimethoprim (co-trimoxazole), p. 714
telithromycin, p. 725

▸▸ **Key drug.**

*Full generic name is given in parentheses. For the purposes of this text, the more common shortened name is used.

Glossary

Antibiotic Having or pertaining to the ability to destroy or interfere with the development of a living organism. The term used most commonly to refer to antibacterial drugs. (p. 709)

Bactericidal antibiotic An antibiotic that kills bacteria. (p. 715)

Bacteriostatic antibiotic An antibiotic that does not actually kill bacteria but rather inhibits their growth. (p. 712)

β-Lactam The name for a broad, major class of antibiotics that includes four subclasses: penicillins, cephalosporins, carbapenems, and monobactams. (p. 715)

β-Lactamase Any of a group of enzymes produced by bacteria that catalyze the chemical opening of the crucial β-lactam ring structures in β-lactam antibiotics. (p. 715)

β-Lactamase inhibitors Drugs combined with certain penicillin drugs to block the effect of β-lactamase enzymes. (p. 715)

Empirical antibiotic therapy Administration of antibiotics based on the practitioner's judgement of the pathogens most likely to be causing an apparent infection; it involves the presumptive treatment of an infection to avoid treatment delay, before specific culture information has been obtained. (p. 710)

Glucose-6-phosphate dehydrogenase (G6PD) deficiency An inherited disorder in which the red blood cells are partially or completely deficient in glucose-6-phosphate dehydrogenase, a critical enzyme in the metabolism of glucose. (p. 712)

Host factors Factors that are unique to the body of a particular patient that affect the patient's susceptibility to infection and response to antibiotic drugs. (p. 711)

Infection The invasion and multiplication of microorganisms in body tissues. (p. 708)

Microorganisms Microscopic living organisms (also called *microbes*). (p. 708)

Prophylactic antibiotic therapy Antibiotics taken before anticipated exposure to an infectious organism in an effort to prevent the development of infection. (p. 710)

Slow acetylator A common genetic host factor in which the rate of metabolism of certain drugs is reduced. (p. 712)

Subtherapeutic Referring to antibiotic treatment that is ineffective in treating a given infection. Possible causes include inappropriate drug therapy, insufficient drug dosing, or bacterial drug resistance. (p. 708)

Superinfection (1) An infection occurring during antimicrobial treatment for another infection, resulting from overgrowth of an organism not susceptible to the antibiotic used. (2) A secondary microbial infection that occurs in addition to an earlier primary infection, often because of weakening of the patient's immune system function by the first infection. (p. 710)

Teratogens Substances that can interfere with normal prenatal development and cause one or more developmental abnormalities in the fetus. (p. 711)

Therapeutic Referring to antibiotic therapy that results in sufficient concentrations of the drug in the blood or other tissues to render it effective against specific bacterial pathogens. (p. 710)

MICROBIAL INFECTION

A person is normally able to remain healthy and resistant to infectious **microorganisms** because of the existence of certain host defences. These defences take various forms. They can be actual physical barriers such as intact skin or the ciliated respiratory mucosa. They can be physiological defences such as the gastric acid in the stomach and immune factors such as antibodies. They can also be the phagocytic cells (macrophages and polymorphonuclear neutrophils) that are part of the reticuloendothelial system.

Microorganisms are everywhere, both in the external environment and in many parts of the internal environment of our bodies. They can be intrinsically harmful to humans, or they can be innocuous and even beneficial under normal circumstances but can become harmful when conditions are altered in some way. An example of an intrinsically harmful microorganism is *Rickettsia rickettsii*, which causes Rocky Mountain spotted fever (RMSF). In contrast, certain species of Streptococcus are normally present on the body skin surface and usually do not cause harm. However, a common streptococcal throat infection ("strep throat") can cause endocarditis in patients whose heart valves have been damaged as a result of rheumatic fever. Rheumatic fever is a condition that is often a result of a previous streptococcal infection. Every known major class of microbes has member organisms that can infect humans, including bacteria, viruses, fungi, and protozoans. The focus of this chapter is common bacterial **infections**.

Recall from microbiology that bacteria come in a number of different shapes. This property of bacteria is called their *morphology* (Figure 38-1). Bacteria may also be grouped according to other common recognizable characteristics (Figure 38-2). One of the most important ways of categorizing different bacteria is on the basis of their response to the *Gram-stain* procedure (Figure 38-3). Bacterial species that stain purple with the Gram-stain dyes are classified as gram-positive organisms. Those bacteria that stain red are classified as gram-negative organisms.

Bacterial Morphology Shapes

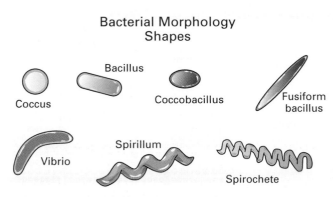

FIG. 38-1   Bacterial morphologies. (From Murray, P. R., Rosenthal, K. S., Kobayashi, G. S., & Pfaller, M. A. (2002). *Medical microbiology.* St. Louis, MO: Mosby.)

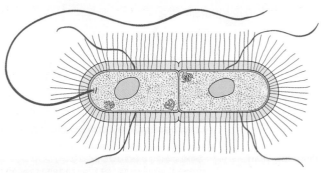

FIG. 38-2   A dividing bacterial cell with a single flagellum, four sex pili, numerous common fibriae, a cell wall, a cytoplasmic membrane, two nuclear bodies, three mesosomes, and numerous ribosomes. (From Greenwood, D., Slack, R., & Peutherer, J. (2002). *Medical microbiology* (16th ed.). Edinburgh: Elsevier Science.)

This seemingly simple difference proves to be significant in guiding the choice of **antibiotic** therapy.

Gram-positive organisms have cell walls with a much thicker constituent known as *peptidoglycan,* which refers to the protein (peptido-) and sugar (-glycan) components of its chemical structure. In addition, gram-positive organisms have a thicker outer cell *capsule.* In contrast, gram-negative organisms have a cell wall structure that is more complex, with a smaller outer capsule and peptidoglycan layer than that of gram-positive bacteria but with two cell membranes: an outer and inner membrane (Figures 38-4 and 38-5). These differences usually make gram-negative bacterial infections more difficult to treat because the drug molecules have a harder time penetrating the more complex cell walls of gram-negative organisms.

When a person's normal host defences are breached or somehow compromised, that person becomes susceptible to infection. The microorganisms invade and multiply in the body tissues, and if the infective process overwhelms the body's defence system, the infection becomes clinically apparent. The patient then usually manifests the following classic signs and symptoms of infection: fever, chills, sweats, redness, pain and swelling, fatigue, weight loss, increased white blood cell (WBC) count, and the formation of pus. Not all patients will exhibit signs of infection. This is especially true in older adults and patients who are immunocompromised.

To help the body and its normal host defences combat an infection, antibiotic therapy is often required. Antibiotics are most effective when their actions are combined with functioning bodily defence mechanisms. Before specific types of drug therapy are discussed here, some general principles are reviewed.

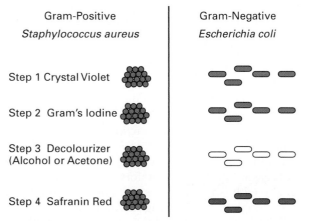

FIG. 38-3   Gram-stain morphology of bacteria. The crystal violet of Gram stain is precipitated by Gram iodine and is trapped in the thick peptidoglycan layer in gram-positive bacteria. The decolourizer disperses the gram-negative outer membrane and washes the crystal violet from the thin layer of peptidoglycan. Gram-negative bacteria are visualized by the red counterstain. (From Murray, P. R., Rosenthal, K. S., Kobayashi, G. S., & Pfaller, M. A. (2002). *Medical microbiology.* St. Louis, MO: Mosby.)

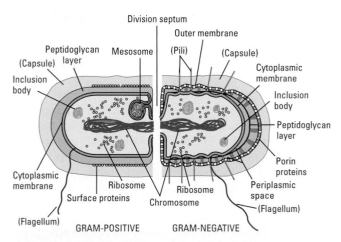

FIG. 38-4   Gram-positive and gram-negative bacteria. A gram-positive bacterium has a thick layer of peptidoglycan *(left).* A gram-negative bacterium has a thin peptidoglycan layer and an outer membrane *(right).* Structures in parentheses are not found in all bacteria. (From Murray, P. R., Rosenthal, K. S., Kobayashi, G. S., & Pfaller, M. A. (2002). *Medical microbiology.* St. Louis, MO: Mosby.)

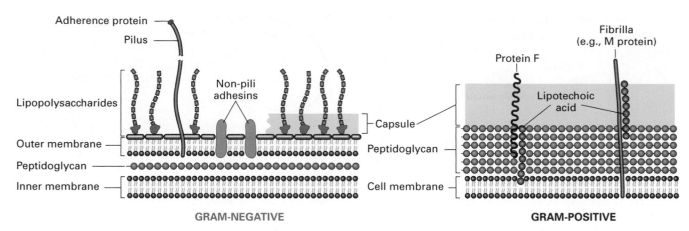

FIG. 38-5   Molecules on the surface of gram-negative and gram-positive bacteria involved in pathogenesis. Not shown is the type 3 secretory apparatus of gram-negative bacteria. (From Cotran, R. S., Kumar, V., & Collins, T. (1999). *Robbins pathologic basis of disease* (6th ed.). Philadelphia: Saunders.)

GENERAL PRINCIPLES OF ANTIBIOTIC THERAPY

Antibiotic drug therapy should begin with a clinical assessment of the patient to determine whether the common signs and symptoms of infection are present. The patient should also be assessed during and after antibiotic therapy to evaluate the effectiveness of the drug therapy, to monitor for adverse drug effects, and to ensure that the infection does not recur.

Often the signs and symptoms of an infection appear long before an organism can be identified. When this happens and the risk of life-threatening or severe complications is high (e.g., suspected acute meningitis), an antibiotic is given to the patient immediately. The antibiotic selected is one that can best kill the microorganisms known to be the most common causes of infection. This type of treatment is called **empirical antibiotic therapy**. Before the start of empirical antibiotic therapy, specimens from suspected areas of infection should be cultured in an attempt to identify a causative organism. It must be emphasized that culture specimens should be obtained before drug therapy is initiated whenever possible. Otherwise, the presence of antibiotics in the tissues may result in misleading culture results. If an organism is identified in the laboratory, it is then tested for susceptibility to antibiotics. The results of these tests can confirm whether the empirical therapy chosen is appropriate for eradicating the organism identified. If not, therapy can be adjusted to optimize its efficacy against the specific infectious organism(s).

Antibiotics are also given for prophylaxis. This is often the case, for example, when patients are scheduled to have a procedure in which the likelihood of dangerous microbial contamination is high during or after the procedure. **Prophylactic antibiotic therapy** is used to prevent an infection. However, the risk of infection varies depending on the procedure being performed. For example, the risk of infection in a patient undergoing coronary artery bypass surgery (with standard preoperative

cleansing of the body) is relatively low compared with that in a person undergoing intra-abdominal surgery for the treatment of open wounds from a motor vehicle crash. In the latter case, contamination of the abdominal cavity with bacteria from the gastrointestinal tract is more likely to occur. This would constitute a contaminated, or "dirty," surgical field, and thus the likelihood of clinically serious infection would be much higher. Antibiotic therapy would likely be required for a longer period after the procedure.

To optimize antibiotic therapy, the patient should be continuously monitored for both **therapeutic** efficacy and adverse drug effects. A therapeutic response to antibiotics is one in which there is a decrease in the specific signs and symptoms of infection compared with the baseline findings (e.g., fever, elevated white blood cell [WBC] count, redness, inflammation, drainage, pain). Antibiotic therapy is said to be **subtherapeutic** when these signs and symptoms do not improve. This can result from use of an incorrect route of administration, inadequate drainage of an abscess, poor drug penetration to the infected area, insufficient serum levels of the drug, or bacterial resistance to the drug. Antibiotic therapy is considered toxic when the serum levels of the antibiotic are too high or when the patient has an allergic or other major adverse reaction to the drug. These reactions include rash, itching, hives, fever, chills, joint pain, difficulty breathing, or wheezing. Relatively minor adverse drug reactions such as gastrointestinal discomfort and diarrhea are quite common with antibiotic therapy and are usually not severe enough to require drug discontinuation.

Superinfections and antibiotic interactions with food and other drugs are other problems to watch for in patients taking antibiotics. **Superinfections** can occur when antibiotics reduce or completely eliminate the normal bacterial flora, which consists of certain bacteria and fungi that are needed to maintain normal function in organs. When these bacteria or fungi are killed by antibiotics, other bacteria or fungi are permitted to take over and cause infection. An example of a superinfection caused by antibiotics is the development of vaginal yeast infections when the normal vaginal bacterial flora are reduced and yeast growth is no longer kept in balance.

Another type of superinfection occurs when a second infection closely follows an initial primary infection from an external source (as opposed to normal body flora), which may still be ongoing. A common example is a case in which a patient who already has a viral respiratory infection develops a secondary bacterial infection, probably because of weakening of the patient's immune system function by the primary viral infection. Although the viral infection will not respond to antibiotic therapy, antibiotics may be needed to treat the secondary bacterial infection. This situation calls for some diagnostic finesse on the part of prescribers (physicians or nurse practitioners), who should avoid prescribing unnecessary antibiotics for a viral infection. The presence of coloured sputum (e.g., green or yellow) is one sign of a bacterial superinfection during a viral respiratory illness. Patients will often expect to receive an antibiotic prescription even when they show no signs of a bacterial superinfection. From their perspective, they know they are "sick" and want "some medicine" to expedite their recovery from illness. This expectation can create both diagnostic confusion and an emotional dilemma for the prescriber.

Over the decades since antibiotics were first developed in the 1940s, many formerly treatable bacterial infections have become increasingly resistant to antibiotic therapy. One major cause of this phenomenon is the overprescribing of antibiotics, often in the clinical situations described earlier. Antibiotic resistance is now considered one of the world's most pressing public health problems. *Emerging infections*, such as those with drug-resistant bacteria, are major culprits. Inappropriate antibiotic prescribing has had the effect of selecting out the most drug-resistant bacteria. Another factor that contributes to this problem is the tendency of many patients not to complete their antibiotic regimen. Patients should be counselled to take the entire course of prescribed antibiotic drugs, even if they feel that they are no longer ill. This increases the likelihood of a more complete bacterial kill, while reducing the chance of recurrent illness and survival of drug-resistant bacteria. The only usual exceptions are cases in which culture results indicate that the chosen antibiotic therapy is not ideal for a particular type of bacterial infection or major drug intolerance occurs. Patients should be educated as needed regarding such matters.

The chemical makeup of antibiotics can cause the body to react in many ways. Food–drug and drug–drug interactions are common problems when antibiotics are taken. One of the more common food–drug interactions is that between milk or cheese and tetracycline, which results in decreased gastrointestinal absorption of tetracycline. An example of a drug–drug interaction is that between quinolone antibiotics and antacids, resulting in decreased absorption of quinolones.

Other important factors that must be understood to use antibiotics appropriately are host-specific factors, or **host factors.** These are factors that pertain specifically to a given patient, and they can have an important impact on the success or failure of antibiotic therapy. Some of these host factors are age, allergy history, kidney and liver function, pregnancy, genetic characteristics, site of infection, and host defences.

Age-related host factors are those that apply to patients at either end of the age spectrum. For example, infants and children may not be able to take certain antibiotics such as tetracyclines, which affect developing teeth or bones; fluoroquinolones, which may affect bone or cartilage development in children; and sulfonamides, which may displace bilirubin from albumin and precipitate kernicterus (hyperbilirubinemia) in neonates. The aging process affects the functioning of organ systems. As people age, there is a gradual decline in the functioning of the kidneys and liver, the organs primarily responsible for metabolizing and eliminating antibiotics. Therefore, depending on the level of the kidney or liver function of an older adult, dosage adjustments may be necessary. Pharmacists often play a significant role in evaluating the dosages of antibiotics and other medications to ensure optimal dosing for a patient's level of organ function.

A patient history of allergic reaction to an antibiotic plays an important role and must also be considered in the selection of the most appropriate antibiotic for that patient selecting an antibiotic. Penicillins and sulfonamides are two broad classes of antibiotics to which many people have allergic anaphylactic reactions. The most dangerous of these reactions is anaphylactic shock, in which a patient can suffocate from drug-induced respiratory arrest. Although this outcome is the most extreme, the potential for it underscores the importance of consistently assessing patients for drug allergies and documenting any known allergies clearly in the medical record. All reported drug allergies should be taken seriously and investigated further before making a final decision about administering a given drug. Many patients will say that they are "allergic" to a drug when, in fact, what they have had was a common mild adverse effect such as stomach upset or nausea. Patients who report drug allergies should be asked open-ended questions to elicit descriptions of prior allergic reactions so that the actual severity of the reaction can be assessed. The most common severe reactions to any medication that need to be noted in the patient's chart include any difficulty breathing; significant rash, hives, or other skin reaction; and severe gastrointestinal intolerance. Although some antibiotics are ideally taken on an empty stomach, eating a small amount of food with the medication may be sufficient to help the patient tolerate it and realize its therapeutic benefits.

Pregnancy-related host factors are also important to the selection of appropriate antibiotics because several antibiotics can pass through the placenta and cause harm to the developing fetus. Drugs that cause development abnormalities in the fetus are called **teratogens**. Their use in pregnant women can result in birth defects.

Some patients have certain genetic abnormalities that result in enzyme deficiencies. These conditions can adversely affect drug actions in the body. Two of the most common examples of such genetic host factors are **glucose-6-phosphate dehydrogenase (G6PD) deficiency** and **slow acetylators.** The administration of antibiotics such as sulfonamides, nitrofurantoin, and dapsone to a person with G6PD deficiency may result in the hemolysis, or destruction, of red blood cells (RBCs). Patients who are slow acetylators have a physiological makeup that causes certain drugs to be metabolized more slowly than usual in a chemical step known as *acetylation.* This can lead to toxicity from drug accumulation. The most common example of such toxic effects is the development of a peripheral neuropathy in a patient who is a slow acetylator and is given typical adult dosages of the antituberculosis drug isoniazid (Chapter 41). Enzyme deficiencies such as G6PD deficiency are discussed in Chapter 2.

The anatomical site of the infection is another important host factor to consider when determining not only which antibiotic to use but also the dosage, route of administration, and duration of therapy.

Consideration of these host factors helps prescribers and pharmacists to ensure optimal drug selection for each patient. Continued patient assessment and proper monitoring of antibiotic therapy increase the likelihood that this therapy will be safe and effective.

ANTIBIOTICS

Antibiotics are classified into many broad categories on the basis of their chemical structures. Some of the more common of these categories are sulfonamides, penicillins, cephalosporins, macrolides, fluoroquinolones, aminoglycosides, and tetracyclines. In addition to chemical structure, the characteristics that distinguish one class of drugs from the next include antibacterial spectrum, mechanism of action, potency, toxicity, and pharmacokinetic properties. The four most common mechanisms of antibiotic action are interference with bacterial cell wall synthesis, interference with protein synthesis, interference with replication of nucleic acids (deoxyribonucleic acid [DNA]) and ribonucleic acid [RNA]), and antimetabolite action that disrupts critical metabolic reactions inside the bacterial cell. Figure 38-6 portrays these mechanisms of action in combating bacterial infections and indicates which mechanisms are used by several major antibiotic classes.

Perhaps the greatest challenge in understanding antimicrobial therapy is remembering the types and species of microorganisms against which a given drug can act. The list of individual microorganisms against which a given drug has activity can be quite extensive and can seem daunting to the inexperienced practitioner. Most antimicrobials have activity against only one *type* of microbe (e.g., bacteria, viruses, fungi, protozoans). However, a few drugs do have activity against more than

one class of organisms. Understanding antimicrobial therapy will deepen with clinical experience. The field of infectious disease treatment is continually evolving, largely because of the continual emergence of resistant bacterial strains. For this reason, drug indications change frequently, often from year to year, as bacterial species become resistant to previously effective anti-infective therapy. It is always appropriate to check the most current reference materials or consult with colleagues (e.g., nurses, pharmacists, physicians) when questions remain.

This chapter concentrates on the sulfonamides, penicillins, cephalosporins, carbapenems, monobactams, macrolides, and tetracyclines. The remaining antibiotic classes are discussed in Chapter 39.

SULFONAMIDES

Sulfonamides are a chemically related group of antibiotics that are all synthetic derivatives of sulfanilamide, the first sulfonamide to be discovered. They were one of the first groups of drugs used as antibiotics. Some of the commonly prescribed single-drug sulfonamides are sulfadiazine, sulfamethoxazole, and sulfisoxazole. However, in most cases, the sulfonamide is combined with another antibiotic known as trimethoprim for a synergistic drug effect. Sulfasalazine, another sulfonamide, is used to treat ulcerative colitis and rheumatoid arthritis and is not used as an antibiotic.

Mechanism of Action and Drug Effects

Sulfonamides do not actually destroy bacteria but inhibit their growth. For this reason, they are considered **bacteriostatic antibiotics.** They inhibit the growth of susceptible bacteria by preventing bacterial synthesis of folic acid, a B-complex vitamin that is required for the proper

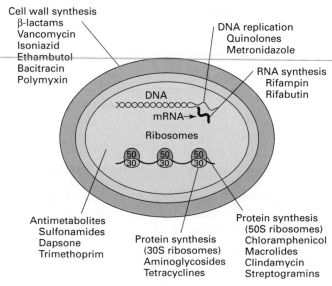

FIG. 38-6 Basic sites of antibiotic activity. (From Murray, P. R., Rosenthal, K. S., Kobayashi, G. S., & Pfaller, M. A. (2002). *Medical microbiology.* St. Louis, MO: Mosby.)

synthesis of purines, one of the chemical components of nucleic acids (DNA and RNA). Chemical components of folic acid include para-aminobenzoic acid (PABA), pteridine, and glutamic acid. Specifically, in a process known as competitive inhibition, sulfonamides compete with PABA for the bacterial enzyme tetrahydropteroic acid synthetase, which incorporates PABA into the folic acid molecule during biosynthesis. Because sulfonamides are capable of blocking a specific step in a biosynthetic pathway, they are also considered *antimetabolites*. However, those microorganisms that require exogenous folic acid (not synthesized by the bacterium itself) are not affected by sulfonamide antibiotics.

Trimethoprim is a nonsulfonamide antibiotic that is given in combination with sulfamethoxazole in the most common type of sulfonamide therapy. The resulting combination is called co-trimoxazole and is often abbreviated as SMX-TMP to reflect the generic names of the two component drugs. Although trimethoprim is also sometimes given as a single drug, sulfamethoxazole is currently available only in the combination drug co-trimoxazole. Trimethoprim blocks the action of bacterial tetrahydrofolate reductase, another enzyme required for bacterial folic acid synthesis. The step involving this enzyme occurs immediately after the step inhibited by sulfonamide drugs. Thus, when sulfamethoxazole and trimethoprim are given in combination, they inhibit two successive steps in the bacterial folic acid pathway. This action enables an additive antibacterial effect with greater anti-infective efficacy (e.g., against urinary tract infections [UTIs]).

In summary, microorganisms that synthesize their own folic acid are inhibited by sulfonamides. These drugs do not affect folic acid metabolism in human cells and cells of other organisms that require exogenous folic acid.

Indications

Sulfonamides have a broad spectrum of antibacterial activity, including activity against both gram-positive and gram-negative organisms. These antibiotics achieve high concentrations in the kidneys, through which they are eliminated. In particular, co-trimoxazole is often used in the treatment of UTIs. Commonly susceptible organisms include strains of *Enterobacter* species (spp.), *Escherichia coli*, *Klebsiella* spp., *Proteus mirabilis*, *Proteus vulgaris*, and *Staphylococcus aureus*. Unfortunately, resistant bacterial strains are a growing problem, as is the case with other antibiotic classes. Results of culture and sensitivity testing help optimize drug selection in individual cases. Co-trimoxazole is also used for treating respiratory tract infections. However, it is now less effective against streptococci infecting the upper respiratory tract and the pharynx. Another specific use for co-trimoxazole is prophylaxis and treatment of opportunistic infections in patients with pneumonia associated with human immunodeficiency virus [HIV] infection, especially infection by *Pneumocystis jirovecii* (formerly known as *Pneumocystis carinii*),

a common cause of HIV] (Chapter 40). There are also several less common uses for co-trimoxazole. The drug is used to treat nocardiosis, a bacterial infection caused by *Nocardia* spp. This infection usually occurs as pneumonia but can lead to skin and brain abscesses. Co-trimoxazole is also a drug of choice for infections caused by the bacterium *Stenotrophomonas maltophilia*. Although an uncommon infection, it is associated with prolonged hospitalization.

Contraindications

Use of sulfonamides is contraindicated in cases of known drug allergy to sulfonamides or to chemically related drugs such as the sulfonylureas (used to treat diabetes, Chapter 32), thiazide and loop diuretics, and carbonic anhydrase inhibitors (Chapter 26), and cyclooxygenase-2 inhibitors such as celecoxib (Chapter 45). Their use is also contraindicated in pregnant women at term and in infants younger than 2 months of age.

Adverse Effects

Sulfonamide drugs are a common cause of allergic reactions. Patients sometimes refer to this as "sulfa allergy" or even "sulfur allergy." Although immediate reactions can occur, sulfonamides typically cause delayed cutaneous reactions. Such reactions frequently begin with fever followed by a rash (morbilliform eruptions, erythema multiforme, or toxic epidermal necrolysis). Photosensitivity reactions are another type of skin reaction that is induced by exposure to sunlight during sulfonamide drug therapy. In some cases, such reactions can result in severe sunburn. These reactions are also common with the tetracycline class of antibiotics discussed later in this chapter, as well as with other drug classes (see Index) and may occur immediately or have a delayed onset. Other reactions to sulfonamides include mucocutaneous, gastrointestinal, liver, kidney, or hematological complications, all of which may be fatal in severe cases. It is believed that sulfonamide reactions are immune mediated and involve the production of reactive metabolites in the body.

It is important to differentiate between sulfites and sulfonamides. Sulfites are commonly used as preservatives in many products ranging from wine to food to injectable drugs. A person allergic to sulfonamide drugs may or may not also be allergic to sulfite preservatives. Sulfonamides should not be given to women at 32 weeks of pregnancy because of the possible association of severe jaundice leading to kernicterus (damage to the brain) in newborns. Reported adverse effects to the sulfonamides are listed in Table 38-1.

Interactions

Sulfonamides can have clinically significant interactions with a number of other medications. Sulfonamides can potentiate the hypoglycemic effects of sulfonylureas in diabetes, the toxic effects of phenytoin, and the anticoagulant effects of warfarin, which can lead to hemorrhage. There is also limited case-report evidence that

TABLE 38-1

Sulfonamides: Reported Adverse Effects

Body System	Adverse Effects
Blood	Agranulocytosis, aplastic anemia, hemolytic anemia, thrombocytopenia
Gastrointestinal	Nausea, vomiting, diarrhea, pancreatitis
Integumentary	Epidermal necrolysis, exfoliative dermatitis, Stevens–Johnson syndrome, photosensitivity
Other	Convulsions, crystalluria, toxic nephrosis, headache, peripheral neuritis, urticaria

sulfonamides can inhibit the immunosuppressant effects of cyclosporine used in patients who received a transplant and can also increase the likelihood of cyclosporine-induced nephrotoxicity. Patients receiving any of these drug combinations may require more frequent monitoring to ensure optimal drug effects. Sulfonamides may also reduce the efficacy of oral contraceptives. Patients should be advised to use additional contraceptive methods.

Dosages

For recommended dosages of selected sulfonamides, see the Dosages table below.

 DRUG PROFILES

Sulfonamides act by interfering with bacterial synthesis of the essential nutrient folic acid. Most sulfonamide therapy today uses the combination drug co-trimoxazole. However, a few other sulfonamide drugs remain on the market for specific uses. These include sulfadiazine (in opthalamic and topical formulations), sulfacetamide (in opthalamic formulations), sulfapyridine, and sulfisoxazole (with and without erythromycin).

sulfamethoxazole-trimethoprim (co-trimoxazole)

Co-trimoxazole (Apo-Sulfatrim, Novo-Trimel, Nu-Cotrimox, Septra Injection) is a fixed-combination drug product containing a 5:1 ratio of sulfamethoxazole to trimethoprim. It is available in both oral and injectable forms.

PHARMACOKINETICS

Half-Life	Onset	Peak	Duration
7–12 hr	Variable	2–4 hr (plasma)	Up to 12 hr

DOSAGES Selected Sulfonamides and Combination Drug Products

Drug (Pregnancy Category)	Pharmacological Class	Usual Dosage Range	Indications
*erythromycin/sulfisoxazole (Pediazole) (C)	Macrolide/ sulfonamide	*Children older than 2 mo only* PO: Fixed combination of erythromycin 200 mg and sulfisoxazole 600 mg/5 mL oral suspension Liquid dose range: 2.5–10 mL q6h based on weight	*Haemophilus influenzae, Streptococcus pneumoniae, Staphylococcus pyogenes, Branhamella catarrhalis* otitis media
*sulfamethoxazole-trimethoprim (co-trimoxazole), (Apo-Sulfatrim, Novo-Trimel, Nu-Cotrimox, Septra Injection) (C)	Sulfonamide and folate antimetabolite	*Children/Adult* IV: 5–20 mg/kg/day (trimethoprim component) divided bid–qid *Children* PO: 5–20 mg /kg/day (trimethoprim component) bid–qid *Adult* PO: 160 mg trimethoprim/800 mg sulfamethoxazole bid–qid	Meningitis, pyleonephritis, *Pneumocystis jirovecii* pneumonia, UTIs, acute exacerbation of chronic bronchitis UTIs, otitis media, sinusitis, *P. jirovecii* pneumonia *P. jirovecii* prophylaxis, otitis media, acute exacerbation of chronic bronchitis
sulfisoxazole (generic) (C)	Sulfonamide	*Children older than 2 mo* PO: 75 mg/kg load, then 150 mg/kg/day divided q4–6h *Adult* PO: 2–4 g load, then 4–8 g/day divided q4–6h	Otitis media, UTI, *Haemophilus influenzae* meningitis, nocardiosis, toxoplasmosis (with pyrimethamine)

IV, intravenous; *PO*, oral; *UTI*, urinary tract infection.

*Dosage ranges are typical but are not necessarily exhaustive because of space limitations. Clinical variations may occur.

β-LACTAM ANTIBIOTICS

β-lactam antibiotics are commonly used drugs, named because of the β-lactam ring that is part of the chemical structure (Figure 38-7). This broad group of drugs includes four major subclasses: penicillins, cephalosporins, carbapenems, and monobactams. Some bacterial strains produce the enzyme β-**lactamase**. This enzyme provides a mechanism for bacterial resistance to these antibiotics: the enzyme can break the chemical bond between the carbon (C) and nitrogen (N) atoms in the structure of the β-lactam ring. When this occurs, all β-lactam drugs lose their antibacterial efficacy. Thus, additional drugs known as β-**lactamase inhibitors** are added to the dosage forms of several different penicillin β-lactam antibiotics to make the drug more powerful against β-lactamase–producing bacterial strains. Each of the four classes of β-lactam antibiotics is examined in detail in the following sections.

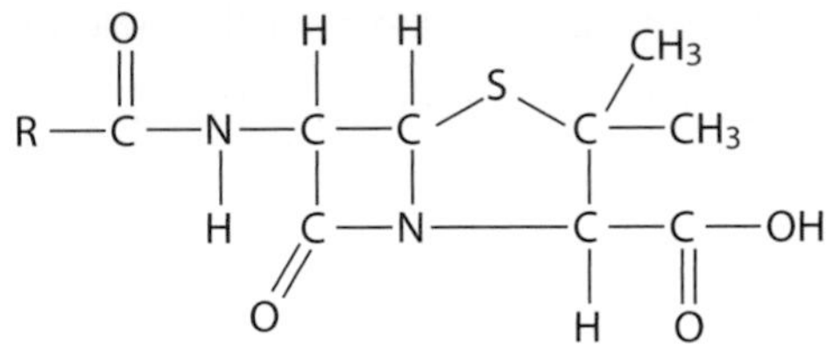

PENICILLINS

The penicillins are a large group of chemically related antibiotics that are derived from a mould fungus often seen on bread or fruit. The penicillins can be divided into four subgroups based on their structure (see Figure 38-7) and the spectrum of bacteria that they can kill: natural penicillins, penicillinase-resistant penicillins, aminopenicillins, and extended-spectrum penicillins. Examples of antibiotics in each subgroup and a brief description of their characteristics are given in Table 38-2.

Broad-spectrum natural penicillins were first introduced in the early 1940s during World War II, and to this day they have remained effective and safe antibiotics. They are **bactericidal antibiotics** and can kill a wide variety of gram-positive and some gram-negative bacteria. Penicillins act by inhibiting bacterial cell wall synthesis. However, some bacteria have acquired the capacity to produce β-lactamases capable of destroying penicillins. These enzymes can inactivate the penicillin molecules by opening

FIG. 38-7   Chemical structure of penicillins. *R,* Variable portion of drug chemical structure.

the β-lactam ring. There are many types of β-lactamase enzymes with differing abilities to resist β-lactam antibiotics. The β-lactamases that specifically inactivate penicillin molecules are called *penicillinases.* Bacterial strains that produce these drug-inactivating enzymes were a therapeutic obstacle until drugs were synthesized to inhibit these enzymes. Two of these β-lactamase inhibitors are clavulanic acid (also called *clavulanate*) and tazobactam. These drugs bind with the β-lactamase enzyme to prevent the enzyme from breaking down the penicillin molecule, although they are not always effective.

The following are examples of currently available combinations of penicillin and β-lactamase inhibitor:
- amoxicillin + clavulanic acid = Clavulin
- ticarcillin + clavulanic acid = Timentin
- piperacillin + tazobactam = Tazocin

Mechanism of Action and Drug Effects

The mechanism of action of penicillins involves the inhibition of bacterial cell wall synthesis. Once distributed by the patient's bloodstream to infected areas, penicillin molecules slide through the bacterial cell walls to arrive at their site of action. Some penicillins, however, are too large to pass through these openings in the cell walls, and because they cannot get to their site of action, they cannot kill the bacteria. By contrast, some bacteria can make the openings in their cell walls smaller so that the penicillin cannot gain entry to kill them. The penicillin molecules that do pass through into the bacteria must then find the appropriate binding sites. These are known as *penicillin-binding proteins.*

TABLE 38-2

Penicillin Classification

Subclass	Generic Drug Names	Description
Broad-spectrum	amoxicillin, ampicillin pivmecillinam	Have an amino group attached to the basic penicillin structure that enhances their activity against gram-negative bacteria compared with that of narrow-spectrum penicillins
Extended-spectrum	piperacillin, ticarcillin	Have wider spectra of activity than those of all other penicillins
Narrow-spectrum	penicillin G, penicillin V	Although many modifications of the original broad-spectrum natural (mould-produced) structure have been made, these are the only two in current clinical use. Penicillin G is the injectable form for IV or IM use; penicillin V is a PO dosage form (tablet and liquid).
Penicillinase-resistant	cloxacillin	Stable against hydrolysis by most staphylococcal penicillinases (enzymes that normally break down the broad-spectrum natural penicillins)

IM, intramuscular; *IV,* intravenous; *PO,* oral.

By binding to these proteins, the penicillin molecules interfere with the normal cell wall synthesis, causing the formation of defective cell walls that are unstable and easily broken down (see Figure 38-6). Bacterial death usually results from lysis (rupture) of the bacterial cells because of this drug-induced disruption of cell wall structure.

Indications

Penicillins are indicated for the prevention and treatment of infections caused by susceptible bacteria. The microorganisms most commonly destroyed by penicillins are gram-positive bacteria, including the *Streptococcus* spp., *Enterococcus* spp., and *Staphylococcus* spp. Most penicillins have little if any ability to kill gram-negative bacteria, although some of the extended-spectrum penicillins can do so.

Contraindications

Penicillins are usually safe and well-tolerated drugs. The only usual contraindication is known drug allergy.

Adverse Effects

Allergic reactions to penicillin occur in 0.7% to 4% of treatment courses. The most common reactions are urticaria, pruritus, and angioedema. A wide variety of idiosyncratic (unpredictable) drug reactions can occur, such as maculopapular eruptions, eosinophilia, Stevens–Johnson syndrome, and exfoliative dermatitis. Maculopapular rash occurs in approximately 2% of treatment courses with natural penicillin and in 5.2% to 9.5% with ampicillin. Anaphylactic reactions are much less common, occurring in 0.004% to 0.015% of patients. They are fatal in only 0.001% to 0.003% of cases (1 in 32,000 to 1 in 100,000 cases). Severe reactions are much more common with injected than with orally administered penicillin, as is the case with most other antibiotics that come in oral and injectable forms.

A common clinical scenario is one in which a prescriber wants to administer a cephalosporin to a patient reporting a penicillin allergy. Patients who are allergic to penicillins have a fourfold to sixfold increased risk of allergy to other β-lactam antibiotics. The incidence of cross-reactivity between cephalosporins and penicillins is reported as between 1% and 18%. Patients reporting penicillin allergy should be asked to describe their prior allergic reaction. The decision to continue with cephalosporin therapy in such cases is often a matter of clinical judgement, based on the severity of reported prior reactions to penicillin drugs, the nature of the infection and the drug susceptibility of the infective organism if known, and the availability and patient tolerance of other alternative antibiotics. Macrolide antibiotics, discussed later in this chapter, are a commonly used alternative class of medications for patients reporting allergy to penicillins or cephalosporins.

As mentioned earlier, penicillins are generally well tolerated and associated with few adverse effects. As with many drugs, the most common adverse effects involve the gastrointestinal system. The most common adverse effects of the penicillins are listed in Table 38-3.

TABLE 38-3

Penicillins: Reported Adverse Effects

Body System	Adverse Effects
Central nervous	Lethargy, hallucinations, anxiety, depression, twitching, coma, convulsions
Gastrointestinal	Nausea, vomiting, diarrhea, increased AST and ALT levels, abdominal pain, colitis
Hematological	Anemia, increased bleeding time, bone marrow depression, granulocytopenia
Metabolic	Hyperkalemia, hypokalemia, alkalosis
Other	Taste alterations; sore mouth; dark, discoloured, or sore tongue; hives; rash

ALT, alanine aminotransferase; *AST,* aspartate aminotransferase.

Interactions

Many drugs interact with penicillins; some have positive effects, while others have harmful effects. The most common and clinically significant drug interactions associated with penicillin use are listed in Table 38-4.

Dosages

For dosage information on selected penicillins, see the Dosages table on p. 718.

CEPHALOSPORINS

Cephalosporins are semisynthetic antibiotic derivatives of cephalosporin C, a substance produced by a fungus but synthetically altered to produce an antibiotic. These chemically altered derivatives of the fungus are structurally and pharmacologically related to penicillins. Similar to the penicillins, cephalosporins are bactericidal and act by interfering with bacterial cell wall synthesis. They also bind to the same penicillin-binding proteins inside bacteria that were described earlier for the penicillins. Although there are a variety of such proteins, they are collectively referred to as penicillin-binding regardless of the type of β-lactam drug involved.

Cephalosporins can destroy a broad spectrum of bacteria, and this ability is directly related to the chemical changes that have been made to their basic cephalosporin structure. Modifications to this chemical structure by pharmaceutical scientists have given rise to four generations of cephalosporins. Depending on the generation, these drugs may be active against gram-positive, gram-negative, or anaerobic bacteria. They are not active against fungi and viruses. The different drugs of each generation have certain chemical similarities, thus they can kill similar spectra of bacteria. In general, the level of gram-negative coverage increases with each successive generation. However, anaerobic coverage and gram-positive coverage are both more variable among the different generations. Cefepime is the only fourth-generation cephalosporin available in Canada, although some references classify cefepime with the other third-generation drugs. The currently

TABLE 38-4

Penicillins: Drug Interactions

Drug	Mechanism	Result
Aminoglycosides (IV)	Synergistic, but possible inactivation of penicillin by aminoglycosides if mixed in same IV bag	Reduced penicillin efficacy when mixed in same bag; mix drugs in separate IV bags, and, if using same IV line for both, flush line with normal saline between doses
Aminoglycosides (IV) and clavulanic acid	Additive	More effective killing of bacteria
Macrolides (e.g., erythromycin)	Uncertain	Have both synergism (which can be beneficial) and antagonism with penicillins (clinical judgement call)
neomycin (an oral aminoglycoside)	Reduced absorption of penicillin in gastrointestinal tract when both drugs are given orally	Reduced penicillin efficacy; avoid concurrent use or consider injectable penicillin instead
NSAIDs	Compete for protein binding	More free and active penicillin (may be beneficial)
Oral contraceptives	Uncertain	May decrease efficacy of the contraceptive
Potassium supplements, table salt	Penicillin G potassium has 1.7 mmol of potassium ion per million units; penicillin G sodium has 2 mmol of sodium ion per million units	Effects unlikely for most patients, but may precipitate or worsen hyperkalemia and hypernatremia; monitor sodium and potassium levels as needed in at-risk patients and choose alternative drugs if indicated
probenecid	Competes for elimination	Prolongs the effects of penicillins
rifampin	Inhibition	May inhibit the killing activity of penicillins
Tetracyclines	Uncertain	May reduce efficacy of penicillins; avoid concurrent use
warfarin	Reduced vitamin K from gut flora	Enhanced anticoagulant effect of warfarin

IV, intravenous; *NSAIDs*, nonsteroidal anti-inflammatory drugs.

 DRUG PROFILES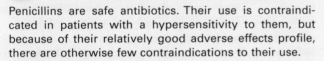

Penicillins are safe antibiotics. Their use is contraindicated in patients with a hypersensitivity to them, but because of their relatively good adverse effects profile, there are otherwise few contraindications to their use.

NATURAL PENICILLINS

▶▶ penicillin G and penicillin V potassium

Penicillin G has three salt forms: benzathine, potassium, and sodium. All of these forms are given by injection, either intravenously (IV) or intramuscularly (IM). The benzathine and procaine salts are used as longer-acting IM injections. They are formulated into a thick, white, pastelike material designed for prolonged dissolution and absorption from the IM site of injection. These preparations should never be given IV, however, because their consistency is too thick for IV administration; such use can be lethal. The IM formulations can be especially helpful for treating the sexually transmitted infection syphilis because often only one injection is needed, thus it can be given one time at a clinic that treats sexually transmitted infections.

Penicillin V potassium is available only for oral use.

PHARMACOKINETICS

Half-Life	Onset	Peak	Duration
30 min	Variable	30–60 min (plasma)	4–6 hr

PENICILLINASE-RESISTANT PENICILLINS

cloxacillin sodium

Cloxacillin sodium is the only penicillinase-resistant penicillin currently available in Canada. This penicillinase-resistant penicillin is able to resist breakdown by the penicillin-destroying enzyme (penicillinase) commonly produced by bacteria such as staphylococci. For this reason, such drugs may also be referred to as antistaphylococcal penicillins. The chemical structure of these drugs features a large, bulky side chain near the β-lactam ring. This side chain serves as a barrier to the penicillinase enzyme, preventing it from breaking the β-lactam ring, which would inactivate the drug. There are, however, certain strains of staphylococci, specifically *Staphylococcus aureus*, that are resistant to cloxacillin. Such bacteria require alternative antibiotic regimens.

Cloxacillin is available in oral and injectable forms.

PHARMACOKINETICS

Half-Life	Onset	Peak	Duration
20–30 min	Variable	30–60 min	6 hr (IV)

AMINOPENICILLINS

There are two aminopenicillins: amoxicillin and ampicillin. They are so named because of the presence of a free amino group ($-NH_2$) in their chemical structure. This structural feature gives aminopenicillins enhanced activity against gram-negative bacteria that the natural and penicillinase-resistant penicillins are relatively ineffective against. Amoxicillin is an analogue of ampicillin.

▶▶ amoxicillin

Amoxicillin (Amoxil, Novamoxin, others) is a commonly prescribed aminopenicillin. Amoxicillin is used to treat infections caused by susceptible organisms in the ears, nose, throat, genitourinary tract, skin, and skin structures.

Continued

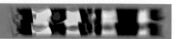

DRUG PROFILES (cont'd)

Pediatric dosages are sometimes higher than those used in the past because of the development of increasingly resistant *Streptococcus pneumoniae* organisms. The traditional adult dosage continues to be adequate in most cases. The drug is available only for oral use.

PHARMACOKINETICS

Half-Life	Onset	Peak	Duration
PO: 1–1.3 hr	PO: 0.5–1 hr	PO: 1–2 hr	PO: 6–8 hr

ampicillin

Ampicillin (generic) is the prototypical aminopenicillin. It differs from penicillin G only in that it has the amino group on its molecular structure. It is available in two different salt forms: trihydrate and sodium. As with penicillin G, each salt form allows it to be administered by a different route. Ampicillin trihydrate is administered orally, whereas ampicillin sodium is given parenterally. This drug is still currently available, although it is now used less frequently than before because many other newer drug options are being marketed to prescribers.

PHARMACOKINETICS

Half-Life	Onset	Peak	Duration
PO: 0.7–1.4 hr	PO: Variable	PO: 1–2 hr (serum)	PO: 4–6 hr

EXTENDED-SPECTRUM PENICILLINS

By making a few changes in the basic penicillin structure, drug developers have produced another generation of penicillins that have a wider spectrum of activity than that of either of the other two classes of semisynthetic penicillins (penicillinase-resistant penicillins and aminopenicillins) or of the natural penicillins. Currently, two extended-spectrum penicillins are available: piperacillin and pivmecillinam. Ticarcillin, also an extended-spectrum antibiotic, is only available as a combination drug product (described later).

These extended-spectrum drugs have activity against some bacteria that the other classes of penicillins cannot kill, such as the *Pseudomonas* spp. They also have stability against the β-lactamase enzymes produced by *Proteus* spp. Infections with both of these bacterial genera are generally among the more difficult infections to treat.

pivmecillinam hydrochloride and piperacillin sodium

Piperacillin is given only intravenously, whereas pivmecillinam is given only orally. The only usual contraindication is drug allergy. Both ticarcillin and piperacillin are available in fixed-combination products that include β-lactamase inhibitors. The ticarcillin fixed-combination product (Timentin) includes clavulanate potassium. Piperacillin is available in combination with with tazobactam (in a product called Tazocin). These β-lactamase–inhibiting products allow for enhanced multiorganism coverage, especially against anaerobic organisms that are common in intestinal infections.

PHARMACOKINETICS

pivmecillinam hydrochloride: 185 mg tablets

Half-Life	Onset	Peak	Duration
PO: 0.8–1 hr	PO: Variable	PO: 0.5–2 hr (serum)	PO: 6 hr

piperacillin sodium: 2, 3, and 4 g vials for injection

Half-Life	Onset	Peak	Duration
IV: 0.9–1.3 hr	IV: Variable	IV: 5 min (serum)	IV: Variable

DOSAGES Selected Penicillins

Drug (Pregnancy Category)	Pharmacological Class	Usual Dosage Range	Common Indications
amoxicillin (Amoxil, Novamoxin, others) (B)	Aminopenicillin	*Children older than 3 mo* PO: 20–90 mg/kg/day divided q8–12h *Adult* PO: 250 mg–2g q8–12h	Otitis media; sinusitis; susceptible respiratory, skin, and urinary tract infections; dental prophylaxis for bacterial endocarditis; *Helicobacter pylori* infection
ampicillin (generic) (B)	Aminopenicillin	*Children* 25–200 mg/kg/day divided q4–6h *Adult* PO/IV/IM: 1–14 g/day divided q4–6h	Primarily gram-negative infections such as *Shigella, Salmonella, Escherichia, Haemophilus, Proteus,* and *Neisseria* spp.; infection with some gram-positive organisms
cloxacillin sodium (generic only) (B)	Penicillinase-resistant penicillin	*Children* PO/IM/IV: 50–200 mg/kg/day divided q6–12h *Adult* PO/IM/IV: 250–500 mg q4–6h	Infection with penicillinase-producing staphylococci
penicillin V potassium (Penicillin V) (B)	Natural penicillin	*Children under 12 yr* PO: 150–500 mg in 3–6 divided doses IM/IV (children 1 mo– 12 yr): 25,000–400,000 units/kg/day, divided q4–6h *Children older than 12 yr/Adult* PO: 300 mg q6–8h IM/IV: 1–20 million units/day, divided q4–6h	Primarily infection with gram-positive organisms such as *Streptococcus* (including *Streptococcus pneumoniae*) and *Staphylococcus* spp.

IM, intramuscular; *IV,* intravenous; *PO,* oral; *spp.,* species.

available parenteral and oral cephalosporin antibiotics are listed in Table 38-5. As is often the case, injectable drugs produce higher serum concentrations than those administered by the oral route, and they are needed to treat more serious infections.

The safety profiles, contraindications, and pregnancy ratings of the cephalosporins are similar to those of the penicillins. The most commonly reported adverse effects include mild diarrhea, abdominal cramps, rash, pruritus, redness, and edema. Because cephalosporins are chemically similar to penicillins, a person who has had an allergic reaction to penicillin may also have an allergic reaction to a cephalosporin. This is referred to as *cross-sensitivity*. Investigators have observed that the incidence of cross-sensitivity between penicillins and cephalosporins is between 1% and 18%. However, only those patients who have had a serious anaphylactic reaction to penicillin should definitely not be given cephalosporins. As a class, the cephalosporins are safe and effective antibiotics, and

they should not be unnecessarily avoided out of over-cautiousness about possible cross-sensitivity.

Penicillins and cephalosporins are practically identical in their mechanisms of action, drug effects, therapeutic effects, adverse effects, and drug interactions. For this reason, this information is not repeated for the cephalosporins, and the reader is referred to the pertinent discussion in the Penicillins section. Cephalosporins of all generations are safe drugs. Their use is contraindicated in patients who have shown a hypersensitivity to them and any patient with a history of life-threatening allergic reaction to penicillins. Drug interactions are listed in Table 38-6. The prototypical first-, second-, third-, and fourth-generation cephalosporins are described in the following Drug Profiles section.

Dosages

For the recommended dosages of selected cephalosporin drugs, see the Dosages table on p. 722.

TABLE 38-5

Cephalosporins: Parenteral and Oral Preparations

First Generation		Second Generation		Third Generation		Fourth Generation	
IV	PO	IV	PO	IV	PO	IV	PO
cefazolin	cefadroxil	cefoxitin	cefaclor	cefotaxime	cefixime	cefepime	
	cephalexin	cefuroxime	cefuroxime	ceftazidime			
axetil*			axetil*				
			cefprozil	ceftriaxone			

IV, intravenous; *PO*, oral.

*Prodrug salts that aid in drug delivery into the gastrointestinal tract.

TABLE 38-6

Cephalosporins: Drug Interactions

Drug	Mechanism	Result
Aminoglycosides	Potentiation of nephrotoxic effect of aminoglycosides by cephalosporins (especially cephalothin)	Avoid concurrent use, but this is a clinical judgement call. Monitor patient's kidney function carefully if concurrent drug therapy is indicated
ethanol (alcohol)	Accumulation of acetaldehyde metabolite of ethanol	Acute alcohol intolerance (disulfiram-like reaction) after drinking alcoholic beverages within 72 hr of taking the following cephalosporins: cefazolin, cefmetazole, cefoperazone. Symptoms include stomach cramps, nausea, vomiting, diaphoresis, pruritus, headache, and hypotention.
Oral contraceptives (OCs)	Enhanced OC metabolism	Increased risk for unintended pregnancy
probenecid	Reduction of clearance of cephalosporins	No toxic effects reported

DRUG PROFILES

FIRST-GENERATION CEPHALOSPORINS

First-generation cephalosporins are usually active against gram-positive bacteria and have limited activity against gram-negative bacteria. They are available in

both parenteral and oral forms. Currently available first-generation cephalosporins include cefadroxil, cefazolin, and cephalexin.

Continued

DRUG PROFILES (cont'd)

▸▸ *cefazolin sodium*

Cefazolin sodium (generic only) is a prototypical first-generation cephalosporin. As with all first-generation cephalosporins, it provides excellent coverage against gram-positive bacteria but limited coverage against gram-negative bacteria. It is available only for parenteral use.

PHARMACOKINETICS

Half-Life	Onset	Peak	Duration
1.2–2.2 hr	Variable	1–2 hr	Variable

▸▸ *cephalexin*

Cephalexin (Keflex, Novo-Lexin, others) is a prototypical oral first-generation cephalosporin. It also provides excellent coverage against gram-positive bacteria but limited coverage against gram-negative bacteria. It is available only for oral use.

PHARMACOKINETICS

Half-Life	Onset	Peak	Duration
0.5–1.2 hr	Variable	1 hr	6–12 hr

SECOND-GENERATION CEPHALOSPORINS

Second-generation cephalosporins have coverage against gram-positive organisms that is similar to that of the first-generation cephalosporins but have enhanced coverage against gram-negative bacteria. Both parenteral and oral formulations are available. Like the first-generation drugs, second-generation cephalosporins are also excellent prophylactic antibiotics because of their favourable safety profile, the broad range of organisms they can kill, and the relatively low cost. Currently available second-generation cephalosporins include cefaclor, cefoxitin, cefuroxime, and cefprozil. These drugs differ slightly with regard to their antibacterial coverage. Cefoxitin may have better coverage against anaerobic bacteria such as *Bacteroides fragilis*, *Peptostreptococcus* spp., and *Clostridium* spp. than the other drugs in this class. Cefoxitin differs structurally from the other drugs in the class by having a methoxy group rather than a hydrogen group on the β-lactam ring of the cephalosporin nucleus. These drugs are called *cephamycins*. Their unique structure enables them to kill certain bacteria known as anaerobes that the other second-generation drugs cannot.

▸▸ *cefoxitin sodium*

Cefoxitin sodium (generic only) is a parenteral second-generation cephalosporin. It has excellent gram-positive coverage and better gram-negative coverage than the first-generation drugs. Because it is a cephamycin, it can also kill anaerobic bacteria. Cefoxitin has been used extensively as a prophylactic antibiotic in patients undergoing abdominal surgery because it can effectively kill intestinal bacteria. Normal intestinal flora include gram-positive, gram-negative, and anaerobic bacteria. Cefoxitin is available only in injectable form.

PHARMACOKINETICS

Half-Life	Onset	Peak	Duration
30–60 min	Variable	20–30 min	Variable

cefuroxime sodium

Cefuroxime sodium (generic only) is the parenteral form of this second-generation cephalosporin. The oral form is a different salt of cefuroxime, cefuroxime axetil (Ceftin). Cefuroxime is a versatile second-generation cephalosporin. It is also widely used as a prophylactic antibiotic for surgical procedures. It has more activity against gram-negative bacteria than do first-generation cephalosporins but a narrower spectrum of activity against gram-negative bacteria than do third-generation cephalosporins. It differs from the cephamycins such as cefoxitin in that it does not kill anaerobic bacteria. Cefuroxime axetil is a prodrug. It has little antibacterial activity until it is hydrolyzed in the liver to its active cefuroxime form. It is available only for oral use. Cefuroxime sodium is available only in injectable form.

PHARMACOKINETICS

Half-Life	Onset	Peak	Duration
1.2 hr	Variable	2.2–3 hr	6–8 hr

THIRD-GENERATION CEPHALOSPORINS

The currently available third-generation cephalosporins include cefotaxime, cefixime, ceftazidime, and ceftriaxone. These are the most potent of the three generations of cephalosporins in fighting gram-negative bacteria, but they generally have less activity than first- and second-generation drugs against gram-positive organisms. As with all of the different classes of both penicillins and cephalosporins, slight modifications in the chemical structure have endowed specific drugs with certain advantages over the others against some bacteria.

Because of specific changes in its basic cephalosporin structure, ceftazidime has significant activity against *Pseudomonas* spp. In fact, this third-generation drug has the best activity of all the cephalosporins against this gram-negative bacterium that is notoriously difficult to treat. Cefixime is currently the only third-generation cephalosporin available for oral use. All the other third-generation drugs are only available in parenteral forms.

ceftazidime pentahydrate

Ceftazidime pentahydrate (Fortaz) is a parenterally administered third-generation cephalosporin with excellent coverage against difficult-to-treat gram-negative bacteria such as *Pseudomonas* spp. It is the third-generation cephalosporin of choice for many indications because of its excellent spectrum of activity and safety profile. It is available only in injectable form. One idiosyncrasy of this particular drug is that gas builds up in the medication vial when its powder is reconstituted with diluent. The quantity of gas produced can be so great that it expels the needle right out of the vial.

Continued

DRUG PROFILES (cont'd)

PHARMACOKINETICS

Half-Life	Onset	Peak	Duration
2 hr	Variable	1 hr	8–12 hr

▶▶ ceftriaxone sodium

Ceftriaxone sodium (Rocephin) is an extremely long-acting third-generation drug that can be given only once a day in the treatment of most infections. It also has the unique characteristic of being able to pass easily through the blood–brain barrier. For this reason, it is one of the few cephalosporins that is indicated for the treatment of meningitis, an infection of the meninges of the brain.

Structurally, it resembles other third-generation drugs such as cefotaxime, but it has an acidic enol group that distinguishes it from these other drugs. This is believed to be responsible for the long serum half-life of the drug. It can be given both IV and IM. In some cases of infection, one IM injection can eradicate the infection. Ceftriaxone is 93% to 96% bound to plasma protein, a proportion higher than that of many of the other cephalosporins. This drug is also unique in that its elimination is primarily hepatic. For this reason, it should not be given to neonates with hyperbilirubemia or to patients with severe liver dysfunction. This drug is only available for injection.

PHARMACOKINETICS

Half-Life	Onset	Peak	Duration
4.3–8.7 hr	Variable	IM: 2–4 hr	24 hr

FOURTH-GENERATION CEPHALOSPORINS

There is currently one fourth-generation cephalosporin: cefepime. Some references classify this drug with the third-generation drugs. Cefepime has a broader spectrum of antibacterial activity, especially against gram-positive bacteria, than do the third-generation drugs. It may also be more resistant to β-lactamase enzymes.

cefepime hydrochloride

Cefepime hydrochloride (Maxipime) is the prototypical fourth-generation cephalosporin. Cefepime is a broad-spectrum cephalosporin that most closely resembles ceftazidime in its spectrum of activity. It differs from ceftazidime in that it has increased activity against many *Enterobacter* spp. (gram-negative) as well as gram-positive organisms. Cefepime is indicated for the treatment of uncomplicated and complicated UTIs, uncomplicated skin and skin structure infections, and pneumonia. Cefepime is available only in injectable form.

PHARMACOKINETICS

Half-Life	Onset	Peak	Duration
2 hr	0.5 hr	0.5–1.5 hr	8–12 hr

Carbapenems

Carbapenems have among the broadest antibacterial action of any antibiotics to date. Because of this, they are often reserved for complicated body cavity and connective tissue infections in acutely ill hospitalized patients.

One hazard of carbapenem use is drug-induced seizure activity, which occurs in a relatively small percentage of patients but is obviously undesirable and explains why carbapenem therapy is not normally the first-line drug therapy. However, the risk of seizures can be reduced by proper dosage adjustment in truly impaired patients. Currently available carbapenems include imipenem-cilastatin, meropenem, and ertapenem.

▶▶ imipenem-cilastatin

Imipenem-cilastatin (Primaxin) is a fixed combination of imipenem, which is a semisynthetic carbapenem antibiotic similar to β-lactam antibiotics, and cilastatin, an inhibitor of an enzyme that breaks down imipenem. Imipenem has a wide spectrum of activity against gram-positive and gram-negative aerobic and anaerobic bacteria. Cilastatin is a unique drug in that it inhibits an enzyme in the kidneys called *dihydropeptidase*, which would otherwise quickly break down the imipenem. Cilastatin also blocks the kidney tubular secretion of imipenem, which prevents imipenem from being excreted from the kidneys, the primary route of excretion of the drug.

Imipenem-cilastatin exerts its antibacterial effect by binding to penicillin-binding proteins inside bacteria, which, in turn, inhibits bacterial cell wall synthesis. It also kills bacteria and is therefore bactericidal. Unlike many of the penicillins and cephalosporins, imipenem-cilastatin is resistant to the antibiotic-inhibiting actions of β-lactamases. Drugs with which it potentially interacts include cyclosporine, ganciclovir, and probenecid, all of which may potentiate the CNS adverse effects (including seizures) of imipenem. Concurrent use with these drugs should be avoided whenever clinically feasible. The most serious adverse effect associated with imipenem-cilastatin therapy is seizures, which have been reported to occur in up to 1.5% of patients receiving more than 500 mg every 6 hours. In patients receiving high dosages of the drug (more than 500 mg every 6 hours), however, there is about a 10% incidence of seizures. Seizures are more likely in the older adult and in patients with renal disease. Seizures have also been associated with the use of both meropenem and ertapenem, but data suggest that they are less likely to occur than with imipenem-cilastatin.

Imipenem-cilastatin is indicated for the treatment of bone, joint, skin, and soft tissue infections; bacterial endocarditis caused by *S. aureus*; intra-abdominal bacterial infections; pneumonia; UTIs and pelvic infections; and bacterial septicemia caused by susceptible bacterial organisms. All dosage forms contain the same number of milligrams of both imipenem and cilastatin.

meropenem and ertapenem

Meropenem (Merrem) is the second drug in the carbapenem class of antibiotics. Compared with imipenem-cilastatin, meropenem appears to be somewhat less active against gram-positive organisms, more active against Enterobacteriaceae, and equally active against

Continued

DRUG PROFILES (cont'd)

Pseudomonas aeruginosa. However, meropenem is the only carbapenem currently indicated for the treatment of bacterial meningitis.

The newest carbapenem is ertapenem (Invanz), which has a spectrum of activity comparable with that of imipenem-cilastatin, although it is not active against *Enterococcus* or *Pseudomonas* spp. Note that only imipenem is combined with the dehydropeptidase inhibitor cilastatin. Neither meropenem nor ertapenem is susceptible to this bacterial enzyme, which gives these drugs one advantage over imipenem-cilastatin.

PHARMACOKINETICS (CARBAPENEMS)

Half-Life	Onset	Peak	Duration
2–3 hr	Variable	2 hr	6–8 hr

MONOBACTAMS

Monobactams are synthetic β-lactam antibiotics that are primarily active against aerobic gram-negative bacteria, including *E. coli*, *Klebsiella* spp., and *Pseudomonas* spp. Currently, there are no monobactam antibiotics marketed in Canada.

DOSAGES   Selected Cephalosporins

Drug (Pregnancy Category)	Pharmacological Class	Usual Dosage Range	Indications
▶▶ **cefazolin sodium (generic) (B)**	First-generation cephalosporin	*Children* IM/IV: 25–100 mg/kg/day divided q6–8h *Adult* IM/IV: 1–2 g q8h	Comparable with those for cephalexin, plus active against some penicillinase-producing and more gram-negative organisms; preoperative and postoperative prophylaxis
cefepime hydrochloride (Maxipime) (B)	Fourth-generation cephalosporin	*Children 2 mo–12 yr* IV: 50 mg/kg q8–12h *Children 12 yr and older (weighing more than 40 kg)/Adult* IM/IV: 0.5–2 g q8–12 h	Comparable with those for cefditoren, plus provides more extensive coverage of gram-negative organisms, including those causing intra-abdominal infections
▶▶ **cefoxitin sodium (generic) (B)**	Second-generation cephalosporin	*Children 3 mo and older* IV/IM: 80–160 mg/kg/day divided q4–6h, not to exceed 12 g/day *Adult* IM/IV: 1–2 g/day q8–12h; max 12 g/day	Less coverage of gram-positive organisms, greater coverage of gram-negative and anaerobic organisms; preoperative and postoperative prophylaxis
ceftazidime pentahydrate (Fortaz) (B)	Third-generation cephalosporin	*Children* IM/IV: 25–50 mg/kg/day q8–12h *Adult* IM/IV: 250–2000 mg q8–12h	More extensive coverage of gram-negative organisms, including *Pseudomonas* spp.
▶▶ **ceftriaxone sodium (Rocephin, generic) (B)**	Third-generation cephalosporin	*Children* IM/IV: 50–100 mg/kg/day once–bid *Adult* IM/IV: 1–2 g/day once–bid	Comparable with those for ceftazidime; postexposure prophylaxis for meningococcal meningitis, Lyme disease
cefuroxime sodium (Zinacef); ceruroxime axetil* (Ceftin, tablet form) (B)	Second-generation cephalosporin	*Children 3 mo–12 yr* PO oral suspension: 10–15 mg/kg/day divided bid *Adult 12 yr and older* PO (tabs): 250–500 mg bid *Children 1 mo–12 yr* IM/IV: 30–240 mg/kg/day, divided q6–8h *Adult* IM/IV: 750–3000 mg q8h	Comparable with those for cephalexin, plus provides more coverage of gram-negative organisms
▶▶ **cephalexin (Keflex, Novo-Lexin, others) (B)**	First-generation cephalosporin	*Children* PO: 25–100 mg/kg/day, divided q6h bid *Adult* PO: 250–500 mg bid	Infections of respiratory and GU tracts, skin, and bone; otitis media caused by susceptible gram-positive and gram-negative organisms

GI, gastrointestinal; *GU*, genitourinary; *IM*, intramuscular; *IV*, intravenous; *PO*, oral; *spp.*, species.

*Cefuroxime axetil and cefditoren pivoxil are both prodrugs for PO use that are hydrolyzed into the active ingredient in the fluids of the gastrointestinal tract.

MACROLIDES

Macrolides are a large group of antibiotics that first became available in the early 1950s with the introduction of erythromycin. Macrolides are considered bacteriostatic; however, in high enough concentrations they may be bactericidal to some susceptible bacteria. There are three main macrolide antibiotics: azithromycin, clarithromycin, and erythromycin. Azithromycin and clarithromycin are two of the newer drugs in the class and, together with the original drug, erythromycin, are currently the most widely used of the macrolides. Although the spectra of antibacterial activities of both azithromycin and clarithromycin are similar to that of erythromycin, the former have longer durations of action, which allows them to be given less often. They produce fewer and milder gastrointestinal adverse effects than does erythromycin, and azithromycin is usually dosed over a shorter length of time than many of the erythromycin products. They also exhibit better efficacy in eradicating some species of bacteria and are capable of better tissue penetration. Because erythromycin has a bitter taste and is quickly degraded by the acidity of the stomach, several salt forms and many dosage formulations have been developed to circumvent these problems. The salts and dosage formulations and the benefits of each are briefly summarized in Table 38-7.

Mechanism of Action and Drug Effects

The mechanism of action of macrolide antibiotics is similar to that of other antibiotics. They work by inhibiting protein synthesis in susceptible bacteria. For this synthesis to occur, transfer RNA must bind to the messenger RNA ribosome. The macrolides obstruct this synthesis by binding to the portion of the ribosome called the *50S* subunit inside the cells of bacteria. This prevents the production of the bacterial protein needed for the bacteria to grow, and so they eventually die (see Figure 38-6). This action

TABLE 38-7	
Erythromycin Formulations	
Formulation	**Benefit**
SALT FORMS	
Estolate	Developed to overcome bitter
Ethylsuccinate ester	taste of erythromycin
Stearate salt	
DOSAGE FORMULATION	
Enteric coated (pellets and particles)	Developed to overcome bitter taste and to protect erythromycin from acid degradation in the stomach
Film coated	
STRUCTURAL CHANGES	
Semisynthetic Macrolides	
Azide group (azithromycin)	Developed to improve resistance to acid degradation in the stomach and increase
Methylation of hydroxyl group (clarithromycin)	tissue penetration to improve antibiotic efficacy

can immediately kill some susceptible strains of bacteria if the concentration of the macrolide is high enough. Macrolides are effective in the treatment of a wide range of infections. These include infections of the upper and lower respiratory tract, skin, and soft tissue caused by some strains of *Streptococcus* and *Haemophilus*; spirochetal infections such as syphilis and Lyme disease; gonorrhea; and *Chlamydia, Mycoplasma,* and *Corynebacterium* infections. Gonorrheal infections have become increasingly difficult to treat with macrolide monotherapy, so these drugs are sometimes used in combination with other antibiotics such as cephalosporins.

Because of its gastrointestinal tract–irritating properties, erythromycin affects the motility of the gastrointestinal tract. This characteristic has been studied experimentally and may prove to be of benefit in increasing gastrointestinal motility in conditions such as delayed gastric emptying in patients with diabetes (known as diabetic gastroparesis). Macrolides are also somewhat unique among antibiotics in that they are especially effective against several bacterial species that often reproduce inside host cells instead of just in the bloodstream or interstitial spaces. Common examples of such bacteria, some of which were previously listed, are *Listeria, Chlamydia, Legionella* (one species of which causes Legionnaire's disease), *Neisseria* (one species of which causes gonorrhea), and *Campylobacter.*

Indications

The therapeutic effects of macrolide antibiotics are mostly limited to their antibacterial actions. Infections caused by *Streptococcus pyogenes* (group A β-hemolytic streptococci) are inhibited by macrolides, as are mild to moderate upper and lower respiratory tract infections caused by *Haemophilus influenzae.* Spirochetal infections treated with erythromycin and other macrolides are syphilis and Lyme disease. Various forms of gonorrhea and *Chlamydia* and *Mycoplasma* infections are also susceptible to the effects of macrolides.

As previously noted, a therapeutic effect of erythromycin outside its antibiotic actions is its ability to irritate the gastrointestinal tract, which stimulates smooth muscle and gastrointestinal motility. This action may be of benefit to patients who have decreased gastrointestinal motility. It has also been shown to be helpful in facilitating the passage of feeding tubes from the stomach into the small bowel. Azithromycin and clarithromycin have both been recently approved for the treatment of *Mycobacterium avium-intracellulare complex* infections. This is a common *opportunistic infection* often associated with HIV/AIDS (Chapter 40). Clarithromycin also has another new indication: is has been approved for use in combination with omeprazole for the treatment of patients with active ulcer associated with *Helicobacter pylori* infection.

Contraindications

The only usual contraindication to macrolide use is known drug allergy. In fact, as indicated earlier, macrolides are often used as alternative drugs for patients with allergies to β-lactam antibiotics.

Adverse Effects

Many of the older macrolide products, primarily erythromycin formulations, have a number of adverse effects. Most of these affect the gastrointestinal tract, although the two newest macrolides, azithromycin and clarithromycin, seem to be associated with a lower incidence of these gastrointestinal tract complications. Reported adverse effects are listed in Table 38-8.

Interactions

There are a number of potential drug interactions with the macrolides. Examples of some especially common drugs that compete for liver metabolism with the macrolides are carbamazepine, cyclosporine, digoxin, theophylline, and warfarin. When these drugs are given with macrolides, the results are enhanced effects and possible toxicity of the second drug. Azithromycin is not as prone to such interactions as are other macrolides because of its minimal effects on the cytochrome P450 enzymes in the liver. These drug combinations should be avoided when possible. When a macrolide is given together with any of these drugs, the patient should be observed for signs of drug toxicity, and appropriate laboratory measurements (e.g., blood drug levels) should be conducted as indicated. These interactions may occasionally be beneficial by allowing smaller dosages of the interacting drugs to be given and thereby reducing the likelihood of other worse adverse effects.

Two properties of macrolides that are the source of many of these interactions are that they are highly protein bound and they are metabolized in the liver. Drugs that are bound to protein are usually bound to albumin in the blood, making them inactive. When they are

TABLE 38-8

Macrolides: Reported Adverse Effects

Body System	Adverse Effects
Cardiovascular	Palpitations, chest pain
Central nervous	Headache, dizziness, vertigo, somnolence
Gastrointestinal	Nausea, hepatotoxicity, heartburn, vomiting, diarrhea, stomatitis, flatulence, cholestatic jaundice, anorexia
Integumentary	Rash, pruritus, urticaria, thrombophlebitis (at intravenous site)
Other	Hearing loss, tinnitus

displaced from these binding sites on albumin and are then free and unbound, they become active. Therefore, when a patient is given two or more drugs that compete for the same binding sites on albumin in the blood, one will not bind successfully, but will circulate in the blood as free drug and remain active. That drug will then have a greater effect in the body. For drugs metabolized by the liver, drug interactions commonly arise from competition between the different drugs for metabolic enzymes, specifically the *cytochrome P450 complex*. Such enzymatic effects generally lead to more pronounced drug interactions than does competition for protein binding. The result is a delay in the metabolic clearance of one or more interacting drugs and thus a prolonged and possibly toxic drug effect. Macrolides can also reduce the efficacy of oral contraceptives.

Dosages

For dosage information on selected macrolide antibiotics, see the Dosages table on p. 725.

 DRUG PROFILES

Macrolide antibiotics are used to treat a variety of infections ranging from Lyme disease to Legionnaire's disease. Of the three macrolide drugs currently available, erythromycin has been available for the longest period and has provided the anchor of treatment for various infections for more than four decades. Azithromycin and clarithromycin have fewer adverse effects and better pharmacokinetics profiles than those of the older drugs.

Macrolides use is contraindicated in patients with known drug allergy. As previously noted, because macrolides are significantly protein bound to varying degrees and are metabolized in the liver, they may interact with other drugs that are also highly protein bound or metabolized in the liver.

▶▶ erythromycin

Erythromycin, which has many product names, was for many years the most commonly prescribed macrolide antibiotic. However, other macrolides are now more commonly used. The drug is available in several different salt and dosage forms for oral use that were developed to circumvent some of the chmical disadvantages. (These benefits are summarized in Table 38-7.) A parenteral form is available for intravenous use. Erythromycin is also available in topical forms for dermatological use (Chapter 57) and in ophthalmic dosage forms (Chapter 58). The absorption of oral erythromycin is enhanced if it is taken on an empty stomach, but because of the high incidence

Continued

DRUG PROFILES (cont'd)

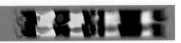

of stomach irritation associated with its use, many of these drugs are taken after a meal or snack. Erythromycin is classified as pregnancy category B. The salt forms and dosage formulations, their strengths, and product names are listed in Table 38-9.

▶▶ azithromycin and clarithromycin

Azithromycin (Zithromax) and clarithromycin (Biaxin) are semisynthetic macrolide antibiotics that differ structurally from erythromycin and, as a result, have several advantages over erythromycin. These include better adverse effect profiles, including less gastrointestinal tract irritation, and more favourable pharmacokinetic properties. Both have a similar range of activity that differs only slightly from that of erythromycin. The two drugs are used for the treatment of both upper and lower respiratory tract and skin structure infections.

Azithromycin has excellent tissue penetration, so it can reach high concentrations in infected tissues. It also has a long duration of action, which allows it to be dosed once daily. Taking the drug with food decreases both the rate and extent of gastrointestinal absorption. The drug is available in oral and injectable forms.

Clarithromycin can be given only twice daily and is recommended for use in adults and children 12 years of age and older. Its safety and efficacy in younger patients has not been established. It is also available only for oral use.

PHARMACOKINETICS

azithromycin

Half-Life	Onset	Peak	Duration
PO: 6–8 hr	PO: Variable	PO: 2.5 hr	PO: Up to 24 hr

clarithromycin

Half-Life	Onset	Peak	Duration
3–7 hr	Variable	2 hr	Up to 12 hr

DOSAGES   Selected Macrolides and Ketolides

Drug (Pregnancy category)	Pharmacological Class	Usual Dosage Range	Indications
▶▶ azithromycin (Zithromax) (B)	Semisynthetic macrolide	*Children* PO: 30 mg/kg × 1 dose or 10 mg/kg/day × 3 days or 10 mg/kg × 1 dose, then 5 mg/kg/day × 4 days *Adult older than 16* PO: 500 mg × 1 dose, then 250 mg/day × 4 days PO: 500 mg daily × 3 days, or 2 g × 1 dose	Comparable with those for erythromycin, but especially GU and respiratory tract infections, including MAC infections
▶▶ clarithromycin (Biaxin) (C)	Semisynthetic macrolide	*Children* PO: 15 mg/kg/day bid (max 500 mg/dose) *Adult* PO: 250–500 mg q12h	Comparable with erythromycin, but especially GI and respiratory tracts, including MAC infections
▶▶ erythromycin (generic) (B)	Natural macrolide	*Children** 30–100 mg/kg/day divided q6h *Adult** PO: 250–500 mg q6h	Infections of respiratory and GI tracts and skin caused by gram-positive, gram-negative, and miscellaneous organisms
telithromycin (Ketek) (C)	Ketolide	*Children 13 yr and older only/Adult* PO: 800 mg once daily × 5–10 days	CAP, bacterial sinusitis, and exacerbations of chronic bronchitis

CAP, community-acquired pneumonia; *GI*, gastrointestinal; *GU*, genitourinary; *MAC, Mycobacterium avium* complex; *PO*, oral.

*There are many types of dosage forms, and dosages may vary from those listed.

 ## DRUG PROFILES

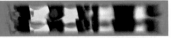

telithromycin

Telithromycin (Ketek) is currently the only drug in a new class known as ketolides. It is derived from erythromycin A and has better acid stability and better antibacterial coverage compared with macrolides. Its mechanism of

action is also similar to that of macrolides—that is, inhibition of bacterial protein synthesis by binding to the 50S ribosomal subunit. The drug is active against the majority of gram-positive bacteria, including multidrug-resistant

Continued

DRUG PROFILES (cont'd)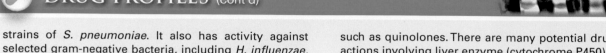

strains of *S. pneumoniae*. It also has activity against selected gram-negative bacteria, including *H. influenzae*, *Moraxella catarrhalis*, and *Bordetella pertussis*. It is indicated for treatment of community-acquired pneumonia, acute bacterial sinusitis, and bacterial exacerbations of chronic bronchitis.

Telithromycin is available only for oral use. For dosage information, see the Dosages table on p. 725.

Use of this drug is contraindicated in cases of drug allergy. Adverse reactions are similar to those of macrolide antibiotics and include headache, dizziness, gastrointestinal discomfort, hypokalemia or hyperkalemia, and prolongation of the QT interval on the electrocardiogram. Avoidance of the drug is recommended in patients with a history of heart disease that already includes prolonged QT interval, bradycardia, or electrolyte disturbances, and in those receiving antidysrhythmic drugs (Chapter 23) or other drugs known to prolong the QT interval

such as quinolones. There are many potential drug interactions involving liver enzyme (cytochrome P450) effects, which can increase or decrease the concentrations (and therefore the effectiveness) of either drug. Some of the interacting drugs are benzodiazepines, calcium channel blockers, cyclosporine, statins (for hypercholesterolemia), antidepressants, protease inhibitors (for HIV), doxycycline, erythromycin, verapamil, and imatinib (an antineoplastic [Chapters 48 and 49]). In complicated cases, a clinical pharmacist will be asked to evaluate complex medication regimens and make recommendations to the prescriber regarding the safest and most effective drug combinations and dosages.

PHARMACOKINETICS

Half-Life	Onset	Peak	Duration
9–10 hr	Unknown	1 hr	Unknown

TABLE 38-9

Erythromycin Dosage Forms and Product Names

Dosage Form Name	Strength	Product Name
ERYTHROMYCIN BASE (PO)		
Capsules		
Delayed-release (enteric-coated)	250 mg and 333 mg	Apo-Erythro E-C, Eryc
Tablets	250, 333, 500, and 600 mg	Nu-Erythromycin-S, PCE Tab, Erythro-Base Tab, Erythro-ES, E.E.S. 600, Erythromycine, Erybid
Capsules		
Delayed-release (enteric-coated pellets)	250 and 333 mg	Eryc
ERYTHROMYCIN ESTOLATE (PO)		
Oral suspension	250 mg/5 mL	Novo-Rythro
ERYTHROMYCIN ETHYLSUCCINATE (PO)		
Tablets		
Film-coated	600 mg	Apo Erythro-ES tab
Powder for oral suspension	40 mg/mL and 200 and 400 mg/5 mL	Novo-Rythro, EryPed 200, E.E.S. 200 Granules, EryPed 400
ERYTHROMYCIN LACTOBIONATE		
Intravenous	500 and 1 g	erythromycin lactobionate (generic only)
ERYTHROMYCIN STEARATE (PO)		
Tablets		
Film-coated	250 and 500 mg	Nu-Erythromycin-S, Erythro-500
Oral suspension	50 mg/mL	Erythrocin

TETRACYCLINES

The tetracyclines are a small chemically related group of three antibiotics, one of which is naturally occurring and two of which are semisynthetic. They are derivatives of *Streptomyces* organisms. Although the tetracyclines are bacteriostatic, the body's own host defence mechanisms assist in killing the bacteria as well. The naturally occurring tetracycline is oxytetracycline, and the two semisynthetic tetracyclines are doxycycline and minocycline. The available tetracycline antibiotics and brief descriptions of them are given in Table 38-10.

Tetracyclines are chemically and pharmacologically similar to one another. The most significant chemical characteristic of these drugs is their ability to chelate (combine with) divalent (Ca^2, Mg^2) and trivalent (Al^3) metallic ions to form insoluble complexes. Therefore, when coadministered with milk, antacids, or iron salts, their oral absorption is considerably reduced. In addition, their strong affinity for calcium usually precludes their use in children younger than 8 years of age because they can result in significant tooth discoloration. Tetracyclines should also be avoided in pregnant women and nursing mothers. The drugs pass into breast milk;

TABLE 38-10	
Available Tetracycline Antibiotics	
Generic Name	**Description**
NATURAL TETRACYCLINES	
tetracycline	Chemically derived from *Streptomyces* spp. by a fermentation process
SEMISYNTHETIC TETRACYCLINES	
doxycycline	Chemical derivative of oxytetracycline
minocycline	Chemical derivative of tetracycline

this can be another route of exposure leading to tooth discoloration.

Tetracyclines differ from one another in the following ways:

- *Oral absorption rates:* All are adequately absorbed, but doxycycline and minocycline are absorbed the most.
- *Body tissue penetration:* Doxycycline and minocycline have the best penetration potential (brain and cerebrospinal fluid).
- *Half-life and resulting dosage schedule:* See the Dosages table on p. 728 and the pharmacokinetics information in the Drug Profiles section.

Mechanism of Action and Drug Effects

Tetracyclines act by inhibiting protein synthesis in susceptible bacteria. For this synthesis to occur, transfer RNA must bind to the messenger RNA ribosome. Tetracyclines obstruct this synthesis by binding to that portion of the ribosome called the *30S subunit* (Figure 38-6). This action is comparable with the mechanism of the macrolides, which bind to the 50S subunit. Consequently, many of the bacterium's essential functions shut down, such as growth and repair, so that eventually the bacterium stops growing and dies.

Tetracyclines are used primarily for their antibiotic effects. They inhibit the growth of and kill a wide range of *Rickettsia, Chlamydia,* and *Mycoplasma* organisms, as well as a variety of gram-negative and gram-positive bacteria (see Indications). They are also useful in the treatment of spirochetal infections such as syphilis and Lyme disease. Another drug effect of tetracyclines is their ability to cause inflammation that results in fibrosis in the lungs. This property is useful in patients with pleural or pericardial effusions caused by metastatic tumours, thoracentesis, or thoracostomy tubes because when instilled into the pleural space of the lungs, tetracyclines cause scar tissue to form and thereby reduce fluid accumulation.

Indications

Tetracyclines have a wide range of activity, and all drugs in this class are effective against essentially the same range of microbes. They inhibit the growth of many gram-negative and gram-positive organisms and even some protozoa. Traditionally used to treat acne in adolescents and adults, they are also considered the drugs of choice for the treatment of the following infections caused by susceptible organisms:

- *Chlamydia:* Lymphogranuloma venereum; psittacosis; and nonspecific endocervical, rectal, and urethral infections
- *Mycoplasma:* Mycoplasma pneumonia
- *Rickettsia:* Q fever, rickettsial pox, Rocky Mountain spotted fever, scrub typhus, and typhus
- *Other bacteria:* Acne, brucellosis, chancroid, cholera, granuloma inguinale, shigellosis, spirochetal relapsing fever, Lyme disease, *H. pylori* infections associated with peptic ulcer disease (used as part of the treatment regimen), and syphilis (used as an alternative drug to treat patients with penicillin allergy). Tetracyclines are now unreliable in treating gonorrhea because of resistant bacterial strains.
- *Protozoa:* Balantidiasis

Contraindications

The only usual contraindication is known drug allergy. However, tetracyclines should also be avoided by pregnant and nursing women and should not be given to children under the age of 8 years.

Adverse Effects

All tetracyclines cause similar adverse effects. They can cause discoloration of the permanent teeth and tooth enamel hypoplasia in fetuses and children and possibly retard fetal skeletal development if taken during pregnancy. Other clinically significant undesirable effects include photosensitivity, and alteration of the intestinal flora, which can result in the following:

- Overgrowth of nonsusceptible organisms (superinfection), especially candidiasis and staphylococcal enteritis in children
- Diarrhea
- Pseudomembranous colitis

The tetracyclines can also alter the vaginal flora, which results in vaginal moniliasis. They can cause reversible bulging fontanelles in neonates; precipitate thrombocytopenia, possible coagulation irregularities, and hemolytic anemia; and exacerbate systemic lupus erythematosus. Other effects include gastric upset, enterocolitis, and maculopapular rash.

Interactions

Several significant drug interactions are associated with the use of tetracyclines. When tetracyclines are taken with antacids, antidiarrheal drugs, dairy products, or iron preparations, the oral absorption of the tetracycline is reduced. Tetracyclines can potentiate the effects of oral anticoagulants, which necessitates more frequent monitoring of the anticoagulant effect and possible dose adjustment. They can also antagonize the effects of bactericidal antibiotics and oral contraceptives. Depending on the dosage, they can cause the blood urea nitrogen levels to be increased.

Dosages

For dosage information for selected tetracyclines, see the Dosages table on p. 728.

DRUG PROFILES

Tetracyclines were one of the first classes of antibiotics capable of providing coverage against a broad spectrum of microorganisms. They are also unusual in that they are useful in the treatment of conditions other than bacterial infections. They are used as sclerosing (tissue-hardening) drugs in the treatment of pleural effusions. They are prescription-only drugs that are potentially harmful to children younger than 8 years of age. Tetracyclines should not be given to pregnant women; by binding to calcium, they can prevent normal bone growth and cause tooth enamel hypoplasia in the fetus. Their use is also contraindicated in patients who have had previous hypersensitivity reactions and in lactating women. Resistance to one tetracycline implies resistance to all tetracyclines.

▶▶ *doxycycline hyclate*

Doxycycline hyclate (Apo-Doxy, Atridox, Doxycin Cap, Doxytab, Vibramycin) is a semisynthetic tetracycline antibiotic that was made by altering the naturally occurring tetracycline *oxytetracycline*. Doxycycline is available in Canada in the salt form hyclate. It is useful in the treatment of rickettsial infections, *Clostridium difficile*, chlamydial, and mycoplasmal infections, spirochetal infections, and many infections with gram-negative organisms. Doxycycline may also be used as a sclerosing drug in the treatment of pleural effusions. It is available in oral forms.

PHARMACOKINETICS

Half-Life	Onset	Peak	Duration
14–24 hr	Variable	1.5–4 hr	Up to 12 hr

DOSAGES Selected Tetracyclines

Drug (Pregnancy Class)	Pharmacological Class	Usual Dosage Range	Indications
▶▶ doxycycline* hyclate (Apo-Doxy, Atridox, Doxycin Cap, Doxytab, Vibramycin, others) (D)	Tetracycline	*Children older than 8 yr*** PO: 2–4 mg/kg/day, divided daily or bid *Adult* PO: 200 mg first day, then 100 mg daily thereafter	Broad antibacterial coverage, including treatment of skin infections and respiratory, GI, and GU tract infections

GI, gastrointestinal; *GU*, genitourinary; *PO*, oral.

*A parenteral form of doxycline is available through the Special Access Programme, Health Canada.

**Use of tetracyclines is contraindicated in children younger than 8 yr and in pregnant women because of risk of significant tooth discoloration in children.

NURSING PROCESS

 Assessment

To ensure effective treatment, in general, before the administration of any antibiotic, it is crucial to assess for a history of or symptoms indicative of hypersensitivity or allergic reactions (mild reactions with rash, pruritus, or hives; severe reactions with laryngeal edema, bronchospasms, hypotension, and possible cardiac arrest). Further assessment should include the patient's age, weight, and baseline vital signs with body temperature as well as examination of the results of any laboratory studies that have been ordered, including liver function studies (aspartate aminotransferase [AST] level and alanine aminotransferase [ALT] level), kidney function studies (usually blood urea nitrogen and creatinine levels), heart function studies and tests (pertinent laboratory tests, electrocardiogram, or ultrasonography if indicated), culture and sensitivity tests, and complete blood count (CBC) with hemoglobin/hematocrit (Hgb/Hct) levels and platelet/clotting values. Intake and output values should also be noted (e.g., more than 30 mL/hr or 600 mL/day). A neurological assessment is important

because of possible CNS adverse effects, as is an assessment of bowel sounds and patterns because of possible drug-related gastrointestinal adverse effects. Contraindications, cautions, and drug interactions should be assessed with a complete list of all medications, including over-the-counter drugs and natural health products.

Ethnocultural assessment is important because of racial and ethnic differences in responses to certain drugs and the use of folk remedies or alternative therapies to try to alleviate infections. Learning preparedness, willingness to learn, and educational level should also be assessed because of the importance of patient education in taking these (and all) medications. The nurse should assess oral mucosa and the respiratory, gastrointestinal, and genitourinary tracts because of the risk of superinfection. Superinfections are often evidenced by fever, lethargy, mouth sores, perineal itching, and other anatomically related symptoms (discussed previously under General Prinicples of Antibiotics). Because antibiotic resistance is so prevalent, the patient or caregiver should be asked about long-term use, overuse, or abuse of antibiotics. Assessment information related to each group of antibiotics is presented in the following discussion.

For patients taking sulfonamides, a careful assessment for drug allergies to sulfa-type drugs, such as the oral sulfonylureas (antihyperglycemic drugs), and thiazide diuretics, is critical to patient safety. A thorough skin assessment during drug therapy is also important because Stevens–Johnson syndrome is a possible adverse effect of these drugs. Blood counts, specifically RBCs, need to be assessed before the initiation of drug therapy because of the possibility of drug-related anemias and other blood dyscrasias. Kidney function should be assessed because of the potential for drug-related crystalluria.

Given the association with the highest incidence of allergic reactions, penicillins require astute assessment of hypersensitivity. In addition, the patient must be assessed for a history of asthma, sensitivity to multiple allergens, aspirin allergy, and sensitivity to cephalosporins because these conditions place the patient at higher risk for penicillin allergy. If procaine penicillin is to be given, the patient should be assessed for procaine hypersensitivity. Liver and kidney functioning should be assessed, and results of culture and sensitivity tests on any specimens should be noted. Because of possible CNS and gastrointestinal adverse effects, thorough neurological, abdominal, and bowel assessments should be completed. Especially important for patients with electrolyte disturbances, heart disease, or kidney disease is an assessment of serum sodium and potassium levels because of the high sodium and potassium ion concentrations in some penicillins. For example, penicillin G contains 1.7 mmol of potassium ion per million units and 2 mmol of sodium ion per million units (see Table 38-4). In these situations, hypernatremia and hyperkalemia could lead to complications such as congestive heart failure, fluid overload, or cardiac dysrhythmias. With any dosage forms of the penicillins, it is important to patient safety to assess for the possibility of an immediate, accelerated, or delayed allergic reaction. A small percentage of patients taking penicillins may develop serious superinfections manifested by antibiotic-associated pseudomembranous colitis; therefore, thorough bowel and gastrointestinal-tract assessment should be ongoing for this potential complication.

Cephalosporins require a thorough assessment of allergies, including allergy to penicillins because of possible cross-sensitivity. Baseline vital sign measurements, blood count, bleeding time and clotting studies, and kidney and liver function tests should be assessed as ordered. Assessment for signs and symptoms of pseudomembranous colitis, such as severe diarrhea, bloody stools, and abdominal pain, is needed in patients taking this group of drugs. It is also important to obtain information about the specific drug and to note what generation of cephalosporins is being taken because each of the four drug generations has distinctive adverse effects and complications in addition to commonalities with the other groups.

Carbapenems are similar to penicillins, thus assessment for allergy to the penicillin group (see previous discussion on penicillins) is needed. Neurological functioning, seizure disorders, and baseline hearing levels need to be assesed because of possible CNS adverse effects such as CNS stimulation and tinnitus (ringing in the ears). Gastrointestinal functioning should also be assessed because these drugs may worsen any existing diarrhea, nausea, and vomiting.

With macrolides, assessment of heart function (because of the risk of exacerbation of heart disease) and a thorough assessment of kidney and liver function may help identify adverse effects early on in therapy. Drug interactions need to be noted, particularly the concurrent prescribing or use of a macrolide and warfarin because the interaction of these drugs can be detrimental to clotting ability, thus platelet counts and results of clotting studies (e.g., international normalized ratio, prothrombin time, partial thromboplastin time) must be examined. In addition, there is always concern for use of antibiotics with oral contraceptives as this may lead to contraceptive failure.

With tetracyclines, careful assessment of culture and sensitivity reports, CBC counts, and results of kidney and liver function tests is needed. These drugs should not be used in patients younger than 8 years of age because of the adverse effect of permanent mottling and discoloration of the teeth. Use of these drugs in pregnancy may also pose problems for the fetus, as previously discussed. Assessment for any whitish, sore patches on the oral mucosa (due to candidiasis or yeast infection) as well as any vaginal itching, pain, or cottage cheese–like discharge (because of vaginal candidiasis) is important for early identification and early treatment of superinfections.

Nursing Diagnoses

- Risk for infection related to the patient's compromised immune system status before treatment due to bacterial invasion
- Risk for injury (compromised organ function) related to the adverse effects of drugs (e.g., anemias, liver and kidney toxicity) and the weakened physical state
- Acute pain related to infection and adverse reaction to drugs
- Deficient knowledge related to lack of information about the disease process and the drug regimen
- Nonadherence to the treatment regimen because of lack of information about the proper use of antibiotics

Planning

Goals

- Patient will remain free of the signs and symptoms of infection once therapy is completed.
- Patient will experience minimal adverse effects as well as full therapeutic effects of antibiotic therapy.
- Patient will remain adherent to antibiotic therapy regimen for the full duration of treatment.
- Patient will experience improvement in any discomfort or pain related to the infection.
- Patient will remain informed about the drug therapy as well as about other treatment modalities and alternative therapies.
- Patient will return for follow-up visits to the health care provider as recommended.

■ Outcome Criteria

- Patient states the signs and symptoms of an infection or its worsening, such as fever, pain, malaise, chills, joint pain, and increase in site-related symptoms.
- Patient describes improvement in the body's response to a resolving infection with subsequent increase in energy level and ability to carry out activities of daily living.
- Patient states the adverse effects of antibiotic therapy, such as gastrointestinal upset, nausea, and diarrhea (specific to each class), and the effects to report to the physician, such as severe gastrointestinal symptoms, jaundice (yellowish discoloration of skin and sclera), and severe skin rashes.
- Patient implements actions to minimize the gastrointestinal distress and other adverse effects associated with antibiotic therapy, such as forcing fluids and eating dairy products like yogourt and buttermilk as appropriate.
- Patient experiences increased periods of comfort related to a resolving infectious process.
- Patient keeps all follow-up appointments and takes appropriate measures after completing antibiotic therapy, as explained by the health care provider.

■ Implementation

Nursing interventions that apply to all antibiotics are as follows:

- Oral antibiotics should be given within the recommended time frames and with the appropriate fluids or foods.
- Therapy should be completed in full unless otherwise instructed by the physician.
- Drugs should be administered round the clock to maintain effective blood levels.
- Avoid giving oral antibiotics at the same time as antacids, calcium supplements, iron products, laxatives containing magnesium, or some of the antilipemic drugs (see previous discussion of individual drugs for a listing of drug interactions).
- Natural health products should be used only if they do not interact with the antibiotic.
- Continual monitoring for hypersensitivity reactions past the initial assessment phase is important because immediate reactions may not occur for up to 30 minutes, accelerated reactions may occur within 1 to 72 hours, and delayed responses may occur after 72 hours. Hypersensitivity reactions may be manifested by wheezing; shortness of breath; swelling of the face, tongue, or hands; itching; or rash.

Sulfonamides should always be taken as directed and with increased intake of fluids (2000 to 3000 mL/24 hr) to prevent drug-related crystalluria. Oral dosage forms should be taken with food to minimize gastrointestinal upset. It is also important to encourage patients to immediately report the following to their physician: worsening abdominal cramps, stomach pain, diarrhea, blood in the urine, severe or worsening rash, shortness of breath, and fever.

With penicillins, as with other antibiotics, the natural flora in the gastrointestinal tract may be killed off by the antibiotic. Unaffected gastrointestinal bacteria such as *Clostridium difficile* may overgrow (see Penicillins section). This process may be prevented by the consumption of probiotics, such as products containing lactobacillus, supplements, or cultured dairy products like yogurt, buttermilk, and kefir. Kefir is prepared with milk from sheep, goats, and cows, and soy milk kefirs are now commercially available. Some specific nursing considerations for penicillin formulations include the following:

- Oral penicillins should be taken with at least 180 mL of water (not juices) because acidic juices nullify the drug's antibacterial action.
- Penicillin V, amoxicillin, and amoxicillin-clavulanate should be taken with water 1 hour before or 2 hours after meals to help decrease gastrointestinal upset while maximizing absorption.
- Procaine and benzathine salt penicillins are thick solutions that should be administered as ordered; they should be given IM using at least a 21-gauge needle and should be injected into a large muscle mass with rotation of sites as needed.
- IM imipenem-cilastatin should be reconstituted in sterile saline, with plain lidocaine—as ordered and if the patient has no allergy to it—and then injected deep into a large muscle mass.
- When IV penicillins (e.g., ampicillin) are administered, as with any IV therapy, the proper diluent should be used and the medication infused over the recommended time. The IV rate and site should be checked and changed as appropriate, and the compatibility of solutions and drug(s) should be checked thoroughly.
- IV sites should be checked for infiltration (swelling and tenderness at the IV site) and for irritation of the vein (phlebitis), manifested by heat, redness, and pain over the vein.
- Should the patient experience an anaphylactic reaction to a penicillin, epinephrine and other emergency drugs should be given as ordered. Supportive treatment should be on hand (e.g., oxygen).

Orally administered cephalosporins should be given with food to decrease gastrointestinal upset. Alcohol and alcohol-containing products should be avoided because of the potentiation of a disulfiram-like reaction associated with some of the cephalosporins. With the newer cephalosporins, as with many drug groups, the nurse must check the drug names carefully to ensure patient safety because many drug names sound alike, and this can lead to medication errors. Cephalosporin use may also predispose the patient to pseudomembranous colitis, especially if pre-existing gastrointestinal disease is documented.

Macrolides should be administered with the same precautions as those used for other antibiotics. To avoid interaction with the drug, macrolides should not be given with or immediately before or after fruit juices. The patient should be informed about the many drug interactions (discussed in the pharmacology section of this chapter), including those with over-the-counter drugs and natural health products. Patients should report severe rash, itching, hives, difficulty swallowing, jaundice, dark urine, or pale stools to their physician immediately.

Tetracyclines cause photosensitivity, so patients should take precautions to avoid sun exposure and tanning bed use. Oral doses should be given with at least 240 mL of fluids and food to minimize gastrointestinal upset. However, tetracyclines should not be given with dairy products, antacids, sodium bicarbonate, kaolin-pectin, or iron, because these chelate or bind with the antibiotic and decrease the antibiotic effect.

These interacting foods and drugs may be given 2 hours before or 3 hours after the tetracycline to avoid the interaction. IV doxycycline is irritating to the veins, and the IV infusion site should be checked frequently. Patients should be encouraged to report abdominal pain, nausea, vomiting, visual changes, or jaundice.

Teaching guidelines for patients receiving antibiotics are listed in Patient Education.

Evaluation

Evaluation should include monitoring of goals, outcome criteria, and therapeutic effects and adverse effects. The therapeutic effects of antibiotics include a decrease in the signs and symptoms of the infection; a return to normal vital signs, including temperature, and negative results on culture and sensitivity tests; normal results for CBC; and improved appetite, energy level, and sense of well-being. Evaluation for adverse effects includes monitoring for the specific drug-related adverse effects (see each drug profile).

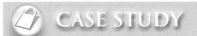 CASE STUDY

Antibiotic Therapy

Mr. G. has been a resident of an assisted care facility since experiencing a left-side stroke 5 years previousy. Presently, his cardiovascular status and cerebrovascular status are stable. However, he has had a productive cough and a low-grade fever for 2 days. After physical assessment and chest radiographic examination, the physician diagnoses him with pneumonia of the left lower lobe of the lung. The physician orders intravenous piperacillin-tazobactam (Tazocin) 2.25 g every 8 hours and oral theophylline (Pulmophylline Elx) 300 mg every 12 hours. Mr. G. also takes warfarin (Coumadin) 2 mg every evening. Maalox 30 mL has been ordered as needed for gastrointestinal upset and oral ibuprofen 400 mg to be given as needed for pain.

1. Explain the rationale behind the use of tazobactam with piperacillin in Tazocin.
2. What assessments does the nurse need to make prior to starting the antibiotic?
3. What concerns or drug interactions should the nurse be aware of with the use of Tazocin and the other medications ordered for Mr. G.?
4. What parameters should be monitored to determine whether Tazocin is acting? Explain your answer.

For answers see http://evolve.elsevier.com/Canada/Lilley/pharmacology/.

 IN MY FAMILY

French Canadian Home Remedies

(as told by M.F., of French-Canadian descent)

"Onion for ear infection: Chop onions and stuff them into socks. Fasten one to each ear (pulling a hat over the head and socks works well), and keep them there for the duration of the pain.

Mustard plaster for congestion: Mix crushed seed or powdered mustard with flour, and add a little lukewarm water to make a paste. This mixture is spread between two pieces of cotton or linen and wrapped in flannel, then placed on the chest. Use on the chest should not exceed 10 minutes, with a maximum of 3 to 5 minutes for children, and it should never be used on the face."

PATIENT EDUCATION

- Patients should be educated about foods and beverages that may interact negatively with antibiotics, such as alcohol, acidic fruit juices, and dairy products.
- Patients should be instructed to report severe adverse effects to the physician. In addition, patients should be conscientious about follow-up visits to the health care provider because of the need to monitor the infection and its treatment. Laboratory tests may also be performed at these visits.
- Patients should be instructed to increase fluid intake to up to 3000 mL/day unless contraindicated. Reporting of the following is also important because these symptoms may indicate superinfection: fever, black hairy tongue, stomatitis, loose or foul-smelling stools, vaginal discharge, or cough.
- Patients should be educated about foods that may help prevent superinfections (e.g., vaginal yeast infections), such as yogourt, buttermilk, and kefir. New yogourts, termed probiotics, are available that help re-establish the natural flora of the gastrointestinal tract.
- Patients taking oral contraceptives for birth control should be educated about interactions between certain antibiotics and oral contraceptives. Effectiveness of oral contraceptives may be decreased with these antibiotics. The patient should be informed to use a backup method of contraception to avoid pregnancy.
- Patients should be encouraged to wear a medical alert bracelet or necklace if allergic to antibiotics (or to any other medication) and to keep this information available at all times.
- With sulfonamides, patients should be instructed to take the antibiotic with plenty of fluids (2000 to 3000 mL/24 hr) to prevent drug-related crystalluria or precipitation in the kidneys and to take these drugs with food. Patients should report the following to their health care provider immediately: worsening abdominal cramps, stomach pain, diarrhea, blood in the urine, severe or worsening rash, shortness of breath, or fever.
- With penicillins, patients should take the medication exactly as prescribed for the full duration indicated, with doses spaced at regularly scheduled intervals. The patient should take oral dosage forms with water and should avoid taking them with caffeine-containing foods or beverages, citrus fruit, cola beverages, fruit juices, or tomato juice because the drug will be inactivated. If the patient must take a penicillin drug four times a day, the patient should set up a reminder system so that blood levels will remain steady. Reminders may be set up using a watch or even a cell phone alarm so that the patient will be sure to take the drug exactly as directed.
- For cephalosporins, patients should be encouraged to report diarrhea, flulike symptoms, blistering or peeling of the skin, hearing loss, breathing difficulty, or seizures to the health care provider immediately. The patient should also report any foul-smelling, loose, frequent, or bloody stools.
- With macrolides, patients should be instructed to take the drug as directed and to check for interactions with other drugs being taken at the same time, especially interactions between erythromycin and other medications. The nurse should always be sure that the patient knows the proper dosage and instructions for the drug being taking.
- With tetracyclines, patients should be advised to avoid exposure to tanning beds and direct sunlight or to use sunscreen and wear protective clothing because of drug-related photosensitivity. These photosensitive effects may be noticed within a few minutes to hours after taking the drug and may last up to several days after the drug has been discontinued.

POINTS TO REMEMBER

- Antibiotics can be either bacteriostatic or bactericidal. Bacteriostatic antibiotics inhibit the growth of bacteria but do not directly kill them. Bactericidal antibiotics directly kill the bacteria.
- Most antibiotics work by inhibiting bacterial cell wall synthesis in some way. Bacteria have survived over the ages because they can adapt to their surroundings. If a bacterium's environment includes an antibiotic, over time it can mutate in such a way that it can survive an attack by the antibiotic. The production of β-lactamases is one way in which bacteria can fend off the effects of antibiotics.
- Nurses need to be aware of the most common adverse effects of antibiotics, which include nausea, vomiting, and diarrhea. Nurses should inform patients that antibiotics should be taken for the prescribed length of time.
- Each class of antibiotics is associated with specific cautions, contraindications, drug interactions, and adverse effects that must be carefully assessed for and monitored by the nurse.
- Because normally occurring bacteria are killed during antibiotic therapy, superinfections may arise during treatment. These may be manifested by the following signs and symptoms: fever, perineal itching, oral lesions, vaginal irritation and discharge, cough, and lethargy.

EXAMINATION REVIEW QUESTIONS

1 Your patient is scheduled for colorectal surgery tomorrow. He does not have sepsis, his WBC count is normal, he has no fever, and he is otherwise in good health. However, the nurse notes that there are orders to administer an antibiotic on call before he goes to surgery. What is the rationale for this antibiotic order?
   a. To provide empirical therapy
   b. To treat for a superinfection
   c. To provide prophylactic therapy
   d. To reduce the number of resistant organisms

2 A teenage patient is taking a tetracycline drug as part of treatment for severe acne. When the nurse teaches this patient about drug-related precautions, what is the most pertinent information that must be conveyed?
   a. When the acne clears up, the medication may be discontinued.
   b. This medication should be taken with antacids to reduce gastrointestinal upset.
   c. The teeth should be observed closely for signs of mottling or other colour changes.
   d. The patient should use sunscreen or avoid exposure to sunlight because this drug may cause photosensitivity.

3 A newly admitted patient reports a penicillin allergy. The physician has ordered a second-generation cephalosporin as part of the therapy. Which of the following nursing actions is appropriate?
   a. Give the medication, and monitor for adverse effects.
   b. Call the physician to clarify the order because of the patient's allergy.
   c. Ask the pharmacy to change the order to a first-generation cephalosporin.
   d. Administer the drug with a nonsteroidal anti-inflammatory to reduce adverse effects.

4 During patient education regarding an oral macrolide such as erythromycin, which of the following points is appropriate to make?
   a. The patient should take each dose with a sip of water.
   b. If gastrointestinal upset occurs, the drug will have to be stopped.
   c. The drug should be taken with an antacid to avoid gastrointestinal problems.
   d. The patient may take the drug with a small snack to reduce gastrointestinal irritation.

5 A woman who has been taking an antibiotic for a urinary tract infection calls the nurse practitioner to complain of severe vaginal itching. She has also noticed a thick, whitish vaginal discharge. Which of the following does the nurse practitioner suspect is occurring?
   a. A superinfection has developed.
   b. This is an expected response to antibiotic therapy.
   c. The urinary tract infection is resistant to the antibiotic.
   d. The urinary tract infection has become worse instead of better.

For answers see http://evolve.elsevier.com/Canada/Lilley/pharmacology/.

CRITICAL THINKING ACTIVITIES

1 Explain the rationale for not taking dairy products, iron, or calcium with tetracycline. What would be recommended if these products are not omitted from the diet?
2 What symptoms would alert the nurse to the fact that a patient is suffering from a superinfection or overgrowth of normal flora stemming from the use of tetracycline?
3 If a person is allergic to penicillin, then is that person also allergic to cephalosporins? Explain your answer.

For answers see http://evolve.elsevier.com/Canada/Lilley/pharmacology/.

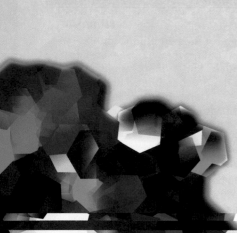

Antibiotics Part 2: Aminoglycosides, Fluoroquinolones, and Other Drugs

Learning Objectives

After reading this chapter, the successful student will be able to do the following:

1 Review the general principles of antibiotic therapy.

2 Review all of the previously discussed antibiotics in Chapter 38 in preparation for discussion of the following antibiotics or antibiotic classes: aminoglycosides, fluoroquinolones, clindamycin, metronidazole, nitrofurantoin, vancomycin, and several other miscellaneous antibiotics.

3 Review the advantages and disadvantages associated with use of antibiotics with discussion of overuse and abuse of antibiotics, development of drug resistance, superinfections, and antibiotic-associated colitis.

4 Discuss the indications, cautions, contraindications, mechanisms of action, adverse effects, toxic effects, routes of administration, and drug interactions associated with aminoglycosides, fluoroquinolones, clindamycin, metronidazole, nitrofurantoin, vancomycin, and miscellaneous antibiotics.

5 Develop a collaborative plan of care that includes all phases of the nursing process for the patient receiving antibiotics.

e-Learning Activities

Web site
(http://evolve.elsevier.com/Canada/Lilley/pharmacology/)

- Animations
- Answers to chapter questions, activities, and case studies
- Calculators and Category Catchers
- Glossary with audio pronunciations
- IV Therapy and Medication Error Checklists
- Multiple-Choice Review Question quizzes
- Nursing Care Plans
- Online Appendices and Supplements
- WebLinks

Drug Profiles

amikacin (amikacin sulfate)*, p. 738
▸▸ **ciprofloxacin (ciprofloxacin hydrochloride)***, p. 741
▸▸ **clindamycin,** p. 741
dapsone, p. 742
▸▸ **gentamicin (gentamicin sulfate)***, p. 738
levofloxacin, p. 741
linezolid, p. 742
▸▸ **metronidazole,** p. 743
nitrofurantoin, p. 743
quinupristin, dalfopristin, p. 743
tobramycin, p. 738
▸▸ **vancomycin,** p. 743

▸▸ Key drug.

*Full generic name is given in parentheses. For the purposes of this text, the more common shortened name is used.

Glossary

Concentration-dependent killing A property of some antibiotics, especially aminoglycosides and vancomycin, of achieving a relatively high, even if brief, plasma drug concentration that results in the most effective bacterial kill (see *time-dependent killing*). (p. 736)

Facultative anaerobic metabolism A property of certain bacteria (e.g., enterococci) that allows them to adapt to low tissue oxygen concentrations and still thrive, even though they normally thrive in oxygen-rich environments. (p. 736)

Microgram   One millionth of a gram. (p. 736)

Minimum inhibitory concentration (MIC)   A laboratory measurement of the lowest drug concentration needed to kill a certain standard amount of bacteria. (p. 735)

MRSA   Originally, this abbreviation stood exclusively for methicillin-resistant *Staphylococcus aureus*, to describe an *S. aureus* species that was resistant to the β-lactamase–resistant penicillin known as methicillin. It now more commonly refers to strains of *S. aureus* that are resistant to several drug classes, thus it may also stand for (depending on context or health facility) multidrug-resistant *S. aureus*. (p. 739)

Nephrotoxicity   Toxicity to the kidneys, often drug induced and manifesting in compromised kidney function. (p. 735)

Ototoxicity   Toxicity to the ears, often drug induced and manifesting in varying degrees of hearing loss that is more likely to be permanent than nephrotoxicity. (p. 735)

Postantibiotic effect (PAE)   A period of continued bacterial suppression that occurs after brief exposure to certain antibiotic drug classes, especially aminoglycosides and carbapenems (Chapter 38). (p. 736)

Pseudomembranous colitis   A necrotizing, inflammatory bowel condition that is often associated with antibiotic therapy. A more general term used is antibiotic-associated colitis. (p. 742)

Synergistic effect   In the context of antibiotics, refers to a stronger bacterial kill with two antibiotics given together than with either given alone. (p. 736)

Therapeutic drug monitoring   Ongoing monitoring of plasma drug concentrations and dosage adjustment based on these values as well as on other laboratory indicators such as kidney and liver function tests. (p. 735)

Time-dependent killing   A property of most antibiotic classes, in contrast to concentration-dependent killing (see above), in which prolonged high plasma drug concentrations are required for effective bacterial kill. (p. 736)

OVERVIEW

This chapter is a continuation of Chapter 38 and focuses on additional classes of antibiotics. In general, the antibiotics used for more serious and harder-to-treat infections are described in Chapter 39. Many of the drugs in this chapter are administered by the parenteral (injectable) route only, a route generally reserved for treating more clinically serious infections in the hospital setting. Also included are miscellaneous drugs that are unique in their class, as well as newer drugs and drug classes. Since the previous edition of this textbook, the number of antibiotic drugs available has increased to the point that they are best covered over two chapters.

AMINOGLYCOSIDES

The aminoglycosides are a group of natural and semi-synthetic antibiotics classified as bactericidal drugs (see Chapter 38). They are similar to the tetracyclines in that they are derived from *Streptomyces* organisms. Although they are potent antibiotics, they have been replaced to varying degrees (depending on the institution) with fluoroquinolones, which have somewhat safer adverse-effect profiles. Nonetheless, bacterial resistance may be less common than with fluoroquinolones, making aminoglycosides the better choice for particularly virulent infections. The aminoglycoside antibiotics available for clinical use are listed in Table 39-1. These drugs can be given by several different routes, but they are not given orally because of their poor oral absorption.

The three aminoglycosides most commonly used for the treatment of systemic infections are amikacin, gentamicin, and tobramycin. Serum levels of these drugs are routinely monitored from patients' blood samples. Dosages are then adjusted to maintain known optimal levels that maximize drug efficacy and minimize the risk for toxicity. This process is known as **therapeutic drug monitoring**. Aminoglycoside therapy is commonly monitored in this way because of its associated nephrotoxicity and ototoxicity. **Ototoxicity** (toxicity to the ears) often manifests as some degree of temporary or permanent hearing loss. **Nephrotoxicity** (toxicity to the kidneys) manifests in varying degrees of reduced kidney function. This is generally indicated by laboratory test results such as serum creatinine level. A rising serum creatinine suggests reduced creatinine clearance by the kidneys and is indicative of declining kidney function. Most commonly, dosing is adjusted for the patient's level of kidney function, based on calculated estimates of creatinine clearance from serum creatinine values. This function is often carried out by a hospital pharmacist consulting for the prescriber.

The **minimum inhibitory concentration (MIC)** for any antibiotic is a measurement of the lowest concentration of drug needed to kill a certain standard amount of bacteria. This value is determined in vitro (in the laboratory) for each drug. It has been shown that other classes of antibiotics, such as β-lactams, work on

TABLE	39-1

Available Aminoglycoside Antibiotics

Origin	Product	Description
Natural	gentamicin neomycin paromomycin streptomycin tobramycin	All chemically derived from *Streptomyces* spp. by a fermentation process
Semisynthetic	amikacin	Chemical derivative of kanamycin

time-dependent killing—that is, the amount of time above MIC that is crucial for maximal bacterial kill. However, aminoglycosides work primarily on the basis of **concentration-dependent killing**, where achieving an increase in plasma concentration above MIC, but for no particular length of time, enhances the bacterial kill of the drug. For this reason, although originally given in three daily intravenous doses, the current predominant practice is once-daily aminoglycoside dosing. Several clinical studies have shown that once-daily dosing provides a sufficient plasma drug concentration for bacterial kill, along with equal or less risk for toxicity than multiple-daily dosage regimens. A once-daily regimen, versus the traditional three times daily regimen, also reduces the required nursing care time and often allows for outpatient or even home-based aminoglycoside drug therapy. Table 39-2 lists the traditional desired drug levels for these drugs. Note that peak (the highest) levels for once-daily regimens are usually not measured, as it is assumed that the peak level for a single daily dose will be short-lived and decline within a reasonable time frame. However, trough (the lowest) levels are routinely measured to ensure adequate kidney clearance of the drug and to avoid toxicity. Dosage information appears in the designated Dosages table on p. 739. Dosage regimens and ranges for serum levels may vary between institutions.

The trough blood sample should be drawn at least 18 hours after completion of the dose and closer to 24 hours afterward for patients with impaired kidneys. The therapeutic goal is a trough concentration ("trough") at or below 1 mcg/mL (which is considered undetectable) because troughs above 2 mcg/mL are associated with greater risk for both ototoxicity and nephrotoxicity. Trough levels are normally monitored once every 3 days until drug therapy is discontinued. The patient's serum creatinine should also be measured at least twice weekly as an index of kidney function, and drug dosages should be adjusted as needed for any changes in kidney function.

Mechanism of Action and Drug Effects

Aminoglycosides work similarly to the tetracyclines in that they also bind to ribosomes and thereby prevent protein synthesis in bacteria (see Figure 38-6). Specifically, they do this by binding to a structure known as the 30S ribosomal subunit. Protein synthesis is then disrupted by genetic misreadings of messenger RNA (mRNA) molecules,

leading to cell death. Often aminoglycosides are used in combination with other antibiotics such as β-lactams or vancomycin in the treatment of select infections because the combined effect of the two antibiotics is greater than that of either drug alone. This effect is known as a **synergistic effect**. Aminoglycosides also have a property known as **postantibiotic effect (PAE)**, which is a period of continued bacterial growth suppression that occurs after short-term antibiotic exposure as in once-daily aminoglycoside dosing (see above). Carbapenems are another antibiotic class having a PAE. The PAE is enhanced with higher peak drug concentrations, smaller bacterial inocula, and concurrent use of β-lactam antibiotics.

As with most antibiotic drug classes, bacterial mechanisms of resistance have emerged among gram-positive and gram-negative species that were previously more susceptible to aminoglycosides. The prevalence and intensity of such resistance vary with specific drugs, organisms, patient populations, disease states, and geographic prescribing patterns. Aminoglycoside resistance is less likely to develop during the course of a given patient's drug therapy, unlike the resistance of β-lactam drugs, especially cephalosporins. Instead, it is usually a longer process or occurs in response to an especially large bacterial inoculum, as is common with patients having serious burns or cystic fibrosis. In addition, concurrent use of aminoglycosides with cephalosporins does not prevent the development of resistance to the cephalosporins. In general, resistant bacterial strains produce drug-impeding enzymes. These proteins result from adaptive changes at the genetic level (DNA, RNA, or both) within the bacterial cells. Such enzymes may work through chemical interactions with the drug molecules themselves or by altering the permeability of the bacterial cell wall membrane to the drug molecules. One common example is resistance among enterococcal bacterial strains. This species has a characteristic known as **facultative anaerobic metabolism**—these bacteria can adaptively function metabolically in the absence of oxygen. When this occurs, the anaerobic biochemical reactions alter the cell membrane electrical potentials in such a way as to make it chemically more difficult for the drug molecules to enter the cell to reach their site of action.

Indications

The toxicity associated with aminoglycosides normally limits their use to treatment of serious gram-negative

TABLE 39-2					
Desired Traditional Serum Drug Levels of the Aminoglycoside Antibiotics					
	Peak			**Trough**	
Serum Drug Levels	**Multi-daily dosing***	**Once-daily dosing**		**Multi-daily dosing**	**Once-daily dosing**
amikacin	20–30 mcg/mL[†]	Usually not measured		5–10 mcg/mL	Less than 10 mcg/mL
gentamicin and tobramycin	5–10 mcg/mL	Usually not measured		Less than 2 mcg/mL	Less than 2 mcg/mL

*q8h or q12h.

[†]mcg = **microgram**; note that one microgram = 1/1000 (one thousandth) of a milligram or 1/1,000,000 (one millionth) of a gram. Also note that microgram is abbreviated *mcg*, whereas milligram is abbreviated *mg*.

infections and specific conditions involving gram-positive cocci, in which case gentamicin is usually given in combination with a penicillin. Commonly treated gram-negative infections include *Pseudomonas* spp. and several organisms belonging to the Enterobacteriaceae family (facultatively anaerobic gram-negative rods), including *Escherichia coli*, *Proteus* spp., *Klebsiella* spp., and Serratia spp. Such infections are often treated with a suitable aminoglycoside and an extended-spectrum penicillin, third-generation cephalosporin, or a carbapenem. Gram-positive infections may include *Enterococcus* spp., *Staphylococcus aureus*, and bacterial endocarditis, which is usually streptococcal in origin. A three-daily dose regimen is more common when treating gram-positive infections, as this often enhances synergy with other antibiotics used. Aminoglycosides are also used for prophylaxis in procedures involving the gastrointestinal or genitourinary tract, as such procedures have a high risk for enterococcal bacteremia. They are also commonly given in combination with either ampicillin or vancomycin (for penicillin-allergic patients) for surgical patients with a history of valvular heart disease because diseased heart valves are more prone to enterococcal infection.

Aminoglycosides should be administered with caution in premature and full-term neonates because of the immaturity of the kidneys in these patients; prolonged actions of the aminoglycosides and a greater risk for toxicities may result. In children, serious infections for which aminoglycosides are commonly used include pneumonia, meningitis, and urinary tract infections. Drug selection for both children and adults is based on the susceptibility of the causative organism. Refer to Table 39-3 for more information on the antibacterial spectra of specific aminoglycosides. A few aminoglycosides have even more specific indications. Streptomycin is active against *Mycobacterium* spp. (Chapter 41), whereas paromomycin is used to treat amebic dysentery, a protozoal intestinal disease (Chapter 43). Aminoglycosides are relatively inactive against fungi, viruses, and most anaerobic bacteria.

Contraindications

The only usual contraindication is known drug allergy. Aminoglycosides have been shown to cross the placenta and cause fetal harm when administered to pregnant women. There have been several case reports of total, irreversible bilateral congenital deafness in the children of women receiving aminoglycosides during pregnancy. Therefore, aminoglycosides should be used in pregnant women only in the event of life-threatening infections when safer drugs are ineffective. These drugs are also distributed in breast milk. Their use should be avoided in lactating women to avoid risk for drug toxicity in nursing infants.

Adverse Effects

Because aminoglycosides are potent antibiotics, they are capable of potentially serious toxicities, particularly to the kidneys (nephrotoxicity) and to the ears in terms of hearing and balance functions (ototoxicity). Duration of drug therapy should be as short as possible; sound clinical judgement is required as well as monitoring of the patient's progress. Nephrotoxicity typically occurs in 5% to 25% of patients and is usually manifests as urinary casts (visible remnants of destroyed kidney cells), proteinuria, and increased blood urea nitrogen and serum creatinine levels. It is usually reversible, but the patient's kidney function tests should be monitored throughout therapy. In contrast, ototoxicity is less common and occurs in 3% to 14% of patients, and is often not reversible. It can result in varying degrees of permanent hearing loss, depending on the dosage and duration of drug therapy. It is believed to result from damage to the eighth cranial nerve (CN VIII; cochleovestibular nerve or auditory nerve) and involves both cochlear damage (hearing loss) and vestibular damage (disrupted sense of balance). Symptoms include dizziness, tinnitus, a sense of fullness in the ears, and hearing loss. Preventive monitoring may include audiometry screenings to detect high-frequency hearing loss, assuming that the patient is mentally fit to interact with the audiologist to complete the exam. However, because aminoglycosides are often used to treat serious infections in critically ill patients, this is one example in which the risk for drug toxicity may become a secondary consideration to the risk for death or disability from the infection itself.

Other less common effects include headache, paresthesia, dizziness, vertigo, skin rash, fever, overgrowth

TABLE 39-3

Aminoglycosides: Comparative Spectra of Antimicrobial Activity

Aminoglycoside	Spectrum
amikacin sulfate	*Acinetobacter* spp., *Enterobacter aerogenes*, *Escherichia* coli, *Klebsiella pneumoniae*, *Proteus* spp., *Providencia* spp., *Pseudomonas* spp., *Serratia* spp., *Staphylococcus* infections
gentamicin sulfate	*E. aerogenes*, *E. coli*, *K. pneumoniae*, *Proteus* spp., *Pseudomonas* spp., *Salmonella* spp., *Serratia* spp. (nonpigmented), *Shigella* spp.
neomycin sulfate	Used as a topical antibacterial
paromomycin sulfate	Amebic dysentery
streptomycin sulfate	Granuloma inguinale, plague, tularemia, tuberculosis, nonhemolytic streptococcal endocarditis
tobramycin sulfate	*Citrobacter* spp., *Enterobacter* spp., *E. coli*, *Klebsiella* spp., *Proteus* spp., *Providencia* spp., *P. aeruginosa*, *Serratia* spp.

of nonsusceptible organisms, and neuromuscular paralysis (very rare and reversible). The risk for these toxicities is greatest in patients with pre-existing kidney impairment, patients already receiving other renally toxic drugs, and patients on high doses of or prolonged aminoglycoside therapy.

Interactions

Several significant drug interactions are associated with aminoglycoside use. The risk for nephrotoxicity can be increased with concurrent use of other nephrotoxic drugs such as vancomycin, cyclosporine, and amphotericin B.

Concurrent use with loop diuretics increases the risk for otoxoticity. In addition, because aminoglycosides, like many other antibiotics, also kill normal intestinal bacterial flora, they reduce the amount of vitamin K produced by these gut bacteria. These normal flora serve to balance the effects of oral anticoagulants such as warfarin (Coumadin). Therefore, aminoglycosides can potentiate warfarin toxicity.

Dosages

For recommended dosages of selected aminoglycosides, see the Dosages table on p. 739.

 DRUG PROFILES

Historically, the aminoglycoside antibiotics were used primarily for gram-negative infections. However, they are now used much more commonly than before for gram-positive infections because of the increased incidence of resistant gram-positive organisms. Aminoglycosides are normally given intravenously or intramuscularly. However, neomycin is only used topically in Canada (Chapter 57). Topical dosage forms of both gentamicin and tobramycin are available for dermatological (Chapter 57) and ophthalmic (Chapter 58) use. Currently available aminoglycosides include amikacin, gentamicin, paromomycin, streptomycin, and tobramycin. The variations in the suffixes of some of the drug names, in particular –mycin versus –micin, denote different bacterial origins of the aminoglycosides. Dosage and other information appear in the designated Dosages table on p. 739.

amikacin sulfate

Amikacin sulfate (generic) is a semisynthetic aminoglycoside antibiotic derived by chemically altering kanamycin, a naturally occurring aminoglycoside derived from *Streptomyces* spp. It is often used for infections that are resistant to gentamicin or tobramycin. It is only available in injectable form.

PHARMACOKINETICS

Half-Life	Onset	Peak	Duration
2.2 hr	Variable	1 hr	8–12 hr

▶▶ *gentamicin sulfate*

Gentamicin sulfate (generic) is a naturally occurring aminoglycoside obtained from cultures of *Micromonospora* spp. It is one of the most commonly used aminoglycosides in clinical practice today. It is usually administered intramuscularly. The intravenous route is recommended when the intramuscular route is not feasible, such as in patients in shock, with severe burns, with hemorrhagic disorders, or with low muscle mass. The dosage is the same for both routes. It is indicated for the treatment of several susceptible gram-positive and gram-negative bacteria. Gentamicin is available in several forms, including injections, topical ointments, and eye drops and ointments.

PHARMACOKINETICS

Half-Life	Onset	Peak	Duration
IV: 2 hr	IV: Variable	IV: 0.5–2 hr	IV: 8–12 hr

tobramycin

Tobramycin (generic) is also derived from *Streptomyces* spp. Its dosages, routes of administration, and indications are comparable with those of gentamicin for generalized infections. In addition, it is commonly used to treat recurrent pulmonary infections in cystic fibrosis by both parenteral and inhaled dosing. It is also available in topical and ophthalmic dosage forms.

PHARMACOKINETICS

Half-Life	Onset	Peak	Duration
IV: 2–3 hr	IV: Variable	IV: 30 min	IV: Up to 24 hr

FLUOROQUINOLONES

Fluoroquinolones are potent, bactericidal, broad-spectrum antibiotics. The first of these drugs to become available were the original quinolones, cinoxacin and nalidixic acid. These two drugs have narrower spectra of antibacterial activity than the newer, more potent, and less toxic fluoroquinolones and are therefore seldom used anymore. A fluorine atom was added onto the basic quinolone structure to create these newer drugs, which

increased their antibacterial potency and spectra. However, both generations of drugs are commonly referred to as *quinolones* for brevity. Currently available quinolone antibiotics include norfloxacin, ciprofloxacin, levofloxacin, moxifloxacin, gatifloxacin, and gemifloxacin.

Mechanism of Action and Drug Effects

Quinolone antibiotics destroy bacteria by altering their DNA (see Figure 38-6). They accomplish this by interfering with the bacterial enzymes DNA gyrase and

DOSAGES	Selected Aminoglycosides		
Drug (Pregnancy Category)	**Pharmacological Class**	**Usual Dosage Range**	**Indications**
amikacin sulfate (generic) (D)	Aminoglycoside	*Neonates/Children/Adult* IIM/V: 15 mg/kg/day divided bid administered over 30–60 min	Primarily gentamicin- and tobramycin-resistant gram-negative infections along with severe staphylococcal infections
▸▸**gentamicin sulfate (generic) (C)**	Aminoglycoside	*Neonates/Children* IM: 3–6 mg/kg/day divided q8h IV: 3 mg/kg/day divided q8h *Adult* IM: 3–5 mg/kg/day divided IV: 3 mg/kg/day divided q8h	Primarily gram-negative infections along with severe staphylococcal infections
tobramycin (generic) (D)	Aminoglycoside	*Neonates* IV: 4 mg/kg q12h *Children* IV: 6–7.5 mg/kg/day divided tid–qid *Adult* IV: 3–5 mg/kg/day divided tid–qid or 5–7 mg/kg once daily	Primarily gram-negative infections along with severe staphylococcal infections

topoisomerase IV. Quinolones do not seem to affect the corresponding mammalian enzymes and thus do not inhibit the production of human DNA.

The drug effects of quinolone antibiotics are mostly limited to their effects on bacteria. They kill susceptible strains of mostly gram-negative and some gram-positive organisms. Some quinolones are also believed to diffuse into and concentrate themselves in human neutrophils, killing such bacteria as *S. aureus*, *Serratia marcescens*, and *Mycobacterium fortuitum* that sometimes accumulate in these cells. Nonetheless, bacterial resistance to quinolone antibiotics has been identified among several bacterial species, including *Pseudomonas aeruginosa*, *S. aureus*, *Pneumococcus* spp., *Enterococcus* spp., and the broad Enterobacteriaceae family that includes *E. coli*. Mechanisms for such resistance include altered DNA gyrase and topoisomerase enzymes, as well as altered cell membrane permeability to reduce entry of drug molecules into cells and speed efflux of such molecules out of cells.

Indications

Quinolones are active against a wide variety of gram-negative and selected gram-positive bacteria. Most are excreted primarily by the kidneys, which contain a high percentage of unchanged drug. Because of this trait and their extensive gram-negative coverage, they are suitable for treating complicated urinary tract infections. Exceptions include moxifloxacin and gemifloxacin, which are excreted less by the kidneys. They are also commonly used for respiratory, skin, gastrointestinal, bone, and joint infections, and sexually transmitted infections (STIs).

Levofloxacin is somewhat more active than older quinolones against gram-positive organisms such as *S. pneumoniae*, including penicillin-resistant strains, as well as *Enterococcus* and *S. aureus*. Gatifloxacin and moxifloxacin are also effective against *S. pneumoniae* and some

strains of *S. aureus* and enterococci. However, multidrug-resistant *S. aureus* (**MRSA**; see the Glossary definition in this chapter) and vancomycin-resistant enterococci (VRE) are generally also resistant to gatifloxacin and moxifloxacin. The activity of gatifloxacin and moxifloxacin against many enteric gram-negative bacteria and *P. aeruginosa* is similar to that of levofloxacin and less than that of ciprofloxacin. Moxifloxacin often has stronger anaerobic bacterial coverage. Norfloxacin has limited oral absorption but is only available in oral form, so its use is limited to genitourinary infections, including STIs. Quinolones are often combined with aminoglycosides to treat *P. aeruginosa*. Gatifloxacin and moxifloxacin also have some in vitro activity against anaerobes. Gemifloxacin, the newest quinolone, is primarily indicated for gram-negative respiratory infections such as bacterial exacerbations of chronic bronchitis and community-acquired pneumonia (CAP) and is effective against resistant strains of *S. pneumoniae*.

The use of quinolones in prepubescent children is still not generally recommended because these drugs have been shown to affect cartilage development in laboratory animals. However, more recent evidence suggests that judicial use in children might be less of a risk than previously thought. There is some variance in spectra between drugs; Box 39-1 lists selected microbes commonly susceptible to quinolone therapy in general. Table 39-4 lists common indications by individual drug.

Contraindications

The most common contraindication is known drug allergy. However, quinolones also have some unique contraindications related to heart function. Dangerous cardiac dysrhythmias are more likely to occur when quinolones are taken by patients receiving class IA and class III antiarrhythmic drugs such as disopyramide and amiodarone. Therefore these drug combinations should be avoided.

TABLE   39-4

Quinolones: Common Indications for Specific Drugs

Generic Name (Brand Name)	Antibacterial Spectrum	Common Indications
ciprofloxacin (Cipro)	Comparable with norfloxacin	Anthrax (inhalational, postexposure); respiratory, skin, urinary tract, prostate, intra-abdominal, gastrointestinal, bone and joint infections; typhoid fever; STIs; selected nosocomial pneumonias
gatifloxacin (Zymar)	Comparable with norfloxacin	Respiratory and urinary tract infections
gemifloxacin (Factive)	Comparable with norfloxacin	Acute bacterial exacerbation of chronic bronchitis; CAP
levofloxacin (Levaquin)	Comparable with norfloxacin	Respiratory and urinary tract infections; prophylaxis in transrectal and transurethral prostate surgical procedures
moxifloxacin hydrochloride (Avelox)	Comparable with norfloxacin	Respiratory and skin infections; CAP caused by PRSP; plus anaerobic infections
norfloxacin (Apo-Norflox)	Extensive gram-negative and selected gram-positive coverage	Urinary tract infections; prostatitis; STIs

CAP, community-acquired pneumonia; *PRSP*, penicillin-resistant streptococcal pneumonia; *STI*, sexually transmitted infection.

BOX   39-1

Overview of Quinolone-Susceptible Microbial Spectra

- Gram-positive: *Streptococcus* (including *S. pneumoniae*), *Staphylococcus*, enterococci, *Listeria monocytogenes*
- Gram-negative: *Neisseria gonorrhea*, *N. meningitidis*, *Haemophilus influenzae*, *H. parainfluenzae*, *Enterobacteriaceae* (including *Escherichia coli*, *Enterobacter*, *Klebsiella*, *Proteus mirabilis*, *Salmonella*, *Shigella*), *Acinetobacter*, *P. aeruginosa*, *Pastorella multocida*, *Legionella*, *Mycoplasma pneumoniae*, *Chlamydia*
- Anaerobes: *Bacteroides fragilis*, *Peptococcus*, *Peptostreptococcus* (moxifloxacin strongest)
- Other: Rickettsia (ciprofloxacin only)

TABLE   39-5

Quinolones: Reported Adverse Effects

Body System	Adverse Effects
Central nervous	Headache, dizziness, fatigue, insomnia, depression, restlessness, convulsions
Gastrointestinal	Nausea, constipation, increased AST and ALT levels, flatulence, heartburn, vomiting, diarrhea, oral candidiasis, dysphagia, pseudomembranous colitis
Integumentary	Rash, pruritus, urticaria, flushing
Other	Fever, chills, blurred vision, tinnitus

ALT, alanine aminotransferase; *AST*, aspartate aminotransferase.

Adverse Effects

Fluoroquinolones are capable of causing a variety of adverse effects, the most common of which are listed in Table 39-5. Bacterial overgrowth is another possible complication of quinolone therapy, but this is more commonly associated with long-term use. More worrisome is a heart effect that involves prolongation of the QT interval on the electrocardiogram (ECG). Although there is some debate regarding this effect, cases are still reported. Also, tendonitis and even tendon rupture have been reported. This effect is more common in the older adult, patients with kidney failure, and those on concurrent glucocorticoid therapy (e.g., prednisone).

Interactions

With the exception of norfloxacin, quinolones have excellent oral absorption. In many cases, the extent of oral absorption is comparable with that of intravenous injection. However, the concurrent use of antacids with quinolones causes their oral absorption to be greatly reduced. There are several drugs that interact with quinolones—antacids, iron or zinc preparations, or sucralfate causes the oral absorption of the fluoroquinolone to be greatly reduced. In contrast, presence of a quinolone can reduce the oral absorption of multivalent cations, such as calcium and magnesium, whether dietary or medicinal. Patients should take calcium and magnesium supplements at least 1 hour before or after taking quinolones. Probenecid can reduce kidney excretion of quinolones, and the use of some quinolones with theophylline may increase the toxicity of the bronchodilator. Nitrofurantoin, discussed later in this chapter, can antagonize the antibacterial activity of the quinolones. Oral anticoagulants should be used with caution in patients receiving quinolones because of the antibiotic-induced alteration of the intestinal flora, which affects vitamin K synthesis.

Dosages

For recommended dosages of selected fluoroquinolones, see the Dosages table on p. 741.

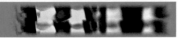

 DRUG PROFILES

Two of the most commonly prescribed quinolones include ciprofloxacin and levofloxacin. Dosage information appears in the designated Dosages table below.

▶▶ ciprofloxacin hydrochloride

Ciprofloxacin hydrochloride (Cipro, many generics) was one of the first of the newer broad-coverage, potent fluoroquinolones to become available. It was first marketed in an oral form and, as such, has the advantage and convenience of an oral medication. Also, because of its excellent bioavailability, it can work as well as many intravenous antibiotics. It is capable of killing a wide range of gram-negative bacteria and is even effective against traditionally difficult-to-kill gram-negative bacteria such as Pseudomonas. Some anaerobic bacteria as well as atypical organisms such as *Chlamydia*, *Mycoplasma*, and *Mycobacterium* can also be killed by ciprofloxacin. It is also a drug of choice for anthrax infection (*Bacillus*

anthracis). It is available in oral, injectable, ophthalmic (Chapter 58), and otic (Chapter 59) forms.

PHARMACOKINETICS

Half-Life	Onset	Peak	Duration
3–4.8 hr	Variable	1–2.3 hr	Up to 12 hr

levofloxacin

Levofloxacin (Levaquin) is one of the newer quinolones. It has a broad spectrum of activity similar to that of ciprofloxacin, but it has the advantage of once-daily dosing, as does gatifloxacin. Levofloxacin is available in both oral and injectable forms.

PHARMACOKINETICS

Half-Life	Onset	Peak	Duration
6–8 hr	Variable	1–2 hr	Up to 24 hr

DOSAGES   Selected Fluoroquinolones ("Quinolones")

Drug (Pregnancy Category)	Pharmacological Class	Usual Dosage Range	Indications
▶▶ ciprofloxacin hydrochloride (Cipro)	Fluoroquinolone	*Adult** IV: 200–400 mg q8–12h PO: 250–750 mg q12h	Broad gram-positive and gram-negative coverage for infections throughout the body
levofloxacin (Levaquin)	Fluoroquinolone	*Adult only* IV/PO: 250–750 mg once daily	Various susceptible bacterial infections

IV, intravenous; *PO*, oral.

*Not normally recommended for children under 8 years because of adverse musculoskeletal effects shown in studies of immature animals.

 DRUG PROFILES

MISCELLANEOUS ANTIBIOTICS

There are a number of antibiotics that do not fit into any of the previously described broad categories. Most of these antibiotics have somewhat unique indications or are especially preferred for a particular type of infection. Although they may not be used as commonly as drugs from the other major classes, they are still of clinical importance. Several of these drugs are described individually as follows. See the Dosages table on p. 744 for dosing information.

▶▶ clindamycin

Clindamycin (Dalacin C) is a semisynthetic derivative of lincomycin, an older antibiotic. Like many semisynthetic derivatives, it was improved over its predecessor drugs through the addition of certain chemical groups to the basic structure, with the result that it is more effective and causes fewer adverse effects than its parent compound.

Clindamycin can be either *bactericidal* or bacteriostatic (Chapter 38), depending on the concentration of the drug

at the site of infection and on the infecting bacteria. It inhibits protein synthesis in bacteria by binding to the 50S ribosomal subunit, the same site that erythromycin binds to (see Figure 38-6 in Chapter 38). Clindamycin is indicated for the treatment of chronic bone infections, genitourinary tract infections, intra-abdominal infections, anaerobic pneumonia, septicemia caused by streptococci and staphylococci, and serious skin and soft-tissue infections caused by susceptible bacteria. Most aerobic gram-positive bacteria, including staphylococci, streptococci, and pneumococci, are susceptible to clindamycin's actions. It also has the special advantage of being active against several anaerobic organisms and is most often used for this purpose. However, resistant strains of gram-positive, gram-negative, and anaerobic organisms do occur. All *Enterobacteriaceae* strains are resistant to clindamycin.

Clindamycin is contraindicated in patients with a known hypersensitivity to it and those with ulcerative colitis or enteritis. Gastrointestinal tract adverse effects are the most common ones and include nausea, vomiting,

Continued

DRUG PROFILES (cont'd)

abdominal pain, diarrhea, pseudomembranous colitis, and anorexia. **Pseudomembranous colitis** is a necrotizing inflammatory bowel condition that is often associated with antibiotic therapy, especially clindamycin. With regard to drug interactions, clindamycin has been shown in the laboratory (in vitro) to antagonize the antibiotic effects of both erythromycin and aminoglycoside drugs. However, this has not been confirmed in vivo (in people or animals). Patients receiving these drug combinations should be appropriately monitored to ascertain their clinical progress. Clindamycin is also known to have some neuromuscular blocking properties that may enhance the actions of neuromuscular drugs used in perioperative and critical care settings (Chapter 12), such as vecuronium. Patients receiving both drugs should be monitored for excessive neuromuscular blockade and respiratory paralysis, with appropriate ventilatory support as needed. Clindamycin is available in oral, injectable, and topical forms (Chapter 57).

PHARMACOKINETICS

Half-Life	Onset	Peak	Duration
3.5–4.5 hr	Variable	45 min	6 hr

dapsone

Dapsone (generic only) is an antibiotic of the sulfone class, which is structurally different from the sulfonamides described earlier. It has been used clinically for several decades. Dapsone works by competitive antagonism of a compound known as para-aminobenzoic acid (PABA), which is essential to bacterial synthesis of folic acid. Bacteria die when they cannot synthesize this vitamin compound. Its official indications include leprosy and a skin condition known as dermatitis herpetiformis, an idiopathic (cause unknown) recurring inflammatory skin condition with lesions resembling herpes blisters but that is not caused by a herpes virus. Leprosy is an infectious disease also known as Hansen's disease. It is characterized by disfiguring nodular skin lesions and is caused by *Mycobacterium leprae*, a bacterium of the same genus that causes tuberculosis (*Mycobacterium tuberculosis*). Dapsone is also used for the prophylactic treatment of *Pneumocystis jirovecii* pneumonia (associated with HIV/AIDS) for individuals who are unable to tolerate sulfamethaxazole-trimethoprim.

Dapsone is contraindicated in cases of drug allergy. Adverse effects include stomach pain, loss of appetite, nausea, vomiting, headache, and skin rash. More serious adverse effects include tingling of the hands or feet, dizziness, incoordination, muscle weakness, blurred vision, ringing in the ears, fever, sore throat, weakness, fatigue, jaundice, and rapid heartbeat. This medication can also cause serious anemias. Patients should have ongoing blood counts while taking this medication. With regard to drug interactions, both the antituberculosis drug

rifampin (Chapter 41) and the anti-HIV drug didanosine (Chapter 40) can chemically reduce the efficacy of dapsone, whereas the sulfonamide antibiotic trimethoprim (Chapter 38) can enhance its therapeutic effects. Dapsone can also reduce the efficacy of oral contraceptives. It is currently available only in tablet form.

PHARMACOKINETICS

Half-Life	Onset	Peak	Duration
10–50 hr	Unknown	4–8 hr	>3 wk

linezolid

Linezolid (Zyvoxam) is the first antibacterial drug in a new class of antibiotics known as *oxazolidinones*. This drug acts by inhibiting bacterial protein synthesis by binding to bacterial ribosomal RNA subunits. Linezolid is used to treat infections associated with vancomycin-resistant *Enterococcus faecium* (VREF), more commonly referred to as VRE. VRE is a notoriously difficult infection to treat and often occurs as a nosocomial (acquired during hospitalization) infection. Linezolid has also received approval for the treatment of hospital-acquired pneumonia, gram-positive infections in infants and children, and complicated skin and skin structure infections, including cases caused by MRSA. Methicillin-resistant *S. aureus*, better known as *MRSA*, is another virulent nosocomial infection. This bacterium is notorious for causing serious infections, especially in the hospital setting. Although methicillin, a penicillinase-resistant penicillin, has been removed from the Canadian market, largely because of bacterial resistance to it, *MRSA* is still the term used to describe the bacterium. Although oxacillin is now the test drug for this organism, linezolid is still used for treatment of community-acquired pneumonia and uncomplicated skin and skin structure infections.

The most commonly reported adverse effects attributed to linezolid are headache, nausea, diarrhea, and vomiting. It has also been shown to decrease platelet count. It is contraindicated in patients with a known hypersensitivity to it. In terms of drug interactions, linezolid has the potential to strengthen the vasopressor (prohypertensive) effects of vasopressive drugs (Chapter 18) such as dopamine through an unclear mechanism. Also, there have been postmarketing case reports of this drug causing serotonin syndrome (Chapter 16) when used concurrently with serotonergic drugs such as the serotonin-selective reuptake inhibitor (SSRI) antidepressants (Chapter 16). Finally, tyramine-containing foods, such as aged cheese or wine, soy sauce, smoked meats or fish, and sauerkraut, can interact with linezolid to raise blood pressure. Linezolid is available in oral and injectable forms.

PHARMACOKINETICS

Half-Life	Onset	Peak	Duration
5 hr	1–2 hr	1–2 hr	12 hr

Continued

DRUG PROFILES (cont'd)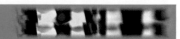

▶▶ *metronidazole*

Metronidazole (Flagyl, generic) is an antimicrobial drug of the class nitroimidazole. It has especially good activity against anaerobic organisms and is widely used for intra-abdominal and gynecological infections caused by such organisms. Examples of the anaerobes include *Peptostreptococcus* spp., *Eubacterium* spp., *Bacteroides* spp., and *Clostridium* spp. Metronidazole is also indicated for treatment of protozoal infections such as amebiasis and trichomoniasis (Chapter 43). Like the quinolones, it works by interfering with microbial DNA synthesis (see Figure 38-6 in Chapter 38).

Metronidazole is contraindicated in cases of drug allergy. Although it is classified as a pregnancy category B drug, it is not recommended for use during the first trimester of pregnancy. Adverse effects include dizziness, headache, gastrointestinal discomfort, nasal congestion, and reversible neutropenia and thrombocytopenia. Drug interactions include acute alcohol intolerance when taken with alcoholic beverages, due to accumulation of acetaldehyde, the principal alcohol metabolite. Metronidazole may also increase the toxicity of lithium, benzodiazepines, cyclosporine, calcium channel blockers, antidepressants (e.g., venlafaxine), and other drugs. In contrast, phenytoin and phenobarbital may reduce the effects of this drug. These interactions occur through enzymatic effects among the cytochrome P450 liver enzymes that result in altered metabolism of the drugs listed above, when taken concurrently. Metronidazole is available in both oral and injectable forms.

PHARMACOKINETICS

Half-Life	Onset	Peak	Duration
8 hr	Unknown	1–2 hr	Unknown

nitrofurantoin

Nitrofurantoin (MacroBID, Macrodantin) is an antibiotic drug of the class nitrofuran. It is indicated primarily for urinary tract infections caused by *E. coli*, *S. aureus*, *Klebsiella* spp., and *Enterobacter* spp. The drug is believed to work by interfering with the activity of enzymes that regulate bacterial carbohydrate metabolism and by disrupting bacterial cell wall formation. It is contraindicated in cases of drug allergy and in cases of significant kidney function impairment because the drug concentrates in the urine. Adverse effects include gastrointestinal discomfort, dizziness, headache, skin reactions (mild to severe reported), blood dyscrasias, ECG changes, possibly irreversible peripheral neuropathy, and hepatotoxicity. This drug is nonetheless very commonly used, even in the frail older adult, and is usually well tolerated as long as the patient is kept well hydrated, which facilitates urinary elimination of the drug. Drug interactions are few and include probenecid, which can reduce kidney excretion of nitrofurantoin, and

antacids, which can reduce the extent of its gastrointestinal absorption. The drug is available for oral use only.

PHARMACOKINETICS

Half-Life	Onset	Peak	Duration
20–60 min*	Unknown	Unknown	Unknown

*This is the plasma half-life, depending on kidney function. The primary site of drug action is in the lumen of the urinary tract, including the bladder.

quinupristin and dalfopristin

Quinupristin and dalfopristin (Synercid) are two *streptogramin* antibacterials marketed in a 30:70 combination. They are approved for intravenous treatment of bacteremia and life-threatening infection caused by vancomycin-resistant *Enterococcus* (VRE) and for the treatment of complicated skin and skin structure infections caused by *S. aureus* and *S. pyogenes*. These two streptogramin antibacterials work synergistically on the bacterial ribosome to disrupt protein synthesis (see Figure 38-6 in Chapter 38). In Canada, this drug combination is available through the Special Access Programme, Health Canada.

Common adverse effects are arthralgias and myalgias, which may become severe. Adverse effects related to the infusion site, including pain, inflammation, edema, and thrombophlebitis, have developed in approximately 75% of patients treated through a peripheral intravenous line. The drug is contraindicated in patients with a known hypersensitivity to it. Drug interactions are limited, the most serious being potential increase of cyclosporine levels, which can be addressed by laboratory monitoring and dosage adjustment of cyclosporine. The drug is available only in injectable form.

PHARMACOKINETICS

Half-Life	Onset	Peak	Duration
1–3 hr	1–2 hr	3–4 hr	8–12 hr

▶▶ *vancomycin*

Vancomycin (Vancocin, generic) is a natural bactericidal antibiotic structurally unrelated to any other commercially available antibiotics. It destroys bacteria by binding to the bacterial cell wall, producing immediate inhibition of cell wall synthesis and death (see Figure 38-6 in Chapter 38). This mechanism differs from that of β-lactam antibiotics.

Vancomycin is the antibiotic of choice for the treatment of MRSA infection and infections caused by many other gram-positive bacteria. It is not active against gram-negative bacteria, fungi, or yeast. Oral vancomycin is indicated for the treatment of antibiotic-induced pseudomembranous colitis (*Clostridium difficile*) and staphylococcal enterocolitis. Because the oral formulation is poorly absorbed from the gastrointestinal tract, it is used for its local effects on the surface of the gastrointestinal tract. The parenteral form is indicated

Continued

DRUG PROFILES (cont'd)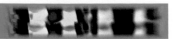

for the treatment of bone and joint infections and bacterial bloodstream infections caused by *Staphylococcus* spp. Resistance to vancomycin has been noted with increasing frequency in patients with infections caused by *Enterococcus* organisms. Although these strains have been isolated most often from gastrointestinal tract infections, they have also been isolated from skin, soft tissue, and bloodstream infections. Federal, provincial, and institution guidelines are available for the management and treatment of MRSA, VRE, and *C. difficile*.

Vancomycin is contraindicated in patients with known hypersensitivity to it. It should be used with caution in those with pre-existing kidney dysfunction or hearing loss, as well as in the older adult and neonates. Vancomycin is similar to the aminoglycosides in that specific drug levels in the blood are required in order for it to be effective and safe. If the levels are too low (less than 5 mg/mL), the dosage may be subtherapeutic with reduced antibacterial efficacy. If the blood levels are too high (over 50 mg/mL), this may cause toxicities, the two most severe being ototoxicity (hearing loss) and nephrotoxicity (kidney damage). Nephrotoxicity is more likely to occur with concurrent therapy with other nephrotoxic drugs such as aminoglycosides and cyclosporine. Vancomycin can also cause additive neuromuscular blocking effects with patients receiving neuromuscular blockers. The patient's respiratory function must therefore be appropriately monitored and supported as needed. Another common adverse effect that is bothersome but usually not harmful is known as "red man syndrome". This involves flushing and itching of the head, face, neck, and upper trunk area. It can usually be alleviated by slowing the rate of infusion of dose to at least 1 hour. Optimal blood levels of vancomycin should be a peak level of 20 to 40 mcg/mL and a trough level of 5 to 15 mcg/mL. Vancomycin is available in both oral and injectable forms.

PHARMACOKINETICS

Half-Life	Onset	Peak	Duration
4–6 hr	Variable	1 hr	Up to 12 hr

DOSAGES Selected Miscellaneous Antibiotics

Drug (Pregnancy Category)	Pharmacological Class	Usual Dosage Range	Indications
▸▸clindamycin (Dalacin C) (B)	Lincosamide	*Neonates under 1 mo* IM/IV: 10–20 mg/kg/day divided tid–qid *Children older than 1 mo* IM/IV: 10–40 mg/day, divided tid–qid PO: 8–20 mg/kg/day divided tid–qid *Adult* IM/IV: 600–2700 mg/day, divided bid–tid–qid PO: 150–450 mg q6h	Anaerobes; streptococcal and staphylococcal infections of bone, skin, respiratory, and GU tract
dapsone (generic only) (C)	Sulfone	*Children/Adult* PO: 50–300 mg once daily	Leprosy (*Mycobacterium leprae*); dermatitis herpetiformis
linezolid (Zyvoxam) (C)	Oxazolidinone	*Adults only* IV/PO: 400–600 mg q12h	VRE; skin and respiratory infections caused by *Staphylococcus* and *Streptococcus* spp.
▸▸metronidazole (Flagyl, generic) (B)	Nitroimidazole	*Children* IV/PO: 15–50 mg/kg/day divided tid *Adult* IV/PO: 250–500 mg q6–12h	Primarily anaerobic and gram-negative infections of abdominal cavity, skin, bone, and respiratory and GU tracts
nitrofurantoin (MacroBID, Macrodantin) (B)	Nitrofuran	*Children* PO: 5–7 mg/kg/day divided qid *Adult* PO: 50–100 mg qid	Primarily UTIs caused by gram-negative organisms and *Staphylococcus aureus*
quinupristin/dalfopristin*(Synercid) (B)	Streptogramins	*Children/Adult* IV: 7.5 mg/kg q8–12h	VRE; skin infections caused by streptococcal and staphylococcal infections
▸▸vancomycin (Vancocin, generic) (B, oral; C injection)	Tricyclic glycopeptide	*Neonates, Infants, and Children* IV/PO: 10–15 mg/kg q6–12h *Adult* IV/PO: 500–2000 mg q12–24h	Severe staphylococcal infections, including MRSA; other serious gram-positive infections, including *Streptococcus* spp.

GU, genitourinary; *IM*, intramuscular; *IV*, intravenous; *MRSA*, methicillin-resistant *S. aureus*; *PO*, oral; *spp.*, species; *UTIs*, urinary tract infections; *VRE*, vancomycin-resistant *Enterococcus*.

*Available through Special Access Programme, Health Canada

NURSING PROCESS

Assessment

Many of the antibiotics discussed in this chapter are often reserved for more virulent infections and are mainly administered by parenteral routes (as compared with the drugs discussed in Chapter 38), thus demanding more astute and thorough assessment of the patient and for the specific drug. The groups of antibiotics in this chapter require critical assessment for any history of or current symptoms that are indicative of hypersensitivity or allergic reactions (from mild reactions with rash, pruritus, hives to severe reactions with laryngeal edema, bronchospasms, hypotension, and possible cardiac arrest). Further assessment should include a nursing physical assessment, age, weight, baseline vital signs, and body temperature. Diagnostic and laboratory studies that may be ordered include some of the following:

- For assessing liver function: aspartate aminotransferase (AST), alanine aminotransferase (ALT)
- For kidney function: urinalysis, blood urea nitrogen (BUN), and serum creatinine
- For heart function: Electrocardiogram (ECG), echocardiogram, ultrasound, and heart enzymes
- For sensitivity of antibiotic to the bacteria: culture and sensitivity tests of the infected tissue, site, or blood
- For baseline blood counts: white blood count (WBC), hemoglobin (Hgb), hematocrit (Hct), red blood cells (RBCs), and platelet/clotting values

A baseline neurological assessment should include baseline sensory and motor intactness and assessment of any alterations in neurological functioning—for example, altered sensorium and level of consciousness because of potential central nervous system adverse effects. Baseline abdominal and gastrointestinal assessments are important with focus on bowel patterns and bowel sounds because of possible gastrointestinal adverse effects. Contraindications, cautions, and drug interactions should also be noted, including a complete list of the patient's medications, including over-the-counter drugs and natural health products. An ethnocultural assessment is important because of certain racial and ethnic groups' responses to specific drugs and the potential use of alternative healing practices.

As with any antibiotic, it is important for the nurse to assess for superinfection or a secondary infection that occurs with the destruction of "normal" flora during antibiotic therapy (Chapter 38). Fungal infections (e.g., superinfections) are evidenced by fever, lethargy, perineal itching, and other anatomically related symptoms. The status of the patient's immune system and overall condition is important to assess; if there is a deficiency (e.g., patients with cancer, autoimmune disorders such as lupus erythematosus, acquired immune deficiency syndrome (AIDS), or any chronic illness), the patient's ability to physically resist infection may be diminished. Antibiotic resistance is a continual concern with antibiotic drug therapy, especially with children and in large health care institutions and long-term care facilities. This resistance to certain antibiotics should be considered when assessing patients for symptoms of infection and superinfection. Once a thorough assessment has been done and follow-up to therapy considered, the nurse should share information about antibiotic resistance prevention (see Implementation).

With aminoglycosides, hypersensitivity, pre-existing conditions and diseases, and the patient's other medications need to be assessed because of the many cautions, contraindications, and possible drug interactions. The aminoglycosides are known for their ototoxicity and nephrotoxicity; therefore, baseline hearing tests with audiometry and vestibular function as well as kidney function studies (BUN, urinalysis, serum and urine creatinine levels) should be performed and all results documented. If kidney baseline functioning is decreased or abnormal, dosage amounts may need to be adjusted by the physician to address the nephrotoxicity. A thorough neuromuscular assessment should be performed because of possible drug-related neurotoxicity and the higher risk for complications in those with impaired neurological functioning. For example, patients with myasthenia gravis and Parkinson's disease may experience worsening of muscle weakness because of the drug's neuromuscular blockade. Neonates (because of an immature nervous system and kidneys) and older adults (because of decreased neurological and kidney functioning) are at highest risk for nephrotoxicity, neurotoxicity, and ototoxicity and thus require careful assessment before and during drug therapy. Hydration status should also be assessed.

Fluoroquinolones, such as ciprofloxacin, require careful assessment for drug allergies. Pre-existing central nervous system disorders (e.g., seizures or history of strokes) may be exacerbated with the concurrent use of these drugs, thus a careful history is needed before administering this group of drugs. Assessment of bowel activity is necessary, as is assessment of neuromuscular functioning because of the potential for dizziness, headache, and visual changes. It is also necessary to assess the timing of medication dosing. Most other drugs should not be administered at the same time because of the interaction with antacids (see earlier discussion on drug interactions). Fluoroquinolines have a preferred dosing time of 2 hours after meals. It is also important to remember the many drug interactions with these antibiotics, including that with iron, multivitamin products, and zinc. These drugs may be used but should not be given within 2 hours of the fluoroquinolones because the drug absorption is decreased. Blood glucose levels and kidney and liver function tests should also be assessed and documented.

Hypersensitivity to either clindamycin or related compounds should be assessed and documented as well as any allergy to aspirin. These drugs should never be given at the same time as neuromuscular blocking drugs. In addition, because of the risk for antibiotic-associated colitis, blood dyscrasias, and nephrotoxicity, it is critical to patient safety to assess gastrointestinal patterns, presence of abdominal pain, frequency and consistency of stools, WBC, platelets, BUN, and serum creatinine levels.

With dapsone, the indication for its use is important in assessment. If it is used for malaria, it may be taken for 3 to 5 years instead of for a shorter period with other indications (e.g., *Pneumocystis carinii* pneumonia [PCP] or what is now often referred to as *Pneumocystis jirovecii* pneumonia), thus changing the focus of an assessment. Gastrointestinal status and bowel patterns, including bowel sounds, gastrointestinal upset, nausea, and vomiting, are important to assess because of the drug's adverse effects. Baseline neurological assessment with concentration on sensory and motor functioning and any pre-existing neurological abnormalities, such as numbness, tingling, dizziness, muscle weakness, blurred vision, or tinnitus (ringing in the ears), is needed because of central nervous system–related adverse effects. Seizures may be indicative of dapsone overdose, thus it is important to assess for any past or present seizure activity. In addition, assessment of vital signs with close attention to the patient's temperature and pain status is important in order to establish baseline parameters against which other vital signs may be compared during therapy. This assessment may call attention to any unusual adverse effects, including fever or sore throat. Because of the drug's potential for causing tachycardia and other heart adverse effects and the potential for serious anemias, assessment of pulse rate, blood pressure, and auscultation of heart sounds is important. Monitoring of complete blood counts with focus on RBCs, WBC, Hgb, and Hct is also appropriate. Skin colour should be noted because a bluish discoloration of the skin may indicate toxicity or overdosage with these drugs.

Linezolid is used for diabetic foot infections, community-acquired infections, vancomycin-resistant *Enterococcus faecium* (VRE), nosocomial pneumonias, and other severe infections. An astute and careful assessment of the patient's underlying immune status and kidney, liver, gastrointestinal, and hematological functioning is critical to patient safety and to early identification of adverse or toxic effects. A systems-related nursing assessment includes a history of infections and response to infections, overall immune status, intake and output, bladder functioning, jaundice, liver enlargement (noted on abdominal palpation and percussion), bowel sounds, bowel patterns, and any complaints of gastrointestinal-related symptoms (e.g., nausea, vomiting, diarrhea, abdominal pain). The related laboratory or diagnostic testing may include the following:

- For immune and hematological status: immunoglobulin levels, WBC, RBCs, platelets, Hgb, and Hct
- For kidney and liver status: BUN, creatinine, urinalysis, ALT, AST, alkaline phosphatase (AP), and gamma-glutamyltransferase (GGT)

The above lab value assessments are all important to the safe use of linezolid, to the prevention of possible adverse and toxic effects, and to the patient's overall well-being. Should the patient be immune compromised and present with kidney or liver dysfunction, adverse effects may be exacerbated, with the potential for complications and toxicity.

Patients taking metronidazole need to be assessed for allergy to the drug and to other nitroimidazole derivatives. Culture and sensitivity reports should be known prior to starting this therapy. There should also be a baseline assessment of neurological (dizziness, numbness, tingling, and other sensory and motor abnormalities), gastrointestinal (bowel sounds, bowel problems and patterns), and genitourinary (urinary patterns, colour of urine, intake and output) systems. Pregnancy status, even with topical applications, is important to assess and document because these would be contraindications. In addition, concurrent intake of alcohol should be noted and subsequent information given in relation to interaction with the drug. A disulfiram-like (Antabuse) reaction may occur, leading to flushing of the face, tachycardia, palpitations, nausea, and vomiting.

Assessment of allergies and a history of asthma (which puts a patient at risk for drug allergy) are important with use of nitrofurantoin. Kidney and liver functions should be assessed. Patients with a history of glucose-6-phosphate dehydrogenase (G6PD) deficiency are of concern because they have a greater risk for hemolytic anemia. Patients who are debilitated are at greater risk for peripheral neuropathies. Other medications that are neurotoxic should be avoided because of an additional risk for neurological adverse effects (e.g., irreversible peripheral neuropathy). The patient's skin and its colour, turgor, and intactness should be noted because of the drug-related risk for Stevens–Johnson syndrome. Assessment should also include respiratory patterns and breath sounds and noting cough if present.

With quinupristin-dalfopristin, vital signs should be noted along with baseline liver and kidney function tests and complete blood count (CBC). Gastrointestinal functioning is important to assess, with a focus on bowel patterns, bowel sounds, and abdominal pain, because of drug-related antibiotic-associated colitis.

With vancomycin, patient assessment should include enquiry about other medications the patient is taking, especially if the drugs are nephrotoxic and ototoxic. Vital signs should be assessed with close attention to blood pressure during infusion of the drug. Bowel patterns and sounds need to be assessed because of the risk for gastrointestinal and abdominal adverse effects. Because of the risk for ototoxicity, baseline hearing status should be assessed, as should urinary patterns because of the risk for nephrotoxicity. The colour of the patient's skin should be noted to assess the risk for red man syndrome. Given the multiple incompatibilities, as with several of the previously mentioned parenteral antibiotics in this chapter, the nurse should always assess for potential fluid–medication interactions.

Nursing Diagnoses

- Risk for infection related to the patient's compromised immune system status before and during treatment
- Risk for injury (compromised organ function) related to adverse effects of medications (e.g., ototoxicity and nephrotoxicity) and from a weakened physical state
- Pain related to infection, adverse reaction to medications, or both
- Deficient knowledge related to lack of information and experience with the medication regimen
- Ineffective therapeutic regimen management related to lack of information about the proper use of antibiotics and the lack of patient's experience with the therapy

Planning

Goals

- Patient will be free of the signs and symptoms of infection once therapy is completed.
- Patient will experience minimal adverse effects of antibiotic therapy.
- Patient will remain adherent to therapy.
- Patient will return for follow-up visits as recommended.
- Patient will complete the entire course of antibiotics as ordered.

Outcome Criteria

- Patient experiences increased sense of well-being related to resolving infection.
- Patient states the signs and symptoms of an infection (e.g., fever, pain, malaise) and reports them if they occur while on antibiotics.
- Patient identifies the adverse effects of antibiotic therapy such as gastrointestinal upset, nausea, and diarrhea (specific to each class).
- Patient experiences increased periods of comfort and improved energy levels related to a resolving infectious process and experiences minimal adverse effects of therapy.
- Patient states the reasons for adherence to therapy (i.e., to adequately eradicate bacteria).
- Patient states the measures to take to minimize the gastrointestinal distress associated with antibiotic therapy, such as taking with yogourt or other foods, as appropriate.
- Patient keeps follow-up appointments with the physician or other health care provider to be evaluated for therapeutic effects or complications of therapy.

Implementation

Aminoglycosides should be given exactly as ordered and with adequate hydration. Unless contraindicated, fluids up to 3000 mL/day should be encouraged, unless contraindicated, especially with oral dosage forms. Parenteral dosage forms are most common. To address potential nephrotoxicity, intake and output should be calculated with constant monitoring of urine specific gravity. Consumption of yogourt or buttermilk may help prevent antibiotic-induced superinfections (Chapter 38). The patient should be encouraged to report to the health care provider any changes in hearing, ringing in the ears (tinnitus), or a full feeling in the ears. Nausea, vomiting with motion, ataxia, nystagmus, or dizziness should also be reported immediately. Redness, burning, and itching of eyes may indicate an adverse reaction to ophthalmic forms, and redness over the skin area may indicate an adverse reaction to topical forms. Intramuscular sites should be checked for induration. If noted, it should be reported immediately to the physician, and the site should not be reused. Intravenous sites should be checked for heat, swelling, redness, pain, or red streaking over the vein (phlebitis) per protocol or policy.

Gentamicin sulfate comes in intrathecal, ophthalmic, topical, and parenteral dosage forms. Special considerations for each of these routes include the following:

- Intramuscular: Give deeply and slowly to minimize discomfort.
- Intravenous: Check for other drug incompatibilities and only give clear or only slightly yellow solutions that have been diluted with either NaCl or D5W, infusing as prescribed.
- Intrathecal: This dosage form should be "preservative" free and, as a point of information, mixed with 10% estimated cerebral spinal fluid (CSF) or NaCl and given over a period of 3 to 5 minutes.
- Ophthalmic: Refer to Chapter 10 and Figures 10-81 through 10-83 for specific instructions on administering eye drops and ointments. Additionally, it is important to assess serum levels; peak levels range from 5 to 10 mcg/mL, trough levels are less than 2 mcg/mL, and toxic peak levels are over 10 mcg/mL. Toxic trough levels are values over 2 mcg/mL.

Neomycin, another aminoglycoside, is available only topically in opthalamic and otic drugs, often in combinations and as an over-the-counter drug. Nursing considerations associated with the use of tobramycin are similar to those discussed with parenteral, ophthalmic, and topical dosage forms of gentamicin.

Fluoroquinolones should be taken exactly as prescribed and for the full course of treatment. The patient should not take antacids at the same time as oral fluoroquinolones in order to prevent inactivation of the antibiotic. It is recommended that oral fluoroquinolones be given 2 hours before antacids or ferrous sulfate to avoid alteration in the antibiotic's absorption. Alkaline foods and fluids, such as dairy products, peanuts, and sodium bicarbonate, may lead to a higher incidence of crystalluria from a more alkaline urinary pH and thus should be avoided. It is recommended, however, that the patient force fluids and increase intake of fluids and foods high in ascorbic acid (e.g., cranberry juice and citrus fruits) to prevent crystalluria. See Patient Education for more information.

Clindamycin should be administered as ordered whether by oral, topical, intravaginal, intravenous, or intramuscular routes. Oral forms should be taken with 240 mL of water or fluids and dosed evenly over 24 hours, as with other dosage forms. Once oral solutions are reconstituted, they should never be refrigerated because of the tendency of the solution to thicken. With topical forms, it is important to avoid simultaneous use of peeling or abrasive acne products, soaps, or alcohol-containing cosmetics so that there are no cumulative effects. Topical forms should be applied in a "thin" layer to the affected area. Intravaginal doses are usually given via an applicator—for example, one full applicator at bedtime for 3 to 7 days, or one suppository at bedtime for 3 days. Bedtime use is recommended for comfort reasons, and perineal pads may be worn to catch any leakage of the medicine from the vagina. Intravenous (IV) dosage forms should be infused by piggyback technique and as ordered. Most references state to never give IV push. Doses of the drug should be diluted and infused per manufacturer guidelines and as ordered. Too rapid IV infusion could lead to severe hypotension and possible cardiac arrest. Intramuscular (IM) dosage forms should be given as deep IM injections.

Dapsone should be taken with food or milk to reduce gastrointestinal upset. Alternative methods of contraception should be used if the patient is taking oral contraceptives because of lack of effectiveness when taken with dapsone.

Linezolid is generally given orally or intravenously. Oral dosages should be evenly spaced and given with food or milk to decrease possible gastrointestinal upset. Oral suspension forms should be given within 21 days of reconstitution. IV dosages should be protected from light and infused over 30 to 120 minutes and should not be mixed with any other medication. Because of the risk for antibiotic-associated colitis, superinfections, and myelosupression, it is important to watch for the occurrence of frequent, loose, and foul-smelling stools; severe genital or anal pruritus; and severe mouth soreness. In addition, complete blood counts should be watched closely (e.g., weekly) during therapy.

Oral forms of metronidazole should be given with food or meals to decrease gastrointestinal upset. It is recommended that intravaginal doses be given at bedtime, and topical creams, ointments, or lotions are to be applied thinly to the affected area. An applicator is required for intravaginal dosages. Generally speaking, gloves are worn to protect the hands from unnecessary exposure to medication; the nurse should always wear gloves as a means of standard precautions. Topical forms should not be applied close to the eyes, to avoid irritation. IV dosage forms are supplied in a "ready-to-use" infusion bag and should be stored at room temperature.

Nitrofurantoin is available in oral forms and should be given with sufficient fluids, food, or milk to reduce gastrointestinal upset. Because of the risk for superinfection, hepatotoxicity, and peripheral neuropathy (which may be irreversible), it is necessary to document findings from constant monitoring of their respective signs and symptoms. Jaundice, itching, rash, and liver enlargement may indicate toxic effects to the liver, whereas numbness and tingling may occur with peripheral neuropathy. In addition, constant monitoring of breath sounds, breathing patterns, and any cough is important because of the risk for permanent lung function impairment.

For quinupristin and dalfopristin, IV dosage forms should be reconstituted as recommended by the drug manufacturer; these are stable for only 1 hour at room temperature. A diluted infusion bag is stable for up to 6 hours at room temperature and 54 hours if refrigerated. These characteristics are important to know in order to prevent untoward complications. When reconstituting the drug, use only the recommended diluents; 0.9% NaCl is an incompatible solution. Use a gentle swirling action to mix the drug instead of shaking it (to help minimize foaming). Generally, infusions are given over at least 60 minutes. As with other antibiotics, the same measures should be implemented with superinfection, hepatotoxicity, and antibiotic-associated colitis. It is important to report any of the following symptoms to the physician: diarrhea with fever, abdominal pain, and mucus or blood in the stools. If these symptoms occur, the patient should be monitored and the drug withheld until further orders are received from the physician.

Vancomycin may be used orally but is poorly absorbed, thus parenteral dosage forms are used more frequently. For *C. difficile*, the drug may be given orally for better therapeutic effect. A powder-reconstituted dose form may be used via a nasogastric tube, and oral solutions are only stable for 2 weeks if refrigerated. Powder forms for oral dosage forms are not to be used with IV administration. IV dosages should be reconstituted as recommended (e.g., with either D5W or 0.9% NaCl) and should be infused over at least 60 minutes. Too rapid administration of IV vancomycin may lead to red man syndrome with a subsequent decrease in blood pressure and flushing of neck, face, and upper body. Extravasation may cause local skin irritation and damage; therefore frequent monitoring of the infusion and, more specifically, the IV site, is needed. Constant monitoring for drug-related neurotoxicity, nephrotoxicity, ototoxicity, and superinfection is critical to patient safety. Adequate hydration (at least 2 litres of fluids/24 hr unless contraindicated) is especially important to prevent nephrotoxicity. When monitoring serum drug levels, it is important to remember that therapeutic or optimal "peak" levels range from 20 to 40 mg/mL with a trough at less than 15 mg/mL. Levels higher than these optimum levels are considered toxic.

◪ Evaluation

Evaluation of goals, outcome criteria, therapeutic effects, and adverse effects should be ongoing at the start of, during, and after antibiotic therapy. Patients should report a decrease in symptoms (e.g., infection) as well as no injury and a decrease in pain. Therapeutic goals include all of those previously mentioned as well as a return to normal for all complete blood counts and vital signs, negative reports of culture and sensitivity, and improved appetite, energy level, and sense of well-being.

Signs and symptoms of the infection should be resolved, and the patient should have knowledge levels sufficient to enhance the success of treatment. Another aspect of evaluation includes monitoring for adverse effects of therapy, such as superinfections, antibiotic-associated colitis, nephrotoxicity, ototoxicity, neurotoxicity, hepatotoxicity, and other drug-specific adverse effects.

 IN MY FAMILY

Silk of the Corn Cob

(as told by K.C., of Portuguese descent)

"Both my parents grew up on a small Portuguese island named Madeira. . . . [A] traditional remedy used for individuals with urinary infection would be silk from corn picked from their garden. . . . The silk would be boiled in water to become a form of tea. . . . While drinking the tea, the individual would place some of the warm water and silk in a container and sit on it because they believed the steam coming from the silk and water would together cure the infection."

PATIENT EDUCATION

Aminoglycosides

❖ Patients should be educated about the drug, its purpose, and adverse effects and that hearing loss may occur even after therapy has been completed. Patients need to be aware that any change in hearing must be reported immediately to the health care provider.

❖ Patients should be instructed that forcing fluids up to 3000 mL/day, unless contraindicated, is important with any medication, and especially with antibiotics.

❖ Patients should be informed to report any of the following to their physician: tinnitus, high-frequency hearing loss, persistent headache, nausea, and vertigo. They also need to know about the signs and symptoms of superinfection, as with any antibiotic, such as diarrhea; vaginal discharge; stomatitis; glottitis; black, hairy tongue; loose and foul-smelling stools; and cough.

Fluoroquinolones

❖ Patients should be educated about avoiding exposure to sun and tanning beds. Use of sunglasses and sunscreen protection is recommended.

❖ Patients should be informed about signs and symptoms that need to be reported, including dizziness, restlessness, stomach distress, diarrhea, unusual emotional behaviour, confusion, and an irregular or rapid heartbeat.

❖ Drug interactions occur between these antibiotics and oral anticoagulants (e.g., warfarin [Coumadin]), and patients should be educated about the need for frequent coagulation studies (INR) so that clotting ability is monitored and appropriate action can be taken as needed.

Clindamycin

❖ Patients should be encouraged not to use topical forms near the eyes or near any abraded areas, to avoid irritation.

❖ With use of vaginal dosages, patients should be informed not to engage in sexual intercourse for the duration of the therapy and that the entire course of treatment must be completed as ordered for maximal therapeutic effects.

❖ Patients should be informed that in the event of accidental contact of creams with the eyes, the eyes need to be rinsed immediately with copious amounts of cool tap water.

Dapsone

❖ Patients should be instructed to contact the physician if any tingling of hands or feet, dizziness, lack of coordination, muscle weakness, blurred vision, ringing of the ears (tinnitus), fever, fatigue, jaundice, or rapid heartbeat is experienced.

❖ If a dose is missed and remembered within a short time frame, patients may be instructed to take the dose; however, they should be reminded to NOT take the missed dose if it is time for the next dose. They should not double-up on the dose to "catch up."

❖ If overdose is suspected (e.g., nausea, vomiting, seizures, and a bluish discoloration of the skin), patients should be encouraged to contact a local poison control centre or emergency room immediately. This phone number is important to be kept at hand for any drug overdose.

❖ Female patients should be informed that backup contraception is indicated with this drug.

Linezolid

❖ Patients should be instructed that medication must be taken for the full length of treatment (as with all antibiotics) and that they must avoid tyramine-containing foods (e.g., red wine, aged cheeses).

❖ Patients should immediately report any of the following to their physician: severe abdominal pain, fever, severe diarrhea, or worsening of signs and symptoms of infection.

Continued

Metronidazole

❖ Patients should be warned about the red-brown or darker coloured urine that may occur with this drug and to avoid any alcohol and alcohol-containing products (e.g., cough preparations and elixirs) because of the risk for an disulfiram-like reaction (e.g., severe vomiting).

❖ Patients should be encouraged to understand the purpose of the drug, such as its use as either an antibacterial drug or as an antifungal drug because knowing about medications is crucial to achieve its therapeutic effect and to prevent adverse effects.

Nitrofurantoin

❖ Patients should be informed that their urine may become dark yellow or brown with drug therapy. They should also be educated about avoiding exposure to the sun and ultraviolet light because of photosensitivity and about wearing protective clothing and sunscreen if they will be exposed to the sun.

❖ Patients should be encouraged to notify their physician or health care provider if they experience cough, fever, chest pain, difficulty breathing, numbness or tingling of extremities, or alopecia.

Vancomycin

❖ Patients should report any changes in hearing such as ringing in the ears, feeling of fullness in the ears, any nausea, vomiting with motion, unsteady gait, or dizziness. Other adverse effects that should be reported immediately include a generalized "tingling" (usually after IV dosing), chills, fever, rash, or hives.

❖ Patients should be informed that follow-up appointments are important for monitoring serum drug levels and possible toxicity. Therapeutic serum levels need to be monitored throughout therapy and are critical to prevention of toxicity.

POINTS TO REMEMBER

❖ There are various classes of antibiotics with different mechanisms of actions and spectrums of activity.

❖ Over the years, bacteria have developed enzymes and mechanisms to interact with antibiotics and render the antibiotic ineffective. A significant condition is methicillin-resistant *Staphylococcus aureus* (MRSA).

❖ The aminoglycosides are a group of natural and semisynthetic antibiotics that are classified as bactericidal drugs, which are extremely potent, and are capable of potentially serious toxicities (e.g., nephrotoxicity, ototoxicity).

❖ Fluoroquinolones are extremely potent bactericidal, broad-spectrum antibiotics and include norfloxacin, ciprofloxacin, levofloxacin, moxifloxacin, gatifloxacin, and gemifloxacin.

❖ Clindamycin is a semisynthetic derivative of lincomycin, an older antibiotic.

❖ Dapsone is an antibiotic of the sulfone class and structurally different from the sulfonamides.

❖ Linezolid (Zyvoxam) is an antibacterial drug used to treat infections associated with vancomycin-resistant *Enterococcus faecium* (VREF), more commonly referred to as VRE. VRE is a difficult infection to treat and often occurs as a nosocomial (acquired while hospitalized) infection.

❖ Metronidazole (Flagyl) is an antimicrobial drug of the class nitroimidazole, has good activity against anaerobic organisms, and is widely used to treat intra-abdominal and gynecological infections, as well as protozoal infections (e.g., amebiasis, trichomoniasis).

❖ Nitrofurantoin (MacroBID, Macrodantin) is an antibiotic drug of the class nitrofuran. It is indicated primarily to treat urinary tract infections caused by the following bacteria: *E. coli*, *S. aureus*, *Klebsiella* spp., and *Enterobacter* spp.

❖ Quinupristin and dalfopristin (Synercid) are two streptogramin antibacterials approved for intravenous treatment of bacteremia and life-threatening infection caused by VRE and for treatment of complicated skin and skin-structure infections caused by *S. aureus* and *S. pyogenes*.

❖ Antibiotics require critical assessment for any history of or current symptoms indicative of hypersensitivity or allergic reactions (mild reactions with rash, pruritus, and hives, to severe reactions with laryngeal edema, bronchospasms, hypotension, and possible cardiac arrest). Further assessment includes a nursing physical assessment and data on age, weight, and baseline vital signs, especially body temperature and laboratory studies (e.g., culture and sensitivity, kidney and liver function tests, and complete blood count).

❖ With any antibiotic, it is important for the nurse to assess for superinfection, or a secondary infection that occurs with the destruction of "normal" flora during antibiotic therapy. Superinfections may occur in the mouth, respiratory tract, gastrointestinal and genitourinary tracts, and the skin. Fungal infections are evidenced by fever, lethargy, perineal itching, and other anatomically related symptoms.

EXAMINATION REVIEW QUESTIONS

1 While assessing a woman who is receiving an antibiotic for community-acquired pneumonia, the nurse notes that the patient has a thick, white vaginal discharge. The patient is also complaining about perineal itching. Which of the following problems does the nurse suspect that the patient has?
a. A superinfection
b. An allergic reaction
c. Resistance to the antibiotic
d. An adverse effect to the antibiotic

2 The nurse is preparing to administer the first dose of an aminoglycoside to a patient. In addition to assessing for allergies, which laboratory results would be of greatest concern at this time?
a. Decreased serum creatinine level
b. Increased serum creatinine level
c. Decreased red blood cell count
d. Increased white blood cell count

3 While administering vancomycin, which of the following would the nurse know is the most important assessment before giving a dose?
a. Liver function
b. Platelet count
c. Kidney function
d. White blood cell count

4 During therapy with an intravenous aminoglycoside, the patient calls the nurse and says, "I am hearing some odd sounds, like ringing, in my ears." Which is the best action of the nurse at this time?
a. Reduce the rate of the intravenous infusion
b. Increase the rate of the intravenous infusion
c. Stop the infusion immediately and notify the physician
d. Reassure the patient that these are expected adverse effects

5 When giving intravenous quinolones, which drugs that may have serious interactions with quinolones does the nurse need to keep in mind?
a. Diuretics
b. NSAIDs
c. Antihypertensives
d. Oral anticoagulants

For answers see http://evolve.elsevier.com/Canada/Lilley/pharmacology/.

CRITICAL THINKING ACTIVITIES

1 During an infusion of vancomycin, a patient complains of flushing of the face and neck and itching over those same areas. Is this an allergic reaction, or is there another reason for this? Explain.

2 During therapy with the aminoglycoside tobramycin, you note that the latest trough drug level was 3 mg/mL. This drug is given daily, and the next dose is due in 1 hour. On the basis of this trough drug level, should you give the drug? Explain your actions.

3 Discuss what measures are used to monitor for nephrotoxicity and ototoxicity.

For answers see http://evolve.elsevier.com/Canada/Lilley/pharmacology/.

CHAPTER 40

Antiviral Drugs

Learning Objectives

After reading this chapter, the successful student will be able to do the following:

1 Discuss the effects of the immune system with attention to the different types of immunity.

2 Discuss the effects of viruses in the human body.

3 Discuss the process of immunosuppression in patients with viral infections, specifically those with HIV.

4 Discuss the pathophysiology, including the stages, of HIV/AIDS and the drugs used to manage and treat the illness.

5 Discuss the mechanism of action, indications, contraindications, cautions, routes of administration, adverse effects, and toxic effects associated with antiviral and antiretroviral drugs.

6 Develop a collaborative plan of care that includes all phases of the nursing process for patients receiving antiviral and antiretroviral drugs.

e-Learning Activities

Web site
(http://evolve.elsevier.com/Canada/Lilley/pharmacology/)

- Animations
- Answers to chapter questions, activities, and case studies
- Calculators and Category Catchers
- Glossary with audio pronunciations
- IV Therapy and Medication Error Checklists
- Multiple-Choice Review Question quizzes
- Nursing Care Plans
- Online Appendices and Supplements
- WebLinks

Drug Profiles

▸▸ **acyclovir,** p. 761
amantadine (amantadine hydrochloride)*, p. 761
enfuvirtide, p. 770
▸▸ **ganciclovir (ganciclovir hydrochloride)*,** p. 762
▸▸ **indinavir (indinavir sulfate)*,** p. 770
▸▸ **maraviroc,** p. 771
▸▸ **nevirapine,** p. 771
oseltamivir (oseltamivir phosphate)*, zanamivir, p. 762
▸▸ **raltegravir (raltegravir potassium)*,** p. 771
ribavirin, p. 762
tenofovir (tenofovir disoproxil)*, p. 771
▸▸ **zidovudine,** p. 771

▸▸ Key drug.

*Full generic name is given in parentheses. For the purposes of this text, the more common shortened name is used.

Glossary

Acquired immune deficiency syndrome (AIDS) Infection caused by the human immunodeficiency virus (HIV) that weakens the host's immune system, giving rise to opportunistic infections by pathogens that normally coexist in the body with minimal health effects. (p. 754)

Antibody An immunoglobulin molecule that has an antigen-specific amino acid sequence and is synthesized by the humoral immune system (antibodies produced from B lymphoctes) in response to exposure to a specific antigen; the antibody's purpose is to attack and destroy molecules of this antigen. (p. 755)

Antigen A substance, usually a protein, that is foreign to a host (e.g., human) and causes the formation of an antibody and reacts specifically with that antibody. (p. 755)

Antiretroviral drug A more specific term for antiviral drugs that target retroviruses such as HIV (see *retrovirus*). (p. 757)

Antiviral drug   A general term for any drug that destroys viruses, either directly or indirectly, by suppressing their replication. (p. 755)

Cell-mediated immunity (CMI)   One of two major parts of the immune system. CMI consists of nonspecific immune responses mediated primarily by T lymphocytes (T cells) and other immune system cells (e.g., monocytes, macrophages, neutrophils), but not antibody-producing cells (B lymphocytes). (p. 755)

Deoxyribonucleic acid (DNA)   A nucleic acid composed of *nucleotide* units that contain molecules of the sugar deoxyribose, phosphate groups, and purine and pyrimidine bases. DNA molecules transmit genetic information and are found primarily in the nuclei of cells. (Compare with *RNA*). (p. 754)

Fusion   The process by which viruses attach themselves or fuse with the cell membranes of host cells in preparation for infecting the cell for purposes of viral replication (see *replication*). (p. 754)

Genome   The complete set of genetic material of any organism; it may be multiple chromosomes (groups of DNA or RNA molecules) in higher organisms; a single chromosome as in bacteria; or a one- or two-DNA or RNA molecule, as in viruses. (p. 754)

Herpesvirus   Any of several different types of viruses of the family Herpesviridae that causes any form of herpes infection. (p. 758)

Host   Any organism (human, animal, or plant) that is infected with a microorganism such as bacteria or viruses. (p. 753)

Human immunodeficiency virus (HIV)   The retrovirus that causes AIDS. (p. 754)

Humoral immunity   The second of two major parts of the immune system. It consists of specific immune responses in the form of antigen-specific antibodies produced from B lymphocytes (B cells). (p. 755)

Immunoglobulin   (Synonymous with *immune globulin.*) A glycoprotein (sugar protein) synthesized and used by the humoral immune system to attack and kill any substance (antigen) that is foreign to the body. (p. 755)

Influenza virus   The virus that causes influenza, an acute viral infection of the respiratory tract. (p. 755)

Nucleic acids   A general term referring to DNA and RNA. These complex biomolecules contain the genetic material of all living organisms, which is passed to future generations during reproduction. (p. 754)

Nucleoside   A structural component of nucleic acid molecules (DNA or RNA) that consists of a purine or pyrimidine base attached to a sugar molecule. (p. 756)

Nucleotide   A nucleoside that is attached to a phosphate unit, which makes up the side chain "backbone" of a DNA or RNA molecule. (p. 756)

Opportunistic infections   Infections caused by any type of microorganism and occurring in an immunocompromised host that normally would not occur in an immunocompetent host. (p. 756)

Protease   An enzyme that breaks down the amino acid structure of protein molecules by chemically cleaving the peptide bonds that link together the individual amino acids. (p. 764)

Protease inhibitors (PIs)   Antiretroviral drugs that act by inhibiting the *protease* retroviral enzyme, thus interrupting viral replication. (p. 769)

Replication   Any process of duplication or reproduction, such as that involved in the duplication of nucleic acid molecules (DNA or RNA) during the reproduction processes of all living organisms. This term is also used to describe the entire process of viral reproduction, which occurs only inside the cells of an infected host organism. (p. 754)

Retrovirus   Any virus belonging to the family Retroviridae. These viruses contain RNA (as opposed to DNA) as their genome and replicate using the enzyme *reverse transcriptase*. The most clinically significant retrovirus is HIV. (p. 764)

Reverse transcriptase   An RNA-directed DNA-polymerase enzyme. Such an enzyme promotes the synthesis of a DNA molecule from an RNA molecule, which is the "reverse" of the usual process. HIV replicates in this manner. (p. 764)

Reverse transcriptase inhibitors (RTIs)   Antiretroviral drugs that act by blocking activity of the enzyme *reverse transcriptase*; there are currently three subclasses of RTIs: nucleoside RTIs, or NRTIs; non-nucleoside RTIs, or NNRTIs; and nucleotide RTIs, or NTRTIs. (p. 769)

Ribonucleic acid (RNA)   A nucleic acid composed of nucleotide units (see *nucleotide*) that contain molecules of the sugar ribose, phosphate groups, and purine and pyrimidine bases. RNA molecules transmit genetic information and are found in both the nuclei and cytoplasm of cells. (Compare with *DNA.*) (p. 754)

Virion   A mature virus particle. (p. 753)

Virus   The smallest class of microorganisms; it can replicate only inside host cells. (p. 753)

GENERAL PRINCIPLES OF VIROLOGY

Viruses are tiny microorganisms, usually many times smaller than bacteria. They are visible only with the strongest microscopes, such as an electron microscope. Unlike bacteria, viruses can reproduce, or replicate, inside the cells of their **host**, which can be human, animal, plant, or even other types of microorganisms (e.g., bacteria, protozoans). In this respect, all viruses are *obligate intracellular parasites.* Viruses are not cells, per se, but are particles that infect and replicate inside cells. A mature virus particle, or **virion**, has a relatively simple structure that consists of the genome, the capsid, and the envelope. The **genome** is the inner core of the virion, which consists of single- or double-stranded deoxyribonucleic acid (DNA) or ribonucleic acid (RNA) molecules, but not both. Viruses have the least complicated genome of all organisms; the cells of more complex organisms have either much larger nucleic acid strands or multiple strands, which make up *chromosomes*. The latter is the case with higher organisms, including humans. The viral *capsid* is a protein coat that serves to surround and protect the genome. It also plays a role in the fusion between the virions and host cells. **Fusion** occurs when virions attach themselves to host cells in preparation for infecting the cells. The *envelope* is the outermost layer of the virion and is seen in some, but not all, viruses. It has a lipoprotein (lipid and protein) structure containing viral antigens that are often chemically specific for proteins on the surface of the host cell membranes (*cell surface proteins*). This biochemical specificity, when present, also facilitates fusion. The **human immunodeficiency virus (HIV)** functions in this manner.

Viruses can enter the body through at least four routes: inhalation through the respiratory tract, ingestion via the gastrointestinal tract, transplacentally from the mother to infant, and inoculation via skin or mucous membranes. Inoculation occurs through sexual contact, blood transfusions, sharing of syringes or needles (as in injection drug use [IDU]), organ transplants, or animal bites (including human, animal, insect, spider, and others). Once inside the body, the virus particles, or virions, begin to attach themselves to the outer membranes of host cells (*cell membranes* or *plasma membranes*) as illustrated in Figure 40-1.

The viral genome then passes through the plasma membrane into the cytoplasm of the host cell. It later enters the cell nucleus, where the **replication** process begins. The virion may use its own or host enzymes (or both) to direct the replication process. In the host cell nucleus, the viral genome uses the cell's genetic material, the **nucleic acids ribonucleic acid (RNA)** and **deoxyribonucleic acid (DNA)**, to synthesize viral nucleic acids and proteins. These are then used to construct complete new virions, including genome, capsid, and envelope (if applicable). These new virions then exit the infected host cell by budding through the plasma membrane and proceed to infect other host cells, where the replication process repeats. This process is called the *cytopathic effect* and usually results in the destruction of the host cell. Repeated over time, cumulative host cell destruction produces the pathological effects of the virus, which can eventually impair or kill the host organism.

Although this cytopathic effect is the most common outcome, there are other possible outcomes of viral infection. *Viral transformation* involves mutation of the host cell DNA or RNA, which can result in malignant (cancerous) host cells. Viruses that can induce cancer in this way are *oncogenic* viruses. More common than viral transformation is *latent*, or dormant, infection, in which the virions remain inside host cells but do not actively replicate to any significant degree. For example, HIV infection may have a lengthy dormant phase of 10 years or more before developing into **acquired immune deficiency syndrome (AIDS)** in an infected person. HIV infection is discussed in greater detail later in this chapter in the section on retroviruses. Viruses are pervasive in the environment, and most viral infections may not be noticed before they are eliminated by the host's immune system. Such infections are referred to as "silent" viral

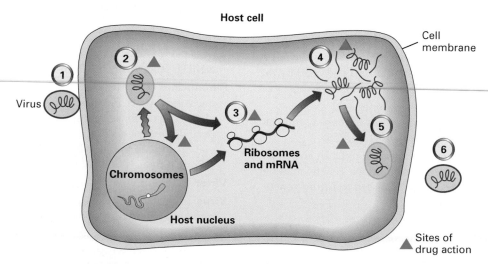

1. Attachment to host cell
2. Uncoating of virus and entry of viral nucleic acid into host cell nucleus
3. Control of DNA, RNA, and protein production
4. Production of viral subunits
5. Assembly of virions
6. Release of virions

FIG. 40-1 Virus replication. Some viruses integrate into host chromosomes with development of latency. (Modified from Brody, T. M., Larner, J., & Minneman, K. P. (1998). *Human pharmacology: Molecular to clinical* (3rd ed.). St. Louis, MO: Mosby.)

infections. Although the host's immune system does act to neutralize a viral infection, the host can become overwhelmed, depending on the strength, or *virulence*, of the virus and how rapidly it replicates inside host cells. In most cases, however, a person's immune system is able to arrest and eliminate the virus.

Host immune responses to viral infections are classified as nonspecific or *specific*. *Nonspecific* immune responses include *phagocytosis* (process of engulfing and killing the engulfed particle) of viral particles by leukocytes (white blood cells [WBCs]) such as neutrophils, macrophages, monocytes, and T lymphocytes (T cells). Another important nonspecific immune response is the release of cytokines from these leukocytes. *Cytokines* are biochemical substances (e.g., histamine, tumour necrosis factor) that stimulate other protective immune functions. Additionally, these *activated* immune system cells may also phagocytize infected host cells to curb the growth and spread of infection. These types of immune responses are collectively referred to as **cell-mediated immunity (CMI)**. CMI is nonspecific in the sense that it does not involve **antibodies** that are specific for a given **antigen**. In contrast, specific immune responses include the production from B lymphocytes (B cells) of antibodies. These antibodies are immune-system proteins (immunoglobulins) that are chemically specific for viral antigens. This type of immune response is also called **humoral immunity**. Immune system function is discussed in further detail in Chapters 46 and 50.

OVERVIEW OF VIRAL ILLNESSES AND THEIR TREATMENT

There are, at a minimum, 6 classes of DNA viruses and no fewer than 14 classes of RNA viruses known to infect humans. Some of the more prominent viral illnesses include smallpox (poxviruses), sore throat and conjunctivitis (adenoviruses), warts (papovaviruses), influenza (orthomyxoviruses), respiratory infections (coronaviruses, rhinoviruses), gastroenteritis (rotavirus, Norwalk-like viruses), HIV/AIDS (retroviruses), herpes (herpesviruses), and hepatitis (hepadnaviruses). Effective drug therapy is currently available for a relatively small number of active viral infections. Drug therapy for hepatitis is discussed further in Chapter 50 on immunomodulating drugs.

Fortunately, many viral illnesses are survivable (e.g., chicken pox), even if bothersome and uncomfortable. The incidence of some of these illnesses has been reduced by the development of effective vaccines (e.g., polio, smallpox, measles, chicken pox). Vaccines are discussed in more detail in Chapter 47. However, many other viral illnesses, such as hepatitis and HIV, can be fatal or have severe long-term outcomes.

Antiviral drugs kill or suppress viruses through either destroying virions or inhibiting their ability to replicate. Even the best medications currently available probably never fully eradicate a virus completely

from its host. Nonetheless, the body's immune system has a better chance of controlling or eliminating a viral infection when the ability of the virus to replicate is suppressed. Drugs that destroy virions include disinfectants and immunoglobulins. Disinfectants such as povidone-iodine (Betadine) are *virucides*, commonly used to disinfect medical equipment, as well as parts of the body during invasive procedures. Such drugs are discussed further in Chapter 44.

Immunoglobulins are concentrated antibodies that attack and destroy viruses. They are isolated and pooled from human or animal blood. They may be nonspecific (e.g., human gamma globulin) or specific (e.g., rabies immunoglobulin, varicella-zoster immunoglobulin) in their activity. Although such substances can technically be thought of as antiviral drugs, they are more commonly thought of as immunizing drugs and thus are discussed in further detail in Chapter 47. Some antiviral drugs, such as interferons, stimulate the body's immune system to kill the virions directly. These drugs are discussed in Chapter 50. In contrast to the antiviral drugs described earlier, the current antiviral drugs are synthetic compounds that work indirectly by inhibiting viral replication instead of directly destroying mature virions. As noted earlier, relatively few of the numerous known viruses can be controlled by the current drug therapy. Some of these viruses are as follows:

- Cytomegalovirus (CMV)
- Hepatitis viruses
- Herpes viruses
- HIV
- **Influenza viruses** ("the flu")
- Respiratory syncytial virus (RSV)

Active viral infections are usually more difficult to eradicate than those by other microbes such as bacteria because viruses can replicate only inside host cells instead of independently replicating in the bloodstream or other tissues. Therefore, antiviral drugs must gain entry to the cells to disrupt viral replication. Historically, the difficulty of developing antiviral drugs that are not overly toxic to host cells has been one reason for the relatively few effective antiviral medications on the market. However, the HIV/AIDS pandemic that began in the early 1990s strongly boosted antiviral drug research, resulting in more available antiviral drugs for HIV than for other viral infections, such as influenza, CMV, and varicella zoster virus (VZV).

Another major reason why viral illnesses are difficult to treat is that the virus has often replicated many thousands or possibly millions of times before symptoms of illness appear. This replication amplifies the challenge of eradicating the virus, even with potent drugs. Therefore, one goal in the field of infectious disease treatment is to be able to diagnose viral illnesses before an infecting virus has undergone widespread replication in a human host. Early diagnosis would theoretically allow the dual benefit of both early drug therapy and easier elimination of the virus by the host's immune system. This has happened to some degree with HIV infection, with relatively early diagnosis made possible by blood tests to screen for HIV antibodies. Of course, the patient must also be alert to the need to seek medical care before serious illness develops.

As described earlier, for a virus to replicate, virions must first attach themselves to host cell membranes through fusion. Once inside the cell, the viral genome makes use of cellular genetic processes to generate viral nucleic acids and proteins, which are then used to build new viral particles, or virions (see Figure 40-1). All virions contain a genome that consists of DNA or RNA, but not both. However, both molecules may temporarily occur simultaneously during viral replication. Antiviral drugs inhibit this replication in various ways. Most antiviral drugs enter the same cells that the viruses enter. Once inside, the antiviral drugs interfere with viral nucleic acid synthesis. Other antiviral drugs work by preventing the fusion process. If a virion cannot fuse with and enter into host cell, it cannot replicate, and dies.

The best responses to antiviral drug therapy are usually seen in patients with a competent immune system. Such an immune system can work synergistically with the drug to eliminate or effectively suppress viral activity. Patients who are already *immunocompromised* because of illnesses are at greater risk for **opportunistic infections** (OIs) that would not normally harm an *immunocompetent* person. The most common examples of such patients include cancer patients with leukemia or lymphoma, organ transplant recipients, and patients with AIDS. These patients are prone to frequent and often severe OIs of many types, including other viruses, bacteria, fungi, and protozoans. Such OIs often require long-term prophylactic anti-infective drug therapy to control the infection and prevent recurrence because of compromised host immune functions.

Recall that there are two types of nucleic acid found in living organisms: DNA and RNA. These are also five organic bases that are major structural components of these nucleic acids. DNA consists of long chains of *deoxyribose* sugar molecules, phosphate groups, together with *purine* (*adenine* or *guanine*) and *pyrimidine* (*cytosine* or *thymine*) bases. RNA consists of long chains of *ribose* sugar molecules linked to phosphate groups, together with *purine* (*adenine* or *guanine*) and *pyrimidine* (*cytosine* or *uracil*) bases. A **nucleoside** is a single unit consisting of a base and its attached sugar molecule. Nucleosides have names similar to their bases with minor spelling modifications (e.g., adenosine, guanosine, cytidine, thymidine). A **nucleotide** is a nucleoside with an attached phosphate molecule. Most antiviral drugs are synthetic purine or pyrimidine nucleoside or nucleotide analogues. These drugs are listed in Table 40-1 along with their specific antiviral activities. In addition, several non-nucleoside drugs whose chemical structures are not based on DNA or RNA components are listed in Table 40-2.

Antiviral drugs are used to treat a variety of viral infections ranging from herpes to AIDS, but their effectiveness varies widely among patients and over time for the same patient. The specific antiviral activities, indications, and therapeutic effects for several of the currently available antiviral drugs are summarized in Table 40-3.

TABLE 40-1

Characteristics of Nucleoside Analogues

Antiviral Drug	Nucleoside Analogue	Antiviral Activity
PURINE NUCLEOSIDE ANALOGUES		
acyclovir, valacyclovir	Guanosine	HSV-1 and -2, VZV
adefovir	Adenosine	HBV
didanosine (ddI), tenofovir	Adenosine	HIV
entecavir	Guanosine	HBV
famciclovir, penciclovir	Guanosine	HSV-1 and -2, VSV
ganciclovir (DHPG), valganciclovir	Guanosine	CMV retinitis and CMV disease
ribavirin (RTCD)	Guanosine	Influenza type A and B, RSV, LV, HV
PYRIMIDINE NUCLEOSIDE ANALOGUES		
emtricitabine	Cytidine	HIV
idoxuridine (IDU)	Thymidine	HSV
lamivudine (3TC)	Cytidine	HIV
stavudine (d4T), zidovudine (AZT)	Thymidine	HIV
trifluridine	Thymidine	HSV
MISCELLANEOUS NUCLEOSIDE OR NUCLEOTIDE ANALOGUES		
abacavir	Unspecified	HIV
cidofovir*	Unspecified	CMV

CMV, cytomegalovirus; *HBV*, hepatitis B virus; *HIV*, human immunodeficiency virus; *HSV*, herpes simplex virus (types 1 and 2); *HV*, Hantavirus; *LV* Lassa virus; *RSV*, respiratory syncytial virus; *VZV*, varicella zoster virus.

*Available through the Special Access Programme, Health Canada.

TABLE 40-2

Examples of Non-nucleoside Analogue Antiviral Drugs

Drug	Antiviral Activity
amantadine	Influenza A
foscarnet	CMV
NEURAMINIDASE INHIBITORS	
zanamivir, oseltamivir	Influenza A
NON-NUCLEOSIDE REVERSE TRANSCRIPTASE INHIBITORS	
delavirdine, efavirenz, nevirapine	HIV
PROTEASE INHIBITORS	
amprenavir, atazanavir, darunavir, fosamprenavir, indinavir, nelfinavir, ritonavir, saquinavir	HIV
enfuvirtide	HIV

CMV, cytomegalovirus; *HIV*, human immunodeficiency virus.

*Available through the Special Access Programme, Health Canada.

Antiviral medications are broadly subdivided into the following two major categories:

- *Antiviral drugs,* now commonly used as a general term for those medications used to treat infections of viruses other than HIV
- **Antiretroviral drugs,** indicated specifically for the treatment of infections caused by HIV. Although antiretroviral drugs also fall under the broader category of antiviral drugs, their mechanisms of action are unique to the HIV virus. Thus they are more commonly referred to by their subclassification as antiretroviral drugs.

Both classes of drugs are discussed in separate sections of this chapter. To provide a summary, however, the indications, adverse effects, and interactions for several common antiviral drugs for both classes are listed in Table 40-3, Table 40-4, and Box 40-1, respectively. Before examining these two major drug classes in detail, one common viral illness will be examined as an example.

TABLE 40-3

Antiviral Drugs: Viral Spectra, Indications, and Therapeutic Effects

Drugs	Antiviral Activity	Indications and Therapeutic Effects
abacavir, didanosine, emtricitabine, lamivudine, stavudine, zidovudine	HIV	Approved for the treatment of HIV infections, these drugs produce a significant reduction in mortality and incidence of opportunistic infections, improve physical performance, and significantly improve T-cell counts. Lamivudine is also used for HBV (Epivir-HBV).
acyclovir, famciclovir, penciclovir, valacyclovir	HSV-1 and -2, VZV	Herpes simplex encephalitis, disseminated or CNS herpes infections in the newborn, herpes keratitis (topically), and herpes zoster. Acyclovir is used topically, PO, and IV, for treatment of herpes simplex, encephalitis, and most other significant herpes infections. Administration as soon as possible produces the best results. These drugs reduce viral shedding, decrease local symptoms, and decrease severity and duration of illness. Valacyclovir is also indicated for herpes labialis (perioral cold sores). Penciclovir is a topical drug for this same condition.
adefovir, entecavir	HBV	Both drugs inhibit HBV nucleic acid enzymes to reduce HBV viral replication.
amantadine	Influenza A	Used for the treatment and prophylaxis of influenza A, but ineffective against influenza B. Most effective if given before exposure or within 48 hr of development of symptoms. Reduces fever and palliates symptoms of influenza. As described in Chapter 15, amantadine is also used in the treatment of Parkinson's disease.
amprenavir, atazanavir, fosamprenavir, indinavir, lopinavir-ritonavir, nelfinavir, ritonavir, saquinavir	HIV	Newer class of drugs for the treatment of HIV infection when antiretroviral therapy is warranted. Used in combination with nucleoside analogues. Ritonavir and indinavir may be used as monotherapy. All are potent inhibitors of the HIV protease enzyme.
cidofovir, ganciclovir, foscarnet, ganciclovir	CMV	Ganciclovir is the older and more studied of these drugs. Ganciclovir has been shown to be effective for not only CMV retinitis but also other CMV infections such as gastrointestinal infection and pneumonitis and for prevention of CMV in recipients of solid organ transplants and in patients with HIV infection. Primary dose-limiting toxicity of ganciclovir is bone marrow toxicity. Cidofovir is less toxic to the bone marrow but can cause kidney failure. This effect can be minimized with the administration of probenecid tablets and hydration on the day of infusion.
delavirdine, efavirenz, nevirapine	HIV	In combination with nucleoside analogues, these two NNRTI are used to treat HIV-infected patients, including newly infected asymptomatic patients.
enfuvirtide	HIV	First and currently only fusion inhibitor

Continued

TABLE 40-3

Antiviral Drugs: Viral Spectra, Indications, and Therapeutic Effects cont'd

Drugs	Antiviral Activity	Indications and Therapeutic Effects
idoxuridine, trifluridine	HSV	Used to treat herpes simplex keratitis. It is used only topically because of significant liver and bone marrow toxicity.
ribavirin	HCV, RSV	Nonaerosol form used for HCV. Severe RSV bronchopneumonia can be treated using an aerosol (ribavirin) or an IV infusion (RSV immunoglobulin). These products have been shown to improve oxygenation, decrease viral shedding, and alleviate pneumonia symptoms. Inhalation treatment with ribavirin has also been shown to be effective in influenza A and B infections.
tenofovir	HIV	First and currently only nucleotide reverse transcriptase inhibitor

CNS, central nervous system; *CMV*, cytomegalovirus; *HBV*, hepatitis B virus; *HCV*, hepatitis C virus; *HIV*, human immunodeficiency virus; *HSV*, herpes simplex virus; *IV*, intravenous; *NNRTI*, non-nucleoside reverse transcriptase inhibitors; *RSV*, respiratory syncytial virus; *VZV*, varicella zoster virus.
*Available through the Special Access Programme, Health Canada.

TABLE 40-4

Selected Antiviral Drugs: Adverse Effects

Antiviral Drug	Adverse Effects
acyclovir	Most common: nausea, vomiting, diarrhea, headache, transient burning when topically applied
amantadine	CNS: insomnia, nervousness, lightheadedness Gastrointestinal: anorexia, nausea, anticholinergic effects
didanosine	CNS: peripheral neuropathies, seizures Gastrointestinal: pancreatitis
foscarnet	CNS: headache, seizures Gastrointestinal: nausea, vomiting, diarrhea Genitourinary: acute kidney failure Hematological: bone marrow suppression Metabolic: hypocalcemia, hypophosphatemia, hyperphosphatemia, hypokalemia
ganciclovir	CNS: headache, seizures Gastrointestinal: nausea, anorexia, vomiting Hematological: bone marrow toxicity
indinavir	Nausea, abdominal pain, headache, diarrhea, vomiting, weakness or fatigue, insomnia, flank pain, taste changes, acid regurgitation, back pain, indirect hyperbilirubinemia, nephrolithiasis
nevirapine	Rash, fever, nausea, headache, fatigue, increases in liver function tests
ribavirin	Rash, conjunctivitis, anemia, mild bronchospasm
trifluridine	Burning, swelling, stinging, photophobia, pain
zalcitabine	Peripheral neuropathy, rash, ulcers
zidovudine	Bone marrow suppression, nausea, headache

*Available through the Special Access Programme, Health Canada.

OVERVIEW OF HERPES SIMPLEX VIRUSES AND VARICELLA-ZOSTER VIRUS INFECTION

The family of viruses known as *Herpesviridae* includes those viruses that cause any type of herpes infections. There are several specific types of such viruses. Herpes simplex virus type 1 (HSV-1) causes mucocutaneous herpes, usually in the form of perioral blisters ("fever blisters" or "cold sores"). Herpes simplex virus type 2 (HSV-2) causes genital herpes. Human **herpesvirus** 3 (HHV-3) causes both chicken pox and shingles. This virus is more commonly known as herpes zoster virus or varicella zoster virus (VZV). Human herpesvirus 4 (HHV-4) is more commonly known as Epstein-Barr virus

(EBV) and is associated with such illnesses as infectious mononucleosis ("mono") and chronic fatigue syndrome. Human herpesvirus 5 (HHV-5) is more commonly known as cytomegalovirus (CMV), the cause of CMV retinitis and CMV disease. The latter is simply a generalized CMV infection, most often occurring in immunocompromised patients (e.g., patients who have AIDS or are receiving cancer chemotherapy or other immunosuppressive drugs, and organ transplant patients). Human herpesviruses 6 and 7 are not especially clinically significant, but may be more likely to occur in immunocompromised patients. Additionally, human herpesvirus 8 is also known as Kaposi's sarcoma herpesvirus and is an oncogenic (cancer-causing) virus believed to cause Kaposi's sarcoma, an AIDS-associated cancer. All of these viruses occur, often asymptomatically, in varying percentages of

acyclovir with the following:
- interferon: additive antiviral effects
- probenecid: increased acyclovir levels by decreasing kidney clearance

amantadine with the following:
- Anticholinergic drugs: increased adverse anticholinergic effects
- CNS stimulants: additive CNS stimulant effects

didanosine with the following:
- Antacids: increased absorption of didanosine, which is a positive effect
- dapsone: may interfere with gastrointestinal absorption of dapsone
- itraconazole and ketoconazole: didanosine decreases their absorption; give 2 hours apart
- Quinolones: didanosine decreases absorption of some quinolone antibiotics
- Tetracyclines: decreased absorption of tetracyclines; give 2 hours before tetracyclines
- zidovudine: additive and synergistic effect against HIV

ganciclovir with the following:
- imipenem-cilastatin: increased risk of seizures
- zidovudine: increased risk of hematological toxicity (i.e., bone marrow suppression)

indinavir with the following:
- Drugs metabolized by the CYP3A4 liver microsomal enzyme system (alprazolam, amiodarone, ergot derivatives, midazolam, pimozide, and triazolam): competition for metabolism, resulting in elevated blood levels and potential toxicity

- ketoconazole: increased plasma concentrations of indinavir
- HMG-CoA reductase inhibitors: increased risk of myopathy and rhabdomyolysis (breakdown of muscle fibres)
- itraconazole: increased plasma concentrations of indinavir
- rifampin: increased metabolism of indinavir
- St. John's wort: potential loss of virological response and possible resistance to indinavir or to the class of protease inhibitors
- sildenafil: increased sildenafil concentrations and may increase sildenafil-associated adverse effects (hypotension, visual changes, priapism)

nevirapine with the following:
- Drugs metabolized by the CYP3A4 liver microsomal enzyme system: increased metabolism of these drugs
- Oral contraceptives: decreased plasma concentrations of oral contraceptives
- Protease inhibitors: decreased plasma concentrations of protease inhibitors
- rifampin and rifabutin: decreased nevirapine serum concentration

zidovudine with the following:
- acyclovir: increased neurotoxicity
- interferon beta: increased serum levels of zidovudine
- Cytotoxic drugs: increased risk for hematological toxicity
- didanosine: additive or synergistic effect against HIV
- ganciclovir and ribavirin: antagonize the antiviral action of zidovudine
- probenecid: increased serum levels of zidovudine

the population. Types 3 through 7 normally do not cause diseases that require medication, except in the case of immunocompromised patients. However, the herpes simplex viruses (types 1 and 2) and the varicella zoster virus (VZV, or HHV-3) commonly cause illnesses that are now routinely treated with prescription medications. These viruses are the focus of this section.

Herpes Simplex Viruses

Although there can be anatomical overlap between the two types of herpes simplex virus (HSV), HSV-1 is most commonly associated with perioral blisters and is therefore often thought of as "oral herpes." In contrast, HSV-2 is most commonly associated with blisters on both male and female genitalia and is therefore commonly referred to as "genital herpes." Although usually not causing serious or life-threatening illness, both infections are certainly annoying and highly transmissible through close physical contact (e.g., kissing, sexual intercourse). Outbreaks of painful skin lesions occur intermittently (come and go) with periods of latency (no sores or other symptoms) occurring between acute outbreaks. Although antiviral medications are not always clinically required and are not curative, they can speed up the process of remission and reduce the duration of painful symptoms. This

is particularly true if the medications are started early in an outbreak. Patients may also be prescribed an ongoing lower dose of antiviral drug for prophylaxis (prevention) of outbreaks.

Situations in which HSV infections can become especially serious, even life threatening, involve immunocompromised patients and virus transmission to a newborn infant. Neonatal herpes can be a life-threatening infection, and babies with this disease are often treated in neonatal intensive care units (NICUs) with intravenous (IV) antiviral drugs. However, these treatments fail in many cases, with infant death or permanent disability being common. Therefore, the best strategy is to prevent transmission of HSV to the newborn infant. Obstetricians will usually recommend delivery by cesarean section ("C-section") for any mother with active genital herpes lesions. Unlike VZV, there is currently no specific HSV immune globulin available for treating infected infants, so prevention is key. The medications used for HSV are the same as those for VZV and are discussed in the section on antiviral drugs.

Varicella Zoster Virus

Both HIV and HSV infections are associated with latency periods, described earlier. Another significant and common example of latent viral infection involves the varicella zoster virus (VZV). As noted earlier, this is a type of herpesvirus (HHV-3) that most commonly causes *chicken pox (varicella)* in childhood, remains dormant for many years, and can then re-emerge in later adulthood as painful *herpes zoster* lesions, known as *shingles*.

Chicken pox is usually an uncomfortable but self-limiting disease of childhood. However, it is highly contagious and easily spread by either direct contact with weeping lesions or via droplet inhalation. It can also lead to significant scarring. The serious condition *Reye's syndrome* (fatty liver damage with encephalopathy) may also complicate varicella, as can other viral infections such as influenza. The end course of a primary infection with varicella does not result in its complete removal from the body. Some virus remains dormant in nerve ganglia. Reactivation of VZV from its dormant state, often decades after a case of childhood chicken pox, results in *herpes zoster* or *shingles,* with lesions occurring in the *dermatome* supplied by that particular nerve. Grouped vesicles, typical of a solitary chicken pox vesicle, develop in that dermatome. The most common site of the vesicles is around the side of the trunk, although they can appear in other areas (e.g., along the trigeminal nerve dermatomes of the face). Zoster lesions are often quite painful and patients may require opioids for pain control. In addition, postherpetic neuralgias (long-term nerve pain) remain following shingles outbreaks in as many as 50% of older adults. Early administration of antiviral drugs such as acyclovir may speed recovery, but this effect is usually not dramatic. The best results are usually seen when the antiviral drug is started within 72 hours of symptom onset.

Active childhood varicella (chicken pox) infections are usually self-limiting and are not normally treated with antiviral drugs, except in high-risk (e.g., immunocompromised) children. Varicella virus vaccine was Health Canada approved in 1998 and is now routinely recommended for healthy children between 12 and 18 months of age who have not had chicken pox, for susceptible older children and adolescents, children and adolescents on chronic salicylate acid therapy or with cystic fibrosis, and susceptible household contacts of immunocompromised persons. The vaccine has been shown effective for producing VZV immunity in HIV-positive children who are reasonably healthy. As this newly vaccinated population ages, it remains to be seen whether the VZV vaccine also protects against shingles in adulthood. There is currently no specific vaccine for shingles. Approximately 95% of pregnant women have VZV antibodies, which protect the fetus from viral infection. However, first-time exposure to VZV infection can pose a teratogenic risk in pregnant women, especially during the first trimester. If the infection manifests in a pregnant woman within 5 days of delivery, one dose of varicella zoster immunoglobulin (VZIG) is recommended for the infant. It may also be beneficial to both mother and infant when given to the mother during pregnancy, preferably as soon as

possible after diagnosis of infection. Both varicella virus vaccine and VZIG are discussed further in Chapter 47.

In a small percentage of shingles cases, skin lesions may progress beyond the usual dermatome regions, and the virus can cause solid organ infections such as pneumonitis, hepatitis, encephalitis, and optic neuritis (infection of the optic nerve). Such infections are uncommon, but the older adult and immunocompromised patients (e.g., those with HIV/AIDS, organ transplants, or cancer) are the most vulnerable to these more serious VZV exacerbations. These infections can also result from first-time exposure to varicella (chicken pox). In general, these more serious infections require IV antiviral drugs, especially in high-risk patients. Intravenous acyclovir is the most commonly used drug, and its use can occasionally prevent fatalities or disability in the most serious infections. Less serious infections are usually treated orally with acyclovir, valacyclovir, or famciclovir. Topical dosage forms of some of these drugs are also available and are discussed further in Chapter 57. Although VZV reactivation is comparable in pathology to that caused by herpes simplex virus (HSV; e.g., oral or genital herpes lesions), VZV reactivation occurs much less regularly than HSV because of a lack of reactivation genes. Because secondary bacterial infections (e.g., group A *Streptococcus* skin infection) are common with VZV exacerbations, antibiotics may also be needed. This is especially true in cases of ophthalmic involvement.

ANTIVIRAL DRUGS (NONRETROVIRAL)

The drugs discussed in this section include those used to treat non-HIV viral infections such as those caused by influenza viruses, HSV, VZV, and CMV. There are also antiviral drugs used for hepatitis A, B, and C viruses (HAV, HBV, and HCV). Hepatitis treatment is discussed in further detail in Chapter 47 because it involves some additional unique drug therapy.

Mechanism of Action and Drug Effects

Most of the current antiviral drugs work by blocking the activity of a polymerase enzyme, which normally catalyzes the synthesis of new viral genomes. The result is impaired viral replication, which ideally results in viral concentrations small enough to be eliminated by the patient's immune system. If this does not occur, the virus may either enter a dormant state or remain at a low level of replication with continuous drug therapy. For some of the more serious viral infections, such as HIV or HCV, long-term drug therapy is often necessary. Pertinent information for specific drugs is also listed in Table 40-3.

Indications

Indications for several commonly used antiviral drugs, including antiretroviral drugs, are summarized in Table 40-3.

Contraindications

Most of the nonretroviral antiviral drugs are surprisingly well tolerated. The only usual contraindication for most of these drugs is known severe drug allergy, keeping in mind that the seriousness of a given patient's illness may leave few treatment options.

However, there are a small number of listed contraindications for a few of the antiviral drugs. Amantadine is contraindicated in lactating women, children younger than 12 months of age, and patients with an eczematic rash. Famciclovir, the orally administered prodrug of penciclovir, is contraindicated in cases of allergy to famciclovir or to penciclovir, which is used topically for *herpes labialis* (perioral sores). Because cidofovir has such a strong propensity for kidney toxicity, it is contraindicated in patients who already have severely compromised kidney function as well as those receiving concurrent drug therapy with other highly nephrotoxic drugs. It is also contraindicated in cases of allergy to probenecid (a sulfa drug) or other sulfa-containing medications. As noted in Table 40-3, probenecid is recommended as concurrent drug therapy with cidofovir, to help alleviate its nephrotoxicity.

Ribavirin has additional specific contraindications besides drug allergy. Its oral dosage forms, tablets, capsules, and oral solution, are contraindicated in patients with pre-existing hemoglobinopathies such as sickle-cell anemia because anemia is also a common adverse effect of ribavirin. This drug is contraindicated in cases of *autoimmune* hepatitis, as it can worsen this condition. Because of the drug's teratogenic potential, it is contraindicated in pregnant women and even their male sexual partners. The aerosol form should not be used in pregnant women or in women who may become pregnant during exposure to the drug. This includes health providers administering the drug in aerosol form because of the potential for second-hand inhalation on the part of the health provider.

Adverse Effects

The adverse effects of the antiviral drugs are as different as the drugs themselves. Each has its own specific adverse-effect profile. Because viruses reproduce in human cells and, therefore, have many of the same features as these cells, it is hard to target a unique enzyme or other feature of the virus. Selective killing is difficult, thus many healthy human cells, in addition to virally infected cells, may be killed in the process, resulting in more serious toxicities. However, this effect is usually not as pronounced as in cancer chemotherapy, which often kills many more healthy cells. The more serious adverse effects are listed by drug in Table 40-4.

Interactions

Significant drug interactions that occur with the antiviral drugs most often develop when antiviral drugs are administered via systemic routes, such as intravenously and orally. However, many of these drugs are also applied topically to the eye or body, and the incidence of drug interactions associated with these routes of administration is much lower. Selected common drug interactions for both antiviral and antiretroviral drugs are listed in Box 40-1.

Dosages

See the corresponding Dosages table on p. 763 for doses of all of the commonly used nonretroviral antiviral drugs.

 DRUG PROFILES

Antiviral drugs are now commonly used to treat active infection with several viruses, including influenza viruses, HSV, VZV, CMV, HBV, HCV, and RSV. More effective methods of drug development have resulted in many new antiviral drugs over the past few decades.

▸▸ *acyclovir*

Acyclovir (Zovirax) is a synthetic nucleoside analogue of the nucleic acid nucleoside *guanosine* that is mainly used to suppress the replication of HSV-1 and -2 and VZV. Acyclovir is considered the drug of choice for the treatment of both initial and recurrent episodes of viral infections by these viruses.

Acyclovir is available in oral, topical, and parenteral formulations. Its topical use is discussed in Chapter 57. Other similar antiviral drugs include valacyclovir and famciclovir. However, the latter two drugs are currently available for oral use only and are indicated for the treatment of shingles and the suppression of genital herpes in immunosuppressed patients. Note the slight differences in the spelling of these drug names. Valacyclovir is a prodrug that is metabolized to acyclovir in the body. It has the advantage of greater oral bioavailability and less frequent dosing (three times daily versus five times daily for acyclovir). It may also provide more effective relief of pain from herpes zoster lesions.

PHARMACOKINETICS

Half-Life	Onset	Peak	Duration
PO: 2.5–3 hr	PO: Unknown	PO: 1.5–2 hr	PO: 4–5 hr

amantadine hydrochloride

One of the earliest antiviral drugs, amantadine hydrochloride (Dom-Amantidine) has a narrow antiviral spectrum in that it is only active against influenza A viruses. It is used both prophylactically and therapeutically. It has been shown to be effective, if not lifesaving, when used prophylactically in the older adult or in chronically ill

Continued

DRUG PROFILES (cont'd)

and immunocompromised patients, in whom influenza A infection can be particularly devastating. It may also be used prophylactically when influenza vaccine is either not available or is contraindicated for a given patient. When used therapeutically to treat active influenza A infections, it can reduce recovery time.

Amantadine is contraindicated in patients with a known hypersensitivity to it, lactating women, children under 12 months of age, and patients with an eczematic rash. Amantadine is available only for oral use.

PHARMACOKINETICS

Half-Life	Onset	Peak	Duration
PO: 17 hr	PO: Unknown	PO: 1–4 hr	PO: 12–24 hr

▶▶ ganciclovir hydrochloride

Like acyclovir, ganciclovir hydrochloride (Cytovene, Valcyte) is a synthetic nucleoside analogue of guanosine, but with a much different spectrum of antiviral activity. Ganciclovir is the antiviral drug most often used in the treatment of CMV infection. The *cytomegalovirus* is carried by up to 50% of the adult population and normally causes no harm. However, in immunocompromised patients (including premature infants), it can cause life-threatening or disabling opportunistic infections. A common site of CMV infections in the immunocompromised patient involves the eye, the result being CMV retinitis, a devastating viral infection that can lead to blindness. Valganciclovir (Valcyte), foscarnet (Foscavir), and cidofovir (Vistide) are three other antiviral drugs used in the treatment of CMV infection, but they are not used as often as ganciclovir. These drugs also have activity against HSV-1 and -2, Epstein–Barr virus (HSV-4), and VZV, but they are not normally used for these infections because there are other effective and less toxic drugs available.

Ganciclovir is also administered to *prevent* CMV disease (generalized infection) in high-risk patients, such as those receiving organ transplants. A dose-limiting toxicity of ganciclovir treatment is bone marrow suppression whereas that of foscarnet and cidofovir is kidney toxicity. Such toxicities should be remembered when deciding which drug is more appropriate in a particular patient. For example, a heart transplant recipient who contracts CMV retinitis is immunocompromised because of immunosuppressant drug therapy and is presumably taking cyclosporine, a nephrotoxic drug. Therefore, using foscarnet in this patient may be more dangerous than using ganciclovir. A patient who contracts a CMV infection and is immunocompromised because of a bone marrow transplant, by contrast, might be better treated using foscarnet.

Ganciclovir is most commonly administered intravenously or orally. Hence it is available in both oral and parenteral forms. Valganciclovir is a prodrug of ganciclovir, for oral use, that is metabolized to ganciclovir in the body. Like the prodrug valacyclovir, valganciclovir allows greater oral bioavailability and reduced frequency of

daily dosing. Cidofovir and foscarnet are available only in injectable form.

PHARMACOKINETICS

Half-Life	Onset	Peak	Duration
PO: 2.5–3.6 hr	PO: Unknown	PO: 24 hr	PO: Variable

oseltamivir phosphate and zanamivir

Oseltamivir phosphate (Tamiflu) and zanamivir (Relenza) belong to one of the newest classes of antiviral drugs, known as *neuraminidase inhibitors*. Both drugs are active against influenza virus types A and B. They are indicated for the treatment of uncomplicated acute illness caused by influenza infection in adults. They have been shown to reduce the duration of influenza infection by several days. The neuraminidase enzyme enables budding virions to escape from infected cells and spread throughout the body. Neuraminidase inhibitors are designed to stop this process in the body, speeding recovery from infection.

The most commonly reported adverse events with oseltamivir are nausea and vomiting; those with zanamivir are diarrhea, nausea, and sinusitis. Oseltamivir is only available for oral use. Oseltamivir is indicated for both prophylaxis and treatment of influenza infection. Zanamivir is available in blister packets of 5 mg of dry powder for inhalation. It is currently indicated only for treatment of active influenza illness. Ideally, treatment with oseltamivir or zanamivir should begin within 2 days of influenza symptom onset.

PHARMACOKINETICS

oseltamivir

Half-Life	Onset	Peak	Duration
PO: 1–3 hr	PO: Unknown	PO: 1–2 hr	PO: 5–15 hr

zanamivir

Half-Life	Onset	Peak	Duration
PO: 2.1–5 hr	PO: Unknown	PO: 1–2 hr	PO: 10–24 hr

ribavirin

Ribavirin (Pegetron, Copegus) is a unique antiviral drug in that it can be given either orally or by nasal inhalation. It is a synthetic nucleoside analogue of guanosine, similar to other antiviral drugs, but it has a broader spectrum of antiviral activity. Ribovirin interferes with both RNA and DNA synthesis and, consequently, inhibits both protein synthesis and viral replication.

The inhalational form (Virazole) is used primarily in hospitalized infants for treatment of severe lower respiratory tract infections caused by RSV.

PHARMACOKINETICS

Half-Life	Onset	Peak	Duration
Inhal: 1.4–2.5 hr*	Inhal: Unknown	Inhal: End of inhalation period	Inhal: Variable

*In respiratory secretions.

DOSAGES   Antiviral Drugs (Nonretroviral)

Drug (Pregnancy Category)	Pharmacological Class	Usual Dosage Range	Indications
▸▸acyclovir (Zorvirax) (B)	Anti-herpesvirus	*Children 12 yr and under* IV: 10 mg/kg q8h × 7 days *Adolescents 12 yr and older/Adult* IV: 5 mg/kg q8h × 7 days *Children/Adult* PO: 200–800 mg q4h 5×/day × 7–10 days *Children/Adult* PO: 20 mg/kg (max 800 mg/dose) qid × 5 days	HSV-1 and HSV-2, including genital herpes, mucocutaneous herpes, and herpes encephalitis; herpes zoster (shingles); higher dose therapy for acute episodes; lower dose therapy for viral suppression Chicken pox (varicella)
adefovir dipivoxil (Hepsera) (C)	Anti-HBV	*Adult* PO: 10 mg daily	Chronic HBV infection
amantadine hydrochloride (Dom-Amantidine) (C)	Anti-influenza	*Children 1–9 yr* PO: 4.5–9 mg/kg/day divided bid–tid, max 150 mg/day *Children 9–12 yr* PO: 100 mg bid *Adult* PO: 200 mg divided once or twice daily	Influenza A virus
cidofovir (Vistide) (C)	Anti-CMV	*Adult* IV: 5 mg/kg q14d (must be given with PO probenecid)	CMV retinitis
entecavir (Baraclude) (C)	Anti-HBV	*Adolescents older than 16 yr/Adult* PO: 0.5–1 mg once daily	Chronic HBV infection
famciclovir (Famvir) (B)	Anti-herpesvirus	*Adult* PO: 125 mg bid–500 mg tid × 5–7 days	Herpes zoster (shingles); recurrent genital herpes
foscarnet* (Foscavir) (C)	Anti-CMV, anti-HSV	*Adult* IV: 40–120 mg/kg divided in one to three daily doses	CMV retinitis; HSV infections that are resistant to standard drug therapy
▸▸ganciclovir hydrochloride (Cytovene, Valcyte) (C)	Anti-CMV	*Adult* IV: 5 mg/kg q12h × 2–3 wk PO: 900 mg once daily–bid with food	CMV retinitis; CMV prevention
oseltamivir phosphate (Tamiflu) (C)	Anti-influenza	*Children 1–12 yr less than 15 kg†* PO: 30 mg bid *Children 15–23 kg* PO: 45 mg bid *Children 23–40 kg* PO: 60 mg bid *Adolescents 13 yr or over 40 kg/Adult* PO: 75 mg bid × 5 days	Influenza A or B infection
ribavirin (Pegetron, Copegus) (X)	Anti-HCV	*Adult* PO: 800–1200 mg divided bid	Chronic HCV
ribavirin (Virazole) (X)	Anti-RSV	*Children* Aerosol: 6 g reconstituted to 20 mg/mL via continuous aerosol × 12 hr/day × 3–7 days	Severe RSV infection in hospitalized infants and toddlers
valacyclovir (Valtrex) (B)	Anti-herpesvirus	*Adult* PO: 500–1000 mg bid–tid × 3–10 days	Herpes zoster (shingles); genital herpes
valganciclovir hydrochloride (Valcyte) (C)	Anti-CMV	*Adult* PO: 900 mg bid × 3 wk with food	CMV retinitis; CMV disease prevention

Continued

Drug (Pregnancy Category)	Pharmacological Class	Usual Dosage Range	Indications
zanamivir (Relenza) (C)	Anti-influenza	*Children 7 yr and older/Adult* Inhalation‡: 10 mg (2 × 5-mg powder doses) bid; first day's doses must be at least 2 hr apart and q12h thereafter	Influenza A or B infection

CMV, cytomegalovirus; *HBV*, hepatitis B virus; *HCV*, hepatitis C virus; *HSV*, herpes simplex virus (types 1 and 2); *IV*, intravenous; *PO*, oral; *RSV*, respiratory syncytial virus.

*Available through the Special Access Programme, Health Canada. Used for salvage.
†Use liquid oral suspension for doses less than 75 mg.
‡Use bronchodilator inhaler first if applicable.

Note: Where children's doses are not provided, dosing guidelines for children are not firmly established for the drug in question and should be based on the careful clinical judgement of a qualified prescriber.

OVERVIEW OF HIV INFECTION AND THE AIDS PANDEMIC

The first cases of AIDS were recognized in 1981 in 31 previously healthy homosexual men in Los Angeles and New York City; the first case in Canada was reported in 1982. These first patients had mysteriously developed *Pneumocystis carinii* pneumonia (PCP) or Kaposi's sarcoma, both normally extremely rare illnesses. (PCP is now known as *Pneumocystis jirovecii* pneumonia.) Within months, similar disease patterns were recognized in intravenous drug users and in patients with hemophilia who had been transfused with blood-derived clotting factors. Other cases began to occur in hospitalized patients transfused with a variety of blood-derived products. In 1983, the *human T-cell lymphotropic virus type 3* (HTLV-3) was isolated from a patient with lymphadenopathy (swollen lymph nodes), and in 1984, this virus was demonstrated to be the cause of AIDS. This virus was later renamed *human immunodeficiency virus (HIV)*, a member of the **retrovirus** family. There are two recognized types of HIV: HIV-1 and HIV-2. Both cause AIDS, but HIV-2 is primarily localized in western Africa, and HIV-1 causes the majority of the HIV pandemic in the rest of the world. By 1985, a laboratory technique known as *enzyme-linked immunosorbent assay* (ELISA) was developed. This technique allowed the detection of HIV exposure through the presence of human antibodies to the virus in blood samples. This diagnostic breakthrough led to an appreciation of the enormity of HIV prevalence both in high-risk groups and as an emerging world pandemic, especially in developing countries. This laboratory screening technique also helped restore the safety of the transfusion blood supply, although it is not 100% reliable. In addition to HIV-1 and HIV-2, there are two other retroviruses known to infect humans: HTLV-1 and HTLV-2. HTLV-1 is an oncogenic virus capable of causing certain types of leukemia, whereas HTLV-2 is not associated with any specific disease.

The retrovirus family was named after the discovery of a unique feature of its replication process. Retroviruses are RNA viruses, unique in their use of the enzyme **reverse transcriptase** during their replication process. This enzyme promotes the synthesis of complementary ("mirror image") DNA molecules from the viral RNA genome. A second enzyme, *integrase*, promotes the integration of this viral DNA into the host cell DNA, a hybrid DNA complex, or a provirus. It produces new viral RNA genomes and proteins, which, in turn, combine to make mature HIV virions that infect other host cells. Another important enzyme is **protease**, which chemically separates new viral RNA from viral protein molecules. These components are initially synthesized into one large macromolecular strand, and the protease enzyme breaks up this strand into its key components. Figure 40-2 illustrates the major structural features of the HIV virion, and Figure 40-3 illustrates the steps in its replication process.

In contrast with retroviruses, nonretroviruses primarily use host cell enzymes (DNA or RNA polymerases) to synthesize viral nucleic acids. Reverse transcriptase is actually an RNA-dependent DNA polymerase and is sometimes also referred to by this name. However, reverse transcriptase is not normally found in host cells; both reverse transcriptase and integrase are carried by the virus. This "reversal" of the usual replication processes led to the enzyme name *reverse transcriptase* and to the *retrovirus* name for the family of viruses. Furthermore, retroviruses' synthesis of DNA from viral RNA molecules is a reversal of the norm because in most other organisms, RNA molecules are synthesized from DNA molecules as part of the reproductive process. Reverse transcriptase differs from host cell nucleic acid polymerases in yet another significant way: It has a higher rate of errors when stringing together the purine and pyrimidine bases (A, T, G, C) during transcription of the viral RNA genome into a DNA molecule during the replication process. These errors allow more frequent genetic mutations among HIV virions and often result in viral strains that are resistant both to drugs and to the patient's immune system. Such mutations also hamper the development of an effective vaccine against the virus.

The primary modes of infection with HIV are sexual, parenteral, and perinatal. Sexual intercourse, primarily receptive anal and vaginal intercourse, is the most

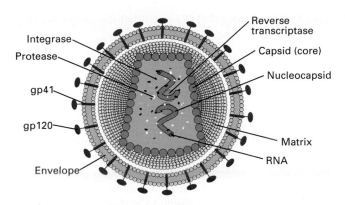

FIG. 40-2 Human immunodeficiency virus (HIV). Within the core capsid, the diploid, single-stranded, positive-sense RNA is complexed to nucleoprotein. *gp,* glycoprotein. (From Newman, W.A. (2003). *Dorland's illustrated medical dictionary* (30th ed.). Philadelphia: Saunders.)

common means of infection. Probability of transmission risk increases after seroconversion and if the partner is in the advanced disease stage (has a high viral load). The risk of heterosexual transmission is highest among those with ulcerative sexually transmitted infections, those with multiple sex partners, and sexual partners of intravenous drug users. Risk of transmission is increased in women who have vaginal bleeding during intercourse. Heterosexual transmission is most common in Africa and Asia. In Canada, the highest incidence of new cases is among men who have unprotected sex with men (39.6%),

followed by injection drug users (17%) and women (28%). Canadians who emigrated from countries with high rates of HIV account for an increasing number of HIV-positive tests. Young people aged 15 to 29 years make up 28% of all positive HIV tests. Aboriginal peoples in Canada have higher rates of HIV than those among the general population. Although HIV can be isolated from almost any body fluid, including tears, sweat, saliva, and urine, its concentrations in these fluids are much lower than those in blood and genital secretions. In approximately 6% of cases, specific risk factors cannot be determined. The risk of transmission to health care workers from percutaneous (needle-stick) injuries is currently approximately 0.3%. The observance of standard precautions in avoiding contact with all body fluids during patient care dramatically reduces the risk of caregiver infection (see Box 10-1).

The rate of new infections is rising more rapidly in minority populations, especially among Blacks and Aboriginal people. Worldwide, there are now more than 40 million cases of HIV/AIDS, with more than 80% of these cases in developing countries. People in these countries often lack access to adequate drug therapy, resulting in millions of orphaned children each year. Untreated pregnant woman infected with HIV transmit the virus to their infant in 15% to 30% of pregnancies. Transmission can occur transplacentally, causing infection in utero, or during birth. When the first antiretroviral drugs were developed in the 1980s, it was feared that they would be too toxic and teratogenic if given

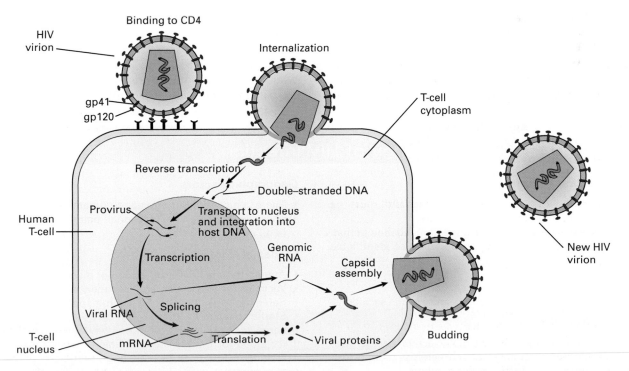

FIG. 40-3 Life cycle of the HIV virus. The extracellular envelope protein gp120 binds to CD4 on the surface of T lymphocytes or mononuclear phagocytes, while the transmembrane protein glycoprotein 41 (gp41) mediates the fusion of the viral envelope with the cell membrane. (From Newman, W.A. (2003). *Dorland's illustrated medical dictionary* (30th ed.). Philadelphia: Saunders.)

to pregnant women. However, prophylactic antiretroviral treatment of infected mothers has been shown to reduce infant infection by at least two thirds and is not normally harmful to either the mother or infant. Medication may also be given prophylactically to the newborn infant, typically for the first 6 weeks of life. Of course, infants and children with established HIV infection must usually continue on drugs indefinitely. Prescribers are encouraged to register patients with the designated Antiretroviral Pregnancy Registry (http://www.apregistry.com), an international collaborative project that monitors maternal and fetal outcomes of antiretroviral drug therapy. Breast milk can transmit the virus to the infant in 10% to 20% of cases, thus breastfeeding is contraindicated in developed countries. In developing countries, however, breastfeeding may be the only available source of nutrition for the infant and, consequently, worth the risk. This is especially true if drugs and other health services are lacking, as is often the case. Box 40-2 summarizes key epidemiological concepts related to HIV/AIDS.

HIV infection that is untreated or treatment resistant eventually leads to immune system failure, with death occurring secondary to opportunistic infections. The infection often progresses over a period of several years. Health organizations, including the U.S. Centers for Disease Control and Prevention (CDC) and the World Health Organization (WHO), have published classification systems describing the "stages" of HIV/AIDS infection. In 1993, the CDC model listed five stages. A 2005 WHO model lists four stages as follows:

- Stage 1: Asymptomatic infection
- Stage 2: Early, general symptoms of disease
- Stage 3: Moderate symptoms
- Stage 4: Severe symptoms, often leading to death

Stage 1 refers to the first few weeks or months after initial exposure to the virus. Patients may be asymptomatic but may show signs of persistent generalized lymphoadenopathy (PGL), or swollen lymph nodes. PGL is more specifically defined as inflammation of the lymph nodes in at least two sites outside the inguinal (groin) area that lasts for some months. During this time, the virus is present in the blood at low levels and has a low rate of replication. CD4 cell counts are usually still within normal limits at 350 cells/microlitre of blood. CD4 refers to the protein on the cell surface of helper T lymphocytes, to which HIV virions attach. Helper T cells normally function by releasing cytokines, chemicals that activate and modulate cell-mediated immunity, a general term for all immune system actions other than those of antibodies. Immune system function is described further in Chapter 50. Helper T lymphocytes circulate in the blood and are the primary target cells for HIV. However, HIV may also infect macrophages, which are usually stationary (noncirculating) CD4-positive cells that remain in various tissues (e.g., lungs, skin, brain) to prevent infection. But it is ultimately through widespread destruction of helper T cells in the blood that HIV infection eventually weakens the patient's immune system.

Stage 2 involves continued lymphadenopathy and other symptoms, including fever, rash, sore throat, night sweats, malaise, diarrhea, idiopathic thrombocytopenia, oral candidiasis, and herpes zoster (shingles). In the early years of the epidemic (early 1980s), this stage was also known as AIDS-related complex, or ARC. These symptoms may actually resolve spontaneously about the time of seroconversion, which is when the patient's own antibodies to the virus (HIV antibodies) begin to appear in blood samples. Seroconversion usually occurs 3 weeks to 3 months after exposure. At this point, the patient is said to be HIV positive. However, the patient may not have further progression of symptoms for 1 to 10 years. During this stage, the CD4+ T-cell count begins to drop, while HIV antibody levels rise as part of an attempt by the patient's own immune system to neutralize the virus.

BOX 40-2 Epidemiology of HIV Infection

Disease Viral Factors

- Developed virus is easily inactivated and must be transmitted in body fluids.
- The disease has a long prodromal or incubation period.
- Virus can be shed before development of identifiable symptoms.

Transmission

- Virus is present in blood, semen, and vaginal secretions.

Who Is At Risk?

- Intravenous drug users; sexually active people with many partners (homosexual and heterosexual); prostitutes; newborns of HIV-positive mothers
- Blood and organ transplant recipients and individuals with hemophilia who received transfusions before 1985 (prescreening programs)

Geographic Factors

- There is a continuously expanding pandemic.
- There is no particular seasonal pattern of infection (e.g., unlike influenza).

Modes of Control

- Antiviral drugs limit progression of disease.
- Vaccines for prevention and treatment are in trials.
- Safer, monogamous sex helps limit spread.
- Sterile injection needles should be used.
- Large-scale screening programs have been developed for blood for transfusions, organs for transplants, and clotting factors used by individuals with hemophilia.

Source: Health Canada HIV/AIDS Web site. Available at http://www.hc-sc.gc.ca/hl-vs/iyh-vsv/diseases-maladies/hiv-vih-eng.php

The virus begins to multiply in the body but does not necessarily produce disabling symptoms. This stage is often the first presenting sign of HIV infection, and stage 1 may not have been noticed or reported by the patient.

During Stage 3, the infection progresses to a moderately symptomatic state. Continued weight loss and chronic diarrhea and fever manifest, and CD4+ count continues to drop. Opportunistic infections (OIs) begin, including oral candidiasis (thrush), severe bacterial pneumonias, and pulmonary tuberculosis (TB). Pulmonary TB is usually more severe in persons with AIDS and is currently the leading cause of death worldwide among HIV-infected patients. Dually infected patients have a greater likelihood of developing active TB and becoming infectious. OIs are so named because the destruction by HIV of the patient's immune system provides the "opportunity" for normally harmless microorganisms in the body to proliferate into serious infections. They may become life threatening or produce significant disability (e.g., blindness from CMV retinitis).

In Stage 4 (formerly called "full-blown AIDS"), viral replication increases dramatically, resulting in increasing destruction of helper T cells and a corresponding decrease in CD4 counts. At this point, there is a major decline in immune system function, and the effects of the illness begin to seriously affect the entire body. When the CD4+ count drops below 200 cells/microlitre, multiple, severe OIs often begin to occur. Fever, night sweats, and malaise resume and are now accompanied by increasingly severe OIs, such as *Mycobacterium avium* complex (MAC) and *Pneumocystis jirovecii* pneumonia. Other common OIs include parasitic infections such as cryptosporidial diarrhea and toxoplasmosis encephalitis; viral infections such as HSV mouth ulcers,

disseminated extrapulmonary tuberculosis, esophagitis, pneumonitis, CMV pneumonia, and CMV retinitis; and fungal infections such as candidiasis of the gastrointestinal and respiratory tracts and invasive aspergillosis of the lungs. A similar opportunistic situation occurs with HIV-associated neoplasms. The most common of these include Kaposi's sarcoma and various types of lymphoma. In HIV-infected women, there is some evidence that cervical cancer is more likely to be in advanced stages upon diagnosis. HIV wasting syndrome is yet another defining condition of the disease and involves major weight loss, chronic diarrhea, more frequent or even constant fever, and chronic fatigue. In addition to its attack on helper T cells and macrophages, the HIV virus itself can also cause additional pathology in such organs as the brain (HIV-induced encephalopathy and dementia), bone marrow, lungs (recurrent pneumonia), and skin. Death is most likely when the CD4+ count falls below 50 cells/microlitre. The viral load, which is measured as the number of viral RNA copies per millilitre of blood, also continues to rise uncontrollably. If this condition continues, death often ensues. All of these manifestations are said to be the defining conditions of AIDS. Box 40-3 lists several such conditions. Figure 40-4 illustrates the events that roughly correlate with these four stages of HIV infection.

Figure 40-4 refers to the hypothetical natural course of the disease, through the four stages, without treatment. Patients who are effectively treated with drug therapy usually do not progress through all of these stages—at least such progression is slowed considerably (years). In fact, advances in antiretroviral drug therapy have given rise to increasingly greater numbers of long-term survivors of HIV infection. Antiretroviral therapy (ART) refers

BOX 40-3   Indicator Diseases of AIDS

Opportunistic Infections

Protozoal
- Toxoplasmosis of the brain
- Cryptosporidiosis with diarrhea
- Isosporiasis with diarrhea

Fungal
- Candidiasis of the esophagus, trachea, and lungs
- *Pneumocystis jirovecii* pneumonia
- Cryptococcosis (extrapulmonary)
- Histoplasmosis (disseminated)
- Coccidioidomycosis (disseminated)

Viral
- Cytomegalovirus disease
- HSV infection (persistent or disseminated)
- Progressive multifocal leukoencephalopathy
- Hairy leukoplakia caused by Epstein–Barr virus

Bacterial
- *Mycobacterium avium intracellularae* complex (MAC) (disseminated)

- Any "atypical" mycobacterial disease
- Extrapulmonary TB
- *Salmonella* septicemia (recurrent)
- Pyogenic bacterial infections (multiple or recurrent)

Opportunistic Neoplasias
- Kaposi's sarcoma
- Primary lymphoma of the brain
- Other non-Hodgkin's lymphomas

Others
- HIV wasting syndrome
- HIV encephalopathy
- Lymphoid interstitial pneumonia

HIV, human immunodeficiency virus; HSV, herpes simplex virus; TB, tuberculosis.

Modified from Mandell, G. L., Bennett, J. E., & Dolin, R. (2008). *Principles and practice of infectious diseases* (7th ed.). Philadelphia: Churchill Livingstone.

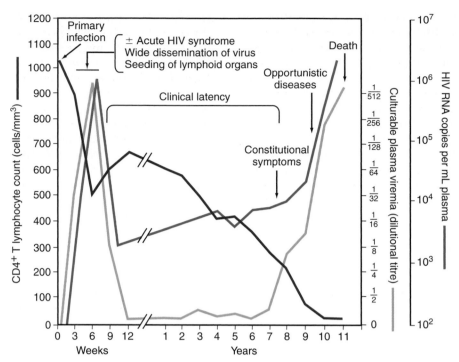

FIG. 40-4 Natural history of HIV infection in the absence of therapy in a hypothetical patient. (From Fauci, A. S., Pantaleo, G., Stanley, S., & Weissman, D. (1996). Immunopathogenic mechanisms of HIV infection. *Annals of Internal Medicine*, 124, 654-663. In Mandell, G. L., Bennett, J. E., & Dolin, R. (2008). *Principles and practice of infectious diseases* (7th ed.). St. Louis, MO: Elsevier, Churchill Livingstone.)

to a combination of at least three antiretroviral drugs to provide maximal suppression of HIV and stop the progression of AIDS. ART is normally started immediately upon confirmation of HIV infection. Opportunistic infections are treated with infection-specific antimicrobial drugs (see corresponding chapters) as they arise. OIs are treated prophylactically, most commonly when a patient's CD4+ count falls below 200. Opportunistic malignancies, such as Kaposi's sarcoma and lymphomas, are treated with specific antineoplastic medications, which are discussed in Chapters 48 and 49, as well as with radiation and surgery as indicated.

Long-term survival is defined as living with HIV infection for at least 10 to 15 years after infection. Some particularly remarkable patients have lived for several years with CD4 counts remaining at the often fatal level of 200 cells/mm3 or less. Improved drug therapy against both HIV and OIs is thought to play an important role in these unusual cases. Other remarkable patients are the *long-term nonprogressors*, or long-term survivors who have maintained normal CD4 counts and low HIV viral loads despite not receiving any anti-HIV drug treatment! These patients are usually able to mount especially strong cell-mediated and humoral immune responses that prevent progression of the viral infection. These individuals are also the subject of much research in order to identify the mechanisms of their survival and find ways to share these advantages with other patients.

Research attempts to develop an effective anti-HIV vaccine are under way throughout the world. There have

been several preclinical (animal) studies using monkeys. Human clinical trials have been conducted since 1990, primarily on non–HIV-infected research volunteers. However, vaccines are also being studied in HIV-positive patients, with some data suggesting the possibility of a vaccine-induced enhanced immune response that could retard disease progression. A variety of laboratory techniques have been used to manufacture the vaccines used in these research studies. Examples of these include attenuated HIV virions, HIV components (e.g., RNA alone), or other virus particles with HIV components attached (e.g., envelope proteins). Despite encouraging data regarding potential benefits, the design of an effective HIV vaccine continues to remain elusive.

ANTIRETROVIRAL DRUGS

There have been significant advances in medical science since HIV was first identified in the early 1980s. The increasing urgency and public awareness of the AIDS epidemic has stimulated much research in the fields of immunology and pharmacology, resulting in the development of several increasingly effective antiretroviral drugs, as well as antiviral drugs in general. Although new drug combinations have definitely prolonged lives and offered hope to many people, these medications often have significant toxicities. Furthermore, HIV/AIDS is still not considered a curable disease, although there have been some remarkable recoveries and apparent cures in a small number of individuals.

Currently, there are six classes of antiretroviral drugs: three distinct classes of reverse transcriptase inhibitors (RTIs); the single class of protease inhibitors (PIs); and the two newest classes, (1) the *fusion inhibitors*, which, to date, include only one medication, a CCR5 antagonist, maraviroc (Celsentri); and (2) the *integrase inhibitors*, of which there is also only one drug, raltegravir (Isentress).

Mechanism of Action and Drug Effects

Although HIV/AIDS is a complex illness, the mechanisms of action of the drug classes are straightforward and distinct. The name of each drug class provides a reminder of its role in suppressing the viral replication process. For example, the **reverse transcriptase inhibitors (RTIs)** act by blocking activity of the enzyme reverse transcriptase, which promotes the synthesis of new viral DNA molecules from the RNA genome of the parent virion. There are currently three subclasses of RTIs: nucleoside RTIs, or NRTIs; non-nucleoside RTIs, or NNRTIs; and nucleotide RTIs, or NTRTIs.

The **protease inhibitors (PIs)** act by inhibiting the *protease* retroviral enzyme. This enzyme promotes the breakup of chains of protein molecules at designated points, a process necessary for viral replication. There is one combination PI that includes both lopinavir and ritonavir (Kaletra). The ritonavir component also serves to inhibit cytochrome P450–mediated enzymatic metabolism of the lopinavir component.

Currently, there is one fusion inhibitor, enfuvirtide, which acts to inhibit viral fusion. Recall that fusion is the process by which an HIV virion attaches to (fuses with) the membrane of a host cell (T lymphocyte) before infecting it in preparation for viral replication.

As the class name implies, the integrase inhibitor raltegravir inhibits the enzyme integrase. This enzyme promotes the integration of viral DNA into the host cell DNA, thus the inhibitor acts to prevent this integration process.

All of these medications are listed in the corresponding Dosages table on p. 772, in addition to the NRTI combination drug products.

Single-drug therapy was most common in the early years of the HIV epidemic, partly because of a lack of treatment options. However, with the development of multiple antiretroviral drugs and the emergence of resistant viral strains, combination drug therapy is now the current standard of care and the most effective treatment to date. Combination drug treatment, referred to as *antiretroviral therapy (ART),* usually includes at least three medications. The most commonly recommended drug combinations include two or three NRTIs; two NRTIs plus one or two PIs; or an NRTI plus an NNRTI with one or two PIs. Atripla is a combination of three widely used antiretroviral drugs (efavirenz, emtricitabine, tenofovir) into one tablet to be taken once daily. Despite the effectiveness of ART, prescribers may still need to alter a patient's drug regimen if there is major drug intolerance (see Adverse Effects) or drug resistance. A given patient's HIV strain can still evolve and mutate over time, allowing it to adaptively become resistant to any drug therapy, especially when used for a prolonged period of time, as is usually the case with HIV treatment. Evidence for drug resistance includes a falling CD4+ count and increased viral load in a patient for whom a given drug regimen previously kept those symptoms under control.

To varying degrees, all antiretroviral drugs have similar therapeutic effects. They reduce the viral load, which is the number of viral RNA copies per millilitre of blood. A viral load of less than 50 copies/mL is considered to be an undetectable viral load and is a primary goal of antiretroviral therapy. Ideally, HIV-infected patients should be monitored by practitioners with extensive training in drug therapy for infectious diseases. These practitioners must often make careful choices and changes in drug therapy over time, based on a given patient's clinical response and severity of any drug-related toxicities. When effective, treatment leads to a significant reduction in mortality and the incidence of opportunistic infections, improves patient's physical performance, and significantly improves T-cell counts.

Indications

As indicated in Table 40-3, the only usual indication for the current antiretroviral drugs is active HIV infection. Prophylactic therapy (Table 40-5) is also administered to individuals (e.g., health care workers and high-risk infants) with known potential exposure to HIV (e.g., via needle-stick injuries in hospitals).

TABLE 40-5

Recommendation for Occupational HIV Exposure Chemoprophylaxis

Type of Exposure	Source	Prophylaxis	Therapy
Percutaneous	Blood	Recommended	zidovudine + lamivudine + indinavir;
	Fluid containing visible blood or other potentially infectious fluid or tissue		zidovudine + lamivudine +/- indinavir
Mucous membrane	Blood	Offer	zidovudine + lamivudine
	Fluid containing visible blood or other potentially infectious fluid or tissue	Offer	zidovudine + lamivudine +/- indinavir
		Offer	zidovudine +/- lamivudine
Skin (i.e., prolonged contact, extensive area, area without skin integrity)	Blood	Offer	zidovudine + lamivudine +/- indinavir

Contraindications

Keeping in mind the potentially fatal outcome of HIV infection, the only usual contraindication to a given medication is known severe drug allergy or other intolerable toxicity. Fortunately, over the past 25 years, with the rise of the HIV pandemic, several categories of antiretroviral medications have been developed. Most of the current antiretroviral drug classes have several alternative drugs to choose from, should a patient be particularly intolerant of a given drug.

Adverse Effects

Common adverse effects of selected antiretroviral drugs are listed in Table 40-4. A few key adverse effects are discussed in more detail later in the chapter. It is not uncommon to need to modify drug therapy because of adverse effects. The goal is to find a regimen that will best control infection, with as tolerable an adverse-effect profile as possible. Different patients may vary widely in their drug tolerance, and individual drug tolerance may change over time. Thus, drug regimens often must be strategically individualized and evolve with the course of the patient's illness.

ART, although certainly an effective treatment against HIV infection, also has a significant downside that involves hepatitis C virus (HCV) infections. Approximately 20% of HIV-infected patients in Canada are also infected with HCV, which tends to be more severe in HIV patients. The most common route of transmission of HCV is through needle sharing; sexual and perinatal routes are much less common. HCV is the most important cause of chronic liver disease in Canada. HCV-induced liver failure is the most common reason for liver transplantation, and liver cancer may occur secondary to HCV infection. Unfortunately, because of the pharmacological strain that it places on the liver, ART is strongly correlated with increased mortality from HCV-induced liver disease.

A major adverse effect of protease inhibitors involves lipid abnormalities, including lipodystrophy, or redistribution of fat stores under the skin. This condition often results in cosmetically undesirable outcomes for the patient, such as a "hump" at the posterior base of the neck, and a skeletonized (bony) appearance of the face. In addition, dyslipidemias, such as hypertriglyceridemia, can occur, even resulting in insulin resistance and type 2 diabetes symptoms. In these cases, switching a patient from a PI to an NNRTI such as nevirapine may help reduce such symptoms without undermining antiretroviral efficacy.

With increasing long-term antiretroviral drug therapy because of prolonged disease survival, another emerging long-term adverse effect associated with these drugs is bone demineralization and possible osteoporosis. When this condition occurs, it may require treatment with standard medications for osteoporosis, such as calcium, vitamin D, and bisphosphonates (Chapter 34).

Interactions

Common drug interactions involving selected antiretroviral drugs are listed in Box 40-1.

Dosages

Dosage information for all of the currently available antiretroviral medications, including combination drug products, is listed in the Dosages table on p. 772.

 ## DRUG PROFILES

enfuvirtide

Enfuvirtide (Fuzeon) is a newer drug, classed as a *fusion inhibitor*. It acts by suppressing the fusion process whereby a virion is attached to the outer membrane of a host T cell before entry into the cell and subsequent viral replication. This mechanism of action serves as yet another example of how antiretroviral drugs are strategically designed to interfere with specific steps of the viral replication process. Enfuvirtide is indicated for treatment of HIV infection in combination with other antiretroviral drugs. Use of this drug in combination with other standard antiretroviral drugs has been associated with markedly reduced viral loads, compared with drug regimens that did not include this drug. Adults and children have shown comparable tolerance of the drug. The drug is currently available only in injectable form.

PHARMACOKINETICS

Half-Life	Onset	Peak	Duration
SC: 4 hr	SC: Unknown	SC: 6 hr	SC: Unknown

▶▶ indinavir sulfate

Indinavir sulfate (Crixivan) belongs to the *protease inhibitor* (PI) class of antiretroviral drugs. Others include ritonavir (Norvir), saquinavir mesylate (Invirase), nelfinavir mesylate (Viracept), atazanavir sulfate (Reyataz), fosamprenavir calcium (Telzir), and the combination product lopinavir/ritonavir (Kaletra). Indinavir can be taken in combination with other anti-HIV therapies or alone. Indinavir is best dissolved and absorbed in an acidic gastric environment, and the presence of high-protein and high-fat foods reduces its absorption. Therefore, it is recommended that it be administered in a fasting state. Indinavir therapy produces increases in CD4+ cell counts. It also produces significant reductions in viral load. PIs are commonly given in combination with two RTIs to maximize efficacy and decrease the likelihood of viral drug resistance.

Indinavir is relatively well tolerated in most patients. Nephrolithiasis (kidney stones) can occur in approximately

Continued

DRUG PROFILES (cont'd)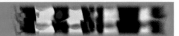

4% of patients. Patients who take indinavir are encouraged to drink at least 1.5 L of liquids every day to maintain hydration and help avoid nephrolithiasis. Indinavir is contraindicated in patients with clinically significant hypersensitivity to any of its components. Indinavir and all other PIs are available only for oral use.

PHARMACOKINETICS

Half-Life	Onset	Peak	Duration
PO: 1.5–2.5 hr	PO: 2 wk*	PO: 0.5–1 hr	PO: 6 mo

*Therapeutic effects.

▸▸ maraviroc

Maraviroc (Celesentri) is a new class of drug, a CCR5 antagonist, that is unique in its action. Whereas other oral HIV drugs target the virus within the white blood cells, CCR5 inhibitors prevent the virus from entering uninfected CD4 T lymphocytes by blocking the main entry point. CCR5 is the chemokine (C-C motif) receptor 5 that HIV uses to gain entry into CD4 cells. When CCR5 "sees" the HIV virus, it signals to the main CD4 cell receptor to allow the HIV antigen into the target T cell. Researchers believe that maraviroc may be most useful in treatment-naïve patients, as the CCR5-tropic HIV-1 receptor seems to be dominant early in the disease process. As the disease progresses, HIV appears to adapt and use an alternative entry point, the CXR4 receptor. Currently, however, maraviroc is indicated for adult patients who are treatment experienced with resistance to multiple antiretroviral drugs. Maraviroc is available in oral form.

PHARMACOKINETICS

Half-Life	Onset	Peak	Duration
PO: 14–18 hr	PO: 2 wk*	PO: 0.5–4 hr	PO: 6 mo

*Therapeutic effects.

▸▸ nevirapine

Nevirapine (Viramune) is *a* non-nucleoside reverse transcriptase inhibitor *(NNRTI)*. This is the second class of antiviral drugs indicated for the treatment of HIV infection. Other currently available NNRTIs include delavirdine mesylate (Rescriptor) and efavirenz (Sustiva). These drugs are often used in combination with nucleoside reverse transcriptase inhibitors *(NRTIs)* such as zidovudine. Nevirapine is well tolerated compared with other therapies for HIV. The most common adverse effects are rash, fever, nausea, headache, and abnormal liver function tests. Efavirenz is available in a fixed-dose combination of efavirenz, emtricitabine, and tenofovir disoproxil fumarate (Atripla). Nevirapine and the other NNRTIs are available only for oral use.

PHARMACOKINETICS

Half-Life	Onset	Peak	Duration
PO: 25–30 hr	PO: 2 hr*	PO: 2–4 hr	PO: 24 hr

*Therapeutic effects.

▸▸ raltegravir potassium

Raltegravir potassium (Isentress) is the first of another new class of HIV drugs, *integrase inhibitors,* approved under the Notice of Compliance. Integrase is one of three enzymes, the other two being reverse transcriptase and protease, required for HIV to replicate in the body. Raltegravir prevents HIV from inserting its genes into DNA, thereby limiting viral replication. It is to be used for treatment-experienced adult patients who show evidence of viral replication and HIV-1 strains resistant to multiple antiretroviral agents. Raltegravir is available only in oral form.

PHARMACOKINETICS

Half-Life	Onset	Peak	Duration
PO: 9 hr	PO: Unknown	PO: 3 hr	PO: 12 hr

tenofovir disoproxil

Tenofovir disoproxil (Viread) is the first and currently the only nucleotide reverse transcriptase inhibitor *(NTRTI)*. It is an analogue of adenine but has an attached phosphate group, which distinguishes this drug class from the nucleoside RTIs. Tenofovir is indicated for use against HIV infection in combination with other antiretroviral drugs. It is currently available only for oral use.

PHARMACOKINETICS

Half-Life	Onset	Peak	Duration
PO: Unknown	PO: Unknown	PO: 1 hr	PO: Unknown

▸▸ zidovudine

Zidovudine (AZT, Retrovir) is a synthetic nucleoside analogue of thymidine that has had an enormous impact on the treatment and quality of life of HIV-infected patients who have AIDS. It was the first, and for a long time the only, anti-HIV medication that offered patients with AIDS any hope in the early years of the pandemic. Other NRTIs include lamivudine (3TC, Heptovir), didanosine (Videx EC), stavudine (Zerit), abacavir sulfate (Ziagen), and emtricitabine (Emtriva). Zidovudine, along with other antiretroviral drugs, is given to HIV-infected pregnant women and to newborns to prevent maternal transmission of the virus to the infant. The major dose-limiting adverse effect of zidovudine is bone marrow suppression; this is often the reason for a patient with an HIV infection being switched to another anti-HIV drug such as zalcitabine or didanosine. Some patients may receive a combination of two of these drugs, in lower doses, to maximize their combined actions. This strategy may decrease the likelihood of toxicity. Zidovudine is available in both oral and injectable formulations.

PHARMACOKINETICS

Half-Life	Onset	Peak	Duration
1.1 hr	Unknown	0.5–1.5 hr	3–5 hr

DOSAGES Antiretroviral Drugs

Drug (Pregnancy Category)	Pharmacological Class	Usual Dosage Range	Indications
abacavir sulfate (Ziagen) (C)	Nucleoside reverse transcriptase inhibitor	*Children 3 mo–12 yr* PO: 8 mg/kg bid (max 300 mg/dose) *Adolescents older than 12 yr/Adult* PO: 300 mg bid	HIV infection
atazanavir (Reyataz) (B)	Protease inhibitor	*Children 6–18 yr* PO: 150–300 mg once daily *Adult* PO: 300–400 mg once daily	HIV infection
delavirdine mesylate (Rescriptor) (C)	Non-nucleoside reverse transcriptase inhibitor	*Adult* PO: 400 mg tid	HIV infection
didanosine (Videx EC) (C)	Nucleoside reverse transcriptase inhibitor	*Adult* PO: 250–400 mg once day	HIV infection
efavirenz (Sustiva) (C)	Non-nucleoside reverse transcriptase inhibitor	*Children older than 3 yr/Adult* PO: 200–600 mg once daily based on weight	HIV infection
emtricitabine (Emtriva) (B)	Nucleoside reverse transcriptase inhibitor	*Adult older than 18 yr* PO: 600 mg once daily	HIV infection
enfuvirtide (Fuzeon) (B)	Fusion inhibitor	*Children 6–16 yr* SC: 2 mg/kg bid (max 90 mg/dose) *Adult* SC: 90 mg bid	HIV infection
fosamprenavir (Telzir) (C)	Protease Inhibitor	*Adult* PO: 700 mg bid to 1400 mg qd–bid	HIV infection
▸▸indinavir sulfate (Crixivan) (C)	Protease inhibitor	*Children older than 3 yr* PO: 500 mg/m² q8h *Adult* PO: 800 mg q8h	HIV infection
lamivudine (Heptovir, Epivir-HBV, 3TC) (C)	Nucleoside reverse transcriptase inhibitor	*Adult 16 yr and older* PO: 100 mg daily	HIV infection
maravinoc (Celsentri) (B)	CCR5 antagonist	*Adult older than 16 yr* PO: 300 mg bid	HIV infection
nelfinavir mesylate (Viracept) (B)	Protease inhibitor	*Children 2–13 yr* PO: 25–30 mg/kg tid *Adolescents 14 yr and older/Adult* PO: 1250 mg divided bid–tid	HIV infection
▸▸nevirapine (Viramune) (C)	Non-nucleoside reverse transcriptase inhibitor	*Adult* PO: 200 mg daily × 14 days, then bid	HIV infection
▸▸raltegravir (Isentress) (C)	Integrase strand transfer inhibitor	*Adult* PO: 400 mg bid	HIV infection
ritonavir (Norvir) (B)	Protease inhibitor	*Children 2–12 yr* PO: 400 mg/m² bid *Adult* PO: 600 mg bid (max 1200 mg)	HIV infection
saquinavir (Invirase) (B)	Protease inhibitor	*Adult 16 yr and older* PO: 1000 mg bid	HIV infection
stavudine (Zerit, d4T) (C)	Nucleoside reverse transcriptase inhibitor	*Children older than 3 mo* PO: 2 mg/kg day *Adult* PO: 30–40 mg q12h	HIV infection
tenofovir disoproxil (Viread) (B)	Nucleoside reverse transcriptase inhibitor	*Adult* PO: 300 mg once daily	HIV infection

Continued

DOSAGES Antiretroviral Drugs (cont'd)

Drug (Pregnancy Category)	Pharmacological Class	Usual Dosage Range	Indications
▸zidovudine (Retrovir, AZT) (C)	Nucleoside reverse transcriptase inhibitor	*Infants 0–6 wk** PO: 2 mg q6h starting within 12 hr after birth IV: 1.5 mg/kg q6h *Children 3 mo–12 yr* PO: 180 mg/m² q6h IV: 120 mg/m² q6h (max 160 mg/dose) *Adult* PO: 600 mg/day divided q12h or 300 mg q8h IV: 1–2 mg/kg q4h *Pregnant women* PO: 100 mg 5×/day until start of labour, then give IV bolus dose of 2 mg/kg over 1 hr followed by an IV infusion of 1 mg/kg/hr until the umbilical cord is clamped	HIV infection
COMBINATION DRUG PRODUCTS abacavir/lamividine (Kivexa) (C)	Double-drug combination nucleoside reverse transcriptase inhibitor	*Adult older than 18 and more than 40 kg* PO: 1 tab daily (1 tab = 60 mg abacavir/300 mg lamuvidine)	HIV infection
abacavir/lamivudine/ zidovudine (Trizivir) (C)	Triple-drug combination nucleoside reverse transcriptase inhibitor	*Adolescent/Adult more than 50 kg* PO: 1 tab bid (1 tab = 300 mg abacavir/150 mg lamivudine/300 mg zidovudine)	HIV infection
emtricitabine/tenofovir disoproxil fumarate (Truvada) (C)	Double-drug combination nucleoside reverse transcriptase inhibitor	*Adult* PO: 1 tab daily (1 tab = 200 mg emtricitabine/300 mg tenofovir disoproxil fumarate)	HIV infection
efavirenz/emtricitabine/ tenofovir disoproxil fumarate (Atripla)	Triple-drug combination nucleoside reverse transcriptase inhibitor	*Adult* PO: 1 tab daily (1 tab = 600 mg efavirenz/200 mg) emtricitabine/300 mg tenofovir disoproxil fumarate)	HIV infection
lamivudine/zidovudine (Combivir) (C)	Double-drug combination nucleoside reverse transcriptase inhibitor	*Adolescents older than 12/Adult* PO: 1 tab bid (1 tab = 150 mg lamivudine/300 mg zidovudine)	HIV infection
lopinavir/ritonavir (Kaletra) (C)	Double-drug combination protease-inhibitor	*Children 7 to less than 15 kg* PO: 12 mg/kg bid *Children 15–40 kg* PO: 10 mg/kg bid *Adult older than 18 and more than 40 kg* PO: 2 tabs, 3 caps,5 mL bid or 4 tabs, 6 caps, 10 mL daily (lopinavir/ritonavir 1 tab = 200 mg/50 mg; 1 cap = 133.3 mg/33.3 mg; oral solution, 1 mL = 80 mg/20 mg)	HIV infection HIV infection

*Drug should be continued either IV or PO through at least 6 weeks of age.

Note: Where children's doses are not provided, dosing guidelines for children are not firmly established for the drug in question and should be based on the careful clinical judgement of a qualified prescriber.

ADDITIONAL SIGNIFICANT VIRAL ILLNESSES

There are numerous other viral infections that could be discussed in this chapter. Four of recent significance are avian influenza, West Nile virus (WNV), sudden acute respiratory syndrome (SARS), and H1N1. These viral infections have resulted in significant morbidity and mortality, sometimes requiring aggressive supportive care in a critical care unit (CCU) setting.

In 1999, the first North American cases of WNV occurred in New York City, and it was not until 2001 that the first documented cases of WNV in humans occurred in Canada. WNV is a member of the arbovirus family and is transmitted to humans by mosquitoes. It also infects animals, primarily birds, and has been detected in horses and cows. By 2007, the U.S. Centers for Disease Control and Prevention (CDC) indicated that the virus had been found in more than 130 species of birds. In humans, WNV can progress to meningitis and encephalitis. The virus can also be transmitted through blood transfusions and has been detected in breast milk. There is new evidence that health care workers may develop WNV via needle-sticks or cuts. It is currently being investigated for maternal–fetal transmission during pregnancy. In June 2003, Health Canada began screening blood donations for WNV using a test developed by the Canadian Blood Services. In Canada, there were 38 reported cases of WNV in 2008, a significant drop from previous years. This decline may be attributed to cool spring temperatures that reduced mosquitoes' ability to breed and expand their population such that the number of mosquitoes infected with the virus was possibly lower. Nevertheless, there are currently no specific antiviral drugs or vaccines available for treatment of human WNV infection. In the more severe cases of encephalitis, aggressive supportive measures such as monitoring and control of intracranial pressure (ICP) can be crucial. Prevention focuses on mosquito control strategies to reduce reproduction and on individual risk reduction strategies.

In November 2002, a new, serious viral infectious disease known as sudden acute respiratory syndrome, or SARS, emerged in China. Cases later appeared in Europe and North America, with the first case in Canada reported on February 23, 2003. The Canadian outbreak was traced to a traveller returning from Hong Kong. A large outbreak later occurred in Singapore in March of 2003 and was eventually traced to three travellers who had stayed at the same Hong Kong hotel during the same period as the individual involved in the Canadian outbreak, indicating the high contagiousness of this virus. The SARS illness can range from a mild to a life-threatening respiratory syndrome. The illness is self-limiting in that it usually resolves on its own within 3 to 4 weeks. However, 10% to 20% of patients required mechanical ventilation and critical care support, with an overall fatality rate of 3%. Although standard antiviral drugs were used, including oseltamivir, no specific drug therapy proved to be definitively helpful. Thanks to a global public health response coordinated by the World Health Organization (WHO), transmission of this virus was apparently halted worldwide as of July 2003. At that point, however, there had been at least 8100 cases of SARS, including more than 800 deaths. The cause of SARS was determined to be a coronavirus, which was named the SARS coronavirus (SARS-CoV). Coronaviruses commonly cause mild to moderate upper respiratory illnesses in humans, including the common cold. The CDC, along with a Canadian laboratory, was able to sequence the genome of this virus.

Avian influenza, or "bird flu," is an influenza virus infection that has been shown to infect birds in Europe as well as birds and humans in Asia. This disease is caused by an influenza A virus known as avian influenza A, subtype H5N1. The virus is carried in the intestines of many wild birds worldwide, often without causing any serious illness. The most common bird symptoms include ruffled feathers and reduced egg production. However, more serious infections can be fatal and spread rapidly among an entire flock of birds. Usually, these viruses do not infect humans. However, since 1997, there have been cases of human infection, mostly following contact with infected birds or their secretions or excrement (e.g., poultry workers). The majority of these cases have occurred in Europe and Asia. Human-to-human transmission has been especially rare and normally occurred no further than between two people. Human symptoms have ranged from typical flulike symptoms, such as fever, cough, sore throat, and muscle aches, to eye infections and acute respiratory illness, with even life-threatening complications. Most cases have occurred in previously healthy children and young adults. This virus is resistant to amantadine and rimantadine, although it is believed (but remains to be confirmed) that zanamivir and oseltamivir would likely offer some therapeutic benefit for this condition. Although vaccine trials are in progress, there is currently no commercially available vaccine against this virus.

Many health experts fear a flu pandemic with this virus, should it mutate to a more easily transmissible form. This occurs frequently with influenza viruses in general, which is why a new seasonal flu vaccine must be developed each year. Although no one can predict if and when such a pandemic might occur with the H5N1 virus, the WHO and other health agencies, including the CDC, are continuously monitoring H5N1 activity patterns as well as its resistance to other antiviral drugs. In 2005, some countries placed a ban on live birds imported from Canada after an outbreak of H7N3 avian flu at a commercial poultry farm in British Columbia. This ban was later lifted. However, more recently, countries have implemented a ban on the import of birds from countries where avian influenza has been shown to be prevalent.

In April 2009, H1N1, a subtype of influenza virus A, emerged in Mexico. H1N1 is composed of genetic elements from four different influenza viruses and is now referred to as the pandemic H1N1 influenza virus. In June 2009, the World Health Organization declared an H1N1 level 6 pandemic, the first since the Hong Kong influenza pandemic in 1968. Initial surveillance indicates that H1N1 is affecting significantly higher numbers of young and healthy people up to age 25 than the number of older adults, as well as young children who are commonly affected by the seasonal influenza. Those at greater risk for severe illness are those with underlying medical conditions and pregnant women.

The H1N1 influenza virus is spread via coughing or sneezing. The virus can also survive on hard surfaces such as doorknobs. Consequently, H1N1 can be transferred to hands and transmitted to the respiratory system. It is thought that infectivity occurs for 1 day before the onset of symptoms and continues for 7 days. Cough and fever are the most common symptoms with other general flulike symptoms such as fatigue, muscle aches, sore throat, headache, and decreased appetite. Antivirals such as oseltamivir phosphate (Tamiflu) and zanamivir (Relenza) are recommended for the treatment of the influenza. The H1N1 vaccine was initiated across Canada the week of October 26, 2009.

NURSING PROCESS

Assessment

Prior to administering an antiviral drug, the nurse should perform a thorough medical and physical assessment and medication history in order to ensure safe medication use. Any known allergies to the medication should be noted. It is also important for the nurse to assess the patient's nutritional status and baseline vital signs because of the profound effects viral illnesses have, particularly if the patient is immunosuppressed. Contraindications, cautions, and drug interactions associated with an antiviral drug need to be considered (as discussed previously in the pharmacology section).

Assessment related to the use of antivirals includes inquiry about the patient's allergy to medications and a listing of any prescription and over-the-counter drugs and natural health products. Assessment of energy levels, weight loss, vital signs, and the characteristics of any visible lesions should be documented for baseline comparison once therapy is initiated. Age is also important to consider, because safety and efficacy have not been proved in children younger than 2 years of age. The older adult may require dosage adjustments because of altered kidney and liver functioning. Patients who are taking other medications that are nephrotoxic and those with underlying dehydration or mineral and electrolyte imbalances need to have these conditions managed before initiation of antiviral therapy. The nurse should assess information about the drug being used to ensure its safe use.

A blood test for HIV antibodies should also be done; with undiagnosed or untreated HIV infections, there is risk for possible HIV resistance. Results of related laboratory testing should always be assessed, including white blood cell (WBC) count, red blood cell (RBC) count, blood urea nitrogen (BUN), creatinine clearance, and liver function studies. Drugs being used for influenza A viral infections (e.g., amantadine hydrochloride) should be used with caution if there is a history of heart failure or orthostatic hypotension because of cardiovascular adverse effects. Assessment of the patient's cardiac system is important, with attention to heart sounds, heart rate, and blood pressure, as is documentation of any underlying edema, such as pedal edema. Specimens from blood, feces, throat, and urine may also be ordered prior to drug therapy. With the antiviral drug ribavirin, respiratory secretions should be obtained for diagnostic purposes and given only after baseline

kidney, liver, heart, and pulmonary functioning have been documented. Breath sounds, respiratory rate and patterns, cough, and sputum production should also be assessed and noted.

Antiretrovirals include a variety of drugs that fall within the six different classes of drugs previously discussed, each with their own cautions, contraindications, and drug interactions. Use of the PIs requires assessment of the patient's medical history, vital signs, baseline weight, allergies, medication history, and baseline laboratory tests such as complete blood counts and kidney and liver studies. These laboratory tests should also be conducted, as ordered, throughout the phases of treatment. Age is an important assessment factor because many of these drugs (e.g., abacavir) cannot be used safely in children between ages 3 months and 13 years. Dosages may need to be reduced in the older adult. With some of the antiretrovirals, specifically didanosine, the patient should be assessed for alcoholism and elevated serum triglycerides. T-cell counts must also be assessed; if the count is less than 100 cells/microlitre, didanosine should not be used.

Ritonavir requires specific attention to blood glucose levels, serum lipase, alanine aminotransferase (ALT), and aspartate aminotransferase (AST), serum triglyceride levels, and allergy to sulfonamide drugs because of cross-sensitivity. With nevirapine, information about the patient's use of oral contraceptives is important because of decreased effectiveness of birth control with this drug. Combination therapy with ritonavir and nucleosides (e.g., stavudine, zalcitabine) may lead to gastrointestinal disturbances, so assessing the patient for any pre-existing gastrointestinal illnesses is important. It has been recommended that ritonavir be initiated first, with the nucleosides added before completing 2 weeks of the ritonavir. Peripheral neuropathies may occur with stavudine, so a thorough neurological assessment is important prior to starting drug therapy. With the use of zidovudine, baseline complete blood cell counts with attention to RBCs, WBCs, and platelets are needed because of the risk for myelosuppression. These hematological tests should continue to be taken during therapy.

With any of the drugs presented in this chapter, especially those used for treatment and management of HIV, assessment of the patient's knowledge about his or her illness and the need for long-term and lifelong therapy is crucial. In addition, the patient's educational and reading levels, the best means of learning, and knowledge about community resources are important to determine in order to effectively implement patient education. Assessment of mental health status and emotional state is important because of the psychological impact of chronic illness. Value systems, social patterns, hobbies, values, support systems, knowledge of community resources, and spiritual beliefs should also be noted and documented. With chronic illnesses, the synthesis of this information will help ensure the development of a collaborative plan of care that is complete and holistic.

Nursing Diagnoses

- Acute pain related to the signs and symptoms associated with viral infections and HIV and related illnesses
- Risk for injury related to falls caused by the adverse effects of antiviral and antiretroviral drugs
- Risk for injury related to the immunosuppressive effects of viral disease processes and their treatment
- Deficient knowledge related to a lack of information about and experience with long-term drug therapy and lack of information about viral infections, their transmission, and treatment
- Activity intolerance related to weakness secondary to decreased energy from pathology of viral infections
- Risk for impaired tissue integrity from a break in skin due to viral lesions

Planning

Goals

- Patient will be free of symptoms of viral infection once therapy is completed.
- Patient will remain adherent to prescribed therapy.
- Patient will experience improved energy and appetite and improved ability to engage in activities of daily living for the duration of therapy.
- Patient will state the rationale for treatment of self and for any of their active sexual partners if diagnosed with genital herpes or other viral sexually transmitted infections.
- Patient will experience minimal adverse effects of antivirals and antiretrovirals.
- Patient will state diminished signs and symptoms of viral infection with drug therapy.
- Patient will state healing of lesions and restoration of intact skin integrity.

Outcome Criteria

- Patient experiences increased periods of comfort as a result of successful treatment of viral infection.
- Patient states the physical impact and effect of a viral infection on their overall state of health (e.g., compromised immune system) and the consequences and impact of appropriate therapy with either antivirals or antiretrovirals.
- Patient states the rationale for his or her own treatment as well as for treatment of any partners with whom the patient has been sexually involved in order to prevent worsening of symptoms and decrease severity of episodes related to genital herpes and other viral diseases.
- Patient identifies the possible adverse effects of antivirals, such as diarrhea, headache, nausea, and insomnia.
- Patient identifies the possible adverse effects of antiretrovirals such as gastrointestinal upset, peripheral neuropathies, immunosuppression, malaise, loss of energy, and loss of strength.
- Patient communicates the appropriate and recommended measures to prevent spread of viral infection as well as means of containment, prevention of spread, and promotion of healing of lesions during and after antiviral or antiretroviral therapy.

Implementation

Nursing interventions pertinent to patients receiving antivirals include use of the appropriate standard precautions with techniques of application or administration of ointment, aerosol powders, or intravenous or oral forms of medication (see Box 10-1 in Chapter 10). Wearing gloves and thorough hand washing, before and after administration of the drug, are necessary to prevent contamination of the site and spread of infection. Strict adherence to standard precautions is important to the safety of both the patient and the nurse. The antivirals (and antiretrovirals) may lead to superimposed infection or superinfections, which must be constantly monitored for, and measures must be implemented for their prevention (Chapters 38 and 39).

Oral antivirals should be given with meals to help prevent gastrointestinal upset. Capsules should be stored at room temperature, and they should not be crushed or broken. Topical dosage forms (e.g., acyclovir) should be applied using a finger cot or rubber glove to prevent autoinoculation, and contact with eyes should be avoided. IV acyclovir is stable for 12 hours at room temperature and will often precipitate when refrigerated. IV infusions should be diluted as recommended (e.g., with D5W or 0.9% NaCl) and infused with caution. Infusions over 1 hour are suggested to avoid the kidney tubule damage seen with more rapid infusions. Adequate hydration should be encouraged during and for several hours after the infusion to prevent drug-related crystalluria. The IV site should be continually assessed; any redness, heat, pain, swelling, or red streaks indicate possible phlebitis.

For patients with viral lesions, the characteristics of the lesions should be documented. Appropriate isolation of individuals with chicken pox or herpes zoster should be implemented, and analgesics should be given for comfort. With the use of all antivirals, laboratory testing for kidney and liver functioning should be ongoing, and monitoring of the patient's complete blood count, including platelets, neutrophils, and thrombocytes, should be performed periodically during therapy. Vital signs with attention to blood pressure should be monitored throughout therapy with these medications, especially acyclovir and amantadine, because of drug-related orthostatic hypotension.

Amantadine and other antivirals should be taken for the entire course of therapy. If a dose is missed, it is important for the patient to take the dose as soon as it is remembered or to contact the health care provider for further instructions. Should dry mouth occur, sugarless candy and gum might be helpful. Daily mouth care, including the use of dental floss, and regular dental preventive visits are encouraged. Saliva substitutes may be needed; should dry mouth continue for more than 2 weeks, the health care provider should be contacted for further management. Livedo reticularis, a red–blue network mottling of skin caused by congestion of the superficial capillaries, may occur; thus patient education about this is important. Discontinuation of amantadine hydrochloride will reverse this effect. It is often recommended that the second dose of drug be given several hours before bedtime to prevent insomnia.

Famciclovir should be taken for the full course of therapy. For patients who have genital herpes, the directions are usually to provide evenly spaced doses round the clock. IV Ganciclovir should be diluted with D5W or 0.9% NaCl and at a concentration and time frame noted by the physician and authoritative sources. Large veins are recommended to provide the dilution needed to minimize the risk for vein irritation. If handling the solution of ganciclovir, avoid exposure of eyes, mucous membranes, or skin to the drug, and use latex gloves and safety glasses for handling and preparation. Should the drug come in contact with these areas, wash and rinse the affected areas thoroughly with soap and water, and rinse and flush the eyes with plain water. Ribavirin may be given by nasal or oral inhalation.

Aerosol generators are available from the drug manufacturer. Reservoir solutions should be discarded if levels are low or empty and changed every 24 hours. Patients taking ribavirin and similar drugs for RSV treatment via a Small Particle Aerosol Generator (SPAG-2) device should be taught how to properly mix and administer the drug. It should be reconstituted (e.g., ribavirin powder) as instructed by manufacturer guidelines. Old solutions that are residual in the equipment should be discarded before adding fresh medication. Drugs administered via SPAG equipment are usually administered 12 to 18 hours daily for up to 7 days, beginning within 3 days of the onset of symptoms. There is also much controversy about use of this drug in patients on ventilators; only those who are specially trained on the use of this drug should administer it. Any "rainout" in the tubing of ventilators should be emptied frequently, and the nurse should always monitor breath sounds in patients receiving inhaled forms of this drug, whether they are ventilator-dependent or not. Zanamivir is inhaled using a Diskhaler device. It is important that the patient exhale completely first. Then, while holding the mouthpiece 1 inch away from the patient's lips, instruct the patient to inhale deeply and hold the breath as long as possible prior to exhaling the drug and breath. Rinsing of the mouth with water is needed to prevent irritation and dryness.

Antiretrovirals include numerous drugs, thus a review of general types of nursing actions related to these drugs' use is presented here, as well as specific drug-related information as appropriate. In regard to dosage forms, there are special administration and handling guidelines for some of the antiretroviral drugs. Delavirdine mesylate should first be dispersed in 180 mL of water prior to administration. Didanosine in tablet forms should be dispersed in water, where it remains stable for 1 hour at room temperature. The oral solution remains stable for approximately 4 hours. Give the oral dosage form 1 hour before or 2 hours after meals to help with absorption of this drug. If chewable dosage forms are given, make sure that the drug is thoroughly crushed and dispersed in at least 30 mL of water before having the patient swallow the mixture. The mixture must be mixed well and then taken immediately. DO NOT mix didanosine with any form of acidic liquid, such as fruit juice, because it will become unstable in the acidic pH. Enteric-coated forms should be taken on an empty stomach, if tolerated. Always check manufacturer guidelines for any specific information regarding dosage administration.

With didanosine, lamivudine, and zidovudine, it is important to continually be aware of liver-related adverse effects, such as abdominal pain, elevated serum amylase or triglycerides, nausea, and vomiting, and to report these immediately to the health care provider, as they may indicate pancreatitis. Monitoring for peripheral neuropathies during therapy is important, with attention to any restless leg syndrome or burning of the feet or lack of muscle coordination. If the patient should experience signs and symptoms of opportunistic infections (e.g., respiratory signs and symptoms, fever, changes in oral mucosa), the physician should be contacted immediately. Weigh patients or encourage them to weigh themselves at least 2 times a week and report a gain of 1 kg or more in 24 hours or 2 kg or more in 1 week. Visual or hearing changes with didanosine should be reported as well. Headaches may occur with some of these drugs; thus be sure to provide analgesia as ordered.

With some of the antiretrovirals, avoidance of high-fat meals and an altered dosage amount for the older adult are recommended, but only as ordered. Film-coated oral dosage forms should not be altered in any way. The taste of ritonavir may be improved by mixing it with chocolate milk or a nutritional beverage within 1 hour of its dosing. Ritonavir's dosage form should be protected from light. The absorption of oral dosages of zidovudine is not disturbed by simultaneous ingestion of food or milk, but it is important to keep the patient upright when giving the medication and for up to 30 minutes afterward to prevent esophageal ulceration. IV dosages should only be given if clear and not containing any particulate matter, using the appropriate dosage, diluents, and infusion time. Because these drugs often come in oral dosage forms, it is usually recommended that they be given with food. Zidovudine and other antiretrovirals are generally given in evenly spaced intervals round the clock, as ordered, to ensure steady-state levels. With all oral and parenteral dosage forms of antiretrovirals, be sure to observe for nausea and vomiting as well as any changes in weight, occurrence of anorexia, and changes in bowel activities and patterns.

Other nursing interventions associated with these drugs include the following:

- Continual monitoring of adverse effects throughout therapies with a focus on the gastrointestinal, neurological, renal, and hepatic systems.
- With oral forms of indinavir and nevirapine, patients should drink at least 1400 mL of fluids every day to maintain adequate hydration and to prevent nephrolithiasis.
- Nevirapine, zidovudine, and similar drugs may be associated with a rash; however, if the rash appears on the extremities, face, or trunk of the body and is accompanied by blistering, fever, malaise, myalgias, oral lesions, swelling or edema, and conjunctivitis, the physician should be contacted immediately.
- If drug therapy results in worsening of peripheral neuropathies, the specific drug may be discontinued by the physician.

- Blood cell counts with attention to complete blood count, hemoglobin, and HIV RNA levels may be required throughout and after the drug regimen.

See Patient Education for more information on both antivirals and antiretrovirals.

Evaluation

The therapeutic effects of antivirals and antiretrovirals include elimination of the virus or a decrease in the symptoms of the viral infections. There may be a delayed progression of HIV infection and AIDS, as well as a decrease in flulike symptoms and in the frequency of herpetic flare-ups and other lesion breakouts. Herpetic lesions should crust over, and the frequency of recurrence should decrease. In addition, there should be constant evaluation for the occurrence of adverse effects and toxicity to specific antiviral and antiretroviral drugs. These adverse reactions are listed in Table 40-4. The nurse must always re-evaluate the collaborative plan of care to ensure that the goals and outcome criteria have been met. It is also the nurse's responsibility to be constantly attentive to reports from the CDC, Health Canada, other provincial health care agencies, and public health care agencies on new strains of viruses and flu syndromes.

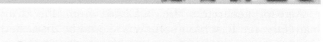

CASE STUDY

Antiviral Therapy

One of your patients, Z.K., a 33-year-old biology professor, has just started therapy with lamivudine/zidovudine (Combivir) for an opportunistic infection. She has many questions about this medication therapy, and you are meeting with her to review her questions.

1. She asks you why there are two drugs in this particular therapy. What is your explanation?

2. Develop a patient teaching guide for Z.K., emphasizing any specific cautions and symptoms to report to the health care provider.

3. At what level of platelets and white blood cells would there probably be a change or discontinuation of this drug?

For answers see http://evolve.elsevier.com/Canada/Lilley/pharmacology/.

IN MY FAMILY

Lemon and Dandelion Jam

(as told by K.S., of Ukrainian descent)

"There are many doctors in Ukraine that have medical degrees but practise only natural medicine (acupuncture, herbal/natural remedies, etc.). . . . Many people also go to people that have no medical degrees but who practise the remedies that were [taught] to them by their parents and grandparents. The beliefs that my culture has about illness are that each problem has to be given a holistic approach. . . . Lemon and dandelion jam [is] made in the spring and eaten throughout the fall and winter (a teaspoon per day) to prevent getting the flu, and cold. It can also be used to cure the flu, but it is slower than Western medicine. When my mother was pregnant, she got a very bad flu. . . . There was no medication she could take that wouldn't hurt the baby, so my grandmother treated my mother with dandelion jam, and my mom recovered."

PATIENT EDUCATION

- Patients should be educated about taking their medication exactly as prescribed and for the full course of therapy. Alert patients to risk of dizziness and to use caution while driving or participating in activities requiring alertness.
- Patients should consult the physician before taking any other prescribed or over-the-counter drugs.
- Patients who are immunocompromised should be advised to avoid crowds and persons with infections.
- Patients with sexually transmitted viral infections, for example, those who are HIV positive, should be advised about standard precautions and safer sex practices. Condom use is a necessity in the prevention of these viral infections, and presence of genital herpes requires sexual abstinence.
- Female patients with genital herpes should be advised to have a Pap test done every 6 months or as ordered by their health care provider to monitor the virus and especially its improvement with treatment. Cervical cancer has been found to be more prevalent in women with genital herpes simplex.
- Patients should be informed that with long-term use of some of these antivirals, oral hygiene is needed several times a day because of drug-related gingival hyperplasia, with red and swollen oral mucosa and gums. Encourage patients to report the following adverse reactions to their health care provider, should they occur: decrease in urinary output, changes in sensorium and central nervous system function, dizziness, confusion, syncope, nausea, vomiting, and diarrhea.
- Patients should be educated with demonstrations and pictures or other teaching aids about special application procedures (e.g., eye drops, use of finger cots or gloved hand with application to lesions).
- Patients should be warned that touching the lesions promotes their spread, so use of a gloved hand or finger cots for application and cleansing is important.
- Patients should be instructed to drink fluids (e.g., 3000 mL/24 hr) unless contraindicated.

- Patients should be encouraged to take the medication round the clock and in evenly spaced doses as ordered.
- Patients should be educated that antiviral drugs provide suppression of the virus and are not a cure.
- With respiratory inhalation forms (e.g., zanamivir), patients should be given clear and simple educational instructions, with demonstrations on proper use of the delivery device for the dosage form.
- Patients should be informed that they need to start therapy with drugs such as valacylcovir (or other antivirals) at the first sign of a recurrent episode of genital herpes or herpes zoster. Additionally, explain that early treatment within 24 to 48 hours is needed for the full therapeutic results.
- Patients should be informed about specific drug interactions (e.g., with prescription or over-the-counter drugs and natural health products).
- Patients should be encouraged to immediately report to their physicians any difficulty breathing, drastic changes in blood pressure, bleeding, new symptoms, worsening of infection, fever, chills, or other unusual problems. Educate about the importance of follow-up appointments.
- Patients should be educated about drug-specific instructions (e.g., with didanosine, avoid alcohol because of the disulfiram-type reaction; take indinavir with water only and without food for the most optimal effects, although a light meal, skim milk, tea, or juice are acceptable and help decrease gastrointestinal adverse effects; stavudine is associated with adverse effects such as abdominal discomfort, fatigue, dyspnea, numbness, nausea, tingling, vomiting, and weakness; with zidovudine, the patient should report any bleeding from their gums, nose, or rectum and should notify the physician if there is difficulty breathing, headache, insomnia, muscle weakness, or worsening of infection).

POINTS TO REMEMBER

- Viruses are difficult to kill and to treat because they live inside human cells, and most antiviral drugs act by inhibiting replication of the viral cell. Antiviral drugs include synthetic purine and pyrimidine nucleoside analogues.
- Most antiviral drugs "trick" the virus into mistaking the drugs for either a purine (a human amino acid [adenosine or guanosine]) or a pyrimidine (another amino acid [cytosine or thymine]) so that the virus cannot replicate.
- Purine analogue antivirals include drugs such as acyclovir, didanosine, and ganciclovir. Pyrimidine analogue antiretroviral drugs include zidovudine. Protease inhibitors are also considered to be antiretrovirals.

- Antiretroviral drugs should be administered only after physician orders are read and understood and after a thorough nursing assessment that includes an examination of the patient's nutritional status, weight, baseline vital signs, and kidney and liver functioning, as well as assessment of heart sounds, neurological status, and gastrointestinal or abdominal tract functioning.
- Comfort measures and supportive nursing care should accompany drug therapy. Patients should be encouraged to drink plenty of fluids and to space medications round the clock, as ordered, for maintaining steady blood levels of the drug.

EXAMINATION REVIEW QUESTIONS

1 During treatment with zidovudine, which potential adverse effect does the nurse need to monitor for?
a. Retinitis
b. Deep vein thromboses
c. Kaposi's sarcomas
d. Bone marrow suppression

2 After giving an injection to a patient with HIV infection, the nurse accidentally receives a needle-stick from a too-full needle-disposal box. Which of the following recommendations for occupational HIV exposure can she use?
a. Acyclovir
b. Didanosine
c. Lamivudine and enfuvirtide
d. Zidovudine, lamivudine, and indinavir

3 When teaching a patient who is taking acyclovir for genital herpes, which statement by the nurse is accurate?
a. "Acyclovir will eradicate the herpes virus."
b. "This drug will help the lesions to dry and crust over."
c. "This drug will prevent the spread of this virus to others."
d. "Acyclovir does not reduce the frequency of genital herpes outbreaks."

4 A patient who has been newly diagnosed with HIV has many questions about the effectiveness of drug therapy. After a teaching session, which statement by the patient reflects a need for more education?
a. "There is no cure for HIV."
b. "These drugs will eventually eliminate the virus from my body."
c. "I will be monitored while on this medicine for adverse effects and improvements."
d. "These drugs do not eliminate HIV, but hopefully the amount of virus in my body will be reduced."

5 During hospitalization for dehydration, an older adult patient is also receiving several doses of amantadine. Which statement explains the rationale for this medication therapy?
a. The drug is given intravenously to treat shingles.
b. Amantadine is used to prevent potential exposure to the HIV virus.
c. This medication is given prophylactically to prevent influenza A infection.
d. Amantadine works synergistically with antibiotics to reduce superinfections.

For answers see http://evolve.elsevier.com/Canada/Lilley/pharmacology/.

CRITICAL THINKING ACTIVITIES

1 A 19-year-old male transfer university student from Germany to Canada was diagnosed with HIV approximately 7 months ago. He has been going through several treatment regimens but the infectious disease physician is about to change his drugs. He has been on several anti-HIV drugs and is now being treated with didanosine. He has experienced some bone marrow depression periodically over the last few months. Which condition(s) and health concern(s) would most likely lead to a change to didanosine? Discuss your answer.

2 One of your young adult female patients underwent a bone marrow transplantation and less than 1 year later contracted cytomegalovirus. If this client were pregnant, would antiviral drugs be problematic for her? Explain why or why not.

3 Discuss the use of rimantadine and amantadine in the older adult. Is there a benefit of one drug over the other? Explain.

For answers see http://evolve.elsevier.com/Canada/Lilley/pharmacology/.

CHAPTER 41

Antituberculosis Drugs

Learning Objectives

After reading this chapter, the successful student will be able to do the following:

1 Briefly explain the pathophysiology of tuberculosis.

2 Identify the first-line and second-line drugs used for the treatment of tuberculosis.

3 Discuss the mechanisms of action, dosages, adverse effects, routes of administration, special dosing considerations, indications for treatment, cautions, contraindications, and drug interactions associated with the antituberculosis drugs.

4 Develop a collaborative plan of care that includes all phases of the nursing process for patients receiving antituberculosis drugs.

5 Develop a comprehensive teaching guide for patients and families affected by the diagnosis of tuberculosis and treatment with antituberculosis drugs.

e-Learning Activities

Web site
(http://evolve.elsevier.com/Canada/Lilley/pharmacology/)

- Animations
- Answers to chapter questions, activities, and case studies
- Calculators and Category Catchers
- Glossary with audio pronunciations
- IV Therapy and Medication Error Checklists
- Multiple-Choice Review Question quizzes
- Nursing Care Plans
- Online Appendices and Supplements
- WebLinks

Drug Profiles

ethambutol (ethambutol hydrochloride)*, p. 786
▸▸ **isoniazid**, p. 787
pyrazinamide, p. 787
rifabutin, p. 787
rifampin, p. 787
streptomycin (streptomycin sulfate)*, p. 787

▸▸ Key drug.

*Full generic name is given in parentheses. For the purposes of this text, the more common shortened name is used.

Glossary

Aerobic Requiring oxygen for the maintenance of life. (p. 782)

Antituberculosis drugs Drugs used to treat infections caused by *Mycobacterium* bacterial species. (p. 783)

Bacillus Rod-shaped bacteria. (p. 782)

Granuloma Any small nodular aggregation of inflammatory cells (e.g., macrophages, lymphocytes); usually characterized by clearly delimited boundaries, as found in *tuberculosis*. (p. 782)

Isoniazid The primary and most commonly prescribed tuberculostatic drug. (p. 783)

Multidrug-resistant tuberculosis (MDR-TB) Tuberculosis (TB) that demonstrates resistance to two or more drugs. (p. 782)

Slow acetylator Someone with a genetic defect that causes a deficiency in the enzyme needed to metabolize isoniazid, the most widely used TB drug, thus reducing the rate of metabolism of the drug. (p. 787)

Tubercle The characteristic lesion of tuberculosis; a small, round, grey, translucent *granulomatous* lesion, usually with a *caseated* (cheesy) consistency in its interior. (See *granuloma*.) (p. 782)

Tubercle bacilli Rod-shaped TB bacteria. (p. 782)

Tuberculosis (TB) Any infectious disease caused by species of *Mycobacterium*; usually *M. tuberculosis* (adjectives: *tuberculous*, *tubercular*). (p. 782)

TUBERCULOSIS

Tuberculosis (TB) is the medical diagnosis of any infectious disease caused by a bacterial species known as *Mycobacterium*. TB is most commonly characterized by **granulomas** in the lungs, nodular accumulations of inflammatory cells (e.g., macrophages, lymphocytes) that are *delimited* ("walled off" with clear boundaries). The characteristic lesion of tuberculosis, a *tubercle*, is a small, round, grey, translucent *granulanatous* lesion, usually with a centre of a cheesy, or *caseated*, consistency. (Casein is the name of a protein that is prevalent in cheese and milk.) Although there are technically two mycobacterial species that can cause TB, *M. tuberculosis* and *M. bovis*, infections caused by *M. tuberculosis* (abbreviated MTB) are far more common. There are also several other mycobacterial species (e.g., *M. leprae*, which causes leprosy) that have varying susceptibility to different drugs used for TB. Infections with these bacteria are much less of a public health problem and hence not the focus of this chapter. MTB is an *aerobic bacillus*, which means that it is a long and slender rod-shaped microorganism (**bacillus**) that requires a large supply of oxygen for it to grow and flourish (**aerobic**). This bacterium's need for a highly oxygenated body site explains why *Mycobacterium* infections most commonly affect the lungs. However, other common sites of infection include the growing ends of bones and the brain (cerebral cortex). Less common sites of infection include the kidney, liver, and genitourinary tract, as well as virtually every other tissue and organ in the body.

These **tubercle bacilli** (a common synonym for MTB) are transmitted from one of three sources: humans, cows (bovine; hence the species name *M. bovis*), or birds (avian), although bovine and avian transmissions are much less common than is human transmission. Tubercle bacilli are conveyed in droplets expelled by infected people or animals during coughing or sneezing and then inhaled by the new host. After these infectious droplets are inhaled, the infection spreads to the susceptible organ sites by means of the blood and lymphatic system. MTB is a slow-growing organism, which makes it more difficult to treat than most other bacterial infections. The MTB bacterium is also surrounded by a unique cell wall made up of mycolic acid, a unique lipid substance found only in mycobacteria. Thus MTB cells are hydrophobic, requiring a specific staining technique to distinguish the bacterium.

Generally, most bactericidal (bacterium cell-killing) drugs act by disrupting critical cellular metabolic processes in the organism. Therefore, the most drug-susceptible organisms are those with faster metabolic activity. Slow-growing microorganisms such as MTB, by contrast, are less metabolically active and thus more difficult to kill and less susceptible to drug treatment. Many of the antibiotics used to treat TB work by inhibiting growth rather than directly killing the organism.

At the most clinically serious end of the TB patient spectrum are infected persons whose host defences have been broken down as the result of immunosuppressive drug therapy, chemotherapy for cancer, or an immunosuppressive disease such as AIDS. In these persons, TB can inflict devastating and irreversible damage. The first infectious episode is considered the *primary* TB infection; *reinfection* represents the more chronic form of the disease. However, TB does not develop in all people who are exposed to it. In some cases, the bacteria become dormant and walled off by calcified or fibrous tissues. These patients may test positive for exposure, but not necessarily be infectious because of this dormancy process.

Canada has one of the lowest reported incidence rates of TB in the world. From 1997 through 2004, there was an average yearly decline in MTB cases of 3%. This is attributed to intensified public health efforts aimed at preventing, diagnosing, and treating TB as well as HIV infection, including more effective antiretroviral drug therapy (Chapter 40). In Canada, drug therapy continues to regularly reduce the number of TB cases every year. Of increasing concern is the number of cases of **multidrug-resistant tuberculosis (MDR-TB)**. In 2004, approximately 12.4% of MTB isolates were resistant to one or more of the antituberculosis drugs: isoniazid, rifampin, ethambutol, pyrazinamide, or streptomycin. These numbers are expected to decline with stronger TB-related public health efforts. Nonetheless, the prevalence and growth of TB continues to be greater in the larger global community and is considered a pandemic, as TB infects one third of the world's population. It is currently second only to HIV in the number of deaths caused by a single infectious organism.

While several factors have contributed to this health care crisis, one important source of the problem is the increasing number of people in vulnerable groups that are particularly susceptible to the infection. These include the homeless, the undernourished or malnourished, individuals infected with HIV, those who misuse drugs, those with cancer, those taking immunosuppressant drugs, and those who live in crowded and poorly sanitized housing facilities. Because *M. tuberculosis* is carried in airborne particles, or droplet nuclei, it can be easily transmitted during sneezing, coughing, or spitting and even while talking. The particles are tiny (1–5 microns in size); consequently, they can remain airborne and can be easily spread throughout a room or building.

All of these factors also favour the acquisition of a drug-resistant infection. Members of racial and ethnic minority groups are at greater risk than White populations, accounting for two-thirds of new cases. Foreign birth is noted to be a significant risk factor associated with drug resistance in Canada. MDR-TB occurs when a *Mycobacterium tuberculosis* strain is resistant to isoniazid and rifampin, two of the most powerful first-line drugs. To cure MDR-TB, health care providers must turn to a combination of second-line drugs. Unfortunately, many of the second-line drugs have more adverse effects, the treatment may last much longer, and the cost may be substantially more than that of first-line therapy. In addition, MDR-TB strains can grow resistant to second-line drugs, further complicating treatment. Directly observed therapy (DOT) is an internationally recognized health strategy identified as the most effective approach to controlling TB and preventing the development of MDR-TB. The strategy includes observing the ingestion of medication by a patient who has active TB.

ANTITUBERCULOSIS DRUGS

The drugs used to treat infections caused by all forms of *Mycobacterium* are called **antituberculosis drugs**. These drugs fall into two categories: *primary* or *first-line* (Figure 41-1) and *secondary* or *second-line* drugs. As these designations imply, primary drugs are those tried first, whereas secondary drugs are reserved for more complicated cases, such as those resistant to primary drugs. The antimycobacterial activity, efficacy, and potential adverse and toxic effects of the drugs determine the class to which they belong. **Isoniazid** (INH) is a primary antituberculosis drug and is most widely used. It can be used either as the sole drug in the prophylaxis of TB or in combination with other antituberculosis drugs. Rifabutin is used in special situations, such as in cases of HIV/AIDS and drug resistance.

The first- and second-line antibiotic drugs are listed in Box 41-1. There are also two miscellaneous TB-related injections—one diagnostic, the other a vaccine. These are described in Box 41-2.

An important consideration during drug selection is the relative likelihood of drug-resistant organisms and drug toxicity. Following are other key elements important to the planning and implementation of effective therapy:

- Drug-susceptibility tests should be performed on the first *Mycobacterium* sp. that is isolated from a patient specimen (to prevent the development of MDR-TB).

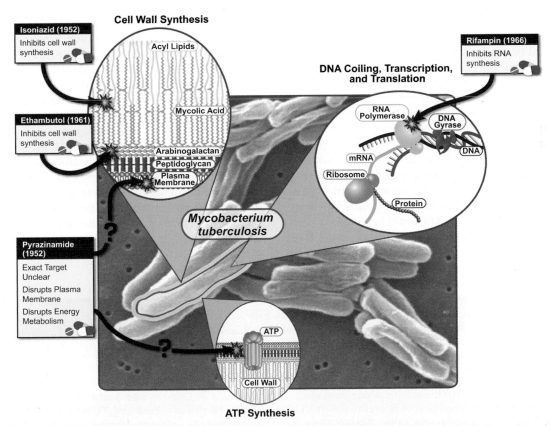

FIG. 41-1 Four drugs in the standard regimen of primary or first-line antituberculosis drugs and their modes of action. Also shown are the dates these four drugs were discovered—all more than 40 years ago. (Source: National Institute of Allergy and Infectious Diseases. (2007). *First-line treatment of tuberculosis (TB) for drug-sensitive TB*. Retrieved August 4, 2009, from http://www3.niaid.nih.gov/topics/tuberculosis/Understanding/WhatIsTB/ScientificIllustrations/firstLineIllustration.htm. Courtesy of the National Institute of Allergy and Infectious Diseases (NIAID); illustrator: Krista Townsend. The photo of *Mycobacterium tuberculosis* was obtained from the Centers for Disease Control and Prevention, CDC/Dr. Ray Butler; Janice Carr).

- Before the results of the susceptibility tests are known, the patient should be started on a four-drug regimen consisting of isoniazid, rifampin, pyrazinamide (PZA), and ethambutol, which together are 95% effective in combating the infection. The use of multiple medications reduces the possibility of the organism becoming drug resistant.
- Once drug susceptibility results are available, the regimen should be adjusted accordingly.
- Patient adherence to, and the adverse effects of, the prescribed drug therapy should be monitored closely because the incidence of both patient nonadherence and adverse effects is high.

Mechanism of Action and Drug Effects

The mechanisms of action of the antituberculosis drugs vary depending on the drug. These drugs act on *M. tuberculosis* in one of the following ways: they inhibit either protein synthesis or cell wall synthesis, or they work by other mechanisms (see Figure 41-1). The antituberculosis drugs are listed in Table 41-1 by their mechanism of action. The major effects of drug therapy include reduction of cough and, therefore, infectiousness of the patient. This outcome normally occurs within 2 weeks of starting drug therapy, assuming that the patient's TB strain is drug sensitive.

Indications

Antituberculosis medications are indicated for TB infections, including both pulmonary and extrapulmonary TB. While most antituberculosis drug effects have not been fully tested in pregnant women, the combination of isoniazid and ethambutol has been used to treat pregnant women with clinically apparent TB without teratogenic complications. Rifampin is another drug that is often safe during pregnancy and is a more likely choice for more advanced disease.

Besides being used for the initial treatment of TB, antituberculosis drugs have proved effective in the management of treatment failures and relapses. Infection with species of *Mycobacterium* other than *M. tuberculosis* (MOTT) and atypical mycobacterial infections have also been successfully treated with these drugs. Nontuberculous mycobacteria (NTM) may also be susceptible to antituberculosis drugs. However, in general, antituberculosis drugs are not as effective against other species of *Mycobacterium* as they are against *M. tuberculosis*. Some of these other species that may be of particular concern in immunocompromised patients such as AIDS patients are *Mycobacterium avium-intracellulare*, *M. flavescens*, *M. marinum*, and *M. kansasii*. Additional *Mycobacterium* infections that may respond to antituberculosis drugs are those caused by *Mycobacterium fortuitum*, *M. chelonae*, *M. smegmatis*, *M. xenopi*, and *M. scrofulaceum*. Treatment regimens for these non-TB mycobacterial infections often include the macrolide antibiotics clarithromycin or azithromycin (Chapter 38), either alone or in combination with one or more antituberculosis drugs.

In summary, antituberculosis drugs are used primarily for the prophylaxis or treatment of TB. The effectiveness of these drugs depends on the type of infection, adequate dosing, sufficient duration of treatment, drug adherence, and the selection of an effective drug combination. The indications of the different antituberculosis drugs are listed in Table 41-2.

TABLE 41-1

Antituberculosis Drugs: Mechanisms of Action

Drugs	Description
INHIBIT PROTEIN SYNTHESIS rifabutin, rifampin, streptomycin	Streptomycin acts by interfering with normal protein synthesis and production of faulty proteins. Rifampin acts at a different point in the protein synthesis pathway. Rifampin inhibits RNA synthesis and may also inhibit DNA synthesis. Human cells are not as sensitive as mycobacterial cells and are not affected by rifampin except at high drug concentrations.
INHIBIT CELL WALL SYNTHESIS isoniazid	Isoniazid acts at least partly to inhibit the synthesis of wall components, but the mechanism of this drug is still not clearly understood.
OTHER MECHANISMS ethambutol, isoniazid, pyrazinamide	Other proposed mechanisms of action for isoniazid exist. Isoniazid is taken up by mycobacteria cells and undergoes hydrolysis to isonicotinic acid, which reacts with cofactor NAD to form a defective NAD that is no longer active as a coenzyme for certain life-sustaining reactions in the *Mycobacterium tuberculosis* organism. Ethambutol affects lipid synthesis, resulting in the inhibition of mycolic acid incorporation into the cell wall, thus inhibiting protein synthesis. The mechanism of action of pyrazinamide (PZA) in the inhibition of TB is unknown. It can be either bacteriostatic or bactericidal, depending on the susceptibility of the particular *Mycobacterium* organism and the concentration of the drug attained at the site of infection.

NAD, nicotinamide adenine; *TB*, tuberculosis.

Contraindications

Contraindications to the use of antituberculosis drugs include severe drug allergy and major kidney or liver dysfunction. However, it must be recognized that the urgency of treating a potentially fatal infection may have to be balanced against any prevailing contraindications. In extreme cases, patients are sometimes given a drug to which they have some degree of allergy along with supportive care that enables them to at least tolerate the medication. Examples of such supportive care might include antipyretic (e.g., acetaminophen), antihistamine (e.g., diphenhydramine), or even corticosteroid (e.g., prednisone or methylprednisolone) therapy.

One relative contraindication to ethambutol is optic neuritis. Chronic alcohol use, especially when associated with major liver damage, may also be a contraindication to any antituberculosis drug therapy, keeping in mind the caveats mentioned earlier. Other contraindications for specific drugs, if any, may be found in the Drug Profiles listed later in the chapter.

Adverse Effects

Antituberculosis drugs are fairly well tolerated. Isoniazid, one of the mainstays of treatment, is noted for causing pyridoxine deficiency and liver toxicity. For this reason, supplements of pyridoxine (vitamin B_6; Chapters 8 and 55)

TABLE 41-2

Antituberculosis Drugs: Indications

Drug	Indications
ethambutol	First-line drug for treatment of TB
isoniazid	Used alone or in combination with other antituberculosis drugs in the treatment and prevention of clinical TB
pyrazinamide	Used with other antituberculosis drugs in the treatment of clinical TB
rifabutin	Used to prevent or delay development of *M. avium-intracellulare* bacteremia and disseminated infections in patients with advanced HIV infection
rifampin	Used with other antituberculosis drugs in the treatment of clinical TB
	Used in the treatment of diseases caused by mycobacteria other than *M. tuberculosis*
	Used for preventive therapy in patients exposed to isoniazid-resistant *M. tuberculosis*
	Used to eliminate meningococci from the nasopharynx of asymptomatic *Neisseria meningitidis* carriers when the risk of meningococcal meningitis is high
	Used for chemoprophylaxis in contacts of patients with *Haemophilus influenzae* type B (Hib) infection
	Used in the treatment of endocarditis caused by methicillin-resistant staphylococci, chronic staphylococcal prostatitis, and multiple-anti-infective–resistant pneumococci
streptomycin	Used in combination with other antituberculous drugs in the treatment of clinical TB and other mycobacterial diseases

are often given concurrently with isoniazid with a common oral dose of 50 mg daily. The most problematic drugs and their associated adverse effects are listed in Table 41-3.

Interactions

The drugs that can interact with antituberculosis drugs can cause significant effects. See Table 41-4 for a listing of selected interactions. Besides these drug interactions, isoniazid can cause false-positive urine glucose test (e.g., Clinitest) readings and an increase in the serum levels of the liver function enzymes alanine aminotransferase (ALT) and aspartate aminotransferase (AST).

Dosages

For the recommended dosages of selected antituberculosis drugs, see the Dosages table on p. 788.

TABLE 41-3

Antituberculosis Drugs: Common Adverse Effects

Drug	Adverse Effects
ethambutol	Retrobulbar neuritis, blindness
isoniazid	Peripheral neuritis, hepatotoxicity, optic neuritis and visual disturbances, hyperglycemia, red–orange–brown discoloration of bodily secretions (e.g., urine, sweat, tears, sputum)
levofloxacin, moxiflozacin hydrochloride	Dizziness, headache, gastrointestinal disturbances, visual disturbances, insomnia
pyrazinamide	Hepatotoxicity, hyperuricemia
rifabutin	Gastrointestinal tract disturbances, rash, neutropenia, red–orange–brown discoloration of urine, sputum, sweat, tears
rifampin	Hepatitis; hematological disorders; red–orange–brown discoloration of urine, tears, sweat, sputum
streptomycin	Ototoxicity, nephrotoxicity, blood dyscrasias

TABLE 41-4

Antituberculosis Drugs: Drug Interactions

Drug	Mechanism	Results
ISONIAZID		
antacids	Reduces absorption	Decreased isoniazid levels
rifampin	Additive effects	Increased CNS and liver toxicity
RIFAMPIN		
β-Blockers		
Benzodiazepines		
Cyclosporine, oral anticoagulants, oral antihyperglycemics, oral contraceptives, phenytoin, quinidine, theophylline	Increase metabolism	Decreased therapeutic effects of these drugs
STREPTOMYCIN		
Nephrotoxic and neurotoxic drugs	Additive	Increased toxicity
Oral anticoagulants	Alter intestinal flora	Increased bleeding tendencies

CNS, central nervous system.

 DRUG PROFILES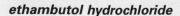

ethambutol hydrochloride

Ethambutol hydrochloride (Etibi) is a first-line bacteriostatic drug used in the treatment of TB that is believed to work by diffusing into the mycobacteria and suppressing ribonucleic acid (RNA) synthesis, thereby inhibiting protein synthesis. Ethambutol is included with isoniazid, pyrazinamide, and rifampin in many TB combination-drug therapies because resistance develops quickly if used as a single drug. It may also be used to treat other mycobacterial diseases.

It is contraindicated in patients with a hypersensitivity to it and those with optic neuritis as it can both exacerbate and cause this condition, resulting in varying degrees of vision loss. It is also contraindicated in children younger than 13 years of age. It is available only in oral form.

PHARMACOKINETICS

Half-Life	Onset	Peak	Duration
3–4 hr	Variable	2–4 hr	Up to 24 hr

Continued

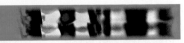

 DRUG PROFILES (cont'd)

▶▶ *isoniazid*

Isoniazid (Isotamine) is not only the mainstay in the treatment of TB but also the most widely used antituberculosis drug. It may be given as a single drug for prophylaxis or in combination with other antituberculosis drugs for the treatment of active TB. It is a bactericidal drug that kills the mycobacteria by disrupting cell-wall synthesis and essential cellular functions. Isoniazid is metabolized in the liver through a process called acetylation, which requires a certain enzymatic pathway to break down the drug. However, some people have a genetic deficiency of the liver enzymes needed for this to occur; Such individuals are referred to as **slow acetylators.** More than 50% of individuals in Caucasian populations are homozygous for this recessive trait and are of the "slow acetylator" phenotype. When isoniazid is taken by slow acetylators, isoniazid accumulates because there are not enough enzymes to break down isoniazid. Therefore, the dosages of isoniazid may need to be adjusted downward in these patients.

Isoniazid is currently available in oral formulations, although the drug may be given by intramuscular injection when oral therapy is not possible. There is also a combination oral formulation of isoniazid, pyrazinamide, and rifampin (Rifater). Isoniazid is contraindicated in patients with a hypersensitivity to it and in those with previous isoniazid-associated liver injury or acute liver disease.

PHARMACOKINETICS

Half-Life	Onset	Peak	Duration
PO: 1–4 hr	PO: Variable	PO: 1–2 hr	PO: Up to 24 hr

pyrazinamide

Pyrazinamide (Tebrazid) is an antituberculosis drug that can be either bacteriostatic or bactericidal, depending on its concentration at the site of infection and the particular susceptibility of the mycobacteria. It is commonly used in combination with other antituberculosis drugs for the treatment of TB. Its mechanism of action is unknown, but it is believed to work by inhibiting lipid and nucleic acid synthesis in the mycobacteria. Pyrazinamide is available in oral form. It is contraindicated in patients with severe liver disease or acute gout. In Canada, it is also not normally used in pregnant patients because of the lack of teratogenicity data, although it may be considered when there is resistance to isoniazid, rifampin, or ethambutol.

PHARMACOKINETICS

Half-Life	Onset	Peak	Duration
PO: 9–10 hr	PO: Variable	PO: 2 hr	PO: Up to 24 hr

rifabutin

Rifabutin (Mycobutin) is the second of two currently available rifamycin antibiotics, the other being rifampin. It is commonly used to prevent infections caused by *Mycobacterium avium* complex (MAC), which includes several non-TB mycobacterial species, in patients with advanced HIV infection. This is also the case with rifampin. A notable adverse effect of rifabutin is that it can turn urine, feces, saliva, skin, sputum, sweat, and tears a red–orange to red–brown colour. Rifabutin is currently available only for oral use.

rifampin

Rifampin (Rifadin, Rofact) is the first of the *rifamycin* class of synthetic macrocyclic antibiotics, which also includes rifabutin. The term *macrocyclic* connotes the large and complex hydrocarbon ring structure included in all the rifamycin compounds. Rifampin has activity against many *Mycobacterium* spp., as well as against meningococcus, *Haemophilus influenzae* type B, and leprosy. It is a broad-spectrum bactericidal drug that kills the offending organism by inhibiting protein synthesis. Rifampin is used concomitantly with at least one other antituberculosis drug in the treatment of TB. Rifampin is available in oral formulations and, as previously mentioned, in combination with isoniazid (Rifater). The parenteral form is available through the Special Access Programme, Health Canada. Rifampin is contraindicated in patients with a known drug allergy to it or any other rifamycin (i.e., rifabutin).

PHARMACOKINETICS

Half-Life	Onset	Peak	Duration
PO: 3 hr	PO: Variable	PO: 2–4 hr	PO: Up to 24 hr

streptomycin sulfate

Streptomycin sulfate is an aminoglycoside antibiotic currently available only in generic form. Introduced in 1944, it was the first drug that could effectively treat TB. Because of its toxicities, it is used most commonly today in combination-drug regimens for the treatment of MDR-TB infections. Streptomycin is currently available only in injectable form. It is usually not given to pregnant patients because of risk of fetal harm.

PHARMACOKINETICS

Half-Life	Onset	Peak	Duration
IM: 2–3 hr	IM: Variable	IM: 1–2 hr	IM: Up to 24 hr

NURSING PROCESS

▨ Assessment

Before administering any of the first-line and second-line antituberculosis drugs and to ensure the safe and effective use of these drugs, the nurse should obtain a thorough medical history, medication profile, and nursing history of the patient as well as perform a complete head-to-toe physical assessment. It is important to note any specific history of diagnoses or symptoms of tuberculosis, as well as the patient's last PPD (purified protein derivative) tuberculin skin test, with assessment of the reaction at the site of the intradermal injection. The most recent chest X-ray and results should also be noted. Liver function studies (e.g., bilirubin, liver enzymes, and blood urea nitrogen

DOSAGES   Selected Antituberculosis Drugs

Drug (Pregnancy Class)	Pharmacological Class	Usual Dosage Range	Indications
ethambutol hydrochloride (Etibi) (B)	Synthetic first-line antimycobacterial	*Adolescents 13 yr and older/Adult* PO: 15–25 mg/kg/day; may also be divided in 2×/wk (max 2.5 g) and 3×/wk (max 2.5 g) dosage regimens with higher doses	Active TB
⇉isoniazid (Isotamine) (C)	Synthetic first-line antimycobacterial	*Children* PO: 10–20 mg/kg/day (max 300 mg) or 20–40 mg/kg 2–3×/wk (max 900 mg/dose) *Adult* PO: 5–10 mg/kg daily (max 300 mg) or 15 mg/kg 1–3×/wk (max 900 mg/dose)	Active TB
pyrazinamide (Tebrazid)	Synthetic first-line antimycobacterial	*Children* PO: 30 mg/kg/day (max 2 g) or 2–3×/wk (max 3–4 g/dose) *Adolescent/Adult* PO: 15–30 mg/kg/day (max 2 g) or 50–70 mg/kg 2–3×/wk (max 3–4 g/dose)	Active TB
rifabutin (Mycobutin) (B)	Semisynthetic second-line antimycobacterial antibiotic	*Adult* PO: 300 mg daily or 150 mg bid	Active TB
rifampin (Rifadin, Rofact) (C)	Semisynthetic first-line antimycobacterial antibiotic	*Children* IV/PO: 10–20 mg/kg daily or 2×/wk (max 600 mg) *Adult* IV/PO: 10 mg/kg daily or 2–3×/wk (max 600 mg)	Active TB, latent TB in patients with advanced HIV
streptomycin	Antimycobacterial aminoglycoside antibiotic	*Children* IV: 20–40 mg/kg 1–2×/wk (max 1 g) *Adult* IM: 15–25 mg/kg 2–3×/wk (max 1 g/dose)	Active TB

[BUN]) need to be considered because of the contraindication of severe liver dysfunction. Not only are these values important for assessing liver function, they also provide a comparative baseline throughout therapy. Because use of some drugs leads to peripheral neuropathies, baseline neurological functioning should also be noted prior to therapy. Hearing status should be assessed, especially with use of streptomycin because of its drug-related ototoxicity.

Assessment of age is important because of the increased likelihood of adverse reactions or toxicity with liver dysfunction in the older adult and the fact that the safety of use in children 13 years of age or younger has not been established. It is also important for the nurse to check the patient's complete blood count (CBC) before administering isoniazid because of potential drug-related hematological disorders. Kidney studies, such as the serum creatinine and BUN, as well as urinalysis should be performed both at the start of antituberculin therapy and throughout, as ordered. Uric acid baseline levels should be noted because there may be an increase in these values and precipitation of gout. Sputum specimens are usually ordered to help in the determination of the appropriate drug regimen. Baseline eye function and exams should be performed prior to therapy with isoniazid and ethambutol. Pyrazinamide requires careful assessment of allergic reactions to other antituberculosis drugs because of close cross-sensitivity.

Contraindications, cautions, and drug interactions need to be considered with use of all of these drugs (as discussed previously in the pharmacology section).

◼ Nursing Diagnoses

- Risk for injury related to neurological adverse effects of antituberculosis drugs, nonadherence to drug therapy, and an overall status of poor health
- Ineffective therapeutic-regimen management of TB related to poor adherence to therapy and lack of knowledge about and experience with long-term therapies
- Ineffective family therapeutic regimen management related to poor adherence and poor housing and living conditions
- Deficient knowledge related to the disease process and treatment protocol

◼ Planning

◼ Goals

- Patient will experience minimal adverse effects of drug therapy for TB.
- Patient will take medication regularly and for the length of time prescribed.

- Patient will remain free of injury related to adverse effects (e.g., peripheral neuropathies) and drug interactions with the antituberculosis drugs.
- Patient will remain free of drug-related toxic effects and states the importance of reporting any symptoms of toxic effects to the physician immediately.
- Patient will remain adherent to the drug therapy.

Outcome Criteria

- Patient reports therapeutic effects (improved signs and symptoms) and possible adverse effects (neuropathies, gastrointestinal upset) of drug regimens.
- Patient takes medication as ordered and regularly with acknowledgement of more effective therapy and prevention of complications, relapses, or recurrences.
- Patient states the drugs that interact with antituberculosis drugs, such as salicylates, antacids, and anticoagulants, and maintains drug safety.
- Patient reports toxic effects, such as jaundice, kidney problems, hearing loss, severe neuropathies, or blindness, to the physician, should they occur.
- Patient shows improvement of disease state with drug adherence and has a decrease in cough, fever, and sputum production as well as a return of normal laboratory values.

Implementation

Because drug therapy is the mainstay of treatment for TB and often lasts for up to 24 months, patient education is critical, with a special emphasis on adherence. Simple, clear, and concise instructions should be given to the patient with appropriate use of audiovisuals and take-home information. This education should include the fact that multiple drugs are often used to improve cure rates. All antituberculosis drugs should be given exactly as ordered and at the same time every day. Consistent use and dosing around the clock are critical to maintaining steady blood levels and for minimizing the chances of resistance to the drug therapy. Instructions to the patient should always emphasize the need for strict adherence to the therapeutic regimen.

Although many drugs are to be given without food for maximum absorption, antituberculosis drugs may need to be taken with food to minimize gastrointestinal upset. There should be constant monitoring of any signs and symptoms of liver dysfunction, such as fatigue, jaundice, nausea, vomiting, dark urine, and anorexia, with reporting of any of these to the physician. If vision changes occur (e.g., altered colour perception, changes in visual acuity), in particular with ethambutol, these changes should be reported immediately to the physician. Uric acid levels will need to be monitored during therapy, as will symptoms of gout such as hot, painful, or swollen joints of the big toe, knee, or ankle. In addition, the physician should

be notified if there are signs and symptoms of peripheral neuropathy (e.g., numbness, burning, and tingling of extremities). Pyridoxine (vitamin B$_6$) may be beneficial with isoniazid-induced peripheral neuropathy. If the physician has ordered sputum collections for acid-fast bacilli, the specimen must be collected early in the morning on each of 3 consecutive days with a repeat several weeks later. All drugs should be taken as ordered and without any omission of doses, for maximal therapeutic results.

Follow-up visits to the health care provider are important in the monitoring of therapeutic effects and in detecting adverse effects and toxicity. If intravenous (IV) dosing of an antituberculosis drug is ordered, the appropriate diluent needs to be used and the drug infused over the recommended time. The IV site should be monitored every hour during the infusion for extravasation with possible tissue inflammation (e.g., redness, heat, and swelling at the IV site). See Patient Education for more information on use of antituberculosis drugs.

As part of ethnocultural considerations associated with these drugs, patients with active tuberculosis and all family members require thorough patient teaching, including the point that some family members may need prophylactic therapy for up to 1 full year. Because some ethnocultural practices involve living in close-knit communities and living quarters, this teaching is critical to ensuring that there is adequate prevention of the spread of this highly infectious disease. All family members or those in close contact with the patient must receive the same thorough instructions about maintaining their health and improving hygiene practices while taking their medications appropriately, and adherence should be emphasized.

Evaluation

The nurse should always document patient responses, or lack of them, to therapy. The therapeutic response to antituberculosis therapy is reflected by a decrease in the symptoms of tuberculosis, such as cough and fever, and by weight gain. The results of laboratory studies (culture and sensitivity tests) and chest X-ray findings should confirm the clinical findings of resolution of the infection. The meeting of goals and outcome criteria should also be evaluated to see if the infection is being adequately treated and if the drug therapy is providing therapeutic relief without complications or toxicity and with minimal adverse effects. Patients also need to be monitored for the occurrence of adverse reactions to antituberculosis drugs, such as fatigue, nausea, vomiting, fever, loss of appetite, depression, and jaundice; numbness, tingling, or burning of extremities; abdominal pain; changes in vision; and easy bruising. Because of the need for long-term therapy and possible treatment of family members or those in close contact with the patient, further evaluation of the home setting is also needed.

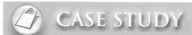 CASE STUDY

Tuberculosis

For a project that received new funding, you and five of your community health nursing peers have been asked to give some mini-presentations to large work settings in the community. One place is in your health department with the nurses who work in the adult clinic.
1. What are some key Internet resources you can share with staff regarding TB infections, control guidelines, and CCOHS recommendations?
2. What information could then be used or shared with patients in the adult clinic?

3. What conditions in the community are considered high risk for transmission of diseases such as TB?
4. What precautions should the nurse take when assessing patients who present with undiagnosed or potential TB?

CCOHS, Canadian Centre for Occupational Health and Safety; *TB*, tuberculosis.

For answers see http://evolve.elsevier.com/Canada/Lilley/pharmacology/.

PATIENT EDUCATION

❖ Patients should take medications exactly as ordered by the physician, with attention to long-term therapy and strict adherence. Ineffective treatment may occur if drugs are taken intermittently or stopped once the patient begins to feel better.
❖ Patients should be encouraged to keep all follow-up appointments with the health care provider so that the infection may be closely monitored.
❖ Patients should be instructed to avoid alcohol while taking antituberculosis drugs and to check with the physician before taking any other type of drug.
❖ Patients should be informed that they will most likely be taking pyridoxine (vitamin B_6) to prevent isoniazid-precipitated peripheral neuropathies and numbness, tingling, or burning of extremities.
❖ Patients taking isoniazid or rifampin should be instructed to report the following adverse effects to the physician immediately, should they occur: fever, nausea, vomiting, loss of appetite, unusual bleeding, numbness, and tingling of extremities.
❖ Patients should be informed to wear sunscreen and protective clothing and to avoid ultraviolet light exposure or prevent exposure to the sun because of drug-related photosensitivity reactions.
❖ Patients should be encouraged to report any flulike symptoms, gastrointestinal upset, or rash to the physician immediately.

❖ Patients should be educated about preventing spread of the infection and that during the initial period of the illness and its diagnosis, they should make every effort to wash their hands and cover their mouths when coughing or sneezing. They should also be careful about disposal of secretions.
❖ Patients should be educated about the need for rest, good sleep habits, adequate nutrition, and maintenance of general health. They should be instructed to keep these and other medications away from children.
❖ Patients should be encouraged to wear a medical alert tag or bracelet with a list of allergies, drugs being taken, and medical conditions. This information should also be kept in written form on their person at all times.
❖ Patients should be informed about the importance of reporting to their health care provider any increase in fatigue, cough, sputum production, bloody sputum, chest pain, unusual bleeding, yellow skin, or yellow eyes.
❖ Patients taking rifampin or rifabutin should be warned that they may experience red–orange–brown discoloration of the skin, sweat, tears, urine, feces, sputum, saliva, cerebrospinal fluid, and tongue as an adverse effect of the drug. The discoloration reverses with discontinuation of the drug; however, contact lenses may be permanently stained.

POINTS TO REMEMBER

❖ All drug therapeutic regimens should be taken exactly as prescribed, with emphasis on adherence and long-term dosing combined with healthy living practices.
❖ Therapeutic effects include resolving of pulmonary and extrapulmonary *M. tuberculosis* infections.
❖ Vitamin B_6 is needed to combat peripheral neuritis associated with isoniazid.
❖ Women taking oral contraceptive therapy who are prescribed rifampin should be counselled on other

forms of birth control because of the ineffectiveness of oral contraception while on rifampin.
❖ Patients and their families need to be educated about the importance of strict adherence to the drug regimen for improvement of condition or cure. Education about drug interactions and the need to avoid alcohol while taking any of these medications should be provided in written and oral formats.

EXAMINATION REVIEW QUESTIONS

1 When teaching a patient who is starting antituberculosis therapy with isoniazid, which of the following adverse effects would the nurse expect to see?
 a. Headache and neck pain
 b. Glaucoma and gynecomastia
 c. Reddish-brown urine and tears
 d. Numbness or tingling of extremities

2 During antituberculosis therapy with isoniazid, the patient received a prescription for pyridoxine. Which statement by the nurse best explains the rationale for this second medication?
 a. "This drug will help to improve your energy level."
 b. "This drug helps to prevent neurological adverse effects."
 c. "This drug works to protect your heart from toxic effects."
 d. "This drug works to reduce gastrointestinal adverse effects."

3 When counselling a woman who is beginning antituberculosis therapy with rifampim, which statement by the nurse is most important regarding potential drug interactions?
 a. "Your birth control pills will remain effective while you are taking rifampin."
 b. "You will need to switch to a stronger brand of oral contraceptive while on rifampin."
 c. "If you are taking birth control pills, you will need to switch to another form of birth control."
 d. "You can take the birth control pills with the rifampin without problems, but it may cause your urine to turn reddish-orange."

4 When counselling a patient who has a new diagnosis of tuberculosis, the nurse should make sure that the patient realizes that the patient is contagious during a specific time period. Which of the following is the correct period to be advised about?
 a. During all phases of the illness
 b. During the postictal phase of TB
 c. Any time up to 18 months after therapy
 d. During the initial period of the illness and its diagnosis

5 While monitoring a patient, which of the following therapeutic responses should a nurse know is related to antituberculosis drugs?
 a. The patient states feelings of improved well-being.
 b. The patient reports a decrease in cough and night sweats.
 c. The patient's laboratory results reflect a lower white blood cell count.
 d. There is a decrease in symptoms, along with improved chest X-ray and sputum culture results.

For answers see http://evolve.elsevier.com/Canada/Lilley/pharmacology/.

CRITICAL THINKING ACTIVITIES

1 What is considered a therapeutic response to antituberculosis drugs?

2 What are some important teaching points for family members of patients with TB that would assist them in supporting successful pharmacological therapy?

3 Explain why drug adherence and resistance to antituberculosis drugs is an issue in Canada.

For answers see http://evolve.elsevier.com/Canada/Lilley/pharmacology/.

CHAPTER 42

Antifungal Drugs

Learning Objectives

After reading this chapter, the successful student will be able to do the following:

1 Briefly discuss fungal infections.

2 Identify the antifungal drugs.

3 Describe the mechanisms of action, indications, contraindications, routes of administration, adverse and toxic effects, and drug interactions associated with the use of antifungal drugs.

4 Develop a collaborative plan of care that includes all phases of the nursing process for patients receiving antifungal drugs.

e-Learning Activities

Web site
(http://evolve.elsevier.com/Canada/Lilley/pharmacology/)

- Animations
- Answers to chapter questions, activities, and case studies
- Calculators and Category Catchers
- Glossary with audio pronunciations
- IV Therapy and Medication Error Checklists
- Multiple-Choice Review Question quizzes
- Nursing Care Plans
- Online Appendices and Supplements
- WebLinks

Drug Profiles

▸▸ **amphotericin B,** p. 797
   caspofungin (caspofungin acetate*), p. 797
▸▸ **fluconazole,** p. 797
   nystatin, p. 798
   terbinafine (terbinafine hydrochloride*), p. 798
   voriconazole, p. 798

▸▸ Key drug.

*Full generic name is given in parentheses. For the purposes of this text, the more common shortened name is used.

Glossary

Antimetabolite A drug or other substance that either is a receptor antagonist or resembles a normal human metabolite and interferes with the metabolite's function in the body, usually by competing for the metabolite's usual receptors or enzymes. (p. 794)

Dermatophyte One of several fungi, often found in soil, that infect skin, nails, or hair of humans. (p. 793)

Ergosterol An unsaturated hydrocarbon of the vitamin D group isolated from yeast, mushrooms, ergot, and other fungi; the main sterol in fungal membranes. (p. 794)

Fungi A large, diverse group of eukaryotic microorganisms that require an external carbon source and form a plant structure known as a *thallus*. Fungi consist of *yeasts* and *moulds*. (p. 793)

Moulds Multicellular fungi characterized by long, branching filaments called *hyphae*, which entwine to form a complex branched structure known as a *mycelium*. (p. 793)

Mycosis The general term for any fungal infection. (p. 793)

Pathological fungi Fungi that cause mycoses. (p. 793)

Sterol The substance in the cell membranes of fungi to which polyene antifungal drugs bind. (p. 794)

Yeasts Single-celled fungi that reproduce by *budding*. (p. 793)

FUNGAL INFECTIONS

Fungi are a large and diverse group of microorganisms that include all yeasts and moulds. **Yeasts** are single-celled fungi that reproduce by *budding* (i.e., a daughter cell forms by pouching out of and breaking off from a mother cell). These organisms have common practical uses in the baking of breads and the processing of alcoholic beverages. **Moulds** are multicellular and are characterized by long, branching filaments called *hyphae*, which entwine to form a "mat" called a *mycelium*. Yeast or fungi colonies are part of the normal flora of the skin, mucous membranes, intestines, and vagina. The body's normal bacterial flora and its intact immune mechanisms and competition for nutrients control colonizing fungi. Diseases or antibiotic therapy can disrupt this balance, resulting in fungal overgrowth and opportunistic infections. The infection caused by a fungus is called a **mycosis**. A variety of fungi can cause clinically significant mycoses; such fungi are called **pathological fungi.** The infections they cause can range in severity from being mild infections with annoying symptoms (e.g., athlete's foot) to systemic mycoses, which are serious, deep-tissue fungal infections that can become life threatening. These infections are acquired by various routes: they can be ingested orally; they can grow on or in the skin, hair, or nails; and, if the fungal spores are airborne, they can be inhaled.

There are four general types of mycotic infections: *systemic, cutaneous, subcutaneous,* and *superficial.* The latter three types describe the layers of *integumentary* (skin, hair, or nail) infections. Fungi that cause integumentary infections are known as **dermatophytes,** and such infections are known as *dermatomycoses.* The most severe systemic fungal infections generally afflict people whose host immune defences are compromised. Commonly, these are patients who have received organ transplants and are on immunosuppressive drug therapy, cancer patients who are immunocompromised as the result of chemotherapy, and patients with AIDS. In addition, the use of antibiotics, antineoplastics, or immunosuppressants such as corticosteroids may result in colonization of *Candida albicans,* followed by the development of a systemic infection. When this condition affects the mouth, it is referred to as *oral candidiasis,* or *thrush.* It is common in newborns and immunocompromised patients. Vaginal candidiasis, commonly called a *yeast infection,* often burdens pregnant women, women with diabetes mellitus, women taking antibiotics, and women taking oral contraceptives. The characteristics of some of the systemic, cutaneous, and superficial mycotic infections are summarized in Table 42-1.

ANTIFUNGAL DRUGS

Fungal infections are treated with antifungal drugs. Systemic mycotic infections and some cutaneous or subcutaneous mycoses are treated with oral or parenteral drugs, but these constitute a fairly small group of drugs, only three or four of which are commonly used. There are few

TABLE 42-1					
Mycotic Infections					
Mycosis	Fungus	Endemic Location	Reservoir	Transmission	Primary Tissue Affected
SYSTEMIC INFECTION					
Aspergillosis	*Aspergillus* spp.	Universal	Soil	Inhalation	Lungs
Blastomycosis	*Blastomyces dermatitidis*	North America	Soil, animal droppings	Inhalation	Lungs
Coccidioidomycosis	*Coccidioides immitis*	Great Lakes, Canada	Soil, dust	Inhalation	Lungs
Cryptococcosis	*Cryptococcus neoformans*	Universal	Soil, pigeon droppings	Inhalation	Lungs, meninges of brain
Histoplasmosis	*Histoplasma capsulatum*	Universal	Soil, droppings of chickens and other birds	Inhalation	Lungs
CUTANEOUS INFECTION					
Candidiasis	*Candida albicans*	Universal	Humans	Direct contact, nonsusceptible antibiotic overgrowth	Mucous membrane or skin disseminated (may be systemic)
Dermatophytes, tinea	*Epidermophyton* spp., *Microsporum* spp., *Trichophyton* spp.	Universal	Humans	Direct and indirect contact with infected persons	Scalp, skin (e.g., groin, feet)
SUPERFICIAL INFECTION					
Tinea versicolor	*Malassezia furfur*	Universal	Humans	Unknown*	Skin

*Malassezia spp. are a usual part of the normal human flora and appear to cause infection only in certain individuals.

such drugs because the fungi have proved difficult to kill, and research into new and improved drugs has occurred at a slow pace, with relatively few important advances to date. One difficulty that has slowed the development of new antifungal drugs is that often the chemical concentrations required for these experimental drugs to be effective cannot be tolerated by human beings. Those drugs that have met with success in the treatment of systemic mycoses and severe dermatomycoses are amphotericin B, caspofungin acetate, fluconazole, flucytosine, griseofulvin, itraconazole, ketoconazole, micafungin, nystatin, terbinafine hydrochloride, and voriconazole. These drugs are the focus of this chapter.

The antifungal drugs discussed here fall into four specific chemical classes: *polyenes* (amphotericin B and nystatin); *azoles*, which include the *imidazoles* (ketoconazole) and *triazoles* (fluconazole, itraconazole, and voriconazole); *echinocandins* (caspofungin, anidulafungin and micafungin); and *allyamines* (allylamine terbinafine hydrochloride). The imidazoles and triazoles are sometimes referred to by the more general term azole *antifungals*. Also included in some of these classes are drugs for topical use, which are described further in Chapter 57. The other two antifungal drugs, flucytosine and griseofulvin, are individually listed and not specifically classified according to their chemical structure.

Topical antifungal drugs are by far the most commonly used antifungal drugs and are most often used without prescription for the treatment of dermatomycoses as well as oral and vaginal mycoses. Although topical drug therapy is usually sufficient for these conditions, systemic oral medications are also sometimes used, especially for more severe or recurrent cases.

Mechanism of Action and Drug Effects

The mechanisms of action of the antifungal drugs vary among drug subclasses. Flucytosine, also known as *5-fluorocytosine* (5-FC), available through the Special Access Programme, Health Canada, acts in much the same way as the antiviral drugs. It is an **antimetabolite**, which is a drug that is taken up into critical cellular metabolic pathways of the fungal cell. Once inside a susceptible fungal cell, the drug is deaminated by the enzyme *cytosine deaminase* to 5-fluorouracil (5-FU). Because human cells do not have this enzyme, they are not harmed by this antimetabolite. Once the 5-FU is generated inside the fungal cell, it interferes with fungal DNA synthesis, resulting in cell death and inhibition of both cell growth and reproduction. 5-FU is also available as an antineoplastic (anticancer) drug and is discussed in more detail in Chapter 48.

Griseofulvin, like flucytosine, is one of the older types of antifungal drugs. It works by preventing susceptible fungi from reproducing. It enters the fungal cell through an energy-dependent transport system and inhibits fungal mitosis (cell division) by binding to key structures known as *microtubules*. This action in turn disrupts the *mitotic spindle* structure, which arrests the metaphase of cell division. Griseofulvin may also cause

the production of defective DNA, which is then unable to replicate. Although griseofulvin and flucytosine are still currently available on the Canadian market, their clinical use has largely been supplanted by the newer antifungal drug classes.

The polyenes act by binding to molecules called **sterols** in the cell membranes of fungi; the main sterol in fungal membranes is **ergosterol**. Human cell membranes are abundant with cholesterol instead of ergosterol. Because polyene antifungals have a strong chemical affinity for ergosterol rather than cholesterol, they do not bind to human cell membranes and, therefore, do not kill human cells. Once the polyene drug molecule binds to the ergosterol, a channel forms in the fungal cell membrane that allows potassium and magnesium ions to leak out of the cell. This loss of ions causes fungal cellular metabolism to be altered, leading to the death of the cell.

Imidazoles and triazoles act as either fungistatic or fungicidal drugs, depending on their concentration in the fungus. They are most effective in combatting rapidly growing fungi and act by inhibiting fungal cell cytochrome P450 enzymes, which are needed to produce ergosterol. The allylamine terbinafine hydrochloride is believed to act by means of a similar mechanism. When the production of ergosterol is inhibited, other sterols, called *methylsterols*, are produced. This production of methylsterols results in a problem similar to that caused by the polyene antifungals—specifically, a leaky cell membrane allows needed electrolytes to escape. The fungal cells die because they cannot carry on cellular metabolism.

The echinocandins—caspofungin, anidulafungin, and micafungin—act by preventing the synthesis of *glucans*, essential components of fungal cell walls that are not present in mammalian cells. This action also contributes to fungal cell death. Some of the fungi that are susceptible to these drugs are the pathogens involved in the mycoses listed in Table 42-1.

Indications

Indications for the use of antifungal drugs are specific to both the antifungal drug and the type of infection being treated. The adverse effects of the newer antifungals are fewer and less serious than those of the older drugs. However, the drug of choice for the treatment of many severe systemic fungal infections remains one of the oldest antifungals, amphotericin B, which often does have major adverse effects. Amphotericin B is effective against a wide range of fungi. It is given with flucytosine in the treatment of serious systemic *Candida* and cryptococcal infections because of the synergy of the two drugs. Amphotericin B is effective for treating aspergillosis, blastomycosis, candidiasis, coccidioidomycosis, cryptococcosis, fungal endocarditis, histoplasmosis, zygomycosis, fungal septicemia, and many other systemic fungal infections. The activity of nystatin is similar to that of amphotericin B, but its usefulness is limited because of its toxic effects when given in the doses required to accomplish the same antifungal actions as those of amphotericin B. It is also not available in a parenteral form. Nystatin is most commonly used for treating oropharyngeal candidiasis, commonly referred to as *thrush*.

Fluconazole and itraconazole are synthetic imidazole antifungals, as are all of the drugs with an "-azole" suffix. Fluconazole can pass into the cerebrospinal fluid (CSF) and inhibit cryptococcal fungi, making it effective in the treatment of cryptococcal meningitis. Both drugs are active against oropharyngeal and esophageal *Candida* infections. Itraconazole, by contrast, has poor CSF penetration but can be widely distributed throughout other areas of the body. It is indicated for the treatment of fungal infections in immunocompromised and nonimmunocompromised patients with disseminated candidiasis, histoplasmosis, blastomycosis, and aspergillosis. The other systemic imidazole, ketoconazole, inhibits many dermatophytes and fungi that cause systemic mycoses, but it is not active against *Aspergillus* organisms or *Phycomycetes* (common moulds) such as *Mucor* spp. Fortunately, the newest imidazole antifungal drug, voriconazole, does have activity against some of these more tenacious fungal infections, including invasive aspergillosis, *Scedosporium* spp., and *Fusarium* spp.

Of the azol antifungals, fluconazole is the most effective for combating infections with *Candida*, *Cryptococcus*, *Blastomyces*, and *Histoplasma* organisms. Fluconazole is also effective against vaginal candidiasis; one 150 mg dose can cure many vaginal candidal infections.

Griseofulvin inhibits dermatophytes of *Microsporum*, *Trichophyton*, and *Epidermophyton* spp. It has no effect on filamentous fungi such as *Aspergillus*, yeasts such as *Candida* spp., or dimorphic species such as *Histoplasma*. Terbinafine hydrochloride is a synthetic allylamine derivative used in a systemic oral form for treatment of *onychomycoses*, or fungally infected fingernails or toenails. The imidazole itraconazole is also sometimes used for this purpose. Topical forms of terbinafine are used for skin infections (Chapter 57).

Contraindications

Drug allergy, liver failure, kidney failure, and griseofulvin in patients with porphyria are the most common contraindications for antifungal drugs. Amphotericin B should not be used in combination with other neurotoxic drugs such as nonsteroidal anti-inflammatory drugs (NSAIDs), aminoglycosides, and cyclosporine because of the risk for increased toxicity. Itraconazole should not be used for treating onychomycoses in patients with severe heart problems. Prior treatment with itraconazole may reduce or inhibit the activity of polyenes such as amphotericin B. Voriconazole can cause fetal harm in pregnant women.

Adverse Effects

The major adverse effects and clinical problems with antifungal drugs are encountered most commonly in conjunction with amphotericin B treatment. While drug interactions and hepatotoxicity are the primary concerns in patients receiving other antifungal drugs, intravenous (IV) administration of amphotericin B is associated with a multitude of adverse effects. The most common and problematic adverse effects are listed in Table 42-2. With amphotericin B treatment in particular, prescribers commonly order premedications (including antiemetics, antihistamines, antipyretics, and corticosteroids) to prevent or minimize infusion-related reactions. The likelihood of such reactions can also be reduced by using longer-than-average drug infusion times (i.e., 2 to 6 hours) with this particular drug.

Interactions

There are many important drug interactions associated with antifungal drugs, some of which can be life threatening. A common underlying source of the problem is that many of the antifungal drugs, as well as other drugs, are metabolized by an abundantly used enzyme system in the liver, the cytochrome P450 system. When two drugs that are both broken down by this system are coadministered, they compete for the limited number of enzymes, and one of the drugs ends up accumulating in the body. Key drug interactions with systemic antifungal drugs are summarized in Table 42-3.

Dosages

For the recommended dosages of selected antifungal drugs, see the Dosages table on p. 798.

TABLE 42-2

Antifungals: Common Adverse Effects and Cautions

Body System	Adverse Effects	Caution
AMPHOTERICIN B		Recheck dosage and type of amphotericin B being administered
Cardiovascular	Cardiac dysrhythmias	
Central nervous	Neurotoxicity; visual disturbances; hand or feet numbness, tingling, or pain; convulsions	
Kidneys	Kidney toxicity, potassium loss, hypomagnesemia	
Pulmonary	Pulmonary infiltrates, other respiratory difficulties	
Other (infusion related)	Fever, chills, headache, malaise, nausea, occasionally hypotension	
FLUCONAZOLE		Use with caution in patients with kidney dysfunction or bone marrow depression
Gastrointestinal	Nausea, vomiting, diarrhea, stomach pain	
Other	Increased AST and ALT levels	

Continued

TABLE 42-2		

Antifungals: Common Adverse Effects and Cautions (cont'd)

Body System	Adverse Effects	Caution
GRISEOFULVIN		Avoid during pregnancy
Central nervous	Headache, peripheral neuritis, paraesthesia, confusion, dizziness, fatigue, insomnia, psychosis	
Ears, eyes, nose, and throat	Blurred vision, oral candidiasis, furry tongue, transient hearing loss	
Gastrointestinal	Nausea, vomiting, anorexia, diarrhea, cramps, dry mouth, flatulence, increased thirst, dysgeusia	
Genitourinary	Proteinuria, precipitate porphyria	
Hematological	Leukopenia, granulocytopenia, neutropenia, monocytosis	
Integumentary	Rash, urticaria, photosensitivity, angioedema, systemic lupus erythematosus	
ITRACONAZOLE		Can trigger rare episodes of serious cardiovascular adverse effects
Central nervous	Headache, dizziness, insomnia, somnolence, depression	
Gastrointestinal	Nausea, vomiting, anorexia, diarrhea, cramps, abdominal pain, flatulence, hepatotoxicity	
Genitourinary	Gynecomastia, erectile dysfunction, decreased libido	
Integumentary	Pruritus, fever, rash	
Other	Edema, fatigue, malaise, hypertension, hypokalemia, tinnitus, hypertriglyceridemia, adrenal insufficiency	
KETOCONAZOLE		Avoid contact with eyes
Central nervous	Headache, dizziness, somnolence, SIADH	
Gastrointestinal	Nausea, vomiting, anorexia, diarrhea, abdominal pain, hepatotoxicity	
Genitourinary	Gynecomastia, erectile dysfunction, vaginal burning	
Hematological	Thrombocytopenia, leukopenia, hemolytic anemia	
Integumentary	Pruritus, fever, chills, photophobia, rash, dermatitis, purpura, urticaria	
Other	Hypoadrenalism, hyperuricemia, hypothyroidism	
NYSTATIN		Local irritation may occur
Gastrointestinal	Nausea, vomiting, anorexia, diarrhea, cramps	
Integumentary	Rash, urticaria	
TERBINAFINE HYDROCHLORIDE		Rarely causes irritation
Central nervous	Headache, dizziness	
Gastrointestinal	Nausea, vomiting, diarrhea	
Integumentary	Rash, pruritus	
Other	Alopecia, fatigue	

ALT, alanine aminotransferase; *AST*, aspartate aminotransferase; *SIADH*, syndrome of inappropriate antidiuretic hormone.

TABLE 42-3	

Antifungal Drugs: Drug Interactions

Drug	Possible Effects
AMPHOTERICIN B	
Digitalis glycosides	Amphotericin B–induced hypokalemia may increase the potential for digitalis toxicity
Nephrotoxic drug	Additive nephrotoxicity
Thiazide diuretics	Severe hypokalemia or decreased adrenal cortex response to corticotropin
FLUCONAZOLE, ITRACONAZOLE, AND MICONAZOLE	
cyclosporine, phenytoin	Increased plasma concentrations of both drugs
Oral anticoagulants	Increased effects of anticoagulants seen as increases in PT
Oral antihyperglycemics	Reduced metabolism of antihyperglycemic drugs

Continued

TABLE 42-3

Antifungal Drugs: Drug Interactions (cont'd)

Drug	Possible Effects
GRISEOFULVIN	
Oral anticoagulants	Decreased effects of anticoagulants seen as decreases in PT
Oral contraceptives, estrogen-containing products	Decreased effectiveness of these drugs
KETOCONAZOLE AND MICONAZOLE	
Alcohol and other hepatotoxic drugs	Increased risk of hepatotoxicity
Antacids, anticholinergics, H$_2$ receptor blockers, omeprazole	Increased gastrointestinal tract pH, which can reduce absorption of ketoconazole
cyclosporine	Increased cyclosporine levels and potential for nephrotoxicity
isoniazid, rifampin	Decreased serum levels of ketoconazole
VORICONAZOLE	
quinidine	Prolongation of QT interval on ECG

ECG, electrocardiograph; *PT*, prothrombin time; *QT* interval, time interval between the start of the Q wave and the end of the T wave in the electrical cycle of the heart.

 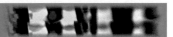

DRUG PROFILES

▶▶ amphotericin B

Amphotericin B (Fungizone) remains the drug of choice for the treatment of severe systemic mycoses. It may be given with flucytosine in the treatment of many types of fungal infections because the two drugs work synergistically. The main drawback of amphotericin B therapy is that use of the drug results in many adverse effects. Almost all patients given the drug intravenously experience fever, chills, hypotension, tachycardia, malaise, muscle and joint pain, anorexia, nausea and vomiting, and headache. For this reason, pretreatment with an antipyretic (acetaminophen), antihistamines, and antiemetics may be given to decrease the severity of this infusion-related reaction.

Lipid formulations of amphotericin B have been developed in an attempt to decrease the incidence of adverse effects and increase its efficacy. There are currently three lipid preparations of amphotericin B: amphotericin B lipid complex (Abelcet), amphotericin B cholesteryl complex (Amphotec), and liposomal amphotericin B (AmBisome). These lipid dosage forms have a higher cost than conventional amphotericin B and thus are often used only when patients are intolerant of or refractory to nonlipid amphotericin B.

Amphotericin B is available as a sterile lyophilized powder in vials providing 50 mg amphotericin B for intravenous injection. It is contraindicated in patients who have shown hypersensitivity reactions to it and in those with severe bone marrow suppression or kidney impairment. However, patients who have life-threatening fungal infections may still be treated with this drug if cultures indicate that no other drug will kill the infection. Often a 1 mg test dose is given over 20 to 30 minutes to check if the patient will tolerate the amphotericin. It has been used as a local irrigant (bladder irrigation) for the treatment of candidal cystitis and has been used intrapleurally and intraperitoneally for the treatment of fungal infections in these body cavities.

PHARMACOKINETICS*

Half-Life	Onset	Peak	Duration
IV: 1–15 days	IV: Variable	IV: 1 hr	IV: 18–24 hr

*For conventional (nonlipid) injection; lipid formulations have prolonged half-lives.

caspofungin acetate

Caspofungin acetate (Cancidas) was the first echinocandin antifungal drug, approved in 2003. It is used for treating severe *Aspergillus* infection (invasive and aspergillosis) in patients who are intolerant of or refractory to other drugs. It is only available in injectable form. Two additional echinocandins, micafungin sodium (Mycamine) and anidulafungin (Eraxis), have since been approved.

PHARMACOKINETICS

Half-Life	Onset	Peak	Duration
IV: 9–50 hr	IV: Unknown	IV: Unknown	IV: Unknown

▶▶ fluconazole

Fluconazole (Diflucan) has proven to represent a significant improvement in the area of antifungal treatment. It has a much better adverse-effect profile than that of amphotericin B, and it has excellent coverage against many fungi. In fact, it is often preferred to amphotericin B because of these qualities. Oral fluconazole has excellent

Continued

DRUG PROFILES (cont'd)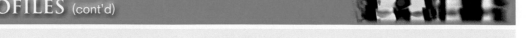

bioavailability, which means that almost the entire dose administered is absorbed into the circulation. Fluconazole is available in both oral and parenteral forms.

PHARMACOKINETICS

Half-Life	Onset	Peak	Duration
PO: 22–50 hr	PO: Less than 1 hr	PO: 1–2 hr	PO: Variable

nystatin

Nystatin (Dom-Nystatin, Nyaderm, Ratio-Nystatin) is a polyene antifungal drug that is often applied topically for the treatment of candidal diaper rash, taken orally as prophylaxis against candidal infections during periods of neutropenia in patients receiving immunosuppressive therapy, and used for the treatment of oral and vaginal candidiasis. It is not available in a parenteral form but does come in several oral and topical formulations. It is currently available for oral, topical, and vaginal use. It is also available with metronidazole (Flagyl) in a vaginal ovule or topical cream (Flagstatin) for the treatment of mixed *Trichomonas vaginalis* and *C. albicans* infections. Another available combination is nystatin, gramicidin (antiobiotic), neomycin sulfate (antibiotic), and triamcinolone acetonide (corticosteroid) compound (Thermaderm, Viaderm) for topical application.

PHARMACOKINETICS

Half-Life	Onset	Peak	Duration
PO: Unknown	PO: 2 hr	PO: Unknown	PO: Unknown

terbinafine hydrochloride

Terbinafine hydrochloride (Lamisil) is classified as an allylamine antifungal drug and is currently the only drug in its class. It is available in a topical cream and spray for treating superficial dermatological infections, including tinea pedis (athlete's foot), tinea cruris (jock itch), and tinea corporis (ringworm). A tablet form is also available for systemic use and is used primarily to treat onychomycoses of the fingernails or toenails.

PHARMACOKINETICS

Half-Life	Onset	Peak	Duration
PO: 22–26 hr	PO: Unknown	PO: 2 hr	PO: Unknown

voriconazole

Voriconazole (VFEND) is also a newer antifungal drug on the Canadian market, approved by Health Canada in 2004. It is used for treating severe fungal infections caused by *Aspergillus* spp. (invasive aspergillosis) and systemic *Candida* in non-neutropenic patients, as well as the following *Candida* infections: disseminated infections in skin and infections in the abdomen, kidney, bladder wall, and wounds. Voriconazole is contraindicated in patients with a known drug allergy to it and when coadministered with certain other drugs metabolized by the cytochrome P450 enzyme CYP3A4 (e.g., quinidine) because of the risk of serious cardiac dysrhythmias. It is also the only antifungal drug contraindicated in pregnancy. The drug is available in oral and injectable forms.

PHARMACOKINETICS

Half-Life	Onset	Peak	Duration
PO: Unknown due to nonlinear kinetics	PO: Unknown	PO: 1–2 hr	PO: Unknown

DOSAGES   Selected Antifungal Drugs

Drug (Pregnancy Category)	Pharmacological Class	Usual Dosage Range	Indications
▶▶amphotericin B (Fungizone) (B)	Polyene antifungal	*Children/Adult* IV: Initial daily dose, 0.25 mg/kg; titrate up to 1–1.5 mg/kg/day	Broad spectrum of systemic fungal infections
amphotericin B lipid complex (ABLC); doses vary with product as follows:	Polyene antifungal	*Children/Adult*	Systemic fungal infections
Abelcet (B)		IV: 5 mg/kg once daily, infused at 2.5 mg/kg/hr	
AmBisome (B)		IV: 3–6 mg/kg/day, infused over 1–2 hr	
Amphotec (B)		IV: 3–4 mg/kg/day, infused at 1 mg/kg/hr	
caspofungin (Cancidas) (C)	Echinocandin antifungal	*Adult* IV: 70 mg loading dose on day 1, followed by 50 mg/day thereafter; infuse doses over 1 hr	Esophageal candidiasis, invasive candidiasis, invasive aspergillosis in patients intolerant of or refractory to other drugs

Continued

DOSAGES   Selected Antifungal Drugs (cont'd)

Drug (Pregnancy Category)	Pharmacological Class	Usual Dosage Range	Indications
▸▸fluconazole (Diflucan) (C)	Synthetic triazole antifungal	*Children* IV/PO: 6–12 mg/kg/day 10–12 wk after negative CSF cultures	Cryptococcal meningitis
		Adult IV/PO: 200–400 mg daily	Oropharyngeal and esophageal candidiasis, systemic candidiasis
		Children IV/PO: 3–12 mg/kg, (dose and duration depend on severity of infection)	
		Adult IV/PO: 100–400 mg/day × 2–5 wk (dose and duration depend on severity of infection)	
nystatin (Dom-Nystatin, Nyaderm, Ratio-Nystatin) (C)	Polyene antifungal	*Infant* PO: 100,000 units (2 mL) oral suspension in oral cavity tid–qid	Oral candidiasis, intestinal moniliasis
		Children/Adult PO: 400,000–600,000 units (4–6 mL) oral suspension in oral cavity qid	
		Adult PO (tab): 500,000–1,000,000 units (1–2 tabs) tid	Intestinal candidiasis
		Topical (cream, lotion, or powder): Apply bid	Topical candidiasis
		Vaginal: Insert one vaginal tablet or applicator of cream once to twice daily ×2 wk	Vaginal candidiasis
terbinafine hydrochloride (Lamisil) (B)	Synthetic allylamine antifungal	*Adult* PO: 250 mg/day × 2–6 wk	Onychomycosis (fungal infection of finger- or toenails)
		Topical cream or solution: apply bid to affected area × 1–2 wk	Athlete's foot (tinea pedis), jock itch (tinea cruris), or ringworm (tinea corporis)
voriconazole (VFEND) (D)	Synthetic triazole antifungal	*Adult over 40 kg* PO: loading dose of 400 mg × 2 doses q12h, then 200 mg bid maintenance *Adult less than 40 kg* PO: loading dose of 200 mg × 2 doses q12h, then 100 mg bid maintenance IV: loading dose of 6 mg/kg/ mL × 2 doses q12h, then 3–4 mg/kg bid	Invasive aspergillosis; candidemia and other invasive candidiasis

CSF, cerebrospinal fluid; *IV,* intravenous; *PO,* oral.

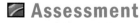

NURSING PROCESS

⬛ Assessment

Although topical dosage forms are discussed in detail in Chapter 57, it is still important to discuss these forms and related nursing process issues here. Vital signs, weight, hemoglobin (Hgb), hematocrit (Hct), red blood cell counts (RBCs), complete blood counts (CBCs) with differential, liver and kidney function tests, and confirmation of culture and sensitivity test results should all be assessed and noted prior to beginning antifungal

therapy. Before administering amphotericin B (or any other antifungal drug), it is important for the nurse to identify any contraindications, cautions, and drug interactions (discussed previously in the pharmacology section). Allergy to amphotericin B or sulfites should be noted and considered a contraindication, and any other nephrotoxic drugs need to be avoided if at all possible. Baseline kidney function studies would be warranted in this situation. Because there is a risk for severe adverse reactions with intravenous (IV) antifungal administration (e.g., amphotericin B), assessment of any special premedication orders for use of antiemetics, antihistamines, antipyretics, and anti-inflammatory drugs should be completed. Caspofungin and other antifungals require recording of baseline vital signs, liver function tests, and CBCs. Patients receiving griseofulvin should be assessed thoroughly for allergy to penicillin because of possible higher risk for allergic reactions to the antifungal. Griseofulvin may also precipitate severe blood dyscrasias, thus baseline CBCs are needed. Patients receiving ketoconazole should have their liver function assessed because of possible drug-related hepatotoxicity.

Because miconazole use is associated with adverse cardiovascular effects, pulse, blood pressure, and electrocardiogram (ECG) interpretation should be noted, as should any history of heart disease. Terbinafine hydrochloride requires close monitoring of liver function tests, especially in patients receiving treatment for longer than 6 weeks, and voriconazole should be given only after baseline liver and kidney function tests have been noted. Voriconazole is contraindicated if the patient is taking drugs such as quinidine and other drugs metabolized in the same pathway. Voriconazole undergoes metabolism by the cytochrome P450 enzyme CYP3A4 and could induce serious cardiac dysrhythmias.

Nursing Diagnoses

- Acute pain related to symptoms of the infectious process
- Deficient knowledge related to lack of information about and experience with antifungal drug therapy
- Risk for injury related to drug interactions or adverse effects of the medication treatment regimen

Planning

Goals

- Patient will state the rationale for adherence to antifungal therapy.
- Patient will state the common adverse effects and ways to prevent injury associated with antifungal drug therapy.
- Patient will experience minimal adverse effects and signs and symptoms of the infection.
- Patient will exhibit relief of the symptoms previously associated with the fungal infection.
- Patient will state the importance of follow-up appointments.

Outcome Criteria

- Patient is free of the complications or suffers minimal adverse effects of the antifungal drug therapy for the duration of treatment (e.g., nausea, vomiting, gastrointestinal upset).
- Patient remains adherent to the drug regimen without omissions or skipping of doses and experiences relief of infection with a return to normal vital signs and normal culture and sensitivity reports after full course of therapy.

- Patient experiences improved appetite, energy level, and physical strength and stamina and a decrease of other symptoms such as pain or itching after taking the antifungal drugs for the prescribed period.
- Patient returns to the physician regularly as recommended by the health care provider for constant monitoring of the infection and of drug therapy with blood tests (e.g., CBC with differential, RBC, Hgb, Hct, kidney and liver function tests).

Implementation

The nursing interventions appropriate to patients receiving antifungal drugs vary depending on the particular drug. With all antifungals, however, the nurse needs to monitor the intake and output amounts, urinalysis results, liver and kidney function tests, and CBCs during therapy. It is also important for the nurse to weigh patients weekly (or encourage them to do this at home) and document weights (even if in the home setting), because a gain of 1 kg or more in a 24-hour period or 2 kg or more in 1 week may indicate possible medication-induced kidney damage, with the need for prompt medical attention. For IV dosages, manufacturer guidelines and the physician's order should be followed for specific solutions and rates of IV administration.

With IV amphotericin B, solutions that are cloudy or with precipitates should not be used. IV infusion pumps are recommended. Monitoring of vital signs should be done every 15 minutes or as needed to assess for adverse reactions, with notation of abdominal pain, anorexia, chills, fever, nausea, shaking, and vomiting. Should these adverse effects or a severe reaction occur, the infusion should be discontinued (while closely monitoring the patient) and the physician contacted. The IV site should be monitored for signs of phlebitis (e.g., heat, pain, and redness over the site or vein). Intake and output should be monitored and the skin checked for burning, itching, and irritation. See Patient Education for further information.

Only clear solutions of caspofungin should be used, diluted with NaCl. Liver function studies need to be monitored closely over the duration of therapy. Fluconazole may be given either orally or intravenously; IV dosage forms are used if there is a specific indication or if the oral dosage forms are poorly tolerated. The IV dosage forms should be used only if clear, and no other medication should be added to the solution. Itching or a rash should be reported immediately, and the patient's temperature, bowel activity, and stool consistency need to be monitored.

Griseofulvin is associated with photosensitivity, thus patients should be instructed to use sunscreen and protective clothing; however, avoiding exposure to the sun is preferred. They should also be monitored for complaints of headaches, and oral dosage forms should be given with food to minimize gastrointestinal upset. Oral dosages of itraconazole should also be given with food to avoid gastrointestinal upset. Intravenous itraconazole should be administered using an IV bag and tubing equipment provided by the manufacturer, with infusions usually given over 60 minutes.

When nystatin suspension is used, the patient needs to "swish" the medication solution thoroughly in the mouth for as long as possible prior to swallowing. Terbinafine may be given orally or topically. Local skin reactions that need to be reported include blistering, itching, oozing, redness, and swelling. Oral dosing of voriconazole should be given 1 hour before or 1 hour after a meal. IV doses may be diluted with D5W or NaCl, and the accurate dosage should be infused over the recommended time frame. Visual acuity must be monitored with this drug

(especially if ordered for longer than 28 days) and any changes reported to the health care provider.

Evaluation

The therapeutic effects of antifungals include improvement and eventual resolution of the signs and symptoms of the fungal infection. An improved energy level and overall sense of well-being as well as baseline normal temperature and vital signs also indicate a therapeutic response. Specific adverse effects to monitor for in patients receiving these drugs are listed in Table 42-2. Goals and outcome criteria should be evaluated in the context of the collaborative plan of care.

IN MY FAMILY

When Grandma's Remedies Don't Work

(as told by M., of Serbian descent)

"[M]y dad had a fungal infection on his big toe, and instead of going to see a doctor he called my grandma for advice. She gathered a leaf called "bocvica" in a nearby forest and then wrapped it several times over my dad's toe. He would change the leaves twice a day. The remedy did not help and a few months later my dad ended up in the emergency room because his whole leg was numb . . . due to the swelling. . . . Home remedies interfere with [medical treatment] mainly because most individuals do not turn to approved medications until their disease is advanced. . . . [Moreover,] Serbia does not make their own medications most of the time, thus they import various medications from surrounding countries. . . . [T]he citizens that do not turn to the health care system do not understand how to use the medications that they buy over the counter or the ones that are prescribed to them. The instructions are often in Swedish or in English, making it difficult to use them."

PATIENT EDUCATION

- ❖ Female patients taking antifungal medications for the treatment of vaginal infections should abstain from sexual intercourse until the treatment is completed and the infection is resolved. They should be instructed to continue to take the medication even if actively menstruating. Patients should notify the physician if symptoms persist after treatment is completed.
- ❖ Some patients receiving amphotericin B may need long-term treatment (i.e., over weeks to months). If so, patients should be advised of the adverse effects, including tinnitus, blurred vision, burning and itching at the infusion site, headache, rash, fever, chills, hypokalemia, gastrointestinal upset, and anemias. Patients should weigh themselves weekly and notify the physician if they gain more than 1 kg in a 24-hour period or 2 kg or more in 1 week. Muscle weakness may occur from hypokalemia, thus serum potassium needs to be monitored.
- ❖ Patients taking caspofungin should report immediately to the appropriate physician or health care provider any problems with shortness of breath, itching, facial swelling, or a rash.
- ❖ Patients taking fluconazole need to be informed that it may cause dizziness; they should not drive

until adverse effects are resolved. Good hygiene is recommended.
- ❖ Patients should be instructed to take griseofulvin exactly as prescribed, which is usually over weeks or months. Patients should be informed of its interaction with alcohol, with resultant flushing of the face and tachycardia. Photosensitivity may occur, thus patients should use sunscreen, wear protective clothing, and avoid exposure to the sun. Patients should also be advised to take the drug with foods high in fat (e.g., milk, ice cream) because they reduce gastrointestinal upset and encourage drug absorption.
- ❖ Patients should be educated about proper dosing instructions related to nystatin; they should be fully informed about how to apply the drug. If vaginal troches are used, the appropriate applicator should be used with a gloved hand and inserted high into the vagina, followed by hand washing. Advise patients to avoid sexual intercourse until treatment is completed. With oral nystatin, patients should rinse with 5 mL of the medication for 2 minutes after meals and at bedtime and then spit it out. Patients should not eat or drink for 30 minutes after treatment. Patients with pharyngeal involvement may be directed to rinse the mouth and then swallow.

Continued

❖ Patients should be instructed to take itraconazole capsules with food. If therapy lasts 3 months or longer, patients should be encouraged to continue with the medication. Patients should also be instructed to report any occurrence of anorexia, dark orange urine, nausea, vomiting, yellow skin, or unusual fatigue.

❖ Patients should be educated that ketoconazole requires an "acidic" environment. If taking antacids, anticholinergics, or H_2 receptor blockers, they should take the ketoconazole 2 hours after dosing. Shampoo forms should be applied to wet hair, massaged for a full minute, rinsed thoroughly, and reapplied for 3 minutes, as ordered, followed by rinsing. Topical dosing should be applied carefully, preventing contact to eyes, mucous membranes, and the mouth. If there are new symptoms or if the patient develops dark orange urine, irritation at topical site, onset of new symptoms, or pale stool or yellow skin or eyes, the physician should be contacted immediately.

❖ Patients should be encouraged to keep affected body areas clean and dry and to wear light and cool clothing. Patients should avoid contact of the topical dosage form with their eyes, mouth, nose, or other mucous membranes, and they need to report any adverse effects such as skin irritation and diarrhea.

❖ Patients should be instructed to take voriconazole 1 hour before or 1 hour after meals. Because voriconazole can cause visual changes, for example, blurred vision or photophobia, patients should be encouraged to avoid driving at night. Patients should also be advised to avoid direct sunlight and to use effective contraception.

POINTS TO REMEMBER

❖ Fungi are a large and diverse group of microorganisms and consist of yeast and moulds. Yeasts are single-celled fungi that may be harmful (e.g., causing infections) or helpful (e.g., when baking or brewing beer). Moulds are multicellular and characterized by long, branching filaments called *hyphae.*

❖ Candidiasis is an opportunistic fungal infection caused by *Candida albicans* and occurs in patients taking broad-spectrum antibiotics, antineoplastics, or immunosuppressants, and in immunocompromised persons. When candidiasis occurs in the mouth, it is commonly termed *oral candidiasis* or *thrush.* It is more commonly seen in newborns or immunocompromised persons.

❖ Vaginal candidiasis is a yeast infection that occurs primarily in women with diabetes mellitus, women taking oral contraceptives, and pregnant women.

❖ Antifungals may be administered either systemically or topically. Some of the most common systemic antifungal drugs are amphotericin B, fluconazole, itraconazole, and ketoconazole; some of the most common topical antifungals are clotrimazole, miconazole, and nystatin. Several chemical categories of antifungal drugs include both topical and systemic drugs, each with its own unique way of killing fungi.

❖ Before administering antifungals, the nurse must thoroughly assess for allergies and other drugs that patients are taking, including prescription drugs, over-the-counter drugs, and natural health products.

❖ Amphotericin B must be properly diluted according to the manufacturer's guidelines and administered using an intravenous infusion pump. Tissue extravasation of fluconazole at the intravenous infusion site leads to tissue necrosis; therefore, the site should be checked hourly and the assessment documented.

EXAMINATION REVIEW QUESTIONS

1 The nurse is assessing a patient who is about to receive antifungal drug therapy. Which problem would be of most concern?
   a. Heart disease
   b. Liver disease
   c. Endocrine disease
   d. Pulmonary disease

2 While monitoring a patient who is receiving intravenous amphotericin B, which adverse effect should the nurse expect to see?
   a. Bradycardia
   b. Hypertension
   c. Fever and chills
   d. Diarrhea and stomach cramps

3 Which of the following is a common underlying source of many of the drug interactions with antifungals?
   a. Polyuria
   b. Bone distribution
   c. Gallbladder metabolism
   d. Cytochrome P450 enzyme system

4 When monitoring the patient who is receiving griseofulvin, which potentially serious adverse effect should the nurse look for?
   a. Hypotension
   b. Blood dyscrasias
   c. Heart palpitations
   d. Gastrointestinal bleeding

5 When instructing a patient who is taking nystatin orally for oral candidiasis, which instruction by the nurse is correct?
   a. "Rinse for 5 minutes after meals and then spit out."
   b. "Rinse for 2 minutes after meals and then spit out."
   c. "Dissolve the medication in a glass of juice, then swallow."
   d. "The drug should be swallowed, followed by a glass of water."

For answers see http://evolve.elsevier.com/Canada/Lilley/pharmacology/.

CRITICAL THINKING ACTIVITIES

1 What laboratory data and other assessment data should be considered before administering any of the systemic antifungals? Specify the data and give the reason for their importance.

2 Explain the rationale for giving doses of antipyretics, antihistamines, and antiemetics to a patient who is receiving an amphotericin B infusion. When are these drugs given?

3 What instructions should accompany a prescription of ketoconazole?

For answers see http://evolve.elsevier.com/Canada/Lilley/pharmacology/.

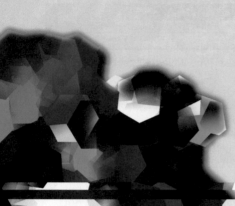

CHAPTER 43

Antimalarial, Antiprotozoal, and Anthelmintic Drugs

Learning Objectives

After reading this chapter, the successful student will be able to do the following:

1 Briefly discuss the infection process associated with malaria, protozoal infestations, and helminths.

2 Compare the signs and symptoms associated with malaria, protozoal, and helminthic infection processes.

3 Identify the more commonly used antimalarial, antiprotozoal, and anthelmintic drugs.

4 Discuss the mechanisms of action, indications, cautions, contraindications, adverse effects, dosages, and routes of administration associated with each antimalarial, antiprotozoal, and anthelmintic drug.

5 Develop a collaborative plan of care that includes all phases of the nursing process for patients receiving antimalarial, antiprotozoal, or anthelmintic drugs.

e-Learning Activities

Web site
(http://evolve.elsevier.com/Canada/Lilley/pharmacology/)

- Animations
- Answers to chapter questions, activities, and case studies
- Calculators and Category Catchers
- Glossary with audio pronunciations
- IV Therapy and Medication Error Checklists
- Multiple-Choice Review Question quizzes
- Nursing Care Plans
- Online Appendices and Supplements
- WebLinks

Drug Profiles

   atovaquone, p. 814
▸▸ chloroquine (chloroquine diphosphate)*, hydroxychloroquine (hydroxychloroquine sulfate)*, p. 808
▸▸ mebendazole, p. 817
   mefloquine (mefloquine hydrochloride)*, p. 808
▸▸ metronidazole, p. 814
   paromomycin (paromomycin sulfate)*, p. 814
   pentamidine (pentamidine isetionate)*, p. 814
   praziquantel, p. 817
▸▸ primaquine (primaquine phosphate)*, p. 809
   pyrantel pamoate, p. 817
   pyrimethamine, p. 809

▸▸ Key drug.

*Full generic name is given in parentheses. For the purposes of this text, the more common shortened name is used.

Glossary

Anthelmintics Drugs that destroy or prevent the development of parasitic worm (helminthic) infections; also called *antihelmintics* or *vermicides;* the terms for the drug categories are usually spelled with only one "h," in the second syllable, whereas the term for worm infection (*helminthic*) is spelled with two "h's," appearing in both the second and third syllables of the term. (p. 805)

Antimalarials Drugs that destroy or prevent the development of the malaria parasite (*Plasmodium* spp.) in human hosts. Antimalarial drugs are a subset of the antiprotozoal drugs, a broader drug category. (p. 805)

Antiprotozoals Drugs that destroy or prevent the development of protozoa in human hosts. (p. 805)

Helminthic infection A parasitic worm infection. (p. 812)

Malaria A widespread protozoal infectious disease caused by four species of the genus *Plasmodium*. (p. 805)

Parasite Any organism that feeds on another living organism (known as a *host*) in a way that results in varying degrees of harm to the host organism. (p. 805)

Parasitic protozoa Harmful protozoa that live on or in human beings or animals and cause disease in the process. (p. 805)

Protozoa Single-celled organisms that are the smallest and simplest members of the animal kingdom. (p. 805)

OVERVIEW

There are more than 28,000 known types of **protozoa,** which are single-celled organisms. Those that live on or in humans are termed **parasitic protozoa.** Billions of people worldwide are infected with these organisms; as a result, these infections are considered a serious health problem. Some of the more common protozoal infections are malaria, leishmaniasis, trypanosomiasis, amoebiasis, giardiasis, and trichomoniasis. Protozoal diseases are particularly prevalent among people living in tropical climates because it is easier for protozoa to survive and be transmitted in these year-round warm and humid environments. Although the population of Canada is relatively free of many of these protozoal infections, international travel and the immigration of people from other countries where such infections are endemic are providing opportunities for increased exposure. Also, the more common protozoal infections are becoming increasingly prevalent in Canada among immunocompromised persons, including those with AIDS.

The broad category of drugs used to destroy or prevent the development of protozoa in human hosts is called the **antiprotozoals. Antimalarials** are a subset of the antiprotozoals, specific for the destruction of the malaria protozoa (*Plasmodium* spp.). This chapter deals with the drugs that destroy or prevent the growth of malaria and nonmalarial protozoa, as well as the **anthelmintics** that are used against the larger multicellular human **parasites** such as tapeworms, flukes, and roundworms.

MALARIA

Malaria is the most significant parasitic disease. It was once thought possible it could be eradicated with the use of both antimalarial drugs and pesticides (specifically DDT, or dichloro-diphenyl-trichloroethane), but DDT was found to be environmentally hazardous, and the mosquito vector became resistant to the insecticide. Worldwide, it is estimated that 250 to 500 million people are infected, resulting in an annual death rate of 750,000 to 2 million people. Malaria is most prevalent in sub-Saharan Africa, Southeast Asia, and Latin America. In Africa, malaria accounts for more than 1 million infant deaths a year. Approximately 1.7 million Canadians travel annually to tropical countries that are potentially malaria endemic. As many as 400 to 1000 cases a year of imported malaria are reported to Health Canada. Some of these cases are severe and can result in death. Risks to Canadians for malaria infection are twofold: first, inappropriate recommendations for malaria prevention, and second, lack of knowledge about or adherence to appropriate recommendations for malaria prevention by the travelling public.

Malaria is caused by a particular genus of protozoa called *Plasmodium*. There are four species of organisms within this genus—*Plasmodium vivax, P. falciparum, P. malariae,* and *P. ovale*—each with its own characteristics and its own ability to resist being killed by antimalarial drugs. Although *P. vivax* is the most widespread of the four species, *P. falciparum* is almost as widespread and causes greater problems with drug resistance. The two remaining species are much less common and geographically limited in their occurrence, but they can still cause serious malarial infections. Most commonly, malaria is transmitted by the bite of an infected female *Anopheline* mosquito. This type of mosquito is endemic to many tropical regions of the world. Malaria can also be transmitted via blood transfusions, congenitally from mother to infant via an infected placenta, or through the use of contaminated needles by drug misusers. Despite the combined efforts of many countries to eradicate malaria, it remains the most devastating infectious disease in the world. As is also the case with tuberculosis (Chapter 41) and AIDS (Chapter 40), many lives are lost to malaria, and the cost of treating and preventing the disease imposes a tremendous economic burden on the often poor countries where the disease is prevalent.

The *Plasmodium* life cycle is quite complex and involves many stages. There are two interdependent life cycles: the *sexual cycle*, which takes place inside the mosquito, and the *asexual cycle*, which occurs in the human host. In addition, the asexual cycle of the parasite consists of a phase outside the erythrocyte (occurring primarily in liver tissues) called the *exoerythrocytic phase* (also called the *tissue phase*) and a phase inside the erythrocyte called the *erythrocytic phase* (also called the *blood phase*). The malarial parasite undergoes many changes during these two phases (Figure 43-1). Malaria signs and symptoms are often described in terms of the *classic malaria paroxysm*. A *paroxysm* is a sudden recurrence or intensification of symptoms. Symptoms include chills and rigor, followed by fever up to 40°C, and diaphoresis, often leading to extreme fatigue and prolonged sleep. This syndrome often repeats itself periodically in 48- to 72-hour cycles. Other common symptoms include headache, nausea, and joint pain.

ANTIMALARIAL DRUGS

Antimalarial drugs administered to humans do not affect the parasite during its sexual cycle when it resides in the mosquito. Rather, these drugs act against the parasite

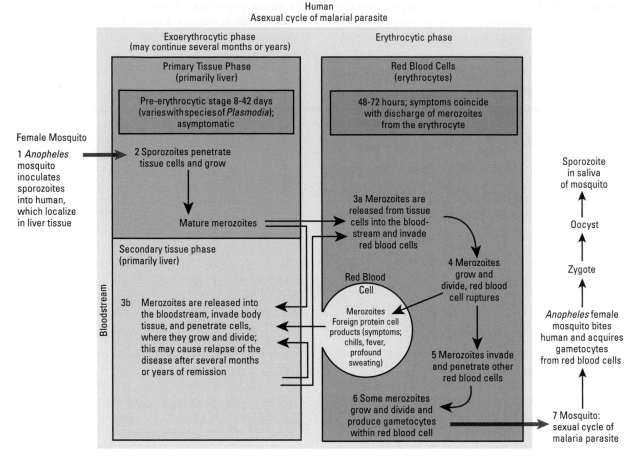

FIG. 43-1 The life cycle of the malaria parasite. (From McKenry, L., Tessier, E., & Hogan, M. (2006). *Mosby's pharmacology in nursing* (22nd ed.). St. Louis, MO: Elsevier Mosby.)

during its asexual cycle, which takes place within the host, the human body. Often antimalarial drugs are given in combinations to achieve an additive or synergistic antimalarial effect. One example is the combination of the two antiprotozoal drugs atovaquone and proguanil hydrochloride (Malarone). Malaria management is changing as the prevalence of drug-resistant malaria increases. For example, in Canada, doxycycline may be used to treat cases of drug-resistant malaria.

Mechanism of Action and Drug Effects

The mechanisms of action of the antimalarial drugs differ depending on the chemical family of drugs to which they belong. The *4-aminoquinoline derivatives* (chloroquine and hydroxychloroquine) act by inhibiting DNA and RNA polymerase, an enzyme essential to DNA and RNA synthesis by the parasite cells. Parasite protein synthesis is also disrupted because protein synthesis is dependent on functioning nucleic acid (DNA and RNA). Antimalarial drugs are believed to raise the pH within the parasite, which interferes with the parasite's ability to metabolize and utilize erythrocyte hemoglobin. This action accounts for the ineffectiveness of antimalarial drugs during the exoerythrocytic phase (tissue phase) of infection. All of these actions contribute to the destruction of the parasite. Quinine, quinidine, and mefloquine comprise another

family known as the *connexin 36 blockers*—these drugs block the action of the neuronal gap junction protein connexin 36, which is important for maintaining central nervous system homeostasis (state of equilibrium), particularly of the extracellular pH. These three connexin 36 blockers are thought to be similar to the 4-aminoquinoline derivatives in their actions in that both classes are believed to raise the pH within the parasite.

The *diaminopyrimidines* (pyrimethamine and trimethoprim [Chapter 38]) act by inhibiting dihydrofolate reductase, an enzyme essential for the production of certain vital substances in malarial parasites. Specifically, inhibition of this enzyme blocks the synthesis of tetrahydrofolate, a precursor of purines and pyrimidines (nucleic acid components), and certain amino acids (protein components) essential for the growth and survival of *Plasmodia* parasites. These two drugs are also only effective during the erythrocytic phase and are often used with a sulfonamide (sulfadoxine, Chapter 38) or sulfone (dapsone, Chapter 39) for synergistic effects exerted by such drug combinations. Tetracyclines such as doxycycline (Chapter 38) and lincomycins such as clindamycin (Chapter 39) may also be used in combination with some of the other antimalarial drugs described earlier, once again because of the synergistic effects resulting from these drug combinations.

Primaquine, an *8-aminoquinoline* that is structurally similar to the 4-aminoquinolines, has the ability to bind to and alter parasitic DNA and is one of the few drugs effective in the exoerythrocytic phase. Atovaquone/proguanil also works by interfering with nucleic acid synthesis.

The drug effects of the antimalarial drugs are typically limited to their ability to kill parasitic organisms, primarily *Plasmodium* spp. Some of these drugs have other drug effects as well. Chloroquine and hydroxychloroquine have anti-inflammatory effects and may be used in the treatment of rheumatoid arthritis and systemic lupus erythematosus. Quinine and quinidine, two plant alkaloids from the bark of the South American cinchona tree, can decrease the excitability of both heart and skeletal muscles. Quinidine is currently used to treat certain types of cardiac dysrhythmias (Chapter 23).

Indications

Antimalarial drugs are used to kill *Plasmodium* parasites. As previously indicated, different antimalarial drugs act during different phases of the parasite's growth inside the human. Those antimalarials exerting the greatest effect on all four *Plasmodium* organisms during the erythrocytic or blood phase are chloroquine phosphate, hydroxychloroquine sulfate, and pyrimethamine. Other drugs known to work in the blood phase are quinine sulfate, quinidine, halofantrine, and mefloquine hydrochloride. Halofantrine is not available in Canada. Because these drugs are ineffective during the exoerythrocytic phase, they cannot *prevent* infection. Health Canada, however, recommends the use of mefloquine hydrochloride for prevention and not as routine treatment for malaria because of the drug's adverse-effect profile.

The most effective antimalarial drug for eradicating the parasite during the exoerythrocytic or tissue phase is primaquine, which actually works during both phases; however, it is indicated specifically for *P. vivax*. Dormant forms of *P. vivax* remain in the liver, thus malaria can relapse after 2 or more years; primaquine is the drug of choice for preventing relapse. Chloroquine and related compounds (the 4-aminoquinolines) remain the drugs of choice for the prevention and treatment of susceptible strains of malarial parasites. They are highly toxic to all *Plasmodium* spp., except in resistant cases of *P. falciparum*, which occur in many areas of the world, including Asia, Africa, and South America. Chloroquine must be combined with primaquine for the treatment of malaria caused by *P. vivax* or *P. ovale*. According to the Canadian Recommendations for the Prevention and Treatment of Malaria Among International Travellers, individuals who are unable to tolerate chloroquine should use atovaquone/proguanil, doxycycline, or mefloquine.

Quinine sulfate is indicated orally for uncomplicated chloroquine-resistant *P. falciparum*, which can cause a type of malaria that affects the cerebral hemispheres. Quinine is commonly used in combination with a second drug such as pyrimethamine, a sulfonamide, or a tetracycline (such as doxycycline). Pyrimethamine is another antimalarial antibiotic that is commonly used in combination with

the fast-acting schizonitides chloroquine or quinine for treatment of acute attacks of malaria. Other antimalarial drugs are usually preferred for treatment of active disease. Mefloquine is a newer antimalarial drug that may be used for both prophylaxis and treatment of malaria caused by *P. falciparum* or *P. vivax*. The drug combination atovaquone and proguanil (Malarone) is also used for the prevention and treatment of *P. falciparum* infection.

Contraindications

Contraindications to the antimalarial drugs include drug allergy, tinnitus, and pregnancy (quinine). Severe renal, hepatic, or hematological dysfunction may also contraindicate the use of antimalarial drugs. Other drug-specific contraindications are noted in the Drug Profiles on p. 809.

Adverse Effects

Antimalarial drugs cause diverse adverse effects. The adverse effects for each drug are listed in Table 43-1.

TABLE 43-1

Antimalarial Drugs: Common Adverse Effects

Body System	Adverse Effects
CHLOROQUINE AND HYDROXYCHLOROQUINE	
Central nervous	Dizziness, vertigo, anxiety, headache
Gastrointestinal	Diarrhea, anorexia, nausea, vomiting, abdominal distress
Other	Alopecia, rash, pruritis, stomatitis, blurred vision, retinopathy, hair bleaching
MEFLOQUINE	
Central nervous	Headache, dizziness, vertigo, abnormal dreams, convulsions, depression, psychosis, anxiety
Dermatological	Rash, pruritis
Gastrointestinal	Abdominal discomfort, nausea, vomiting, diarrhea
PRIMAQUINE	
Gastrointestinal	Nausea, vomiting, epigastric distress, abdominal pain
Hematological	Leukopenia, hemolytic anemia primarily in individuals with G6PD deficiency, methemoglobinemia
PYRIMETHAMINE	
Gastrointestinal	Nausea, colic, vomiting, diarrhea, dryness of mouth and throat
Other	Fever, malaise, rash, leukopenia, anemia, thrombocytopenia, insomnia
QUININE	
Cardiovascular	Conduction disturbances, ventricular tachycardia, angina
Central nervous	Visual disturbances, dizziness, severe headaches, tinnitus, hearing loss
Gastrointestinal	Diarrhea, nausea, vomiting, abdominal pain or discomfort
Other	Rash, pruritus, hives, respiratory difficulties, wheezing, hypoglycemia

Interactions

Some common drug interactions associated with antimalarial drugs are listed in Table 43-2.

Dosages

For the recommended dosages for selected antimalarial drugs, see the Dosages table on p. 809.

TABLE 43-2

Antimalarial Drugs: Drug Interactions

Drug	Mechanism	Result
CHLOROQUINE		
cimetidine	Decreased metabolism of chloroquine	Increased serum chloroquine levels
Hepatotoxic drugs, alcohol	Increased chloroquine levels in liver	Increased hepatotoxicity
MEFLOQUINE		
β-blockers, calcium channel blockers, phenothiazines, nonsedating antihistamines, tricyclic antidepressants, quinidine, quinine	Unknown	Increased risk of dysrhythmia, cardiac arrest, seizures
PRIMAQUINE		
Other hemolytic drugs	Unknown	Increased risk for myelotoxic effects (monitor for muscle weakness)

💊 DRUG PROFILES

The dosing instructions for several of the antimalarial drugs can be confusing because tablet strengths on the medication packaging often indicate the strength of the tablet in terms of the entire salt form of the drug, not just the active ingredient, referred to as the *base ingredient*. Dosing guidelines often list recommended dosages for the base ingredient and not the entire salt. For example, chloroquine tablets come in a 250 mg strength of the salt form of the drug, but actually only have 150 mg of the active ingredient or base. The reader is advised to be mindful of this distinction.

▶▶ chloroquine diphosphate and hydroxychloroquine sulfate

Chloroquine diphosphate (generic only) is a synthetic antimalarial drug that is chemically classified as a 4-aminoquinoline derivative. It is also indicated for the treatment of other parasitic infections, such as extraintestinal amoebiasis. Hydroxychloroquine sulfate (Plaquenil) is another synthetic 4-aminoquinoline derivative that differs from chloroquine by a single hydroxyl group ($^-$OH). Its efficacy in treating malaria is comparable to that of quinine. Both medications also possess anti-inflammatory actions and have been used to treat rheumatoid arthritis and systemic lupus erythematosus since the 1950s. However, hydroxychloroquine is considered to be preferable to quinine for inflammatory illnesses because of its reduced risk of causing ocular toxicity at the high doses required.

Contraindications include known drug sensitivity and visual field changes, keeping in mind that sound clinical judgement may still warrant the use of the medication in urgent clinical situations.

Chloroquine and hydroxychloroquine are available in oral formulations. Both drugs are classified as pregnancy category C; it is recommended that use in pregnant women should occur only in truly urgent situations. These drugs are also distributed into breast milk, with one study demonstrating about one-third the level of chloroquine in breast milk as in the mother's bloodstream.

PHARMACOKINETICS

chloroquine diphosphate

Half-Life	Onset	Peak	Duration
PO: 3–5 days	PO: 8–10 hr	PO: 1–2 hr	PO: Variable

hydroxychloroquine sulfate

Half-Life	Onset	Peak	Duration
PO: 32–50 days	PO: Several hr*	PO: Few hr*	PO: Variable
	PO: 4–6 wk†	PO: Several mo†	

*For malaria.
†For rheumatic diseases.

mefloquine hydrochloride

Mefloquine hydrochloride (Lariam) is an analogue of quinine that is indicated for the management of mild to moderate acute malaria and for the prevention and treatment of chloroquine-resistant malaria and multidrug-resistant strains of *P. falciparum*, which is a difficult species of *Plasmodium* to kill. The drug is commonly used prophylactically by travellers to prevent malarial infection while visiting malaria-endemic areas. The tetracycline antibiotic doxycycline (Chapter 38) is also commonly used for this purpose. Recently, resistance to mefloquine has emerged in some regions, so mefloquine may not be used as primary prophylaxis of malaria in all cases. Mefloquine is available only for oral use.

PHARMACOKINETICS

Half-Life	Onset	Peak	Duration
PO: Days to weeks	PO: Less than 24 hr	PO: 7–24 hr	PO: Variable

Continued

DRUG PROFILES (cont'd)

◆◆ *primaquine phosphate*

Primaquine phosphate (generic only) is similar in chemical structure and antimalarial activity to the 4-amino-quinolines, but it is classified as an 8-aminoquinoline. However, as previously noted, it is one of the few drugs that can destroy malarial parasites in their exoerythrocytic phase (tissue phase). It is indicated for curative therapy in acute cases of *P. vivax*, *P. ovale*, and, to a lesser degree, *P. falciparum* infection.

Primaquine is contraindicated in patients with a known hypersensitivity to it, as well as in those with anemia, lupus erythematosus, and rheumatoid arthritis. It is available for oral use.

PHARMACOKINETICS

Half-Life	Onset	Peak	Duration
PO: 3–6 hr	PO: Less than 2 hr	PO: 1–3 hr	PO: 24 hr

pyrimethamine

Pyrimethamine (Daraprim) is a synthetic antimalarial drug that is structurally related to trimethoprim (Chapter 38). Both drugs are chemically subclassified as *diaminopyrimidines*. Pyrimethamine is contraindicated in patients with known drug allergy to it or with megaloblastic anemia caused by folate deficiency. It is available only for oral use.

PHARMACOKINETICS

Half-Life	Onset	Peak	Duration
PO: 4 days	PO: Less than 6 hr	PO: 2–6 hr	PO: Up to 2 wk

DOSAGES   Selected Antimalarial Drugs

Drug (Pregnancy Category)	Pharmacological Class	Usual Dosage Range	Indications
atovaquone/ proguanil hydrochloride* (Malorone) (C)	Antimalarial	*Children* PO: 11–20 kg: 1 tab/day 21–30 kg: 2 tabs/day 31–40 kg: 3 tabs/day For all weights: Start 1–2 days before entering endemic area and continuing × 7 days after leaving endemic area† *Adult over 40 kg* PO: 1 tab/day start 1–2 days before entering endemic area and continuing × 7 days after leaving endemic area†	Malaria prophylaxis of *P. falciparum*
		Children PO: 11–20 kg: 1 adult tab/day 21–30 kg: 2 adult tabs/day 31–40 kg: 3 adult tabs/day × 3 days *Adult over 40 kg* PO: 4 tabs daily × 3 days	Malaria treatment of *P. falciparum*
◆◆ chloroquine diphosphate (C)	Synthetic antimalarial and antiamoebic	*Children* PO: 8.3 mg base/kg weekly beginning 2 wk before exposure, or 10 mg base/kg in 2 divided doses 6 hr apart at exposure, and continuing for 8 wk after leaving endemic area *Adult* PO: 500 mg (300 mg base) weekly, beginning 2 wk before exposure, or 800 mg at exposure, and continuing for 8 wk after leaving endemic area	Malaria prophylaxis
		Children PO: 25 mg base/kg followed by 5 mg base/kg given 6, 24, and 48 hr later *Adult* PO: 1000 mg day 1, followed by 500 mg 6–8 hr later and daily for days 2 and 3	Malaria treatment

Continued

DOSAGES Selected Antimalarial Drugs (cont'd)

Drug (Pregnancy Category)	Pharmacological Class	Usual Dosage Range	Indications
▸▸hydroxychloroquine sulfate (Plaquenil) (C)	Synthetic antimalarial	*Infants and Children* PO: 5 mg base/kg 2 wk before exposure and 8 wk after, taken on exactly same day each wk *Adult* PO: 400 mg 2 wk before exposure and 8 wk after, taken on exactly same day each wk	Malaria prophylaxis
		Infants and Children Dosage calculated by body weight is preferred; total dose representing 25 mg base/kg given over 3 days as follows: PO: 10 mg base/kg (not to exceed 620 mg base), then 5 mg base/kg (not to exceed 310 mg base) 6 hr later, then 5 mg base/kg 18 hr later, then 5 mg base/kg 24 hr later	Malaria treatment
		Adult PO: Loading dose of 800 mg day 1, followed by 400 6–8 hr later and daily for days 2 and 3. Single dose of 800 mg also effective. Dosage may be calculated by body weight	Treatment of acute malaria attack
mefloquine hydrochloride (Lariam) (C)	Synthetic antimalarial	*Children/Adult 45 kg or less* PO: Weekly dosing, beginning 1 wk before travel and continuing until 4 wk after leaving endemic area, based on weight as follows: 5 to less than 20 kg: $\frac{1}{4}$ tab 20 to less than 30 kg: $\frac{1}{2}$ tab 30 to less than 45 kg: $\frac{3}{4}$ tab Over 45 kg: 1 tab (250 mg) *Adult over 45 kg* PO: 250 mg base weekly beginning 1 wk before travel and continuing until 4 wk after leaving endemic area	Malaria prophylaxis
		Children/Adult PO: 15–25 mg/kg in a single dose, not to exceed 1250 mg	Malaria treatment of mild to moderate malaria caused by susceptible strains of *P. falciparum* or *P. vivax* or chloroquine-resistant *P. falciparum*
▸▸primaquine phosphate (C)	Synthetic antimalarial	*Children* 0.39 mg base/kg/day daily × 14 days *Adult* PO: 15 mg base daily × 14 days	For cure or relapse prevention of malaria infection with *P. vivax, P. ovale*; may also be used for *P. vivax* or *P. ovale* prophylaxis in patients intolerant of chloroquine or if chloroquine is not available
pyrimethamine (Daraprim) (C)	Folic acid antagonist, antimalarial, antitoxoplasmotic drug	*Children 4–10 yr* PO: 25 mg daily × 2 days *Children older than 10 yr/Adult* PO: 50 mg daily × 2 days	Malaria treatment

*Each tablet of Malarone contains atovaquone 250 mg and proguanil hydrochloride 100 mg. Each Malarone Pediatric tablet contains atovaquone 62.5 mg and proguanil hydrochloride 25 mg.

†In addition to endemic areas, prophylaxis should be given for any other nonendemic area where prophylaxis for malaria is recommended by international travel health authorities.

OTHER PROTOZOAL INFECTIONS

Although malaria is the most common protozoal infection, there are several others, including amoebiasis, giardiasis, pneumocystosis, toxoplasmosis, and trichomoniasis. Like malaria, these infections are also more prevalent in tropical regions. The corresponding protozoal parasites that most often cause these infections are, respectively, *Entamoeba histolytica*, *Giardia lamblia*, *Pneumocystis jirovecii* (formerly *P. carinii*), *Toxoplasma gondii*, and *Trichomonas vaginalis*.

These protozoal infections can be transmitted in a number of ways: from person to person (e.g., via sexual contact), through the ingestion of contaminated water or food, through direct contact with the parasite, or by the bite of an insect vector (mosquito or tick). Parasitic infections can be systemic and occur throughout the body or they can be localized to a specific region. For example, amoebiasis most commonly affects the gastrointestinal tract (e.g., amoebic dysentery), whereas pneumocystosis is predominantly a pulmonary infection.

The more common protozoal infections are listed in Table 43-3, accompanied by a brief description of the infection and the antiprotozoal drugs commonly used in its treatment. Only selected drugs are discussed here. Patients whose immune system is compromised, such as those with leukemia, those with transplanted organs who are on immunosuppressive drugs, and those with AIDS, are at particular risk for acquiring a protozoal infection. Often such infections are fatal in these patients.

NONMALARIAL ANTIPROTOZOAL DRUGS

Several drugs are used to treat nonmalarial protozoal infections. Some of these (chloroquine, primaquine, pyrimethamine, and atovaquone) are also used in malaria treatment, as previously noted. Other antiprotozoal drugs normally used for nonmalarial parasites include metronidazole, paromomycin, and pentamidine.

Mechanism of Action and Drug Effects

Antiprotozoal drugs work by several different mechanisms. The most commonly used antiprotozoal drugs and a brief description of their mechanisms of action are provided in Table 43-4. Pyrimethamine and chloroquine were discussed earlier in this chapter in the section on malaria. The drug effects of these antiprotozoal drugs are primarily limited to their ability to kill various forms of protozoal parasites.

Indications

Antiprotozoal drugs are used to treat protozoal infections ranging from intestinal amoebiasis to pneumocystosis. Indications for selected drugs are summarized in Table 43-5. Atovaquone and pentamidine are used for the treatment of *P. jirovecii* infection. Metronidazole and paromomycin are used to treat intestinal amoebiasis, the usual causative organism being *Entamoeba histolytica*. Metronidazole is also effective against several forms

TABLE 43-3

Types of Protozoal Infections

Protozoal Infection	Description	Antiprotozoal Drug
Amoebiasis	Infection that resides mainly in the large intestine but can also migrate to other parts of the body, such as the liver. Produced by the protozoal parasite *Entamoeba histolytica*. It is usually transmitted in contaminated food or water.	chloroquine, metronidazole, paromomycin sulfate, tinidazole
Giardiasis	Caused by *Giardia lamblia*. The most common intestinal protozoal infection, usually residing in the intestinal mucosa (most commonly the duodenum). May cause diarrhea, bloating, and foul-smelling stools. Transmitted by contaminated food or water or by contact with stool from infected persons. In Canada is referred to as "beaver fever."	metronidazole, paromomycin sulfate, tinidazole
Pneumocystosis	Pneumonias caused by *Pneumocystis jirovecii* that occur almost exclusively in immunocompromised people. They are always fatal if left untreated.	atovaquone, dapsone, primaquine phosphate, pentamidine isethionate, sulfamethoxazole/trimethoprim, trimetrexate
Toxoplasmosis	Caused by *Toxoplasma gondii*. Can produce systemic infection in both immunocompetent and immunocompromised hosts. Domesticated animals, usually cats, serve as the intermediate host for parasites, passing infective oocysts in their feces.	dapsone, sulfamethoxazole/trimethoprim, sulfonamides with pyrimethamine, sulfadiazine
Trichomoniasis	Sexually transmitted infection caused by *Trichomonas vaginalis*	metronidazole, tinidazole

TABLE 43-4

Antiprotozoal Drugs: Mechanisms of Action

Antiprotozoal Drug	Mechanism of Action
atovaquone	Selectively inhibits mitochondrial electron transport, reducing ATP synthesis (required for cellular energy). It also inhibits nucleic acid synthesis.
metronidazole	Bactericidal, amoebicidal, and trichomonacidal. It can also kill anaerobic bacteria, which it accomplishes by disrupting nucleic acid synthesis.
paromomycin sulfate	Also a luminal or contact amoebicide. This direct-acting drug kills by inhibiting protein synthesis in susceptible bacteria by binding to the 30S ribosomal subunit.
pentamidine isethionate	Inhibits production of much-needed substances such as DNA and RNA. Can bind to and aggregate ribosomes. It is directly lethal to *Pneumocystis jirovecii* by inhibiting glucose metabolism, protein and RNA synthesis, and intracellular amino acid transport.
tinidazole	Possibly reaction involving a nitrogen free radical

ATP, adenosine triphosphate.

TABLE 43-5

Indications for Selected Antiprotozoal Drugs

Antiprotozoal Drug	Drug Effects
atovaquone	Used for the treatment of acute mild to moderately severe *Pneumocystis jirovecii* pneumonia in patients who cannot tolerate trimoxazole/sulfamethoxazole
dapsone	Used in the prophylaxis of *Pneumocystis jirovecii* pneumonia in patients who cannot tolerate trimoxazole/sulfamethoxazole
metronidazole	An antibacterial (including anaerobes), antiprotozoal, and anthelmintic drug
paromomycin	Indicated for the treatment of acute and chronic intestinal amoebiasis
pentamidine isethionate	Used for the prevention and treatment of *P. jirovecii* pneumonia
sulfamethoxazole-trimethoprim	Drug of choice for the prevention and treatment of *P. jirovecii* pneumonia
tinidazole	Indicated for giardiasis, trichomoniasis, and amoebiasis

of bacteria, including anaerobic bacteria (Chapter 39), as well as against protozoa and helminths (parasitic worms). Worm infection (helminthiasis) is discussed later in this chapter.

Contraindications

Contraindications to the use of antiprotozoal drugs include known drug allergy. Additional contraindications may include serious renal, liver, or other illnesses, weighing the seriousness of the infection against the patient's overall condition.

Adverse Effects

The adverse effects of antiprotozoal drugs vary depending on the drug. The specific adverse effects to common antiprotozoal drugs are listed in Table 43-6.

Interactions

The common drug and laboratory test interactions associated with the use of antiprotozoal drugs are listed in Table 43-7. Some of these interactions can result in severe

toxicities, thus it is important to know them and to understand the mechanism involved.

Dosages

For dosage information on selected antiprotozoal drugs, see the Dosages table on p. 815.

HELMINTHIC INFECTIONS

Parasitic **helminthic infections** (worm infections) are a worldwide problem. No country is spared. It has been estimated that one third of the world's population is infected with parasitic helminths. Those who live in developing countries where sanitary conditions are often poor are by far the most common victims. The incidence of worm infections in the inhabitants of developed countries where sewage treatment is adequate is much lower; usually only a few select helminthic diseases occur under these conditions. The most prevalent helminthic infection in Canada is enterobiasis, caused by one genus of roundworm, *Enterobius*.

TABLE 43-6

Adverse Effects for Selected Antiprotozoal Drugs

Body System	Adverse Effects
ATOVAQUONE	
Cardiovascular	Hypotension
Central nervous	Dizziness, headache, anxiety
Gastrointestinal	Anorexia, increased AST and ALT levels, acute pancreatitis, nausea, vomiting, diarrhea, constipation, abdominal pain, dyspepsia
Hematological	Anemia, neutropenia
Integumentary	Pruritus, urticaria, rash, oral candidiasis
Metabolic	Hypoglycemia
Respiratory	Sinusitis, rhinitis, cough
Other	Sweating, fever
METRONIDAZOLE	
Cardiovascular	Palpitation, chest pain
Central nervous	Headache, dizziness, confusion, fatigue, convulsions, peripheral neuropathy, transient ataxia, insomnia
Gastrointestinal	Nausea, vomiting, diarrhea, anorexia, dyspepsia, constipation, dry mouth, glossitis, stomatitis, oral candidiasis, unpleasant metallic taste, *C. difficile* colitis (rare)
Genitourinary	Darkened urine, dysuria, vaginal *C. albicans*
Hematological	Leukopenia, transient eosinophilia
Integumentary	Rash, pruritus
PAROMOMYCIN	
Central nervous	Hearing loss, dizziness, tinnitus
Gastrointestinal	Stomach cramps, nausea, vomiting, diarrhea
PENTAMIDINE ISETIONATE	
Cardiovascular	Hypotension, dysrhythmias
Central nervous	Disorientation, hallucinations, dizziness, confusion
Gastrointestinal	Increased AST and ALT levels, acute pancreatitis, metallic taste, nausea, vomiting, diarrhea
Genitourinary	Acute kidney failure
Hematological	Anemia, leukopenia, thrombocytopenia
Integumentary	Pain at injection site, pruritus, urticaria, rash
Metabolic	Hyperkalemia, hypocalcemia, hypoglycemia followed by hyperglycemia
Respiratory	Cough, shortness of breath, bronchospasm
Other	Fatigue, chills, night sweats

AST, aspartate aminotransferase; *ALT*, alanine aminotransferase.

TABLE 43-7

Antiprotozoal Drugs: Drug and Laboratory Test Interactions

Antiprotozoal Drug	Mechanism	Result
atovaquone	Compete for binding on protein, resulting in free, active atovaquone	Highly protein-bound drugs (e.g., warfarin, phenytoin): may increase atovaquone drug concentrations and risk of adverse reactions
metronidazole	Increased plasma acetaldehyde concentration after ingestion of alcohol by decreasing the absorption of vitamin K from the intestines as a result of eliminating the bacteria needed to absorb vitamin K	Alcohol: causes a disulfiram-like reaction warfarin: may increase action of warfarin (increased bleeding risk)
paromomycin pentamidine	Additive nephrotoxic effects	Use with an aminoglycoside, amphotericin B, colistin, cisplatin, methoxyflurane, polymyxin B, or vancomycin may result in nephrotoxicity

DRUG PROFILES

Antiprotozoal drugs are used for a number of infectious diseases, including infections with *Pneumocystis jirovecii* and *Trichomonas vaginalis*, amoebic dysentery (*Entamoeba histolytica*), toxoplasmosis, and giardiasis, among many others. All require a prescription and are available in a number of dosage forms, including oral, injectable, and inhalation aerosol.

atovaquone

Atovaquone (Mepron) is a synthetic antiprotozoal drug indicated for the treatment of mild to moderate *P. jirovecii* pneumonia in patients who cannot tolerate sulfamethoxazole/trimethoprim (Chapter 38). It is only available for oral use.

PHARMACOKINETICS

Half-Life	Onset	Peak	Duration
PO: 2–3 days	PO: 8–24 hr	PO: 24–96 hr	PO: Unknown

▶▶ *metronidazole*

Metronidazole (Flagyl) is an antiprotozoal drug that also has fairly broad antibacterial activity as well as anthelmintic activity. The therapeutic uses of metronidazole are varied and range from the treatment of trichomoniasis, amoebiasis, and giardiasis to that of anaerobic bacterial infections, and antibiotic-induced pseudomembranous colitis (Chapters 38 and 39). However, it can sometimes also cause pseudomembranous colitis. Metronidazole is believed to directly kill protozoa by causing free-radical reactions that damage their DNA and other vital biomolecules. Tinidazole is a newer, similar drug, available as Fasigyn through the Special Access Programme, Health Canada.

Contraindications to metronidazole use include known drug allergy and the first trimester of pregnancy. It is available in oral and parenteral form as well as topical preparations.

PHARMACOKINETICS

Half-Life	Onset	Peak	Duration
PO: 8–12 hr	PO: More than 1.5 hr	PO: 1–2 hr	PO: Variable

paromomycin sulfate

Paromomycin sulfate (Humatin) is an aminoglycoside antibiotic used for the treatment of intestinal amoebiasis. It directly kills intestinal protozoa when it comes into contact with them. Its bactericidal activity appears to be related to its ability to inhibit protein synthesis in susceptible organisms by binding to the 30S ribosomal subunit. Contraindications include known drug allergy and gastrointestinal obstruction. The drug is only available for oral use.

PHARMACOKINETICS

Half-Life	Onset	Peak	Duration
PO: Unknown	PO: Unknown	PO: Unknown	PO: Unknown

pentamidine isetionate

Pentamidine isetionate (generic only) is an antiprotozoal drug used mainly for the management of *P. jirovecii* pneumonia. It acts by inhibiting protein and nucleic acid synthesis. Hypersensitivity to the drug is the sole contraindication to its use. The drug should be used with caution in patients with blood dyscrasias, liver or kidney disease, diabetes mellitus, heart disease, hypocalcemia, or hypertension. Pentamidine is available solely for parenteral use. Intramuscular injections of pentamidine have been associated with pain, tenderness, redness, and induration at the site and should be used only in patients with sufficient muscle mass and when intravenous infusion is not feasible.

PHARMACOKINETICS

Half-Life	Onset	Peak	Duration
IV: 9–13 hr	IV: 0.5–1 hr	IV: Under 1 hr	IV: Variable

Helminths that are parasitic in humans are classified as follows:

- Platyhelminthes (flatworms)
- Cestodes (tapeworms)
- Trematodes (flukes)
- Nematoda (roundworms)

The characteristics of a few of the most common of the many helminthic infections are summarized in Table 43-8. Such infections usually begin in and reside in the intestines of their host, but they can sometimes also migrate to other tissues.

ANTHELMINTIC DRUGS

Unlike protozoa, which are single-celled members of the animal kingdom, helminths are larger and have complex multicellular structures. Anthelmintic drugs (also spelled *anthelminthic)* work to destroy these organisms by disrupting their structures. The currently available anthelmintic drugs in Canada are specific in the worms that they can kill. For this reason, the causative worm in an infected host should be accurately identified before the start of treatment. However, there are some scenarios in which the suspected worm will be treated. Worm identification can usually be done by analyzing a sample of feces, urine, blood, sputum, or tissue from the infected host for the presence of the particular parasite ova or larvae.

There are three anthelmintics that are commercially available in Canada for human use:

- mebendazole (Vermox)
- praziquantel (Biltricide)
- pyrantel pamoate (Combantrin, Jaa Pyral)

Other drugs, such as niclosamide and piperazine, may be available either in other countries or by special request to Health Canada. As previously mentioned, anthelmintics are specific in their actions. Mebendazole can be used to treat both tapeworms and roundworms. Praziquantel is a drug that can kill flukes (trematodes).

DOSAGES   Selected Antiprotozoal Drugs

Drug	Pharmacological Class	Usual Dosage Range	Indications
atovaquone* (Mepron) (C)	Synthetic antipneumocystis drug	*Adult* PO: 750 mg bid with meal × 21 days	Treatment of active PJP
▸▸metronidazole (Flagyl) (X, first trimester; B, second and third trimesters)	Amoebicide, antibacterial, trichomonacide	*Children* PO: 35–50 mg/kg tid × 5–7 days *Adult* PO: 500–750 mg tid 3× 5–10 days	Amoebiasis, including amoebic liver abscess
		Children PO: 25–35 mg/kg/day divided bid × 5–7 days *Adult* PO: 250 mg bid × 5–7 days	Giardiasis
		Adult-only 1-day treatment PO: 2 g × 1 dose after a meal *Adult 10-day treatment* PO: 250 mg tid × 10 days	Trichomoniasis
paromomycin sulfate (Humatin) (C)	Antiamoebic aminoglycoside antibiotic (also has antibacterial properties, but is not normally used for this purpose)	*Children/Adult* PO: 25–35 mg/kg/day divided tid with meals × 5–10 days	Acute and chronic intestinal amoebiasis
pentamidine iestionate (generic) (C)	Synthetic antipneumocystis drug	*Children/Adult* IV/IM: 4 mg/kg/day by slow infusion × 14 days	Treatment of active PJP

PJP, Pneumocystis jirovecii pneumonia.

*A combination product containing atovaquone and proguanil is also used against malaria.

TABLE 43-8

Helminthic Infections

Infection	Organism and Other Facts
NEMATODA (INTESTINAL AND TISSUE ROUNDWORMS)	
Ascariasis	Caused by *Ascaris lumbricoides* (giant roundworm); resides in small intestine; treated with pyrantel or mebendazole
Enterobiasis	Caused by *Enterobius vermicularis* (pinworm); resides in large intestine; treated with pyrantel or mebendazole
PLATHELMINTHES (INTESTINAL TAPEWORMS OR FLATWORMS)	
Diphyllobothriasis	Caused by *Diphyllobothrium latum* (fishworm); acquired from fish; treated with niclosamide,* paromomycin sulfate, or praziquantel
Hymenolepiasis	Caused by *Hymenolepis nana* (dwarf tapeworm); treated with niclosamide, paromomycin, or praziquantel
Taeniasis	Caused by *Taenia saginata* (beef tapeworm); acquired from beef; treated with niclosamide, paromomycin, or praziquantel Caused by *Taenia solium* (pork tapeworm); acquired from pork; treated with niclosamide, paromomycin, or praziquantel

*Niclosamide is not available in Canada.

The most commonly used anthelmintics and the specific class of worms they can effectively kill are summarized in Table 43-9.

Mechanism of Action and Drug Effects

The mechanisms of action of the anthelmintics vary greatly from drug to drug, although there are some similarities among the drugs used to kill similar types of worms. The anthelmintic drugs and their respective mechanisms of action are listed in Table 43-10. The drug effects of the anthelmintic drugs are limited to their ability to kill various forms of worms and flukes.

TABLE 43-9

Anthelmintics: Class of Worms Killed

Anthelmintic Drug	Cestodes	Nematodes	Trematodes
mebendazole	Yes	Yes	No
niclosamide	Yes	No	No
pyrantel	No	Yes (giant roundworm and pinworm)	No
praziquantel	Yes	No	Yes

TABLE 43-10

Anthelmintics: Mechanisms of Action

Anthelmintic Drug	Mechanism of Action
mebendazole	Selectively and irreversibly inhibits the uptake of glucose and other nutrients. This results in depletion of endogenous glycogen stores, eventual autolysis of the parasitic worm, and death.
niclosamide	Inhibits mitochondrial oxidative phosphorylation; also decreases generation of ATP by inhibiting the uptake of glucose. Cestodes are then dislodged from the GI wall. The worm is digested in the intestine and subsequently expelled from the GI tract by normal peristalsis.
praziquantel	Increased permeability of the cell membrane of susceptible worms to calcium, resulting in a large influx of calcium. This causes the worms to be dislodged from their usual site of residence in the mesenteric veins to the liver, where they are killed by host tissue reactions. Dislodgement of worms is the result of contraction and paralysis of their musculature and subsequent immobilization of their suckers, which causes the worms to detach from the blood vessel wall and be passively dislodged by normal blood flow.
pyrantel	Blocks ACh at the neuromuscular junction, resulting in paralysis of the worm. The paralyzed worms are then expelled from the GI tract by normal peristalsis.

ACh, acetylcholine; *ATP*, adenosine triphosphate; *GI*, gastrointestinal.

TABLE 43-11

Anthelmintics: Indications

Anthelmintic Drug	Indications
mebendazole	Trichuriasis (whipworm), enterobiasis, ascariasis, *Ancylostoma* infection (common hookworm), *Necator* infection (American hookworm)
niclosamide	*Taenia saginata* infection, diphyllobothriasis, hymenolepiasis
praziquantel	Schistosomiasis, opisthorchiasis (liver fluke), clonorchiasis (Chinese or Oriental liver fluke), fishworm, dwarf tapeworm, neurocysticercosis
pyrantel pamoate	Ascariasis, enterobiasis, other helminthic infections

Indications

Anthelmintic drugs are used to treat roundworm, tapeworm, and fluke infections. Anthelmintic drugs and the particular helminthic infections they are used to treat are listed in Table 43-11.

Contraindications

The only usual contraindication to a specific anthelmintic drug product is known drug allergy. Pyrantel is contraindicated in patients with liver disease.

Adverse Effects

The anthelmintic drugs show a remarkable diversity in their drug-specific adverse effects. Common adverse effects are listed in Table 43-12.

Interactions

The anthelmintics are generally well tolerated. Pyrantel is not recommended in children under 1 year of age. The presence of the anticonvulsants (Chapter 14) carbamazepine and phenytoin may reduce the blood levels of mebendazole. Histamine H$_2$-antagonists (e.g., cimetidine, ranitidine) may raise blood levels of praziquantel.

Dosages

For dosage information for selected anthelmintic drugs, see the Dosages table on p. 817.

TABLE 43-12

Anthelmintics: Common Adverse Effects

Body System	Adverse Effects
MEBENDAZOLE	
Gastrointestinal	Diarrhea, abdominal pain
Hematological	Myelosuppression
PRAZIQUANTEL	
Central nervous	Dizziness, headache, drowsiness
Gastrointestinal	Abdominal pain, nausea
Other	Malaise
PRIMAQUINE	
Gastrointestinal	Nausea, vomiting, abdominal distress
Other	Headaches, pruritus, dark discoloration of urine, hemolytic anemia due to G6PD deficiency
PYRANTEL	
Central nervous	Headache, dizziness, insomnia
Dermatological	Skin rash
Gastrointestinal	Anorexia, abdominal cramps, diarrhea, nausea, vomiting

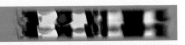

 DRUG PROFILES

Anthelmintics are available only as oral preparations and, with the exception of pyrantel, require a prescription. As illustrated in Table 43-11, different drugs are selected to treat infection with different helminthic species.

▶▶ *mebendazole*

Mebendazole (Vermox) is a synthetic anthelmintic drug that may be used in the treatment of several types of roundworm and a few types of tapeworm infections. It is available only for oral use.

PHARMACOKINETICS

Half-Life	Onset	Peak	Duration
PO: 3–6 hr	PO: Less than 2 hr	PO: 2–4 hr	PO: Variable

praziquantel

Praziquantel (Biltricide) is one of the primary anthelmintic drugs used for the treatment of fluke infections. It is also useful against many species of tapeworm. It is

contraindicated in patients who are hypersensitive to it and in patients with ocular worm infestation (*ocular cysticercosis*). It is available only for oral use.

PHARMACOKINETICS

Half-Life	Onset	Peak	Duration
PO: 0.8–1.5 hr	PO: Less than 1 hr	PO: 1–3 hr	PO: Variable

pyrantel pamoate

Pyrantel pamoate (Combantrin, Jaa Pyral) is a pyrimidine-derived anthelmintic drug indicated for the treatment of infection with intestinal roundworms, including ascariasis, enterobiasis, and other helminthic infections. It is available in Canada for oral use and can be purchased over the counter.

PHARMACOKINETICS

Half-Life	Onset	Peak	Duration
PO: Unknown	PO: Less than 1 hr	PO: 1–3 hr	PO: Unknown

DOSAGES   Selected Anthelmintic Drugs

Drug	Pharmacological Class	Usual Dosage Range	Indications
▶▶mebendazole (Vermox) (C)	General anthelmintic	*Children older than 2 yr/Adult* PO: 100 mg single dose, repeat in 2–4 wk PO: 100 mg bid × 3 days	Enterobiasis Trichuriasis, ascariasis, ankylostomiasis, strongyloidiasis, taeniasis, mixed infections
praziquantel (Biltricide) (B)	Trematode anthelmintic	*Children older than 4 yr/Adult* PO: approx 25 mg/kg tid × 1 day	Fluke infections, schistosomiasis
pyrantel pamoate (Combantrin, Jaa Pyral) (C)	Nematode anthelmintic	*Children older than 1 yr/Adult* PO: 11 mg/kg in a single dose (max dose 1 g)	Single or mixed infections of roundworm, pinworm, threadworm, and hookworm

NURSING PROCESS

▨ Assessment

Before beginning treatment with an antimalarial drug, the nurse should obtain a thorough medication history, head-to-toe physical assessment, and vital signs. Special attention should be paid to the manifestations of malaria (e.g., chills, profound sweating, headache, nausea, joint aching, and fatigue to exhaustion) and any symptoms documented. Other signs and symptoms include periodic diaphoresis and a remittent fever as high as 40° to 40.5°C. Baseline visual acuity, kidney function tests, gastrointestinal status, and electrocardiogram (ECG) are also important to assess and document because of drug-related adverse effects of cranial nerve VIII involvement (quinine and chloroquine), kidney impairment (quinine),

and cardiovascular problems (quinine). Contraindications, cautions, and drug interactions should be assessed for and noted prior to use of any of the antimalarials, antiprotozoals, or anthelmintics.

The contraindications, cautions, and drug interactions for the antiprotozoal drugs (discussed previously in the pharmacology section) should be noted and the patient should be assessed for kidney, heart, or liver dysfunction and for thyroid diseases. The patient's baseline visual acuity should be determined and documented prior to initiation of therapy. Metronidazole should be given only after there has been assessment of allergy to any of the nitroimidazole derivatives and to parabens with the topical dosage forms. Appropriate specimens should be obtained prior to treatment. Patients with blood dyscrasias, central nervous system disorders, and liver dysfunction require thorough assessment prior to use of antiprotozoal drugs.

With any of the anthelmintic drugs, a thorough history of foods eaten, especially meat and fish, and their means of preparation should be obtained. Other individuals in the family household should also be assessed for helminth infestation. Stool specimens are also indicated. Assessment of the patient's energy level, activities of daily living, weight, appetite, and any other symptoms should be noted. Along with contraindications and cautions, the nurse should assess for possible drug interactions (see Tables 43-2 and 43-7).

Nursing Diagnoses

- Risk for injury related to drug adverse effects
- Risk for impaired tissue integrity related to infestation-related lesions
- Risk for infection related to a break in skin integrity from infestation-related lesion
- Imbalanced nutrition, less than body requirements, related to the disease process and adverse effects of drugs
- Deficient knowledge related to the infection and its drug treatment
- Ineffective therapeutic regimen management related to poor adherence to treatment and lack of knowledge about the infection and its treatment

Planning

Goals

- Patient will be free of injury related to the adverse effects of medication.
- Patient will remain free of injury throughout the prescribed drug regimen.
- Patient will remain free of infection for the duration of therapy.
- Patient will maintain normal body weight during drug therapy.
- Patient will remain adherent to drug therapy for the prescribed length of time.
- Patient will experience minimal body image changes related to disease.
- Patient will state adverse effects of the medication, as well as symptoms or adverse reactions to report to the physician.

Outcome Criteria

- Patient states measures to minimize injury related to the adverse effects of drugs, such as dosing, time of day, and drug interactions.
- Patient states measures to prevent worsening of lesions and to minimize tissue injury, such as washing hands

thoroughly, reporting worsening of lesions as well as drainage, fever, or joint pain, and taking medication as prescribed.
- Patient lists foods according to the food guide pyramid that can be included in the patient's diet to improve overall health.
- Patient states the symptoms of the infection, such as fever, lethargy, and loss of appetite.
- Patient understands the rationale for treatment for the prescribed length of time.
- Patient states the symptoms to report to the physician, such as worsening of infection, anorexia, and fever.
- Patient conveys feelings about altered body image to the health care professional.
- Patient states the importance of adhering to therapy and returning for follow-up visits to the physician to monitor progress and for occurrence of adverse reactions.

Implementation

With antimalarials, the nurse needs to monitor, or have the patient monitor, urinary output (more than 600 mL/day). Liver function with attention to liver enzymes should also be assessed as ordered throughout the drug regimen. Antimalarials will concentrate in the liver first; therefore, baseline liver functions and subsequent blood tests should be assessed. This is especially true if the patient has a history of alcohol misuse or drinks a considerable amount of alcohol. Chloroquine and hydroxychloroquine are administered orally and should be given exactly as prescribed. Dosaging with specific attention to the loading doses, subsequent doses, prophylactic dosing, cautions, contraindications, and drug interactions should be followed as prescribed. Antimalarials should be taken with sufficient amounts of fluids, that is, 180 to 240 mL, with each dose, and fluids should be forced throughout the day. See Patient Education for further information.

Most of the antiprotozoal drugs (e.g., metronidazole) should be given with food when given orally. Quinine sulfate, an antiprotozoal, must be administered intact because it is very irritating to the gastrointestinal mucosa. Oral dosage forms of metronidazole should be given with food to decrease gastrointestinal upset. Intravenous (IV) infusions should infuse over more than 30 to 60 minutes and should never be given as IV bolus. During use of this drug, changes in neurological status should be reported to the health care provider.

All anthelmintic drugs should be administered as ordered and for the prescribed length of time. Any syrup forms of these drugs should be stored in tight and closed containers to prevent chemical changes in the drug. Stool specimens, if indicated with the anthelmintics or other antiparasitic drugs, should be collected with use of a clean container, and the stool should not come in contact with water, urine, or chemicals because of possible risk of destroying the parasitic worms. See Patient Education for more information on anthelmintic drugs.

◪ Evaluation

The nurse should monitor the patient for the therapeutic effects of the antimalarial, antiprotozoal, or anthelmintic drug being taken, such as improved energy level and decrease in or resolution of all symptoms. Evaluation of proper hygiene and prevention of spread of the infestation is also necessary. With these three groups of drugs, it is important to assess for the adverse effects associated with each of the drug groups: gastrointestinal upset, liver problems, anemias, thrombocytopenia, heart irregularities, or visual changes, including the risk for retinal damage, which may be irreversible. Antimalarial medications may precipitate hemolysis in patients with G6PD deficiency (mostly Black patients and those of Mediterranean ancestry); therefore, such patients should be closely monitored for this complication during the treatment protocol. With antiprotozoal drugs, the patient should be monitored for visual disturbances, gastrointestinal distress, blurred vision, and altered hearing. For those patients being treated with anthelmintics, adverse effects such as fever, pallor, anorexia, and sudden decrease in red blood cells (RBCs), white blood cells (WBCs), and hemoglobin (Hgb) should be noted.

PATIENT EDUCATION

❖ Antimalarials are known to cause gastrointestinal upset; however, this may be decreased if the medication is taken with food. Patients should be encouraged to contact their health care provider if they experience prolonged nausea, vomiting, profuse diarrhea, or abdominal pain. Patients should also be encouraged to immediately report any changes in vision or visual disturbances, dizziness, or pruritus or jaundice or yellowing of skin or sclera of the eye.

❖ Patients should be educated about the need for prophylactic doses, once prescribed, of antimalarials before visiting malaria-infested countries as well as receiving appropriate treatment upon return.

❖ With antimalarials, patients should be advised to avoid consuming alcohol.

❖ As with all medications, patients should be advised to keep antimalarials out of the reach of children.

❖ Patients should be informed about the adverse effects associated with quinine-containing drugs, such as dizziness, visual blurring, or yellow discoloration of the skin (often referred to as "cinchonism"). Patients should be instructed to take the entire course of medication.

❖ Patients should be instructed to take antiprotozoals exactly as prescribed, and the importance of adherence should be emphasized, as with any of the three groups of drugs.

❖ Patients should be encouraged to take metronidazole with food. Alcohol should be avoided when taking this drug, and any cough syrups or elixirs (they contain alcohol) should also be avoided.

❖ Patients should be informed to avoid activities that require mental alertness or quick motor responses while on metronidazole until their neurological responses have been determined to be back within normal limits.

❖ Patients taking metronidazole for a sexually transmitted infection should avoid sexual intercourse until the physician states otherwise. It should be stressed that this helps prevent transmission of the disease.

❖ Patients who are taking metronidazole for amoebiasis should be instructed in how to check stool samples correctly and safely and in proper disposal.

❖ Patients should be instructed that topical forms of the drug should be applied with a finger-cot or gloved hand and to avoid contact with the eyes. Patients may apply makeup or cosmetics after topical drug application.

❖ Patients with rosacea should be instructed to avoid alcohol as well as exposure to sunlight and to hot and cold temperatures and to hot and spicy foods.

❖ Metronidazole may precipitate dizziness, so patients should be instructed to be cautious with all activities until a response to the drug is noted and consistent.

❖ Patients should be instructed to take anthelmintics exactly as prescribed, and the importance of adherence should be emphasized. Patients should also be encouraged to notify the physician immediately if they experience fatigue; fever; pallor; anorexia; darkened urine; or abdominal, leg, or back pain, which could indicate a sudden decrease in RBCs, Hgb, or WBCs.

POINTS TO REMEMBER

❖ Malaria is caused by *Plasmodium*, a particular genus of protozoa, and is transmitted through the bite of an infected female mosquito. The drug primaquine attacks the parasite when it is outside the red blood cell (exoerythrocytic phase).

❖ Other common protozoal infections are amoebiasis, giardiasis, pneumocystosis, toxoplasmosis, and trichomoniasis. The most toxic protozoal infections are those caused by *Cryptosporidium* spp., *Isospora belli*, *P. jirovecii*, and *Toxoplasma gondii*.

❖ Protozoa are parasites that are transmitted through the following means: person-to-person contact, ingestion of contaminated water or food, direct contact with the parasite, and the bite of an insect (mosquito or tick).

❖ Antiprotozoals such as pentamidine are commonly used to treat *P. jirovecii* infections. Metronidazole is an antibacterial, antiprotozoal, and anthelmintic.

❖ Paromomycin directly kills protozoa such as *Entamoeba histolytica*.

❖ Anthelmintics are drugs used to treat parasitic worm infections caused by cestodes (tapeworms), nematodes (roundworms), and trematodes (flukes).

❖ Nursing considerations include assessment of contraindications, cautions, and drug interactions with the use of any of the antimalarials, antiprotozoals, and anthelmintics. Contraindications related to antimalarials include pregnancy, psoriasis, porphyria, G6PD deficiency, and a history of drug allergy. Contraindications to the use of antiprotozoals include hypersensitivity; underlying kidney, heart, thyroid, or liver disease; and pregnancy. Contraindications to the use of anthelmintics include a history of hypertension; hypersensitivity; visual difficulty; intestinal obstruction; inflammatory bowel disease; malaria; severe liver, kidney, or heart disease; and pregnancy.

EXAMINATION REVIEW QUESTIONS

1 The nurse is reviewing the medication history of a patient who is taking chloroquine. However, the patient's history does not reveal a history of malaria or travel out of the country. For which of the following conditions is the patient most likely taking this medication?
a. *Plasmodium*
b. Roundworms
c. Thyroid disorders
d. Rheumatoid arthritis

2 Which of the following would be appropriate to include in teaching patients about the adverse effects of antimalarials?
a. Antimalarials may cause increased urinary output.
b. Skin may turn "blotchy" while the patient is on these medications.
c. The patient may experience periods of diaphoresis, chills, and fever.
d. Antimalarials may leave a metallic taste in the patient's mouth and cause anorexia.

3 Which of the following should the nurse include information about when teaching a patient about the potential drug interactions with antimalarials?
a. warfarin
b. Antibiotics
c. Decongestants
d. acetaminophen

4 Before administering antiprotozoal drugs, which baseline assessment should the nurse review?
a. Prothrombin time
b. Hemoglobin level
c. Arterial blood gas
d. Serum magnesium

5 Which genus and species of protozoa is the target of antimalarial drugs?
a. *Plasmodium* spp.
b. *Candida albicans*
c. *Pneumocystis jirovecii*
d. *Mycobacterium tuberculosis*

For answers see http://evolve.elsevier.com/Canada/Lilley/pharmacology/.

CRITICAL THINKING ACTIVITIES

1 One of your patients has been taking the antiprotozoal drug metronidazole (Flagyl) for intestinal amoebiasis. What drug–food interaction is important to warn the patient about during therapy with this drug?

2 Your roommate is travelling to a country where there is high risk for malaria infection. She asks you what you

think the physician will order for her, if anything at all. After researching this, what would you most likely tell her that the physician will do or suggest?

3 A patient with a history of AIDS has a severe *Pneumocystis jirovecii* pneumonia. Discuss the treatment options for this infection.

For answers see http://evolve.elsevier.com/Canada/Lilley/pharmacology/.

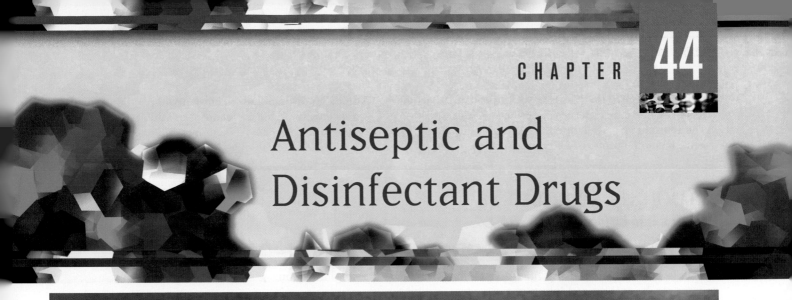

CHAPTER 44

Antiseptic and Disinfectant Drugs

Learning Objectives

After reading this chapter, the successful student will be able to do the following:

1 Identify the differences between antiseptics and disinfectants.

2 Identify the most commonly used and prescribed antiseptics and disinfectants.

3 Develop a collaborative plan of care that includes all phases of the nursing process related to the administration of antiseptics and disinfectants.

e-Learning Activities

Web site
(http://evolve.elsevier.com/Canada/Lilley/pharmacology/)

- Animations
- Answers to chapter questions, activities, and case studies
- Calculators and Category Catchers
- Glossary with audio pronunciations
- IV Therapy and Medication Error Checklists
- Multiple-Choice Review Question quizzes
- Nursing Care Plans
- Online Appendices and Supplements
- WebLinks

Drug Profiles

Acid agents, p. 825
Alcohol agents, p. 825
Aldehyde agents, p. 825
Biguanide agents, p. 825
Chlorine compounds, p. 825
Dyes, p. 825
Iodine compounds, p. 825
Mercurial drugs, p. 825
Oxidizing drugs, p. 826
Phenolic compounds, p. 826
Surface-active agents, p. 826

Glossary

Acid A compound that yields hydrogen ions when dissociated in solution. (p. 825)

Aldehyde Any of a large category of organic compounds derived from a corresponding alcohol by the removal of two hydrogen atoms, as in the conversion of ethyl alcohol to acetaldehyde. (p. 825)

Antiseptic One type of *topical antimicrobial* agent; a chemical that can be applied to the surfaces of both living tissue and nonliving objects that inhibits the growth and reproduction of microorganisms without necessarily killing them; also called a *static agent*. (p. 822)

Community-acquired infection An infection acquired from the environment, including infections acquired indirectly through the use of medications. (p. 822)

Disinfectant A second type of *topical antimicrobial* agent; a chemical applied to nonliving objects to kill microorganisms; also called a *cidal agent*. (p. 822)

Nosocomial infection An infection acquired at least 72 hours after hospitalization, often caused by *Candida albicans*, *Escherichia coli*, hepatitis viruses, herpes zoster virus, *Pseudomonas* organisms, or *Staphylococcus* spp.; also called *hospital-acquired infection*. (p. 822)

821

Spore (1) A resistant (hard to kill), dormant structure formed by certain bacterial species (e.g., *Bacillus* spp.). (2) The reproductive structure of certain lower microorganisms, including protozoa and fungi. (p. 823)

Topical antimicrobial A substance applied to any surface that either kills microorganisms or inhibits their growth or replication. (p. 822)

COMMUNITY-ACQUIRED AND NOSOCOMIAL INFECTIONS

Infectious organisms—bacteria, fungi, and viruses—can be acquired from a number of different sources, such as hospitals, workplaces, nursing homes, and home. These sources can be categorized into two main sites of origin: the community and the hospital. **Community-acquired infections** are defined as those infections that are contracted either in the home or any place in the community outside a health care facility. Hospital-acquired infections, more commonly known as **nosocomial infections**, are defined as those contracted in a hospital or institutional setting such as a nursing home and that were not present or incubating in the patient on admission to the hospital.

The particular organisms that cause these infections have changed over time. Of the two types of infections, nosocomial infections are much more difficult to treat, primarily because these causative microorganisms have been exposed to many strong antibiotics in the past, and those that are left alive in the hospital or institutional setting are the most drug-resistant and the most virulent ones. These pathogens and the reasons for their prevalence are summarized by different time periods in Table 44-1.

Nosocomial infections develop in 5% to 10% of hospitalized patients. The cost of treating them because of the extra hospitalization required amounts to nearly $3.9 million annually in Canada. Most of these infections (70% or more) are either urinary tract infections (UTIs) or postoperative wound infections. Often they are acquired from devices such as mechanical ventilators, intravenous (IV) infusion lines, catheters, and dialysis equipment. Areas of the hospital where the risk of acquiring a nosocomial infection is particularly high are the critical care, dialysis, oncology, transplant, and burn units. The host defences of patients in these areas are typically compromised, making them more vulnerable to infection.

TOPICAL ANTIMICROBIALS

Topical antimicrobials are agents that can be used to reduce the risk for nosocomial infections. They are substances that are applied to any surface for the purpose of either inhibiting or killing as many microorganisms as possible in a given pathogen population. There are two categories of these agents: antiseptics and disinfectants. **Disinfectants** are able to kill organisms and are used only on nonliving objects to destroy organisms that may be present on them. They are sometimes called *cidal agents*. **Antiseptics** generally only inhibit the growth of microorganisms but do not necessarily kill them and are applied exclusively to living tissue. They are also called *static agents*. The differences between disinfectants and antiseptics in a clinical sense are summarized in Table 44-2. Some antiseptic agents differ from disinfectants in their chemical makeup; others may simply be a diluted version of a disinfectant. Table 44-3 contains a list of these agents classified according to their chemical structure.

Mechanism of Action and Effects

Antimicrobial agents either inhibit the growth of microorganisms or destroy them, but the extent to which they do this depends on the number and type of microorganisms present, the concentration of the agent, the patient's temperature, and the time of exposure to the agent. The mechanisms of action of the antiseptics and disinfectants are summarized in Table 44-4.

TABLE 44-1

Changing Prevalence of Nosocomial Pathogens

Period	Cause for Change	Pathogen
Before 1940	No antibiotics	Group A streptococci
Mid-1950s	Antibiotic era	Coagulase-positive *Staphylococcus aureus*
Today	New antibiotics	Gram-negative bacilli (*Pseudomonas* spp.), fungi or yeast (*Candida albicans*), herpesvirus, MRSA, VRE spp.

MRSA, multidrug-resistant *Staphylococcus aureus*; *VRE*, vancomycin-resistant *Enterococcus*.

TABLE 44-2

Antiseptics Versus Disinfectants

	Antiseptics	Disinfectants
Activity against organisms	Primarily inhibits growth (bacteriostatic)	Kills (bactericidal)
Potency	Less	More
Toxic?	No	Yes
Where used	Living tissue	Nonliving tissue

TABLE 44-3

Disinfectants and Antiseptics: Chemical Categories

Drug	Antiseptic	Disinfectant
ACIDS		
Acetic	X	X
Benzoic	X	
Boric	X	
Lactic	X	
ALCOHOLS		
Ethanol	X	X
Isopropanol	X	X
ALDEHYDES		
Formaldehyde		X
Glutaraldehyde		X
BIGUANIDES		
Chlorhexidine gluconate	X	
DYES		
Carbol-fuchsin	X	
Gentian violet	X	
HALOGENS		
Chlorine Compounds		
Halazone		X
Sodium hypochlorite	X	X
Iodine Compounds		
Iodine (tincture and solution)	X	
Iodophors (povidone)	X	
Mercurials		
Merbromin	X	X
Thimerosal	X	
Yellow mercuric oxide	X	
Silver		
Silver nitrate	X	
NITROFURAZONE		
OXIDIZING AGENTS		
Benzoyl peroxide	X	
Hydrogen peroxide	X	X
Potassium permanganate	X	
PHENOLIC COMPOUNDS		
Cresol		X
Hexachlorophene	X	
Hexylresorcinol	X	
Resorcinol	X	
SURFACE-ACTIVE AGENTS		
Benzalkonium chloride	X	
Cetylpyridinium chloride	X	

Indications

Living tissue such as skin and mucous membranes cannot be sterilized. However, the risk of infection can be minimized by reducing the number of microorganisms on such tissues. Antiseptics are applied to these living tissues to inhibit the growth of the microorganisms that typically reside on the tissue surfaces (normal flora) and

that can do harm if they get into the body through an incision in the skin or by means of an injection. For example, these antiseptic agents are contained in the presurgical scrubs (soaps) used by members of surgical teams to wash their hands in preparation for surgery. They are also applied to the patient's skin before the incision is made. The degerming action is only temporary, however, and is limited to the skin surface. Antiseptics are also contained in ointments, mouthwashes, and douches.

Chapter 38 also describes how systemic drugs (e.g., cefazolin, 1 g intravenously preoperative) are often administered to surgical patients as prophylaxis against infection. Antimicrobial drugs, including antiseptics, are also commonly used to irrigate body cavities either directly during surgery or through transdermal catheter devices designed for irrigation purposes.

Inanimate objects such as tabletops and surgical equipment may be treated with disinfectants, as well as by autoclaving, radiation, and heat. These instruments acquire microbes by being placed on or inserted into anatomic sites in patients where many organisms naturally dwell (e.g., thermometers, which are placed orally, rectally, or under the axilla, and colonoscopes, which are used in examinations of the lower gastrointestinal tract [colonoscopy]). Before their use in other patients, the bacteria, fungi, viruses, and **spores** (dormant or reproductive structures of certain microorganisms) that may have been acquired from the previous patient's tissues must be removed from the instrument surfaces to prevent their transmission to others. The therapeutic effects of the antiseptics and disinfectants are listed in Table 44-5.

Contraindications

The only usual contraindication to the use of a particular antiseptic drug is known patient allergy to a specific product.

Adverse Effects

Antiseptics and disinfectants are normally safe agents, with the most common adverse effects, if any, being mild skin irritation. Although quite uncommon, other adverse effects that may occur are summarized in Table 44-6.

Interactions

Few drugs interact with the antiseptics, although other topical agents that also irritate the skin may produce an additive effect when given in combination with one of them. Two topical agents used together may also increase one another's rate of absorption, raising the risk for systemic toxicity, and should be administered separately when possible.

Dosages

For information on the recommended dosages and concentrations for selected antimicrobial drugs, see the Dosages table on p. 827.

TABLE 44-4

Antiseptics and Disinfectants: Mechanisms of Action

Drug	Mechanism of Action	Comments
Alcohols	Denature or essentially destroy the microorganism's protein; some may directly lyse the microorganism	60%–70% concentration, most effective; more than 90% or less than 60% concentration, ↓bactericidal activity
Aldehydes	Act via alkylation, inhibiting the formation of the essential amino acid methionine	Bacteriostatic or bactericidal depending on concentration
Biguanides	Disrupt bacterial cytoplasmic membranes and inhibit membrane-bound ATPase (inhibit cell wall synthesis)	Chlorhexidine
Halogens	Precipitate protein and oxidize essential enzymes by binding to and changing structure of proteins	Iodine compounds: bactericidal; mercurials: bacteriostatic; chlorine compounds: bactericidal
Oxidizing agents	Attack membrane lipids, DNA, and other essential components of the cell	3%–6% concentration: bactericidal and virucidal; 10%–25% concentration: sporicidal
Phenolic compounds	Interrupt bacterial electron transport (cellular respiration of microorganisms) and inhibit other membrane-bound enzymes; high concentrations rupture bacterial membranes	Bacteriostatic or bactericidal depending on concentration
Surface-active agents	Denature or essentially destroy the microorganism's protein, cell membrane, and cytoplasm components	↓Concentrations: bacteriostatic; ↑concentrations: bactericidal and fungicidal

ATPase, adenosine triphosphatase.

TABLE 44-5

Antiseptics and Disinfectants: Therapeutic Effects

Drug	Therapeutic Effects				
	Bacteria	Tubercle Bacilli	Fungi	Viruses	Spores
Alcohols	X	X	X	X	
Aldehydes	X	X	X	X	X
Chlorhexidine	X		X		
Chlorine compounds	X	X	X	X	
Dyes	X				
Iodine compounds	X	X	X	X	O
Mercurial compounds	X				
Oxidizing drugs	X			X	O
Phenolic compounds	X	X	X	X	
Silver compounds	X				
Surface-active agents	X		X	O	

X, static or cidal activity; *O,* some activity if high concentrations of drug and lengthy exposure are employed.

TABLE 44-6

Antiseptic and Disinfectant Drugs: Adverse Effects

Body System	Adverse Effects
ALCOHOLS	
Integumentary	Excessive dryness of the skin
ALDEHYDES	
Integumentary	Burns to skin or mucous membranes
CHLORHEXIDINE GLUCONATE	
Central nervous	Use as a preoperative scrub or as a wash for neonates and burn patients has been stopped because absorption from the skin into systemic circulation has resulted in serious CNS toxicity.
HEXYLRESORCINOL	
Cardiovascular	Myocardial toxicity resulting from systemic absorption from the skin
Hepatic	Toxicity resulting from systemic absorption from the skin
Integumentary	May produce burns on skin or mucous membranes
IODINE COMPOUNDS	
Integumentary	Iodine at concentrations greater than 3% may produce skin blistering. Burns may appear with *tincture of iodine* when the treated area is covered with an occlusive dressing. It may stain skin and cause irritation and pain at wound sites.
SURFACE-ACTIVE AGENTS	
Integumentary	Chemical burns if left in contact with skin for too long, as in wet packs for occlusive dressings

CNS, central nervous system.

DRUG PROFILES

Following are descriptions of the chemical categories of antimicrobials.

ACID AGENTS

Acetic (vinegar), benzoic, boric, and lactic acids are all members of the **acid** (H⁺ ion yielding) family of antiseptic and disinfectant agents. They are commonly used because of their practicality, availability, and low cost. All of these acid agents either kill microorganisms or inhibit their growth by creating an acidic environment for organisms that require a neutral or alkaline medium in order to live and grow. Acetic acid in a 5% solution kills many organisms. In this concentration, it is used as a vaginal douche for antisepsis and as a mild antiseptic-deodorant for the collection containers of indwelling urinary drainage catheters, for bladder irrigation, and for diaper soaks. The 1% solution may be used as a topical antiseptic for certain surgical wounds and burns.

ALCOHOL AGENTS

Isopropanol (isopropyl alcohol) and ethanol are both members of the alcohol category of antiseptics. The alcohol solutions are most effective at a concentration of 60% to 70%; at a concentration of more than 95% or less than 60%, their "cidal" activity dramatically decreases. These agents kill microorganisms by either denaturing their cellular proteins or directly lysing their cell membranes. Both isopropyl and ethyl alcohol are able to kill bacteria, tubercle bacilli, fungi, and viruses.

ALDEHYDE AGENTS

Formaldehyde and glutaraldehyde are members of the **aldehyde** (terminal carboxyl (O=CH) group containing) category of agents. Aldehyde disinfectants act by means of alkylation, inhibiting the formation of the essential amino acid methionine. This action either kills organisms or inhibits their growth, depending on the concentration of the solution. The aldehydes are active against all types of microorganisms, including bacteria, tubercle bacilli, fungi, viruses, and spores. Because these agents are somewhat caustic, they can cause burns to the skin or mucous membranes if used as antiseptics. For this reason they are used mostly as disinfectants. Formaldehyde comes in 5% and 23% concentrations and glutaraldehyde (Cidex) in 2.4% and 3.4% solutions. Both agents are commonly used as disinfectants for instruments, with glutaraldehyde preferred for disinfecting and sterilizing surgical equipment.

BIGUANIDE AGENTS

Chlorhexidine gluconate (Hibiclens, Hibitane) is a biguanide agent with antiseptic activity. Biguanides act by disrupting bacterial cytoplasmic membranes and inhibiting membrane-bound adenosine triphosphatase (ATPase), which results in the inhibition of cell wall synthesis. Chlorhexidine is active against both Gram-positive and Gram-negative bacteria. It is used as a bactericidal skin cleansing solution and is useful as a surgical scrub, a hand-washing agent for health care personnel, and a skin wound cleanser. It may also be used to treat aphthous ulcers of the mouth and for the prevention of dental caries, and is available in a prescription mouthwash for this purpose.

CHLORINE COMPOUNDS

Chlorine compounds actively kill bacteria, tubercle bacilli, and viruses but are only partially active against fungi. They have no activity against spores. Dilute sodium hypochlorite (Dakin's solution) is one of the chlorine compounds commonly used clinically as an antiseptic irrigation. Its antibacterial action is due to the hypochlorous acid that forms when chlorine reacts with water. Hypochlorous acid is rapidly antibacterial.

Sodium hypochlorite is available in many strengths, from 12% to 10.8% in a solution commonly used to disinfect utensils, walls, furniture, floors, and swimming pools, to a 0.5% solution used on skin surfaces for the treatment of fungous infections such as athlete's foot (tinea pedis). The strength of most household bleach solutions such as Javex or Clorox is 5.25% sodium hypochlorite. Intravenous drug users, who frequently share needles and are thus at increased risk for acquiring HIV, are given small bottles of bleach by public health outreach programs to use as a disinfectant for their injection equipment to help prevent the spread of HIV and other dangerous microbes.

Chloramines are chlorine-related compounds that are more stable, less irritating, and slower and more prolonged in their action than their chlorine cousins. The only chloramine product used in Canada, Chloramine T, is a whirlpool antiseptic, available in powder form, for sanitizing whirlpool water, in which it can kill water-borne pathogens within 30 to 60 minutes.

DYES

Gentian violet, crystal violet, methyl violet, brilliant green, and fuchsin are all rosaniline dyes. These are basic dyes that are currently used only occasionally as antiseptic or antiprotozoal agents. Gentian violet is used topically as a 1% preparation, and it has both antibacterial and antifungal activity.

IODINE COMPOUNDS

Iodine (tincture and solution) is a nonmetallic element that readily forms salts when combined with many other elements. Although it is a nonmetallic element, it has a bluish-black metallic lustre and a characteristic odour. It is only slightly soluble in water but is completely soluble in alcohol and in aqueous solutions of sodium iodide and potassium iodide. Iodine tincture and solution are both active against and kill all forms of microorganisms—bacteria, tubercle bacilli, fungi, viruses, and spores. Their activity against spores depends on the concentration and on the timing of administration. There are actually many forms of iodine, some of which are listed in Table 44-7.

MERCURIAL DRUGS

Topical mercurial antiseptics are relatively weak in their actions. They are primarily bacteriostatic drugs whose

Continued

DRUG PROFILES (cont'd)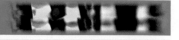

effectiveness is enhanced by the vehicle in which they are contained. Inorganic mercury compounds such as ammoniated mercury ointment owe their effectiveness primarily to these vehicles, which sustain the bacteriostatic action of the agent. Organic mercurial agents such as thimerosal are more bacteriostatic, less irritating, and less toxic than inorganic mercurials. Other examples of mercury compounds used as topical anti-infectives include merbromin, yellow mercuric oxide, and triclosan (Bacti-stat, Teraseptic), the anti-infective found in many over-the-counter antiseptic hand soaps.

Mercurial antiseptics probably act by inhibiting bacterial sulfhydryl enzymes, but they may also inhibit tissue enzymes as well, which reduces their usefulness. Ammoniated mercury is used for the treatment of psoriasis, impetigo, dermatomycoses, pediculosis pubis (crabs), seborrheic dermatitis, and superficial pyodermas (pus-producing skin infections). Skin irritations, as well as hypersensitivity to the agents, have been reported as adverse effects of these compounds.

OXIDIZING DRUGS

Hydrogen peroxide is one of three members of the oxidizing family of antiseptic agents; the other agents are benzoyl peroxide and potassium permanganate. Oxidizing drugs act by attacking membrane lipids, DNA, and other essential components of the microorganism's cell. In concentrations of 3% to 6%, they are bactericidal and virucidal; at 10% to 35%, they are sporicidal.

The use of hydrogen peroxide as a solution to irrigate wounds is controversial. Its use may be detrimental to wounds in that it can destroy newly forming cells as well as bacteria.

PHENOLIC COMPOUNDS

Cresol, carbolic acid (phenol), and Lysol are phenolic compounds used primarily as disinfectants. Because these agents cause burning and possibly blistering, they should not be allowed to come in contact with the skin in concentrations stronger than 2% and never in contact with areas where the skin is broken.

Phenolic compounds work by interrupting bacterial electron transport (cellular respiration of microorganisms) and inhibiting other membrane-bound enzymes. At high concentrations, they rupture bacterial membranes. Depending on the concentration of the phenolic compounds, they can be either bacteriostatic or bactericidal in their actions. The phenolic compounds are active against bacteria, tubercle bacilli, fungi, and viruses, but not spores. See the Dosages table on p. 827 for concentration information on carbolic acid. Hexachlorophene and resorcinol are two other phenolic compounds. Hexachlorophene is available by prescription only and is used as a surgical scrub as well as a bacteriostatic skin cleanser. Its use should be avoided with infants because they are particularly susceptible to transdermal absorption of this agent, with the risk of such serious neurotoxic effects as seizures. Resorcinol is bactericidal and fungicidal and is about one-third as effective as carbolic acid. It is used to treat acne, ringworm, eczema, psoriasis, seborrheic dermatitis, and similar skin lesions.

SURFACE-ACTIVE AGENTS

Benzalkonium chloride and cetylpyridinium chloride are surface-active agents. They act by denaturing the microorganism or essentially destroying its protein, cell membrane, and cytoplasm components. At low concentrations they are bacteriostatic, and at high concentrations they are bactericidal and fungicidal. These agents are used to treat bacteria, fungi, and some viral topical infections.

Certain substances, when used in combination with surface-acting agents, will absorb the active ingredient and consequently weaken the surface-acting agent. Substances such as organic matter, soaps, anionic detergents, and tap water that contain metallic ions are a few examples.

TABLE 44-7

Iodine Formulations

Iodine Formulation	Composition	Uses
Aqueous solution	5% iodine and 5% potassium iodide	These forms of iodine are used preoperatively to disinfect the skin. They are applied topically for their antimicrobial effects against bacteria, fungi, viruses, protozoa, and yeasts.
Iodine tincture	2% iodine in alcohol solution	
Iodine topical solution	2.5% iodine	
Strong iodine solution	5% iodine in alcohol	
Iodophors (Betadine, Rapidyne)	Iodine compounds with a carrier that acts as a sustained-release pool of iodine	Widely used as antiseptics
Povidone-iodine (Betadine)	Iodine with polyvinylpyrrolidone	Used as a 10% or 20% applicator solution or as a 2% scrub, spray, foam, vaginal gel, ointment, mouthwash, perineal wash, or whirlpool concentrate
Tincture of iodine	2% iodine and 2.5% potassium iodide in 83.7% ethyl alcohol	For cutaneous infections caused by bacteria and fungi. Even a 1% tincture will kill almost an entire bacterial population in 1.5 min. Three drops in 1 L of drinking water will reduce amoeba and bacteria counts in 15 min without impairing palatability.

DOSAGES   Selected Antiseptic and Disinfectant Drugs

Agent	Pharmacological Class	Usual Concentration or Dosage Range	Indications
acetic acid	Antibacterial, antifungal acid, antimicrobial	Solution: 2%, 4%–5% (vinegar)	Antibacterial, antifungal
benzalkonium chloride (Amino-Prophyl, Antimicrobe, Bac Liq, Bactol, others)	Broad-spectrum cationic detergent, surface-active antimicrobial	Solution: 2%, 5.12%, 9.4%, 10%, 14.8%, 0.13% Antiseptic towel/wipe: 0.4% Topical spray Topical liquid: 0.3% Otic solution/powder	Skin cleanser, instrument storage, surface cleaner
carbolic acid (phenol)	Phenolic antiseptic	Solution: 3%, 4% (combined with other agents)	Topical disinfectant
chlorhexidine gluconate (Hibiclens, Hibitane)	Broad-spectrum biguanide antimicrobial	Liquid: 0.05%, 2%, 4% Buccal: 0.12% Lotion: 2%	Cleanser, surgical scrub
formaldehyde (Formaline, Vapofene)	Broad-spectrum aldehyde antimicrobial	Solution: 0.05%, 0.23%, 37%	General disinfectant
gentian violet	Antibacterial, antifungal dye	Liquid: 1%, 2%; apply qd–bid	Topical antifungal
hydrogen peroxide (Accel, Vaprox, others)	Oxidizing drug	Buccal: 1.5% Solution: 2%, 3%, 3.95%, 6%, 7%, 35% Wipes: 0.5%	Wound cleansing, antiseptic
iodine	Broad-spectrum iodine antimicrobial	Solution/tincture: 2.5%, apply once to twice daily Mouthwash: 1% Topical: 10%	Topical antiseptic
isopropanol	General alcohol antiseptic, disinfectant, astringent	Solution: 62%, 70%, 75%, 99%	Skin astringent, cleansing drug, utensil disinfectant
povidone-iodine	Broad-spectrum iodine antimicrobial	Topical stick: 0.75%, 10% Topical ointment: 1% Solution: 10% Mouthwash: 1.0% Surgical scrub: 7.5% Prep pad: 10%	Topical antiseptic
sodium hypochlorite	Broad-spectrum antimicrobial, disinfective	Solution: 3.5%, 10.3%, 12% and others	Topical antiseptic

NURSING PROCESS

Assessment

When any type of topical medication such as an antiseptic is to be administered, the concentration of the medication, length of exposure to the skin, condition of the skin, size of area affected, and hydration status of the skin must be taken into consideration, because these factors have a significant influence on the action of the medication. Before applying any topical medication, it is important for the nurse to question the patient about any drug allergies or any previous sensitivity to antiseptics, disinfectants, related compounds, and any additive within the solution, ointment, or other topical dosage form. If the drug is iodine based, for example, povidone-iodine, the nurse should question the patient about

allergies to iodine or seafood (because of iodine concentrations), because these are contraindications to the use of these drugs. Patients being treated with peroxide and other antiseptics and disinfectants should be questioned thoroughly about any previous allergic and local reaction to any of these drugs and their ingredients. Allergies to alcohol, chlorine, mercurial, and phenolic compounds should be noted and the drugs or ingredients avoided. It is also important to understand that there is a higher risk of reactions of antiseptics and disinfectants if there has been an allergic reaction to antibacterial topical drugs. Should a patient have an allergy to a particular type of antibacterial drug, that specific drug or ingredient should not be used at all, regardless of the dosage form. Culture and sensitivity reports will identify appropriate therapy with antiseptics or disinfectants. In addition, specific compounds within an antiseptic or disinfectant are used for particular bacteria or viruses based on known previous sensitivity.

Nursing Diagnoses

- Risk for infection related to compromised skin integrity
- Risk for infection related to skin trauma or injury resulting from adverse reactions to the topical agent
- Deficient knowledge related to topical agents and their proper use

Planning

Goals

- Patient will remain free of adverse reactions to the agent when used for the treatment of skin injury or infection.
- Patient will show evidence of resolution of infection.
- Patient will be adherent to the medication regimen.
- Patient will experience minimal to no adverse reactions to the medication.
- Patient will return for follow-up visits with physician.

Outcome Criteria

- Patient experiences minimal discomfort (such as stinging, itching, burning) resulting from the use of the agent in the treatment of a skin injury or infection.
- Patient experiences maximal therapeutic effects of medication once therapy is complete, with resolution of symptoms such as intact skin, no redness, or drainage.
- Patient demonstrates proper technique for applying topical antiseptic with applicator, tongue blade, gloved hand, and proper hand-washing technique.
- Patient states those situations (adverse reactions to medication or worsening of symptoms of infection) when the physician should be notified immediately.

Implementation

Before applying any topical agent, the nurse should check the physician's order to validate the order, route of administration, equipment needed, and application procedure. Standard precautions should be followed for any situation requiring direct contact with a patient or possible exposure situations (see Box 10-1 in Chapter 10). If the skin is intact and if it is not otherwise indicated, the nurse should wear nonsterile gloves; however, if the skin is not intact or the nurse judges it appropriate, sterile gloves and sterile technique should be used. Often there are specific directions regarding the application of the antiseptic or disinfectant. The order may specify that the agent be applied with a tongue depressor or sterile cotton-tipped applicator or that an occlusive dressing be placed. The nurse should follow the directions if they are within standards of care. As with any procedure, the nurse should always ensure patient privacy, dignity, and level of comfort. The skin site should be thoroughly cleansed and any other specific directions, such as removing water- or alcohol-based topicals with soap and water or normal saline (NS), should be followed. Before application or administration of additional doses of the antiseptic or disinfectant, the site should be cleansed of any debris (e.g., pus, drainage) and of any residual medication. If using an antiseptic or disinfectant for preparing the skin, exact instructions should be followed. Cross-contamination can be avoided through adherence to technique and hand washing. For dressing of the wound, the physician's order or wound care protocol (e.g., use of occlusive, wet, or wet-to-dry dressings) needs to be followed. The nurse should make sure to document the site of application and any drainage from the site, whether there is any swelling, the temperature and colour of the site, and any painful or other sensations that may occur.

Evaluation

When antiseptics are used, the patient's therapeutic response may be manifested by improved healing of the affected area, decreased symptoms of inflammation or infection, or prevention of infection for which the agent was ordered, such as preoperative. In addition, when using these agents on inanimate objects, the nurse must constantly monitor for patient safety from exposure to the agent. It is also important for the nurse to assess patients for any adverse effects (see Table 44-6) and to evaluate him- or herself for any reaction to the compound used for hand washing.

PATIENT EDUCATION

- Patients using antiseptics should be instructed to wash their hands before and after applying any topical medication. Hand-washing technique should also be emphasized and demonstrated.
- Patients should be instructed about proper application of medication and dressings and be provided hands-on demonstrations. Along with oral instructions, they should be provided written instructions, pamphlets, and any other aids to reinforce the importance of the procedure. Make sure patients have all the supplies needed for at-home care. A tongue blade, cotton-tipped applicator, or gloved finger may be used to apply the medication. Encourage hand washing and noting of any unusual colour of the skin, odour, or drainage.
- Patients should be encouraged to report any increase in redness, drainage, pain, swelling, or fever.

POINTS TO REMEMBER

❖ Topical antimicrobials (antiseptics and disinfectants) are used to reduce the risk for nosocomial infections and are applied to topical surfaces to inhibit or kill as many microorganisms as possible.

❖ Disinfectants are antimicrobials that are used only on nonliving objects, and they kill any organisms on these objects. They are *not* the same as antiseptics.

❖ Antiseptics are defined as antimicrobials that are used only on living tissues and primarily inhibit growth and reproduction of microorganisms.

❖ Antiseptics and disinfectants are categorized by their chemical makeup and include such agents as

alcohols, aldehydes, phenolic compounds, biguanides, surface-active agents, acid agents, dyes, oxidizing drugs, chlorine, mercurial, and iodine.

❖ Nurses should always observe standard precautions whenever applying antiseptics or disinfectants and apply these drugs to clean, dry skin unless otherwise ordered or specified. They should also ensure that patients receive adequate instructions about their medication, its application, and hand-washing technique.

EXAMINATION REVIEW QUESTIONS

1 Which of the following statements best describes the purpose of disinfectants?
 a. Used to sterilize the skin before surgery
 b. Bactericidal function and used in open wounds
 c. Applied to nonliving objects to kill microorganisms
 d. Used to inhibit growth of microorganisms on the skin surface

2 Which of the following is considered to be a property of an antiseptic agent?
 a. Bactericidal
 b. Bacteriostatic
 c. Useful on nonliving tissues
 d. More potent than a disinfectant

3 Which patient is most susceptible to a nosocomial infection?
 a. A teenager who has a sports injury
 b. An older adult patient admitted for cataract surgery
 c. A woman who has delivered her baby via vaginal delivery
 d. A middle-aged woman who has had two courses of chemotherapy for cancer

4 Which statement most correctly describes sodium hypochlorite?
 a. Sterilizes all surfaces
 b. Used as a topical antiseptic for wound care
 c. A 5.25% concentration is used for skin surfaces
 d. Contains the same active ingredient as vinegar

5 During a health history, a patient cites an allergy to iodine. Which antiseptic preparation would be contraindicated for this patient?
 a. Isopropyl alcohol
 b. Betadine solution
 c. Sodium hypochlorite
 d. Chlorhexidine gluconate

For answers see http://evolve.elsevier.com/Canada/Lilley/pharmacology/.

CRITICAL THINKING ACTIVITIES

1 What is the primary purpose for using antiseptics and disinfectants?

2 Can disinfectants and antiseptics be used interchangeably? Why or why not?

3 For a patient who is receiving an antiseptic as part of wound care, how would you know that a patient is having a therapeutic response to an antiseptic?

For answers see http://evolve.elsevier.com/Canada/Lilley/pharmacology/.

Anti-inflammatory, Antiarthritic, and Related Drugs

Learning Objectives

After reading this chapter, the successful student will be able to do the following:

1 Discuss the inflammatory response and the role it plays in the generation of pain.

2 Compare the disease processes that are often identified as inflammatory in nature, such as rheumatoid arthritis, osteoarthritis, degenerative joint disorders, and gout.

3 Compare nonsteroidal anti-inflammatory drugs (NSAIDs), antigout drugs, and antiarthritic drugs in relation to their mechanisms of action, indications, adverse effects, dosage ranges, routes of administration, cautions, contraindications, drug interactions, and toxicities.

4 Develop a collaborative plan of care that includes all phases of the nursing process for the patient receiving NSAIDs, antigout drugs, antiarthritic drugs, and other anti-inflammatory drugs.

e-Learning Activities

Web site
(http://evolve.elsevier.com/Canada/Lilley/pharmacology/)

- Animations
- Answers to chapter questions, activities, and case studies
- Calculators and Category Catchers
- Glossary with audio pronunciations
- IV Therapy and Medication Error Checklists
- Multiple-Choice Review Question quizzes
- Nursing Care Plans
- Online Appendices and Supplements
- WebLinks

Drug Profiles

▸▸ **acetylsalicylic acid,** p. 837
▸▸ **allopurinol,** p. 841
    auranofin, p. 842
▸▸ **celecoxib,** p. 838
    colchicine, p. 841
    gold sodium thiomalate, p. 842
▸▸ **ibuprofen,** p. 837
▸▸ **indomethacin,** p. 837
▸▸ **ketorolac (ketorolac tromethamine)*,** p. 837
    leflunomide, p. 842
    probenecid, sulfinpyrazone, p. 841

▸▸ Key drug.

*Full generic name is given in parentheses. For the purposes of this text, the more common shortened name is used.

Glossary

Arthritis Inflammation of one or more joints. (p. 840)

Disease-modifying antirheumatic drugs (DMARDs) Drugs used in the treatment of arthritic diseases that have the potential to arrest or slow the actual disease process. (p. 842)

Done nomogram A standard plot of graphic data for rating the severity of aspirin toxicity following overdose. (p. 835)

Gout Hyperuricemia (elevated uric acid); the arthritis caused by tissue buildup of uric acid crystals. (p. 834)

Inflammation   A localized protective response stimulated by injury to tissues that serves to destroy, dilute, or wall off (sequester) both the injurious agent and the injured tissue. (p. 831)

Nonsteroidal anti-inflammatory drugs (NSAIDs)   A large and chemically diverse group of drugs that possess analgesic, anti-inflammatory, antiarthritic, and antipyretic activity. (p. 831)

Rheumatism   General term for any of several disorders characterized by inflammation, degeneration, or metabolic derangement of connective tissue structures, especially joints and related structures. (p. 831)

Salicylism   The syndrome of salicylate toxicity, including such symptoms as tinnitus, nausea, and vomiting. (p. 835)

OVERVIEW

Nonsteroidal anti-inflammatory drugs (NSAIDs) are among the most commonly prescribed drugs. Each year, approximately 10 million prescriptions are written for NSAIDs in Canada, representing over 5% of all prescriptions. There are currently more than 15 different NSAIDs available in Canada. Some NSAIDs are used more frequently than others, and a patient may respond better to some NSAIDs than others, whether for symptom relief or in terms of adverse-effect profile. NSAIDs are generally taken for **inflammation**, defined as a localized protective response stimulated by injury to tissues. This response serves to destroy, dilute, or wall off (sequester) both the injurious agent and the injured tissue. Classic signs and symptoms of inflammation include pain, fever, loss of function, redness, and swelling. These symptoms result from arterial, venous, and capillary dilation; enhanced blood flow and vascular permeability; exudation of fluids, including plasma proteins; and leukocyte migration into the inflammatory focus. NSAIDs are also taken for **rheumatism**, a general term for any of several disorders characterized by inflammation, degeneration, or metabolic derangement of connective tissue structures, especially joints and related structures such as muscles, tendons, bursae, fibrous tissue, and ligaments. Rheumatic symptoms are similar to and often concurrent with inflammatory symptoms and include pain, stiffness, and reduced range of motion.

NSAIDs are a large and chemically diverse group of drugs that possess analgesic, anti-inflammatory, antiarthritic, and antipyretic activities. They are also used for the relief of mild to moderate headaches, myalgia, neuralgia, and arthralgia; alleviation of postoperative pain; inhibition of platelet aggregation; relief of pain associated with arthritic disorders such as rheumatoid arthritis, juvenile arthritis, ankylosing spondylitis, and osteoarthritis; and treatment of *gout* and *hyperuricemia* (discussed later in this chapter). Steroidal anti-inflammatory drugs (e.g., prednisone, dexamethasone), discussed in Chapter 33, are also used for similar purposes. Generally, NSAIDs have a more favourable adverse-effect profile than that of steroidal anti-inflammatory drugs.

In 1899, acetylsalicylic acid (ASA; aspirin) was marketed and rapidly became the most widely used drug in the world. The success of aspirin established the importance of drugs with antipyretic, analgesic, anti-inflammatory, and antirheumatic properties, properties that all NSAIDs share. However, the widespread use of aspirin also yielded evidence of its potential for causing some major adverse effects. Gastrointestinal intolerance, bleeding, and kidney impairment became major factors limiting its long-term administration. As a result, efforts were mounted to develop drugs that did not have the adverse effects of aspirin. This led to the discovery of other NSAIDs, which in general are associated with a lower incidence of and less serious adverse effects and are often better tolerated than aspirin in patients with chronic diseases.

Before proceeding to the in-depth discussion of the NSAID drugs, it is important to explain the body's arachidonic acid metabolic pathway. The beneficial effects of NSAIDs are thought to result primarily from their inhibition of this pathway.

ARACHIDONIC ACID PATHWAY

The inflammatory response is mediated by a host of endogenous compounds, including proteins of the complement system, histamine, serotonin, bradykinin, leukotrienes, and prostaglandins, the latter two being major contributors to the symptoms of inflammation.

Arachidonic acid is released from phospholipids in cell membranes in response to a triggering event (e.g., an injury). It is metabolized by either the *prostaglandin (PG)* pathway or the *leukotriene (LT)* pathway, both of which are branches of the arachidonic acid pathway, as shown in Figure 45-1. Both of these pathways result in inflammation, edema, headache, and other pain characteristic of the body's response to injury or inflammatory illnesses such as arthritis. Such symptoms are also observed when research subjects are injected with PG compounds.

In the PG pathway, arachidonic acid is converted by the enzyme *cyclooxygenase (COX)* into PGs such as *prostacyclin (PGI$_2$)*, as well as into *thromboxane A$_2$ (TXA$_2$)*. PGs indirectly mediate and perpetuate inflammation by inducing vasodilation and enhancing vasopermeability. These effects in turn potentiate the action of proinflammatory substances, such as histamine and bradykinin, in the production of edema and pain. These symptoms arise

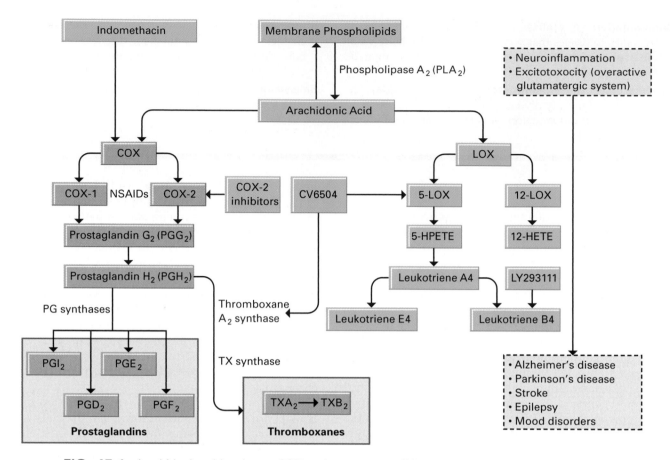

FIG. 45-1 Arachidonic acid pathway. *COX,* cyclooxygenase; *CV6504,* a 5-lipoxygenase inhibitor; *5-HPETE,* 5-hydroperoxyeicosatetraenoic acid; *LOX,* lipoxygenase; *LY293111,* a leukotriene B4 receptor antagonist; *PG,* prostaglandin; *TX,* thromboxane; *12-HETE,* 12-hydroxyeicosatetraenoic acid.

as a result of PG-induced hyperalgesia (excessive motor sensitivity). In this situation, stimuli that would normally not be painful, such as simply moving a joint through its natural range of motion, become painful because of the inflammatory process at work. Fever results when PGE_2 is synthesized in the preoptic hypothalamic region, the area of the brain that regulates temperature.

The LT pathway utilizes lipoxygenases to metabolize arachidonic acid and convert it into LTs. Although LTs are more newly discovered than PGs and not as well studied, they are also mediators of inflammation, promoting vasoconstriction, bronchospasms, and vascular permeability with resultant edema.

NONSTEROIDAL ANTI-INFLAMMATORY DRUGS

As a single class of drugs, NSAIDs constitute an exceptional variety of drugs, and they are used for an equally wide range of indications. Box 45-1 lists these drugs among seven distinct chemical classes. The carboxylic acid drugs are more commonly called *salicylates* and, as previously noted, were the first NSAIDs to be isolated and used therapeutically.

Currently, at least one NSAID has been approved for each of the therapeutic indications listed in Box 45-2; an

NSAID is considered the drug of choice for the treatment of most of these conditions. Almost all NSAIDs are used for the treatment of rheumatoid arthritis and degenerative joint disease (osteoarthritis). Several of these drugs are available in sustained-release formulations, allowing for once- or twice-daily dosing, which is known to improve patients' adherence to prescribed drug therapy regimens.

Mechanism of Action and Drug Effects

NSAIDs act through inhibition of the LT pathway, the PG pathway, or both. More specifically, NSAIDs relieve pain, headache, and inflammation by blocking the chemical activity of either or both of the enzymes cycooxygenase (PG pathway) and leukotriene (LT pathway). Both of these mechanisms differ from that of the opioids, which relieve pain by interfering with pain recognition in the brain. Furthermore, we now know that there are at least two types, or isoforms, of COX. COX-1 is the isoform of the enzyme that promotes the synthesis of homeostatic PGs, which have primarily beneficial effects on various body functions. One example is their role in maintaining an intact gastrointestinal mucosa. In contrast, the COX-2 isoform promotes the synthesis of PGs that are involved in inflammatory processes. In 1999, the newest class of NSAIDs, the COX-2 inhibitors, appeared on the Canadian market. These NSAIDs work by specifically inhibiting

---

BOX 45-1   Chemical Categories of NSAIDs

Acetic Acid Derivatives

diclofenac potassium (Apo-Diclo Rapide, Voltaren Rapide)
diclofenac sodium (Apo-Diclo SR, Voltaren)
sodium indomethacin (Indocid P.D.A.)
sulindac (Apo-Sulin)

Carboxylic Acids

Acetylated

acetylsalicylic acid (many brands)
diflunisal (Apo-Diflunisal)
etodolac (Apo-Etolac)

Nonacetylated

ketorolac tromethamine (Toradol)
magnesium salicylate (Herbogesic)
sodium salicylate (generic only)

COX-2 Inhibitors

celecoxib (Celebrex)

Fenamates

floctafenine (Apo-Floctafenine)
mefenamic acid (Apo-Mefenamic)

Napthylalkanones (nonacidic)

nabumetone (Apo-Nabumetone)

Oxicams

meloxicam (Apo-Meloxicam)
piroxicam (Apo-Piroxicam)

Propionic Acid Derivatives

flurbiprofen (Ansaid)
ibuprofen (Advil, Motrin)
ketoprofen (Apo-Keto-E)
naproxen (Naprosyn E)
naproxen sodium (Aleve, Anaprox, Naprelan)
oxaprozin (Daypro)
tiaprofenic acid (Apo-Tiaprofenic)

COX-2, cyclooxygenase-2.

BOX 45-2

NSAIDs: Health Canada–Approved Indications

- Acute gout
- Acute gouty arthritis
- Acute painful shoulder
- Ankylosing spondylitis
- Bursitis
- Fever
- Juvenile rheumatoid arthritis
- Mild to moderate pain
- Osteoarthritis
- Primary dysmenorrhea
- Rheumatoid arthritis
- Tendinitis
- Various ophthalmic uses

NSAID, nonsteroidal anti-inflammatory drug.

the COX-2 isoform of cyclooxygenase and have limited or no COX-1 effects. Previous NSAID groups functioned nonspecifically by inhibiting both COX-1 and COX-2 activities. The greater enzyme specificity of the COX-2 inhibitors allows for the beneficial anti-inflammatory effects associated with all other NSAIDs while reducing the prevalence of adverse effects, such as gastrointestinal ulceration, associated with the anti–COX-1 activity of the more nonspecific NSAIDs.

The LT pathway is inhibited by some anti-inflammatory drugs, but not by salicylates. Several anti-inflammatory drugs block both the PG pathway and the LT pathway, whereas others only weakly inhibit COX but primarily inhibit lipoxygenase.

The main drug effects of NSAIDs are those of analgesic, anti-inflammatory, and antipyretic effects. NSAIDs reduce fever by inhibiting PGE_2, specifically by inhibiting its biosynthesis within the preoptic hypothalamic region of the brain, which regulates body temperature. One notable effect of the salicylates, especially aspirin, is their inhibition of platelet aggregation, also known as its *antiplatelet activity.* Although all NSAIDs can be ulcerogenic and induce gastrointestinal bleeding, most of these effects are due to drug activity against tissue COX-1. Aspirin has the unique property among NSAIDs of being an irreversible inhibitor of COX-1 receptors within platelets. This effect in turn results in reduced formation by the platelets of TXA_2, a substance that normally promotes platelet aggregation. For this reason, aspirin is often used both prophylactically and following myocardial infarction to aid in the prevention of platelet aggregation, which unopposed, could lead to fibrin clot formation and reinfarction.

Indications

Some of the more noted therapeutic uses of this broad class of drugs are listed in Table 45-1. Nevertheless, they are used primarily for their analgesic, antigout, anti-inflammatory, and antipyretic effects; for the relief of vascular headaches; and for platelet inhibition.

NSAIDs are also widely used for the treatment of rheumatoid arthritis and osteoarthritis, as well as for other inflammatory conditions, rheumatic fever, and mild to moderate pain. They have proved beneficial as adjunctive pain relief medications in patients with persistent pain

Suggested NSAIDs for Patients with Various Medical Conditions

Medical Condition	Recommended NSAID
Ankylosing spondylitis	indomethacin, naproxen, flurbiprofen
Diabetic neuropathy	sulindac
Dysmenorrhea	Fenamates, naproxen, ibuprofen
Gout	indomethacin, naproxen, sulindac
Headaches	aspirin, ibuprofen, naproxen
Hepatotoxicity	naproxen, ibuprofen, piroxicam, fenamates
History of aspirin or NSAID allergy	Avoid NSAIDs if possible; if deemed necessary, consider a nonacetylated salicylate
Hypertension	sulindac, nonacetylated salicylate, ibuprofen, etodolac
Osteoarthritis	diclofenac, oxaprozin, indomethacin
Risk for gastrointestinal toxicity	All COX-2 inhibitors: celecoxib, nonacetylated salicylate, enteric-coated aspirin, diclofenac, nabumetone, etodolac, ibuprofen, oxaprozin
Risk for nephrotoxicity	sulindac, nonacetylated salicylate, nabumetone, etodolac, diclofenac, oxaprozin
Warfarin therapy	sulindac, naproxen, ibuprofen, oxaprozin

syndromes, such as pain from bone cancer and persistent back pain. For the relief of pain, they are sometimes combined with an opioid. They do not cause many of the undesirable effects of opioids, particularly respiratory depression. However, unlike opioids, their effectiveness is limited by a ceiling effect in that any further increase in the dose beyond a certain level increases the risk of adverse effects without a corresponding increase in the therapeutic effect. In contrast, opioid doses may be titrated almost indefinitely to increasingly higher levels, especially for terminally ill patients with severe pain.

As noted earlier, salicylates have an additional beneficial property of opposing the aggregation properties of platelets. For this reason, they are commonly used for both prophylaxis and treatment of arterial, and possibly venous, thrombosis, an effect known as the *antithrombotic effect* of aspirin. This antiplatelet action has made aspirin, along with thrombolytic drugs (Chapter 28), a primary drug in the treatment of acute myocardial infarction (MI) and many other thromboembolic disorders. Other NSAIDs generally lack these antiplatelet effects. However, salicylates can be ulcerogenic, with possible blood loss, by inhibition of the synthesis of protective PGs, which normally function to protect the gastrointestinal mucosa. Other NSAIDs are commonly used in the treatment of **gout**, which is caused by the overproduction of uric acid, decreased uric acid excretion, or both processes. This can often result in hyperuricemia (too much uric acid in the blood), a condition that causes joint pain as a result of the deposition of needlelike crystals of urate precipitate in tissues and the joints.

The appropriate selection of an NSAID is made through clinical judgement based on consideration of the patient's history, including any previous medical conditions, the intended use of the drug, the patient's previous experience with NSAIDs, the patient's preference, and the cost.

Contraindications

Contraindications to NSAIDs include known drug allergy and conditions that place the patient at risk for bleeding. These conditions include rhinitis (risk of

epistaxis [nosebleed]), vitamin K deficiency, and peptic ulcer disease. Other common contraindications apply to most drugs and include severe kidney or liver disease. All NSAIDs are generally rated as pregnancy category C drugs for use during the first two trimesters of pregnancy. They are rated pregnancy category D (not recommended) during the third trimester because NSAID use has been associated with both excessive maternal bleeding and neonatal NSAID toxicity during the perinatal period. Because the ongoing presence of NSAIDs may hinder the desired natural synthesis of PGs in an infant's body, these drugs are also not recommended for nursing mothers, as they are excreted into human milk.

Adverse Effects

One of the more common complaints and potentially serious adverse effects of the NSAIDs is gastrointestinal distress, ranging from mild symptoms such as heartburn to the most severe gastrointestinal complication, gastrointestinal bleeding. In fact, the adverse effects of salicylates mainly involve the gastrointestinal tract and, besides bleeding, include symptomatic gastrointestinal disturbances and mucosal lesions (e.g., erosive gastritis, gastric ulcer). While the potential adverse effects of NSAIDs listed in Table 45-2 do not necessarily apply to all drugs, they do apply to many of them.

Many of the adverse effects of NSAIDs are secondary to their inactivation of protective PGs that help maintain the normal integrity of the stomach lining. The drug misoprostol has proved successful in preventing the gastric ulcers and hence gastrointestinal bleeding that can occur in patients receiving NSAIDs. Misoprostol is a synthetic PGE_1 analogue that potently inhibits gastric acid secretion, by directly inhibiting the function of *parietal cells* that secrete the stomach's acid content. It also has a cytoprotective component, although the mechanism responsible for this action is unclear. Because of this action, misoprostol has been combined with the NSAID diclofenac sodium as a combination product (Arthrotec). Kidney function also depends on PGs, which stimulate vasodilation and increase kidney blood flow. Disruption of this PG function

TABLE 45-2

NSAIDs: Adverse Effects

Body System	Adverse Effects
Cardiovascular	Moderate to severe noncardiogenic pulmonary edema
Gastrointestinal	Most frequent: dyspepsia, heartburn, epigastric distress, nausea
	Less frequent: vomiting, anorexia, abdominal pain, gastrointestinal bleeding, mucosal lesions (erosions or ulcerations)
Hematological	Altered hemostasis through effects on platelet function
Hepatic	Acute reversible hepatotoxicity
Renal	Reduction in creatinine clearance, acute tubular necrosis with kidney failure
Other	Skin eruption, sensitivity reactions, tinnitus, hearing loss

TABLE 45-3

Acute or Chronic Salicylate Intoxication: Signs and Symptoms

Body System	Signs and Symptoms
Cardiovascular	Increased heart rate
Central nervous	Tinnitus, hearing loss, dimness of vision, headache, dizziness, mental confusion, lassitude, drowsiness
Gastrointestinal	Nausea, vomiting, diarrhea
Metabolic	Sweating, thirst, hyperventilation, hypo- or hyperglycemia

- Little or no toxicity: less than 150 mg/kg
- Mild to moderate toxicity: 150–300 mg/kg
- Severe toxicity: 300–500 mg/kg
- Life-threatening toxicity: greater than 500 mg/kg

It should be noted, however, that even doses lower than 150 mg/kg have resulted in fatal toxicity, whereas some patients have survived aspirin overdoses as high as 130 g. A serum salicylate concentration measured 6 hours or more after the ingestion may be used in conjunction with the **Done nomogram** to estimate the severity of intoxication and help guide treatment. The Done nomogram is a graphic plot of serum salicylate levels (in millimoles per litre [mmol/L]) as a function of elapsed time following salicylate ingestion. It was first published in a 1960 issue of the journal *Pediatrics* and is still widely used for gauging acute salicylate toxicity. However, this nomogram is intended only for estimating the severity of acute intoxications, not that of chronic salicylate intoxication or for enteric-coated or sustained-release products. Table 45-4 describes, in general terms, treatment for cases of varying severity. Treatment goals include removing salicylate from the gastrointestinal tract and preventing its further absorption; correcting fluid, electrolyte, and acid–base disturbances; and implementing measures to enhance salicylate elimination. Treatment goals are summarized in Table 45-5.

Toxicity and Management of Overdose

There are both chronic and acute manifestations of salicylate toxicity. *Chronic salicylate intoxication* is known as **salicylism** and results from either short-term high doses or prolonged therapy with high or even lower doses. The most common signs and symptoms of acute or chronic salicylate intoxication are listed in Table 45-3.

The most common manifestations of chronic intoxication in adults are tinnitus and hearing loss. Those in children are hyperventilation and central nervous system effects such as dizziness, drowsiness, and behavioural changes. These effects usually arise when serum salicylate concentrations exceed 2.89 to 4.3 mmol/L. Metabolic complications such as metabolic acidosis and respiratory alkalosis often occur to varying degrees in cases of chronic salicylate intoxication. Metabolic acidosis can also occur with acute intoxication, but it is usually less severe than that in patients with chronic intoxication. Hypoglycemia may also occur and can be life threatening. The treatment of chronic intoxication is based on the presenting symptoms. Serum salicylate concentrations may be determined but are not as useful in estimating the severity because severe intoxication can occur with a concentration as low as 150 mg/kg.

The signs and symptoms of *acute salicylate toxicity* are similar to those of chronic intoxication, but the effects are often more pronounced and occur more quickly. Acute salicylate overdose usually results from the ingestion of a single toxic dose. When higher doses of salicylate are ingested (more than 4 g), the half-life becomes much longer as the biotransformation pathways become overloaded. The severity of acute salicylate overdose can be assessed on the basis of the estimated amount ingested (in mg/kg of body weight), as follows:

TABLE 45-4

Acute Salicylate Intoxication: Treatment

Severity	Treatment
Mild	1. Dosage reduction or discontinuation of salicylates
	2. Symptomatic and supportive therapy
Severe	1. Discontinuation of salicylates
	2. Intensive symptomatic and supportive therapy
	3. Dialysis if: high salicylate levels, unresponsive acidosis (pH less than 7.1), impaired kidney function or kidney failure, pulmonary edema, persistent CNS symptoms (e.g., seizures, coma), progressive deterioration despite appropriate therapy

CNS, central nervous system.

An acute overdose of nonsalicylate NSAIDs (e.g., ibuprofen) causes effects similar to those of salicylate overdose, but they are generally not as extensive or as dangerous. These symptoms include central nervous system toxicities such as drowsiness, lethargy, mental confusion, paraesthesias (abnormal touch sensations), numbness, aggressive behaviour, disorientation, seizures, and gastrointestinal toxicities such as nausea, vomiting, and gastrointestinal bleeding. Intense headache, dizziness, cerebral edema, cardiac arrest, and death have also been known to occur in extreme cases. For suspected overdose, consultation with a Poison Control Centre is recommended. Treatment should consist of the immediate removal of the ingested drug by inducing emesis with gastric lavage. This should be followed by the administration of activated charcoal, with supportive and symptomatic treatment initiated thereafter. Unlike with salicylates, hemodialysis appears to be of no value in enhancing the elimination of NSAIDs.

Interactions

The drug interactions associated with the use of salicylates and other NSAIDs can result in significant complications and morbidity. Some of the more common interactions are listed in Table 45-6.

NSAIDs can also interfere with laboratory test results. Specifically, salicylates can cause what are usually minor and transient elevations in liver enzymes (alanine aminotransferase [ALT], aspartate aminotransferase [AST]), but cases of severe hepatotoxicity are rare. Hematocrit (Hct), hemoglobin (Hgb), and red blood cell (RBC) levels can drop if any drug-induced gastrointestinal bleeding does occur. There can also be NSAID-induced hyperkalemia or hyponatremia.

Dosages

For the recommended dosages of NSAIDs, see the Dosages table on p. 839.

TABLE 45-5

Acute Salicylate Intoxication: Treatment Goals

Treatment Goal	Measure
Reduce salicylate absorption	Gastric lavage* Activated charcoal
Treat fluid and electrolyte imbalance	Appropriate fluid replacement and electrolyte therapy should be implemented promptly, based on fluid, acid–base, and electrolyte status. Therefore, arterial pH and blood gases and electrolytes, serum creatinine, BUN, and blood glucose should be determined.
Enhance salicylate elimination	Alkaline diuresis: intravenous administration of sodium bicarbonate to alkalinize the urine to a pH of greater than 7.5 with sufficient urine flow Hemodialysis: the same considerations as those that apply to chronic intoxication
Provide symptomatic and supportive measures	Hypotension and hemorrhagic complications: fluids and transfusions, along with possible vitamin K injections Respiratory depression: may require assisted pulmonary ventilation and oxygen Seizures: intravenous administration of a benzodiazepine or short-acting barbiturate

BUN, blood urea nitrogen.

*Effective up to 3–4 hr after acute ingestion and maybe up to 10 hr after ingestion in the event of massive overdose.

TABLE 45-6

Salicylates and Other NSAIDs: Drug Interactions

Drug	Mechanism	Result
Alcohol	Additive effect	Increased GI bleeding
Anticoagulants	Platelet inhibition, hypoprothrombinemia	Increased bleeding tendencies
Antihyperglycemic drugs	Increased antihyperglycemic response to sulfonureas	Reduced blood glucose
ASA and other salicylates with NSAIDs	Reduce NSAID absorption, additive GI toxicities	Increased GI toxicity with no therapeutic advantage
Corticosteroids and other ulcerogenic drugs	Additive toxicities	Increased ulcerogenic effects
cyclosporine	Inhibits kidney prostaglandin synthesis	May increase the nephrotoxic effects of cyclosporine
Hypotensive drugs and diuretics	Inhibit prostaglandin synthesis	Reduced hypotensive and diuretic effects
phenytoin	Inhibit phenytoin metabolism	Increase phenytoin serum levels
Protein-bound drugs	Compete for binding	More pronounced drug actions
Uricosurics	Antagonism	Decreased uric acid excretion

ASA, acetylsalicylic acid; *GI*, gastrointestinal; *NSAID*, nonsteroidal anti-inflammatory drug.

DRUG PROFILES

NONSTEROIDAL ANTI-INFLAMMATORY DRUGS

On the basis of their chemical profiles, the broad drug category of NSAIDs can be subdivided into four major categories of carboxylic acids—acetic acids, propionic acids, pyranocarboxylic acids, and pyrrolizine carboxylic acids—and the newest class of NSAIDs, the COX-2 inhibitors.

ACETIC ACIDS

Salicylates are chemically classified as carboxylic acids. Although aspirin is the most commonly used of all these drugs, the others possess many of the same beneficial effects as aspirin. In Canada, aspirin is available without a prescription with the exception of diflunisal (Apo-Diflunisal, others). Salicylates are most commonly used in solid oral dosage forms (i.e., tablets, capsules). Other available dosage forms include a chewing gum tablet (Aspergum) and rectal suppositories. Aspirin is contained in many combination products (see Box 45-3 for a list of the combinations). Many of the combinations contain caffeine, considered to provide an adjunctive analgesic effect. Aspirin is also available in special dosage forms, such as enteric-coated aspirin (Adasol), designed to protect the stomach mucosa by dissolving in the duodenum.

Indomethacin (Indocid P.D.A.) is one of the commonly used acetic acid, or *acetylated,* NSAIDs; the others are aspirin, diflunisal (Apo-Diflunisal, others), diclofenac sodium (Apo-Diclo), etodolac (Apo-Etolac, others), and sulindac (Apo-Sulin, others). There is debate in the literature over whether acylated or nonacetylated NSAIDs provide better pain relief. Because patients vary in their drug responses, it is usually a matter of clinical trial and error to find the ideal drug(s) for a given patient.

▶▶ acetylsalicylic acid

Acetylsalicylic acid (ASA, aspirin) is the prototype salicylate and NSAID and is the most widely used drug in the world. First introduced in the late 1800s, it remains a pillar of many drug treatment regimens. A daily aspirin tablet (81 mg or 325 mg) is now routinely recommended as prophylactic therapy for adults who have strong risk factors for developing coronary artery disease or stroke, even if they have no prior history of such an event. The 81 mg (which is traditionally thought of as "children's" aspirin) and the 325 mg strengths appear to be equally beneficial for the prevention of thrombotic events. For this reason, the lower strength is often chosen for patients who have any elevated risk of bleeding, such as those with prior stroke history or a history of peptic ulcer disease and those taking the anticoagulant warfarin (Coumadin). Aspirin is also often used to treat pain associated with headache, neuralgia, myalgia, and arthralgia, as well as other pain syndromes resulting from inflammation, which include arthritis, pleurisy, and pericarditis. Patients with systemic lupus erythematosus may benefit from ASA therapy because of its antiarthritic effects.

Aspirin and other salicylates all have one specific contraindication to their use. This drug class is contraindicated in children with flulike symptoms, as its use has been strongly associated with Reye's syndrome (see Special Populations: Children). This is an acute and potentially life-threatening condition involving progressive neurological deficits that can lead to coma and may involve liver damage. It is believed to be triggered by viral illnesses such as influenza and by salicylate therapy itself in the presence of a viral illness. Survivors of this condition may or may not suffer permanent neurological damage.

PHARMACOKINETICS

Half-Life	Onset	Peak	Duration
PO: 2–30 hr	PO: 15–30 min	PO: 1–2 hr	PO: 4–6 hr

▶▶ indomethacin

As with the other NSAIDs, indomethacin (Indocid P.D.A.) has analgesic, anti-inflammatory, antiarthritic, and antipyretic properties. Its therapeutic actions are of particular use in the treatment of rheumatoid arthritis, osteoarthritis, acute bursitis or tendinitis, ankylosing spondylitis (spinal arthritis), and acute gouty arthritis. The drug is available for both oral and rectal use. An injectable form of the drug is used intravenously to promote closure of patent ductus arteriosus (PDA), a heart defect that sometimes occurs in premature infants.

PHARMACOKINETICS

Half-Life	Onset	Peak	Duration
PO: 1.5–2 hr	PO: Less than 30 min	PO: 0.5–3 hr	PO: 4–6 hr

PROPIONIC ACIDS

▶▶ ibuprofen

Ibuprofen (Motrin, Advil) is the prototype NSAID in the propionic acid category, which also includes flurbiprofen (Advil, Motrin), ketoprofen (Apo-Keto), naproxen (Naprosyn E), and oxaprozin (Daypro). Ibuprofen is the most commonly used of the propionic acid drugs because of its numerous indications and relatively safe adverse-effect profile. It is often used for rheumatoid arthritis, osteoarthritis, primary dysmenorrhea, dental pain, and musculoskeletal disorders. Naproxen is the second most commonly used of the propionic acid NSAIDs with a somewhat improved reported adverse-effect profile over that of ibuprofen, including fewer drug interactions with angiotensin-converting enzyme (ACE) inhibitors for hypertension. Evidence indicates that ibuprofen is more likely than naproxen to interact with these drugs to hinder their desired hypotensive effects. Ibuprofen is available only for oral use in over-the-counter strengths, whereas naproxen is available in prescription strengths; naproxen sodium (Aleve) is available over the counter.

PHARMACOKINETICS

Half-Life	Onset	Peak	Duration
PO: Less than 30 min	PO: 0.5–2 hr	PO: 1–2 hr	PO: 4–6 hr

▶▶ ketorolac tromethamine

Ketorolac tromethamine (Acular, Toradol) is classified as a pyrrolizine carboxylic acid, currently the only drug in this category. Ketorolac has a somewhat unique chemical

Continued

DRUG PROFILES (cont'd)

structure. Although it does have some anti-inflammatory activity, it is used primarily for its powerful analgesic effects, which are comparable to those of narcotic drugs such as morphine. Oral dosages are indicated for the short-term management (up to 5 days) of moderate post-surgical acute pain or for up to 7 days for patients with moderate-to-severe acute pain that requires analgesia at the opioid level, such as, pain resulting from orthopedic injuries, postpartum uterine cramping, and postsurgical pain. It is not indicated for minor or persistent painful conditions. The opioid-level analgesic potential of the drug can make it a particularly desirable choice for patients with acute pain control needs who are opiate addicted, because ketorolac lacks the addictive properties of the true opioids. Ketorolac is not administered for more than 7 days because of the risk for gastrointestinal bleeding. It is recommended that the lowest possible dose be given for the shortest duration possible. Ketorolac is the only NSAID that can be given orally or by injection; there is also a dosage form for ophthalmic use (Chapter 58).

Ketorolac is available only by prescription. It is a potent NSAID with many contraindications.

PHARMACOKINETICS

Half-Life	Onset	Peak	Duration
IM/IV: 5–7 hr	IM/IV: 0.5 hr	IM/IV: 1–2 hr	IM/IV: 4–6 hr

COX-2 INHIBITORS

COX-2 inhibitors were designed primarily to cause fewer gastrointestinal adverse effects than those with other NSAIDs because of their COX-2 selectivity. However, they are not totally devoid of gastrointestinal toxicity. Gastritis and upper gastrointestinal bleeding have been reported

with their use, although much less frequently than with older NSAIDs. Specific adverse effects of this NSAID subclass include fatigue, dizziness, lower extremity edema, and hypertension.

COX-2 inhibitors have little effect on platelet function.

▶▶ *celecoxib*

Celecoxib (Celebrex) was the first COX-2 inhibitor, approved in 1999. It is indicated for the treatment of osteoarthritis, rheumatoid arthritis, acute pain symptoms, and primary dysmenorrhea. It recently was approved by Health Canada for symptoms associated with ankylosing spondylitis. Celecoxib is also approved for reduction of colon polyps in patients with an inherited condition known as *familial adenomatous polyposis*. It is available only for oral use.

Since 1999, two other COX-2 inhibitors were marketed and have since been recalled: rofecoxib (Vioxx), recalled by Merck in 2004, and valdecoxib (Bextra), recalled by Pfizer in 2005. The recall occurred following several case reports indicating an increased risk for adverse cardiovascular events, including blood clots during medical and surgical procedures, MI, cardiovascular accident, and death. Valdexocib has also been associated with severe skin reactions known as *toxic epidermal necrolysis* and Stevens–Johnson syndrome. There is evidence that celecoxib may pose similar risks. While it currently remains on the Canadian market, its use is now being monitored more closely by Health Canada.

PHARMACOKINETICS

Half-Life	Onset	Peak	Duration
PO: 11 hr	PO: 0.75–1 hr	PO: 3 hr	PO: 4–8 hr

BOX 45-3 Combination Products of Acetylsalicylic Acid

Aspirin Combination	Brand Name	Pharmacological Action	Indications
acetylsalicylic acid, butalbital, caffeine	Fiorinal, Trianal	Butalbital is a sedative (barbiturate); used when analgesic and sedative effects are required	Tension headache, mixed migraine headache, menstrual and postpartum headache and pain
acetylsalicylic acid, butalbital, caffeine, codeine phosphate	Fiorinal C, Trianal-C	Codeine is a narcotic analgesic.	Acute and persistent pain accompanied by tension or anxiety
acetylsalicylic acid, citric acid, sodium bicarbonate	Alka-Seltzer*	Antacid, analgesic	Analgesic plus neutralizes stomach acids
acetylsalicylic acid, codeine phosphate, methocarbamol	Robaxisal C	Methocarbamol is a centrally acting muscle relaxant.	Pain associated with skeletal muscle spasm
acetylsalicylic acid, dipyridamole	Aggrenox	Antiplatelet	Prevention of stroke in those with previous stroke or transient ischemic attack
acetylsalicylic acid, nifedifine	Adalat XL Plus	Calcium channel blocker, antiplatelet	Antianginal, antihypertensive
acetylsalicylic acid, oxycodone hydrochloride	Percodan	Oxycodan is an opioid analgesic.	Mild to moderate and severe pain
acetylsalicylic acid, pravastatin sodium	PravAsa	HMG-CoA reductase inhibitor used for lipid regulation, antiplatelet	Patients requiring lipid level reduction plus anti-inflammatory, antiplatelet effect

*Alka-Seltzer is the only drug available over the counter. All the other products listed are available by prescription only, depending on the amount of codeine in the drug.

SPECIAL POPULATIONS: CHILDREN

Reye's Syndrome

Reye's syndrome is associated with the administration of aspirin in children and teenagers and is a potentially life-threatening illness. Encephalopathy and liver damage are a few of the serious complications resulting from Reye's syndrome. It usually occurs after a viral infection, such as chicken pox or influenza B, during which time aspirin is often given for fever. To reduce the risk for Reye's syndrome, aspirin or medications that contain aspirin should not be given to children or teenagers to treat viral illnesses or fever. Other names for aspirin include acetylsalicylic acid, acetylsalicylate, salicylic acid, and salicylate. Other drugs that can be used instead include acetaminophen and ibuprofen to reduce fever and relieve pain. Check the label on any medication to be given to a child, because aspirin is in many over-the-counter drugs, for example, Alka-Seltzer, some Anacin products, and Pepto-Bismol.

Signs and Symptoms
- Altered liver function
- Causes encephalopathy and fatty degeneration of the viscera, primarily in children and teenagers
- Changes in level of consciousness
- Coma, flaccid paralysis, loss of deep tendon reflexes
- Hypoglycemia
- Seizures
- Vomiting

Medical Management
- Supportive treatment in the critical care unit
- Maintain life functions, regain metabolic balance, and control cerebral edema
- IV glucose (10% or higher) for the treatment of hypoglycemia
- Monitor blood sugars; insulin may be needed

- Vitamin K for clotting problems
- Fresh-frozen plasma may be needed if there is significant bleeding
- Prophylactic antiepileptic drugs
- Monitor intracranial pressure
- Cautious fluid administration
- Osmotic diuretics may be needed with steroids for cerebral edema

Nursing Management
- Critical care setting is often indicated.
- Assess neurological status, vital signs, and arterial and central venous pressures.
- Monitor blood gases and intracranial pressure.
- Control temperature to prevent elevations and increased O_2 demands.
- Elevate head of bed.
- Record intake and output.
- Hyperventilation may be needed with intubation to reduce intracranial pressure by lowering CO_2 levels and increasing O_2 levels.
- Monitor O_2 levels for seizure activity.
- Maintain quiet environment.
- Handle patient gently.
- Provide family support.
- Provide physical and emotional support for the child and family with recovery.
- Offer spiritual care.
- Educate the public about Reye's syndrome and the life-threatening complications.

Source: Health Canada. (2006). *Reye's syndrome.* Retrieved January 1, 2009, from http://www.hc-sc.gc.ca/hl-vs/iyh-vsv/diseases-maladies/reye-eng.php

---

DOSAGES   Most Commonly Used NSAIDs

Drug (Pregnancy Category)	Pharmacological Class	Usual Dosage Range	Indications
▸▸acetylsalicylic acid (ASA, Aspirin) (C/D)	Salicylate	*Children 2 to under 12 yr* PO/PR: 10–15 mg/kg q6h (max 65 mg/day)	Analgesic, antipyretic
		PO/PR: 60–90 mg/kg divided q4–6h (max 100 mg/kg)	Anti-inflammatory
		Adult PO/PR: 325–650 mg q4h (max 4 g/day)	Analgesic, antipyretic
		PO: 3.6–5.4 g/day, divided	Anti-inflammatory
		PO: 80–650 mg daily based on patient needs	Platelet antiaggregant
▸▸celecoxib (Celebrex) (C/D)	COX-2 inhibitor	*Adult older than 18 yr* PO: 100–200 mg bid	Rheumatoid arthritis, osteoarthritis, ankylosing spondylitis
		PO: Initial 400 mg (day 1); then 200 mg/day × 7 days	Acute pain
		PO: 400 mg bid	Reduction of number of hereditary colon polyps in familial adenomatous polyposis

Continued

DOSAGES Most Commonly Used NSAIDs (cont'd)

Drug (Pregnancy Category)	Pharmacological Class	Usual Dosage Range	Indications
▶▶ ibuprofen (Motrin, Advil, others) (C/D)	Propionic acid	*Children under 2 yr* PO (drops): 5 mg/kg tid–qid *Children under 12 yr* PO (suspension): 120–375 mg q6–8h *Children older than 12 yr/Adult* 200–400 mg q4h (max 1200 mg/day)	Fever, pain Arthritis, fever, pain, dysmenorrhea
▶▶ indomethacin (Indocid P.D. A., Nu-Indo) (C/D)	Acetic acid	*Children* PO/PR: 2–4 mg/kg/day divided bid–qid (max 200 mg/day) *Adult* PO/PR: 25–50 mg bid–tid (max 200 mg/day)	Rheumatoid arthritis, ankylosing spondylitis, osteoarthritis, acute gouty arthritis, acute shoulder pain (bursitis or tendinitis)
▶▶ ketorolac tromethamine (Acular, Toradol) (C/D)	Pyrrolizine carboxylic acid	*Adult* PO: 10 mg q4–6h (max 40 mg/day) IM: 10–30 mg q6–12h (max 120 mg/day if under 65 yr; max 60 mg/day if older than 65 yr)	Acute painful conditions that would otherwise require opioid-level analgesia; PO form is recommended only in transition from injectable form to oral form

IM, intramuscular; *PO,* oral; *PR,* rectal.

Pregnancy categories: C/D = C, first and second trimester; D, third trimester.

ENOLIC ACIDS, FENAMIC ACIDS, AND NONACIDIC COMPOUNDS

The last three chemical categories of NSAIDs consist of the smallest number of drugs, and the indications for their use are more limited. The drugs are profiled briefly here. Pregnancy category information is essentially the same as that for other NSAIDs. Both piroxicam (Nu-Pirox, others) and meloxicam (Mobicox) belong to the enolic acid family of NSAIDs. These compounds are more commonly called *oxicams*. They are potent drugs that can produce severe gastrointestinal toxicities. Oxicams are commonly used in the treatment of mild to moderate osteoarthritis, rheumatoid arthritis, and gouty arthritis. Both are available only in oral dosage formulations and have contraindications similar to those of the other NSAIDs.

Mefenamic acid (Apo-Mefenamic, others) belongs to the category of fenamic acid NSAIDs, an older drug, and is not used as commonly as the other NSAIDs. It is indicated for the treatment of mild to moderate pain, osteoarthritis, and rheumatoid arthritis.

Nabumetone (Apo-Nabumetone, others) is a relatively new NSAID that is better tolerated by patients who cannot tolerate the gastrointestinal adverse effects of other NSAIDs. It is classified as a naphthylalkanone and is currently the only drug in its class. It is relatively nonacidic compared with most of the other NSAIDs, which probably accounts for its improved gastrointestinal tolerance. Currently, it is indicated only for the treatment of osteoarthritis and rheumatoid arthritis.

ANTIARTHRITIC DRUGS

Arthritis is a general term that can include numerous identified subtypes. The most common of these are *gout, rheumatoid arthritis,* and *osteoarthritis.* As defined at the beginning of this chapter, *arthritic* illnesses involve inflammation, degeneration, or metabolic derangement of joints and other connective tissue structures, with symptoms including pain, stiffness, and reduced range of motion. As previously emphasized in this chapter, all NSAIDs have some antiarthritic activity. However, there are several non-NSAID medications recognized primarily for their antiarthritic properties, in contrast to the analgesic, anti-inflammatory, and antipyretic properties associated with NSAIDs. These drugs are referred to here as *antiarthritic* drugs, and they are further subdivided into the *antigout* and *antirheumatoid arthritis* drugs. Although some of these drugs have additional medical uses, they are commonly used to treat the prevalent rheumatic conditions of gout and arthritis.

Because each drug is unique in its mechanism of action, these drugs are not described in grouped format. Additional antiarthritic drugs with different mechanisms of action are discussed in Chapter 50.

GOUT AND ANTIGOUT DRUGS

Urate crystals are like small needles that jab and stick into sensitive tissues and joints, a condition known as *gouty arthritis.* Persons with gout either overproduce or underexcrete uric acid, an end product of purine metabolism. Purines are part of the normal dietary intake and are used to make the essential nucleoside and nucleotide structural units of DNA and RNA. During their metabolism, they are converted from hypoxanthine to xanthine and eventually to uric acid. The normal pathway for purine metabolism is depicted in Figure 45-2. This pathway is overactive in patients with gout and is reduced by antigout drug therapy.

Antigout drugs include such drugs as allopurinol, colchicine, probenecid, and sulfinpyrazone. They target the underlying defect in uric acid metabolism—that is, the overproduction or underexcretion of uric acid.

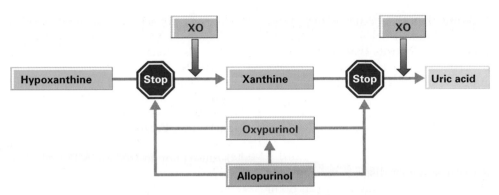

FIG. 45-2   Uric acid production. *XO,* xanthine oxidase.

 DRUG PROFILES

▶ *allopurinol*

The mechanism of action of allopurinol (Alloprin, Zyloprim) in the relief of gout is through the inhibition of the enzyme xanthine oxidase, which thereby prevents uric acid production. Allopurinol is rapidly absorbed and rapidly metabolized when administered orally. Oxypurinol, the main metabolite of allopurinol, also prevents uric acid production and has a half-life of 18 hours, which allows allopurinol to achieve a therapeutic effect with once-a-day dosage. Normal serum urate levels are usually achieved in 1 to 3 weeks.

Allopurinol is contraindicated in patients with a hypersensitivity to it. Significant adverse effects of the drug include agranulocytosis, aplastic anemia, and serious and potentially fatal skin conditions such as exfoliative dermatitis, Stevens–Johnson syndrome, and toxic epidermal necrolysis. Azathioprine and mercaptopurine both interact with allopurinol; because of the important interactions that can result, their doses may have to be adjusted. Allopurinol is available only for oral use. The recommended adult dosage is 400 to 600 mg/day, to a maximum of 800 mg/day. It is classified as pregnancy category C.

▶ *colchicine*

Colchicine (Colchicine-Odam) is an antigout medication with weak anti-inflammatory activity, no effect on the urinary excretion of uric acid, and no analgesic activity. It is effective in the treatment of gout apparently by reducing the inflammatory response to the deposits of urate crystals in joint tissue. Although there are many possible explanations for its ability to do this, the one most favoured is that it inhibits polymorphonuclear leukocyte metabolism, mobility, and *chemotaxis* (chemical attraction of these cells to the site of inflammation, which worsens an inflammatory response). Colchicine is a powerful inhibitor of cell mitosis and can cause short-term leukopenia. Thus it is generally used for the treatment of acute attacks of gout.

Colchicine's more severe adverse effects can include bleeding into the gastrointestinal or urinary tracts; the drug should be stopped should such effects appear. Colchicine can also cause kidney failure. There is no specific antidote for colchicine poisoning. Hypersensitivity is the only contraindication to its use. The drug is available in oral form. The usual adult dosage is an initial dose of 1 to 1.2 mg initially, then 0.5 or 0.6 mg every 2 hours until the gout pain disappears or until nausea, vomiting, or diarrhea develops. It is classified as pregnancy category D.

probenecid and sulfinpyrazone

The beneficial effect of probenecid (Benuryl) in the treatment of gout is the increased excretion of uric acid in the urine by inhibiting its reabsorption by the kidney. Drugs that promote uric acid excretion are known as *uricosurics*. In patients whose gout is due to the underexcretion of uric acid, urate crystals form because uric acid is not being excreted in the urine in sufficient quantities. Instead, most of the uric acid is being reabsorbed from the kidney tubules back into the bloodstream and then conveyed throughout the body. Probenecid acts by preferentially binding to the special transporter protein in the proximal convoluted kidney tubule that takes uric acid from the urine and places it back into the blood. Probenecid is then reabsorbed into the bloodstream while the uric acid remains in the urine and is excreted. In addition to its use for the treatment of the hyperuricemia associated with gout and gouty arthritis, probenecid also has the ability to delay the kidney excretion of penicillin, thus increasing the serum levels of penicillin and prolonging its effect (Chapter 38). Probenecid is available as a 500 mg oral tablet. The usual adult dosage is 250 mg twice a day with food, milk, or antacids for 1 week, followed by 500 mg twice daily thereafter. This dose may be adjusted as needed to maintain desirable serum uric acid levels. Contraindications include peptic ulcer disease. It is classified as pregnancy category B.

Sulfinpyrazone's (Apo-Sulfinyrazone) action is similar to that of probenecid. It is also a uricosuric drug. Despite its generic name, it is not a sulfonamide drug per se, but is chemically related to phenylbutazone, an early NSAID, which is no longer available on the Canadian market. As with other NSAIDs, however, sulfinpyrazone can be ulcerogenic and is therefore contraindicated in patients with peptic ulcer disease. Sulfinpyrazone is available only for oral use. The usual adult dosage is 100 to 200 mg twice a day for 1 week. The subsequent adjusted maintenance dosage can range from 200 to 800 mg daily. It is classified as pregnancy category C during the first and second trimesters, category D during the third trimester.

Although not all gouty deposits occur within joints, gouty arthritis is the condition of one or more inflamed joints resulting from gouty deposits that collect inside the joint anatomy. This is also called *articular gout*, whereas gout that occurs in tissues outside of the joints is called *abarticular gout*.

ANTIRHEUMATOID ARTHRITIS DRUGS

Rheumatoid arthritis is a systemic disease characterized by symmetrical inflammation of the joints; it can occur as early as childhood. It is believed to be an autoimmune disorder, possibly triggered by a viral infection. Osteoarthritis, another arthritic condition, affects the weight-bearing joints in the body and is characterized by increased destruction of cartilage and resulting proliferation of adjacent bone. The prevalence and severity increase with age. The most common symptom of osteoarthritis is pain, which leads to reduced function, strength, and motion. Heredity and activities involving repetitive motion or injury increase the risk for developing osteoarthritis. It is commonly exacerbated by comorbid obesity.

Antirheumatoid arthritis drugs suppress the specific types of inflammation associated with rheumatoid arthritis (hereafter referred to as *arthritis*) and are therefore used in its treatment. These drugs are considered to be more powerful than the NSAIDs in that they not only provide anti-inflammatory and analgesic effects but can also arrest or slow the degenerative disease processes associated with arthritis. For these reasons, this class of medications is also referred to as the **disease-modifying antirheumatic drugs (DMARDs)**. DMARDs often have a slow onset of action of several weeks, instead of minutes to hours for NSAIDs. Consequently, DMARDs are sometimes also referred to as *slow-acting antirheumatic drugs (SAARDs)*. They are also commonly thought of as second-line drugs for the treatment of arthritis because they can have much more toxic adverse effects than those of the NSAIDs. However, use of the term *second-line drugs* can be misleading because DMARDs are more frequently used as first-line drug therapy, in spite of their greater toxicity. Because joint destruction is thought to occur early in the disease process, early and aggressive treatment is often warranted and recommended for people with rheumatoid arthritis to achieve disease control, slow down or reduce joint destruction, and alleviate pain. Grading of the severity of a case of arthritis often depends on careful evaluation by the prescriber of such factors as radiographic (X-ray) evidence and laboratory indicators such as serum *rheumatoid factor* and *antinuclear antibody*.

DMARDs act by inhibiting the movement of cells into an inflamed, damaged area, such as a joint. These inflammatory cells (neutrophils, monocytes, and macrophages) are responsible for causing many of the deleterious effects of chronic rheumatoid arthritis. By preventing the accumulation of the inflammatory cells in the area of the diseased joint, antiarthritic drugs prevent progression of the disease, in addition to decreasing pain. One of these drugs, hydroxychloroquine (Plaquenil), is also used to treat malaria, and was discussed in Chapter 43. Another, sulfasalazine (Salazopyrin), is used for colitis. Some additional DMARDs, such as the newer drug etanercept (Enbrel), are designed and known especially for their immunomodulating effects. These drugs are discussed in Chapter 50.

 DRUG PROFILES

auranofin

Auranofin (Ridaura) is an orally active antiarthritic drug. Twenty-nine percent of it is gold, and as with all antiarthritic drugs, it possesses anti-inflammatory, antiarthritic, and immunomodulating effects. It is poorly absorbed orally — only about 25% percent of the drug is absorbed from the gastrointestinal tract into the blood. Auranofin is contraindicated in patients with a history of gold-induced necrotizing enterocolitis, pulmonary fibrosis, exfoliative dermatitis, bone marrow aplasia, or other types of blood dyscrasia. It is available for oral use. The normal recommended adult dosage is 6 mg once per day or 3 mg twice per day. The dosage can be increased to 9 mg after 6 months of therapy if the response is inadequate. It is classified as pregnancy category C.

gold sodium thiomalate

Gold sodium thiomalate (Myochrysine) is a parenterally administered antiarthritic drug. It is approximately 50% gold and currently available only in an injectable form. It is made by complexing gold with thiomalate via a sulfur linkage. It is administered by the intramuscular route only, with weekly injections ranging from 10 to 100 mg. It requires regular monitoring with either dose reduction or discontinuation if symptoms of toxicity appear, detected by complete blood count, urinalysis, and kidney and liver function tests.

leflunomide

Leflunomide (Arava) is a new drug indicated for the treatment of active rheumatoid arthritis. It modulates or alters the response of the immune system to rheumatoid arthritis. It has antiproliferative, anti-inflammatory, and immunosuppressive activities. Its most common adverse effects are diarrhea, respiratory tract infection, alopecia, elevated liver function tests, hypertension, and rash. It is contraindicated in women who are or may become pregnant, and it should not be used by nursing mothers or those with hypersensitivity to it. Leflunomide is most commonly given as a loading dose of 100 mg daily for 3 days, followed by a maintenance dose of 20 mg daily. ASA, NSAIDs, and low-dose corticosteroids may be continued during leflunomide therapy. It is available only for oral use and is classified as pregnancy category X.

NURSING PROCESS

Assessment

Before administering any of the anti-inflammatory, anti-rheumatoid, and related drugs, it is critical to patient safety and drug effectiveness to assess for drug allergies, contraindications, cautions, and drug interactions associated with each drug within each of these major groups of drugs (discussed previously in the pharmacology section and drug profiles). The nurse should conduct a thorough head-to-toe physical assessment, vital signs assessment, and medication history, noting the patient's use of prescription and over-the-counter drugs and natural health products (see Natural Health Products: Glucosamine and Chondroitin). Laboratory tests reflecting hematological, kidney, and liver functioning should be analyzed, including red blood cells, Hgb, Hct, white blood cells, platelets, blood urea nitrogen, and liver enzymes, before NSAIDs, antigout, DMARDs, or other drugs in these categories are used. In addition, laboratory studies that assess the status of inflammatory-type diseases may be ordered, with attention to rheumatoid factors, sedimentation rate values, and immunoglobulin levels.

With aspirin, NSAIDs, and other drugs in this chapter, it is important for the nurse to assess the duration, onset, location, and type of inflammation and pain that the patient is experiencing, with documentation of precipitating or exacerbating and relieving factors as well as interference with activities of daily living (ADLs). Inspection of all joints with attention to deformities, immobility, or limitations in mobility, overlying skin condition, and any heat or swelling over the joint should be noted. Age is important to consider because drugs such as celecoxib and aspirin are not to be used in children and teenagers because of the increased risk for Reye's syndrome. The odour of the aspirin should be checked because a vinegary smell is associated with a chemical breakdown of the drug. With aspirin it is also important to assess for a history of asthma, wheezing, or other respiratory problems because of increased incidence of allergic reactions to aspirin in these individuals. Patients who have been diagnosed with "aspirin triad," which includes asthma, nasal polyps, and rhinitis, should not be given aspirin because of the risk for reactions to it. It is important to remember that salicylic acid, aspirin, and NSAIDs have anti-inflammatory, antipyretic, analgesic, and antiplatelet properties as well as pose a risk for ulcerogenic and bleeding tendencies. NSAIDs require close assessment not only for gastrointestinal upset but also for any pre-existing peripheral edema. Baseline complete blood count (CBC), blood chemistries with electrolytes, BUN, creatinine, liver function tests, and bleeding/clotting times should be noted prior to initiation of drug therapy. Ketorolac requires assessment of the prescription because it must be for short-term use (e.g., no more than 5 days) and ordered for patients experiencing severe acute pain. Underlying signs of infection should be assessed prior to use of indomethacin because it may mask them with its use.

With *antigout* drugs, it is necessary to obtain a history of gastrointestinal distress, ulcers, and heart, kidney, or liver disease as well as an assessment of baseline hydration status. Serum uric acid levels are generally measured prior to therapy for baseline comparisons, as ordered. Urinary output should also be closely assessed prior to and during the drug therapy to ensure at least 30 to 60 mL/hour output. BUN, serum creatinine, alkaline phosphatase (ALP), aspartate aminotransferase (AST), alanine aminotransferase (ALT), and lactate dehydrogenase (LDH) are some of the more common blood tests done prior to therapy for baseline comparisons. Antigout drugs (e.g., allopurinol, colchicine, probenicid) are indicated for

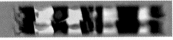

NATURAL HEALTH PRODUCTS

GLUCOSAMINE AND CHONDROITIN

Overview
Glucosamine is chemically derived from glucose. Its chemical name is 2-amino-2-deoxyglucose sulfate. Chondroitin is a protein usually isolated from bovine (cow) cartilage. To date, there are no reports of disease transmission to humans.

Common Uses
These two supplements are often used in combination, and sometimes individually, to treat pain from osteoarthritis. Although most commonly taken orally, injectable forms are commercially available (e.g., for administration by a naturopathic physician).

Adverse Effects
Glucosamine: Usually mild adverse effects comparable to placebo in clinical studies. These include gastrointestinal discomfort, drowsiness, headache, and skin reactions.

Chondroitin: No major ill effects in studies lasting from 2 months to 6 years. Gastrointestinal discomfort is the most common adverse effect, but it is usually well tolerated. Clinical trials have reported cases of lower extremity edema, alopecia, and extracardiac systoles.

Potential Drug Interactions
Both supplements: Possible enhanced anticoagulant effects of warfarin. Measure the patient's INR more frequently during glucosamine or chondroitin therapy, and adjust warfarin dose if indicated.

Contraindications
Both supplements: No specific contraindications are listed, but avoidance in pregnancy is recommended because of lack of firm safety data.

INR, international normalized ratio.

either acute, chronic, or both actions. Thus it is important to note, for example, the presence of acute versus chronic gout because use of colchicine is initiated only after an acute attack has subsided. Consequently, the order and indication of the antigout drug must be assessed to ensure that the patient is receiving the appropriate treatment.

With the use of *DMARDs,* all contraindications, cautions, and drug interactions need to be noted. Administration of *auranofin* (29% gold) and *gold products* requires assessment for pregnancy status prior to beginning therapy as well as results of CBC, BUN, Hct, Hgb, platelet, serum alkaline phosphatase, creatinine, AST, and ALT tests. After injections of gold products, it is common practice to continue to assess the patient for a possible hypersensitivity or allergic reaction with the first or second injection. This reaction would most commonly occur within 10 to 15 minutes after the injection of the gold.

Nursing Diagnoses

- Acute pain related to disease process or injury to joints and injury- or disease-affected areas
- Activity intolerance related to the disorder, condition, or disease process causing the pain, and diminished performance of ADLs
- Risk for injury related to the influence of the disease and its treatment on mobility
- Ineffective health maintenance related to lack of knowledge about pharmacological and nonpharmacological measures of treatment
- Deficient knowledge related to first-time drug therapy for treatment of a pain or disease process.

Planning

Goals

- Patient will be able to describe the use of the medication as it relates to the relief of inflammation and pain.
- Patient will experience pain relief or relief of symptoms within an expected period or time frame.
- Patient will use nonpharmacological measures to enhance drug therapy in order to decrease inflammation so that the patient can increase ADLs, including walking.
- Patient will report adverse effects to the physician as indicated.
- Patient will remain adherent to drug therapy.

Outcome Criteria

- Patient states that pain and changes in joints and mobility are characteristic of inflammation, injury, or related disease processes and will decrease with an effective therapy.

- Patient identifies factors that aggravate or alleviate pain, such as movement, activity, exercising, and change in weather or atmosphere.
- Patient states nonpharmacological measures to promote comfort, increase joint function and mobility, and ADLs (e.g., biofeedback, imagery, massage, hot or cold packs, physical therapy, and relaxation therapy).
- Patient states adverse effects associated with the specific group of drugs being taken.
- Patient identifies symptoms to report to the physician immediately.
- Patient states the importance of correct dosing and consistency in the self-administration of medication.
- Patient returns for follow-up visits with the physician and states the importance of returning for monitoring of success of treatment as well as for occurrence of adverse or toxic effects.

Implementation

If aspirin is used, oral dosage forms should be given with food, milk, or meals. Sustained-released or enteric-coated tablets should not be crushed or broken. Aspirin rectal suppositories should be refrigerated prior to use. Serum levels of aspirin should be monitored if aspirin therapy is used for its antiarthritic effect. Serum aspirin levels are also important to monitor for determining mild versus moderate to severe toxicity. Although aspirin therapy is generally not recommended or used because of its toxicity, the nurse should remain current about its possible use. It is important to be alert to signs of toxicity, such as bleeding, gastric ulcers, and gastric bleeding, and to report these to the physician for immediate treatment. If aspirin is used as an antipyretic, the patient's temperature should begin to decrease within 1 hour. For more information, see Patient Education.

NSAIDs may come in enteric-coated or sustained-release preparations and should not be crushed or chewed. In oral dosage forms, these drugs, including ketorolac, may be taken with antacids or food to decrease gastrointestinal upset or irritation. Moderate to severe gastrointestinal upset, dyspepsia with nausea, vomiting, abdominal pain, and blood in the stool or emesis should be reported to the physician immediately. Other ulcerogenic substances (e.g., alcohol, prednisone, aspirin-containing products, other NSAIDs) should be avoided to help minimize risk for gastrointestinal mucosal breakdown. During therapy with NSAIDs, bowel patterns, stool consistency, and the occurrence of dizziness should be monitored and documented, as should CBC and BUN levels, platelet, bilirubin, serum alkaline phosphatase, and AST and ALT levels. Additionally, with indomethacin, suppository use should be administered with instructions similar to those for aspirin suppositories. Other dosage forms include powder for IV injection and oral liquid or suspension. Intravenous (IV) dosages should be clear and administered as per manufacturer guidelines for dilutional solutions and infusion rates or over 5 to 10 seconds. Safe ambulation should always be emphasized with NSAID use. With ketorolac, it is important that dosing not exceed a 5-day time period with either the oral, intramuscular (IM) (deep IM and slowly injected into a large muscle mass), or IV (infused over at least 15 seconds) dosage forms. COX-2 inhibitors should be taken only as ordered with the same concern for avoiding alcohol, aspirin, other NSAIDs, and over-the-counter medication containing these drugs (e.g., NSAIDs, aspirin, salicylates). Any stomach or abdominal pain, gastrointestinal problems, unusual bleeding, blood in the stool or emesis, chest pain, or palpitations should be reported immediately to the physician.

The antigout drugs are somewhat different from the NSAIDs and have some different types of nursing considerations. Colchicine should be taken on an empty stomach for more complete absorption, which means 1 hour before meals or 2 hours after meals. Alcohol and any over-the-counter cold-relief products that contain alcohol should be avoided while taking colchicine. In addition, patients with gout must be instructed that adherence to the entire medical regimen is critical to successful treatment. Allopurinol should be given with meals to try to prevent the occurrence of gastrointestinal symptoms (nausea, vomiting, anorexia). If allopurinol is administered in conjunction with chemotherapy (in an attempt to decrease hyperuricemia associated with the malignancy and cell death from successful treatment), it is recommended that it be given a few days before the antineoplastic therapy. Patients taking allopurinol should be informed to increase fluid intake to 3 L/day, avoid hazardous activities if dizziness or drowsiness occurs with the medication, and avoid the use of alcohol and caffeine because these drugs will increase uric acid levels and decrease the levels of allopurinol.

DMARDs, specifically gold sodium thiomalate, should never be given intravenously. When given intramuscularly, it should be given into deep muscle. The patient needs to remain recumbent for at least 10 minutes after the injection, and special precautions should be taken for the patient with bleeding disorders or thrombocytopenia. Daily checks of the patient's skin for pruritis, purpura, rash, or ecchymoses are required, as well as examinations of the oral mucosa, palate, pharynx, and borders of the tongue for any ulcerations. The nurse should be attentive to any complaints of a metallic taste in the mouth as this may indicate stomatitis. With any drugs used for rheumatoid arthritis, the patient should be constantly watched and questioned about improved mobility, increased grip strength and joint flexibility, and a decrease in joint pain, stiffness, and swelling. Fluids should be forced, as ordered, and only if not contraindicated. Leflunomide may be given with meals or food to minimize gastrointestinal upset should it occur. See Patient Education for more information on these drugs.

Evaluation

Aspirin and NSAIDs may vary in their potency and anti-inflammatory and analgesic effects. Therapeutic responses to NSAIDs include the following: decrease in acute pain; decrease in swelling, pain, and stiffness and tenderness of a joint or muscle area; improved ability to conduct ADLs; improved muscle grip and strength; reduction in fever; return to normal laboratory values (CBC, RBC, Hgb level, Hct, and sedimentation rates); and return to a less inflamed state as evidenced by improved sedimentation rates, X-ray examination, computed tomography scan, or magnetic resonance imaging. The COX-2 inhibitor should result in improved joint function and fewer inflammation-based signs and symptoms. Patients should begin to show improvement in ADLs and mobility with any of these drugs but within their respective time frame, which may be up to 2 to 3 months, depending on the drug. Monitoring for the occurrence of adverse effects and toxicity is essential to the safe and effective use of aspirin, NSAIDs, antigout drugs, and the COX-2 inhibitor (see Table 45-2).

Evaluation of therapeutic responses to all other antiarthritics and DMARDs includes monitoring for the increased ability to move joints with less discomfort and an overall increased sense of improvement in the condition. Toxicity to gold products is evident with a decreased Hgb level, a white blood cell count of less than 4.0×10^9/L, platelet count of less than 150×10^9/L, hematuria, severe diarrhea, itching, and proteinuria. An elevation of ALT level (if more than 2 but less than or equal to 3, a liver biopsy may be needed) indicates toxicity to DMARDs.

A therapeutic response to antigout drugs (e.g., colchicine) includes decreased pain in affected joints and increased sense of well-being. The patient should be monitored closely for and report to the physician the occurrence of increased pain, blood in the urine, excessive fatigue and lethargy, and chills or fever. A therapeutic response to allopurinol, another antigout drug, includes a decrease in pain in the joints, a decrease in uric acid levels, and a decrease of stone formation in the kidneys.

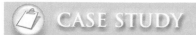 **CASE STUDY**

Postoperative Pain

One of your patients who had abdominal surgery is complaining of abdominal pain, nausea, and breakthrough pain after receiving the pain protocol for hydromorphone hydrochloride (Dilaudid-HP-Plus) patient-controlled analgesia (PCA) and ketorolac tromethamine (Apo-Ketorolac) intramuscularly. She has received ketorolac for 7 days and in multiple doses. A gastrointestinal ulcer is now diagnosed and has been attributed to the ketorolac; however, the patient has a past history of gastritis and reflux disease and a 5-year history of ulcer disease.

1. What is the action of ketorolac and its purpose in this case?

2. What could have been done to prevent the gastrointestinal bleeding and ulcer formation with the ketorolac?

3. What concerns would you have regarding the past history of gastrointestinal disorders, and how could you have handled this potential risk to the patient? Was there any problem with the number of days ordered? Is ketorolac available orally, or only in injectable forms?

For answers see http://evolve.elsevier.com/Canada/Lilley/pharmacology/.

PATIENT EDUCATION

❖ Patients should be instructed not to crush or chew any sustained-release or enteric-coated aspirin. Make sure patients know that the anti-inflammatory effect of the drug may take up to 1 to 3 weeks.

❖ Patients should be advised that they need to inform other health care professionals and dentists that they are taking aspirin or NSAIDs prior to any treatment, specifically if they are taking high doses of aspirin or have been taking aspirin for prolonged periods. Aspirin and NSAIDs should also be discontinued, as per physician's orders, 3 to 7 days prior to surgery, including oral or dental surgery.

❖ Patients should be advised to keep aspirin and other drugs out of the reach of children. If a child (or adult) has consumed large or unknown quantities of aspirin or NSAIDs, the Poison Control Centre should be contacted immediately and emergency medical attention sought. Children and teenagers should not be taking aspirin because of the risk of Reye's syndrome. Acetaminophen is usually preferred in the recommended dosage range.

❖ Patients should be educated about adverse effects of aspirin such as gastrointestinal upset, flushing of the face, dizziness, tinnitus, drowsiness, visual changes, seizures, gastrointestinal bleeding, heartburn, and any bleeding tendencies or easy bruising. Any black or tarry stools, bleeding around the gums, petechiae (tiny red–brown spots), ecchymosis (easy bruising), and purpura (large red spots) should be reported to the physician immediately.

❖ Patients should understand that NSAIDs are used for the treatment of pain, injuries, or inflammatory disease–related processes and work by decreasing the inflammation that leads to pain.

❖ Patients should be educated about the most common adverse effects of NSAIDs: heartburn, gastrointestinal upset, ulcers, nausea, vomiting, hemorrhage, hemolytic anemias, epistaxis, blurred vision, rash, leukopenia, vertigo, and tinnitus. Patients should also be informed to take NSAIDs with food, milk, or antacids to help minimize gastrointestinal distress. Patient education should convey the many drug interactions with NSAIDs, including anticoagulants, aspirin, steroids, corticosteroids, salicylates, oral antihyperglycemic drugs, insulin, penicillin, sulfonamides, and barbiturates. In addition, it is important to educate the patient about the difference between the onset of action of the medication for the relief of acute pain and its more delayed effect when used for the relief of arthritis pain; in the latter case, the therapeutic effects may not be realized for 3 to 4 weeks. In addition, NSAIDs (as well as salicylates and other drugs) come in enteric-coated dosage forms and should not be crushed or chewed.

❖ With gold product injections, patients should be encouraged to report any adverse effects, such as headache, local pain at the injection site, lethargy, and joint pain. Other adverse effects are pruritic dermatitis, stomatitis, ulcers of the oral mucous membranes, sore throat, diarrhea, and abdominal pain. Gold sodium thiomalate is usually given once weekly, as ordered.

❖ Patients should be informed that it may take 3 to 6 months for the full therapeutic response to DMARDs.

POINTS TO REMEMBER

* NSAIDs are one of the most commonly prescribed categories of drugs. The first drug in this category to be synthesized was salicylic acid, or aspirin. Aspirin is often included in the discussion of anti-inflammatory drugs. NSAIDs have analgesic, anti-inflammatory, antipyretic activities; aspirin also has antiplatelet activity. NSAIDs are often used in the treatment of gout, osteoarthritis, juvenile arthritis, rheumatoid arthritis, dysmenorrhea, and musculoskeletal injuries such as strains and sprains.

* The three main adverse effects of NSAIDs are gastro-intestinal intolerance, bleeding (often gastrointestinal bleeding), and kidney impairment. Misoprostol (Apo-Misoprostol) may be given to prevent gastrointestinal intolerance and ulcers resulting from NSAIDs. It is classified as a prostaglandin analogue. There are many contraindications to the use of NSAIDs, such as gastrointestinal tract lesions, peptic ulcers, and bleeding disorders.

* All NSAIDs have a ceiling effect, meaning that they become ineffective after a certain dose.

* Most NSAIDs are better tolerated orally if taken with food to minimize gastrointestinal upset.

* Patients on NSAIDs should be closely monitored for the occurrence of bleeding, such as blood in the stools or emesis. When NSAIDs are used to decrease inflammation in the joints of arthritis patients, thera-peutic effects usually take up to 3 to 4 weeks.

* Antigout drugs are indicated for either acute or chronic or prophylactic gout. Diarrhea and abdominal pain are common adverse effects. Antigout drugs are often used in patients with cell death during cancer chemotherapy to avoid gout-like syndromes and pain.

* DMARDs alter or modify the disease process of rheumatoid arthritis but are not curative. It may take up to 3 to 6 months for the full therapeutic effects, depending on the specific drug used. Because a stepped approach to treating rheumatoid arthritis is no longer commonly used, it is important to empha-size the individualization of each treatment protocol for patients with this disease. DMARDs include gold sodium thiomalate, leflunomide, and sulfasalazine.

EXAMINATION REVIEW QUESTIONS

1 When a patient is receiving long-term NSAID therapy, which may be given to prevent the gastrointestinal adverse effects of NSAIDs?
   a. magnesium sulfate ($MgSO_4$)
   b. metoprolol tartrate (Betaloc)
   c. misoprostol (Apo-Misoprostol)
   d. metoclopramide hydrochloride (Apo-Metoclop)

2 Which of the following manifestations would the nurse recognize as NSAID toxicity?
   a. Tremors
   b. Constipation
   c. Urinary retention
   d. Nausea and vomiting

3 By which mechanism do antigout drugs act?
   a. Increasing blood oxygen levels
   b. Decreasing serum uric acid levels
   c. Decreasing leukocytes and platelets
   d. Increasing protein and rheumatoid factors

4 When teaching about antigout drugs, which statement by the nurse is accurate?
   a. "Colchicine is best taken on an empty stomach."
   b. "Drink only limited amounts of fluid with the drug."
   c. "There are few drug interactions with these medications."
   d. "This drug may cause limited movements of your joints."

5 A mother calls the clinic to ask about what medication to give her 5-year-old child, who has chicken pox and a fever. Which of the following would be the nurse's best response?
   a. "It is best to wait to let the fever break on its own without medication."
   b. "Start with acetaminophen or ibuprofen, but if those do not work, then you can try aspirin."
   c. "Since your child is 5 years old, it would be okay to use children's aspirin to treat his fever."
   d. "You can use children's dosages of acetaminophen or ibuprofen, but aspirin is not recommended."

For answers see http://evolve.elsevier.com/Canada/Lilley/pharmacology/.

CRITICAL THINKING ACTIVITIES

1 Is the following statement true or false? Acetaminophen is an NSAID and exerts anti-inflammatory, antipyretic, analgesic, and antiplatelet effects. Explain your answer. You may need to refer to the chapter on analgesic drugs (Chapter 11).

2 What are the drug interactions for NSAIDs? What problems may occur if these drugs are used with other NSAIDs?

3 Describe the protocol for treating salicylate intoxication of a chronic nature.

For answers see http://evolve.elsevier.com/Canada/Lilley/pharmacology/.

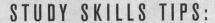

PART EIGHT

Immune and Biological Modifiers and Chemotherapeutic Drugs

STUDY SKILLS TIPS:

- TIME MANAGEMENT
- EVALUATE PRIOR PERFORMANCE
- ANTICIPATE THE TEST
- PLAN FOR DISTRIBUTED STUDY

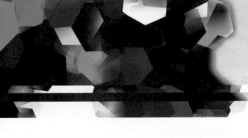

TIME MANAGEMENT

The first step in preparing for a chapter or section exam is to plan for the time needed. Begin by assuming that the next test you have will cover the chapters in Part Eight. First look at how much there is to cover. This will help you determine just how big a task you face. Also consider how much study time you have been devoting to these chapters in the days before the exam. If you have been doing regular study with frequent review sessions, then the demand on your time in the day or two just before the exam will be less than if you have to do a major cram session to try to catch up on study that has been put off. The basic question to answer here is a simple one: "How much time do I need to schedule for exam preparation?" The answer varies for each student. Some will need 6, 8, or more hours of preparation time in the 2 to 3 days before the exam. Others will find that 3, 4, or 5 hours will be adequate. Assess your own learning and prior success to determine how much time is necessary for you.

One factor that should play a major role in determining how much time you need is your performance on prior exams. How have you been doing and how much time have you been spending to achieve that level? If you are not achieving according to your capabilities, then you should think about spending more time preparing for the next exam. If you are achieving at a satisfactory level, then plan on devoting about the same amount of time to test preparation.

The next step in preparing for an exam is to organize the time. Write down what you are going to study and when, and how much time you will spend. Consider the following example based on the material in Chapters 46 and 47:

1 Review Chapter 46 objectives. Monday, 4:00 to 4:30 P.M. Note objectives that are unclear for further review.
2 Question and Answer review, Monday, 4:30 to 5:15 P.M.
3 Self-test, Chapter 46 glossary. Monday, 6:30 to 7:00 P.M. Note terms that need further review for mastery.
4 Review Chapter 47 objectives. Monday, 7:00 to 7:30 P.M.
5 Question and Answer review, Monday, 7:30 to 8:00 P.M.
6 Self-test, Chapter 47 glossary. Monday, 8:00 to 8:30 P.M.

The advantage to this test preparation model is that you now know where you must focus in the days before the exam.

EVALUATE PRIOR PERFORMANCE

As you begin preparing to review for any exam, take some time to look back at previous exams. Evaluate your performance, and use that evaluation to improve on subsequent tests. As you look at prior tests consider the following factors.

What Type of Errors Did I Make?

Students often find that they miss certain types or forms of questions. Assess your errors and try to pinpoint any recurring patterns in your mistakes. Did you miss questions that contained an exemption in the multiple-choice stem? Questions that state "all of the following except" or ask "Which of the following would not be. . ." are exemption questions. Students often choose one of the apparently correct responses. Read the question carefully to see whether you are looking for a correct or an incorrect answer. An exemption stem is asking for the response choice that is "wrong."

Did I Have Trouble with Questions That Required Mastery of Terminology?

Look at questions that demanded mastery of the terms from the chapters. If you missed more than one or two questions of that type, then you know you need to spend more time reviewing terminology.

Did I Miss Concept Questions?

If the question asked you to apply a principle, evaluate a drug response, or in some other way apply knowledge from the course, you are dealing with concepts rather than facts. If you missed a number of concept questions, then you should spend more of your review time studying applications and principles than memorizing facts and terms.

Did I Make Errors Because I Did Not Know the Material?

This question focuses on the quality of your learning. If you miss one or two questions on an exam because you did not learn (or did not remember) the material, it is not a major problem. There will almost always be one or two questions that you do not know how to answer because you do not remember the material.

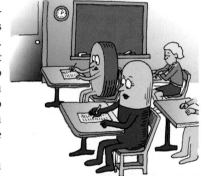

However, if you had to guess on several questions because you did not recall any information that seemed relevant, you may need to put more time into review. It is essential that you acknowledge to yourself that you have missed questions because you did not know the material, so that you can take steps to correct the situation. You may need to do more oral rehearsal so that the material is stored in long-term memory.

ANTICIPATE THE TEST

Do not wait until exam time to find out what you should know. As you review, try to come up with questions you think might be on the test. This does not mean you need to try to write multiple-choice questions; just try to focus your review to help you keep the information in your long-term memory.

Here are some examples of questioning that you might use that is based on material found in Chapter 50.

1 What are immunomodulators (IMs)?
2 What is the role of IMs in the care of patients with cancer?
3 What is the role of the immune system in treating cancer?

The sample questions were drawn from just the first few pages of the chapter. The first question focuses on literal comprehension. This type of question is easy to generate, and being able to answer these questions is important, but if all of your questions are literal, it may be difficult to answer questions that require application of principles and concepts. It is essential that some questions require analysis, synthesis, and evaluation of the material. Question 3 is an example of this type of question.

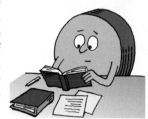

PLAN FOR DISTRIBUTED STUDY

Many students wait too long to begin the review for a test and are forced into a pattern of long hours of intensive study all packed into the last day or two before the exam. Although cramming does work to some degree, it is not the most effective way to learn. It is better to distribute your review over a period of several days with short, 30-minute to 1-hour study sessions several times each day. Distributing practice in this way allows time for you to think about what you have been learning, and it fosters long-term memory.

Spend more of your review time doing oral rehearsal (asking and answering questions) than simply rereading material. Oral rehearsal encourages active learning, which enhances your ability to concentrate, improves comprehension and memory, and thus improves test performance.

CHAPTER 46

Immunosuppressant Drugs

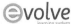

Learning Objectives

After reading this chapter, the successful student will be able to do the following:

1 Discuss the role of immunosuppressive therapy in organ transplant recipients and in the treatment of autoimmune diseases.

2 Discuss the mechanisms of action, contraindications, cautions, adverse effects, routes of administration, drug interactions, and toxicity associated with the most commonly used immunosuppressants.

3 Develop a collaborative plan of care that includes all phases of the nursing process for the patient receiving immunosuppressants either for an organ transplant or for the treatment of autoimmune diseases.

e-Learning Activities

Web site
(http://evolve.elsevier.com/Canada/Lilley/pharmacology/)

- Animations
- Answers to chapter questions, activities, and case studies
- Calculators and Category Catchers
- Glossary with audio pronunciations
- IV Therapy and Medication Error Checklists
- Multiple-Choice Review Question quizzes
- Nursing Care Plans
- Online Appendices and Supplements
- WebLinks

Drug Profiles

▸▸ **azathioprine (azathioprine sodium)*, mycophenolate mofetil**, p. 854
basiliximab, daclizumab, p. 854
▸▸ **cyclosporine**, p. 854
glatiramer (glatiramer acetate)*, p. 854
sirolimus, tacrolimus, p. 855

▸▸ Key drug.

*Full generic name is given in parentheses. For the purposes of this text, the more common shortened name is used.

Glossary

Autoimmune diseases A large group of diseases characterized by the subversion or alteration of the function of the immune system wherein the immune response is directed against normal tissue(s) of the body, resulting in pathological conditions. (p. 852)

Graft The term used for a transplanted tissue or organ. (p. 854)

Immune-mediated diseases A large group of diseases that result when the cells of the immune system react to a variety of situations, such as transplanted organ tissue or drug-altered cells. (p. 852)

Immunosuppressant A drug that decreases or prevents an immune response. (p. 852)

Immunosuppressive therapy A drug treatment used to suppress the immune system. (p. 852)

IMMUNOSUPPRESSANT DRUGS

The human body is under constant attack by invading microorganisms. It possesses several mechanisms with which to fight off these foreign invaders, one being the *immune system*. This system defends the body against invading pathogens, foreign antigens, and its own cells that become cancerous or *neoplastic*. Besides performing this beneficial function, however, this highly sophisticated system can also sometimes attack itself and cause what are known as **autoimmune diseases** or **immune-mediated diseases**. It also participates in hypersensitivity, or anaphylactic, reactions, which can be life threatening. The rejection of kidney, liver, and heart (whole organ) transplants is also directed by the immune system. From all of these responses it is easy to see that the immune system is capable of having many beneficial and detrimental effects. Drugs that decrease or prevent an immune response and, consequently, suppress the immune system are known as **immunosuppressants**. Treatment with such drugs is referred to as **immunosuppressive therapy;** it is used to selectively eradicate certain cell lines

that play a major role in the rejection of a transplanted organ. These cell lines must be targeted and selectively altered or suppressed, otherwise organ rejection will occur. The primary immunosuppressant drugs are the corticosteroids (Chapter 33), cyclophosphamide (Chapter 49), azathioprine, cyclosporine, tacrolimus, glatiramer acetate, daclizumab, basiliximab, and sirolimus.

Mechanism of Action and Drug Effects

All immunosuppressants have similar mechanisms of action because they all selectively suppress certain T-lymphocyte cell lines, thereby preventing their involvement in the immune response. This action results in a pharmacologically immunocompromised state similar to that in a patient with cancer whose bone marrow and immune cells have been destroyed as the result of chemotherapy, or that in a patient with AIDS whose immune cells have been destroyed by the HIV. Each drug differs in the exact way in which it suppresses certain cell lines involved in an immune response. See Table 46-1 for pharmacological classifications, mechanisms of action, and indications of the immunosuppressant drugs.

TABLE 46-1

Classification and Mechanisms of Action for Available Immunosuppressant Drugs

Drug Names	Pharmacological Class and Mechanism of Action	Indications
azathioprine sodium (Imuran)	Blocks metabolism of purines, inhibiting the synthesis of T-cell DNA, RNA, and proteins, thereby blocking immune response	Organ rejection prevention in kidney transplantation; rheumatoid arthritis
basiliximab* (Simulect)	Suppresses T-cell activity by blocking the binding of the cytokine mediator IL-2 to a specific receptor	Organ rejection prevention in kidney transplantation
cyclosporine (Atopica, Neoral, Sandimmune)	Inhibits activation of T cells by blocking the production and release of the cytokine mediator IL-2	Organ rejection prevention in kidney, liver, and heart transplantation; rheumatoid arthritis; psoriasis. Unlabelled uses† include pancreas, bone marrow, and heart or lung transplantation.
daclizumab* (Zenapax)	Suppresses T-cell activity by blocking the binding of the cytokine receptor IL-2 to a specific receptor	Organ rejection prevention in kidney transplantation.
glatiramer acetate (Copaxone)	Precise mechanism unknown. Believed to somehow modify immune system processes that are associated with MS symptoms	Reduction of relapse frequency in patients with RRMS
mycophenolate mofetil (CellCept)	Prevents proliferation of T cells by inhibiting intracellular purine synthesis	Organ rejection prevention in kidney, liver, and heart transplantation
sirolimus (Rapamune)	Inhibits T-cell activation by a unique mechanism: binding to an intracellular protein known as FKBP-12, creating a complex that subsequently binds to a cellular component known as the mTOR, which prevents cellular proliferation	Organ rejection prevention in kidney transplantation
tacrolimus (Advagraf, Prograf)	Inhibits T-cell activation, possibly by binding to an intracellular protein known as FKBP-12	Organ rejection prevention in liver and kidney transplantation; active rheumatoid arthritis. Unlabelled uses† include kidney, bone marrow, heart, pancreas, pancreatic islet cell, and small intestine transplantation; autoimmune diseases; and severe psoriasis.

DNA, deoxyribonucleic acid; *IL-2*, interleukin-2; *MS*, multiple sclerosis; *mTOR*, mammalian target of rapamycin; *RRMS*, relapsing-remitting multiple sclerosis; *RNA*, ribonucleic acid.

*Note that "ab" in any drug name usually indicates that it is a monoclonal antibody synthesized using recombinant DNA technology.
†A use not approved by Health Canada but under investigation.

Indications

The therapeutic uses of immunosuppressants are multiple and vary from drug to drug, as illustrated in Table 46-1. These drugs are indicated primarily for the prevention of organ rejection, which is the focus of this chapter. However, some are also used for other immunological illnesses, such as rheumatoid arthritis and multiple sclerosis. The four newer drugs (basiliximab, daclizumab, sirolimus, and mycophenolate mofetil), all immunosuppressants used in transplant patients, are all indicated for organ rejection prophylaxis. Azathioprine is used as an adjunct medication to prevent the rejection of kidney transplants and to ameliorate severe rheumatoid arthritis. Cyclosporine is the primary immunosuppressant drug used in the prevention of kidney, liver, heart, and bone marrow transplant rejection. It may also have beneficial effects in the treatment of other conditions with an immunological cause, such as certain types of arthritis and psoriasis, and in adults and children with steroid-dependent nephrotic syndrome.

Tacrolimus has many of the same therapeutic effects as those of cyclosporine, but it is currently indicated only for the prevention of liver and kidney transplant rejection, although it has shown promise in preventing the rejection of other transplanted organs as well. It is also used for monotherapy treatment of active rheumatoid arthritis for patients in whom antirheumatic (DMARD) therapy has been unsuccessful.

Glatiramer acetate is the only immunosuppressant currently indicated for treatment of multiple sclerosis (MS). Specifically, it is indicated for reduction of the frequency of MS relapses (exacerbations) in a type of MS known as *relapsing-remitting multiple sclerosis* (RRMS). This is currently its sole indication.

Contraindications

The main contraindication for all immunosuppressants is known drug allergy. Relative contraindications, depending on the patient's condition, may include kidney or liver failure, hypertension, and concurrent radiation therapy. While pregnancy is not necessarily a contraindication to these drugs, immunosuppressants should be used in pregnant women only in urgent situations.

Adverse Effects

Many of the adverse effects of the immunosuppressants can be devastating, especially to a transplant patient. Although not strictly an adverse effect, a heightened susceptibility to opportunistic infections is a major risk for immunosuppressed patients. Other adverse effects are limited to the particular drugs. Some of the most common of these are listed in Table 46-2.

Interactions

Cyclosporine, tacrolimus, and sirolimus are capable of many drug interactions, several of which can be harmful. Drugs that may increase their actions are diltiazem,

verapamil, fluconazole, itraconazole, clarithromycin, allopurinol, metoclopramide, amphotericin B, cimetidine, and ketoconazole. Grapefruit, including its juice, because of its inhibition of key metabolizing enzymes, can also increase the bioavailability of these three immunosuppressants. For example, cyclosporine can have a profound interaction with grapefruit juice; when taken together, there is an increase in the bioavailability of cyclosporine by 20% to 200%. Drugs that may reduce the effects of these immunosuppressants include carbamazepine, phenobarbital, phenytoin, and rifampin. The drug interactions occur because of some of the same cytochrome P450 metabolizing enzymes are shared among these drugs and the immunosuppressant drugs. Although these are the most significant interactions, there are many more of less significance.

It is also recommended that azathioprine not be given with allopurinol because allopurinol inhibits azathioprine's metabolism and thereby increases its effects. The coadministration of angiotensin-converting enzyme (ACE) inhibitors with azathioprine may result in severe leukopenia, whereas azathioprine may reduce the effectiveness of anticoagulants (e.g., warfarin). Azathioprine may also reduce the serum levels of cyclosporine, which may require an increase in dosage of desired

TABLE	46-2

**Immunosuppressant Drugs:
Common Adverse Effects**

Body System	Adverse Effects
AZATHIOPRINE	
Hematological	Leukopenia, thrombocytopenia
Hepatic	Hepatotoxicity is a common adverse effect.
CYCLOSPORINE	
Cardiovascular	Moderate hypertension in as many as 50% of patients
Central nervous	Neurotoxicity, including tremors in approximately 20% of patients
Hepatic	Hepatotoxicity with cholestasis and hyperbilirubinemia
Renal	Nephrotoxicity is common and dose limiting
Other	Hypersensitivity reactions to the vehicle, gingival hyperplasia, and hirsutism
TACROLIMUS	
Central nervous	Agitation, anxiety, confusion, hallucinations, neuropathy
Renal	Albuminuria, dysuria, acute kidney failure, kidney tubular necrosis
ANTIBODY IMMUNOSUPPRESSANTS	
basiliximab, daclizumab	*Cytokine release syndrome*, which includes such immune-mediated symptoms as fever, dyspnea, tachycardia, sweating, chills, headache, nausea, vomiting, diarrhea, muscle and joint pain, and general malaise

immunosuppressant effects. Mycophenolate absorption may be reduced with the use of antacids, iron preparations, and cholestyramine resins. Mycophenolate may also reduce the protein binding of both theophylline and phenytoin, increasing their free plasma levels, and it may reduce the efficacy of oral contraceptives as well as live-virus vaccines.

Because the antibodies basiliximab and daclizumab are generally given in a relatively short single course of therapy, they have few recognized drug interactions. However, the potential interactions between immunosuppressant drugs and natural health products should not be overlooked. For example, the enzyme induction properties of St. John's wort have been demonstrated in case reports to reduce the therapeutic levels of cyclosporine and cause organ rejection. The immunostimulant properties of cat's claw and echinacea may be similarly undesirable in transplant recipients.

Dosages

For the recommended dosages of selected immunosuppressant drugs, see the Dosages table on p. 855.

DRUG PROFILES

▸▸ azathioprine sodium and mycophenolate mofetil

Azathioprine sodium (Imuran) is a chemical analogue of the physiological purines, such as adenine and guanine. It blocks T-cell proliferation by inhibiting purine synthesis, which in turn prevents deoxyribonucleic acid (DNA) synthesis. The immunosuppressant drug mycophenolate mofetil (CellCept) acts with a mechanism similar to that of azathioprine. Both drugs are used for prophylaxis of organ rejection concurrently with other immunosuppressant drugs, such as cyclosporine and corticosteroids. Both drugs are available in both oral and injectable forms.

PHARMACOKINETICS

azathioprine

Half-Life	Onset	Peak	Duration
PO: 5 hr	PO: 2–4 days*	PO: 1–2 hr	PO: Unknown

mycophenolate mofetil

Half-Life	Onset	Peak	Duration
PO: 18 hr	PO: Unknown	PO: 0.75–1 hr	PO: Unknown

*6–8 wk for rheumatoid arthritis.

basiliximab and daclizumab

Basiliximab (Simulect) and daclizumab (Zenapax) are monoclonal antibodies that act by inhibiting the binding of the cytokine mediator interleukin-2 (IL-2) to what is known as the high-affinity IL-2 receptor. Both drugs are used to prevent rejection of transplanted (**graft**) kidneys and are most often used as part of a multidrug immunosuppressive regimen that includes cyclosporine and corticosteroids. They are both prone to cause the allergic-like reaction known as *cytokine release syndrome*, which can be severe and even involve anaphylaxis. Patients are often premedicated with corticosteroids (e.g., intravenous methylprednisolone) in an effort to avoid or alleviate this problem. Both drugs are available only in injectable form.

PHARMACOKINETICS

basiliximab

Half-Life	Onset	Peak	Duration
IV: 7–9 days	IV: 1 day	IV: 3–4 days	IV: Unknown

daclizumab

Half-Life	Onset	Peak	Duration
IV: 20 days	IV: < 1 day	IV: 3–5 days	IV: Unknown

▸▸ cyclosporine

Cyclosporine (Atopica, Neoral, Sandimmune) is an immunosuppressant drug indicated for the prevention of organ rejection. It is a potent immunosuppressant and the principal drug in numerous immunosuppressive drug protocols. Cyclosporine is used in the prevention of graft rejection in bone marrow transplants and the prevention or treatment of graft-versus-host disease. As with azathioprine, it may also be used for the treatment of other immunological disorders, such as rheumatoid arthritis, psoriasis, and nephrotic syndrome.

Cyclosporine is available in oral and injectable forms. Although Neoral and Sandimmune contain the same active ingredient (cyclosporine), the oral and injectable forms cannot be used interchangeably. When changing from Neoral to Sandimmune, the dosage is usually started with a 1:1 mg amount, but dosage adjustments may be necessary to account for the greater bioavailability of Neoral. It is recommended that cyclosporine blood concentration be monitored in patients changing from one product to another. Cyclosporine has a narrow therapeutic index, thus laboratory monitoring of drug levels may be used to ensure therapeutic plasma concentrations and avoid toxicity.

PHARMACOKINETICS*

Half-Life	Onset	Peak	Duration
PO: 1–2 hr (parent compound), then 10–27 hr (metabolites)	PO: 1–3 hr	PO: Unknown	PO: Unknown

*May vary somewhat between brand names.

glatiramer acetate

Glatiramer acetate (Copaxone) is a mixture of random polymers of four different amino acids. This mixture results in a compound that is antigenically similar to myelin basic protein, which is a protein found on the myelin sheath of nerves. The drug is believed to work by blocking T-cell autoimmune activity against this protein, which reduces the frequency of the neuromuscular exacerbations associated with multiple sclerosis. As this drug is mixed in the sugar mannitol, it is contraindicated in patients who are allergic to that component. It is available only in injectable form.

Continued

DRUG PROFILES (cont'd)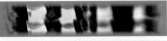

sirolimus and tacrolimus

Sirolimus (Rapamune) and tacrolimus (Advagraf, Prograf) are macrocyclic immunosuppressive, antifungal, and antitumour drugs, produced by fermentation of the fungus *Streptomyces hygroscopicus*. Other macrocyclic immunosuppressive drugs are cyclosporine and tacrolimus. Sirolimus and tacrolimus are structurally related and act through similar mechanisms. Sirolimus is available only for oral use, whereas tacrolimus is available in both oral and injectable forms.

PHARMACOKINETICS

sirolimus

Half-Life	Onset	Peak	Duration
PO: 57–68 hr	PO: Unknown	PO: 1–3 hr	PO: Unknown

tacrolimus

Half-Life	Onset	Peak	Duration
PO: 35 hr	PO: Unknown	PO: 1.5 hr	PO: Unknown

DOSAGES   Selected Immunosuppressant Drugs

Drug (Pregnancy Category)	Pharmacological Class	Usual Dosage Range	Indications
▸▸azathioprine sodium (Imuran) (D)	Purine antagonist	*Children/Adult* IV/PO: 3–5 mg/kg/day to start, then 1–3 mg/kg/day maintenance *Adult* PO: 1 mg/kg/day as a single or divided dose for 6–8 wk, dose increments by 0.5 mg/kg/day q4 wk to a maximum of 2.5 mg/kg/day	Kidney homotransplantation Rheumatoid arthritis
basiliximab (Simulect) (B)	Monoclonal antibody	*Children older than 2 yr*/Adult* IV: Bolus injection of 20 mg given 2 hr prior to transplant surgery; then 20 mg 4 days post-transplant	Prevention of rejection of kidney transplants
▸▸cyclosporine (Atopica, Neoral, Sandimmune) (C)	Polypeptide antibiotic	*Children/Adult* PO: 10–15 mg/kg divided within 12 hr preoperative; continue same dose postoperative for 1–2 wk, then reduce to a maintenance dose of 2–6 mg/kg/day IV: 3–5 mg/kg as a single dose within 12 hr preoperative and continued daily postoperative (up to 12 wk) until patient can be switched to PO dosing	Kidney, liver, heart transplants
daclizumab (Zenapax) (C)	Monoclonal antibody	*Adolescents older than 17*/Adult* IV: Bolus injection of 1 mg/kg 24 hr before transplant; 4 additional post-transplant doses, spaced 14 days apart	Prevention of rejection of kidney transplants
glatiramer acetate (Copaxone) (B)	Miscellaneous biological	*Adult only* SC: 20 mg once daily	RRMS
▸▸mycophenolate mofetil (CellCept) (C)	Miscellaneous	*Children and Adolescents 2–18 yr* IV/PO: 400 mg/m2 twice daily (maximum daily dose: 1.5–2 g daily) *Adult* IV/PO: 1–1.5 g twice daily	Prevention of organ rejection of kidney, heart, or liver transplants
sirolimus (Rapamune) (C)	Fungus-derived	*Children/Adult* PO: Loading dose of 6 mg on day 1, followed by maintenance dose of 2 mg/day	Prevention of rejection of kidney transplants
tacrolimus (Advagraf, Prograf) (C)	Fungus-derived	*Children/Adult* IV: 0.03–0.05 mg/kg/day as continuous IV infusion; then PO: 0.1–0.2 mg/kg/day divided q12h	Prevention of rejection of liver and kidney transplants

IV, intravenous; *PO*, oral; *RRMS*, relapsing-remitting multiple sclerosis; *SC*, subcutaneous.

*Safety and efficacy have not been established in children.

NURSING PROCESS

Assessment

Before administering any immunosuppressant, the nurse should perform a thorough patient assessment with baseline vital signs, history of medical conditions, and documentation of pre-existing chronic diseases affecting immune status (e.g., diabetes, hypertension, cancer). Assessment should also include documentation of weight; urinalysis and urinary patterns; jaundice; edema and ascites; history of heart disease and dysrhythmias; chest pain or hypertension; central nervous system assessment with attention to occurrence of seizure disorders and alteration of motor or sensory function; paresthesias; changing levels of consciousness; occurrence of any inflammatory processes with attention to duration, location, onset, and specific type of inflammation; appearance of joints with noting of deformities; ability to carry out full range of motion and perform ADLs; and the condition of skin over an inflamed joint or area. Respiratory assessment should include questioning about any complaints such as wheezing, cough, activity intolerance, or sputum production. In addition, the following laboratory and diagnostic tests may be ordered and the results analyzed: kidney function tests with blood urea nitrogen (BUN) and creatinine levels; liver function tests with alkaline phosphatase, aspartate aminotransferase (AST), alanine aminotransferase (ALT), and bilirubin levels; and cardiovascular function with baseline electrocardiogram (ECG). See Table 46-2 for information on other systems affected by the immunosuppressant drugs.

As discussed earlier, several of the immunosuppressant drugs are metabolized by cytochrome CYP3A isoenzymes and interact with a specific group of medications such as antifungals, antibiotics, and calcium channel blockers. In addition, there are several natural health product interactions, as noted with St. John's wort, as well as interactions with grapefruit juice. Such interactions may be severe with some of the immunosuppressants. Thus it is important to get a thorough drug history profile, and other prescription and over-the-counter drugs and natural health products should be used with caution.

Azathioprine requires assessment of platelet counts and bleeding tendencies because of related thrombocytopenia. As with other drugs, with cyclosporine, contraindications, cautions, and drug interactions need to be taken into account; however, specific to cyclosporine, it is important to know that the natural health product St. John's wort may alter the absorption of the drug, and grapefruit juice may increase the absorption of cyclosporine and lead to increased risk for toxicity. Lovastatin, a commonly used antilipemic drug, may increase the risk for kidney failure and rhabdomyolysis, both of which may be serious complications. Nephrotoxicity and liver and heart toxicity may occur with the

related organ transplant process, thus it is critical to continuously monitor organ function preoperatively and postoperatively with this drug and any other immunosuppressants that are indicated. Serum potassium and uric acid levels should also be assessed, for increased and toxic levels. As with most organ transplants, mild nephrotoxicity generally occurs within about 2 to 3 months, whereas severe toxicity occurs more immediately after the transplantation. Other conditions that require careful assessment include heart, liver, or kidney impairment and malabsorptive syndromes.

Daclizumab requires assessment of baseline vital signs with specific attention to blood pressure and pulse rate. Any immune-compromised disorders should also be noted as well as infectious disease processes. Laboratory studies (e.g., hemoglobin [Hgb] level, hematocrit [Hct] values, white blood cell [WBC], and platelet counts) should be performed and the results documented before, during (monthly), and after therapy. If the leukocyte count should drop below 3×10^9 mm/L, the drug should be discontinued, but only after the physician is contacted.

With the use of sirolimus, the patient should be asked about any history of chicken pox, herpes zoster infection, hyperlipidemia, or malignancy because immunosuppressed patients are at increased risk for opportunistic infections, including the activation of latent viral infections and herpes zoster infection, and chicken pox (including recent exposure) can be worsened. The possible development of lymphoma can also occur with the use of sirolimus, and hyperlipidemia can be increased. Thus baseline CBC levels and lipid profile levels should be assessed prior to administering sirolimus. For use of tacrolimus, a thorough patient history and physical assessment are needed with attention to the patient's drug history, BUN levels, CBC, liver enzymes, serum creatinine, and serum electrolytes. Upon administration of this drug, the patient requires very close assessment for the first 30 minutes and with the first dosage of the medication. An anaphylactic reaction can occur past this first 30 minutes and first dose, thus resuscitative equipment should be readily available, and its functioning checked, along with appropriate doses of epinephrine and oxygen.

Nursing Diagnoses

- Risk for injury related to the physiological influence of the disease, overall weakness, and adverse effects of immunosuppressants
- Risk for injury, allergic reaction, and subsequent systemic responses, due to hypersensitivity reactions to immunosuppressants
- Risk for infection related to altered immune status from chronic disease and from medication regimen with immunosuppressants
- Acute pain, myalgias, and arthralgias related to adverse effects of immunosuppressant drugs
- Nonadherence related to undesired adverse effects of drug treatment and lack of knowledge

Planning

Goals

- Patient will experience minimal complications and injuries during drug therapy.
- Patient will state feelings of maximal comfort during drug therapy.
- Patient will remain adherent to drug therapy and return for follow-up visits with the physician.
- Patient will identify the symptoms of adverse reactions to therapy and signs of exacerbation of illness that need to be reported to the physician, should they occur.
- Patient will state the importance of reporting any signs and symptoms of allergic reactions to the nurse, physician, or other health care provider.

Outcome Criteria

- Patient states measures to help minimize adverse effects such as taking acetaminophen for fever and joint pain, reporting unusually high blood pressure readings, and participating in relaxation therapy, massage, and biofeedback.
- Patient expresses an improvement in energy levels, decrease in disease-related symptoms, increased ability to perform ADLs, and overall mental health status improvement.
- Patient has follow-up visits with the physician and other health care professionals to monitor therapeutic effects (decreased symptomatology) and any adverse effects or toxic reactions to immunosuppressants (e.g., myalgias, arthralgias).
- Patient notifies physician immediately if fever, rash, sore throat, fatigue, or other unusual problems or symptoms develop.
- Patient states measures to enhance comfort while on immunosuppressant therapy (e.g., use of nonaspirin analgesics, rest, biofeedback, therapeutic touch or massage, imagery, diversional activities, hypnosis).
- Patient notifies appropriate health care personnel, or emergency medical services (EMS) personnel if in a home setting, in the case of difficulty breathing, shortness of breath, flushing of the face, urticaria, rash or whelps, dizziness, or syncope.
- Patient states appropriate measures to be taken, after contacting the physician or EMS personnel, to help alleviate risk for further systemic symptoms of hypersensitivity, such as taking diphenhydramine or related drugs to alter an allergic reaction, as ordered.

Implementation

It is important that oral immunosuppressants be taken with food to minimize gastrointestinal upset. Given the immunosuppressed condition of patients receiving immunosuppressants, oral forms of the drugs should be used whenever possible to decrease the risk of infection associated with intramuscular injections. An oral antifungal medication may be ordered to treat the oral candidiasis that occurs as a consequence of the treatment and the disease processes; however, there may be significant drug interactions between the immunosuppressant and antifungal drug. Therefore, this possible interaction should be considered and avoided prior to giving the medications. It is also important to ensure that supportive treatment equipment and drugs are available in case of an allergic reaction with use of the immunosuppressants; nurses need to be aware of the high risk for this occurrence. With antihistamines and anti-inflammatory drugs, it is common to see premedication protocols.

Cyclosporine is now available in two oral formulations, but they are not to be used interchangeably. Oral liquid dosage forms are available with a calibrated liquid measuring device. Oral solutions may be mixed in a glass container with chocolate milk, regular milk, or orange juice and served at room temperature. Once the solution is mixed, the patient must drink it immediately. Use of Styrofoam containers should be avoided because the drug has been found to adhere to the inside wall of the cup or container. Oral solutions should not be refrigerated.

When administered intravenously, cyclosporine should be diluted as recommended in the manufacturer guidelines and given according to the standards of care and institutional policy regarding its administration. Cyclosporine is usually diluted with normal saline (NS) or 5% dextrose in water (D5W) and infused over the recommended time frame. The patient should be closely monitored during the infusion, especially for the first 30 minutes, for any allergic reactions, such as facial flushing, urticaria, wheezing, dyspnea, and rash. Vital signs need to be frequently recorded. It is also important to closely monitor the patient's BUN, lactate dehydrogenase (LDH), AST, and ALT levels during therapy for possible kidney and liver impairment. Oral hygiene should be performed frequently to prevent gum hyperplasia. The nurse needs to know that therapeutic serum levels of cyclosporine are 50 to 300 ng/mL and toxic levels are 400 ng/mL or greater.

Both sirolimus and tacrolimus have long half-lives, thus toxicity is an added concern because of possible cumulative effects. Basiliximab and daclizumab are administered parenterally. Dilutional solutions and amounts should be followed as per manufacturer guidelines and the intravenous (IV) drip closely monitored. Use of an IV infusion pump may help administer the proper dosage. Sirolimus and tacromilus should be administered as ordered by either IV or oral routes. If IV tacrolimus is to be discontinued to be replaced by maintenance dosing, oral tacrolimus is usually ordered to be given 8 to 12 hours after discontinuation of the IV drug. IV solution should not be stored in polyvinyl chloride containers and should be given in an appropriately designed container and tubing. Oral dosages of tacrolimus should be given on an empty stomach and in a glass container. The same concerns of not using Styrofoam and eating no grapefruit within 2 hours of taking the drug apply (as with cyclosporine). Complete blood counts (CBC), liver enzymes, and serum potassium levels need to be monitored throughout the duration of therapy with these drugs as well.

Evaluation

The nurse should continually evaluate and re-evaluate the goals and outcome criteria as related to the nursing process and administration of drug therapy. In addition, therapeutic responses to the immunosuppressants should be evaluated and may include acceptance of the transplanted organ or graft and improved symptoms in those with autoimmune disorders. CBC levels; erythrocyte sedimentation rates (ESR); C-reactive protein levels; liver, kidney, and heart function tests; pulmonary function; chest X-ray; and plasma levels of T-lymphocyte surface phenotyping are a few of the tests that may be evaluated during and after drug therapy. Evaluation of drug-specific adverse effects and toxicity (see Table 46-2) and specific therapeutic drug levels (as indicated) should be ongoing.

PATIENT EDUCATION

- ❖ Patients taking immunosuppressants should be encouraged to avoid crowds to minimize the risk for infection. Educate patients to report any fever, sore throat, chills, joint pain, or fatigue to the physician because these symptoms may indicate severe infection and require immediate medical attention.
- ❖ Female patients receiving immunosuppressants should be educated about the use of contraception during treatment and for up to 12 weeks after therapy.
- ❖ Patients taking cyclosporine should be informed to take the drug at the same time every day (as with most immunosuppressants) and that if a dose is omitted, they should contact the physician for further instructions.
- ❖ Patients should be informed that blood work will be performed during therapy, so routine follow-up appointments are encouraged.
- ❖ Patients should be educated about the adverse effects of cyclosporine, which include headache and tremor, and advised to avoid consumption of grapefruit and grapefruit juice because of the potential for increase in blood concentrations of cyclosporine.
- ❖ Patients should be educated to keep gel caps in a cool, dry environment and avoid their exposure to light, and that the dosage form should be kept in its original packaging. Also, patients should be reminded

- to avoid prolonged exposure to the sun and to wear sunscreen and protective clothing when outdoors.
- ❖ Patients who are to undergo transplant surgery and who are receiving cyclosporine should know that several days before surgery, they may be told to take it with corticosteroids, and they may also be given an oral antifungal as prophylaxis for *Candida* infections.
- ❖ Patients taking the oral form of cyclosporine should be told to take their medication with meals or mixed with milk to minimize gastrointestinal upset.
- ❖ Patients taking azathioprine should be informed that several days before transplant surgery they should take all their medication by the oral route if possible and avoid intramuscular injection, which carries the risk for infection.
- ❖ Patients should be informed to take sirolimus or tacrolimus exactly as ordered and at the same time every day and to avoid crowds and those with infections. Patients need to be educated about the adverse effects of chest pain, dizziness, headache, problems with urination, rash, and respiratory and other infections.
- ❖ Patients should be told to avoid grapefruit when taking sirolimus or tacrolimus. Patients should also know the importance of follow-up visits to the physician for laboratory tests.

POINTS TO REMEMBER

- ❖ Immunosuppressants decrease or prevent the body's immune response and include drugs such as azathioprine, cyclosporine, sirolimus, and tacrolimus.
- ❖ Some of the indications for immunosuppressants include suppression of immunodeficiency disorders and malignancies and improvement of short-term and long-term allograft survival and outcomes in the treatment of autoimmune disease processes. Nursing considerations associated with the immunosuppressants include monitoring laboratory studies (e.g., Hgb level, Hct values, WBC, and platelet count). Studies should be performed and the results documented

before, during (monthly), and after therapy. Should the leukocyte count drop below 3.0×10^9/L, the drug should be discontinued.
- ❖ Nursing considerations include the possible administration of oral antifungals often given with immunosuppressants to treat oral candidiasis that occurs as a result of immunosuppression and fungal overgrowth. The nurse should inspect the oral cavity as often as necessary (at least once every shift) for any white patches on the tongue, mucous membranes, and oral pharynx. These patches may indicate oral candidiasis.

EXAMINATION REVIEW QUESTIONS

1 When assessing a patient who is to begin therapy with cyclosporine, which of the following patient conditions should the nurse recognize as one with which the drug must be used cautiously?
   a. Anemia
   b. Myalgia
   c. Glaucoma
   d. Kidney dysfunction

2 Which of the following would be a contraindication for glatiramer acetate?
   a. Acute myalgia
   b. Fluid overload
   c. Polycythemia
   d. Allergy to mannitol

3 During therapy with azathioprine (Imuran), which adverse effect must the nurse monitor for?
   a. Diarrhea
   b. Vomiting
   c. Bradycardia
   d. Thrombocytopenia

4 During a patient teaching session for a patient receiving an immunosuppressant drug, which statement should the nurse include?
   a. "You will remain on antibiotics to prevent infections."
   b. "Be sure to take your medications with grapefruit juice to enhance its effects."
   c. "It is better to use oral forms of these drugs to prevent the occurrence of thrush."
   d. "It is important to use some form of contraception during treatment and for up to 12 weeks after the end of therapy."

5 During drug therapy with basiliximab (Simulect), the nurse monitors for signs of cytokine release syndrome. Which of the following are signs of this condition?
   a. Hepatotoxicity
   b. Neurotoxicity
   c. Polycythemia
   d. An allergic-type reaction

For answers see http://evolve.elsevier.com/Canada/Lilley/pharmacology/.

CRITICAL THINKING ACTIVITIES

1 A 58-year-old recipient of a heart transplant is currently taking cyclosporine to prevent his immune system from rejecting his transplanted heart. How does cyclosporine prevent this patient's immune system from attacking his transplanted heart?

2 Explain why infection is important to avoid in a patient on immunosuppressive therapy.

3 Mr. G. is about to undergo a right lung transplant. Why should intramuscular injections be kept to a minimum during the time before his surgery?

For answers see http://evolve.elsevier.com/Canada/Lilley/pharmacology/.

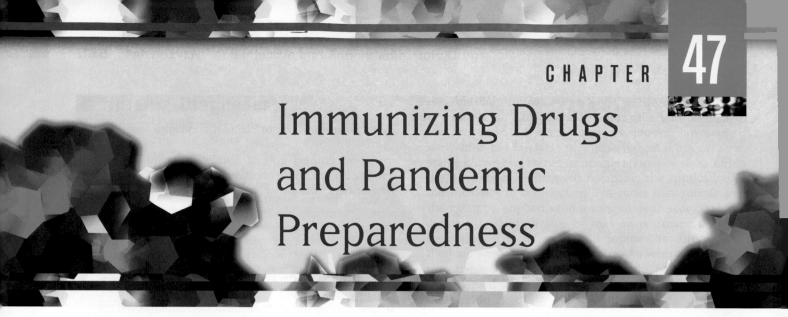

CHAPTER 47

Immunizing Drugs and Pandemic Preparedness

Learning Objectives

After reading this chapter, the successful student will be able to do the following:

1 Discuss the importance of immunity as it relates to immunizing drugs and their use in patients of all ages.

2 Identify the diseases that are prevented or treated with toxoids or vaccines.

3 Compare the mechanisms of action, indications, cautions, contraindications, adverse effects, toxicity, and routes of administration for toxoids and vaccines.

4 Develop a collaborative plan of care that includes all phases of the nursing process related to the administration of immunizing drugs across the lifespan.

5 Develop a collaborative plan of care covering aspects of the nursing process that relate to pandemic preparedness with emphasis on the nurse's role.

e-Learning Activities

Web site
(http://evolve.elsevier.com/Canada/Lilley/pharmacology/)

- Animations
- Answers to chapter questions, activities, and case studies
- Calculators and Category Catchers
- Glossary with audio pronunciations
- IV Therapy and Medication Error Checklists
- Multiple-Choice Review Question quizzes
- Nursing Care Plans
- Online Appendices and Supplements
- WebLinks

Drug Profiles

diphtheria and tetanus toxoids, acellular
  pertussis vaccine, p. 867
Haemophilus influenzae type b vaccine, p. 868
▸▸ hepatitis B immune globulin, p. 871
▸▸ hepatitis B virus vaccine, p. 868
▸▸ human papillomavirus vaccine, p. 868
▸▸ immune globulin, p. 871
▸▸ influenza virus vaccine, p. 869
▸▸ measles, mumps, rubella virus vaccine, p. 870
  meningococcal C conjugate vaccine, p. 870
▸▸ pneumococcal vaccine, polyvalent and 7-valent,
  p. 870
▸▸ poliovirus vaccine, p. 870
  rabies immune globulin, p. 872
  rabies virus vaccine, p. 870
  Rh₀(D) immune globulin, p. 872
▸▸ rotavirus oral vaccine, p. 871
  tetanus immune globulin, p. 872
▸▸ varicella virus vaccine, p. 871
  varicella zoster immune globulin, p. 872

▸▸ Key drug.

Glossary

Active immunization A type of immunization that causes development of a complete and long-lasting immunity to a certain infection through exposure of the body to the associated disease antigen; it can be natural active immunization (i.e., having the disease) or artificial active immunization (i.e., receiving a vaccine or toxoid). (p. 862)

Active immunizing drugs Toxoids or vaccines that are administered to a host (human or animal) to stimulate host production of antibodies. (p. 864)

Antibodies Immunoglobulin molecules that have an antigen-specific amino acid sequence and are synthesized by the humoral immune system (B cells) in response to exposure to a specific antigen (foreign substance), with the purpose of attacking and destroying molecules of this antigen. (p. 861)

Antibody titre Amount of an antibody required to react with a given volume of a specific antigen and protect the body against the particular pathogen. (p. 865)

Antigens Substances, usually proteins and foreign to a host (human or animal), that stimulate the host to produce antibodies and react specifically with antibodies; allergens (e.g., dust, pollen, mould) are also antigens that can produce an immediate-type hypersensitivity reaction or allergy. (p. 861)

Antiserum A serum that contains antibodies. (p. 864)

Antitoxin An antiserum against a toxin (or toxoid). (p. 864)

Antivenin An antiserum against a venom (poison produced by an animal), used to treat humans or other animals that have been envenomed (e.g., by snakebite or spider bite). (p. 864)

Biological antimicrobial drugs Substance of biological origin (e.g., vaccines, toxoids, immunoglobulins) used to prevent, treat, or cure infectious diseases. These drugs are often simply referred to as *biologics*. (p. 862)

Booster shot A repeat dose of an antigen, such as a vaccine or toxoid, usually administered in an amount smaller than that used in the original immunization. (p. 865)

Cell-mediated immune system The immune response mediated by T cells (as opposed to B cells, which produce antibodies). (p. 862)

Herd immunity An entire community or population's resistance to a disease, resulting from a very large proportion of its members being immune to the disease. (p. 866)

Immune response A cascade of biochemical events that occurs in response to entry into the body of an antigen (foreign substance). (p. 861)

Immunization The induction of immunity by administration of a vaccine or toxoid (active immunization) or antiserum (passive immunization). (p. 862)

Immunizing biologics Toxoids, vaccines, or immune globulins targeted against specific infectious microorganisms or toxins. (p. 862)

Immunoglobulins Glycoproteins synthesized and used by the humoral immune system (B cells) to attack and kill all substances foreign to the body. (p. 861)

Passive immunization A type of immunization in which immunity to infection is conferred by bypassing the host's immune system; it can be natural passive immunization (i.e., antibodies are transferred from mother to infant) or artificial passive immunization (i.e., receiving a serum or concentrated immunoglobulins). (p. 862)

Passive immunizing drugs Drugs containing antibodies or antitoxins that can kill or inactivate pathogens by binding to the associated antigens. (p. 863)

Recombinant Relating to or containing a combination of genetic material from two or more organisms. (p. 868)

Reticuloendothelial system Specialized cells located in the liver, spleen, lymphatics, and bone marrow that remove miscellaneous particles from the circulation, such as aging antibody molecules. (p. 865)

Toxin Any poison produced by a plant, animal, or microorganism that is highly toxic to other living organisms. (p. 862)

Toxoids Bacterial exotoxins that are modified or inactivated (by chemicals or heat) so that they are no longer toxic but can still bind to host B cells in order to stimulate the formation of antitoxin. (p. 862)

Vaccines Suspension of live, attenuated, or killed microorganisms that can promote an artificially induced active immunity against a particular microorganism. (p. 862)

Venom A poison secreted by an animal (e.g., snake, insect, or spider). (p. 864)

IMMUNITY AND IMMUNIZATION

Centuries ago, it was noticed that people who contracted certain diseases acquired an immune tolerance to the disease so that, when exposed to the disease again, they did not suffer a second incident of illness. This basic observation prompted scientists to investigate ways of artificially producing this tolerance. Along with this came an understanding of the way in which the normal immune system functions, knowledge important to an understanding of how immunizing drugs work. Briefly, when the body first comes in contact with **antigens,** or proteins foreign to the body, specific information is imprinted into a cellular "memory bank" of the immune system so that the body can effectively fight any future invasion by mounting an immune response. This cellular memory bank consists of specialized immune cells known as *memory cells*. When an antigen presents itself to a person's humoral immune system by binding to B lymphocytes (B cells), the B cells differentiate into two types of cells: memory cells and *plasma cells*, whose role is to produce large volumes of antibodies against the invading antigen. **Antibodies** are immunoglobulin molecules that have antigen-specific amino acid sequences. **Immunoglobulins**, or *immune globulins*, are glycoprotein molecules synthesized by the humoral immune system for the purpose of destroying all substances that the body recognizes as foreign. Immunoglobulins can be general or specific. A general immunoglobulin lacks a specific amino acid sequence that would allow it to recognize a specific antigen; an immunoglobulin with a specific amino acid sequence (or antibody) can recognize a specific antigen. Because of this process, people rarely suffer twice from certain diseases, such as mumps, chicken pox, and measles. Instead, those who have developed the relevant antibodies have a complete and long-lasting immunity to those infections.

In contrast to the humoral immune system, which is the focus of this chapter, the **cell-mediated immune system** is the branch of the immune system that does not synthesize antibodies. Instead, it is driven by T cells (T lymphocytes) and works via the release of *cytokines* (chemicals that promote other immune system functions such as inflammatory responses, runny nose, etc.) from these T cells and through *phagocytosis* (the engulfing and destruction of antigens by the T cells). To varying degrees, these two immune-system branches work simultaneously or even interdependently, with the humoral immune system also being activated and driven partly by cytokines from the cell-mediated immune system.

There are two ways of developing immunity to certain infections: through **active immunization** and through **passive immunization**. Either of these can be an artificial or natural process. In *artificial active immunization*, the body is clinically exposed to a relatively harmless form of an antigen (foreign invader) that does not cause an actual infection. Information about the antigen is then imprinted into the memory of the immune system, and the body's defences are stimulated to resist any subsequent exposure (by producing antibodies). In contrast, *natural active immunization* occurs when a person acquires immunity by surviving the disease itself and producing antibodies to the disease-causing organism. *Artificial passive immunization* involves clinical administration of serum, or concentrated immunoglobulins obtained from humans or animals, which directly gives the inoculated individual the substance needed to fight off the invading microorganism. This type of **immunization** bypasses the host's immune system. Finally,

natural passive immunization occurs when antibodies are transferred in breast milk from the mother to her infant or through the bloodstream via the placenta during pregnancy. The major differences between active and passive immunity are summarized in Table 47-1 and are discussed in greater depth in subsequent sections.

ACTIVE IMMUNIZATION

In general, **biological antimicrobial drugs** (also simply referred to as *biologics*) are substances such as antitoxins, antisera, toxoids, and vaccines used to prevent, treat, or cure infectious diseases. Toxoids and vaccines are known as **immunizing biologics** that target a particular infectious microorganism.

Toxoids

Toxoids are substances that contain antigens, most often in the form of bacterial (usually Gram-positive bacterial) exotoxins. These substances have been detoxified or weakened (attenuated) with chemicals or heat, rendering them nontoxic and unable to regress to a toxic form. Nonetheless, they remain highly antigenic and can stimulate an artificial active immune response (production of antitoxin antibodies) when injected into a host patient. These antibodies can then neutralize the same exotoxin upon any future exposure. Toxoids were first developed in 1923 at the Pasteur Institute by Ramon and his associates. Modern versions are effective against diseases such as diphtheria and tetanus that are caused by **toxin**-producing bacteria.

Vaccines

Vaccines are suspensions of live, attenuated (weakened), or killed (inactivated) microorganisms that can stimulate antibody production against the particular organism. As with toxoids, these slight alterations in the bacteria and viruses prevent the person injected with the vaccine from

---

TABLE 47-1

Active Versus Passive Immunity

Differences	Active	Passive
ARTIFICIAL		
Type of immunization	Toxoid or vaccine	Immune globulin or antitoxin
Mechanism of action	Causes an antigen–antibody response, similar to that with exposure to natural disease process	Results from direct administration of exogenous antibodies. Antibody concentration will decrease over time, so if re-exposure is expected, it is wise to continue passive immunizations.
Use	To prevent development of active disease in the event of exposure to a given antigen in people who have at least a partially functioning immune system	To provide temporary protection against disease in people who are immunodeficient, those for whom active immunization is contraindicated, or those who have been exposed to or anticipate exposure to the disease. An antibody response is not stimulated in the host.
NATURAL		
Mechanism of action	Production of own antibodies during actual infection	Transmission of antibodies from mother to infant through the placenta or during breastfeeding

contracting the disease, but the vaccine is still able to promote active immunization against the organism, including an antibody response. People vaccinated with live bacteria or virus (as well as those who recover from an actual infection) enjoy lifelong immunity against that particular disease. Only partial immunity is conferred on those vaccinated with killed bacteria or virus, thus they must be given periodic booster shots to maintain immune system protection against infection with the specific organism.

One exception is the smallpox vaccine because it uses live cowpox virus (*vaccinia* virus) instead of the more virulent smallpox virus. Edward Jenner, an English physician born in 1749, noticed that milkmaids who had suffered cowpox infections were rarely victims of smallpox and was the first to study the relationship of cowpox to smallpox immunity. His observation led to the development of the smallpox vaccine, using the cowpox virus. In 1796, Jenner successfully immunized a young boy against smallpox by vaccinating him with cowpox virus obtained from a cowpox vesicle on an infected cow. With the help of the modern version of this vaccine, smallpox was eradicated by 1980. Routine smallpox vaccination of Canadians was discontinued in 1972. However, following the terrorist attacks in the United States on September 11, 2001, fears arose of a large-scale bioterrorism attack using the smallpox virus. These fears have subsided and there is currently no evidence to support routine smallpox immunization of the general Canadian population. The Canadian Smallpox Contingency Plan is updated as necessary by the Office of Emergency Preparedness, the Centre of Emergency Preparedness and Response, and the Public Health Agency of Canada, with recommendations for action to be taken if a case of smallpox occurs in Canada or elsewhere in the world. Also listed are several high-priority high-risk groups, including direct health care personnel, who should be vaccinated first if a suspected outbreak occurs.

Today there are more than 20 infectious diseases for which vaccines are available. New vaccines appear periodically but not with the rapidity of other types of drugs because of the complexities of developing a safe and effective vaccine. Most modern vaccines are produced in a laboratory by genetic-engineering methods and contain some extract of the pathogen, or a synthetic extract, rather than the microbe. This extract gives the vaccine its ability to stimulate an antibody response in host patients against a particular bacterial or viral infection without causing active disease. Some vaccines, such as influenza vaccine, may contain actual whole or split virus particles. Most, however, contain a smaller fraction of the organism, such as the bacterial capsular polysaccharides used to make pneumococcal vaccine. The attenuating or killing agent is usually a chemical such as formaldehyde or a physical mechanism such as heat. Attenuation may also be accomplished with the repeated passage of the microbe through some medium, such as a fertile hen egg or a special tissue culture.

The search for new and better drugs will never end. Current goals include finding vaccines against HIV/AIDS

and malaria; the ultimate goal is to develop an effective vaccine against all infectious diseases. The currently available immunizing vaccines are listed in Box 47-1. Note that the drug given to prevent serious respiratory syncytial virus (RSV) infection in high-risk infants and children, palivizumab (Synagis), is a humanized monoclonal antibody and is considered a passive immunizing drug. It is discussed in Chapter 50. The RSV immunoglobulin is no longer available.

The current childhood immunization schedule published by the National Advisory Committee on Immunization (NACI) is shown in Figure 47-1. The NACI provides the Public Health Agency of Canada with ongoing medical, scientific, and public health advice regarding vaccines approved for use in humans in Canada and recommendations for immunization. All recommendations on vaccine use are published every 4 years in *The Canadian Immunization Guide* (available online at http://www.phac-aspc.gc.ca/publicat/cig-gci/). Within the immunization guide is detailed information about vaccines. There is also a catch-up schedule for children who may have missed scheduled immunizations as well as an adult immunization schedule. Recently, in Canada and the United States, there have been some unusual outbreaks of mumps and measles. Situations such as these, although relatively uncommon, serve as a reminder of the reality of vaccine-preventable illnesses.

PASSIVE IMMUNIZATION

In passive immunization, the host's immune system is bypassed and the person is inoculated with serum containing immune globulins obtained from humans or animals. This is called *artificially acquired passive immunity* and it confers temporary immunity against a particular antigen following exposure to the antigen. It differs from active immunization in that it produces a comparatively transitory (short-lived) immune state and the antibodies are already prepared for the host; the host's immune system does not have to synthesize its own antibodies. This allows for more rapid prevention or treatment of disease. Important examples include immunization with tetanus immune globulin, hepatitis immune globulin, rabies immune globulin, and snakebite antivenin.

As noted earlier, passive immunization occurs naturally between mother and fetus or nursing infant when the mother passes maternal antibodies directly to the fetus, through the placenta or to the nursing infant through breast milk. This type of immunity is called *naturally acquired passive immunity*.

Specific populations that can benefit from passive immunization but not from active immunization (see Table 47-1) include people who have been rendered immunodeficient for any reason (e.g., by drugs or disease) and who therefore cannot mount an immune response to a toxoid or vaccine injection because their immune systems are too suppressed to do so. People who already have the disease targeted by the **passive immunizing drug** are

BOX 47-1 Available Immunizing Drugs

Active Immunizing Drugs	Abbreviations	Active Immunizing Drugs	Abbreviations
Bacillus Calmette-Guérin	BCG	Measles, mumps, and rubella	MMR
Cholera—Oral	Chol-O	Measles, rubella	MR
Cholera–*E. coli*—Oral	Chol-Ecol-O	Pneumococcal—conjugate-valent	Pneu-C-7
Diphtheria, tetanus, acellular pertussis— children	DTaP	Pneumococcal—polysaccharide-valent	Pneu-P-23
		Rabies	Rab
Diphtheria, tetanus, acellular pertussis, *Haemophilus influenzae* type b	DTaP-Hib	Rotavirus	ROT
		Tetanus	T
Diphtheria, tetanus, acellular pertussis, inactivated polio— children	DTaP-IPV	Tetanus, diphtheria—adult	Td
Diphtheria, tetanus, acellular pertussis, inactivated polio, *Haemophilus influenzae* type b—children	DTaP-IPV-Hib	Tetanus, diphtheria, acellular pertussis— adult	Tdap
		Tetanus, diphtheria, inactivated polio— adult	Td-IPV
Diphtheria, tetanus, acellular pertussis, inactivated polio, *Haemophilus influenzae* type b, hepatitis B—children	DTaP-IPV-Hib-HB	Tick-borne encephalitis	TBE
		Typhoid—injection	Typh-I
		Typhoid—oral	Typh-O
Diphtheria, tetanus, acellular pertussis, inactivated polio, hepatitis B—children	DTaP-IPV-HB	Varicella	Var
		Yellow fever	YF
Diphtheria, tetanus, polio—children	DT-IPV	**Passive Immunizing Drugs**	
Haemophilus influenzae type b	Hib	Botulism antitoxin	BAtx
Hepatitis A	HA	Cytomegalovirus immunoglobulin	CMV-IGIV
Hepatitis A and B	HAHB	Diptheria antitoxin	DAtx
Hepatitis A and typhoid—injection	HA-Typh-I	Hepatitis B immunoglobulin	HBIg
Hepatitis B	HB	Immune globulin	Ig
Human papillomavirus	HPV	palivizumab	RSVAB
Inactivated polio	IPV	Rabies immunoglobulin	RabIg
Influenza	Inf	Tetanus immunoglobulin	TIg
Japanese encephalitis	JE	Varicella immunoglobulin	VarIg
Meningococcal—conjugate	Men-C		
Meningococcal—polysaccharide	Men-P-AC		
	Men-P-ACWY		

Note: Smallpox virus vaccine is not currently on the Canadian market, but a supply is available in the event of bioterrorism threats.

also candidates for these drugs, especially individuals with diseases that are rapidly harmful or fatal, such as rabies, tetanus, and hepatitis. Because these diseases can progress rapidly, the body does not have time to mount an adequate immune defence against them before death occurs. The passive immunization of such individuals confers a temporary protection that is usually sufficient to keep the invading organism from killing them, even though it does not stimulate an antibody response.

The passive immunizing drugs are divided into three groups: antitoxins, immune globulins, and snake and spider antivenins. An **antiserum** is a serum containing antibodies, usually obtained from an animal that has been immunized against a specific antigen, either by injection with the antigen or by infection with specific microorganisms that produce the antigen. When the antigen is a toxin or toxoid, the purified antiserum produced is called an **antitoxin;** antitoxins provide artificial passive immunity to humans exposed to a given toxin (e.g., tetanus immune globulin). When the antigen is a **venom,** such as a poison secreted by a reptile, insect, or arthropod (spider), the antibody-containing antiserum is called an **antivenin,** often referred to as *antivenom*. An *immune globulin* is a concentrated preparation containing predominantly immunoglobulin G and is harvested from a large pool of blood donors.

IMMUNIZING DRUGS

Mechanism of Action and Drug Effects

Active immunizing drugs consist of vaccines and toxoids that may be administered either orally or intramuscularly and that work by stimulating the humoral immune system. The system synthesizes *immunoglobulins,* or *antibodies,* of which there are five distinct types: M, G, A, E, and D. These immunoglobulins attack and kill antigenic foreign substances that invade the body. Vaccines contain an actual live or attenuated pathogen or a killed pathogen that triggers the formation of antibodies against the specific pathogen. The amount of antibodies that the altered pathogens in the vaccine cause to be produced can be measured in the blood.

Age at Vaccination	DTaP-IPV	Hib	MMR	Var	HB	Pneu-C-7	Men-C	Tdap	Inf
Birth									
2 months	O	□				✦	⊙		
4 months	O	□				✦	(⊙)		
6 months	O	□			Infancy 3 doses	✦	⊙ or		6–23 months ■
12 months			△	◇	❖ or Pre-teen/ teen 2–3 doses	✦ 12–15 months	⊙ If not yet given		1–2 doses
18 months	O	□	△ or △						
4–6 years	O								
14–16 years							⊙ If not yet given	●	

( ) Symbols with brackets around them imply that these doses may not be required, depending on the age of the child or adult.
O Diphtheria, tetanus, acellular pertussis, and inactivated polio virus vaccine (DTaP-IPV): DTaP-IPV (± Hib) vaccine is the preferred vaccine for all doses in the vaccination series, including completion of the series in children who have received one or more doses of DPT (whole-cell) vaccine (e.g., recent immigrants).
□ *Haemophilus influenzae* type b conjugate vaccine (Hib): The Hib schedule shown is for the *Haemophilus* b capsular polysaccharide polyribosylribitol phosphate (PRP) conjugated to tetanus toxoid (PRP-T).
△ Measles, mumps, and rubella vaccine (MMR): A second dose of MMR is recommended for children at least 1 month after the first dose for the purpose of better measles protection. For convenience, options include giving it with the next scheduled vaccination at 18 months of age or at school entry (4–6 years) (depending on the provincial/territorial policy) or at any intervening age that is practical.
◇ Varicella vaccine (Var): Children aged 12 months to 12 years should receive one dose of varicella vaccine. Susceptible individuals 13 years of age and older should receive two doses at least 28 days apart.
❖ Hepatitis B vaccine (HB): Hepatitis B vaccine can be routinely given to infants or preadolescents, depending on the provincial/territorial policy. For infants born to chronic carrier mothers, the first dose should be given at birth (with hepatitis B immunoglobulin), otherwise the first dose can be given at 2 months of age to fit more conveniently with other routine infant immunization visits. The second dose should be administered at least 1 month after the first dose, and the third at least 2 months after the second dose, but these may fit more conveniently into the 4- and 6-month immunization visits. A two-dose schedule for adolescents is an option (see the *Canadian Immunization Guide,* Seventh Edition, 2006, "Hepatitis B Vaccine" chapter).
✦ Pneumococcal conjugate vaccine—7-valent (Pneu-C-7): Recommended for all children under 2 years of age.
⊙ Meningococcal C conjugate vaccine (Men-C): Recommended for children under 5 years of age, adolescents and young adults.
● Diphtheria, tetanus, acellular pertussis vaccine—adult/adolescent formulation (Tdap): A combined adsorbed "adult type" preparation for use in people 7 years of age and older, Tdap contains less diphtheria toxoid and fewer pertussis antigens than preparations given to younger children and is less likely to cause reactions in older people.
■ Influenza vaccine (Inf): Recommended for all children 6 to 23 months of age and all persons 65 years of age and older.

FIG. 47-1 Recommended Childhood Immunization Schedule in Canada. (Source: Public Health Agency of Canada. (2008). *Immunization schedules.* Available at http://www.phac-aspc.gc.ca/im/is-cv/index-eng.php. Adapted and reproduced with the permission of the Minister of Public Works and Government Services Canada, 2009.)

An **antibody titre** is the amount of antibody that must be present in the blood to effectively protect the body against the particular pathogen. Sometimes the levels of these antibodies decline over time. When this occurs, another dose, or **booster shot**, of vaccine is given to restore the antibody titres to a level that can protect the person against the infection. Usually the dose administered is an amount smaller than that used in the original immunization. Toxoids are altered forms of bacterial toxins that stimulate the production of antibodies in the same way as vaccines.

Because both toxoids and vaccines rely on the immunized host to mount an immune response, the host's immune system must be intact. Therefore, patients who are immunocompromised (i.e., who cannot mount an immune response), such as those undergoing immunosuppressive cancer chemotherapy, those receiving immunosuppressive therapy to prevent the rejection of transplanted organs, and those with immunosuppressive diseases such as AIDS, may not benefit from receiving vaccines or toxoids. Instead, their clinical situations may warrant giving them passive immunizing drugs such as immune globulins. Recall that passive immunizing drugs are the actual antibodies (immunoglobulins) that can kill or inactivate the pathogen. The process is called *passive* because the person's immune system does not participate in the synthesis of antibodies; they are provided by the immunizing drug. Immunity acquired in this way generally lasts for a much shorter time than that produced by active immunization, persisting only until the injected immunoglobulins are removed from the person's immune system by the **reticuloendothelial system**. The reticuloendothelial system is composed of specialized cells in the liver, spleen, lymphatics, and bone marrow.

Indications

Vaccines and toxoids are the active immunizing drugs that have been developed for the prevention of many illnesses caused by bacteria and their toxins, as well as those caused by viruses. Antivenins, antitoxins, and immune globulins comprise the passive immunizing drugs. Such drugs can inactivate spider and snake venom, bacterial toxins (exotoxins), and potentially lethal viruses. (See Box 47-1 for a list of the currently available immunizing drugs.) The successful immunization of 95% or more of a population confers protection on the entire population, which is called **herd immunity**.

Antivenins, also known as *antisera*, are used to prevent or minimize the effects of poisoning by venoms of crotalids (rattlesnakes, copperheads, cottonmouths, water moccasins), black widow spiders, and coral snakes. Of concern in Canada are the crotalids (rattlesnakes found in northern Ontario, Manitoba, Alberta, and some parts of British Columbia) and black widow spiders, whose poison can be lethal. Most healthy adults do not die from the bites of spiders or snakes if they receive the appropriate treatment (administration of the appropriate antivenin). Young children and older persons with health problems, however, are particularly susceptible to the effects of venom of some of these animals. In either situation, an antivenin is needed to neutralize the venom.

Certain viruses are potent and even potentially lethal (e.g., hepatitis B virus, rabies virus). Consequently, they can do major harm quickly before the infected person can mount an effective immune response against them. Passive immunization of the person with the appropriate immune globulin provides the individual the antibodies needed to defend against the harmful effects of the virus. Immune globulins are also available for protection against some bacterial infections (e.g., diphtheria, tetanus). In addition, antitoxins are used to provide active immunity against certain harmful bacteria, such as those that cause diphtheria and tetanus.

Contraindications

Contraindications to the administration of immunizing drugs include drug allergy and allergy to egg products because some vaccines are derived from such products. In the case of a potentially fatal illness such as rabies, however, the corresponding drugs may still need to be given, depending on the likelihood of actual exposure to the disease-causing organism, and any allergic reaction controlled with other medications. Some vaccines may contain trace elements of still other products (e.g., the measles, mumps, and rubella vaccine contains trace amounts of neomycin and gelatin), so anyone who is allergic to such products should not receive the vaccine. Administration of some immunizing drugs is best deferred until after recovery from a febrile illness or temporary immunocompromised state (e.g., following cancer chemotherapy), if possible. This is often a matter of clinical judgement, and the individual patient's condition and risk factors for serious illness may be arguments for or against administration of a given immunizing drug at a given time.

Adverse Effects

The undesirable effects of immunizing drugs, listed in Table 47-2, can range from mild and transient to more serious and potentially life threatening. Minor reactions can be treated with acetaminophen and rest. More severe reactions, such as fever higher than 39.4°C, should be treated with acetaminophen and cooling baths. Serum sickness may occur after repeated injections of equine-made immunizing drugs. Signs and symptoms consist of edema of the face, tongue, and throat, as well as rash, urticaria, arthritis, adenopathy, fever, flushing, itching, cough, dyspnea, cyanosis, vomiting and cardiovascular collapse. Serum sickness is best treated with analgesics, antihistamines, epinephrine, or corticosteroids. In such instances, hospitalization may be required.

Any serious or unusual reactions to immunizing drugs should be reported to the Canadian Adverse Events Following Immunization Surveillance System (CAEFISS). This is a voluntary (except in Ontario and Québec, where reporting is mandatory) national vaccine safety surveillance program monitored by the Vaccine Safety Unit (VSU) of the Immunization and Respiratory Infections Division of the Public Health Agency of Canada. A reporting form can be printed from the Public Health Agency of Canada Web site (http://www.phac-aspc.gc.ca/dird-dimr/pdf/hc4229e.pdf). Health Canada also collaborates with the Canadian Paediatric Society (CPS) and pediatric infectious disease specialists on IMPACT (Immunization Monitoring Program ACTive), a pediatric hospital–based, national active surveillance system, to monitor serious adverse events following immunization, vaccination failures, and selected infectious diseases. IMPACT was established in 1990 to further support the timely reporting of adverse events, particularly for the most serious reactions in children. The Public Health Agency of Canada Web site (http://www.phac-aspc.gc.ca/im/vs-sv/caefiss-eng.php) provides extensive information

TABLE 47-2

Immunizing Drugs:
Minor and Severe Adverse Effects

Body System	Adverse Effects
MINOR EFFECTS	
Central nervous	Fever, adenopathy
Integumentary	Minor rash, soreness at injection site, urticaria, arthritis
SEVERE EFFECTS	
Central nervous	Fever higher than 39.4°C, encephalitis, convulsions, peripheral neuropathy, anaphylactic reaction, shock, unconsciousness
Integumentary	Urticaria, rash
Respiratory	Dyspnea
Other	Cyanosis

on these reporting systems and the data collected by them. Such data are used to improve the quality of immunizing drugs and can even be possible grounds for a Health Canada recall of biologics that demonstrate adverse effects exceeding acceptable safety thresholds.

In the early 1980s, in response to vaccine-related injuries, many parents became reluctant to immunize their children against common, and even potentially fatal, childhood illnesses. There has also been recent controversy linking immunizations to autism in children. Most of the concern is associated with the mercury-based preservative thimerosal. The Public Health Agency of Canada's Web site provides a summary statement by the National Advisory Committee on Immunization (NACI) on the safety of vaccines containing thimersol, at http://www.phac-aspc.gc.ca/publicat/ccdr-rmtc/07vol33/acs-06/index-eng.php.

Interactions

Drug interactions are generally not a problem with most immunizing drugs, probably because immunizing drugs are normally given in a single dose or a relatively small number of doses. One drug class of note that can potentially reduce the efficacy of immunizing drugs is immunosuppressive drugs, such as corticosteroids, transplant antirejection drugs, and cancer chemotherapy drugs. All of these drugs can hinder, to varying degrees, the generation of active immunity that would normally occur following vaccine or toxoid administration. The BCG (*Bacillus* Calmette-Guérin) vaccine for tuberculosis (used in certain vulnerable groups in Canada and in developing countries) can cause false-positive results on the tuberculin skin test (Chapter 41).

Some vaccines should not be given in close temporal proximity. For example, the meningococcal vaccine, whole-cell pertussis vaccine, and typhoid vaccine together have an undesirably large bacterial endotoxin content and should not be administered simultaneously. The effectiveness of measles, mumps, and rubella vaccines may be reduced by concurrent interferon therapy. Influenza vaccine may also theoretically lose efficacy if given while antiviral influenza drugs are being taken (Chapter 40). Recommendations are to give the influenza vaccine at least 48 hours after stopping such antiviral drug therapy. In general, immunizations requiring intramuscular injection should be given with particular caution (and with appropriate monitoring) to patients receiving anticoagulant drugs such as warfarin (Chapter 28). The nurse should review the package insert for any immunizing drugs given to obtain the latest information and identify other specific drug interactions that may occur. Hepatitis B immunoglobulin interacts with live vaccines; administration of such vaccines should be deferred until 3 months after the dose of immunoglobulin is given.

Dosages

For the recommended dosages of selected immunizing drugs, see the Dosages table on p. 872.

 ## DRUG PROFILES

Some of the more commonly used vaccines, toxoids, and immunoglobulins are described in the following sections. The immunizing drugs currently available commercially in Canada, including several combination vaccines for prevention of more than one disease, are listed in Box 47-1. Combination vaccines obviously reduce the number of injections that the patient receives, thus their use is desirable when possible, especially for children.

ACTIVE IMMUNIZING DRUGS

diphtheria and tetanus toxoids, acellular pertussis vaccine (adsorbed)

The active immunizing drugs include diphtheria and tetanus toxoids and the acellular pertussis vaccine (adsorbed). *Adsorption* refers to the laboratory techniques used to make most vaccines and toxoids. These toxoids are obtained from the bacteria *Clostridium tetani* and *Corynebacterium diphtheriae*. To make the drugs, diphtheria and tetanus toxins are taken from the bacteria, attenuated into toxoids, and adsorbed onto plates of carrier media such as aluminum hydroxide, aluminum phosphate, or potassium alum. From these plates of dried toxoid and carrier media, specific quantities are removed and placed in dosing containers to provide toxoids of uniform dose. The process is similar for other toxoids and vaccines.

While diphtheria, tetanus, and pertussis are different disorders, an injection that combines all three vaccines (DTP; also commonly called DPT) has been routinely given to children since the 1940s. More recently, a new vaccine combination containing diphtheria and tetanus toxoids with acellular pertussis vaccine adsorbed (DTaP) was approved for the full childhood immunization series and has replaced DPT. It uses a different form of the pertussis component, *acellular pertussis*, which is a more purified product containing only specific proteins and consists of a single weakened toxoid; previous pertussis vaccines contained multiple toxoids. Acellular vaccines have reduced the frequency and severity of local and systemic hypersensitivity reactions compared with those with DTP, particularly in older patients who are more prone to such reactions, thus allowing adults to receive a pertussis booster. Pertussis vaccine is only available in combined form with other agents such as diphtheria (D) and tetanus (T) toxoids with or without inactivated polio vaccine (IPV) and Hib conjugate vaccine (Hib). Currently, diphtheria, tetanus, acellular pertussis, and inactivated polio virus vaccine (DTaP-IPV [Quadrecel]) and Quadrecel combined with *Haemophilus influenzae* b conjugate

Continued

DRUG PROFILES (cont'd)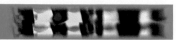

vaccine (Pentacel) are the preferred preparations for all doses in the vaccination series (refer to Figure 47-1). (Two formulations of acellular pertussis vaccine are available, an infant/child formulation (aP) and an adolescent/adult formulation [ap]). The combination product containing pertussis, tetanus, and diphtheria toxoids (Tdap [Adacel]) is administered to persons 7 years of age and older who require a tetanus booster. Emergency booster doses of Td (for adult use) are unnecessary when the wound is clean and minor (not tetanus prone) and the patient has received a primary or booster immunization, adminis-tered as Td, against tetanus within the previous 10 years. Tetanus, diphtheria and pertussis are prevalent in popula-tions of many developing countries, thus the risk of con-tracting one of these diseases may be higher elsewhere than in Canada.

Pertussis is much less common in children older than 7 years of age and in adults. The combination of tetanus and diphtheria toxoids adsorbed (Td) is generally given to children 7 years of age and older and to adults with func-tioning immune systems. It promotes immunity to diph-theria and tetanus by inducing the production of specific antitoxins (antibodies to toxin) by the patient's immune system. However, there is recent evidence that pertus-sis is actually recurring among adolescents and adults (whose previous vaccine-induced immunity has waned), who in turn are passing it on to their children. For this rea-son, prescribers may elect to give adults Tdap (described earlier) instead of the more traditional adult drug Td.

These toxoids (DTaP, Tdap, and Td) are available only as parenteral preparations to be given as deep intramuscular injections. Their use is contraindicated in persons who have had a prior systemic hypersensitivity reaction or a neurological reaction to one of the ingredients. Some manufacturers state that use is contraindicated in cases of concurrent acute or active infections but not in cases of minor illness. Although there have been few, if any, studies documenting the safety of their use in pregnant women, it is generally considered safe to give diphtheria, tetanus, and pertussis toxoids after the first trimester.

Haemophilus influenzae *type b vaccine*

Haemophilus influenzae type b (Hib) vaccine (Act-HIB, Liquid PedvaxHIB) is a noninfectious, bacteria-derived vaccine. It is made by extracting *H. influenzae* particles that are antigenic and by chemically attaching the par-ticles to a protein carrier for use in injections. All Can-adian provinces and territories include Hib conjugate vaccine in their immunization program for children. The vaccine is given by injection to previously unimmunized adults and children 5 years of age or older considered at high risk for acquiring *H. influenzae* infection. Conditions that may predispose an individual to Hib infection are septicemia, pneumonia, cellulitis, arthritis, osteomyelitis, pericarditis, sickle cell anemia, an immunodeficiency syn-drome, or Hodgkin's disease.

Before this vaccine was developed, infections caused by Hib were the leading cause of bacterial meningitis in children 3 months to 5 years of age. This bacterium can also cause several other serious infections in children and adults. This form of bacterial meningitis has a mortality rate of 5% to 10%. Of those who survive, 20% to 45% suf-fer serious morbidity in the form of neurological deficits. All Hib vaccine products are parenteral formulations that are administered intramuscularly.

▶▶ *hepatitis B virus vaccine*

Hepatitis B virus (HBv) is a double-stranded DNA virus with three major antigens, known as hepatitis B surface antigen (HBsAg), hepatitis B e antigen (HBeAg), and hepatitis B core antigen (HBcAg). The antigen HBsAg is detected in serum 30 to 60 days after HBv exposure and persists until the infection resolves. The HBv vaccine inactivated (Recombivax HB, Engerix-B) is a noninfec-tious viral vaccine containing HBsAg. It is made from viral particles and yeast using **recombinant** deoxyribonucleic acid (DNA) technology (a method that combines genetic material from different organisms). In this technique, DNA from two or more organisms is combined. Yeast cells then produce this viral antigenic substance in mass quantities. The substance is attached to a carrier medium (alum) and made into a vaccine injection preparation. This antigenic HBsAg is used to promote active immunity to hepatitis B infection in persons considered at high risk for potential exposure to the hepatitis B virus or HBsAg-positive materials (e.g., blood, plasma, serum). Health care workers and staff and inmates of correctional insti-tutes, for example, are persons considered at high risk, as are injection drug users and men who have sex with men. Universal immunization against HBv is now part of the publicly funded vaccine programs offered in all Canadian provinces and territories.

Use of the vaccine is contraindicated in people who are hypersensitive to yeast. Pregnancy is not considered a contraindication to use. The potential for exposure of a pregnant woman to hepatitis B infection and for the development of chronic infection in the neonate are both good reasons to give the vaccine. It is adminis-tered by intramuscular injection. Hepatitis B vaccines are approved for use in Canada for pre-exposure and postexposure prophylaxis. There is also a formulation for patients over 19 years old in hemodialysis. A combina-tion with hepatitis A vaccine (Twinrix, Twinrix Junior) is preferred for individuals travelling to countries where both hepatitis A and hepatitis B are endemic, such as cer-tain parts of Africa, Asia, and the Americas; individuals who use illicit drugs; men who have sex with men; and in those individuals with chronic liver disease.

▶▶ *human papilomavirus vaccine*

The human papillomavirus (HPV) vaccine (Gardasil) is a recombinant quadrivalent vaccine that protects against four types (6, 11, 16, and 18) of human papillomavirus. It is made from highly purified recombinant major capsid (L1) particle proteins of each of the four types of viruses. The proteins are separately produced through yeast

Continued

DRUG PROFILES (cont'd)

fermentation, and they self-assemble into the viral protein particles.

Human papillomavirus infection is the most common sexually transmitted infection, spread primarily through skin-to-skin contact. It affects approximately 550,000 Canadians yearly. Because this virus is so common, most women are exposed at some point in their lives. Prevalence increases with the onset of sexual activity and decreases with age. HPV types 16 and 18 are the cause of 70% of cervical cancer cases while types 6 and 11 are responsible for 90% of anorectal wart cases. Cervical cancer is the second most common form of cancer in women between the ages of 20 and 44.

For optimum effectiveness, the Canadian National Advisory Committee on Immunization (NACI) recommends the vaccine for females between 9 and 13 years of age, before the onset of sexual intercourse, which can begin at an early age, often by grade six. Universal vaccination is offered to females in many of the provinces and territories at different grades (e.g., grade eight in Ontario and grade five in the Yukon). It is also offered to females between the ages of 14 and 26, even if they already are sexually active, have had previous Pap abnormalities, or have had a previous HPV infection. The vaccine is administered for prevention of HPV infection and is endorsed by the Canadian Paediatric Society and the Society of Obstetrics and Gynecology of Canada. The approved vaccine has generated enormous media attention in addition to debate among some health care professionals. The vaccine is considered safe with mild injection site reactions. The vaccine is supplied in single-dose vials or prefilled single-use syringes.

▶▶ influenza virus vaccine

The influenza virus vaccine (Flurival, Influvac, Vaxigrip) is used to prevent influenza. Each year before the influenza season, this vaccine is administered to persons at high risk of contracting influenza. Such inoculation is the single most important influenza control measure. Each year, a new influenza vaccine is developed by virology researchers. The vaccine usually contains three different influenza virus strains (usually two of type A and one type B strain), chosen from among the hundreds of influenza virus strains in the environment on the basis of the latest epidemiological data indicating which influenza viruses will most likely circulate in North America in the upcoming winter. The vaccine is made from highly purified, egg-grown viruses that have been rendered noninfectious (inactivated).

Influenza is characterized by abrupt onset of fever, myalgia, sore throat, and nonproductive cough. Severe malaise may last several days. More severe illness can occur in certain populations such as older individuals, children, and adults with underlying serious health problems (e.g., HIV infection, asthma, cardiopulmonary disease, cancer, diabetes). Health care personnel are also considered a high-risk group. Many health care institutions make influenza immunization a condition

of employment. If health care workers become ill with influenza, they are more likely than the general population to require hospitalization. Increased mortality results not only from influenza and pneumonia but also from cardiopulmonary and other chronic diseases exacerbated by influenza. More than 90% of the deaths attributed to pneumonia and influenza occur among persons 65 years of age or older. Another fairly unusual but important risk group is children and teenagers, aged 6 months to 18 years, who are receiving long-term aspirin therapy (e.g., for juvenile arthritis) and who therefore might be at risk for developing Reye's syndrome after influenza (Chapter 45). New recommendations for influenza vaccination include healthy children aged 6 to 23 months and contacts capable of transmitting influenza to those at high risk of influenza-related complications. Another unique risk group is individuals involved in the culling of poultry infected with avian influenza. Immunization may prevent influenza with human strains in these individuals and prevent human–avian reassortment of genes.

The effectiveness of influenza vaccine in preventing illness varies. Factors that may alter its effectiveness are the age and immunocompetence of the vaccine recipient and the degree of similarity between the virus strains included in the vaccine and those that actually predominate during a given influenza season. Healthy individuals under the age of 65 have a 70% chance of preventing illness caused by influenza when there is a good match between the vaccine and the circulating viruses.

Older persons, especially those residing in nursing homes, can avoid severe illness, secondary complications, and death by receiving the influenza vaccine. In frail older persons, the vaccine can prevent hospitalization and pneumonia up to 50% to 60% of the time and death up to 80% of the time. Achieving a high rate of vaccination among nursing home residents can reduce the spread of infection in a facility, thus preventing disease through herd immunity.

Influenza vaccine may be administered to any healthy child, adolescent, or adult for whom contraindications are not present. To reduce the morbidity and mortality associated with influenza and the impact of illness in our communities, immunization programs should focus on those at high risk of influenza-related complications, those capable of transmitting influenza to individuals at high risk of complications, and those who provide essential community services. Significant morbidity and societal costs are also associated with seasonal interpandemic influenza illness and its complications occurring in healthy children and adults. For this reason, healthy children and adults should be encouraged to receive the vaccine. For those individuals who developed Guillain–Barré syndrome within 8 weeks of a previous influenza vaccination, the NACI recommends that they not be revaccinated.

In April 2009, the H1N1 influenza virus emerged in North America. H1N1 is a new strain of pandemic influenza that previously affected pigs. H1N1 is particularly dangerous, as individuals have little to no natural

Continued

DRUG PROFILES (cont'd)

immunity to H1N1 and it can cause serious illness. Those most susceptible to more serious illness and complications are children under the age of 5 (especially children under the age of 2), pregnant women, and those with underlying medical conditions.

▶▶ measles, mumps, and rubella virus vaccine (live, attenuated)

The measles, mumps, and rubella vaccine (M-M-R, Priorix) is a live, attenuated virus preparation consisting of live measles, mumps, and rubella viruses that are weakened (attenuated). The vaccine promotes active immunity to these diseases by inducing the production of virus-specific immunoglobulin G and immunoglobulin M antibodies. The antibody response to initial vaccination resembles that caused by primary natural infection.

Administration of the measles vaccine or any of the combination products that includes the measles virus is contraindicated in people with a history of anaphylactic, anaphylactoid, or some other immediate reaction to egg ingestion. Use of these products is also contraindicated in persons who have had an anaphylactic reaction to topically or systemically administered neomycin because this antibiotic is used as a preservative in some of the vaccine preparations. These vaccines should not be administered to pregnant women, and pregnancy should be avoided for 3 months after measles virus vaccination and 30 days after vaccination with a rubella-containing (measles-rubella [MR] or MMR) measles virus vaccine. This precaution is based on the theoretical risk that the live virus vaccine may cause a fetal infection.

meningococcal C conjugate vaccine

Two available types of meningococcal vaccine are available in Canada that protect against meningococcal meningitis. In Canada, there are five types of meningococci responsible for disease: A, B, C, Y, and W 135. Meningitis is endemic in Canada with outbreaks occurring every 10 to 15 years, more often during the winter months. Those individuals most susceptible are infants under the age of 12 months and adolescents between the age of 15 and 19 years. Serogroups B and C cause the majority of cases of endemic disease in Canada; serogroup B is responsible for most of the outbreaks. Meningococcal C protein–polysaccharide conjugate vaccine (Meningitec, Menjugate, NeisVac-C) is recommended for routine immunization of infants and for immunization of children aged 1 to 4 years old and for adolescents and young adults. The purified capsular polysaccharide vaccine (Menomune) is recommended for international travellers and for outbreaks.

▶▶ pneumococcal vaccine, polyvalent and 7-valent

Two available forms of vaccine against pneumococcal pneumonia protect against bacteremia, meningitis, bacterial pneumonia, and acute otitis media caused by *Streptococcus pneumonia,* commonly referred to as *pneumococcus.* Invasive pneumococcal disease (IPD)

affects most commonly the young, the older adult, and certain groups at high risk, such as individuals with functional or anatomical asplenia and individuals with congenital or immunosuppressed diseases. The polyvalent type of vaccine (Pneumovax 23, Pneumo 23) is used primarily in adults. (The term *polyvalent* refers to the vaccine being designed to be effective against the 23 strains of pneumococcus most commonly implicated in adult cases of pneumonia.) This vaccine may also be recommended for children at higher risk for pneumonia as a result of serious chronic illnesses, especially those who are immunocompromised. The 7-valent vaccine, 7-valent conjugate vaccine (Prevnar), is routinely recommended for children. It is made using a special type of protein isolated from *C. diphtheriae,* the bacterium that causes diphtheria. The name *7-valent* refers to the vaccine's immunization against the top seven pneumococcal strains found in pneumonia cases in children. The pneumococcal conjugate vaccine is a publicly funded immunization program of all provinces and territories in Canada.

Contraindications to the use of either vaccine include known drug allergy to components of the vaccine itself, as well as the presence of current significant febrile illness or immunosuppressed state as a result of drug therapy (e.g., cancer chemotherapy). In these cases, the vaccine may sometimes still be given if it is felt that withholding the vaccine poses an even greater risk to the patient.

▶▶ poliovirus vaccine (inactivated)

The use of live oral polio vaccine (OPV) is no longer routine in Canada. Since 1980, the only indigenous cases of poliomyelitis reported in Canada (11 cases) have been associated with use of the live OPV; the last reported indigenous wild case occurred in 1977. Injected doses of inactivated polio vaccine (IPV) are instead recommended for routine use. All provinces and territories use IPV as part of routine immunization programs.

rabies virus vaccine

Although vaccination against the rabies virus is not normally a routine immunization, situations requiring vaccination occur periodically in many practice settings. Rabies is a virus that can infect a variety of mammals, including skunks, foxes, raccoons, bats, dogs, and cats. The virus is usually transferred to humans by an animal bite and almost universally causes fatal brain tissue destruction if the patient is not treated with rabies vaccine and immunoglobulin. Rabies virus vaccine (Imovax, RabAvert) is produced using laboratory techniques involving infected human cell cultures and selected antimicrobial drugs. Current recommendations call for a total of five intramuscular injections on days 0, 3, 7, 14, and 28 following an animal bite that raises concern for rabies transmission. This includes bites by any animal whose rabies immunization status is unknown or that escapes and cannot be observed for signs of rabies. This type of treatment is known as *postexposure prophylaxis.* *Pre-exposure prophylaxis* is recommended for persons

Continued

DRUG PROFILES (cont'd)

at high risk for exposure to the rabies virus (e.g., veterinarians). The pre-exposure course consists of only three injections on days 0, 7, and 21. Periodic booster shots are also recommended for such individuals approximately every 2 to 5 years, or based on the levels of the patient's rabies virus antibody titres. Previously immunized patients who have a new bite may need only two booster shots on days 0 and 3.

Contraindications to the administration of rabies vaccine include a history of allergic reaction to the vaccine itself or to the drugs neomycin, gentamicin, or amphotericin B. Given the life-threatening nature of rabies infection, however, treatment may still be required, with supportive therapy (e.g., epinephrine, diphenhydramine, corticosteroids) provided to minimize allergic reactions. Patients with any kind of febrile illness should delay occupational pre-exposure prophylaxis treatment until the illness has subsided. Rabies vaccine is administered intramuscularly into the edges surrounding the wound, if possible. For pre-exposure prophylaxis, according to the World Health Organization, the intradermal route may be used because it requires less vaccine and the protection derived is similar.

▶▶ rotavirus oral vaccine

The live, oral, rotavirus vaccine (RotaTeq) protects infants and children from five of the six most common strains of rotavirus infection in Canada. *Rotavirus* is a common virus spread through person-to-person contact (fecal–oral) that infects the stomach and intestines, resulting in gastroenteritis and potential dehydration from fever and profuse watery diarrhea. Infants between the age of 16 and 24 months are most frequently affected. In Canada, it is the major cause for serious diarrhea illness in young children. It is estimated that one in five cases of all childhood gastroenteritis is caused by rotavirus and that almost all children will be infected at least once by 5 years of age.

The vaccine is a liquid given orally in three doses at 2, 4, and 6 months of age and can be administered at the same time as other childhood immunizations. The first dose must be given between 6 weeks and 12 weeks of age. Doses should be spaced 1 to 2 months apart. If a dose is missed, all doses should be given by 32 weeks of age.

▶▶ varicella virus vaccine

The live attenuated varicella virus vaccine (Varivax III, Varilrix) is used to prevent varicella (chicken pox) and herpes zoster (shingles) infections. Varicella occurs primarily in children younger than 5 years of age or in individuals with compromised immune systems, such as the older adult or HIV-infected patients. It is estimated that only 10% of children older than 12 years of age are still susceptible to varicella. Only 2% of adults develop varicella virus infections. However, 50% of the deaths associated with varicella infections are in adults. Half of these are in immunocompromised patients. In 2006, the United States adopted a goal to eliminate varicella. In order to

achieve this goal, a varicella vaccine combined with MMR (MMVR) became available for a routine two-dose schedule for children. To date, no such goal exists in Canada; however, the NACI recommends a single-dose administration of varicella vaccine as part of routine vaccination, given at the same time as MMR.

The virus in varicella vaccine is attenuated by the passage of virus particles through human and embryonic guinea pig cell cultures. Varicella vaccine is stored in a refrigerator, not the freezer. It is administered by subcutaneous injection. Generally, the vaccine should not be administered to immunodeficient patients or to patients who have received high doses of systemic steroids in the previous month. However, the vaccine is recommended for select individuals with immunosuppressed immune systems who meet certain criteria, such as those with intact T-cell systems. It is also recommended that salicylates be avoided for 6 weeks after vaccination with varicella vaccine because of the possibility of Reye's syndrome (Chapter 45).

PASSIVE IMMUNIZING DRUGS

The currently available antivenins, antitoxins, and immunoglobulins that comprise the passive immunizing drugs are listed in Box 47-1. Those that are more commonly used are described in the following profiles.

▶▶ hepatitis B immune globulin

Hepatitis B immune globulin (Hepagam B, Hyperhep B) is used to provide passive immunity against hepatitis B infection in the postexposure prophylaxis and treatment of persons exposed to hepatitis B virus or HBsAg-positive materials (e.g., blood, plasma, serum). It is prepared from the plasma of human donors with high titres of antibody to HBsAg. All donors are tested for the antibody to HIV to prevent transmission.

Because of the possible devastating consequences of exposure to hepatitis B infection, pregnancy is not considered a contraindication to the use of H-BIg when there is a clear need for it.

▶▶ immune globulin

Immune globulin (Gamastan S/D, Gammagard, Igivnex, others) is available in both intramuscular or intravenous dosage forms. Two types of immune globulin preparations are available. The first type is a standard immune globulin (Ig) of human origin, often referred to as *immune serum globulin* or *gamma globulin*. The second type is a preparation of either human or animal sera that contains high titres of specific antibodies to a particular microorganism or its toxin. Immune globulin provides passive immunity by increasing antibody titre and antigen–antibody reaction potential. Immunoglobulins are given to help prevent certain infectious diseases in susceptible persons or to ameliorate the diseases in those already infected. Immunoglobulins are pooled from the blood of at least 1000 human donors. This plasma is prepared by cold alcohol fractionation and usually washed with a

Continued

DRUG PROFILES (cont'd)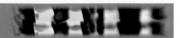

detergent to destroy any harmful viruses, such as hepatitis or HIV. Health Canada–approved uses for immunoglobulins are primary humoral immunodeficiency syndrome, HIV in children, idiopathic thrombocytopenic purpura, B-cell chronic lymphocytic leukemia, and allogenic bone marrow transplant.

rabies immune globulin

Rabies immune globulin (Imogam Rabies Pasteurized, HyperRab S/D) is a passive immunizing drug that is used concurrently with rabies virus vaccine following suspected exposure to the rabies virus. In humans this usually occurs following an animal bite. Rabies immune globulin is derived from human cells harvested from persons who have been immunized with rabies vaccine. The only contraindication to its use is drug allergy, although an allergic patient may still need to be dosed rather than face infection with the almost universally fatal rabies virus. The decision to dose a patient in such a case would be based on the probability of rabies infection, given the particular circumstances surrounding the animal bite.

Rh$_0$(D) immune globulin

Rh$_0$(D) immune globulin (WinRho SDR) is used to suppress the active antibody response and the formation of anti-Rh$_0$(D) antibodies in an Rh$_0$(D)-negative person exposed to Rh-positive blood. Because an Rh$_0$(D)-negative person reacts to Rh-positive blood as if it were a foreign, "non-self" substance, an immune response develops against it and an antigen–antibody reaction occurs. This reaction can be fatal. The administration of this immune globulin helps prevent the reaction and, hence, this outcome. The most common use of this product is in cases of maternal–fetal Rh incompatibility (postpartum). Normally, only the mother is dosed. The treatment objective is to prevent a harmful maternal immune response to a fetus during a future pregnancy should an Rh-negative mother become pregnant with an Rh-positive child.

Rh$_0$(D) immune globulin is prepared from the plasma or serum of adults with a high titre of anti-Rh$_0$(D) antibody to the red blood cell antigen Rh$_0$(D). Administration of immune globulin is contraindicated in persons who have been previously immunized with this drug and in Rh$_0$(D)-positive and Du-positive patients. It is normally given postpartum.

tetanus immune globulin

Tetanus immune globulin (Hypertet S/D) is a passive immunizing drug effective against tetanus. It contains tetanus antitoxin antibodies that neutralize the bacterial exotoxin produced by *Clostridium tetani,* the bacterium that causes tetanus. Tetanus immune globulin is prepared from the plasma of adults hyperimmunized with the tetanus toxoid and is given as prophylaxis to people with tetanus-prone wounds. It may also be used to treat active tetanus.

varicella zoster immune globulin

Varicella zoster immune globulin (VariZIG [VZIG]) can be used to modify or prevent chicken pox in susceptible individuals who have had recent significant exposure to the disease. VZIG is prepared from the plasma of normal blood donors with high antibody titres to varicella zoster virus (VZV). VZIG should be administered within 96 hours of exposure. Candidates for therapy with VZIG are those at high risk of serious disease or complications if they become infected with the varicella zoster virus. Two examples are newborn children, including premature infants with significant exposure, pregnant women, and immunocompromised adults. Healthy adults, including pregnant women, should be evaluated on a case-by-case basis. The duration of protection against infection provided by VZIG is at least 3 weeks.

DOSAGES   Selected Immunizing Drugs

Drug (Pregnancy Category)	Pharmacological Class	Usual Dosage Range*	Indications
ACTIVE IMMUNIZING DRUGS			
diphtheria, tetanus, and acellular pertussis (DTaP [Quadracel or Pentacel with *Haemophilus influenzae* b conjugate vaccine])	Mixed toxoid/ vaccine	*Children* IM: Series of three 0.5 mL injections at 2, 4, and 6 mo; booster at 4–6 yr; booster of adult (ap) at 14–16 yr	Prophylaxis against diphtheria, tetanus, pertussis, and polio with or without *Haemophilus influenzae* b
Haemophilus influenzae type b conjugate vaccine (Act-HIB, Liquid PedvaxHIB) (C)	Bacterial capsular antigenic extract vaccine	*Infants 2–6 mo/Children* IM: Series of three injections (0.5 mL each) at 2, 4, and 6 mo *Previously Unvaccinated Children 7–17 yr* IM: Two injections 2 mo apart; booster at 15–18 yr *Adolescents/Adult 18–59 yr* IM: 1 injection	*H. influenzae* type b prophylaxis

Continued

DOSAGES   Selected Immunizing Drugs (cont'd)

Drug (Pregnancy Category)	Pharmacological Class	Usual Dosage Range*	Indications
▸▸hepatitis B virus vaccine, recombinant (Energix, Recombivax HB) (C)	Viral surface antigen	*Children to 10 yr* Recombivax HB IM: 2.5–5 mcg at birth then at 1 mo and 6 mo *Adult 19 yr and older* IM: Three 10 mcg doses: day 0, 1 mo, and 2 mo	Hepatitis B virus prophylaxis
▸▸human papillomavirus vaccine (Gardasil) (C)	Live, attenuated viral vaccine	*Girls/Women 9–26 yr* IM: 0.5 mL at 0, 2, and 6 mo	Prophylaxis against human papillomavirus types 6, 11, 16, 18
▸▸influenza virus vaccine (Flurival, Influvac, Vaxigrip) (C)	Viral surface antigen	*Infants and Children 6 mo to less than 9 yr* IM: Single yearly dose (0.25–0.5 mL; two doses given at least 1-mo interval if receiving influenza vaccine for first time) *Children 9 yr and older/Adult* IM: Single yearly dose (0.5 mL)	Influenza prophylaxis
▸▸measles, mumps, and rubella virus vaccine, live (M-M-R, Priorix)	Live, attenuated viral vaccine	*Children older than 12 mo/Adult* SC: 0.5 mL single dose; booster at 18 mo or 4–6 yr	Prophylaxis against measles, mumps, and rubella
meningococcus C conjugate vaccine (Meningitec, Menjugate) (C)	Conjugate vaccine	*Infants under 12 mo* IM: 0.5 mL at 2, 3, and 4 mo	Meningococcal meningitis prophylaxis
pneumococcal polysaccharide vaccine (Pneumo 23) (C)	Bacterial capsular antigenic extract vaccine	*Children 5 yr and older/Adult* IM/SC: 0.5 mL	*Streptococcus pneumoniae* prophylaxis
▸▸poliovirus vaccine, inactivated (IPV) (C)	Inactivated viral vaccine	*Infants and Children* SC: Four 0.5 mL doses: 2 mo, 4 mo, and 18 mo, and 4–6 yr, usually in combination with other routine vaccinations	Polio prophylaxis
rabies virus vaccine (Imovax, RabAvert) (C)	Inactivated viral vaccine	*Children/Adult* *Postexposure prophylaxis* IM: 1 mL on days 0, 3, 7, 14, and 28 (with one dose of rabies immune globulin [see p. 874] on day 0) *Pre-exposure prophylaxis for those at high risk for rabies exposure (e.g., veterinarians)* IM/ID: 1 mL IM or 0.1 mL ID on days 0, 7, and 21, q2–5 yr, depending on antibody titres	Rabies prophylaxis
tetanus and diphtheria toxoids, adsorbed (Td)	Mixed toxoid	*Adult/Unvaccinated Children older than 7 yr* IM: 0.5 mL on day 0; second dose 2 mo later; third dose 6–12 mo later; booster 10 yr after third dose	Prophylaxis against diphtheria and tetanus
▸▸varicella virus vaccine (Varivax III, Varilrix) (C)	Live, attenuated viral vaccine	*Children 1–12 yr* SC: One 0.5-mL dose *Adolescents 13 yr and older/Adult* SC: Two 0.5 mL doses given 4–8 wk apart	Prophylaxis against varicella virus (causes chicken pox and shingles)

Continued

DOSAGES Selected Immunizing Drugs (cont'd)

Drug (Pregnancy Category)	Pharmacological Class	Usual Dosage Range*	Indications
PASSIVE IMMUNIZING DRUGS			
▸▸**hepatitis B immune globulin (Hepagam B, Hyperhep B) (C)**	Pooled human immune globulin	*Infant (of known hepatitis B–positive mother)* IM: 0.5 mL at birth *Children/Adult* IM: 0.06 mg/kg within 24 hr after exposure	Passive hepatitis B prophylaxis
▸▸**immune globulin intravenous (Gamastan S/D, Gammagard, Igivnex, others) (C)**	Pooled human immune globulin	Dosages vary widely; refer to current manufacturer's dosage information regarding specific indications	Primary humoral immunodeficiency syndrome, HIV in children, idiopathic thrombocytopenic purpura, B-cell chronic lymphocytic leukemia, allogenic bone marrow transplant
rabies immune globulin (Imogam Rabies Pasteurized, HyperRab S/D) (C)	Pooled human immune globulin	*Children/Adult* Single dose 20 units/kg; infiltrate as much of dose as possible into bite wound area and give remainder IM in gluteal region; do not give into same site as rabies vaccine	Rabies prophylaxis
Rh$_0$(D) immune globulin (Windro SDF) (C)	Immunosuppressant globulin	*Women* IM/IV (full dose): 1500 units at 28 wk gestation; 600 units within 72 hr after delivery IM: 600 units after spontaneous or elective abortion of pregnancy 12 wk gestation	Prophylaxis of Rh immunization
tetanus immune globulin (Hypertet S/D) (C)	Pooled human immune globulin	*Children/Adult* IM: 250 units as a single dose	Postexposure tetanus prophylaxis Tetanus treatment
varicella zoster immune globulin (VariZIG) (C)	Human immune globulin	*Children/Adult* IM/IV: 125–625 units within 96 hr varicella exposure	Prophylaxis against varicella zoster virus

ID, intradermal; *IM*, intramuscular; *SC*, subcutaneous.

*Note: Dosages given are only for brands listed. Dosing amounts and regimens may vary for different brands. The user should always follow the manufacturer's current dosing directions.

PANDEMIC PREPAREDNESS AND RESPONSE

In anticipation of an influenza pandemic in the near future, pandemic planning for the health care sector involves a federal, provincial, and territorial framework to provide a planned, coordinated, efficient, and effective public health response—the Canadian Pandemic Influenza Plan for the Health Sector (CPIP). The plan is a collaborative effort put forth by public health and emergency preparedness and response experts from the government of Canada, provincial and territorial governments, and other expert stakeholders. The Canadian pandemic plan has two overall goals: (1) to minimize overall illness and deaths, and (2) to minimize societal disruption associated with an influenza pandemic. The plan offers guidance and information to help support planning for and responding to an influenza pandemic. The original plan is regularly updated to reflect current thinking and new knowledge. Two key components to the plan are *preparedness* and *response*. *Preparedness* involves prevention strategies and activities to prepare for the pandemic, including guidelines for planning activities that would aid in managing an influenza pandemic. Surveillance, vaccine programs, the use of antivirals, health services, public health measures, and communications are all examples of such activities. *Response* involves high-level operational activities for an effective national health sector response, including roles and responsibilities for health care workers. A *recovery* plan would focus on the coordination of a postpandemic response for health care and emergency response sectors. Additional information about the CPIP is available at http://www.phac-aspc.gc.ca/cpip-pclcpi/s01-eng.php. SafeCanada.ca also offers access to a wide range of information and resources on all types of influenza-related information.

NURSING PROCESS

Assessment

Before administering a toxoid or vaccine, the nurse should gather complete information about the patient's health history, including medications taken, present and past health status, previous reactions and responses to these types of drugs, previous allergy test results, use of any immunosuppressants, presence of autoimmune or immunosuppressing diseases or infections, pregnancy or lactation status, and any unusual reaction to other drugs, food, or other substances. When children are to receive a vaccine or toxoid, the immunization schedule and the dose ordered by the physician must be followed. In collaboration with the Public Health Agency of Health Canada, the NACI provides the latest recommendations for adult and child immunizations in Canada. These recommendations are easily accessible on the Internet at http://www.phac-aspc.gc.ca/naci-ccni/index.html and should be referred to and kept close at hand in any facility that administers these drugs. It is crucial for the nurse to keep current on immunization cautions and contraindications; this Web site and other published materials from the NACI and Health Canada on immunization are important sources of information.

Because passive immunizing drugs may precipitate a hypersensitivity reaction to proteins in antiserum derived from an animal source, the older adult and those who have chronic illnesses or are debilitated must be assessed carefully before treatment (i.e., vital signs taken, intake and output recorded, and electrocardiogram and baseline assessment performed). All relevant contraindications, cautions, and drug interactions (discussed in the pharmacology section of this chapter) need to be taken into account, and special care is required when these drugs are considered for patients who have active infections or who may be immunocompromised.

Contraindications, cautions, and drug interactions need to be considered with the use of active immunizing drugs as well. Pregnant patients and patients with current infections (especially infections caused by the same pathogen or by organisms producing the same toxin), severe febrile illnesses (which exclude minor illnesses such as a cold, mild infection, ear infection, or low-grade fever), or a history of reactions or serious adverse effects to one or more of these drugs require special assessment regarding their use. Patients who are already immunosuppressed (e.g., those with AIDS, the older adult, those with chronic diseases or cancer, neonates) are at increased risk for serious adverse effects to toxoids or vaccines; therefore, cautious use of these drugs is indicated in such patients. Many adults assume that the vaccines they received as children will protect them for a lifetime, and this is usually the case. However, some adults were never vaccinated as children, or newer vaccines were not available at the time they were vaccinated.

An influenza pandemic is a future reality. The nurse's role may range from aiding in the preparations for a coordinated response and performing triage to carrying out the nursing process during a pandemic. The nurse's role may also include assessing individuals, groups, and communities and providing related education to help people understand the benefits of being informed, making plans, and maintaining a state of preparation at all times to the degree that is possible. In such assessment, ethnocultural background, knowledge and educational levels, age, motor skills, cognitive abilities, awareness of extended family members and their level of preparedness, and ability to manage stress and to think during a crisis are just a few of the areas worthy of consideration. Nurses also have a responsibility to ensure that, regardless of the situation, they maintain a calm, reassuring, compassionate, caring, and empathic manner during the assessment phase (and all other phases of the nursing process) in the care of those in need and that they avoid excessively anxiety-provoking comments or actions.

Nursing Diagnoses

- Risk for injury related to possible adverse effects of or allergic reactions to an immunizing drug
- Acute pain related to local or systemic effects of the injection of a toxoid, vaccine, or passive immunizing drug
- Deficient knowledge related to the use of toxoids, vaccines, or passive immunizing drugs
- Anxiety related to suspected risk of influenza pandemic

Planning

Goals

- Patient will state the adverse effects of the drug.
- Patient will experience minimal discomfort from the administration of a toxoid, vaccine, or passive immunizing drug.
- Patient will remain adherent to the therapeutic regimen.
- Patient will return for follow-up injections and booster injections and for follow-up visits with the physician.
- Patient will state the importance of proactive behaviour and education related to the risk of influenza.

Outcome Criteria

- Patient experiences minimal adverse effects of or allergic reactions to the immunizing drug, such as fever, chills, myalgia, and bronchospasms (allergic), and is able to manage these effects with the use of acetaminophen and diphenhydramine, if ordered.
- Patient uses measures such as the application of cold or heat packs to the site of injection, as indicated and as ordered by the physician, to help relieve localized discomfort or alleviate any localized reactions.

- Patient remains adherent to the therapeutic regimen for the prevention of illness or disease through follow-up visits with physician.
- Patient states any problems or concerns to report immediately to the physician, such as fever higher than 38.3°C, infection, wheezing, increasing weakness, or any other unusual reaction.
- Patient states methods of remaining well informed about the possibility of an influenza pandemic and specific actions for self-protection, including reading reliable sources and staying abreast of local and national news.

Implementation

When administering immunizing drugs, the nurse must always recheck the specific protocols and schedules of administration. In addition, it is always important to read and follow the manufacturer's recommendations for storage and administration of the drug, routes and site of administration, dosage, and precautions and contraindications to its use. Parents of young children must be encouraged and taught how to maintain an accurate journal of the child's immunization status with dates of immunization and the reaction(s), if any, to avoid gaps in the child's immunization schedule. To this end, Canada is working toward the development of a national electronic Immunization Tracking System.

If the patient experiences discomfort at the injection site, use of warm compresses or acetaminophen may help. Patients on tumour necrosis factor–blocking agents such as adalimumab (Humira) or the monoclonal antibody infliximab (Remicade) should not receive live vaccines because of the suppressant effect of these drugs on the immune system. With the possibility of an influenza pandemic, patients need to be kept well informed, and the nurse must be constantly aware of the need to minimize anxiety. (See http://evolve.elsevier.com/Canada/Lilley/pharmacology/ for more information on specific agencies, policy development issues, and online resources related to pandemic planning.)

Evaluation

The therapeutic response in patients receiving immunizing drugs is the prevention or amelioration of the specific disease being targeted. While adverse reactions are specific to the immunizing drug, the nurse should monitor for a localized reaction, including swelling, redness, discomfort, and heat at the site of injection. A more serious reaction should be reported immediately to the physician (e.g., high fever, lymphadenopathy, rash, itching, joint pain, severe flulike symptoms, decreased level of consciousness, or shortness of breath). For a complete list of expected reactions or adverse effects, including minor and severe ones, see Table 47-2. As immunizing drugs improve and newer ones are developed, it is hoped that fewer adverse effects and fewer adverse drug events and complications will occur.

PATIENT EDUCATION

- ❖ A localized reaction to the injection sometimes occurs when toxoids and vaccines are administered. Patients should be told that they can relieve the discomfort by placing warm compresses on the injection site, resting, and taking acetaminophen or diphenhydramine, as directed by the physician. Instructions for the care of infants or children experiencing such reactions are generally given by the child's health care provider when the immunizing drug is administered.
- ❖ Patients, parents, or caregivers should be instructed to notify the physician if high or prolonged fever,

rash, itching, or shortness of breath occurs after the vaccination.
- ❖ Patients, parents, or caregivers should be encouraged to always keep a double record (two copies kept in separate places) of all of the medications being taken, particularly all vaccinations received.
- ❖ Patients should be informed that a vaccine adverse event reporting system is available through Health Canada (http://www.phac-aspc.gc.ca/im/vs-sv/caefiss-eng.php).

POINTS TO REMEMBER

- ❖ A foreign substance in the body is termed an *antigen;* the body creates a substance called an *antibody* to specifically bind to it.
- ❖ B lymphocytes (B cells), when stimulated by the binding of an antigen molecule, begin to differentiate into memory cells and plasma cells.
- ❖ Memory cells remember the characteristics of a particular antigen in case the body is exposed to the same antigen in the future.

- ❖ Plasma cells manufacture antibodies and will massproduce clones of antibodies upon re-exposure to a particular antigen.
- ❖ The two types of immunity are active and passive immunity. Different types of drugs are used to induce each, and these drugs are indicated for different populations, as follows:
  - Active immunization involves administration of a toxoid or a vaccine that exposes the body to a

relatively harmless form of the antigen (foreign invader) to imprint cellular memory and stimulate the body's defences to fight any subsequent exposure. It provides long-lasting or permanent immunity. The recipient must have an active, functioning immune system to benefit from immunization.

- Passive immunization involves the administration of immune globulins, antitoxins, or antivenins. Serum or concentrated immune globulins are obtained from humans or animals and, after screening and testing, are injected into the patient, directly giving the patient the ability to fight off the invading microorganism. Passive immunization provides temporary protection and does not stimulate an antibody response in the host. It is used in patients who are immunocompromised or who have been exposed or anticipate exposure to the disease.

❖ Patients who should not receive immunizing drugs include those with active infections, febrile illnesses, or a history of a previous reaction to the drug. Use of these drugs in pregnant women is also usually contraindicated.

❖ Patients who are immunocompromised are at greater risk for suffering serious adverse effects from immunizing drugs.

❖ Parents should keep updated records of their children's and their own immunizations with any toxoids or vaccines.

EXAMINATION REVIEW QUESTIONS

1 When assessing a patient who will be receiving a passive immunizing drug, which condition will the nurse consider to be a possible contraindication?
a. Anemia
b. Pregnancy
c. Ear infection
d. Common cold

2 When giving a vaccination to an infant, which adverse effect should the nurse tell the mother to expect?
a. Chills
b. Dyspnea
c. Fever over 39.4°C
d. Soreness at the injection site

3 After a suspected hepatitis B exposure, prophylactic doses of which of the following would be given to the individual?
a. Immune serum globulin
b. Hepatitis B virus vaccine
c. Hepatitis B immune globulin
d. $Rh_0(D)$ immune globulin

4 During a routine checkup, a 72-year-old patient is advised to receive an influenza vaccine injection. He questions this, saying, "I had one last year. Why do I need another one?" What is an appropriate response from the nurse?
a. "The effectiveness of the vaccine wears off after 6 months."
b. "When you reach age 65, you need boosters on an annual basis."
c. "Taking the flu vaccine each year allows you to build your immunity to a higher level each time."
d. "Each year a new vaccine is developed on the basis of flu strains that are likely to be in circulation."

5 A patient is in the urgent care centre after stepping on a rusty tent nail. The nurse evaluates the patient's immunity status. Which of the following is true to necessitate a tetanus booster?
a. It has been a year since his last booster shot.
b. It has been 2 years since his last booster shot.
c. It has been 5 years since his last booster shot.
d. It has been 10 years since his last booster shot.

For answers see http://evolve.elsevier.com/Canada/Lilley/pharmacology/.

CRITICAL THINKING ACTIVITIES

1 Compare and contrast active and passive immunization.

2 Within 2 hours after a tetanus booster vaccination, your patient is showing signs of a serious adverse reaction. Describe the process for reporting this adverse event after you address the patient's needs for physical care.

3 You are working as a staff nurse on a medical–surgical unit in a suburban area. In the event of a pandemic of influenza, what are your responsibilities?

For answers see http://evolve.elsevier.com/Canada/Lilley/pharmacology/.

CHAPTER **48**

Antineoplastic Drugs Part 1: Cancer Overview and Cell Cycle–Specific Drugs

Learning Objectives

After reading this chapter, the successful student will be able to do the following:

1 Briefly describe the concepts related to carcinogenesis.

2 Define the different types of malignancy.

3 Discuss the purpose and role of the treatment modalities in the management of cancer.

4 Define *antineoplastic*.

5 Discuss the role of antineoplastic therapy in the treatment of cancer.

6 Contrast the cell cycle of normal cells and malignant cells with regard to growth, function, and response of the cell to chemotherapeutic drugs and other treatment modalities.

7 Compare the characteristics of highly proliferating normal cells (including cells of the hair follicles, gastrointestinal tract, and bone marrow) with the characteristics of highly proliferating cancerous cells.

8 Briefly describe the differences between cell cycle–specific and cell cycle–nonspecific antineoplastic drugs (cell cycle–nonspecific drugs and miscellaneous other antineoplastics are presented in Chapter 49).

9 Identify the drugs that are categorized as cell cycle–specific, including mitotic inhibitors, topoisomerase inhibitors, and antineoplastic enzymes.

10 Describe the common adverse effects and toxic reactions associated with the antineoplastic drugs, including the causes for their occurrence and methods of treatment, such as antidotes for toxicity.

11 Discuss the mechanisms of action, indications, dosage, routes of administration, cautions, contraindications, and drug interactions of cell cycle–specific drugs, mitotic inhibitors, topoisomerase inhibitors, and antineoplastic enzymes.

12 Apply knowledge about the antineoplastic drugs to the development of a comprehensive collaborative plan of care for patients receiving cell cycle–specific drugs, mitotic inhibitors, topoisomerase inhibitors, and antineoplastic enzymes.

13 Briefly describe extravasation and other major adverse effects associated with the antineoplastics, including discussion of protocols and antidotes.

e-Learning Activities

Web site
(http://evolve.elsevier.com/Canada/
Lilley/pharmacology/)

- Animations
- Answers to chapter questions, activities, and case studies
- Calculators and Category Catchers
- Glossary with audio pronunciations
- IV Therapy and Medication Error Checklists
- Multiple-Choice Review Question quizzes
- Nursing Care Plans
- Online Appendices and Supplements
- WebLinks

Drug Profiles

▶▶ **asparaginase**, p. 899
   capecitabine, p. 893
   cladribine, p. 893
▶▶ **cytarabine**, p. 893
▶▶ **etoposide**, p. 893
   fludarabine, p. 893
   fluorouracil, p. 893
   gemcitabine (gemcitabine hydrochloride)*, p. 893
   irinotecan (irinotecan hydrochloride)*, p. 898
▶▶ **methotrexate**, p. 893
▶▶ **paclitaxel**, p. 893
   pegaspargase, p. 899
   raltitrexed (raltitrexed disodium)*, p. 893
   topotecan (topotecan hydrochloride)*, p. 898
▶▶ **vincristine**, p. 893

▶▶ Key drug.

*Full generic name is given in parentheses. For the purposes of this text, the more common shortened name is used.

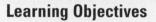

878

Glossary

Analogue   A chemical compound with a structure similar to that of another compound but differing from it with respect to some other component; it may have a similar or opposite metabolic or other action in the body. (p. 890)

Anaplasia   The absence of the cellular differentiation that is part of the normal cellular growth process (see *differentiation*; adjective: *anaplastic*). (p. 885)

Antineoplastic drugs   Drugs used to treat cancer. Also called *cancer drugs, anticancer drugs, cancer chemotherapy,* and *chemotherapy*. (p. 883)

Benign   Term denoting a neoplasm that is noncancerous and therefore not an immediate threat to life, even though treatment eventually may be required for health or cosmetic reasons. (p. 880)

Cancer   A term encompassing a group of neoplastic diseases characterized by uncontrolled cellular growth and possible invasion into surrounding tissue and metastasis to other tissues or organs; its natural course is fatal (see *neoplasm*). (p. 880)

Carcinogen   Any cancer-producing substance or organism. (p. 882)

Carcinomas   Malignant epithelial neoplasms that tend to invade surrounding tissue and metastasize to distant regions of the body. (p. 880)

Cell cycle–nonspecific   Term denoting antineoplastic drugs that are cytotoxic in any phase of the cellular growth cycle. (p. 885)

Cell cycle–specific   Term denoting antineoplastic drugs that are cytotoxic during a specific cell cycle phase. (p. 885)

Clone   A cell or group of cells that is genetically identical to a given parent cell. (p. 880)

Differentiation   An important part of normal cellular growth processes involving changes in immature cells that allow them to mature into different types of more specialized cells, each having different functions. (p. 880)

Dose-limiting adverse effects   Adverse effects that prevent an antineoplastic drug from being given in higher doses, often limiting the effectiveness of the drug. (p. 887)

Emetic potential   The potential of the drug to irritate the cells of the stomach or stimulate the vomiting centre in the central nervous system, which results in nausea and vomiting. (p. 887)

Extravasation   The leakage of any intravenously or intra-arterially administered medication into the tissue space surrounding the vein or artery. (p. 888)

Growth fraction   The percentage of cells in mitosis at any given time. (p. 883)

Intrathecal   A route of drug injection through the theca of the spinal cord and into the subarachnoid space. (p. 893)

Leukemias   Malignant neoplasms of blood-forming tissues characterized by the diffuse replacement of normal bone marrow cells with proliferating leukocyte precursors,

which, in turn, results in abnormal numbers and forms of immature white blood cells in the circulation, and the infiltration of lymph nodes, spleen, and liver. (p. 881)

Lymphomas   Neoplasms of lymphoid tissue that are usually malignant but in rare cases may be benign. (p. 881)

Malignant   Tending to worsen and cause death; anaplastic, invasive, and metastatic. (p. 880)

Metastasis   The process by which a cancer spreads from the original site of growth to a new and remote part of the body (adjective: *metastatic*). (p. 880)

Mitosis   The process of cell reproduction occurring in somatic (nonsexual) cells and resulting in the formation of two genetically identical daughter cells containing the diploid (complete) number of chromosomes characteristic of the species. (p. 883)

Mitotic index   The number of cells per unit (usually 1000) undergoing mitosis during a given time. (p. 883)

Mutagen   A chemical or physical agent that induces or increases genetic mutations by causing changes in deoxyribonucleic acid (DNA) or ribonucleic acid (RNA). (p. 882)

Mutation   A permanent change in cellular genetic material (DNA or RNA) that is transmissible to future cellular generations. (p. 880)

Myelosuppression   Suppression of bone marrow function, which can result in dangerously reduced numbers of red and white blood cells and platelets. Also referred to as *bone marrow suppression* or *bone marrow depression*. (p. 887)

Nadir   Lowest point in any fluctuating value over time, such as the white blood cell count after it has been depressed by chemotherapy. (p. 888)

Neoplasm   Any new and abnormal growth, specifically growth that is uncontrolled and progressive; a synonym for *tumour*. (p. 880)

Nucleic acids   Molecules of DNA and RNA in the nucleus of every cell (hence the name *nucleic acid*); they contain the genetic material of all living organisms. (p. 882)

Oncogenic   Giving rise to tumours, either benign or malignant; the term is applied especially to tumour-inducing viruses. (p. 882)

Paraneoplastic syndromes (PNSs)   Symptom complexes arising in patients with cancer that cannot be explained by local or distant spread of their tumours. (p. 881)

Primary lesion   The original site of growth of a tumour; opposite of a metastatic lesion. (p. 880)

Sarcomas   Malignant neoplasms of the connective tissues arising in bone, fibrous, fatty, muscular, synovial, vascular, or neural tissue; often first presenting as a painless swelling. (p. 881)

Tumour   A new growth of tissue characterized by a progressive, uncontrolled proliferation of cells. (p. 880)

Tumour lysis syndrome   A common metabolic complication of chemotherapy for rapidly growing tumours. (p. 890)

OVERVIEW

Cancer is a broad term encompassing a group of diseases characterized by cellular transformation (e.g., by genetic **mutation**), uncontrolled cellular growth, and possible invasion into surrounding tissue and metastasis (spread) to other tissues or organs distant from the original body site. Lack of cellular **differentiation** or maturation into specialized, productive cells is also a common characteristic of cancer cells. Figure 48-1 illustrates the multiple steps involved in the development of cancer. This cellular growth differs from normal cellular growth in that cancerous cells do not possess a growth control mechanism. Cancerous cells will continue to grow and invade adjacent structures, and they may break away from the original tumour mass and travel by means of the blood or lymphatic system to establish a new clone of cancer cells and create a metastatic growth elsewhere in the body. A **clone** is a cell or group of cells that is genetically identical to a given parent cell. For the remainder of this and the next chapter, the term *cancer* will generally be used to refer to any type of malignant neoplasm.

Metastasis refers to the spread of a cancer (uncontrolled cell growth) from the original site of growth (**primary lesion**) to a new and remote part of the body (secondary *or metastatic lesion*). The terms *malignancy, neoplasm,* and *tumour* are often used as synonyms for cancer; however, each has its own meaning. A **neoplasm** ("new tissue") is a mass of new cells that exhibit uncontrolled cellular reproduction. It is another term for **tumour**. There are two types of tumours: benign and malignant. A **benign** tumour is of a uniform size and shape and displays no invasiveness (in terms of infiltrating other tissues) or metastatic properties. The terms *nonmalignant* and *benign* suggest that these tumours may be harmless, which is true in most cases. However, a benign tumour

can be lethal if it grows large enough to mechanically interrupt the normal function of a critical tissue or organ (e.g., brain, heart, lung). **Malignant** neoplasms typically consist of cancerous cells that invade (infiltrate) surrounding tissues at the cellular level and metastasize to other tissues and organs, where they form metastatic tumour deposits. Some of the characteristics of benign and malignant neoplasms, or tumours, are listed in Table 48-1.

Over 100 types of cancers affect humans. They are usually classified by their primary anatomic location (organ or tissue) and the type of cell from which the cancer develops. Common body sites for growth of such tumours include the following:

- Blood-producing tissue
- Breast
- Colon
- Kidney
- Liver
- Lung
- Lymphatic system
- Ovary
- Prostate gland
- Rectum
- Skin
- Uterus

Tumour types based on tissue categories include sarcomas, carcinomas, lymphomas, leukemias, and tumours of nervous tissue origin. Examples of these common malignant tumours are listed in Table 48-2. It is important to know the tissue of origin because this determines the type of chemotherapy used, the likely response to therapy, and the prognosis.

Carcinomas arise from epithelial tissue, which is located throughout the body. It covers or lines all body surfaces, both inside and outside the body. Examples are the skin, the mucosal lining of the entire gastrointestinal

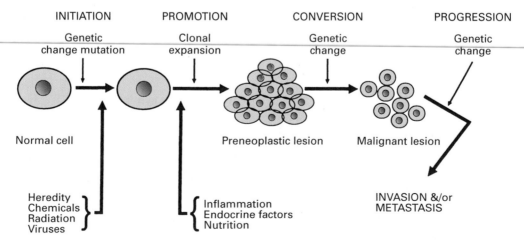

FIG. 48-1 Schematic model of multistep carcinogenesis. *Genetic change* refers to events such as the activation of protooncogenes or drug-resistance genes or the inactivation of tumour suppressor genes, antimetastasis genes, or apoptosis (normal cell death). Genetic change may be relatively minimal, as with the translocations seen in leukemias, or it may involve multiple sequential genetic alterations, as exemplified by the development of colon cancer. (From Haskell, C. M. (2001). *Cancer treatment* (5th ed.) Philadelphia: Saunders.)

TABLE 48-1

Tumour Characteristics: Benign and Malignant

Characteristics	Benign	Malignant
Encapsulated	Yes	No
Potential to metastasize	No	Yes
Similar to tissue of origin	Yes	No
Rate of growth	Slow	Unpredictable and unrestrained
Recurrence after surgical removal	Rare	Common

TABLE 48-2

Tumour Classification Based on Specific Tissue of Origin

Tissue of Origin	Malignant Tissue
EPITHELIAL = CARCINOMAS	
Glands or ducts	Adenocarcinomas
Kidney	Kidney cell carcinoma
Respiratory tract	Small- and large-cell carcinomas
Skin	Squamous cell, epidermoid, and basal cell carcinoma; melanoma
CONNECTIVE = SARCOMAS	
Blood vessels	Kaposi's sarcoma
Bone	Osteogenic sarcoma (Ewing's tumour)
Cartilage	Chondrosarcoma
Fibrous tissue	Fibrosarcoma
Mesothelium	Mesothelioma
Synovia	Synoviosarcoma
LYMPHATIC = LYMPHOMAS	
Bone marrow	Multiple myeloma
Lymph tissue	Lymphomas (e.g., Hodgkin's, non-Hodgkin's)
NERVE	
Adrenal medulla nerves	Pheochromocytoma
Glia	Glioma
BLOOD	
White blood cells	Leukemia

tract, and the bronchial tree (lungs). The purpose of these epithelial tissues is to protect the body's vital organs. **Sarcomas** are malignant tumours that arise primarily from connective tissues, although some sarcomas are tumours of epithelial cell origin. Connective tissue is the most abundant and widely distributed of all tissues and includes bone, cartilage, muscle, lymphatic, and vascular structures. Its purpose is to support and protect other tissues. **Lymphomas** are cancers within the lymphatic tissue. **Leukemias** arise from the various types of leukocytes in the blood. These two types of tumours differ from carcinomas and sarcomas in that the cancerous cells do not form solid tumours but are interspersed throughout the lymphatic or circulatory system and interfere with the normal functioning of these systems. For this reason, they are sometimes referred to as *circulating tumours,* although *hematological malignancy* is a more precise term.

Nerve or *neural tissue tumours* are those arising in and affecting the cells of the central or peripheral nervous systems.

Cancer patients may also experience groups of symptoms that cannot be directly attributed to the spread of a cancerous tumour. Such symptom complexes are referred to as the **paraneoplastic syndromes (PNSs).** They are estimated to occur in up to 15% of patients with cancer and may even be the first sign of malignancy, with *cachexia* (general ill health and malnutrition) being the most common symptom complex. Examples of other common PNSs are listed in Table 48-3. These syndromes are believed to result from the effects of biologically or immunologically active substances, such as hormones and antibodies, secreted by the tumour cells. Many patients also exhibit more generalized symptoms, such as anorexia, weight loss, fatigue, and fever.

ETIOLOGY OF CANCER

The etiology of cancer remains a mystery for the most part, and cancer researchers have made slow progress toward identifying possible causes. In recent years, however, certain etiological factors have come to light, some of these and the cancers they are causally associated with are listed in Table 48-4. Radiation, oncogenic viruses, and immunological, ethnic, genetic, age-related, and gender-related characteristics are among the causative factors identified.

AGE- AND GENDER-RELATED DIFFERENCES

The probability that a neoplastic disease will develop generally increases with advancing age. However, acute lymphocytic leukemia and Wilms' tumour are exceptions to this pattern, and the incidence of these disorders decreases with age. Chronic lymphocytic and myelocytic leukemia, colon cancer, and lung cancer, by contrast, usually develop during middle and old age and are rare in young children. (Note that the terms *lymphocytic* and *myelocytic* are synonymous in the literature with the terms *lymphoblastic,* and *myeloblastic* and *myelogenous,* respectively.)

TABLE 48-3

Paraneoplastic Syndrome Associated with Some Cancers

Paraneoplastic Syndrome	Associated Cancer
Addison's syndrome	Adrenal, lymphomas
Cushing's syndrome	Lung, thyroid, testes, adrenal
Disseminated intravascular coagulation	Leukemia
Hypercalcemia, sensory neuropathies, SIADH	Lung

SIADH, syndrome of inappropriate antidiuretic hormone secretion.

TABLE 48-4

Cancer: Proposed Etiological Factors

Risk Factor	Associated Cancer
ENVIRONMENT	
Radiation (ionizing)	Leukemia, breast, thyroid, lung
Radiation (ultraviolet)	Skin, melanoma
Viruses	Leukemia, lymphoma, nasopharyngeal
FOOD	
Aflatoxin	Liver
Dietary factors	Colon, breast, endometrial, gallbladder
LIFESTYLE	
Alcohol	Esophageal, liver, stomach, laryngeal
Tobacco	Lung, oral, esophageal, laryngeal, bladder
MEDICAL DRUGS	
Alkylating drugs	Leukemia, bladder
Diethylstilbestrol (DES)	Vaginal in offspring, breast, testicular, ovarian
Estrogens	Endometrial
OCCUPATIONAL	
Aniline dye	Bladder
Asbestos	Lung, mesothelioma
Benzene	Leukemia
Vinyl chloride	Liver
REPRODUCTIVE HISTORY	
Late first pregnancy, early menses	Breast
Multiple sexual partners	Cervical, uterus
No children	Ovarian

DES, diethylstilbestrol.

With the exception of cancers affecting the reproductive system, few cancers exhibit a sex-related difference in incidence. Lung and urinary cancers are more common in men than in women, but this may have more to do with exogenous factors such as smoking and occupational exposure to environmental toxins than to gender-related characteristics. The incidence of colon, rectal, pancreatic, and skin cancers, as well as leukemia, is comparable for the two genders.

GENETIC AND ETHNIC FACTORS

Few cancers have been confirmed to have a hereditary basis (some types of breast, colon, and stomach cancers are exceptions). The understanding of tumour biology has nonetheless helped guide therapy tremendously. Two such advancements are determination of hormone receptor status and identification of specific gene expression in various types of tumour cells. For example, some tumour cells have been shown to express on their cell membrane surfaces either estrogen receptors or progesterone receptors, and some tumour cells express specific genes such

as the *HER2/neu* gene. Because these indicators aid in the classification of a patient's tumour, they also help in choosing appropriate drug therapy, predicting response to therapy, and anticipating a prognosis. The tendency to develop tumours with identifiable gene expression patterns often shows a familial pattern of inheritance. Burkitt's lymphoma is an example of a cancer that shows a racial predilection; the disease is more common in young Black children. Another example of ethnic predisposition is the high incidence of nasopharyngeal cancer in Chinese individuals.

ONCOGENIC VIRUSES

Extensive research has indicated that there are cancer-causing (**oncogenic**) viruses that can affect most mammalian species. Examples include human papilloma virus, the cat leukemias, the Rous* sarcoma virus in chickens, and the Shope* papilloma virus in rabbits.

The herpesviruses are common examples of oncogenic viruses. Epstein–Barr virus, a type of herpesvirus, is most commonly recognized as the cause of infectious mononucleosis (commonly referred to as "mono" or the "kissing disease"). However, it is also associated with the development of Burkitt's lymphoma and nasopharyngeal cancer. There also seems to be a link between the development of cervical cancer and infection with the herpes simplex type 2 virus (herpes genitalis). Infection with human papilloma virus (HPV) is the cause of almost all cases of cervical cancer and is linked to anal cancer.

OCCUPATIONAL AND ENVIRONMENTAL CARCINOGENS

A **carcinogen** is any substance that can induce the development of a cancer or accelerate its growth. In the nucleus of every cell there are molecules of **nucleic acids**, so named because of their location in the cell nucleus. The two types of nucleic acids are *deoxyribonucleic acid (DNA)* and *ribonucleic acid (RNA)*. DNA molecules are the master molecules of genetic material within cells. They reproduce, or *replicate*, by making RNA molecules, which in turn gather *amino acids* to make the protein molecules necessary for cellular reproduction. This process is discussed further in the section on alkylating drugs in Chapter 49. A **mutagen** is any substance or physical agent (e.g., radiation) that enhances the rate of genetic mutations by inducing changes, primarily in DNA molecules, but that can also damage RNA. Mutations in cellular genetic material (DNA) often *transform* normal cells into cancer cells whose growth is unrestrained. Thus, *mutagenicity* is associated with and often (but not always) leads to carcinogenicity. Health Canada regulations mandate that carcinogenic studies be performed before any new drug is approved for use. However, no amount of

---
*Doctors P. Rous and R. Shope were early investigators of oncogenic viruses.

clinical testing can fully reveal all of the possible carcinogenic effects because testing for drug carcinogenic activity is difficult and current test methods are often not satisfactory. In addition, with any given drug there can be species-related differences in carcinogenic potential. Carcinogenic effects may not have been observed in the laboratory animals on which the drug was tested and may become obvious only when the drugs are used in human subjects. The hope is that such effects become apparent before the medication is marketed. However, given the relatively small number of subjects in clinical research trials, it is possible that the carcinogenic potential of a drug is not be observed until after the drug is marketed for use in the general population. If patterns of carcinogenicity begin to emerge during this period of postmarketing surveillance (or postmarketing studies), the drug may be recalled from the market. This recall can be either initiated voluntarily by the manufacturer or mandated by Health Canada.

IMMUNOLOGICAL FACTORS

The immune system plays an important role in the body in cancer surveillance and the elimination of neoplastic cells. While neoplastic cells are believed to routinely develop in everyone, in healthy persons the immune system recognizes them as abnormal and eliminates them by means of cell-mediated immunity (cytotoxic T lymphocytes; Chapter 50). It has also been shown that the incidence of cancer is much higher in immunocompromised individuals, such as patients undergoing cancer chemotherapy, organ transplant patients receiving immunosuppressive therapy, and patients suffering from immunological impairment or disease, including AIDS. This relationship between cancer and a suppressed immune system has also been noted in cancer patients being treated with immunotherapy consisting of interferon derivatives (Chapter 50), the *bacillus Calmette-Guérin (BCG)* vaccine (used to treat bladder cancer, Chapter 47), and *lymphokines* (immune-modulating molecules; Chapter 50).

CANCER DRUG NOMENCLATURE

As mentioned earlier, a more technical term for cancer is *malignant neoplasm*. Drugs used to treat cancer are therefore known as **antineoplastic drugs** but are also called *cancer drugs, anticancer drugs,* and, most commonly, *cytotoxic chemotherapy* or just *chemotherapy*. The nomenclature (naming system) of cancer drugs can be somewhat more complex and confusing than that for other drug classes. Cancer treatment is an intensively researched area in health care, with many ongoing research protocols. Often more new drugs are approved by Health Canada and the U.S. Food and Drug Administration (FDA) for cancer treatment in any given year than drugs approved for treatment of other disease categories. Further complicating matters is the fact that multiple names are often used for the same drug, depending on its stage of development.

The following text and Table 48-5 provide examples of the various names for antineoplastic medications that may be encountered in clinical practice.

CELL GROWTH CYCLE

Normal cells in the body *proliferate* (grow by dividing) in a controlled and organized fashion, and this growth is regulated by means of various mechanisms. In contrast, cancer cells lack regulatory mechanisms and proliferate uncontrollably, although some modulation of cancer cell proliferation may occur if blood flow to the cancer is disrupted. Often, the growth of cancer cells is also more constant or continuous than that of nonmalignant cells. Thus, one important growth index for malignant tumours is the time it takes for the tumour to double in size. This *doubling time* varies greatly for different types of cancers and is directly related to and important in determining the prognosis for a particular patient. Cancer treatment that cannot destroy every neoplastic cell does not prevent the regrowth of the tumour, and the time it takes for regrowth to occur depends on the doubling time of the particular cancer. For example, Burkitt's lymphoma has an extremely short doubling time, whereas multiple myeloma has one of the longest doubling times. A cancer with a shorter doubling time is often more difficult to treat and more likely to have a poorer prognosis.

The cell growth characteristics for normal and neoplastic cells are similar. Both types of cells pass through five distinct growth phases: G_0, the *resting* phase; G_1, the first growth phase; S, the *synthesis* phase; G_2, the second growth phase; and M, the **mitosis** phase. During mitosis, one cell divides into two genetically identical *daughter* cells. Mitosis is further subdivided into four distinct subphases related to the time periods before and during the alignment and separation of the chromosomes (DNA strands): *prophase, metaphase, anaphase,* and *telophase*. A complete cycle from one mitosis to the next is called the *generation time* (this is the same as doubling time), which is different for all tumours, ranging from hours to days. The cell growth cycle and the events that occur in the different phases are summarized in Table 48-6. Figure 48-2 shows the point in the general phases of the cell cycle at which the cell cycle–specific chemotherapeutic drugs show their greatest proportional kill of cancer cells.

The growth activity in a mass of tumour cells can also be characterized and has an important bearing on the killing power of chemotherapy drugs. The *percentage* of cells undergoing mitosis (M) at any given time is called the **growth fraction** of the tumour mass. The *actual number* of cells that are in the M phase of the cell cycle is called the **mitotic index.** Chemotherapy is most effective when the greatest number of cells are dividing, that is, when both the growth fraction and mitotic index are high; a tumour in which both these indicators are high is known as a *highly proliferative* tumour.

Any cell that is a precursor to another cell is known as a *stem cell.* In the bone marrow, stem cells eventually

TABLE 48-5

Common Names for Selected Cell Cycle–Specific Antineoplastic Drugs

Generic Name	Trade Names	Other Names
ANTIMETABOLITES		
Folic Acid Antagonist Analogue		
methotrexate	Apo-Methotrexate, Metoject	MTX
Purine Analogues		
cladribine	Leustatin	2-chloro-2-deoxyadenosine, 2-CdA, CdA
fludarabine	Fludara	FAMP, NSC-312887, *9-B-D*-arabinofuranosyl-2-fluoroadenine-5′-monophosphate, 2-fluoro-ara-A monophosphate
mercaptopurine	Purinethol	6-mercaptopurine, 6-MP
thioguanine	Lanvis	6-TG, TG, 2-amino-6-mercaptopurine
Pyrimidine Analogues		
capecitabine	Xeloda	
cytarabine, conventional	Cytosar	1-B-arabinofuranosylcytosine, ara-C, cytosine arabinoside
cytarabine, liposomal	DepoCyt	
fluorouracil	Efudex Cream, Fluoroplex Cream, Fluorouracil	5-fluorouracil, 5-FU, NSC-19893
gemcitabine	Gemzar	2,2-difluorodeoxycytidine, dFdC, LY188011
NATURAL PRODUCTS		
Camptothecin Analogues (From a Chinese Shrub)		
irinotecan	Camptosar	CPT-11
topotecan	Hycamtin	NSC-609699
Enzymes		
asparaginase (from *Escherichia coli* bacteria)	Kidrolase	A-ase, ASN-ase, Colaspase, Crasnitin, Elspar, L-asparagine amidohydrolase
pegaspargase (from *E. coli* bacteria)	Oncaspar	PEG-L-asparaginase, Pegaspargasa, Pegaspargasum
Epipodophyllotoxins (From Mandrake Plant or May Apple)		
etoposide	VePesid	VP-16
teniposide	Vumon	VM-26, PTG
Taxanes (From Yew Trees)		
docetaxel	Taxotere	RP56976
paclitaxel	Abraxane, Taxol	NSC-125973
Vinca Alkaloids (From Periwinkle Plant)		
vinblastine sulfate	Vinblastine Sulfate Injection	Vincaleukoblastine sulfate, VLB
vincristine	Vincristine Sulfate Injection	VCR, leurocristine, LCR
vinorelbine tartrate	Navelbine	VRL, VNL, NVB

TABLE 48-6

Cell Cycle Phases

Phase	Description
G_0: Resting phase	Most normal human cells exist predominantly in this phase. Cancer cells in this phase are not susceptible to the toxic effects of cell cycle–specific drugs.
G_1: First growth phase or *postmitotic* phase	Enzymes necessary for DNA synthesis are produced.
S: DNA synthesis phase	DNA synthesis takes place, from DNA strand separation to replication of each strand to create duplicate DNA molecules.
G_2: Second growth phase or *premitotic* phase	RNA and specialized proteins are made.
M: Mitosis phase	This phase is divided into four subphases: prophase, metaphase, anaphase, and telophase; the cell divides (reproduces) into two *daughter* cells.

DNA, deoxyribonucleic acid; *RNA*, ribonucleic acid.

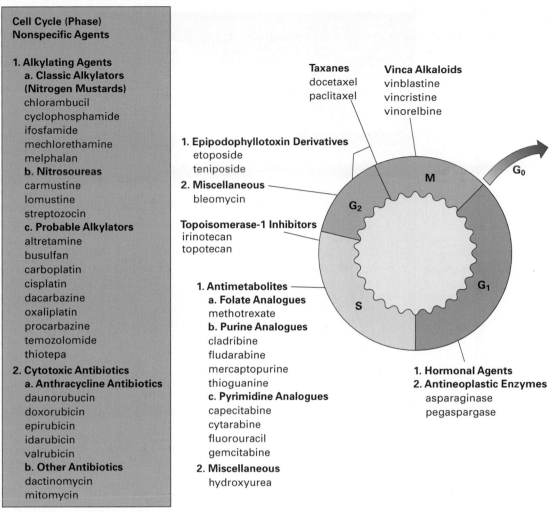

Cell Cycle (Phase) Nonspecific Agents

1. Alkylating Agents
   a. Classic Alkylators (Nitrogen Mustards)
   chlorambucil
   cyclophosphamide
   ifosfamide
   mechlorethamine
   melphalan
   b. Nitrosoureas
   carmustine
   lomustine
   streptozocin
   c. Probable Alkylators
   altretamine
   busulfan
   carboplatin
   cisplatin
   dacarbazine
   oxaliplatin
   procarbazine
   temozolomide
   thiotepa
2. Cytotoxic Antibiotics
   a. Anthracycline Antibiotics
   daunorubicin
   doxorubicin
   epirubicin
   idarubicin
   valrubicin
   b. Other Antibiotics
   dactinomycin
   mitomycin

Taxanes
docetaxel
paclitaxel

Vinca Alkaloids
vinblastine
vincristine
vinorelbine

1. Epipodophyllotoxin Derivatives
   etoposide
   teniposide
2. Miscellaneous
   bleomycin

Topoisomerase-1 Inhibitors
irinotecan
topotecan

1. Antimetabolites
   a. Folate Analogues
   methotrexate
   b. Purine Analogues
   cladribine
   fludarabine
   mercaptopurine
   thioguanine
   c. Pyrimidine Analogues
   capecitabine
   cytarabine
   fluorouracil
   gemcitabine
2. Miscellaneous
   hydroxyurea

1. Hormonal Agents
2. Antineoplastic Enzymes
   asparaginase
   pegaspargase

M G_0 G_2 G_1 S

FIG. 48-2   General phase of the cell cycle in which the cell cycle–specific chemotherapeutic drugs have their greatest proportionate kill of cancer cells.

change into more mature and specialized cells through differentiation. The level of differentiation within a tumour, whether solid or circulating, becomes important in the treatment of neoplasms because more highly differentiated tumours generally have a better therapeutic response (tumour shrinkage) to treatments such as chemotherapy and radiation. In contrast, some cancers, such as leukemia, involve proliferation of immature white blood cells (WBCs) known as *blast cells*. Cancers with a larger proportion of such *undifferentiated* cells are often less responsive to chemotherapy or radiation and are thus more difficult to treat. Lack of normal cellular differentiation is known as **anaplasia**, and such undifferentiated cells are said to be *anaplastic* cells.

DRUG THERAPY

Cancer is normally treated with one or more of three major medical approaches: surgery, radiation therapy, and chemotherapy. *Chemotherapy* is a general term that technically can refer to chemical (drug) therapy for any kind of illness. In practice, however, this term usually refers to the pharmacological treatment of cancer. Normal cells in the body divide (proliferate) in a controlled and organized fashion, and this growth is regulated by means of various mechanisms. In contrast, cancer cells lack regulatory mechanisms and proliferate uncontrollably. Figure 48-3 shows what is termed the *Gompertzian tumour growth curve*, which illustrates the effects on patient clinical status of tumour growth over time. Figure 48-4 shows how combinations of cancer treatment may succeed, or fail, over time.

Cancer chemotherapy drugs can be subdivided into two main groups on the basis of where in the cellular life cycle they have their effects. Antineoplastic drugs that are cytotoxic, or cell killing, in any phase of the cycle are called **cell cycle–nonspecific** drugs. Those drugs that are cytotoxic during a specific cell cycle phase are called **cell cycle–specific** drugs. It should be noted, however, that these are broad categories that describe the *predominant* activity of a drug with regard to cell cycle. Individual drugs may have actions that fall into both

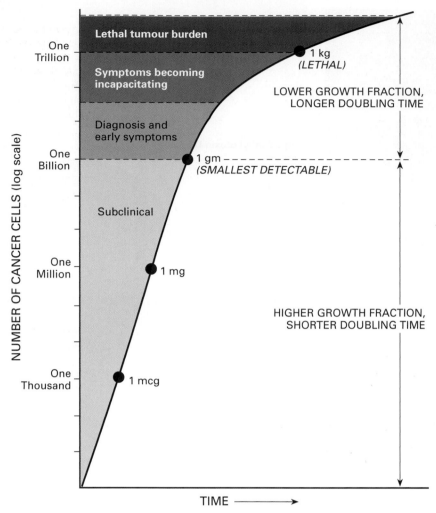

FIG. 48-3 Gompertzian tumour growth curve showing the relationship between tumour size and clinical status. (From Lehne, R. A. (2007). *Pharmacology for nursing care* (6th ed.). St. Louis, MO: Elsevier Saunders.)

these categories. Cell cycle–nonspecific drugs are more effective against large, slowly growing tumours. Cell cycle–specific drugs are more effective against rapidly growing tumours. This chapter has described the individual phases of the cell cycle and discusses the corresponding cell cycle–specific drugs. Chapter 49 focuses on cell cycle–nonspecific drugs as well as miscellaneous antineoplastic drugs.

The ultimate goal of any anticancer regimen is to kill every neoplastic cell and produce a cure, yet this goal is not achieved in most cases. One reason for this is that antineoplastic drugs are usually only cytotoxic and not tumouricidal; that is, they usually only kill a portion of the cells in a tumour, such as those that are dividing, and not all the cells in the tumour. Other factors that affect the chances of cure and the length of patient survival include the cancer stage at the time of diagnosis, type of cancer and its doubling time, efficacy of the cancer treatment, development of drug resistance, and general health of the patient. When total cure is not possible, the primary goal of therapy is to control the growth of the cancer while maintaining the best quality of life for the patient,

with the least possible level of discomfort, compromise (in performing the activities of daily living), and adverse effects of treatment.

Cancer care and treatment involve many rapidly evolving medical sciences. Cancer is an intensively researched area, the ultimate goal being to prevent cancer and prevent premature death in those diagnosed. Chemotherapy medications are often dosed as part of complex, specific treatment protocols that are subject to frequent revision by oncology clinicians and researchers. For these reasons, the drug dosing information provided in this chapter is offered as representative of current cancer treatment and is not absolute or comprehensive. Oncology nursing is a highly specialized area of practice with focused, ongoing continuing education requirements that may vary among provinces and territories. Furthermore, the indications listed for each specific drug are the current primary Health Canada–approved indications. These, too, may change as a given drug is determined to be more (or less) effective for treating certain types of cancer. Also, in clinical practice, patients are often treated by their supervising oncologists with one or more antineoplastic

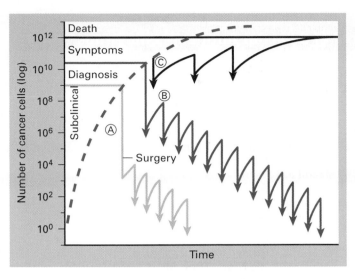

FIG. 48-4 Relationship of tumour burden to treatment strategies and outcome with systemic chemotherapy. Human tumours grow in accordance with the Gompertzian curve (*dashed line*), with a decreasing doubling time as tumour burden increases. Treatment interventions relate to tumour type and extent of disease. *A*, Surgery followed by pulse courses of adjuvant chemotherapy. Combined modality has curative potential with the addition of chemotherapy after surgery. *B*, Systemic chemotherapy for stage III Hodgkin's disease. Cure is possible with prolonged administration of combination chemotherapy. *C*, Palliative chemotherapy for advanced non–small cell cancer. The patient's tumour burden is too great, and the potency of the drugs for this specific form of cancer too inadequate because of the development of drug resistance, to allow cure. (Source: Modified from Salmon, S. E., & Sartorelli, A. C. Cancer chemotherapy. In Katzung, B. G. (Ed.). (1989). *Basic and clinical pharmacology* (4th ed., p. 685). Norwalk, CT: Appleton & Lange.)

medications for "off-label" uses; that is, the drug is not currently approved for this particular use by Health Canada. This use is often a judgement made by the attending oncologist. Such decisions may be based on case studies or simply trial and error in the final efforts to treat patients for whom other drug therapies have failed. This process is one way in which new information is discovered. As noted earlier, however, only the current Health Canada–approved indications will be mentioned in this chapter.

No antineoplastic drug is effective against all types of cancer. Most cancer drugs also have a *low therapeutic index,* meaning that a narrow margin exists between the therapeutic effect and toxicity. However, one important discovery yielded by clinical experience is that a combination of drugs is usually more effective than single-drug therapy. Because drug-resistant cells often develop in tumours as the result of the tumour's genetic instability, exposure to multiple drugs with multiple mechanisms and sites of action will destroy more subpopulations of cells. The delayed onset of resistance to a particular antineoplastic drug is thus one benefit of combination drug therapy. To be most effective, however, the drugs used in such a combination regimen should possess the following characteristics:

- Some efficacy even as single drugs in the treatment of the particular type of cancer
- Different mechanisms of action so that the cytotoxic effect is maximized; this includes differences in cell cycle specificity
- Different cytotoxic properties so that each drug in the combination can be administered in a full therapeutic dose (in other words, have minimal or no overlapping toxicities)

One major drawback to the use of antineoplastic drugs is that their use usually results in adverse effects. Many of these effects are severe or toxic; antineoplastic drugs are harmful to all rapidly growing cells, including harmful cancer cells and healthy, normal human cells. Three types of such rapidly dividing beneficial human cells are cells of hair follicles, gastrointestinal tract cells,

and bone marrow cells. Because most antineoplastic drugs cannot differentiate between the cancer cells and the healthy cells, the latter are also destroyed, with the undesirable consequences of hair loss, nausea and vomiting, and bone marrow toxicity. These effects are called **dose-limiting adverse effects** because they often prevent the antineoplastic drug from being administered in sufficiently high doses to kill the entire population of cancer cells, which would be curative.

Hair follicle cells are continually in a rapidly dividing state, which results in the normal growth and replacement of head and body hair. Cancer drugs that affect these cells often cause the adverse effect of *alopecia,* or hair loss. Many patients, particularly women, choose to wear wigs, hats, or scarves to disguise this adverse effect. Some antineoplastic drugs are more harmful to the epithelial cells of the stomach and intestinal tract, which often leads to nausea, vomiting, and diarrhea. The likelihood that a given drug will produce vomiting is known as its **emetic potential**. Other anticancer drugs cause nausea and vomiting by stimulating the cells of the *vomiting centre* in the medulla, also known as the *chemoreceptor trigger zone*. Chemoreceptors located in the stomach, jejunum, and ileum are involved with the detection of toxic stimuli in the gastrointestinal tract. Preventing these adverse effects entirely would likely require subtherapeutic drug dosages and more limited cancer treatment. Box 48-1 lists the relative emetic potential of selected chemotherapy drugs.

Myelosuppression, also known as *bone marrow suppression* or *bone marrow depression*, is another unwanted adverse effect of certain antineoplastics. It commonly results from drug- or radiation-induced destruction of certain rapidly dividing cells in the bone marrow, primarily the cellular precursors of WBCs, red blood cells (RBCs), and platelets. This can also occur secondary to the disease processes of the cancer itself. Myelosuppression, in turn, leads to leukopenia, anemia, and thrombocytopenia. The cancer patient is often at great risk for infection because of *leukopenia* (reduced WBC counts) secondary

BOX 48-1 — Relative Emetic Potential of Selected Antineoplastic Drugs*

Low (Less Than 10% to 30%)

asparaginase
bleomycin
busulfan
capecitabine
chlorambucil
cladribine
cytarabine (less than 1000 mg/m^2)
daunorubicin, liposomal
docetaxel
doxorubicin (less than 20 mg/m^2)
doxorubicin, liposomal
estramustine
etoposide
fludarabine
fluorouracil (less than 1000 mg/m^2)
gefitinib
gemcitabine
hydroxyurea
imatinib
melphalan
mercaptopurine
methotrexate (less than 250 mg/m^2)
mitomycin
paclitaxel
pegaspargase
rituximab
teniposide
thioguanine
thiotepa
topotecan
trastuzumab
tretinoin
vinblastine
vincristine
vinorelbine

Moderate (30% to 60%)

altretamine
cyclophosphamide (less than 750 mg/m^2)
dactinomycin
daunorubicin (less than 50 mg/m^2)
doxorubicin (20 to 60 mg/m^2)
epirubicin (less than 90 mg/m^2)
idarubicin
ifosfamide (less than 1500 mg/m^2)
irinotecan
methotrexate (250 to 1000 mg/m^2)
mitoxantrone (less than 15 mg/m^2)
temozolomide

High (60% to More Than 90%)

carboplatin
carmustine
cisplatin
cyclophosphamide (750 to more than 1500 mg/m^2)
cytarabine (more than 1000 mg/m^2)
dacarbazine
dactinomycin
daunorubicin (more than 50 mg/m^2)
doxorubicin (more than 60 mg/m^2)
ifosfamide (more than 1500 mg/m^2)
lomustine
mechlorethamine
methotrexate (more than 1000 mg/m^2)
mitoxantrone (more than 15 mg/m^2)
oxaliplatin
procarbazine
streptozocin

*Drugs in this list that are not covered in this chapter are described in Chapter 49.

to chemotherapy. Patients tend to need large dosages of antibiotics, often intravenously, to either prevent or treat bacterial infections. Drug-induced *anemia* (reduced RBC count) often leads to hypoxia and fatigue, whereas *thrombocytopenia* (reduced platelet count) makes the patient more susceptible to bleeding. The lowest level reached by bone marrow cells following a chemotherapy (or radiation) treatment is the **nadir**. The time until the nadir is reached in a patient may become shorter and the recovery time for the bone marrow may become longer with multiple courses of antineoplastic treatment. The nadir normally occurs approximately 10 to 28 days after dosing, depending on the particular cancer drug or combination of drugs that is used to treat the patient. Anticipation of this nadir based on known cancer drug data can be used to guide the timing of prophylactic (preventative) administration of antibiotics as well as blood stimulants known as *biological response modifiers* (see Chapter 50).

Common specific indications for the use of drugs in the antineoplastic classes are listed in the Dosages table

provided for selected drugs in each class. Also provided in this chapter and in Chapter 49 are tables and boxes containing drug-specific guidelines for the treatment of **extravasation** (Box 48-2), or unintended leakage of a chemotherapy drug (with vesicant potential) into the surrounding tissues outside of the intravenous line used for administration.

Because of the often severe toxicity of cancer medications, a current major focus of cancer drug research is the development of *targeted* drug therapy—that is, drugs that chemically recognize and act against only cancer cells, while sparing healthy cells. One example of such targeted therapy is the newer class of cancer drugs known as *monoclonal antibodies* (Chapter 50).

Pharmacokinetic data for antineoplastic medications are challenging to obtain. It is difficult to determine precise values for onset of action, peak effect, and duration of action when treating malignant tumours that often have erratic growth kinetics of their own. Response to therapy is usually determined by clinical evaluation of

BOX 48-2   Extravasation of Antineoplastics

Extravasation is one of the more devastating complications of antineoplastic therapy and may lead to extensive tissue damage, need for skin grafting, other problems to surrounding areas, and even loss of a limb. Because many cell cycle–specific and cell cycle–nonspecific drugs are given intravenously (IV), there is a constant danger of extravasation of vesicants and subsequent injury, including permanent damage to nerves, tendons, and muscles. Astute nursing care may help to prevent extravasation or to identify it early if it does occur, which can reduce the severity of tissue damage. There are important reasons for using central venous IV catheters rather than peripheral catheters when long-term treatment is anticipated. Infiltration may occur with any IV catheter; it is the specific drug and its characteristics, such as irritant or vesicant properties, that pose the greater danger. Because peripheral veins are small and offer minimal dilution of the IV drug with blood flow, there is greater risk of severe and irreversible damage if a substance infiltrates and spreads to surrounding tissues, including muscles, tendons, and ligaments. If the drug is a vesicant, extravasation may lead to massive tissue injury, whereas extravasation of an irritant results in significantly less damage. Central venous access is needed for administration of vesicants to avoid the problems associated with extravasation.

Should extravasation of a vesicant be suspected, immediate action should be taken, and the antidote, if known, should be given following strict procedures. Steps to help manage extravasation include the following: (1) Stop the infusion immediately and contact the physician, but leave the IV catheter in place. (2) Usually, aspiration of any residual drug and blood from the catheter is performed next. (3) Consult institutional policy or guidelines or the pharmacist regarding the use of antidotes, application of hot or cold packs and sterile occlusive dressings, and elevation and rest of the affected limb. The extravasation incident must be thoroughly documented with attention to all phases of the nursing process related to the problem.

Data from the National Cancer Institute Web site, available at http://www.nci.hih.gov. Internet resources for additional information: http://www.bccancer.bc.ca/; http://www.OncoLink.com

the patient, blood sampling to determine cell counts and measure the presence of tumour marker proteins, and imaging scans (e.g., computed tomography, magnetic resonance imaging) to assess the extent of tumour response to cancer treatment. For these reasons, pharmacokinetic data are not included with the drug profiles in this chapter.

In spite of their toxicity, and given the often fatal outcome of neoplastic diseases, most cancer drugs are only rarely considered to be absolutely contraindicated for a given patient. Even if a patient has a known allergic reaction to a given antineoplastic medication, the urgency of treating the patient's cancer may still necessitate administering the medication and treating any allergic symptoms with supportive medications such as antihistamines and acetaminophen. These latter medications are often given before chemotherapy treatment with many drugs known to have potential for allergic-type reactions. For these reasons, no specific contraindications are listed for any of the drugs in this chapter.

Common relative contraindications for all cancer drugs include weakened status of the patient as manifested by indicators such as extremely low WBC count, any ongoing infectious process, or severe compromise in nutritional and hydration status, kidney or liver function, or the function of any other organ system that may be affected by a given drug. These are situations in which chemotherapy treatment is commonly delayed until the patient's status improves. Alternatively, dosages are often reduced for frail older adult patients or others with significantly compromised organ system function, depending on the drugs used. Thus all of the cancer drugs described in this chapter have no absolute contraindications.

Reduction in fertility is often a major concern in postpubertal adolescents. Cancer also complicates 1 in 1000 pregnancies. Prepubertal patients are more resilient, however, and can have normal puberty and fertility.

In the older adult, *frailty* refers to loss of most of the patient's functional reserve and limited ability to tolerate even minimal physiological stress (e.g., chemotherapy treatment). More robust older adult patients are certainly better candidates for cancer treatment, although frail patients often benefit as well, especially in terms of *palliative* (noncurative) symptom control.

Both radiation and chemotherapy treatments can cause significant, permanent fetal harm or death. The greatest risk is during the first trimester. Chemotherapy treatment during the second or third trimester is more likely to improve maternal outcome without significant fetal risk. However, radiation poses great risk to the fetus throughout pregnancy and should be reserved for the postpartum period if possible. Patients are usually examined (and laboratory blood tests performed) by qualified specialists before each chemotherapy treatment. At that time, a clinical judgement is made regarding each patient's fitness for receiving specific antineoplastic drugs.

CELL CYCLE–SPECIFIC ANTINEOPLASTIC DRUGS

Cell cycle–specific drug classes include antimetabolites, mitotic inhibitors, topoisomerase I inhibitors, and antineoplastic enzymes. These drugs are collectively used to treat a variety of solid and circulating tumours, although some drugs have much more specific indications than others. See Table 48-5 for the nomenclature for these drugs.

ANTIMETABOLITES

An **analogue** is a compound that is structurally similar to a normal cellular metabolite. Analogues may have agonist or antagonist activity relative to the corresponding cellular compounds. An antagonist analogue is also known as an *antimetabolite*.

Mechanism of Action and Drug Effects

Antineoplastic antimetabolites are cell cycle–specific analogues that work by antagonizing the actions of key cellular metabolites. More specifically, antimetabolites inhibit cellular growth by interfering with the synthesis or actions of three classes of compounds critical to cellular reproduction: the vitamin *folic acid*, and *purines* and *pyrimidines*, the two classes of compounds that make up the bases contained in *nucleic acid* molecules (DNA and RNA). These drugs work via two mechanisms: (1) by falsely substituting for purines, pyrimidines, or folic acid, or (2), by inhibiting critical enzymes involved in the synthesis or function of these compounds. Thus, they ultimately inhibit the synthesis of DNA, RNA, and proteins, all of which are necessary for cellular reproduction. Antimetabolites work primarily in the S phase of the cell cycle, when DNA synthesis occurs. The available antimetabolites and the metabolites they antagonize are as follows:

Folate antagonists
- methotrexate raltitrexed disodium

Purine antagonists
- allopurinol
- cladribine
- fludarabine phosphate
- mercaptopurine thioguanine
- rasburicase

Pyrimidine antagonists
- capecitabine
- cytarabine fluorouracil
- gemcitabine

Folic Acid Antagonism

The antimetabolite methotrexate is an analogue of folic acid and inhibits dihydrofolate reductase, an enzyme responsible for converting folic acid to a chemically reduced form normally used in the biosynthesis of other molecules. This inhibition prevents the formation of folate, the reduced or anionic form of folic acid, which is needed for the synthesis of DNA and cell reproduction. The result is that DNA is not produced and the cell dies. In practice, the terms *folic acid* and *folate* are often used interchangeably. Pemetrexed disodium is a newer folate antagonist with a mechanism of action similar to that of methotrexate.

Purine Antagonism

The purine bases present in DNA and RNA are adenine and guanine (discussed further in Chapter 49), which are required for the synthesis of the purine nucleotides that are incorporated into the nucleic acid molecules.

Mercaptopurine and fludarabine are synthetic analogues of adenine, and thioguanine is a synthetic analogue of guanine. Cladribine is a more general purine antagonist. Cladribine is unique in that it actually lacks cell cycle specificity relative to other drugs in its class. It is included in this section because of its similar pharmacology and mechanism of action. All of these drugs work by ultimately interrupting the synthesis of both DNA and RNA. Although allopurinol and rasburicase are chemically similar to purines, they do not disrupt DNA synthesis, unlike the other drugs in this class. Instead, both work by reducing serum and urinary levels of *uric acid*. Uric acid is a common waste product that often accumulates in the blood following lysis of tumour cells, part of a condition known as **tumour lysis syndrome** (see Adverse Effects on p. 891).

Pyrimidine Antagonism

Of the pyrimidine bases, cytosine and thymine occur in the structure of DNA molecules, and cytosine and uracil are part of the structure of RNA molecules. These bases are essential for DNA and RNA synthesis. Fluorouracil is a synthetic analogue of uracil and cytarabine is a synthetic analogue of cytosine. Capecitabine is actually a prodrug of fluorouracil and is converted to that drug in the liver and other body tissues. Its prodrug form allows it to be given orally. Gemcitabine inhibits the action of two essential enzymes, *DNA polymerase* and *ribonucleotide reductase*. Overall, these drugs act in a way that is similar to that of the purine antagonists, incorporating themselves into the metabolic pathway for the synthesis of DNA and RNA and thereby interrupting synthesis of both of these nucleic acids.

Indications

Antimetabolite antineoplastic drugs are used for the treatment of a variety of solid tumours and some hematological cancers. They may also be used in combination chemotherapy regimens to enhance the overall cytotoxic effect. Methotrexate is also used to treat severe cases of psoriasis (a skin condition) as well as rheumatoid arthritis (Chapter 45). Because some of these drugs are available in both oral and topical preparations, they are sometimes used for low-dose maintenance and palliative cancer therapy. Allopurinol and rasburicase are both indicated for the hyperuricemia associated with tumour lysis syndrome and are usually given in anticipation of this condition during chemotherapy regimens associated with the syndrome. Allopurinol is also used commonly in oral form to treat gout (Chapter 45). Rasburicase is used for the treatment and prophylaxis of hyperuricemia in children and adult cancer patients. It is a recombinant urate-oxidase enzyme that oxidizes uric acid into an inactive and soluble metabolite (allantoin) that is easily excreted by the kidneys. The commonly used drugs and their common specific therapeutic uses are listed in the Dosages table on p. 894.

Adverse Effects

As with all antineoplastic drugs, antimetabolites cause hair loss, nausea, vomiting, diarrhea, and myelosuppression. The relative emetic potentials for some of these drugs are listed in Box 48-1. In addition, these and other antineoplastic drug classes are associated with other major types of toxicity, including neurological, cardiovascular, pulmonary, hepatobiliary, gastrointestinal, genitourinary, dermatological, ocular, otic, and metabolic toxicity. Manifestations of these toxicities are listed in Table 48-7, in order of increasing severity, and are described in general terms for each drug in Table 48-8.

Note that a single drug may not cause all of the specific symptoms that are listed for each toxicity category, and actual symptoms may vary widely in severity among individual patients. The most common general symptoms are fever and malaise. Metabolic toxicity also includes tumour lysis syndrome, a common post-chemotherapy condition. This syndrome is often associated with *induction* (initial) chemotherapy for rapidly growing malignancies. It may include hyperphosphatemia, hyperkalemia, and hypocalcemia. These electrolyte abnormalities are often treated with diuretics such as mannitol, intravenous calcium supplementation, oral or rectal potassium exchange resin (for hyperkalemia; Chapter 27), and oral aluminum hydroxide (for hyperphosphatemia; Chapter 52). Hyperuricemia can lead to nephropathy, and hemodialysis may be required in severe cases of tumour lysis syndrome.

A severe, but usually reversible, form of dermatological toxicity is known as *palmar-plantar dysesthesia* or *paresthesia* (also called *hand-foot syndrome*). It can range from mild symptoms such as painless swelling and erythema to painful blistering of the patient's palms

TABLE 48-7

Common Manifestations of Antineoplastic Toxicity

Type of Toxicity	Common Manifestations
Cardiovascular	Hot flushes, edema, thrombophlebitis and bleeding (e.g., near infusion site), chest pain, tachycardia, bradycardia, other dysrhythmias, angina, venous or arterial thrombosis, transient ischemic attacks, heart failure, myocardial ischemia, pericarditis, pericardial effusion, pulmonary embolism, aneurysm, cardiomyopathy, myocardial infarction, stroke, cardiac arrest, sudden cardiac death
Dermatological	Rash, erythema, pruritus, ecchymosis, dryness, edema, photosensitivity, sweating, discoloration (pigmentation changes), freckling, petechiae, purpura, numbness, tingling, hypersensitivity, fissuring, scaling, seborrhea, acne, eczema, psoriasis, skin hypertrophy, subcutaneous nodules, alopecia, nail disorder including onycholysis (loss of nails), dermatitis, cellulitis, excoriation, maceration, ulceration, urticaria, abscesses, benign skin neoplasm, hemorrhage (at injection site), palmar-plantar dysesthesia-paresthesia, toxic epidermal necrolysis, Stevens–Johnson syndrome
Gastrointestinal (GI)	Dyspepsia (heartburn), hiccups, gingivitis (inflamed gums), glossitis (inflamed tongue), abdominal pain, nausea, vomiting, diarrhea, constipation, gastroenteritis, stomatitis (painful mouth sores), oral candidiasis (thrush), ulcers, proctalgia (rectal pain), hematemesis, GI hemorrhage, melena (blood in stool), toxic intestinal dilation, ileus (bowel paralysis), ascites, necrotizing enterocolitis
Genitourinary	Oliguria, nocturia, dysuria, proteinuria, crystalluria, hematuria, urinary retention, abnormal kidney function test results, hemorrhagic cystitis, kidney failure
Hepatobiliary	Increased bilirubin and liver enzyme levels, jaundice, cholestasis, acalculic cholecystitis (inflamed gallbladder without stones), hepatitis, sclerosis, fibrosis, fatty liver changes, veno-occlusive liver disease, cirrhosis, hepatic coma
Metabolic	Weight loss or gain, anorexia, dehydration, hypokalemia, hypocalcemia, hypomagnesemia, hypertriglyceridemia, hyperglycemia, syndrome of inappropriate secretion of antidiuretic hormone, hypoadrenalism, protein-losing enteropathy, hyperuricemia, tumour lysis syndrome
Musculoskeletal	Back pain, limb pain, bone pain, myalgia, joint stiffness, arthralgia, muscle weakness, fibromyositis
Neurological	Fatigue, weakness, depression, agitation, euphoria, insomnia, sedation, headache, reduced libido, confusion, amnesia, hallucinations, dizziness, loss of taste or altered taste sensations, dysarthria (joint pain), polyneuropathy (e.g., numbness in extremities), neuritis, paresthesia (abnormal touch sensations), facial paralysis, migraine, tremor, hemiplegia, loss of consciousness, seizures, ataxia, stroke, encephalopathy
Ocular	Eye irritation, increased lacrimation, nystagmus, photophobia, visual changes, visual hallucinations, conjunctivitis, keratitis, dacryostenosis (narrowing of lacrimal duct)
Otic	Hearing loss, auditory hallucinations
Pulmonary–respiratory	Cough, rhinorrhea (runny nose), sore throat, sinusitis, bronchitis, pharyngitis, laryngitis, epistaxis (nosebleed), abnormal breath sounds, asthma, bronchospasms, atelectasis, pleural effusion, hemoptysis, hypoxia, respiratory distress, pneumothorax, diffuse interstitial pneumonitis, fibrosis, hemorrhage, anaphylaxis and generalized allergic reactions

TABLE 48-8

Selected Antimetabolites: Common Drug-Specific Adverse Effects

Antimetabolite Drug	Adverse Effects
capecitabine	Neurological, hepatobiliary, heart, GI, GU, ocular, musculoskeletal
cladribine	Neurological, GU, GI, dermatological, heart, pulmonary, musculoskeletal, metabolic
cytarabine	Liver, pulmonary, CV, GI, GU, neurological, ocular
fludarabine	Kidney and stomach
fluorouracil	GI, GU, liver, CV, neurological, ocular
gemcitabine	Neurological, pulmonary, GI, GU, CV, liver, dermatological
mercaptopurine	Liver, GI, GU
methotrexate	Liver, GI, CV, pulmonary, dermatological
thioguanine	Liver, GI

CV, cardiovascular; *GI*, gastrointestinal; *GU*, genitourinary.

and soles. Other severe, but fortunately uncommon, dermatological syndromes that can similarly affect the skin in more generalized regions include *Stevens–Johnson syndrome* and *toxic epidermal necrolysis*.

Interactions

As is true with cancer drugs in general, the administration of one antimetabolite drug with another that causes similar toxicities may result in additive toxicities. Therefore, the respective risks and benefits should be weighed carefully before therapy is initiated with either another antimetabolite or any other drug possessing a similar toxicity profile. Table 48-9 lists some known common examples of drugs that cause interactions with antimetabolites.

Dosages

For information on the dosages of selected antimetabolite chemotherapeutic drugs, see the Dosages table on p. 894.

TABLE 48-9

Selected Antimetabolites: Common Drug Interactions

Antimetabolite	Interacting Drug/Observed and Reported Effects*
capecitabine	leucovorin: potentiation of capecitabine with possible toxicity phenytoin: reduced phenytoin clearance and toxicity warfarin: altered coagulation test results with potential for fatal bleeding
cladribine	None listed
cytarabine	Aminoglycoside antibiotics: reduced antibiotic efficacy against *Klebsiella pneumoniae* infections digoxin: reduced absorption likely due to cytarabine-induced damage to intestinal mucosa; elixir form may be better absorbed
floxuridine	None listed
fludarabine	cytarabine: reduction of fludarabine metabolism, which reduces its antineoplastic effects pentostatin: potentially fatal pulmonary toxicity; do not use together
fluorouracil	warfarin: enhanced anticoagulant effects
gemcitabine	None listed
mercaptopurine (6-MP)	allopurinol: inhibition of 6-MP metabolism by inhibition of xanthine oxidase enzyme, with possible enhanced 6-MP toxicity Hepatotoxic drugs: increased risk of liver toxicity warfarin: 6-MP reported to both enhance and inhibit its effects
methotrexate (MTX)	folic acid: reduced MTX efficacy (theoretical only) Hepatotoxic drugs: increased risk of liver toxicity Live virus vaccines: viral infection (true for any immunosuppressive drug) penicillins, NSAIDs: possible reduced kidney elimination of MTX with potentially fatal hematological and GI toxicity Protein-bound drugs and weak organic acids (e.g., salicylates, sulfonamides, sulfonylureas, phenytoin, tetracyclines): possible displacement of MTX from protein-binding sites, enhancing its toxicity theophylline: reduced theophylline clearance
thioguanine	busulfan: reports of hepatotoxicity, esophageal varices, and portal hypertension Other cytotoxic drugs in general: reports of hepatotoxicity

GI, gastrointestinal; *NSAIDs*, nonsteroidal antiinflammatory drugs.

*Note that not all mechanisms of these drug interactions have been clearly identified. The information in this table is based on reported clinical observations, with mention of known or theorized mechanisms when available.

DRUG PROFILES

FOLATE ANTAGONISTS

▶▶ methotrexate

Methotrexate (Apo-Methotrexate) is the prototypical anti-metabolite antineoplastic of the folate antagonist group and is currently one of three antineoplastic folate antagonists used clinically. It has proved useful for the treatment of solid tumours such as breast, head and neck, as well as lung cancers and the management of acute lymphocytic leukemia and non-Hodgkin's lymphomas. Methotrexate also has immunosuppressive activity because it can inhibit lymphocyte multiplication. For this reason, it may be useful for the treatment of rheumatoid arthritis (Chapter 45). Its combined immunosuppressant and anti-inflammatory properties also make it useful for the treatment of psoriasis.

The bone marrow suppression associated with high-dose methotrexate (doses of more than 500 mg/m^2) is always tempered with "rescue" dosing of its antidote drug *leucovorin*. Methotrexate is available in both injectable and oral (tablet) forms. A preservative-free injectable formulation is required for **intrathecal** (spinal) administration, used in treatment of some cancers. One other folate antagonist is a newer drug called *pemetrexed disodium (Altima),* which has an action similar to that of methotrexate. However, it is much less widely used because of its limited indications for treatment of certain types of lung cancer.

raltitrexed disodium

Raltitrexed sodium (Tomudex) is a quinazoline folate analogue that selectively inhibits a key enzyme (thymidylate synthase) required for the synthesis of deoxyribonucleic acid (DNA), resulting in DNA fragmentation and cell death. It is actively transported into the cells via a reduced folate carrier and then extensively metabolized to polyglutamate forms without metabolic degradation. This particular property of raltitrexed facilitates a convenient dosing schedule of an infusion every 3 weeks. Raltitrexed is cell-cycle phase-specific for the S phase and is also a radiation-sensitizing agent. Raltitrexed is currently indicated for the treatment of advanced colorectal cancer.

PURINE ANTAGONISTS

The currently available purine antagonists are cladribine, fludarabine, mercaptopurine, and thioguanine. Of the four, mercaptopurine and thioguanine are administered orally. The other two are available only in injectable form. These drugs are not currently widely used because of their specific indications. Those not profiled in the following paragraph are listed in the Dosages table on p. 894 with their corresponding indications.

cladribine

Cladribine (Leustatin) is a newer drug first marketed in the early 1990s. It is indicated for the treatment of a specific type of leukemia known as *hairy-cell leukemia,* so named because of the appearance of its cancerous cells under the microscope.

fludarabine

Fludarabine (Fludara) was also approved by Health Canada in the early 1990s. As with cladribine, it also has a specific single indication, chronic lymphocytic leukemia.

PYRIMIDINE ANTAGONISTS

The currently available antimetabolite antineoplastics that are members of the pyrimidine antagonist family are capecitabine, cytarabine, fluorouracil, and gemcitabine. These drugs are used more commonly than the purine antagonists. They are available only in parenteral formulations, except for capecitabine, which is currently available only in tablet form. Dosage and other information appears in the Dosages table on p. 894.

capecitabine

Capecitabine (Xeloda) was approved by Health Canada in 2000. It is indicated primarily for the treatment of metastatic breast cancer and metastatic colorectal cancer.

▶▶ cytarabine

Cytarabine (Cytosar) is used primarily in the treatment of leukemias (acute myelocytic and lymphocytic and meningeal leukemia) and non-Hodgkin's lymphomas. As previously noted, it is available only in injectable form and may be administered intravenously, subcutaneously, or intrathecally. It is also now available in a special encapsulated liposomal form (Depocyt) for intrathecal use only in treating meningeal leukemia.

fluorouracil

Fluorouracil (5-FU) is used in a variety of treatment regimens, including the palliative treatment of cancers of the colon, rectum, stomach, breast, and pancreas.

gemcitabine hydrochloride

Gemcitabine hydrochloride (Gemzar) is an antineoplastic drug structurally related to cytarabine. Gemcitabine is believed to have antitumour activity superior to that of cytarabine. Gemcitabine was approved for marketing in 2001 by Health Canada. Approved indications include first-line therapy for locally advanced or metastatic cancer of the pancreas, for treatment of non–small cell lung cancer, and for advanced bladder cancer.

DOSAGES Selected Antimetabolites

Drug (Pregnancy Category)	Pharmacological Class	Usual Dosage Range*	Indications
allopurinol (Zyloprim, Alloprin) (C)	Purine antagonist analogue	IV: 200–400 mg/m²/day PO: 300–600 mg daily	Prevention of uric acid nephropathy during chemotherapy; gout
capecitabine (Xeloda) (D)	Pyrimidine antagonist (analogue)	PO: 1250 mg/m² bid for 2 wk, followed by 1-wk rest period; this 3-wk cycle repeatable as ordered	Metastatic colorectal and breast cancer
cladribine (Leustatin) (D)	Purine antagonist analogue	IV: 0.09 mg/kg/day by continuous infusion for 7 consecutive days	Hairy-cell leukemia
▸▸cytarabine (Cytosar) (D)	Pyrimidine antagonist (analogue)	IV: 100 mg/m²/day by continuous infusion × 7 days (other regimens as well)	Leukemias (several varieties), NHL
fludarabine (Fludara) (D)	Purine antagonist analogue	IV: 25 mg/m²/day for 5 consecutive days; repeatable every 28 days	Acute and chronic leukemias, NHL
fluorouracil (5-FU) (D)	Pyrimidine antagonist (analogue)	IV: 12 mg/kg once daily for 14 days initial dose; dose varies afterward depending on patient response	Colon, rectal, breast, esophageal, head and neck, cervical, and kidney cancer
gemcitabine hydrochloride (Gemzar) (D)	Pyrimidine antagonist (analogue)	IV: 1000 mg/m² once weekly or as protocol dictates; cycle may be repeated or modified according to patient tolerance	Pancreatic, non–small cell lung, and bladder cancer
▸▸methotrexate (Apo-Methotrexate, Metoject) (X)	Folate antagonist analogue	IV: 30–40 mg/m²/week PO: 15–30 mg/day 5 days, repeated every 7 days, 3–5 courses	Acute lymphocytic[†] leukemia; gestational choriocarcinoma; breast, head and neck, and many other cancers
pemetrexed (Alimta) (D)	Folate antagonist analogue	IV: 500–600 mg/m² on day 1 of each 21-day cycle	Malignant pleural mesothelioma, non–small cell lung cancer
raltitrexed disodium (Tomudex) (D)	Folate antagonist analogue	IV: 3 mg/m²/every 3 weeks	Advanced colorectal cancer
rasburicase (Fasturtec) (C)	Urocolytic agent	*Children/Adult* IV: 0.2 mg/kg over 30 min once daily for up to 7 days	Prevention and treatment of uric acid nephropathy during chemotherapy

IV, intravenous; *NHL*, non-Hodgkin's lymphoma; *PO*, oral.

*All dosages are for adults, unless indicated otherwise.

[†]The term *lymphocytic* is synonymous in the literature with the term *lymphoblastic*.

MITOTIC INHIBITORS

Mitotic inhibitors include natural products obtained from the periwinkle plant (*Catharenthus roseus,* formerly called *Vinca rosea*) and semisynthetic drugs obtained from the mandrake plant (also known as the *may apple*). The periwinkle plant contains antineoplastic alkaloids, including vinblastine, vincristine, and vinorelbine. They are known as *vinca alkaloids*. Etoposide and teniposide are semisynthetic derivatives of *epipodophyllotoxin*, which is obtained from the resinous extract of the mandrake plant. Two newer plant-derived drugs are the *taxanes.* These include paclitaxel, derived from the bark of the slow-growing Western (Pacific) yew tree, and docetaxel, a semisynthetic taxoid produced from the needles of the European yew tree. Docetaxel is pharmacologically similar to paclitaxel. The mitotic inhibitors and their plant sources can be summarized as follows:

Epipodophyllotoxin derivatives (mandrake plant)
- etoposide
- teniposide

Taxanes
- doxetaxel (European yew tree: needles)
- paclitaxel (Western yew tree: bark)

Vinca alkaloids (periwinkle)
- vinblastine
- vincristine
- vinorelbine

Dosage and other information appear in the Dosages table on page 896.

Mechanism of Action and Drug Effects

Depending on the particular drug, these plant-derived compounds can work in various phases of the cell cycle (late S phase, throughout G_2 phase, and M phase), but they all work shortly before or during mitosis and thus retard cell division. Each different subclass inhibits mitosis in a unique way.

The vinca alkaloids (vincristine, vinblastine, and vinorelbine) bind to the protein *tubulin* during the metaphase of mitosis (M phase). This action prevents the assembly of key structures called *microtubules,* which in turn results in the dissolution of other important structures, *mitotic spindles.* Without these mitotic spindles, cells cannot reproduce properly. The result is an inhibition of cell division and synthesis of DNA, RNA, and protein. The epipodophyllotoxin derivatives (etoposide and teniposide) exert their cytotoxic effects by inhibiting the enzyme *topoisomerase II,* which causes breaks in DNA strands. These drugs exert their effects during the late S phase and the G_2 phase of the cell cycle.

The yew tree derivatives (taxanes) paclitaxel and docetaxel both act in the late G_2 phase and M phase of the cell cycle. They bring about the formation of nonfunctional microtubules, which halts mitosis in metaphase.

Indications

Mitotic inhibitors are used to treat a variety of solid tumours and some hematological malignancies. They are often used in combination chemotherapy regimens to enhance the overall cytotoxic effect. The commonly administered drugs and some of their specific therapeutic uses are listed in the Dosages table on p. 896.

Adverse Effects

Like many of their antineoplastic counterparts in other classes, mitotic inhibitor antineoplastic drugs can cause hair loss, nausea and vomiting, and myelosuppression.

TABLE 48-10

Mitotic Inhibitors: Adverse Effects

Antibiotic Drug	Adverse Effects
docetaxel	Neurological, CV, GI, dermatological, musculoskeletal
etoposide	GI, CV, dermatological, neurological
paclitaxel	Neurological, CV, GI, GU, dermatological, musculoskeletal, liver, pulmonary, ocular
vincristine	Neurological, pulmonary, dermatological, CV, GI, otic, metabolic

CV, cardiovascular; *GI,* gastrointestinal; *GU,* genitourinary.

The emetic potential of some of the drugs is given in Box 48-1. Major adverse effects specific to these drugs are summarized in Table 48-10. (Review also the more general adverse effects of antineoplastic drugs in Table 48-7).

Toxicity: Management of Extravasation

Most of the mitotic inhibitor antineoplastics are administered intravenously, which makes extravasation of the drugs and its serious consequences a constant threat. Measures to be taken for the treatment of extravasation of the mitotic inhibitors are given in Table 48-11.

Interactions

A variety of drug interactions are possible with most antineoplastic drugs, some more significant than others. A few basic principles that apply to all antineoplastic drug classes should be kept in mind. When a drug interacts with warfarin, resulting in enhanced anticoagulation, this can generally be assumed to be due to the displacement of warfarin from its plasma protein-binding sites by the drug in question. Any drug that reduces the clearance of another drug also increases the risk of toxicity for the second drug. Also, because most antineoplastic drugs cause bone marrow depression, with increased risk of infection, it can usually be assumed that this risk is greater for patients receiving multiple antineoplastic drugs. Patients should be monitored and treated accordingly for hematological toxicity and infections. Observed drug interactions specific for mitotic inhibitor drugs are summarized in Table 48-12.

Dosages

For the recommended dosages of selected mitotic inhibitors, see the Dosages table on p. 896.

TABLE 48-11

Mitotic Inhibitor Extravasation

Mitotic Inhibitor Drug	Method
etoposide teniposide vinblastine vincristine	1. Elevate limb and apply gentle pressure to the site. 2. Apply *warm* compresses to the site for one hour.* Take care to avoid excessive heat that may cause more tissue injury. 3. The antidote hyaluronidase (Hyalase) is available through the Special Access Programme Canada (1500 units/mL: add 1 mL NaCl (1500 units/mL). It is given subcutaneously in a clockwise rotation around the site.

*Important: Corticosteroids and topical cooling appear to worsen toxicity.

TABLE 48-12

Selected Mitotic Inhibitors: Common Drug Interactions

Mitotic Inhibitor	Interacting Drug/Observed and Reported Effects*
docetaxel	CYP3A4 inducers (e.g., carbamazepine, nafcillin, phenytoin): reduced docetaxel effect
	CYP3A4 inhibitors (azole antifungals, ciprofloxacin, clarithromycin, imatinib, verapamil, many others): enhanced docetaxel effect (possible toxicity)
etoposide	cyclosporine: reduced etoposide clearance
	warfarin: enhanced anticoagulation
paclitaxel	azole antifungals: reduced paclitaxel clearance
	CNS depressants: enhanced sedation due to alcohol in paclitaxel formulation
vincristine	asparaginase: reduced vincristine clearance (give vincristine 12–24 hr before asparaginase)
	azole antifungals: increased risk of severe neuromuscular toxicity (consider reduction of vincristine dose during azole therapy)
	mitomycin: increased risk of pulmonary toxicity
	phenytoin: reduced phenytoin concentrations, enhancing seizure risk

CNS, central nervous system; *CYP3A4*, cytochrome P450 liver enzyme subtype 3A4.

*Note that not all mechanisms of these drug interactions have been clearly identified. The information in this table is based on reported clinical observations, with mention of known or theorized mechanisms when available.

DRUG PROFILES

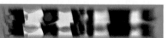

▸▸ *etoposide*

Etoposide (Etoposide Injection, VePesid) is a semisynthetic epipodophyllotoxin derivative. Its structure, mechanism of action, and adverse-effect profile are similar to those of teniposide. As previously noted, it is believed to kill cancer cells in the late S phase and the G_2 phase of the cell cycle. Etoposide is indicated for the treatment of small cell and non–small cell lung cancer, histiocytic lymphoma, and testicular cancer. It is available in oral and injectable forms.

▸▸ *paclitaxel*

Paclitaxel (Abraxane, Toxol) is a natural mitotic inhibitor obtained from the bark of the Pacific yew tree. The European yew tree is the source of another mitotic inhibitor, docetaxel (Taxotere). Paclitaxel is currently approved for the treatment of breast cancer, non–small cell lung

cancer, and Kaposi's sarcoma, among other cancers. Paclitaxel is extremely water insoluble (hydrophobic), thus it is put into a solution containing oil rather than water. The particular oil is a type of castor oil called *Cremophor EL,* the same oil with which cyclosporin is formulated. Many patients cannot tolerate this oil and show hypersensitivity responses similar to anaphylactic reactions. For this reason, before patients receive paclitaxel they may be premedicated with a steroid, antihistamine, and histamine-2 (H_2) antagonist (e.g., ranitidine). One formulation (Abraxane) does not require premedication. Paclitaxel is available only in injectable form.

▸▸ *vincristine*

Vincristine is an alkaloid isolated from the periwinkle plant and is indicated for the treatment of acute leukemia and other cancers. It is available only in a parenteral form.

DOSAGES   Selected Mitotic Inhibitors

Drug (Pregnancy Category)	Pharmacological Class	Usual Dosage Range*	Indications
EPIPODOPHYLLOTOXIN DERIVATIVE			
▸▸ etoposide (Etoposide Injection, VePesid) (D)	Topoisomerase II inhibitor	IV: 50–100 mg/m²/day for 5 days PO: 100–200 mg/m²/day for 5 days	Testicular, small cell and non–small cell lung cancer, histiocytic lymphoma
TAXANES			
docetaxel (Taxotere) (D)	Mitotic spindle inhibitor	IV: 75–100 mg/m² q3wk	Advanced breast, non–small cell lung, ovarian, and prostate cancer, squamous cell carcinoma of the head and neck
▸▸ paclitaxel (Abraxane, Toxol) (D)	Inhibitor of tubulin depolymerization	IV (Abraxane): 260 mg/m² q3wk) IV (Toxol): 175 mg/m² q3wk	Metastatic breast cancer Breast and lung cancer
VINCA ALKALOID			
▸▸ vincristine	Inhibitor of tubulin polymerization	*Children* IV: 2 mg/m² *Adult* IV: 1.4 mg/m² weekly	Acute leukemia

IV, intravenous; *PO*, oral.

*Note that dosages may vary widely among treatment protocols. Unless otherwise indicated, all dosages are for adults.

TOPOISOMERASE I INHIBITORS (CAMPTOTHECINS)

Topoisomerase I inhibitors are a relatively new class of chemotherapy drugs. The two drugs currently available in this class are topotecan and irinotecan. Both are semisynthetic analogues of the compound camptothecin, which was originally isolated in the 1960s from *Camptotheca acuminata*, a Chinese shrub. For this reason, they are also referred to as *camptothecins*.

Mechanism of Action and Drug Effects

The Chinese shrub–derived camptothecins inhibit DNA function in the S phase by binding to the DNA–topoisomerase I complex. This complex normally allows DNA strands to be temporarily cleaved and then reattached in a critical step known as *religation*. The binding of the camptothecin drugs to this complex retards the religation process.

Indications

The two currently available topoisomerase I inhibitors are used primarily to treat ovarian and colorectal cancers. Topotecan has been shown to be effective in metastatic cases of ovarian cancer that have failed to respond to platinum-containing regimens (i.e., cisplatin, carboplatin) and paclitaxel. Topotecan is also sometimes used to treat small-cell lung cancer. Irinotecan is currently approved for the treatment of metastatic colorectal cancer, small-cell lung cancer, and cervical cancer.

Adverse Effects

As with many cancer chemotherapeutic drugs, the main adverse effect of topotecan is suppression of blood cell production in the bone marrow. This bone marrow suppression is predictable, noncumulative, reversible, and manageable. Topotecan should not be given to patients with baseline neutrophil counts of less than 1.5×10^9/L. Other adverse effects are relatively minor compared with those of the other antineoplastic drug classes. These effects include mild to moderate nausea, vomiting, and diarrhea, headache, rash, muscle weakness, and cough.

Irinotecan causes more severe adverse effects than those of topotecan. In addition to producing similar hematological adverse effects, it has been associated with severe diarrhea, known as *cholinergic diarrhea*, which may occur during irinotecan infusion. It is recommended that this condition be treated with atropine unless use of this drug is strongly contraindicated. Delayed diarrhea may occur 2 to 10 days after infusion of irinotecan. This diarrhea can be severe and even life threatening. Delayed diarrhea should be treated aggressively with loperamide. Severe cardiovascular toxicity, including thrombosis, pulmonary embolism, stroke, and acute fatal myocardial infarction, has been reported during irinotecan therapy. Such effects have been seen particularly when irinotecan is given with intravenous fluorouracil and leucovorin. These drug combinations should be given with careful monitoring or avoided whenever possible. Severe nausea and vomiting are also seen with irinotecan, requiring appropriate supportive care such as intravenous rehydration and antiemetic drug therapy.

Interactions

The *granulocyte colony-stimulating factor* filgrastim (Chapter 50), used to enhance WBC recovery after chemotherapy, has actually been shown to worsen myelosuppression when given concurrently with topotecan. It is recommended that filgrastim be administered 24 hours after completion of the topotecan infusion. Laxatives and diuretics should not be given concomitantly with irinotecan because of the potential to worsen the dehydration resulting from the severe diarrhea that this drug can produce. Several additional recognized drug interactions occur with irinotecan, which are summarized in Table 48-13.

Dosages

For recommended dosages of selected topoisomerase I inhibitors, see the Dosages table on p. 898.

TABLE 48-13

Irinotecan: Common Drug Interactions

Interacting Drug	Observed and Reported Effects*
CYP2B6 inducers (e.g., carbamazepine, phenytoin, nevirapine)	Reduced effects of irinotecan
CYP2B6 inhibitors (e.g., paroxetine, sertraline)	Increased effects and toxicity of irinotecan
CYP3A4 inducers (e.g., aminoglutethimide, carbamazepine, nafcillin, nevirapine, phenytoin)	Reduced effects of irinotecan
CYP3A4 inhibitors (e.g., azole antifungals, ciprofloxacin, clarithromycin, imatinib, isoniazid, verapamil)	Increased effects and toxicity of irinotecan; concurrent use not recommended
St. John's wort	Reduced effects of irinotecan; stop St. John's wort 2 wk before initiating irinotecan therapy

CYP2B6, cytochrome P450 liver enzyme subtype 2B6; *CYP3A4*, cytochrome P450 subtype 3A4.

*Note that not all mechanisms of these drug interactions have been clearly identified. The information in this table is based on reported clinical observations, with mention of known or theorized mechanisms when available.

DRUG PROFILES

SELECTED TOPOISOMERASE I INHIBITORS
irinotecan hydrochloride

Irinotecan hydrochloride (Camptosar) is usually given with both fluorouracil and leucovorin. It is available only in injectable form.

topotecan hydrochloride

After initial therapy with other antineoplastics, cancer cells commonly become resistant to their effects. The use of topotecan hydrochloride (Hycamtin) to treat ovarian cancer and small-cell lung cancer has been extensively studied. As noted earlier, it produces therapeutic responses even in cases in which powerful drugs such as cisplatin and paclitaxel have failed. It is available only in injectable form.

DOSAGES **Selected Topoisomerase I Inhibitors**

Drug (Pregnancy Category)	Pharmacological Class	Usual Dosage Range*	Indications
irinotecan hydrochloride (Camptosar) (D)	Synthetic camptothecin	IV: 125 mg/m² on days 1, 8, 15, 22 (many other complex regimens are used as well)	Metastatic colorectal cancer
topotecan hydrochloride (Hycamtin) (D)	Semisynthetic camptothecin	IV: 1.5 mg/m² once daily for 5 consecutive days on a repeatable 21-day course	Ovarian and small-cell lung cancer

*Dosages listed are for adults.

ANTINEOPLASTIC ENZYMES

One antineoplastic enzyme, *Escherichia coli*–based asparaginase, is currently commercially available. Two others, pegaspargase and *Erwinia* asparaginase, are available only by special request through the Health Canada Special Access Programme. *Erwinia* asparaginase is available for patients who have developed allergic reactions to *E. coli*–based asparaginase, described in the following drug profile. All three drugs are synthesized from cultures of certain bacteria using recombinant DNA technology. Specifically, a critical segment of DNA that contains the genes for producing the enzyme is inserted into the genetic material of the bacteria, which then mass-produce the enzyme as the bacteria multiply in culture. The enzyme is then isolated from this culture using laboratory techniques and purified for clinical use.

Indications

The antineoplastic enzymes are currently approved exclusively for the treatment of acute lymphocytic leukemia.

Adverse Effects

Of particular note for the antineoplastic enzymes is a fairly unique adverse effect of impaired pancreatic function. This can lead to hyperglycemia and severe or fatal pancreatitis. Other types of adverse effects associated with these drugs are dermatological, liver, genitourinary, neurological, musculoskeletal, gastrointestinal, and cardiovascular effects.

Interactions

Commonly reported drug interactions involving the antineoplastic enzymes are summarized in Table 48-14.

Dosages

Dosages for the antineoplastic enzymes are given in the Dosages table on p. 899.

TABLE **48-14**

Selected Antineoplastic Enzymes: Common Drug Interactions

Enzyme	Interacting Drug/Observed and Reported Effects*
asparaginase	cyclophosphamide, mercaptopurine, vincristine: interference with efficacy or clearance
	mercaptopurine, methotrexate, prednisone: enhanced liver toxicity
	methotrexate: reduced antineoplastic effect when given concurrently, but possibly enhanced antineoplastic effect when given 9–10 days before or shortly after methotrexate
	prednisone: hyperglycemia (give asparaginase after prednisone)
	vincristine: neuropathy (give asparaginase after vincristine)
pegaspargase	Same as above, plus the following: aspirin, other NSAIDs, dipyridamole, heparin, warfarin: coagulation factor imbalances
	cyclophosphamide: reduced clearance of cyclophosphamide

NSAIDs, nonsteroidal anti-inflammatory drugs.

*Note that not all mechanisms of these drug interactions have been clearly identified. The information in this table is based on reported clinical observations, with mention of known or theorized mechanisms when available.

DRUG PROFILES

▸▸ *asparaginase*

Asparaginase (Kidrolase) is used to induce remissions in acute lymphoblastic leukemia. Its mechanism of action is slightly different from that of traditional antineoplastics in that it is an enzyme that catalyzes the conversion of the amino acid asparagine to aspartic acid and ammonia. Leukemic cells are then unable to synthesize the asparagine required for synthesis of DNA and proteins needed for cell survival.

The only commercially available asparaginase product in Canada is the Kidrolase INJ PWS product manufactured by OPI S.A. in France. This product is derived from the *E. coli* bacterium, and it is common for patients to develop allergic reactions to it. When this occurs, one alternative is to use the asparaginase synthesized from the *Erwinia* bacteria. This product is not commercially available in Canada; however, it is available by special request from the Health Canada Special Access Programme. Another treatment alternative is pegaspargase, also available only

through the Special Access Programme. All antineoplastic enzymes are available only in injectable form.

pegaspargase

Pegaspargase (Oncaspar) has a mechanism of action, indications, and contraindications similar to those of asparaginase. It is essentially the same enzyme that has been formulated so as to reduce its allergenic potential. This process involves chemical conjugation of the enzyme with units of a relatively inert compound known as monomethoxypolyethylene glycol. Because polyethylene glycol is abbreviated PEG, this process is known as *pegylation*. It is a relatively new process that is increasingly used in formulating other drugs described in other chapters (e.g., Chapter 50). These drugs are recognized by the prefix *peg* in their generic names. Pegaspargase is usually prescribed for patients who have developed an allergy to asparaginase, a common occurrence, especially with repeated treatment.

DOSAGES   Selected Antineoplastic Enzymes

Drug (Pregnancy Category)	Pharmacological Class	Usual Dosage Range*	Indications
▸▸ **asparaginase (Kidrolase) (C)**	*Escherichia coli*–derived L-asparagine amidohydrolase enzyme	IM/IV: 200–1000 units/kg/day for 28 successive days, may continue for an additional 14 days if remission not induced	Acute lymphoblastic leukemia
pegaspargase (Oncaspar) (C)	Pegylated version of asparaginase	IV/IM: 2500 units/m² q14d	Acute lymphocytic leukemia (usually in patients who have developed an allergy to asparaginase)

IM, intramuscular; *IV*, intravenous.

*All dosages listed are for adults.

NURSING PROCESS

▨ Assessment

A patient should undergo thorough assessment before any antineoplastic drug is administered. The assessment should include taking a complete and thorough nursing history; performing a head-to-toe physical examination; measuring height, weight, and vital signs; testing hearing and vision; taking a complete medical history and family history; and noting any food and drug allergies. A complete assessment of ethnocultural, emotional, spiritual, sexual, and financial influences, concerns, or issues should also be carried out. Ability to perform the activities of daily living is important to consider, as are mobility and gait patterns. Bowel and bladder patterns, neurological status, heart sounds, heart rhythm, and breath sounds and lung function should also be assessed. In examining the skin and mucosa, the nurse should note turgor,

hydration, colour, and temperature. Signs and symptoms of fear and anxiety should also be noted with attention to communication of feelings, insomnia, irritability, shakiness, restlessness, palpitations, and any unusual problems that could be attributed to stress and anxiety.

Contraindications, cautions, drug interactions, and drug allergies should be assessed for and documented prior to use of any antineoplastic drug. A number of laboratory tests are usually ordered as well and need to be reviewed. These tests may include complete blood counts, platelet counts, and bleeding times, as well as liver, kidney, and heart function tests and pulmonary function tests. In addition, measurement of tumour markers and related blood work may be ordered to help monitor baseline levels and determine the impact of the disease on the patient, confirm the diagnosis, and help determine the patient's response to different drug therapies. Further discussion of laboratory studies specific to antineoplastic therapy is provided in Lab Values Related to Drug Therapy: Antineoplastic Therapy. Another area of importance is information regarding the specific antineoplastic drug(s) being used for the treatment protocol and the nurse's responsibility in implementing the protocol. Many of the adverse effects and toxic effects associated with antineoplastic drugs are attributed to the killing of not only rapidly dividing malignant cells but also normal cells. See Box 48-3 for more information about the specific adverse effects associated with destruction of populations of normal cells.

Areas of assessment related to some of the more common effects of antineoplastic therapy on normal, rapidly dividing cells include the following:

- For *altered nutritional status* and *impaired oral mucosa*: Assess for signs and symptoms of altered nutrition with a focus on weight loss, abnormal serum protein-albumin and blood urea nitrogen levels (negative nitrogen status due to low protein levels is indicated by a decreasing blood urea nitrogen level), weakness, fatigue, lethargy, poor skin turgor, and pale conjunctiva. Assess oral mucosa for signs and symptoms of *stomatitis,* such as pain or burning in the mouth, difficulty swallowing, taste changes, viscous saliva, dryness, cracking, and fissures with or without bleeding of mucosa.
- For *effects on the gastrointestinal mucosa*: Assess for signs and symptoms of *diarrhea,* such as frequent, loose stools (more than three stools per day), urgency, abdominal cramping, and hyperactive bowel sounds, and obtain information about the presence of blood, consistency, colour, odour, and amount of stool. Assess for *nausea and vomiting* and determine whether symptoms are acute, delayed, or anticipatory; if vomiting occurs, determine the colour, amount, consistency, frequency, and odour and whether blood is present. The severity of nausea and vomiting may be rated using a scale of 1 to 10 (where 10 is the worst) or using the terms *mild, moderate,* and *severe.*
- For *alopecia*: Consider the patient's views, concerns, and emotions about potential hair loss. Assess the patient's need to prepare for hair loss: the patient may leave the hair as it is and allow it to fall out on its own; have the hair cut short; wear a scarf, hat, bandanna, or hair wrap; or purchase a wig and have it styled before the hair is actually lost so that the hairstyle is similar to that before chemotherapy.
- For *bone marrow suppression*: Assess for signs and symptoms of *anemia* (decrease in RBC, hemoglobin, and hematocrit), such as pallor of skin, oral mucous membranes, and conjunctiva; fatigue; loss of interest in activities; shortness of breath and other intolerance

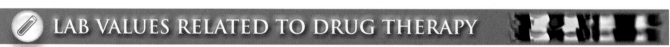

🔬 LAB VALUES RELATED TO DRUG THERAPY

Antineoplastic Therapy: Rationales for Assessment and Monitoring of Blood Cell Counts

Because antineoplastics kill both normal and abnormal rapidly dividing cells, the bone marrow and its rapidly dividing cellular constituents are negatively affected. Given this characteristic of chemotherapeutic drugs, red blood cells (RBCs), white blood cells (WBCs), and platelets are suppressed and thus require frequent monitoring. Presented here is information specifically on RBCs and subsequent hemoglobin (Hgb) and hematocrit (Hct) levels as well as platelet levels. Chapter 49 presents more information on WBCs, including neutrophil counts and nadir levels.

Laboratory Test	Normal Ranges	Rationale for Assessment
Hct	M: 0.4%–0.5% F: 0.38%–0.47%	Hct measures the amount of space or volume of RBCs in the blood; if the RBC value is low, the Hct is also low. The impact of this low value is discussed in the section on RBCs (see below).
Hgb	M: 135–180 g/L F: 120–160 g/L	Hgb is the major substance in RBCs, carries oxygen, and is responsible for the blood cell colour of red. With low levels of Hgb, the consequence to the patient is the same as that noted with RBCs.
Platelets	$150–400 \times 10^9$/L	Platelets are the smallest type of blood cell and play a large role in the process of blood coagulation and clotting. When bleeding occurs, the platelets swell, clump, and form a plug that helps stop the bleeding. Therefore, if platelet levels drop to 10×10^9/L, the patient is at high risk for uncontrolled bleeding or hemorrhage.
RBCs	M: $4.5–6 \times 10^{12}$/L F: $4.2–5.4 \times 10^{12}$/L	Bone marrow suppression from antineoplastics also affects RBC values, leading to severe anemia. Red blood cells carry oxygen from the lungs, with oxygen attached to the Hgb, to the rest of the body. RBCs also help carry carbon dioxide back to the lungs for it to be exhaled. Therefore, if RBC counts are low (e.g., with anemia), the body does not receive sufficient oxygen, leading to lack of energy, fatigue, intolerance for activity, shortness of breath, and hypoxemia. For the cancer patient who may already be experiencing the impact of bone marrow suppression from either the disease or the treatment, this loss of oxygen may be exacerbated, producing even more of an impact on the patient. The ability to get up and about and perform activities of daily living may be decreased, and the patient may even lose the ability to eat meals and visit with family and friends.

F, female; *M,* male.

BOX 48-3   Effects of Antineoplastic Drugs on Normal Cells and Related Adverse Effects

Antineoplastic drugs are designed to kill rapidly dividing *cancer* cells, but they also kill rapidly dividing *normal* cells. Such normal cells include cells of the oral and gastrointestinal mucous membranes, hair follicles, reproductive germinal epithelium, and components of bone marrow (e.g., white blood cells [WBCs], red blood cells [RBCs], and platelets). The more common adverse effects of normal cell kill are as follows:

- Killing of normal cells of the gastrointestinal mucous membranes may result in adverse effects such as *altered nutritional status*, *stomatitis* with inflammation and ulcerations of the oral mucosa and throughout the gastrointestinal tract, *altered bowel function*, *poor appetite*, *nausea*, *vomiting* (often intractable and requiring aggressive antiemetics treatment), and *diarrhea*.

- Killing of the normal cells of hair follicles leads to *alopecia* (loss of hair).

- Killing of normal cells in the bone marrow results in dangerously low (life-threatening) blood cell counts. Because of the negative impact on these normal cells, the nurse must carefully assess the patient's WBC counts (leukocytes, neutrophils, and band neutrophils), RBC counts, hemoglobin level, hematocrit, and platelet (thrombocyte) counts (see Lab Values Related to Drug Therapy on p. 900 in this chapter and on p. 925 in Chapter 49, for discussion of *anemia, leukopenia*, and *neutropenia*, and of *thrombocytopenia* [a low platelet count]). In addition, monitoring of the patient's absolute neutrophil count (ANC) is needed (ANC is the WBC count multiplied by the percentage of neutrophils). By following the ANC values, the nurse and other health care providers can identify the nadir (see Lab Values Related to Drug Therapy on p. 925 in Chapter 49)—the time of the lowest count when the patient is most vulnerable. An ANC of 1×10^9/L or below indicates severely impaired immune function and high risk for immunosuppression and infection.

- Killing of germinal epithelial cells (also rapidly dividing) leads to *sterility* (irreversible) in males and to *teratogenic* effects with possible fetal death, as well as damage to the ovaries with *amenorrhea* in females.

---

of activity; lethargy; and an inability to concentrate (see Lab Values Related to Drug Therapy on p. 900 in this chapter). Assess for signs and symptoms of *leukopenia* or *neutropenia* (decrease in WBC and an absolute neutrophils count below 1×10^9/L), including fever; chills; tachycardia; abnormal breath sounds; productive cough with purulent, green, or rust-coloured sputum; change in colour of urine; lethargy or fatigue; and acute confusion. (For more information, see Lab Values Related to Drug Therapy on p. 925 in Chapter 49). Assess for signs and symptoms of *thrombocytopenia* (decrease in thrombocyte or platelet counts and abnormal clotting test results), including indications of unusual bleeding such as petechiae, purpura, ecchymosis, gingival (gum) bleeding, excessive or prolonged bleeding from puncture sites (e.g., intramuscular or intravenous sites or laboratory draw sites), unusual joint pain, or blood in stool, urine, or vomitus; and a decrease in blood pressure with elevated pulse rate (see Lab Values Related to Drug Therapy on p. 900 in this chapter and on p. 541 in Chapter 28).

- For possible *sterility, teratogenesis*, damage to ovaries with *amenorrhea*: For the adult male patient, assess baseline reproductive history with attention to sexual functioning, fathering of children, and past and current reproductive or sexual problems or concerns. For the female adult patient, inquire about reproductive history with attention to sexual functioning, fertility, childbearing history, menstrual history with focus on menstrual irregularities, and age at the onset of menses and menopause, if applicable.

Assessing for *pain* is also an important part of the care of patients with cancer. Patient reports of oral, pharyngeal, esophageal, or abdominal pain; painful swallowing; epigastric or gastric pain, especially after eating spicy or acidic foods; achiness in joints or lower extremities; and numbness, tingling, and any burning or sharp pain that is general or localized need to be noted and addressed. Pain should be assessed using an intensity rating scale (e.g., 0 to 10 with 0 = no pain and 10 = worse pain ever). The pattern of pain should also be noted, with a focus on the location, quality, onset, duration, and precipitating or alleviating factors. The nurse should inquire about past experiences with pain and any drug, nondrug, or alternative therapies used and successes or failures with its treatment. Ethnocultural beliefs and background as they relate to pain are important to assess because the individual's ethnoculture may affect how pain is perceived, communicated, and treated (Chapter 11).

With *cell cycle–specific drugs*, once allergies, cautions, contraindications, and drug interactions have been documented, a baseline assessment of the patient's general health status is an important starting point in development of a plan of care. A thorough baseline and physical assessment should include weight, height, vital signs, and pain assessment, as well as a complete nursing history with attention to the liver, kidney, and gastrointestinal, male and female genitourinary, cardiac, and respiratory systems. Laboratory testing associated with these systems (e.g., uric acid level, complete blood cell counts, platelets, RBCs, hemoglobin/hematocrit, fluid/electrolyte levels, clotting studies) is generally performed before, during, and after chemotherapy (see Lab Values

Related to Drug Therapy on p. 900 in this chapter and on p. 541 in Chapter 28). For antimetabolites, most of the drugs do not produce severe emesis (i.e., in fewer than 10% of cases); however, some of the pyrimidine analogues have emetic potential and thus require assessment of baseline gastrointestinal functioning. Folate antagonists are not as likely to cause emesis but may be associated with gastrointestinal abnormalities (e.g., peptic ulcer disease, ulcerative colitis, stomatitis), and genitourinary abnormalities requiring baseline assessment of bowel patterns, bowel sounds, and bladder patterns. Because these drugs are generally administered parenterally (intravenously), assessment of peripheral access areas or central venous sites is critical to prevent possible damage to surrounding tissue, joints, and tendons.

Specific assessment features associated with use of the antimetabolite cytarabine include monitoring for the occurrence of *cytarabine syndrome*. This syndrome occurs usually within 6 to 12 hours after drug administration and is characterized by fever, myalgia, bone pain, nausea, vomiting, occasional chest pain, and rash. In addition, a thorough assessment of heart and breath sounds, with a complete nursing assessment of cardiac and respiratory systems, is warranted with the use of cytarabine (as well as other antimetabolites) because it may cause cardiac or pulmonary toxicity.

Patients receiving *mitotic inhibitors* (e.g., vinblastine, vincristine, etoposide) should undergo thorough assessment for baseline fluid and electrolyte levels and blood counts (see Lab Values Related to Drug Therapy on p. 900 in this chapter and on p. 925 in Chapter 49). Liver and kidney toxicities are a concern, so liver and kidney function studies should be performed frequently. Because serum uric acid levels generally increase with cell death (related to the therapeutic effects as well as adverse effects of these drugs), the patient should be observed for first-time appearance of gout or exacerbation of existing gout once therapy is initiated. Bowel and bladder patterns should be noted, and baseline neurological functioning should be assessed with attention to muscle tone and reflexes. Because these drugs have multiple incompatibilities and are either irritants (irritating the intravenous site and vein) or vesicants (causing cell death with extravasation and necrosis with ulcerations), the nurse should know all potential solution and drug interactions and should document initial and follow-up assessments of the intravenous site.

Other mitotic inhibitors, docetaxel and paclitaxel, are drugs in the *taxane* family and are also associated with severe neutropenia (see Lab Values Related to Drug Therapy on p. 925 in Chapter 49); thus, blood counts must be performed before drug therapy. The patient should be assessed for severe hypersensitivity reactions—characterized by dyspnea, severe hypotension, angioedema, and generalized urticaria—during treatments and in the home setting. Results of all blood cell counts should also be examined. The nurse should be alert to the smallest clues to a hypersensitivity reaction, which may indicate the potential for severe reactions. Platelet and neutrophil levels are of most concern with these drugs, thus close examination of baseline levels and assessment for a decrease in these levels with therapy are important. Drops in these blood cell counts may occur before there is any clinical evidence of the actual anemia or other blood-related adverse effect. Because peripheral neuropathies may occur, any abnormal sensations in the extremities or other abnormalities that are present before treatment need to be noted.

Topoisomerase inhibitors are associated with hematological adverse effects, thus baseline WBC counts need to be performed. Specifically, topotecan may produce severe neutropenia due to bone marrow suppression. This bone marrow suppression is predictable, noncumulative, reversible, and manageable, so topotecan should not be given to patients with baseline neutrophil counts of less than $1.5 \times 10^9/L$. Assessment of gastrointestinal functioning and bowel patterns is important with these drugs because of the related adverse effects of mild to moderate nausea, vomiting, and diarrhea. Irinotecan causes more severe adverse effects than does topotecan, thus related systems should be assessed and findings noted. During irinotecan infusion, *cholinergic diarrhea* may occur, so it needs to be watched for. This diarrhea may also occur 2 to 10 days after the irinotecan infusion and may require further medical treatment, especially with severe forms of diarrhea. Severe cardiovascular toxicity, thrombosis, pulmonary embolism, stroke, and acute fatal myocardial infarction are related adverse effects and require astute assessment of related systems. These adverse effects have been seen particularly when irinotecan is given with intravenous fluorouracil and leucovorin. Such drug combinations should be given with careful monitoring or avoided whenever possible. Severe nausea and vomiting is also seen with irinotecan and should be assessed for and documented, as appropriate.

Patients being given *natural enzyme* drugs (e.g., asparaginase, pegaspargase) require assessment for allergies and gout. The results of complete blood counts and kidney and liver function tests need to be examined because of the associated damage to these systems. The nurse should also determine whether the patient has a history or concurrent outbreak of chicken pox or herpes zoster because the virus can become active and create problems for the patient. Any recent cytotoxic treatment or radiation therapy should be noted because of the potential for worsening of adverse effects and toxicity. Baseline neurological functioning should be assessed, with a focus on any history of seizures; the presence of numbness or tingling in the extremities, nervousness, irritability, or confusion; and evaluation of level of mobility, muscle strength, and gait. As with any drug therapy, measurement of vital signs is an important aspect of assessment with these drugs. In particular, hyperthermia may be an adverse effect, so temperature should be measured and checked frequently. Because of the risk of pancreatitis, patients should be assessed for moderate to severe abdominal pain, which often occurs in the left quadrant, and for nausea and vomiting. Coagulopathies may also occur, so baseline blood cell counts need to be performed and documented (see Lab Values Related to Drug Therapy on p. 900 in this chapter and on p. 541 in Chapter 28). It is also important to assess for high serum ammonia levels and complaints of headache.

Ethnocultural assessment should be thorough and the results respected by everyone involved in the care of the cancer patient because members of different ethnocultural groups have different interpretations of health, illness, and pain. They may talk about illnesses and convey symptoms in different ways and may even differ in how they respond to a given drug. Cancer and its treatment may affect the patient's body image, coping mechanisms, and emotional status, so the nurse must constantly assess mental health status and support systems and remain alert to clues that the patient may need more support before, during, and after chemotherapy. Genetic considerations are an additional area of importance in the treatment of cancer with antineoplastics as well as with all drug therapy. Individuals should be assessed for the presence of the following characteristics before chemotherapy is initiated: (1) genetic markers for oral cancers, (2) genetic determinants of testosterone or estrogen metabolism, and (3) genetically linked enzyme system abnormalities, such as those involving specific cytochrome P450 enzymes that metabolically convert nicotine to a carcinogenic substance. These genetic factors are very complex; nevertheless, the nurse should be aware of the possible influence of genetic differences and should look to those involved in drug research and administration for additional information.

Nursing Diagnoses

- Activity intolerance related to drug-induced anemia with fatigue and lethargy caused by cell cycle–specific and related antineoplastic drugs
- Anxiety and ineffective coping related to the unknowns of therapy and cancer illness and the fear of death
- Disturbed body image related to drug-induced alopecia, darkening of skin, and sexual dysfunctioning
- Constipation related to the adverse effects of antineoplastic drugs
- Diarrhea related to the adverse effects of antineoplastic drugs
- Risk for infection related to drug-induced bone marrow suppression with possible leukopenia and neutropenia.
- Imbalanced nutrition, less than body requirements, related to loss of appetite, nausea, vomiting, stomatitis, and changes in taste as a result of antineoplastic therapy
- Impaired oral mucous membranes related to the adverse effects of stomatitis, leukopenia, and neutropenia
- Nausea (and vomiting) related to the adverse effects of antineoplastic therapy
- Acute pain related to the disease process and drug-induced joint pain, stomatitis, nausea and vomiting,

and other discomforts associated with antineoplastic cell cycle–specific therapy (e.g., neuropathies)
- Impaired physical mobility related to drug-induced anemia and fatigue
- Disturbed self-concept related to the adverse effects of alopecia, muscle wasting, weight loss, amenorrhea, and other physical changes caused by antineoplastic therapy

Planning

Goals

- Patient will maintain levels of activity and mobility, as tolerated and without major muscle mass loss, during drug treatment.
- Patient will remain calm and comfortable without moderate or severe anxiety during therapy.
- Patient will maintain an intact and healthy body image and effective coping mechanisms while experiencing alopecia, skin changes, and sexual dysfunction associated with antineoplastic drugs.
- Patient will experience minimal problems from oral and gastrointestinal adverse effects, specifically stomatitis, constipation, diarrhea, nausea, and vomiting, while taking antineoplastic drugs.
- Patient will experience minimal risks for infection as well as minimal breaks in skin integrity and oral mucous membranes (possibly due to the occurrence of stomatitis) while receiving antineoplastic drugs.
- Patient will remain safe and free from injury with minimal neurological, sensory, and motor deficits due to the adverse effects of antineoplastic drugs.
- Patient's nutritional status will return to normal during the recovery period and after completion of the antineoplastic protocol.
- Patient will regain normal urinary patterns during and after antineoplastic therapy.

Outcome Criteria

- Patient states measures to maximize activity levels and mobility, such as conserving energy with planned activities, seeking assistance, and maintaining range of motion daily.
- Patient uses nonpharmacological, complementary, and alternative therapies (e.g., relaxation, music therapy, pet therapy, biofeedback, massage, therapeutic touch, diversion) as well as prescribed drug therapy to control pain and discomfort related to the adverse effects of antineoplastic drugs or the disease process itself.
- Patient states measures to enhance levels of comfort during drug therapy, such as managing pain; taking antiemetics as prescribed; keeping skin clean, dry, and moist; and maintaining range of motion daily.
- Patient openly expresses any anxieties, fears, concerns, or feelings of being upset or of depression about changes in body image and self-concept to help in coping.

- Patient states measures to assist in maintaining healthy breathing and respiratory patterns as well as measures to prevent respiratory infections, such as deep breathing exercises, frequent hand washing, forcing of fluids, consumption of a well-balanced diet, avoidance of malls and other crowded places, and avoidance of persons with colds, flu, or communicable respiratory illnesses while undergoing chemotherapy.
- Patient states and demonstrates ways to minimize oral mucosal breakdown, such as performing frequent mouth care and dental hygiene measures using mild toothpaste, gentle sponge-type toothettes, and non–alcohol-based mouthwash, and taking fluid frequently while undergoing drug therapy.
- Patient demonstrates the use of measures to enhance skin integrity while undergoing antineoplastic therapy, such as keeping skin clean, dry, and lubricated.
- Patient understands the importance of daily measures to help minimize the risk of injury related to the adverse effects of bone marrow suppression, such as avoiding crowds, monitoring temperature daily or as needed, not using straight razors, and avoiding venipuncture and injections, if possible.
- Patient uses nonpharmacological methods (e.g., consumption of a well-balanced diet with fibre and roughage as allotted, intake of fluids, exercise) and pharmacological methods (e.g., use of stool softeners or bulk-forming laxatives) to regain or maintain normal or prechemotherapy bowel elimination patterns.
- Patient adheres to daily regimen for increasing urinary health, such as forcing fluids, consuming fluids that minimize urinary infections (e.g., cranberry juice), and maintaining daily hydration while undergoing antineoplastic therapy.
- Patient states ways to minimize risk for injury from neurological adverse effects of chemotherapy by establishing a safety plan that includes removal of throw rugs or furniture that may lead to falls, use of assistive devices such as a walker or cane, having a bedside commode, use of night lights, and instituting other measures to ease mobility.

Note that the nursing diagnoses, goals, and outcome criteria presented here are appropriate to treatment with many antineoplastic drugs as well as to treatment with the cell cycle–specific and other drugs discussed in this chapter.

Implementation

Antineoplastic drugs are some of the most toxic medications given to patients. Because of their toxicity, serious complications and adverse effects may occur. With the possibility of such adverse effects and toxicities, astute nursing care must be based on critical thinking and careful assessment. General considerations in nursing implementation applicable to most antineoplastic drugs as well as specific aspects of implementation related to cell cycle–specific drugs are discussed here. Other nursing

process information related to cell cycle–nonspecific drugs is presented in Chapter 49.

For antineoplastic therapy in general, nursing considerations related to *reducing fear and anxiety* include establishing a therapeutic relationship with the patient that begins with trust and empathy. In addition, the nurse should always maintain a calm, warm, empathic, and supportive manner while projecting confidence in providing nursing care. The nurse should give thorough yet appropriate explanations of the tests as well as specific instructions as ordered. Collaboration with all members of the health care team is needed, and the nurse should reinforce the physician's explanations while clarifying any misconceptions about treatment protocols. The patient should be encouraged to consider relaxation techniques such as listening to music, doing yoga, or engaging in guided imagery. It may be necessary to call on other sources of support, such as social services, counselling services, or members of the patient's religious denomination or belief community, while respecting the patient's emotional or other support systems. Appropriate consults with other practitioners may be necessary (e.g., clinical psychiatrist, mental health nurse, nurse practitioner, oncology nurse specialist, psychologist or psychiatrist, clergy).

A variety of interventions can assist in the management of *stomatitis* or excessive oral mucosa dryness and irritation, including the following:
- Performance of oral hygiene measures before and after eating or as needed may help provide cleanliness and comfort. Products containing lemon, glycerin, undiluted peroxide, or alcohol should be avoided because of their drying and irritating effects on the oral mucosa.
- Use of a soft-bristle toothbrush or soft-tipped toothette or swab with solutions of diluted, warm saline is recommended. Chlorhexidine gluconate (Peridex) in a spray bottle with warm saline solution can be used to mist the oral cavity as needed.
- Dentures, if used, should be removed and cleaned frequently and, if stomatitis is severe, replaced only at mealtimes.
- The lips should be kept moist, and sugarless candy or gum used to stimulate saliva production; over-the-counter saliva substitutes can also be used.
- Spicy, acidic, or hot foods should be avoided.
- Oral antifungal suspensions (e.g., nystatin) may be ordered if stomatitis worsens or if white patches are noted on the oral mucosa.
- Other oral suspensions may be mixed by the pharmacy to help with the pain associated with stomatitis (e.g., lidocaine to swish and swallow).
- Smoking, tobacco chewing, and alcohol consumption should be avoided because of the irritation to the oral mucosa.

Nausea and vomiting occur commonly with antineoplastic drugs. Emetic potential varies depending on the drug or treatment protocol (see earlier discussion and Box 48-1). Measures to enhance comfort during times of nausea and vomiting include restricting oral intake; removing noxious odours or sights to avoid stimulating the vomiting centre; performing oral hygiene measures as needed; promoting relaxation through slow, deep breathing and other techniques; consuming small, frequent meals and eating slowly; and consuming clear liquids and a bland diet. Use of intravenous fluids may be indicated if nausea and vomiting are severe. Antiemetics are also a vital part of antineoplastic therapy (see Chapter 54 for more specific drug-related information). Granisetron, ondansetron, and dolasetron are a few of the drugs used; however, H_2 antagonists, metoclopramide, prochlorperazine, methylprednisolone, or lorazepam may also be used. Dronabinol and nabilone (synthetic cannabinoids) may also be prescribed. Premedication with antiemetics 30 to 60 minutes before administration of the antineoplastic(s) is the preferred treatment protocol to help reduce nausea and vomiting, prevent dehydration and malnutrition, and promote comfort. Combination antiemetic drug therapy may be more effective than single-drug therapy. Intravenous hydration may also be helpful in preventing complications.

Diarrhea is also a common adverse effect of antineoplastic therapy. The following nursing interventions may be helpful:

- Restrict oral intake of irritating, spicy, and gas-producing foods; caffeine; high-fibre foods; alcohol; extremely hot or cold foods or beverages; and lactose-containing foods and beverages. Foods high in nonabsorbable sugars (e.g., sorbitol) may be helpful.
- Appropriate resource personnel should be consulted, as ordered, to help the patient and family plan meals and arrange ways to meet the patient's dietary and bowel elimination needs.
- Cheese is a constipating food and may be consumed if tolerated.
- Opioids (e.g., paregoric) or synthetic opioids (e.g., loperamide, diphenoxylate hydrochloride) may be ordered as antidiarrheals.

Adsorbents-protectants and antisecretory drugs may also help reduce gastrointestinal upset and diarrhea (Chapter 53).

To address *nutritional concerns*, meals and snacks consumed over a 24-hour period should be monitored to determine if nutritional intake is adequate. The following measures may help to improve oral intake and nutritional status:

- Antiemetic therapy, pain management, mouth care, and hydration may reduce the adverse effects of therapy.
- Taste alterations caused by antineoplastic drugs may be eased with consumption of mild-tasting foods and use of cold chicken, turkey, or cheese for protein sources. Consumption of iced protein drinks or protein bars may be helpful.
- Eating meat at breakfast may be helpful for those who find meat distasteful at dinnertime.
- Using extra honey or other sweeteners; marinating meats in bland wine, sauces, or flavourings; and

serving foods cold or at room temperature may help with taste changes.
- Plastic rather than metal utensils may be used if the patient complains of a metallic taste.
- Difficulty with swallowing should be reported to the physician immediately, and lidocaine swish-and-swallow solutions may be prescribed.
- The patient should be encouraged to eat foods that are easy to swallow, such as custards; gelatins; puddings; mashed white or sweet potatoes; blended drinks with crushed ice, fruit, and yogourt; nutritional supplement drinks and snacks; and frozen Popsicles or lactose-free ice cream.
- Sticky or dry foods should be avoided, whereas the use of gravy or cream sauces to moisten food items should be encouraged.
- Small, frequent meals are recommended and should be consumed in an environment that is conducive to eating (e.g., free of odours, excess noise, etc.).
- Appetite stimulants such as megestrol acetate or dronabinol may be prescribed.
- The patient should be encouraged to rest before and after meals for energy conservation.
- Snacks containing protein and extra calories (e.g., milkshakes, eggnog with cream, and commercially prepared dietary supplement shakes, ice creams, and breakfast drinks) should be used frequently.

Alopecia, a common adverse effect of antineoplastic drugs, may be disturbing to patients regardless of age or gender. Ensuring that the patient is informed about this effect is crucial to helping the patient feel in control because the illness and its treatment take away the control a patient has over other parts of his or her life. Nursing interventions that may be helpful in dealing with alopecia include the following:

- The patient and family should be informed that hair loss is reversible and usually begins 7 to 10 days after treatment. New hair growth is often a different colour and texture from that of the hair lost.
- The patient should be given the option of acquiring a wig or hairpiece, or scarves or hats, before actual hair loss; the Canadian Cancer Society is a resource for these items and possibly for financial assistance.

Antineoplastic-induced bone marrow suppression leads to *anemias, leukopenia, neutropenia,* and *thrombocytopenia* (see previous discussions regarding myelosuppression caused by antineoplastic drugs). Anemias lead to fatigue and loss of energy and are common adverse effects of therapy and the disease process. Anemias may require blood transfusions, peripheral blood stem cell treatment, or treatment with prescribed medications such as iron preparations, folic acid, or erythropoietic growth factors (e.g., epoetin or darbepoetin alfa). These injections may be given at home and may be administered at the first sign of a decrease in RBC levels. Other nursing measures include having the patient drink fluids to at least 2500 mL/day unless contraindicated, allowing activity as tolerated and scheduling several rest periods during the day, providing assistance with personal care, limiting the number of visitors or their length of stay, organizing the patient's personal space so that necessary items (e.g., phone, light, call bell, and personal items) are close at hand, and encouraging sleep (the use of sedative hypnotics may be needed, as ordered). Energy-saving measures should be encouraged and include, for example, use of a chair or bench when showering, and sitting while carrying out the activities of daily living (e.g., hair brushing, oral care).

Risk of infection from *leukopenia* or *neutropenia* and from immunosuppression is one of the more significant adverse effects that requires close attention. The patient, family, and caregivers need to understand that when WBC counts are low, the patient is at high risk for infection and that defences remain low until the counts recover. Following standard precautions and using good hand-washing technique are the most important practices toward preventing transmission of infection in the hospital and home settings. Because fever is a principal early sign of infection, oral or axillary temperature should be taken at least every 4 hours during periods when the patient is at risk. Taking the temperature rectally should be avoided to minimize tissue trauma, breaks in skin integrity, and, thus, loss of the first line of defence. Temperatures of 38.1°C or above should be reported immediately to the physician so that appropriate treatment can be initiated and complications avoided. Invasive procedures such as urinary catheterization, venipunctures, and injections should be avoided if possible to prevent introduction of bacteria. Intravenous sites should be monitored and sites and tubing changed as per policy, and all drainage systems (wound or urinary) should be kept sterile. Minimizing exposure to contagions is critical to preventing infections; therefore, if a patient is hospitalized (and some physicians avoid hospitalization because of the risk of nosocomial infections), every precaution must be taken to minimize infection. WBC and differential counts should be monitored weekly, and therapy may be postponed temporarily if the WBC count is lower than $3.5 \times 10^9 / \text{L}$ (this value may vary depending on the physician, drug, and patient).

The onset of neutropenia is rapid, with the lowest neutrophil count, or nadir, reached between days 10 and 14. Recovery occurs within 3 or 4 weeks or longer depending on the drug(s) used. Delayed neutropenia may occur with some drugs in about 2 weeks, with the nadir for these drugs being reached in 3 to 4 weeks and recovery occurring in about 7 weeks. Monitoring neutrophil counts is essential to safe nursing care and prevention of infections; normal ranges are between 2.5 and $7 \times 10^9/\text{L}$. Should counts fall below $5 \times 10^9/\text{L}$, the physician should be contacted immediately so that protective or neutropenic precautions can be instituted (see Lab Values Related to Drug Therapy on p. 925 in Chapter 49). These precautions include having nurses, health care workers, and visitors wear gloves, mask, and gown to decrease the patient's exposure to bacteria and viruses.

Other interventions may include intravenous antibiotic therapy based on laboratory test results, and culture and sensitivity reports. It is important to inform the patient and those involved in the patient's care that fever in the presence of neutropenia is a primary early sign of infection, and frequent temperature monitoring is indicated.

If needed, and ordered, administration of colony-stimulating factors may be beneficial. Filgrastim and pegfilgrastim are examples of drugs given to accelerate WBC recovery during antineoplastic drug therapy. These drugs may be used to minimize neutropenia. They specifically act on the bone marrow to enhance neutrophil production; help decrease the incidence, severity, and duration of neutropenia; and possibly help to decrease the incidence of hospitalization and the need for intravenous antibiotic therapy. These medications must be administered within a certain time frame; they are discussed further in Chapter 50. Patients with *immune suppression* should be encouraged to do the following:

- Be aware of environments and persons to avoid, such as individuals who have been recently vaccinated (who may have a subclinical infection), or who have a cold or flu or other symptoms of an infection
- Hydrate with up to 3000 mL/day of fluid unless contraindicated and maintain adequate nutrition
- Adhere to a "low-microbe" diet by washing fresh fruits and vegetables and making sure foods are well cooked
- Maintain intact oral and gastrointestinal mucosa (see discussion of stomatitis)
- Turn, cough, and deep breathe to help prevent stasis of respiratory secretions
- Report temperatures of 38.3°C or higher, sore throat, cough, or flulike symptoms to the health care provider immediately

Thrombocytopenia may also be a consequence of antineoplastic therapy and puts the patient at risk for bleeding (because of a decrease in circulating platelets). Platelet counts, coagulation studies, RBC counts, hemoglobin levels, and hematocrit values should be monitored and should be reported if decreased (see Lab Values Related to Drug Therapy on p. 900 in this chapter). Injections should be avoided, if possible, and alternative routes of administration sought if available. If injections or venipunctures are absolutely necessary, the nurse should use the smallest gauge needle possible and apply gentle, prolonged pressure to the site. Patients undergoing bone marrow aspiration should be monitored closely after the procedure for bleeding at the aspiration site. Blood pressure monitoring should be performed only if necessary and should be done quickly without overinflation of the cuff.

The nurse should monitor the patient for bleeding from the mouth, gums, and nose, and bleeding after brushing of the teeth. If bleeding occurs with oral care, the nursing measures discussed earlier for stomatitis should be used. Bleeding times and results of coagulation studies need to be closely monitored during and after therapy. It is also important that patients know that bleeding may be increased by drugs that affect coagulation, such as anticoagulants, aspirin, and other nonsteroidal anti-inflammatory drugs (NSAIDs). If an analgesic is needed, a non-NSAID should be selected (e.g., acetaminophen). Dosages of acetaminophen should not exceed recommendations because of the possibility of liver toxicity.

Shaving with a straight-edge razor is discouraged. The use of electric razors is encouraged for both men and women to prevent trauma, breaks in the skin, and bleeding. Rectal temperature measurement and use of rectal suppositories or enemas should be avoided to prevent trauma and bleeding. The risk for falls should be reduced. The patient should be instructed to avoid clutter in the room and to wear slippers or shoes with nonskid or nonslip soles. If ordered, platelets or estrogen-progestin preparations (to suppress any menses and bleeding) may be given or oprelvekin may be used to stimulate platelet production as ordered.

The patient should be aware that antineoplastics also have a negative impact on the reproductive tract; they cause destruction of the germinal epithelium of the testes and are associated with sterility, amenorrhea, and teratogenesis. Patients should be educated about the possibility of these adverse effects as well as the risk for decreased libido and for impotence. Male patients should be counselled about the risk for sterility, which is often irreversible. Sperm banking before chemotherapy may be an option. Female patients of childbearing age who are sexually active should protect themselves against pregnancy because of the risk of embryonic death. Use of contraceptive measures is encouraged during chemotherapy and up to at least 8 weeks after discontinuation of therapy. With some antineoplastic therapy, patients may be instructed to use contraception for up to 2 years after completion of treatment because of the risk of genetic abnormalities. Should pregnancy occur, termination of the pregnancy may have to be considered. Some antineoplastic drugs may cause reversible amenorrhea because of their effect on the ovaries, and damage to the ovaries may lead to premature menopausal symptoms (e.g., hot flashes, decreased vaginal secretions, irritability). Water-soluble lubricants may be used during intercourse to prevent tissue trauma.

With *antimetabolites*, the physician's orders should always be followed regarding premedication with antiemetics and antianxiety drugs. Orders or protocol for the use of other symptom-control medication should be followed as well. Fluid intake of up to 3000 mL/24 hours should be encouraged, or intravenous hydration should be used as needed or as ordered. All drugs should be handled carefully and direct contact with skin, eyes, and mucous membranes avoided. All protocols for chemotherapy administration, as well as any hospital or facility policies or manufacturer guidelines, should be followed. If in doubt about any order for any drug, the nurse should stop and consult appropriate resources for further information. Drug incompatibilities are common, and the nurse should check for these before infusions are given

to prevent more adverse reactions. Oral hygiene should be performed frequently; a soft toothbrush should be used and, if flossing, waxed dental floss should be used. Nutritional intake should be constantly monitored and weight measured daily or weekly. Generally speaking, with antimetabolites, gastrointestinal adverse effects occur around the fourth day. This situation requires preplanning for special medication assistance, if needed, and dietary changes to meet the patient's specific needs. Antibiotic therapy may be ordered prophylactically for infection, as well as analgesics for pain and antispasmodics for diarrhea. See earlier discussion of nursing considerations regarding treatment of stomatitis, loss of appetite, diarrhea, nausea, and vomiting as well as for the blood disorders that may occur.

Cytarabine should be used with extreme caution in handling and administration by the various routes (intravenous, subcutaneous, or intrathecal). Major concerns related to therapy with this drug include bone marrow suppression and cytarabine syndrome, which is manifested by fever, joint pains, chest pain, conjunctivitis, and overall malaise. If high dosages are used, cytarabine may also cause central nervous system, gastrointestinal, or pulmonary toxicity, so the patient must be continually monitored for these system-related adverse effects. For intrathecal administration, the drug may be reconstituted with NaCl, or the physician may use the patient's spinal fluid. With fluorouracil, the solution is colourless to slightly yellow, and the drug should not be added to any other intravenous infusions; it should only be given by itself in the appropriate diluent. If an infusion port is not used, intravenous sites should not be over joints, tendons, or small veins, or in extremities that are edematous.

Intravenous dosages should be given exactly as ordered with constant monitoring of the intravenous site, infusion port, and infusion solution and equipment. If intravenous infiltration occurs, the protocol for management should be followed and will most likely include the application of an ice pack. All hospital or infusion protocols should be followed without exception because treatment of extravasation is handled differently depending on the specific drug (see related discussions in the pharmacology section). If topical forms of the drug are used, the patient should be told to apply the drug exactly as ordered and to the affected area only. Gloves or fingercots should be used to apply the topical dosage form.

Gemcitabine, another antimetabolite, is dosed on the basis of absolute granulocyte counts and platelet nadirs and is given if the counts exceed 1.5×10^9/L and 1×10^9/L, respectively. Intravenous solutions should be kept at room temperature to avoid crystallization and used within 24 hours. Infusions are to be given as ordered. Antiemetics as well as antidiarrheals may be needed. Mercaptopurine is available in oral dosage forms and should not be given with meals.

The antimetabolite methotrexate has numerous toxicities and adverse effects, which may be minimized by appropriate medical treatment. Preplanning for therapy includes consideration of boosting the immune status and blood cell counts before aggressive therapy is initiated. Patients must be encouraged to drink up to 2000 to 3000 mL/day if tolerated and not contraindicated. The nurse should continue to monitor creatinine clearance, as ordered, to detect any nephrotoxicity. Nutritional status may be enhanced by increasing the intake of bran, dried beans, nuts, fruits, asparagus, and other fresh vegetables (thoroughly washed and if tolerated) because these foods are high in folic acid. While these food items may not be tolerated during the actual drug therapy, their consumption is encouraged when the patient is able to tolerate them because it is yet another measure to help minimize the possibility of methotrexate toxicity. Should gastrointestinal upset or stomatitis occur, the patient may need to decrease any sources of irritation (e.g., high-fibre food) and take the other measures noted earlier.

Methotrexate is usually given orally, intramuscularly, or intravenously. The nurse should wear gloves when giving the drug, and if any of the powder comes in contact with the skin, the area should be washed immediately and thoroughly with soap and water. Intravenous administration of fluids should accompany therapy to insure adequate hydration. Bicarbonate may be ordered to help alkalinize the urine and encourage excretion of the drug. Intramuscular injections and other procedures that induce bleeding or trauma should be avoided until blood counts return to acceptable limits, as noted by the physician. If venipunctures are performed, pressure should be applied firmly to the site for up to 5 minutes or longer, if needed. As with many antineoplastics, there are numerous incompatibilities, and the nurse must be aware of these and check for them.

Methotrexate can cause life-threatening bone marrow toxicity. As a "rescue" treatment, leucovorin is used, which helps to limit the toxic effects of methotrexate on bone marrow cells. It is often ordered to be used within 1 hour of accidental overdosage of folic acid antagonists such as methotrexate; it may also be prescribed in conventional cytoprotective dosages. For a listing of other types of drugs used as antagonists to antineoplastics or given for their cytoprotective actions, see the discussion of methotrexate in the pharmacology section.

For the *mitotic inhibitors*, which include docetaxel, paclitaxel, vincristine, and vinblastine, some nursing considerations are similar to those for other antineoplastic drug categories, whereas others are unique to this drug class. For the taxane family of drugs, particularly docetaxel, there are generally premedication protocols that may include administration of drugs such as oral corticosteroids (e.g., dexamethasone), beginning several days before day 1 of therapy to help decrease the risk of hypersensitivity and reduce the severity of fluid retention. Solutions should be protected from light and are stable only for approximately 8 hours either at room temperature or under refrigeration. Manufacturers generally send information about diluents. Any solutions should be gently rolled to mix. During the infusion, the patient must be closely monitored for the sudden onset of bronchospasms, flushing of the face, and localized skin reactions; these may indicate a hypersensitivity response requiring immediate treatment. These symptoms may occur within just a few minutes of beginning the infusion. In addition, any dyspnea, abdominal distension, crackles in the lungs, or dependent edema during therapy should be tended to immediately by medical personnel. Cutaneous reactions may also appear during therapy, such as rash on the hands and feet, and need immediate attention and treatment. With paclitaxel, the patient may also be premedicated with diphenhydramine, corticosteroids, and H_2 antagonist drugs.

Nurses should wear gloves when giving these antineoplastics. Reconstituted solutions are stable for a short period of time; refer to authoritative sources for exact information. Polyvinyl chloride (PVC) plasticized tubing and equipment should not be used, and the drug should be mixed with the proper diluent and administered at the proper rate as ordered. The patient's vital signs should be watched closely, especially during the first hour of infusion. If there is any evidence of hypersensitivity, the physician should be contacted immediately, the patient should be monitored, and treatment protocols should be initiated to prevent harm to the patient. Intramuscular injections, rectal temperature measurement and rectal administration of medications, and other traumas that might induce bleeding should be avoided. All other measures to help avoid bleeding should be implemented, including application of gentle, firm pressure to the site of any bleeding.

With the *topoisomerase inhibitors* irinotecan and topotecan, blood counts should be monitored closely with every treatment. Diarrhea or a drop in blood counts may cause a temporary postponing of therapy. Extravasation of the solution should be treated immediately, and the intravenous site should be flushed with sterile water and ice applied. Ensuring that intravenous sites remain patent and without any indications of infiltration is critical to preventing damage to tissue from extravasation. Nausea and vomiting may lead to dehydration and electrolyte disturbances, so patients should be aware of the need to report these symptoms immediately before negative consequences occur (see previous discussion for specific interventions). Intravenous incompatibilities are numerous for both these drugs and should be an area of constant concern. With topotecan, intravenous extravasation is usually accompanied by only a mild local reaction such as erythema or bruising and, if noted, should be managed immediately to avoid further trauma and risk for loss of skin integrity. Headaches and difficulty breathing may be more common with topotecan; therefore, the patient should be monitored closely for these symptoms with every administration. The nurse should be ready to implement appropriate interventions.

The *enzyme antineoplastics* asparaginase and pegaspargase should be handled with extreme caution and care. An intradermal test dose of asparaginase may be given before therapy has begun or when a week or longer has passed between doses. With asparaginase, the solution and powder may be irritants to the skin, and washing is required after contact (as described later for pegaspargase). During therapy, if there are signs and symptoms of oliguria, anuria (kidney failure), or pancreatitis, the drug will most likely be discontinued. Pegaspargase requires cautious handling and administration, and inhalation of its fumes should be avoided at all costs. This drug is an irritant; should it come in contact with the skin, the area should be washed with copious amounts of water for a minimum of 15 minutes. The intramuscular route of administration is usually preferred because it carries a lower risk of clotting abnormalities, gastrointestinal disorders, and kidney and liver toxicity. If solutions are cloudy, they should not be used. If more than 2 mL is required for a dose, two injections should be used. Pancreatitis is problematic with this drug and can be serious, so close attention should be given to symptoms such as severe abdominal pain with nausea and vomiting. Serum lipase and amylase levels should be constantly monitored. If any signs or symptoms of pancreatitis occur, the drug is generally discontinued immediately.

Intravenous infusions also require close monitoring for extravasation. The site should be monitored every hour for pain, erythema, heat, swelling, and a bluish discoloration. Intravenous infusions of vesicant drugs (which, if extravasated, lead to tissue death, necrosis, and sloughing) and irritant drugs (which, if extravasated, lead to irritation but not tissue death) should always be carefully administered via a patent intravenous infusion line or through an infusion port. Severe necrosis from vesicant extravasation may require surgical intervention and possibly skin grafting. The use of an infusion port helps prevent the severe tissue damage that occurs with peripheral intravenous infusion extravasations, so these ports are commonly placed before therapy. If extravasation is suspected, the specific antineoplastic drug should be discontinued immediately, the intravenous catheter left in place, and any residual drug or blood aspirated from the intravenous catheter if possible and if indicated. The requisite antidote must then be prepared and instilled through the existing intravenous catheter, after which the needle should be removed. Antidotes and other substances may also be injected around the intravenous site to reach affected issues. A sterile occlusive dressing may be ordered to be placed on the entire area and warm or cold compresses may be indicated, depending on the extravasated drug and recommended protocol. The affected limb should then be elevated and allowed to rest to help minimize the amount of tissue damage from further spread of the drug. Appropriate and timely treatment of extravasation of vesicants may help to prevent some of the most devastating consequences of chemotherapy, such as loss of a limb or the need for multiple surgeries.

Many of the common adverse effects associated with antineoplastic therapy are presented in earlier sections of the chapter and may be referred to for review. Use of cytoprotective drugs, briefly discussed in the pharmacology section of this chapter, is discussed further in Chapter 49.

Evaluation

Evaluation of nursing care should focus on reviewing whether goals and outcomes are being met as well as monitoring for therapeutic responses and adverse effects and toxic effects of the antineoplastic therapy. Therapeutic responses may manifest as clinical improvement, decrease in tumour size, and decrease in metastatic spread. Evaluation of nursing care with reference to goals and outcomes may reveal improvements related to a decrease in adverse effects and a decrease in the impact of cancer on the patient's well-being, with increases in comfort, nutrition, hydration, energy levels, ability to carry out the activities of daily living, and quality of life. Goals and outcomes should be revisited to identify more specific areas to monitor. In addition, certain laboratory studies such as measurement of tumour markers levels, levels of carcinoembryonic antigens, and RBC, WBC, and platelet counts may be performed to aid in determining how well the treatment protocol has worked. As part of the evaluation, physicians may also order additional radiographs, computed tomographic scans, magnetic resonance images, tissue analysis, or other studies appropriate to the diagnosis both during and after antineoplastic therapy has been completed, at time intervals related to the anticipated tumour response.

CASE STUDY

Facing Chemotherapy

Mrs. D., a 48-year-old married mother of two teenaged daughters, has been diagnosed with breast cancer. She has had lumpectomy surgery to remove the tumour and is about to start chemotherapy. She states that she has "faced the facts" about her disease and the threat to her life but says, "I know this is silly, but I hate the thought of losing my hair to this disease."

1. What measures can be taken to help her deal with her hair loss?
2. Ten days after the chemotherapy, her neutrophil count drops to 2×10^9/L. She is hospitalized because she has

developed a cough, and her friends send a fruit basket to the hospital. What actions should be taken to protect her from infection?
3. During rounds, the nurse finds Mrs. D. curled up in the bed and sobbing. Mrs. D. states that she feels "so afraid" and is worried about who will care for her family if she dies. Discuss some nursing actions that the nurse might perform.

For answers see http://evolve.elsevier.com/Canada/Lilley/pharmacology/.

PATIENT EDUCATION

* To help minimize gastrointestinal adverse effects and decrease irritation to the oral and gastrointestinal mucosa, patients should be encouraged to avoid consuming foods that are high in fibre, are spicy, contain citric acid, are hot or cold, or have a rough texture. Alcohol use and smoking are also irritating to the oral and gastrointestinal mucosa and should be avoided.
* Patients should be informed that examining their mouth daily is important and to report any problems (e.g., sores, pain, white patches) to the health care provider immediately. They should also report, at the first sign, symptoms such as headache, fatigue, faintness, and shortness of breath (possibly indicative of anemia); bleeding and easy bruising (possibly indicative of a drop in platelet count); and sore throat and fever (possibly indicative of infection). Fever and chills may be the first sign of an oncoming infection.
* Women of childbearing age should be encouraged to use nonpharmacological forms of contraception for the duration of antineoplastic therapy and for up to several months or years after treatment. Sperm conservation through sperm donor or banking may be an option for men treated with these drugs, to allow fathering a child at a later time.
* Patients should be educated about medications to avoid while receiving antineoplastics, including aspirin, ibuprofen, and products containing these drugs, in order to help prevent excessive bleeding.
* Patients receiving antineoplastics should be informed about the risk of alopecia (hair loss) before drug therapy begins. Patients should have the opportunity to discuss options for hair and scalp care, including the option of having their hair cut short before treatment and selecting and purchasing or renting a wig

or hairpiece comparable to their existing hair in colour, texture, length, and style, or having bandannas, scarves, or hats on hand before the hair is actually lost. Although hair loss is temporary, patients need to be informed that it will occur and should also be aware that wigs and hairpieces are available through the Canadian Cancer Society.
* Patients should be informed about the following Web sites as helpful online resources for the patient and significant others: http://www.hc-sc.gc.ca/dc-ma/cancer, http://www.hc-sc.gc.ca/fn-an/food-guide-aliment, http://www.nih.gov, http://www.wellspring.ca, http://www.bccancer.bc.ca, http://www.who.int/en, and http://www.oncolink.upenn.edu
* With *cytarabine*, patients should be encouraged to increase fluid intake to help decrease the risk of dehydration and hyperuricemia. It is important that patients report any signs of easy bruising, fever, infection, or unusual bleeding from any site; that they not receive vaccinations during treatment; and that they avoid individuals who have recently received a live-virus vaccine.
* With *fluorouracil* and *gemcitabine*, patients should be encouraged to practise frequent oral hygiene and to report bleeding, bruising, chest pain, diarrhea, nausea or vomiting, heart palpitations, infection, or changes in vision to their physician immediately. For fluorouracil, patients should be encouraged to avoid overexposure to sun or ultraviolet light and to wear protective clothing, sunscreen, and sunglasses when in the sun. The use of topical ointment may leave the affected area looking somewhat unsightly for several weeks after therapy, and the hands should be washed thoroughly after its application.

Continued

❖ With *mercaptopurine*, patients should be advised to avoid alcohol consumption because it increases the risk of drug toxicity. The same concerns regarding vaccination and precautions for infection and bleeding apply as were noted earlier.

❖ With *methotrexate*, patients should be told to notify the physician if nausea and vomiting are problematic or uncontrollable, or if fever, sore throat, muscle aches and pains, or unusual bleeding occurs. Alcohol, salicylates, NSAIDs, and exposure to sunlight or ultraviolet light should be avoided. Both male and female patients should use contraceptive measures for up to 3 months or longer after therapy.

❖ With *taxanes*, drug-induced alopecia is reversible, but patients should be warned that new hair growth will most likely differ in colour and texture from that of the hair lost. Hair growth usually resumes 2 to 3 months after the last dose of chemotherapy. Oral hygiene must be thorough, and patients should avoid individuals with infections or those who have received live-virus vaccines. Patients should use contraceptive measures until otherwise advised by the physician. Nausea and vomiting should be reported immediately so that appropriate treatment can be rendered—especially if the patient is at home, to prevent hospitalizations. For paclitaxel, patients should also be told to report any signs or symptoms of neuropathy (e.g., numbness or tingling of extremities).

❖ With *etoposide* and *teniposide*, patients should be cautioned to avoid individuals who have received live-virus vaccines or who are ill and to avoid crowds when the patient's blood cell counts are low. Patients should be encouraged to contact the physician if they experience easy bleeding, bruising, difficulty breathing, fever, sore throat, or chills. Contraception should be used. Hair loss is reversible.

❖ With *asparaginase* and *pegaspargase*, patients should be encouraged to drink fluids and to report immediately to the physician any severe nausea or vomiting as well as any bleeding, excessive fatigue, fever, or other signs or symptoms of infection.

POINTS TO REMEMBER

❖ Cancers are diseases that are characterized by uncontrolled cellular growth.

❖ *Malignancy* refers specifically to a neoplasm that is anaplastic, invasive, and metastatic, as opposed to benign. Malignant tumours typically consist of cancerous cells that infiltrate surrounding tissues and spread to other tissues and organs, where they form metastatic tumour deposits. Tumours are generally classified by tissue of origin: epithelial (carcinoma), connective (sarcoma), lymphatic (lymphoma), and leukocytes (leukemia).

❖ Antineoplastics are drugs used to treat cancer. They may be either cell cycle–specific or cell cycle–nonspecific drugs or have miscellaneous actions.

❖ Cell cycle–specific drugs kill cancer cells during specific phases of the cell growth cycle. Cell cycle–nonspecific drugs kill cancer cells during any phase of the cell growth cycle.

❖ Chemotherapy, or antineoplastic therapy, requires astute nursing care, and the nurse must act prudently and make critical decisions about the nursing care of patients receiving these drugs. Knowledge of the adverse effects and toxic effects of antineoplastic drugs is important to ensure patient safety and to protect the patient from such effects of these drugs.

❖ Cell cycle–specific drug classes include antimetabolites, mitotic inhibitors, topoisomerase I inhibitors, and antineoplastic enzymes. These drugs are collectively used to treat a variety of solid and circulating tumours, although some drugs have much more specific indications than others.

❖ Antineoplastic antimetabolites are cell cycle–specific antagonistic analogues that work by inhibiting the actions of key cellular metabolites. They interfere with the biosynthesis of precursors essential to cellular growth by inhibiting the synthesis or actions of three classes of compounds: the vitamin folic acid, and purines and pyrimidines, and the two classes of compounds that make up the bases contained in nucleic acid molecules (DNA and RNA).

❖ Two plant-derived antineoplastic drugs are the taxanes, which include paclitaxel, derived from the bark of the slow-growing Western (Pacific) yew tree, and docetaxel, a semisynthetic taxoid produced from the needles of the European yew tree. Docetaxel is pharmacologically similar to paclitaxel.

❖ Topoisomerase I inhibitors are a relatively new class of chemotherapy drugs. The two drugs currently available in this class are topotecan and irinotecan.

❖ Antineoplastic enzymes include asparaginase and pegaspargase. A third, *Erwinia* asparaginase, together with pegaspargase, is available only by special request from Health Canada's Special Access Programme, for patients who have developed allergies to *E. coli*–based asparaginase.

❖ Several drugs that are available are classified as cytoprotective drugs. These medications help to reduce the toxicity of antineoplastics. The decision of whether to use them is often patient-specific, as is the case with chemotherapy regimens.

❖ Extravasation of vesicants may lead to severe tissue injury with complications such as permanent damage to muscles, tendons, and ligaments, and possible loss of a limb.

EXAMINATION REVIEW QUESTIONS

1 Which nursing intervention is appropriate for a patient suffering from stomatitis?
 a. Keep dentures in the mouth between meals.
 b. Use lemon-glycerin swabs to keep the mouth moist.
 c. Rinse the mouth with commercial mouthwash twice a day.
 d. Clean the mouth with a soft-bristle toothbrush and warm saline solution.

2 Which intervention is most appropriate in caring for a patient who is very nauseated during chemotherapy?
 a. Hold all fluids during chemotherapy to avoid vomiting.
 b. Encourage light activity during chemotherapy as a distraction.
 c. Provide antiemetic medications only upon the request of the patient.
 d. Provide antiemetic medications 30 to 60 minutes before chemotherapy begins.

3 For which of the following will the nurse monitor the patient who is experiencing thrombocytopenia from severe bone marrow suppression?
 a. Decreased skin turgor
 b. Elevated body temperature
 c. Increased bleeding and bruising
 d. Complaints of severe weakness and fatigue

4 A patient receiving chemotherapy is experiencing severe bone marrow suppression. Which nursing diagnosis is most appropriate at this time?
 a. Acute pain
 b. Activity intolerance
 c. Disturbed body image
 d. Impaired physical mobility

5 Should extravasation of an antineoplastic medication occur, which intervention should the nurse perform first?
 a. Apply cold compresses to the site and elevate the arm.
 b. Inject subcutaneous doses of epinephrine around the intravenous site every 2 hours.
 c. Stop the infusion immediately while leaving the catheter in place, and notify the physician.
 d. Inject the appropriate antidote through the intravenous catheter after stopping the intravenous infusion.

For answers see http://evolve.elsevier.com/Canada/Lilley/pharmacology/.

CRITICAL THINKING ACTIVITIES

1 Two broad categories of drugs used to treat cancer are cell cycle–specific drugs and cell cycle–nonspecific drugs. Explain the difference between the two categories of drugs, based on their mechanisms of action.

2 Your patient is experiencing stomatitis. What kinds of food would you encourage her to avoid? Explain your answer.

3 Your patient is taking irinotecan as part of his chemotherapy regimen. He has received the dose and is about to be discharged. Discuss a potential problem he may face at home as a result of this chemotherapy, and how it can be treated.

For answers see http://evolve.elsevier.com/Canada/Lilley/pharmacology/.

Antineoplastic Drugs Part 2: Cell Cycle–Nonspecific and Miscellaneous Drugs

Learning Objectives

After reading this chapter, the successful student will be able to do the following:

1. Review the concepts related to carcinogenesis, the types of malignancies and related terminology, and the different treatment modalities, including the use of cell cycle–nonspecific and miscellaneous antineoplastic drugs (see also Chapter 48).

2. Identify the drugs classified as cell cycle–nonspecific or hormonal or that are considered miscellaneous drugs.

3. Discuss the common adverse effects and toxic effects of the cell cycle–nonspecific and miscellaneous antineoplastic drugs, including the reasons for their occurrence and methods of treatment, such as use of any antidotes.

4. Describe the mechanisms of action, indications, dosages, routes of administration, cautions, contraindications, and drug interactions of the cell cycle–nonspecific drugs, hormonal drugs, and miscellaneous antineoplastic drugs.

5. Apply knowledge about the cell cycle–nonspecific, hormonal agonist–antagonist, and other miscellaneous antineoplastic drugs and their characteristics to the development of a comprehensive collaborative plan of care for patients with cancer.

6. Briefly describe extravasation and other major adverse effects associated with the antineoplastics in this chapter.

e-Learning Activities

Web site
(http://evolve.elsevier.com/Canada/Lilley/pharmacology/)

- Animations
- Answers to chapter questions, activities, and case studies
- Calculators and Category Catchers
- Glossary with audio pronunciations
- IV Therapy and Medication Error Checklists
- Multiple-Choice Review Question quizzes
- Nursing Care Plans
- Online Appendices and Supplements
- WebLinks

Drug Profiles

bevacizumab, p. 922
▸▸ cisplatin, p. 919
▸▸ cyclophosphamide, p. 919
▸▸ doxorubicin (doxorubicin hydrochloride)*, p. 921
hydroxyurea, p. 922
imatinib (imatinib mesylate)*, p. 922
▸▸ mechlorethamine (mechlorethamine hydrochloride)*, p. 919
mitotane, p. 922
mitoxantrone (mitoxantrone hydrochloride)*, p. 921
octreotide, p. 922

▸▸ Key drug.

*Full generic name is given in parentheses. For the purposes of this text, the more common shortened name is used.

Glossary

Alkylation A chemical reaction in which an alkyl group is transferred from an alkylating drug. (p. 914)

Bifunctional Referring to alkylating drugs composed of molecules that have two reactive alkyl groups and are thus able to alkylate two cancer cell DNA molecules per drug molecule. (p. 917)

Extravasation The leakage of any intravenously or intra-arterially administered medication into the tissue space surrounding the vein or artery. (p. 918)

Mitosis The process of cell reproduction occurring in somatic (nonsexual) cells and resulting in the formation of two genetically identical daughter cells containing the diploid (complete) number of chromosomes characteristic of the species. (p. 917)

Polyfunctional Referring to the action of alkylating drugs that can engage in several alkylation reactions with cancer cell DNA molecules per single molecule of drug. (p. 917)

OVERVIEW

This chapter is a continuation of Chapter 48 and focuses on additional classes of antineoplastic drugs. Two new chapters on antineoplastic drugs were created for this textbook edition because of the complexity of drug classes and the large and ever-increasing numbers of individual drugs. Chapter 48 describes the antineoplastic drugs that are effective against cancer cells during specific phases in the *cell growth cycle*. In contrast, this chapter focuses on drugs that have antineoplastic activity regardless of the phase of the cell cycle. Also discussed in this chapter are drugs classified as *miscellaneous* antineoplastics due to their lack of clear cell-cycle specificity or their unique or *novel* (new) mechanisms of action. Table 49-1 summarizes the nomenclature for these drug classes. For a description of the cell growth cycle, see Chapter 48.

CELL CYCLE–NONSPECIFIC ANTINEOPLASTIC DRUGS

There are currently two broad classes of cell cycle–nonspecific cancer drugs: alkylating drugs and cytotoxic antibiotics.

ALKYLATING DRUGS

Records of the use of drugs to treat cancer date back several centuries. However, not until the 1940s were truly successful systemic cancer chemotherapy treatments documented. At this time, the first alkylating drugs were developed from mustard gas agents used for chemical warfare before and during World War I. The first drug to be developed was mechlorethamine, also known as *nitrogen mustard*. It is the prototypical drug of this class and is still used for cancer treatment. Since its antineoplastic activity was discovered in the mid-twentieth century, many analogues have been synthesized for use in the treatment of cancer, collectively referred to as *nitrogen mustards*. *Alkylation* is the chemical process by which these drugs work in cancer cells (see Mechanism of Action on this page).

The alkylating drugs commonly used in clinical practice in Canada fall into three categories: *classic alkylators*

(also called *nitrogen mustards*); *nitrosoureas*, which have a different chemical structure than that of the nitrogen mustards but also work by alkylation; and *probable alkylators*, which also have a different chemical structure than that of the nitrogen mustards but are known to work at least partially by alkylation. These drugs are used to treat a wide spectrum of malignancies. The drugs in each category are as follows:

Classic alkylators (nitrogen mustards)
- chlorambucil
- cyclophosphamide
- ifosfamide
- mechlorethamine
- melphalan
- thiotepa

Nitrosoureas
- carmustine
- lomustine
- streptozocin

Probable alkylators
- altretamine
- busulfan
- carboplatin
- cisplatin
- dacarbazine
- oxaliplatin
- procarbazine
- temozolomide

Mechanism of Action and Drug Effects

The alkylating drugs act by preventing cancer cells from reproducing, and they have a unique way of accomplishing this. Specifically, they alter the chemical structure of deoxyribonucleic acid (DNA), which is essential to the reproduction of any cell, by causing alkyl groups rather than hydrogen atoms to be attached to the nucleic acid. This process is called **alkylation**. Recall from chemistry that alkyl groups are composed of both hydrogen and carbon atoms linked by covalent bonds. Examples include a methyl group ($-CH_3$) and an ethyl group ($-CH_2CH_3$). DNA molecules consist of two adjacent strands, each consisting of alternating sequences of phosphate and sugar molecules (Figure 49-1). These components

TABLE 49-1

Common Names for Selected Antineoplastic Drugs

Generic Name	Trade Names	Other Names
CELL CYCLE–NONSPECIFIC DRUGS		
Alkylating Drugs		
Classic Alkylators		
busulfan	Myleran, Busulfex	BSF
chlorambucil	Leukeran	chlorbutinum, CB-1348, NSC-3088
cyclophosphamide	Cytoxan, Procytox	cyclo, CPA, CPM, CTX, CYC, CYT
ifosfamide	Ifex	isophosphamide, iphosphamide
mechlorethamine	Mustargen	chlormethine, nitrogen mustard, HN2, mustine
melphalan	Alkeran	L-sarcolysin, phenylalanine mustard, L-PAM
Nitrosoureas		
carmustine	BiCNU	BCNU
lomustine	CeeNU	CCNU
streptozocin	Zanosar	streptozotocin
Probable Alkylators		
altretamine	Hexalen	hexamethylmelamine, HMM, HXM, NSC-13875
carboplatin	Carboplatin	CBDCA, JM-8, NSC-241240
cisplatin	Cisplatin	*cis*-diamminedichloroplatinum (II), *cis*-platinum-II; CDDP
dacarbazine	Dacarbazine	DTIC, DIC
oxaliplatin	Eloxatin	ACT-078, 1-OHP, LOHP, oxalotoplatin, oxaliplatinum
procarbazine hydrochloride	Matulane	
temozolomide	Temodal	TMZ, SCH S2 365, NSC-362856
thiotepa		TSPA, TESPA
Cytotoxic Antibiotics		
Anthracyclines		
daunorubicin hydrochloride	Cerubidine	daunomycin, rubidomycin, DNR
doxorubicin hydrochloride, conventional	Adriamycin	DDR, daunorubicin, rubidomycin
doxorubicin hydrochloride, liposomal	Caelyx, Myocet	
epirubicin hydrochloride	Ellence	4'-epidoxorubicin, IMI 28, NSC-256942
idarubicin	Idamycin	Imi 30, NSC-256439
valrubicin	Valtaxin	NSC-246131
Other Cytotoxic Antibiotics		
bleomycin	Blenoxane	BLM, Bleo, NSC-125066
dactinomycin	Cosmegen	actinomycin-D
mitomycin	Mitomycin (generic)	mitomycin-C, MTC
mitoxantrone hydrochloride	Mitoxantrone (generic)	DHAD, dihydroxyanthracenedione
MISCELLANEOUS ANTINEOPLASTICS (CELL CYCLE–SPECIFICITY UNCLEAR)		
bevacizumad	Avastin	NSC704865
bortezomib	Velcade	MLN341, PS-341
gefitinib	Iressa	ZD1839
imatinib mesylate	Gleevec	STI-571
mitotane	Lysodren	o,p'-DDD
porfimer sodium	Photofrin	dihaematoporphyrin ether, porphyrins
CELL CYCLE–SPECIFIC DRUGS		
Cytoprotective Drugs		
amifostine (available through Special Access Programme, Health Canada)	Ethyol	ethiofos, gammaphos, WR2721, ethanethiol, NSC-296961
dexrazoxane	Zinecard	ICRF-187
leucovorin calcium	Lederle Leucovorin (generic)	calcium folinate, citrovorum factor, folinic acid, 5-formyl tetrahydrofolate
mesna	Uromitexan	sodium 2-mercaptoethane sulfonate
HORMONAL AND RELATED DRUGS		
Adrenocorticosteroids		
dexamethasone	Dexasone, generic	
hydrocortisone	Solu-Cortef	
methylprednisolone	Depo-Medrol, Medrol, Solu-Medrol	
prednisone	Winpred, generic	

Continued

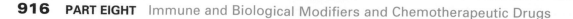

TABLE 49-1

Common Names for Selected Antineoplastic Drugs (cont'd)

Generic Name	Trade Names	Other Names
HORMONAL AND RELATED DRUGS—cont'd		
Androgens		
testosterone propionate		
Antiandrogens		
bicalutamide	Casodex	
flutamide	Euflex	
nilutamide	Anadron	
Aromatase Inhibitors		
anastrozole	Arimidex	
exemestane	Aromasin	
letrozole	Femara	
Estrogens		
diethylstilbestrol	Stilbestrol	DES
ethinyl estradiol		
Estrogen–Nitrogen Mustard Combination		
estramustine (estradiol 1 nornitrogen mustard)	Emcyt	
Antiestrogens		
fulvestrant	Faslodex	
tamoxifen	Nolvadex, Tamofen	
Gonadotropin-Releasing Hormone Analogues		
goserelin acetate	Zoladex	
leuprolide acetate	Eligard, Lupron, Lupron Depot	
triptorelin pamoate	Trelstar, Trelstar LA	
Progestins		
medroxyprogesterone acetate	Medroxy-5, Provera, Depo-Provera	
megestrol acetate	Megace	
MISCELLANEOUS CELL CYCLE–SPECIFIC DRUGS		
hydroxyurea	Hydrea, generic	hydroxycarbamide
OTHER TOXICITY INHIBITORS		
allopurinol	Alloprin	
rasburicase	Fasturtec	
RADIOACTIVE ANTINEOPLASTICS		
chromic phosphate P 32		
samarium SM 153 lexidronam		samarium 153, 153SM-EDTMP
sodium iodide I 131		I-131
sodium phosphate P 32	Sodium Phosphate P 32	
strontium 89 Sr chloride		strontium-89

DTIC, dimethyltriazenoimidazolecarboxamide.

make up the "backbone" of the DNA strands. These two strands are cross-linked to each other by the third DNA structural element—nitrogen-containing bases (adenine, guanine, thymine, and cytosine, abbreviated A, G, T, and C, respectively). These bases are bound to the sugar molecules of the DNA backbone, and two bases, linked to each other by covalent hydrogen bonds, form the molecular bridges between the two DNA strands that bring them into the double helix structure. A *nucleotide*, which consists of one molecule each of base, sugar, and phosphate that are bound together, is the structural unit of molecules of both DNA and ribonucleic acid (RNA), another nucleic acid that is important in cellular reproduction. A *nucleoside* consists of a base molecule and sugar molecule only. RNA molecules are produced by DNA molecules during the complex process of cellular reproduction. RNA molecules differ from DNA molecules in at least three ways: they are single stranded (versus double stranded), the thymine base is replaced by another base known as *uracil* (U), and the sugar molecule is *ribose*, which has a slightly different structure than that of the *deoxyribose* molecules of DNA.

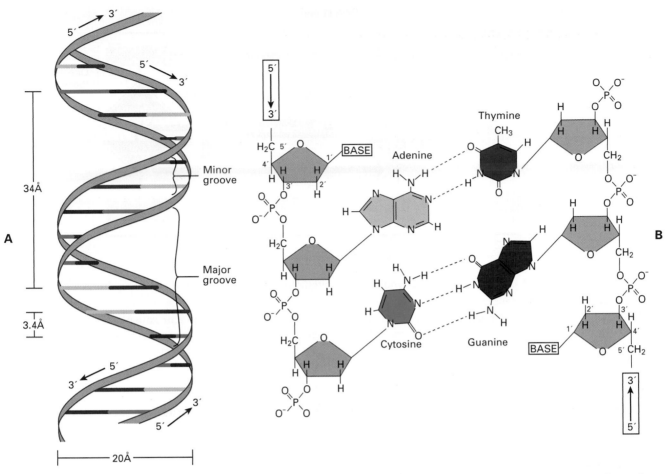

FIG. 49-1   Deoxyribonucleic acid (DNA) double helix. *A,* Diagrammatic model of the helical structure, showing its dimensions, the major and minor grooves, the periodicity of the bases, and the antiparallel orientation of the backbone chains (represented by ribbons). The base pairs (represented by rods) are perpendicular to the axis and lie stacked one on another. *B,* The chemical structure of the backbone and bases of DNA, showing the sugar–phosphate linkages of the backbone and the hydrogen bonding between the base pairs. There are two hydrogen bonds between adenine and thymine, and three between cytosine and guanine. (From *Dorland's illustrated medical dictionary* (30th ed.) (2003). Philadelphia: Saunders.)

During the normal process of reproduction, the double helix uncoils and its two strands separate. A strand of RNA is then assembled next to each single DNA strand in a process known as *transcription*. RNA strands, in turn, are involved in both protein synthesis (*translation*) and replication of the original DNA structure before cell division, or **mitosis**. These processes ultimately result in the creation of a new cell with the same DNA sequence, and thus the same characteristics, as its parent cell.

Alkyl groups that are part of the chemical structure of antineoplastic alkylating drugs attach to DNA molecules by forming covalent bonds with the bases described earlier. As a result, abnormal chemical bonds form between the adjacent DNA strands. This action leads to the formation of defective nucleic acids that are then unable to perform the normal cellular reproductive functions, resulting in cell death.

Alkylating drugs can also be characterized by the number of alkyl groups they possess and thus the number of alkylation reactions in which they can participate

per single molecule of drug. **Bifunctional** alkylating drugs have two reactive alkyl groups that are able to alkylate two DNA molecules. **Polyfunctional** alkylating drugs can participate in several alkylation reactions. Figure 49-2 shows the location along the DNA double helix where the alkylating drugs work.

Indications

The most commonly used alkylating drugs are effective against a wide spectrum of malignancies, including both solid and hematological tumours. Common examples of the types of cancer that different alkylating drugs are used to treat are listed in the Dosages table on p. 919.

Adverse Effects

Alkylating drugs are capable of causing all of the dose-limiting adverse effects described in Chapter 48. Additional adverse effects are described in Table 49-2. The relative emetic potential of the alkylating drugs is given in Box 48-1 on p. 888 of Chapter 48. The adverse effects

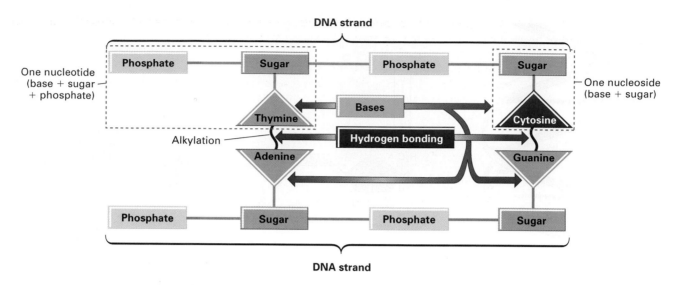

FIG. 49-2 Organization of deoxyribonucleic acid (DNA) and site of action of alkylating drugs.

of these drugs are important because of their severity, although they can be prevented by prophylactic measures. For instance, nephrotoxicity can often be prevented or minimized by adequately hydrating the patient with intravenous fluids. Drug **extravasation** (see Box 48-2 in Chapter 48) occurs when an intravenous catheter punctures the vein and medication leaks (infiltrates) into the surrounding tissues. With cancer chemotherapy in

particular, this leakage can cause severe tissue damage and even *necrosis* (tissue death) if the drug has vesicant properties. Extravasation antidotes for select alkylating drugs are listed in Table 49-3.

Interactions

Only a few alkylating drugs are capable of causing significant drug interactions. The most important rule for preventing such drug interactions is to avoid administering an alkylating drug with any other drug capable of causing similar toxicities. For example, a major adverse effect of cisplatin is nephrotoxicity. Therefore, if possible, it should not be administered with a drug such as an aminoglycoside antibiotic (gentamicin, tobramycin, or amikacin) because of the resulting additive nephrotoxic effect and hence increased likelihood of kidney failure. Mechlorethamine and cyclophosphamide, both of which have significant bone marrow–suppressing effects, ideally should not be administered with radiation therapy or with other drugs that suppress the bone marrow. These two drugs, as well as cisplatin, should not be given with probenecid or sulfinpyrazone, both of which

TABLE 49-2

Commonly Used Alkylating Drugs: Severe Adverse Effects

Alkylating Drug	Severe Adverse Effects
busulfan	Pulmonary fibrosis
carboplatin	Less nephrotoxicity and neurotoxicity but more bone marrow suppression
cisplatin	Nephrotoxicity, peripheral neuropathy, ototoxicity
cyclophosphamide	Hemorrhagic cystitis

TABLE 49-3

Alkylating Drug Extravasation: Specific Antidotes

Alkylating Drug	Antidote Preparation	Method
carmustine	Mix equal parts 1 mmol/mL sodium bicarbonate (premixed) with sterile NS (1:1 solution); resulting solution is 0.5 mmol/mL.	1. Inject 2–6 mL IV through the existing line with multiple SC injections into the extravasated site. 2. Apply cold compresses. 3. Total dose should not exceed 10 mL of 0.5 mmol/mL solution.
mechlorethamine	Mix 4 mL 10% sodium thiosulfate with 6 mL sterile water for injection.	1. Inject 5–6 mL IV through the existing line with multiple SC injections into the extravasated site. 2. Repeat SC injections over the next few hours. 3. Apply cold compresses. 4. No total dose has been established.

IV, intravenous; *NS*, normal saline; *SC*, subcutaneous.

are *uricosuric drugs* used to treat gout. This combination can result in hyperuricemia or exacerbation of gout because of competition for kidney elimination between these drugs and the molecules of normal body uric acid waste product. In general, the nurse should work with available pharmacy and oncology staff to proactively anticipate (and avoid, if possible) undesirable drug and treatment interactions.

Dosages

For the recommended dosages of selected alkylating drugs, see the Dosages table below.

 DRUG PROFILES

The most widely used alkylating drugs, based on standard treatment protocols, are profiled here. Information for these and for some of the less commonly used drugs also appears in the Dosages table below.

▶▶ cisplatin

Cisplatin (generic only) is an antineoplastic drug that contains platinum in its chemical structure. It is classified as a probable alkylating drug because it is believed to destroy cancer cells in the same way as the classic alkylating drugs, by forming cross-links with DNA and thereby preventing its replication. It is also considered a bifunctional alkylating drug.

Cisplatin is used for the treatment of many solid tumours, such as bladder, testicular, and ovarian tumours. It is available only in injectable form. Cisplatin has a half-life of approximately 30 minutes after a bolus or intravenous infusion (over 2 to 7 hours). The platinum complexes of cisplatin become bound to plasma proteins and have a half-life of approximately 5 days. Platinum may be present in body tissues for 180 days after the final administration.

▶▶ cyclophosphamide

Cyclophosphamide (Procytox) is a nitrogen mustard derivative that was discovered during the course of research to improve mechlorethamine. It is a polyfunctional alkylating drug and is used in the treatment of cancers of the bone and lymph, as well as solid tumours. Various leukemias, Hodgkin's and non-Hodgkin's lymphomas, multiple myeloma, and some sarcomas may also respond to cyclophosphamide therapy. It is available in both oral and injectable dosage forms. Cyclophosphamide has an average half-life of 7 hours for adults and 4 hours for children.

▶▶ mechlorethamine hydrochloride

Mechlorethamine hydrochloride (nitrogen mustard) (Mustargen) is the prototypical alkylating drug. It is a nitrogen analogue of sulfur mustard (mustard gas) that was used for chemical warfare in World War I. As noted earlier, mechlorethamine was the first alkylating antineoplastic drug discovered, and its beneficial effects in the treatment of cancers were discovered after the war. Some of the cancers it is used to treat are Hodgkin's lymphoma, other lymphomas, and chronic leukemia.

Mechlorethamine is a bifunctional alkylating drug capable of forming cross-links between two DNA nucleotides, which interferes with RNA transcription and prevents cell division and protein synthesis. It is effective on rapidly proliferating cells. It is available in a parenteral form only, for administration intravenously or by an intracavitary route, such as intrapleurally or intraperitoneally.

DOSAGES   Selected Alkylating Drugs

Drug (Pregnancy Category)	Pharmacological Subclass	Usual Dosage Range*	Indications
altretamine (Hexalen) (D)	Methylmelamine	PO: 260 mg/m²/day, divided into 4 doses, for 14–21 consecutive days for 28-day cycles	Recurrent ovarian cancer
carmustine (BiCNU) (D)	Nitrosourea	IV: 200 mg/m² q6wk	Brain tumours, multiple myeloma, HL, NHL, melanoma, gastrointestinal carcinoma
▶▶ cisplatin (generic only) (D)	Platinum coordination complex	*Children/Adult* IV: 50–75 mg/m² q3–4 wk or 15–20 mg/m² daily × 5 days q3–4 wk	Palliation for metastatic testicular and ovarian cancers, and bladder cancer. Other off-label uses: brain tumours, esophageal, head, neck, lung, and cervical cancer
▶▶ cyclophosphamide (Procytox) (D)	Classic alkylator	IV: 100 mg/m² daily × 14 days (many other regimens as well)	HL, NHL; leukemia, breast and ovarian cancer; retinoblastoma; almost every solid tumour
▶▶ mechlorethamine hydrochloride (Mustargen) (D)	Classic alkylator	IV: 0.4 mg/kg each cycle of chemotherapy	HL, NHL, leukemia, bronchogenic carcinoma, others

Continued

DOSAGES	Selected Alkylating Drugs (cont'd)		
Drug (Pregnancy Category)	Pharmacological Subclass	Usual Dosage Range*	Indications
temozolomide (Temodal) (D)	Imidazotetrazine derivative	PO: 150 mg/m² once daily for 5 consecutive days per 28-day treatment cycle	Recurrent anaplastic astrocytoma, glioblastoma
thiotepa (D) Available through Special Access Programme	Ethylenimines	IV: 0.3–0.4 mg/kg at 1- to 4-wk intervals	Breast, ovarian, or bladder cancer; HL, NHL

HL, Hodgkin's lymphoma; *IV*, intravenous; *NHL*, non-Hodgkin's lymphoma; *PO*, oral.

*Dosages listed are for adults unless indicated otherwise.

CYTOTOXIC ANTIBIOTICS

The cytotoxic antibiotics consist of natural substances produced by the mould *Streptomyces* as well as synthetic substances not produced by this mould. Although they all have the ability to kill bacteria and, in some cases, even viruses, they are normally used only for the treatment of cancer because of their toxicity. While cytotoxic antibiotics differ from other antineoplastic drugs in the toxicities they cause, all of them can produce bone marrow suppression, except bleomycin, which can cause pulmonary toxicity (pulmonary fibrosis and pneumonitis). Other severe toxicities associated with the use of cytotoxic antibiotics are heart failure (daunorubicin) and, rarely, acute left ventricular failure (doxorubicin). The available cytotoxic antibiotics, categorized according to the specific subclass to which they belong, are as follows:

Anthracyclines
- daunorubicin
- doxorubicin hydrochloride
- epirubicin
- idarubicin
- valrubicin

Other cytotoxic antibiotics
- bleomycin (which is actually a cell cycle–specific drug)
- dactinomycin
- mitomycin
- mitoxantrone

Mechanism of Action and Drug Effects

Cytotoxic antibiotic antineoplastic drugs are primarily cell cycle–nonspecific drugs, although some, such as daunorubicin, are more active in the S phase. In most cases, however, the drugs are active during all phases of the cell cycle. Most act either through alkylation or by a process called *intercalation*, in which the drug molecule is inserted between the two strands of a DNA molecule; this process is very similar to the way in which antineoplastic antimetabolites work (Chapter 48) and ultimately blocks DNA synthesis. Specifically, the drug binds to the nucleotide base pairs of the DNA helix, causing the shape of the DNA helix to change

into an unstable structure. The result is the blockade of DNA, RNA, and protein synthesis. Some cytotoxic antibiotic drugs can block all three, but others affect DNA synthesis only.

Indications

Cytotoxic antibiotics are used to treat a variety of solid tumours and some hematological malignancies as well. Common examples of these drugs and the malignancies they are used to treat are given in the Dosages table on p. 921.

Adverse Effects

As with all of the antineoplastic drugs, cytotoxic antibiotics have the undesirable effects of hair loss, nausea and vomiting, and myelosuppression. The emetic potential of the drugs in this category is given in Box 48-1. Major adverse effects specific to the cytotoxic antibiotics are listed in Table 49-4.

Toxicity and Management of Overdose

Severe cases of cardiomyopathy are associated with large cumulative doses of doxorubicin. Routine monitoring of cardiac ejection fraction with multiple-gated acquisition (MUGA) scans, cumulative dose limitations, and the use of cytoprotectant drugs such as dexrazoxane can decrease the incidence of this devastating

TABLE   49-4

Cytotoxic Antibiotics: Severe Adverse Effects

Cytotoxic Antibiotic Drug	Severe Adverse Effects
bleomycin	Pulmonary fibrosis, pneumonitis
dactinomycin, daunorubicin	Liver toxicity, tissue damage in the event of extravasation, heart failure
doxorubicin, idarubicin	Liver and cardiovascular toxicities
mitomycin	Liver, kidney, and lung toxicities
mitoxantrone	Cardiovascular toxicity
plicamycin	Tissue damage secondary to extravasation

toxicity. Box 49-1 outlines the management of doxorubicin extravasation.

Interactions

The cytotoxic antibiotics used in chemotherapy interact with many drugs. They all tend to produce increased toxicities when used in combination with other chemotherapeutic drugs or with radiation therapy. Some drugs, most notably bleomycin and doxorubicin, have been known to cause serum digoxin levels to increase. Patients receiving one of these drugs along with digoxin should be observed for signs of digoxin toxicity. Dosage reduction or elimination of digoxin therapy may be indicated (Chapter 22).

Dosages

For recommended dosages of selected cytotoxic antibiotic drugs, see the Dosages table below.

BOX 49-1

Treatment of Doxorubicin Hydrochloride Extravasation

1. Cool the site to patient tolerance for 24 hours.
2. Elevate and rest the extremity for 24 to 48 hours, then have the patient resume normal activity as tolerated.
3. If pain, erythema, or swelling persists beyond 48 hours, discuss with the physician the need for surgical intervention or other treatment options.

Data from the National Cancer Institute Web site, available at http://www.nci.hih.gov; http://www.bccancer.bc.ca. Internet resources for additional information: http://www. OncoLink.com; http://www.vhpharmsci.com/

 ## DRUG PROFILES

▸▸ doxorubicin hydrochloride

Doxorubicin hydrochloride (Adriamycin) is used in many combination chemotherapy regimens. Its use is contraindicated in patients with a known hypersensitivity to it, patients with severe myelosuppression, and patients who are at risk for severe cardiac toxicity because they have already received a large cumulative dose of any of the anthracycline antineoplastics. It is available only in injectable form. Doxorubicin is also now available in a liposomal drug delivery system (Caelyx, Myocet). In this dosage formulation, the drug is encapsulated in a lipid molecule bilayer called a *liposome*. The advantages of liposomal encapsulation are reduced systemic toxicity and increased duration of action. Liposomal encapsulation extends the biological half-life of doxorubicin to 50 to 60 hours and increases its affinity for cancer cells. The liposomal dosage formulation is currently indicated for the treatment of Kaposi's sarcoma, which primarily affects individuals infected with HIV that causes AIDS, and for metastatic breast cancer.

mitoxantrone hydrochloride

Mitoxantrone hydrochloride (generic) is indicated for the initial treatment of acute nonlymphocytic leukemia and metastatic carcinoma of the breast. It is also indicated for relapsed adult leukemia and for patients with lymphoma or hepatoma. It is available only in injectable form.

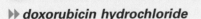

DOSAGES   Selected Cytotoxic Antibiotics

Drug (Pregnancy Category)	Pharmacological Subclass	Usual Dosage Range*	Indications
ANTHRACYCLINE ANTIBIOTICS			
▸▸doxorubicin hydrochloride, conventional (Adriamycin) (D)	Anthracycline	IV: 60–75 mg/m² as a single injection given q21 days	Multiple cancers, including breast, bone, and ovarian, and leukemia, neuroblastoma, HL, NHL
doxorubicin hydrochloride, liposomal (Caelyx, Myocet) (D)	Anthracycline	IV: 20 mg/m² q3 wk for as long as tolerated and responsive to treatment IV: 50 mg/m² q4 wk	AIDS-related Kaposi's sarcoma when other chemotherapy drugs have failed or patient is intolerant to them Recurrent metastatic ovarian cancer
ANTHRACENEDIONE ANTIBIOTICS			
mitoxantrone hydrochloride (generic) (D)	Anthracenedione	IV: 12 mg/m² q3 wk	Metatastic breast cancer, acute myelocytic leukemia, lymphoma, hepatoma

AIDS, acquired immunodeficiency syndrome; *HL*, Hodgkin's lymphoma; *IV*, intravenous; *NHL*, non-Hodgkin's lymphoma.

*Dosages listed are for adults.

MISCELLANEOUS ANTINEOPLASTICS

The miscellaneous antineoplastic drugs are those that, because of their unique structure and mechanism of action, cannot be classified into the previously described categories. However, some drugs that are originally classified as miscellaneous drugs are later reclassified as more is learned about their mechanisms of action and other characteristics. Drugs currently in the miscellaneous category include bevacizumab, hydroxyurea, imatinib, mitotane, hormonal drugs, and radioactive and related antineoplastic drugs. Selected drugs are profiled in the following sections.

 ## DRUG PROFILES

The drugs in the miscellaneous category of antineoplastics are used to treat a wide range of neoplasms. Hydroxyurea is administered orally. Bevacizumab, imatinib, and mitotane are available only in injectable form.

bevacizumab

Bevacizumab (Avastin) is the first, and currently the only, approved antineoplastic drug in a new category—*angiogenesis inhibitors*. It was approved in 2005 by Health Canada. *Angiogenesis* is the creation of new blood vessels that supply oxygen and other blood nutrients to growing tissues. In the case of malignant (and even benign) tumours, angiogenesis that occurs within the tumour mass promotes continued tumour growth. As a tumour enlarges, its central tissues gradually die off (*necrosis*). However, its outer portion continues to grow, often to fatal proportions, with blood supplied through angiogenesis. Thus, inhibiting this process offers a promising new mechanism for antineoplastic drug action. Bevacizumab is a recombinant "humanized" monoclonal immunoglobulin G1 antibody derived from mouse, or *murine,* antibodies. (The scientific name for any compound derived from mouse tissue is *murine.*) *Humanization* refers to the use of recombinant DNA techniques to make animal-derived antibody proteins more genetically similar to those of humans. Immunoglobulin G1 is a subtype of *immunoglobulin G*, the principal class of antibodies produced by mammalian immune systems (Chapter 47). This drug works by binding to and inhibiting the biological activity of human *vascular endothelial growth factor (VEGF)*. VEGF is an endogenous protein that normally promotes angiogenesis in the body.

Bevacizumab in combination with paclitaxel is currently indicated for the treatment of patients with metastatic HER2-negative breast cancer who are palliative. There are no data indicating that disease-related symptoms are improved or that survival results are increased by use of bevacizumab. Bevacizumab in combination with carboplatin/paclitaxel chemotherapy regimen is indicated for the treatment of patients with unresectable advanced, metastatic or recurrent nonsquamous, non–small cell lung cancer. It is also used for metastatic colorectal cancer.

Bevacizumab is available only in injectable form. The only recognized contraindication is severe drug allergy or allergy to other murine products. Adverse reactions include those affecting the cardiovascular system (hypertension or hypotension, thrombosis), central nervous system (CNS) (pain, headache, dizziness), skin (alopecia, dry skin), metabolism (weight loss, hypokalemia), gastrointestinal tract (nausea, vomiting, diarrhea), kidneys (nephrotoxicity with proteinuria), and respiratory tract (infection). More severe effects can occur in any of these systems but are much less common than those listed. Reported drug interactions are limited but include potentiation of the cardiotoxic effects of the anthracycline antibiotics such as doxorubicin.

hydroxyurea

Hydroxyurea (Hydrea) most closely resembles the antimetabolite antineoplastics in its actions. It interferes with the synthesis of DNA by inhibiting the incorporation of thymidine into DNA. It works primarily in the S and G_1 phases of the cell cycle, which makes it a cell cycle–specific drug. It is indicated for concomitant use with irradiation therapy in the treatment of primary squamous cell (epidermoid) carcinomas of the head and neck, excluding the lip. Hydroxyurea may also be used to treat melanoma and resistant chronic myelocytic leukemia. The drug is available only in oral form. Adverse reactions include edema, drowsiness, headache, rash, hyperuricemia, nausea, vomiting, dysuria, myelosuppression, elevated liver enzyme levels, muscular weakness, peripheral neuropathy, nephrotoxicity, dyspnea, and pulmonary fibrosis. Drugs with which it interacts include the anti-HIV drugs zidovudine, zalcitabine, and didanosine (Chapter 40), all of which can actually have a synergistic effect with hydroxyurea. Concurrent use with fluorouracil increases the risk of neurotoxic symptoms. Because hydroxyurea can reduce the clearance of cytarabine, dosage reduction of cytarabine is recommended when the two are used concurrently. Peak plasma levels are reached in 1 to 4 hours after an oral dose.

imatinib mesylate

Imatinib mesylate (Gleevec) is indicated for the treatment of chronic myeloid leukemia (CML), particularly after failure of interferon alfa therapy. It is one of the newest available antineoplastic drugs, approved by Health Canada Notice of Compliance with Conditions on the basis of promising evidence of clinical effectiveness in 2007. It works by inhibiting the action of a key enzyme (protein-tyrosine kinase) that plays an important role in the CML disease process. Although its name sounds similar to those of some monoclonal antibody drugs, imatinib is not a monoclonal antibody. It is available only in oral form.

Common adverse reactions include fatigue, headache, rash, fluid retention, gastrointestinal and hematological effects, musculoskeletal pain, cough, and dyspnea; more severe effects occur less commonly for most body

Continued

systems. Potential drug interactions are quite numerous because they primarily involve drugs metabolized by the cytochrome P450 group of liver enzymes. Concurrent use of acetaminophen increases the risk of hepatotoxicity, for example. There are also many other potentially interacting drugs, too numerous to list here. Major examples include amiodarone, verapamil, warfarin, azole antifungals, antidepressants, and antibiotics. A pharmacist may be needed to review the patient's medication regimen and adjust dosages or delete medications accordingly, in collaboration with the patient's prescriber.

mitotane

Mitotane (Lysodren) is an adrenal cytotoxic drug that is indicated specifically for the treatment of inoperable adrenal corticoid carcinoma. It is available only in oral form. Adverse reactions include CNS depression, rash, nausea, vomiting, muscle weakness, and headache. Reported drug interactions include enhanced CNS depressive effects when taken concurrently with other CNS depressants (e.g., benzodiazepines). Mitotane may also increase the clearance of both warfarin and phenytoin, reducing their effects. The potassium-sparing diuretic spironolactone may negate the effects of mitotane.

octreotide

Octreotide (Sandostatin) is a unique medication used for control of symptoms in patients with metastatic carcinoid and vasoactive intestinal peptide-secreting tumours. It is also used in patients with acromegaly (Chapter 30).

DOSAGES   Miscellaneous Antineoplastics

Drug (Pregnancy Category)	Pharmacological Class	Usual Dosage Range*	Indications
bevacizumab (Avastin) (D)	Angiogenesis inhibitor	IV: 5 mg/kg once q14 days	Metastatic colorectal cancer
		IV: 10 mg/kg given wk 1 and 3 of each 4-wk cycle	Metastatic breast cancer
		IV: 15 mg/kg given once q3wk	Locally advanced, metastatic or recurrent non–small cell lung cancer
hydroxyurea (Hydrea) (D)	Antineoplastic agent	PO: 80 mg/kg as single dose every third day	Solid tumours and concomitant use with irradiation therapy
imatinib mesylate (Gleevec) (D)	Protein kinase inhibitor	*Children* PO: 340 mg/m²/day (rounded to the nearest 100 mg (not to exceed 600 mg/day) *Adult* PO: 400 mg/day *Adult* PO: 400–600 mg/day	Chronic myeloid leukemia (CML) Gastrointestinal stromal tumours
mitotane (Lysodren) (D)	Antineoplastic agent	PO: 2–6 g/day, divided tid–qid, increased as quickly as possible to 8–10 g/day or higher	Inoperable adrenal cortical carcinoma
octreotide (Sandostatin) (D)	Synthetic octapeptide analogue of somatostatin	SC: 100–600 mcg/day divided bid–qid	Carcinoid tumours
		SC: 200–300 mcg divided bid–qid during initial 2 wk of therapy to control symptoms, adjusted to therapeutic range	Vasoactive intestinal peptide-secreting tumours
		SC: 200–300 mcg/day	Acromegaly

IV, intravenous; *PO,* oral; *SC,* subcutaneous.

*Dosages listed are for adults unless indicated otherwise.

HORMONAL ANTINEOPLASTICS

Hormonal drugs are used in the treatment of a variety of neoplasms in both males and females. The rationale is that sex hormones act to accelerate the growth of some common types of malignant tumours, especially certain types of breast and prostate cancers. Therefore, therapy may involve administration of hormones with opposing effects (i.e., male vs. female hormones) or drugs that block the body's sex hormone receptors. These drugs are used most commonly as palliative and adjuvant therapy. For certain types of cancer they may also be used as drugs of first choice. Some of the more commonly used hormonal drugs for female-specific neoplasms such as breast cancer are tamoxifen, megestrol, medroxyprogesterone, and fulvestrant. For male-specific neoplasms such as prostate cancer, bicalutamide, flutamide, nilutamide, leuprolide, goserelin, and estramustine are used (see Table 49-1).

RADIOPHARMACEUTICALS AND RELATED ANTINEOPLASTICS

Antineoplastic drugs that are usually administered only by physicians include porfimer sodium and various radioactive pharmaceuticals (radiopharmaceuticals). Porfimer sodium is used to treat esophageal or bronchial tumours that are present on the surface mucosa. The medication is given intravenously and is followed by one or more sessions of laser light therapy to the esophageal or bronchial mucosa for direct tumour lysis and manual debridement. Radiopharmaceuticals are used to treat a variety of cancers or symptoms caused by cancers. Five commonly used radiopharmaceuticals are chromic phosphate P 32 (for cancer-induced peritoneal or pleural effusions), samarium SM 153 lexidronam (for bone cancer pain), sodium iodide I 131 (for thyroid cancer and hyperthyroidism), sodium phosphate P 32 (for various leukemias and palliative treatment of bone metastases), and strontium Sr 89 chloride (for bone cancer pain). These medications are usually administered by nuclear medicine physician specialists.

CYTOPROTECTIVE DRUGS AND MISCELLANEOUS TOXICITY INHIBITORS

Several drugs are available that are classified as cytoprotective drugs. These medications help to reduce the toxicity of antineoplastics. The decision of whether to use them is often very patient specific, as is the case with chemotherapy regimens. Such decisions are generally made by patients' oncologists. All of these drugs are normally administered intravenously with the exception of allopurinol, which may also be given orally. These medications are listed in Table 49-1 on p. 916; extravasation of irritants versus vesicants was discussed in Chapter 48. For more information related to extravasation and the handling and administration of antineoplastics, see Box 48-2 in Chapter 48, and Boxes 49-1 and 49-2. Also see Lab Values Related to Drug Therapy on p. 925 in this chapter.

NURSING PROCESS

As discussed in Chapter 48, antineoplastic drugs are some of the most toxic medications given to patients. Because of their toxicities, serious complications and adverse effects may occur. Nursing care must be based on a thorough knowledge of cancer and its treatment and the subsequent effects of different treatment modalities, specifically antineoplastic drug therapy, on the patient. The nurse should also bear in mind the potential of medication errors occurring with administration of some of these drugs, such as errors that occur from confusing drugs with "sound-alike" names (see Preventing Medication Errors: Sound-Alike Drugs: "Rubicins"). Whereas Chapter 48 discusses the general adverse effects that occur with most antineoplastic drugs, cell cycle–specific drugs, and antineoplastic enzymes, this discussion relates to cell cycle–nonspecific, hormonal, and miscellaneous antineoplastic drugs.

Assessment

For patients receiving any of the *alkylating drugs*, such as cisplatin and cyclophosphamide, baseline fluid and electrolyte levels, kidney and liver function test results, and

---

BOX 49-2 Concerns in the Handling and Administration of Vesicant Antineoplastic Drugs

The handling and administration of antineoplastic drugs is controversial because the nurse mixing and giving the drug may experience negative consequences. In most institutions, the pharmacy department is responsible for mixing these drugs, and preparation is carried out carefully in an appropriate environment with use of a laminar airflow hood and personal protective equipment (mask, gown, gloves). Many facilities recommend taking special precautions during the care of a patient who is receiving chemotherapy, such as double-flushing the patient's bodily secretions in the commode and using special hampers for the disposal of all items that come into contact with the patient, including used personal protective equipment. Special spill kits are employed to clean up even the smallest chemotherapy spills. These precautions are necessary to protect the health care provider from the cytotoxic effects of these drugs. In addition, appropriate and updated knowledge about these drugs is important to safe and appropriate nursing care.

All nurses must be certified to administer chemotherapy and must remain current in their level of practice and competencies related to this treatment modality. All equipment and containers should be handled appropriately once the infusion is completed, and the hands and any exposed area must be washed to ensure the safety of the health care provider. The British Columbia Cancer Agency (http://www.bccancer.bc.ca/default.htm) and the Canadian Association of Nurses in Oncology (http://www.cano-acio.ca/) offer exceptional resources for individuals involved in the care of patients receiving chemotherapy.

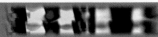

LAB VALUES RELATED TO DRUG THERAPY

Antineoplastic Therapy: Assessment and Monitoring of White Blood Cells and Nadir*

Laboratory Test	Normal Ranges	Rationale for Assessment
Leukocytes (WBCs)	5–10 × 10⁹/L	WBCs are protection against infection, and when an infection develops, the WBCs attack and destroy the causative bacteria, virus, or other organism. In response to the infection, WBCs increase in number dramatically. If WBCs are decreased from antineoplastic treatment and subsequent bone marrow suppression, and should they decrease to levels below 3.5 × 10⁹/L (leukopenia), there is a high risk for severe infection and immunosuppression.

WBC components:
  Neutrophils
  Band neutrophils
	47%–77% or above
	2 × 10⁹/L
	0–3%
		The major types of WBCs are neutrophils, lymphocytes, monocytes, eosinophils, and basophils. Immature neutrophils are called *band neutrophils;* with neutrophil counts, they provide a picture of the patient's immune system. If neutrophils are decreased to levels below 1.8–2 × 10⁹/L (neutropenia), there is risk for severe infection. If band neutrophils are included in the WBC differential count, then the abnormally low value reinforces the risk for severe infection.

Nadir	See normal range of each blood cell	*Nadir* refers to the point in time at which bone marrow cells reach their lowest levels. This time frame may become shorter and recovery longer with successive courses of antineoplastic treatment, with a general estimate of time frame between 10 and 28 days. Anticipation of the nadir allows the oncologist and health care team to develop a preventative treatment plan that may include biological response modifiers and antibiotics.

WBCs, white blood cells.

*Information on red blood cells (RBCs) and platelets is presented in Chapter 48.

complete blood cell counts should be assessed. Specific to alkylating drugs is a loss of vision for light and colour, emesis, nephrotoxicity, and bone marrow suppression; therefore, assessment should include a baseline vision test and determination of any changes in near or far vision or colour vision, which can be accomplished using a Snellen or colour chart. In addition, a baseline abdominal assessment should be performed, with auscultation of bowel sounds and questioning of the patient about any problems with nausea and vomiting. Hyperactive or hypoactive bowel sounds—or none at all—are important to report, and skin turgor, moistness of mucosa, urinary output, and urine colour should be noted. Loss of turgor, dryness, or cracking of the oral mucosa and lips, and decrease in urinary output and dark amber urine are indicative of dehydration as a consequence of nausea and vomiting. Baseline neurological status should be assessed with documentation of level of consciousness, mental clarity, memory, attention, and cognition, and the patient should be questioned about any history of seizures or other CNS disorders because of the potential for drug-related seizures and neurological changes. In addition, peripheral neuropathies are often associated with these drugs, thus the presence of any numbness or tingling of the extremities should be noted. Because of the possibility of loss of or changes in motor function, a thorough assessment of baseline motor function should be performed, with a rating of deep tendon reflexes, gait characteristics, mobility, and degree of independence in activity. Cisplatin may be ototoxic, so baseline hearing should be documented.

Because alkylating drugs may have a profound impact on the patient's nutritional status, this should also be assessed (Chapter 48). Serum levels of albumin and protein as well as fluid and electrolyte values (e.g., sodium, potassium, chloride, magnesium, calcium) should be

PREVENTING MEDICATION ERRORS

Sound-Alike Drugs: "Rubicins"

The anthracycline chemotherapy drugs have the same sound-alike suffix and are often nicknamed the "rubicins." These drugs include daunorubicin, doxorubicin, epirubicin, idarubicin, and valrubicin. Even though these drugs are in the same class, their use and drug effects are different. Medication errors have occurred because one "rubicin" was mistaken for another. It is important to refer to these drugs by their complete names rather than as a "rubicin."

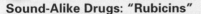

noted. The use of alkylating drugs may also result in hepatotoxicity and kidney damage, so the results of liver and kidney function tests should be assessed. Because bone marrow suppression and pulmonary toxicity may also occur, it is important to know the patient's baseline blood cell counts and to assess for the presence of abnormal to absent breath sounds, irregular breathing patterns, difficulty breathing, cyanosis around the lips or in the fingernails, chest pain, cough with or without sputum, and any other respiratory symptoms. Because of the risk of drug-related cardiac toxicity, it is important to assess for any heart disease. Chest pain; abnormal heart rate and rhythm; abnormal heart sounds, including gallops or murmurs; edema; and other signs or symptoms of heart disorder should be noted.

Some of the major adverse effects associated with the use of *cytotoxic antibiotics* (e.g., doxorubicin) are pulmonary fibrosis and liver toxicity. To determine the impact of the medication on the lungs, assessment should include taking a nursing history with a focus on respiratory functioning (in the past and present); examining the results of pulmonary function studies and the values for arterial blood gas levels and partial pressures of CO_2 and O_2; evaluating breath sounds, breathing rate, rhythm, and depth; and noting the results of radiographic examination of the chest. When intravenous sites are not patent and become infiltrated from *extravasation*, or leakage of the drug into surrounding tissues, necrosis may occur, with sloughing of the layers of skin and underlying supportive structures (e.g., muscles, ligaments). (See previous discussion of extravasation in the pharmacology section, including Table 49-3 and Box 49-2.) Because tissue necrosis can be severe, prevention of infiltration is critical to patient safety, and the intravenous site should be assessed frequently, with attention to the patency of the intravenous line and the appearance of any redness, red streaking above the intravenous site, warmth, or swelling. Assessment of nutritional status, reproductive system, cardiac system, pulmonary system, immune system, and bone marrow functioning is needed before and during drug therapy (see previous discussion for specific information). When doxorubicin is given, patients with documented heart disease may need further diagnostic testing, including electrocardiograms and MUGA scans, to assess cardiac ejection fraction. These tests may also aid in evaluating the effectiveness of the cytoprotective drug dexrazoxane, which is used to help decrease the risk of life-threatening cardiac toxicities.

Hormonal antineoplastics require a thorough assessment of specific systems. These antineoplastics include drugs such as corticosteroids, estrogens, estrogen-mustards, selective estrogen receptor modulators (SERMs) or estrogen antagonists (antiestrogens), progestins, androgens, androgen antagonists, gonadotropin-releasing hormone agonists, and aromatase inhibitors. Many of these drugs are discussed in Chapters 34 and 35; the use of these drugs in cancer treatment protocols and their implications for the nursing process are also presented in detail online at http://evolve.elsevier.com/Canada/Lilley/pharmacology/.

Assessment associated with the use of *estrogen antagonists* such as fulvestrant, tamoxifen, and toremifene citrates (SERMs) often begins with the review of any tumour estrogen receptor assays, computed tomographic scans, and other X-rays. Results of complete blood cell counts, clotting studies, liver function studies, lipid profiles, and serum cholesterol and calcium levels should be noted before and during drug therapy so that drug-related changes can be identified early and any appropriate action taken. With the adverse effect of hypercalcemia, signs and symptoms may include constipation, confusion, lethargy, weakness, and changes in urinary patterns. A neurological assessment of sensation, motor strength, and gait is important because of possible asthenia, or loss of strength, in the extremities. Heart function should be assessed and notation made of baseline weight and any existing edema or congestive heart failure. Patients may experience flare-ups of bone pain, so the nurse should be alert to these complaints and note their severity and duration. Should these complaints continue for a prolonged period, the physician should be contacted.

Blood cell counts, hemoglobin level, hematocrit, blood pressure, and weight should be measured before and during the use of *androgens* (e.g., testosterone). Serum cholesterol level, lipid levels, and levels of electrolytes and liver enzymes should be measured before the initiation of therapy, if ordered. Assessment of urinary patterns and any complaints should be noted. It is also important to understand the reason for the use of these hormones in cancer patients, such as the administration of androgens in cases of advanced breast cancer to promote tumour regression. The emotional turmoil that may be associated with advanced disease is, in itself, important to consider, as are the patient's feelings about treatment with a hormone that leads to masculine secondary sexual characteristics such as growth of body hair, lowering of the voice, and muscle growth in female patients (with long-term treatment). See Chapter 35 and http://evolve.elsevier.com/Canada/Lilley/pharmacology/ for more information.

Flutamide and leuprolide are *antiandrogens* and require assessment of baseline kidney and liver function and blood cell counts. Because flutamide may cause liver failure, the nurse needs to watch for nausea, vomiting, jaundice or yellowish discoloration of the skin or eye area, dark yellow urine, flulike symptoms, abdominal pain, extreme fatigue, and loss of appetite. Weight and height are important to note, and a nutritional assessment should be carried out (Chapter 48). Urinary patterns and sexual functioning are also important to assess with attention to any existing problems or difficulties. Existing heart disease and any edematous conditions should be noted because edema may occur with these drugs and the extra fluid volume could exacerbate existing disease states. The patient's history should be examined for the presence of glucose-6-phosphate dehydrogenase deficiency because this disorder would be a possible contraindication to the use of flutamide. Documentation of the use of a reliable form of birth control is important because of the possibility of teratogenic effects with use of these drugs. Male sperm production may be affected (Chapter 48), and men may experience a decline in sexual functioning, desire, and ability.

With the use of *gonadotropin-releasing hormone agonists*, such as leuprolide and goserelin, the patient must be assessed for any allergies to the drugs. It is important to know the patient's contraceptive history because women who are taking these drugs must use a nonhormonal contraceptive. Often the physician will order laboratory tests for male patients for serum testosterone level and prostatic acid phosphatase level before and during therapy; an increase is normally noted during the initial week of therapy and then levels return to baseline by 4 weeks. Assessment of the cardiac system should include evaluation of heart sounds, pulse rate and rhythm, blood pressure, weight, and presence of edema. Difficulty in passing urine may worsen for a short period with initiation of goserelin therapy, so urinary patterns need to be documented prior to therapy.

Exemestane is a drug used in women whose breast cancer has progressed during treatment with tamoxifen. Baseline respiratory and heart function is important to document because the drug can cause cough, hoarseness, laboured breathing, shortness of breath, edema of the extremities, and tightness in the chest.

For patients taking *antiadrenal drugs* (e.g., mitotane), basic assessment includes recording drug allergies, measuring vital signs, taking a medical and medication history, and identifying conditions that represent cautions or contraindications to drug use as well as possible drug interactions. Because of the common adverse effects of skin darkening, diarrhea, loss of appetite, mental depression, and nausea and vomiting, it is important to complete an assessment and to document baseline findings such as bowel sounds, skin colour and turgor, results of a mental health status examination, and patient 24-hour recall of dietary intake.

◪ Nursing Diagnoses

- Activity intolerance related to drug-induced anemia with fatigue and lethargy
- Anxiety related to the unknowns of therapy and illness
- Disturbed body image related to drug-induced alopecia, darkening of the skin, and sexual dysfunction (such as is seen with cyclophosphamide, nitrosoureas, and other alkylating drugs)
- Decreased cardiac output related to the cardiotoxicity associated with cytotoxic antibiotics
- Diarrhea related to the adverse effects of antineoplastic drugs
- Disturbed sensory perception (hearing loss, optic neuritis) as a result of ototoxicity associated with cisplatin

- Imbalanced nutrition, less than body requirements, related to loss of appetite, nausea, vomiting, stomatitis, and changes in taste as a result of antineoplastic therapy
- Impaired urinary elimination related to the adverse effects of cyclophosphamide (hemorrhagic cystitis and nephrotoxicity)
- Ineffective breathing pattern related to the pulmonary toxicity associated with some antineoplastic drugs
- Risk for injury due to loss of reflexes, numbness of the hands and feet, and ataxia from cisplatin-related neurotoxicity

◪ Planning

◧ Goals

- Patient will maintain as healthy a diet as possible, with adequate intake of protein, vitamins, and other nutrients, to increase energy and stamina and allow continued performance of the activities of daily living during antineoplastic treatment.
- Patient will maintain an intact and healthy body image and effective coping mechanisms while experiencing alopecia, skin changes, and sexual dysfunction associated with antineoplastic therapy.
- Patient will express concerns, fears, and anxieties associated with changes in body image.
- Patient's cardiac output will remain within normal limits while the patient is taking antineoplastics.
- Patient will state the foods and fluids that should be avoided to prevent further gastrointestinal irritation and is able to identify foods that help bulk up stool and minimize problems from diarrhea.
- Patient will remain safe and free from injury with minimal neurological, sensory, and motor deficits from the adverse effects of antineoplastic therapy.
- Patient will receive consultation regarding appropriate dietary intake and fluid and electrolyte needs, help with meal planning, grocery shopping tips, and information on the use of food groups and medications, as ordered, to prevent problems of nutritional imbalance.
- Patient will regain normal urinary patterns during and after antineoplastic therapy.

◧ Outcome Criteria

- Patient openly expresses any anxieties, fears, concerns, or feelings of being upset or depressed about changes in body image and self-concept and seeks out appropriate resources for help in coping, such as spiritual support, therapeutic touch, counselling, and talking with family, friends, and other individuals with cancer who are trained to visit cancer patients. Such individuals can be located through the Canadian Cancer Society and community support groups.
- Patient adheres to a daily "heart-healthy" regimen of conserving energy, planning activities, and monitoring

pulse rate and blood pressure in a consistent routine and asks for assistance with care and activities as needed.

- Patient adheres to a daily regimen for increasing urinary health, such as forcing fluids, consuming fluids that minimize urinary infections (e.g., cranberry juice), and maintaining daily hydration while on antineoplastic therapy.
- Patient states measures to follow for pulmonary health, such as avoiding individuals with influenza, colds, fever, or other illnesses; avoiding smoking and exposure to second-hand smoke; coughing and performing deep breathing frequently during waking hours; forcing fluids; and taking prophylactic antibiotic therapy, if deemed necessary.
- Patient states ways to minimize risk for injury (from neurological adverse effects), such as removing throw rugs and furniture that may lead to falls in the home, using assistive devices such as a walker or cane, having a bedside commode available, installing night lights, and instituting other measures to aid mobility.

See Chapter 48 for additional nursing diagnoses, goals, and outcome criteria that may be relevant to the discussion here.

Implementation

With *alkylating* drugs, such as cisplatin and cyclophosphamide, the patient should expect problems related to bone marrow suppression, such as anemia, leukopenia, and thrombocytopenia. Stomatitis is common, as are nausea, vomiting, and diarrhea. Nursing considerations related to these adverse effects are discussed in Chapter 48; however, there are other interventions that can be used with this group of antineoplastic drugs. Vital signs should be measured every 1 to 2 hours during infusion of these drugs (vital signs should be measured for all antineoplastic drugs). Hydration is critical to prevention of adverse effects; if output is less than 100 mL/hr, the physician should be contacted. Patients at home after treatment with alkylating drugs should be reminded of the importance of hydration and should be told to contact the physician if they experience dry mucous membranes, dark amber urine, vomiting of large amounts over a period of 8 hours or less or little or no urinary output. Intravenous infusions are to be administered per guidelines and policy, and solutions must be protected from light. Any ringing or roaring in the ears or hearing loss should be reported because of the potential for ototoxicity associated with several alkylating drugs. Peripheral neuropathies may occur, so numbness, tingling, or pain in the extremities should be reported immediately to prevent complications and enhance comfort. Cyclophosphamide is known to cause all of the symptoms mentioned here as well as hemorrhagic cystitis. Hydration before and during therapy is important to prevent a negative impact on the bladder and minimize the adverse effect. Because

of its possible carcinogenic, mutagenic, and teratogenic properties, the drug should be handled and administered with extreme caution.

Some alkylating drugs may be nephrotoxic, thus frequent monitoring of kidney function test results is required after therapy has begun. Hydration should be encouraged, with intake of up to 3000 mL/day if not contraindicated. Drug-induced neuropathies may occur, so the patient should be encouraged to avoid extremely cold temperatures or the handling of cold objects during the infusion because this may exacerbate the toxicity. Pulmonary toxicity may occur with some of the alkylating drugs, so the nurse should be alert to cough, shortness of breath, and abnormal breath sounds. These adverse effects should be reported immediately to the physician.

Aluminum needles or administration sets should not be used with many of these drugs because aluminum can degrade the platinum compounds in them; it is important that the nurse ensure that the proper infusion equipment is used. Other drugs in this group may be given by various routes, such as intrapericardial, intratumoural, and intravesical routes, so appropriate interventions will need to be performed per the manufacturer's guidelines or hospital policy. Parenteral reconstitution of any of these drugs should be performed according to the manufacturer's guidelines and suggestions because not all diluents are compatible.

As with all antineoplastic drugs, the nurse should take sufficient time to discuss the therapy's protocol—times, frequency, and duration of therapy—with the patient, family, and significant others or caregivers. For example, therapy may be given at an outpatient facility for 1 day every 3 weeks, but it may take 8 hours for completion of therapy. Patient assistance with planning, transportation, and meals or snacks is needed for the entire protocol. This treatment can last 3 to 6 months or even longer depending on the drug and the cancer. Community resources are available through social service departments, hospice organizations, home health services, Meals on Wheels programs, church volunteer organizations, and chapters of the Canadian Cancer Society.

Therapy with *cytotoxic antibiotics* is associated with bone marrow suppression, nausea, vomiting, and diarrhea, as well as with most of the other adverse effects discussed earlier for the alkylating drugs. Patients experiencing adverse effects of interstitial pneumonitis may require more frequent monitoring of pulmonary function, such as having chest radiographs taken every 1 to 2 weeks during therapy. Liver and kidney function tests should be monitored throughout therapy. Because hyperuricemia may occur, provision of fluids and hydration are important to minimize this adverse effect (see previous discussion). With daunorubicin in particular, the patient should be informed that the urine may turn a reddish colour for a few days after the treatment. Knowing about this effect will help ease any fears or anxieties. Stomatitis is more severe with some of these drugs, and ulceration of the mucous membranes may occur within 2 or 3 days. See Chapter 48 for further information about stomatitis, alopecia, diarrhea, nausea, vomiting, fatigue, various anemias, neutropenia, and thrombocytopenia. Cardiac toxicity may also occur, so heart and breath sounds should be checked frequently and daily weights recorded (with reporting of an increase of 2 pounds or more in 24 hours or 5 pounds or more in a week).

Use of *estrogens*, *progestins*, *testosterone*, and hormone antagonists in the treatment of various neoplasms is somewhat common. Associated nursing interventions and patient education for the use of these hormones are discussed in depth in Chapters 34 and 35. *Corticosteroids* and related nursing considerations are presented in Chapter 33. Further information and discussion regarding the use of hormones and hormone antagonists in the treatment of patients with various types of cancer can also be found online at http://evolve.elsevier.com/Canada/Lilley/pharmacology/.

Hydroxyurea is used in a variety of treatment protocols. When this drug is given and throughout therapy, platelet and leukocyte counts should be monitored in order to avoid harm to the patient. If the platelet count falls below $100 \times 10^9/L$ or leukocyte count falls below $2.5 \times 10^9/L$, the therapy may need to be temporarily interrupted until counts rise toward the normal values. See earlier discussion of nursing considerations associated with treatment of anemias, fatigue, weakness, bleeding tendencies, and infection.

Etoposide is given intravenously, so the precautions for handling and administering other antineoplastics also apply here. The drug should be given with proper diluents and at the appropriate rate. During therapy, the patient should be closely monitored for signs and symptoms of infection, anemia, bleeding tendencies, and stomatitis, with appropriate interventions implemented (Chapter 48). Nursing considerations for teniposide are similar to those for the previous enzyme, but the drug should be prepared and administered in glass or polyolefin containers; PVC containers should be avoided. Intravenous infusions should be given slowly and as ordered with supportive measures available should allergic reaction occur.

In addition to the nursing interventions discussed earlier and in Chapter 48, it is highly recommended that epinephrine, antihistamines, and anti-inflammatories be kept available in case of an allergic or anaphylactic reaction. Each antineoplastic drug has its own peculiarities and its own set of cautions, contraindications, nursing implementations, and toxicities. Cytoprotective drugs are useful in reducing certain toxicities, such as the use of intravenous amifostine to reduce kidney toxicity associated with cisplatin, or the use of intravenous or oral allopurinol to reduce hyperuricemia (see Tables 48-7 and 48-8). Other major concerns related to the care of patients receiving chemotherapy are the oncological emergencies that arise because of the damage that occurs to rapidly dividing normal cells as well as rapidly dividing cancerous cells. Some of the complications identified as emergencies are infections, pulmonary toxicity, allergic reactions, stomatitis with severe ulcerations; bleeding; metabolic aberrations; bowel irritability with diarrhea; and kidney, liver, and cardiac toxicity (Box 49-3).

Evaluation

Evaluation of nursing care should centre on determining whether goals and outcomes have been met, as well as on monitoring for therapeutic responses and adverse effects or toxic effects of antineoplastic therapy. Therapeutic responses may manifest as clinical improvement, decrease in tumour size, and decrease in metastatic spread. Evaluation of nursing care with reference to goals and outcomes may reveal improvements related to a decrease in adverse effects; a decrease in the impact of cancer on the patient's well-being; an increase in comfort, nutrition, and hydration; improved energy levels and ability to carry out the activities of daily living; and improved quality of life. The goals and outcomes can be revisited to identify more specific areas to monitor. In addition, certain laboratory studies such as measurement of tumour marker levels, levels of carcinoembryonic antigens, and red blood cell, white blood cell, and platelet counts may also be used to determine how well the goals and outcomes have been met. As part of the evaluation, physicians may order additional radiographs, computed tomographic scans, magnetic resonance images, tissue analyses, and other studies appropriate to the diagnosis during and after antineoplastic therapy, at time intervals related to anticipated tumour response.

> **BOX 49-3**
>
> ### Indications of an Oncological Emergency
>
> - A cough that is new and persistent
> - Bleeding gums
> - Blood in the stools
> - Blood in the urine
> - Changes in bladder function or patterns
> - Changes in gastrointestinal or bowel patterns, including "heartburn" or nausea, vomiting, constipation, or diarrhea lasting longer than 2 or 3 days
> - Dry, burning, "scratchy," or "swollen" throat
> - Fever and chills with a temperature higher than 38.1°C
> - New sores or white patches in the mouth or throat
> - Swollen tongue with or without cracks and bleeding
>
> Note: The patient should contact the physician immediately if any of the listed signs or symptoms occurs. If the physician is not available, the patient should seek medical treatment at the closest emergency department.

PATIENT EDUCATION

❖ Patients should be educated about avoiding aspirin, ibuprofen, or products containing these drugs to help prevent excessive bleeding.

❖ Patients should be educated about the risk of alopecia (hair loss) before drug therapy begins. They should be provided the opportunity to discuss options for hair and scalp care, including the option of having their hair cut short before treatment and selecting and purchasing or renting a wig or hairpiece comparable to the existing hair in colour, texture, length, and style, or having bandannas, scarves, or hats on hand before the hair is actually lost. Although hair loss is temporary, patients need to be informed that it will occur and that wigs and hairpieces are available through the Canadian Cancer Society.

❖ Patients should be encouraged to increase fluid intake to up to 3000 mL/day, if not contraindicated, to prevent dehydration and further weakening and,

in the case of cyclophosphamide, to prevent or help manage hemorrhagic cystitis.

❖ Patients should be informed about ways to help manage constipation or diarrhea depending on the specific antineoplastic drug given, as well as the use of certain narcotics for pain management. To help avoid constipation, forcing of fluids and consumption of a balanced diet are important; however, the oncologist generally orders either a stool softener or a mild noncramping laxative to prevent the problem. Diarrhea is generally treated by dietary restrictions and use of antidiarrheals as ordered.

❖ Patients should be informed of the following helpful online resources for the patient and significant others: http://www.bccancer.bc.ca/; http://www.hc-sc.gc.ca/hl-vs; http://www.who.int/en; and http://www.oncolink.upenn.edu.

POINTS TO REMEMBER

❖ *Antineoplastics* are drugs used to treat malignancies and are classified as cell cycle–specific drugs, cell cycle–nonspecific drugs, miscellaneous antineoplastics, and hormonal drugs.

❖ Cell cycle–specific drugs kill cancer cells during specific phases of the cell growth cycle, whereas the cell cycle–nonspecific drugs discussed in this chapter kill cancer cells during any phase of the growth cycle.

❖ Chemotherapy, or antineoplastic drug therapy, requires very astute nursing care, and the nurse must act prudently and make critical decisions about the nursing care of patients receiving these drugs.

❖ Pertinent knowledge is important to ensure patient safety and to protect the nurse from the adverse effects of antineoplastics. Extreme caution must be exercised in the handling and administration of cell cycle–nonspecific (and cell cycle–specific) drugs.

❖ Hormonal drugs, both agonists and antagonists as well as female and male hormones, are used to treat a variety of malignancies. Some of the more common hormonal drugs for the treatment of female-specific neoplasms such as breast cancer are tamoxifen, megestrol, medroxyprogesterone, and fulvestrant. For male-specific neoplasms such as prostate cancer, the following drugs are used: bicalutamide, flutamide, nilutamide, leuprolide, goserelin, and estramustine. More information is presented at http://evolve.elsevier.com/Canada/Lilley/pharmacology/.

❖ Oncological emergencies occur as a consequence of cell death and may be life threatening. Astute assessment and immediate intervention may help to decrease the severity of the problem or even reduce the occurrence of such emergencies.

EXAMINATION REVIEW QUESTIONS

1 A patient who is receiving chemotherapy with cisplatin has developed pneumonia. The nurse would be concerned about nephrotoxicity if which type of antibiotic was ordered as treatment for the pneumonia at this time?
   a. Sulfa drug
   b. Penicillin
   c. Aminoglycoside
   d. Fluoroquinolone

2 During treatment with doxorubicin, which potentially life-threatening adverse effect must the nurse monitor closely for?
   a. Ototoxicity
   b. Nephrotoxicity
   c. Cardiomyopathy
   d. Peripheral neuritis

3 While teaching a patient who is about to receive cyclophosphamide chemotherapy, which of the following potential adverse effects should the nurse instruct the patient to watch for?
   a. Ototoxicity
   b. Cholinergic diarrhea
   c. Peripheral neuropathy
   d. Hemorrhagic cystitis

4 When chemotherapy with alkylating drugs is planned, which intervention may help to prevent nephrotoxicity?
   a. Limiting fluids before chemotherapy
   b. Monitoring drug levels during chemotherapy
   c. Assessing creatinine clearance during chemotherapy
   d. Hydrating the patient with intravenous fluids before chemotherapy

5 During therapy with the cytotoxic antibiotic bleomycin, which of the following must be assessed to monitor for a potentially serious adverse effect?
   a. Respiratory function
   b. Cranial nerve function
   c. Cardiac ejection fraction
   d. Blood urea nitrogen and creatinine levels

For answers see http://evolve.elsevier.com/Canada/Lilley/pharmacology/.

CRITICAL THINKING ACTIVITIES

1 Compare the management of extravasation of doxorubicin and that of mechlorethamine.

2 Describe bevacizumab (Avastin) and discuss the process of angiogenesis. What is different about the mechanism of action of this drug?

3 How are cytotoxic antibiotics different from regular antibiotics?

For answers see http://evolve.elsevier.com/Canada/Lilley/pharmacology/.

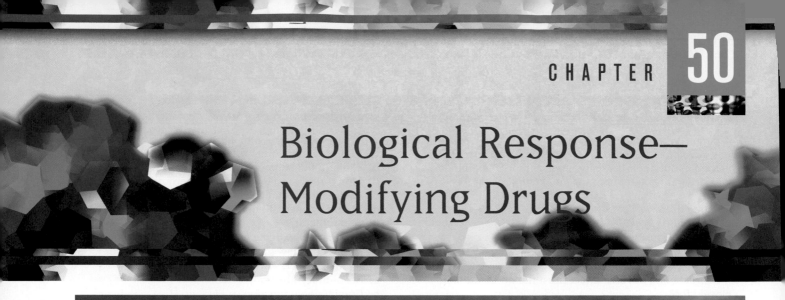

CHAPTER 50

Biological Response– Modifying Drugs

Learning Objectives

After reading this chapter, the successful student will be able to do the following:

1 Describe the basic anatomy, physiology, and functions of the immune system.

2 Compare and discuss the two major classes of biological response– modifying drugs (e.g., hematopoietic drugs, immunomodulating drugs) with regard to their mechanisms of action, indications, dosages and routes of administration, adverse effects, cautions, drug interactions, and contraindications.

3 Develop a collaborative plan of care that includes all phases of the nursing process for patients receiving hematopoietic drugs and immunomodulating drugs.

e-Learning Activities

Web site
(http://evolve.elsevier.com/Canada/Lilley/pharmacology/)

- Animations
- Answers to chapter questions, activities, and case studies
- Calculators and Category Catchers
- Glossary with audio pronunciations
- IV Therapy and Medication Error Checklists
- Multiple-Choice Review Question quizzes
- Nursing Care Plans
- Online Appendices and Supplements
- WebLinks

Drug Profiles

    adalimumab, p. 943
▸▸ **aldesleukin,** p. 946
    alemtuzumab, p. 943
    anakinra, p. 946
    bevacizumab, p. 943
    cetuximab, p. 943
▸▸ **epoetin alfa,** p. 937
▸▸ **filgrastim,** p. 938
    infliximab, p. 943
▸▸ **interferon alfa-2b, interferon alfacon-1, peginterferon alfa-2a, peginterferon alfa-2b,** p. 940
▸▸ **interferon beta-1a, interferon beta-1b,** p. 940
    natalizumab, p. 943
    palivizumab, p. 944
▸▸ **rituximab,** p. 944
    sargramostim, p. 938
    tositumomab (iodine I 131 tositumomab), p. 944
    trastuzumab, p. 944

▸▸ Key drug.

*Full generic name is given in parentheses. For the purposes of this text, the more common shortened name is used.

Glossary

Adjuvant A nonspecific *immunostimulant*—that is, an immunostimulant that somehow enhances overall immune function, rather than stimulating the function of a specific immune system cell or cytokine through specific chemical reactions. (p. 947)

Antibodies Immunoglobulin molecules (Chapter 47) having the ability to bind to and inactivate antigen molecules through formation of an antigen–antibody complex. (p. 934)

Antigen A biological or chemical substance that is recognized as foreign by the body's immune system. (p. 934)

Biological response–modifying drugs A broad class of drugs that includes hematopoietic drugs and immunomodulating drugs. They are also known as biological response modifiers (BRMs). (p. 933)

B lymphocytes (B cells) Leukocytes of the humoral immune system that develop into plasma cells, which produce the antibodies that bind to and inactivate antigens. (p. 934)

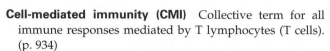

Cell-mediated immunity (CMI)   Collective term for all immune responses mediated by T lymphocytes (T cells). (p. 934)

Colony-stimulating factors (CSFs)   Cytokines that regulate the growth, differentiation, and function of bone marrow stem cells. (p. 936)

Cytokines   The generic term for nonantibody proteins released by specific cell populations (e.g., activated T cells) on contact with antigens. (p. 935)

Cytotoxic T cells   Differentiated T cells that can recognize and lyse (rupture) target cells that bear foreign antigens on their surfaces. (p. 935)

Differentiation   The process of cellular development from a simplified into a more complex and specialized cellular structure. (p. 936)

Hematopoiesis   The collective term for all of the body's processes originating in the bone marrow that result in the formation of various types of blood components. (p. 933)

Humoral immunity   The collective term for all immune responses mediated by B cells, which ultimately work through the production of antibodies against specific antigens. (p. 934)

Immunoglobulins   Complex immune system glycoproteins synthesized by the humoral immune system (B cells) that bind to and inactivate foreign antigens. The term is synonymous with *immune globulins*. (p. 934)

Immunomodulating drugs (IMDs)   Collective term for subclasses of biological response–modifying drugs that specifically or nonspecifically enhance or reduce immune responses (Chapter 46). (p. 934)

Immunostimulant   A drug that enhances immune response through specific and nonspecific chemical interactions with particular immune system components. (p. 947)

Immunosuppressant   A drug that reduces immune response through specific chemical interactions with particular immune system components (Chapter 46). (p. 939)

Interferon (IFN)   One type of cytokine that promotes resistance to viral infection in uninfected cells and can strengthen the body's immune response to cancer cells. (p. 938)

Leukocytes   The collective term for all subtypes of white blood cells. (p. 935)

Lymphokine-activated killer (LAK) cell   Cytotoxic T cells that have been further activated by interkeukin-2 and therefore have a stronger and more specific response against cancer cells. (p. 945)

Lymphokines   Cytokines produced by sensitized T lymphocytes on contact with antigen particles; they serve as chemical mediators of the immune system. (p. 935)

Memory cells   Cells involved in the humoral immune system that remember the exact characteristics of a particular foreign invader or antigen for the purpose of expediting immune response in the event of future exposure to this antigen. (p. 934)

Monoclonal   Term denoting a group of identical cells or organisms derived from a single cell. (p. 934)

Plasma cells   Cells derived from B cells found in the bone marrow, connective tissue, and blood. (p. 934)

T-helper cells   Cells that promote and direct the actions of other cells of the immune system. (p. 935)

T lymphocytes (T cells)   Leukocytes of the cell-mediated immune system. (p. 934)

T-suppressor cells   Cells that regulate and limit the immune response, balancing the effects of T-helper cells. (p. 935)

Tumour antigens   Chemical compounds expressed on the surfaces of tumour cells that label these cells as abnormal. (p. 934)

OVERVIEW OF IMMUNOMODULATORS

Formerly, care of patients with cancer required an understanding of only three treatment modalities: surgery, radiation, and chemotherapy. Although these are highly sophisticated methods of cancer treatment, many cancer patients still are not cured. Surgery and radiation therapy are, at best, local or regional treatments. As discussed in the preceding chapters, adjuvant drug therapy is needed to destroy undetected distant micrometastases. The advantage of cytotoxic chemotherapy with antineoplastic drugs is that these drugs attack tumour cells throughout the body. However, this advantage is also the greatest limitation because all normal cells are exposed to the cytotoxic drug as well. This capability accounts for the severe adverse effects that can occur with chemotherapy, which often require the administration of other types of drugs for their control (e.g., antiemetics, intravenous

hydration, pain medications for drug-induced stomatitis). Antineoplastic drug dosage reduction (or discontinuation) may also be required, which unfortunately will also limit their ability to cure or arrest cancer.

Over the last two decades, through medical technology a group of drugs have been developed whose primary site of action is the immune system. These new additions to the class of drugs known as **biological response–modifying drugs**, or biological response modifiers (BRMs), can enhance or restrict the patient's immune response to disease, stimulate a patient's hematopoietic (blood-forming) function, and prevent disease. **Hematopoiesis** is the collective term for all of the blood component–forming processes of the bone marrow. Current BRMs have three common mechanisms by which they act against cancer cells in particular. The first mechanism is enhancement of the host's immune system defences against the tumour. The second is a direct toxic effect of the molecules of a particular BRM on tumour cells that causes them to *lyse*, or rupture. The third mechanism involves adverse modification of the tumour's biology, which makes it harder for the tumour cells to survive and reproduce. Two broad classes of BRMs are *hematopoietic drugs (HDs)* and *immunomodulating drugs (IMDs)*; the majority of BRMs fall into the latter category. Subclasses of IMDs include interferons, monoclonal antibodies, interleukin receptor agonists and antagonists, and miscellaneous IMDs.

Immunomodulating drugs are defined as medications that therapeutically alter a patient's immune response. In cancer treatment, they make up the fourth type of cancer therapy, along with surgery, chemotherapy, and radiation. The human immune system, in addition to being the body's defence against primarily pathogenic bacteria and viruses, has effective antitumour capabilities; an intact immune system can identify malignant cells and destroy them. In contrast to chemotherapeutic drugs, a healthy immune system can distinguish between tumour cells and normal body tissues. People develop cancerous cells in their bodies on a regular basis, and normally the immune system is able to eliminate these cells before they multiply to uncontrollable levels. It is only when these natural immune responses fail to keep pace with these initially microscopic cancer cell growths that a person develops a true "cancer" that requires clinical intervention. IMDs work to strengthen the body's natural defence system against this cancer.

Some IMDs are also used to treat autoimmune, inflammatory, and infectious diseases. In these instances, the IMDs ideally function to either reduce the patients' inappropriate immune responses (in the case of inflammatory and autoimmune diseases, such as rheumatoid arthritis) or strengthen the immune responses against microorganisms (especially viruses) and cancer cells. To better understand this important class of anticancer drugs, a quick review of the immune system is useful.

IMMUNE SYSTEM

The immune system is an intricate biological defence network of cells that are capable of distinguishing an unlimited variety of substances as being either foreign ("nonself") or a natural part of the host's or patient's body ("self"). When a foreign substance such as a bacterium or virus enters the body, the cells of the immune system recognize it as being nonself and mount an immune response to eliminate or neutralize the invader. Tumours are not truly foreign substances because they arise from cells of normal tissues whose genetic material (deoxyribonucleic acid [DNA] and ribonucleic acid [RNA]) has somehow mutated, causing uncontrolled cell growth. However, tumour cells do express chemical compounds on their surfaces that signal to the immune system that these cells are a threat to the body. These chemical markers, called **tumour antigens** or *tumour markers*, label the tumour cells as abnormal cells. An **antigen** is any substance that the body's immune system recognizes as foreign. This recognition of antigens varies among individuals, which is why some people are more prone than others to immune-related diseases such as allergies, inflammatory diseases, and cancer.

The two major components of the body's immune system are **humoral immunity**, mediated by B-cell functions (primarily through *antibody* production), and **cell-mediated immunity (CMI)**, which is mediated by T-cell functions. The two systems act together to recognize and destroy foreign particles and cells in the blood or other body tissues. Communication between these two divisions is vital to the success of the immune system as a whole. Attack against tumour cells by antibodies produced by the **B lymphocytes (B cells)** of the humoral immune system prepares tumour cells for destruction by the **T lymphocytes (T cells)** of the cell-mediated immune system. This is just one example of the effective way that the two divisions communicate with each other for a collaborative immune response.

Humoral Immune System

The primary functional cells of the humoral immune system are the B lymphocytes. They are also called *B cells* because they originate in the bone marrow. Antigens that enter the body send a biochemical signal to B lymphocytes when antigen molecules bind to the antigen receptors located on the B cells. The B cells that are capable of generating a particular antibody normally remain dormant until the corresponding antigen is detected in this manner. These B cells then mature or differentiate into **plasma cells**, which, in turn, produce antibodies. **Antibodies** are **immunoglobulins** (large glycoprotein molecules; glyco = sugar; protein = amino acid chain) that bind to specific antigens, forming an antigen–antibody complex that ideally inactivates disease-causing antigens.

The immune system in a healthy individual is genetically preprogrammed to be able to mount an antibody response against literally millions of different antigens. This ability results from the lifetime antigen exposure of all of a person's ancestors, and an acquired immune response capability is further developed through exposure to new antigens passed down through many generations. The antibodies that a single plasma cell makes are all identical; thus they are called **monoclonal** antibodies. They are active against the single specific antigen that was originally recognized by their ancestor B cell as foreign. Since the 1980s, monoclonal antibodies have also been prepared synthetically using recombinant DNA (rDNA) technology, which has resulted in newer drug therapies.

There are five major types of naturally occurring immunoglobulins in the body: immunoglobulins A, D, E, G, and M. These unique immunoglobulins have different structures and functions and are found in various areas of the body. During an immune response, when B lymphocytes differentiate into plasma cells, some of these B cells become **memory cells**. Memory cells "remember" the exact characteristics of a particular foreign invader or antigen, which allows for a stronger and faster immune response in the event of re-exposure to the same antigen. The cells of the humoral immune system are shown in Figure 50-1.

Cell-Mediated Immune System

The primary functional cells of the cell-mediated (in contrast to antibody-mediated) immune system are the T lymphocytes. They are also referred to as *T cells* because, although they originate in the bone marrow similar to their B-cell counterparts, they mature in a mediastinal gland, the *thymus.* There are three distinct populations of T cells—cytotoxic T cells, helper T cells, and suppressor T cells—which are distinguished by the different functions they perform. **Cytotoxic T cells** directly kill their targets by causing cell lysis, or rupture. **T-helper cells,** considered the master controllers of the immune system, direct the actions of many other components, such as lymphokines and cytotoxic T cells. **Lymphokines** are a subset of a broader category of blood proteins known as cytokines. **Cytokines** are nonantibody proteins that serve as chemical mediators of a variety of physiological functions. Lymphokines are specifically those cytokines that are released by T lymphocytes upon contact with antigens and serve as chemical mediators of the immune response. **T-suppressor cells** have an effect on the immune system that is opposite to that of T-helper cells and serve to limit or control the immune response. A healthy immune system has approximately twice as many T-helper cells as T-suppressor cells at any given time.

The cells of the cell-mediated immune system are believed to be the major cells involved in the destruction of cancer cells. The cancer-killing cells of the cellular immune system include macrophages (derived from monocytes), natural killer (NK) cells (another type of lymphocyte), and polymorphonuclear **leukocytes** (not lymphocytes), which are also called *neutrophils.* In contrast, T-suppressor cells have the most important negative influence on antitumour actions of the immune system. Overactive T-suppressor cells may be

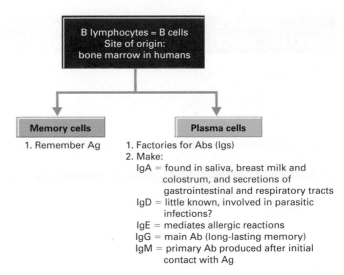

FIG. 50-1   Cells of the humoral (antibody-mediated) immune system. *Ab*, antibody; *Ag*, antigen; *Ig*, immunoglobulin.

responsible for clinically significant cancer cases by permitting tumour growth beyond immune system control. Figure 50-2 shows the components of the cellular immune system.

Therapy with BRMs combines the knowledge of several disciplines, including general biology, genetics, immunology, pharmacology, medicine, and nursing. The general therapeutic effects of BRMs are as follows:
- Enhancement of hematopoietic function (hematopoietic BRMs)
- Regulation or augmentation (enhancement) of the immune response, including cytotoxic or cytostatic activity against cancer cells
- Inhibition of metastases, prevention of cell division, or inhibition of cell maturation

Box 50-1 lists the currently available BRM drugs used in the treatment of cancer or other illnesses that have varying levels of immune system–related pathophysiology. The drugs are classified according to biological effects.

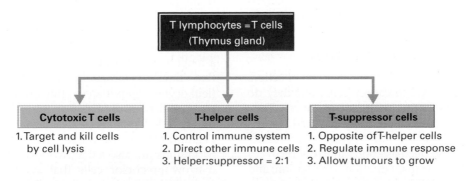

FIG. 50-2   Cells of the cellular immune system.

BOX 50-1 Biological Response Modifiers

Hematopoietic Drugs

Colony-Stimulating Factors
filgrastim (R-Methug-CSF)
pegfilgrastim
sargramostim GM-CSF†

Other
darbepoetin alfa epoetin alfa

Immunomodulating Drugs

Interferons
IFN alfa-2a
IFN alfa-2b*
pegIFN alfa-2a
pegIFN alfa-2b
IFN alfacon-1
IFN beta-1a
IFN beta-1b

Monoclonal Antibodies
alemtuzumab
bevacizumab
palivizumab
rituximab
tositumomab
trastuzumab

Interleukin Receptor Agonist and Antagonists

Agonist
aldesleukin (IL-2)

Antagonist
anakinra

Miscellaneous Immunomodulators

Tumour Necrosis Factor Receptor Antagonist
etanercept

Retinoid Receptor Agonist
tretinoin

Adjuvants (Nonspecific Immunostimulants)
BCG vaccine
leflunomide
mitoxantrone
thalidomide†

BCG, Bacillus Calmette-Guérin, *G-CSF*, granulocyte colony-stimulating factor; *IFN*, interferon; *IL*, interleukin.

*Also available in combination with the antiviral drug ribavirin.
†Available only through Health Canada's Special Access Programme.

HEMATOPOIETIC DRUGS

Hematopoietic drugs (HDs) include several newer medications developed over the past 10 to 15 years. Within this category are two erythropoietic drugs (epoetin alfa and darbepoetin alfa) and three **colony-stimulating factors (CSFs)** (filgrastim, pegfilgrastim, and sargramostim) available in Canada. Currently, the sole platelet-promoting drug (oprelvekin) is not available in Canada. All of these drugs promote the synthesis of various types of major blood components by promoting the growth, **differentiation** (development into mature specialized cells), and function of their corresponding precursor cells in the bone marrow.

Mechanism of Action and Drug Effects

All of the HDs have the same basic mechanism of action. They are not directly toxic to cancer cells, but they do have beneficial effects in the treatment of cancer. They decrease the duration of chemotherapy-induced anemia and neutropenia and enable administration of higher doses of chemotherapy; decrease bone marrow recovery time after bone marrow transplantation or radiation; and stimulate other cells in the immune system to destroy or inhibit the growth of cancer cells as well as that of virus- or fungus-infected cells.

All of these drugs are produced by rDNA technology, which allows them to be essentially identical to their endogenously produced counterparts in the body.

These substances work by binding to receptors on the surfaces of specialized progenitor *cells* in the bone marrow. Progenitor cells are responsible for the production of three particular cell lines: red blood cells (RBCs), white blood cells (WBCs), and platelets. When a HD binds to a progenitor cell surface, the progenitor cell is stimulated to mature, proliferate (reproduce itself), differentiate (transform into its respective type of specialized blood component), and become functionally active. HDs may enhance certain functions of mature cell lines as well.

Epoetin alfa, also called *EPO*, is a synthetic derivative of the human hormone *erythropoietin*, which is produced primarily by the kidney. It promotes the synthesis of erythrocytes (RBCs) by stimulating RBC progenitor cells in the bone marrow. Darbepoetin alfa, a newer drug, is a longer-acting form of epoetin alfa. Filgrastim is a CSF that stimulates progenitor cells for the subset of WBCs (leukocytes), *granulocytes* (including basophils, eosinophils, and neutrophils). For this reason, it is also commonly called *granulocyte colony-stimulating factor* (G-CSF). Pegfilgrastim is a newer, longer-acting form of filgrastim. Sargramostim, also a CSF, works by stimulating the bone marrow precursor cells that synthesize both granulocytes and the phagocytic (cell-eating) cells known as monocytes, some of which become macrophages. Because of this action, it is also called granulocyte-macrophage colony-stimulating factor (GM-CSF). Oprelvekin, which is not available in Canada, is the newest drug and is also classified as an interleukin, specifically interleukin-11

(IL-11). Other interleukins are discussed later in this chapter. Oprelvekin stimulates the bone marrow cells, specifically megakaryocytes, that eventually give rise to platelets.

Indications

HDs have many therapeutic uses. Neutrophils are the most important granulocytes for fighting infection. Because administration of CSFs reduces the duration of low neutrophil counts, they reduce the incidence and the duration of infections. Infections normally appear in patients who have experienced destruction of bone marrow cells as a result of cytotoxic chemotherapy. CSFs stimulate these cells to grow and mature and thus directly oppose the detrimental bone marrow actions of chemotherapeutic drugs (see Interactions later). CSFs also enhance the functioning of mature cells of the immune system, such as macrophages and granulocytes. This effect increases the ability of the body's immune system to kill cancer cells, as well as virus- and fungus-infected cells. Ultimately, these CSF properties allow patients to receive higher dosages of chemotherapy, which results in the destruction of greater numbers of cancer cells. Similar benefits occur with epoetin alfa on RBC counts.

The effect of HDs on the bone marrow cells also reduces their recovery time after bone marrow transplantation and radiation therapy. Bone marrow transplantation chemotherapy dosages are often much higher than those of conventional chemotherapy. Both bone marrow transplantation chemotherapy and radiation therapy are toxic to the bone marrow. When one or more HDs are administered as part of the drug therapy for bone marrow transplantation, bone marrow cell counts return to normal in a significantly shortened time. This shortened recovery helps increase the likelihood of a successful bone marrow transplantation and, therefore, patient survival. Specific drug indications are listed in the Dosages table on p. 939.

Contraindications

Contraindications for HDs include drug allergy. Use of epoetin and darbepoetin is contraindicated in cases of uncontrolled hypertension. Use of G-CSF, GM-CSF, and pegfilgrastim is also contraindicated in the presence of more than 10% myeloid blasts (immature tumour cells in the bone marrow) because CSF may stimulate malignant growth of these myeloid tumour cells.

Adverse Effects

Adverse effects associated with the use of HDs are mild. The most common adverse effects are fever, muscle aches, bone pain, and flushing. Table 50-1 lists additional adverse effects.

Interactions

Of the currently available HDs, G-CSF (filgrastim) and GM-CSF (sargramostim) are the two drugs that have significant drug interactions. The most significant drug interaction occurs when *myelosuppressive* (bone marrow depressant) antineoplastic drugs are given with these two drugs. G-CSF and GM-CSF are administered to enhance the production of bone marrow cells; therefore, when myelosuppressive antineoplastics are given with them, the drugs directly antagonize each other. Typically, BRMs would not be given within 24 hours of myelosuppressive antineoplastics. However, they are often given soon after this time to help prevent the WBC nadir from dropping to dangerous levels and to speed WBC recovery. It is also recommended that these drugs be used with caution or not given with other medications that can potentiate their *myeloproliferative* (bone marrow–stimulating) effects. Two examples are lithium and corticosteroids.

Dosages

For the recommended dosages of HDs, see the Dosages table on p. 939.

TABLE 50-1	
Hematopoietic Drugs: Common Adverse Effects	
Body System	**Adverse Effects**
Cardiovascular	Hypertension (epoetin alfa), edema
Gastrointestinal	Anorexia, nausea, vomiting, diarrhea
Integumentary	Alopecia, rash
Respiratory	Cough, dyspnea, sore throat
Other	Fever, blood dyscrasias, headache, bone pain

EPO, erythropoietin.

 DRUG PROFILES

▶▶ *epoetin alfa*

Epoetin alfa (Eprex) is a biosynthetic form of the natural hormone erythropoietin, which is normally secreted by the kidneys in response to a decrease in RBCs and many other stimuli. Epoetin is synthetically manufactured in mass quantities using rDNA technology. Although epoetin alfa is not technically classified as a CSF, its actions in promoting erythrocyte synthesis are functionally similar to the leukocyte-enhancing functions of G-CSF and GM-CSF.

Epoetin alfa is used to correct deficiencies of endogenous erythropoietin production. These conditions are common in patients with anemia resulting from end-stage kidney disease, human immunodeficiency virus (HIV) infection, and cancer. More recently, epoetin has been approved for use in both critically ill and preoperative

Continued

patients to reduce the need for blood transfusions. Epoetin stimulates the progenitor cells in the bone marrow to manufacture large numbers of immature RBCs and to greatly speed up their maturation. If therapy is not stopped when the hemoglobin level reaches the goal of 120 g/L or if the level rises too quickly, hypertension and seizures can result. Epoetin is also ineffective without adequate body iron stores.

Pertinent laboratory values to be monitored before and during therapy include transferrin saturation (which should be at least 20%), and ferritin level (which should be at least 100 ng/mL). A newer, longer-acting form of epoetin called darbepoetin is available that reduces the required number of injections, although one cost study found that there is no significant difference in overall cost between the two. Both drugs are available for injection only.

PHARMACOKINETICS

Half-Life	Onset	Peak	Duration
4–13 hr	7–10 days	5–24 hr (serum)	Variable

▶▶ filgrastim

Filgrastim (Neupogen) is a synthetic analogue of human G-CSF and is commonly referred to as *G-CSF*. G-CSF promotes the proliferation, differentiation, and activation of the cells that make granulocytes. Granulocytes are the body's primary defence against bacterial and fungal infections. Filgrastim has the same pharmacological effects as those of endogenous human G-CSF, which is normally secreted by specialized leukocytes, the *monocytes*, *macrophages*, and mature *neutrophils*.

Filgrastim is indicated for the prevention or treatment of febrile neutropenia in patients receiving myelosuppressive antineoplastics for nonmyeloid (non–bone marrow) malignancies. It should be given before a patient develops an infection, but not within 24 hours before or after myelosuppressive chemotherapeutic drug, because doing so tends to cancel out the therapeutic benefits of the filgrastim. Pegfilgrastim (Neulasta) is a long-acting

form of filgrastim that reduces the number of required injections. Both drugs are available for injection only.

PHARMACOKINETICS

Half-Life	Onset	Peak	Duration
3.5 hr	1 hr	2–8 hr	12–24 hr

sargramostim

Sargramostim (Leukine) is a synthetic analogue of human GM-CSF and is commonly referred to as GM-CSF. Granulocytes are one of three major subsets of leukocytes, the other two being monocytes and lymphocytes (B cells and T cells). As noted earlier, granulocytes are further subdivided into basophils, eosinophils, and neutrophils, with neutrophils being the most important in fighting infection. Macrophages are tissue-based (as opposed to circulating) cells derived from monocytes, which circulate in the blood. Neutrophils, monocytes, and macrophages make up the three main categories of phagocytic (cell-eating) blood cells, and they literally ingest foreign cells and other antigens as part of their immune system function. Sargramostim has the same effects as those of endogenous human GM-CSF. It stimulates the proliferation, differentiation, and activation of the cells in the bone marrow that eventually become granulocytes, monocytes, and macrophages.

Sargramostim is indicated for promoting bone marrow recovery after autologous (own marrow) or allogenic (donor marrow) bone marrow transplantation in patients with various types of leukemia and lymphoma. It is even used for bone marrow reconstitution after failure of bone marrow transplantation. This drug is available for injection only. Sargramostim is only available through the Special Access Programme, Health Canada, on a case-by-case basis.

PHARMACOKINETICS

Half-Life	Onset	Peak	Duration
2 hr	4 hr*	2 hr	10 days

*Therapeutic effect.

INTERFERONS

Before the commercial use of CSFs, **interferons (IFNs)** were the best studied and most widely used BRMs. *Interferons* are proteins that have three basic properties: antiviral, antitumour, and immunomodulating. Chemically they are glycoproteins. There are three different groups of IFN drugs, each with its own antigenic and biological activity: the alfa, beta, and gamma IFNs. IFNs are most commonly used in the treatment of certain viral infections and certain types of cancer. They can be manufactured using genetically modified *Escherichia coli* bacteria with rDNA technology. In addition, IFNs are also obtained from pooled human leukocytes that have

been stimulated (challenged) with natural and synthetic inducers (antigens).

Mechanism of Action and Drug Effects

IFN drugs are recombinantly manufactured substances that are identical to the IFN cytokines naturally present in the human body. Therefore, they have the same properties. IFNs protect human cells from virus attack by enabling human cells to produce proteins (enzymes) that arrest virus replication and prevent viruses from penetrating healthy cells. Their effects on cancer cells are thought to be caused by a combination of direct inhibitory effects on DNA and protein synthesis within cancer cells (antitumour effects) and multiple immunomodulatory

DOSAGES Hematopoietic Drugs

Drug (Pregnancy Category)	Pharmacological Class	Usual Dosage Range*	Indications
darbepoetin alfa (Aranesp) (C)	Long-acting human recombinant hormone (erythropoietin) analogue	IV/SC: 6.25–200 mcg/wk based on previous epoetin alfa dose	Chemotherapy-induced anemia, anemia associated with chronic kidney failure
»epoetin alfa (Eprex) (C)	Human recombinant hormone (erythropoietin) analogue	IV/SC: 50–100 units/kg 3×/wk	Chemotherapy-induced anemia; anemia associated with chronic kidney failure, zidovudine therapy (for HIV infection); reduction of need for blood transfusions in surgical patients
»filgrastim (Neupogen) (C)	Colony-stimulating factor	IV/SC: 5–10 mcg/kg/day	Chemotherapy-induced neutropenia, severe chronic neutropenia, prevention of neutropenia in HIV
pegfilgrastim (Neulasta) (C)	Long-acting colony-stimulating factor	SC: 6 mg once per chemotherapy cycle	Reduce febrile neutropenia
sargramostim (Leukine) (C)	Colony-stimulating factor	IV: 250 mcg/m²/day	Bone marrow recovery

IL, interleukin; *IV*, intravenous; *SC*, subcutaneous.

*Dosages listed are for adults unless indicated otherwise.

effects on the host's immune system. That is, IFNs prevent cancer cells from dividing and replicating, and they increase the activity of other cells in the immune system, such as the phagocytic ability of macrophages, the cytotoxic activity of NK cells, and the activity of neutrophils.

Unlike with conventional cytotoxic antineoplastics, the optimal biological dose of IFNs is not necessarily the maximum dose tolerated by the patient, although some newer studies support the use of higher IFN dosages. IFNs are also believed to increase the expression of cancer cell antigens on the cell surface, which enables the immune system to recognize cancer cells more easily, specifically marking them for destruction.

Overall, IFNs have three different effects on the immune system: they can (1) restore its function if it is impaired, (2) augment (amplify) the immune system's ability to function as the body's defence, and (3) inhibit the immune system. This latter function may be particularly useful when the immune system has become dysfunctional, causing an *autoimmune* disease. This is believed to be the case in multiple sclerosis (MS), for example, for which two IFN drugs are specifically indicated. Inhibiting the dysfunctional immune system prevents further damage to the body.

Indications

The beneficial actions of IFNs (antiviral, antineoplastic, and immunomodulatory) make them excellent drugs for the treatment of viral infections, various cancers, and some autoimmune disorders. Currently accepted indications for IFNs are listed in the Dosages table on p. 941.

Contraindications

Contraindications to the use of IFNs include known drug allergy as well as autoimmune disorders, hepatitis or liver failure, concurrent use of **immunosuppressant** drugs, Kaposi's sarcoma of acquired immune deficiency syndrome (AIDS), and severe liver disease.

Adverse Effects

The most common adverse effects can be broadly described as flulike symptoms: fever, chills, headache, malaise, myalgia, and fatigue. The major dose-limiting adverse effects of IFNs are listed in Table 50-2.

TABLE 50-2

Interferons: Adverse Effects

Body System	Adverse Effects
General	Flulike syndrome, fatigue
Cardiovascular	Tachycardia, cyanosis, ECG changes, MI (rare), orthostatic hypotension
Central nervous	Mild confusion, somnolence, irritability, poor concentration, seizures, hallucinations, paranoid psychoses
Gastrointestinal	Nausea, diarrhea, vomiting, anorexia, taste alterations, dry mouth
Hematological	Neutropenia, thrombocytopenia
Renal and hepatic	Increased BUN and creatinine levels, proteinuria, abnormal liver function test results (transaminases)

BUN, blood urea nitrogen; *ECG*, electrocardiogram; *MI*, myocardial infarction.

Interactions

Drug interactions are seen with both IFN alfa-2a and IFN alfa-2b when they are used with drugs such as aminophylline that are metabolized in the liver via the cytochrome P450 enzyme system. The combination results in decreased metabolism and increased accumulation of these drugs, which leads to drug toxicity. There is also some evidence that concomitant use of IFNs, in general, with antiviral drugs such as zidovudine enhances the activity of both but may lead to toxic levels of zidovudine. IFNs can also interact with angiotensin-converting enzyme (ACE) inhibitors to produce blood abnormalities such as anemia and diminished WBC and platelet counts. IFN beta products can enhance the anti-coagulant effects of warfarin, which may be undesirable and place the patient at greater risk for bleeding.

Dosages

For the recommended dosages of IFNs, see the Dosages table on p. 941.

 ## DRUG PROFILES

The three major classes of IFNs include alfa, beta, and gamma (gamma products are not available in Canada), which are sometimes also written using the lowercase Greek letters α, β, and γ, respectively. The "alfa" designation is synonymous with the Greek letter "alpha," but "alfa" is now more commonly used clinically. The IFNs vary in their antigenic makeup, biological actions, and pharmacological properties. The best known IFN class is IFN alfa. As noted earlier, IFNs can be produced by *E. coli* bacteria using rDNA laboratory techniques, and some IFNs can also be collected from pooled human leukocytes. In the body, IFNs are naturally produced by activated T cells and by other cells in response to viral infection.

IFN products are BRMs that can be broadly classified as cytokines. Cytokines are immune system proteins that serve two essential functions: They direct the actions and communication between the cell-mediated and humoral divisions of the immune system, and they augment or enhance the immune response. Other cytokines include tumour necrosis factor, interleukins, and CSFs. IFNs were first found to have antiviral activity in 1957. Their beneficial effects in treating cancer were discovered much later. With the exception of the CSFs, IFNs are the most well studied and most widely used of the BRMs.

INTERFERON ALFA PRODUCTS

▶▶ *interferon alfa-2b, interferon alfacon-1, peginterferon alfa-2a, peginterferon alfa-2b*

The most commonly used IFN products are in the IFN alfa class. They are also referred to as *leukocyte IFNs* because they are produced from human leukocytes. IFN alfa-2b is a pure clone of single α-subtypes manufactured by rDNA technology. This means that they are consistent from lot to lot. Two newer types of IFN alfa include peginterferon (pegIFN) alfa-2a and pegIFN alfa-2b. The *peg* refers to the attachment of a polymer chain of the hydrocarbon polyethylene glycol (PEG). This "pegylation" process increases the size of the IFN molecule and confers upon it several advantageous properties, including prolonged drug absorption, with increased half-life and decreased plasma clearance rate, which prolongs its therapeutic effects. In addition, pegylation is believed to reduce the immunogenicity of the IFN and thus delay its recognition and destruction by the immune system, as it is still a foreign substance to the body. This action may also help enhance and prolong its therapeutic effect. Similarly, pegfilgrastim, mentioned previously in this chapter, is a pegylated form of filgrastim and is also longer acting.

Alfa-2b IFNs are indicated for the following: chronic active hepatitis B and chronic hepatitis C, chronic myelogenous leukemia, multiple myeloma, non-Hodgkin's lymphoma, hairy-cell leukemia, basal cell carcinoma, AIDS-related Kaposi's sarcoma, and condylomata acuminata. PegIFN alfa-2b is currently indicated only for the treatment of chronic hepatitis C, whereas pegIFN alfa-2a is indicated for treatment of chronic hepatitis B and C. IFN alfacon-1 is a purely synthetic (i.e., non-naturally occurring) recombinant product that is currently indicated only for hepatitis C. All IFNs are most commonly given by either intramuscular or subcutaneous injection. However, IFNs have sometimes been given by intravenous and intraperitoneal routes as well.

INF alfa-2b (Intron A) is dosed in millions of units and these doses are often abbreviated "MU." For example, a dose of 10 million units might be written as "10 MU." The nurse should always double-check to make sure that this is the correct dose, however, because the prescriber's writing of "MU" can sometimes be mistaken for "mg" or "μg" (an older abbreviation for micrograms, which is better abbreviated as "mcg"). If there is any question in the nurse's mind about the dose of any medication, it should be double-checked with the prescriber, pharmacist, or other experienced colleague before administering the medication to the patient. Although this practice is true for all medications, it is a special consideration for IFNs and other BRMs because of their potency and their dosage variability.

INTERFERON BETA PRODUCTS

▶▶ *interferon beta-1a and beta-1b*

IFN beta-1a and IFN beta-1b are the two currently available IFN beta products. They interact with specific cell receptors found on the surface of human cells and possess antiviral and immunomodulatory activities. Both are produced by rDNA techniques and are indicated for the treatment of relapsing multiple sclerosis to slow the progression of physical disability and decrease frequency of clinical exacerbations. Drug allergy, including allergy to human albumin, is currently the only contraindication. Both drugs are available for injection only.

DOSAGES   Currently Available Interferons

Drug (Pregnancy Category)	Pharmacological Class	Usual Dosage Range*	Indications
▸▸IFN alfa-2b (Intron A) (C)	Immunomodulator, antiviral, antineoplastic	IM/SC: 1–30 million units 3x/wk[†]	Hairy-cell leukemia, malignant melanoma, follicular lymphoma, condylomata acuminata (venereal/genital warts), AIDS-related Kaposi's sarcoma, chronic hepatitis C, chronic active hepatitis B
▸▸IFN alfacon-1 (Infergen) (C)	Immunomodulator, antiviral	SC: 9 mg 3x/wk for 24 wk	Chronic hepatitis C
▸▸pegIFN alfa-2a (Pegasys) (C)	Immunomodulator, antiviral	SC: 180 mcg weekly for 48 wk	Chronic hepatitis C and B, HIV-HCV co-infection
▸▸pegIFN alfa-2b (Unitron Peg) (C)	Immunomodulator, antiviral	SC: 1 mcg/kg/wk for 1 yr[‡]	Hepatitis C
▸▸IFN beta-1a (Avonex, Avonex PS, Rebif) (C)	Immunomodulator	IM (Avonex): 30 mcg 1x/wk SC (Rebif): 44 mcg 3x/wk	Multiple sclerosis
▸▸IFN beta-1b (Betaseron) (C)	Immunomodulator	SC: 0.25 mg every other day	Multiple sclerosis

IM, intramuscular; *SC,* subcutaneous.

*Dosages listed are for adults unless indicated otherwise.

[†]May also be given by intravenous infusion for melanoma. Route and dose vary depending on indication.

[‡]Dose is IFN alfa-2b 1.5 mcg/kg/wk if given with ribavirin capsules (see Chapter 40).

MONOCLONAL ANTIBODIES

Monoclonal antibodies (MABs) are quickly becoming standards of therapy in many areas of medicine, including the treatment of cancer (Chapter 49), rheumatoid arthritis and other inflammatory diseases, and multiple sclerosis (MS) and organ transplantation (Chapter 46). In cancer treatment, they have advantages over traditional antineoplastics in that they can target cancer cells and have minimal effect on healthy cells, unlike conventional cancer treatments. This targeting reduces many of the adverse effects traditionally associated with antineoplastics. There are currently several commercially available MABs used to treat cancer and rheumatoid arthritis, which are listed in the Dosages table on p. 944. As mentioned in Chapter 46, the *mab* suffix in a drug name is usually an abbreviation for "monoclonal antibody."

Mechanism of Action, Drug Effects, and Indications

Because these drugs are so diverse, specific information for each appears in the individual drug profiles provided later in this chapter. Figure 50-3 shows the general mechanism of action of a monoclonal antibody.

Contraindications

The only clear contraindication to the use of MABs thus far is drug allergy to a specific product. The use of MABs is also usually contraindicated in patients with known active infectious processes because of their

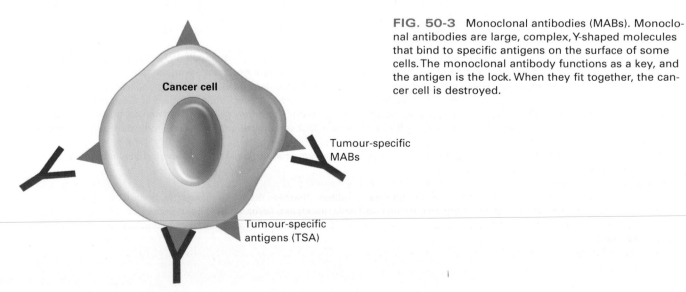

FIG. 50-3 Monoclonal antibodies (MABs). Monoclonal antibodies are large, complex, Y-shaped molecules that bind to specific antigens on the surface of some cells. The monoclonal antibody functions as a key, and the antigen is the lock. When they fit together, the cancer cell is destroyed.

Cancer cell

Tumour-specific MABs

Tumour-specific antigens (TSA)

immunosuppressive qualities. Although known drug allergy is a contraindication, depending on the urgency of the clinical situation, a MAB may be the only viable treatment option for a seriously ill patient. In such situations, allergic symptoms may be controlled with supportive medications such as diphenhydramine and acetaminophen (for fever control). Infliximab has been shown to worsen severe cases of heart failure and should be dosed at no more than 5 mg/kg and only after considering other treatment options for its indications. Use of alemtuzumab is also contraindicated in patients with active systemic infections and immunodeficiency conditions, including AIDS.

Adverse Effects

Many, if not most, patients receiving these very potent drugs manifest acute symptoms that are comparable with classic allergy or flulike symptoms, such as fever, dyspnea, and chills. The primary objective is to administer the medication and control such symptoms as well as possible. Because of their mechanisms of action working through augmentation (or inhibition) of the human immune response, these drugs can have a variety of adverse effects, some mild, some severe, that affect several body systems. Drug-specific adverse effects with the highest reported incidence (10% to 50% or more) are listed in Table 50-3. Again, the risk of such adverse effects must be weighed against the severity of the patient's underlying illness, which itself may be fatal, especially in the case of malignancies. It should be noted that many of these adverse effects may also be associated with the patient's disease process (e.g., infections) and even with life in general (e.g., headache, depression). This is especially true for the milder effects.

Dosages

For the recommended dosages of the antineoplastic MABs, see the Dosages table on p. 944.

TABLE 50-3

Common Adverse Effects Associated with Specific Immunomodulating Drugs

Drug	Adverse Effects
adalimumab	Localized inflammatory reaction at the injection site, infectious processes such as upper respiratory tract and urinary tract infections, and higher rates of various malignancies. Although such effects are likely related to the immunosuppressive properties of this drug, patients with rheumatoid arthritis, especially those with more severe disease, are known to have higher rates of cancer.
alemtuzumab	Rash, pruritus (itching), nausea, vomiting, diarrhea, dyspnea, cough, rigors (muscle spasms), fever, fatigue, pain (especially skeletal pain), and myelosuppression.
bevacizumab	Deep vein thrombosis, hypertension, diarrhea, abdominal pain, constipation, vomiting, GI hemorrhage, leukopenia, asthenia (muscular fatigue and weakness), headache, dizziness, dry skin, proteinuria, hypokalemia, epistaxis, and weight loss
cetuximab	Headache, insomnia, skin rash, conjunctivitis, GI discomfort, anemia, leukopenia, dehydration, edema, weight loss, dyspnea, asthenia, back pain, and fever
infliximab	Headache, rash, GI discomfort, dyspnea, and upper and lower respiratory tract infection
natalizumab	Depression, fatigue, headache, GI discomfort, urinary tract infection, lower respiratory tract infection, and joint pain. Of even greater concern are four case reports from 2005 and 2006 of a rare, potentially fatal brain disorder known as progressive multifocal leukoencephalopathy (PML) occurring with use of this drug. PML usually occurs in individuals with weakened immune systems. At the time of this writing, the drug remains on the Canadian market but is under scrutiny by Health Canada.
palivizumab	Upper respiratory infection, otitis media, rhinitis, rash, pain, hernia, increased aspartate aminotransferase, pharyngitis
rituximab	Fever, chills, and headache are commonly reported with the use of rituximab. Potentially fatal infusion-related events can also occur with rituximab, including severe bronchospasm, dyspnea, hypoxia, pulmonary infiltrates, adult respiratory distress syndrome, hypotension, and angioedema; tumour lysis syndrome (Chapter 48) with acute kidney failure has also been reported. Because of these potentially fatal adverse effects, this drug should be used only after consideration of other treatment options. The drug should be stopped immediately if any of these reactions appears imminent and indicated supportive care provided.
tositumomab and iodine I 131 tositumomab	Headache, rash, GI discomfort, muscle pains, dyspnea, pharyngitis, asthenia, fever, chills, and infection
trastuzumab	Fever, chills, headache, infection, nausea, vomiting, diarrhea, dizziness, headache, insomnia, rash, GI discomfort, edema, dyspnea, rhinitis, asthenia, back pain, fever, chills, and infection

GI, gastrointestinal.

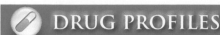
DRUG PROFILES

The design and use of pharmaceutical MABs is now considered part of the leading edge in drug therapy for several diseases, including cancer, inflammatory conditions, and multiple sclerosis (MS). All of these drugs are synthesized using rDNA technology. Because of the complexities of this technology, these drugs tend to be much more expensive than most other medications, with prices in the hundreds or thousands of dollars per single dose. Given this cost, other, less costly medications may be tried first. Most MABs are used to treat various forms of cancer. Their advantage is that they offer greater cell-killing specificity aimed at cancer cells instead of all body cells. Nonetheless, these drugs are all associated with significant adverse effects and, therefore, risk, which must be weighed against the severity and associated risks of the patient's underlying disease, using expert clinical judgement.

Severe allergic inflammatory-type infusion reactions occur in varying percentages of patients. Patients may therefore be premedicated with acetaminophen or diphenhydramine to reduce such reactions. Reactions that do occur may also be treated with diphenhydramine and other drugs such as epinephrine and corticosteroids. Conventional pharmacokinetic data are not listed for most of these drugs because they do not follow standard pharmacokinetic models owing to their unique behaviour in the body. It is known, however, that they may remain in the affected tissues for many weeks or months. The elimination half-life is listed in the following profiles when known.

adalimumab

Adalimumab (Humira) works through its specificity for human tumour necrosis factor-α (TNF-α). TNF-α is a naturally occurring cytokine involved in normal inflammatory and immune responses. It is indicated for the treatment of severe cases of rheumatoid arthritis that have failed to respond to other medications, including methotrexate. It can be used either alone or concurrently with such medications. In patients with rheumatoid arthritis, elevated levels of TNF are found in the synovial fluid in the spaces of affected joints. In addition to preventing TNF-α molecules from binding to TNF cell-surface receptors as part of the rheumatoid arthritis disease process, adalimumab also modulates the inflammatory biological responses that are induced or regulated by TNF. Adalimumab is also used in the treatment of psoriatic arthritis, ankylosing spondylitis, Crohn's disease, and psoriasis. Use of adalimumab is contraindicated in patients with any active infectious process, whether localized or systemic, acute or chronic.

alemtuzumab

Alemtuzumab (MabCampath) was approved by Health Canada to treat chronic lymphocytic leukemia caused by B cells (abbreviated B-CLL). It is classified as a recombinant humanized antibody that is directed against the CD52 glycoprotein that appears on the surfaces of virtually all B and T lymphocytes, thus making it useful for treating B-CLL. It is used specifically in patients for whom other first-line chemotherapy treatments, including treatment with alkylating drugs and the antimetabolite fludarabine, have failed. Its contraindications are drug allergy, active systemic infection, and documented immunodeficiency disease such as HIV-positive status. Its half-life is 10 hours to 30 days.

bevacizumab

Bevacizumab (Avastin) was approved for the treatment of metastatic colon or rectal cancer in combination with the first-line antineoplastic drug 5-fluorouracil (Chapter 48). It is unique in that it binds to and inhibits vascular endothelial growth factor, a protein that promotes development of new blood vessels in tumours (as well as in normal body tissues). It has no listed contraindications but may complicate surgical wound healing because of its antivascular effects. Its half-life is 11 to 50 days.

cetuximab

Cetuximab (Erbitux) was approved for the treatment of metastatic colorectal cancer and squamous cell carcinoma of the head and neck. It is a recombinant MAB made from both human and mouse (murine) genetic material and is designed for concurrent use with the second-line antineoplastic drug irinotecan (Chapter 48). It binds to epidermal growth factor on the surface of tumour cells, where it hinders cell growth through interference with cell metabolism. It is used either in combination with irinotecan (Chapter 48) or alone in patients who are intolerant of the latter drug. It has no listed contraindications but is known to cause severe infusion reactions in up to 3% of patients receiving it. Its half-life is 97 to 114 hours.

infliximab

Infliximab (Remicade) is one of the earliest MABs. It works through an anti–TNF-α action, similar to adalimumab, but it is approved for the treatment of ankylosing spondylitis and Crohn's disease, in addition to rheumatoid arthritis. It has the special contraindication of severe heart failure (grade III or IV on the New York Heart Association scale) because it may worsen this condition. It also has a Health Canada warning reporting cases of fatal tuberculosis and fungal infections associated with use of this drug. It is recommended that patients be tested for latent tuberculosis before infliximab is administered. Its half-life is 8 to 9 days.

natalizumab

Natalizumab (Tysabri) was approved for the treatment of MS. It is a humanized MAB derived from murine myeloma cells. Humanization involves the insertion of human DNA sequences during drug production to make the drug better tolerated by human patients. Natalizumab works

Continued

DRUG PROFILES (cont'd)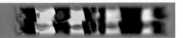

by binding to the α_4 subunits of integrins, proteins found on leukocyte surfaces (with the exception of neutrophils). While these proteins are implicated in the MS disease process, the exact mechanism by which this drug exerts its therapeutic effects is unknown. The drug is known to inhibit the leukocyte adhesion that is mediated by these α_4 protein subunits and is believed to be part of the MS disease process. Natalizumab has no listed contraindications. Its half-life is 11 days.

palivizumab

Palivizumab (Synagis) is a passive immunizing agent (humanized monoclonal antibody). It is indicated for the prevention of serious lower respiratory tract disease caused by the highly contagious respiratory syncytial virus (RSV) in children who are at high risk of RSV disease. The recommended dose of palivizumab administered intramuscularly is 15 mg/kg of body weight. It is administered monthly during peak times (generally November to April) of RSV risk. The first dose should be administered prior to the beginning of the RSV season, with subsequent doses administered monthly during the RSV season. The mean half-life is 20 days.

▶▶ rituximab

Rituximab (Rituxan) specifically binds to antigen CD20. This antigen is a protein on the membranes of both normal and malignant B cells found in patients with non-Hodgkin's lymphoma. Antigen CD20 is expressed in more than 90% of B-cell non-Hodgkin's lymphomas. Once rituximab binds to these B cells, a host immune response causes lysis of the cells. Rituximab has become a standard drug for the treatment of patients with follicular low-grade non-Hodgkin's lymphoma for whom previous therapy has failed. It is recommended that patients be premedicated with acetaminophen and diphenhydramine before each infusion of the drug to reduce its well-known infusion-related adverse effects.

tositumomab and iodine I 131 tositumomab

Tositumomab and iodine I 131 tositumomab or I 131 tositumomab (Bexxar) are used for the treatment of non-Hodgkin's lymphoma. This drug is a murine MAB with dual radioactive and nonradioactive components. Both components bind to the CD20 antigen, a transmembrane protein expressed on the cell membranes of more than 90% of B-cell non-Hodgkin's lymphoma cells. Theoretical mechanisms of action include induction of apoptosis (programmed cell death), complement-dependent cytotoxicity, or antibody-dependent cytotoxicity mediated by the drug itself. *Complement* is a collective term for about 20 different proteins normally present in plasma that aid other immune system components (e.g., B cells and T cells) in mounting an immune response.

trastuzumab

Trastuzumab (Herceptin) kills tumour cells by mediating antibody-dependent cellular cytotoxicity. It accomplishes this by inhibiting proliferation of human tumour cells that overexpress HER2 protein. This protein is overexpressed in 25% to 30% of primary malignant breast tumours. The overexpression of the *HER2* gene has been established as an adverse prognostic factor for early-stage breast cancer. Because of the relatively selective expression of HER2 on cancer cells, it has been an appealing target for antineoplastic therapy. The combination of trastuzumab and paclitaxel has produced encouraging results.

Ventricular dysfunction and heart failure have been associated with this drug. Patients should be monitored for signs and symptoms of heart failure and ventricular dysfunction before and during treatment. In addition, fatal hypersensitivity reactions, infusion reactions, and pulmonary events have occurred in association with it use; therefore, careful clinical judgement, risk evaluation, and informed patient consent are called for in its use. Its half-life is 10 to 30 days.

DOSAGES Monoclonal Antibodies

Drug (Pregnancy category)	Pharmacological Class	Usual Dosage Range*	Indications
adalimumab (Humira) (B)	Anti-TNF-α monoclonal antibody	*Adult only* SC: 40 mg every other week	Moderate to severe, RA, psoriatic arthritis, ankylosing spondylitis, Crohn's disease, psoriasis
alemtuzumab (MabCampath) (C)	Anti–glycoprotein CD52	IV: 3–10 mg daily until maximum dose tolerated, then 30 mg 3×/wk (alternate days) for up to 12 wk	B-cell chronic lymphocytic leukemia
bevacizumab (Avastin) (C)	Anti–human vascular endothelial growth factor	IV: 5 mg/kg q14d	Metastatic colorectal cancer
cetuximab (Erbitux) (C)	Anti–human epidermal growth factor	IV: 400 mg/m² loading dose, then 250 mg/m² weekly	Metastatic colorectal cancer, squamous cell carcinoma of head and neck

Continued

DOSAGES   Monoclonal Antibodies (cont'd)

Drug (Pregnancy category)	Pharmacological Class	Usual Dosage Range*	Indications
infliximab (Remicade) (B)	Anti–TNF-α	*Children* IV: 5 mg/kg at 0, 2, and 6 wk, then q8 wk	Crohn's disease
		Adult IV: 3–5 mg/kg at 0, 2, and 6 wk, then every 6 wk	Ankylosing spondylitis, Crohn's disease, RA, ulcerative colitis, psoriatic arthritis
natalizumab (Tysabri) (C)	Anti–α⁴ integrin subunit	IV: 300 mg every 4 wk	Multiple sclerosis
palivizumab (Synagis)	Passive immunizing agent (humanized monoclonal antibody)	*Children* IM: 15 mg/kg/month during peak RSV season	Prevention of serious lower respiratory tract disease caused by RSV
▶▶rituximab (Rituxan) (C)	Anti-CD20 surface antigen	IV: 375 mg/m² 1×/wk × 4 doses on days 1, 8, 15, and 22 IV: 1000 mg, 2 wk apart	Non-Hodgkin's lymphoma Rheumatoid arthritis
tositumomab and iodine I 131 tositumomab (Bexxar) (X)	Radioactive MAB	IV: Complex dosing regimen involving both drug components; follow instructions in package insert as ordered	Non-Hodgkin's lymphoma
trastuzumab (Herceptin) (B)	Anti–HER2 protein MAB	IV: Loading dose, 4–8 mg/kg IV: Maintenance dose, 2 mg/kg/wk	Breast cancer

IM, intramuscular; *IV*, intravenous; *MAB*, monoclonal antibodies; *RA*, rheumatoid arthritis; *RSV*, respiratory syncytial virus; *SC*, subcutaneous; *TNF*, tumour necrosis factor.

*Dosages listed are for adults unless indicated otherwise.

INTERLEUKINS AND RELATED DRUGS

Interleukins are a natural part of the immune system. They are classified as lymphokines, which are soluble proteins released from activated lymphocytes such as NK cells. There are several known interleukins in the body (IL-2, IL-3, IL-4, IL-5, IL-6, and IL-11) and more are being identified as knowledge of the immune system increases.

The sole interleukin receptor agonist currently commercially available in Canada is aldesleukin. Two additional interleukin receptor agonists, oprelvekin and denileukin diftitox, are available in the United States. Aldesleukin is synthesized using rDNA technology and is patterned after corresponding natural interleukins in the body. Another drug, anakinra, is actually an IL-1 receptor antagonist. It is also a recombinant product that is patterned after its natural counterpart in the body.

Mechanism of Action and Drug Effects

Interleukins cause multiple effects in the immune system, one of which is beneficial antitumour action. Aldesleukin is produced by activated T cells in response to macrophage-"processed" antigens and secreted IL-1. It was formerly called *T-cell growth factor* because, among other actions, it aids in the growth and differentiation of T lymphocytes. Aldesleukin acts indirectly to stimulate or restore immune response. Aldesleukin binds to receptor sites on T cells, which stimulates the T cells to multiply. One type of cell that results from this multiplication is the **lymphokine-activated killer (LAK) cell**. LAK cells recognize and destroy only cancer cells and ignore normal cells, which allows some of the toxic effects of standard antineoplastics to be avoided. A detailed list of aldesleukin's specific immunomodulating effects appears in Box 50-2.

BOX 50-2

Interleukin-2: Drug Effects

Modulating Effects

Increased production of B cells (antibodies)
Proliferation and activation of LAK cells
Proliferation and activation of NK cells
Proliferation of T cells
Synthesis and secretion of cytokines

Enhancing Effects

Amplification of the effects of cytokines
Enhancement of killer T-cell activity
Enhancement of the cytotoxic actions of NK cells and LAK cells

LAK, lymphokine-activated killer; NK, natural killer.

Anakinra is a recombinant form of the natural human IL-1 receptor antagonist. It competitively inhibits the binding of IL-1 to its corresponding receptor sites, which are expressed in many different tissues and organs.

Indications

Aldesleukin was previously indicated for metastatic kidney cell carcinoma, a malignancy that originates in kidney tissues. It is now also approved for the treatment of metastatic malignant melanoma. Anakinra is indicated for symptom control in patients with rheumatoid arthritis when other therapy has failed.

Contraindications

Contraindications to the administration of aldesleukin include drug allergy, organ transplantation, and abnormal results on thallium heart stress tests or pulmonary function tests. For anakinra, the only usual contraindication is drug allergy.

Adverse Effects

Unfortunately, therapy with aldesleukin is commonly complicated by severe toxicity. A syndrome known as *capillary leak syndrome* is responsible for the severe toxicities of aldesleukin. As the name implies, capillary leak syndrome refers to a condition in which capillaries lose their ability to retain vital colloids such as albumin, protein, and other essential components of blood vessels.

When the capillaries become "leaky," these substances migrate into surrounding tissues. This migration results in massive fluid retention (10–15 kg), which can lead to the life-threatening problems of respiratory distress, heart failure, dysrhythmias, and myocardial infarction. Fortunately, these conditions are all reversible after discontinuation of interleukin therapy. Close monitoring and vigorous supportive care are essential for the patient receiving aldesleukin therapy. Other adverse effects are fever, chills, rash, fatigue, hepatotoxicity, myalgias, headaches, and eosinophilia. Anakinra has a much milder adverse-effect profile that includes local reactions at the injection site, respiratory infections, and headache.

Interactions

When given with antihypertensives, aldesleukin can have additive hypotensive effects. Coadministration of corticosteroids with aldesleukin can reduce its antitumour effectiveness. The toxic effects of aldesleukin are increased when it is administered with aminoglycosteroids, indomethacin, cytotoxic chemotherapeutic drugs, methotrexate, asparaginase, and doxorubicin. No particular drug interactions have been reported, to date, for anakinra.

Dosages

For the recommended dosages of the interleukin agonists and antagonists, see the Dosages table below.

DRUG PROFILES

The interleukins are a group of naturally occurring cytokines in the body that originally were believed to be produced by and act primarily on leukocytes (WBCs). They are now recognized as multifunctional cytokines that are produced by a variety of cells but act at least partly within the lymphatic system. As is the case with MABs, pharmacokinetic data may not have been ascertained for these drugs.

▶▶ *aldesleukin*

Aldesleukin (Proleukin) is a human IL-2 derivative that is manufactured using rDNA technology. It is a cytokine produced by lymphocytes and is therefore classified as a lymphokine. Aldesleukin is currently approved only for the

treatment of metastatic kidney cell carcinoma and metastatic malignant melanoma, despite its activity in other cancers. Aldesleukin is contraindicated in patients with drug allergy, abnormal thallium stress test or pulmonary function tests (because of potential drug effects on cardiopulmonary function), and organ transplants (because of the immunostimulating qualities of the drug, which may cause organ rejection). It is only available for injection.

anakinra

Anakinra (Kineret) is an IL-1 receptor antagonist that is also rDNA synthesized. It is used to control symptoms of rheumatoid arthritis. Its only current contraindication is drug allergy. It is available for injection only.

DOSAGES   Interleukins and Related Drugs

Drug (Pregnancy Category)	Pharmacological Class	Usual Dosage Range*	Indications
▶▶aldesleukin [IL-2] (Proleukin) (C)	Human recombinant IL-2 analogue	IV: 600,000 units/kg (0.037 mg/kg) q8h × 14 doses; rest for 9 days, repeat × 14 doses	Metastatic kidney cell carcinoma, metastatic malignant melanoma
anakinra (Kineret) (B)	Interleukin-1 receptor antagonist	SC: 100 mg/day	Rheumatoid arthritis

IV, intravenous; *SC*, subcutaneous.

*Dosages listed are for adults.

MISCELLANEOUS IMMUNOMODULATING DRUGS

In addition to the major drug classes discussed, several additional medications can be broadly classified as miscellaneous IMDs. They work by specific and nonspecific mechanisms. A special term used for **immunostimulant** drugs that work by a nonspecific mechanism is **adjuvant**. These medications, including some that are classified as adjuvants, are outlined in Table 50-4.

NURSING PROCESS

Assessment

Before administering any of the BRMs, nurses must review and update their own knowledge about these drugs, including (1) hematopoietic drugs, (2) IFNs, (3) MABs, (4) interleukins, and (5) miscellaneous drugs, in order to have a complete knowledge base. The patient must be assessed for any contraindications, cautions, or drug interactions, as well as for hypersensitivity to the drug, egg proteins, or immunoglobulin G (such patients will most likely have an allergic reaction to these drugs). Cautious use of these drugs with close monitoring is recommended for pregnant and lactating women, children, and patients with heart disease, angina, heart failure, chronic obstructive pulmonary disease, diabetes mellitus, bleeding disorders, bone marrow depression, or convulsive disorders. The nursing history should be reviewed

and analyzed for any of these conditions. Head-to-toe examination should include thorough assessment of breath sounds and listening for any crackles in the lungs; evaluation of heart sounds and heart rate and rhythm; assessment for edema, shortness of breath, decrease in partial pressure of oxygen, or increase in partial pressure of carbon dioxide; inspection for any cyanotic discoloration around the mouth or nail beds; assessment for the presence of chest pain, hypotension, or hypertension; evaluation of mental health status; and assessment for any seizure-like activity. Height, weight, uric acid levels, electrolyte levels, skin condition, ability to carry out activities of daily living, nutritional status (see Nursing Process in Chapters 48 and 49), presence or absence of underlying diseases, and symptoms and success or failure of drug regimens in the past should also be documented before therapy is initiated. In addition, baseline vital signs and complete blood count (CBC) should be determined and documented. For therapy with any of the drugs in this chapter, baseline assessment should also include data about the patient's emotional status, educational level, learning needs, desire and ability to learn, past coping strategies, support systems, and self-care abilities.

For hematopoietic BRMs, in addition to elements assessed with use of all BRMs, specific drugs require special considerations. For *epoetin alfa* and similar drugs, the patient should be assessed for a history of hypertension, seizure activity, thrombosis, and chest pain because these may be exacerbated by the drug. Kidney function should be evaluated because patients with chronic kidney failure (and receiving these drugs) may have transient rises in blood pressure. Iron stores should be assessed by

TABLE 50-4			
Miscellaneous Immunomodulating Drugs			
Drug	**Classification**	**Indications**	**Mechanism of Action**
BCG vaccine (Immuncyst, OncoTIST)	Live virus vaccine, adjuvant	Localized bladder cancer	Promotes local inflammation and immune response in bladder mucosa
etanercept (Enbrel)	TNF receptor antagonist	Rheumatoid arthritis (including juvenile), active ankylosing spondylitis, plaque and psoriatic arthritis	Blocks effects of TNF, a major inflammatory mediator
leflunomide (Arava)	Antimetabolite	Rheumatoid arthritis	Exerts anti-inflammatory effects via inhibition of cellular DNA synthesis.
mitoxantrone hydrochloride	Anthracycline antibiotic (also an antineoplastic drug)	Metastatic breast cancer, relapsed leukemia	Inhibits cellular RNA and DNA synthesis and alters chromosome structure
thalidomide[†] (Thalomid)	Immunostimulant	Multiple myeloma, erythema nodosum*	Exact mechanism unclear, but may have anti-TNF properties, which counter the disease process
tretinoin[†] (Vescanoid)	Retinoid receptor agonist	Acute promyelocytic leukemia	Induces differentiation and maturation of leukemic cells, reducing proliferation of immature, disease-causing cells.

DNA, deoxyribose nucleic acid; *RNA*, ribose nucleic acid; *TNF*, tumour necrosis factor.

*An inflammatory reaction in the subcutaneous fat, often following a bacterial infection or reaction to drugs such as oral contraceptives or sulfonamides.

[†]Available through Health Canada's Special Access Programme.

measuring transferrin saturation, which must be at least 20%, and ferritin level, which should be at 100 ng/mL. These levels allow appropriate erythropoietin stimulation. Possible subcutaneous and intravenous sites should be assessed and blood pressures measured before starting therapy and early in treatment.

For CSFs, CBCs should be assessed; for example, with filgrastim and sargramostim, counts should be determined before therapy and throughout therapy to monitor for problems with leukocytosis and thrombocytosis. Levels of liver enzymes should be measured to assess liver function. Potential intravenous and subcutaneous sites should be noted, and, if appropriate, chemotherapy-induced absolute neutrophil nadir (low point) should be watched for, because timing of the dose is critical to boosting blood cell counts. For example, with filgrastim, the drug should not be given within 24 hours before or after the chemotherapy (see discussion in pharmacology section). In addition, any existing pain, especially joint or bone pain, is important to document because of the possible mild, moderate, or severe bone pain with filgrastim.

Before IFNs (e.g., IFN alfa-2b) are given, the patient's CBC should be documented to monitor for bone marrow suppression, an adverse effect of long-term therapy with these drugs. Other serum laboratory values such as platelet counts, blood urea nitrogen (BUN) and creatinine levels, urinalysis results, and levels of aspartate aminotransferase and alkaline phosphatase should be checked before treatment and twice weekly during therapy or as ordered. Before aldesleukin is administered, it is important for the nurse to document baseline measurements of vital signs, neurological functioning, bowel status, and results of liver and kidney studies in order to monitor for possible drug-related impaired kidney and liver functions. Because capillary leak syndrome is also associated with interleukin drugs, it is important to document any edema and assess baseline vital signs and baseline heart, respiratory, kidney, and liver status. The symptoms of this potentially fatal syndrome include hypotension; reduced organ perfusion; extravasation of plasma proteins and fluid; and symptoms of angina and respiratory, kidney, and liver insufficiency. Because of heart concerns, the interleukins may not be administered to patients with heart diseases or symptoms (e.g., hypotension, hypertension, angina). Any allergy to proteins of *E. coli* should be noted because of cross-sensitivity to interferon. Attention to the timing of these drugs is important, because they are not usually given at the same time as antineoplastics; instead, they are usually given at least 24 hours after chemotherapy.

With use of the MAB drugs (e.g., alemtuzumab, rituximab, trastuzumab), blood pressure should be monitored and any gastrointestinal signs and symptoms, fatigue, weakness, or malaise watched for. With use of trastuzumab, liver, kidney, and heart function should be

assessed. For any of these drugs, the medication order should be examined for timing of the dose because of different protocols. Intravenous sites should also be assessed. For rituximab, withholding of antihypertensives for 12 hours before infusion may be considered, as ordered, to avoid any transient hypotensive episodes.

◩ Nursing Diagnoses

- Acute pain related to the adverse effects of BMRs
- Altered nutrition, less than body requirements, related to the adverse effects of BRMs
- Impaired skin integrity (rash) related to the adverse effects of BMRs
- Risk for falls related to weakness and fatigue from the disease process and from drug therapy
- Risk for caregiver stress related to the demands of therapy and need for assistance in the care of a loved one or significant other

◩ Planning

◼ Goals

- Patient will experience adequate control of pain during drug treatment.
- Patient will regain prechemotherapy (and as near normal as possible) nutritional status.
- Patient will experience minimal weight loss during therapy.
- Patient will maintain or regain normal bowel and bladder patterns.
- Patient's mucous membranes will maintain or regain intactness during therapy.
- Patient will be free of injury related to drug therapy.
- Patient's family, caregiver, and significant other will experience minimal stress and anxiety and maximal rest and relaxation.

◼ Outcome Criteria

- Patient describes nutritional needs and daily meal planning reflecting dietary needs, such as consumption of a high-calorie, low-residue, high-protein diet and adequate fluids; patient identifies grocery-shopping tips.
- Patient eats appropriate foods that provide high energy content through protein and complex carbohydrates.
- Patient states measures to minimize gastrointestinal adverse effects, such as eating small, frequent meals and avoiding spicy foods.
- Patient drinks fluids up to 3000 mL/day, unless contraindicated, using creative means such as consumption of flavoured water, decaffeinated iced tea, lemonade, sugar-free juices (if appropriate), and cranberry juice, with adequate urinary output noted.

- Patient's skin and mucous membranes remain intact and clean through daily bathing, skin care with moisturizing products, and daily oral hygiene with a soft toothbrush and gentle flossing as well as follow-up care with a dental professional.
- Patient states ways to minimize injury related to weakness and fatigue from the disease process and related BRM treatment, such as using assistive devices and grab bars or rails; removing rugs, mats, or other obstacles in the bedroom and bathroom; maintaining muscle mass and energy; and obtaining assistance in performing the activities of daily living, if needed.
- Patient's family members, significant others, loved ones, and caregivers attend appropriate seminars or are able to obtain information and community resources designed to assist in stress management, rest, relaxation, and respite.

Implementation

In general, BRMs should be given exactly as prescribed and in keeping with manufacturer guidelines to minimize all expected and untoward adverse effects. Vital signs, with special attention to temperature, should also be measured throughout drug therapy. Premedication with acetaminophen and diphenhydramine may be necessary when any of the BRMs is administered. With some of the BRMs, treatment with narcotics, antihistamines, or anti-inflammatory drugs may be required for the management of bone pain and chills if treatment with acetaminophen or diphenhydramine is not successful. Meperidine may be the narcotic of choice if the patient is in the hospital setting or in a physician's office for treatment. Antiemetics may also be needed for any drug-related nausea or vomiting and may be administered before a specific BRM is taken. Antiemetics may be dosed round the clock should nausea and vomiting occur.

The patient should be encouraged to rest when tired, not to overexert during therapy, and to contact the physician if profound fatigue or loss of appetite is experienced. The patient should drink fluids up to 3000 mL/day (unless contraindicated) to promote excretion of the byproducts of cellular breakdown. Consultation with a dietitian or nutritionist may be helpful to the patient to learn about a healthy diet (e.g., foods high in protein, complex carbohydrates, and necessary natural health products) to boost health and wellness. Menu planning and grocery shopping may also be discussed, with specific suggestions provided according to each patient's needs. Many grocery stores support Internet shopping with pickup at the store on the same day, and many stores deliver groceries at no or minimal cost. Community resources (e.g., Meals on Wheels, respite-care organizations, physical and occupational therapists) should be shared with patients as needed. A social services agency should be contacted if the patient needs assistance in covering the cost of treatments or other services.

Other nursing interventions include giving the drug at night or at bedtime to decrease daytime fatigue. IFNs are administered parenterally by subcutaneous, intravenous, or intramuscular routes, depending on the drug (e.g., IFN alfa-2a is given subcutaneously or intramuscularly). Epoetin alfa may be given intravenously or subcutaneously, and the dose may change depending on hematocrit values. If there is no response to the drug, the patient should undergo a workup for iron deficiency; underlying infection, inflammation, or malignancies; occult blood loss; hematological disease; hemolysis; folic acid or vitamin B_{12} deficiency; and aluminum intoxication. Recommendations for the administration of epoetin alfa are to give the drug without shaking the vial and with only one use per vial; use the smallest possible amount per injection (e.g., 1 mL or less per injection), always as ordered; change the needle once the medication has been withdrawn from the vial; and apply ice to numb the injection site. With sargramostim, only one dose should be withdrawn per vial, and as with all vials and packages, expiration dates should be checked. Vials should not be shaken but instead rolled between the hands. Filgrastim drug vials contain single-dose-only portions and should be stored in the refrigerator.

For drugs administered subcutaneously, the injection site should be rotated. See Patient Education for more information. See also Legal and Ethical Principles: The Nurse and Patient Care regarding the nursing code of ethics required in the treatment of cancer patients.

Evaluation

Therapeutic responses to BRMs include a decrease in the growth of the lesion or mass, decreased tumour size, and an easing of symptoms related to the tumour or disease process. Other therapeutic responses are an improvement in WBC, RBC, and platelet counts or a return to normal levels, absence of infection, anemia, and hemorrhage. Journalling may help provide health care providers with more data from which to evaluate the patient's response during and after therapy. Possible adverse effects for which to evaluate are presented in Tables 50-1, 50-2, and 50-3.

LEGAL & ETHICAL PRINCIPLES

The Nurse and Patient Care

The nurse should never neglect or be deceptive with a patient despite any conflict with the nurse's ethnocultural, racial, spiritual, or personal belief systems. This dilemma is often encountered with various types of treatment modalities for cancer patients or those needing drugs that alter the patient's biological responses. The nurse does have the right to refuse to participate in any treatment or aspect of a patient's care that violates personal ethical principles, but it is important to understand that this refusal of care can in *no* way be through desertion or neglect of the patient. In this situation, the nurse should inform the appropriate supervisory personnel about the conflict and transfer the patient to the safe care of another qualified professional before the start of nursing care by another nurse. As detailed in the Canadian Nurses Association *Code of Ethics*, nurses are bound by the profession to always remain ethical in the administration of their care to patients. This may include participation in the care of a patient who needs the nurse's care but who may be receiving treatment or care that is not "acceptable" according to the nurse's own standards or ethics.

PATIENT EDUCATION

- ❖ Patients should avoid hazardous tasks because the central nervous system changes noted with several BRMs could compromise physical ability. Fatigue is also a common adverse effect, so the patient should report excessive fatigue.
- ❖ Patients should report signs of infection, such as sore throat, fever, diarrhea, vomiting, or a fever of 37.8°C or higher.
- ❖ Women taking BRMs should be encouraged to avoid getting pregnant. Education should include information about contraceptive choices and the need to use contraception for up to 2 years after completion of therapy.
- ❖ Patients should be told that the adverse effects associated with BRMs usually disappear within 72 to 96 hours after therapy has been discontinued. Patients should be encouraged to have follow-up appointments.

- ❖ Interleukins may be self-administered; therefore, patients should learn the self-injection technique and proper disposal of equipment (e.g., needles, syringes). A corresponding instruction sheet should be provided to patients, and they should keep a daily journal to record the site of injection and an overall rating of how they feel.
- ❖ Patients should be informed that bone pain and flu-like symptoms often occur with some of the BRMs, and the use of nonopioid or, in some cases, opioid analgesics may be required. Some patients may find relief with ibuprofen.
- ❖ Patients should report any adverse effects (e.g., hair loss, fever, joint pain, chills, diarrhea, edema, anemia, anorexia, fatigue, hypotension, thrombocytopenia) to the physician immediately so that the dosage can be adjusted or reconsidered.

POINTS TO REMEMBER

- ❖ Cancer treatment has traditionally involved surgery, radiation, and chemotherapy. Surgery and radiation are usually local or regional. Chemotherapy is usually systemic, but it often does not completely eliminate all of the cancer cells in the body. Adjuvant therapy is frequently used to destroy undetected distant micrometastases.
- ❖ BRMs provide another treatment option for patients who have malignancies and for those receiving chemotherapy and need to boost their blood cell counts. BRMs include hematopoietics and IMDs. IFNs, interleukins, MABs, and miscellaneous drugs are the categories of IMDs.
- ❖ In BRM therapy, the body's immune system is used to destroy cancerous cells, and the drugs may augment, restore, or modify host defences against the tumour.

- ❖ The humoral and cellular immune systems act together to recognize and destroy foreign particles and cells. The humoral immune system is composed of lymphocytes known as B cells, which are transformed into plasma cells when they come in contact with an antigen (foreign substance). The plasma cells then manufacture antibodies to that antigen.
- ❖ Nursing management associated with the administration of BRMs focuses on the use of careful aseptic technique and other measures to prevent infection; proper nutrition, oral hygiene, and monitoring of blood counts; and management of the adverse effects of BRMs, including joint and bone pain and flulike effects.

EXAMINATION REVIEW QUESTIONS

1 Which of the following best describes the action of IFNs in the management of malignant tumours?
  a. Increase the production of specific anticancer enzymes
  b. Have antiviral and antitumour properties and strengthen the immune system
  c. Stimulate the production and activation of T lymphocytes and cytotoxic T cells
  d. Help improve the cell killing action of T cells because they are retrieved from healthy donors

2 During therapy with IFNs, which is the major dose-limiting factor that the nurse must keep in mind?
  a. Fever
  b. Fatigue
  c. Nausea and vomiting
  d. Bone marrow suppression

3 Which of the following is an appropriate nursing intervention for the patient receiving a BRM?
  a. Limit fluids to 1000 mL/day.
  b. Avoid acetaminophen products during therapy.
  c. Encourage a low-protein, high-carbohydrate diet during therapy.
  d. Premedicate with acetaminophen and diphenhydramine if beneficial.

4 In caring for a patient receiving therapy with a myelosuppressive antineoplastic drug, the nurse notes an order to begin filgrastim after the chemotherapy is completed. Which of the following statements correctly describes when the nurse should begin the filgrastim therapy?
  a. Filgrastim therapy can begin during chemotherapy.
  b. Filgrastim therapy should begin immediately after chemotherapy is completed.
  c. Filgrastim therapy should not be initiated until 24 hours after chemotherapy is completed.
  d. Filgrastim therapy should not be begun until at least 72 hours after chemotherapy is completed.

5 A patient with kidney failure has severe anemia, and there is an order for darbepoetin. As the nurse assesses the patient, which condition listed below should the nurse consider a contraindication to use of this medication?
  a. Angina
  b. Diabetes mellitus
  c. Hypothyroidism
  d. Uncontrolled hypertension

For answers see http://evolve.elsevier.com/Canada/Lilley/pharmacology/.

CRITICAL THINKING ACTIVITIES

1 Your patient is to receive filgrastim (Neupogen) after therapy with carmustine and radiation for treatment of a brain tumour. The patient weighs 60 kg. The protocol that the oncologist has given you states that filgrastim should be dosed at 5 mcg/kg. Filgrastim (Neupogen) is available as 300 mcg/mL. What dose should the patient receive?

2 What is so important about the timing of the dose of a CSF, such as filgrastim or pegfilgrastim, in the treatment of neoplasms?

3 Many drugs, particularly chemotherapeutic drugs, may lead to bone marrow suppression of various blood cell components. What symptoms would you expect to see if your patient had diminished production of platelets? RBCs? WBCs? Explain your answers.

For answers see http://evolve.elsevier.com/Canada/Lilley/pharmacology/.

CHAPTER 51

Gene Therapy and Pharmacogenomics

Learning Objectives

After reading this chapter, the successful student will be able to do the following:

1 Describe the terms related to genetics and drug therapy.

2 Briefly discuss the major concepts of genetics as an evolving segment of health care, such as principles of genetic inheritance; deoxyribonucleic acid (DNA), ribonucleic acid (RNA), and their functioning; the relationship of DNA to protein synthesis; and the significance of amino acids.

3 Describe the Human Genome Project and its impact on the role of genetics in health care.

4 Discuss the gene therapies currently available for patients and those that are undergoing Health Canada–approved clinical trials.

5 Differentiate between the direct and indirect forms of gene therapy.

6 Identify the regulatory and ethical issues related to gene therapy, drug therapy, and the health care professions.

7 Briefly discuss the concept of pharmacogenomics.

8 Contrast pharmacogenetics and pharmacogenomics.

e-Learning Activities

Web site
(http://evolve.elsevier.com/Canada/
Lilley/pharmacology/)

- Animations
- Answers to chapter questions, activities, and case studies
- Calculators and Category Catchers
- Glossary with audio pronunciations
- IV Therapy and Medication Error Checklists
- Multiple-Choice Review Question quizzes
- Nursing Care Plans
- Online Appendices and Supplements
- WebLinks

Glossary

Acquired disease Any disease acquired through external factors and not *directly* caused by a person's genes (e.g., an infectious disease, noncongenital cardiovascular diseases). (p. 954)

Alleles Any alternative forms of a gene that can occupy a specific locus (location) on a chromosome (see *chromosome*) and vary with regard to a specific genetic trait (p. 853)

Chromatin A collective term for all chromosomal material within a given cell. (p. 955)

Chromosome Structure in the nuclei of cells that contains linear threads of deoxyribonucleic acid (DNA), which transmits genetic information, and is associated with ribonucleic acid (RNA) molecules and synthesis of protein molecules. (p. 953)

Gene The biological unit of heredity; a segment of a DNA molecule that contains all of the molecular information

required for the synthesis of a biological product such as an RNA molecule or an amino acid chain (protein molecule). (p. 953)

Gene therapy New therapeutic technologies that directly target human genes in the treatment or prevention of illness. (p. 955)

Genetic disease Any disorder caused by a genetic mechanism. (p. 954)

Genetic material DNA or RNA molecules or portions of them. (p. 953)

Genetic polymorphisms Allele variants that occur in the chromosomes of 1% or more of the general population (i.e., they occur too frequently to be caused by recurrent mutations). (p. 957)

Genetic predisposition The presence of certain factors in a person's genetic makeup or *genome* that increases the likelihood of developing one or more diseases. (p. 954)

Genetics The study of the structure, function, and inheritance of genes. (p. 954)

Genome The complete set of genetic material of any organism. (p. 955)

Genomics The study of the structure and function of the genome, including DNA sequencing, mapping, and expression, and of the way genes and their products work in both health and disease. (p. 955)

Genotype The alleles present at a given site (locus) on the chromosomes of an organism (e.g., human, animal, plant) that determine a specific genetic trait for that organism (see *phenotype*). (p. 953)

Inherited disease A genetic disease that results from defective alleles passed from parents to offspring. (p. 954)

International Human Genome Project (IHGP) A project by an international group of scientists to describe in detail the entire genome of a human being. (p. 955)

Nucleic acids Molecules of DNA or RNA in the nucleus of every cell. DNA makes up the chromosomes and encodes the genes. (p. 953)

Penetrance The measurement of the proportion of individuals in a population who carry a disease-causing allele and express the disease phenotype. (p. 954)

Personalized medicine The use of tools such as molecular-level and genetic characterizations of disease processes and the patient for the customization of drug therapy. (p. 957)

Pharmacogenetics A general term for the study of the genetic basis for variations in the body's response to drugs, with a focus on variations related to a single gene. (p. 957)

Pharmacogenomics A branch of pharmacogenetics that involves the survey of the entire genome to detect multigenic (multiple-gene) determinants of drug response. (p. 957)

Phenotype The expression in the body of a genetic trait that results from a person's genotype (see *genotype*). (p. 954)

Proteome The entire set of proteins produced by an organism's genome. (p. 955)

Proteomics The detailed study of the proteome, including all biological actions of proteins. (p. 955)

Recombinant DNA (rDNA) DNA molecules that have been artificially synthesized or modified in a laboratory setting. (p. 956)

Variable expressivity The variability in expression of inherited diseases, in which individuals with the same mutation may not all express the disorder in the same way. (p. 954)

OVERVIEW

Genetic processes are a highly complex part of physiology and are far from being completely understood by scientists. Given the importance of such processes to human health, genetic research has become one of the most intensely active branches of science, involving many health care professionals, including nurses. Expected outcomes of this research include a deeper knowledge of the genetic influences on disease, along with the development of gene-based therapies. The practice of nursing will also increasingly require an understanding of genetic concepts, health issues, and therapeutic techniques (see Box 51-1). The goal of this chapter is to introduce some of the major concepts of this complex and emerging branch of health science. In 1996, in the United States, the National Coalition for Health Professional Education in Genetics (NCHPEG) was founded (http://www.nchpeg.org). The purpose of NCHPEG is to promote the education of health professionals and the public regarding advances in applied genetics. In February 2005, the NCHPEG endorsed a revised set of core competencies for health professionals related to genetics. These guidelines, relevant to all health care professionals, including nurses, continue to be expanded and can be viewed on the NCHPEG Web site at http://www.nchpeg.org/core/Corecomps2005.pdf. Any practising nurse may be expected to develop these skills, in varying degrees, depending on the practice setting and the needs of the presenting patient population.

BASIC PRINCIPLES OF GENETIC INHERITANCE

Nucleic acids are biochemical compounds consisting of molecules of deoxyribonucleic acid (DNA) and ribonucleic acid (RNA). These DNA molecules make up the **genetic material** that is passed between all types of organisms during reproduction. In some organisms (e.g., HIV), it is the RNA molecules that pass the organism's genetic material between generations; however, this is an exception to the norm. A **chromosome** is basically a long strand of DNA contained in the nuclei of cells. DNA molecules, in turn, act as the template for the formation of RNA molecules, from which proteins are synthesized. Humans normally have 23 pairs of chromosomes in each of their *somatic cells*. Somatic cells are all the cells in the body other than the sex cells (sperm cells or egg cells), which have only 23 single (unpaired) chromosomes. One pair of chromosomes in each cell is called the *sex chromosomes* and is normally XX for females and XY for males. One member of each pair of chromosomes comes from the father's sperm cell and one from the mother's egg. **Alleles** are the alternative forms of a **gene** that can vary with regard to a specific genetic trait. Genetic traits can be desirable (e.g., lack of allergies) or undesirable (e.g., predisposition to a specific disease). Alleles are dominant or recessive. Every person has two alleles for every gene-coded trait: one allele from the mother, the other from the father. The particular combination of alleles, or **genotype**, for a given trait normally determines whether a person manifests

---

BOX 51-1 — Application of Genetics, Genomics, and Pharmacogenomics in Nursing and Health Care

Competencies and outcome criteria for professional nursing practice are well integrated into the goals of educational programs in nursing. With the use of technology in health care accelerating, these defined competencies and outcomes must reflect contemporary health care practices. Genetics and the knowledge gained through the Human Genome Project need to be included in nursing education programs. The application of human genetics to pharmacology is important to achieving high-quality care of patients in a variety of settings. The nurse must integrate knowledge, skills, and attitudes related to genetics into everyday nursing practice with individuals, groups, and communities.

Since the beginning of genetic research and the subsequent definition of core competencies in genetics for health care professionals in early 2001, the world has witnessed a number of advances in genetics and genomics, including completion of the sequencing of the human genome, the use of microarray technology to determine gene expression, the use of genetics in the treatment of selected cancers, the increasing application of pharmacogenomics in the research and development of new drugs, and the application of pharmacogenomics in treatment with drugs already on the market. Genetics, genomics, and, specifically concerning the topic of this textbook, pharmacogenomics promise to transform the nursing care of patients with diseases such as diabetes, cancer, and mental health disorders. Therefore, professional nurses must remain current in their knowledge and skills related to genetics and pharmacogenomics. At some level, nurses may be involved with their patients in research and in new and experimental treatment protocols. In these situations, as with all nursing care, they should always behave in a professional, ethical, compassionate, and sensitive manner. The citations that follow represent just a few readings relating to the current core competencies in genetics that are essential for nurses and other health care professionals.

Bottorff, J. L., McCullum, M., Balneaves, L. G., Esplen, M. J., Carroll, J. C., Kelly, M., et al. (2005). Canadian nursing in the genomic era: A call for leadership. *Nursing Leadership, 18*(2), 56–72.

Conley, Y. P., & Tinkle, M. B. (2007). The future of genomic nursing research. Genomics to health. *Journal of Nursing Scholarship, 39*(1), 17–24.

Feetham, S. L., & Williams, J. K. (2004). *Nursing and 21st century genetics: Leadership for global health.* Geneva, Switzerland: International Council of Nurses.

International Council of Nurses. (2009). *Genetics and nursing.* Retrieved January 15, 2009, from http://www.icn.ch/matters_genetics.htm

International Society of Nurses in Genetics. (2006). *About ISONG.* Retrieved January 15, 2009, from http://www.isong.org/about/index.cfm

Kirk, M., Tonkin, E., & Gaff, C. (2006). Genetics. Primary care nursing and genetics: It isn't part of your role . . . is it? *Primary Health Care, 16*(7), 34–38.

Westwood, G., Pickering, R. M., Latter, S., Lucassen, A., Little, P., & Temple, I. K. (2006). Feasibility and acceptability of providing nurse counsellor genetics clinics in primary care. *Journal of Advanced Nursing, 53*(5), 591–604.

---

that trait, the person's **phenotype**. Genetic traits that are passed on differently to male and female offspring are said to be *sex-linked traits* because they are carried on either the X or Y chromosome. For example, hemophilia genes are carried by females but usually manifest as a bleeding disorder only in males. This is also an example of an **inherited disease**—that is, a disease passed from parents to offspring because of genetic defects. A more general term is **genetic disease**, which is any disease caused by a genetic mechanism. Note, however, that not all genetic diseases are inherited disease, because chromosomal abnormalities (aberrations) can also occur spontaneously during embryonic development. In contrast, an **acquired disease** is any disease that develops in response to external factors and is not directly related to a person's genetic makeup. Genetics can play an indirect role in acquired disease, however. For example, atherosclerotic heart disease is often acquired in mid- or later life. Many people have certain genes in their cells that increase the likelihood of this condition. This is known as a **genetic predisposition**. In some cases, as in the example given here, a person may be able to offset a genetic predisposition by making lifestyle choices, such as healthy diet and exercise, to avoid developing heart disease.

For many inherited diseases, the same mutation may not always be expressed in all individuals who carry it; furthermore, when the mutation is expressed, it may vary in its expression. This quality is referred to as **variable expressivity.** *Expressivity* measures the extent to which a genotype shows its phenotypical expression (e.g., extent of signs and symptoms or disease severity). Huntington's disease, for example, may vary in the age of onset and severity of symptoms. **Penetrance** is the measurement of the proportion of individuals in a population who carry a disease-causing allele and express the disease phenotype. If some people with the mutation do not develop features of the disorder, the condition is said to have reduced (or incomplete) penetrance. For example, not all females with a mutation in the *BRCA1* or *BRCA2* gene will develop cancer during their lifetime.

THE DISCOVERY, STRUCTURE, AND FUNCTION OF DNA

A major turning point in the current understanding of **genetics** came in 1953, when Drs. James Watson and Francis Crick first reported the chemical structures of human genetic material and named the primary biochemical compound *deoxyribonucleic acid (DNA)*. They later received a Nobel Prize for their discovery. It is now recognized that DNA is the primary molecule in the body that serves to transfer genes from parents to offspring. It exists in the nucleus of all body cells as strands of chromosomes, collectively called **chromatin**. As described in Chapter 49, DNA molecules contain four different organic bases, each with its own letter designation: *adenine (A), guanine (G), thymine (T),* and *cytosine (C)*. These bases are linked to a type of sugar molecule known as *deoxyribose*. Finally, these sugar molecules are linked to a "backbone" chain of phosphate molecules, which results in the classic *double-helix* structure of two side-by-side, spiral macromolecular chains. An important related biomolecule is *ribonucleic acid (RNA)*. RNA has a chemical structure similar to that of DNA, except that its sugar molecule is the compound *ribose* rather than deoxyribose and it contains the base *uracil (U)* in place of thymine. RNA more commonly occurs as a single-stranded molecule, although in some genetic processes it can also be double stranded. In double-stranded nucleic acid structures, the base of each strand binds (via hydrogen bonds) to that of the other strand in the space between the two strands (see Figure 49-1). This binding is based on complementary base pairing determined by the chemistry of the base molecules themselves. Specifically, adenine can only bind with guanine, whereas cytosine can only bind with thymine or uracil.

A *nucleotide* is the structural unit of DNA and consists of a single base and its attached sugar and phosphate molecules. A *nucleoside* is the base and its attached sugar and phosphate molecules. A relatively small sequence of nucleotides is called an *oligonucleotide* (the prefix *oligo-* means "a small number of"). Certain new drug therapies involve synthetic analogues of both nucleosides and nucleotides (see Chapters 40, 48, and 49). One of these, the ophthalmic antiviral drug fomivirsen (not currently available in Canada), is an oligonucleotide with a chemical structure that is opposite (complementary) to that of a critical part of the messenger RNA (mRNA) of the cytomegalovirus. For this reason, it is called an *antisense oligonucleotide* and is the first of this new class of drugs. Other types of antisense oligonucleotide drugs are anticipated in the near future as one type of gene therapy. An organism's entire DNA structure is its **genome**. **Genomics** is the relatively new science of determining the location (mapping) and structure (DNA base sequencing) of individual genes among the entire genome and identifying their functions in both health and disease processes.

Protein Synthesis

Protein synthesis is the primary function of DNA in human cells. In the cell nuclei, the double strands of DNA uncoil and separate, and a strand of mRNA forms on each strand through complementary base pairing, as described earlier. This process is called *transcription* of the DNA. These mRNA molecules then detach from their corresponding DNA strands, leave the cell nucleus, and enter the cytoplasm, where they are then "read," or

translated, by the ribosomes. Ribosomes are composed of a second type of RNA known as *ribosomal RNA* (rRNA), as well as several accessory proteins. Individual sequences of three bases at a time along the mRNA molecule serve to code for specific amino acid molecules. This translation process involves molecules of a third type of RNA, *transfer RNA* (tRNA). The tRNA molecules transport the corresponding amino acid molecules to the site of ribosomal translation along the mRNA strand in sequence according to the three-base codes along the mRNA strand. This process, in turn, results in the creation of chains of multiple amino acid molecules (*polypeptide chains*), which are known as protein molecules. The specificity of this code is important for proper protein synthesis.

There are numerous specific amino acid sequences (polypeptides) that result in the synthesis of many thousands of types of protein molecules. Proteins include hormones, enzymes, immunoglobulins, and numerous other biochemical molecules that regulate processes throughout the body. They are involved in both healthy (normal) physiological processes and the pathophysiological processes of many diseases. Biomedical researchers continue to identify and describe, from both scientific and clinical perspectives, many proteins that are part of disease processes. Manipulation of genetic material, as in *gene therapy* (see Gene Therapy section later in this chapter), can theoretically modify the synthesis of these proteins and thus help in the treatment of disease. This emerging science continues to give rise to novel terminology and discoveries. The entire set of proteins produced by a genome is now known as the **proteome**. **Proteomics,** the newest genetic science, is the study of the proteome, including protein expression, modification, localization, and function, as well as the protein–protein interactions that are part of biological processes. This science is expected to provide new drug therapies in the future.

The Human Genome Project

In the mid-1980s, there was discussion in the scientific community of a bold new project that would seek to map the entire DNA sequence (genome) of a human being. This project, officially begun in 1990, was known as the **International Human Genome Project (IHGP)** and was a worldwide research initiative. Sequencing was not expected to be finished until 2005 but was completed ahead of schedule in 2003. The goals of this project were to identify the estimated 30,000 genes in human DNA and determine the approximately three *billion* base pairs that make up human DNA. Related goals were to develop new tools for genetic data analysis and storage, transfer newly developed technologies to the private sector, and address inherent ethical, legal, and social issues involved in genetic research and clinical practice.

GENE THERAPY

One result of the availability of information from the IHGP is the continued development of **gene therapy**.

This therapy involves the treatment or prevention of disease by transferring exogenous (foreign) genetic material (DNA or RNA) into the body of an individual. The primary driving force of gene therapy research is the ongoing discovery of new details regarding cellular processes, including biochemical processes that occur at the molecular level. In addition, the increasing understanding of allelic variation and its role in disease susceptibility can be used to guide attempts at preventive therapy based on a person's genotypical risk factors.

Currently, there are numerous Health Canada–approved clinical trials in progress using gene therapy techniques. However, to date, no gene therapy has received approval for routine treatment of disease. The general goal of gene therapy is to transfer to the patient exogenous genes that will either provide a temporary substitute for or initiate permanent changes in the patient's own genetic functioning in order to treat a given disease. Originally expected to provide treatment primarily for inherited genetic diseases, gene therapy techniques are now being researched for the treatment of acquired illnesses such as cancer, cardiovascular diseases, diabetes, infectious diseases, and substance misuse. In the more distant future, in utero gene therapy may be used to prevent the development of serious diseases as part of the prenatal care of the unborn infant.

During gene therapy, segments of DNA are usually injected into a patient's body in a process called *gene transfer*. These DNA splices, also known as **recombinant DNA (rDNA),** must usually be inserted into some kind of vector for the gene transfer process. Current vectors being evaluated by researchers include spherical lipid compounds known as *liposomes*, free DNA splices known as *plasmids*, DNA conjugates in which DNA splices are linked (conjugated) to either protein or gold particles, and various types of viruses. Viruses are the most widely studied rDNA vectors thus far. One commonly used group of viruses is that of the adenoviruses, which includes human influenza ("flu") viruses. If the desired rDNA segment can be inserted into the viral genome, the virus can then be injected into the patient to therapeutically infect human cells. If this planned infectious process is successful, the viral genome will be combined with the human host cell genome and specific proteins will be produced to counter a disease process. Ideally, this would result in a permanent positive physiological change in the host. However, viruses used in this way can also induce viral disease and be immunogenic in the human host. The proteins produced by such artificial methods can also be immunogenic. Even in the absence of significant virus-induced disease, the positive effects (e.g., supplemented protein synthesis) may only be temporary; therefore, future treatments may be required. Consequently, viruses must be carefully chosen and modified in an effort to optimize therapeutic effects while minimizing undesirable adverse effects. The determination of an ideal gene transfer method remains a major challenge for gene therapy researchers. Figure 51-1 provides a clinical example of the potential use of gene therapy.

One indirect form of gene therapy is already well established. It involves the use of rDNA vectors in the laboratory to make recombinant forms of drugs, especially biological drugs such as hormones, vaccines, antitoxins, and monoclonal antibodies (discussed in Chapters 47 and 50). One of the most widespread examples is the use of the *Escherichia coli* bacterial genome to manufacture a recombinant form of human insulin. When the human insulin gene is inserted into the genome of bacterial cells, the resulting culture growth artificially generates human insulin on a large scale. Although this insulin must be isolated and purified from its bacterial culture source, most of the world's medical insulin supply has been produced by this method for well over a decade.

Regulatory and Ethical Issues Regarding Gene Therapy

Gene therapy research is inherently complex, and this therapy can carry great risk for its recipients. Research subjects who receive gene therapy often have a life-threatening illness, such as cancer, which may justify the risks involved. However, case reports of patient deaths in gene therapy trials have underscored these risks and raised awareness of patient safety among researchers. The Biologics and Genetic Therapies Directorate (BGTD) of Health Canada is assigned the responsibility for oversight of gene therapy research in Canada. It reviews clinical trials involving human gene transfer and schedules public forums to discuss pertinent issues. The Food and Drug Regulations, Health Canada, must also review and

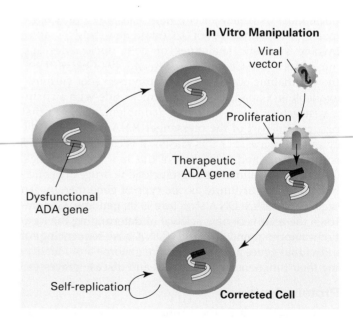

FIG. 51-1   Gene therapy for adenosine deaminase (ADA) deficiency attempts to correct this immunodeficiency state. The viral vector containing the therapeutic gene is inserted into the patient's lymphocytes. These cells can then make the ADA enzyme. (From Lewis, S. M., Heitkemper, M. M., & Dirksen, S. R. (2009). *Medical-surgical nursing: Assessment and management of clinical problems* (2nd ed.). (Canadian Eds. S. Goldsworthy & M. Barry). St. Louis, MO: Elsevier Mosby.)

approve all human clinical gene therapy trials, as it does with any type of drug therapy.

The federal government also plays a significant role as a research funder through the Canadian Institutes of Health Research (CIHR) and the National Research Council's Genomics and Health Initiative. Any institution that conducts any type of research involving human subjects must have a research ethics board (REB), whose purpose is to protect research subjects from unnecessary risks. The guiding requirements are outlined in Health Canada's *Tri-Council Policy Statement: Ethical Conduct for Research Involving Humans (TCPS)*. Also required for gene therapy research is an institutional biosafety committee (IBC). The role of the IBC is to ensure compliance with the Medical Council of Canada (MRC)'s *Guidelines for the Handling of Recombinant DNA Molecules and Animal Viruses and Cells*. This document was revised in 1986 by the MRC and Health and Welfare Canada and in 1990 published as *Laboratory Biosafety Guidelines*, now in its third edition.

A major ethical issue related to gene therapy techniques is the fear of *eugenics*, which is the intentional selection, before birth, of genotypes that are considered more desirable than others. For similar reasons, the prospect of manipulating genes in human *germ cells* (sperm and eggs), even at a pre-embryonic stage, is also cited as a potential hazard of gene therapy experimentation. Theoretically, even cosmetic modifications could be attempted using such techniques as a part of routine family planning. Because of such ethical concerns, Canadian gene therapy research is limited to somatic cells. Gene therapy in germline (reproductive) cells is currently illegal in Canada. This limitation remains despite arguments from those who believe that human germ-cell research would likely yield cures for many serious chronic illnesses and disabilities, such as Parkinson's disease and spinal paralysis.

PHARMACOGENOMICS

Pharmacogenetics is the most general term for the study of genetic variations in drug response and focuses on single-gene variations. In addition to gene therapy, a second important branch of health science related to the IHGP is **pharmacogenomics**. This newer branch of pharmacogenetics involves working with the whole genome to determine multiple individual genetic factors that influence a person's response to specific medications. For example, one patient may be more likely than another to benefit from (or suffer toxicity from) a certain type of drug therapy, depending on the presence or absence of specific alleles in the individual's genome. The relationship between the terms *pharmacogenetics* and *pharmacogenomics* can be difficult to understand intuitively, and they are sometimes used interchangeably in the literature.

The individual differences in alleles are known as **genetic polymorphisms** if the alleles are common enough to occur in at least 1% of the population (i.e., they occur too frequently to be caused by recurrent mutation). Genetic polymorphisms that alter the amount or functioning of drug-metabolizing enzymes can, therefore, alter the body's reactions to medications. Known examples include genetic polymorphisms that affect the metabolism of certain antimalarial drugs, the antituberculosis drug isoniazid, and drugs metabolized by several subtypes of cytochrome P450 enzymes. Study of both the genome of the patient and the presenting genetics of the disease (e.g., tumour cells, infectious organisms) before treatment could theoretically allow customized drug selection and dosing. Such analysis could help identify drugs less likely to be effective as well as optimal drug doses, in order to minimize the risk of adverse drug effects for a given patient. This application of pharmacogenomics is known as **personalized medicine**.

To this end, researchers have developed an analytical tool known as a high-density microarray. This technology applies methods used in computer chip manufacture to design amazingly small microchip plates that contain thousands of DNA samples. A patient's blood sample can then be screened for thousands of corresponding DNA sequences (which bind to the sequences on the chip) to determine the presence or absence of genes, such as those related to drug metabolism. Such technology is currently used primarily in nonclinical research laboratories. However, it is expected within 5 years to become more readily available and affordable for routine use in the clinical setting. With the expanding availability of comprehensive genetic testing, proactive customization of drug therapy is expected to become increasingly more frequent over the next one to two decades. However, it is not yet a part of routine clinical practice; most drug dosage changes are still usually made on a trial-and-error basis by monitoring patient response. Table 51-1 lists some current clinical applications of pharmacogenomics.

SUMMARY

Increasing scientific understanding of genetic processes is expected to revolutionize modern health care in many ways. The artificial manipulation and transfer of genetic material, although not a standard treatment for disease, is the focus of numerous current human clinical gene therapy trials. The spectrum of diseases that may eventually be treatable by gene therapy includes inherited diseases that are present from birth, disabilities such as paralysis from spinal cord injuries, life-threatening illnesses such as cancer, and even other chronic illnesses acquired later in life for which a person may have a genetic predisposition. The science of pharmacogenomics has already identified some of the genetic nuances in how different people's bodies metabolize and experience benefit or harm from drugs. Continued study in this area is expected to result in proactive customization of drug therapy to promote therapeutic benefits while minimizing or eliminating toxic effects. Genetic procedures and therapeutic techniques will likely become a growing part of nursing practice, as well as of health care delivery in general. As the impact of genetics on drug therapy increases, so will its role in the nursing process (see Box 50-1).

TABLE 51-1

Current Clinical Applications of Pharmacogenomics

Genotyping for presence of CYP2D6 enzyme and for the CYP2D6 alleles to determine whether patients are poor, intermediate, extensive, or ultrarapid metabolizers with these enzymes (under study)	Psychiatry and general medicine: helps guide prescribing of selected medications such as anticoagulants, immunosuppressants, antidepressants, antipsychotics, anticonvulsants, β-blockers, and antidysrhythmics
Genotyping for presence of the *p-glycoprotein* drug transport protein (under study)	Cardiology, infectious diseases, oncology, and other practice areas: assists in drug selection and dosing for drugs such as digoxin, antiretrovirals, and antineoplastics
Genotyping for presence of thiopurine methyltransferase enzyme	Oncology: used to temper toxicity through more careful dosing of the cancer drug 6-mercaptopurine in children with leukemia
Genotyping for variations in β-adrenergic receptors (under study)	Pulmonology: Determines which asthma patients are more or less responsive to β-agonist therapy (e.g., albuterol) and which patients might benefit from other types of drug therapy
Genotyping for presence of the Philadelphia chromosome	Oncology: identifies those patients with chronic myelogenous leukemia who can benefit from the cancer drug imatinib (Gleevec)
Genotyping for presence of the *HER2* proto-oncogene	Oncology: identifies a subset of breast cancer patients whose tumours express this gene, which indicates their suitability for treatment with the cancer drug trastuzumab (Herceptin)
Viral genotyping of hepatitis C viruses (under study)	Infectious diseases: can determine whether a particular infection warrants 26 versus 48 weeks of drug therapy (thereby reducing both costs and adverse drug effects)

CYP2D6, cytochrome P450 enzyme subtype 2D6.

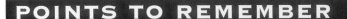

POINTS TO REMEMBER

❖ Genetic processes are a highly complex facet of human physiology, and genetics is becoming an integral part of health care that holds much promise in the form of new treatments for alterations in health.

❖ The IHGP described in detail the entire genome of a human individual.

❖ Basic genetic inheritance begins with 23 pairs of chromosomes in each of the somatic cells; one pair of chromosomes in each cell is called the *sex chromosomes,* identified as XX for females and XY for males.

EXAMINATION REVIEW QUESTIONS

1 In the creation of which of the following is an indirect form of gene therapy most appropriately seen?
   a. Insulin
   b. Stem cells
   c. Antigen substitution
   d. Platelet inhibitors or stimulators

2 Use of gene therapy may be immunogenic in the human host. To which of the following can immunogenicity in the human host possibly lead?
   a. Biological vaccines
   b. Antitoxin formation
   c. Temporary reduction of a disease process
   d. Cures of almost any type of antigen-related disease process

3 Which of the following is the responsibility of the Biologics and Genetic Therapies Directorate?
   a. Approving all forms of clinical gene therapy
   b. Analyzing genomes and determining whether they appear mutagenic
   c. Identifying all major risks to the human subjects in a specific research protocol
   d. Reviewing clinical trials involving human gene transfer and scheduling public forums

4 Which one of the following describes factors in a person's genetic makeup that increases the likelihood of eventually developing one or more diseases?
   a. Genotype
   b. Genetic mutation
   c. Genome predisposition
   d. Genetic polymorphism

5 Which of the following is a commonly studied adenovirus?
   a. *Genovirum*
   b. *Genovirum pallodium*
   c. Human influenza
   d. Hepatitis A and C

For answers see http://evolve.elsevier.com/Canada/Lilley/pharmacology/.

CRITICAL THINKING ACTIVITIES

1 "An indirect form of gene therapy is already seen in contemporary health care practices." Explain this statement and provide examples.

2 Explain how the use of gene therapy could also be immunogenic. How would this affect patients? Give examples.

3 Analyze the process for producing human insulin, and present a few examples of how this same process could be used in other areas of health care.

For answers see http://evolve.elsevier.com/Canada/Lilley/pharmacology/.

PART NINE

Drugs Affecting the Gastrointestinal System and Nutrition

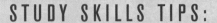

STUDY SKILLS TIPS:

- ACTIVE QUESTIONING
- DETERMINING THE RIGHT QUESTIONS
- KINDS OF QUESTIONS
- QUESTIONING APPLICATION

ACTIVE QUESTIONING

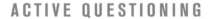

One study technique that cannot be overemphasized is active questioning. In the PURR model, it is critical that you be able to generate questions in the Plan, Rehearsal, and Review steps. The questions you generate will help maintain concentration as you study, improve your comprehension as you read assigned material, and develop long-term memory. Active questioning is a strategy that develops with practice.

DETERMINING THE RIGHT QUESTIONS

Some questions generated during the Plan step will be useful in that they will focus on exactly the right issues for maximum learning. Some questions will seem logical and important when you are working with the limited amount of information available using the Plan step, but as you read the chapter you will find that they miss the mark. Do not worry about whether each question you ask is perfectly focused. As you read, rehearse, and review the material, you can and should revise questions

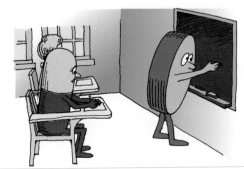

on the basis of your growing understanding of the material. Ask many questions to maintain active involvement in the learning process and anticipate questions that will appear on exams. The more questions you ask, the more effective you will become as both an active questioner and an active learner.

KINDS OF QUESTIONS

First, you must realize that more than one kind of question can be asked. Over the years, educators have proposed many questioning hierarchies, comprising three to eight different types of questions. Following is a simple approach that focuses on two types of questions.

Literal Questions

Literal questions are those that are answered directly and specifically by the text. If you were reading a Canadian history text and found a topic heading, "The First Prime Minister," an obvious question would be, "Who was the first prime minister?" The answer would be stated clearly and directly in the text under this heading. This is an example of a literal question. A literal question usually has a single correct response. The answer is stated directly in the text, and every reader will find the same information.

Interpretive Questions

Interpretive questions are more challenging because they require the reader to interpret, synthesize, evaluate, and analyze the material. They require not only knowledge of the literal information but also enough understanding to select several different bits of data and put them together. In Canadian history, an interpretive question might be, "Why was Lester Pearson considered an exemplary prime minister?" This question requires you to not only know the facts about Pearson but also evaluate and judge those facts in order to reach a conclusion that can be supported by the literal information. Some interpretive questions have only one correct response; others have more than one correct response. Both kinds of questions are essential in the learning process.

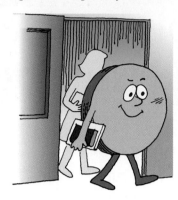

QUESTIONING APPLICATION

In Chapter 52, the terms *pepsinogen* and *proenzyme* are italicized. Italics are used to gain the reader's attention and to indicate that the material is especially noteworthy.

Emphasized material should always be considered a potential source of questions. What is pepsinogen? What is a proenzyme? Again, we can begin the questioning with simple, literal questions, but it is essential that interpretive questions also be asked. What do pepsinogen and proenzyme have in common? How are the terms related in the broader topic of acid-related pathophysiology? These questions require that you read for broader general understanding.

At the end of each chapter, a section entitled "Critical Thinking Activities" is given. Even though this information is stated in question form, you should consider generating additional questions of your own. The first question in Chapter 52 is, "What is the purpose of adding simethicone to drugs used to treat gastrointestinal disorders?" In answering it, some additional questions will help you focus your learning. What adverse affects are there with drugs used to treat gastrointestinal disorders? What is simethicone? To what class of drugs does it belong? What are its mechanisms of actions and indications?

The more active you become as a questioner, the easier it will become to ask the kinds of questions that are necessary for your learning.

CHAPTER 52

Acid-Controlling Drugs

Learning Objectives

After reading this chapter, the successful student will be able to do the following:

1 Obtain a brief overview of the gastrointestinal system and the role of hydrochloric acid in digestion.

2 Discuss the physiological influences of pathologies such as peptic ulcer disease, gastritis, spastic colon, gastroesophageal reflux disease, and hyperacidic states on the health of patients and on their gastrointestinal tracts.

3 Describe the mechanisms of action, indications, cautions, contraindications, drug interactions, adverse effects, dosages, and routes of administration for the following classes of acid-controlling drugs: antacids, histamine-2 (H_2)–blocking drugs (H_2 antagonists), proton pump inhibitors, and acid suppressants.

4 Develop a collaborative plan of care that includes all phases of the nursing process related to the administration of acid-controlling drugs.

e-Learning Activities

Web site
(http://evolve.elsevier.com/Canada/Lilley/pharmacology/)

- Animations
- Answers to chapter questions, activities, and case studies
- Calculators and Category Catchers
- Glossary with audio pronunciations
- IV Therapy and Medication Error Checklists
- Multiple-Choice Review Question quizzes
- Nursing Care Plans
- Online Appendices and Supplements
- WebLinks

Drug Profiles

    antacids, general, p. 969
➞ **cimetidine**, p. 970
    misoprostol, p. 972
➞ **omeprazole (omeprazole magnesium)***, p. 972
    simethicone, p. 973
➞ **sucralfate**, p. 973

➞ Key drug.

*Full generic name is given in parentheses. For the purposes of this text, the more common shortened name is used.

Glossary

Antacids Basic compounds composed of different combinations of acid-neutralizing ionic salts. (p. 966)

Chief cells Cells in the stomach that secrete the gastric enzyme pepsinogen (a precursor to pepsin). (p. 964)

Gastric glands Secretory glands in the stomach containing the following cell types: parietal, chief, mucus, endocrine, and enterochromaffin. (p. 964)

Gastric hyperacidity The overproduction of stomach acid. (p. 964)

Hydrochloric acid (HCl) An acid secreted by the *parietal cells* in the lining of the stomach that maintains the environment of the stomach at a pH of 1 to 4. (p. 964)

Mucous cells Cells whose function in the stomach is to secrete mucus that serves as a protective mucous coat against the digestive properties of HCl. (p. 964)

Parietal cells Cells in the stomach that produce and secrete HCl. (p. 964)

Pepsin An enzyme in the stomach that breaks down proteins. (p. 964)

OVERVIEW

One of the conditions of the stomach that requires drug therapy is *hyperacidity,* or excessive acid production. Left untreated, this condition can lead to such serious conditions as acid reflux, ulcer disease, esophageal damage, and even esophageal cancer. Overproduction of stomach acid is also referred to as **gastric hyperacidity**. Before the acid-controlling drugs are discussed, an overview of the gastrointestinal system is provided.

ACID-RELATED PATHOPHYSIOLOGY

For a more complete understanding of the large family of drugs used to treat acid-related disorders of the stomach, a brief overview of gastrointestinal system function and the role of **hydrochloric acid (HCl)** in digestion is beneficial. The stomach secretes many substances with physiological functions:

- HCl (an acid that aids digestion and serves as a barrier to infection)
- Bicarbonate (a base that is a natural mechanism to prevent hyperacidity)
- Pepsinogen (an enzymatic precursor to *pepsin,* an enzyme that digests dietary proteins)
- Intrinsic factor (a glycoprotein that facilitates gastric absorption of vitamin B_{12})
- Mucus (for protection of the stomach lining from both HCl and digestive enzymes)
- Prostaglandins (PGs) (have a variety of anti-inflammatory and protective functions; Chapter 45)

The stomach, although one structure, can be divided into three functional areas. Each area has specific glands with which it is associated. These glands are composed of different cells, and these cells secrete different substances. Figure 52-1 shows the three functional areas of the stomach and the distribution of the associated types of stomach glands.

The three primary glands in the stomach are cardiac, pyloric, and gastric glands. These glands are named for their positions in the stomach. *Cardiac glands* are located around the cardiac sphincter (also known as the gastroesophageal sphincter); *gastric glands* are in the fundus (hence also known as the *fundic* gland or zone), the greater part of the body of the stomach; and *pyloric glands* are in the pyloric region and in the transitional zone between the pyloric and the fundic (or gastric) zones. Gastric glands are the most numerous and are of primary importance to the discussion of acid-related disorders and drug therapy.

Gastric glands are highly specialized secretory glands composed of several different types of cells: parietal, chief, mucous, endocrine, and enterochromaffin. Each cell secretes a specific substance. The three most important cell types are parietal cells, chief cells, and mucous cells (see Figure 52-1).

Parietal cells produce and secrete HCl. They are the primary sites of action for many of the drugs used to treat acid-related disorders. The parietal cells contain receptors for histamine, gastrin, and acetylcholine. **Chief cells** secrete *pepsinogen,* which is a proenzyme (enzyme precursor) that becomes **pepsin** when activated by exposure to acid. Pepsin breaks down proteins and is therefore referred to as a *proteolytic* enzyme. **Mucous cells** are mucus-secreting cells that are also called *surface epithelial cells.* The secreted mucus serves as a protective coating against the digestive action of HCl and digestive enzymes.

These three cell types play an important role in the digestive process. When the balance between these three cells and their secretions is impaired, acid-related diseases can occur. While the most harmful of these involve acid hypersecretion and *peptic ulcer disease (PUD)* and *esophageal cancer,* the most common condition is mild to moderate hyperacidity. Many lay terms (e.g., *indigestion, sour stomach, heartburn, acid stomach*) have been used to describe this condition of overproduction of HCl by the parietal cells. Hyperacidity is often associated with *gastroesophageal reflux disease (GERD),* which refers to the tendency of excessive and acidic stomach contents to back up, or *reflux,* into the lower (and even upper) esophagus. Over time, this condition can lead to more serious disorders such as *erosive esophagitis* and *Barrett's esophagus,* a precancerous condition. Besides patient discomfort, its potential for becoming a serious diorder is one of the major reasons for aggressively treating GERD with one or more of the medications described in this section.

HCl is an acid that, as noted earlier, is secreted by the parietal cells in the lining of the stomach. It is the primary substance secreted in the stomach that maintains the environment of the stomach at a pH of 1 to 4. This acidity aids in the proper digestion of food and serves as one of the body's defences against microbial infection via the gastrointestinal tract. Several substances stimulate HCl secretion by the parietal cells, such as food, caffeine, chocolate, and alcohol. In moderation, any of these is usually not problematic. However, excessive consumption of large, fatty meals or alcohol, as well as emotional stress, may result in the hyperproduction of HCl from the parietal cells, which lead to hypersecretory disorders such as PUD. Sight, taste, and smell are also stimulants for HCl secretion. Acid secretion follows a circadian rhythm with higher acid secretion occurring at night and the lowest level in the morning.

Because the parietal cell is the source of HCl production, it is the primary target for many of the most effective drugs for the treatment of acid-related disorders. A closer look at how the parietal cell receives signals to produce and secrete HCl will enhance the understanding of the mechanism of action of many of the drugs used to treat acid-related disorders.

The wall of the parietal cell has three types of receptors: acetylcholine (ACh), histamine, and gastrin. When any one of these is occupied by its corresponding chemical stimulant (ACh, histamine, or gastrin, which can all be considered first messengers), the parietal cell will

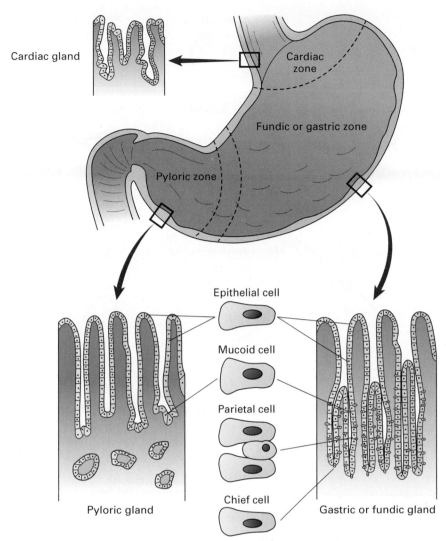

FIG. 52-1 The three specific zones of the stomach and the different glands.

produce and secrete HCl. Figure 52-2 shows the parietal cell with its three receptors. Once these receptors have become occupied, a *second messenger* is sent inside the cell. In the case of histamine receptors, occupation results in the production of adenylate cyclase. Adenylate cyclase converts adenosine triphosphate (ATP) to cyclic adenosine monophosphate (cAMP), which provides energy for the *proton pump* to work. The proton pump or, more precisely, the hydrogen–potassium–adenosine triphosphatase (ATPase) pump, is a pump for the transport of hydrogen ions and is located in the parietal cells. If energy is present, the proton pump will be activated, and the pump will be able to transport hydrogen ions needed for the production of HCl.

In the case of both ACh and gastrin receptors on the parietal cell surfaces, the second messenger that drives the proton pump is not cAMP but, instead, calcium ions. Anticholinergic drugs (Chapter 21) such as atropine block ACh receptors; this action also results in decreased hydrogen ion secretion from the parietal cells. However, these drugs are now rarely used for this purpose and

have been superseded by other drug classes discussed in this chapter. There is currently no drug to block the binding of the hormone gastrin to its corresponding receptor on the parietal cell surface.

Peptic ulcer disease (PUD) is a general term for gastric or duodenal ulcers caused by the digestion of the gastrointestinal mucosa by the enzyme pepsin, which normally serves to break down only food proteins. As noted earlier, pepsin is the activated form of pepsinogen, which is produced by the chief cells of the stomach in response to HCl released from the parietal cells. Because the process of ulceration is driven by the proteolytic (protein breakdown) actions of pepsin together with the caustic effects of HCl, PUD and related problems are also referred to by the more general term *acid–peptic disorders*.

In 1983, a certain gram-negative spiral bacterium, *Campylobacter pylori*, was isolated from several patients with gastritis. Over the next 6 years, this bacterium was further studied, and it gradually came to be implicated in the pathophysiology of PUD. At that time, the official name of this bacterium was changed to *Helicobacter pylori*

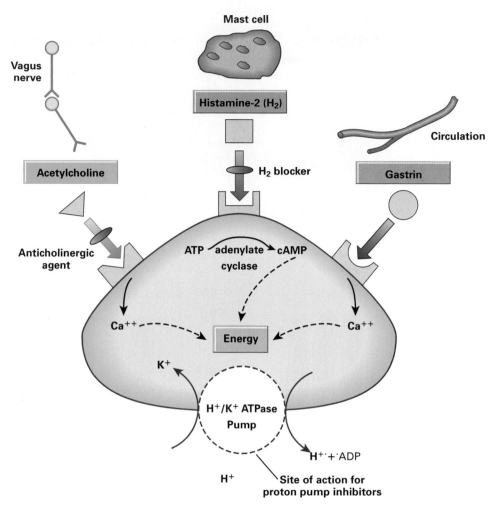

FIG. 52-2 Parietal cell stimulation and secretion. *ATP*, adenosine triphosphate; *cAMP*, cyclic adenosine monophosphate.

because it was felt to have more characteristics of the *Helicobacter* genus. The prevalence of *H. pylori* as measured by serum antibody tests is approximately 40% to 60% for patients older than 60 years of age and only 10% for those younger than 30 years of age. The bacterium is found in the gastrointestinal tracts of approximately 90% of patients with duodenal ulcers and 70% of those with gastric ulcers. However, this bacterium is also found in many patients who do not have PUD, and its presence is not associated with acute, perforating ulcers. These latter observations suggest that more than one factor is involved in ulceration. Table 52-1 lists standard treatment options for *H. pylori* infection.

ANTACIDS

Antacids are basic compounds used to neutralize stomach acid. Most commonly, they are nonprescription salts of aluminum, magnesium, calcium, or sodium (Box 52-1). Antacids have been used for centuries in the treatment of patients with acid-related disorders. Ancient Greeks used crushed coral (calcium carbonate) in the first century AD

to treat patients with dyspepsia. The use of antacids was the principal antiulcer treatment until the introduction of histamine-2 (H_2) antagonists in the late 1970s. For decades before that, the classic treatment for acid-related disorders was a combination regimen that included an antacid and an anticholinergic drug such as atropine. H_2 antagonists, proton pump inhibitors, surface-protective drugs, and mucus-producing prostaglandins have generally replaced anticholinergics for the treatment of acid-related gastrointestinal disease. However, antacids, particularly, over-the-counter formulations, are still used extensively. They are available in a variety of dosage forms, some including more than one antacid salt. In addition, many antacid preparations also contain the *antiflatulent* (antigas) drug simethicone (see Miscellaneous Acid-Controlling Drugs, p. 972), which reduces gas and bloating. Many aluminum- and calcium-based formulations also contain magnesium, which contributes to the acid-neutralizing capacity and counteracts the constipating effects of aluminum and calcium. There are multiple salts of calcium. Calcium carbonate is the most commonly used salt of calcium when calcium is used

TABLE 52-1	
Current Health Canada–Approved Regimens for Eradicating *Helicobacter pylori* **Infection in Adults**	
Suggested Treatment Regimens: Triple Therapies (PPI plus Two Antibiotics)	**Recommended Doses**

A. Proton Pump Inhibitor (PPI) + amoxicillin + clarithromycin
B. Proton Pump Inhibitor (PPI) + metronidazole + clarithromycin
  Alternative Treatment Regimen*
  Quadruple Therapy (PPI plus BMT)
C. Proton Pump Inhibitor (PPI) + bismuth subsalicylate + metronidazole + tetracycline (BMT)
  Treatment adherence is imperative.
  Duration of therapy for adults is 7 days for all regimens.
  Some experts recommend a 14-day regimen.
  Eradication rates are approximately 90%.
  Metronidazole is appropriate for patients with penicillin allergies.
  The alternative treatment regimen is appropriate for patients with clarithromycin intolerance. It may also be used for triple-therapy failures.
	Proton Pump Inhibitor:
	esomaprazole 40 mg bid
	or
	lansoprazole 30 mg bid
	or
	omeprazole 20 mg bid
	or
	pantoprazole 40 mg bid
	or
	rabeprazole 20 mg bid
	amoxicillin = 1 g bid
	clarithromycin = 500 mg bid
	metronidazole = 500 mg bid **or** 250 mg qid in PPI + BMT protocol
	bismuth subsalicylate = 2 tablets qid
	tetracycline = 500 mg qid

*Tetracycline is substituted in this regimen for those patients with intolerance to clarithromycin.

as an antacid. It is not prescribed as frequently as other antacids because its use may result in kidney stones and increased gastric acid secretion. Sodium bicarbonate is a highly soluble antacid form with a rapid onset but a short duration of action.

Mechanism of Action and Drug Effects

Antacids work primarily by neutralizing gastric acidity. They do nothing to prevent the overproduction of acid but instead help neutralize acid secretions. It is also thought that antacids promote gastric mucosal defensive mechanisms, particularly at lower dosages. They do this by stimulating the secretion of mucus, prostaglandins, and bicarbonate secretion from the cells inside the gastric glands. Mucus serves as a protective barrier against the destructive properties of HCl. Bicarbonate helps buffer the acidity of HCl. Prostaglandins prevent histamine from binding to its corresponding parietal cell receptors, thereby preventing the production of adenylate cyclase. Without adenylate cyclase, no cAMP is formed and no second messenger is available to activate the proton pump (see Figure 52-2).

The primary drug effect of antacids is the reduction of symptoms associated with acid-related disorders, such as pain and reflux ("heartburn"). One dose of antacid that raises the gastric pH from 1.3 to 1.6 (only 0.3 point) reduces gastric acidity by 50%; acidity is reduced by 90% if the pH is raised one entire point (e.g., 1.3 to 2.3). Antacid-associated pain reduction is thought to be a result of base-mediated inhibition of the protein-digesting ability of pepsin, increase in the resistance of the stomach lining to irritation, and increase in the tone of the cardiac sphincter, which reduces reflux from the stomach.

BOX 52-1

Antacids: Salt Content

Magnesium Salts	Aluminum Salts	Calcium Salts	Sodium Salts
carbonate hydroxide oxide trisilicate	carbonate hydroxide	carbonate	bicarbonate citrate

COMMONLY AVAILABLE ANTACID PRODUCTS
Aluminum-Containing Antacids
Hydroxide salt: Almagel (with magnesium hydroxide)
Combination products: Maalox, Mylanta

Calcium-Containing Antacids
Carbonate salt: Tums, Rolaids Antacid, Extra Strength
  Calcium Antacid Chewable, Antacid 2, Gastrocalm,
  Bismuth + Antacid, Trial Antacid

Magnesium-Containing Antacids
Carbonate salt: Magmix
Hydroxide salt: milk of magnesia
Oxide salt: magnesium oxide
Trisilicate salt: Gasulsol Tablets
Combination product: Calmax, Maalox

Sodium-Containing Antacids
Bicarbonate salt and citrate salt: Alka-Seltzer, Bromo
  Madelon, E-Z-Gas 2

Note: Most of the antacids listed above contain a mixture of antacids, not just one single ingredient.

Indications

Antacids are indicated for the acute relief of symptoms associated with peptic ulcer, gastritis, gastric hyperacidity, and heartburn.

Calcium acetate, calcium liquid, and calcium carbonate are often used to prevent or treat calcium deficiency. Aluminum hydroxide, calcium acetate, calcium carbonate, calcium liquid, and sevelamer (Renagel) bind dietary phosphate; these may be used in patients with kidney failure to reduce the amount of phosphorus absorbed from food. Magnesium-containing antacids may also be used for magnesium replacement.

Contraindications

The usual contraindication to antacid use is known allergy to a specific drug product. Other contraindications may include severe kidney failure or electrolyte disturbances (because of the potential toxic accumulation of electrolytes in the antacids themselves) and gastrointestinal obstruction (antacids may stimulate gastrointestinal motility when it is undesirable on account of an obstructive process requiring surgical intervention).

Adverse Effects

The adverse effects of antacids are limited. Magnesium preparations, particularly milk of magnesia, can cause diarrhea. Both aluminum- and calcium-containing formulations can result in constipation. Calcium products can also cause kidney stones. Excessive use of these drugs can theoretically result in systemic alkalosis. This condition is more common with sodium bicarbonate. Another adverse effect that is more common with the calcium-containing products is rebound hyperacidity, or acid rebound, in which the patient experiences hyperacidity when antacid use is discontinued. Long-term self-medication with antacids may mask the symptoms of serious underlying diseases such as bleeding ulcers or malignancy. Patients with ongoing symptoms should undergo regular medical evaluations because additional medications or other interventions may be needed. Box 52-2 lists several specific nursing concerns for patients taking antacids.

Interactions

Antacids are capable of causing several drug interactions when administered with other drugs. There are four basic mechanisms by which antacids cause such interactions:

- *Adsorption* of other drugs to antacids, which reduces the ability of the other drug to be absorbed into the body
- Chemical inactivation of other drugs by *chelation*, which produces insoluble complexes
- *Increased stomach pH*, which increases the absorption of basic drugs and decreases the absorption of acidic drugs
- *Increased urinary pH*, which increases the excretion of acidic drugs and decreases the excretion of basic drugs

Most drugs are either weak acids or weak bases. Therefore, pH conditions, both in the gastrointestinal and urinary tracts, will affect the extent to which drug molecules are ionized (charged). Ionized drug molecules are generally more water soluble and thus more likely to be excreted (at the kidney) or not absorbed (from the gastrointestinal tract). Nonionized drug molecules are more likely to be absorbed in the gastrointestinal tract because they are usually more fat soluble than their ionized counterparts. This quality allows them to be better absorbed through the lipid-based cell membranes of the gastrointestinal tract and ultimately into the bloodstream. Common examples of drugs whose effects may be chemically enhanced by the presence of antacids (because of pH effects) include benzodiazepines, sulfonylureas (may also be reduced, depending on the drugs involved), sympathomimetics, and valproic acid. More commonly, the presence of antacids reduces the efficacy of interacting drugs by interfering with their gastrointestinal absorption. These drugs include allopurinol, tetracycline, thyroid hormones, captopril, corticosteroids, digoxin R, histamine antagonists, phenytoin, isoniazid, ketoconazole, methotrexate, nitrofurantoin, phenothiazines, and salicylates. Patients are advised to take any interacting drugs at least 2 hours before or after antacids are taken.

Dosages

For information on dosages for selected antacid drugs, see the Dosages table on p. 969.

BOX 52-2 Nursing Concerns for Patients Taking Antacids

Aluminum, when used to reduce gastric acid, binds to phosphate and may lead to hypercalcemia. Early hypercalcemia is characterized by constipation, headache, increased thirst, dry mouth, decreased appetite, irritability, and a metallic taste in the mouth. Later signs and symptoms of hypercalcemia include confusion, drowsiness, increase in blood pressure, irregular heart rate, nausea, vomiting, and increased urination. Use of aluminum-based antacids may also produce hypophosphatemia, which is characterized by loss of appetite, malaise, muscle weakness, and bone pain. The use of calcium-containing antacids (e.g., calcium carbonate) may lead to milk-alkali

syndrome, which is associated with headache, anorexia, nausea, vomiting, and unusual tiredness. Use of sodium bicarbonate may lead to metabolic alkalosis if the drug is misused or used over the long term. Alkalosis is manifested by irritability, muscle twitching, numbness and tingling, cyanosis, slow and shallow respirations, headache, thirst, and nausea. Acid rebound occurs with the discontinuation of antacids that have high acid-neutralizing capacity and with overuse or misuse of antacid therapy. If acid neutralization is sudden and high, the result is an immediate elevation in pH to alkalinity and just as rapid a decline in pH to a more acidic state in the gut.

DRUG PROFILES

ANTACIDS, GENERAL

Some of the available aluminum, magnesium, calcium, and sodium salts used in many of the antacid formulations are listed in Box 52-1. There are far too many individual antacid products on the market to mention all formulations. Briefly, over-the-counter antacid formulations are available as capsules, chewable tablets, effervescent granules and tablets, powders, suspensions, and plain tablets, giving patients a variety of options for self-medication. While pharmacokinetic parameters are not normally listed for antacids, these drugs are generally excreted quickly through the gastrointestinal tract and the electrolyte homeostatic mechanisms of the kidneys.

Antacids are generally considered safe for use in pregnancy if prolonged administration and high dosages are avoided. However, it is recommended that pregnant women consult their physicians before taking an antacid. Aluminum- and sodium-based antacids are often recommended for patients with kidney compromise because these antacids are more easily excreted than are antacids of other categories. Calcium-containing antacids are currently advertised as an extra source of calcium. Calcium carbonate neutralization will produce gas and possibly belching. For this reason, it may be combined with an antiflatulent drug such as simethicone (see Miscellaneous Acid-Controlling Drugs). Magnesium-containing antacids commonly have a laxative effect; frequent administration of these antacids alone often cannot be tolerated.

DOSAGES   Selected Antacid Drugs*

Drug (Pregnancy Category)	Pharmacological Class	Usual Dosage Range	Indications
aluminum hydroxide and magnesium hydroxide (Alumag, Gelusil, Maalox, Mylanta) (A)	Combination antacid	*Adult* PO: 400–2400 mg 3–6×/day	Hyperacidity
calcium carbonate (Tums) (A)	Calcium-containing antacid	*Adult* PO: 0.5–1.5 g prn	Hyperacidity
magnesium hydroxide (generic) (A)	Magnesium-containing antacid	*Adult* PO: 0.65–1.3 g prn, up to qid	Hyperacidity (more commonly used as a laxative)

*Many more antacid products are available than appear in this table. Dosages given are approximate dosages of active ingredients; there may be variations among different products and different dosage forms of the same product.

H₂ ANTAGONISTS

H_2 antagonists (HAs), also called H_2 receptor blockers, are the prototypical acid-secretion antagonists. These drugs reduce but do not eliminate stimulated acid secretion. They have become the most popular drugs for the treatment of many acid-related disorders, including peptic ulcer disease (PUD), because of their efficacy, patient acceptance, and excellent safety profile. The four available HAs are cimetidine, ranitidine, famotidine, and nizatidine. There is little difference among these four HAs from the standpoint of efficacy. Ranitidine and famotidine are available over the counter.

Mechanism of Action and Drug Effects

H_2 antagonists competitively block the H_2 receptor of acid-producing parietal cells, rendering the cells less responsive to not only histamine but also the stimulation of ACh and gastrin. This process is shown in Figure 52-2. Up to 90% inhibition of vagal- and gastrin-stimulated acid secretion occurs when histamine is blocked. However, complete inhibition has not been shown. The drug effect of H_2 antagonists is reduced hydrogen ion secretion from the parietal cells, which results in an increase in the pH of the stomach and relief of many of the symptoms associated with hyperacidity-related conditions.

Indications

H_2 antagonists have several therapeutic uses, including treatment of GERD, PUD, erosive esophagitis, and pathological gastric hypersecretory conditions such as *Zollinger-Ellison syndrome,* and as adjunct therapy to control upper gastrointestinal tract bleeding. Zollinger-Ellison syndrome is one form of *hyperchlorhydria,* or excessive gastric acidity.

Contraindications

The only usual contraindication to the use of H_2 antagonists is a known drug allergy. Liver and kidney dysfunction are relative contraindications that may warrant dosage reductions. If in doubt, the nurse should review applicable laboratory values and check with the pharmacist.

Adverse Effects

H_2 antagonists have a remarkably low incidence of adverse effects (less than 3% of cases). The four available H_2 antagonists are similar in many respects but have some differences in adverse-effect profiles. Table 52-2 lists the adverse effects seen with these drugs. While central nervous system adverse effects occur in less than 1% of patients taking H_2 antagonists, such effects are sometimes seen in the older adult in particular, such as confusion and disorientation. The nurse should be alert for mental health status changes when giving these drugs, especially if they are new to the patient. Cimetidine may cause erectile dysfunction and gynecomastia. This effect is the result of cimetidine's inhibition of estradiol metabolism and displacement of dihydrotestosterone from peripheral androgen-binding sites. All four H_2 antagonists may increase the secretion of prolactin from the anterior pituitary.

Interactions

Cimetidine carries a higher risk of drug interactions than that of the other three H_2 antagonists, particularly in the older adult. These interactions may be of clinical importance. Cimetidine binds enzymes of the liver cytochrome P450 microsomal oxidase system. This is a group of enzymes in the liver that metabolize many different drugs by oxidation. By inhibiting the oxidation of drugs metabolized via this pathway, cimetidine may raise the blood concentrations of these drugs. Ranitidine has only 10% to 20% of the binding action of cimetidine on the P450 system, and nizatidine and famotidine have essentially no effect. This interaction has little clinical significance for most drugs; problems are more likely to arise with medications having a narrow therapeutic-to-toxic ratio, such as theophylline, warfarin, lidocaine, and phenytoin. All H_2 antagonists may inhibit the absorption of certain

TABLE	52-2

H_2 ANTAGONISTS: ADVERSE EFFECTS

Body System	Adverse Effects
Cardiovascular	Hypotension (monitor for this effect with intravenous administration)
Central nervous	Headache, lethargy, confusion, depression, hallucinations, slurred speech, agitation
Endocrine	Increased prolactin secretion, gynecomastia (with cimetidine)
Gastrointestinal	Diarrhea, nausea, abdominal cramps
Genitourinary	Impotence, increased blood urea nitrogen, creatinine levels
Hematological	Agranulocytosis, thrombocytopenia, neutropenia, aplastic anemia
Hepatobiliary	Elevated liver enzyme levels, jaundice
Integumentary	Urticaria, rash, alopecia, sweating, flushing, exfoliative dermatitis

drugs such as ketoconazole that require an acidic gastrointestinal environment for gastric absorption. Smoking has been shown to decrease the effectiveness of H_2 antagonists. For optimal results, H_2 antagonists should be taken 1 hour before antacids.

Dosages

For dosage information for the H_2 antagonists, see the Dosages table below.

 DRUG PROFILES

Histamine-2 (H_2) antagonists are the prototypical acid-secretion antagonists. These drugs reduce but do not eliminate stimulated acid secretion. They are among the most commonly used drugs in the world because of their efficacy, patient acceptance, and excellent safety profile. However, this drug class has been partially supplanted by proton pump inhibitors (see the next section).

▶▶ cimetidine

Cimetidine was the first drug in this class to be released on the market. It is the prototypical H_2 antagonist. Other

drugs in this class now include ranitidine (Zantac), famotidine (Pepcid, Ulcidine), and nizatidine (Axid). All four drugs are available in oral form, and famotidine and ranitidine are also available in parenteral dosage form.

PHARMACOKINETICS

Half-Life	Onset	Peak	Duration
2 hr	15–60 min	1–2 hr	4–8 hr

DOSAGES Selected H_2 Antagonists

Drug (Pregnancy Category)	Pharmacological Class	Usual Dosage Range	Indications
▶▶ cimetidine (generic) (B)	Histamine H_2 receptor antagonist	*Adult* PO: 200 mg bid PO: 800–1200 mg/day or divided bid PO: 300 mg bid or 400 mg at bedtime PO: 1200 mg/day PO: 300 mg qid; do not exceed 2400 mg/day PO: 800 mg/day or divided bid PO: 300 mg qid	Dyspepsia, heartburn Treatment of ulcers Prophylaxis of recurrent ulcer GERD Pathological hypersecretion NSAID-induced lesions and symptoms Zollinger–Ellison syndrome

Continued

DOSAGES   Selected H₂ Antagonists   (cont'd)

Drug (Pregnancy Category)	Pharmacological Class	Usual Dosage Range	Indications
famotidine (Pepcid, Pepcid AC) (B)	Histamine H₂ receptor antagonist	*Adult* PO: 10 mg daily–bid PO: 40 mg/day at bedtime or 20 mg at bedtime PO: 20 mg q6h IV: 20 mg q12h PO: 20–40 mg bid	Dyspepsia, heartburn Ulcers Pathological hypersecretion GERD
nizatidine (Axid) (B)	Histamine H₂ receptor antagonist	*Adult* PO: 300 mg at bedtime or 150 mg bid PO: 150 mg bid	Ulcers GERD
ranitidine (Zantac) (B)	Histamine H₂ receptor antagonist	*Adult* PO: 75 mg bid PO: 150 mg bid or 300 mg at bedtime PO: 150 mg tid PO: 150 mg qid IM/IV: 50 mg q6–8h	Dyspepsia, heartburn Ulcers Pathological hypersecretion, GERD Erosive esophagitis Any indications

IM, intramuscular; *IV*, intravenous; *PO*, oral.

PROTON PUMP INHIBITORS

The newest drugs introduced for the treatment of acid-related disorders are the proton pump inhibitors *(PPIs)*. These include lansoprazole (Prevacid, Prevacid FasTab), omeprazole magnesium (Losec), rabeprazole, rabeprazole sodium (Pariet), pantoprazole (Pantoloc), and esomeprazole (Nexium). These drugs are even more powerful than the H₂ antagonists. PPIs bind directly to the hydrogen–potassium–ATPase pump mechanism itself and irreversibly inhibit the action of this enzyme, which results in a total blockage of hydrogen ion secretion from the parietal cells.

Mechanism of Action and Drug Effects

The action of the hydrogen–potassium–ATPase pump is the final step in the acid-secretory process of the parietal cell (see Figure 52-2). If chemical energy is present to run the pump, it will transport hydrogen ions out of the parietal cell, which increases the acid content of the surrounding gastric lumen and lowers the pH. Because hydrogen ions are protons (positively charged hydrogen atoms), this ion pump is also called the proton pump. PPIs bind irreversibly to the proton pump. The binding of this enzyme prevents the movement of hydrogen ions out of the parietal cell into the stomach and thereby blocks all gastric acid secretion. Although H₂ antagonists may block almost 90% of all acid secretion, PPIs effectively stop over 90% of acid secretion over 24 hours, making most patients temporarily *achlorhydric* (without acid). For acid secretion to return to normal after a PPI has been stopped, the parietal cell must synthesize new hydrogen–potassium–ATPase. Although there are other proton pumps in the body, hydrogen–potassium–ATPase is structurally and mechanically distinct from other hydrogen-transporting enzymes and appears to exist only in the parietal cell. Thus the action of PPIs is specific for the proton pump and limited to its effects on gastric acid secretion.

Indications

PPIs are currently indicated as first-line therapy for erosive esophagitis, symptomatic GERD that is poorly responsive to other medical treatment such as therapy with H₂ antagonists, short-term treatment of active duodenal ulcers and active benign gastric ulcers, gastric hypersecretory conditions (e.g., Zollinger–Ellison syndrome), and nonsteroidal anti-inflammatory drug (NSAID)-induced ulcers. Long-term therapeutic uses include the maintenance of healing of erosive esophagitis and pathological hypersecretory conditions, including both GERD and Zollinger–Ellison syndrome. Several PPIs may also be given through a nasogastric or percutaneous enterogastric (PEG) tube. This is commonly done to prevent stress ulcers, which may be associated with coma or other severely compromising conditions. For example, esomeprazole capsules may be opened, the granules dissolved in 50 mL of water, and then this liquid given through the tube. Similar tubal administration is listed by the manufacturer for lansoprazole capsules and tablets and for omeprazole powder for oral suspension. Consult the drug packaging for drug-specific instructions.

Many treatment regimens involving PPIs have emerged to cure *H. pylori*–induced ulcers; these regimens are listed in Table 52-1. *H. pylori* eradication has been shown to reduce the risk of duodenal ulcer recurrence as well.

Contraindications

The only usual contraindication to the PPIs is known drug allergy.

Adverse Effects

PPIs are generally well tolerated. The frequency of adverse effects has been similar to that for placebo or H₂ antagonists. There was some early concern that long-term use of PPIs might promote malignant gastric tumours. This has not been the case, however, and the initial concern has subsided. There are some newer concerns that these drugs may be overprescribed and may predispose patients to gastrointestinal tract infections because of the reduction of the normal acid-mediated antimicrobial protection.

Interactions

Few drug interactions occur with PPIs. PPIs may increase serum levels of diazepam and phenytoin. There may be an increased chance for bleeding in patients who are taking both a PPI and warfarin. Other possible interactions include interference with ketoconazole, ampicillin, iron salts, and digoxin absorption. Sucralfate may delay absorption of PPIs. The PPI may be given 30 minutes before sucralfate to avoid this interaction.

Dosages

For recommended dosages see the Dosages table below.

MISCELLANEOUS ACID-CONTROLLING DRUGS

There are a few other acid-controlling drugs that are unique in terms of their mechanisms and other features. These include sucralfate, misoprostol, and simethicone. They are profiled individually in the following paragraphs. Other acid-controlling drugs include bismuth subsalicylate (Bismuth, Pepto-Bismol) and metoclopramide (Chapter 54).

DRUG PROFILES

▸▸ omeprazole magnesium

Omeprazole magnesium (Losec) was the first drug to become available in this breakthrough class of antisecretory drugs. Pantoprazole is the sole PPI available in injectable form. Orally administered PPIs (and H₂ antagonists) often work best when taken 30 to 60 minutes before meals.

PHARMACOKINETICS

Half-Life	Onset	Peak	Duration
40 min	2 hr*	4 hr	up to 72 hr

*50%–86% acid secretion reduction.

DOSAGES   Selected Proton Pump Inhibitors

Drug (Pregnancy Category)	Pharmacological Class	Usual Dosage Range	Indications
esomeprazole (Nexium) PPI	Proton pump inhibitor	*Child, 1-11 yr* PO:10–20 mg/day for 8 wk **Adolescents 12-17 yr** PO: 20–40 mg/day for 2–8 wk *Adult* PO: 20–40 mg/day for 2–8 wk	Esophagitis Nonerosive reflux disease Prevention and treatment of NSAID-associated gastric ulcers
lansoprazole (Prevasid, Prevasid FasTab) (C)	Proton pump inhibitor	*Child, 1–11 yr* PO: 15–30 mg/day for 12 wk *Adolescents 12–17 yr/Adult* PO: 15–30 mg/day for 2–8 wk PO: 15 mg	Esophagitis Duodenal ulcer, gastric ulcer, esophagitis Long-term management of healed esophagitis
▸▸ omeprazole magnesium (Losec) (C)	Proton pump inhibitor	*Adult* PO: 20 mg/day for 4–8 wk PO: 20–40 mg/day	Esophagitis, duodenal ulcer Hypersecretory conditions
pantoprazole sodium (Pantoloc, Panto IV)	Proton pump inhibitor	*Adult* PO/IV: 40 mg/day PO: 20 mg/day A.M.	GERD, gastric and duodenal ulcer Prevention of NSAIDs lesions

---

DRUG PROFILES

misoprostol

The use of misoprostol (generic), a prostaglandin E analogue, has been shown to effectively reduce the incidence of gastric ulcers in patients taking NSAIDs. Prostaglandins have a wide variety of biological activities. They are thought to inhibit gastric acid secretion. They are also believed to protect the gastric mucosa from injury (cytoprotective function), possibly by enhancing the local production of mucus or bicarbonate, promoting local cell regeneration, and helping to maintain mucosal blood flow. Use of misoprostol is contraindicated in patients with known drug allergy and in pregnant women. Adverse effects include headache, gastrointestinal distress, and vaginal bleeding. There are no major drug interactions, although antacids may reduce drug absorption.

Although some studies show that synthetic analogues of prostaglandins promote the healing of duodenal ulcers, they must be used in dosages that usually produce more disturbing adverse effects, such as abdominal cramps and

Continued

diarrhea. Thus, they are not believed to be as effective as H₂ antagonists and PPIs for this indication. Misoprostol has been used for its abortifacient properties. For this reason, it is a pregnancy category X drug. The usual dosage is 200 mcg four times daily with meals for the duration of NSAID therapy in patients at high risk for ulceration.

PHARMACOKINETICS

Half-Life	Onset	Peak	Duration
PO: 20–40 min	PO: 2 days	PO: 12 min	PO: 1–2 days

simethicone

Simethicone (Oval Drops, Pediacol, Phazyme) is used to reduce the discomforts of gastric or intestinal gas (flatulence) and aid in its release via the mouth or rectum. It is therefore classified as an antiflatulent drug. Gas commonly appears in the gastrointestinal tract as a consequence of the swallowing of air as well as normal digestive processes. Gas in the upper gastrointestinal tract is composed of swallowed air and thus consists largely of nitrogen. It is usually expelled from the body by belching. The composition of flatus, however, is determined largely by the dietary intake of carbohydrates and the metabolic activity of the bacteria in the intestines. These bacteria are anaerobic and cause fermentation with the production of hydrogen (H_2), carbon dioxide (CO_2), and methane (CH_4) gases.

Some foods, including legumes (beans) and cruciferous vegetables (e.g., cauliflower, broccoli), are well known for their gas-producing properties. Gas can also result from disorders such as diverticulitis, dyspepsia (heartburn), peptic ulcers, and spastic or irritable colon, and gaseous distention can occur postoperatively. Simethicone works by altering the elasticity of mucus-coated gas bubbles, which causes them to break into smaller ones. This action reduces gas pain and facilitates the expulsion of gas via the mouth or the rectum. Simethicone has no listed adverse effects, drug interactions, or pharmacokinetic parameters. It is available only for oral use. The usual simethicone dosage is one to two tablets four to six times daily as needed. A variety of different over-the-counter products are currently available.

▶▶ sucralfate

Sucralfate (Sulcrate) is a drug used as a mucosal protectant in the treatment of active stress ulcerations and in long-term therapy for PUD. Sucralfate acts locally, not systemically, binding directly to the surface of an ulcer.

Sucralfate's basic structure is a sugar, sucrose. Sulfate and aluminum hydroxide groups are attached to this sugar in places where there are normally hydroxyl groups. Once sucralfate comes into contact with the acid of the stomach, it begins to dissociate into aluminum hydroxide (an antacid) and sulfate anions. The aluminum salt stimulates secretion of both mucus and bicarbonate base. The sulfated sucrose molecules of sucralfate are attracted to and bind to positively charged tissue proteins at the bases of ulcers and erosions, forming a protective barrier that can be thought of as a liquid bandage. By binding to the exposed proteins of ulcers and erosions, sucralfate also limits the access of pepsin. This enzyme normally breaks down proteins in food but can have the same effect on gastrointestinal epithelial tissue, either causing ulcers or making them worse. Sucralfate also binds and concentrates epidermal growth factor, which is present in the gastric tissues and promotes ulcer healing. In addition, the drug stimulates the gastric secretion of prostagladin molecules, which serve a mucoprotective function.

Despite its many beneficial actions, sucralfate has fallen out of common use because its effects are transient, and multiple daily dosing (up to four times daily) is therefore needed. It is indicated for stress ulcers, esophageal erosions, and PUD. Because sucralfate binds phosphates in the gastrointestinal tract, it has also been used for this purpose in patients who have kidney failure with hyperphosphatemia. However, the aluminum in the drug can also accumulate to hazardous levels in patients with kidney failure. Aluminum toxicity can result in bone disease and encephalopathy. Its use in these patients is based on clinical judgement best made by a nephrologist.

The only usual contraindication to sucralfate use is drug allergy. Adverse effects are uncommon but include nausea, constipation, and dry mouth. Only minimal systemic absorption occurs, and the drug is virtually inert. Drug interactions mainly involve physical interference with the absorption of other drugs, which can be alleviated by taking other drugs at least 2 hours ahead of sucralfate. Sucralfate is also best given 1 hour before meals and at bedtime. It is a pregnancy category B drug that is normally dosed at 1 g orally four times daily.

PHARMACOKINETICS

Half-Life	Onset	Peak	Duration
PO: 6–20 hr	PO: 1 hr	PO: 2–4 hr	PO: 3–6 hr

NURSING PROCESS

Assessment

Before administering an acid-controlling drug, the nurse should assess the patient and obtain the medical history, with particular attention to gastrointestinal tract–related illnesses and signs and symptoms of ulcer disease, GERD,

and other conditions discussed earlier in this chapter. Any change in bowel patterns or gastrointestinal tract functioning, and gastrointestinal tract–related pain should also be assessed and documented. Results of baseline serum chemistry laboratory tests, as ordered, should be examined with specific attention to liver function (e.g., serum alkaline phosphatase level, serum glutamic-oxaloacetic transaminase [aspartate aminotransferase] level, serum glutamic-pyruvic transaminase [alanine aminotransferase] level) and kidney function (serum creatinine level). The nurse should thoroughly assess for any contraindications, cautions, and drug interactions (discussed in the pharmacology section). Because acid-controlling drugs have many interactions, all medications the patient is taking should be noted; in taking the medication history, it is important to ask the patient about prescription drugs, over-the counter drugs, and natural health products. Other components of assessment include a physical examination and a thorough cardiac history, with close attention to a history of heart failure, hypertension, or other heart diseases; the presence of edema, fluid and electrolyte imbalances; or kidney disease. One reason it is important to assess for these conditions is that the high sodium content of antacids may lead to exacerbation of heart problems, kidney dysfunction, and fluid–electrolyte problems.

When *aluminum-containing antacids* are taken, all other medications the patient is taking should be identified, and information about cautions and contraindications should be noted. With *magnesium-containing antacids*, related cautions, contraindications, and drug interactions should also be noted. Combination products containing both magnesium and aluminum may have fewer adverse effects than either antacid by itself. For example, aluminum-containing antacids are associated with constipation, whereas magnesium-containing antacids lead to diarrhea. The net effect of a combination of these antacids is a balancing out of both adverse effects and fewer problems with altered bowel patterns. *Calcium-based antacids* may also be used, especially as a source of calcium; however, they carry the risks of rebound hyperacidity, milk-alkali syndrome, and changes in systemic pH, especially if the patient has abnormal kidney function (see Box 52-2). Sodium bicarbonate is generally not recommended as an antacid because of the high risk for systemic electrolyte disturbances and alkalosis. The sodium content of sodium bicarbonate is high and is problematic for patients who have hypertension, heart failure, or kidney insufficiency.

Patients using *H₂ antagonist* drugs should be assessed for kidney and liver function as well as level of consciousness because of drug-related adverse effects. The older adult may react to these drugs with more disorientation and confusion. Drugs such as cimetidine and famotidine should not be administered simultaneously with antacids. These drugs may be spaced 1 hour apart if both drugs need to be given. Patients taking nizatidine or ranitidine require assessment of baseline blood chemistry results, with attention to levels of blood urea nitrogen, creatinine, alkaline phosphatase, bilirubin, alanine aminotransferase, and aspartate aminotransferase to assess kidney and liver functions before treatment is initiated.

For *PPIs* (e.g., omeprazole, pantoprazole), the patient's swallowing capacity needs to be assessed because of the size of some of the oral capsules. Assessment of kidney and liver functions and a complete blood count are also required before initiation of long-term therapy. Because of possible drug interactions, the patient's medication list should always be checked before giving this or any other type of medication. Other drugs used by patients with gastrointestinal disorders include *sucralfate* and

simethicone. With use of simethicone (an antiflatulent) and sucralfate (an ulcer-adherent), the patient's bowel patterns and bowel sounds should be noted, and abdominal distention and rigidity evaluated. Treatment of PUD involves the use of antibiotics (to attack the *H. pylori* bacteria) along with frequent dosing of other drugs as listed in Table 52-1. The gastrointestinal tract should be assessed, and signs and symptoms should be noted.

Nursing Diagnoses

- Acute pain related to gastric hyperacidity and other gastrointestinal disorders such as ulcer disease
- Constipation related to the adverse effects of aluminum-containing antacids and other drugs used to treat hyperacidity
- Diarrhea related to the adverse effects of magnesium-containing antacids and other drugs used to treat hyperacidity
- Deficient knowledge related to lack of information about antacids, H₂ antagonists, or PPIs, including their use and potential adverse effects

Planning

Goals

- Patient will experience minimal to no pain during therapy with antacids or other acid-controlling drugs.
- Patient will experience minimal adverse effects while using antacids or acid-controlling drugs.
- Patient will remain adherent to the therapeutic regimen.

Outcome Criteria

- Patient experiences increased comfort related to the use of acid-controlling drugs, abdominal massage, application of heat, if appropriate, and frequent repositioning.
- Patient states adverse effects of antacids, H₂ antagonists, and PPIs, such as constipation, diarrhea, headache, and confusion, and seeks advice from the health care provider if adverse effects worsen or are not relieved after several days.
- Patient states the importance of adherence to the drug regimen and strict adherence to medication instructions regarding the use of acid-controlling drugs to adequately resolve symptoms of the hyperacidity or other gastrointestinal disorder.

Implementation

When giving acid-controlling drugs, the nurse should be sure that chewable tablets are well chewed and that liquid forms are thoroughly shaken before they are taken. These drugs should be taken between meals for best effect. Antacids should be given with at least 240 mL of water to enhance absorption of the antacid in the stomach, except for newer forms that are rapid-dissolve drugs. Should constipation or diarrhea occur with single-component drugs, the nurse should suggest a combination aluminum and magnesium product to the physician and educate the patient about the adverse effects of aluminum-only or magnesium-only products. It is also recommended that antacids be given as ordered but not within 1 to 2 hours of other medications because of the effect of antacids on the absorption of oral medications. This dosing schedule can be implemented safely by the nurse without interrupting safe dosing of the other medications. The dosing will differ if the physician has ordered the drug to be given with antacids. Antacid overuse or misuse, or the rapid discontinuation of antacids with high acid-neutralizing capacity may lead to acid rebound. Therefore, antacids should be used only as prescribed or directed.

Because H$_2$ antagonists and other acid-controlling drugs are now available over the counter, it is critical to patient safety that patients be educated about proper medication use and administration (see Patient Education). For example, cimetidine should be taken with meals, and antacids, if also used, should be taken 1 hour before or after the cimetidine. Famotidine may be given orally without regard to meals or food. Ranitidine should be given as ordered and, if administered with antacids, should be given 1 hour before or after the antacid. Intravenous forms of famotidine or ranitidine should be diluted with appropriate solutions and given within the documented time frame. With intravenous ranitidine, heart irregularities and hypotension may occur with rapid infusion. The nurse should refer to appropriate sources for information on other specific drugs and their intravenous administration. For all these H$_2$ antagonists, blood pressure readings should be monitored as needed during intravenous infusion because of the risk of hypotension. Patients with a diagnosis of ulcers or gastrointestinal irritation should be continually monitored for gastrointestinal tract bleeding. Blood in the stool or the occurrence of black, tarry stool or hematemesis should be reported. The nurse should also listen to bowel sounds and examine the abdomen to assess for the effectiveness of therapy and to monitor for possible complications.

Lansoprazole oral dosage forms should be given as ordered and with fluids. If the patient has difficulty swallowing these capsules, a delayed-release capsule may be opened and the granules sprinkled over at least one tablespoon of apple sauce, which should be swallowed immediately. For patients who have a nasogastric tube, lansoprazole delayed-release capsules can be opened and the granules mixed in 40 mL of apple juice or water

and injected through the nasogastric tube, followed with 30 mL of apple juice or water to flush. Delayed-release tablets are also available and should be placed on the tongue and allowed to dissolve. The tablet usually dissolves in approximately 1 minute. The nurse should monitor for abdominal pain, distention, and abnormal bowel sounds.

Omeprazole should be administered before meals, and the capsule should be taken whole and not crushed, opened, or chewed. Omeprazole may also be given with antacids if ordered. Omeprazole and most of the other PPIs are given for the short term, with specific patient instructions. The nurse should always double-check the names and dosages of these drugs to ensure that they are not confused with similarly named drugs. Pantoprazole may be given orally without crushing or splitting of the tablet. Intravenous pantoprazole should be given exactly as ordered, using the correct dilutional fluids and over the recommended time frame.

Simethicone may also be added to the oral medication protocol with PPIs and is usually well tolerated. It is to be taken after meals and at bedtime. Tablets should be chewed thoroughly and suspensions shaken well before use. Sucralfate is usually given 1 hour before meals and at bedtime. Tablets may be crushed or dissolved in water, if needed. Antacids should be avoided for 30 minutes before or after taking sucralfate. Suggestions for patient education for all of these drugs are presented in Patient Education.

Evaluation

Therapeutic response to the administration of antacids, H$_2$ antagonists, PPIs, and other related drugs includes the relief of symptoms associated with peptic ulcer, gastritis, esophagitis, gastric hyperacidity, or hiatal hernia (i.e., decrease in epigastric pain, fullness, and abdominal swelling). Adverse effects for which to monitor include nausea, vomiting, abdominal pain, hypotension, and heart irregularities. Milk-alkali syndrome, acid rebound, hypercalcemia, and metabolic alkalosis are known complications associated with antacids; the patient must also be evaluated for these adverse effects and measures taken to prevent or resolve them. Therapeutic response to all of the drugs in the categories discussed in this chapter is also measured by evaluating whether the identified goals and outcome criteria have been met.

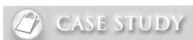 

Gastroesophageal Reflux Disease

A 47-year-old attorney has just undergone an endoscopy to rule out gastroesophageal reflux disease (GERD) and gastritis secondary to stress-induced hyperacidity. The physician has prescribed omeprazole (Losec) 20 mg once a day and informed the patient to stop taking excessive amounts of liquid antacids.

1. What laboratory studies are indicated for patients receiving omeprazole? Explain the significance of

these studies. How long is therapy with this proton pump inhibitor (PPI) indicated?

2. What is the rationale for the use of PPIs in GERD?

3. Why are antacids no longer the mainstay of treatment for acid-related gastric ulcers and reflux disease?

For answers see http://evolve.elsevier.com/Canada/Lilley/pharmacology/.

PATIENT EDUCATION

- Patients should be instructed not to take any other medications within 1 to 2 hours after taking an antacid because of its influence on the absorption of many medications in the stomach and lower peak serum levels.
- Patients should be encouraged to contact the physician immediately if they experience severe or prolonged constipation or diarrhea, an increase in abdominal pain, abdominal distension, nausea, vomiting, hematemesis, or black tarry stools (a sign of possible gastrointestinal tract bleeding).
- Patients should be instructed to take over-the-counter medications for no longer than 2 weeks, unless otherwise prescribed.
- Patients should be informed that if they are taking enteric-coated medications, it is important to know that use of antacids may promote premature dissolving of the enteric coating. Enteric coatings are used to diminish the stomach upset caused by irritating medications, and if the coating is destroyed early in the stomach, gastric upset may occur.
- Patients should be encouraged to take H_2 antagonists exactly as prescribed. They need to be informed that smoking decreases the drug's effectiveness. H_2 antagonists should not be taken within 1 hour of antacids. Patients need to know that occurrence of a prolonged headache with therapy should be reported to the physician immediately. Patients requiring treatment with these drugs should also

be encouraged to avoid aspirin, NSAIDs, alcohol, and caffeine because of these agents' ulcerogenic or gastrointestinal tract–irritating effects.
- Patients taking omeprazole and other PPIs should be instructed to take the drugs before meals. If they are taking lansoprazole, the granules may be sprinkled from the capsule in a tablespoon of apple sauce if needed. If lansoprazole is taken with sucralfate, it should be taken 30 minutes before the latter drug.
- Patients should be instructed to follow manufacturer's directions when taking simethicone. Chewable forms must always be chewed thoroughly; liquid preparations should be shaken thoroughly before administration. Patients with gas problems, or flatulence, should be encouraged to avoid problematic foods (e.g., spicy, gas-producing foods) and carbonated beverages.
- Patients taking sucralfate should be instructed to do so on an empty stomach, and antacids should be avoided or, if indicated, taken 2 hours before or 1 hour after sucralfate administration. Taking sips of tepid water, keeping fluids nearby, and using sugarless or sour hard candy may help alleviate dry mouth.
- Patients taking the drug regimen for the treatment of *H. pylori* infection–PUD should be informed of the need to take each drug, including the antibiotics, exactly as prescribed and without fail to guarantee success of the treatment. If treatment protocols are not followed appropriately, the condition will recur.

POINTS TO REMEMBER

- The stomach secretes many substances (hydrochloric acid, pepsinogen, mucus, bicarbonate, intrinsic factor, and prostaglandins).
- The parietal cell is responsible for the production of acid.
- In acid-related disorders, the balance among the substances secreted by the stomach is impaired.
- The most common impairment is hyperacidity, or the overproduction of acid. The most harmful effects are PUD and esophageal cancer.
- Antacids were used for centuries and were the mainstays of antiulcer therapy until the 1970s, when other drugs were developed.
- H_2 antagonists are H_2 blockers that bind to and block histamine receptors located on parietal cells. This blocking renders these cells less responsive to stimuli, and thus acid secretion occurs. Up to 90% inhibition of acid secretion can be achieved with the H_2 antagonists.
- PPIs block the final step in the acid production pathway, the hydrogen–potassium–ATPase pump, and hence block all acid secretion.
- Sucralfate is used for the treatment of PUD and stress-related ulcers. It binds to tissue proteins in

eroded areas and prevents exposure of the ulcerated area to stomach acid.
- Misoprostol is a synthetic prostaglandin analogue that inhibits gastric acid secretion and is used to prevent NSAID-related ulcers.
- Cautious use of antacids is recommended in patients who have heart failure, hypertension, or other heart diseases or who require sodium restriction, especially if the antacid is high in sodium content. Other conditions that require cautious antacid use include fluid imbalances, dehydration, gastrointestinal tract obstruction, kidney disease, and pregnancy.
- Many drug interactions occur with acid-controlling drugs, primarily because these drugs alter the absorption of other medications in the stomach. Other medications should not be taken within 1 to 2 hours after an antacid is taken. Simultaneous use of antacids and other acid-controlling drugs should be avoided sometimes.
- Magnesium–aluminum combination antacids are used to prevent the adverse effects of constipation and diarrhea.
- Some of the more serious concerns with antacids include acid rebound, hypercalcemia, milk-alkali syndrome, and metabolic alkalosis.

EXAMINATION REVIEW QUESTIONS

1 A 30-year-old business executive is taking simethicone for excessive flatus associated with diverticulitis. Which of the following best describes simethicone's mechanism of action that reduces flatus?
   a. It neutralizes gastric pH, thereby preventing gas.
   b. It buffers the effects of pepsin on the gastric wall.
   c. It causes mucus-coated gas bubbles to break into smaller ones.
   d. It decreases gastric acid secretion and thereby minimizes flatus.

2 With which of the following would H_2 antagonists most likely adversely interact?
   a. Codeine
   b. Penicillin
   c. Ketoconazole
   d. Acetaminophen

3 Digoxin preparations and adsorbents should not be given simultaneously. Which of the following will occur if a proton pump inhibitor and an antacid are given simultaneously?
   a. Altered absorption of the antacid
   b. Increased risk of electrolyte imbalance
   c. Enhanced action of the proton pump inhibitor
   d. Altered absorption of the proton pump inhibitor

4 A patient with a history of kidney problems is asking for advice about which antacid he should use. Which of the following should the nurse recommend?
   a. Antacids that are calcium based
   b. Antacids that are aluminum based
   c. Antacids that are magnesium based
   d. None. Antacids should not be used by patients who have kidney problems

5 A patient who is taking oral tetracycline complains of heartburn and requests an antacid. Which of the following is the nurse's best action?
   a. Administering both medications together
   b. Giving the tetracycline, but delaying the antacid for 1 to 2 hours
   c. Giving the antacid, but delaying the tetracycline for at least 4 hours
   d. Explaining that the antacid cannot be given while the patient is taking the tetracycline

For answers see http://evolve.elsevier.com/Canada/Lilley/pharmacology/.

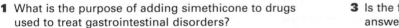

CRITICAL THINKING ACTIVITIES

1 What is the purpose of adding simethicone to drugs used to treat gastrointestinal disorders?
2 Are there any concerns regarding the use of antacids in patients with decreased kidney functioning? Explain your answer.

3 Is the following statement true or false? Explain your answer.
"Antacids coat the stomach and are therefore beneficial to patients with ulcers."

For answers see http://evolve.elsevier.com/Canada/Lilley/pharmacology/.

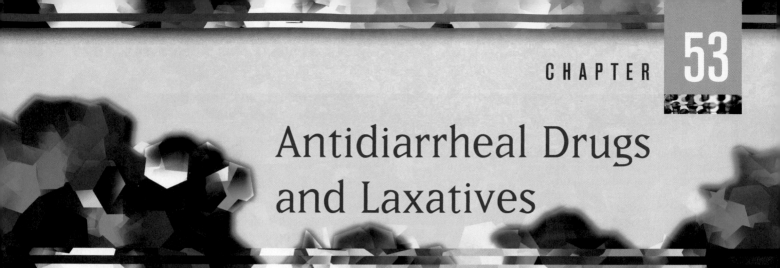

CHAPTER 53

Antidiarrheal Drugs and Laxatives

Learning Objectives

After reading this chapter, the successful student will be able to do the following:

1 Discuss the anatomy and physiology of the gastrointestinal tract, including the process of peristalsis.

2 Identify the factors affecting bowel elimination and bowel patterns.

3 List the groups of drugs used to treat alterations in bowel elimination, specifically diarrhea and constipation.

4 Discuss the mechanisms of action, indications, cautions, contraindications, drug interactions, adverse effects, routes of administration, and dosages associated with the use of antidiarrheal and laxative drugs.

5 Develop a collaborative plan of care that includes all phases of the nursing process for patients taking antidiarrheals or laxatives.

e-Learning Activities

Web site
(http://evolve.elsevier.com/Canada/Lilley/pharmacology/)

- Animations
- Answers to chapter questions, activities, and case studies
- Calculators and Category Catchers
- Glossary with audio pronunciations
- IV Therapy and Medication Error Checklists
- Multiple-Choice Review Question quizzes
- Nursing Care Plans
- Online Appendices and Supplements
- WebLinks

Drug Profiles

attapulgite, p. 981
belladonna alkaloids, p. 981
bismuth subsalicylate, p. 981
▸▸ **diphenoxylate with atropine (diphenoxylate hydrochloride with atropine sulfate)***, p. 981
▸▸ **docusate salts**, p. 986
▸▸ **glycerin**, p. 986
Lactobacillus acidophilus–Lactobacillus rhamnosus, p. 982
▸▸ **lactulose**, p. 986
▸▸ **loperamide (loperamide hydrochloride)***, p. 981
magnesium salts, p. 987
methylcellulose, p. 986
mineral oil, p. 986
polyethylene glycol (polyethylene glycol 3350)*, p. 987
▸▸ **psyllium (psyllium hydrophilic mucilloid)***, p. 986
▸▸ **senna**, p. 987

▸▸ Key drug.

*Full generic name is given in parentheses. For the purposes of this text, the more common shortened name is used.

Glossary

Antidiarrheal drugs Drugs that counter or combat diarrhea. (p. 979)

Constipation A condition of abnormally infrequent and difficult passage of feces through the lower gastrointestinal tract. (p. 983)

Diarrhea The abnormal frequent passage of loose stools. (p. 979)

Irritable bowel syndrome (IBS) A recurring condition of the intestinal tract characterized by bloating, flatulence, and often periods of diarrhea that alternate with periods of constipation. (p. 979)

Laxatives Drugs that promote bowel evacuation, such as by increasing the bulk of the feces, softening of the stool, or lubricating the intestinal wall. (p. 983)

OVERVIEW

The key symptoms of gastrointestinal disease are abdominal pain, nausea or vomiting, and diarrhea. **Diarrhea** is defined as the abnormal frequent passage of loose stools or, more specifically, the abnormal passage of stools with increased frequency, fluidity, and weight, or with increased stool water excretion. *Acute diarrhea* refers to diarrhea that is of sudden onset in a previously healthy individual. It lasts from 3 days to 2 weeks and is self-limiting, resolving without sequelae. *Chronic diarrhea* lasts for longer than 3 to 4 weeks and is associated with recurrent passage of diarrheal stools, possible fever, loss of appetite, nausea, vomiting, weight reduction, and chronic weakness.

Diarrhea and the diseases with which it is commonly associated account for 5 to 8 million deaths per year in infants and small children and are among the leading causes of death and morbidity in developing nations. Diarrheal disorders also have a financial impact on our society, with outpatient costs and loss of time from work because of acute infectious diarrhea. Children in Canada experience approximately one to three episodes of diarrhea per year.

The probable cause of diarrhea should be taken into consideration when designing a drug regimen to treat it. Causes of acute diarrhea include drugs, bacteria, viruses, nutritional factors, and protozoa. Causes of chronic diarrhea include tumours, acquired immune deficiency syndrome (AIDS), diabetes mellitus, hyperthyroidism, Addison's disease, and **irritable bowel syndrome (IBS)**, a condition characterized by bloating, flatulence, and periods of diarrhea that alternate with periods of constipation. Treatment is directed at the cessation of the increased stool frequency associated with diarrhea, alleviation of abdominal cramps, fluid resuscitation and electrolyte replacement, and prevention of weight loss and nutritional deficits from malabsorption.

ANTIDIARRHEALS

The drugs used to treat diarrhea are called **antidiarrheal drugs**. They are divided into different groups based on specific mechanism of action: adsorbents, antimotility drugs (anticholinergics and opiates), and intestinal flora modifiers (also known as probiotics and bacterial replacement drugs). The specific classes and the drugs in each class are listed in Table 53-1.

Mechanism of Action and Drug Effects

Antidiarrheal drugs have varying mechanisms of action; knowing how these drugs produce their effects gives the nurse greater insight into the treatment needs and responses of a given patient. *Adsorbents* act by coating the walls of the gastrointestinal tract. They bind the causative bacteria or toxin to their adsorbent surface for elimination from the body through the stool. Adsorption is similar to absorption but differs in that it involves the chemical binding of substances (e.g., ions, bacterial toxins) onto the surface of an adsorbent. In contrast, absorption generally refers to the *penetration* of a substance into the interior structure of the absorbant or the uptake of a substance across a surface (e.g., the absorption of dietary nutrients into the intestinal villi). The adsorbent bismuth subsalicylate is a form of aspirin, or acetylsalicylic acid, thus it also has many of the same drug effects as aspirin (Chapter 45). Activated charcoal is not only helpful in coating the walls of the gastrointestinal tract and adsorbing bacteria but is also useful in cases of overdose because of its drug-binding properties. The antilipemic drugs colestipol and cholestyramine (Chapter 29) are anion exchange resins that are sometimes prescribed as antidiarrheal adsorbents and lipid-lowering drugs. Besides binding to diarrhea-causing toxins, they have the additional benefit of decreasing cholesterol levels.

Anticholinergic drugs work to slow peristalsis by reducing the rhythmic contractions and smooth muscle tone of the gastrointestinal tract. They are often used in combination with adsorbents and opiates (see later). Anticholinergics are discussed in detail in Chapter 21.

Intestinal flora modifiers are products obtained from bacterial cultures, most commonly *Lactobacillus* organisms. They make up the majority of the body's normal bacterial flora and are the organisms most commonly destroyed by antibiotics. Intestinal flora modifiers work by exogenously replenishing these bacteria, which help restore the balance of normal flora and suppress the growth of diarrhea-causing bacteria. *Saccharomyces boulardii* (Florastor) is another intestinal flora modifier that destroys *Clostridium difficile* toxins, as well as other bacterial toxins that try and attach to intestinal tract receptor sites.

The primary action of *opiates* (Chapter 9) in diarrhea treatment is to decrease bowel motility. A secondary effect that makes opiates beneficial in the treatment of diarrhea is reduction of the pain associated with diarrhea by relief of rectal spasms. Because they increase the transit time of food through the gastrointestinal tract, they enable longer contact of the intestinal contents with the absorptive

TABLE	**53-1**
Antidiarrheals: Drug Categories and Selected Drugs	
Category	**Antidiarrheal Drugs**
Adsorbents	activated charcoal, aluminum hydroxide, attapulgite, bismuth subsalicylate, cholestyramine, kaolin-pectin, polycarbophil
Anticholinergics	atropine, hyoscyamine, hyoscine
Intestinal flora modifiers	*Lactobacillus acidophilus*, *Saccharomyces boulardii* (Florastor)
Opiates	opium tincture, paregoric, codeine, diphenoxylate, loperamide

surface of the bowel, which increases the absorption of water, electrolytes, and other nutrients from the bowel and reduces stool frequency and net volume.

Indications

Antidiarrheal drugs are indicated for the treatment of diarrhea of various types and levels of severity. Adsorbents are more likely to be used in milder cases, whereas anticholinergics and opiates tend to be used in more severe cases. Intestinal flora modifiers are often helpful in patients with antibiotic-induced diarrhea.

Contraindications

Contraindications to the use of antidiarrheals include known drug allergy and any major acute gastrointestinal condition, such as intestinal obstruction or colitis, unless prescribed by the patient's physician after careful consideration of the specific case.

Adverse Effects

The adverse effects of the antidiarrheals are specific to each drug family. Most of these potential effects are minor and are not life threatening. The major adverse effects of specific drugs within each drug class are listed in Table 53-2. Intestinal flora modifiers do not have any listed adverse effects.

Interactions

Many drugs are absorbed from the intestines into the bloodstream, where they are delivered to their respective sites of action. A number of the antidiarrheals have the potential to alter this normal process, by either increasing or decreasing the absorption of these other drugs.

The adsorbents can decrease the effectiveness of many drugs when given concurrently, primarily by decreasing the absorption of antidiarrheal drugs. Examples include digoxin, clindamycin, quinidine, probenecid, and antihyperglycemic drugs. Oral anticoagulants are more likely to cause increased bleeding times or bruising when they are coadministered with adsorbents. This effect is thought to be primarily due to the adsorbents binding to vitamin K, which is needed to make certain clotting factors. Vitamin K is synthesized by the normal bacterial flora in the bowel. In addition, the toxic effects of methotrexate are more likely to occur when it is given with adsorbents.

The therapeutic effects of the anticholinergic antidiarrheals can be decreased by coadministration with antacids. Amantadine, tricyclic antidepressants, monoamine oxidase inhibitors, and antihistamines, when given with anticholinergics, can result in increased anticholinergic effects. The opiate antidiarrheals have additive central nervous system (CNS)–depressant effects if they are given with CNS depressants, alcohol, narcotics, sedative–hypnotics, antipsychotics, and skeletal muscle relaxants.

Bismuth subsalicylate can lead to increased bleeding times and bruising when administered with oral anticoagulants as well as with aspirin and other NSAIDs. It can also cause confusion in older adults.

Dosages

For the recommended dosages of antidiarrheal drugs, see the Dosages table on p. 982.

TABLE 53-2

Selected Antidiarrheals: Adverse Effects

Drug	Body System	Adverse Effects
ADSORBENTS		
bismuth subsalicylate	Central nervous	Confusion, twitching
	Gastrointestinal	Constipation, dark stools
	Hematological	Increased bleeding time
	Other	Hearing loss, tinnitus, metallic taste, blue gums
ANTICHOLINERGICS		
atropine, hyoscyamine, hyoscine	Cardiovascular	Hypotension, hypertension, bradycardia, tachycardia
	Central nervous	Headache, dizziness, confusion, anxiety, drowsiness
	Eye, ear, nose, throat	Blurred vision, photophobia, increased pressure in the eye
	Genitourinary	Urinary retention and hesitancy, erectile dysfunction
	Integumentary	Dry skin, rash, flushing
OPIATES		
codeine	Cardiovascular	Bradycardia, palpitations, hypotension
	Central nervous	Drowsiness, sedation, dizziness, lethargy
	Gastrointestinal	Nausea, vomiting, anorexia, constipation
	Genitourinary	Urinary retention
	Integumentary	Flushing, rash, urticaria
	Respiratory	Respiratory depression

DRUG PROFILES

Drug therapy for diarrhea depends on the specific cause of the diarrhea, if known, and the antidiarrheal drug that will best combat it. All antidiarrheal drugs are orally administered drugs available as suspensions, tablets, or capsules. Some antidiarrheals are over-the-counter (OTC) medications, whereas others require a prescription.

ADSORBENTS
attapulgite

Attapulgite (Kaopectate) has replaced the use of kaolin-pectin in the newer forms of this preparation. Kaolin is a naturally hydrated aluminum compound that is now less commonly used as an antidiarrheal agent. Pectin, however, which is extracted from apples or citrus fruit, is used in many combination products. Attapulgite is a clay-like powder believed to work by adsorbing the bacteria or germ that may be causing the diarrhea. It is indicated for quick relief of diarrhea and cramping. It should not be used for more than 2 days or if a high fever is present. Attapulgite is also an OTC antidiarrheal. It is available for oral use.

PHARMACOKINETICS

Half-Life	Onset	Peak	Duration
Unknown	12 hr	14–20 hr	Unknown

bismuth subsalicylate

Bismuth subsalicylate (Bismuth, Maalox Multi Action, Pepto-Bismol) is a salicylate by chemical structure; therefore, it should be used with caution in children and teenagers who have or are recovering from chicken pox or influenza because of the risk of Reye's syndrome (see Special Populations: Children on p. 982 in this chapter and on p. 839 in Chapter 45). It can also cause all of the adverse effects that are associated with an aspirin-based product. Two alarming but harmless adverse effects are temporary darkening of the tongue or the stool. Bismuth subsalicylate is available OTC for oral use.

PHARMACOKINETICS

Half-Life	Onset	Peak	Duration
24–33 hr*	0.5–2 hr	2–5 hr	Variable

*For bismuth.

ANTICHOLINERGICS
belladonna alkaloids

The anticholinergics atropine, hyoscyamine, and hyoscine are used either alone or in combination with other antidiarrheals because they slow gastrointestinal tract motility. These drugs are commonly referred to as *belladonna alkaloids* and are discussed in Chapter 21. Their safety margin is not as wide as that of many of the other antidiarrheals because they can cause serious adverse effects if used inappropriately. For this reason they are available only by prescription. In Canada, belladonna is available only in combination with opium (see next section). No products with combinations of belladonna with

phenobarbital, hyoscyamine, or scopolamine are available in Canada.

OPIATES

There are four opiate-related antidiarrheal drugs: codeine, diphenoxylate hydrochloride with atropine sulfate, loperamide, and opium with belladonna. The only opiate-related antidiarrheal that is available as an OTC medication is loperamide; all others are prescription-only drugs because of the risks of respiratory depression and dependency associated with opiate use.

▶▶ diphenoxylate hydrochloride with atropine sulfate

Diphenoxylate hydrochloride (Lomotil) is a synthetic opiate agonist that is structurally related to meperidine. It acts on the smooth muscle of the intestinal tract, inhibiting gastrointestinal motility and excessive gastrointestinal propulsion. It has little or no analgesic activity. Diphenoxylate is combined with subtherapeutic quantities of atropine sulfate to discourage recreational opiate drug use. The amount of atropine present in the combination is too small to interfere with the conjugated diphenoxylate. However, when taken in large doses, the combination results in extreme anticholinergic effects (e.g., dry mouth, abdominal pain, tachycardia, blurred vision).

Use of the combination of diphenoxylate and atropine is contraindicated in patients experiencing diarrhea associated with pseudomembranous colitis or toxigenic bacteria because the drug's anticholinergic effects might be problematic in such conditions. This drug is available only for oral use.

PHARMACOKINETICS*

Half-Life	Onset	Peak	Duration
2.5–4 hr	40–60 min	2–3 hr	3–4 hr

*Diphenoxylate component.

▶▶ loperamide hydrochloride

Loperamide hydrochloride (Imodium) is a synthetic antidiarrheal that is similar to diphenoxylate. It inhibits both peristalsis in the intestinal wall and intestinal secretion, thereby decreasing the number of stools and their water content. Although the drug exhibits many characteristics of the opiate class, physical dependence on loperamide has not been reported. Because of its safety profile, it is the only opiate antidiarrheal drug that is available as an OTC medication. It is also available as a combination product containing 2 mg of loperamide and 125 mg of antiflatulent simethicone. Loperamide use is contraindicated in patients with severe ulcerative colitis, pseudomembranous colitis, and acute diarrhea associated with *Escherichia coli*.

PHARMACOKINETICS

Half-Life	Onset	Peak	Duration
7–15 hr	1–3 hr	4 hr	40–50 hr

Continued

DRUG PROFILES (cont'd)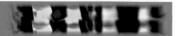

INTESTINAL FLORA MODIFIERS

Intestinal flora modifiers suppress the growth of diarrhea-causing bacteria and re-establish the normal flora that reside in the intestine. They are bacterial cultures of *Lactobacillus* organisms.

Lactobacillus acidophilus–Lactobacillus rhamnosus

Lactobacillus acidophilus–Lactobacillus rhamnosus (Lacidofil) is a combination of two acid-producing bacteria prepared in a concentrated, dried culture for oral administration. These two probiotic strains of live

lactic acid bacteria balance the intestinal flora. They are normal inhabitants of the gastrointestinal tract where, through the fermentation of carbohydrates (which produces lactic acid), they create an unfavourable environment for the overgrowth of harmful fungi and bacteria. Preliminary research shows that Lactofil may enhance the eradication of *H. pylori* as an adjunct to conventional treatment.

PHARMACOKINETICS

Half-Life	Onset	Peak	Duration
Unknown	Unknown	Unknown	Unknown

SPECIAL POPULATIONS: CHILDREN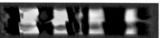

Antidiarrheal Preparations

- Always check with the physician before administering antidiarrheal preparations to a child at home and report the symptoms in case further assessment or medical management is needed. If diarrhea is accompanied by fever, malaise, or abdominal pain, contact the physician immediately because of the possibility of excessive fluid and electrolyte loss. Dehydration and electrolyte loss occur rapidly in children because of their small size and their sensitivity to loss of fluid volume and electrolytes through the stool.

- Always contact the physician or pharmacist for the proper dosage of antidiarrheals if the child is 6 years of age or younger or if there is any doubt as to proper dosing. Never hesitate to contact the physician, pediatrician, or nurse practitioner with any concern or question regarding any medication recommended for the child.

- Bismuth subsalicylate (Pepto-Bismol, Kaopectate) is a salicylate by chemical structure; therefore, it should be used with caution in children and teenagers because of the risk of Reye's syndrome.

- Immediately report to the physician abdominal distention, firm abdomen, painful abdomen, and worsening of or no improvement in diarrhea 24 to 48 hours after medication administration. Measurement of the amount of diarrhea by the number of soiled diapers or number of stools per day provides important information.

- Antidiarrheal preparations should always be used with caution in children. If symptoms persist or dehydration occurs (e.g., no tears and decreased urine output in the child), contact the physician.

- If the child is sluggish, lethargic, or confused or the diarrhea is bloody, contact the physician immediately, or go to the closest emergency facility.

DOSAGES   Selected Antidiarrheal Drugs

Drug (Pregnancy Category)	Pharmacological Class	Usual Dosage Range	Indications
attapulgite (Kaopectate) (C)	Adsorbent antidiarrheal	*Children 3–6 yr* PO (regular strength): 7.5 mL q4h *Children 6–12 yr* PO: 15 mL q4h *Children over 12 yr/Adult* PO: 30 mL q4h	Diarrhea
bismuth subsalicylate (Bismuth, Maalox Multi Action, Pepto-Bismol) (D)	Antimicrobial, antidiarrheal	Doses repeated q30–60 min, not to exceed 8/day; all doses PO *Children 3–5 yr* 5 mL or ⅓ tab *Children 6–9 yr* 10 mL or ⅔ tab *Children 10–12 yr* 15 mL or 1 tab	Diarrhea

Continued

DOSAGES   Selected Antidiarrheal Drugs   (cont'd)

Drug (Pregnancy Category)	Pharmacological Class	Usual Dosage Range	Indications
▸▸diphenoxylate hydrochloride with atropine sulfate (Lomotil) (C)	Antidiarrheal	*Children 2–12 yr* PO: 2.5 mg bid–qid *Adult* PO: 5 mg tid–qid until control of symptoms	Diarrhea
Lactobacillus acidophilus– Lactobacillus rhamnosus (Lacidofil) (A)	Intestinal flora modifier	*Children over 12 yr/Adult* PO: 1 cap bid	Dietary supplement Restore and maintain normal flora of intestinal tract after diarrhea
▸▸loperamide hydrochloride (Imodium) (B)	Opiate antidiarrheal	*Children 2–12 yr* PO: 1–2 mg bid–tid *Children over 12 yr/Adult* PO: 4 mg followed by 2 mg after each BM (not to exceed 16 mg/day)	Diarrhea

BM, bowel movement; *PO*, oral.

LAXATIVES

Laxatives are used for the treatment of **constipation**, defined as the abnormally infrequent and difficult passage of feces through the lower gastrointestinal tract. Individuals may complain of constipation if they think they defecate too infrequently or with too much effort, if their stools are too hard or too small, if defecation is painful, or if they have a sense of incomplete evacuation. Constipation is a symptom, not a disease; it is a disorder of movement through the colon or rectum that can be caused by a variety of diseases or drugs. Some of the more common causes of constipation are noted in Table 53-3.

The gastrointestinal tract is responsible for the digestive process, which involves (1) ingestion of dietary intake, (2) digestion of dietary intake into basic nutrients, (3) absorption of basic nutrients, and (4) storage and removal of fecal material via defecation.

Ingestion → Digestion → Absorption → Storage and removal

The usual time span between ingestion and defecation is 24 to 36 hours. The last segment of the gastrointestinal tract, the large intestine (colon), is responsible for (1) forming the stool by removing excess water from the fecal material, (2) temporarily storing the stool until defecation, and (3) extracting essential vitamins from the intestinal bacteria (particularly vitamin K).

The colon is 120 to 150 cm long and is separated from the small intestine by the ileocecal valve. The colon extends into the rectum, which terminates at the anus. The rectum is the temporary storage site for the stool, which is composed of water and unabsorbed and indigestible material. Evacuation of the rectal contents is accomplished by bowel movements.

A *bowel movement* (*defecation*) is a reflex act that involves both smooth and skeletal muscles. The entry of feces into the rectum stimulates mass peristaltic movement that results in a bowel movement. However, voluntary initiation or inhibition of defecation is also possible via skeletal muscle pathways.

Treatment of constipation must involve an understanding of the whole patient, with special attention given to the underlying causes for the constipation. Treatment should be individualized, taking into consideration the patient's age, concerns, and expectations; duration and severity of constipation; and potential contributing factors. Treatment can be either surgical

TABLE   53-3

Causes of Constipation

Causes	Examples
Adverse drug effects	Analgesics, anticholinergics, iron supplements, aluminum antacids, calcium antacids, opiates, calcium channel blockers, vinca alkaloids
Lifestyle	Poor bowel movement habits: deliberate refusal to defecate, which results in constipation
	Diet: poor fluid intake and low-residue (low roughage) diet or excessive consumption of dairy products
	Physical inactivity: lack of proper exercise, especially in older adults
	Psychological: anxiety, stress, hypochondria
Metabolic and endocrine disorders	Diabetes mellitus, hypothyroidism, pregnancy, hypercalcemia, hypokalemia
Neurogenic disorders	Autonomic neuropathy, intestinal pseudo-obstruction, multiple sclerosis, spinal cord lesions, Parkinson's disease, stroke

(in extreme cases) or nonsurgical. Nonsurgical treatments can be separated into three broad categories of approach: dietary (e.g., fibre supplementation), behavioural (e.g., increased physical activity), and pharmacological. The focus in this chapter is on pharmacological treatment.

Laxatives are among the most misused OTC medications. Chronic and often inappropriate use of laxatives may result in laxative dependence, produce damage to the bowel, or lead to previously nonexistent intestinal problems. With the exception of the bulk-forming type, laxatives should not be used for long periods. Laxatives are divided into five major groups based on their mechanisms of action: bulk-forming, emollient, hyperosmotic, saline, and stimulant laxatives. Table 53-4 lists the currently available laxative drugs by the respective drug family.

Mechanism of Action and Drug Effects

All laxatives promote bowel movement, but each class of laxative has a different mechanism of action. Laxatives may act by (1) affecting fecal consistency, (2) increasing fecal movement through the colon, or (3) facilitating defecation through the rectum. *Bulk-forming laxatives* act in a manner similar to that of the fibre naturally contained in the diet. They absorb water into the intestine, which increases bulk and distends the bowel to initiate reflex bowel activity, thus promoting a bowel movement.

Emollient laxatives are also referred to as stool softeners (docusate salts) and lubricant laxatives (mineral oil). Fecal softeners work by lowering the surface tension of gastrointestinal fluids so that more water and fat are absorbed into the stool and the intestines. The lubricant type of emollient laxatives works by lubricating the fecal material and the intestinal wall and thus preventing absorption of water from the intestines. Rather than being absorbed, this water content in the bowel softens and expands the stool. This effect promotes bowel distension and reflex peristaltic actions, which ultimately lead to defecation.

Hyperosmotic laxatives work by increasing fecal water content, which results in distention, increased peristalsis, and evacuation. Their site of action is limited to the large intestine. *Saline laxatives* increase osmotic pressure in the small intestine by inhibiting water absorption and increasing both water and electrolyte (sodium) secretions from the bowel wall into the bowel lumen. This action results in watery stools. The increased distention promotes peristalsis and evacuation. Rectal enemas of sodium phosphate, a saline laxative, produce defecation 2 to 5 minutes after administration.

As the name implies, *stimulant laxatives* stimulate the nerves that innervate the intestines, which results in increased peristalsis. They also increase fluid in the colon, which increases bulk and softens the stool. Table 53-5 summarizes the specific drug effects of the different classes of laxatives.

Indications

The therapeutic uses for laxatives range from common constipation to bowel preparation before surgery. The therapeutic effects vary by category. Laxatives are helpful in relieving constipation, in preparing for some medical procedures, and in removing unwanted substances from the body. The following are some of the more common uses of laxatives:

- Removal of intestinal parasites
- Facilitation of bowel movement in patients with inactive colon
- Reduction of ammonia absorption in hepatic encephalopathic conditions (lactulose only)
- Treatment of drug-induced constipation
- Treatment of constipation associated with pregnancy or postobstetric period
- Treatment of constipation caused by reduced physical activity
- Removal of toxic substances from the body

TABLE 53-4

Laxatives: Drug Categories and Selected Drugs

Category	Laxative Drugs
Bulk forming	psyllium, polycarbophil, methylcellulose
Emollient	docusate salts, mineral oil
Hyperosmotic	polyethylene glycol, lactulose, sorbitol, glycerin
Saline	magnesium sulfate, magnesium phosphate, magnesium citrate, sodium phosphate
Stimulant	castor oil, senna, anthraquinones

TABLE 53-5

Laxatives: Drug Effects

Drug Effect	Bulk	Emollient	Hyperosmotic	Saline	Stimulant
Acts only in large bowel	N	N	Y	N	N
Causes increased secretion of water and electrolytes in small bowel	Y	Y	N	Y	Y
Increases peristalsis	Y	Y	Y	Y	Y
Inhibits absorption of water in small bowel	Y	Y	N	Y	Y
Increases wall permeability in small bowel	N	Y	N	N	Y
Increases water in fecal mass	Y	Y	Y	Y	Y
Softens fecal mass	Y	Y	Y	Y	Y

- Treatment of constipation associated with poor dietary habits
- Facilitation of defecation in megacolon
- Preparation for colonic diagnostic procedures or surgery
- Facilitation of bowel movements with reduced pain in anorectal disorders

See Table 53-6 for specific therapeutic indications for each laxative drug class.

Contraindications

All categories of laxatives share the same general contraindications and precautions, including drug allergy and the need for cautious use in the presence of the following: acute surgical abdomen; appendicitis symptoms such as abdominal pain, nausea, and vomiting; fecal impaction (mineral oil enemas excepted); intestinal obstruction; and undiagnosed abdominal pain.

Adverse Effects

As is true for the therapeutic effects of laxatives, the adverse effects of the drugs are specific to the laxative group. Most of the adverse effects from laxatives are confined to the intestine; however, the overuse and misuse of laxatives can lead to many effects that are not expected or designed to occur with appropriate use. The major adverse effects of the laxative drugs are listed in Table 53-7.

Interactions

Many drugs are absorbed in some part of the intestine. Because laxatives alter intestinal function, they can interact with other drugs quite readily. Bulk-forming laxatives can decrease the absorption of antibiotics, digoxin, nitrofurantoin, salicylates, tetracyclines, and oral anticoagulants. Mineral oil can decrease the absorption of fat-soluble vitamins (A, D, E, and K). Hyperosmotic laxatives can cause increased CNS depression if they are given with barbiturates, general anesthetics, opioids, or antipsychotics. Oral antibiotics can decrease the effects of lactulose. Stimulant laxatives decrease the absorption of antibiotics, digoxin, nitrofurantoin, salicylates, tetracyclines, and oral anticoagulants.

Dosages

For the recommended dosages of selected laxatives, see the Dosages table on p. 988.

TABLE 53-6

Laxatives: Indications

Category	Indication
Bulk forming	Acute and chronic constipation, irritable bowel syndrome, diverticulosis
Emollient	Acute and chronic constipation, softening of fecal impacts, facilitation of bowel movements in anorectal conditions
Hyperosmotic	Chronic constipation, bowel preparation for diagnostic and surgical procedures
Saline	Constipation, removal of helminths and parasites, bowel preparation for diagnostic and surgical procedures
Stimulant	Acute constipation, bowel preparation for diagnostic and surgical procedures

TABLE 53-7

Laxatives: Adverse Effects

Category	Adverse Effects
Bulk forming	Impaction above strictures, fluid overload, electrolyte imbalances, gas formation, esophageal blockage, allergic reaction
Emollient	Skin rashes, decreased absorption of vitamins, lipid pneumonia, electrolyte imbalances
Hyperosmotic	Abdominal bloating, rectal irritation, electrolyte imbalances
Saline	Magnesium toxicity (with kidney insufficiency), electrolyte imbalances, cramping, diarrhea, increased thirst
Stimulant	Nutrient malabsorption, skin rashes, gastric irritation, electrolyte imbalances, discoloured urine, rectal irritation

 DRUG PROFILES

The treatment of constipation with laxatives must involve an understanding of the whole patient. Many drugs in the five major groups of laxatives are available as OTC medications, whereas others require a prescription for use. The following text describes the prototypical drugs in each of the laxative groups.

BULK-FORMING LAXATIVES

Bulk-forming laxatives are composed of water-retaining (hydrophilic) natural and synthetic cellulose derivatives. Psyllium is an example of a natural bulk-forming laxative, and methylcellulose is an example of a synthetic cellulose derivative. Other bulk-forming laxatives are malt soup extract preparations and polycarbophil preparations. Bulk-forming drugs increase water absorption, which results in greater total volume (bulk) of the intestinal contents. Unlike some of the other laxatives, bulk-forming laxatives tend to produce normal, formed stools, as opposed to liquid stools. Their action is limited to the gastrointestinal tract, so there are few, if any, systemic effects. However, they should be taken with liberal amounts of water to prevent esophageal obstruction and fecal impaction. The

Continued

DRUG PROFILES (cont'd)

bulk-forming laxatives, which are all available over the counter, are among the safest laxatives and the only ones that are recommended for long-term use.

methylcellulose

Methylcellulose (Entrocel solution) is a synthetic bulk-forming laxative that attracts water into the intestine and absorbs excess water into the stool, stimulating the intestines and increasing peristalsis. Specific contraindications include gastrointestinal obstruction and hepatitis. Methylcellulose is an oral drug available in powdered form that provides approximately 2 g of fibre per heaping tablespoon.

PHARMACOKINETICS

Half-Life	Onset	Peak	Duration
Unknown	12–24 hr	Unknown	Unknown

▶▶ psyllium hydrophilic mucilloid

Psyllium hydrophilic mucilloid (Metamucil Preparations) is a natural bulk-forming laxative obtained from the dried seed of the *Plantago psyllium* plant. It has many of the characteristics of methylcellulose. Psyllium use is contraindicated in patients with intestinal obstruction or fecal impaction. Its use is also contraindicated in patients experiencing abdominal pain or nausea and vomiting. Psyllium is available for oral use in powder form.

PHARMACOKINETICS

Half-Life	Onset	Peak	Duration
Unknown	12–24 hr	Unknown	Unknown

EMOLLIENT LAXATIVES

Emollient laxatives either directly lubricate the stool and the intestines, as with mineral oil, or act as fecal softeners. By lubricating the fecal material and the intestinal walls, lubricant emollient laxatives prevent water from leaking out of the intestines, thus softening and expanding the stool. Stool softeners (docusate salts) work by lowering the surface tension of fluids, allowing more water and fat to be absorbed into the stool and the intestines.

▶▶ docusate salts

As noted earlier, docusate salts (calcium and sodium) are stool-softening emollient laxatives that facilitate the passage of water and fats into the fecal mass. These drugs are used to treat constipation, soften fecal impactions, and facilitate easy bowel movements in patients with hemorrhoids and other painful anorectal conditions. In addition to the docusate salt formulations, combination products are also available. Docusate use is contraindicated in patients with intestinal obstruction, fecal impaction, or nausea and vomiting.

PHARMACOKINETICS

Half-Life	Onset	Peak	Duration
Unknown	1–3 days	Unknown	1–3 days

mineral oil

Mineral oil (Fleet Enema Mineral Oil, Lansoyl) eases the passage of stool by lubricating the intestines and preventing water from escaping the stool. Mineral oil is the only lubricant laxative in the emollient category. It is a mixture of liquid hydrocarbons derived from petroleum and is most commonly used to treat constipation associated with hard stools or fecal impaction.

Mineral oil use is contraindicated in patients with intestinal obstruction, abdominal pain, or nausea and vomiting. Mineral oil drugs are available as enemas and in products for oral use.

PHARMACOKINETICS

Half-Life	Onset	Peak	Duration
Unknown	6–8 hr	Unknown	Unknown

HYPEROSMOTIC LAXATIVES

The hyperosmotic laxatives glycerin, lactulose, sorbitol, and polyethylene glycol (PEG) relieve constipation by increasing the water content of feces, which results in distention, peristalsis, and evacuation. They are most commonly used to treat constipation and to evacuate the bowels before diagnostic and surgical procedures.

▶▶ glycerin

Glycerin (Glycerin Suppositories) promotes bowel movements by increasing osmotic pressure in the intestine, which draws fluid into the colon. Because it is a mild laxative, it is often used in children. Glycerin has properties similar to those of sorbitol, another hyperosmotic laxative. Glycerin use is contraindicated in patients who have shown a hypersensitivity reaction to it. It is available as rectal suppositories. A combination product of glycerin/sodium citrate/sodium lauryl sulfoacetate/sorbic acid/sorbitol (Microlax) is commonly used as a rectal enema.

PHARMACOKINETICS

Half-Life	Onset	Peak	Duration
30–45 min	16–36 min	1 hr	2–4 hr

▶▶ lactulose

Lactulose is a disaccharide sugar containing one molecule of galactose and one molecule of fructose. It is a synthetic derivative of the natural sugar lactose, which is not digested in the stomach or absorbed in the small bowel. Consequently, it is passed unchanged into the large intestine, where it is metabolized. Colonic bacteria digest lactulose to produce lactic acid, formic acid, and acetic acid, which creates a hyperosmotic environment that draws water into the colon and produces a laxative effect. This drug-induced acidic environment also reduces blood ammonia levels by converting ammonia to ammonium. Ammonium is a water-soluble cation that is trapped in the intestines and cannot be reabsorbed into the systemic circulation. This effect has proved helpful

Continued

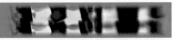

in reducing serum ammonia levels in patients with hepatic encephalopathy. Lactulose use is contraindicated in patients who have shown a hypersensitivity reaction to it and in patients on a low-galactose diet. It is available as a powder for either oral or rectal use.

PHARMACOKINETICS

Half-Life	Onset	Peak	Duration
Unknown	24 hr	24–48 hr	Variable

polyethylene glycol 3350

Polyethylene glycol 3350 (Klean-Prep, PegLyte [PEG]) is most commonly used before diagnostic or surgical bowel procedures because it is a potent laxative that induces total cleansing of the bowel. The 3350 designation refers to the osmolality of the drug. It is usually available in a powdered dosage form that contains a balanced mixture of electrolytes that also helps stimulate bowel evacuation. The powder is reconstituted to a large volume of fluid (4 L) that is then gradually ingested by the patient in the afternoon of the day before the procedure. Use of PEG is contraindicated in patients with gastrointestinal obstruction, gastric retention, bowel perforation, toxic colitis, toxic megacolon, or ileus. A common sample product composition is as follows:

- PEG-3350, 59 g/L
- Potassium chloride 0.74 g/L
- Sodium bicarbonate 1.68 g/L
- Sodium chloride 1.46 g/L
- Sodium sulfate 5.68 g/L

Diarrhea usually occurs within 30 to 60 minutes after ingestion; complete evacuation and cleansing of the bowel is accomplished within 4 hours.

PHARMACOKINETICS

Half-Life	Onset	Peak	Duration
Unknown	1 hr	2–4 hr	4 hr

SALINE LAXATIVES

Saline laxatives consist of magnesium or sodium salts. They increase osmotic pressure and draw water into the colon, producing a watery stool usually within 3 to 6 hours of ingestion. The currently available saline laxatives are listed in Box 53-1.

magnesium salts

The magnesium saline laxatives magnesium citrate, magnesium hydroxide, and magnesium sulfate (Epsom salts) are commonly used, even though unpleasant-tasting, OTC laxative preparations. They should be used with caution

or not at all in patients with kidney insufficiency because they can be absorbed into the systemic circulation in sufficient quantities to cause hypermagnesemia. They are most commonly used for rapid evacuation of the bowel in preparation for endoscopic examination and to remove unabsorbed poisons from the gastrointestinal tract.

Use of magnesium salts are contraindicated in patients with kidney disease, abdominal pain, nausea and vomiting, intestinal obstruction, acute surgical abdomen, or rectal bleeding. Magnesium hydroxide, more commonly referred to as milk of magnesia, is available in oral liquid and tablet forms. It is also found in a variety of combination products, such as Dioval and Pepsid. Other magnesium products are listed in the discussion of saline laxatives earlier in this chapter.

PHARMACOKINETICS

Half-Life	Onset	Peak	Duration
Unknown	0.5–3 hr	3 hr	Variable

STIMULANT LAXATIVES

Stimulant laxatives, including natural plant products and synthetic chemical drugs, induce intestinal peristalsis through their irritant effect on the lining of the colon that stimulates the muscles of the colon. Plant-derived laxatives include bisacodyl, dicacodyl tannex, and phenolphthalein (white and yellow). The anthraquinones make up another plant-derived subgroup of stimulant laxatives; these include drugs such as cascara sagrada, senna, aloe (casanthranol), and danthron. Their site of action is the entire gastrointestinal tract. The action of the stimulant laxatives is proportional to the dose. The stimulant class is the most likely of all laxative classes to cause dependence.

▶▶ senna

Senna (Senokot) is a commonly used OTC stimulant laxative. Senna is obtained from the dried leaves of the *Cassia acutifolia* plant. It may be used for relief of acute constipation or for bowel preparation for surgery or examination. Because of its stimulating action on the gastrointestinal tract, it may cause abdominal pain. It can produce complete bowel evacuation in 6 to 12 hours. Senna is available in a variety of dosages as tablets and syrup. One product, Senokot-S, includes both senna and the stool softener docusate sodium.

PHARMACOKINETICS

Half-Life	Onset	Peak	Duration
Variable	6–24 hr	24 hr	24–36 hr

DOSAGES Selected Laxatives

Drug (Pregnancy Category)	Pharmacological Class	Usual Dosage Range	Indications
▸▸docusate sodium (Colace) (C)	Stool softener, emollient laxative	*Children 3–12 yr** PO: 20–120 mg/day divided *Adult* PO: 100–200 mg/day divided	Facilitation of defecation (e.g., postpartum period or in any condition involving painful defecation because of hardened stools)
▸▸glycerin (Glycerin Suppositories) (C)	Hyperosmotic laxative	*Children/Adult* PR only: Insert one adult, child, or infant suppository PR daily–bid prn; attempt to retain 15–30 min; suppository does not have to dissolve to induce BM	Constipation
▸▸lactulose (generic) (B)	Disaccharide, hyperosmotic laxative	*Child–Adolescent†* PO: 1–3 mL/kg/day divided *Adult†* PO: 15–30 mL daily–bid	Constipation
magnesium citrate, anhydrous (Citro-Mag, Citrodan) (C)	Saline laxative	*Children under 6 yr* 0.5 mL/kg (max 200 mL); may repeat q4–6h until stools clear *Children 6–11 yr* 100–150 mL × 1 dose *Adult* 120–300 mL × 1 dose	Constipation; bowel cleansing before diagnostic procedure or surgery
methylcellulose (Entrocel solution) (B)	Bulk-forming laxative	*Children 6–11 yr* ½ 12 yr–adult dose *Children over 12 yr/Adult* PO: 1 heaping teaspoon in 240 mL cold water daily–tid	Constipation
mineral oil (Fleet Enema Mineral Oil) (B)	Emollient laxative	*Children 2–12 yr* PR: 60 mL × 1 *Adult* PR: 120 mL × 1	Constipation
polyethylene glycol (Klean-Prep, PegLyte) (C)	Hyperosmotic laxative	*Adult* PO: 4 L solution, usually evening before procedure; patient should fast at least 4 hr before drinking solution	Bowel cleansing before diagnostic procedure or surgery
▸▸psyllium hydrophilic mucilloid (Metamucil Preparations) (B)	Bulk-forming laxative	*Children 6 yr and older* ½ 12 yr–adult dose daily–tid *Adult* PO: 10.2 g/day divided in 240 mL water or juice	Constipation; often used as part of a daily maintenance program
▸▸senna (Senokot Preparations) (C)	Stimulant/irritant laxative	*Children 2–5 yr‡* PO (syrup): 3–5 mL at bedtime (max 5 mL bid) *Children 6–12 yr‡* PO (tabs): 1–2 tabs at bedtime (max 2 tabs bid) PO (syrup): 5–10 mL at bedtime (max 10 mL bid) *Adult‡* PO (tabs): 2–4 tabs at bedtime (max 4 tabs bid) PO (syrup): 10–15 mL at bedtime (max 15 mL bid)	Constipation

PO, oral; *PR,* rectal.

*Docusate sodium is available in both capsule and liquid forms.
†Rectal route is sometimes used to reverse hepatic coma.
‡There are many dosage forms; consult product labelling if in doubt. Most common dosage forms consist of 187 mg senna in tablet form and 1.7 mg/mL of sennosides in liquid form.

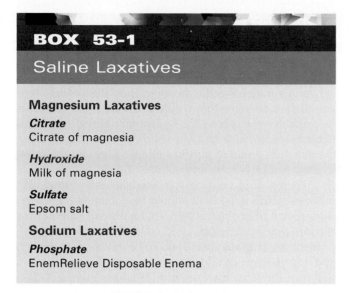

BOX 53-1

Saline Laxatives

Magnesium Laxatives

Citrate
Citrate of magnesia

Hydroxide
Milk of magnesia

Sulfate
Epsom salt

Sodium Laxatives

Phosphate
EnemRelieve Disposable Enema

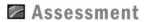

NURSING PROCESS

Assessment

Before administering antidiarrheal preparations, the nurse should obtain a thorough history of bowel patterns, general state of health, and recent history of illness and dietary changes and document this information. Abdominal assessment should include auscultation of bowel sounds in all four quadrants after inspection of the entire abdomen but before percussion and palpation. This practice avoids stimulation of peristalsis or bowel sounds that would not be there otherwise. When the frequency of bowel sounds ranges from 6 to 32 per minute, it is important to describe exactly what is heard and the amount of activity in each of the four quadrants. Terms such as high-pitched, low-pitched, gurgling, or tinkling may be used to describe the character or the sounds, whereas activity may be described as *hypoactive* (less than 6 per minute), *normoactive* (a range of 6 to 32 sounds per minute), or *hyperactive* (greater than the normal range). The abdominal assessment should be performed for any patient with gastrointestinal complaints, including altered bowel status. The presence of tenderness, rigidity, changes in contour, bulges, and obvious peristaltic waves across the abdomen should be noted. Also, the frequency, consistency, amount, colour, and odour (if present) of stools should be noted and documented. It is critical to patient safety and health to rule out the possibility of *Clostridium difficile* infection or other infectious diarrhea.

The use of some antidiarrheals (e.g., bismuth subsalicylate, diphenoxylate hydrochloride, loperamide) requires consideration of the history of bowel patterns and contraindications, cautions, and drug interactions. With diphenoxylate, there is an additional concern for use in patients with respiratory problems because of the risk for respiratory depression. Loperamide is not tolerated well by older adults. Patients in this age group are also more susceptible to fluid and electrolyte depletion; thus, hydration status needs to be closely monitored in addition to assessment of abdominal and bowel patterns. With any of these drugs, if an assessment shows bloody stools, abdominal rigidity, severe abdominal pain, or no bowel sounds, the drug should not be used and the physician should be contacted immediately.

Laxative use requires assessment beyond taking the history of abdominal and bowel patterns, described earlier. For example, questions should focus on changes in bowel habits or patterns, long-term use of laxatives (because patients may become laxative dependent), and dietary and fluid intake. Vital signs, particularly blood pressure; daily weight measurements; intake and output; fluid and electrolyte levels; and the presence of any weakness should be assessed because of the possibility of hypotension and volume or electrolyte depletion with chronic laxative use. The type of laxative and the related mechanism of action dictate specific assessments, as there are differences in how strongly the patient reacts to the laxative drugs. While the bulk-forming laxatives are often used to treat chronic constipation and have few adverse effects, they still require a basic abdominal and bowel pattern assessment and related history. Contraindications, cautions, and drug interactions should be assessed and documented. Docusate products must also be used with caution in older adults and require the same thorough assessment.

Magnesium-based laxatives act as osmotics, so assessment should include specific attention to baseline fluid and electrolyte levels to identify any deficits before their use. All of the previously mentioned assessment data regarding abdominal examination and bowel patterns are appropriate for these drugs, but the patient should also be assessed for abdominal pain, the degree of peristalsis, history of any recent abdominal surgery, nausea, vomiting, or weight loss. Serum magnesium, blood urea nitrogen, and creatinine levels should also be evaluated. Older adults react more negatively to this class of laxatives, so their use in this patient group should be avoided. Patients who have diabetes or are on a low-sodium diet should be assessed carefully because of drug-related elevation in blood glucose and serum sodium with use of magnesium laxatives. Lactulose is also an osmotic laxative; in addition to collecting the assessment data required for use of laxatives, the nurse should document baseline mental health status and ammonia levels.

Assessment of patients taking cascara sagrada requires evaluation of the abdomen and bowel status. Senna should be used with caution in the older adult because of possible dehydration and electrolyte loss. Patients taking a PEG-electrolyte solution, often used for gastrointestinal cleansing or preparation, should be assessed for the presence of ulcerative colitis because the solution may be given differently and only in specific situations in these patients. The nurse should note whether other medications are to be given to the patient; if so, they should be given 1 hour before the polyethylene solution so that absorption of other oral medications is not decreased.

Nursing Diagnoses

- Constipation related to improper diet and fluid intake
- Diarrhea related to gastrointestinal irritation from food, bacteria or viruses, or pathology
- Fluid volume deficit related to excessive diarrhea and loss of fluids and electrolytes through frequent, loose stools
- Risk for injury related to the adverse effects of drugs
- Nonadherence related to lack of knowledge of or experience with the medication regimen

Planning

Goals

- Patient will regain normal bowel patterns.
- Patient will remain free of fluid and electrolyte disturbances related to changes in bowel patterns and lack of proper management of bowel alterations.
- Patient will be free from injury related to possible weakness and dizziness or the adverse effects of medications.
- Patient will remain adherent to the medication regimen and nonpharmacological measures.

Outcome Criteria

- Patient reports the signs and symptoms of constipation or diarrhea to the health care provider if recommended measures and medications do not correct altered bowel patterns within a specified period.
- Patient reports the signs and symptoms of fluid and electrolyte loss, such as weakness, lethargy, decreased urinary output, and dizziness.
- Patient states measures to avoid adverse effects and injuries related to change in bowel patterns, changes in fluid and electrolyte status, or treatment, such as changing positions slowly, increasing intake of fluids, asking for assistance with ambulation as needed, and ambulating slowly.
- Patient states methods of administration that enhance effective and safe use of recommended drugs, including following proper dosing, taking oral doses with water or fluids as appropriate, and reporting undesired adverse effects.
- Patient states nonpharmacological measures to relieve constipation or diarrhea, such as forcing fluids, increasing intake of fibre or bulk for constipation, removing irritating food from the diet, and increasing bulk for diarrhea.

Implementation

Antidiarrheals should be taken exactly as prescribed, with strict adherence to the recommended dose, frequency, and duration of treatment. The nurse should encourage patients to be aware of their fluid intake and any dietary changes that would affect their health status or possibly exacerbate the symptoms already present. Patients should also be aware of the factors precipitating the diarrhea, and if symptoms persist, they should know to contact a physician immediately. Bowel pattern changes, weight, fluid volume status, intake and output, and mucous membrane status should be documented before, during, and after the initiation of treatment, whether for constipation or diarrhea.

Bismuth subsalicylate should be taken as directed, and the patient should be aware that this medication will turn the stool black or grey. If tablets are used, they should be chewed thoroughly before swallowing with at least 180 mL of fluid. This medication is a salicylate, and it should not be taken with other salicylates to avoid risk of toxicity. Diphenoxylate hydrochloride may be given without regard to food intake but should be given with adequate fluid. Loperamide should be taken as directed and with specific directions followed (e.g., take the specific number of tablets as recommended by the manufacturer after the first loose stool and the total number of tablets within a 24-hour time frame). Maximum amounts should not be exceeded, and if diarrhea continues or other symptoms occur (e.g., fever, abdominal pain, bloody stools), the health care provider should be contacted immediately. See Patient Education for more information.

Bulk-forming laxatives, such as methylcellulose and polycarbophil, must be administered as specified by package insert or as ordered. Methylcellulose should be taken with at least 240 mL or 1 full glass of liquid after the powder form has been thoroughly stirred into it. The fluid must be taken immediately to avoid choking or swelling of the product in the throat or esophagus. The medication should not be taken in its dry form. Polycarbophil, used both as a bulk-forming laxative and as an antidiarrheal, should be given every one-half hour up to the maximum daily dosage, and it should be given with 240 mL of liquid as directed. See Patient Education for more information.

Docusate is available in a variety of oral dosage forms (e.g., capsules, tablets, drops), and all should be taken with at least 180 mL of water or other fluid. An additional 180 mL to 240 mL of water a day should be ingested to help with stool softening. Milk or fruit juices may be used to disguise the taste, if needed.

Bisacodyl should be taken on an empty stomach for faster action, and whole tablets should not be chewed or crushed. Milk, antacids, or juices should not be taken with the dose or within 1 hour of taking the medication. Rectal suppositories, if too soft, can be placed in a medicine cup with ice to harden them before insertion. Once the wrapper is removed, a water-soluble lubricant should be applied and the suppository inserted immediately into the rectum. The patient should attempt to keep the suppository in place by lying still and on the left side for at least 15 to 30 minutes to allow the drug to dissolve. Cascara sagrada should be only given with water because, like bisacodyl, it interacts with milk and antacids. Lactulose may be taken with juice, milk, or water to increase palatability. The normal colour of the oral solution is pale yellow. Rectal dosage forms are administered as a retention enema with dilution as ordered and retained for 30 to 60 minutes. For a retention enema, the tip of the apparatus should be well lubricated and inserted carefully with the nozzle pointed toward the umbilicus of the patient, who should be lying on the left side. Fluid should be released gradually, and administration should be discontinued if the patient experiences severe abdominal pain. If long-term use is indicated, electrolyte levels should be monitored.

Magnesium-based laxatives should be used only as ordered and in certain situations. Fluids should be forced and other instructions followed per the physician's order or the package instructions. Refrigeration may help increase the palatability of the oral solution. It is important that this type of drug be taken exactly as prescribed for constipation, with consumption of plenty of fluids and careful attention to adverse effects. PEG-electrolyte solution should be mixed with water as directed and shaken well before taken. Chilled solutions are tolerated better, and rapid drinking is recommended.

Evaluation

Therapeutic responses to antidiarrheals and laxatives include an improvement in the gastrointestinal-related signs and symptoms reported by the patient (e.g., decrease in diarrhea or constipation), return to normal bowel patterns with normal bowel sounds, and absence of abnormal findings from an assessment of the abdomen and bowel patterns. Adverse effects for which to monitor patients vary according to each drug. Goals and outcome criteria should also serve as a means to evaluate the collaborative plan of care related to each problem, whether it is constipation or diarrhea.

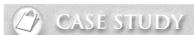 

CASE STUDY

Constipation

Mrs. M. is a 66-year-old retired school teacher. She enjoys good health and exercises three times a week with a senior citizens' group in a supervised arthritis swim class at the local recreation centre. She arrives at the physician's office with complaints of "constipation" and states that in the past 3 months she has been having only one bowel movement every 3 days, whereas she used to have one every day. In the assessment of this patient, you discover that she has been taking a laxative up to twice a day and is also now feeling "weak." She also states that she is experiencing "a lot of tummy cramping."

1. What are at least five questions you, as the nurse, should ask Mrs. M.? Provide reasons for each question.
2. What types of problems are generally related to chronic use of laxatives? Explain your answer.
3. If the nurse practitioner suggested an OTC drug to prevent constipation, what would be your choice(s), and why?

For answers see http://evolve.elsevier.com/Canada/Lilley/pharmacology/.

 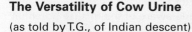

IN MY FAMILY

The Versatility of Cow Urine

(as told by T.G., of Indian descent)

"In Punjab, India . . . it is believed that natural remedies are more curable of an illness, whereas prescribed medications are not only more costly but they cause the severity of the illness to increase. . . . The most common natural remedy that helps with various conditions such as skin diseases, hypertension, endocrine disorders and many more is cow urine. Cow urine has [been] known to eliminate signs and symptoms of these disorders. . . . The best results have been seen with gastrointestinal disorders such as anorexia, constipation, nausea, and ulcers. It is believed that many elements of the urine are antibacterial and help to purify the blood by helping to excrete toxins from the body."

PATIENT EDUCATION

❖ Patients should be encouraged to take antidiarrheals exactly as prescribed, with close attention to indicated dosages and how not to exceed them. Stool frequency, consistency, and amount should be recorded for comparison and evaluation purposes. Patients should be told to contact their health care provider if they experience abdominal pain, bloody stools, fever, or abdominal distention. If diarrhea does not stop within 3 days, they should know to contact the physician.

❖ Patients should be reminded that antidiarrheal drugs have sedating adverse effects, so patients should be cautious with tasks that require mental alertness or motor skills until it is clear how they are affected by the drug.

❖ Patients taking either antidiarrheals or laxatives should be instructed to report abdominal distention, firm abdomen, pain, worsening (or no improvement) of symptoms, and other gastrointestinal-related signs and symptoms such as rectal bleeding to the physician immediately.

❖ Patients taking laxatives should be encouraged to contact their physician if they experience muscle weakness, cramps, or dizziness, which may indicate possible fluid or electrolyte loss.

❖ Patients should be encouraged to treat dry mouth with frequent mouth care, fluid intake, or use of sugarless gum or candy.

❖ Patients should be informed that bismuth subsalicylate may turn the stool tarry black, and they should report any bloody stools to the physician. Encourage

patients to avoid other drugs containing salicylates at this time and to always check for age-related cautions and contraindications.

❖ Patients with constipation should be encouraged to increase their intake of fluids; high-fibre, whole-grain products; green, leafy vegetables; and fruits, as well as increase their amount of exercise and try non-pharmacological methods of treatment.

❖ Patients should be encouraged to be honest with their health care provider about their bowel elimination patterns and be informed that what is normal for one person is not normal for another.

❖ Patients should be warned to not take a laxative if they are experiencing nausea, vomiting, or abdominal pain. If symptoms are not resolved and worsen, the patient should contact the health care provider.

❖ Patients should be warned to keep all antidiarrheals and laxatives out of the reach of children.

❖ Patients should be given specific instructions for certain drugs (e.g., powder forms of methylcellulose should be thoroughly mixed with at least 180 mL of liquid, stirred, and ingested immediately to avoid esophageal or throat obstruction). Senna may turn the urine pink-red, red-violet, red-brown, or yellowish brown. Patients should also be informed that other medications should not be taken within 1 hour of taking senna and that it often takes 6 to 12 hours for the laxative effect of the oral drug to occur.

❖ Patients should be advised that PEG solutions are more palatable if chilled and swallowed quickly.

POINTS TO REMEMBER

❖ Diarrhea is a leading cause of morbidity and mortality in developing countries.

❖ Drug therapy for diarrhea includes adsorbents, anticholinergics, opiates, and intestinal flora modifiers.

❖ Most acute diarrhea is self-limiting, subsiding in 3 days to 2 weeks.

❖ Fluid and electrolyte replacement is vital while a patient is experiencing diarrhea.

❖ Patients should be encouraged to check and recheck dosage instructions before taking medications and note any drug–food and drug–drug interactions.

❖ Anticholinergics work by decreasing gastrointestinal peristalsis through their parasympathetic blocking effects. Adverse effects include urinary retention, headache, confusion, dry skin, rash, and blurred vision.

❖ Adsorbents work by coating the walls of the gastrointestinal tract. They remain in the intestine and bind the causative bacteria or toxin to the adsorbent surface so that it can be eliminated through the stool. They may increase bleeding and cause constipation, dark stools, and black tongue.

❖ Intestinal flora modifiers are used to manage diarrhea and consist of bacterial cultures of *Lactobacillus*. They re-establish normal intestinal flora destroyed by infection or antibiotics and suppress the growth of diarrhea-causing bacteria.

❖ Opiates are used as antidiarrheals and help decrease bowel motility and thus permit longer contact of intestinal contents with the absorptive surface of the bowel. Opiates also help reduce the pain associated with rectal spasms.

❖ Laxatives, especially osmotic medications, may cause fluid and electrolyte loss.

❖ Patients must be made aware of the misuse potential of laxatives and the problems associated with such misuse.

❖ Stool softeners and bulk-forming drugs are often preferred in the treatment of constipation because they are not as problematic in terms of fluid and electrolyte loss.

EXAMINATION REVIEW QUESTIONS

1 A patient is being prepared for a colonoscopy. Which laxative is most appropriate as preparation for this procedure?
   a. Psyllium
   b. Methylcellulose
   c. Docusate sodium
   d. Polyethylene glycol (PEG)

2 What is the major concern regarding the administration of oral methylcellulose?
   a. Dehydration
   b. Tarry stools
   c. Kidney calculi
   d. Possible obstruction

3 Which of the following is the nurse's best response when educating the patient about prokinetic drugs?
   a. "These drugs stop acid production in the stomach."
   b. "The faster the food travels out of the stomach, the less chance there is for it to be refluxed."
   c. "They work by covering your stomach contents with foam to prevent reflux acid production."
   d. "They work by temporarily neutralizing the acid that is in the stomach at the time they are taken."

4 When the nurse teaches a patient about taking bisacodyl tablets, which instruction is correct?
   a. "Take this medication with juice or milk."
   b. "Take this medication on an empty stomach."
   c. "Chew the tablet for quicker onset of action."
   d. "Take this medication with an antacid if it upsets your stomach."

5 A patient has been on long-term antibiotic therapy as part of treatment for an infected leg wound. He tells the nurse that he has had "spells of diarrhea" for the past 1 week. Which medication is most appropriate for him at this time?
   a. Codeine
   b. Bismuth subsalicylate
   c. *Lactobacillus acidophilus*
   d. Diphenoxylate with atropine

For answers see http://evolve.elsevier.com/Canada/Lilley/pharmacology/.

CRITICAL THINKING ACTIVITIES

1 You are explaining to a group of older adults the importance of seeking treatment for diarrhea. During your discussion with the group, the following questions are posed to you:
   a. "What are some nondrug therapies I can use once I have begun to recover from diarrhea caused by a virus or the flu?"
   b. "If I have eaten something 'bad,' does it matter if I take something to stop the diarrhea?"
Provide answers that are appropriate for this older adult population, and provide a rationale for each response.

2 A woman calls the clinic because her 4-month-old daughter who is your patient has had diarrhea for approximately 8 hours. What would you recommend, and why?

3 Why is it important that the older adult be monitored closely while taking any type of bowel preparation medication before diagnostic studies such as a colonoscopy? Explain your answer.

For answers see http://evolve.elsevier.com/Canada/Lilley/pharmacology/.

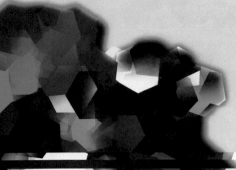

CHAPTER **54**

Antiemetic and Antinausea Drugs

Learning Objectives

After reading this chapter, the successful student will be able to do the following:

1 Discuss the pathophysiology of nausea and vomiting, including specific precipitating factors and diseases.

2 Identify antiemetic and antinausea drugs and their drug classifications.

3 Identify the mechanisms of action, indications for use, contraindications, cautions, drug interactions, adverse effects, routes of administration, and dosages associated with the antiemetic and antinausea drugs.

4 Develop a collaborative plan of care that includes all phases of the nursing process for patients taking antiemetic and antinausea drugs.

e-Learning Activities

Web site
(http://evolve.elsevier.com/Canada/Lilley/pharmacology/)

- Animations
- Answers to chapter questions, activities, and case studies
- Calculators and Category Catchers
- Glossary with audio pronunciations
- IV Therapy and Medication Error Checklists
- Multiple-Choice Review Question quizzes
- Nursing Care Plans
- Online Appendices and Supplements
- WebLinks

Drug Profiles

  aprepitant, p. 1000
  dronabinol, p. 1000
▸▸ **meclizine (meclizine hydrochloride)*,** p. 999
▸▸ **metoclopramide (metoclopramide hydrochloride)*,** p. 999
▸▸ **ondansetron (ondansetron hydrochloride dihydrate)*,** p. 999
▸▸ **prochlorperazine,** p. 999
  scopolamine, p. 998

▸▸ Key drug.

*Full generic name is given in parentheses. For the purposes of this text, the more common shortened name is used.

Glossary

Antiemetic drugs Drugs given to relieve nausea and vomiting. (p. 995)

Chemoreceptor trigger zone (CTZ) The area of the brain that is involved in the sensation of nausea and the action of vomiting. (p. 995)

Emesis The forcible emptying or expulsion of gastric and, occasionally, intestinal contents through the mouth; also called *vomiting.* (p. 995)

Nausea Sensation often leading to the urge to vomit. (p. 995)

Vomiting centre (VC) The area of the brain that is involved in stimulating the physiological events that lead to nausea and vomiting. (p. 995)

994

NAUSEA AND VOMITING

Nausea and vomiting are two gastrointestinal disorders that not only can be extremely unpleasant but also can lead to more serious complications if not treated promptly. **Nausea** is an unpleasant feeling that often precedes vomiting. If nausea does not subside spontaneously or is not relieved by medication, it can lead to vomiting. *Vomiting*, which is also called **emesis,** is the forcible emptying or expulsion of gastric and, occasionally, intestinal contents through the mouth. A variety of stimuli can induce nausea and vomiting, including foul odours or tastes, unpleasant sights, irritation of the stomach or intestines, and certain drugs (e.g., antineoplastic drugs). The **vomiting centre (VC)** is an area in the brain that is responsible for initiating the necessary physiological events that lead to nausea and, eventually, vomiting. Neurotransmitter signals are sent to the VC from the **chemoreceptor trigger zone (CTZ)**, another area in the brain involved in the induction of nausea and vomiting. These signals alert these areas of the brain to the existence of nauseating substances (nauseous stimuli) that need to be expelled from the body. Once the CTZ and VC are stimulated, they initiate the events that trigger the vomiting reflex. The neurotransmitters involved in this process and their respective receptors are listed in Table 54-1. The pathways and the areas of the body that send the signals to the VC via these pathways are illustrated in Figure 54-1.

ANTIEMETIC DRUGS

The drugs used to relieve nausea and vomiting are called **antiemetic drugs**. The discovery of new drugs coupled with a better understanding of how the older drugs work has had a dramatic impact on how nausea and vomiting are now treated. All antiemetic drugs work at some site in the vomiting pathways. There are six categories of antiemetics with varying mechanisms of action. When drugs from the various categories are combined, the

TABLE	54-1

Neurotransmitters Involved in Nausea and Vomiting

Neurotransmitter	Site in the Vomiting Pathway
Acetylcholine	VC in brain; vestibular and labyrinth pathways in inner ear
Dopamine (D$_2$)	GI tract and CTZ in brain
Histamine (H$_1$)	VC in brain; vestibular and labyrinth pathways in inner ear
Prostaglandins (PGs)	GI tract
Serotonin (5-HT$_3$)	GI tract; CTZ and VC in brain

CTZ, chemoreceptor trigger zone; *D$_2$*, dopamine-2 receptor; *GI*, gastrointestinal; *H$_1$*, histamine-1 receptor; *5-HT$_3$*, 5-hydroxytriptamine-3; *VC*, vomiting centre.

antiemetic effectiveness of the resulting preparation is increased because it can then block more than just one of the pathways. Some of the more commonly used antiemetics in the various categories are listed in Table 54-2, and the sites at which some of them work in the vomiting pathway are shown in Figure 54-2.

Mechanism of Action and Drug Effects

The numerous drugs used to prevent or treat nausea and vomiting have many different mechanisms of action. Most work by blocking one of the vomiting pathways, as shown in Figure 54-2, and in doing so block the neurological stimulus that induces vomiting. The mechanisms of action of the drugs in the six antiemetic drug categories are summarized in Table 54-3.

Anticholinergic drugs, discussed in Chapter 21, have several uses. As antiemetics, they act by binding to and blocking acetylcholine (ACh) receptors on the vestibular nuclei, which are located deep within the brain. When ACh is prevented from binding to these receptors, these drugs prevent nausea-inducing signals in this area that cannot be transmitted to the CTZ. Anticholinergics also block receptors located in the reticular formation and

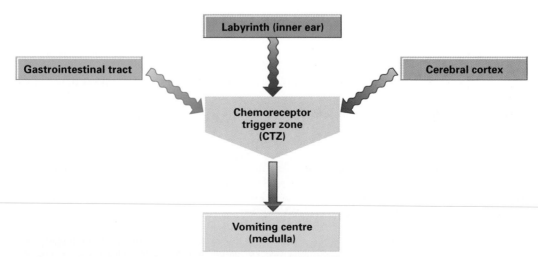

FIG. 54-1   The pathways and areas in the body sending signals to the vomiting centre.

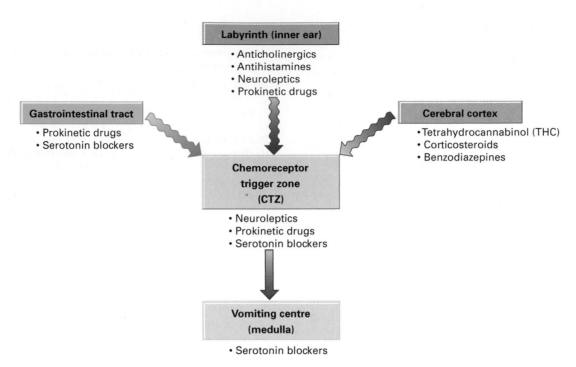

FIG. 54-2 Sites of action of selected antinausea drugs.

thus prevent ACh from binding to these receptors so that nausea-inducing signals originating in this area cannot be transmitted to the VC. Anticholinergics also tend to dry gastrointestinal secretions and reduce smooth muscle spasms, which is often helpful in reducing acute gastrointestinal symptoms, including nausea and vomiting.

Antihistamines (histamine-1 [H₁] receptor blockers) act by inhibiting vestibular stimulation similar to how anticholinergics work. Although they bind primarily to H₁ receptors, they also have potent anticholinergic activity as an adverse effect, including antisecretory and antispasmodic effects. They thus prevent cholinergic stimulation in the vestibular and reticular systems. Nausea

and vomiting occur when these areas of the brain are stimulated. These drugs are not to be confused with histamine-2 [H₂] receptor blockers used for gastric acid control (Chapter 52). Although the latter drugs are also technically a type of antihistamine, the term "antihistamine" is usually applied to histamine H₁ blockers, often in reference to their use in treating allergy symptoms (Chapter 36).

TABLE 54-3

Antiemetic Drugs: Mechanisms of Action

Category	Mechanism of Action
Anticholinergics	Block ACh receptors in the vestibular nuclei and reticular formation
Antihistamines	Block H₁ receptors, thereby preventing ACh from binding to receptors in the vestibular nuclei
Neuroleptics	Block dopamine in the CTZ and may also block ACh
Prokinetics	Block dopamine in the CTZ or stimulate ACh receptors in the GI tract
Serotonin blockers	Block serotonin receptors in the GI tract, CTZ, and VC
Tetrahydrocannabinoids	Have inhibitory effects on the reticular formation, thalamus, and cerebral cortex

ACh, acetylcholine; *CTZ,* chemoreceptor trigger zone; *GI,* gastrointestinal; *H₁,* histamine-1; *VC,* vomiting centre.

TABLE 54-2

Antiemetic Drugs: Common Drug Categories

Category	Antiemetic Drugs
Anticholinergics (ACh blockers)	scopolamine
Antihistamines (H₁ receptor blockers)	dimenhydrinate, diphenhydramine, meclizine, promethazine
Neuroleptics	chlorpromazine, perphenazine, prochlorperazine, promethazine, trimeprazine
Prokinetics	metoclopramide
Serotonin blockers	dolasetron, granisetron, ondansetron
Tetrahydrocannabinoids	dronabinol, nabilone

ACh, acetylcholine.

Neuroleptic drugs, although traditionally used for their antipsychotic effects (Chapter 16), also prevent nausea and vomiting by blocking dopamine receptors on the CTZ. Many of the neuroleptics have anticholinergic actions similar to those of anticholinergic drugs. In addition, neuroleptic drugs calm the central nervous system (CNS), an effect beneficial in treating the symptoms of psychiatric disorders (anxiety, tension, and agitation).

Prokinetic drugs, in particular metoclopramide, also act as antiemetics by blocking dopamine receptors in the CTZ, which desensitizes the CTZ to impulses it receives from the gastrointestinal tract. Their primary action, however, is to stimulate peristalsis in the gastrointestinal tract. This action enhances the emptying of stomach contents into the duodenum, as well as intestinal movements.

Serotonin blockers work by blocking serotonin receptors located in the gastrointestinal tract, CTZ, and VC. There are many subtypes of serotonin receptors, and these receptors are located throughout the body (CNS, smooth muscles, platelets, and gastrointestinal tract). The receptor subtype involved in the mediation of nausea and vomiting is the 5-hydroxytryptamine 3 (5-HT3) receptor. These receptors are the site of action for the serotonin blockers such as ondansetron and granisetron.

Tetrahydrocannabinol (THC), in a drug class by itself, is the major psychoactive substance in marihuana. Nonintoxicating doses in the form of the drugs dronabinol and nabilone are occasionally used as antiemetics because of their inhibitory effects on the reticular formation, thalamus, and cerebral cortex. These effects cause an alteration in mood and the body's perception of its surroundings, which may be beneficial in relieving nausea and vomiting. Although this particular category of antiemetics is less commonly prescribed, there are occasionally unusual cases of nausea and vomiting that respond well to THC. Examples include nausea and vomiting in patients being treated for cancer or acquired immune deficiency syndrome (AIDS), who can also be prone to having nutritional wasting syndromes. In such patients, dronabinol and nabilone may stimulate the appetite. The drug also demonstrates some benefit in controlling symptoms of glaucoma. There is a large, but highly controversial, political movement that is in favour of legalization of the marihuana plant for medical use in cancer, AIDS, and glaucoma patients.

Indications

The therapeutic uses of antiemetic drugs vary depending on the drug category. There are several indications for the drugs in each class. These indications are listed in Table 54-4.

Contraindications

The primary contraindication for all antiemetics is known drug allergy. Other contraindications for specific drugs are mentioned in the drug profiles.

TABLE 54-4

Antinausea Drugs: Indications

Antinausea Category	Indications
Anticholinergic drugs	Motion sickness, secretion reduction before surgery, nausea and vomiting
Antihistamine drugs	Motion sickness, nonproductive cough, sedation, rhinitis, allergy symptoms, nausea and vomiting
Neuroleptic drugs	Psychotic disorders (mania, schizophrenia, anxiety), intractable hiccups, nausea and vomiting
Prokinetic drugs	Delayed gastric emptying, gastroesophageal reflux, nausea and vomiting
Serotonin blockers	Nausea and vomiting associated with cancer chemotherapy, postoperative nausea and vomiting
Tetrahydrocannabinoids	Nausea and vomiting associated with cancer chemotherapy, anorexia and associated weight loss in AIDS patients

Adverse Effects

Most of the adverse effects of antiemetics stem from their nonselective blockade of receptors. For example, antihistamines bind not only to H$_1$ receptors in the vestibular nuclei, consequently preventing ACh from acting on them, but also to histamine receptors located elsewhere in the body, thus causing secretions to become dry. Some of the more common adverse effects associated with the various categories of antinausea drugs are listed in Table 54-5.

Interactions

The drug interactions associated with antiemetic drugs are also specific to individual drug categories. Anticholinergic antiemetics have additive drying effects when given with antihistamines and antidepressants. Antihistamine antiemetics, when administered with barbiturates, opioids, hypnotics, tricyclic antidepressants, or alcohol, can increase CNS depression. Neuroleptic antiemetics, when given with levodopa, may cancel the beneficial effects of the latter. Increased CNS depression can be seen when alcohol or other CNS depressants are given with neuroleptic drugs. Combining quinidine and neuroleptic drugs may result in increased adverse heart effects. When given with alcohol, prokinetic drugs can cause additive CNS depression. Anticholinergics and analgesics can block the motility effects of metoclopramide. Serotonin blockers and THC have no significant drug interactions.

Dosages

For the recommended dosages of selected antiemetic drugs, see the Dosages table on p. 1000.

TABLE 54-5	
Antinausea Drugs: Adverse Effects	
Body System	**Adverse Effects**
ANTICHOLINERGICS	
Cardiovascular	Tachycardia
Central nervous	Dizziness, drowsiness, disorientation
Ears, eyes, nose, throat	Blurred vision, dilated pupils, dry mouth
Genitourinary	Difficult urination, constipation
Integumentary	Rash, erythema
ANTIHISTAMINES	
Central nervous	Dizziness, drowsiness, confusion
Ears, eyes, nose, throat	Blurred vision, dilated pupils, dry mouth
Genitourinary	Urinary retention
NEUROLEPTIC DRUGS	
Cardiovascular	Orthostatic hypotension, electrocardiographic changes, tachycardia
Central nervous	Extrapyramidal symptoms, pseudoparkinsonism, akathisia, dystonia, tardive dyskinesia, headache
Ears, eyes, nose, throat	Blurred vision, dry eyes
Gastrointestinal	Dry mouth, nausea and vomiting, anorexia, constipation
Genitourinary	Urinary retention
PROKINETIC DRUGS	
Cardiovascular	Hypotension, supraventricular tachycardia
Central nervous	Sedation, fatigue, restlessness, headache, dystonia
Gastrointestinal	Dry mouth, nausea and vomiting, diarrhea
SEROTONIN BLOCKERS	
Central nervous	Headache
Gastrointestinal	Diarrhea, transient increased AST and ALT levels
Other	Rash, bronchospasm
TETRAHYDROCANNABINOIDS	
Central nervous	Drowsiness, dizziness, anxiety, confusion, euphoria
Ears, eyes, nose, throat	Visual disturbances
Gastrointestinal	Dry mouth

ALT, alanine aminotransferase; *AST*, aspartate aminotransferase.

 ## DRUG PROFILES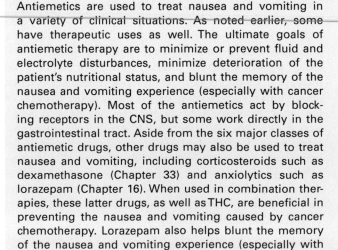

Antiemetics are used to treat nausea and vomiting in a variety of clinical situations. As noted earlier, some have therapeutic uses as well. The ultimate goals of antiemetic therapy are to minimize or prevent fluid and electrolyte disturbances, minimize deterioration of the patient's nutritional status, and blunt the memory of the nausea and vomiting experience (especially with cancer chemotherapy). Most of the antiemetics act by blocking receptors in the CNS, but some work directly in the gastrointestinal tract. Aside from the six major classes of antiemetic drugs, other drugs may also be used to treat nausea and vomiting, including corticosteroids such as dexamethasone (Chapter 33) and anxiolytics such as lorazepam (Chapter 16). When used in combination therapies, these latter drugs, as well as THC, are beneficial in preventing the nausea and vomiting caused by cancer chemotherapy. Lorazepam also helps blunt the memory of the nausea and vomiting experience (especially with cancer chemotherapy). Chemotherapy-induced nausea

and vomiting and postoperative nausea and vomiting can be especially difficult to treat. The serotonin blockers have proved to be effective in preventing these types of nausea and vomiting.

ANTICHOLINERGICS
scopolamine

Scopolamine (Transderm-V) is the primary anticholinergic drug used as an antiemetic. It has potent effects on the vestibular nuclei, which, as previously noted, are within the area of the brain that controls balance. It works by blocking the binding of ACh to the cholinergic receptors in this region, thereby correcting an imbalance between the neurotransmitters ACh and norepinephrine. These effects make scopolamine one of the most commonly used drugs for the treatment and prevention of the nausea and vomiting associated with motion sickness. It is also used as an adjunct to anesthesia to inhibit salivation and excessive respiratory secretions. Scopolamine produces

Continued

DRUG PROFILES (cont'd)

amnesia and sedation, and it may be used for palliative control of secretions. Scopolamine use is contraindicated in patients with glaucoma. Scopolamine is available in injectable and transdermal forms. The most commonly used formulation for nausea is the 72-hour transdermal patch, which releases a total of 1 mg of the drug.

PHARMACOKINETICS

Half-Life	Onset	Peak	Duration
TP: 9.5 hr	TP: 1–2 hr	TP: 6–8 hr	TP: 72 hr

TP, transdermal patch.

ANTIHISTAMINES

Antihistamine antiemetics are some of the most commonly used and safest antiemetics. Some of the popular antihistamines are promethazine hydrochloride (Histantil), meclizine hydrochloride (Bonamine), dimenhydrinate (Dinate, Gravol, Nauseatol, others), and diphenhydramine hydrochloride (Aller-Aide, Allerdryl, Benadryl). Many of the antihistamines are available over the counter, and some others are prescription drugs.

▶▶ *meclizine hydrochloride*

Meclizine hydrochloride (Bonamine) is most commonly used to treat the dizziness, vertigo, and nausea and vomiting associated with motion sickness. Contraindications include shock and lactation. It is available for oral use only.

PHARMACOKINETICS

Half-Life	Onset	Peak	Duration
PO: 6 hr	PO: 1 hr	PO: Variable	PO: 8–24 hr

NEUROLEPTIC DRUGS

Prochlorperazine (Nu-Prochlor), chlorpromazine hydrochloride, perphenazine, promethazine hydrochloride (Histantil), droperidol, and trifluoperazine hydrochloride (Terfluzine) are antiemetics in the neuroleptic class. These drugs have antidopaminergic as well as antihistaminergic and anticholinergic properties. Many of these drugs are used to treat psychotic disorders such as mania and schizophrenia and the associated anxiety, intractable hiccups, as well as nausea and vomiting.

▶▶ *prochlorperazine*

Prochlorperazine (Nu-Prochlor), particularly in the injectable form, is one of the more commonly used antiemetics in the hospital setting. Its use is contraindicated in patients with hypersensitivity to phenothiazines, those in a coma, and those who have seizures, encephalopathy, or bone marrow depression. It is available for both injection and oral use.

PHARMACOKINETICS

Half-Life	Onset	Peak	Duration
IM: 6–8 hr	IM: 30–40 min	IM: 2–4 hr	IM: 3–4 hr

PROKINETIC DRUGS

Prokinetic drugs promote the movement of substances through the gastrointestinal tract and increase gastrointestinal motility. The prokinetic drug that is also used to prevent nausea and vomiting is metoclopramide.

▶▶ *metoclopramide hydrochloride*

Metoclopramide hydrochloride (Apo-Metoclop, other generic) is the oldest and most commonly used prokinetic drug. It is available only by prescription because it can cause some severe adverse effects if not used correctly. Metoclopramide is used for the treatment of delayed gastric emptying and gastroesophageal reflux and also as an antiemetic. Its use is contraindicated in patients with seizure disorder, pheochromocytoma, breast cancer, or gastrointestinal obstruction, and also in patients with a hypersensitivity to it or to procaine or procainamide. Metoclopramide is available in both oral and parenteral formulations.

PHARMACOKINETICS

Half-Life	Onset	Peak	Duration
PO: 3–5 hr	PO: 30–60 min	PO: 45–90 min	PO: 3–4 hr

SEROTONIN BLOCKERS

The serotonin blockers are also called *5-HT$_3$ receptor blockers* because they block the 5-HT$_3$ receptors in the gastrointestinal tract, CTZ, and vomiting centre. (The chemical name for serotonin is 5-hydroxytryptamine [5-HT]). Because of their specific actions, these drugs cause few adverse effects. They are indicated for the prevention of nausea and vomiting associated with cancer chemotherapy and for the prevention of postoperative or radiation-induced nausea and vomiting. Currently, there are three drugs in this category: dolasetron mesylate (Anzemet), granisetron hydrochloride (Kytril), and ondansetron hydrochloride dihydrate (Zofran).

▶▶ *ondansetron hydrochloride dihydrate*

Ondansetron hydrochloride dihydrate (Zofran) is the prototypical drug in this class. Approved in 1991, it represented a major breakthrough in treating chemotherapy-induced nausea and vomiting and, later, postoperative nausea and vomiting. Its specific mechanism of action in the control of chemotherapy-induced nausea and vomiting is not known, nor is there any certainty whether ondansetron's action is mediated peripherally, centrally, or both. Its only listed contraindication is drug allergy. It is available in both oral (tablets and solution) and injectable forms. Ondansetron (Zofran ODT) is an oral disintegrating tablet.

PHARMACOKINETICS

Half-Life	Onset	Peak	Duration
IV: 3–5.5 hr	IV: 15–30 min	IV: 1–1.5 hr	IV: 6–12 hr

Continued

DRUG PROFILES (cont'd)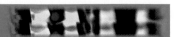

TETRAHYDROCANNABINOIDS

dronabinol

Dronabinol (Marinol) and nabilone (Cesamex) are commercially available tetrahydrocannabinoids. They are synthetic derivatives of THC, the major active substance in marihuana. They are approved for the treatment of nausea and vomiting associated with cancer chemotherapy. They are generally used as second-line drugs after treatment with other antiemetics has failed. They are also used to stimulate appetite and weight gain in patients with AIDS. Dronabinol's only listed contraindication is drug allergy. It is available for oral use only.

PHARMACOKINETICS

Half-Life	Onset	Peak	Duration
PO: 25–36 hr	PO: 30–60 min	PO: 2–4 hr	PO: 4–6 hr

MISCELLANEOUS ANTINAUSEA DRUGS

aprepitant

Aprepitant (Emend) is the first in a new class of antiemetic drugs, approved in 2007. It is an antagonist of substance P–neurokinin-1 receptors in the brain. In contrast to other antiemetics, this drug has little affinity for 5-HT_3 (serotonin) and dopamine receptors. However, studies show that aprepitant augments the antiemetic actions of both ondansetron and the corticosteroid dexamethasone. This drug is specifically indicated for the prevention of nausea and vomiting in *highly and moderately emetogenic* cancer chemotherapy regimens, including high-dose cisplatin or cyclophosphamide and anthracycline. Common adverse effects include dizziness, headache, insomnia, and gastrointestinal discomfort, but these are generally no more common than with other standard antiemetic regimens. Aprepitant has drug interactions with warfarin (international normalized ratio [INR] should be monitored to assess the need for dosage adjustment) and steroids. Because, like aprepitant, steroids such as dexamethasone and methylprednisolone are metabolized by the cytochrome P450 subtype 3A4 isoenzymes, aprepitant can reduce their metabolism, lowering the required steroid dosages by 25% to 50%. It is classified as pregnancy category B.

DOSAGES   Selected Antiemetic and Antinausea Drugs

Drug (Pregnancy Category)	Pharmacological Class	Usual Dosage Range	Indications
ANTICHOLINERGICS			
scopolamine (Transderm-V) (C)	Anticholinergic, belladonna alkaloid	Apply 1 patch (1 mg) behind ear q3d (starting at least 12 hr before desired effect)	Motion sickness prophylaxis
ANTIHISTAMINES			
⇥meclizine hydrochloride (Bonamine) (B)	Anticholinergic, antihistamine	*Adult* PO: 25–50 mg 1 hr before travel and repeated daily during travel PO: 25–100 mg/day, divided	Motion sickness prophylaxis Treatment of vertigo
NEUROLEPTICS			
⇥prochlorperazine (Nu-Prochlor) (C)	Phenothiazine	*Children* PO/rectal: 9–14 kg: 2.5 mg once daily–bid (max 7.5 mg/day) 14–18 kg: 2.5 mg bid–tid (max 10 mg/day) 18–39 kg: 2.5 mg tid or 5 mg bid (max 15 mg/day) IM: 0.13 mg/kg *Adult* PO/rectal: 5–10 mg tid–qid IM/IV: 5–10 mg bid–tid	Antiemetic
PROKINETICS			
⇥metoclopramide hydrochloride (Apo-Metolop) (B)	Dopamine antagonist	*Children* IV: 0.5–1.5 mg/kg q2–3h × 3 doses, then prn (max 10 mg/kg/day) *Adult* IV: 1–2 mg/kg (30 min before chemotherapy; repeat q2h × 2 doses, then q3h × 3 doses) IM: 10–20 mg × 1 dose near end of surgery	Chemotherapy antiemetic Chemotherapy antiemetic Prevention of postoperative nausea and vomiting

Continued

DOSAGES   Selected Antiemetic and Antinausea Drugs (cont'd)

Drug (Pregnancy Category)	Pharmacological Class	Usual Dosage Range	Indications
SEROTONIN BLOCKERS			
▸▸**ondansetron hydrochloride dihydrate (Zofran) (B)**	Antiserotonergic	*Children 4–12 yr* PO: 4 mg tid, after chemotherapy, × up to 5 days IV: 3–5 mg/m² over 15 min, immediately before chemotherapy, then oral as above	Chemotherapy antiemetic
		Adult PO: 8 mg bid up to 5 days after the initial 24-hr IV dose IV: 8 mg over 15 min, given 30 min before chemotherapy, followed by 1 mg/hr continuous infusion up to 24 hr, or one dose of 32 mg over 15 min, given 30 min before chemotherapy	Chemotherapy antiemetic
		PO: 16 mg 1 hr before surgery IV: 4 mg over 2–5 min × 1 dose (second dose not shown to be effective in patients who fail first dose)	Prevention and treatment of postoperative nausea
TETRAHYDROCANNABINOIDS			
dronabinol (Marinol) (C)	Marihuana-derived antiemetic	*Adult* PO: Initially, 5 mg/m² 1–3 hr before chemotherapy, then q2–4h after chemotherapy up to 4–6×/day; if needed, this dose may be increased in 2.5 mg/m² increments to a max dose of 15 mg/m²	Chemotherapy antiemtic
		PO: 2.5–5 mg bid before lunch and before or after dinner, or 2.5 mg as single P.M. or bedtime dose for patients intolerant of 5 mg doses	Appetite stimulation in HIV/AIDS

IM, intramuscular; *IV*, intravenous; *PO*, oral.

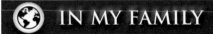
IN MY FAMILY

Traditional Remedy for Upset Stomach

(as told by H.K, of Korean descent)

"When I was young, I got [an] upset stomach (indigestion) after eating [a] very big meal at my grandmother's house. I had stomach ache, felt pressure, bloating, and discomfort. I was pale and my hands were cold and clammy. . . . My grandmother made me drink a pop (carbonated drink) and stroked my back in order to induce a burp. I was encouraged to massage my hand, where the thumb and index finger meets, with pressure. She tied my thumb with a string, and massaged my arm from shoulder toward fingers, like moving the blood toward the fingers. Then she pricked my thumb with a needle, and let out the dark-coloured blood from my thumb. She did the same for my other thumb, and within a few minutes, I belched and felt comfortable. . . . This is a common Korean traditional remedy practised for upset stomach."

NURSING PROCESS

Assessment

Before any antinausea or antiemetic drug is administered, a thorough nursing history and physical assessment of the patient should be completed, with attention to the following: history of the symptoms of nausea and vomiting; medical history and drugs currently being taken, including over-the-counter drugs, natural health products (including herbals), prescription drugs, and social drugs (e.g., cigarettes, alcohol); and any alternative therapies used (see Natural Health Products: Ginger). Any factors precipitating nausea or vomiting should be identified; weight loss should be noted; baseline vital signs should be measured; intake and output should be assessed; the skin and mucous membranes should be examined and turgor and colour noted; and capillary refill (which should be less than 5 seconds) should also be noted. Once laboratory tests are ordered (e.g., serum sodium, potassium, and chloride levels; hemoglobin level; hematocrit; red and white blood cell counts; and urinalysis), the findings should be assessed and documented to establish baseline levels. The patient should be assessed for any contraindications or cautions to the use of these drugs and for drug interactions (discussed previously in the pharmacology section), as well as for any allergies.

The anticholinergic drug scopolamine, which is commonly administered in patch form to prevent motion sickness, should be given only after careful assessment of the patient's health history and medication history. The drug is contraindicated in patients with a hypersensitivity to it and in those with glaucoma. If the patient has a history of narrow-angle glaucoma, a different antiemetic or antinausea drug should be used. Patients with narrow-angle glaucoma should also not take antihistamines (e.g., meclizine). In addition, antihistamines should be used cautiously in children, who may have severe paradoxical reactions, and in older adults, who often develop agitation, mental confusion, hypotension, and even psychotic-type reactions to these drugs. If these reactions occur, alternative medications should be considered for these patients.

Neuroleptic drugs such as prochlorperazine should be used only after cautious assessment for signs and symptoms of dehydration and electrolyte imbalance by evaluation of skin turgor and examination of the tongue for the presence of longitudinal furrows. As with other antiemetic drugs, the contraindications, cautions, and drug interactions for these drugs should be noted. Particularly when they are used in a psychotic patient, the patient's appearance, behaviour, emotional status, responses to the environment and to others, and speech and thought content need to be assessed. The drug name and mechanism of action should be double-checked so that the drug is not confused with chlorpromazine.

Prokinetic drugs (e.g., metoclopramide) are often reserved for the treatment of nausea and vomiting associated with antineoplastic drug therapy or radiation therapy and for the treatment of gastrointestinal motility disturbances. The action of these drugs is decreased, however, when they are taken with anticholinergics or opiates. In addition, children and the older adult are at increased risk of tardive dyskinesia with use of these drugs. Granisetron should be given only after assessment of baseline vital signs and age (its safety in children younger than 2 years of age has not been established). With use of ondansetron, the nurse needs to look for signs and symptoms of dehydration and electrolyte disturbances, with evaluation of skin turgor and examination for dry mucous membranes or longitudinal furrows in the tongue. Serum levels of bilirubin, aspartate aminotransferase, and alanine aminotransferase should also be assessed before initiation of therapy, especially in patients with liver dysfunction.

With use of dronabinol, the drug's contraindications, cautions, and drug interactions need to be noted. Patients taking this drug should be assessed for signs and symptoms of dehydration, with attention to low urine output, dry mucous membranes, poor skin turgor, and overall lethargy, before this medication is given. A thorough assessment of hydration status is important because treatment of volume and electrolyte imbalances may be required in addition to treatment with antinausea or antiemetic drugs. Motor and cognitive abilities should also be assessed and a neurological head-to-toe examination performed before and during drug therapy.

Nursing Diagnoses

- Risk for injury and falls related to weakness and dizziness from vomiting and to the adverse effects of the drugs (e.g., sedation and dizziness)
- Risk for deficient fluid volume related to nausea and vomiting and limited oral intake
- Impaired physical mobility related to weakness from fluid and electrolyte disturbances secondary to vomiting

---

NATURAL HEALTH PRODUCTS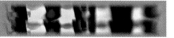

GINGER (*Zingiber officinale*)

Overview
Found naturally in the Asian tropics; now cultivated in other continents, including part of the United States; plant parts used are the rhizome and root; active ingredients include gingerols and gingerdione

Common Uses
Used as an antioxidant; also used for relief of such varied symptoms as sore throat, migraine headache, and nausea and vomiting (including that induced by cancer chemotherapy, morning sickness, and motion sickness); many other varied uses

Adverse Effects
Skin reactions, anorexia, nausea, vomiting

Potential Drug Interactions
Can increase absorption of all oral medications; may theoretically increase bleeding risk with anticoagulants (e.g., warfarin [Coumadin]) or antiplatelet drugs (e.g., clopidogrel [Plavix])

Contraindications
Contraindicated in cases of known product allergy; may worsen cholelithiasis (gallstones); anecdotal evidence of abortifacient properties—some clinicians recommend not using it during pregnancy

Planning

■ Goals

- Patient will remain free of injury and falls from weakness and dizziness secondary to nausea, vomiting, and adverse effects of drug therapy.
- Patient will manage the adverse effects of the drugs and identifies symptoms for which to seek medical care.
- Patient will regain normal fluid volume status and hydration levels.
- Patient will regain normal levels of activity without risk of falls and injury.

■ Outcome Criteria

- Patient states measures to implement to prevent injury, such as obtaining assistance while ill, rising slowly, changing positions slowly, taking medications as ordered, and initiating fluid intake once nausea and vomiting subside.
- Patient states adverse effects of drug therapy such as severe sedation, confusion, lethargy, hypotension, and CNS depression.
- Patient states measures to implement to prevent further fluid volume deficits, such as consumption of oral fluids (e.g., clear liquids) or chilled gelatin along with the drugs.
- Patient increases activity by 10 to 15 minutes each day with cautious rising and walking.

Implementation

Undiluted forms of diphenhydramine should be administered intravenously at the recommended rate of 25 mg/min. Intramuscular forms should be administered into large muscles (e.g., ventral gluteal), and the sites should be rotated if repeated injections are necessary.

Prochlorperazine may be given orally without regard to meals; parenteral doses should be given using the proper dilutional solutions and infusion rates. Because of the hypotensive effects of the drug, the patient should remain lying down for 30 to 60 minutes after the drug has been given parenterally, and the legs should be elevated to help minimize the hypotensive effect. Suppository dosage forms should be moistened with water or water-soluble lubricating gel before inserting deep into the rectum. Patients should be placed on the left side for suppository insertion; they should remain there for several minutes and hold in the suppository as long as possible to increase its absorption. Vital signs should be taken frequently, and the patient should be monitored for extrapyramidal symptoms throughout therapy, whether at home or in the hospital. The patient should be encouraged to avoid other CNS depressants and alcohol and to limit caffeine when this drug is used; they should also avoid driving and other activities that require mental alertness or motor coordination.

Patients taking meclizine should have their blood pressures checked frequently, especially if they are older

adults. Sedation raises a concern for patient safety; as patients may become unsteady on their feet, they should move about with caution at all times. To alleviate dry mouth produced by any of these medications, the patient can chew sugarless gum or suck on hard candy.

Metoclopramide is given orally and should be administered 30 minutes before meals and at bedtime. Intravenous dosage forms should be given within the recommended time frame. In addition, solutions for parenteral dosing should be kept for only 48 hours and protected from light. Metoclopramide should not be given in combination with any other medications such as phenothiazines that would lead to exacerbation of extrapyramidal reactions. Such reactions should be reported immediately to the physician.

The scopolamine transdermal patch is applied behind the ear as directed. The area behind the ear should be cleansed and dried before the patch is applied. If the patch becomes dislodged, the residual drug should be washed off and a fresh patch put in place. The patient should be warned not to engage in tasks requiring mental clarity or motor skill while taking the medication.

Granisetron may be given intravenously or orally. Intravenous doses should be infused within the recommended time frame and diluted as appropriate. A transient taste disorder may occur, especially if the drug is taken with antineoplastic medications, but will pass with continued therapy. The patient should be encouraged to use relaxation techniques and imagery as complementary therapies. Ondansetron may be given orally, intramuscularly, or intravenously. Intramuscular doses should be injected into a large muscle mass. Intravenous push is usually given over 2 to 5 minutes and infusions over 15 minutes as ordered and per manufacturer guidelines. Oral forms are well tolerated regardless of the relation of dosing to meals. The patient should be encouraged to avoid alcohol and other CNS depressants during this therapy and to avoid any activities requiring mental alertness or motor skill. Dronabinol, granisetron, and ondansetron are usually indicated before chemotherapy. Dronabinol should be administered 1 to 3 hours before antineoplastic therapy and may be taken at home before the scheduled appointment for treatment. Relief of nausea and vomiting should occur within approximately 15 minutes of oral drug administration.

Evaluation

The therapeutic effects of antiemetic and antinausea drugs range from a decrease in and the elimination of complaints of nausea to vomiting, to avoidance or elimination of complications such as fluid and electrolyte imbalances and weight loss. The patient should also be monitored for adverse effects such as gastrointestinal upset, drowsiness, lethargy, weakness, extrapyramidal reactions, and orthostatic hypotension during the treatment. Laboratory testing (e.g., electrolyte levels, blood urea nitrogen level, urinalysis with specific gravity) may be ordered for evaluation purposes. Defined goals and outcomes may be used to evaluate therapeutic effectiveness.

CASE STUDY

Nausea Associated with Chemotherapy

Ms. S., a 58-year-old retired seamstress, has started outpatient chemotherapy for a recent diagnosis of breast cancer. She has recovered well from a right modified mastectomy, the incisions are healing well, and she is now physically and emotionally ready for the 3-month regimen of chemotherapy. Her premedication consists of a variety of drugs, including granisetron (Kytril). Her home medication list includes oral ondansetron (Zofran).

1. What is the mechanism of action of granisetron that makes it effective in the management of chemotherapy-induced nausea and vomiting?

2. What patient teaching about ondansetron is important for Ms. S.?

3. After 2 weeks of therapy, the physician discontinues the ondansetron because Ms. S. complained that it did nothing to help her nausea and vomiting. She receives a prescription for dronabinol but expresses concern because she knows "there's marihuana in that pill!" What would you explain to her?

For answers see http://evolve.elsevier.com/Canada/Lilley/pharmacology/.

PATIENT EDUCATION

❖ Patients taking any of the antiemetic or antinausea drugs should be warned about the drowsiness they can cause and told to avoid performing any potentially hazardous tasks or driving while taking these medications. Patients should also be cautioned about taking antiemetic or antinausea drugs with alcohol and other CNS depressants because of the possible toxicity and CNS depression that can occur.

❖ Patients should be educated about the adverse effects of ondansetron, including headache, which may be relieved with a simple analgesic (e.g., acetaminophen).

❖ Patients taking dronabinol should be reminded to change positions slowly to prevent syncope or dizziness resulting from the hypotensive effects of the drug. They should also avoid taking any other CNS depressants with this antiemetic and should be cautious when engaging in activities that require mental alertness.

❖ Patients should be instructed to rotate the application sites for transdermal scopolamine patches and that the patches should be applied to nonirritated areas behind the ear. The hands should be washed thoroughly before and after patch application.

❖ Patients taking antiemetic or antinausea drugs should be cautioned that drowsiness and hypotension may occur, thus they should avoid driving and using heavy machinery while taking these medications.

POINTS TO REMEMBER

❖ Antiemetics help control vomiting, or emesis, and are also useful in relieving or preventing nausea.

❖ Antiemetics are used to prevent motion sickness, reduce secretions before surgery, manage delayed gastric emptying, and prevent postoperative nausea and vomiting.

❖ The categories of antiemetics are anticholinergics, antihistamines, neuroleptic drugs, prokinetic drugs, serotonin blockers, and tetrahydrocannabinoids.

❖ Anticholinergics act by blocking ACh receptors in the vestibular nuclei and reticular formation. This blocking prevents areas in the brain from being activated by nauseous stimuli.

❖ Antihistamines act by blocking H_1 receptors, which has the same effect as that of the anticholinergics.

❖ Neuroleptic antiemetics block dopamine receptors in the CTZ and may also block ACh receptors.

❖ Prokinetic drugs also block dopamine receptors in the CTZ.

❖ The serotonin-blocking drugs may be highly effective antiemetics. They are most commonly used for the prevention of chemotherapy-induced nausea and vomiting and act by blocking $5\text{-}HT_3$ receptors in the gastrointestinal tract, CTZ, and VC.

❖ Antiemetics are often administered 30 minutes to 3 hours before a chemotherapy drug is administered and may also be given during the chemotherapeutic treatment. Because multiple pathways are involved in chemotherapy-induced nausea and vomiting, combination therapy may be the most effective treatment. Prophylaxis of nausea and vomiting is usually the most effective approach.

❖ Most antiemetic and antinausea drugs cause drowsiness.

❖ Granisetron and ondansetron are successful in treating chemotherapy-induced nausea and vomiting.

❖ Dronabinol and nabinol combination therapy is used to prevent antineoplastic-induced nausea and vomiting and is associated with postural hypotension.

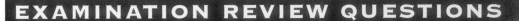

EXAMINATION REVIEW QUESTIONS

1 Which patient teaching instruction is most appropriate for a patient who plans to use scopolamine transdermal patches during a cruise?
a. "Apply the patch the day before travelling."
b. "The patch should be applied to the shoulder area."
c. "Apply the patch at least 12 hours before travelling."
d. "The patch should be applied on the temple just above the ear."

2 A middle-aged woman is experiencing severe vertigo realted to Ménière's disease. Which of the medications listed below is considered the most appropriate treatment for vertigo?
a. dronabinol (Marinol)
b. meclizine (Bonamine)
c. metoclopramide (Apo-Metoclop)
d. prochlorperazine (Nu-Prochlor)

3 A 33-year-old patient is in the outpatient cancer centre for the first round of chemotherapy. When is the best time to administer an intravenous dose of antiemetic?
a. At the first sign of nausea
b. Four hours before chemotherapy begins
c. At the same time as the chemotherapy drugs
d. Thirty minutes before chemotherapy begins

4 The nurse is reviewing various types of antinausea medications, for which of the following conditions are prokinetic drugs also used?
a. Vertigo
b. Motion sickness
c. Delayed gastric emptying
d. Gastrointestinal obstruction

5 A patient who has been receiving chemotherapy tells the nurse that he has been searching the Internet for antinausea remedies and that he found a reference to a product called aprepitant (Emend). He wants to know if this drug would help him. Which of the following would be the nurse's best answer?
a. "This drug is used only after other drugs have not worked."
b. "This may be a good remedy for you. Let's talk to your physician."
c. "This drug is used only to treat severe nausea and vomiting caused by chemotherapy."
d. "This drug may not help the more severe nausea symptoms associated with chemotherapy."

For answers see http://evolve.elsevier.com/Canada/Lilley/pharmacology/.

CRITICAL THINKING ACTIVITIES

1 Explain how ondansetron (Zofran) decreases the nausea and vomiting associated with chemotherapy. Compare its effectiveness to that of prochlorperazine for treatment of chemotherapy-induced nausea and vomiting.

2 Explain why it is important to assess the patient's hydration status when giving antinausea and antiemetic drugs.

3 What general adverse effects of antinausea and antiemetic drugs cause the most concern, especially with older adults?

For answers see http://evolve.elsevier.com/Canada/Lilley/pharmacology/.

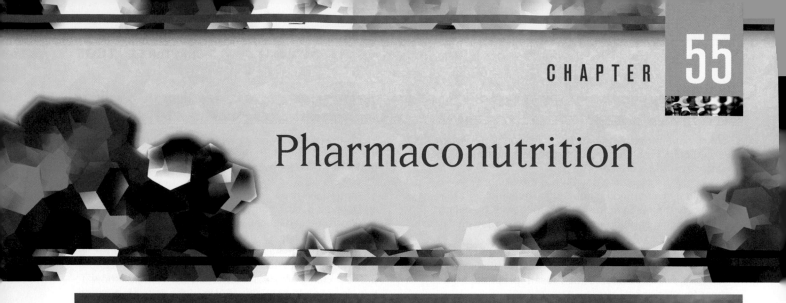

CHAPTER 55

Pharmaconutrition

Learning Objectives

After reading this chapter, the successful student will be able to do the following:

1 Describe the pathophysiological processes and disease states that may lead to nutritional deficiencies and require nutritional support.

2 Discuss enteral and parenteral nutrition used to treat the nutritional deficiencies, including specific ingredients.

3 Describe the nurse's role in the process of initiating and maintaining continuous or intermittent enteral feedings, total parenteral nutrition (TPN), and other forms of nutrition.

4 Compare enteral feeding solutions, including specific uses and the special needs of patients requiring this nutritional support.

5 Discuss the mechanisms of action, cautions, contraindications, routes of administration, drug interactions, adverse effects, and related complications associated with enteral and parenteral nutrition.

6 Develop a collaborative plan of care that includes all phases of the nursing process for patients receiving enteral and parenteral nutrition.

7 Discuss the laboratory values related to nutritional deficits or altered nutritional status and their impact on monitoring the therapeutic effects of the therapy.

e-Learning Activities

Web site
(http://evolve.elsevier.com/Canada/ Lilley/pharmacology/)

- Animations
- Answers to chapter questions, activities, and case studies
- Calculators and Category Catchers
- Glossary with audio pronunciations
- IV Therapy and Medication Error Checklists
- Multiple-Choice Review Question quizzes
- Nursing Care Plans
- Online Appendices and Supplements
- WebLinks

Drug Profiles

amino acids, p. 1010
carbohydrate formulation, p. 1010
carbohydrates, p. 1012
fats, p. 1012
fat formulation, p. 1010
lipid emulsions, p. 1012
protein formulation, p. 1010

Glossary

Anabolism Constructive metabolism characterized by the conversion of simple substances into the more complex compounds of living matter. (p. 1007)

Casein The principal protein of milk and the basis for curd and cheese. (p. 1010)

Catabolism A complex metabolic process in which energy is liberated for use in work, energy storage, or heat production by the destruction of complex substances by living cells to form simple compounds. (p. 1012)

Dumping syndrome A complex bodily reaction to the rapid entry of concentrated nutrients into the jejunum of the small intestine. (p. 1009)

Enteral nutrition The provision of food or nutrients via the gastrointestinal tract, either naturally by eating or through a feeding tube in patients unable to eat. (p. 1007)

Essential amino acids Amino acids that cannot be manufactured by the body. (p. 1012)

Essential fatty acid deficiency A condition that develops if fatty acids that the body cannot produce are not present in the diet or in nutritional supplements. (p. 1012)

Hyperalimentation Term formerly used to refer to parenteral nutrition; it is now discouraged as it may be misinterpreted as overfeeding. (p. 1011)

Malnutrition   Any disorder of undernutrition. (p. 1007)

Multivitamin infusion (MVI)   A concentrated solution containing several water- and fat-soluble vitamins and used as part of an intravenous (parenteral) nutritional source. (p. 1013)

Nonessential amino acids   Those amino acids that the body can produce without extracting from dietary intake. (p. 1012)

Nutrients   Substances that provide nourishment and affect the nutritive and metabolic processes of the body. (p. 1007)

Nutritional supplements   Oral, enteral, or intravenous preparations used to provide optimal nutrients to meet the body's nutritional needs. (p. 1007)

Nutritional support   Refers to the provision of nutrients orally, enterally, or parenterally for therapeutic reasons. (p. 1007)

Parenteral nutrition   The administration of nutrients by a route other than through the alimentary canal, such as intravenously. (p. 1007)

Pharmaconutrition   The science elucidating the role nutrition plays in general health, as well as the key nutrients required by the critically ill. (p. 1007)

Semiessential amino acids   Those amino acids that can be produced by the body but not in sufficient amounts in infants and children. (p. 1012)

Total parenteral nutrition (TPN)   Term that also refers to parenteral nutrition. (p. 1011)

OVERVIEW

The integrity and normal function of all cells within the body require a constant supply of nutrients. **Nutrients** are dietary products that undergo chemical changes when ingested (metabolized) and cause tissue to be enhanced and energy to be liberated. Nutrients are required for cell growth and division; enzyme activity; protein, carbohydrate, and fat synthesis; muscle contraction; neurohormonal secretion (e.g., vasopressin, gastrin); wound repair; immune competence; gut integrity; and numerous other essential cellular functions. Providing for these nutritional needs is known as **nutritional support**. Adequate nutritional support is needed to prevent the breakdown of tissue proteins for use as an energy supply to sustain essential organ systems. This process occurs during starvation and **malnutrition,** a condition in which the body's essential need for nutrients is not met by nutrient intake. Malnutrition can decrease organ size and impair the function of organ systems (e.g., cardiac, respiratory, gastrointestinal, hepatic, renal). The purpose of nutritional support is to prevent, recognize, and manage malnutrition. In order to provide adequate nutritional support to meet the body's needs, dietary products called **nutritional supplements** are used. Recently, a new science called **pharmaconutrition** has emerged that seeks to understand the ways in which nutrition affects health in general and specifically the key nutrients that are required by the critically ill.

Nutritional products can be administered to patients in different ways. They vary in their amounts and the chemical complexity of carbohydrate, protein, and fat. The electrolyte, vitamin, mineral, and osmolality of the specific product can vary as well. These nutrients may be given in a digested form, a partially digested form, or an undigested form. Nutritional supplements can also be tailored for specific disease states.

A wide variety of nutritional supplements is needed because of the wide variety of conditions for which patients require nutritional support. Patients' nutrient requirements vary according to age, gender, size or weight, physical activity, pre-existing medical conditions, nutrition status, and current medical or surgical treatment. Nutritional supplements are classified according to the method of administration: enteral or parenteral. **Enteral nutrition** is the provision of food or nutrients with the gastrointestinal tract as the route of administration. **Parenteral nutrition** is the intravenous administration of nutrients, with the purpose of promoting **anabolism** (tissue building), nitrogen balance, and body weight. It is used when the oral or enteral feeding routes cannot or should not be used (e.g., a postoperative patient or a patient who is cachectic from advanced cancer or acquired immune deficiency syndrome [AIDS]). Parenteral nutrients are delivered directly into the circulation by means of intravenous infusion. The selection of enteral or parenteral nutrition and the specific nutritional composition of the product depend on the patient profile and the clinical situation.

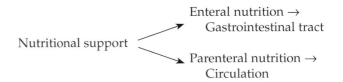

ENTERAL NUTRITION

Many biological processes occur from the beginning of the digestive system in the mouth to the end of the digestive system in the anus. These processes have evolved over time to most effectively digest dietary nutrients. Thus, providing food or nutrition via the enteral route, that is, through the gastrointestinal tract, is considered to be the superior route of administration of pharmaconutrition and should be used whenever possible.

The most common and least invasive route of administration is the oral route. A feeding tube is used in the other five routes (Figure 55-1). The six routes of enteral delivery are listed in Table 55-1.

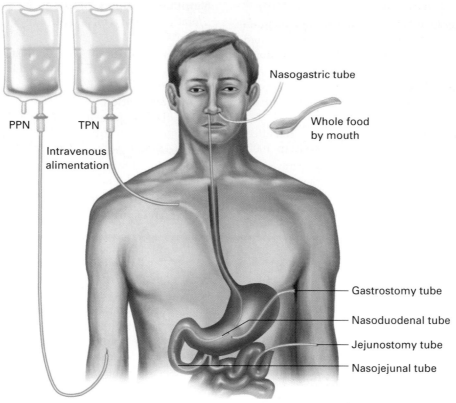

FIG. 55-1 Tube feeding routes. *PPN,* peripheral parenteral nutrition; *TPN,* total parenteral nutrition. (Reproduced with permission from *Routes of Nutrition Support,* available at *http://www.rxkinetics.com/tpntutorial/1_4.html.* Copyright 1984–2008 Rx Kinetics. All rights reserved.)

Patients who may benefit from feeding tube delivery of nutrients include those with abnormal esophageal or stomach peristalsis, altered anatomy secondary to surgery, depressed consciousness, or impaired digestive capacity. Use of the different enteral routes depends on the clinical situation.

Approximately 100 different enteral formulations are available. The enteral nutrients have been divided into five groups according to the basic characteristics of the individual formulations: elemental, polymeric, modular, altered amino acid, and impaired glucose tolerance. These formulations are described in Box 55-1.

Mechanism of Action and Drug Effects

The enteral formula groups provide the basic building blocks for anabolism. Different combinations and amounts of these drugs are used on the basis of an individual patient's anabolic needs. After the body receives and absorbs these nutrients, it must process them into living matter. Enteral nutrition supplies complete dietary needs through the gastrointestinal tract by the normal oral route or by feeding tube.

Indications

Enteral nutrition can be used to support an oral diet that is currently insufficient for a patient's nutrient needs, or it can be used solely to meet all of the patient's nutrient needs. Patients who are unable to consume or digest normal foods, have accelerated catabolic status, or are undernourished because of disease often use enteral nutrition. Box 55-2 lists the main types of enteral nutrients and their indications.

Contraindications

The usual contraindication to nutritional support of any kind is known drug allergy to a specific product or genetic disease that renders a patient unable to metabolize certain types of nutrients.

TABLE 55-1

Routes of Enteral Nutrition Delivery

Route	Description
Gastrostomy	Feeding tube surgically inserted directly into the stomach
Jejunostomy	Feeding tube surgically inserted into the jejunum
Nasoduodenal	Feeding tube placed from the nose to the duodenum
Nasogastric	Feeding tube placed from the nose to the stomach
Nasojejunal	Feeding tube placed from the nose to the jejunum
Oral	Nutritional support delivered by mouth

BOX 55-1

Enteral Formulations

Elemental Formulations

Peptamen Vital HN Vivonex Plus VivonexTEN	**Contents:** dipeptides, tripeptides, or crystalline amino acids, glucose oligosaccharides, and vegetable oil or MCTs **Comments:** minimum digestion; residue is minimal **Indications:** partial bowel obstruction, irritable bowel disease, radiation enteritis, bowel fistulas, and short bowel syndrome

Polymeric Formulations

Complete Ensure Ensure-Plus Isocal Osmolite Portagen Sustagen	**Contents:** complex nutrients (proteins, carbohydrates, and fat) **Indications:** preferred over elemental formulations, for patients with fully functional gastrointestinal tracts and few specialized nutrient requirements

Modular Formulations

Carbohydrate Caloren Moducal Polycose ***Fat*** MCT Oil Microlipid ***Protein*** Casec ProMod Resource Resource Plus	**Contents:** single-nutrient formulas (protein, carbohydrate, or fat) **Indications:** can be added to a monomeric or polymeric formulation to provide a more individual specialized nutrient formulation

Altered Amino Acid Formulations

Criticare High
  Nitrogen
Magnacal Renal
Traumacal
Ultracal High
  Nitrogen
Vital High
  Nitrogen
	Contents: varying amounts of specific amino acids
	Indications: patients with diseases associated with altered metabolic capacities

Formulation for Impaired Glucose Tolerance

Glucerna	**Contents:** protein, carbohydrate, fat, sodium, potassium **Indications:** patients with impaired glucose tolerance (e.g., diabetic patients)

HN, high nitrogen; *MCT,* medium-chain triglyceride; *TEN,* total enteral nutrition.

Note: Not all of the formulations listed here are intended specifically for oral use; some are specifically designed to be delivered by nasogastric tube or percutaneous endoscopic gastrostomy (PEG) and are not orally palatable.

BOX 55-2

Enteral Nutrition: Therapeutic Effects

Complete Nutritional Formulations (i.e., for General Nutritional Deficiencies)

- Unable to consume or digest normal foods
- Accelerated catabolic status
- Undernourished because of disease

Incomplete Nutritional Formulations (i.e., for Specific Nutritional Deficiencies)

- Genetic metabolic enzyme deficiency
- Liver or kidney impairment

Infant Nutritional Formulations

- Sole nutritional intake for premature and full-term infants
- Supplemental nutritional intake for older infants receiving solid foods
- Supplemental nutrition for breast-fed infants

Adverse Effects

The most common adverse effect of nutritional supplements is gastrointestinal intolerance, and the most common result of this intolerance is diarrhea. Infant nutritional formulations are often associated with allergies and digestive intolerance. The other nutritional supplements are most commonly associated with osmotic diarrhea. Rapid feeding or bolus doses can result in **dumping syndrome**, which produces intestinal disturbances. The patient may experience nausea, weakness, sweating, palpitations, syncope, sensations of warmth, and diarrhea. This syndrome can occur when the patient eats after partial gastrectomy or when enteral feedings are administered too rapidly into the stomach or jejunum via a feeding tube. In addition, tube feeding places the patient at significant risk for aspiration pneumonia. This is especially true in patients with compromised mental status, gag reflexes, and general mobility. Rapid changes in laboratory values, including serum magnesium, phosphate, and electrolytes, may be observed.

Interactions

Nutrients can interact with drugs to produce significant food–drug interactions. With some exceptions, food usually delays the absorption of drugs when administered simultaneously. Chemical inactivation with high gastric acid content or prolonged emptying time can result in decreased effects of cephalosporins, erythromycin, and penicillins when these are given with nutritional supplements. An increased absorption rate resulting in increased therapeutic effects can be seen when corticosteroids or vitamins A and D are given with nutritional supplements. Decreased antibiotic effects of tetracyclines and quinolones are seen when they are given with nutritional supplements because chemical inactivation occurs when these drugs complex with calcium.

Dosages

Because nutrient requirements vary greatly, dosages are individualized according to patient needs.

PARENTERAL NUTRITION

Parenteral nutrition (intravenous administration) is the preferred method for patients who are unable to tolerate and maintain adequate enteral or oral intake. Instead of administering partially digested nutrients into the gastrointestinal tract, vitamins, minerals, amino acids, dextrose,

 DRUG PROFILES

Enteral nutrition can be provided by a variety of supplements. The individual patient characteristics determine the appropriate enteral supplement. There are five basic types of enteral formulations: elemental, polymeric, modular, altered amino acid, and for impaired glucose tolerance.

ELEMENTAL FORMULATIONS

Elemental formulations are enteral supplements that contain dipeptides, tripeptides, or crystalline amino acids. Because of the composition of elemental formulation supplements, minimal digestion is required. These supplements are indicated in patients with pancreatitis, partial bowel obstruction, irritable bowel disease, radiation enteritis, bowel fistulas, and short bowel syndrome. These supplements are contraindicated in patients who have had hypersensitivity reactions to them. Elemental formulation supplements are available without a prescription and have no pregnancy category.

POLYMERIC FORMULATIONS

Polymeric formulations are enteral supplements that contain complex nutrients derived from proteins, carbohydrates, and fat. The polymeric formulations are some of the most commonly used enteral formulations because they most closely resemble normal dietary intake. They are preferred over elemental formulations in patients with fully functional gastrointestinal tracts who have no specialized nutrient needs. They are also less hyperosmolar than elemental formulations and therefore cause fewer gastrointestinal problems. They are contraindicated in patients who have had hypersensitivity reactions to them. They are available without a prescription and have no pregnancy category.

Ensure is a commonly used enteral supplement from the polymeric formulation category of enteral nutritional products. It is lactose free and is also available in a higher caloric formula called Ensure-Plus. Other polymeric formulations include Isocal, Magnacal, Meritene, Osmolite, Portagen, and Sustacal. These drugs contain complex nutrients such as **casein** (the principal protein of milk) and soy protein (for protein), corn syrup and maltodextrins (for carbohydrates), and vegetable oil or milk fat (for fat). They are available in liquid formulations only.

MODULAR FORMULATIONS

carbohydrate formulation

Moducal and Polycose are examples of commonly used enteral supplements from the carbohydrate modular-formulation category. Both are carbohydrate supplements that supply carbohydrates only. They are intended to be used as an addition to monomeric or polymeric

formulations to provide a more individual specialized nutrient formulation. They are available in liquid formulations only. These products are available without a prescription, have no pregnancy category, and are contraindicated only if a patient has had a hypersensitivity reaction to them.

fat formulation

Microlipid and MCT Oil are the formulations available in the fat category. Microlipid is a fat supplement supplying solely fats. It is a concentrated source of calories and contains 4.5 kcal/mL. These supplements are used to individualize nutrient formulations. They may be used in malabsorption and other gastrointestinal disorders and in patients with pancreatitis. They are available in liquid formulations only. These products are available without a prescription, have no pregnancy category, and are contraindicated only if a patient has had a hypersensitivity reaction to them.

protein formulation

Casec, ProMod, and Resource are examples of protein modular formulations. They are used to increase and provide additional proteins to enhance patients' protein intake. They are derived from a variety of sources such as *whey* (the thin serum of milk remaining after casein and fat have been removed; it contains proteins, lactose, water-soluble vitamins, and minerals), casein, egg whites, and amino acids. All of the available products are dried powders that have to be reconstituted with water. They may sometimes be reconstituted by placing them in enteral feedings that are already in liquid form. These products are indicated for patients with increased protein needs. They are contraindicated in patients who have had hypersensitivity reactions to them. Protein formulation supplements are available without a prescription and have no pregnancy category.

ALTERED AMINO ACID FORMULATIONS

There are many amino acid formulation nutritional supplements available. Many of the nutritional supplements in this category are also listed as modular formulations because they can be used as both single-nutrient formulas and as nutritional formulations for patients with genetic errors of metabolism. Specialized amino acid formulations are used most commonly in patients who have metabolic disorders such as phenylketonuria, homocystinuria, or maple syrup urine disease. They are also used to supply nutritional support to patients with such illnesses as kidney impairment, eclampsia, heart failure, or liver failure.

and lipids are administered intravenously directly into the circulatory system. This procedure effectively bypasses the entire gastrointestinal system, eliminating the need for absorption, metabolism, and excretion. Parenteral nutrition is also called **total parenteral nutrition (TPN)** or **hyperalimentation**. TPN can supply all of the calories, carbohydrates, amino acids, fats, trace elements, vitamins, and minerals needed for growth, weight gain, wound healing, convalescence, immunocompetence, and other health-sustaining functions.

TPN can be administered through either a peripheral vein or a central vein. Each route of delivery of TPN has specific requirements and limitations. It is generally accepted that TPN should be considered only when oral or enteral support is impossible or when the gastrointestinal absorptive or functional capacity is not sufficient to meet the nutrition needs of the patient. Some of the conditions that must be considered in the decision to place a patient on peripheral versus central TPN are listed in Table 55-2.

PERIPHERAL TOTAL PARENTERAL NUTRITION

In the peripheral route of administration of TPN (PPN) a peripheral vein is used to deliver nutrients to the patient's circulatory system. It is usually a temporary method of administration. The long-term administration of nutritional supplements via a peripheral vein may lead to phlebitis. PPN should be considered a temporary measure to provide adequate nutrient needs in patients with mild deficits or who are restricted from oral intake and have slightly elevated metabolic rates. PPN is most valuable in patients who do not have large nutrition needs, can tolerate moderately large fluid loads, and need nutritional supplements only temporarily. PPN may be used alone or in combination with oral nutritional supplements to provide the necessary fat, carbohydrate, and protein needed by the patient to maintain health.

Mechanism of Action and Drug Effects
PPN provides the basic nutrient building blocks for anabolism. Different combinations and amounts of these drugs are used on the basis of an individual patient's anabolic needs. After the body receives these nutrients, it must process them into living matter.

Indications
PPN is used to supplement nutrients to patients who need more nutrients than their current oral intake can provide or to provide entire daily nutrition. PPN is meant only as a temporary means (less than 2 weeks) of delivering TPN.

Conditions in which patients may benefit from the delivery of PPN are as follows:
• Procedures that restrict oral feedings
• Anorexia caused by radiation or cancer chemotherapy
• Gastrointestinal illnesses that prevent oral food ingestion
• After any type of surgery
• When nutritional deficits are minimal but oral nutrition will not be started for more than 5 days

TABLE 55-2
Peripheral and Central Parenteral Nutrition: Characteristics

Considerations	Peripheral	Central
Goal of nutritional therapy (total vs. supplemental)	Supplemental (total if moderate to low needs)	Total
Length of therapy	Short (less than 14 days)	Long (14 or more days)
Osmolarity	Hyperosmolar (600–900 mOsm/L)	
Fluid tolerance	Must be high	Can be fluid restricted
Amino acids	Less than 3%	More than 3%–7%
Fats	10%–20%	10%–20%
Dextrose	Less than 12.5%	10%–35%
Calories/day	Less than 2000 kcal/day	More than 2000 kcal/day

Contraindications
As mentioned previously for the enteral nutritional products, the only usual contraindication to nutritional supplements of any kind is known drug allergy to a specific product or genetic disease that renders a patient unable to digest certain types of nutrients.

Adverse Effects
The most devastating adverse effect of PPN is phlebitis, which is a vein irritation or inflammation of a vein. If it is severe enough and not treated appropriately, phlebitis can lead to the loss of a limb. However, this is rare. Another potential adverse effect is fluid overload. PPN is limited to lower dextrose-concentrated solutions, generally less than 10%, to avoid sclerosing of the vein. Larger amounts of nutritional supplements are needed with lower concentrated solutions to meet a patient's daily nutritional requirements. Some patients, such as those with kidney or heart failure, cannot tolerate large fluid volume. PPN may be unable to provide adequate calories to these fluid-restricted patients.

Dosages
Dosage requirements vary from patient to patient. Age, gender, weight, and numerous other factors must be considered for proper administration of TPN. Guidelines for amino acids appear in Table 55-3.

TABLE 55-3
Amino Acids: Recommended Daily Dosage Guidelines

Healthy		Malnourished or Trauma/Burn
Adult	Infant or Child	Adult
0.9 g/kg	1.5–3 g/kg	Up to 2 g/kg

DRUG PROFILES

The individual components of peripheral and central TPN are the same. The difference lies in the concentrations and amounts of the components delivered per volume of nutritional supplement. The basic components of peripheral or central TPN are amino acid, carbohydrate, lipid, trace elements, vitamin, fluids, and electrolytes. Many of the electrolyte components are discussed in Chapter 27.

AMINO ACIDS

Amino acids have many roles in the maintenance of normal nutritional status. The primary role is protein synthesis, or anabolism. Adequate amino acids in nutritional supplements reduce the breakdown of proteins (**catabolism**) and also help to promote normal growth and wound healing. Amino acids are commonly classified as essential or nonessential according to whether they can or cannot be produced by the body. **Nonessential amino acids** are those that the body produces and are therefore not needed in dietary intake. The body is able to manufacture, from nutritional nitrogen sources, all but eight of the available amino acids. **Essential amino acids** are those amino acids that cannot be produced by the body. Therefore, they must be included in daily dietary intake. Amino acids are used as building blocks for protein that is needed for normal growth and development. Two amino acids, histidine and arginine, are not manufactured by the body in large enough quantities during rapid growth periods such as infancy or childhood. Thus they are referred to as **semiessential amino acids**. Box 55-3 lists amino acids according to their categories.

amino acids

Amino acid crystalline solutions (Aminosyn, 5%, 7%, 8.5%, and 10%, and Primene 10%) can be used in either peripheral or central TPN. Amino acids are a source of both protein and calories. They provide 4 kcal/g. The two currently available amino acid solutions differ only in their respective concentrations. The dosage of these solutions varies depending on the patient's weight and requirements. These drugs have no restrictions regarding pregnancy and have no contraindications to use. Recommended dosages for healthy and trauma patients are listed in Table 55-3.

carbohydrates

In nutritional support, carbohydrates are usually supplied to patients through dextrose. Hydrous dextrose is normally the greatest source of calories and provides 3.4 kcal/g. However, protein (amino acids) and lipids are also used as calorie sources (see Figure 55-2). Concentrations of dextrose in TPN are important considerations. In peripheral TPN, dextrose concentrations are kept below 10% to decrease the possibility of phlebitis. In central TPN, dextrose concentrations can range from 10% to 50% but are commonly 25% to 35%. Because dextrose is a sugar, supplemental insulin may be given simultaneously in nutritional supplements. A balanced nutrition supplement that contains dextrose and lipids for caloric sources decreases the need for large amounts of insulin.

fats

The average North American diet contains 40% fat. This means that of the total calories supplied, 40% to 50% of the calories are obtained through fat grams. The ideal diet contains 30% fat. Intravenous fat emulsions serve two functions: they supply essential fatty acids, and they are a source of energy or calories. As with the amino acids, certain fatty acids are essential because the body cannot produce them. Linoleic acid cannot be synthesized by the body and is needed to produce linolenic and arachidonic acid. If these fatty acids are not present in dietary or nutritional supplements, an **essential fatty acid deficiency** may develop. Clinical signs of essential fatty acid deficiency are hair loss, scaly dermatitis, growth retardation, reduced wound healing, decreased platelets, and fatty liver (Figure 55-3).

lipid emulsions

The currently available lipid emulsions are Intralipid, available as either 10%, 20%, or 30% emulsions, and Liposyn, available as 10% or 20%. They differ in fat origin. Intralipid is made from soybean oil; Liposyn is made from both soybean and safflower oil. Normally, lipid emulsions should be adjusted to deliver 20% to 30% of the total daily calories, while not exceeding 60% of daily caloric intake. Fat emulsions are most beneficial when combined with dextrose solutions. The use of fat to meet caloric needs prevents potentially harmful conditions, such as hyperglycemia, hyperinsulinemia, and hyperosmolarity, that can occur when a patient's entire caloric needs are being met solely by dextrose.

CENTRAL TOTAL PARENTERAL NUTRITION

In central TPN, a large central vein is used to deliver nutrients directly into the patient's circulation. Usually, the subclavian or internal jugular vein is used. Central TPN is generally indicated for patients who require nutritional supplements for a prolonged period, usually more than 7 to 10 days. It can also be used in the home care setting. The disadvantages of central TPN are the risks associated with venous catheter insertion and use and maintenance of the central vein. There is a greater potential for infection, more serious catheter-induced trauma and related events, metabolic alterations, and other technical or mechanical problems than with peripheral TPN.

The same formulations used in peripheral TPN are used in central TPN. Often the concentrations of fluids administered through the central vein are much higher than those used in peripheral nutrition supplements. Besides these minor differences, the nutrition supplements used are identical (see Drug Profiles above).

BOX 55-3

Amino Acids: Classification

Essential	Nonessential	Semiessential
Isoleucine	Alanine	Arginine
Leucine	Asparagine	Histidine
Lysine	Aspartic acid	
Methionine	Cysteine	
Phenylalanine	Glutamine	
Threonine	Glutamic acid	
Tryptophan	Glycine	
Valine	Proline	
	Serine	
	Tyrosine	

Mechanism of Action and Drug Effects

Central TPN is used to supply nutrients to patients who cannot ingest nutrients by mouth and cannot meet required daily nutritional needs by the enteral or peripheral parenteral routes. Like peripheral TPN, central TPN provides the basic building blocks for anabolism. However, TPN solutions for central intravenous infusion may be more concentrated, especially in terms of carbohydrate content, and may contain as much as 35% dextrose. Different combinations and amounts of liquid nutrients are used, according to the individual patient's anabolic needs. After the body receives these nutrients, it must process them into living matter. Central TPN works by delivering these essential nutrients directly into the circulation via a central vein and provides the necessary fat, carbohydrate, and protein that the patient needs to maintain health.

Indications

Central TPN delivers total dietary nutrients to patients who require nutritional supplementation. Patients who may benefit from the delivery of TPN include the following:
- Patients who have large nutrition requirements (metabolic stress or hypermetabolism)

- Patients who need nutrition support for prolonged periods (more than 7 to 10 days)
- Patients who are unable to tolerate large fluid loads

Contraindications

Central TPN is contraindicated in patients with allergy to any of its components. Rarely, some patients who are allergic to eggs may have cross-sensitivity to lipid formulations. Central TPN should only be used when the gastrointestinal tract cannot or should not be used (e.g., postoperative patients or those otherwise unable to eat or digest and absorb nutrients).

Adverse Effects

The most common adverse effects of central TPN are those surrounding the use of the central vein for delivery of the TPN. The risks associated with the insertion of the infusion line, as well as the use and maintenance of the central vein for administration of TPN, can create some complications. There is a greater potential for infection, more serious catheter-induced trauma and related events, and other technical or mechanical problems than with peripheral TPN. Larger and more concentrated volumes of nutrition supplements are delivered with central TPN, thus there is a greater chance for metabolic complications, such as hyperglycemia.

Dosages

Administration is individualized according to patient needs.

TRACE ELEMENTS

Trace element solutions are available individually or in many different combinations. The following are considered trace elements:
- Chromium
- Copper
- Iodine
- Manganese
- Molybdenum
- Selenium
- Zinc

Specific dosages and frequencies depend on the individual patient's requirements. Vitamins and minerals may also be added accordingly. A common multivitamin combination is **multivitamin infusion (MVI)**.

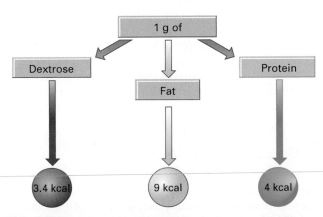

FIG. 55-2 One gram of dextrose, fat, or protein will provide varying amounts of energy as calories.

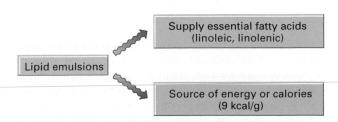

FIG. 55-3 Lipid emulsions supply essential fatty acids and energy.

NURSING PROCESS

Assessment

The nurse should conduct a thorough nutritional assessment with a dietary history, weekly and daily food intakes, weight, and height before beginning any enteral or parenteral nutritional supplementation. A nursing history should include a thorough survey of all systems, with questions about any unusual symptoms, possible nutritional concerns, nausea, vomiting, loss of appetite, and weight gain or loss. Other questions should focus on the patient's medical and health histories; current medical condition; history of any difficulties regarding nutrition, gastrointestinal absorption, or food intolerance; stressors; and a complete medication profile, including a listing of all prescription and over-the-counter drugs and natural health products. Consultation with a registered dietician is crucial to identification of the nutrients missing in a particular patient's diet. Total body metabolic rate, body mass index, muscle mass, and other variables linked to nutritional status should be assessed. Laboratory studies generally include total protein, albumin, blood urea nitrogen (BUN), red blood cells (RBCs), white blood cells (WBCs), vitamin B_{12}, cholesterol, and hemoglobin (Hgb). Other laboratory studies may include cholesterol, electrolytes, total lymphocyte count, serum transferrin, iron levels, urine creatinine clearance, lipid profile, and urinalysis. Anthropometric measurements and weights may also provide much-needed data. All of the objective and subjective data collected will then assist the physician, nutritionist or dietician, and other members of the health care team to select the appropriate nutrition supplements for the patient.

Before beginning an enteral nutritional supplement of elemental formulations, the nurse must also determine if the patient has a history of allergic reaction to any of the contents of the solution. Polymeric formulations such as Ensure are contraindicated in patients with hypersensitivity to any of their ingredients. Contraindications, cautions, and drug interactions must also be assessed for and documented. Of most concern is the patient's heart and kidney status and ensuring that the ingredients and the amount of solution are not too taxing on these systems. In addition, because these solutions are given orally, either by mouth or by tube feedings, it is most important to assess bowel sounds, nausea, vomiting, and ability to swallow. Protein-based formulations are to be avoided in patients with allergies to egg whites and whey.

Parenteral nutrition (PN) requires assessment of allergies to any of the ordered components of the intravenous (IV) solution as well as attention to age and metabolic needs. There are usually multiple combinations of products available, thus allergies to essential proteins, amino acids, carbohydrates, trace elements, minerals, vitamins, lipids, high concentrations of dextrose, and fluids need to

be noted. It is important that nurses assess their own knowledge base about PN and about infusions through a central line, peripherally inserted central lines (PICs), or peripherally inserted midline catheters. (See http://evolve.elsevier.com/Canada/Lilley/pharmacology/ for more information.) Some of the complications of PN include pneumothorax, infection, air emboli or emboli related to protein or lipid aggregation (associated with central catheter IV lines), septicemia related to the nutrient-rich solutions and invasive IV route of administration, and metabolic imbalances because of the solution or ingredients and nausea (seen with lipid administration in PN). A baseline and thorough assessment of the following must also be conducted: (1) central line site, noting its patency, intactness, and appearance; (2) WBC/RBC counts and other laboratory values and parameters listed earlier; (3) vitals signs with attention to temperature; (4) serum glucose levels; and (5) heart rhythm with electrocardiogram readings. Other core patient variables that may need to be assessed include daily weights (same time, same amount of clothing), a fractional urinary analysis, serum glucose levels every 6 to 8 hours, baseline intake and output, and neurological status.

Nursing Diagnoses

- Diarrhea related to a decreased tolerance of enteral feedings and their ingredients
- Ineffective airway clearance related to possible aspiration of enteral feedings
- Deficient fluid volume related to altered nutritional status
- Risk of infection or sepsis, related to parenteral infusions and use of central venous access
- Ineffective individual therapeutic management related to lack of information about therapeutic regimen with enteral or parenteral supplementation

Planning

Goals

- Patient will remain free of complications associated with enteral feedings and parenteral supplements.
- Patient will regain near-normal to normal bowel patterns.
- Patient will remain free of injury and infection during enteral or parenteral nutritional supplementation.
- Patient will remain free of infection during therapy.
- Patient will regain normal fluid volume status.
- Patient will remain adherent to therapy and makes return visits to the physician as needed.

Outcome Criteria

- Patient identifies measures to decrease diarrhea while receiving enteral feedings, such as use of prescribed drugs to decrease motility and use of over-the-counter drugs or natural health products as ordered.

- Patient (or caregiver) demonstrates adequate technique for enteral tube feedings to decrease risk for aspiration, with emphasis on elevating head of the bed and checking tube placement and residuals before feeding is initiated.
- Patient states measures to minimize risk of infection at the PN or TPN site, such as making sure the site is changed as ordered and is assessed frequently for redness, swelling, drainage, or fever, and reporting these signs to the physician or home health care nurse immediately.
- Patient begins to show adequate fluid volume status with improved turgor, improved urinary output to at least 30 mL/hr, and a return to normal laboratory values.
- Patient states symptoms to report to the physician, such as increased lethargy, fever, and shortness of breath.

Implementation

A physician's order must be complete and dated before beginning enteral, parenteral, or total parenteral supplementation. In general, monitoring the status of the patient during and after enteral feedings is crucial to safe and prudent nursing care. Gastric tube placement should always be verified before initiating an enteral feeding. Tinting tube feeding solutions with blue food colouring is used at times to detect aspiration but should not replace checking for tube placement and for residuals. Gastric residual volumes should be obtained and documented before each feeding as well as before each medication is administered. The tube feeding is usually stopped first, and stomach contents are aspirated using a syringe connected to the particular tube to detect any residual. If the volume is more than what has been consistent over the previous 2 hours of continuous feeding, the nurse should return the aspirate, withhold the feeding, and contact the physician; the head of the bed should be kept elevated. For intermittent bolus feedings, if the residual amount is greater than 50% of the volume previously infused, the nurse should return the aspirate, withhold the feeding, and contact the physician. A reduction in the tube feeding volume will probably be ordered by the physician. Always check hospital policy.

Newer tubes for nasogastric and enteral feeding have smaller diameters and are thinner (No. 5 through No. 10 French) and more pliable for better patient tolerance. However, the smaller-diameter tubes make checking for gastric aspiration more difficult. The process of medication administration through a nasogastric tube is reviewed in Chapter 10 with step-by-step guidelines.

To prevent clogging of the feeding tube with formula, it is often helpful to flush the tube with 30 mL of cranberry juice or other designated solution (per policy), followed by 10 mL of water. The juice may help break up the formula residue and unclog certain types of feeding tubes, and the water helps keep the tube clean and free of residue. Percutaneous enteral gastrostomy (PEG) tubes are now commonly used in certain situations but require

surgical insertion (often done under moderate sedation) by a gastroenterologist. Their care includes dressing changes in the initial period and then progresses to checking for residuals. Placement is not checked, but if it appears that the tube has come out of the opening and is longer in length than previously noted, stop the infusion and contact the physician.

Physician-ordered enteral feeding infusion rates and concentrations should be followed carefully. Usually, the initial rate is 50 mL/hr at one-half strength, but this can be increased per patient tolerance to a rate of 25 mL/hr at three-quarter strength concentration. Although more rapid feeding increases the risk of hyperglycemia, dumping syndrome, and diarrhea, the nurse should continue to increase the patient's intake because the total volume amount and amount of calories with recommended daily allowances (RDAs) is important. Tube-feeding formulas should always be at room temperature and never administered cold or warmed. If all the necessary steps to decrease or prevent diarrhea have failed, antidiarrheal medications may be needed. Lactose-free solutions are available and should be used with patients who are lactose intolerant. Patients who suffer from lactose intolerance experience cramping, diarrhea, abdominal bloating, and flatulence with the ingestion of the enteral milk-based feeding.

Infusions of PN and TPN should be assessed every hour or per the facility's policy and procedure. The entire infusion system and equipment as well as the condition of the patient should be documented; the standard of care is to examine the patient first and then check the PN or TPN insertion site, infusion pump, and solution. Tubings with PN and TPN are often ordered to be changed every 24 hours or more frequently in order to prevent infection. It is also recommended that tubing changes occur daily with the beginning of each new infusion. A 1.2 micron filter is used to trap bacteria, including *Pseudomonas* spp. The patient's temperature should be recorded every 4 hours during the infusion, and any increase in temperature over 37.8°C should be reported to the physician immediately. The patient should also be checked frequently for signs and symptoms of hyperglycemia, such as headache, dehydration, and weakness. IV feeding rates should never be accelerated to increase plasma volume because the rapid increase of dextrose solution may precipitate hyperglycemia and other related complications. Insulin replacement may be needed with the increase in dextrose; therefore, serum glucose levels per glucometer readings are important for immediate recognition and treatment of hyperglycemia.

If PN or TPN is discontinued abruptly, rebound hypoglycemia may occur. This can be prevented with providing infusions of 5% to 10% glucose in situations in which PN or TPN must be discontinued immediately. Hypoglycemia is manifested by cold, clammy skin, dizziness, tachycardia, and tingling of the extremities. Hypoglycemia associated with PN and TPN may be prevented by gradual reduction of the IV feeding rate in order to allow the pancreas time to adapt to the changing blood glucose levels. Fluid overload may also occur with PN and TPN, manifested by weak pulse, hypertension, tachycardia, confusion, decreased urine output, and pitting edema. This situation may be prevented by maintaining IV rates as ordered. If signs of fluid overload occur, the nurse should slow the infusion rate, remain with the patient, take a set of vital signs, auscultate breath and heart sounds, and contact the physician immediately. Measurement of intake and output is usually indicated with use of PN or TPN and with enteral supplementation. See Patient Education and http://evolve.elsevier.com/Canada/Lilley/pharmacology/ for more information about related nursing considerations associated with PN and TPN.

Evaluation

Therapeutic responses to nutrition supplementation include improved sense of well-being, energy, strength, and performance of activities of daily living; an increase in weight; and laboratory studies that reflect a more positive nutritional status. Specific laboratory values may include some of the following: albumin, total protein, hemoglobin, hematocrit, RBC and WBC levels, blood urea nitrogen, electrolytes, blood glucose and insulin levels, and iron values. Evaluation should be ongoing and re-evaluation done periodically so that the patient's nutritional needs are met. To this end, frequent physician appointments or monitoring by a home health care nurse may be required. Always refer to goals and outcome criteria to evaluate the effectiveness of therapy.

PATIENT EDUCATION

❖ Because patients are often discharged with various types of tube feedings, patients and their family should receive education, instructions, and demonstrations about the daily care of the tube, preparation of tube feedings, and related procedures, which should be presented in a way that reflects the learning needs of the patient and those involved in their care.

❖ Patients and caregivers should be instructed about the need for correct placement of the tube, which should be checked prior to each tube feeding if a nasogastric tube is used. Signs of incorrect placement of a nasogastric tube are coughing, choking, difficulty speaking, cyanosis, and subsequent respiratory distress. The head of the bed should remain elevated during infusions; this is more critical with nasogastric tube feedings than with gastrostomy tube feedings.

❖ Patients and caregivers should be given contact names and phone numbers of physicians, home health nurses, and other resources to be used in the event that any problems or concerns related to the feeding are experienced. Fever, difficulty breathing, congested lung sounds, high residual amounts, resistance against the flow of the feeding solution, or resistance against checking for residuals are all areas of concern and require appropriate interventions, including seeking emergency medical care if all else fails.

❖ Patients who are homebound and have PN or TPN should be given individualized education as well as support from home health care or related health care services. Practice is critical to the patient's and

family's or caregiver's skill in managing this type of feeding and should be an integral part of patient education. All procedures for storage; cleansing and care of the site; dressing changes; irrigation of the catheter; pump function and care; and changing of the bag, filters, and tubing should be explained, demonstrated, and shown in a return demonstration by the patient (and caregiver) before the patient is discharged. Educate the patient about the fact that PN or TPN will require home health care services by a registered nurse to help prevent complications of infection at the site, sepsis, fever, and pneumonia.

❖ Patients should be educated about checking serum glucose levels at home, as ordered by the physician, if TPN or other infused solutions high in dextrose are being used. The use of a glucometer should be explained and specific steps included in the demonstration to the patient and family or caregiver. Additionally, instructions in self-administration of insulin, based on sliding-scale coverage, may need to be included and reinforced.

❖ Patients and caregivers should be instructed to report signs and symptoms of potential complications of PN and TPN, including fever, cough, chest pains, dyspnea, and chills, all of which are indicative of adverse reactions to lipid infusions. Restlessness, nervousness, fainting, and tachycardia are associated with hypoglycemia and should also be reported, whereas nausea, vomiting, polyuria, and polydipsia may indicate hyperglycemia (which should also be reported).

POINTS TO REMEMBER

- ❖ A thorough nutritional assessment and possible consultation with a registered dietitian or nutritionist are essential for adequate intervention for the malnourished patient.
- ❖ There are various enteral feedings with different nutrition content, including some that are lactose free.
- ❖ Enteral feedings may result in complications such as hyperglycemia, dumping syndrome, and aspiration of feeding.
- ❖ TPN is administered through a central venous catheter because of the hyperosmolarity of substances used and the need for dilution that a larger-diameter

vein can provide; the larger vein and dilution also prevent damage to the vein. PN given through a peripherally inserted central catheter (PICC) line is another option but has a lower concentration of dextrose and other ingredients.
- ❖ Parenteral feedings may result in air embolism, fever, infection, fluid volume overload, hyperglycemia, or hypoglycemia. If discontinued abruptly, rebound hypoglycemia may result.
- ❖ Cautious and astute nursing care with enteral or parenteral nutrition supplementation may prevent or decrease the occurrence of associated complications.

EXAMINATION REVIEW QUESTIONS

1 Which of the following is the route of enteral nutritional delivery with a basic nasogastric feeding tube?
a. Surgical placement into the stomach
b. Placement from the nose into the jejunum
c. Surgical insertion directly into the jejunum
d. Placement from the nose into the stomach

2 With total parenteral nutrition (TPN), the provision of which of the following nutrients is a purpose of intravenous fat (lipid) emulsions?
a. Calories
b. Minerals
c. Amino acids
d. Immunoglobulins

3 When considering the routes of administering nutrition products, which of the following is an example of enteral nutrition?
a. Intralipid infusion
b. PN via a PICC line
c. TPN via a central line
d. Osmolite via a PEG tube

4 In which situation would peripheral parenteral nutrition be most appropriate?
a. Dextrose needs of 20% concentration
b. Nutrition need of 3000 calories per day
c. Therapy that is expected to last over 2 weeks
d. Therapy that is expected to last less than 14 days

5 During the night shift, a patient's infusion of TPN runs out, the pharmacy is closed, and a new bag of TPN will not be available for about 6 hours. Which of the following would be the nurse's most appropriate action at this time?
a. Set up a bag of normal saline.
b. Set up a bag of 10% dextrose.
c. Set up a bottle of intralipid solution.
d. Call the physician for stat TPN orders.

For answers see http://evolve.elsevier.com/Canada/Lilley/pharmacology/.

CRITICAL THINKING ACTIVITIES

1 Which nursing actions will help address the nursing diagnosis of diarrhea as related to enteral feedings?
2 What outcome criteria will address the nursing diagnosis of deficient fluid volume related to insufficient intake?

3 What is the concern about abrupt withdrawal of a 25% glucose TPN solution? Explain your answer.

For answers see http://evolve.elsevier.com/Canada/Lilley/pharmacology/.

PART TEN

Miscellaneous Therapeutics: Hematological, Dermatological, Ophthalmic, and Otic Drugs

STUDY SKILLS TIPS:
- TIME MANAGEMENT
- PURR
- REPEAT THE STEPS

TIME MANAGEMENT

As you plan study time for Part Ten, it should be clear that Chapter 58 will take significantly more time to complete than the other chapters. Do not let the length of the chapter overwhelm you. Apply the principles of time management to this chapter and you will succeed. The most important aspect of time management to apply to this chapter is the use of clear goal statements and action plan steps to achieve the goals.

Goal Statements

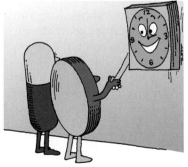

Remember SMART. Goal statements must be Specific, Measurable, Attainable, Realistic and Time limited. "I will study the chapter" is not a very specific goal; "I will master the 33 terms in the chapter glossary" is a more specific goal statement.

Goal statements must be measurable. In the example of studying the glossary, including the number of terms contained in Chapter 58 helps clarify the goal. There must be a time limit to how long you will spend on this goal.

Action Planning

The second segment of time management is the use of action planning. An action plan is a series of smaller, specific activities that you will accomplish to meet your goal statements. Your goal is to master the 33 terms. What will you do to meet that goal?

Action Steps Example

1 I will spend 1 hour making vocabulary drill cards for the terms found in the glossary in Chapter 58 from 3:00 to 4:00 P.M. on Monday.
2 I will spend 15 minutes on rehearsal and review of these cards every day until the exam on this chapter is over.
3 Each time I cannot define and explain a term I will put an "x" on the card to identify it as a term needing more review.
4 I will spend 1 hour the night before the exam doing a comprehensive review of the terms in Chapter 58, with special emphasis on those cards that have one or more "x" marks.

Action steps help ensure that you are spending your study time actively focusing on what you need to learn.

PURR

Prepare Example

Chapter 58, Objective 3: "Discuss the mechanisms of action, indications, dosage forms with application techniques, adverse effects, cautions, contraindications, and drug interactions of ophthalmic preparations."
- Question 1. What does *ophthalmic* mean? (Literal question [LQ])
- Question 2. What are ophthalmic preparations? (LQ)
- Question 3. What is the mechanism of action of ophthalmic preparations? (LQ)

- Question 4. Is there more than one mechanism of action? (LQ)
- Question 5. If there is more than one mechanism of action, how are the mechanisms similar, and how are they different? (Interpretive question)

These questions are only suggestions of generated questions based on the chapter objectives. Many more questions can be asked about Objective 3. These questions are an essential part of the study process. Questions help make you an active reader and an active learner. The more questions you generate, the easier it will be to understand the chapter.

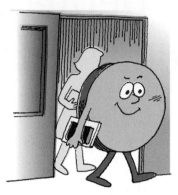

Outline Example

1 *Looking through the chapter, decide how much material is appropriate for a single reading session.* The section headed "Antiglaucoma Drugs" is probably too much material. Looking at the chapter headings, this section could be broken down into six blocks of material. Block one would cover the introductory material under the main heading, as well as the material under the heading "Cholinergic Drugs." Block two would be the material under the heading "Sympathomimetics." The next four blocks would be "β-Adrenergic Blockers," "Carbonic Anhydrase Inhibitors," "Osmotic Diuretics," and "Prostaglandin-$F_{2\alpha}$ Analogues."

2 *Apply the Prepare step to each block.* Beginning with the first block, generate some questions to guide your reading. Remember that it is important to ask questions that will focus on literal information as well as questions that will help you interpret, evaluate, and analyze as you read.

3 *Read the material.* As soon as you have completed generating questions for the first block of material, read the block immediately. Read for understanding. As you read, remember the questions you generated. This approach will help your concentration and comprehension.

4 *Take a short break.* Once you have completed the reading of this section of the chapter, give your mind a chance to reflect and consolidate the learning. Limit the time you allow for a break and use the time for something pleasurable. Give yourself 5 or 10 minutes to read the newspaper, get a snack, or just take a short walk.

5 *Rehearse.* Before going on to the next section of the chapter, it is important to spend a few minutes in rehearsal. Using the questions from Step 2, go back over the material you read and try to respond to those questions. When you find yourself unable to answer a question, put a mark in the text beside the heading that caused the difficulty and move on. The mark will serve as a reminder for future review. At this point, the objective is not complete mastery of the material. The objective is to see what you have learned so that you can move smoothly into the next section. Breaking a chapter into blocks is useful, but it is also imperative to make links between sections as you study.

6 *Review.* After completing two or three major sections of the chapter, it is time to review. Start at the beginning of the chapter. Ask your questions. Try to answer them. If you cannot formulate a clear answer, then some rereading is necessary. Also, pay attention to the marks you made during the rehearsal step. Those marks indicate areas that you have already identified as needing review. When rereading, remember that the object is to read only as much of the material as needed to be able to respond to self-generated questions. There simply is not enough time to read the entire chapter a second or third time.

REPEAT THE STEPS

Prepare, read for understanding, take a short break, and then rehearse the material just read. It may seem that this process takes an excessive amount of time and involves a lot of repetition, but in the long run it will produce better learning. The time spent in Prepare, Understand, and Rehearse will reduce the time needed to review. Frequent review as you move through the chapter will make the final review at exam time go more quickly and enable you to achieve mastery of the material.

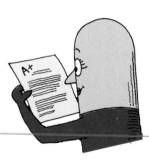

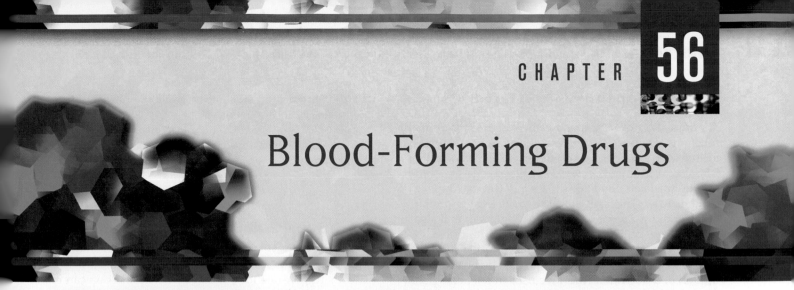

CHAPTER 56

Blood-Forming Drugs

Learning Objectives

After reading this chapter, the successful student will be able to do the following:

1 Discuss the importance of iron, vitamin B_{12}, and folic acid to the formation of blood cells.

2 Discuss the conditions requiring treatment with blood-forming drugs.

3 Discuss the mechanisms of action, cautions, contraindications, drug interactions, uses, dosages, special administration techniques, and measures to enhance the effectiveness of and decrease adverse effects related to the blood-forming drugs.

4 Develop a collaborative plan of care that includes all phases of the nursing process related to the administration of blood-forming drugs.

e-Learning Activities

Web site
(http://evolve.elsevier.com/Canada/Lilley/pharmacology/)

- Animations
- Answers to chapter questions, activities, and case studies
- Calculators and Category Catchers
- Glossary with audio pronunciations
- IV Therapy and Medication Error Checklists
- Multiple-Choice Review Question quizzes
- Nursing Care Plans
- Online Appendices and Supplements
- WebLinks

Drug Profiles

▸▸ **ferrous fumarate**, p. 1025
▸▸ **folic acid**, p. 1026
  iron dextran, p. 1025

▸▸ Key drug.

Glossary

Erythrocyte Another name for red blood cell (RBC). (p. 1022)

Erythropoiesis The process of erythrocyte production. (p. 1022)

Globin Part of the hemoglobin molecule (see below); a protein chain consisting of four different structural chains: α_1 and α_2, and β_1 and β_2. (p. 1022)

Hematopoiesis The normal formation and development of all blood cell types in the bone marrow. (p. 1022)

Heme Part of the hemoglobin molecule; a nonprotein, iron-containing portion of the Hgb molecule. (p. 1022)

Hemoglobin (Hgb) A complex protein–iron compound in the blood that carries oxygen to the cells from the lungs and carbon dioxide away from the cells to the lungs. (p. 1022)

Hemolytic anemia Any anemia resulting from excessive destruction of erythrocytes. (p. 1023)

Hypochromic Pertaining to less-than-normal colour. (p. 1022)

Microcytic Pertaining to smaller-than-normal cells. (p. 1022)

Pernicious anemia A type of megaloblastic anemia, usually seen in older adults, caused by impaired intestinal absorption of vitamin B_{12} due to lack of availability of intrinsic factor. (p. 1022)

Reticulocytes An immature erythrocyte characterized by a meshlike pattern of threads and particles at the former site of the nucleus. (p. 1022)

Spherocytes Small, globular, completely hemoglobinated erythrocytes without the usual central concavity or pallor. (p. 1023)

ERYTHROPOIESIS

The formation of new blood cells is one of the primary functions of bones. This process, known as **hematopoiesis**, includes the production of **erythrocytes** (red blood cells, or RBCs), as well as leukocytes (white blood cells) and thrombocytes (platelets), and takes place in the myeloid tissue or bone marrow. This specialized tissue is located primarily in the ends, or *epiphyses*, of certain long bones and also in the flat bones of the skull, pelvis, sternum, and ribs.

Erythropoiesis, the process of erythrocyte formation, is the focus of this chapter. This process involves the maturation of a nucleated RBC precursor into a hemoglobin-filled, nucleus-free erythrocyte. Erythropoiesis is driven by the hormone erythropoietin, produced by the kidneys.

When RBCs are manufactured in the bone marrow by myeloid tissue, they are released into the circulation as immature RBCs called **reticulocytes**. Once in the circulation, reticulocytes undergo a 24- to 36-hour maturation process to become mature, fully functional RBCs. Mature RBCs have a lifespan of approximately 120 days.

It is important to know the structural components of the RBC in order to understand how anemia develops and why certain drugs are used to correct it. More than one third of the RBC is made of hemoglobin. **Hemoglobin (Hgb)** is composed of two parts: heme and globin. **Heme** is the red pigment. Each molecule of heme contains one atom of iron. **Globin** is a protein chain that consists of four structurally different parts, or globulins: α_1 and α_2, and β_1 and β_2. Together one molecule of heme and one protein chain of globin make one Hgb molecule (Figure 56-1).

TYPES OF ANEMIA

Anemias are classified into four main types based on underlying causes (Figure 56-2). Knowledge of the etiologies of anemias will help understand the therapies used to treat them. Anemias can be caused by maturation defects, or they can be secondary to excessive RBC destruction. Two types of maturation defects cause anemias, depending on the location of the defect within the cell: *cytoplasmic* maturation defects occur in the cell cytoplasm, and *nuclear* maturation defects occur in the cell nucleus.

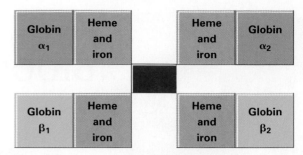

FIG. 56-1 Schematic structure of a hemoglobin molecule.

Factors responsible for excessive RBC destruction can be either intrinsic (internal) or extrinsic (external).

The types of anemias arising from cytoplasmic maturation defects are summarized in Figure 56-3. Major examples include iron-deficiency anemia and genetic disorders such as thalassemia, which result in defective globin synthesis. The RBCs appear **hypochromic** (lighter red than normal) and **microcytic** (smaller than normal) on a blood smear. Cytoplasmic maturation anemias occur as a result of reduced or abnormal Hgb synthesis. Because Hgb is synthesized from both iron and globin, a deficiency in either one can lead to a Hgb deficiency. Some common causes of iron-deficiency anemia are blood loss, surgery, childbirth, gastrointestinal bleeding, and hemorrhoids.

The types of anemias arising from nuclear maturation defects are summarized in Figure 56-4. These anemias occur because of defects in DNA or protein synthesis. Both DNA and protein require vitamin B_{12} and folic acid to be present in normal amounts for their proper production. If either of these two vitamins is absent or deficient, anemias secondary to nuclear maturation defects may develop. RBCs in such anemias actually appear to be *normochromic* (normal in colour) but are *macrocytic* (larger than normal) on a blood smear. One example is **pernicious anemia**. This anemia results from a dietary deficiency of vitamin B_{12}, which is used in the formation of new RBCs. The usual underlying cause is the failure of the stomach lining to produce *intrinsic factor*, a gastric glycoprotein that allows vitamin B_{12} to be absorbed in the intestine (Chapter 8). Another example is the anemia caused by folic acid deficiency. Both pernicious anemia

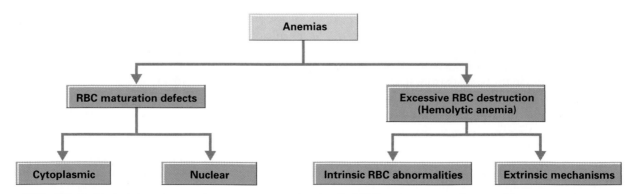

FIG. 56-2 Underlying causes of anemia are red blood cells (RBC) maturation defects and factors secondary to excessive RBC destruction.

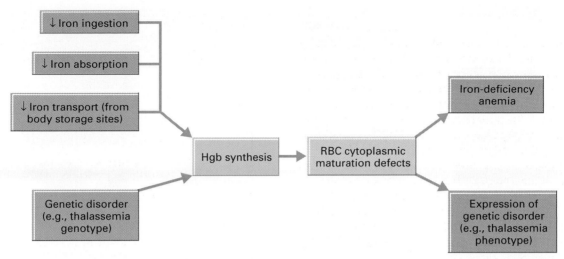

FIG. 56-3 Schematic showing common causes and results of red blood cell (RBC) cytoplasmic maturation anemia.

and folic acid deficiency anemia are known as types of megaloblastic anemia, as they are both characterized by large, immature RBCs. Megaloblastic anemias are usually due to poor dietary intake and are most commonly seen in infancy, childhood, and pregnancy.

The types of anemias arising from excessive RBC destruction, or **hemolytic anemias,** are summarized in Figure 56-5. These anemias can occur from abnormalities within the RBCs (*intrinsic factors*) or as a result of factors outside (*extrinsic* to) the RBCs. The erythrocytes in both cases appear on a blood smear as **spherocytes,** which are small, globular erythrocytes with excessive amounts of hemoglobin and thus lacking the central pallor (paleness) and concavity of normal RBCs. These RBCs also appear to be fragmented when observed on a blood smear. Examples of hemolytic anemia due to intrinsic factors include *sickle-cell anemia, hereditary spherocytosis,* and *glucose-6-phosphate dehydrogenase (G6PD) deficiency.* Examples of extrinsic mechanisms for excessive RBC destruction include drug-induced *antibodies* that target and destroy RBCs, septic shock that produces *disseminated intravascular coagulation (DIC),* and mechanical forces

such as *intra-aortic balloon pumps* and *ventricular assist devices,* commonly used in cardiac critical care units.

IRON

Iron is an essential mineral for the proper function of all biological systems in the body. It is stored in many sites throughout the body (liver, spleen, and bone marrow). It is also the principal nutritional deficiency in Canada, resulting in anemia. Individuals who require the greatest amount of iron are women (particularly pregnant women) and children. Women are most likely to develop iron-deficiency anemia, in part because of ongoing menstrual blood losses. Men, therefore, are less likely to develop this disorder. In fact, most vitamin supplements for men contain little or no iron. Nonetheless, dietary iron is usually sufficient for both men and women in developed countries.

Dietary sources for iron include meats and certain vegetables and grains (see http://evolve.elsevier.com/Canada/Lilley/pharmacology/ for specific examples). These forms of iron must be converted by gastric juices

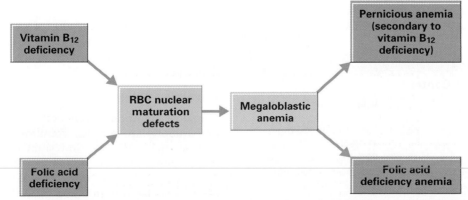

FIG. 56-4 Red blood cell (RBC) nuclear maturation defects occur because of vitamin B$_{12}$ or folate deficiencies.

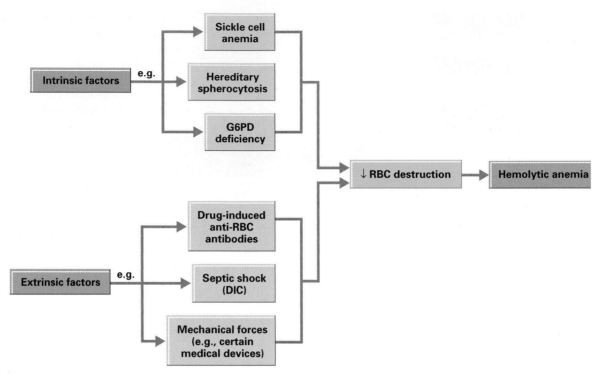

FIG. 56-5 Increased red blood cell destruction occurs as a result of intrinsic and extrinsic factors. *DIC,* disseminated intravascular coagulation; *G6PD,* glucose-6-phosphate dehydrogenase; *RBC,* red blood cell.

before they can be absorbed. Other foods such as orange juice, veal, fish, and ascorbic acid may assist with iron absorption. Conversely, eggs, corn, beans, and many cereal products containing chemicals known as *phytates* may impair iron absorption from either other iron-containing foods or iron supplements. However, it should also be noted that both beans and eggs are themselves common dietary sources of iron. Iron preparations are available as ferrous salts. See Table 56-1 for a list of the currently available iron salts and their respective iron content.

Mechanism of Action and Drug Effects

Iron is an oxygen carrier in both Hgb and *myoglobin* (oxygen-carrying molecule in muscle tissue) and thus is critical for tissue respiration. Iron is also a required component of a number of enzyme systems in the body and is necessary for energy transfer in the cytochrome oxidase and xanthine oxidase enzyme systems. Administration

TABLE 56-1

Ferrous Salts: Iron Content

Ferrous Salts	Iron Content
Ferrous fumarate	33% iron or 330 mg/g
Ferrous gluconate	11.6% iron or 116 mg/g
Ferrous sulfate	20% iron or 200 mg/g
Ferrous sulfate (desiccated, dried, or exsiccated)	30% iron or 300 mg/g

of iron corrects iron-deficiency states such as anemia, dysphagia, dystrophy of the nails and skin, and fissuring of the angles of the lips, as well as maintaining bodily functions, as described earlier.

Indications

Supplemental iron contained in multivitamins plus iron or iron supplements alone are indicated for the prevention and treatment of iron-deficiency syndromes. In all cases, an underlying cause should be identified. After identification of the cause, treatment should be aimed at attempting to correct the cause rather than simply alleviating the symptoms. Iron supplementation is also used in epoetin therapy (Chapter 50) because it is essential for the production of RBCs.

Contraindications

Contraindications to the use of iron products include known drug allergy, *hemolytic anemia, hemochromatosis* (iron overload), and any anemia not associated with iron deficiency.

Adverse Effects

The most common adverse effects associated with iron preparations are nausea, vomiting, diarrhea, constipation, stomach cramps, and stomach pain. Excess iron intake can lead to accumulation and iron toxicity. See Table 56-2 for a more complete listing of the undesirable effects associated with iron preparations.

TABLE 56-2

Iron Preparations: Adverse Effects

Body System	Adverse Effects
Gastrointestinal	Nausea, constipation, epigastric pain, black and tarry stools, vomiting, diarrhea
Integumentary	Temporary discoloration of tooth enamel and eyes, pain upon injection

Toxicity and Management of Overdose

Iron overdose is a leading cause of child poisoning deaths reported to Canadian poison control centres. Many iron supplements are enteric coated and resemble candy. Toxicity from iron ingestion results from a combination of the corrosive effects on the gastrointestinal mucosa and the metabolic and hemodynamic effects caused by the presence of excessive elemental iron.

Treatment is founded on good symptomatic and supportive measures, including suction and maintenance of airway, correction of acidosis, and control of shock and dehydration with intravenous fluids or blood, oxygen, and vasopressors. Abdominal radiographs may be helpful because iron preparations are radiopaque and may be visualized on X-ray film. A serum iron concentration may be helpful in establishing the severity of ingestion; a serum iron concentration of 54 micromol/L places the patient at serious risk for toxicity. In any case of iron overdose, consultation with a Poison Control Centre is recommended. Gastric lavage is not routinely performed but may be considered on advice from the Poison Control Centre. Because many of the iron products are extended-release formulations that release contents in the intestines rather than the stomach, whole-gut irrigation using polyethylene glycol solution is generally believed to be a superior and more effective approach to decontaminating the bowel. In patients with severe symptoms of iron intoxication, such as coma, shock, or seizures, chelation therapy with intravenous deferoxamine should be initiated.

Interactions

The absorption of iron can be enhanced when it is given with ascorbic acid or decreased when it is given with antacids. Iron preparations can decrease the absorption of thyroid drugs, tetracyclines, and quinolone antibiotics.

Dosages

For the recommended dosages of iron preparations, see the Dosages table on p. 1026.

FOLIC ACID

Folic acid is a water-soluble B-complex vitamin. It is also synonymously referred to as *folate,* the name of its anionic form. The human body requires oral intake of folic acid.

 ## DRUG PROFILES

Iron preparations are available by prescription and as over-the-counter medications. They are contraindicated in patients with ulcerative colitis and regional enteritis, conditions of excessive body iron stores (e.g., *hemosiderosis, hemochromatosis*), peptic ulcer disease (PUD), hemolytic anemia, cirrhosis, gastritis, and esophagitis. Goals of therapy include maintenance of normal Hgb and hematocrit (Hct) and energy level.

▸▸ *ferrous fumarate*

The ferrous fumarate iron salts (Palafer CF, others) contain the largest amount of iron per gram of salt consumed. Ferrous sulfate and ferrous gluconate are two other forms of iron that are commonly used. Ferrous fumarate is 33% elemental iron; therefore, a 300 mg tablet of ferrous fumarate provides 100 mg of elemental iron. Ferrous fumarate is available only for oral use.

PHARMACOKINETICS

Half-Life	Onset	Peak	Duration
PO: 6 hr	PO: 3–10 days*	PO: Unknown	PO: Variable

*Increased reticulocyte values.

iron dextran

Iron dextran (Dexiron, Infurer) is a colloidal solution of iron (as ferric hydroxide) and dextran. Sodium ferric gluconate (Ferrlecit) and iron sucrose (Venofer) are other available forms of injectable iron. They are intended for intravenous or intramuscular use for iron deficiency. Anaphylactic reactions to iron dextran, including fatal anaphylaxis, have been reported in 0.2% to 0.3% of patients. Because of this possibile reaction, a test dose of 25 mg of iron dextran should be administered by the chosen route before injecting the full dose. Although anaphylactic reactions usually occur within a few moments after the test dose, it is recommended that a period of at least 1 hour elapse before the remaining portion of the initial dose is given. Individual doses of 2 mL or less may be given on a daily basis until the calculated total amount required has been reached. The product Dexiron is given undiluted at a gradual rate, not exceeding 50 mg (1 mL)/min. Iron dextran is available only for injection.

PHARMACOKINETICS

Half-Life	Onset	Peak	Duration
IM: 5–20 hr	IM: Unknown	IM: 24–48 hr	IM: ≤ 3 wk

Dietary sources of folic acid include dried beans, peas, oranges, and green vegetables. Several conditions can lead to folic acid deficiency. However, because folic acid is absorbed in the upper duodenum, malabsorption syndromes are the most common cause of deficiency.

Mechanism of Action and Drug Effects

Dietary ingestion of folate is required for the production of the nucleic acids DNA and RNA. It is also essential for normal erythropoiesis. Folic acid is not active in the ingested form. It must first be converted in the body to *tetrahydrofolic acid*, which is a cofactor for reactions in the biosynthesis of purines and thymidylates of nucleic acids.

Indications

Folic acid is used primarily to prevent and treat folic acid deficiency. Anemias caused by folic acid deficiency can be treated by exogenous supplementation of folic acid. There is also much evidence to support the use of folic acid in the prevention of neural tube defects such as spina bifida, anencephaly, and encephalocele. It is recommended that administration begin at least 1 month before pregnancy and continue through early pregnancy to reduce the risk for fetal neural tube defects. Indications for folic acid include the following:
- Folic acid deficiency anemia
- Prophylaxis of neural tube defects in pregnant women
- Tropical sprue

Contraindications

Contraindications to the use of folic acid include known allergy to a specific drug product and any anemia not related to folic acid deficiency (e.g., pernicious anemia). Folic acid should not be used to treat anemias until the underlying cause and type of anemia have been determined. For example, administering folic acid to a patient with pernicious anemia may correct the hematological changes of anemia while masking other symptoms of pernicious anemia.

Adverse Effects

Adverse effects associated with folic acid use are rare. Allergic reaction or yellow discoloration of urine may occur.

Interactions

Oral contraceptives (Chapter 34), corticosteroids (Chapter 33), sulfonamides (Chapter 38), and dihydrofolate reductase inhibitors (including the antineoplastic drug methotrexate [Chapter 48] and the antibiotic trimethoprim [Chapter 38]) can all cause signs of folic acid deficiency. Folic acid can also lower the serum levels of phenytoin with possible breakthrough seizures.

Dosages

For recommended dosages of folic acid, see the Dosages table below.

 DRUG PROFILES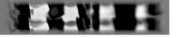

▶▶ folic acid

Folic acid is a water-soluble B-complex vitamin that is used primarily in the treatment and prevention of folic acid deficiency and anemias caused by folic acid deficiency. Folic acid is available as an over-the-counter medication in multivitamin preparations and by prescription as a single drug. It is contraindicated in patients with anemias other than megaloblastic or macrocytic anemia.

These contraindicated conditions include vitamin B$_{12}$ deficiency anemia and uncorrected pernicious anemia. Folic acid is available for both oral and injectable use.

PHARMACOKINETICS

Half-Life	Onset	Peak	Duration
PO: Unknown	PO: Unknown	PO: 60–90 min	PO: Unknown

DOSAGES · Selected Iron Preparations and Folic Acid

Drug (Pregnancy Category)	Pharmacological Class	Usual Dosage Range	Indications
▶▶ferrous fumarate (Palafer CF) (A)	Oral iron salt	*Children** *Infant–4 mo* 0.3 mg/day *Older than 4 mo** 6–8 mg/day *Adolescents/Adult** PO: 8–13 mg/day	Iron deficiency
▶▶folic acid (A)	Vitamin B–complex group; water-soluble B-vitamin	*Children†* PO/IV/IM/SC: 0.1–0.4 mg/day *Adult†* PO/IV/IM/SC: Up to 1 mg/day PO/IV/IM/SC: 3–15 mg/day	Folate deficiency; nutritional supplement; pregnancy supplement; tropical sprue

Continued

DOSAGES   Selected Iron Preparations and Folic Acid   (cont'd)

Drug (Pregnancy Category)	Pharmacological Class	Usual Dosage Range	Indications
iron dextran (Dexiron, Infurer) (C)	Parenteral iron salt	*Infants less than 5 kg†* IM/IV: 25 mg/day elemental iron (0.5 mL/day) *Children less than 10 kg†* IM/IV: 50 mg/day elemental iron (1 mL/day) *Adult†* IM/IV: 100 mg/day elemental iron (2 mL/day)	Iron deficiency when oral iron is unsatisfactory

IM, intramuscular; *IV,* intravenous; *PO,* oral; *SC,* subcutaneous.

*Doses are in terms of elemental iron, not the salt itself.

†Expressed in milligrams of elemental iron. Dosages are calculated for each patient's weight according to manufacturer's label. Doses are approximate.

OTHER BLOOD-FORMING DRUGS

Other drugs that may be used in the prevention and treatment of anemia are cyanocobalamin (vitamin B_{12}) and epoetin alfa ([erythropoietin] Eprex). Cyanocobalamin is discussed in detail in Chapter 8, and epoetin alfa is discussed in Chapter 50.

NURSING PROCESS

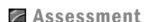 **Assessment**

Before administering any blood-forming drug, it is important for the nurse to assess medical history; current condition; and medication profile, including prescription and over-the-counter drugs and natural health products. Contraindications, cautions, and drug interactions should be assessed thoroughly prior to initiation of drug therapy. Laboratory studies such as Hgb, Hct, reticulocytes, bilirubin levels, and baseline levels of folate and B-complex vitamins should be obtained and documented. A nutritional assessment should also be performed, focusing on the amount of iron intake in the patient's diet and a 24-hour recall of all food intake with serving sizes. Dietary consultation may prove beneficial, if ordered.

Nursing Diagnoses

- Activity intolerance related to fatigue and lethargy associated with anemias
- Risk for injury related to adverse effects of iron products
- Deficient knowledge related to limited exposure to use of drug
- Imbalanced nutrition, less than body requirements, related to disease process

Planning

Goals

- Patient will regain normal level of activity, as ordered.
- Patient will remain free of symptoms related to adverse effects of blood-forming drugs (e.g., iron products).
- Patient will discuss rationale for use, adverse effects, and patient education guidelines related to use of blood-forming drugs.
- Patient will attain normal nutritional status through use of pharmacological and nonpharmacological measures.

🌐 IN MY FAMILY

Home Remedy for Blood Renewal

(as told by S.N., second-generation Canadian of Armenian descent)

"My parents and great grandparents believed that routine renewal of blood was needed to improve the body's circulation and to remove unwanted toxins. In order to remove the "bad blood," tiny cuts would be made on a person's back with a sharp razor and the blood would be left to pour out. Or oxygen would be removed out of a glass jar with a torched stick, and the jar would be placed with the lid pressing against the person's back. Due to the negative pressure, blood would accumulate where the jar was placed. . . . Once enough blood had accumulated, the jar would be removed and a small cut made at the place [of the blood accumulation]. Once enough of the "bad blood" had been removed, the area would be cleansed and dressed. Every single time this procedure was completed, the patient would feel significantly better."

■ Outcome Criteria

- Patient is able to tolerate a gradual increase in activity as ordered (e.g., performing activities of daily living, walking 10 minutes per day with increases as tolerated) while taking the blood-forming drug.
- Patient uses measures to minimize the adverse effects of the blood-forming drug, such as taking it with food.
- Patient takes medication exactly as prescribed to enhance its efficacy.
- Patient reports symptoms related to disease process or to adverse reactions to drugs, such as abdominal distention, cramping, nausea, and vomiting.
- Patient keeps a daily journal of dietary intake to share with the health care provider each week.
- Patient uses examples of a balanced diet for daily menu planning.

◰ Implementation

Liquid oral forms of iron products should be diluted per manufacturer instructions and taken through a plastic straw to avoid discoloration of tooth enamel. Oral forms should be given with juice or with meals, but not with antacids or milk, for maximal absorption. Taking the oral dosages with meals is recommended mainly to avoid the high risk for gastrointestinal distress, even though the food will alter absorption. Iron dextran should be administered only after all oral iron preparations have been discontinued. A test dose of iron may be ordered, with the remaining dose given 1 hour later. Intramuscularly administered iron should be injected deep in a large muscle mass using the Z-track method (see Figures 10-41 and 10-42 in Chapter 10). Intravenous iron dextran should be given after the intravenous line is flushed with 10 mL of normal saline (NS) and should be given with the recommended amount of diluent and per the recommended drip rate. Epinephrine and resuscitative equipment should always be available and its functioning double-checked in case of anaphylactic reaction (to iron or any drug with a greater risk of causing anaphylaxis). In addition, it may be necessary for the patient to remain recumbent 30 minutes after the intravenous injection to prevent drug-induced orthostatic hypotension. When moving about, the patient should be slow and purposeful at this time.

When ferrous salts are given to infants, they should be administered only with vitamin E to prevent the possible occurrence of hemolytic anemia. While ferrous salts are best given between meals for maximal absorption, they are often taken with food or meals to decrease gastrointestinal upset. At least 1 to 2 hours should be allowed between intake of the ferrous drug and the intake of milk or antacids. The drug should be stored in a light-resistant, airtight container. Patients should be cautioned to avoid reclining after ingesting the drug and to remain in an upright or sitting position for up to 30 minutes to minimize esophageal irritation and corrosion. It is important to also inform patients that use of any iron product will turn stools to a black, tarry or dark green colour. Folic acid may be ordered as an additive drug for total parenteral nutritional solutions, and in such cases the patient must be monitored for hypotension and allergic reactions. More information for patients taking blood-forming drugs is presented in Patient Education. Special Populations: The Older Adult lists precautions to take when giving iron products to older adults.

◰ Evaluation

Evaluation of therapeutic responses to blood-forming drugs should stem from goals and outcome criteria as well as from monitoring of therapeutic versus adverse effects. Therapeutic responses to iron products include improved nutritional status, increased weight, increased activity tolerance and well-being, and absence of fatigue. Adverse effects include nausea, constipation, epigastric pain, black and tarry stools, and vomiting. Toxic signs may include nausea, diarrhea (green, tarry stools), hematemesis, pallor, cyanosis, shock, and coma.

SPECIAL POPULATIONS: THE OLDER ADULT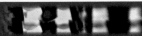

Iron Products

- Instructions on how to take oral forms of iron are crucial to safe administration. All types of teaching strategies should be implemented to reinforce verbal and written instructions. Patient education needs to be individualized and geared for the patient with alterations in sensory perception. Patients should be cautioned about making changes in their medication regimen, such as doubling doses or discontinuing them without a physician's order.
- Older adults and their spouses or caregivers should be informed of food sources high in iron and of ways to include them in their menu planning. Patients need to be instructed to steam vegetables and to not overcook them through excessive boiling. By not overcooking or boiling vegetables and other food items, vitamin, mineral, and elemental content, including iron, is better preserved.
- Older patients need to be reminded that gastrointestinal upset may occur with many drugs, including vitamins and iron. Iron products should be taken with food or a snack to help decrease this upset.
- Always inform older adults, their spouses, family members, significant others, and caregivers about appropriate community resources (e.g., Meals on Wheels, senior citizen community centres, public recreation centres). A list of these community resources is often available through a city Web page, social services, and other outlets.

PATIENT EDUCATION

- ❖ Patients should be instructed to take iron products with caution and to be aware of potential poisoning if taken at amounts greater than what is recommended. Oral dosage forms of iron should be given intact, should not be crushed or altered in any way, and should be taken with at least 120 to 180 mL of water or fluid to minimize gastrointestinal upset and increase absorption.
- ❖ Patients should be informed that an iron product, if ordered, cannot be substituted for another one because each product contains different forms of the iron salt and comes in different amounts.
- ❖ Patients should be reminded to remain upright for up to 15 to 30 minutes and to avoid reclining during this time to prevent esophageal irritation or corrosion. Inform patients that iron products may lead to the occurrence of black and tarry stools.
- ❖ Patients should be encouraged to eat foods high in iron, such as meat, dark green leafy vegetables, dried beans, dried fruits, and eggs (see http://evolve.elsevier.com/Canada/Lilley/pharmacology/ for more information).

POINTS TO REMEMBER

- ❖ Iron and folic acid are important in the treatment of many disorders and diseases (e.g., malignancies), to achieve RBC and Hgb formation that is as adequate as possible, and to prevent nutritional deficits that can affect all body systems, particularly the immune system.
- ❖ Blood-forming drugs are often used in the treatment of pernicious anemia, malabsorption syndromes, hemolytic anemia, hemorrhage, and kidney and liver diseases.
- ❖ Iron products should be taken exactly as ordered. Parenteral dosage forms may cause anaphylaxis and orthostatic hypotension.

EXAMINATION REVIEW QUESTIONS

1 When administering oral iron tablets, which of the following should the nurse keep in mind as being the most appropriate liquid, other than water, to give with these tablets?
a. Milk
b. Pudding
c. Liquid antacid
d. Orange juice

2 When teaching a group of patients about foods that contain iron, which foods should the nurse recommend as good sources of iron?
a. Meats
b. Citrus fruits
c. Tomatoes
d. Yellow vegetables

3 When administering iron dextran intramuscularly, which nursing intervention is correct?
a. Give the entire dosage in one injection.
b. Administer with oral iron supplements.
c. Inject intramuscularly into the deltoid muscle.
d. Inject deep into a large muscle mass using the Z-track method.

4 When assessing a patient who is to receive folic acid supplements, which condition is important to rule out?
a. Pregnancy
b. Tropical sprue
c. Pernicious anemia
d. Malabsorption syndromes

5 A patient who is taking oral iron supplements calls the office, upset about having "very black, shiny stools." What should the nurse's response be?
a. "Are you taking this medication on an empty stomach?"
b. "You may be bleeding and should come to the office immediately."
c. "This is an unusual reaction, and you should stop the tablets immediately."
d. "It is normal for oral iron products to change stools to a black and tarry colour."

For answers see http://evolve.elsevier.com/Canada/Lilley/pharmacology/.

CRITICAL THINKING ACTIVITIES

1 In your clinical area, take a 24-hour dietary intake history from one of your assigned patients. Analyze the iron content of the patient's intake while she is hospitalized. In addition, note the drugs ordered to identify any supplemental vitamins or iron tablets and to identify any drug interactions. Also note any laboratory values, such as RBC, Hgb, Hct, bilirubin levels, and reticulocyte levels.

2 Discuss the importance of monitoring reticulocyte counts, Hgb, and Hct levels once oral iron therapy has been initiated.

3 Discuss teaching that you should share with a patient taking oral iron supplements.

For answers see http://evolve.elsevier.com/Canada/Lilley/pharmacology/.

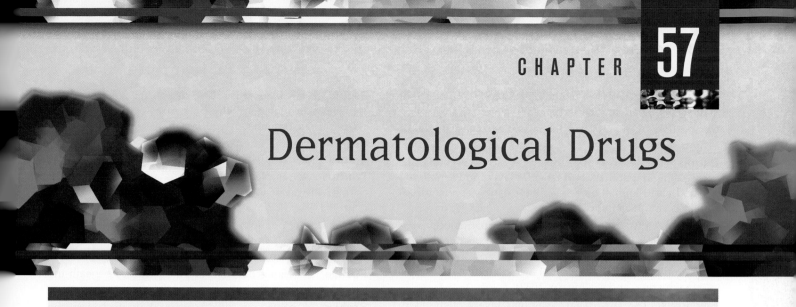

Dermatological Drugs

Learning Objectives

After reading this chapter, the successful student will be able to do the following:

1 Discuss the normal anatomy, physiology, and functions of the skin.

2 Describe the different disorders, infections, and conditions commonly affecting the skin.

3 Identify dermatological drugs used to treat skin disorders, infections, and conditions, with description of the classifications.

4 Discuss the mechanisms of action, indications, contraindications, cautions, application techniques, and adverse effects associated with dermatological drugs.

5 Develop a collaborative plan of care that includes all phases of the nursing process for patients receiving dermatological drugs.

e-Learning Activities

Web site
(http://evolve.elsevier.com/Canada/Lilley/pharmacology/)

- Animations
- Answers to chapter questions, activities, and case studies
- Calculators and Category Catchers
- Glossary with audio pronunciations
- IV Therapy and Medication Error Checklists
- Multiple-Choice Review Question quizzes
- Nursing Care Plans
- Online Appendices and Supplements
- WebLinks

Drug Profiles

anthralin, p. 1041
▶▶ bacitracin, p. 1034
▶▶ benzoyl peroxide, p. 1035
calcipotriol, p. 1041
clindamycin (clindamycin phosphate)*, p. 1036
▶▶ clotrimazole, p. 1037
finasteride, p. 1042
fluorouracil, p. 1043
imiquimod, p. 1043
▶▶ isotretinoin, p. 1036
▶▶ lindane, p. 1042
miconazole (miconazole nitrate)*, p. 1037
minoxidil, p. 1042
mupirocin, p. 1035
neomycin, bacitracin, polymyxin B, p. 1035
pimecrolimus, p. 1043
▶▶ silver sulfadiazine, p. 1035
tar-containing products, p. 1041
tazarotene, p. 1041
tretinoin, p. 1036

▶▶ Key drug.

*Full generic name is given in parentheses. For the purposes of this text, the more common shortened name is used.

Glossary

Acne vulgaris A chronic inflammatory disease of the pilosebaceous glands of the skin, involving lesions such as papules and pustules ("pimples"). (p. 1035)

Actinic keratosis A slowly developing, localized thickening of the outer layers of the skin resulting from long-term, prolonged exposure to the sun. (p. 1043)

Atopic dermatitis A chronic skin inflammation seen in patients with hereditary susceptibility to pruritus. (p. 1032)

Basal cell carcinoma The most common form of skin cancer; arises from epidermal cells known as *basal cells* and is rarely metastatic. (p. 1032)

Carbuncle A necrotizing infection of skin and subcutaneous tissue caused by multiple furuncles (boils). (p. 1034)

Cellulitis An acute, diffuse, spreading infection involving the skin, subcutaneous tissue, and sometimes muscle. (p. 1034)

Dermatitis Any inflammation of the skin. (p. 1032)

Dermatophyte   Any of common groups of fungi that infect skin, hair, and nails. (p. 1037)

Dermatosis   General term for any abnormal skin condition. (p. 1032)

Dermis   The layer of the skin just below the epidermis, consisting of papillary and reticular layers and containing blood and lymphatic vessels, nerves and nerve endings, glands, and hair follicles. (p. 1032)

Eczema   A pruritic, papulovesicular dermatitis occurring as a reaction to many endogenous and exogenous agents and characterized by erythema, edema, and an inflammatory infiltrate of the dermis that includes oozing, vesiculation, crusting, and scaling. (p. 1032)

Epidermis   The superficial, avascular layers of the skin, made up of an outer, dead, cornified portion and a deeper, living, cellular portion. (p. 1032)

Folliculitis   Inflammation of a follicle, usually a hair follicle. (p. 1034)

Furuncle   A painful skin nodule caused by a staphylococcal infection that enters skin through the hair follicles. Also called a *boil*. (p. 1034)

Impetigo   A pus-generating, contagious superficial skin infection, usually caused by staphylococci or streptococci. (p. 1034)

Papule   A small circumscribed, superficial, solid elevation of the skin that is usually pink in colour and less than 0.5 to 1 cm in diameter. (p. 1034)

Pediculosis   An infestation with lice of the family Pediculidae. (p. 1042)

Pruritus   An unpleasant cutaneous sensation that provokes the desire to rub or scratch the skin to obtain relief. (p. 1037)

Psoriasis   A common, chronic squamous cell dermatosis with polygenic (multi-gene) inheritance and a fluctuating pattern of recurrence and remission. (p. 1032)

Pustule   A visible collection of pus within or beneath the epidermis. (p. 1034)

Scabies   A contagious disease caused by *S. scabiei,* the itch mite, characterized by intense itching of the skin and injury to the skin (excoriation) resulting from scratching. (p. 1042)

Tinea   A group of fungal skin diseases caused by dermatophytes of several kinds and characterized by itching, scaling, and, sometimes, painful lesions. *Tinea* is a general term for infections of dermatophytes that occur on several sites. Also called *ringworm.* (p. 1037)

Vesicle   A smaller sac containing liquid; also called a *cyst.* (p. 1034)

SKIN ANATOMY AND PHYSIOLOGY

The largest organ of the body is the skin. It covers the body and serves several functions, most of which are taken for granted. It serves as a protective barrier for the internal organs. Without skin, harmful external forces such as microorganisms and chemicals would gain access to and damage or destroy many of a person's delicate internal organs. Part of this protection includes the skin's ability to maintain a surface pH of 4.5 to 5.5. This weakly acidic environment discourages the growth of microorganisms that grow at a more alkaline pH of 6 to 7.5, which is why infected skin usually has a higher pH than noninfected skin. The skin also has the ability to sense changes in temperature (hot or cold), pressure, or pain information, which is then transmitted along nerve endings. The temperature of the environment changes constantly and can be extremely hot or cold. Despite this, the body maintains an almost constant internal temperature in most environments, thanks, in large part, to the skin, which plays a major role in the regulation of body temperature. Heat loss and conservation are regulated in coordination with the blood vessels that supply blood to the skin and through perspiration. The skin is also able to excrete fluid and electrolytes through sweat glands. It stores fat, synthesizes vitamin D, and provides a site for drug absorption.

The skin is made up of two layers: the dermis and the epidermis (Figure 57-1). The outer skin layer, or **epidermis**, is composed of four layers. From the outermost to innermost layer, the layers are the stratum corneum, stratum lucidum, stratum granulosum, and the stratum germinativum. The respective functions of these layers are described in Table 57-1.

None of these layers has a direct blood supply of its own. Instead, its nourishment is provided through diffusion from the dermis below. The **dermis** lies between the epidermis and subcutaneous fat and differs from the epidermis in many ways. It is approximately 40 times thicker than the epidermis. Traversing the dermis is a rich supply of blood vessels, nerves, lymphatic tissue, elastic tissue, and connective tissue, which provide extra support and nourishment to the skin. Also contained in this layer are the exocrine glands, the eccrine, apocrine, and sebaceous glands, and the hair follicles. The functions of the various types of exocrine glands are explained in Table 57-2.

Below the dermis is a layer of loose connective tissue called the *hypodermis*, which makes the skin flexible. The hypodermis also contains the subcutaneous fat tissue, which provides thermal insulation and cushioning or padding. It is also the source of nutrition for the skin.

TOPICAL DERMATOLOGICAL DRUGS

Reactions or disorders of the skin are common and numerous. A **dermatosis** is any abnormal skin condition. Dermatoses include a variety of types of **dermatitis** (skin inflammation), such as **atopic dermatitis**, **eczema**, and **psoriasis.** In addition, there are a variety of skin cancers, including **basal cell carcinoma**, squamous cell carcinoma, and melanoma. Drugs administered directly

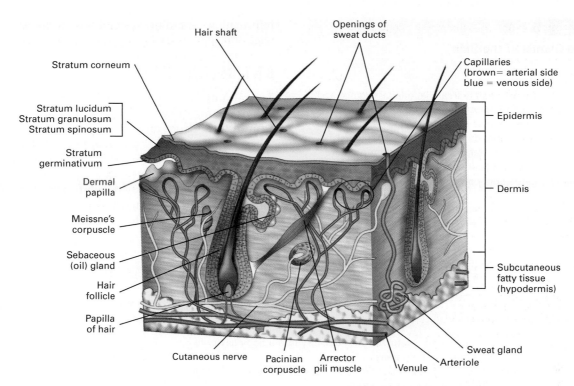

FIG. 57-1 A microscopic view of the skin. The epidermis, shown in longitudinal section, is raised at one corner to reveal the ridges in the dermis. (Modified from Thibodeau, G. A., & Patton, K. T. (2003). *Anatomy and physiology* (5th ed.). St. Louis, MO: Mosby.)

to the site are called topical *dermatological drugs*. A variety of formulations are available that are suitable for specific indications. Each formulation has certain characteristics that make it suitable for specific indications. The formulations, their characteristics, and some examples of them are summarized in Table 57-3. While the focus of this chapter is topically administered medications, systemically administered drugs are also used to treat several skin disorders. Therefore, included in this chapter are cross-references to previous chapters where systemic drug categories are discussed in more detail.

There are also many therapeutic categories of dermatological drugs. Some of the most common ones are as follows:

- Antibacterial drugs
- Antifungal drugs
- Anti-inflammatory drugs
- Antineoplastics
- Antipruritic drugs for treating itching
- Antiviral drugs
- Burn drugs
- Débriding drugs that promote wound healing
- Emollients that soften skin
- Keratolytics that cause softening and peeling of the stratum corneum
- Local anaesthetics
- Sunscreens
- Topical vasodilators

Because there are so many drugs available, the scope of this chapter is limited to some of the most commonly used medications, and its focus is topical medications. At times, the reader may be referred to other chapters for

---

TABLE 57-1

Epidermal Layers

Layer	Description
Stratum corneum ("horny layer," so named because keratin is the same protein that makes up the horns of animals)	Outermost layer consisting of dead skin cells that are made of a converted water-repellent protein known as *keratin;* it is the protective layer for the entire body. After it is desquamated, or shed, it is replaced by new cells from below.
Stratum lucidum ("clear layer")	Layer where keratin is formed; it is translucent and contains flat cells.
Stratum granulosum ("granular layer")	Cells die in this layer; granulated cells are located here, giving this layer the appearance for which it is named.
Stratum germinativum ("germinative layer")	New skin cells are made in this layer; it contains melanocytes, which produce melanin, the skin colour pigment.

TABLE 57-2

Exocrine Glands of the Skin

Gland	Function
Apocrine	Glands mainly in axilla, genital organs, and breast areas; emit an odour; believed to be scent or sex glands
Eccrine	Sweat glands located throughout the skin surface; help regulate body temperature and prevent skin dryness
Sebaceous	Large lipid-containing cells that produce oil or film that covers the epidermis; protects and lubricates skin, and is water repellent and antiseptic

information regarding systemically administered drugs (e.g., oral, injectable) that are indicated for skin conditions.

ANTIMICROBIALS

Topical antimicrobials are antibacterial, antifungal, and antiviral drugs that are applied topically. Systemically administered drugs are discussed in detail in Part Seven, where their specific pharmacological characteristics are also described. Those with available topical dosage forms are discussed here. Although they have many of the same properties as systemic forms, there are some differences in terms of their toxicities and adverse effects. Drugs commonly used to treat acne are also covered in this section.

TABLE 57-3

Dermatological Drug Formulations: Characteristics and Examples

Formulation	Characteristics	Examples
Aerosol foam	Can cover large area; useful for drug delivery into a body cavity (e.g., vagina, rectum) or hair areas	Proctofoam, contraceptive foams
Aerosol spray	Spreads thin liquid or powder film; covers large areas; useful when skin is tender to touch (e.g., burns)	Solarcaine, Tinactin
Cleanser	Nongreasy; used as an astringent (oil remover) or wash with water	Zoderm
Cream	Contains water and can be removed with water; not greasy or occlusive; usually white semisolid; good for moist areas	hydrocortisone cream, Benadryl cream, Triaderm
Gel/jelly	Contains water and possibly alcohol; easily removed and good lubricator; usually clear, semisolid substance; useful when lubricant properties are desirable	K-Y jelly
Lotion	Contains water, alcohol, and solvents; may be a suspension, emulsion, or solution; good for large or hairy areas	Calamine lotion, Lubriderm lotion, Kwellada-P lotion
Oil	Contains little if any water; occlusive, liquid; not removable with water	Many brands
Ointment	Contains no water; not removable with water; occlusive, greasy, and semisolid; desirable for dry lesions because of occlusiveness	petrolatum (Vaseline), zinc oxide ointment, A & D ointment, Triaderm
Paste	Similar properties to those of the ointments; contains more powder than ointments; excellent protectant properties	zinc oxide paste
Pledget (pad)	Moistened pad is applied to or wiped over affected area	Sani-Dex
Powder	Slight lubricating properties; may be shaken on affected area; promotes drying of area where applied	Tinactin powder, Desenex powder
Shampoo	Soapy liquid for washing hair and skin	Nizoral (ketoconazole)
Solution	Nongreasy liquid; dries quickly	Various skin care products
Stick	Spreads thin chalky or viscous liquid film; often better for smaller areas	Benadryl Itch Relief

 DRUG PROFILES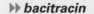

GENERAL ANTIBACTERIAL DRUGS

Common skin disorders caused by bacteria are **folliculitis, impetigo, furuncles, carbuncles, papules, pustules, vesicles**, and **cellulitis**. The bacteria responsible are most commonly *Streptococcus pyogenes* and *Staphylococcus aureus*. Dermatological antibacterial drugs are used to treat or prevent these skin infections, and the most commonly used drugs are bacitracin, polymyxin, and neomycin.

▶▶ **bacitracin**

Bacitracin (Bacitin) is a polypeptide antibiotic that is applied topically for the treatment or prevention of local skin infections caused by susceptible aerobic and anaerobic gram-positive organisms such as staphylococci, streptococci, anaerobic cocci, corynebacteria, and clostridia. Also available in systemic and ophthalmic (Chapter 58) formulations, it works by inhibiting bacterial cell wall synthesis, which leads to cell death. It can

Continued

DRUG PROFILES (cont'd)

be either bactericidal or bacteriostatic, depending on the causative organism.

Bacitracin's antimicrobial spectrum is broadened in several available combination drug products. Most of the products contain neomycin, polymyxin B, or both. Adverse reactions are usually minimal; however, reactions ranging from skin rash to allergic anaphylactoid reactions have occurred. If itching, burning, inflammation, or other signs of sensitivity occur, bacitracin should be discontinued. This drug is available in ointment form, and it is usually applied to the affected area 1 to 3 times daily.

mupirocin

Mupirocin (Bactroban) is an antibacterial product available only by prescription. It is used on the skin for staphylococcal and streptococcal impetigo. A newer indication involves intranasal use for nasal colonization with methicillin-resistant *Staphylococcal aureus* (MRSA). This drug is applied topically three times daily and intranasally twice daily. Adverse reactions are usually limited to local burning, itching, or minor pain.

neomycin, bacitracin, and polymyxin B

Neomycin and polymyxin B are two additional broad-spectrum antibiotics that are available as the popular nonprescription product Neosporin. Neosporin ointment contains bacitracin. Several brand-name and generic combinations of these topical antibiotics are available, and all are commonly used as topical antiseptics for minor skin wounds. (See Evidence-Informed Practice: Honey and Wound Care on p. 1038 for more information on antiseptics and wound care.) Although it is still a popular over-the-counter drug product, there is evidence that neomycin/polymyxin B can actually increase the likelihood of future allergic sensitivity of the skin.

silver sulfadiazine

One of the concerns with burn victims is infection at the burn site. There are two problems posed by the use of either topically or systemically administered antimicrobial drugs in this setting, however. Because of the increased systemic absorption of a drug that can occur in compromised skin areas such as burns, topical burn drugs must not be too potent or toxic to cause dangerous systemic effects. This is especially true for larger burned areas because the drug may be applied over a large surface area of skin and thus absorbed in greater quantities. On the other hand, the blood supply to burned areas is often drastically reduced, such that systemically administered antibiotics either cannot reach the site or do so only in quantities too low to be effective. Therefore, the only way of applying these drugs to ensure that they reach the burn site is to do so topically. One commonly used drug that has proved both effective and safe in the prevention or treatment of infections in burns is silver sulfadiazine (Demazin, Flamazine).

Silver sulfadiazine is a synthetic antimicrobial drug produced when silver nitrate reacts with the chemical

sulfadiazine. It appears to act on the cell membrane and cell wall of susceptible bacteria and is used as an adjunct in the prevention and treatment of infection in second- and third-degree burns. The adverse effects of silver sulfadiazine are similar to those of other topical drugs and include pain, burning, and itching. This medication should not be used in patients who are allergic to sulfonamide drugs. It is available only as a 1% cream and should be applied topically to cleansed, débrided, burned areas once or twice daily using a sterile-gloved hand.

ANTIACNE DRUGS

Other antibacterial drugs are used to treat **acne vulgaris,** the most common skin infection. Its precise cause is unknown and somewhat controversial. Likely causative factors include heredity, stress, drug reactions, hormones, and bacterial infections. Common bacterial causes include staphylococcal species and *Propionibacterium acnes.* Drugs used to treat acne include benzoyl peroxide, clindamycin, erythromycin, and the vitamin A acid known as *retinoic acid.* Many other drugs are also used in the treatment and prevention of acne, including systemic use of the antibiotics minocycline, doxycycline, and tetracycline (Chapter 38). Some practitioners also prescribe oral contraceptives (Chapter 34) for female patients with acne, as beneficial estrogen effects against acne have been shown in some controlled studies, especially hormone-driven acne.

▶▶ benzoyl peroxide

The microorganism that most commonly causes acne, *P. acnes,* is an anaerobic bacterium that needs an environment poor in oxygen to grow. Benzoyl peroxide (Acetoxyl, Adacept, Benzac) is effective in combating such infection because it slowly and continuously liberates active oxygen in the skin, causing antibacterial, antiseptic, drying, and keratolytic actions. These actions create an unfavourable environment for the continued growth of the *P. acnes* bacteria and they soon die. Drugs such as benzoyl peroxide that soften scales and loosen the outer horny layer of the skin are referred to as *keratolytics.*

Benzoyl peroxide generally produces signs of improvement within 4 to 6 weeks. Advese effects tend to be dose related (including overuse) and involve peeling skin, red skin, or a sensation of warmth. Blistering or swelling of the skin is generally considered an allergic reaction to the product and is an indication to stop treatment. Overuse with this drug and with tretinoin is common among adolescent patients who are attempting to quickly cure their acne. The result can be painful, reddened skin, which usually resolves upon return to use of these medications as prescribed.

Benzoyl peroxide is available in multiple topical dosage forms including a cleansing bar, liquid, lotion, mask, cream, gel, and cleanser. It is also available in combination drug products that include the chemical element sulfur, and the antibiotics erythromycin and clindamycin (Chapter 38). It is usually applied topically one to four

Continued

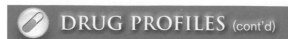

DRUG PROFILES (cont'd)

times daily, depending on the dosage form and the prescriber's instructions. It is classified as pregnancy category C.

clindamycin phosphate

Clindamycin phosphate (Clindasol, Clindets) is a topical form of the systemic antibiotic described in Chapter 38. It is most commonly prescribed for acne. Adverse reactions are usually limited to minor, local skin reactions, including burning, itching, dryness, oiliness, and peeling. The drug is available in cream, gel, lotion, suspension, and pledget form. It is usually applied once or twice daily. This drug is classified as pregnancy category B.

▶▶ isotretinoin

Isotretinoin (Accutane, Clarus) is an oral product indicated for the treatment of severe recalcitrant cystic acne. Isotretinoin inhibits sebaceous gland activity and has anti-keratinizing (anti–skin-hardening) and anti-inflammatory effects. Isotretinoin is one of relatively few medications classified as pregnancy category X drugs. This means that it is a proven human teratogen, or a chemical known to induce birth defects. For these reasons, a risk-management program of unprecedented size and scope, known as "iPLEDGE," was designed and approved by the U.S. Food and Drug Administration (FDA) in 2006 for this drug. Under this program, U.S. federal law requires that any health provider who prescribes this drug be a registered and activated member of this program, and patients must be qualified and registered. Drug wholesalers and pharmacists who dispense this drug are also required to be part of this program. In Canada, the risk-management program called the Accutane Prevention Program (PPP) requires that women of childbearing age taking isotretinoin give written informed consent, receive education about the teratogenicity of the drug, and agree to use two contraceptive methods while on the drug. Also included in the risk-management program are suggestions for an expanded physicians' checklist to include the lists of potentially interacting medications and natrual health products, a toll-free number that both patients and health care providers can use to get information, a Web site with information available on isotretinoin and contraception, improved education for physicians and pharmacists, and the introduction of generic forms of isotretinoin. Additionally, there have been case reports of suicide and suicide attempts in patients receiving this medication. Patients should be educated to report immediately any signs of depression to their health care providers. Follow-up treatment may be needed, and simply stopping the drug may be

insufficient. Despite these rather severe concerns, this drug does prove to be helpful in treating severe acne cases. Isotretinoin is available only for oral use.

tretinoin

Tretinoin (retinoic acid, vitamin A acid) (Rejuva-A, Renova, Retina-A) is a derivative of vitamin A that is used to treat acne and ameliorate the dermatological changes (e.g., fine wrinkling, mottled hyperpigmentation, roughness) associated with photodamage (sun damage). (See Research: Dermatological Preparations on p. 1039 for another new drug, tazarotene, indicated for skin wrinkling and mottled hypo- and hyperpigmentation.) The drug appears to act as an irritant on the skin, in particular the follicular epithelium. Specifically, it stimulates the turnover of epidermal cells, which results in skin peeling. While this is occurring, the free fatty acid levels of the skin are reduced, and the horny cells of the outer epidermis cannot then adhere to one another. Without fatty acids and horny cells, acne and its comedo, or pimple, cannot exist.

Topically administered tretinoin has been shown to enhance the repair of skin damaged by ultraviolet radiation, or sunlight, by increasing the formation of fibroblasts and collagen, both of which are needed to rebuild skin. The drug may also reduce collagen degradation by inhibiting the enzyme collagenase that breaks down collagen.

As with erythromycin, tretinoin's main adverse effects are local inflammatory reactions, which are reversible when therapy is discontinued. Some of the most common adverse effects are excessively red and edematous blisters, crusted skin, and temporary alterations in skin pigmentation. Tretinoin is available in many topical formulations, including creams, gels, and a liquid. Because of its potential to cause severe irritation and peeling, it may initially be applied once every 2 or 3 days, often starting with a lower-strength product.

Retin-A Microis is approved for the treatment of acne vulgaris. This particular acne product contains tretinoin inside a synthetic polymer called a *microsponge system.* This system is made of round microscopic particles of synthetic polymer. The microspheres act as reservoirs for tretinoin, allowing the skin to absorb small amounts of the drug over time. Retin-A Micro is currently available only in gel form. All topical forms of tretinoin are rated pregnancy category C. They are not to be confused with the oral capsule form of tretinoin mentioned in Chapter 48 that is used to treat leukemia and is rated pregnancy category D. Another antiacne retinoid is adapalene (Differiun), available as a topical gel or cream.

Continued

DRUG PROFILES (cont'd)

ANTIFUNGAL DRUGS

A few fungi produce keratinolytic enzymes, which allow them to live on the skin. Topical fungal infections are primarily caused by *Candida* spp. (candidiasis), **dermatophytes**, and *Malassezia furfur* (tinea versicolor). These fungi exist in moist, warm environments, primarily in dark areas such as the feet or groin.

Candidal infections are commonly caused by *Candida albicans*, a yeast-like opportunistic fungus present in the normal flora of the mouth, vagina, and intestinal tract. Two significant factors that can predispose a person to a candidal infection are broad-spectrum antibiotic therapy, which promotes an overgrowth of nonsusceptible organisms in the natural body florae, and immunodeficiency disorders such as those that occur in patients with cancer, acquired immune deficiency syndrome (AIDS), or organ transplants. Because these infections favour warm, moist areas of the skin and mucous membranes, they most commonly occur orally (e.g., thrush in infants), vaginally, and cutaneously, for example, beneath the breasts and in diapered areas. They may also cause nail infections.

Dermatophytes are a group of three closely related genera consisting of *Epidermophyton* spp., *Microsporum* spp., and *Trichophyton* spp. that use the keratin found on the skin to feed their growth. They produce superficial mycotic (fungal) infections of keratinized tissue (hair, skin, and nails). Infections caused by dermatophytes are collectively called **tinea**, or *ringworm*, infections. The name *ringworm* comes from the infection assuming a circular pattern at the site of infection. Tinea infections are further identified by the location where they occur: tinea pedis (foot), tinea cruris (groin), tinea corporis (body), and tinea capitis (scalp). Tinea infections are also known as *athlete's foot* or *jock itch*.

Fungi usually invade the stratum corneum, which is the dead layer of desquamated (shedded) cells. Inflammation occurs when fungi invade this layer; sensitivity (e.g., itching) occurs when they penetrate the epidermis and dermis.

Many of the fungi that cause topical infections are difficult to eradicate. They are slow growing, and antifungal therapy may be required for periods ranging from several weeks to as long as 1 year. Fortunately, many topical antifungal drugs are available for the treatment of both dermatophyte infections and those caused by yeast and yeastlike fungi. Some of these drugs, their dosage forms, and their uses are listed in Table 57-4. Systemically administered antifungal drugs are sometimes used for skin conditions as well. These drugs were discussed in Chapter 42.

The most commonly reported adverse effects of topical antifungals are local irritation, **pruritus**, a burning sensation, and scaling. Ciclopirox olamine (Loprox) and clotrimazole (Canesten) are classified as pregnancy category B drugs, whereas ketoconazole (Ketoderm, Nizoral) and miconazole (Micatin) are classified as pregnancy category C drugs. Hypersensitivity is the sole contraindication to the use of any of these drugs.

▶▶ clotrimazole

Clotrimazole (Canesten) is available both over the counter and with a prescription. It is available in a cream formulation for the treatment of dermatophytoses (e.g., athlete's foot), superficial mycoses, and cutaneous candidiasis. Similar topical preparations (cream and vaginal tablets) are also available for intravaginal administration in the treatment of vulvovaginal candidiasis, commonly called a *yeast infection,* and vaginal trichomoniasis. Different dosages and dosage forms are used for the treatment of different fungal infections. Clotrimazole is classified as pregnancy category B.

miconazole nitrate

Miconazole nitrate (Micatin, Micozole, Monistat) is a topical antifungal drug available in several over-the-counter and prescription products. Miconazole inhibits the growth of several fungi, including dermatophytes and yeast, as well as gram-positive bacteria. This drug is commonly used to treat dermatophytoses, superficial mycoses, cutaneous candidiasis, and vulvovaginal candidiasis. It is present in many remedies for athlete's foot, jock itch, and yeast infections.

For the treatment of athlete's foot, jock itch, ringworm, and other susceptible fungal infections, miconazole should be applied sparingly to the cleansed, dry, infected area twice daily, in the morning and evening. For the treatment of yeast infections, one ovule suppository should be inserted in the vagina once daily at bedtime for 3 consecutive days. Also available is the dual-pack, which contains one 100 mg suppository and 2% cream. The suppository is administered intravaginally once daily at bedtime for 7 days and the cream is applied to the itchy, irritated area. The most common adverse effects of topically administered miconazole are vulvovaginal burning and itching, pelvic cramps and rash, urticaria, stinging, and contact dermatitis. It is available in a variety of topical formulations: a 2% aerosol spray and powder; a 2% cream; a 2% vaginal cream; and a 100, 400, and 500 mg vaginal suppository. It is also available as a 1200 mg vaginal suppository for one-time dosing. Miconazole is classified as pregnancy category C.

EVIDENCE-INFORMED PRACTICE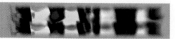

Honey and Wound Care

Review
There is increasing evidence to support the use of honey as a healing modality in wound care. Honey has been recognized for its antibacterial qualities against both gram-positive and gram-negative organisms. This antibacterial activity occurs because of the action of inhibines, which consist of hydrogen peroxide, flavinoids, and phenolic acids, and numerous other unidentified components. Honey has a pH of 3.2 to 4.5, which inhibits bacterial growth.

Type of Evidence
This study, conducted in the United Kingdom, involved 105 patients in a single-centre, open-label, randomized controlled trial. Participants were selected who had a wound healing by secondary intention. Exclusion criteria included patients with diabetes, those who required antibiotics, known allergy to bee or honey products, and specific wound criteria. Participants were treated with either a conventional wound dressing or a honey dressing.

Results of Study
This study by Robson and colleagues provided evidence that there are benefits to the use of honey in wound care and that healing times may be reduced compared with those with conventional management. The honey treatment group experienced a median healing time of 100 days compared with 140 days in the control group, a result demonstrating clinical significance. However, this result was not considered statistically significant because of insufficient patient enrolment in the study.

Link of Evidence to Nursing Practice
Nurses are often faced with challenges in managing complex wounds. The prevalence of multidrug-resistant bacteria and wounds that are difficult to heal increase the desire to look for alternatives to wound management. Honey is a potential alternative, but more research needs to be done to validate its use in wound care.

Based on Robson, V., Dodd, S., & Thomas, S. (2009). Standardized antibacterial honey (Medihoney™) with standard therapy in wound care: Randomized clinical trial. *Journal of Advanced Nursing, 65*(3), 565–575.

TABLE 57-4

Topical Antifungal Drugs

Drug	Trade Names	Dosage Forms	Uses	Legal Status
butoconazole nitrate	Gynazole.1	2% vaginal cream	Candidiasis	Rx
ciclopirox olamine	Loprox, Stieprox Shampoo)	1% cream and lotion, 1.5% shampoo	Cutaneous candidiasis, dermatophytoses, tinea versicolor	Rx
clioquinol	Locatorin (with flumethasone pivalate); Vioform (with hydrocortisone)	3% cream	Dermatophytoses	Rx
clotrimazole	Canesten Combi-Pak Lotriderm	1% vaginal cream, 200 mg and 500 mg vaginal tabs Cream (1% clotrimazole, 0.05% beclamethasone dipropionate)	Candidiasis Dermatophytoses	OTC Rx
clotrimazole	Clotrimaderm	1% topical cream	Candidiasis; dermatophytoses; tinea vesicolor	OTC
clotrimazole	Canesten	1%, 2%, 10% cream	Candidiasis	OTC
ketoconazole	Ketoderm Nizoral	2% cream	Candidiasis, dermatophytoses, tinea versicolor	Rx
		2% shampoo	Dermatophytoses, tinea versicolor	OTC
miconazole nitrate	Micatin	2% cream, powder spray	Candidiasis, dermatophytoses, tinea versicolor	OTC
miconazole nitrate	Micozole	2% cream	Candidiasis, dermatophytoses, tinea versicolor	OTC

Continued

TABLE	57-4

Topical Antifungal Drugs (cont'd)

Drug	Trade Names	Dosage Forms	Uses	Legal Status
miconazole nitrate	Monistat Monistat Pak	100, 400, and 1200 mg vaginal ovules	Candidiasis	OTC
		2% cream and 100, 400, and 1200 mg vaginal suppository	Candidiasis	OTC
naftifine hydrochloride	Naftin	1% cream and gel	Dermatophytoses	OTC
nystatin	Flagistatin, Nyaderm	Cream, ointment, powder	Candidiasis	Rx
nystatin	Generic	Vaginal cream, tab	Candidiasis	Rx
terbinafine hydrochloride	Lamisil	1% cream and spray	Dermatophytoses	Rx
tolnaftate	Pitrex, Tinactin, Zeasorb, many others	1% cream, solution, gel, powder, swab, and spray	Dermatophytoses	OTC
undecylenic acid	Feet Athletes Foot and Antifungal	Powder, spray	Dermatophytoses	OTC

OTC, available over the counter without prescription; *Rx*, currently available by prescription only.

 ## RESEARCH

Dermatological Preparations

A new topical retinoid, tazarotene 0.1%, is available as a cream to reduce fine facial wrinkles and to even out mottled hyper- and hypopigmentation. In two double-blind vehicle-controlled studies, White patients who had mild to severe fine wrinkles, mottled hypo- and hyperpigmentation, or benign lentigines (sun spots, age spots) of the face (from overexposure to the sun) applied either tazarotene 0.1% or a placebo once a day for approximately 24 weeks. Treatment also included the use of sunscreen with an SPF greater than 15. Tazarotene 0.1% was shown to be "significantly superior" to the placebo, with an improvement of at least one grade from baseline. This product is now available by prescription for adults over the age of 12 years for once-daily dosing.

It is recommended that female patients of childbearing age have a pregnancy test with negative results 2 weeks before starting therapy with this drug and that contraceptives be used throughout treatment and for 1 month thereafter. Tazarotene 0.1% must be kept away from the eyes and mouth. It is a "sun-sensitive" product; exposure to ultraviolet (UV) radiation should be avoided, and it is not to be used on broken or sunburned skin. In addition, increased irritation may be noted in cold, wintry weather or extreme weather conditions. For more information visit http://www.tazorac.com/.

Data from *Monthly Prescribing Reference*, pp. A–10, January 2003.

ANTIVIRAL DRUGS

Topical antivirals are now used less frequently than before in dermatology practice as systemic antiviral drug therapy has generally been shown to be superior for controlling such viral skin conditions. Nonetheless, two antiviral ointments are described here. As is the case with systemic drug therapy, these products are best used early in a viral skin lesion outbreak. Topical antivirals are more likely to be used for acute outbreaks only, whereas systemic drugs are used for acute outbreaks and for ongoing prophylaxis against outbreaks. As noted in Chapter 40, viral infections are challenging to manage because they live within the body's healthy cells and use their cell mechanisms to reproduce. This is also true for topical viral infections. Infections caused by herpes simplex types 1 and 2 and the human papillomavirus (which causes anogenital warts) are particularly serious and are becoming more common.

The topical antiviral drugs currently available to treat such viral infections are acyclovir (Zovirax) and penciclovir (Denavir). Acyclovir and penciclovir act by inhibiting the viral enzymes necessary for deoxyribonucleic acid (DNA) synthesis (discussed in more detail in Chapter 40). Acyclovir is available as a 5% topical ointment, whereas penciclovir is available as a 1% topical cream. Acyclovir is applied every 3 hours, or 6 times daily, for 1 week. Penciclovir is applied every 2 hours while the patient is awake, for 4 days. A finger cot or rubber glove should be worn for application of the ointment to prevent the spread of infection. The most common adverse effects are stinging, itching, and rash. Acyclovir is contraindicated in patients with hypersensitivity to it. Acyclovir is classified as a pregnancy category C drug and penciclovir as a pregnancy category B drug.

TOPICAL ANAESTHETIC, ANTIPRURITIC, AND ANTI-INFLAMMATORY DRUGS

Topical anaesthetic drugs are drugs used to numb the skin. They accomplish this by inhibiting the conduction of nerve impulses from sensory nerves, thereby reducing or eliminating the pain or pruritus associated with insect bites, sunburn, and plant allergies such as poison ivy, as well as many other uncomfortable skin disorders. They are also used to numb the skin before a painful injection (e.g., intravenous insertion in a child). Topical anaesthetics are available as ointments, creams, sprays, liquids, and jellies, and are discussed in Chapter 12.

TOPICAL ANTIPRURITICS

Topical antipruritic (anti-itching) drugs contain antihistamines or corticosteroids. Many exert a combined anaesthetic and antipruritic action when applied topically. The antihistamines and their therapeutic effects are covered in Chapter 36. New recommendations for the use of topical antihistamines state that they should not be used for chicken pox or widespread poison ivy or over a large body surface area because of systemic absorption and the risk of toxicity. Topical anti-inflammatory drugs are most commonly corticosteroids (Chapter 33), and they are generally indicated for the relief of inflammatory and pruritic dermatoses. With the use of topically administered corticosteroids, many of the undesirable systemic adverse effects associated with the use of the systemically administered corticosteroids are averted. The beneficial drug effects of topically administered corticosteroids are their anti-inflammatory, antipruritic, and vasoconstrictor actions. The available dosage forms of corticosteroids differ in their relative potency, which often guides their selection for treating various conditions. For example, corticosteroids that are fluorinated are used for the treatment of dermatological disorders such as psoriasis. The vehicle in which the corticosteroid

is contained also has the effect of altering its vasoconstrictor properties and therapeutic efficacy. Ointments are generally the most penetrating, followed by gels, creams, and lotions. Propylene glycol also enhances the penetration of the corticosteroid and its vasoconstrictor effects. Most corticosteroids are available in a variety of topical formulations, thus offering numerous options. The currently available topical corticosteroids, along with their respective potencies, are listed in Table 57-5.

Adverse effects of these drugs include skin reactions such as acne eruptions, allergic contact dermatitis, burning sensation, dryness, itching, skin fragility, hypopigmentation, purpura, hirsutism (usually facial), folliculitis, round and swollen face, and alopecia (usually of the scalp). Another adverse effect is the opportunistic overgrowth of bacterial, fungal, or viral flora as a result of the immunosuppressive effects of this class of drugs. These drugs are also prone to tachyphylaxis (weakening of drug effect over time), especially with persistent use or overuse. They should usually be limited to applications of no more than twice daily as a thin layer over the affected area. The usual adult dosage of these drugs is one or two applications daily, as directed. Less potent topical corticosteroids are used for children but following the same schedule. Corticosteroids are classified as pregnancy category C drugs and are contraindicated in patients with hypersensitivity to them. Because many of these products are available orally as well as topically, the potential exists for both to be administered simultaneously. This practice is not recommended and is potentially harmful; the combined use of topical and oral preparations of the same drug can lead to toxicity.

ANTIPSORIATIC DRUGS

Psoriasis is a common, chronic skin condition involving flat, epidermal-layer skin cells known as squamous cells. It is a condition believed to involve polygenic (multigene) inheritance and has a characteristic fluctuating pattern of recurrence and remission. Although there are many subtypes, the most classic one is known as *plaque psoriasis* and typically involves large, dry, erythematous scaling patches of the skin that are often white or silver on top. Commonly affected skin areas include the nails,

TABLE	57-5

Topical Corticosteroids*

Range of Potency	Corticosteroid
High potency*	betamethasone dipropionate (ointment), clobetasol 17-propionate, halobetasol propionate
Moderate potency*	amcinonide, betamethasone dipropionate (lotion), betamethasone valerate (0.1% cream, ointment, and lotion), desoximetasone , fluocinolone acetonide (cream and ointment), halcinonide, mometasone furoate, triamcinolone acetonide (0.5% cream and ointment)
Mild potency*	desonide, fluocinolone (0.01% solution), hydrocortisone, triamcinolone (0.1% cream, lotion)

*Skin penetration and, thus, potency are enhanced by the vehicle containing the steroid. Ointments, gels, creams, and lotions are given in decreasing order of effectiveness.

scalp, genitals, and lower back. Topical medications with antipsoriatic properties are profiled individually later. In addition to these topical drugs, there are newer, systemically administered antipsoriatic drugs. Those given by systemic injection include etanercept (Enbrel), alefacept (Amevive), efalizumab (Raptiva), and adalimumab (Humira). Etanercept is discussed in more detail in Chapter 50 on biological response modifiers. In addition, the antineoplastic antimetabolite methotrexate (Chapter 48) is used for its antipsoriatic properties.

MISCELLANEOUS DERMATOLOGICAL DRUGS

There are many other topically applied drugs that are available for treating dermatological disorders. Those discussed here are the topical ectoparasiticidal (scabicides and pediculicides), hair growth, antineoplastic, and antimicrobial drugs. Many of these drugs are available over the counter and by prescription. Aloe vera herbal preparations (see Natural Health Products: Aloe) are also available over the counter.

 ## DRUG PROFILES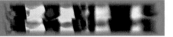

anthralin

Anthralin is a unique drug believed to work by inhibition of DNA synthesis and mitosis within the epidermis, which slows down the high turnover of skin cells and reduces the underlying inflammation. Consequently, the psoriatic lesions are reduced. It is available in ointment and cream forms and usually applied once daily. Adverse reactions are usually limited to minor skin irritation. Anthralin is classified as pregnancy category C.

calcipotriol

Calcipotriol ([also calcipotriene] Dovobet, Dovonex) is a synthetic vitamin D_3 analogue that works by binding to vitamin D_3 receptors in skin cells known as keratinocytes, whose abnormal growth contributes to psoriatic lesions. Calcipotriene helps regulate the growth and reproduction of keratinocytes. Adverse reactions usually include minor skin irritations. However, in some cases more serious reactions can occur, including worsening of psoriasis, dermatitis, skin atrophy, and folliculitis. Calcipotriene is usually applied twice daily. It is classified as pregnancy category C.

tar-containing products

Drug products containing actual coal tar derivatives were among the first medications used to treat psoriasis and are still used today for this purpose. Tar derivatives are known to have antiseptic, antibacterial, and antiseborrheic properties that serve to soften and loosen scaly or crusty areas of the skin. Seborrhea is excessive secretion of sebum, a normal skin secretion containing fat and epithelial cell debris. Tar-containing products are available in a variety of shampoo forms (for scalp psoriasis), as well as solution, oil, ointment, cream, lotion, gel, and even soap forms for bathing. These products typically contain 1% to 10% coal tar. Common product names are Doak Tar oil and TFal shampoo. Adverse reactions usually include minor skin burning, photosensitivity, and other irritations. These products may be applied from 1 to 4 times daily or once or twice weekly as prescribed.

tazarotene

Another drug in the retinoid family is tazarotene (Tazorac). Tazarotene is a receptor-selective retinoid. It is thought to normalize epidermal differentiation, reducing the influx of inflammatory cells into the skin. Synthetic retinoids are vitamin A analogues and are thought to play a role in skin cell differentiation and proliferation. Tazaroene is available in gel form and is approved for the treatment of stable plaque psoriasis and mild to moderately severe facial acne vulgaris. It is also a pregnancy category X drug, requiring appropriate counselling for female patients, as described earlier.

 ## NATURAL HEALTH PRODUCTS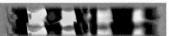

ALOE *(ALOE VERA L.)*

Overview
The dried leaves of the aloe plant contain anthranoids, which give aloe a laxative effect when it is taken orally. The topical application of the plant has been known for years to aid in wound healing.

Common Uses
Wound healing, constipation

Adverse Effects
Diarrhea, nephritis, abdominal pain, dermatitis when used topically

Potential Drug Interactions
Digoxin, antidysrhythmics, diuretics, corticosteroids

Contraindications
Contraindicated in patients who are menstruating or have kidney disease; can increase menstrual blood flow and also cause acute kidney failure

DRUG PROFILES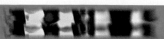

ECTOPARASITICIDAL DRUGS

Ectoparasites are insects that live on the outer surface of the body. The drugs used to kill them are called *ectoparasiticidal drugs*. Lice are transmitted from person to person by close contact with infested people, clothing, combs, or towels. A parasitic infestation on the skin with lice is called **pediculosis**, and such infestations go by one of three different names, depending on the location of the infestation:

- Pediculosis pubis: pubic lice, or "crabs," caused by *Phthirus pubis*
- Pediculosis corporis: body lice, caused by *Pediculus humanus corporis*
- Pediculosis capitis: head lice, caused by *Pediculus humanus capitis*

Common findings in infested persons include itching; eggs of the lice (called nits) attached to the hair shafts; lice on the skin or clothes; and in the case of pubic lice, sky blue macules (discoloured skin patches) on the inner thighs or lower abdomen. Pediculoses are treated with a class of drugs called *pediculicides* (see later). A second common parasitic skin infection known as **scabies** is caused by the itch mite *Sarcoptes scabiei*. Scabies is transmitted from person to person by close contact, such as by sleeping next to an infested person. The scabies mite causes irritation and itching by boring into the horny layers of skin located in cracks and folds. Itching seems to occur most commonly in the evening. The drugs used to treat these infestations are called *scabicides*.

Treatment of parasitic infestations should begin with identification of the source of infestation to prevent reinfestation. Next, the clothing and personal articles of the infested person should be decontaminated by washing them in hot, soapy water or by dry-cleaning them. All close contacts of the person should also be treated to prevent reinfestation.

Crotamiton (Eurax) is an ectoparasiticidal drug with an unclear mechanism of action. It is applied to the whole body, and after 48 hours the patient showers. It is also used to treat the pruritis caused by scabies. Crotamiton produces a counterirritation; upon evaporation from the skin, the drug produces a cooling effect, which distracts the patient from the itching.

▶▶ lindane

Lindane (Hexit) is a chlorinated hydrocarbon originally developed as an agricultural insecticide. It is both a scabicide and a pediculicide because it is effective in treating both scabies and pediculosis. It is available in two topical formulations: a 1% lotion and a 1% shampoo.

For the treatment of pubic or body lice, the cream or lotion is applied in a sufficient quantity to cover the skin and hair of the infested and surrounding areas. It is left on

for 12 hours and then thoroughly washed off. A second application is seldom needed. Head lice can be treated with lindane shampoo, which should be worked into the hair and left on for 4 minutes. The hair should then be rinsed and dried, after which the nits (eggs) should be combed from the hair shafts. The treatment for scabies is similar. It involves the application of lindane over the entire body, from the neck down. It is left on for 8 to 12 hours and washed off. A similar second application is often recommended for 1 week later. The over-the-counter products are applied in similar fashion, although details may vary between individual products.

For many years, lindane was the most widely used pediculocide, but its use has been superceded to some degree by permethrin because of case reports of neurotoxicity, including dizziness, seizures, and deaths, associated with lindane. Most of the adverse events occurred as a result of product misuse (e.g., ingestion) or overuse. Children are at higher risk of neurotoxicity because they have a larger skin surface area to body weight ratio. For this reason, the Canadian Paediatric Society has recommended that topical lindane not be used on infants and children under the age of 6 years. Lindane is still recommended as second-line therapy for eradicating lice and scabies, after failure of one of the over-the-counter preparations.

HAIR GROWTH DRUGS

finasteride

The systemically administered drug finasteride (Proscar, 5 mg) is used for benign prostatic hypertrophy, as discussed in Chapter 35. A smaller-strength version known as Propecia (1 mg) is also used for treating male-pattern alopecia.

minoxidil

Minoxidil (Rogaine) is a vasodilating drug that is administered systemically to control hypertension (see Chapter 25). Topically, it has the same vasodilating effect, and thus it is applied to the scalp to stimulate hair growth. The vasodilation it causes is one possible explanation for its ability to stimulate hair growth. It may also act at the level of the hair follicle, stimulating hair follicle growth directly.

Minoxidil can be used in men who are experiencing baldness or hair thinning. It is not approved by Health Canada for use in women, as it is classified as pregnancy category C. Treatment involves administering the drug to the affected (balding and anticipated balding) area twice daily, usually morning and evening. It generally takes 4 months before results are seen. Systemic absorption of the topically applied minoxidil may occur, with possible adverse effects, including tachycardia, fluid retention, and weight gain. Local effects may include skin irritation,

Continued

DRUG PROFILES (cont'd)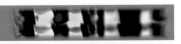

but the drug should not be applied to skin that is already irritated, nor should it be used concurrently with other topical medications applied to the same site. Topically administered minoxidil is available as a 2% solution. Each metered dose delivers 1 mL (20 mg) of the drug. The maximum recommended daily topical dose is 2 mL. The beneficial effects of this drug can be reduced by heat, including the use of a blow dryer.

SUNSCREENS

Sunscreens are topical products used to protect the skin from damage caused by the ultraviolet (UV) radiation of sunlight. There are numerous specific sunscreen products on the market, with none requiring a prescription for use. Each product is made of typically three to five chemical ingredients that work together to provide UV protection and, usually, a moisturizing effect as well. Common examples of these ingredients include titanium dioxide, octyl methoxycinnamate, homosalate, and parabens. Sunscreens are rated with a sun protection factor (SPF). The SPF is the length of time that sunscreen-protected skin can be exposed to UV rays before a minimal redness (erythema) appears, compared with the length of time it takes on unprotected skin. This is a number ranging from 2 to 30 in order of increasing potency of UV protection. Coppertone Sport and Hawaiian Tropic are just two of the many available products. Most sunscreens come in lotion, cream, or gel form. A smaller number of lip balms are also available.

TOPICAL ANTINEOPLASTIC DRUGS

fluorouracil

Premalignant skin lesions and basal cell carcinomas may be treated with the topically applied antineoplastic drug fluorouracil (Efudex). As noted in Chapter 48, this drug is an antimetabolite that acts by interfering with key cellular metabolic reactions and thus destroying rapidly growing cells, such as premalignant and malignant cells. It is also used topically in the treatment of *solar* or **actinic keratosis** and superficial basal cell carcinomas of the skin, often in addition to local surgical excision. More aggressive skin cancers include squamous cell carcinoma and malignant melanoma; these are usually treated with more aggressive surgery, radiation therapy, systemic chemotherapy, or a combination of these treatments (Chapters 48 and 49).

The adverse effects associated with the topical use of this antineoplastic are generally limited to local inflammatory reactions such as dermatitis, stomatitis, and photosensitivity. More serious effects include swelling, scaling, pain, pruritus, burning, soreness, tenderness, suppuration, scarring, and hyperpigmentation.

Fluorouracil is available as a topical cream. It can be applied with a nonmetalic applicator, clean fingertips, or gloved fingers. If fingers are used, they should be washed thoroughly immediately after application. The 1% fluorouracil cream can be used for the treatment of multiple actinic keratoses (AK) of the head and neck. It should be applied twice daily to the lesions. Superficial basal cell carcinoma may be treated with 5% fluorouracil, administered twice daily for at least 2 to 6 weeks. Another topical drug used for actinic keratoses and basal cell carcinomas is the immunomodulator imiquimod, discussed below.

IMMUNOMODULATORS

imiquimod

Imiquimod (Aldara) is an immunomodulating drug that has demonstrated efficacy in treating actinic keratoses, basal cell carcinoma, and anogenital warts. While its exact mechanism of action is unknown, it is believed to enhance the body's immune response to these conditions. It is applied two to five times per week, as prescribed, depending on the condition being treated. Adverse reactions include mild skin reactions (burning, induration [hardness], irritation, pain, bleeding), which can occur both locally (at the site of medication administration) and at skin areas *remote* from the site of administration. More severe adverse skin reactions include edema, erosion or ulceration, scaling, scabbing, exudate, and vesicles. Systemic reactions, likely related to systemic immunomodulating effects, include cough, upper respiratory infection, musculoskeletal reactions (e.g., back pain), and lymphadenopathy. This drug is available only in cream form.

pimecrolimus

The latest immunomodulating dermatological drug, pimecrolimus (Elidel), is available in cream form for treating atopic dermatitis. This condition is caused by a hereditary susceptibility to pruritus and is often associated with allergic rhinitis, hay fever, and asthma. This drug works through a mechanism similar to that of the anti–transplant-rejection drug tacrolimus (Advagraf, Prograf), which was discussed in Chapter 46 on immunosuppressant drugs.

WOUND CARE DRUGS

Although superficial skin wounds often require minimal interventions, deeper skin wounds require more definitive care for optimal healing. Such care includes addressing the systemic issues (e.g., body nutritional status) that are critical to tissue repair. Topical wound care medications are key to one of the fundamental steps of wound care, referred to in the literature as preparation of the wound bed. The concept of wound débridement refers to removal of nonviable tissue and removal of bacteria by suitable cleansing. Table 57-6 lists information on selected, currently available wound care medications.

TABLE 57-6

Select Wound-Care Products

Product Name	Category	Advantages	Disadvantages	Contraindications
collagenase (Santyl)	Selective	Good for patients on anticoagulants or in whom surgery is contraindicated; selectively removes necrotic tissue; does not harm normal tissue; satisfactory for infected wounds	Requires prescriber's order; not for use with other common wound care products such as Dakin's solution; expensive	Clean, well-granulating wound; product allergies
iodine (locidedosorb, others)	Chemical, nonselective	Slow-release; safe for viable cells; absorbs exudates; promotes wound healing	Partly toxic to fibroblast cells; stains tissue	Iodine allergy
sodium hypochlorite (Dakin's solution 0.5% modified)	Chemical, nonselective	Aids débridement; reduces microbial count	Partly toxic and irritating to healing tissue	Clean, noninfected wounds

NURSING PROCESS

Assessment

Before using any of the dermatological preparations, the nurse should assess the patient for allergies (including those to ingredients such as benzoyl or peroxide), contraindications, cautions, and drug interactions (see previous discussion in the pharmacology section). Topical antibacterials are associated with a wide range of reactions because of the generalized sensitivity of patients to antibiotics, even when in a different dosage form; therefore, if a patient is allergic to a systemic antibacterial, the patient will also be allergic to topical dosage forms. The nurse should also assess the completion of an order for culture and sensitivity testing prior to use of the antibacterial to ensure appropriate identification of sensitive drugs. Before administering any type of topical medication (e.g., antimicrobial, corticosteroid, antiacne drug), the nurse should always consider the concentration of the medication, length of exposure to the skin, condition of the skin, size of the area affected, and hydration status of the skin. All of these factors have significant effects on the action of the medication.

The skin or area affected must be inspected thoroughly under an adequate lighting source and the area palpated with a gloved hand. In dark-skinned patients, an erythematous area may not be visible but may be palpated as an area of warmth. Should there be any possibility of systemic absorption of topical drugs (e.g., tretinoin), liver function studies should be assessed prior to drug therapy. For some antibacterial drugs, the possibility of systemic absorption warrants assessment of baseline kidney and liver functioning. Baseline hearing levels with use of drugs known to be ototoxic should also be assessed. Along with physical assessment of the skin, the surrounding structures, including lymph nodes, should be examined.

The patient's overall health status and hygiene practices should also be assessed, including whether the patient has suffered any trauma or if there is a history of any immunosuppression. The skin of very young children and older adults is more fragile and permeable to certain topical dermatological preparations. These characteristics can lead to a higher risk for systemic absorption from the skin. Other possible situations that may result in an effect that is less than therapeutic, such as the use of topical drugs over an area full of pus or debris, should also be noted. Use of natural health products such as topical aloe requires thorough assessment, and any allergies, contraindications, cautions, and drug interactions should be noted (see Natural Health Products: Aloe, on p. 1041).

Nursing Diagnoses

- Impaired skin integrity related to diseases, reactions, conditions, or breaks in skin barrier
- Acute pain related to the skin condition or from adverse effects of the topical drug
- Deficient knowledge related to lack of experience with and exposure to use of topical drugs
- Ineffective therapeutic regimen related to lack of information about importance of adherence to therapy and maintaining frequent dosing

Planning

Goals

- Patient's skin will remain intact and healed in appearance and integrity.
- Patient will remain adherent to therapy and use the correct application technique.
- Patient will remain free of injury to skin while on therapy.
- Patient will experience minimal to no complications of therapy.

■ Outcome Criteria

- Patient's skin improves daily as stated by the patient, with less redness, drainage, discomfort, itching, and rash.
- Patient experiences increased comfort and minimal pain and itching at the site of skin disorder.
- Patient demonstrates how to apply medication as prescribed and per physician's orders, with specific attention to emollient, lotion, solution, spray, cream, and ointment dosage forms.
- Patient states the rationale for treatment, adverse effects of the specific dermatological preparation, and symptoms to report associated with the dermatological therapy.
- Patient remains adherent to the medication therapy with resultant improved condition of skin or affected area within 2 to 4 weeks of treatment.

■ Implementation

In general, before applying any topical medication, the nurse should cleanse the affected site of any debris and residual medication, making sure to follow any specific directions, such as removing water- or alcohol-based topical preparations with soap and water and using standard precautions (see Box 10–1). The nurse or patient should wear gloves, not only to prevent contamination from secretions but also to prevent absorption of the medication through the skin. A finger-cot, tongue depressor, or cotton-tip applicator is recommended. Lotions and solutions should be shaken or mixed thoroughly before use and evenly applied. Creams, ointments, and emollients are often applied with a sterile cotton-tipped applicator, tongue blade, or gloved hand (see earlier for more information and refer to Chapter 10). Hands should be washed before and after application of the medication.

Any dressings should be applied as ordered, with special attention to directions concerning occlusive, wet, or wet-to-dry dressing changes. Most topical dermatological drugs, however, do not require a dressing once the medication is applied. The medication order may also state avoidance of any sort of dressing or coverage of the area. With wound care and use of medications, there is usually a step-by-step protocol for use of a cleansing agent, possible débridement drug, rinsing solution, and final application of anti-infective, antifungal, burn product, antiseptic, or other solution that may have been ordered.

Patient education for wound care and use of topical dermatological drugs should be comprehensive (see Patient Education for more information). If home health care is needed for care at home, arrangements should be made and in place prior to the patient returning home. Information about the site of application, drainage (colour and amount), swelling, temperature, odour, skin colour, pain, or other sensations, as well as the type of treatment rendered and the response should be documented. This information should be documented with each treatment or application and a "before and after" comparison assessment noted. Patients should be encouraged to continue this documentation when they are able to do so.

The manufacturer's guidelines regarding the use of any of the dermatological preparations should always be followed because each medication has a different type of base solution. All dosage forms of medication should be stored as recommended. Specific application procedures may be required for different dosage forms. It is also important to follow any instructions or orders regarding other treatments to the affected area, such as use of an occlusive or wet dressing. Medicated areas may need to be protected from exposure to air or sunlight. Strict adherence to the proper method of application and dosage of any dermatological preparation is important to its effectiveness, and doubling-up of a missed dose is not recommended. After the patient or nurse has completed the medication administration process, all contaminated dressings, gloves, or equipment should be disposed of properly. See http://evolve.elsevier.com/Canada/Lilley/pharmacology/ for more information about the classifications of topical dermatological drugs and associated nursing implications.

■ Evaluation

Evaluation should always begin with monitoring of goals and outcome criteria. Therapeutic responses to the dermatological preparations include improved condition of skin and healing of lesions or wounds; a decrease in the size of the lesions with eventual resolution; and a decrease in swelling, redness, weeping, itching, and burning of the area. The physician, advanced practice registered nurse, or nurse practitioner should be notified if a therapeutic response is not noted within an appropriate time frame (anywhere from 48 to 72 hours or longer, depending on the drug, disorder, skin problem, or chronicity) or if signs and symptoms worsen or new ones appear. Adverse effects to evaluate for include increased severity of symptoms—for example, increased redness, swelling, pain, and drainage; fever; or any other unusual problems at the affected area. Adverse effects may range from slight irritation of the site where the topical drug has been applied, to an allergic reaction, to toxic systemic effects.

PATIENT EDUCATION

❖ Patients should be instructed about keeping the skin clean and dry and maintaining adequate general hygiene, cleanliness, adequate hydration, and proper nutrition during drug therapy. The patient needs to understand how to prepare the skin for application of medication and to follow instructions as provided.

❖ Patient should be informed to avoid exposure to sunlight during drug therapy and to always wear sunscreen if sun exposure is allowed.

❖ If indicated or ordered, patients should be instructed on how to apply dressings to the area after the medication has been applied. Proper disposal of contaminated dressings or equipment should be emphasized. Thorough hand-washing before and after application of medication should also be emphasized and demonstrated to all those involved in the care of the patient. Adherence and its importance should also be stressed.

❖ Patients should be encouraged to notify the physician of any unusual or adverse reactions or if the original problem or condition worsens or shows a lack of improvement within a designated period.

❖ All female patients of childbearing age should be counselled about the birth defect hazards associated with exposure to certain dermatological drugs. All sexually active women must use contraception during treatment and for at least 1 month after use of any teratogenic medication.

POINTS TO REMEMBER

❖ Topical drugs are used to treat dermatological infections.

❖ Common skin disorders caused by bacteria are folliculitis, impetigo, furuncles, carbuncles, and cellulitis.

❖ The bacterium most commonly responsible for acne is *Propionibacterium acnes*. The fungi that are responsible for causing topical fungal infections are *Candida*, dermatophytes, and *Malassezia furfur*.

❖ The most common topical fungal infections are *Candida* infections, for example, yeast infections.

❖ Some of the most common topical viral infections are herpes simplex types 1 and 2 infections.

❖ Topical anaesthetics are used therapeutically to topically numb the skin. Indications for topical anaesthetics include insect bites, sunburn, poison ivy, and painful injections.

❖ Corticosteroids are some of the most widely used topical drugs that are indicated for relief of topical inflammatory and pruritic disorders.

❖ Beneficial effects of corticosteroids include anti-inflammatory, antipruritic, and vasoconstrictor actions.

❖ Adverse and toxic reactions to dermatological drugs can and do occur; therefore, these drugs should be administered cautiously and the physician's orders and manufacturer's guidelines followed. This practice is critical to ensure safe and effective treatment.

❖ Patient education about the medication, its administration, and its effectiveness is important to ensure adherence.

EXAMINATION REVIEW QUESTIONS

1 When performing wound care to a burn area with silver sulfadiazine, which method is correct?
 a. Apply cream to the wound four times a day.
 b. Do not débride the area before application of the cream.
 c. Cleanse the area first, then apply the drug with a clean-gloved hand.
 d. Use a sterile-gloved hand to apply cream to cleansed and débrided areas.

2 Of the variety of over-the-counter topical corticosteroid products, which preparation is considered the most effective?
 a. Gels
 b. Sprays
 c. Lotions
 d. Ointments

3 Which of the following are indications of allergic reactions to topical bacitracin and similar antimicrobials?
 a. Petechiae
 b. Thickened skin
 c. Purulent drainage
 d. Itching and burning

4 When teaching a patient about the mechanism of action of tretinoin, which statement by the nurse is correct?
 a. "This medication actually causes skin peeling."
 b. "This medication has anti-inflammatory actions."
 c. "This medication acts by killing the bacteria that cause acne."
 d. "This medication acts by protecting your skin from UV sunlight."

5 You are providing wound care with Dakin's solution to a patient who has a stage III pressure ulcer, and the patient exclaims, "I smell bleach! Why are you putting bleach on me?" Which statement is the best explanation?
 a. "We would never use bleach on a patient!"
 b. "This is used to dissolve the dead tissue in your wound."
 c. "This is used instead of medication to promote wound healing."
 d. "This is a diluted solution and acts to reduce the bacteria in the wound so that it can heal."

For answers see http://evolve.elsevier.com/Canada/Lilley/pharmacology/.

CRITICAL THINKING ACTIVITIES

1 Develop a teaching plan for a 29-year-old woman who has a 6-year-old child newly diagnosed with head lice. Emphasize the importance of avoiding contaminating others and preventing future episodes.

2 Discuss the major functions of the epidermis that make its intactness critically important to homeostasis.

3 A 22-year-old woman with severe acne is receiving counselling before taking isotretinoin (Accutane) therapy. She has read the Health Canada online information and is shocked to learn that two negative pregnancy tests are required before starting therapy, and a monthly test done during therapy. What should you tell her to explain these requirements?

For answers see http://evolve.elsevier.com/Canada/Lilley/pharmacology/.

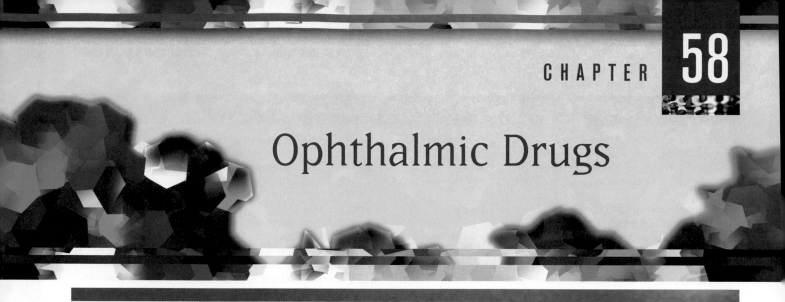

Ophthalmic Drugs

Learning Objectives

After reading this chapter, the successful student will be able to do the following:

1 Discuss the anatomy and physiology of the structures of the eye and how the structures are affected by glaucoma and other disorders and disease processes.

2 List the classifications of ophthalmic drugs, with examples of specific drugs.

3 Discuss the mechanisms of action, indications, dosage forms with application techniques, adverse effects, cautions, contraindications, and drug interactions of ophthalmic preparations.

4 Develop a collaborative plan of care related to the nursing process for patients receiving ophthalmic drugs.

e-Learning Activities

Web site
(http://evolve.elsevier.com/Canada/Lilley/pharmacology/)

evolve learning system

- Animations
- Answers to chapter questions, activities, and case studies
- Calculators and Category Catchers
- Glossary with audio pronunciations
- IV Therapy and Medication Error Checklists
- Multiple-Choice Review Question quizzes
- Nursing Care Plans
- Online Appendices and Supplements
- WebLinks

Drug Profiles

    acetylcholine (acetylcholine chloride)*, p. 1056
    apraclonidine (apraclonidine hydrochloride)*, p. 1057
▸▸ artificial tears, p. 1069
▸▸ atropine sulfate, p. 1068
▸▸ bacitracin, p. 1064
▸▸ betaxolol (betaxolol hydrochloride)*, p. 1058
▸▸ ciprofloxacin (ciprofloxacin hydrochloride)*, p. 1064
    cromolyn (cromolyn sodium)*, p. 1069
    cyclopentolate (cyclopentolate hydrochloride)*, p. 1068
▸▸ dexamethasone, p. 1067
▸▸ dipivefrin (dipivefrin hydrochloride)*, p. 1057
▸▸ dorzolamide, brinzolamide, p. 1060
    emedastine (emedastine difumarate)*, p. 1069
▸▸ erythromycin, p. 1063
    fluorescein, p. 1068
    flurbiprofen (flurbiprofen sodium)*, p. 1067
▸▸ gentamicin (gentamicin sulfate)*, p. 1063
    ketorolac (ketorolac tromethamine)*, p. 1067
▸▸ latanoprost, p. 1062
    mannitol, p. 1061
▸▸ pilocarpine (pilocarpine hydrochloride)*, p. 1056
▸▸ sulfacetamide (sulfacetamide sodium)*, p. 1064
    tetracaine (tetracaine hydrochloride)*, p. 1068
    tetrahydrozoline (tetrahydrozoline hydrochloride)*, p. 1069
▸▸ timolol (timolol maleate)*, p. 1059
    trifluridine, p. 1064

▸▸ Key drug.

*Full generic name is given in parentheses. For the purposes of this text, the more common shortened name is used.

Glossary

Accommodation The adjustment of the lens of the eye to variation in distance. (p. 1052)

Angle-closure glaucoma Glaucoma that occurs as a result of a narrowed anatomical angle between the lens and cornea. (p. 1052)

Anterior chamber The space of the eyeball between the iris and the cornea that contains the aqueous humor. (p. 1049)

Aqueous humor The clear, watery fluid circulating in the anterior and posterior chambers of the eye. (p. 1051)

Bactericidal Describes any substance that kills bacteria. (p. 1063)

Bacteriostatic Describes any substance that inhibits the growth and reproduction of bacteria. (p. 1064)

Canal of Schlemm A tiny circular vein at the angle of the anterior chamber of the eye through which the aqueous humor is drained and ultimately funnelled into the bloodstream. Also called *Schlemm's canal*. (p. 1052)

Cataract An abnormal progressive condition of the lens of the eye, characterized by loss of transparency, with resultant blurred vision. (p. 1051)

Ciliary muscle   The circular muscle between the anterior and posterior chambers behind the iris. It is connected to the *suspensory ligaments* that modulate the curvature of the *lens*. (p. 1051)

Cones   Photoreceptive (light-receiving) cells in the retina of the eye that enable a person to visualize colours and that play a large role in *central* (straight-ahead) vision. (p. 1052)

Cornea   The convex, transparent anterior part of the eye. (p. 1051)

Cycloplegia   Paralysis of the *ciliary muscles*, which prevents the accommodation of the lens to variations in distance. (p. 1052)

Cycloplegics   Drugs that paralyze the ciliary muscles. (p. 1052)

Dilator muscle   A muscle that constricts the *iris* of the eye but dilates the pupil. Also called *dilator pupillae*. (p. 1051)

Glaucoma   An abnormal condition of elevated pressure within the eye because of obstruction of the outflow of aqueous humor. (p. 1052)

Intraocular pressure (IOP)   The internal pressure of all fluids in the eye. (p. 1051)

Iris   A pigmented (coloured) membrane in the eye that controls the amount of light reaching the retina. (p. 1051)

Lacrimal ducts   Small tubes that drain tears from the lacrimal glands into the nasal cavity. (p. 1051)

Lacrimal glands   Glands located at the medial corner of the eyelids that produce *tears*. (p. 1051)

Lens   The transparent crystalline, curved structure of the eye that is located directly behind the iris and the pupil and attached to the ciliary body by ligaments. (p. 1051)

Lysozyme   An enzyme with antiseptic actions that destroys some foreign organisms. It is normally present in tears, saliva, sweat, and breast milk. (p. 1051)

Miotics   Drugs that constrict the pupil. (p. 1052)

Mydriatics   Drugs that dilate the pupil. (p. 1052)

Open-angle glaucoma   A type of glaucoma that is often bilateral, develops slowly, is genetically determined, and does not involve a narrow angle between the *iris* and the *cornea*. (p. 1052)

Optic nerve   A major nerve that connects the posterior end of each eye to the brain, to which it transmits visual signals. (p. 1052)

Posterior chamber   The part of the eye that is behind the iris but in front of the vitreous body. Includes the lens and its suspensory ligaments, as well as aqueous humor. (p. 1052)

Pupil   A circular opening in the iris of the eye, located slightly to the nasal side of the centre of the iris. (p. 1051)

Retina   The layer of the eye that forms the visual image. (p. 1052)

Rods   Tiny cylindrical photoreceptive elements arranged perpendicularly to the surface of the retina that produce black-and-white vision and help provide peripheral vision. (p. 1052)

Sphincter pupillae   A muscle that expands the iris while constricting or narrowing the diameter of the *pupil*. (p. 1051)

Tears   Watery saline or alkaline fluid secreted by the lacrimal glands to moisten the conjunctiva. (p. 1051)

Uvea   The fibrous tunic beneath the sclera that includes the *iris*, the ciliary body, and the choroid of the eye. Also called *tunica vasculosa bulbi* or *uveal tract*. (p. 1051)

Vitreous humor   A transparent, semigelatinous substance contained in a thin membrane filling the cavity behind the lens of the eye. Also called the *corpus vitreum* or *vitreous body*. (p. 1051)

OCULAR ANATOMY AND PHYSIOLOGY

To thoroughly understand the drugs used to treat disorders of the eye, it is necessary to understand the structure and normal function of the eye. The eye is the organ responsible for the sense of sight. Figure 58-1 illustrates the structures of the eye, all of which are needed for accurate eyesight. Each eyeball is nearly spherical and approximately 2.5 cm in diameter. Each eye is recessed into a small skull cavity, known as the *orbit*. The exposed anterior chamber of the eye is covered by three layers: the protective external layer (*cornea* and *sclera*), a vascular middle layer known as the *uvea* (which includes the *choroid*, *iris*, and *ciliary body*), and the internal layer, known as the *retina*. All of these layers are protected by the *eyelid*, which serves as an external protection device.

Each eye is held in place and moved by six muscles controlled by cranial nerves. These muscles include the *rectus* and *oblique* muscles. There are four types of rectus muscles: *inferior*, *superior*, *medial*, and *lateral*. These muscles are shown in Figure 58-2. (The medial rectus muscle is not shown in this figure but can be visualized to be directly across from the lateral rectus muscle.) The *levator palpebrae superioris* muscle opens the eyelid (see later). This muscle rests on top of the superior rectus muscle.

There are several other important structures that are either part of or adjacent to the eye. The structures and purposes of each are as follows:

- *Eyebrow:* Rows of short hair above the upper eyelids. The eyebrow protects the eye from direct light, falling dust or other small particles, and perspiration coming from the forehead.
- *Eyelid:* The eyelid consists of an outer layer of skin, a middle layer of muscle, and an inner conjunctiva. The *conjunctiva* is a thin, transparent tissue that covers the outer anterior surface of the eye and that also lines the inside of the eyelids. It can be thought of as a window that sits in front of the lens and allows the passage of light. The eyelid is movable and can open or close. It protects the eye when closed and allows

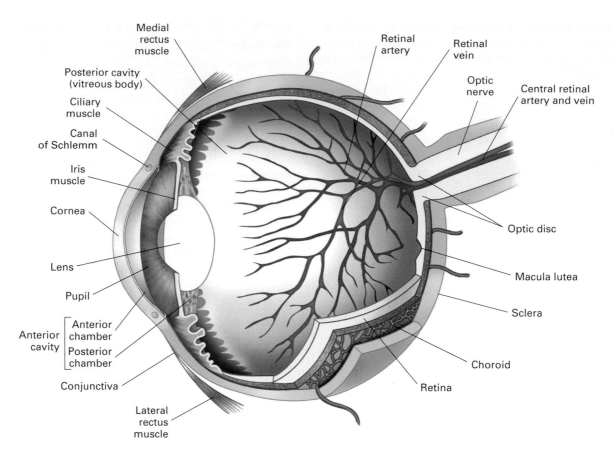

FIG. 58-1 A horizontal section through the left eyeball, looking from the top down. (Modified from Thibodeau, G. A., & Patton, K. T. (2003). *Anatomy and physiology* (5th ed.). St. Louis, MO: Mosby.)

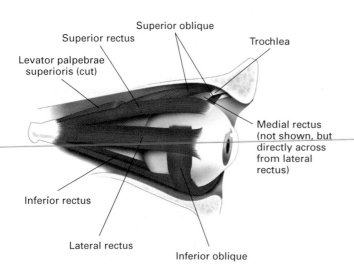

FIG. 58-2 Extrinsic muscles of the right eye. Lateral view. (Modified from Thibodeau, G. A., & Patton, K. T. (2003). *Anatomy and physiology* (5th ed.). St. Louis, MO: Mosby.)

vision when open. The eyelid is raised by contraction of the levator palpebrae superioris muscle and is lowered by relaxation of this muscle (see Figure 58-2).

- *Eyelashes:* Two or three rows of hairs located on the edge (*margin*) of the eyelids. They help prevent small particles from falling into the eye when it is open.

- *Palpebral fissure:* The space between the upper and lower eyelids when the eyelids are open but relaxed.
- *Sclera:* A tough, white coat of fibrous tissue that surrounds the entire eyeball, except the cornea. It helps maintain the shape of the eye. Commonly called the *white* of the eye, the sclera is nonvascular and allows light to pass through it to the lens.
- *Choroid:* One of the middle-layer structures of the eyeball that contains the blood vessels supplying the eye; it also absorbs light.
- *Ciliary body:* The structure that supports the ciliary muscles that control the curvature of the lens via attached suspensory ligaments.
- *Conjunctiva:* The mucous membrane that lines the eyelids and also covers the exposed anterior surface of the eyeball.
- *Iris:* The coloured (*pigmented*) muscular apparatus behind the cornea.
- *Pupil:* The variable-sized opening in the centre of the iris that allows light to enter into the eyeball when the eyelids are open. Its diameter changes with contraction and relaxation of the muscular fibres of the iris as the eye responds to changes in light, emotional states, and other kinds of stimulation. The pupil is the rear portion of the window of the eye through which light passes to the lens and the retina (the cornea being the front part of this "window").

- *Medial canthus:* The site near the nose where the upper and lower eyelids unite.
- *Lacrimal caruncle:* A small, red, rounded elevation covered by modified skin at the medial angle of the eye; the site of the lacrimal glands (see section below).
- *Lateral canthus:* The site away from the nose where the upper and lower eyelids unite.

LACRIMAL GLANDS

The eye is kept moist and healthy by an intricate network of connected canals, ducts, and sacs that work together. The **lacrimal glands** produce tears that bathe and cleanse the exposed anterior portion of the eye. **Tears** are composed of an isotonic, aqueous solution that contains an enzyme called **lysozyme**, which acts as an antibacterial agent to prevent eye infections. Tears drain into the nasal cavity through the **lacrimal ducts**.

LAYERS OF THE EYE

The eye has three separate anatomical layers. The fibrous *outer layer* of the eye has two parts that are continuous with each other: the *sclera* and the *cornea*. The sclera is a tough, fibrous layer that protects and maintains the shape of the eye. The **cornea** is a nonvascular transparent portion of the outer layer that allows light to enter the eye. It is located at the extreme front of the eye and is continuous with the sclera. It is pain sensitive, has a protective function, and obtains nutrition from **aqueous humor,** the clear, watery fluid that circulates in the *anterior* and *posterior chambers* of the eye (see discussion below).

The vascular *middle layer* of the eye is composed of the *iris* (to the anterior), ciliary body, and choroid, to the posterior. These three structures are collectively called the **uvea**. The **iris** gives colour to the eye and has an adjustable-sized opening in the centre called the **pupil.** The main function of the iris is to regulate the amount of light that enters the eye by causing the size of the pupil to vary. Pupil size is controlled by two circular smooth muscles. The **sphincter pupillae** muscle is controlled by the parasympathetic nervous system and constricts (miosis) the diameter of the pupil (Figure 58-3). A *sphincter* is any circular band of muscle fibres that constricts a passage or closes a natural opening in the body (e.g., pyloric sphincter). Impulses from the parasympathetic nervous system operate this muscle. In contrast, the pupil is opened (mydriasis) by a radial smooth muscle called the **dilator muscle**. It is composed of radiating fibres, like spokes of a wheel, that converge from the circumference of the iris toward its centre. Sympathetic nervous system impulses control this muscle (see Figure 58-3).

The anterior portions of both the retina and choroid merge to become the *ciliary body*, which produces aqueous humor. This clear, watery fluid should not be confused with tears (described earlier). Aqueous humor, along with vitreous humor (see later), also contributes to the **intraocular pressure (IOP)** of the eye. The IOP is the internal pressure of all fluids against the tunics (retina, choroid, sclera) of the eye. Obviously, given the already small space of the eye, any change in the volume of aqueous humor present can lead to increased or reduced IOP. The ciliary body also provides a support for the *suspensory ligaments* that support the lens (see later). Normally, the aqueous humor is removed from the anterior chamber via the canal of Schlemm at a rate that balances out its production by the ciliary body. The *choroid* is a thin, dark layer that lines most of the internal side of the sclera. The function of the choroid is to absorb light and prevent its reflection out of the eye. The choroid is also the major location of the network of blood vessels that supply each eye.

The **lens** is the transparent crystalline structure of the eye, located directly behind the iris and the pupil. It has a *biconvex* (oval-spherical) shape and is held in place by *suspensory ligaments* attached to the **ciliary muscles**. Contraction of the ciliary muscles modifies the tension of the suspensory ligaments, which changes the shape of the lens. This function is important for visual accommodation as well as for focusing light (and visual images) onto the retina. These muscles are controlled by the parasympathetic nervous system (PSNS) through the oculomotor cranial nerve (CN-III). Accordingly, the lens divides the interior of the eyeball into posterior and anterior chambers. The larger chamber behind the lens is filled with a jelly-like fluid called **vitreous humor.** The lens is normally transparent to easily allow the passage of light. It is composed of uniform layers of protein fibres encased by a clear connective tissue capsule. A loss of lens transparency results in a visual condition called a **cataract.** This is a grey-white opacity that can be seen within the lens. If cataracts are untreated, sight may eventually be completely lost. At the onset of a cataract, vision is blurred and may be further worsened by the glare of bright lights. Diplopia, or double vision, may also develop.

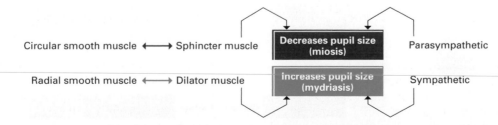

FIG. 58-3   Different nervous systems control pupil size.

Before light images reach the retina, they are focused into a sharp image by the lens of the eye. The elasticity of the lens enables it to change its shape and focusing power. This process is called **accommodation** and is facilitated by the ciliary body. Paralysis of accommodation is called **cycloplegia.** Drugs that paralyze the ciliary body are called **cycloplegics**, but they also have *mydriatic* properties (e.g., atropine, cyclopentolate) (Figure 58-4). **Mydriatics** are drugs that dilate the pupil (e.g., apraclonidine). Those drugs that constrict the pupil are called **miotics** (e.g., acetylcholine, pilocarpine). All of these medications are used to facilitate visualization of the inner eye during ophthalmic examinations.

The third and inner layer of the eye is a thin, delicate layer known as the **retina**. The basic function of the retina is image formation via light-sensitive photoreceptors called *rods* and *cones*. Both types of photoreceptors are located near the surface of the retina. **Rods** produce black-and-white vision, including shades of grey, especially in low light, and **cones** are responsible for colour vision (Figure 58-5). Additionally, rods are more active in providing peripheral ("off-to-the-side") vision, whereas cones are more active in central vision. The posterior centre part of the retina is attached to the **optic nerve**. The function of the optic nerve is to connect the retina with the visual centre of the brain, located within the occipital lobe that extends above and behind the cerebellum. It is this location within the brain that interprets incoming visual stimuli.

OPHTHALMIC DRUGS

In this chapter, the focus is on the medications used to treat disorders of the eye. Such medications can be divided into several major drug groups: antiglaucoma drugs, antimicrobials, anti-inflammatory drugs, topical anaesthetics, diagnostics, antiallergic drugs, and lubricants and moisturizers. There are also a variety of combination drug products that include two or more medications from different subclasses. These products are not discussed further in this chapter; the reader can presume the same therapeutic indications and drug effects as those for the single-ingredient drug products that are discussed here. While the focus of this chapter is on commonly used therapeutic medications, a multitude of other ophthalmic products are also available and used, for example, in

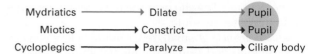

FIG. 58-4 Drug classes and their effects on pupil size.

the care of contact lenses, including contact lens–cleaning enzymes, irrigating solutions, and eye washes. Their use is fairly straightforward with limited risk. The more complex surgical drugs are also beyond the scope of this chapter. The reader is advised to refer to manufacturer information on the package for information on any unfamiliar product encountered in clinical practice.

ANTIGLAUCOMA DRUGS

As noted, the aqueous humor is a nourishing liquid that is produced by the ciliary body and flows from the **posterior chamber** (behind the iris) to the **anterior chamber** (in front of the iris). The liquid is removed via the **canal of Schlemm**, which is located adjacent to the union of the sclera and cornea in the anterior chamber. When the normal flow and drainage of aqueous humor is inhibited, it is not drained through the canal of Schlemm as quickly as it is formed by the ciliary body. The accumulated aqueous humor creates a backward IOP that pushes vitreous humor against the retina. This creates a serious ocular condition called **glaucoma.** The two major types of glaucoma for purposes of this chapter are **angle-closure glaucoma** and **open-angle glaucoma**. Figure 58-6 shows the pathophysiology of each and provides an enlarged view of the involved eye structures. Table 58-1 lists additional characteristic features of each. Glaucoma can be a primary illness (occurring on its own) or secondary to another eye condition or injury (e.g., post-traumatic glaucoma). Congenital glaucoma can occur in infants. Glaucoma can occur even in the absence of increased IOP (normotensive glaucoma). There are a few other more extraordinary forms of glaucoma (e.g., pigmentary glaucoma, pseudoexfoliative glaucoma) that are also beyond the scope of this chapter.

If glaucoma is left untreated, continued pressure on the retina destroys its neurons, leading to impaired vision and eventual blindness (Figure 58-7). Effective treatment of glaucoma involves reducing IOP by either increasing the drainage of aqueous humor or decreasing

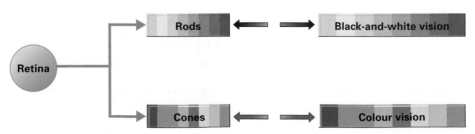

FIG. 58-5 Function of rods and cones in relation to colour vision.

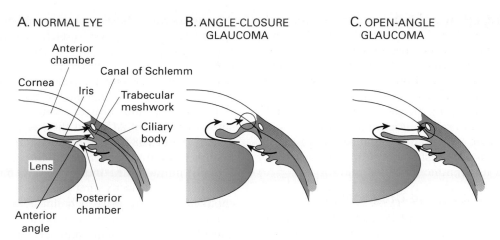

FIG. 58-6 Main structures of the eye and an enlargement of the canal of Schlemm showing an aqueous flow. *A,* Normal eye. *B,* In angle-closure glaucoma, the closure of the anterior angle prevents aqueous humor from exiting through the canal of Schlemm, leading to increased intraocular pressure. *C,* In open-angle glaucoma, the anterior angle remains open, but the canal of Schlemm is obstructed by tissue abnormalities. (Modified from McKenry, L. M., Tessier, E., & Hogan, M. A. (2006). *Mosby's pharmacology in nursing–revised and updated* (22nd ed.). St. Louis, MO: Mosby.)

TABLE 58-1

Glaucoma: Types and Characteristics

	Angle-Closure	Open-Angle
Synonyms	Closed-angle glaucoma, narrow-angle glaucoma, congestive glaucoma, and pupillary closure glaucoma	Chronic glaucoma, wide-angle glaucoma, and simple glaucoma
Chronicity	Acute (can cause rapid vision loss)	Chronic
Major symptoms	Blurred vision, severe headaches, eye pain	Blurred vision, occasional headaches
Most common age of onset and race	Older than 30 yr, White	Older than 30 yr, Black
Nature of angle	Narrow	Larger
Treatment	Topical or systemic drugs, surgery	Topical or systemic drugs, surgery
Relative incidence	Less common	More common

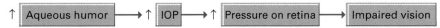

FIG. 58-7 How increased aqueous humor can result in impaired vision. *IOP,* intraocular pressure.

the production of aqueous humor. Some drugs may do both. Effective drug therapy can delay and possibly even prevent the development of glaucoma. Drugs used to reduce IOP include the following:

- Cholinergics, direct-acting (also called miotics and parasympathomimetic drugs)
- Cholinergics, indirect-acting (also called miotics, cholinesterase inhibitors, and parasympathomimetic drugs)
- Adrenergics (also called mydriatics and sympathomimetic drugs)
- Antiadrenergics (β-blockers; also called sympatholytic drugs)
- Carbonic anhydrase inhibitors
- Osmotic diuretics
- Parasympathomimetics, direct-acting
- Prostaglandin agonists

See Table 58-2 for a comparison of drug effects on aqueous humor flow.

TABLE 58-2

Antiglaucoma Drug Effects on Aqueous Humor

Drug Class	Increased Drainage	Decreased Production
MIOTICS		
Direct-acting cholingerics	+++	0
Indirect-acting cholinergics (cholinesterase inhibitors)	+++	0
MYDRIATICS		
Sympathomimetic	++	+++
OTHERS		
β-blockers	+	+++
Carbonic anhydrase inhibitors	0	+++
Osmotic diuretics	+++	0
Prostaglandin agonist	+++	0

0 = no effect; + = minor effect; ++ = moderate effect; +++ = pronounced effect.

CHOLINERGIC DRUGS

There are two categories of ocular parasympathomimetic drugs, more concisely referred to as cholinergic drugs: direct-acting and indirect-acting. Direct-acting cholinergics include acetylcholine, carbachol, and pilocarpine. Indirect-acting drugs, which are also called cholinesterase inhibitors, include echothiophate (currently not available in Canada). Because one primary drug effect is pupillary constriction or miosis (see later), these drugs are also commonly called miotics.

Mechanism of Action and Drug Effects

As discussed in Chapters 20 and 21, acetylcholine (ACh) is the endogenous neurochemical mediator of nerve impulses in the parasympathetic nervous system (PSNS). It stimulates parasympathetic or cholinergic receptors located in the brain and throughout the body along PSNS nerve branches. This action results in several effects on the eye: miosis (pupillary constriction), vasodilation of blood vessels in and around the eye, contraction of ciliary muscles, drainage of aqueous humor, and reduced IOP. The ciliary muscle contraction itself promotes aqueous humor drainage by widening the space where the

drainage occurs. Miosis promotes aqueous humor drainage by causing the iris to stretch, which also serves to widen this space. The action of ACh is normally short lived. It is rapidly hydrolyzed to *choline* and *acetic acid* by two cholinesterase enzymes known as acetylcholinesterase (AChE) and pseudocholinesterase (Figure 58-8).

Both direct- and indirect-acting miotics have effects similar to those of ACh, but their actions are more prolonged (Figure 58-9). The direct-acting miotics are able to directly stimulate ocular cholinergic receptors and actually mimic ACh. Indirect-acting miotics work by binding to and inactivating the cholinesterases (acetylcholinesterase and pseudocholinesterase), the enzymes that break down ACh by hydrolysis, as noted earlier. As a result, ACh accumulates and acts longer at the cholinergic receptor sites. This process leads to drug effects including miosis, ciliary muscle contraction, enhanced aqueous humor drainage, and reduced IOP by an average of 20% to 30% (Figure 58-10). Drug-induced miotic effects may be less pronounced in individuals with dark eyes (e.g., brown or hazel) than in those with lighter eyes (e.g., blue) because the pigment of the iris also absorbs the drug (reducing its therapeutic effects), and dark eyes have more pigment.

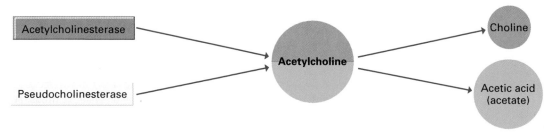

FIG. 58-8 Metabolism of acetylcholine by endogenous enzymes.

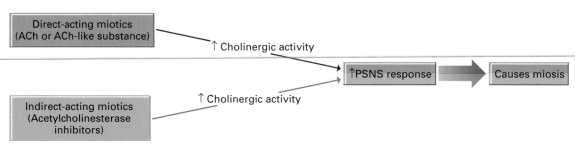

FIG. 58-9 Cholinergic response of miosis to parasympathomimetics. *ACh,* acetylcholine; *PSNS,* parasympathetic nervous system.

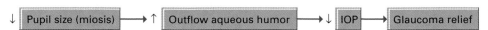

FIG. 58-10 The therapeutic effects of direct- and indirect-acting parasympathomimetics on glaucoma. *IOP,* intraocular pressure.

Indications

The direct- and indirect-acting miotics are used for open-angle glaucoma, angle-closure glaucoma, ocular surgery, and convergent strabismus (a condition in which one eye points toward the other ["cross-eye"]). They are also used to reverse the effect of mydriatic (pupil-dilating) drugs following ophthalmic examination. Specific indications may vary among drugs, as shown in Table 58-3.

Contraindications

Contraindications of miotics include known drug allergy and any serious active eye disorder in which induction of miosis might be harmful. An ophthalmologist will usually make this judgement.

Adverse Effects

Most of the adverse effects associated with the use of the cholinergic drugs and anticholinesterase drugs (miotics) are local and limited to the eye. This quality is an advantage of ocular drug administration. Ocular adverse effects are more likely with indirect-acting miotics as they usually have longer-lasting effects; it takes more time for the ocular tissues to synthesize new cholinesterase enzymes. Effects include blurred vision, drug-induced myopia (nearsightedness), and accommodative spasms. Such effects are secondary to contraction of the ciliary muscle, resulting in spasm (paralysis) of visual accommodation by the lens. Miotic drugs also cause vasodilation of blood vessels supplying the conjunctiva, iris, and ciliary body. This action results in increased permeability of the blood–aqueous barrier, which may lead to vascular congestion and ocular inflammation. The blood–aqueous barrier is the anatomical barrier that normally prevents exchange of fluids between eye chambers and the blood, comparable with the blood–brain barrier mentioned in Chapter 2. Other undesirable effects include temporary stinging upon drug instillation, reduced night-time or low-light vision, conjunctivitis, lacrimation (tearing), twitching eyelids (blepharospasm),

and eye or brow pain. Prolonged use can result in iris cysts, lens opacities, and, rarely, retinal detachment.

As discussed earlier, systemic effects are uncommon with local ocular drug administration but are more likely to occur with cholinesterase inhibitors (indirect-acting miotics). When they do occur, they are due to generalized cholinergic stimulation apart from the eyes, as would be expected with any systemically administered cholinergic drug. Sufficient drug absorption into the general circulation must occur for systemic effects to appear. Possible systemic adverse effects are listed in Table 58-4.

Toxicity and Management of Overdose

Occasionally, toxic effects may develop after the use of topically applied miotic drugs. Toxicity produced by miotics is an extension of their systemic effects and is more common with prolonged use of high doses. Most severe and prolonged effects are seen with long-acting anticholinesterases. Excessive PSNS effects are treated with intravenous or intramuscular atropine. Epinephrine may be used for bronchoconstriction or bradycardia.

Interactions

As with the systemic adverse effects, drug interactions are unlikely due to primarily local drug actions. When given with topical adrenergic, antiadrenergic (e.g., β-blockers), and carbonic anhydrase inhibitors, however, miotic drugs can have additive-lowering effects on IOP. Systemic cholinergic drugs can theoretically have additive effects when given with mitotic drugs. Indirect-acting miotics (cholinesterase inhibitors) may also potentiate the effects of the neuromuscular blocker succinylcholine (Chapter 12), possibly leading to cardio-respiratory arrest.

Dosages

For recommended dosages of miotic drugs, see the Dosages table on p. 1056.

TABLE	58-3

Miotics: Indications

Miotic Drug	Indications
acetylcholine	Complete and rapid miosis after cataract lens extraction, iridectomy
carbachol	Open-angle glaucoma
echothiophate	Accommodative esotropia, obstructive aqueous humor outflow, open- and angle-closure glaucoma after iridectomy
pilocarpine	Open-angle glaucoma, secondary glaucoma after iridectomy, cycloplegic reversal

TABLE	58-4

Miotics: Adverse Effects

Body System	Adverse Effects
Cardiovascular	Hypotension, bradycardia, or tachycardia
Central nervous	Headache
Dermatological	Sweating
Gastrointestinal	Salivation, nausea, vomiting, abdominal cramps, diarrhea
Genitourinary	Urinary incontinence
Respiratory	Bronchoconstriction, including asthma attacks

DRUG PROFILES

DIRECT-ACTING MIOTICS

Direct-acting ocular cholinergics include acetylcholine chloride (Miochol E, Miogan PSW), carbachol (Miostat), and pilocarpine hydrochloride (Akarpine, Diocarpine, Minims). Indirect-acting drugs, also called cholinesterase inhibitors, are not available in Canada. These drugs are used for glaucoma, as adjuncts for ocular surgery, and for other ophthalmic conditions.

acetylcholine chloride

Acetylcholine chloride (Miochol E, Miogan PSW) is a direct-acting parasympathomimetic drug used to produce miosis during ophthalamic surgery. It is a pharmaceutical form of the naturally occurring neurotransmitter in the body. It begins to work almost immediately. When used for ophthalmic indications, acetylcholine is administered directly into the anterior chamber of the eye before and after securing one or more sutures. It is available as 10 and 20 mg powders for intraophthalmic use only.

PHARMACOKINETICS

Half-Life	Onset	Peak	Duration
Short (few minutes)	Instant	Instant	10 min

▶▶ pilocarpine hydrochloride

Pilocarpine hydrochloride (Akarpine, Diocarpine, Minims) is a direct-acting parasympathomimetic drug used as a miotic in the treatment of glaucoma. Pilocarpine is available in many different formulations and strengths as an ophthalmic gel and solution.

PHARMACOKINETICS

Half-Life	Onset	Peak	Duration
Unknown	10–30 min	75 min	4–8 hr

DOSAGES — Selected Miotics (Parasympathomimetics)

Drug (Pregnancy Category)	Pharmacological Class	Usual Dosage Range	Indications
acetylcholine chloride (Miochol E, Miogan PSW) (C)	Direct-acting	0.5 to 2 mL preoperative	Surgical miosis
▶▶ pilocarpine hydrochloride (Akarpine, Diocarpine, Minims) (C)	Direct-acting	Solution: 1–2 drops tid–qid Gel: 0.5 inch into lower conjunctival sac at bedtime (use any other eye drops at least 5 min before gel)	Chronic open-angle and angle-closure glaucoma; acute angle-closure glaucoma; pre- and postoperative intraocular hypertension; reversal of drug-induced mydriasis

SYMPATHOMIMETICS

Sympathomimetic drugs are used for the treatment of glaucoma and ocular hypertension. These drugs include the α-receptor agonists brimonidine (Alphagan) and apraclonidine hydrochloride (Iopidine), epinephrine hydrochloride (Epinrin), and the α- and β-receptor agonist dipivefrin (Propine).

Mechanism of Action and Drug Effects

Because these drugs are sympathomimetic drugs, they mimic the sympathetic neurotransmitters norepinephrine and epinephrine and stimulate the dilator muscle to contract by means of α- or β-receptor interaction or that of both receptors. This stimulation results in increased pupil size, or mydriasis (Figure 58-11). Dilation is seen within minutes of instillation of the ophthalmic drops and lasts for several hours, during which time the IOP is reduced (Figure 58-12). The exact mechanism by which the sympathomimetic drugs lower IOP is unknown. However, α-receptor stimulation is known to reduce IOP by enhancing aqueous humor outflow through the canal of Schlemm. Another possible drug effect is the reduction of aqueous humor production by the ciliary body. All of these effects appear to be dose dependent.

Indications

Both epinephrine and dipivefrin may be used to reduce elevated IOP in the treatment of chronic, open-angle glaucoma, either as initial therapy or as chronic therapy. Apraclonidine is used primarily to inhibit perioperative IOP increases. Increases in IOP during ophthalmic

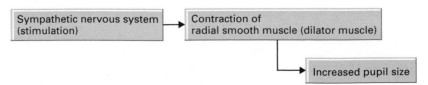

FIG. 58-11 Mechanism of mydriasis.

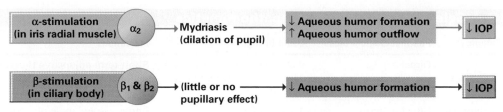

FIG. 58-12 Ocular effects of α- and β-stimulation. *IOP*, intraocular pressure.

surgery are usually mediated via increased catecholamine stimulation of the sympathetic nervous system (SNS). Apraclonidine stimulates the α_2-receptors, which oppose these effects, and thus corrects the surgery-induced changes in IOP. Brimonidine also has primarily α_2-activity but is normally used to lower IOP in patients with open-angle glaucoma or ocular hypertension.

Contraindications

Contraindications for the sympathomimetic ophthalmic drugs include drug allergy and may include active, severe ophthalmic problems that, in the judgement of an ophthalmologist, might be aggravated by the effects of these drugs.

Adverse Effects

The adverse effects of the sympathomimetic mydriatics are primarily limited to ocular effects and include burning, eye pain, and lacrimation. Such effects are usually temporary and may subside as the patient grows accustomed to the medication. Other ocular effects include conjunctival hyperemia, localized melanin deposits in the conjunctiva, and released pigment granules from the iris. Although systemic effects associated with the use

of sympathomimetic mydriatics are uncommon, they are possible, especially in larger doses or prolonged drug therapy. They include cardiovascular effects such as extrasystoles, tachycardia, and hypertension. Other effects that may be noticed are headache and feeling faint.

Toxicity and Management of Overdose

Rare toxic reactions to these drugs are primarily the result of an extension of their therapeutic and adverse effects. The most significant reactions are cardiac dysrhythmias. Discontinuation of the drugs usually eliminates the toxic symptoms.

Interactions

With sufficient topical absorption, sympathomimetic mydriatics have the potential to react with other drugs. Cardiac dysrhythmias are potentiated when mydriatic drugs are given with halogenated anaesthetics, cardiac glycosides, thyroid hormones, or tricyclic antidepressants.

Dosages

For recommended dosages of sympathomimetic drugs, see the Dosages table on p. 1058.

 DRUG PROFILES

Sympathomimetic ophthalmic drugs include dipivefrin (Propine), epinephrine hydrochloride (Epinrin), apraclonidine hydrochloride (Iopidine), and brimonidine tartrate (Alphagan, Alphagan P). These drugs are used for glaucoma, ocular hypertension, and ocular surgery.

apraclonidine hydrochloride

Apraclonidine hydrochloride (Iopidine) is structurally and pharmacologically related to the α_2-stimulant clonidine. It reduces IOP 23% to 39% by stimulating α_2- and β_2-receptors. It also prevents ocular vasoconstriction, which reduces ocular blood pressure as well as aqueous humor formation. Apraclonidine is used primarily to inhibit perioperative IOP increases, rather than for glaucoma. Brimonidine (Alphagen, Alphagan P) is a similar drug but is used primarily for glaucoma.

PHARMACOKINETICS

Half-Life	Onset	Peak	Duration
8 hr	1 hr	3–5 hr	12 hr

▶▶ dipivefrin hydrochloride

Dipivefrin hydrochloride (Propine), a synthetic sympathomimetic miotic drug, is a prodrug of epinephrine. The prodrug has little or no pharmacological activity until hydrolyzed in the eye to two forms of epinephrine. These chemical alterations account for the main advantage of this drug over epinephrine. It has enhanced lipophilicity (fat solubility) and can better penetrate into the anterior chamber of the eye. This quality also reduces the likelihood of any systemic adverse effects. Dipivefrin typically reduces mean IOP approximately 15% to 25%. Dipivefrin is 4 to 11 times as potent as epinephrine in reducing IOP and 5 to 12 times as potent as epinephrine in terms of its mydriatic effects. Epinephryl (Epinal) is a newer drug with similar properties and uses. It is available in a combination format with the β-blocker levobunolol hydrochloride (Probeta).

PHARMACOKINETICS

Half-Life	Onset	Peak	Duration
1–3 hr	30 min	1 hr	12 hr

DOSAGES	Selected Ophthalmic Sympathomimetics			
Drug (Pregnancy Category)	Pharmacological Class	Usual Dosage Range	Indications
apraclonidine hydrochloride (Iopidine) (C)	Direct-acting	0.5% solution: 1–2 drops tid 1% solution: 1 drop in eye preoperative	Short-term adjunctive therapy for glaucoma not controlled with other drugs Anterior-segment laser surgery
▸▸ dipivefrin hydrochloride (Propine) (C)	Direct-acting	1 drop q12h	Chronic open-angle glaucoma

β-ADRENERGIC BLOCKERS

The antiglaucoma β-adrenergic blockers that reduce IOP include the selective β₁-blockers and the nonselective β₁- and β₂-blockers. Recall from Chapter 19 that selective β-blockers are also called cardioselective. Betaxolol hydrochloride (Betoptic) is the only β₁-selective blocker available. The available nonselective ophthalmic β₁- and β₂-blockers are levobunolol hydrochloride (Betagan) and timolol maleate (Apo-Timop).

Mechanism of Action and Drug Effects

The ophthalmic β-blockers reduce both elevated and normal IOP, without affecting pupillary size, accommodation, or night vision. They appear to reduce IOP by minimizing aqueous humor formation. In addition, timolol may produce a minimal increase in aqueous outflow.

Indications

Ophthalmic β-blockers are used to reduce elevated IOP in various conditions, including chronic open-angle glaucoma and ocular hypertension. They may also be used alone or in combination with a topical miotic (e.g., pilocarpine), topical dipivefrin, or systemic carbonic anhydrase inhibitors (CAIs). When used in combination, these drugs may have an additive IOP-lowering effect. They may also be used to treat some forms of angle-closure glaucoma.

Contraindications

Contraindications for ophthalmic β-blockers include known drug allergy and any ocular condition in which β-receptor blockade might be harmful.

Adverse Effects

The adverse effects of antiglaucoma β-blockers are primarily ocular effects and limited systemic effects. The most common ocular effects are transient burning and discomfort. Other adverse effects include blurred vision, pain, photophobia, lacrimation, blepharitis, keratitis (inflammation of the cornea), and decreased corneal sensitivity. Because these drugs are administered topically, few, if any, systemic effects are expected. Theoretical systemic effects include bradycardia, bronchospasm, headache, and dizziness, as described for systemic β-blockers in Chapter 19. However, ophthalmic β-blockers have not been shown to affect glucose metabolism.

Toxicity and Management of Overdose

Toxic reactions to β-blockers are rare and involve primarily the cardiovascular system. Symptoms include bradycardia, heart failure, hypotension, and bronchospasms. Treatment comprises discontinuation of the drug and symptomatic care (e.g., adrenergic and anticholinergic drugs).

Interactions

As is the case with adverse effects, drug interactions with systemic drugs are unlikely because of the primarily localized nature of ocularly administered drugs. Theoretically, ophthalmic β-blockers can have additive therapeutic or adverse effects when given with systemically administered β-blockers or other cardiovascular drugs (e.g., calcium channel blockers), up to and including cardiorespiratory arrest.

Dosages

For recommended dosages of β-adrenergic blockers, see the Dosages table on p. 1059.

 DRUG PROFILES

The currently available ophthalmic β-blocking drugs are betaxolol hydrochloride (Betoptic), levobunolol hydrochloride (Betagan), and timolol maleate (Apo-Timop). These drugs are used for glaucoma and ocular hypertension.

▸▸ *betaxolol hydrochloride*

Betaxolol hydrochloride (Betoptic) is a β₁-selective β-blocker. It is structurally related to the systemic adrenergic β-receptor blocker metoprolol that is used primarily for cardiovascular disorders. Its ability to decrease aqueous humor formation and, consequently, IOP has made it an excellent drug for the treatment of ocular disorders such as open-angle glaucoma and ocular hypertension. Betaxolol is available only in liquid form.

PHARMACOKINETICS

Half-Life	Onset	Peak	Duration
Unknown	0.5–1 hr	2 hr	≥ to12 hr

Continued

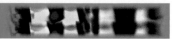

DRUG PROFILES (cont'd)

▶▶ *timolol maleate*

Timolol maleate (Apo-Timop) may differ slightly from the other ophthalmic β-blockers in that it may increase the outflow of aqueous humor as well as its formation. The drug acts at β_1- and β_2-receptors and is indicated for the treatment of open-angle glaucoma and ocular hypertension. It is available in liquid forms, both with preservatives and preservative-free. Preservative-free products were developed for patients with allergies to benzalkonium chloride, a commonly used preservative. Timolol is also available in a gel-forming solution (with preservatives). These gel-forming products are longer acting and allow for once-daily dosing, more convenient than the twice-daily dosing that many patients require of the other timolol formulations. Combination products of timolol are available: with the carbonic anhydrase inhibitor dorzolamide hydrochloride (Cosopt), with the α-adrenergic blocker brimonidine tartrate (Combigan), and with the prostaglandin analogue travoprost (Duotrav).

PHARMACOKINETICS

Half-Life	Onset	Peak	Duration
Unknown	15–30 min	1–2 hr	12–24 hr

DOSAGES   Selected Ophthalmic β-Blockers

Drug (Pregnancy Category)	Pharmacological Class	Usual Dosage Range	Indications
▶▶ **betaxolol hydrochloride (Betoptic) (C)**	Direct-acting	1–2 drops bid	Chronic open-angle glaucoma; ocular hypertension
▶▶ **timolol maleate (Betimol, Timoptic, Tim-AK) (C)**	Direct-acting	Solution: 1 drop bid Gel-forming solution: 1 drop daily	Open-angle glaucoma; ocular hypertension

CARBONIC ANHYDRASE INHIBITORS

Ophthalmic carbonic anhydrase inhibitors (CAIs) include brinzolamide (Azopt) and dorzolamide (Trusopt). Both drugs are also sulfonamides and thus chemically related to sulfonamide antibiotics (Chapter 38). Brinzolamide and dorzolamide are available only in the topical ophthalmic form. Systemic CAIs for oral use, described in Chapter 26 on diuretics, are sometimes used as adjunct drug therapy for glaucoma.

Mechanism of Action and Drug Effects

These drugs work by inhibiting the enzyme *carbonic anhydrase*, which exists throughout the body and is involved in acid–base balance. In the eye, the inhibition of this enzyme results in decreased IOP by reduction of aqueous humor formation.

Indications

Ophthalmic CAIs are used primarily for the treatment of glaucoma, including both open-angle and angle-closure glaucoma. They are also used preoperatively.

Contraindications

Contraindications for ophthalmic CAIs include known drug allergy and any ophthalmic condition in which they might be considered harmful by an ophthalmologist.

Adverse Effects

With these drugs there is systemic absorption, and although systemic adverse effects are unlikely, the same effects of sulfonamide antibiotics, listed in Chapter 38, can theoretically occur with these drugs. Patients with sulfa allergies may develop cross-sensitivities to the CAIs. Specific adverse effects are listed in Table 58-5.

Toxicity and Management of Overdose

Toxicity associated with the use of CAIs is rare. The mechanism by which these drugs work predisposes the patient to possible acidotic states and electrolyte imbalances. These toxic reactions generally require only supportive care, which may include the restoration of electrolytes, especially potassium, and the administration of bicarbonate to correct the CAI-induced acidotic state.

TABLE   58-5

Carbonic Anhydrase Inhibitors: Adverse Effects

Body System	Adverse Effects
Central nervous	Drowsiness, confusion, paraesthesia, seizures
Eyes, ears, nose, throat	Transient myopia, tinnitus
Gastrointestinal	Anorexia, vomiting, diarrhea, liver failure
Genitourinary	Polyuria, hematuria
Hematological	Blood dyscrasias
Integumentary	Urticaria, rare photosensitivity, severe skin reactions (e.g., Stevens–Johnson syndrome)
Metabolic	Acidotic states and electrolyte imbalance with long-term therapy

Interactions

The systemic use of CAIs can result in several significant drug interactions, and ophthalmic CAIs may (but are less likely to) interact with other drugs. CAIs can cause hypokalemia and increase the likelihood of digitalis toxicity. Hypokalemia is more likely to occur when these drugs are coadministered with corticosteroids and diuretics. CAIs increase kidney excretion of lithium, thereby reducing its therapeutic effects. CAIs also tend to increase the effects of basic drugs as a result of decreased kidney excretion.

Dosages

For recommended dosages of selected CAIs, see the Dosages table below.

 DRUG PROFILES

▸▸ dorzolamide and brinzolamide

Dorzolamide (Trusopt) is solely indicated for elevated IOP associated with either ocular hypertension or open-angle glaucoma. It is currently available only as an ophthalmic solution. The other drug in this class, brinzolamide (Azopt), has comparable indications, dosage, and pharmacokinetics.

PHARMACOKINETICS

Half-Life	Onset	Peak	Duration
3–4 mo*	Rapid	Variable	Variable

*Because of red blood cell distribution in plasma.

DOSAGES **Ophthalmic Carbonic Anhydrase Inhibitors**

Drug (Pregnancy Category)	Pharmacological Class	Usual Dosage Range	Indications
brinzolamide (Azopt) (C)	Carbonic anhydrase inhibitor	One drop tid	Open-angle glaucoma; ocular hypertension
▸▸ dorzolamide (Trusopt) (C)	Carbonic anhydrase inhibitor	One drop tid	Open-angle glaucoma; ocular hypertension

OSMOTIC DIURETICS

Osmotic diuretic drugs may be administered either intravenously, orally, or topically to reduce IOP. In Canada, the osmotic diuretic most commonly used for this purpose is mannitol. Glycerin is also an osmotic diuretic found in eye drops.

Mechanism of Action and Drug Effects

Mannitol reduces ocular hypertension by causing the blood to become hypertonic in the presence of both intraocular and spinal fluids. This creates an osmotic gradient that draws water from the aqueous and vitreous humors into the bloodstream, causing a reduction in volume of intraocular fluid, which results in a decrease in IOP (Figure 58-13). Systemic (nonophthalmic) drug effects are discussed in Chapter 26.

Indications

Ocular uses for mannitol include acute glaucoma episodes, and before or after ocular surgery to reduce IOP.

Contraindications

Mannitol is contraindicated in patients with known drug allergy, pronounced anuria, acute pulmonary edema, cardiac decompensation, and severe dehydration, as it can worsen all of these conditions.

Adverse Effects

The most frequent reactions to mannitol are nausea, vomiting, and headache. The most significant adverse effects are fluid and electrolyte imbalance. Other effects are possible irritation and thrombosis at the injection site. A variety of other possible adverse effects are listed in Table 58-6.

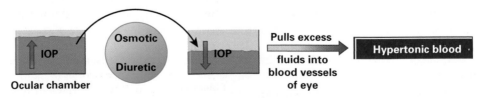

FIG. 58-13 Mechanism and ocular effects of osmotic diuretics.

TABLE 58-6

Osmotic Diuretics (Mannitol): Adverse Effects

Body System	Adverse Effects
Cardiovascular	Edema, thrombophlebitis, hypotension, hypertension, tachycardia, angina-like chest pains, fever, chills
Central nervous	Dizziness, headache, convulsions, rebound increased intracranial pressure, confusion
Electrolytes	Fluid electrolyte imbalances, acidosis, electrolyte loss, dehydration
Eyes, ears, nose, throat	Loss of hearing, blurred vision, nasal congestion
Gastrointestinal	Nausea, vomiting, dry mouth, diarrhea
Genitourinary	Marked diuresis, urinary retention, thirst

Interactions

Increased lithium excretion caused by mannitol is the only significant drug interaction that has been reported.

Toxicity and Management of Overdose

Toxic reactions are primarily a result of the hyperosmolarity of the blood. The most significant toxic reactions include hypovolemia (secondary to diuresis), cardiac dysrhythmias, and hyperosmolar nonketotic coma. If any of these occur, the drug should be discontinued and symptoms treated with fluids and electrolytes.

Dosages

For recommended dosages of mannitol, see the Dosages table below.

DRUG PROFILES

The sole osmotic diuretic used in Canada is mannitol (Osmitrol). It is normally reserved for acute reduction of IOP during glaucoma crises. It is also used perioperatively in ocular surgery.

mannitol

Mannitol (Osmitrol) is used only by intravenous infusion to reduce elevated IOP when the pressure cannot be lowered by other treatments. Mannitol has been shown to be effective in the treatment of acute episodes of angle-closure, absolute, or secondary glaucoma and for lowering IOP before intraocular surgery. Mannitol does not penetrate the eye and may be used when irritation is present.

PHARMACOKINETICS

Half-Life	Onset	Peak	Duration
15–100 min	30–60 min	1 hr	6–8 hr

DOSAGES   Selected Osmotic Diuretics

Drug (Pregnancy Category)	Pharmacological Class	Usual Dosage Range	Indications
mannitol (Osmitrol) (C)	Organic alcohol	IV: 1.5–2 g/kg over at least 30 min; for preoperative use give 1–1.5 hr before surgery	Acute reduction of elevated IOP

PROSTAGLANDIN-F$_{2\alpha}$ ANALOGUES

Latanoprost (Xalatan) is the most popular of the three drugs in this newer class of ophthalmic drugs used to treat glaucoma, the prostaglandin-F$_{2\alpha}$ analogues (PAs). The other two drugs are travoprost (Travatan) and bimatoprost (Lumigan).

Mechanism of Action and Drug Effects

Prostaglandins reduce IOP primarily by increasing the outflow of aqueous fluid, not by decreasing its production. This is believed to occur through an increase in aqueous fluid outflow between the uvea and sclera to the usual exit through the trabecular meshwork, a filter-like structure within the eye (see Figure 58-6). A single dose of ophthalmic PAs lowers the IOP for 20 to 24 hours, allowing a single daily dosage regimen. The drug effects of PAs are primarily limited to these ocular effects.

Indications

Prostaglandins are used in the treatment of glaucoma.

Contraindications

The only usual contraindication to the use of PAs is known drug allergy.

Adverse Effects

PAs are generally well tolerated. Adverse effects reported in clinical trials included foreign body sensation, punctate epithelial keratopathy (dotted appearance of cornea), stinging, conjunctival hyperemia ("bloodshot" eyes), blurred vision, itching, and burning. Systemic effects occur in a small percentage of patients and include skin reactions, upper respiratory infections, and headache. There is one unique adverse effect associated with all PAs. In some people with hazel, green, or bluish-brown eyes, the eye colour will turn permanently brown, even if they stop using the medication. This adverse effect appears to be a cosmetic one, with no known ill effects on the eye. This iris colour change does not affect IOP readings.

Interactions

Concurrent administration of PAs with any other eye drops containing the preservative thimerosal may result in precipitation. It is recommended that the two medications be administered at least 5 minutes apart.

Dosages

For recommended dosages of latanoprost, see the Dosages table below.

 DRUG PROFILES

▶▶ *latanoprost*

Latanoprost (Xalatan) is a prodrug of a naturally occurring prostaglandin known as prostaglandin $F_{2\alpha}$. When this ester prodrug is administered, it is converted by hydrolysis (with water from ocular fluids) to prostaglandin $F_{2\alpha}$, which, in turn, reduces IOP. About 3% to 10% of patients treated with latanoprost have shown increased iris pigmentation after 3 to $4\frac{1}{2}$ months of treatment. This drug is available only in eye drop form.

PHARMACOKINETICS

Half-Life	Onset	Peak	Duration
17 min	30–60 min	2 hr	24 hr

DOSAGES   Selected Prostaglandin Analogues

Drug (Pregnancy Category)	Pharmacological Class	Usual Dosage Range	Indications
▶▶ latanoprost (Xalatan) (C)	Prostaglandin analogue	One drop every day in the evening	Open-angle glaucoma and ocular hypertension, in patients intolerant of or whose condition is uncontrolled by other drugs

---

ANTIMICROBIAL DRUGS

Topical antimicrobials used for treating ocular infections include antibacterial, antifungal, and antiviral drugs. All of these drugs require a prescription. Many of them are also available for systemic administration for infections elsewhere in the body. The choice of a particular ophthalmic antimicrobial drug should be based on the following:

- Clinical experience
- Sensitivity and characteristics of the organisms most likely to cause the infection
- The disease sensitivity and response of the patient
- Laboratory results (cultures and sensitivities)

Some common eye infections that may require antibiotic therapy are listed in Table 58-7.

Mechanism of Action and Drug Effects

The drugs used to treat infections of the eye work in a variety of ways to destroy the invading organism. Their specific antimicrobial actions are similar to those described for systemically administered drugs. These are described in Chapters 38, 39, 40, and 42. The effects of the drugs used to treat ocular infections are focused on the microorganism invading the eye. Some antimicrobials destroy the causative organism, whereas others simply inhibit the organism's growth, allowing the body's immune system to fight the infection.

Indications

Indications for ophthalmic antimicrobials are known or suspected infection with one or more specific microorganisms. Empirical treatment (without culture and sensitivity confirmation) should be based on reasonable clinical evaluation of presenting signs and symptoms. Topical use of antimicrobials helps prevent antimicrobial drug resistance that could arise from unnecessary systemic use. However, systemic antimicrobials may be used in more severe ocular infections.

Contraindications

Contraindications of antimicrobial use include known drug allergy or other severe prior adverse drug reaction. Also, use of any drug class for the wrong infection (e.g., an antibacterial drug for a viral infection) may worsen the infection and delay treatment. This situation should be avoided whenever possible and the patient monitored for signs of progress or treatment failure.

Adverse Effects

The most common adverse effects of ophthalmic antibiotics are local and transient inflammation, burning, stinging, urticaria, dermatitis, angioedema, and drug hypersensitivity. Other effects are listed in the profiles of specific drugs. Topical application of antimicrobial

TABLE 58-7

Common Ocular Infections

Infection	Description
Blepharitis	Inflammation of the eyelids
Conjunctivitis	Inflammation of the conjunctiva, which is the mucous membrane lining the back of the lids and the front of the eye except the cornea. It may be bacterial or viral in nature and is often associated with common colds. When caused by *Haemophilus* organisms, it is commonly called "pink eye." It is highly contagious but usually self-limiting.
Endophthalmitis	Inner eye structure inflammation caused by bacteria
Hordeolum (sty)	Acute localized infection of the eyelash follicles and the glands of the anterior lid; results in the formation of a small abscess or cyst
Keratitis	Inflammation of the cornea often caused by bacterial infection. Herpes simplex keratitis is caused by viral infection.
Uveitis	Infection of the uveal tract or the vascular layer of the eye, which includes the iris, ciliary body, and choroid

drugs may also interfere with growth of the normal bacterial flora of the eye, thus encouraging growth of other more harmful organisms.

Interactions

Systemic drug interactions are unlikely because of the primarily local effects of ophthalmic antimicrobials. One possible interaction is the concurrent use of

corticosteroids (e.g., dexamethasone). Such drugs have immunosuppressive effects, which may impede the therapeutic effects of ophthalmic antimicrobials, as is also the case with systemic antimicrobials.

Dosages

For recommended dosages of ophthalmic antimicrobials, see the Dosages table on p. 1065.

 ## DRUG PROFILES

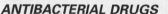

ANTIBACTERIAL DRUGS

A variety of infections can occur in the eye; many are self-limiting (i.e., the body's own immune system fights them). These infections seldom result in harm. However, some infections require elimination through the use of ophthalmic antimicrobials. The most commonly used antimicrobials from the main antimicrobial drug classes are discussed here.

AMINOGLYCOSIDES

Aminoglycosides (Chapter 39) are potent antimicrobials that destroy bacteria by interfering with protein synthesis in bacterial cells by binding to ribosomal subunits, which eventually leads to bacterial death. Aminoglycosides used to treat ocular infections include gentamicin sulfate (Alcomicin, Diogent, others) and tobramycin (Tobrex). Adverse effects include swollen eyelids, mydriasis, and local erythema. Toxic reactions are rare because of poor topical absorption. Another possible toxic reaction is the overgrowth of nonsusceptible organisms, which can lead to eye infections that are resistant to treatment.

▶▶ gentamicin sulfate

Gentamicin sulfate (Alcomicin, Diogent, Garamycin, others) is effective against a wide variety of gram-negative

and gram-positive organisms. It is particularly useful against *Pseudomonas*, *Proteus*, and *Klebsiella* organisms. Gram-positive organisms that are effectively destroyed by gentamicin are staphylococci and streptococci that have developed resistance to other antibiotics. Gentamicin is available as an ophthalmic ointment and a solution.

PHARMACOKINETICS

Half-Life	Onset	Peak	Duration
Unknown	Variable	Immediate	6–12 hr

MACROLIDES

Macrolide antibiotics include erythromycin, azithromycin, and other drugs (Chapter 38). Erythromycin is currently the only macrolide available for ophthalmic use.

▶▶ erythromycin

Erythromycin (AK Mycin) is a macrolide antibiotic indicated for the treatment of ocular infections. It is available only as an ophthalmic ointment. In normal concentrations, it inhibits the growth of an organism but does not destroy it. Erythromycin relies on the body's defence mechanisms to destroy bacteria; however, in high concentrations, it becomes **bactericidal**. It is indicated for the treatment of neonatal conjunctivitis caused by

Continued

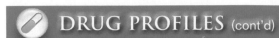

Chlamydia trachomatis and for the prevention of eye infections in newborns that may be caused by *Neisseria gonorrhoeae* or other susceptible organisms.

PHARMACOKINETICS

Half-Life	Onset	Peak	Duration
Unknown	Variable	Immediate	Variable

POLYPEPTIDES

Bacitracin and polymyxin B are polypeptide antibiotics. These drugs are rarely used systemically because of their potent nephrotoxic effects. They are bactericidal antimicrobials that inhibit protein synthesis in susceptible organisms, which leads to cell death. They are most commonly used in the treatment of surface infections caused by gram-positive bacteria.

Polypeptides are often used in combination with other antibiotics to broaden their spectrum of activity. For example, neosporin ophthalmic solution is a combination of gramicidin, neomycin, and polymyxin.

▶▶ bacitracin

Bacitracin is an ophthalmic antimicrobial drug used to treat eye infections. It is available as a single-ingredient product for topical use and as a combination product with polymyxin; or neomycin and polymyxin; or hydrocortisone, neomycin, and polymixin for ophthalmic use. These combinations were developed to make bacitracin a broader-spectrum antibiotic. Bacitracin is available in ointment form.

PHARMACOKINETICS

Half-Life	Onset	Peak	Duration
Unknown	Variable	Immediate	Variable

QUINOLONES

Quinolone antibiotics are effective broad-spectrum antibiotics; they are discussed in detail in Chapter 39. These antibiotics are bactericidal, destroying a wide spectrum of organisms that are often difficult to treat. Currently, four ophthalmic quinolones are available: ciprofloxacin hydrochloride (Ciloxan), gatifloxacin (Zymar), moxifloxacin hydrochloride (Vigamox), and ofloxacin (Apo-Ofloxacin).

Significant adverse effects include corneal precipitates during treatment for bacterial keratitis. Other reactions include corneal staining and infiltrates. Toxic reactions are limited because of poor topical absorption. Those that occur are usually taste disorders and nausea. No significant drug interactions have been found to occur.

▶▶ ciprofloxacin hydrochloride

Ciprofloxacin hydrochloride (Ciloxan) is a synthetic quinolone antibiotic. It is available in ointment and solution forms. Ciprofloxacin is indicated in the treatment of bacterial keratitis and conjunctivitis caused by susceptible gram-positive and gram-negative bacteria. One notable adverse reaction to ophthalmic ciprofloxacin has been the appearance on the corneal surface of a

white, crystalline precipitate occurring within any corneal lesions for which the patient was being treated. This has occurred in about 17% of patients and within 1 to 7 days of starting therapy. However, all cases have been self-limiting, have not required drug discontinuation, and have not adversely affected clinical outcome.

PHARMACOKINETICS

Half-Life	Onset	Peak	Duration
1–2 hr	Variable	Immediate	Variable

SULFONAMIDES

Sulfonamides are synthetic **bacteriostatic** antibiotics that work by blocking the synthesis of folic acid in susceptible bacteria. Sulfacetamide sodium (AK Sulf, Bleph-10, Cetamide) is the sole sulfonamide used to treat conjunctivitis and other ocular infections caused by susceptible bacteria.

The adverse effects are primarily limited to local reactions and include local irritation and stinging. Sulfonamide use can result in the overgrowth of nonsusceptible organisms. No significant topical toxic effects have been reported with its use.

▶▶ sulfacetamide sodium

Sulfacetamide sodium (AK Sulf, Bleph-10, Cetamide) is the most commonly used ophthalmic sulfonamide antibacterial drug. It is available in solution and ointment forms. It is also available in a combination with prednisolone acetate (AK Cide, Dioptimyd).

PHARMACOKINETICS

Half-Life	Onset	Peak	Duration
Unknown	Variable	Immediate	Variable

ANTIVIRALS

The sole available antiviral ophthalmic drug is trifluridine (Viroptic). The dosages for this drug appear in the Dosages table on p. 1065.

trifluridine

Trifluridine (Viroptic) is a pyrimidine nucleoside. Recall from biochemistry that the chemical bases associated with DNA and RNA structure are classified as pyrimidines and purines. A *nucleoside* is a base with its attached sugar molecule from the DNA or RNA "backbone" chain (a *nucleotide* is a nucleoside plus its associated phosphate molecule in the "backbone" chain). Trifluridine inhibits viral replication because its metabolites block viral DNA synthesis by inhibiting viral DNA polymerase, an enzyme required for DNA synthesis. This ophthalmic drug is used against ocular infections (keratitis and keratoconjunctivitis) caused by types 1 and 2 of the herpes simplex virus (HSV). Significant adverse effects include secondary glaucoma, corneal punctate defects, uveitis, and stromal edema (edema in the tough, fibrous, transparent portion of the cornea known as the *stroma*). The drug exhibits no appreciable topical absorption, and no significant drug interactions have been reported.

DOSAGES   Selected Ophthalmic Antimicrobials

Drug (Pregnancy Category)	Pharmacological Class	Usual Dosage Range	Indications
ANTIBACTERIAL DRUGS			
▸▸bacitracin (AK-Tracin) (C)			
bacitracin polymyxin B (Polyoptic) (C)	Miscellaneous antibiotic		
bacitracin polymyxin B neomycin (Diosporin) (C)		Solution: 1–2 drops q1–4h	
▸▸ciprofloxacin (Ciloxan) (C)	Quinolone	Ointment: 12 mm ribbon into	Ocular infections
▸▸erythromycin (AK Mycin) (C)	Macrolide	lower conjunctival sacs tid–qid	
▸▸gentamicin (Alcomicin, Diogent, Garamycin, others) (C)	Aminoglycoside		
▸▸sulfacetamide (Bleph-10) (C)	Sulfonamide		
ANTIVIRAL DRUGS			
trifluridine (Viroptic) (C)		Initially 1 drop q2h while awake (max 9 drops/day); may later decrease to 5 drops/day	Viral ocular infections: HSV type 1- and type 2-induced keratitis, keratoconjunctivitis

HSV, herpes simplex virus.

ANTI-INFLAMMATORY DRUGS

Many of the anti-inflammatory drug classes that are used systemically may also be used ophthalmically to treat ocular inflammatory disorders and surgery-related pain and inflammation. These drugs include both nonsteroidal anti-inflammatory drugs (NSAIDs) and corticosteroids. The anti-inflammatory drugs are listed in Box 58-1.

Mechanism of Action and Drug Effects

Corticosteroids and NSAIDs, as discussed in Chapters 33 and 45, both act to reduce inflammatory responses that result from the body's metabolic pathway (series of biochemical reactions) for the naturally occurring biochemical arachidonic acid. Each of the drug classes acts at different enzymatic sites of this complex metabolic pathway, as illustrated in Figure 58-14.

When tissues are damaged, their cell membranes release phospholipids as a part of the tissue-damaging process. The phospholipids are then broken down by several different enzymes within the arachidonic acid metabolic pathway. Phospholipase is one of the first enzymes involved, and it is this enzyme that is inhibited by corticosteroids. A second enzyme, cyclooxygenase, occurs farther down the pathway and is the site of action of the NSAIDs. Both drug actions reduce the production of inflammatory mediators, such as leukotrienes, prostaglandins, and thromboxanes. This effect, in turn, reduces pain, erythema, and other inflammatory processes.

Indications

Corticosteroids and NSAIDs are applied topically for the symptomatic relief of many ophthalmic inflammatory conditions. They may be used to treat corneal, conjunctival, and scleral injuries from chemical, radiation, or thermal burns or from penetration of foreign bodies. They are also used during the acute phase of the injury process to prevent fibrosis and scarring that results in visual impairment. The immunosuppressant effect is more notable with corticosteroids than with NSAIDs. Consequently, NSAIDs are considered less toxic and are preferred as initial topical therapy for such injuries. NSAIDs are also used in the symptomatic treatment of seasonal allergic conjunctivitis.

Corticosteroids and NSAIDs are used prophylactically before ophthalmic surgery to prevent or reduce intraoperative miosis that may occur secondary to surgery-induced trauma. They are also used prophylactically after ophthalmic surgery, such as cataract extraction, glaucoma surgery, and corneal transplants, to prevent inflammation and scarring.

BOX 58-1

Ophthalmic Anti-inflammatory Drugs

NSAIDs	Corticosteroids
diclofenac sodium (Voltaren Ophtha)	dexamethasone (AK Dex, Doidex, Dioptrol, Maxidex)
flurbiprofen sodium (Ocufen)	fluorometholone (Flarex, FML-Neo)
ketorolac tromethamine (Acular)	medrysone (HMS)
	prednisolone acetate (Diopred)
	rimexolone (Vexol)

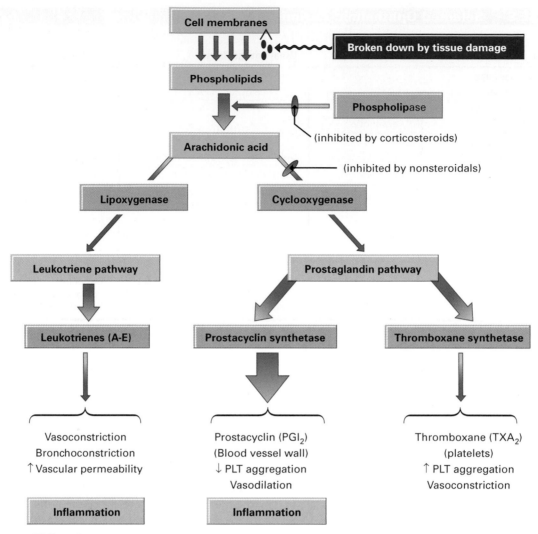

FIG. 58-14 Anti-inflammatory action of corticosteroids and nonsteroidals. *PLT,* platelet.

Contraindications

Aside from known drug allergy, anti-inflammatory drugs should not be used for minor abrasions or wounds because they may suppress the ability of the eye to resist bacterial, viral, or fungal infections. This is especially true of corticosteroids, which have stronger immunosuppressant effects.

Adverse Effects

The most common adverse effect of corticosteroids is transient burning or stinging on application. The extended use of corticosteroids may result in cataracts, increased IOP, and optic nerve damage.

TOPICAL ANAESTHETICS

Topical anaesthetic ophthalmic drugs are local anaesthetics used to alleviate eye pain. The two currently available topical anaesthetics used for ophthalmic purposes are

benoxinate hydrochloride and tetracaine hydrochloride. Benoxinate hydrochloride is only available in combination with fluorescein sodium (Fluress). Fluorescein (see section on diagnostic drugs) is a chemical dye used to identify and locate damage to the surface of the eye. It can only enter damaged cells of the eye. Fluorescein will stain (temporarily) any cells it enters and therefore marks any damaged areas of the eye.

Mechanism of Action and Drug Effects

Local anaesthetics reversibly stabilize the neuronal membranes by binding to sodium channels, resulting in a decrease in the movement of sodium ions into and out of the nerve endings. When nerves are stabilized in this way, they cannot transmit signals about painful stimuli to the brain. Usually, the application of topical anaesthetic drugs to the eye results in local anaesthesia in less than 30 seconds.

Corticosteroids and NSAIDs used to treat ophthalmic inflammatory disorders are listed in Box 58-1. The ophthalmic formulations share many of the characteristics of their systemic drug counterparts. However, the ophthalmic derivatives have limited systemic absorption. Thus the majority of therapeutic and toxic effects are limited to the eye.

▶▶ *dexamethasone*

Dexamethasone (AK Dex, Diodex, Dioptrol, Maxidex) is a synthetic corticosteroid that is available in many ophthalmic formulations. It is used to treat inflammation of the eye, eyelids, conjunctiva, and cornea, and it may also be used in the treatment of uveitis, iridocyclitis (inflammation of both the iris and the ciliary body), allergic conditions, and burns, and in the removal of foreign bodies. Dexamethasone is available in ointment, suspension, and solution forms.

PHARMACOKINETICS

Half-Life	Onset	Peak	Duration
Unknown	Variable	Immediate	Variable

flurbiprofen

Flurbiprofen sodium (Ocufen) is an NSAID used to treat inflammatory ophthalmic conditions, such as postoperative inflammation after a cataract extraction. It is also used to inhibit intraoperative miosis that may be induced by operative trauma and tissue injury. It is available in solution form.

PHARMACOKINETICS

Half-Life	Onset	Peak	Duration
Unknown	30 min	90 min	> 2 hr

ketorolac tromethamine

Ketorolac tromethamine (Acular) is an NSAID available in both oral and injectable formulations for systemic use. The ophthalmic formulation is used to reduce certain manifestations of ocular inflammation caused by trauma, such as ocular surgery, and inflammation secondary to external drugs, such as allergens and bacteria. Ketorolac is contraindicated in patients who have exhibited hypersensitivity to it. It is available in solution form. This drug may delay eye wound healing and lead to corneal epithelial breakdown, so constant monitoring of the eye should continue through the duration of therapy.

PHARMACOKINETICS

Half-Life	Onset	Peak	Duration
Unknown	Rapid	Immediate	4–6 hr

Indications

Ophthalmic anaesthetic drugs are used to produce anaesthesia for short corneal and conjunctival procedures. They prevent pain during the following surgical procedures and certain painful ophthalmic examinations:

- Contact lens fitting
- Corneal scraping for diagnostic purposes
- Examinations of painful eye injuries
- Gonioscopy (an examination technique for measuring the angle of the anterior chamber of the eye and for demonstrating ocular rotation and motility)
- Irrigation of painful injuries
- Minor conjunctival surgery
- Paracentesis (surgical puncture of the eye to remove fluid for diagnostic or therapeutic reasons)
- Removal of foreign bodies
- Removal of sutures
- Tonometry (an external measuring technique involving a puff of air, used to estimate IOP)
- Any other uncomfortable short procedure

Contraindications

Contraindications to local ophthalmic anaesthetics include known drug allergy. These medications are recommended only for short-term use and are not recommended for self-administration.

Adverse Effects

Adverse effects are rare with ophthalmic anaesthetic drugs and are limited to local effects such as stinging, burning, redness, and lacrimation. Some of the more common adverse effects are allergic contact dermatitis, softening and erosion of corneal epithelium, pupillary dilation, cycloplegia, conjunctival congestion and hemorrhage, and stromal edema. The ophthalmic anaesthetic drugs also have mydriatic and cycloplegic effects because they dilate the pupil and paralyze the ciliary muscle, which prevents accommodation of vision. Systemic toxicity is rare but can theoretically lead to central nervous system (CNS) stimulation, or CNS or cardiovascular depression.

Interactions

Because of limited systemic absorption and short duration of action, ophthalmic anaesthetic drugs have no significant drug interactions.

DRUG PROFILES

Topical ophthalmic anaesthetic drugs are a small class of the many available ophthalmic drugs. There are currently two drugs available for this purpose: benoxinate hydrochloride (generic) and tetracaine hydrochloride (Minims). They are similar in their indications and dosing regimens. All have mydriatic and cycloplegic effects because they dilate the pupil and paralyze the ciliary muscle, which prevents accommodation of vision.

tetracaine hydrochloride

Tetracaine hydrochloride (Minims) is a local anaesthetic of the ester type (Chapter 12). It is applied as an eye drop to numb the eye for ophthalmic procedures listed previously under Indications. Tetracaine begins to act in about 25 seconds and lasts for approximately 30 minutes. Additional drops are applied as needed. It is currently available only in solution form.

PHARMACOKINETICS

Half-Life	Onset	Peak	Duration
Short	< 30 sec	1–5 min	15–20 min

DIAGNOSTIC DRUGS

The diagnostic mydriatics are used primarily to dilate the pupils to accommodate more thorough ophthalmic examinations. Drugs that have cycloplegic (paralysis) effects are used to prevent accommodation, which can interfere with the ophthalmic examination. Ophthalmic dyes are used to aid in visualizing defects and foreign objects in the eye.

ANTIALLERGIC DRUGS

As the name implies, these drugs are used to alleviate ocular allergies that arise from eye irritants (such as cosmetics, or industrial and commercial chemical sprays) or general seasonal allergies such as hay fever.

DRUG PROFILES

CYCLOPLEGIC MYDRIATICS
▶▶ *atropine sulfate*

Atropine sulfate solution is used as a mydriatic and cycloplegic drug. It dilates the pupil (mydriasis) and paralyzes the ciliary muscle (cycloplegic refraction), which prevents accommodation. Such drug action may be needed for either eye examination or uveal tract inflammatory states that benefit from pupillary dilation. The usual dose for uveitis (inflammation of the choroid, iris, or ciliary body) in children and adults is 1 to 2 drops of the solution 2 to 3 times daily. The dose for eye examination is 1 drop of solution ideally 1 hour before the procedure.

cyclopentolate hydrochloride

Cyclopentolate hydrochloride solution (Cyclogyl) is used primarily as a diagnostic mydriatic and cycloplegic drug. Unlike atropine, it is not normally used to treat uveitis. The usual adult dose is 1 to 2 drops (0.5% or 1%). This is repeated in 5 to 10 minutes if needed. The dose for children is the same as that for adults. Infants require 1 drop of the 0.5% solution. The drug effects usually subside within

24 hours. Other cycloplegic mydriatics are homatropine (Isopto Homatropine) and tropicamide (Mydriacyl). Both are topical ophthalmic solutions with indications similar to those for atropine and cyclopentolate.

OPHTHALMIC DYE
fluorescein

Fluorescein sodium (AK-Fluor) is an ophthalmic diagnostic dye used to identify corneal defects and to locate foreign objects in the eye. It is also used in fitting hard contact lenses. After the instillation of fluorescein, defects are highlighted. They are distinguished according to the following criteria:
• Corneal defects are coloured bright green.
• Conjunctival lesions are coloured yellow–orange.
• Foreign objects have a green halo around them.
• A contact lens that touches the cornea will appear black in ultraviolet light.
Fluorescein is available for use as an ophthalmic injection, solution, and diagnostic applicator strips. Dosing and drug administration are usually carried out by an ophthalmologist.

DRUG PROFILES

ANTIHISTAMINES
emedastine difumarate

Emedastine difumarate (Emadine) is an ocular antihistamine used to treat symptoms of allergic conjunctivitis ("hay fever"), which can be seasonal or nonseasonal. It acts by competing at the receptor sites of histamine, an inflammatory mediator produced by mast cells. Histamine normally produces such ocular symptoms as itching and tearing. One other antihistamine is levocabastine hydrochloride (Levostin). The antihistamine drugs have similar mechanisms of action, therapeutic and adverse effects, and drug interactions as those of the systemic antihistamines described in Chapter 36, although systemic effects are less likely with ophthalmic administration. Dosages for emedastine can be found in the Dosages table below.

MAST CELL STABILIZERS
cromolyn sodium

Cromolyn sodium (Opticrom) is an antiallergic drug that inhibits the release of inflammation-producing mediators from the sensitized inflammatory cells, *mast cells.* It is used in the treatment of vernal keratoconjunctivitis (springtime inflammation of the cornea and conjunctiva). Other mast cell stabilizers with similar effects are nedocromil sodium (Alocril), lodoxamide (Alomide), and olopatidine hydrochloride (Patanol). Dosages for cromolyn can be found in the Dosages table below.

DECONGESTANTS
tetrahydrozoline hydrochloride

Tetrahydrozoline hydrochloride (Allergy Eye Drops, Visine) is an ophthalmic decongestant. It works by promoting vasoconstriction of blood vessels in and around the eye, thus reducing the edema associated with allergic and inflammatory processes. It is specifically indicated to control redness, burning, and other minor irritations. Other ophthalmic decongestants include phenylephrine hydrochloride (Prefrin), oxymetazoline hydrochloride (Claritin), and naphazoline (Clear Eyes). Dosages for tetrahydrozoline can be found in the Dosages table below.

LUBRICANTS AND MOISTURIZERS
▸▸ artificial tears

An array of over-the-counter products is available to use as lubrication or moisture for the eyes, which is often helpful to patients with dry or otherwise irritated eyes. Artificial tears are isotonic and contain buffers for pH control. In addition, they contain preservatives for microbial control and may contain viscosity drugs for extended ocular activity. Selected over-the-counter brand names include GenTeal Tears, Isopto Tears, Eyestil, Murine, Refresh, and Tears Plus. There are many similar products on the market, available as solution (eye drop) and lubrication ointment. They are often dosed to patient comfort as needed.

DOSAGES   Selected Ophthalmic Antiallergics

Drug (Pregnancy Category)	Pharmacological Class	Usual Dosage Range	Indications
cromolyn sodium (Opticrom) (C)	Mast cell stabilizer	1–2 drops in each eye 4–6 times daily	Vernal (springtime) conjunctivitis and keratitis (corneal inflammation)
emedastine difumarate (Emadine) (B)	Antihistamine	1 drop in the affected eye up to 4 times daily	Allergic conjunctivitis
tetrahydrozoline hydrochloride (Allergy Eye Drops, Visine) (C)	Decongestant	1–2 drops in affected eye(s) up to 4 times daily	Redness, burning, or other minor irritation

NURSING PROCESS

Assessment

Before administering an ophthalmic drug according to the physician's orders, the nurse should perform a baseline assessment of the eye and its structures to document specific data about normal versus abnormal findings. Any redness, swelling, pain, excessive tearing, eye drainage or discharge, decrease in visual acuity, or any other unusual symptoms should be documented. Hypersensitivity to medications or other drug- or disorder-related contraindications, as well as drug interactions should also be documented. Baseline vital signs and a visual acuity test (e.g., Snellen chart) should be documented before, during, and after drug treatment. Loss or change in vision and loss in peripheral vision in one eye or both eyes should be noted. A thorough nursing history should focus on past or present systemic disease processes and exposure to any chemicals that could be topical irritants to the eye, skin, or mucous membranes, including occupational and environmental exposures past and present. All known drug, chemical, and ingredient sensitivities should be documented as well. The systemic effects associated with ophthalmic dosage forms are usually minimal if given as prescribed and directed. If the drug used has access to the circulation, adverse effects should be anticipated.

Because of the frequency of use of the drugs in this chapter, it is important to review the pharmacological profile and specific contraindications, cautions, and drug interactions for each of the drug groups, such as sympathomimetics in Chapter 18, sympatholytics in Chapter 19, and parasympathomimetics in Chapter 20. The pharmacological profiles and related information about antibiotics is presented in Chapters 38 and 39, about antivirals in Chapter 40, and about anti-inflammatory drugs in Chapter 45.

Nursing Diagnoses

- Risk for infection related to eye diseases, conditions, or irritation because of a lack of information about eye problems and lack of motivation to follow directions
- Risk for injury to the eye related to improper use of medications and improper instillation procedures
- Acute pain related to eye disorders, infections, or inflammatory eye conditions
- Deficient knowledge related to lack of information about eye disorders and related medication therapies

Planning

Goals

- Patient will remain free of signs and symptoms of infection or irritation of the eye.
- Patient will remain adherent to therapy.
- Patient will remain free from injury related to adverse effects of therapy.
- Patient will state that eye pain related to the eye disorder is reduced.

Outcome Criteria

- Patient states the signs and symptoms of infection of the eye, such as eye pain, drainage, redness, and decreased activity, and reports them immediately to the physician.
- Patient states ways to become more adherent to therapy by taking medications as prescribed, including proper timing, instillation, and other non-drug therapy aids such as warm or cool compresses as recommended.
- Patient minimizes injury related to the adverse effects of therapy by creating a safe environment at home, such as getting rid of any clutter or moving rugs and furniture; adding more lighting, especially night lights; and using assistive devices as needed for altered vision.
- Patient minimizes eye pain related to the eye disorder by using compresses or analgesics (other than aspirin) as ordered.

Implementation

Because it is important to administer only clean solutions, the nurse should shake the medication container before each use to make sure the solution has mixed well and remains clear and without particulate matter. Most important to instillation of drops and ointment is to avoid touching the eye with the tip of the dropper or the container to prevent contamination of the product. Any excess medication must be removed promptly and pressure must be applied to the inner canthus for 1 minute (or other specified duration) to avoid systemic adverse effects because of absorption into the vasculature. Ointments and any ophthalmic topical drug dosage form should always be applied as a thin layer and applied to the conjunctival sac and never directly onto the eye

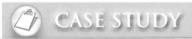 CASE STUDY

Eye Trauma

Mr. P., a construction worker, is being seen in the emergency department because of a possible eye injury. He was working without eye protection, and a gust of wind sprayed metal shavings on his face. The physician has instilled fluorescein sodium and has noted areas in the eyeball with green halos around them.

1. What is the purpose of the fluorescein sodium, and what is indicated by the green halos?

2. Mr. P. is sent to an ophthalmologist for further treatment. What eye medication do you expect will be used for the next procedure?

3. After the procedure, Mr. P. receives a prescription for dexamethasone (AK Dex) ophthalmic ointment, to be taken three times a day. What specific patient teaching should be shared with Mr. P.?

For answers see http://evolve.elsevier.com/Canada/Lilley/pharmacology/.

itself. To facilitate the instillation, the patient needs to tilt the head back and look up at the ceiling during administration. Several ophthalmic drugs with different actions are often ordered, and each drug must be given exactly as ordered and within the specified time frame. Ointments may cause a temporary blurriness to the vision because of the film that bathes over the eye. This film will decrease once absorbed, and vision should become clearer. The nurse should refer to an authoritative drug source for specific instructions and guidelines about specific application techniques, length of time to apply pressure to the inner canthus, and any other specific instructions. See Chapter 10 for the administration technique for ophthalmic drugs.

Directions for antiviral ophthalmic preparations should be followed closely. Topical anaesthetics should be administered as ordered for removal of a foreign body or treatment of eye injury. Repeated and continuous use should be avoided because of the risk for delayed wound healing, corneal perforation, permanent corneal opacification, and vision loss. When there is an injury or abrasion to the eye and appropriate medications ordered, a patch for the affected eye is recommended. This helps prevent further injury resulting from the loss of the blink reflex from overuse of topical anaesthetic. Additional instructions should include appropriate information about any change in eye colour. For example, latanoprost turns the eye colour permanently brown from hazel, green, or bluish-brown. However, there is no known injury to the eye associated with the colour change.

Ophthalmic ketorolac should be given as ordered. Artificial tear solutions are often used in long-term care and are available over the counter. Once therapy has been initiated, the physician may order IOP readings and visual field and funduscopic examinations. The importance of these follow-up visits should be emphasized to the patient (see Patient Education). In addition, a listing of some of the ophthalmic preparations, their mechanisms of action, and related nursing considerations is provided at http://evolve.elsevier.com/Canada/Lilley/pharmacology/.

Evaluation

Therapeutic responses to miotics include decreased aqueous humor of the eye with resultant decreased IOP and decreased signs, symptoms, and long-term effects associated with glaucoma. For possible adverse effects, see Patient Education. β-Adrenergic blockers are therapeutic if there is a resultant decrease in IOP. Possible adverse effects to assess for include weakness, depression, anxiety, nausea, confusion, eye irritation, rash, bradycardia, hypotension, and dysrhythmias. Therapeutic responses to antibiotic and antiviral ophthalmic drugs include elimination of the infection, resolution of symptoms, and prevention of complications. Therapeutic responses to ophthalmic anaesthetics include healing of the eye without permanent damage and a decrease in symptoms associated with the damage. Adverse effects include CNS excitation if the anaesthetic is systemically absorbed, causing blurred vision, dizziness, tremors, nervousness, and restlessness. Drowsiness, dyspnea, and cardiac dysrhythmias may occur secondary to CNS depression. Anti-inflammatory ophthalmic solutions should result in a decrease in allergic reactions such as itching, tearing, redness, and eye discharge. Potential complications of these solutions include swelling of the conjunctiva (chemosis). Further monitoring should include re-evaluation of goals and outcome criteria.

PATIENT EDUCATION

* Patients taking parasympathomimetic ophthalmic drugs should be informed about the correct procedure for instilling eye drops and for applying pressure to the inner canthus. Demonstrations and return demonstrations should be used. Solutions with eye-droppers and other equipment should be kept sterile by avoiding touching any surface of the eye. Long-term therapy is usually necessary and patient education about proper technique is important to prevent eye damage.

* Before being given the drug, patients taking indirect parasympathomimetics should properly demonstrate adequate knowledge of the medication and technique for its administration. They should also be informed of adverse effects associated with most direct- and indirect-acting drugs (e.g., blurred vision, broncho-spasm, nausea, vomiting, bradycardia, hypotension, sweating), as well as other potential adverse effects, including decreased night visual acuity, stinging sensation, dull ache, or tearing upon instillation. Patients should be instructed to call the physician if these symptoms worsen. With sympathomimetic drugs, patients should be reminded to report any stinging, burning, itching, lacrimation, or puffiness of the eye.

* Patients should be cautioned to instill sympatho-lytic drugs as ordered and to apply pressure to the inner canthus with a tissue or 2 × 2 gauze pad for 1 full minute or as directed. Blurred vision, difficulty breathing, wheezing, sweating, flushing, and loss of sight should be reported to the physician.

* Patients should be informed that photosensitivity is an expected adverse effect of mydriatics, and use of sunglasses should be encouraged to help minimize eye discomfort and headaches while in sunlight.

* With topical anaesthetics, patients should be instructed to not rub or touch the eye while it is numb because of possible eye damage. Patients should also wear a patch to protect the eye because of loss of the blink reflex.

* Patients should be encouraged to always report any of the following to the health care provider immediately: increase in eye pain, discharge from the eye, fever, and loss of vision.

* Patients should be instructed to use ophthalmic drugs as ordered and to not misuse them. The medication should not be stopped without consulting the physician because of the possibility of adverse reactions. Contact lenses should not be worn while instilling ophthalmic drugs and for the duration of therapy because the lenses may cause further irritation.

* Patients should be encouraged to use a gloved hand or finger-cot during application and to avoid touching the structures of the eye with any of the equipment (e.g., dropper tip). Once applied, the patient needs to close the eye and apply pressure to the lacrimal sac for 1 to 2 minutes or as ordered to avoid drainage of the medication into the nose or throat and to decrease the risk of systemic adverse effects. Ophthalmic ketorolac, an anti-inflammatory drug, may delay eye wound healing and lead to corneal epithelial breakdown, so any such concerns should be reported if present or suspected.

POINTS TO REMEMBER

* Glaucoma is a disorder of the eye caused by inhibition of the normal flow and drainage of aqueous humor. Treatment of glaucoma helps reduce intra-ocular pressure either by increasing aqueous humor drainage or decreasing its production.

* Drugs that increase aqueous humor drainage are direct parasympathomimetics, indirect parasympathomimetics, and β-blockers.

* A large proportion of the inflammatory diseases of the eye are caused by viruses, and there are many ophthalmic antimicrobials used to treat bacterial and viral infections of the eye.

* Common ocular infections include conjunctivitis, hordeolum (sty), keratitis, uveitis, and endophthalmitis.

* Anti-inflammatory ophthalmic drugs include corticosteroids and are used to inhibit inflammatory responses to mechanical, chemical, or immunological drugs.

* Topical anaesthetics are used to prevent pain in the eye and are beneficial during surgery, ophthalmic examinations, and the removal of foreign bodies.

* All ophthalmic preparations need to be administered exactly as ordered and into the conjunctival sac. Safe and accurate application or instillation technique must be used, while avoiding contact of the dropper or tube with the eye to prevent contamination of the drug.

* Patients should report any increase in symptoms such as eye pain or drainage and fever to the physician immediately.

EXAMINATION REVIEW QUESTIONS

1 The ophthalmologist has given a patient a dose of ophthalmic atropine drops. Which statement by the nurse accurately explains to the patient the reason for these drops?
a. "These drops cause your pupils to dilate, making the eye examination easier."
b. "These drops cause your pupils to constrict, making the eye examination easier."
c. "These drops are used to check for any possible foreign bodies or corneal defects that may be in your eye."
d. "These drops will cause the surface of your eye to become numb, so that the doctor can do the examination."

2 When assessing a patient who is receiving a direct-acting parasympathomimetic eye drop as part of treatment for glaucoma, the nurse notes that the drug has taken effect. Which of the following would she observe on the pupil?
a. It changed the colour of the pupil.
b. It caused no change in pupil size.
c. It caused mydriasis, or pupil dilation.
d. It caused miosis, or pupil constriction.

3 When teaching the patient on self-administration of eye drops, which statement by the nurse is correct?
a. "Hold the eye drops over the cornea and squeeze out the drop."
b. "Be sure to place the drop in the conjunctival sac of the lower eyelid."
c. "Squeeze your eyelid closed tightly after placing the drop into your eye."
d. "Apply pressure against the lacrimal duct area for 5 minutes after administration."

4 Which of the following is correct patient teaching about how miotics help treat glaucoma?
a. They cause pupillary dilation.
b. They increase tear production.
c. They decrease intraocular pressure.
d. They decrease intracranial pressure.

5 During an assessment of a patient with glaucoma who may be receiving a carbonic anhydrase inhibitor (CAI) as part of treatment, which condition would be considered a problem?
a. Hypertension
b. Diabetes mellitus
c. Allergy to penicillins
d. Allergy to sulfa drugs

For answers see http://evolve.elsevier.com/Canada/Lilley/pharmacology/.

CRITICAL THINKING ACTIVITIES

1 Describe the process of glaucoma and explain the value of treatment to preserve vision.

2 Develop a teaching plan for the older adult patient who is already vision impaired and needs instructions for the daily administration of antiglaucoma eye drops.

3 Which patient teaching item is important for the patient who has a prescription for latanoprost (Xalatan) before the patient starts taking this medication?

For answers see http://evolve.elsevier.com/Canada/Lilley/pharmacology/.

CHAPTER 59

Otic Drugs

Learning Objectives

After reading this chapter, the successful student will be able to do the following:

1 Describe the anatomy of the ear and the purposes of each structure located in the outer, middle, and inner ear.

2 List the categories of ear disorders, with explanation of causes and signs and symptoms.

3 List the otic preparations and their indications.

4 Discuss the mechanisms of action, dosage, cautions, contraindications, drug interactions, and specific application techniques related to each of the otic drugs.

5 Develop a collaborative plan of care that includes all phases of the nursing process as it relates to the administration of otic drugs.

e-Learning Activities

Web site
(http://evolve.elsevier.com/Canada/Lilley/pharmacology/)

- Animations
- Answers to chapter questions, activities, and case studies
- Calculators and Category Catchers
- Glossary with audio pronunciations
- IV Therapy and Medication Error Checklists
- Multiple-Choice Review Question quizzes
- Nursing Care Plans
- Online Appendices and Supplements
- WebLinks

Drug Profiles

Antibacterial products (ciprofloxacin/hydrocortisone, gentamicin/betamethasone), p. 1076

▸▸ urea hydrogen peroxide, p. 1076

▸▸ Key drug.

Glossary

Cerumen A yellowish or brownish waxy excretion produced by modified sweat glands in the external ear canal. Also called *earwax*. (p. 1076)

Otitis externa Inflammation or infection of the external auditory canal. (p. 1075)

Otitis media Inflammation or infection of the middle ear. (p. 1075)

OVERVIEW OF EAR PHYSIOLOGY

The ear is made up of four parts: the external, outer, middle, and inner ear. The external ear is composed of the *pinna* (outer projecting part of the ear) and the *external auditory meatus*, or opening of the ear canal. *Auricle* and *ala* are synonyms for the pinna. The outer ear refers primarily to the *external auditory canal*. This is the space between the external auditory meatus and the *tympanic membrane* (eardrum). The middle ear is composed of the *tympanic cavity*, which is the space that begins with the

tympanic membrane and ends with the oval window. Included in the middle ear are three bony appendages of the mastoid bone—the *malleus* ("hammer"), *incus* ("anvil"), and *stapes* ("stirrup")—as well as the *auditory* or *eustachian* tube. The inner ear includes the *cochlea* and *semicircular* canals. The ear and its associated structures are illustrated in Figure 59-1.

Disorders of the ear can be categorized according to the portion of the ear affected. External ear (pinna) disorders are generally the result of physical trauma to the ear and consist of lacerations or scrapes to the skin and

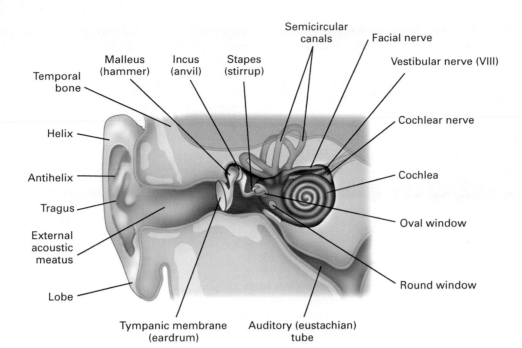

FIG. 59-1 Structure of the ear.

localized infection of the hair follicles that often cause the development of a boil. These disorders also tend to be self-limiting and heal with time. Other examples include contact dermatitis, seborrhea, or psoriasis, as evidenced by itching, local redness, inflammation, weeping, or drainage. These conditions usually respond to the same topical medications used for any other local skin disorders, as discussed in Chapter 57. Those of the outer and middle ear are the disorders usually treated with the drugs discussed in this chapter. In general, the most common disorders of these portions of the ear are bacterial and fungal infections—inflammatory disorders that cause pain and earwax accumulation. Such disorders tend to be self-limiting, and if treatment is needed, it is generally successful. However, if problems persist or are left untreated, more serious problems such as hearing loss may result. Symptoms such as drainage, pain, and dizziness are sometimes also the first signs of a more serious underlying condition (e.g., head trauma, meningitis) and warrant prompt medical evaluation. Medications for disorders affecting the outer (ear canal) and middle ear are the focus of this chapter. Diseases of the inner ear involve highly specialized medical practices that are beyond the scope of this chapter.

By far the most common disorder affecting the outer (ear canal) and middle ear disorder is inflammation or infection caused by microorganisms. Cases affecting the ear canal are known as **otitis externa (OE)**, whereas those affecting the middle ear are known as **otitis media (OM)**. OM is a common affliction of infancy and early childhood. It is often preceded by an upper respiratory tract infection. It may also occur in adults, but it is then generally associated with trauma to the tympanic membrane.

Foreign objects and infection or inflammation from water sports are the usual sources of such trauma. In adults, the condition is also more likely to manifest as OE, involving the ear canal and external tympanic membrane. Common symptoms of both OM and OE include pain, fever, malaise, pressure, a sensation of fullness in the ears, and hearing loss. If left untreated, tinnitus (ringing in the ears), nausea, vertigo, mastoiditis, and even temporary or permanent hearing deficits may occur.

TREATMENT OF EAR DISORDERS

While some of the minor ailments that affect the outer ear can be treated with over-the-counter medications, persistent, painful conditions generally require prescription medications. Drugs used for ear conditions are known as otic drugs, most of which are topically applied to the ear canal. These drugs generally have no drug interactions. Adverse effects are uncommon, but if they do occur, they usually do not extend beyond localized irritation. Otic drugs are normally only contraindicated in cases of known drug allergy. Pertinent drug classes include the following:
- Antibacterials (antibiotics)
- Antifungals
- Anti-inflammatory drugs
- Local analgesics
- Local anaesthetics
- Steroids
- Wax emulsifiers

More serious cases of ear disorders may require treatment with systemic drug therapy such as antimicrobial drugs, analgesics, anti-inflammatory drugs, and antihistamines. These medications have been discussed in detail, by their respective drug classes, in previous chapters.

ANTIBACTERIAL OTIC DRUGS

Antibacterial otic drugs are often combined with steroids to take advantage of the steroidal anti-inflammatory,

antipruritic, and antiallergic drug effects. These drugs are used for outer and middle ear infections (OE and OM). As they all act and are dosed similarly, the products are profiled together below. Systemic antibiotics are also commonly prescribed for these conditions (e.g., amoxicillin; Chapter 38), either alone, or in addition to the otic drugs described in the following sections. Table 59-1 lists several commonly used products and their component amounts.

TABLE 59-1

Common Antibacterial Otic Products

Steroid	Antibiotics	Trade Name
betamethasone sodium phosphate 1 mg/mL	gentamicin sulfate 3 mg/mL	Garasone
dexamethasone 0.1%	ciprofloxacin 0.3%	Ciprodex
dexamethasone sodium phosphate 0.1%		AK Dex
	gentamicin sulfate 3 mg/mL	Garamycin Otic
flumethasone pivaleate 0.02%	clioquinol 1%	Locacorten Vioform
hydrocortisone (1%)	ciprofloxacin 2 mg/mL	Cipro HT Otic
hydrocortisone acetate 10 mg/mL	3.5 mg/mL of neomycin and 10,000 units/mL polymyxin B	Spor-HC Otic Suspension
hydrocortisone acetate 1%	chloramphenicol 1% or 0.2%	Pentamycetin/HC

 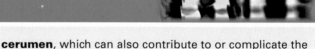

DRUG PROFILES

ANTIBACTERIAL PRODUCTS

Spor-HC Otic Suspension is a three-drug combination that includes hydrocortisone and two antimicrobials, neomycin sulfate (an aminoglycoside; Chapter 39) and polymyxin B sulfate. Hydrocortisone is the steroid most commonly used in otic drugs, although there is one preparation (Ciprodex) containing both ciprofloxacin (a fluoroquinolone; Chapter 39) and dexamethasone sodium phosphate. There is also a single-drug dexamethasone sodium phosphate (AK Dex). In either case, the purpose of the steroid component is to reduce the inflammation and itching associated with ear infections. Gentamicin sulfate (Garamycin Otic) is available as a single-drug product and as a combination product with betamethasone sodium phosphate (Garasone). One additional combination product is flumethasone pivaleate and clioquinol (Locacorten). All of these products are used for the treatment of bacterial OE or OM caused by susceptible bacteria such as *Staphylococcus aureus*, *Escherichia coli*, *Klebsiella* spp., and others. Their usual dosage is 4 drops 3 to 4 times daily. With some otic drugs, a recommended way of dosing the drug is to saturate a retrievable cotton or tissue wick and let this wick soak inside the ear canal. The wick can be periodically remoistened with additional drug, or removed with further ear drops inserted directly into the ear canal. The nurse should follow specific instructions on the drug package or as recommended by the prescriber or pharmacist.

WAX EMULSIFERS

An additional common ear problem is the accumulation and eventual impaction (hardening) of earwax, or

cerumen, which can also contribute to or complicate the infectious and inflammatory conditions described earlier. Wax, or cerumen, is a natural product of the ear and is produced by modified sweat glands in the ear canal. Occasionally, it can build up and become impacted, resulting in pain and temporary deafness. A nonpolar substance is one that is non–water-soluble. Such a substance is said to be emulsified when it is chemically or physically converted to a more water-soluble form. Products that soften and eliminate earwax, referred to as earwax emulsifiers, loosen impacted cerumen, allowing it to be irrigated (with water) out of the ear canal. Often the simple application of olive or almond oil is sufficient to soften wax.

▶▶ *urea hydrogen peroxide*

The only wax removal system is urea hydrogen peroxide (Earoxide). This combination of drugs works to loosen and help remove cerumen. When exposed to moisture such as that on the skin or the mouth, hydrogen peroxide releases oxygen. This release of oxygen imparts a weak antibacterial action to the otic drug. In addition, the *effervescence* (foaming) resulting from the release of oxygen has the mechanical effect of emulsifying impacted cerumen from against the walls of the ear canal. Urea acts as a rehydrating or softening drug to facilitate easier cerumen removal. This drug is an over-the-counter product and should not be used in cases of ear drainage, tympanic membrane rupture, or significant pain or other irritation. After allowing the drug to dissolve the earwax, it can be removed by gentle flushing of the ear canal with warm water from a bulb syringe.

NURSING PROCESS

Assessment

Before administering any of the otic preparations, the nurse should ensure that the patient's baseline hearing or auditory status is evaluated, as appropriate, and the findings documented. There should also be a thorough evaluation of the patient's symptoms, and any other related medical information should be noted. Any drug or food allergies should be documented. The nurse must understand the specific indication for, or the intended use of, the medication so that it can be given exactly as ordered and adverse effects or complications are avoided. It is important to use the administration technique required for the drug being given. A baseline understanding of the anatomy of the ear is also important, especially as it relates to patients in different age groups. Contraindications, cautions, and drug interactions to the use of any of these drugs, chemicals, or solutions should also be noted. A perforated eardrum is usually a contraindication to the use of these drugs.

Nursing Diagnoses

- Impaired verbal communication related to possible hearing impairment or loss stemming from damage due to long-term ear disorders or infections
- Risk for injury related to symptoms of the ear disorder and possible vestibular dysfunction
- Risk for infection related to inadequate treatment
- Disturbed sensory perception related to complications from untreated or undertreated ear infections or disorders.
- Deficient knowledge related to lack of experience with otic drugs and their method of administration
- Nonadherence related to a lack of motivation for using frequent ear drops as ordered

Planning

Goals

- Patient will regain normal patterns of hearing and communicating.
- Patient will state feeling less discomfort and symptoms related to the ear disorder.
- Patient will experience minimal or no signs and symptoms of ear infection with the course of treatment.
- Patient will experience no adverse effects or complications associated with medication therapy.
- Patient will adhere to recommended drug therapy as ordered.

Outcome Criteria

- Patient openly expresses feelings related to problems with communication, such as a decrease in or loss of hearing related to ear infections and disorders or as a consequence of therapy.
- Patient reports increased hearing loss; increased symptoms of ear pain, redness, and swelling of the ear canal; and fever to the physician immediately, should any of these problems occur.
- Patient states measures to take to increase the effectiveness of the medication regimen, such as accurate application or instillation, remaining supine, or sitting with the affected ear facing upward.
- Patient demonstrates accurate medication administration techniques as related to age group and subsequent directions.
- Patient takes medication exactly as ordered and within the guidelines for frequency.

Implementation

Ear drops should be instilled only after the ear has been thoroughly cleansed, all cerumen has been removed (by irrigation if necessary or if ordered), and the dropper cleaned before use. Ear drops, solutions, and ointments should be warmed to room temperature before instillation. Solutions that are too cold may cause a vestibular type of reaction, with vomiting and dizziness. If the solution has been refrigerated, it should be left to warm to room temperature; higher temperatures may affect the potency of these solutions. Normally, corticosteroids, antibiotic drugs, corticosteroid–antibiotic combination drugs, wax emulsifiers, and ear-drying drugs should be administered according to their respective guidelines and as ordered. Adults should receive ear drops while holding the pinna up and back, whereas children younger than 3 years of age need to have the pinna held down and back. Time should be allowed for adequate coverage of the ear by the drug. Gentle massage to the tragus area of the ear may also help increase coverage of the drug. See Patient Education and Chapter 10 for further information on ear drop instillation.

Evaluation

As with all drugs, the therapeutic effects of otic drugs should be gauged by evaluation of goals and objectives. Therapeutic effects should include less pain, redness, and swelling in the ear; a reduction in fever and white blood cell counts; and negative culture findings if the previous culture yielded positive findings. The ear canal should be monitored for the occurrence of rash or any signs of local irritation, such as redness and heat at the site. Adverse effects should also be evaluated with each application or instillation. Any unusual appearance of the outer ear and ear canal should be reported immediately to the physician and documented.

PATIENT EDUCATION

❖ Patients should be properly instructed on the use of ear drops. They should understand and repeat specific instructions and relate further information about the frequency of dosing and the drug's mechanism of action and adverse effects. In addition, the technique of instillation should be thoroughly discussed and the technique re-demonstrated. Patients should be encouraged not to touch the dropper or its tip to the ear. They should also be warned that dizziness may occur after instillation of the medication, thus they should remain supine during instillation and for a few minutes thereafter.

❖ Patients should be instructed to administer ear drops and solutions at body temperature. Running warm water over the bottle can warm a cold solution to this temperature, but care must be taken to not allow water to get into the bottle or to damage the label so that the directions become unreadable. Patients should take care not to actually heat the drops, for example, not to put them in the microwave, because ear drops that are overheated may lose their potency.

If the drug is kept in a refrigerator as indicated by the pharmacy, the drug should be taken out of the refrigerator up to 1 hour before drops are to be instilled so that they can warm up to room temperature. Most otic preparations are usually stored at room temperature.

❖ Patients should be instructed to lie on the side opposite the side of the affected ear for about 5 minutes after instillation of the drug. If the patient prefers, a small cotton ball may be inserted gently into the ear canal to keep the drug there, but the cotton should not be forced into the ear or jammed down into the ear canal.

❖ Patients should be encouraged to show family members how to instill ear drops so that their assistance can be solicited if necessary.

❖ Patients should be informed that the ear drop solution and the placement of cotton balls in the ear may seem to cause some loss of hearing. Any other loss of hearing not resulting from these factors may be due to the ear disorder.

POINTS TO REMEMBER

❖ Otic drugs include the following ingredients, either alone or in combination (depending on physician's order): corticosteroids, antibacterials, anti-inflammatories, and wax emulsifying compounds. Many of the anti-infective drugs are combined with steroids (in solution) to take advantage of their additional anti-inflammatory, antipruritic, and antiallergic drug effects.

❖ Some ear infections require additional drug therapy with systemic dosage forms of corticosteroids, antibiotics, antifungals, and anti-inflammatory drugs, so the patient may need to be reminded of oral and other dosage forms.

❖ Some disorders of the ear are self-limiting to a degree, although appropriate treatment is important to prevent complications to the area and systemic complications. Left untreated, ear infections and disorders may lead to loss or a decrease in hearing.

❖ Wax, or cerumen, is a natural product of the ear and is normally produced by modified sweat glands in the auditory canal; emulsifying otic drugs (such as urea hydrogen peroxide) loosen and help remove this wax.

❖ Single-drug use or combination-drug products are used to treat many ear conditions, and the nurse must know the indications for and specific information about these drugs to ensure their safe use.

EXAMINATION REVIEW QUESTIONS

1 While teaching a patient about treatment of otitis media, which of the following should the nurse mention that untreated otitis media may lead to?
   a. Mastoiditis
   b. Throat infections
   c. Fungal ear infection
   d. Decreased cerumen production

2 During a teaching session about ear drops, the patients tells the nurse, "I know why an antibiotic is in this medicine, but why do I need to take a steroid?" Which statement is the nurse's best answer?
   a. "The steroid also has antifungal effects."
   b. "The steroid will help soften the cerumen."
   c. "The steroid reduces itching and inflammation."
   d. "This medication helps anaesthetize the area to decrease pain."

3 Which technique for administering ear drops is correct?
   a. Warm the solution to 41°C before using.
   b. Massage the tragus before administering the ear drops.
   c. Position the patient so that the unaffected ear is accessible.
   d. Gently insert a cotton ball into the outer ear canal after the drops are given.

4 Which statement about ear wax emulsifiers is true?
   a. These drugs enhance the secretion of earwax.
   b. These drugs are used to rinse out excessive earwax.
   c. These drugs are useful for treatment of ear infections.
   d. These drugs loosen impacted cerumen so that it may be removed by irrigation.

5 During an examination, the nurse notes that a patient has a perforated tympanic membrane. There is an order for ear drops. Which action by the nurse is most appropriate?
   a. Give the medication as ordered.
   b. Administer the drops with a cotton wick.
   c. Check the patient's hearing, then give the drops.
   d. Hold the medication, and check with the prescriber.

For answers see http://evolve.elsevier.com/Canada/Lilley/pharmacology/.

CRITICAL THINKING ACTIVITIES

1 Develop a patient teaching plan for the caregiver who will be administering antibacterial and steroidal otic drops to a 2-year-old child.

2 The mother of child patient tells you that she does not understand why ear infections require treatment with antibiotics. She states, "We used home remedies when I was growing up." What information would you share with the patient's mother, and why?

3 What is the indication for a wax emulsifier? Explain your answer.

For answers see http://evolve.elsevier.com/Canada/Lilley/pharmacology/.

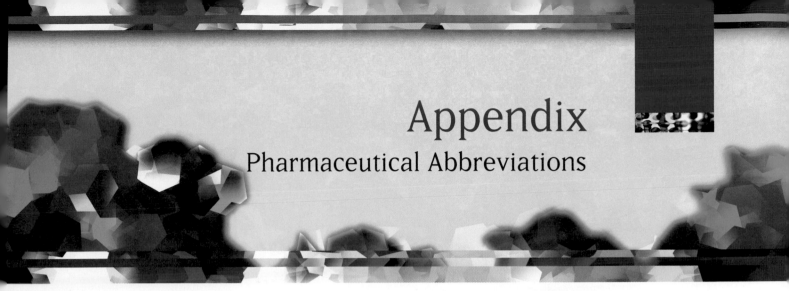

Appendix
Pharmaceutical Abbreviations

Abbreviation	Translation
DRUG DOSAGE	
g or Gm	Gram
gtt	Drop
L	Litre
mEq	Milliequivalent
min	Minute
mL	Millilitre
qs	Quantity sufficient, as much as needed
ss	One half
tbsp	Tablespoon
tsp	Teaspoon
mcg	Microgram
DRUG ROUTE	
AU	Both ears
ID	Intradermal
IM	Intramuscular
IV	Intravenous
NG	Nasogastric
PO	Per orally (by mouth)v
SC	Subcutaneous
SL	Sublingual

Abbreviation	Translation
DRUG ADMINISTRATION	
ac	Before meals
ad lib	As desired, freely
bid	Twice a day
h or hr	Hour
noct	Night
NPO	Nothing by mouth
pc	After meals
prn	When needed
qh	Every hour
qid	Four times a day
qod	Every other day
Rx	Prescribe/take
stat	Immediately
tid	Three times a day

Appendix
Pharmaceutical Abbreviations

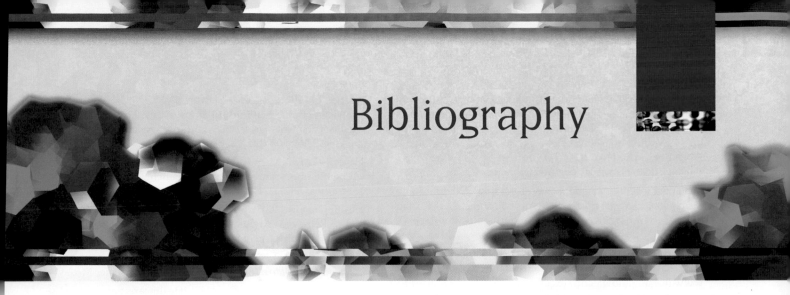

Bibliography

General References

Brown, J. E., Isaacs, J. S., Krinke, U. B., Murtaugh, M. A., Sharbaugh, C., Stag, J., et al. (2007). *Nutrition: Through the life cycle* (3rd ed.). Belmont, CA: Thomson Wadsworth.

Canadian Pharmacists Association. (2003). *Therapeutic choices* (4th ed.). Ottawa, ON: Author.

Canadian Pharmacists Association. (2008). *Compendium of pharmaceuticals and specialties. The Canadian drug reference for health professionals.* Ottawa, ON: Author. [The subscription-based e-CPS is available at http://www.pharmacists.ca.]

DiPiro, J. T., Talbert, R. L., Yee, G. C., Matzke, G. R., Wells, B. G., & Posey, L. M. (2005). *Pharmacotherapy. A pathophysiological approach* (6th ed.) New York: McGraw-Hill.

Katz, D. (2008). *Nutrition in clinical practice: A comprehensive, evidence-based manual for the practitioner* (3rd ed.). Philadelphia: Wolters Kluwer Health/Lippincott Williams & Wilkins.

Lewis, S. M., Heitkemper, M. M., & Dirksen, S. R. (2009). *Medical-surgical nursing in Canada: Assessment and management of clinical problems* (2nd Canadian ed., M. A. Barry, S. Goldsworthy, & D. Goodridge, Canadian Eds.). Toronto, ON: Mosby.

McKendry, L., Tessier, E., & Hogan, M. (2006). *Mosby's pharmacology in nursing* (22nd ed.). St. Louis, MO: Elsevier Mosby.

Mosby. (2009). *Mosby's drug reference for health professions* (2nd ed.). St. Louis, MO: Mosby.

Chapter 1

Alfaro-LeFevre, R. (2009). *Critical thinking and clinical judgment* (4th ed.). St. Louis, MO: Saunders.

Bruccoliere, T. (2000). How to make patient teaching stick. *RN*, 63(2), 34–38.

Canadian Nurses Association (CNA). (2002). *Position statement. Evidence-based decision-making and nursing practice.* Retrieved August 8, 2008, from http://www.cna-nurses.ca/CNA/documents/pdf/publications/PS63_Evidence_based_Decision_making_Nursing_Practice_e.pdf

Canadian Nurses Association. (2006). *Position statement. Nursing information and knowledge management.* Retrieved August 1, 2008, from http://www.cna-nurses.ca/CNA/documents/pdf/publications/PS87-Nursing-info-knowledge-e.pdf

Canadian Nurses Association. (2007). *Framework for the practice of registered nurses in Canada.* Retrieved June 3, 2008, from http://www.cna-aiic.ca/CNA/documents/pdf/publications/RN_Framework_Practice_2007_e.pdf

Canadian Nurses Association. (2008). *Code of ethics for registered nurses (2008 centennial edition).* Retrieved July 14, 2009, from www.cna-aiic.ca/CNA/documents/pdf/publications/Code_of_Ethics_2008_e.pdf

Cullum, N., Ciliska, D., Haynes, R. B., & Marks, S. (2008). *Evidence-based nursing. An introduction.* Malden, MA: Blackwell.

Davies, J. M., Hébert, P., & Hoffman, C. (2003). *The Canadian patient safety dictionary.* Retrieved August 1, 2007, from http://rcpsc.medical.org/publications/PatientSafetyDictionary_e.pdf

Dicenso, A., Guyatt, G., & Ciliska, D. (2005). *Evidence-based nursing. A guide to clinical practice.* St. Louis, MO: Elsevier Mosby.

Dochterman, J., & Bulechek, G. (2008). *Nursing interventions classification (NIC)* (5th ed.). St. Louis, MO: Mosby.

Health Canada. (2008). *Drug product database.* Retrieved August 1, 2008, from http://www.hc-sc.gc.ca/dhp-mps/prodpharma/databasdon/index-eng.php/

Hughes, R., & Edgerton, E.A. (2005). Reducing pediatric medication errors. *American Journal of Nursing*, 105(5), 79–84.

Jackson, M., Ignatavicius, D. D., & Case, B. (2006). *Conversations in critical thinking and critical judgment.* Sudbury, MA: Jones and Bartlett.

Kennedy, M. A., & Hannah, K. (2007). Representing nursing practice: Evaluating the effectiveness of a nursing classification system. *Canadian Journal of Nursing Research*, 39(7), 58–79.

McCaffery, M., & Pasero, C. (1999). *Pain: Clinical manual* (2nd ed.). St. Louis, MO: Mosby.

Michigan Nurses Association. (2008). *Overview of the standardized nursing languages: NANDA, NIC, & NOC.* Retrieved August 1, 2008, from http://www.minurses.org/prac/SNLOverview.shtml

Nagle, L. (2007). Clinical documentation standards: Promise or peril? *Canadian Journal of Nursing Leadership*, 20(4), 33–36.

NANDA International. (2007). *NANDA nursing diagnoses: Definitions and classification 2007–2008.* Philadelphia: Author.

National Coordinating Council for Medication Error Reporting and Prevention. (2008). *About medication errors.* Retrieved August 8, 2008, from http://www.nccmerp.org/aboutMedErrors.html

Pearson, A. (2003). The role of documentation in making nursing work visible. *International Journal of Nursing Practice*, 9(5), 271.

Philpott, M. (1985). *Legal liability & the nursing process.* Toronto, ON: Saunders Canada.

Przybycien, P. (2005). *Safe meds.* St. Louis, MO: Mosby.

Rutherford, M. (2008). Standardized nursing language: What does it mean for nursing practice? *OJIN: The Online Journal of Issues in Nursing, 13*(1). Retrieved August 1, 2008, from http://www.nursingworld.org/MainMenuCategories/ANAMarketplace/ANAPeriodicals/OJIN/TableofContents/Vol31998/Vol3No21998/StandardizedNursingLanguage.aspx

Sigma Theta Tau International Society of Nursing. (2007). *Evidence-based nursing position statement.* Retrieved August 8, 2008, from http://www.nursingsociety.org/aboutus/PositionPapers/Pages/EBN_positionpaper.aspx

University of Iowa College of Nurses. (n.d.). *Nursing interventions classification.* Retrieved August 1, 2008, from http://www.nursing.uiowa.edu/excellence/nursing_knowledge/clinical_effectiveness/index.htm

University of Iowa College of Nurses. (n.d.). *Nursing outcomes classification.* Retrieved August 1, 2008, from http://www.nursing.uiowa.edu/excellence/nursing_knowledge/clinical_effectiveness/index.htm

Wilkinson, J. (2006). *Nursing process and critical thinking* (4th ed.). Upper Saddle River, NJ: Prentice Hall.

Chapter 2

Melnyk, B. M., & Fineout-Overholt, E. (2005). *Evidence-based practice in nursing & healthcare.* Philadelphia: Lippincott Williams & Wilkins.

Chapter 3

Alzheimer Society of Canada. (2008). *Alzheimer disease statistics.* Retrieved August 11, 2008, from http://www.alzheimer.ca/english/disease/stats-people.htm

Ballantine, N. H. (2008). Polypharmacy in the elderly. Maximizing benefit, minimizing harm. *Critical Care Nursing Quarterly, 31*(1), 40–45.

Brager, R., & Sloand, E. (2005). Pediatric and geriatric considerations: The spectrum of polypharmacy. *Nurse Practitioner: American Journal of Primary Health Care, 30*(6), 44–6, 48, 50.

Briggs, G. G., Freeman, R. K., & Yaffe, S. J. (2005). *Drugs in pregnancy and lactation. A reference guide to fetal and neonatal risk* (7th ed.). Philadelphia: Lippincott, Williams & Wilkins.

Canadian Institutes of Health Research. (2004). *Alzheimer's disease.* Retrieved August 11, 2008, from http://www.cihr-irsc.gc.ca/e/24936.html

Canadian Pediatric Society. (2003, currently in revision). Position statement. Drug investigation for Canadian children. The role of the Canadian Pediatric Society. [Electronic version] *Pediatric Child Health, 8*(4), 231–234. Retrieved August 11, 2008, from http://www.cps.ca/ english/statements/DT/dt03-01.pdf

Chandra, A., & Gerwig, J. (2007). Addressing the challenges associated with polypharmacy and adverse drug events: Identifying preventive strategies. *Hospital Topics, 85*(4), 29–34.

Ferrario, C. G. (2008a). Geropharmacology: A primer for advanced practice, acute care, and critical care nurses, Part I. *ACCN Advanced Critical Care, 19*(1), 23–35.

Ferrario, C. G. (2008b). Geropharmacology: A primer for advanced practice, acute care, and critical care nurses, Part II. *AACN Advanced Critical Care, 19*(2), 134–149.

George, J., Elliott, R. A., & Stewart, D. C. (2008). A systematic review of interventions to improve medication taking in elderly patients prescribed multiple medications. *Drugs & Aging, 25*(4), 307–324.

Hayes, B. D., Klein-Schwartz, W., & Barrueto, F. (2007). Polypharmacy and the geriatric patient. *Clinics in Geriatric Medicine, 23*(2), 371–390.

Health Canada. (2008). *MedEffect Canada. Adverse reaction reporting.* Retrieved August 11, 2008, from http://www.hc-sc.gc.ca/dhp-mps/medeff/report-declaration/index-eng.php

Hockenberry, M. J., & Wilson, D., (2007). *Wong's nursing care of infants and children* (8th ed.). St. Louis, MO: Elsevier Mosby.

Jano, E., & Aparasu, R. R. (2007). Healthcare outcomes associated with Beers criteria: A systematic review. *Annuals of Pharmacotherapy, 41,* 438–448.

Laroche, M., Charmes, J., Nouaille, Y., & Merle, L. (2006). Is inappropriate medication use a major cause of adverse drug reaction in the elderly? *British Journal of Clinical Pharmacology, 63*(2), 177–186.

Ligi, I., Arnaud, F., Jouve, E., Tardieu, S., Sambuc, R., & Simeoni, U. (2008). Iatrogenic events in admitted neonates: A prospective cohort study. *Lancet, 371,* 404–410.

Motherisk. (2008). *Drugs in pregnancy.* Retrieved August 10, 2008, from http://www.motherisk.org/women/drugs.jsp

O'Mahony, D., & Gallagher, P. F. (2008). Inappropriate prescribing in the older population: Need for new criteria. *Age and Ageing, 37,* 138–141.

Perhats, C., Valdez, A. M., & St. Mars, T. (2008). Promoting safer medication use among older adults. *Journal of Emergency Nursing, 34*(2), 156–158.

Sari, A. B., Crackwell, A., & Sheldon, T. A. (2008). Incidence, preventability and consequences of adverse events in older people: Results of a retrospective case-note review. *Age and Ageing, 37,* 265–269.

Viktil, K. K., Blix, H. S., Moger, T. A., & Reikvam, A. (2006). Polypharmacy as commonly defined is an indicator of limited value in the assessment of drug-related problems. *British Journal of Clinical Pharmacology, 63*(2), 187–195.

Chapter 4

Bon Bernard, C. (2003). *Cross-cultural profiles.* Updated by Health Care Interpreters, Calgary Health Region. Calgary, AB: Multicultural Awareness Program, Peter Lougheed Hospital. Available at www.calgaryhealthregion.ca/programs/diversity/diversity_resources/library/cross_cultural_profiles_2003.pdf

Canada Gazette. (2003). *Order amending Schedule III to the Controlled Drugs and Substances Act.* Retrieved July 17, 2005, from http://canadagazette.gc.ca/partII/2003/20031231/html/sor412-e.html

Canadian Institute for Health Information. (2005a). *Drug expenditure in Canada 1985 to 2007.* Ottawa, ON: Source. Retrieved August 17, 2008, from http://secure.cihi.ca/cihiweb/products/Drug_Expenditure_in_Canada_1985_2007_e.pdf

Canadian Institute for Health Information. (2005b). *Exploring the 70/30 split: How Canada's health care system is financed.* Re-trieved August 17, 2008, from http://secure.cihi.ca/cihiweb/dispPage.jsp?cw_page=PG_469_E&cw_topic=469&cw_rel=AR_1282_E

Canadian Nurses Association. (2008). *Code of ethics for registered nurses*. Ottawa, ON: Author. Available online at http://www.cna-nurses.ca/CNA/documents/pdf/publications/Code_of_Ethics_2008_e.pdf

Commission on the Future of Health Care in Canada. (2002). *Building on values. The future of health care in Canada—Final report*. Retrieved August 17, 2008, from http://www.cbc.ca/healthcare/final_report.pdf

Department of Justice Canada. (2004). *Narcotic control regulations*. Retrieved August 17, 2008, from http://laws.justice.gc.ca/en/C-38.8/C.R.C.-c.1041/index.html

Health Canada. (2008a). *Clinical trials*. Retrieved August 17, 2008, from http://www.hc-sc.gc.ca/dhp-mps/prodpharma/activit/proj/enreg-clini-info/index-eng.php

Health Canada. (2008b). Natural health products regulations. *Canada Gazette 137*(13). Ottawa, ON: Author. Retrieved August 17, 2008, from http://www.hc-sc.gc.ca/dhp-mps/prodnatur/index-eng.php

Health Canada. (2008c). *Questions and answers: Schedule A and Section 3 regulatory amendments and associated guidance*, 46–51. Retrieved August 11, 2008, from http://www.hc-sc.gc.ca/dhp-mps/prodpharma/applic-demande/guide-ld/scha_qa_qr-eng.php 99(8).

Leininger, M. (2002). *Transcultural nursing: Concepts, theories, research, and practice* (3rd ed.). New York: McGraw-Hill.

McClean, W. (2007). An adherence study of prescription refill data, with and without a periodic patient education program [electronic version]. *CPJ/RPC, 140*(2), 104–106.

Mundoz, C., & Hildenberg, C. (2006). Ethnopharmacology: Understanding how ethnicity can affect drug response is essential to providing culturally competent care. *Holistic Nursing Practice, 20*(5), 227–234.

Pugh, M. J., Rosen, A. K., Montez-Rath, M., Amuan, M. E., Fincke, B. G., Burk, M., et al. (2008). Potentially inappropriate prescribing for the elderly: Effects of geriatric care at the patient and health care system level. *Medical Care, 46*(2), 167–173.

Saul, D. (2004). National pharmacare: A pill not easily swallowed. *University of Toronto Medical Journal, 82*, 14–15.

Spector, R. E. (2000). *Cultural care: Guides to heritage assessment and health traditions* (2nd ed.). Upper Saddle River, NJ: Pearson/Prentice Hall.

Statistics Canada. (2006). *Canada's ethnocultural portrait, mosaic, 2006 census. Summary*. Retrieved August July 17, 2008, from http://www.cerium.ca/Canada-s-Ethnocultural-Mosaic-2006

Chapter 5

Abushaiqa, M. E., Zaran, F. K., Bach, D. S., Smolarek, R. T., & Farber, M. S. (2007). Educational interventions to reduce use of unsafe abbreviations. *American Journal of Health-System Pharmacy, 64*(11), 1170–1173.

Baker, G. R., Norton, P. G., Flintoft, V., Blais, R., Brown, A., Cox, J., et al. (2004). The Canadian adverse events study: The incidence of adverse events among hospital patients in Canada. *Canadian Medical Association Journal, 170* (11), 1678–1686.

Balas, M. C., Scott, L. D., & Rogers, A. E. (2004). Frequency and type of errors and near errors reported by hospital staff nurses. *Applied Nursing Research, 17*(4), 224–230.

Barnsteiner, J. H. (2005). Medication reconciliation: Transfer of medication information across settings—keeping it free from error. *American Journal of Nursing, 105*(3 Suppl), 31–36.

Bartlett, G., Blais, R., Tamblyn, R., & Clermont, R. J. (2008). Impact of patient communication problems on the risk of preventable adverse events in acute care settings. *Canadian Medical Association Journal, 178*(12), 1555–1562.

Baumann, A., O'Brien-Pallas, L., Armstrong-Stausser, M., Blythe, J., Bourbonnais, R., Cameron, S., et al. (2001). *Commitment and care. The benefits of a healthy workplace for nurses, their patients, and the system*. Retrieved August 20, 2008, from http://www.chsrf.ca/nursing_research_fund/pdf/pscomcare_e.pdf

Bournes, D. A., & Flint, F. (2003). Mis-takes: Mistakes in the nurse–person process. *Nursing Science Quarterly, 16*(2), 127–130.

Brunetti, L., Santell, J. P., & Hicks, R. W. (2007). The impact of abbreviations on patient safety. *Joint Commission Journal on Quality and Patient Safety, 33*(9), 576–583. Retrieved August 20, 2008, from http://www.wapatientsafety.org/downloads/Brunetti_JCJQPS_2007.pdf

Canadian Federation of Nurses Unions. (2008). *A renewed call for action. A synthesis report on the nursing shortage in Canada*. Retrieved August 20, 2008, from http://www.nursesunions.ca/media.php?mid=675

Canadian Health Services Research Foundation. (2006). *What's ailing our nurses? A discussion of the major issues affecting nursing human resources in Canada*. Retrieved June 30, 2009, from www.chsrf.ca/research_themes/pdf/What_sailingourNurses-e.pdf

Canadian Institute for Health Information. (2004). *Health care in Canada*. Ottawa, ON: Author.

Canadian Nurses Association. (2002). *Planning for the future: Nursing human resource projections*. Retrieved July 18, 2009, from www.cna-aiic.ca/CNA/documents/pdf/publications/Planning_for_the_future_June_2002_e.pdf

Canadian Nurses Association. (2003). *Position statement. Patient safety*. Retrieved August 20, 2008, from http://www.cna-aiic.ca/CNA/documents/pdf/publications/PS70_Patient-Safety_en.pdf

Canadian Nurses Association. (2008). *Code of ethics for registered nurses*. Retrieved August 20, 2008, from http://www.cna-nurses.ca/CNA/documents/pdf/publications/PS95_Code_of_Ethics_2008_e.pdf

Canadian Nurses Association and Canadian Federation of Nurses Association (2006). *Joint position statement. Practice environments: Maximizing patient, nurse, and system outcomes*. Retrieved August 20, 2008, from http://www.cna-aiic.ca/CNA/documents/pdf/publications/PS88-Practice-Environments-e.pdf

Carlton, G., & Blegen, M. A. (2006). Medication-related errors: A literature review of incidence and antecedents. *Annual Review of Nursing Research, 24*, 19–38.

Catchpole, K., Mishra, A., Handa, A., & McCulloch, P. (2008). Teamwork and error in the operating room: Analysis of skills and roles. *Annals of Surgery, 2447*(4), 699–706.

Cho, J., Laschinger, H. K., & Wong, C. (2006). Workplace empowerment, work engagement and organizational commitment of new graduate nurses. *Canadian Journal of Nursing Research, 19*(3), 43–60.

College of Nurses of Ontario. (2004). *Best practices in disclosing health care error*. Retrieved August 20, 2008, from http://www.cno.org/new/notices/disclosing_error.htm

Cornish, P.L., Knowles, S. R., Marchesano, R., Tam, V., Shadowitz, S., Juurlink, D. N., et al. (2005). Unintended medication discrepancies at the time of hospital admission. *Archives of Internal Medicine, 165*, 424–429.

Davidhizar, R., & Lonser, G. (2003). Strategies to decrease medication errors. *Health Care Manager, 22*(3), 211–218.

Eisenhauer, L. A., Hurley, A. C., & Dolan, N. (2007). Nurses' reported thinking during medication administration. *Journal of Nursing Scholarship, 39*(1), 82–87.

Forster, A. J., Clark, H. D., Menard, A., Dupuis, N., Chernish, R., Chandok, N., et al. (2004). Adverse events among medical patients after discharge from hospital. *Canadian Medical Association Journal, 170*(3), 345–349.

Greenall, J., Hyland, S., Colquhoun, M., & Jelincic, V. (2004). Medication safety alerts. *Canadian Journal of Hospital Pharmacy, 57*(2), 110–113.

Hall, L. M., Doran, D., & Pink, G. (2004). Nurse staffing models, nursing hours, and patient safety outcomes. *Journal of Nursing Administration, 34*(1), 41–45.

Health Canada. (2008). *Canadian medication incident reporting and prevention system (CMIRPS)*. Retrieved August 20, 2008, from http://secure.cihi.ca/cihiweb/dispPage.jsp?cw_page=services_cmirps_e

Horack, C. L., & Taylor, R. M. (2006). Medication reconciliation. *Nursing Critical Care, 1*(2), 26–33.

Hughes, R. (2005). Medication errors: Why they happen, and how they can be prevented. *American Journal of Nursing, 105*(2), 14–24.

Institute for Safe Medication Practices Canada. (2006). Eliminate use of dangerous abbreviations, symbols, and dose designations. *ISMP Canada Safety Bulletin, 6*(4), 1–4. Retrieved August 20, 2008, from http://www.ismp.org/newsletters/acutecare/articles/dangerousabbrev.asp

Institute for Safe Medication Practices. (2008a). *Do not use these dangerous abbreviations or dose designations*. Retrieved August 20, 2008, from http://www.ismp.org/Tools/errorproneabbreviations.pdf

Institute for Safe Medication Practices. (2008b). *ISMP's list of high-alert medications*. Retrieved May 12, 2009, from http://www.ismp.org/Tools/highalertmedications.pdf

Koczmara, C., Jelincic, V., & Dueck, C. (2005). Dangerous abbreviations: "U" can make a difference! *Canadian Association of Critical Care Nurses, 16*(3), 11–15. Retrieved August 20, 2008, from http://www.ismp-canada.org/download/CACCN-Fall05.pdf

Kuhn, I. F. (2007). Abbreviations and acronyms in healthcare: When shorter isn't sweeter. *Pediatric Nursing, 33*(5), 392–398.

LaPointe, N. M., & Jollis, J. G. (2003). Medication errors in hospitalized cardiovascular patients. *Archives of Internal Medicine, 163*, 1461–1466.

Laschinger, H. K., & Leiter, M. P. (2006). The impact of nursing work environments on patient safety outcomes: The mediating role of burnout/engagement. *Journal of Nursing Administration, 5*, 259–267.

Leiter, M. P., & Laschinger, H. K. (2006). A work environment to support professional nursing practice: Implications for burnout. *Nursing Research, 55*, 137–146.

McCleave, S. H. (2001). How to respond to a formal patient complaint. *Journal of Clinical Outcomes Management, 8*(10), 35–42.

Milligan, F. (2003). Adverse health-care events: Part I, the nature of the problem. *Professional Nurse, 18*(9), 502–505.

Paparella, S. (2006). Medication reconciliation. Doing what's right for safe patient care. *Journal of Emergency Nursing, 32*(6), 516–520.

Pastorius, D. (2007). Crime in the workplace. Part I. *Nursing Management, 38*(10), 18–27.

Poloway, L., & Greenall, J. (2006). Medication safety alerts. *Canadian Journal of Hospital Pharmacy, 59*(4), 206–209.

Registered Nurses Association of Ontario. (2006a). *Healthy work environments best practice guidelines. Collaborative practice among working teams*. Retrieved August 20, 2008, from http://www.rnao.org/Storage/23/1776_BPG_Collaborative_Practice.pdf

Registered Nurses Association of Ontario. (2006b). *Healthy work environments best practice guidelines. Developing and sustaining nursing leadership*. Retrieved August 20, 2008, from http://www.rnao.org/Storage/16/1067_BPG_Sustain_Leadership.pdf

Registered Nurses Association of Ontario. (2007a). *Healthy work environments best practice guidelines. Developing and sustaining effective staffing and workload practices*. Retrieved August 20, 2008, from http://www.rnao.org/Storage/35/2935_BPG_Staffing_Workload.pdf

Registered Nurses Association of Ontario. (2007b). *Healthy work environments best practice guidelines. Embracing cultural diversity in health care: Developing cultural competence*. Retrieved August 20, 2008, from http://www.rnao.org/Storage/29/2336_BPG_Embracing_Cultural_Diversity.pdf

Registered Nurses Association of Ontario. (2007c). *Healthy work environments best practice guidelines. Professionalism in nursing*. Retrieved August 20, 2008, from http://www.rnao.org/Storage/28/2303_BPG_Professionalism.pdf

Registered Nurses Association of Ontario. (2008). *Healthy work environments best practice guidelines. Workplace health, safety, and well-being of the nurse*. Retrieved August 20, 2008, from http://www.rnao.org/Storage/36/3089_RNAO_BPG_Health_Safety.pdf

Rich, V. (2005). How we think about medication errors: A model and a change. *American Journal of Nursing, 105*(3), 10–11.

Richardson, W. C., Berwick, D. M., Bisgard, J. C., Bristow, L. R., Buck, C. R., Cassel, C.K., et al. (1999). *To err is human: Building a safer health system*. Washington, DC: National Academy Press.

Rosenstein, A. H., & O'Daniel, M. (2005). Original research: Disruptive behavior and clinical outcomes: Perceptions of nurses and physicians: Nurses, physicians, and administrators say that clinicians' disruptive behavior has negative effects on clinical outcomes. *American Journal of Nursing, 105*(1), 54–64.

Shields, M., & Wilkins, K. (2006). *Findings from the 2005 national survey of the work and health of nurses*. Retrieved July 18, 2009, from www.cihi.ca/cihiweb/en/downloads/NS_SummRep06_ENG.pdf

Stone, P. W., Du, Y., Cowell, R., Amsterdam , N., Helfrich, T. A., Linn, R. W., et al. (2006). Comparison of nurse, system and quality patient care outcomes in 8-hour and 12-hour shifts. *Medical Care, 44*(12), 1099–1106.

Stone, P. W., Mooney-Kane, C., Larson, E. L., Horan, T., Glance, L. G., Zwanziger, J., et al. (2007). Nurse working conditions and patient safety outcomes. *Medical Care, 45*(6), 571–578.

Wilkins, K., & Shields, M. (2008). Correlates of medication error in hospitals. *Health Reports, 19*(2), 1–12.

Wolf, Z. R. (2007). Pursuing safe medication use and the promise of technology. *Medsurg Nursing, 16*(2), 92–100.

Wong, J. (2005). *Medication awareness key to catching errors: Study.* Retrieved August 20, 2008, from http://www.news.utoronto.ca/bin6/050228-1038.asp

World Health Organization. (2008). *World alliance for patient safety.* Retrieved August 20, 2008, from http://www.who.int/patientsafety/en/

Zed, P. J., Abu-Laban, R. B., Balen, R. M., Loewen, P. S., Hohl, C. M., & Brubacher, J. R. (2008). Incidence, severity and preventability of medication-related visits to the emergency department: A prospective study. *Canadian Medical Association Journal, 178*(12), 1563–1569.

Chapter 6

Bass, L. (2005). Health literacy: Implications for teaching the adult patient. *Journal of Infusion Nursing, 28*, 15–22.

Bergman-Evans, B. (2006). AIDES to improving medication adherence in older adults. *Geriatric Nursing, 27*(3), 174–182.

Canobbio, M. M. (2006). *Mosby's handbook of patient teaching* (3rd ed.). St. Louis, MO: Mosby.

Cutilli, C. C. (2005). Do your patients understand? Determining your patient's health literacy skills. *Orthopedic Nursing, 24*(5), 372–377.

Cutilli, C. C. (2008). Teaching the geriatric patient: Making the most of "cognitive resources" and "gains." *Orthopedic Nursing, 27*(3), 195–198.

Erickson, E. (1959). *Identity and the life cycle; Selected papers.* New York: International Universities Press.

George, J., Elliott, R. A., & Stewart, D. C. (2008). A systematic review of interventions to improve medication taking in elderly patients prescribed multiple medications. *Drugs & Aging, 25*(4), 307–324.

Health Canada. (2005). *Medication matters. How you can help seniors use medications wisely.* Retrieved August 21, 2008, from http://www.phac-aspc.gc.ca/seniors-aines/pubs/med_matters/pdf/med_matters_e.pdf

Koelling, T. M., Johnson, M. L., Cody, R. J., & Aaronson, K. D. (2005). Discharge education improves clinical outcomes in patients with chronic heart failure. *Circulation, 111*, 179–185.

Polzien, G. (2007). Prevent medication errors: A New Year's resolution: Teaching patients about their medications. *Home Healthcare Nurse, 25*(1), 59–62.

Public Health Agency of Canada. (2005). *Beyond words. The health–literacy connection.* Retrieved August 21, 2008, from http://www.nald.ca/library/research/cahealth/English.pdf

Shopper's Drug Mart. (2005). *HealthWATCH medication library.* Retrieved July 21, 2005, from http://www.shoppersdrugmart.ca/medispan/en_CA/welcome.htm

Statistics Canada. (2005). *Building on our competencies. Canadian results of the international adult literacy and skills survey.* Retrieved August 21, 2008, from http://www.nald.ca/fulltext/booc/booc.pdf

Winslow, E.H. (2001). Patient education materials. Can patients read them or are they ending up in the trash? *American Journal of Nursing, 101*(10), 33–38.

Chapter 7

Be Medwise. (2005). *Survey on Canadians' use of OTC medications.* Retrieved August 24, 2008, from http://www.bemedwise.ca/english/usagesurvey.html

Blumenthal, M., Goldberg, A., & Busse, W. R. (2001). *The complete German Commission E Monographs: Therapeutic guide to herbal medicines.* New York: Thieme.

Butterweck, V., & Derendorf, H. (2008). Potential of pharmacokinetic profiling for detecting herbal interactions with drugs. *Clinical Pharmacokinetics, 47*(6), 383–397.

Canadian Institute for Health Information. (2008). *Drug expenditure in Canada 1985 to 2007.* Ottawa, ON: Author. Retrieved August 22, 2008, from http://www.cihi.ca

Canadian Interdisciplinary Network for Complementary & Alternative Medicine Research. (2009). *Mission statement.* Retrieved July 18, 2009, from http://www.incamresearch.ca/index.php

Canadian Paediatric Society. (2008). *Canadian Paediatric Surveillance Program.* Retrieved August 24, 2008, from http://www.cps.ca/English/Surveillance/CPSP/index.htm

Cañigueral, S., Tschopp, R., Ambrosetti, L., Vignutelli, A., Scaglione, F., & Petrini O. (2008). The development of herbal medicinal products: Quality, safety, and efficacy as key factors. *Pharmaceutical Medicine, 22*(2), 107–118.

Chan, E. (2008). Quality of efficacy research in complementary and alternative medicine. *Journal of the American Medical Association, 299*(22), 2685–2686.

Dobson, R., Taylor, J. G., & Lynd, L. D. (2004). Are we ready for prescriptive authority? Lessons from the self-care example. *Canadian Pharmacists Journal, 137*(9), 38–39.

Goldman, R. D., Rogovik, A. L., Lai, D., & Vohra, S. (2008). Potential interactions of drug–natural health products and natural health products–natural health products among children. *Journal of Pediatrics, 152*, 521–526.

Harkness, R., & Bratman, S. (2003). *Mosby's handbook of drug–herb and drug–supplement interactions.* St. Louis, MO: Mosby.

Health Canada. (2003a). *Health Canada reminds Canadians of the dangers of Ephedra/ephedrine products.* Retrieved August 24, 2008, from http://www.hc-sc.gc.ca/ahc-asc/media/advisories-avis/_2003/2003_43-eng.php

Health Canada. (2003b). *Natural health products regulations.* Retrieved August 24, 2008, from http://canadagazette.gc.ca/partII/2003/20030618/html/sor196-e.html

Health Canada. (2004). *Overview of the natural health products guidance document*. Retrieved August 26, 2008, from http://www.hc-sc.gc.ca/dhp-mps/prodnatur/legislation/docs/regula-regle_over-apercu-eng.php#45

Health Canada. (2005). *Health Canada baseline natural health products survey among consumers*. Retrieved August 24, 2008, from http://www.hc-sc.gc.ca/dhp-mps/pubs/natur/eng_cons_survey-eng.php

Health Canada. (2006a). *It's your health. Safe use of natural health products*. Retrieved August 24, 2008, from http://www.hc-sc.gc.ca/hl-vs/iyh-vsv/med/nat-prod-eng.php

Health Canada. (2006b). *Marijuana medical access regulations*. Retrieved August 24, 2008, from eng.php http://canadagazette.gc.ca/partII/2001/20010704/html/sor227-e.html

Health Canada. (2007). *Natural health products compliance guide*. Retrieved July 24, 2009, from http://www.hc-sc.gc.ca/dhp-mps/prodnatur/legislation/docs/complian-conform_guide-eng.php

Health Canada. (2008a). *Compendium of monographs*. Retrieved August 24, 2008, from http://www.hc-sc.gc.ca/dhp-mps/prodnatur/applications/licen-prod/monograph/mono_list-eng.php

Health Canada (2008b). *Medical use of marijuana*. Retrieved August 24, 2008, from http://www.hc-sc.gc.ca/dhp-mps/marihuana/index-eng.php

Health Canada (2009a). *Natural health products*. Retrieved July 22, 2009, from www.hc-sc.gc.ca/dhp-mps/prodnatur/index-eng.php

Health Canada. (2009b). *Welcome to the licensed natural health products database (LNHPD)*. Retrieved October 8, 2009, from http://www.hc-sc.gc.ca/dhp-mps/prodnatur/applications/licen-prod/lnhpd-bdpsnh-eng.php

Hulisz, D. T. (2007). *Top herbal products: Efficacy and safety concerns*. Retrieved August 24, 2008, from http://www.medscape.com/viewprogram/8494

International Scientific Association for Probiotics and Prebiotics. (2008). *Introduction to probiotics and prebiotics*. Retrieved August 26, 2008, from http://www.isapp.net/pp_intro.asp

Kligler, B., Hanaway, P., & Cohrssen, A. (2007). Probiotics in children. *Pediatric Clinics of North America, 54*, 949–967.

Koren, G., Oren, D., Rouleau, M., Carmeli, D., & Matsui, D. (2006). Comparison of verbal claims for natural health products made by health food stores staff versus pharmacists in Ontario, Canada. *Canadian Journal of Clinical Pharmacology, 13*(2), e251–e256.

Mertens-Talcott, S. U., Zadezensky, I., De Castro, W. V., Derendorf, H., & Butterweck, V. (2006). Grapefruit–drug interactions: Can interactions with drugs be avoided? *Journal of Clinical Pharmacology, 46*(12), 1390–1416.

Messina, B. A. M. (2006). Herbal supplements: Facts and myths. Talking to your patients about herbal supplements. *Journal of PeriAnesthesia Nursing, 21*(4), 268–278.

Millar, W. (2001). Patterns of use—Alternative health care practitioners. *Health Reports 13*(1), 9–21. Retrieved August 24, 2008, from http://www.statcan.gc.ca/cgi-bin/af-fdr.cgi?l=eng&loc=http://www.statcan.gc.ca/studies-etudes/82-003/archive/2001/6021-eng.pdf&t=Patterns%20of%20use%20-%20Alternative%20health%20care%20practitioners

Munoz, C., & Hilgenberg, C. (2006). Ethnopharmacology: Understanding how ethnicity can affect drug response is essential to providing culturally competent care. *Holistic Nursing Practice, 20*(5), 227–234.

Murty, M. (2007). Postmarket surveillance of natural health products in Canada: Clinical and federal regulatory perspectives. *Canadian Journal of Physiology and Pharmacology, 85*, 952–955.

Natural Health Products Directorate (2009). *Mission statement*. Retrieved July 24, 2009, from http://www.hc-sc.gc.ca/ahc-asc/branch-dirgen/hpfb-dgpsa/nhpd-dpsn/index-eng.php

Nonprescription Drug Manufacturers Association of Canada. (1995). Self-medication: A health care solution for the '90s. *NDMAC Self-Medication Digest, 1*(2). Retrieved July 22, 2009, from www.ndmac.ca/

Reid, G. (2006). Probiotics prevent the need for, and augment the use of, antibiotics. *Canadian Journal of Infectious Diseases and Medical Microbiology, 17*(5), 291–295.

Reid, G., Jass, J., Sebulsky, T., & McCormick, J. K. (2003). Potential uses of probiotics in clinical practice. *Clinical Microbiology Reviews, 16*(4), 658–672.

Singh, S. R., & Levine, M. A. H. (2007). Potential interactions between pharmaceuticals and natural health products in Canada. *Journal of Clinical Pharmacology, 47*, 249–258.

Skalli, S., Zaid, A., & Soulaymani, R. (2007). Drug interactions with herbal medicines. *Therapeutic Drug Monitoring, 29*(6), 679–686.

Soo, I., Madsen, K. L., Tejpar, Q., Sydora, B. C., Sherbaniuk, R., Cinque, B., et al. (2008). VSL#3 probiotic upregulates intestinal mucosal alkaline sphingomyelinase and reduces inflammation. *Canadian Journal of Gastroenterology. 22*(3), 237–242.

Vohra, S., & Cohen, M. H. (2007). Ethics of complementary and alternative medicine use in children. *Pediatric Clinics of North America, 54*, 875–884.

Winslow, L. C., & Kroll, D. J. (1998). Herbs as medicines. *Archives of Internal Medicine, 158*, 2192–2199.

Chapter 8

First Nations, Inuit and Métis Health Committee, Canadian Paediatric Society (CPS). (2007). Vitamin D supplementation: Recommendations for Canadian mothers and infants. *Paediatrics and Child Health, 12*(7), 583–589.

Giovannucci, E., Liu, Y., & Hollis, B. W. (2008). 25-hydroxyvitamin D and risk of myocardial infarction in men: A prospective study. *Archives of Internal Medicine, 168*(11), 1174–1180.

Gordon, C. M., Feldman, H. A., Sinclair, L., Williams, A. L., Kleinman, P. K., Perez Rossello, J., et al. (2008). Prevalence of vitamin D deficiency among healthy infants and toddlers. *Archives of Pediatrics and Adolescent Medicine, 1626*, 505–512.

Health Canada. (2004). *Dietary reference intakes*. Retrieved September 3, 2008, from http://www.hc-sc.gc.ca/fn-an/nutrition/reference/index-eng.php

Health Canada. (2006). *The safety of vitamin E supplements*. Retrieved September 3, 2008, from http://www.hc-sc.gc.ca/hl-vs/iyh-vsv/food-aliment/vitam-eng.php

Health Canada. (2007a). *Drug and health products. Vitamin A.* Retrieved August 29, 2008, from http://www.hc-sc.gc.ca/dhp-mps/prodnatur/applications/licen-prod/monograph/mono_vitamin_a-eng.php

Health Canada. (2007b). *Drug and health products. Vitamin B₁₂.* Retrieved September 1, 2008, from http://www.hc-sc.gc.ca/dhp-mps/prodnatur/applications/licen-prod/monograph/mono_vitamin_b12-eng.php

Health Canada. (2007c). *Drug and health products. Vitamin B₆.* Retrieved September 1, 2008, from http://www.hc-sc.gc.ca/dhp-mps/prodnatur/applications/licen-prod/monograph/mono_vitamin_b6-eng.php

Health Canada. (2007d). *Drug and health products. Vitamin C.* Retrieved September 1, 2008, from http://www.hc-sc.gc.ca/dhp-mps/prodnatur/applications/licen-prod/monograph/mono_vitamin_c-eng.php

Health Canada. (2007e). *Drug and health products. Vitamin D.* Retrieved September 1, 2008, from http://www.hc-sc.gc.ca/ahc-asc/media/advisories-avis/_2007/2007_72-eng.php

Holick, M. F. (2007). Vitamin D deficiency. *New England Journal of Medicine, 357*(3), 266–281.

Katz, D. (2005). *Nutrition in clinical practice: A comprehensive, evidence-based manual for the practitioner* (2nd ed.). Philadelphia: Lippincott Williams & Wilkins.

Lappe, J. M., Travers-Gustafson, D., Davies, K. M., Recker, R. R., & Heaney, R. P. (2007). Vitamin D and calcium supplementation reduces cancer risk: Results of a randomized trial. *American Journal of Clinical Nutrition, 85*(6), 1586–1591.

Moe, S., Wazny, L. D., & Martin, J. E. (2008). Oral calcitriol versus oral alfacalcidol for the treatment of secondary hyperparathyroidism in patients receiving hemodialysis: A randomized cross-over trial. *Canadian Journal of Clinical Pharmacology, 15*(1), 36–42. Retrieved May 22, 2009, from http://www.cjcp.ca/pdf/CJCP07017_wazny_e36-e43V2.pdf.

Munroe, R. W., & Kessenich, C. (2008). Vitamin D deficiency across the lifespan. *Journal for Nurse Practitioners, 4*(6), 448–454.

Roth, D. E., Martz, P., Yeo, R., Prosser, C., Bell, M., & Jones, A. B. (2005). Are national vitamin D guidelines sufficient to maintain adequate blood levels in children? *Canadian Journal of Public Health, 96*, 443–449.

Ward, L. M. (2005). Vitamin D deficiency in the 21st century: A persistent problem among Canadian infants and mothers. *Canadian Medical Association Journal, 172*, 769–70.

Chapter 9

Adlaf, E. M., & Paglia-Boak, A. (2007). *Drug use among Ontario students, 1977–2007: detailed OSDUS findings* [CAMH Research Document series no. 20]. Toronto, ON: Centre for Addiction and Mental Health. Retrieved September 7, 2008, from www.camh.net/Research/Areas_of_research/Population_Life_Course_Studies/OSDUS/OSDUHS2007_DrugDetailed_final.pdf

Buxton, J. A., & Dove, N. A. (2008). The burden and management of crystal meth use. *Canadian Medical Association Journal, 178*(12), 1537–1539.

Canadian Centre on Substance Abuse. (2007a). *A drug prevention strategy for Canada's youth.* Ottawa, ON: Author. Retrieved September 7, 2008, from http://www.ccsa.ca/2007%20CCSA%20Documents/ccsa-011522-2007-e.pdf

Canadian Centre on Substance Abuse. (2007b). *Substance abuse in Canada: Youth in focus.* Ottawa, ON: The Centre. Retrieved September 7, 2008, from http://www.ccsa.ca/2007%20CCSA%20Documents/ccsa-011521-2007-e.pdf

Centre for Addiction and Mental Health. (2008). *Methadone maintenance treatment client handbook.* Revised. Retrieved May 1, 2009, from http://www.camh.net/Care_Treatment/Resources_clients_families_friends/Methadone_Maintenance_Treatment/mmt_client_hndbk.pdf

College of Physicians and Surgeons of Ontario. (2005, Revised 2007). *Methadone maintenance guidelines.* Retrieved September 7, 2008, from http://www.cpso.on.ca/publications/MethGuideNov05revOct07.pdf

Fischer, B., Goldman, B., Rehm, J., & Popova, S. (2008). Non-medical use of prescription opioids and public health in Canada. *Canadian Journal of Public Health, 99*(3), 182–184.

Hamid, H., El-Mallakh, R., & Vandeveir, K. (2005). Substance abuse: Medical and slang terminology. *Southern Medical Journal, 98*(3), 350–362.

Health Canada. (2002). *Best practices—treatment and rehabilitation for seniors with substance use problems.* Retrieved September 7, 2008, from http://www.hc-sc.gc.ca/hl-vs/pubs/adp-apd/treat_senior-trait_ainee/index-eng.php

Health Canada. (2004). *Misuse and abuse of oxycodone-based prescription drugs.* Retrieved September 7, 2008, from http://www.hc-sc.gc.ca/dhp-mps/pubs/precurs/oxycodone/fs-fi/index-eng.php

Health Canada. (2008). *Canadian addiction survey. A national survey of Canadians' use of alcohol and other drugs. Focus on gender.* Retrieved September 7, 2008, from http://www.hc-sc.gc.ca/hl-vs/pubs/adp-apd/cas-etc/gender-sexe/index-eng.php

Levine, D. A. (2007). "Pharming": The abuse of prescription and over-the-counter drugs in teens. *Current Opinion in Pediatrics, 19*, 270–274.

Rehm, J., Ballunas, D., Brochu, S., Fischer, B., Gnam, W., Patra, J., et al. (2006). *The costs of substance abuse in Canada 2002: Highlights.* Retrieved July 27, 2009, from www.ccsa.ca/2006%20CCSA%20Documents/ccsa-011332-2006.pdf

Thomas, G. (2004). *Alcohol-related harms and control policy in Canada.* Retrieved July 27, 2009, from www.ccsa.ca/2004%20CCSA%20Documents/ccsa-004840-2004.pdf

Tjepkema, M. (2002). *Alcohol and illicit drug dependence.* Ottawa, ON: Statistics Canada. Retrieved September 4, 2008, from http://www.statcan.ca/english/freepub/82-003-SIE/2004000/pdf/82-003-SIE20040007447.pdf

United Nations Office on Drugs and Crime. (2007). *World drug report.* Retrieved July 27, 2009, from www.unodc.org/unodc/en/data-and-analysis/WDR-2007.html

Chapter 10

Burkhart, P. V., Ravens, M., & Bowman, R. (2003). An evaluation of children's metered-dose inhaler technique for asthma medications. *Nursing Clinics of North America, 40*(1), 167–182.

Ignatavicius, D. D. (2002). Asking the right questions about medication safety. *Nursing, 30*(9), 51–54.

Institute for Safe Medication Practices. (2002). *Hazard alert! Asphyxiation possible with syringe tip caps.* Retrieved September 10, 2008, from www.ismp.org/hazardalerts/Hypodermic.asp

Institute for Safe Medication Practices. (2007). Patches: What you can't see can harm patients. *Nurse Advise-ERR, 5*(4), 1. Retrieved September 10, 2008, from http://www.ismp.org/newsletters/nursing/Issues/NurseAdviseERR200704.pdf

Kaestli, L. Z., Wasilewski-Rasca, A. F., Bonnabry, P., & Vogt-Ferrier, N. (2008). Use of transdermal drug formulations in the elderly. *Drugs & Aging, 25*(4), 269–280.

Karch, A. (2003). Not so fast! IV push drugs can be dangerous when given too rapidly. *American Journal of Nursing, 103*(8), 71.

Karch, A., & Karch, F. (2000). Practice errors: A hard pill to swallow. *American Journal of Nursing, 100*(4), 25.

Love, G. H. (2005). Clinical do's and don'ts: Administering an intradermal injection. *Nursing 36*(6), 20.

McConnell, E. (2000). Clinical do's and don'ts: Administering an intradermal injection. *Nursing, 30*(2), 50–52.

McConnell, E. (2001). Clinical do's and don'ts: Applying nitroglycerin ointment. *Nursing, 31*(6), 17.

McConnell, E. (2002). Clinical do's and don'ts: Administering medications through a gastrostomy tube. *Nursing, 32*(12), 22.

Miller, D., & Miller, H. (2000). To crush or not to crush? *Nursing, 30*(2), 50–52.

Moshang, J. (2005). Making a point about insulin pens. *Nursing, 35*(2), 46–47.

Perry, A., &, Potter, P. (2008). *Canadian fundamentals of nursing* (2nd ed.). (Canadian Eds. Ross-Kerr, J. C., & Wood, M. J.). Toronto, ON: Mosby.

Pope, B. A. (2002). How to administer subcutaneous and intramuscular injections. *Nursing 32*(1): 50.

Pruitt, W. (2005). Teaching your patient to use a peak flowmeter. *Nursing, 35*(3), 54–55.

Pullen, R. L., Jr. (2003). Managing IV patient-controlled analgesia. *Nursing, 33*(7), 24.

Pullen, R. L., Jr. (2005). Administering medication by the Z-track method. *Nursing, 35*(7), 24.

Pullen, R. L., Jr. (2008). Administering a transdermal patch. *Nursing 38*(5), 14.

Schulmeister, L. (2005). Transdermal drug patches: Medicine with muscle. *Nursing 35*(1), 48–52.

Stein, H. G. (2006). Glass ampules and filter needles: An example of implementing the sixth "r" in medication administration. *Medsurg Nursing, 15*(5), 290–294.

Chapter 11

Canadian Institutes of Health Research. (2005). *Community advisory boards play key role in NAOMI heroin addiction study.* Retrieved September 16, 2008, from http://www.cihr-irsc.gc.ca/e/29084.html

Carbajal, R., Biran, V., Lenclen, R., Epaud, R, Cimerman, P., Thibault, P., et al. (2008). EMLA cream and nitrous oxide to alleviate pain induced by palivizumab (Synagis) intramuscular injections in infants and young children. *Pediatrics, 121*, e1591–e1598.

Centre for Addiction and Mental Health (2008). *What is addiction?* Retrieved August 18, 2009, from www.camh.net

Cregin, R., Rappaport, A. S., Montagnino, G., Sabogal, G., Moreau, H., & Abularrage. (2008). Improving pain management for pediatric patients undergoing nonurgent pain procedures. *American Journal of Health-Systems Pharmacology, 65*, 723–727.

D'Arcy, Y. (2005). Conquering pain: Have you tried these new techniques? *Nursing, 35*(3), 36–41.

Fischer, B., Cruz, M. F., & Rehm, J. (2006). Illicit opioid use and its key characteristics: A select overview and evidence from a Canadian multisite cohort of illicit opioid users (OPICAN). *Canadian Journal of Psychiatry, 51*(10), 624–633.

Fischer, B., Rehm, J., Patra, J., & Cruz, M. F. (2006). Changes in illicit opioid use across Canada. *Canadian Medical Association Journal, 175*(11), 1385–1387.

Gilron, I., Watson, C. P. N., Cahill, C.M., & Moulin, D. E. (2006). Neuropathic pain: A practical guide for the clinician. *Canadian Medical Association Journal, 175*(6), 265–275.

Harrison, D. M. (2008). Oral sucrose for pain management in the paediatric emergency department: A review. *Australasian Emergency Nursing Journal, 11*, 72–79.

Health Canada. (2004). *Fact sheet—Misuse and abuse of oxycodone-based prescription drugs.* Retrieved September 14, 2008, from http://www.hc-sc.gc.ca/dhp-mps/pubs/precurs/oxycodone/fs-fi/index-eng.php

Health Canada. (2005). *Health Canada endorsed important safety information: Duragesic fentanyl transdermal system.* Retrieved September 15, 2008, from http://www.hc-sc.gc.ca/dhp-mps/alt_formats/hpfb-dgpsa/pdf/medeff/duragesic_hpc-cps-eng.pdf

Health Canada. (2006). *Guidance document. Basic product monograph information for nonsteroidal anti-inflammatory drugs (NSAIDs).* Retrieved September 16, 2008, from http://www.hc-sc.gc.ca/dhp-mps/prodpharma/applic-demande/guide-ld/nsaid-ains/nsaids_ains-eng.php

Health Canada. (2008). *The use of opioids in the management of opioid dependence.* Retrieved September 14, 2008, from http://www.hc-sc.gc.ca/dhp-mps/pubs/precurs/opi-treat-trait/index-eng.php

Kim, H. S., Schwartz-Barcott, D., Tracy, S. M., Fortin, J. D., & Sjostrom, B. (2005). Strategies of pain assessment used by nurses on surgical units. *Pain Management Nursing 6*(1), 3–9.

Krenzischek, D. A., Dunwoody, C. J., Polomano, R. C., & Rathwell, J. P. (2008). Pharmacology for acute pain: Implications for practice. *Journal of PeriAnesthesia Nursing, 23*(1), S28–S42.

Ladak, S. S. J., Chan, V. W. S., Easty, T., & Chagpar, A. (2007). Right medication, right dose, right patient, right time, and right route: How do we select the right patient-controlled analgesia (PCA) device? *Pain Management Nursing, 8*(4), 140–145.

McCaffery, M., & Pasero, C. (1999). *Pain—Clinical manual* (2nd ed.). St. Louis, MO: Mosby.

Melzack, R., & Wall, P. D. (1965). Pain mechanisms: A new theory. *Science, 150*, 971–979.

Monsivais, D., & McNeill, J. (2007). Multicultural influences on pain medication attitudes and beliefs in patients with non-malignant chronic pain syndromes. *Pain Management Nursing, 8*(2), 64–71.

Niemi-Murola, L., Poyhia, R., Onkinen, K., Rhen, B., Makela, A., & Niemi, T. T. (2007). Patient satisfaction with postoperative pain management—Effect of preoperative factors. *Pain Management Nursing, 8*(3), 122–129.

North American Opiate Medication Initiative. (2008). *Key issues.* Retrieved September 15, 2008, from http://www.naomistudy.ca/pdfs/naomi_brief.pdf

Richards, J., & Hubbert, A. O. (2007). Experiences of expert nurses in caring for patients with postoperative pain. *Pain Management Nursing, 8*(1), 17–24.

Riley, J. L., & Hastie, B. A. (2008). Individual differences in opioid efficacy for chronic non-cancer pain. *Clinical Journal of Pain, 24*(6), 509–520.

Roman, M., & Cabaj, T. (2005). Epidural analgesia. *Medsurg Nursing, 14*(4), 257–259.

Srivastava, A., & Kahan, M. (2006). Buprenorphine: A potential new treatment option for opioid dependence. *Canadian Medical Association Journal, 174*(13), 1835.

Turk, D., Swanson, K. S., & Gatchel, R. J. (2008). Predicting opioid misuse by chronic pain patients: A systematic review and literature. *Clinical Journal of Pain, 24*(6), 497–508.

Viscusi, E. R. (2008). Patient-controlled drug delivery for acute postoperative pain management: A review of current and emerging technologies. *Regional Anesthesia and Pain Medicine, 33*(2), 146–158.

Wichman, K., & U, D. (2005). Overdose a risk of transdermal patch in diverse settings. Problems even occur with discarded patch. *Canadian Pharmacy Journal, 138*(7), 65–66.

World Health Organization. (2008). *WHO's pain ladder.* Retrieved September 16, 2008, from http://www.who.int/cancer/palliative/painladder/en/index.html

Chapter 12

Drain, C. B., & Odom-Forren, J. (2008). *Perianesthesia nursing: A critical care approach* (5th ed.). St. Louis, MO: Saunders.

Dripps, R. D., Eckenhoff, J. E., & Vandam, L. D. (Eds.). (1988). *Introduction to anesthesia: The principles of safe practice* (7th ed.). Philadelphia: Saunders.

Health Canada. (2002). *Drug interactions with Natural Health Products: A discussion paper (November 2001).* Retrieved September 19, 2008, from http://www.hc-sc.gc.ca/dhp-mps/pubs/complement/interaction_drug-medicament_11-01/interaction_drug-medicament_11-01_9-eng.php

Lennox, P. H., & Henderson, C. L. (2003). Herbal medicine use is frequent in ambulatory surgery patients in Vancouver Canada. *Canadian Journal of Anesthesiology, 50,* 21–25.

Litman, D. O., & Rosenberg, H. (2005). Malignant hyperthermia. *Journal of the American Medical Association, 293*(23), 2918-2924.

Nathan, N., & Odin, I. (2007). Induction of anaesthesia. *Drugs, 67*(5), 701–723.

Chapter 13

Anderson, P. O., Knoben, J. E., & Troutman, W. G. (2002). *Handbook of clinical drug data* (10th ed.). New York: McGraw-Hill/Appleton & Lange.

Bachman, K. A., Lewis, J. D., Fuller, M. A., & Bonfiglio, M. F. (2003). *Lexi-Comp's drug interactions handbook: The new standard for drug and herbal interactions.* Hudson, OH: Lexi-Comp.

Baillargeon, L., Landreville, P., Verreault, R., Beauchemin, J. P., Grégoire, J. P., & Morin, C. M. (2003). Discontinuation of benzodiazepines among older insomniac adults treated with cognitive–behavioural therapy combined with gradual tapering: A randomized trial. *Canadian Medical Association Journal, 169*(10), 1015–1020.

Bradley, W. G., Fenichel, G. M., Jankovic, J., & Daroff, R. B. (2004). *Neurology in clinical practice* (4th ed.). Philadelphia: Butterworth-Heinemann.

Brunton, L. L., Lazo, J. S., & Parker, K. L. (2006). *Goodman and Gilman's the pharmacological basis of therapeutics* (11th ed.). New York: McGraw-Hill.

Ford, M. D. D., Delaney, K., Ling, L., Rutherford, R., & Erickson, T. (2001). *Clinical toxicology.* Philadelphia: Elsevier Saunders.

Katzung, B. G. (2004). *Basic and clinical pharmacology* (9th ed.). New York: Lange Medical Books/McGraw-Hill.

Koda-Kimble, M., Young, L., Bennett, D., Gugliemo, B., & Horgas, A. (2005). *Applied therapeutics: The clinical use of drugs* (8th ed.). Baltimore: Lippincott Williams & Wilkins.

Kryger, M. H., Roth, T., & Dement, W. C. (2005). *Principles and practices of sleep medicine* (4th ed.). St. Louis, MO: Elsevier Saunders.

McEvoy, G. (2008). *AHFS drug information.* Bethesda, MD: American Society of Health-System Pharmacists.

Miller. R. (2005). *Miller's anesthesia* (6th ed.). St. Louis, MO: Elsevier Churchill Livingstone.

Russell, L. C., Goldman, L., & Bennett, J. C. (2007). *Cecil textbook of medicine* (13th ed.). St. Louis, MO: Elsevier Saunders.

Sweetman, S. C. (2007). *Martindale: The complete drug reference* (35th ed.). London: Pharmaceutical Press.

Swiss Pharmaceutical Society. (2008). *Index nominum international drug directory* (19th ed.). Stuttgart: Medpharm GmbH Scientific.

Tariq, S. H., & Pulisetty, S. (2008). Pharmacotherapy for sleep. *Clinics in Geriatric Medicine, 24,* 93–105.

Weiner, C. P., & Buhimschi, C. (2004). *Drugs for pregnant and lactating women.* St. Louis, MO: Elsevier Churchill Livingstone.

Chapter 14

Bergey, G. K. (2004). Initial treatment of epilepsy: Special issues in treating the elderly. *Neurology 63*(10, S4), S40–S48.

Blume, W. T. (2003). Diagnosis and management of epilepsy. *Canadian Medical Association Journal, 168*(4), 441–448.

Brodie, M. J., & Kwan, P. (2005). Clinical review: Epilepsy in elderly people. *British Medical Journal, 331,* 1317–1322.

Canadian Pediatric Society. (1996, reaffirmed 2002). Management of the paediatric patient with generalized convulsive status epilepticus in the emergency department. [Electronic version]. *Paediatrics and Child Health, 1*(2), 151–155. Retrieved July 29, 2005, from http://www.cps.ca/english/statements/EP/ep95-01.htm

Freeman, J. M., Kossoff, E. H., & Hartman, A. L. (2007). The ketogenic diet: One decade later. *Pediatrics, 119*(3), 535–543.

French, J. A., & Pedley, T. A. (2008). Clinical practice: Initial management of epilepsy. *New England Journal of Medicine, 359*(2), 166–176.

Kaplan, P. W. (2004). Reproductive health effects and teratogenicity of antiepileptic drugs. *Neurology, 63*(10, S4), S13–S23.

Kinirons, P., & Doherty, C. P. (2008). Status epilepticus: A modern approach to management. *Medicine, 15*, 187–195.

Kohrman, M. H. (2007). What is epilepsy? Clinical perspectives in the diagnosis and treatment. *Journal of Clinical Neurophysiology, 24*(2), 87–95.

Leppik, I. E., Bergey, G. K., Ramsay, R. E., Rowan, A. J., Gidal, B. E., Birnbaum, A. K., et al. (2004). Advances in antiepileptic drug treatments: A rational basis for selecting drugs for older patients with epilepsy. *Geriatrics 59*(12), 14–18, 22–24.

Lyseng-Williamson, K. A., & Yang, L. P. H. (2007). Topiramate: A review of its use in the treatment of epilepsy. *Drugs, 67*(15), 2231–2256.

Manufacturer's package inserts for Gabitril, Keppra, Lamictal, Lyrica, Neurontin, Trileptal, and Zonegran.

Marson, A. G., Al-Kharusi, A. M., Alwaidh, M., Appleton, R., Baker, G. A., Chadwick, W. D., et al. (2007). The SANAD study of effectiveness of carbamazepine, gabapentin, lamotrigine, oxcarbazepine, or topiramate for treatment of partial epilepsy: An unblinded randomised controlled trial. *Lancet, 369*(9566), 1000–1015.

Ortinski, P., & Meador, K. J. (2004). Cognitive side effects of antiepileptic drugs. *Epilepsy Behavior, 5*(S1), S60–S65.

Prasad, A. N., & Seshia, S. S. (2006). Status epilepticus in pediatric practice: Neonate to adolescent. *Advances in Neurology, 97*, 229–243.

Ramsay, R. E., Rowan, A. J., & Pryor, F. M. (2004). Special considerations in treating the elderly patient with epilepsy. *Neurology, 62*, S24–S29.

Scott, R., & Kirkham, F. (2006). Clinical update: Childhood convulsive status epilepticus. *Lancet, 370*(9589), 724–726.

Sethi, N. K., Torgovnick, J., & Arsura, E. (2007). Comparison of levetiracetam and controlled-release carbamazepine in newly diagnosed epilepsy. *Neurology, 68*(6), 402–408.

Smith, P. E. (2008). Neurology in practice: Epilepsy. *Practical Neurology, 8*(3), 195–202.

Thomas, R. H., & Smith, P. E. M. (2008). Epilepsy in older adults. *Geriatric Medicine, 38*(2), 16–23.

Chapter 15

Brooks, D. J. (2004). Safety and tolerability of COMT inhibitors. *Neurology, 62*(S1), S39–S46.

Lo, K., Leung, K., & Shek, A. (2007). Management of Parkinson disease: Current treatments, recent advances, and future development. *Formulary, 42*(9), 529–532, 535–536, 537.

Olanow, C. W., & Stocchi, F. (2004). COMT inhibitors in Parkinson's disease: Can they prevent and/or reverse levodopa-induced motor complications? *Neurology, 62*(S1), S72–S81.

Welsh, M. (2008). Treatment challenges in Parkinson's disease. *The Nurse Practitioner, 33*(7), 32–38.

Chapter 16

Adis International Limited. (2008). Antidepressants have the central role in the pharmacological treatment of agoraphobia with panic disorder. *Drugs & Therapy Perspectives, 24*(4), 13–16.

Alexander, M. P., Farag, Y. M., Mittal, B.V., Rennke, H. G., & Singh, A. K. (2008). Lithium toxicity: A double-edged sword. *Kidney International, 73*(2), 233–237.

Alexopoulos, G. (2005). Depression in the elderly. *Lancet, 365*, 1961–1970.

Alper, B. S. (2006). Psychotherapy plus antidepressant effective for panic disorder. *Clinical Advisor, 9*(11), 128.

Anghelescu, I. G., Kohnen, R., Szegedi, A., Klement, S., & Kieser, M. (2006). Comparison of *Hypericum* extract WS 5570 and paroxetine in ongoing treatment after recovery from an episode of moderate to severe depression: Results from a randomized multicenter study. *Pharmacopsychiatry, 39*(6), 213–219.

Anonymous. (2008). Combination therapy for panic disorder: Recent analyses reinforce the view that adding psychotherapy to medication improves outcomes. *Preview Harvard Mental Health Letter, 24*(12), 4–5.

Bishara, D., & Taylor, D. (2008). Upcoming agents for the treatment of schizophrenia. Mechanism of action, efficacy and tolerability. *Drugs, 68*(16), 2269–2292.

Buchanan, R. W., Ball, E., Weiner, E., Kirkpatrick, B., Gold, J. M., McMahon, R. P., et al. (2005). Olanzapine: Treatment of residual positive and negative symptoms. *American Journal of Psychiatry, 162*(1), 124–129.

Burdick, K. E., Braga, R. J., Goldberg, J. F., & Malhotra, A. K. (2007). Cognitive dysfunction in bipolar disorder: Future place of pharmacotherapy. *CNS Drugs, 21*(12), 971–981.

Cairney, J., Corna, L. M., Veldhuizen, S., Herrmann, N., & Streiner, D. L. (2008). Comorbid depression and anxiety in later life: Patterns of association, subjective well-being, and impairment. *American Journal of Geriatric Psychiatry, 16*(3), 201–208.

Cheung, A. H., Emslie, G. J., & Mayes, T. L. (2006). The use of antidepressants to treat depression in children and adolescents. *Canadian Medical Association Journal, 174*(2), 193–200.

Cheung, A. H., Zuckerbrot, R. A., Jensen, P. S., Ghalib, K., Laraque, D., Stein, R. E., GLAD-PC Steering Group. (2007). Guidelines for adolescent depression in primary care (GLAD-PC): II. Treatment and ongoing management. *Pediatrics, 120*(5), e1313–e1326.

Cheung, A. H., Zuckerbrot, R. A., Jensen, P. S., Stein, R. E., Laraque, D., GLAD-PC Steering Committee. (2008). Expert survey for the management of adolescent depression in primary care. *Pediatrics, 121*(1), e101–e107.

Corna, L. M., Cairney, J., Herrmann, N., Veldhuizen, S., McCabe, L., Streiner, D., et al. (2008). Update on early intervention in schizophrenia. *Journal of Psychosocial Nursing & Mental Health Services, 46*(6), 19–23.

Côté, S. M., Boivin, M., Liu, X., Nagin, D. S., Zoccolillo, M., & Tremblay, R. E. (2009). Depression and anxiety symptoms: Onset, developmental course and risk factors during early childhood. *Journal of Child Psychology and Psychiatry, 50*(10), 1201–1208.

Emslie, G. J., Mayes, T. L., & Ruberuy, M. (2005). Continuation and maintenance therapy of early-onset major depressive disorder. *Pediatric Drugs, 7*(4), 203–217.

Ghaemi, S. N. (2008). Treatment of rapid-cycling bipolar disorder: Are antidepressants mood destabilizers? *American Journal of Psychiatry, 165*(3), 300–302.

Gill, S. S., Bronskill, S. E., Normand, S. T., Anderson, G. M., Sykora, K., Lam, K., et al. (2007). Antipsychotic drug use and mortality in older adults with dementia. *Annals of Internal Medicine, 146,* 775–786.

Grillon, C., Lissek, S., Rabin, S., McDowell, D., Dvir, S., & Pine, D. S. (2008). Increased anxiety during anticipation of unpredictable but not predictable aversive stimuli as a psychophysiologic marker of panic disorder. *American Journal of Psychiatry, 165*(7), 898–904.

Health Canada. (2005). *Health Canada endorsed important safety information on atypical antipsychotic drugs and dementia.* Retrieved August 29, 2009, from http://www.hc-sc.gc.ca/dhp-mps/medeff/advisories-avis/prof/_2005/atyp-antipsycho_hpc-cps-eng.php

Katz, L. Y., Kozyrskyi, A. L., Prior, H. J., Enns, M. W., Cox, B. J., & Sareen, J. (2008). Effect of regulatory warnings on antidepressant prescription rates, use of health services and outcomes among children, adolescents, and young adults. *Canadian Medical Association Journal, 178*(8), 1005–1011.

Kish-Doto, J., Evans, W. D., Squire, C., Williams, P., Ranney, L. M., & Melvin, C. L. (2008). Patterns of prescribing antiepileptic drugs for bipolar disorder. *Journal of Psychiatric Practice, 14*(Suppl 1), 35–43.

Lotrich, F. E., & Pollock, B. G. (2005). Aging and clinical pharmacology: Implications for antidepressants. *Journal of Clinical Pharmacology, 45,* 1106–1122.

Mackenzie, D. L., & Raymond, M. K. (2008). Deadly serotonin syndrome. *RN, 71*(8), 26–31.

Marchand, W. R. (2007). Self-assessment in psychiatry: Panic disorder. *Hospital Physician, 43*(10), 44–46.

Melvin, C. L., Carey, T. S., Goodman, F., Oldham, J. M., Williams, J. W. Jr., & Ranney, L. M. (2008). Effectiveness of antiepileptic drugs for the treatment of bipolar disorder: Findings from a systematic review. *Journal of Psychiatric Practice, 14*(Suppl 1), 9–14.

Mosholder, A. D., & Willy, M. (2006). Suicidal adverse events in pediatric randomized, controlled clinical trials of antidepressant drugs are associated with active drug treatment: A meta-analysis. *Journal of Child and Adolescent Psychopharmacology, 16*(1–2), 25–32.

National Institute of Mental Health. (2006). Gene influences antidepressant response. *Science Daily.* Retrieved October 3, 2008, from http://www.sciencedaily.com/releases/2006/03/060315174915.htm

National Institute of Mental Health. (2007). *Bipolar disorder.* Retrieved March 4, 2008, from http://www.nimh.nih.gov/health/publications/bipolar-disorder/summary.shtml

Neher, J. O., & Schumann, S. (2007). Combination therapy for panic disorder. *Evidence-Based Practice, 10*(10): 1–3.

Patton, S., & Juby, H. (2008). *A profile of clinical depression in Canada.* Retrieved October 2, 2008, from https://dspace.ucalgary.ca/bitstream/1880/46327/6/Patten_RSS1.pdf

Perlis, R. H. (2008). Pharmacogenetic studies of antidepressant response: How far from the clinic? *Psychiatric Clinics of North America, 30*(1), 125.

Public Health Agency of Canada. (2002). *A report on mental health disorders in Canada. Chapter 4: Anxiety disorders.* Retrieved October 12, 2008, from http://www.phac-aspc.gc.ca/publicat/miic-mmac/chap_4-eng.php

Public Health Agency of Canada. (2003). *Women's health surveillance report: Depression.* Retrieved October 13, 2008, from http://www.phac-aspc.gc.ca/publicat/whsr-rssf/chap_18-eng.php

Rochon, P. A., Normand, S., Gomes, T., Gill, S. S., Anderson, G. M., Melo, M., et al. (2008). Antipsychotic therapy and short-term serious events in older adults with dementia. *Archives of Internal Medicine, 168*(10), 1090–1096.

Roy-Byrne, P. P., Craske, M. G., & Stein, M. B. (2006). Panic disorder. *Lancet, 368*(9540), 1023–1032.

Saeed, S. A., Bloch, R. M., & Antonacci, D. J. (2007). Herbal and dietary supplements for treatment of anxiety disorders. *American Family Physician, 76*(4), 549–556.

Sarris, J. (2007). Herbal medicines in the treatment of psychiatric disorders: A systematic review. *Phytotherapy Research, 21*(8), 703–716.

Schloredt, K., & Varley, C. (2005). Current perspectives on the diagnosis and treatment of adolescent depression in the primary care setting. *Journal of Clinical Outcomes Management, 12*(5), 260–274.

Schmidt, N. B., Mitchell, M. A., & Richey, J. A. (2008). Anxiety sensitivity as an incremental predictor of later anxiety symptoms and syndromes. *Comprehensive Psychiatry, 49*(4), 407–412.

Schneck, C. D., Miklowitz, D. J., Miyahara, S., Araga, M., Wisniewski, S., Gyulai, L., et al. (2008). The prospective course of rapid-cycling bipolar disorder: Findings from the STEP-BD. *American Journal of Psychiatry, 165*(3), 370–377.

Sego, S. (2007). Ginseng. *Clinical Advisor, 10*(11), 125.

Singh, B. (2005). Recognition and optimal management of schizophrenia and related psychoses. *Internal Medicine Journal, 35,* 413–418.

Sree, H. R. V., Raghvendra, R. C., & Yergani, V. K. (2006). A novel technique to evaluate fluctuations of mood: Implications for evaluating course and treatment effects in bipolar/affective disorders. *Bipolar Disorders, 8*(5), 453–466.

Swinson, R. P. and Working Group Members. (2006). Clinical practice guidelines: Management of anxiety disorders. *Canadian Journal of Psychiatry, 51*(Suppl 2), S1–S92.

University of Montreal. (2009, August 30). Depression and anxiety affect up to 15 percent of preschoolers, Canadian study finds. *ScienceDaily.* Retrieved August 31, 2009, from http://www.sciencedaily.com/releases/2009/08/090828104134.htm

Usher, K., Foster, K., & Park, T. (2006). The metabolic syndrome and schizophrenia: The latest evidence and nursing guidelines for management. *Journal of Psychiatric and Mental Health Nursing, 14,* 730–734.

Valente, S. (2008). Suicide risk in elderly patients. *Nurse Practitioner, 33*(8), 34–40.

Vasudev, A., Macritchie, K., Watson, S., Geddes, J. R., & Young, A. H. (2008). Oxcarbazepine in the maintenance treatment of bipolar disorder. *Cochrane Database of Systematic Reviews, 1*, CD005171.

Woo, V., & Harris, S. B. (2005). Canadian Diabetes position paper: Antipsychotic medications and associated risk of weight gain and diabetes. *Canadian Journal of Diabetes, 29*(2), 111–112.

Yan, J. (2008). Canada sees troubling trend in antidepressant prescribing. *Psychiatric News, 43*(10), 14.

Young, A. H., & Newham J. I. (2006). Lithium in maintenance therapy for bipolar disorder. *Journal of Psychopharmacology, 20*(2 Suppl), 17–22.

Zuckerbrot, R. A., Cheung, A. H., Jensen, P. S., Stein, R. E., Laraque, D., GLAD-PC Steering Group. (2007). Guidelines for adolescent depression in primary care (GLAD-PC): I. Identification, assessment, and initial management. *Pediatrics, 120*(5), e1299–e1312.

Chapter 17

Canadian Institutes of Health Research. (2007). *Obesity*. Retrieved May 5, 2009, from http://www.cihr-irsc.gc.ca/e/20406.html

Caputo, F., & Zoli, G. (2007). Treating narcolepsy with cataplexy. *Lancet, 369*(9567), 1080–1081.

Dauvilliers, Y., Arnulf, I., & Mignot, E. (2007). Narcolepsy with cataplexy. *Lancet, 369*(9560), 499–511.

Evans, C., Blackburn, D., Butt, P., & Dattani, D. (2004). Use and abuse of methylphenidate in attention deficit/hyperactivity disorder. *Canadian Pharmaceutical Journal, 137*(6), 30–35.

Fetrow, C. W., & Avila, J. R. (2000). *The complete guide to herbal remedies*. Springhouse, PA: Springhouse.

Kernan, W. N., Viscoli, C. M., Brass, L. M., Broderick, J. P., Brott, T., & Feldmann, E. (2000). Phenylpropanolamine and the risk of hemorrhagic stroke. *New England Journal of Medicine, 343*(25), 1826–1832.

Kuk, J. L., Katzmarzyk, P. T., Nichaman, M. Z., Church, T. S., Blair, S. N., & Ross, R. (2006). Visceral adiposity is an independent predictor of all-cause mortality in men. *Obesity, 14*, 336–341.

Luo, W., Morrison, H., de Groh, M., Waters, C., DesMeules, M., Jones-McLean, E., et al. (2007). The burden of adult obesity in Canada. *Chronic Diseases in Canada, 27*(4), 135–144.

Martin, S. (2001). Prevalence of migraine headache in Canada. *Canadian Medical Association News Pulse, 164*(10), 1481.

Rossi, L. N., Vajani, S., Cortinovis, I., Spreafico, F., & Menegazzo, L. (2008). Analysis of the International Classification of Headache Disorders for diagnosis of migraine and tension-type headache in children. *Developmental Medicine & Child Neurology, 50*(4), 305–310.

Scheffer, R. E. (2006). Psychopharmacology: Clinical implications of brain neurochemistry. *Pediatric Clinics of North America, 53*(4), 767–775.

Shields, M., & Tjepkema, M. (2006). Trends in adult obesity. *Health Reports, 17*(3). Available at http://www.statcan.ca/english/studies/82-003/archive/2006/17-3-d.pdf

Spencer, T. J., Wilens, T. E., Biederman, J., Weisler, R. H., Read, S. C., & Pratt, R. (2006). Efficacy and safety of mixed amphetamine salts extended release (Adderall XR) in the management of attention-deficit/hyperactivity disorder in adolescent patients: A 4-week, randomized, double-blind, placebo-controlled, parallel-group study. *Clinical Therapeutics, 28*(2), 266–279.

Chapter 18

DiGregorio, R.V., & Fung, H. B. (2009). Rapid dosing of critical care infusions: The dopamine and norepinephrine "clock." *Journal of Emergency Nursing, 35*(2), 165–168.

Health Canada. (2002). *Ephedra/ephedrine—frequently asked questions*. Retrieved October 23, 2008, from http://www.hc-sc.gc.ca/ahc-asc/media/advisories-avis/_2002/2002_01bk2-eng.php

Chapter 19

Arnold, J. M. O., Howlett, J. G., Dorian, P., Ducharme, A., Gianetti, N., Haddad, H., et al. (2007). Canadian Cardiovascular Society Consensus Conference recommendations on heart failure, update 2007: Prevention, management during intercurrent illness or acute decompensation, and use of biomarkers. *Canadian Journal of Cardiology, 23*(1), 21–45.

Arnold, J. M. O., Liu, P., Demers, C., Dorian, P., Gianetti, N., Haddad, H., et al. (2006). Canadian Cardiovascular Society consensus conference recommendations on heart failure 2006: Diagnosis and management. *Canadian Journal of Cardiology, 22*(1), 23–45.

Colbert, K., & Greene, M. H. (2003). Nesiritide: A new treatment for acute decompensated congestive heart failure. *Critical Care Nursing Quarterly, 26*(1), 40.

Poole-Wilson, P. A., Swedberg, K., Cleland, J., Di Lenarda, A., Hanrath, P., Komajda, M., et al. (2003). Comparison of carvedilol and metoprolol on clinical outcomes in patients with chronic heart failure in the Carvedilol or Metoprolol European Trial (COMET): Randomised controlled trial. *Lancet 362*(9377), 7–13.

Riggs, J. M. (2004). New therapies for heart failure. *RN, 67*(3), 29–33.

Sauls, J. L., & Rone, T. (2005). Emerging trends in the management of heart failure: Beta blocker therapy. *Nursing Clinics of North America, 40*(1), 135–148.

Tejani, A., Musini, V., Perry Jr., T. L., Mintzes, B., & Wright, J. M. (2006). Benign prostatic hypertrophy. Update on drug therapy. *Canadian Family Physician, 52*(9), 1075–1076, 1077–1078.

Chapter 20

Bird, T. D. (2008). Genetic aspects of Alzheimer disease. *Genetics in Medicine, 10*(4), 231–239.

Blennow, K., de Leon, M. J., & Zetterberg, H. (2006). Alzheimer's disease. *Lancet, 368*(9533), 387–403.

Chertkow, H., Massoud, F., Nasreddine, Z., Belleville, S., Joanette, Y., Bocti, C., et al. (2008). Diagnosis and treatment of dementia: 3. Mild cognitive impairment and cognitive impairment without dementia. *Canadian Medical Association Journal, 178*(10), 1273–1285.

Cummings, J. L., Doody, R., & Clark, C. (2007). Disease-modifying therapies for Alzheimer disease. *Neurology, 69,* 1622–1634.

Downey, D. (2008). Pharmacologic management of Alzheimer disease. *Journal of Neuroscience Nursing, 40*(1), 55–59.

Farlow, M. R., Graham, S. M., & Alva, G. (2008). Memantine for the treatment of Alzheimer's disease. *Drug Safety, 31*(7), 577–585.

Farlow, M. R., Miller, M. L., & Pejovic, V. (2008). Treatment options in Alzheimer's disease: Maximizing benefit, managing expectations. *Dementia and Geriatric Cognitive Disorders, 25,* 408–422.

Gray, S. L., Anderson, M. L., Crane, P. K., Breitner, J. C. S., McCormick, W., Bowen, J. D., et al. Antioxidant vitamin supplementation use and risk of dementia or Alzheimer's disease in older adults. *Journal of the American Geriatric Society, 56,* 291–295.

Hermann, N., & Gauthier, S. (2008). Diagnosis and treatment of dementia: 6. Management of severe Alzheimer disease. *Canadian Medical Association Journal, 179*(12), 1279–1287.

Hogan, D. B., Bailey, P., Black, S., Carswell, A., Chertkow, H., Clarke, B., et al. (2008a). Diagnosis and treatment of dementia: 4. Approach to management of mild to moderate dementia. *Canadian Medical Association Journal, 179*(8), 787–793.

Hogan, D. B., Bailey, P., Black, S., Carswell, A., Chertkow, H., Clarke, B., et al. (2008b). Diagnosis and treatment of dementia: 5. Nonpharmacologic and pharmacologic therapy for mild to moderate dementia. *Canadian Medical Association Journal, 174*(10), 1019–1026.

Jia, X., McNeill, G., & Avenell, A. (2008). Does taking vitamin, mineral, and fatty acid supplements prevent cognitive decline? A systematic review of randomized controlled trials. *Journal of Human Nutrition and Dietetics, 21,* 317–336.

Maidmont, I. D., Fox, C. G., Boustani, M., Rodriguez, J., Brown, R. C., & Katona, C. L. (2008). Efficacy of memantine on behavioral and psychological symptoms related to dementia: A systematic review. *Annals of Pharmacotherapy, 42,* 32–38.

Patterson, C., Feightner, J. W., Garcia, A., Hsiung, G.-Y., MacKnight, C., & Sadovnick, A. D. (2008). Diagnosis and treatment of dementia: 1. Risk assessment and primary prevention of Alzheimer disease. *Canadian Medical Association Journal, 178*(5), 548–556.

Quaseen, A., Snow, V., Cross, T., Forciea, M. A., Hopkins, R., Shekelle, P., et al. (2008). Current pharmacologic treatment of dementia: A clinical practice guideline from the American College of Physicians and the American Academy of Family Physicians. *Annals of Internal Medicine, 148,* 370–378.

Qui, C., De Ronchi, D., & Fratiglioni, L. (2007). The epidemiology of the dementias. *Current Opinion in Psychiatry, 20,* 380–385.

Raina, P., Santaguida, P., Ismaila, A., Patterson, C., Cowan, D., Levine, M., et al. (2008). Effectiveness of cholinesterase inhibitors and memantine for treating dementia: Evidence review for a clinical practice guideline. *Annals of Internal Medicine, 148,* 379–397.

Razay, G., & Wilcock, G. K. (2008). Galantamine in Alzheimer's disease. *Expert Review of Neurotherapeutics, 8*(1), 9–17.

Samanta, M. K., Wilson, B., Santhi, K., Sampath Kumar, K. P., & Suresh, B. (2006). Alzheimer disease and its management: A review. *American Journal of Therapeutics, 13*(6), 516–526.

Van Marum, R. J. (2008). Current and future therapy in Alzheimer's disease. *Fundamental and Clinical Pharmacology, 22,* 265–274.

Winblad, B., Gauthier, S., Scinto, L., Feldman, H., Wilcock, G. K., Truyen, L., et al. (2008). GAL-INT-11/18 study group. *Neurology, 70*(22 Part 1), 2024–2035.

Chapter 21

Anonymous. (2008). Drug news. Urinary incontinence: Anticholinergic drug therapy may tax the memory. *Nursing, 38*(7), 24.

Chancellor, M. B., & Miguel, F. (2007). Treatment of overactive bladder: Selective use of anticholinergic agents with low drug–drug interaction potential. *Geriatrics, 62*(5), 15–17, 24.

Ellsworth, P., & Caldamone, A. (2008). Pediatric voiding dysfunction: Current evaluation and management. *Urologic Nursing, 28*(4), 249–258, 283.

Frascogna, N. (2007). Physostigmine: Is there a role for this antidote in pediatric poisonings? *Current Opinion in Pediatrics, 19*(2), 201–205.

Garely, A. D., Kaufman, J. M., Sand, P. K., Smith, N., & Andoh, M. (2006). Symptom bother and health-related quality of life outcomes following solifenacin treatment for overactive bladder: The VESIcare Open-Label Trial (VOLT). *Clinical Therapeutics, 28*(11), 1935–1946.

Hesch, K. (2007). Agents for treatment of overactive bladder: A therapeutic class review. *Baylor University Medical Center Proceedings, 20*(3), 307–314.

Kosier, J. H., Combest, W., & Newton, M. (2006). Medication minute. Solifenacin succinate (VESIcare): Overactive bladder therapy. *Urologic Nursing, 26*(6), 496–497.

Ramjan, K. A., Williams, A. J., Isbister, G. K., & Elliott, E. J. (2007). "Red as a beet and blind as a bat" anticholinergic delirium in adolescents: Lessons for the paediatrician. *Paediatrics and Child Health, 43*(11), 779–780.

Roxburgh, C., Cook, J., & Dublin, N. (2007). Anticholinergic drugs versus other medications for overactive bladder syndrome in adults. *Cochrane Database of Systematic Reviews, 4,* CD003190.

Rudolph, J. L., Salow, M. J., Angelini, M. C., & McGlinchey, R. E. (2008). The anticholinergic risk scale and anticholinergic adverse effects in older persons. *Archives of Internal Medicine, 168*(5), 508–513.

Shamliyan, T. A., Kane, R. L., Wyman, J., & Wilt, T. J. (2008). Systematic review: Randomized, controlled trials of nonsurgical treatments for urinary incontinence in women. *Annals of Internal Medicine, 148*(6). 459–473.

Sink, K. M., Thomas, J., Xu, H., Craig, B., Kritchevsky, S., & Sands, L. P. (2008). Dual use of bladder anticholinergics and cholinesterase inhibitors: Long-term functional and cognitive outcomes. *Journal of the American Geriatrics Society, 56*(5), 847–853.

Smulders, R. A., Krauwinkel, W. J., Swart, P. J., & Huang, M. (2004). Pharmacokinetics and safety of solifenacin succinate in healthy young men. *Journal of Clinical Pharmacology, 44*(9), 1023–1033.

Zagaria, M. A. E. (2007). Issues in pharmacotherapy. Anticholinergic adverse effects. *American Journal for Nurse Practitioners, 11*(9), 20–22, 25–26.

Chapter 22

Adis International Limited. (2007). Understanding the mechanisms and manifestations of digoxin toxicity helps in its management and treatment. *Drugs & Therapy Perspectives, 23*(2), 20–23.

Ahmed, A. (2007). Digoxin and reduction in mortality and hospitalization in geriatric heart failure: Importance of low doses and low serum concentrations. *Journals of Gerontology Series A: Biological Sciences and Medical Sciences, 62A*(3), 323–329.

Ahmed, A., Rich, M. W., Love, T. E., Lloyd-Jones, D. M., Aban, I. B., Colucci, W. S., et al. (2006). Digoxin and reduction in mortality and hospitalization in heart failure: A comprehensive post hoc analysis of the DIG trial. *European Heart Journal, 27*, 178–186.

Ahmed, A., Young, J. B., & Gheorghiade, M. (2007). The underuse of digoxin in heart failure, and approaches to appropriate use. *Canadian Medical Association Journal, 176*(5), 641–643.

Allen, L. A., & O'Connor, C. M. (2007). Management of acute decompensated heart failure. *Canadian Medical Association Journal, 176*(6), 797–805.

Anderson, K. M. (2008). Clinical uses of brain natriuretic peptide in diagnosing and managing heart failure. *Journal of the American Academy of Nurse Practitioners, 20*, 305–310.

Arnold, J. M. O., Howlett, J. G., Dorian, P., Ducharme, A., Gianetti, N., Haddad, H., et al. (2007). Canadian Cardiovascular Society Consensus Conference recommendations on heart failure update 2007: Prevention, management during intercurrent illness or acute decompensation, and use of biomarkers. *Canadian Journal of Cardiology, 23*(1), 21–45.

Arnold, J. M. O., Howlett, J. G., Ducharme, A., Ezekowitz, J. A., Gardiner, M. J., Gianetti, N., et al. (2008). Canadian Cardiovascular Society Consensus Conference recommendations on heart failure—2008 update: Best practices for the transition of care of heart failure patients, and the recognition, investigation, and treatment of cardiomyopathies. *Canadian Journal of Cardiology, 24*(1), 21–40.

Arnold, J. M. O., Liu, P., Demers, C., Dorian, P., Gianetti, N., Haddad, H., et al. (2006). Canadian Cardiovascular Society Consensus Conference recommendations on heart failure 2006: Diagnosis and management. *Canadian Journal of Cardiology, 22*(1), 23–45.

Bryne, M., Kaye, D. M., & Power, J. (2008). The synergism between atrial fibrillation and heart failure. *Journal of Cardiac Failure, 14*(4), 320–326.

Chavey, W. E., Bleske, B., Harrison, V., Hogikyan, R. V., Kesterosn, S. K., & Nicklas, J. M. (2008). Pharmacologic management of heart failure caused by systolic dysfunction. *American Family Physician, 77*(7), 957–964, 967–968.

Chun, J., & Chodosh, J. (2006). Controversy in heart failure management: Digoxin use in the elderly. *Journal of the American Medical Directors Association, 7*(9), 581–586.

Cottrell, D. B., & Mack, K. J. E. N. (2008). Atrial fibrillation: An emergency nurse's rapid response. *Journal of Emergency Nursing, 34*(3), 207–210.

Digitalis Investigation Group. (1997). The effect of digoxin on mortality and morbidity in patients with heart failure. *New England Journal of Medicine, 336*(8), 525–533.

Fenton, M., & Burch, M. (2008). Understanding chronic heart failure. *Archives of Disease in Childhood, 92*(9), 812–816.

Hardin, S. R., & Steele, J. R. (2008). Atrial fibrillation among older adults: Pathophysiology, symptoms, and treatment. *Journal of Gerontological Nursing, 34*(7), 26–35.

Howlett, J. G. (2008). Current treatment for early management in acute decompensated heart failure. *Canadian Journal of Cardiology, 24*(Suppl B), 9B–14B.

Katz, E. A. (2008). Pharmacologic management of the postoperative cardiac surgery patient. *Critical Care Nursing Clinics of North America, 19*(4), 487–496.

LePage, S. (2008). Acute decompensated heart failure. *Canadian Journal of Cardiology, 24*(Suppl B), 6B–8B.

Miller, A. H., Nazeer, S., Pepe, P., Estes, B., Gorman, A., & Yancy, C. W. (2008). Acutely decompensated heart failure in a county emergency department: A double-blind randomized controlled comparison of nesiritide versus placebo treatment. *Annals of Emergency Medicine, 51*(5), 571–578.

Overgaard, C. B., & Dzavík, V. (2008). Inotropes and vasopressors: Review of physiology and clinical use in cardiovascular disease. *Circulation, 118*(10), 1047–1056.

Prows, C. A., & Beery, T. A. (2008). Pharmacogenetics in critical care: Atrial fibrillation as an exemplar. *Critical Care Nursing Clinics of North America, 20*(2), 223–231.

Prudente, L. A., De Jong, M., & Doering, L. (2008). Atrial fibrillation (AF) and heart failure (HF): To treat the AF, be sure to treat the HF. *Progress in Cardiovascular Nursing, 23*(3), 146–149.

Pruitt, A. L. (2008). Heart failure: It's not just for men. *Critical Care Nursing Clinics of North America, 20*, 327–341.

Quinn, B. (2007). Pharmacological treatment of heart failure. *Critical Care Nurse Quarterly, 30*(4), 299–306.

Rich, M. W. (2008). Multidisciplinary heart failure clinics: Are they effective in Canada? *Canadian Medical Association Journal, 173*(1), 53–54.

Rogers, S. (2208). Management of atrial fibrillation: NICE guidance and its relevance to primary care. *Primary Health Care, 18*(4), 31–35.

Thacker, D., & Sharma, J. (2007). Digoxin toxicity. *Clinical Pediatrics, 46*(3), 276–279.

Waldo, S. W., Beede, J., Isakson, S., Villard-Saussine, S., Fareh, J., Clopton, P., et al. (2008). AS Pro-B-type natriuretic peptide levels in acute decompensated heart failure. *Journal of the American College of Cardiology, 51*(19), 1874–1882.

Woods, S. L., Sivarajan Froelocher, E. S., Underhill Motzer, S., & Bridges, E. J. (2005). *Cardiac Nursing* (5th ed.). Philadelphia: Lippincott Williams & Wilkins.

Yancy, C. W. (2008). Vasodilator therapy for decompensated heart failure. *Journal of the American College of Cardiology, 52*(3), 208–210.

Chapter 23

Anderson, K. P. (2008). The changing epidemiology of ventricular arrhythmias. *Cardiology Clinics, 26*(3), 321–333.

Boriani, G., Diemberger, I., Biffi, M., Martignani, C., & Branzi, A. (2004). Pharmacological cardioversion of atrial fibrillation: Current management and treatment options. *Drugs, 64*(24), 2741–2762.

Cardiac Arrhythmia Suppression Trial (CAST) Investigators. (1989). Preliminary report of the Cardiac Arrhythmia Suppression Trial (CAST): Effect of encainide and flecainide on mortality in a randomized trial of arrhythmia suppression after myocardial infarction. *New England Journal of Medicine, 321*(6), 406–412.

Chapa, D. W., Lee, H., Kao, C., Friedmann, E., Thomas, S. A., Anderson, J., et al. (2008). Reducing mortality with device therapy in heart failure patients without ventricular arrhythmias. *American Journal of Critical Care, 17*(5), 443–453.

Coleman, C. I., Kalus, J. S., Caron, M. F., Kluger, J., & White, C. M. (2004). Model of effect of magnesium prophylaxis on frequency of torsades de pointes in ibutilide-treated patients. *American Journal of Health System Pharmacy, 61*, 685–688.

Cottrell, D. B., & Jones, M. M. (2008). Women with dysrhythmia: A clinical challenge. *Critical Care Nursing Clinics of North America, 20*(3), 311–314.

Das, M. K., Dandamudi, G., & Steiner, H. (2008). Role of ablation therapy in ventricular arrhythmias: *Cardiology Clinics, 26*(3), 459–479.

Franklin, D. E., & Bono, M. J. (2008). Guide to antiarrhythmic therapies. *Emergency Medicine, 40*(1), 36–39.

Goldberger, J. J., Cain, M. E., Hohnloser, S. H., Kadish, A. H., Knight, B, P., Lauer, M.S., et al. (2008). American Heart Association/American College of Cardiology Foundation/Heart Rhythm Society scientific statement on noninvasive risk stratification techniques for identifying patients at risk for sudden cardiac death: A scientific statement from the American Heart Association Council on Clinical Cardiology Committee on Electrocardiography and Arrhythmias and Council on Epidemiology and Prevention. *Circulation, 118*(14), 1497–1518.

Goldstein, R. N., & Stambler, B. S. (2005). New antiarrhythmic drugs for prevention of atrial fibrillation. *Progress in Cardiovascular Diseases, 48*(3), 193–208.

Haïssaguerre, M., Derval, N., Sacher, F., Jesel, L., Deisenhofer, I., de Roy, L., et al. (2008). Sudden cardiac arrest associated with early repolarization. *New England Journal of Medicine, 358*(19), 2016–2023.

Hardin, S. R., & Steele, J. R. (2008). Atrial fibrillation among older adults: Pathophysiology, symptoms, and treatment. *Journal of Gerontological Nursing, 34*(7), 26–35.

Kashima, A., Funahashi, M., Fukumoto, K., Komamura, K., Kamakura, S., Kitakaze, M., et al. (2005). Pharmacokinetic characteristics of amiodarone in long-term oral therapy in Japanese population. *Biological & Pharmaceutical Bulletin,*

28(10), 1934–1938. Retrieved September 14, 2009, from http://www.jstage.jst.go.jp/article/bpb/28/10/1934/_pdf

Keegan, B. (2008). Caring for women undergoing cardiac ablation. *Critical Care Nursing Clinics of North America, 20*(3), 315–319.

Kowalski, M., Huizar, J. F., Kaszala, K., & Wood, M. A. (2008). Problems with implantable cardiac device therapy. *Cardiology Clinics, 26*(3), 441–458.

Kusumoto, F. A. (2008). Comprehensive approach to management of ventricular arrhythmias. *Cardiology Clinics, 26*(3), 481–496.

LaPointe, N. M. A., Sun, J., Kaplan, S., d'Almada, P., & Al-Khatib, S. M. (2008). Rhythm versus rate control in the contemporary management of atrial fibrillation in-hospital. *American Journal of Cardiology, 101*(8), 1134–1141.

Lo, R., & Hsia, H. H. (2008). Ventricular arrhythmias in heart failure patients. *Cardiology Clinics, 26*(3), 381–403.

McNamara, R. L., Tamariz, L. J., Segal, J. B., & Bass, E. B. (2003). Clinical guidelines. Management of atrial fibrillation: Review of the evidence for the role of pharmacologic therapy, electrical cardioversion, and echocardiography. *Annals of Internal Medicine, 139*(12), 1018–1033.

Mitchell, L. B. (2008). Role of drug therapy for sustained ventricular tachyarrhythmias. *Cardiology Clinics, 26*(3), 405–418.

Reising, S., Kusumoto, F., & Goldschlager, N. (2007). Life-threatening arrhythmias in the intensive care unit. *Journal of Intensive Care Medicine, 22*(1), 3–13.

Wojnowski, L. (2004). Genetics of the variable expression of CYP3A in humans. *Therapeutic Drug Monitoring, 26*(2), 192–199.

Woods, S. L., Sivarajan Froelocher, E. S., Underhill Motzer, S., & Bridges, E. J. (2005). *Cardiac nursing* (5th ed.). Philadelphia: Lippincott Williams & Wilkins.

Chapter 24

Crouch, M. A. (2005). Chronic heart failure: Developments and perspectives. *Consultive Pharmacist 20*(9), 751–765.

Frattaroli, J., Weidner, G., Merritt-Worden, T. A., Frenda, S., & Ornish, D. (2008). Angina pectoris and atherosclerotic risk factors in the multisite cardiac lifestyle intervention program. *American Journal of Cardiology, 101*(7), 911–918.

Galderisi, M., & D'Errico, A. (2008). Beta-blockers and coronary flow reserve: The importance of a vasodilatory action. *Drugs, 68*(5), 579–590.

Pilote, L., Dasgupta, K., Guru, V., Humphries, K. H., McGrath, J., Norris, C., et al. (2007). A comprehensive view of sex-specific issues related to cardiovascular disease. *Canadian Medical Association Journal, 176*(6 Suppl.), S1–S44.

Price, J. W., & Price, J. R. (2008). Accuracy and precision of metered doses of nitroglycerin lingual spray. *American Journal of Health-System Pharmacy, 65*(16), 1556–1559.

Wenger, N. K. (2008). Drugs for cardiovascular disease prevention in women. Implications of the AHA guidelines 2007 update. *Drugs, 68*(3), 339–358.

Woods, S. L., Sivarajan Froelocher, E. S., Underhill Motzer, S., & Bridges, E. J. (2005). *Cardiac nursing* (5th ed.). Philadelphia: Lippincott Williams & Wilkins.

Zaman, M. J., Junghans, C., Sekhri, N., Chen, R., Feder, G. S., Timmis, A. D., et al. (2008). Presentation of stable angina pectoris among women and South Asian people. *Canadian Medical Association Journal, 197*(7), 659–667.

Chapter 25

Beckett, N. S., Peters, R., Fletcher, A. E., Staessen, J. A., Liu, L., Dumitrascu, D., et al. (2008). Treatment of hypertension in patients 80 years of age or older. *New England Journal of Medicine, 358*(18), 1887–1898.

Benedict, N., Seybert, A., & Mathier, M. A. (2007). Evidence-based pharmacologic management of pulmonary arterial hypertension. *Clinical Therapeutics, 29*(10), 2134–2153.

Benza, R. L., Rayburn, B. K., Tallaj, J. A., Pamboukian, S. V., & Bourge, R. C. (2008). Treprostinil-based therapy in the treatment of moderate-to-severe pulmonary arterial hypertension: Long-term efficacy and combination with bosentan. *CHEST, 134*(1), 139–145.

Black, H. R., Davis, B., Barzilay, J., Nwachuku, C., Baimbridge, C., Marginean, H., et al. (2008). Metabolic and clinical outcomes in nondiabetic individuals with the metabolic syndrome assigned to chlorthalidone, amlodipine, or lisinopril as initial treatment for hypertension: A report from the Antihypertensive and Lipid-Lowering Treatment to Prevent Heart Attack Trial (ALLHAT). *Diabetes Care, 31*(2), 353–360.

Brown, M. J. (2008). Aliskiren. *Circulation, 11*(7), 773–784.

Canadian Hypertension Education Program. (2007). *2007 CHEP recommendations for the management of hypertension.* Retrieved November 22, 2008, from http://www.hypertension.ca/chep/wp-content/uploads/2007/10/chep-2007-spiral-mar16.pdf

Canadian Hypertension Education Program. (2009). *2009 Canadian hypertension education program recommendations: The short clinical summary—an annual update.* Retrieved September 21, 2009, from http://hypertension.ca/chep/wp-content/uploads/2009/07/2009-short-clinical-summary-final-2.pdf

Daugherty, K. K. (2008). Aliskiren. *American Journal of Health-System Pharmacy, 65*(14), 1323–1332.

Desapriya, E., & Pike, I. (2006). Promotion of traditional lifestyles. *Canadian Medical Association Journal, 175*(8), 919–922.

Fagard, R. H. (2008). Influencing the natural history of hypertension: It is the blood pressure achieved more than the drug. *Journal of Hypertension, 26*(8), 1533–1535.

First Nations Centre. (2005). *First Nations Regional Longitudinal Health Survey (RHS) 2002/03: Results for adults, youth and children living in First Nations communities.* Ottawa, ON: Source. Retrieved November 26, 2008, from http://www.naho.ca/firstnations/english/documents/RHS2002-03TechnicalReport_001.pdf

Flynn, J. T., & Daniels, S. R. (2006). Pharmacologic treatment of hypertension in children and adolescents. *Journal of Pediatrics, 149*(6), 746–754.

Frank, J. (2008). Managing hypertension using combination therapy. *American Family Physician, 77*(9), 1279–1286, 1289.

Galiè, N., Rubin, L., Hoeper, M., Jansa, P., Al-Hiti, H., Meyer, G., et al. (2008). Treatment of patients with mildly symptomatic pulmonary arterial hypertension with bosentan (EARLY study): A double-blind, randomised controlled trial. *Lancet, 371*(9630), 2093–2100.

Henderson, L. S., Tenero, D. M., Baidoo, C. A., Campanile, A. M., Harter, A. H., Boyle, D., et al. (2006). Pharmacokinetic and pharmacodynamic comparison of controlled-release carvedilol and immediate-release carvedilol at steady state in patients with hypertension. *American Journal of Cardiology, 98*(Suppl 7A), 17–26.

Joffres, M. R., Campbell, N. R. C., Manns, B., & Tu, K. (2007). Estimate of the benefits of a population-based reduction in dietary sodium additives on hypertension and its related health care costs in Canada. *Canadian Journal of Cardiology, 23*(6), 437–443.

Khan, N. A., Hemmelgarn, B., Herman, R. J., Rabkin, S. W., McAlister, F. A., Bell, C. M., et al. (2008). *2008 Canadian Hypertension Education Program recommendations.* Retrieved November 22, 2008, from http://www.hypertension.ca/chep/wp-content/uploads/2007/10/chep-2007-spiral-mar16.pdf

Koshy, S., Grisaru, S., & Midgley, J. (2008). The diagnosis and management of hypertension in children. *Hypertension Canada, 95*, 1–2, 5.

Lammers, A. E., Hislop, A. A., Flynn, Y., & Haworth, S. G. (2007). Epoprostenol treatment in children with severe pulmonary hypertension. *Heart, 93*(6), 739–743.

Leenen, F. H. H., Dumais, J., McInnis, N. H., Turton, P., Stratychuk, L., Nemeth, K., et al. (2008). Results of the Ontario survey on the prevalence and control of hypertension. *Canadian Medical Association Journal, 178*(11), 1441–1449.

Lenfant, C. (2008). Can prevention of hypertension work? *American Journal of Therapeutics, 15*, 334–339.

Mann, J. F., Schmieder, R. E., McQueen, M., Dyal L., Schumacher, H., Pogue, J., et al., for the ONTARGET investigators. (2008). Renal outcomes with telmisartan, ramipril, or both, in people at high vascular risk (the ONTARGET study): A multicentre, randomised, double-blind, controlled trial. *Lancet, 372*, 547–553.

McKay, D. W., Myers, M. G., Bolli, P., & Chockalingam, A. (2006). Masked hypertension: A common but insidious presentation of hypertension. *Canadian Journal of Cardiology, 22*(7), 617–620.

McLean, D., Kingsbury, K., Costello, J., Cloutier, L., & Matheson, S. on behalf of Canadian Hypertension Education Program (CHEP). 2007 hypertension education program (CHEP) Recommendations: Management of hypertension by nurses. *Canadian Journal of Cardiovascular Nursing, 17*(2), 10–16.

Mohan, S., & Campbell, N. R. C. (2008). Hypertension management in Canada: Good news, but important challenges remain. *Canadian Medical Association Journal, 178*(11), 1458–1460.

Nolan, R. P. (2008). Device-assisted slow breathing as complementary treatment for hypertension. *Hypertension Canada, 95*(7-8), 1–2, 7.

Pannarale, G. (2008). Optimal drug treatment of systolic hypertension in the elderly. *Drugs & Aging, 25*(1), 1–8.

Penz, E. D., Joffres, M. R., & Campbell, N. R. (2008). Reducing dietary sodium and decreases in cardiovascular disease in Canada. *Canadian Journal of Cardiology, 24*, 497–501.

Poirier, L. (2008). Should we treat hypertension in patients 80 years and older? Results from the HYVET trial. *Hypertension Canada, 96*, 1–2, 7.

Registered Nurses Association of Ontario. (2005). *Nursing management of hypertension.*Retrieved November 29, 2008, from http://www.rnao.org/Storage/11/607_BPG_Hypertension.pdf

Roncesvalles, A., Lee, F. W., Camamo, J., & Priestley, G. (2008). Patient safety challenges in treprostinil therapy. *MEDSURG Nursing, 17*(2), 101–106.

Rosenzweig, E. B., & Barst, R. J. (2008). Pulmonary arterial hypertension in children: A medical update. *Current Opinion in Pediatrics, 20*(3), 288–293.

Salvadori, M., Sontrop, J. M., Garg, A. X., Truong, J., Suri, R. S., Mahmud, F. H., et al. (2008). Elevated blood pressure in relation to overweight and obesity among children in a rural Canadian community. *Pediatrics, 122*(4), e821–e827.

Seikaly, M. G. (2007). Hypertension in children: An update on treatment strategies. *Current Opinion in Pediatrics, 19*(2), 170–177.

Swartz, M. J. (2008). Managing hypertension in women. *Critical Care Nursing Clinics of North America, 20*(3), 305–310.

Tobe, S. W., Pylypchuk, G., Wentworth, J., Kiss, A., Szalai, P., Perkins, N., et al. (2006). Effect of nurse-directed hypertension treatment among First Nations people with existing hypertension and diabetes mellitus: The Diabetes Risk Evaluation and Microalbuminuria (DREAM 3) randomized controlled trial. *Canadian Medical Association Journal, 174*(9), 1267–1271.

Tu, K., Chen, Z., Lipscombe, L. L., for the Canadian Hypertension Education Program. (2008). Prevalence and incidence of hypertension from 1995 to 2005: A population-based study. *Canadian Medical Association Journal, 178*(11), 1429–1435.

Woods, S. L., Sivarajan Froelocher, E. S., Adams Motzer, S., & Bridges, E. J. (2009). *Cardiac nursing* (6th ed.). Philadelphia: Lippincott Williams & Wilkins.

Chapter 26

Anonymous. (2007). Fast facts about loop diuretics. *Nursing, 3*(10), 7–8.

Chu, J. (2008). Elderly men and bone loss with loop diuretics. *American Journal of Nursing, 108*(10), 51.

Khanna, A., Lefkowitz, L., & White, W. B. (2008). Evaluation of recent fixed-dose combination therapies in the management of hypertension. *Current Opinion in Nephrology & Hypertension, 17*(5), 477–483.

Lim, L. S., Fink, H. A., Kuskowski, M. A., Taylor, B. C., Schousboe, J. T., & Ensrud, K. E. (2008). Loop diuretic use and increased rates of hip bone loss in older men: The Osteoporotic Fractures in Men study. *Archives of Internal Medicine, 168*(7), 735–740.

Padilla, M. C., Armas-Hernández, M. J., Hernández, R. H., Israili, Z. H., & Valasco, M. (2007). Update of diuretics in the treatment of hypertension. *American Journal of Therapeutics, 14*(2), 154–160.

Pitt, B., Zannad, F., Remme, W. J., Cody, R., Castaigne, A., Perez, A., et al., for the Randomized Aldactone Evaluation Study Investigators. (1999). The effect of spironolactone on morbidity and mortality in patients with severe heart failure. *New England Journal of Medicine, 341*(10), 709–717.

Sica, D. A., Gehr, T. W. B., & Frishman, W. H. (2007). Use of diuretics in the treatment of heart failure in the elderly. *Clinics in Geriatric Medicine, 23*(1), 107–121.

Sumnall, R. (2007). Fluid management and diuretic therapy in acute renal failure. *Nursing in Critical Care, 12*(1), 27–33.

Wang, D. J., & Gottlieb, S. S. (2008). Diuretics: Still the mainstay of treatment. *Critical Care Medicine, 36*(1 Suppl), S89–S94.

Woods, S. L., Sivarajan Froelocher, E. S., Underhill Motzer, S., & Bridges, E. J. (2005). *Cardiac nursing* (5th ed.). Philadelphia: Lippincott Williams & Wilkins.

Chapter 27

Holcomb, S. (2008). Third-spacing: when body fluid shifts. *Nursing, 38*(7), 50–54.

Chapter 28

Baigent, C., Collins, R., Appleby, P., Parish, S., Sleight, P., & Peto, R., on behalf of the ISIS-2 (Second International Study of Infarct Survival) Collaborative Group. (1998). ISIS-2 10-year survival among patients with suspected acute myocardial infarction in randomised comparison of intravenous streptokinase, oral aspirin, both or neither. *British Medical Journal, 316*, 1337–1343.

Bauer, K. A. (2008). New anticoagulants. *Current Opinion in Hematology, 15*(5), 509–515.

Boden, W. E., Eagle, K., & Granger, C. B. (2007). Reperfusion strategies in acute ST-segment elevation myocardial infarction: A comprehensive review of contemporary management options. *Journal of the American College of Cardiology, 50*(10), 917–929.

DeWood, M. A., Spores, J., Notske, R., Mouser, L. T., Burroughs, R., Golden, M. S., et al. (1980). Prevalence of total coronary occlusion during the early hours of transmural myocardial infarction. *New England Journal of Medicine, 303*(16), 897–902.

Eshaghian, S., Kaul, S., Amin, S., Shah, P. K., & Diamond, G. A. (2007). Role of clopidogrel in managing atherothrombotic cardiovascular disease. *Annals of Internal Medicine, 146*(6), 434–441.

Gori, A. M., Marcucci, R., Migliorini, A., Valenti, R., Moschi, G., Paniccia, R., et al. (2008). Incidence and clinical impact of dual nonresponsiveness to aspirin and clopidogrel in patients with drug-eluting stents. *Journal of the American College of Cardiology, 52*(9), 734–739.

Grines, C., & Cho, L. (2008). Atherothrombotic disease and the role of antiplatelet therapy in women. *Journal of Women's Health, 17*(1), 35–46.

Gumina, R. J., Yang, E. H., Sandhu, G. S., Praspirind, A., Bresnahan, J. F., Lennon, R. J., et al. (2008). Survival benefit with concomitant clopidogrel and glycoprotein IIb/IIIa inhibitor therapy at ad hoc percutaneous coronary intervention. *Mayo Clinic Proceedings, 83*(9), 995–1001.

GUSTO Investigators. (1993). An international randomized trial comparing four thrombolytic strategies for acute myocardial infarction. *New England Journal of Medicine, 329*, 673–682.

Hauer, K. E. (2005). Evolving approaches to the management of venous thromboembolic disease. *Johns Hopkins Advanced Studies in Medicine, 5*(3), 112–113, 140–149.

Hirsh, J., Bauer, K. A., Donati, M. B., Gould, M., Samama, M. M., & Weitz, J. I. (2008). Parenteral anticoagulants: American College of Chest Physicians evidence-based clinical practice guidelines (8th ed.) *CHEST, 133*(6 Suppl), 141S–159S.

Jennings, L. K., & Saucedo, J. F. (2008). Antiplatelet and anti-coagulant agents: Key differences in mechanisms of action, clinical application, and therapeutic benefit in patients with non–ST-segment-elevation acute coronary syndromes. *Current Opinion in Cardiology, 23*(4), 302–308.

Kastrati, A., Neumann, F., Mehilli, J., Byrne, R. A., Iijima, R., Büttner, H. J., et al. (2008). Bivalirudin versus unfractionated heparin during percutaneous coronary intervention. ISAR-REACT 3 (Intracoronary Stenting and Antithrombotic Regimen: Rapid Early Action for Coronary Treatment) Trial Investigators. *New England Journal of Medicine, 359*(7), 688–696.

Lee, S., Ahn, Y., Ahn, S., Doo, H., & Lee, B. (2008). Interaction between warfarin and *Panax gingseng* in ischemic stroke patients. *Journal of Alternative and Complementary Medicine, 14*(6), 715–721.

Lobo, B. L. (2007). Use of newer anticoagulants in patients with chronic kidney disease. *American Journal of Health-System Pharmacy, 64*(19), 2017–2026.

Mannucci, P. M., & Levi, M. (2007). Prevention and treatment of major blood loss. *New England Journal of Medicine, 356*(22), 2301–2311.

McRae, S. J., & Ginsberg, J. S. (2005). New anticoagulants for venous thromboembolic disease. *Current Opinion in Cardiology, 20*(6), 502–508.

Motsch, J., Walther, A., Bock, M., & Böttiger, B. W. (2006). Update in the prevention and treatment of deep vein thrombosis and pulmonary embolism. *Current Opinion in Anaesthesiology, 19*(1), 52–58.

Nappi, J. (2008). Benefits and limitations of current antiplatelet therapies. *American Journal of Health-System Pharmacy, 65*(Suppl 1), S5–S10.

Nutescu, E. A., Shapiro, N. L., & Chevalier, A. (2008). New anticoagulant agents: Direct thrombin inhibitors. *Cardiology Clinics, 26*(2), 169–187.

Schneeweiss, S., Seeger, J. D., Landon, J., & Walker, A. M. (2008). Aprotinin during coronary-artery bypass grafting and risk of death. *New England Journal of Medicine, 358*(8), 771–783.

Shoulders-Odom, B. (2008). Management of patients after percutaneous coronary interventions. *Critical Care Nurse, 28*(5), 26–32, 34–42.

Spinler, S. A., Nutescu, E. A., Smythe, M. A., & Wittkowsky, A. K. (2005). Anticoagulation monitor Part 1: Warfarin and parenteral direct thrombin inhibitors. *Annals of Pharmacotherapy, 39*(6), 1049–1055.

Stehle, S., Kirchheiner, J., Lazar, A., & Fuhr, U. (2008). Pharmacogenetics of oral anticoagulants. A basis for dose individualization. *Clinical Pharmacokinetics, 47*(9), 565–594.

Sullivan, J., & Amarish, N. (2008). Dual antiplatelet therapy with clopidogrel and aspirin. *American Journal of Health-System Pharmacy, 65*, 1134–1143.

Talbert, R. L. (2008). Overview of advances in cardiovascular disease treatment and prevention: The evolving role of antiplatelet therapy. *American Journal of Health-System Pharmacy, 65*(Suppl 1), S1–S5.

Tinmouth, A. T., McIntyre, L. A., & Fowler, R. A. (2008). Blood conservation strategies to reduce the need for red blood cell transfusion in critically ill patients. *Canadian Medical Association Journal, 178*(1), 49–57.

Trudell, J., & McMurdy, N. (2008). Current antifibrinolytic therapy for coronary artery revascularization. *American Association of Nurse Anesthetists Journal, 76*(2), 121–124.

White, H. D., Ohman, E. M., Lincoff, A. M., Bertrand, M. E., Colombo, A., McLaurin, B. T., et al. Safety and efficacy of bivalirudin with and without glycoprotein IIb/IIIa inhibitors in patients with acute coronary syndromes undergoing percutaneous coronary intervention: 1-year results from the ACUITY (Acute Catheterization and Urgent Intervention Triage strategY) trial. *Journal of the American College of Cardiology, 52*(10), 807–814.

Woods, S. L., Sivarajan Froelocher, E. S., Underhill Motzer, S., & Bridges, E. J. (2009). *Cardiac nursing* (6th ed.). Philadelphia: Lippincott Williams & Wilkins.

Zarra, N., Aspirinni, S., & Copp, M. A. (2008). Cardiac care: Managing postoperative bleeding. *RN, 71*(3), 27–33.

Chapter 29

American Heart Association. (2002). Third report of the National Cholesterol Education Program (NCEP) Expert Panel on detection, evaluation, and treatment of high blood cholesterol in adults (Adult Treatment Panel III) final report. *Circulation, 106*, 3143–3420.

Bays, H. E., & Goldberg, R. B. (2007). The "forgotten" bile acid sequestrants: Is now a good time to remember? *American Journal of Therapeutics, 14*(6), 567–580.

Becker, D. J., Gordon, R. Y., Morris, P. B., Yorko, J., Gordon, Y. J., Li, M., et al. (2008). Simvastatin vs. therapeutic lifestyle changes and supplements: Randomized primary prevention trial. *Mayo Clinic Proceedings, 83*(7), 758–764.

Becker, J. (2008). Cardiovascular risk assessment and hyperlipidemia. *Critical Care Nursing Clinics of North America, 20*(3), 277–285.

Berra, K. (2008). Lipid-lowering therapy today: Treating the high-risk cardiovascular patient. *Journal of Cardiovascular Nursing, 23*(5), 414–421.

Blankenhorn, D. H., Johnson, R. L., Nessim, S. A., Azen, S. P., Sanmarco, M. E., & Selzer, R. H. (1987). The Cholesterol Lowering Atherosclerosis Study (CLAS): Design, methods, and baseline results. *Controlled Clinical Trials, 8*(4), 356–387.

Brown, B. G., Brockenbrough, A., Zhao, X-Q., Dowdy, A. A., Monick, E. A., Frechette, E. H., et al. (1998). Very intensive lipid therapy with lovastatin, niacin and colestipol for prevention of death and myocardial infarction: A 10-year familial atherosclerosis treatment study (FATS) follow-up. *Circulation, 98*, I-635.

Cannon, C. P., Braunwald, E., McCabe, C. H., Rader, D. J., Rouleau, J. L., Belder, R., et al., for the Pravastatin or Atorvastatin Evaluation and Infection Therapy–Thrombolysis in Myocardial Infarction 22 Investigators. (2004). Intensive versus moderate lipid lowering with statins after acute coronary syndromes. *New England Journal of Medicine, 350*, 1495–1504.

Castelli, W. P., Garrison, R. J., Wilson, P. W., Abbott, R. D., Kalousdian, S., & Kannel, W. B. (1986). Incidence of coronary heart disease and lipoprotein cholesterol levels:

The Framingham study. *Journal of the American Medical Association, 256*(20), 2835–2838.

Després, J., Lemieux, I., & Robins, S. J. (2004). Role of fibric acid derivative in the management of risk factors for coronary heart disease. *Drugs, 64*(19), 2177–2198.

Elpers, M. (2008). Common obstacles in lipid management. *Critical Care Nursing Clinics of North America, 20*(3), 287–295.

Frick, M. H., Elo, O., Haapa, K., Heinonen, O. P., Heinsalmi, P., Helo, P., et al. (1987). Helsinki Heart Study: Primary-prevention trial with gemfibrozil in middle-aged men with dyslipidemia. Safety of treatment, changes in risk factors, and incidence of coronary heart disease. *New England Journal of Medicine, 317*(20), 1237–1245.

Godfrey, J. R. (2008). Toward optimal health: Strategies for prevention of heart disease in women. *Journal of Women's Health, 17*(8), 1271–1276.

Grady, D., Herrington, D., Bittner, V., Blumenthal, R., Davidson, M., Hlatky, M., et al. HERS Research Group. (2002). Cardiovascular outcomes during 6.8 years of hormone therapy: Heart and Estrogen/progestin Replacement Study Follow-up (HERS II). *Journal of the American Medical Association, 288*, 49–57.

Grover, S. A., Lowensteyn, I., Joseph, L., Kaouache, M., Marchand, S., Coupal, L., et al., and for the Cardiovascular Health Evaluation to Improve Patient Knowledge of Coronary Risk Profile Improves the Effectiveness of Dyslipidemia Therapy. (2008). The CHECK-UP study: A randomized controlled trial. *Archives of Internal Medicine, 167*(21), 2296 – 2303.

Grover, S. A., Palmer, C., & Coupal, L. (1994). Serum lipid screening to identify high-risk individuals for coronary death: the results of the Lipid Research Clinics Prevalence Cohort. *Archives of Internal Medicine, 154*(6), 679–684.

Hausenloy, D. J., & Yellon, D. M. (2008). Targeting residual cardiovascular risk: Raising high-density lipoprotein cholesterol levels. *Heart, 94*(6), 706–714.

Health Canada. (2005). *Health Canada advises patients about the risks of CRESTOR® (rosuvastatin). Advisory.* Retrieved November 7, 2008, from http://www.hc-sc.gc.ca/ahc-asc/media/advisories-avis/_2005/2005_10-eng.php

Heart and Stroke Foundation of Canada. (2008). *Trans fatty acids ("trans fat") and heart disease and stroke. Position paper.* Retrieved October 7, 2009, from http://www.heartandstroke.com/site/c.ikIQLcMWJtE/b.3799313/k.9ED5/Trans_fatty_acids_position_statement.htm#

Hulley, S., Grady, D., Bush, T., Furberg, C., Herrington, D., Riggs, B., et al. (1998). Randomized trial of estrogen plus progestin for secondary prevention of coronary heart disease in postmenopausal women. Heart and Estrogen/progestin Replacement Study (HERS) Research Group. *Journal of the American Medical Association, 280*, 605–613.

Kamanna, V. S., Vo, A., & Kashyap, M. L. (2008). Nicotinic acid: Recent developments. *Current Opinion in Cardiology, 23*(4): 393–398.

Kane, J. P., Malloy, M. J., Ports, T. A., Phillips, N. R., Diehl, J. C., & Havel, R. J. (1990). Regression of coronary atherosclerosis during treatment of familial hypercholesterolemia with combined drug regimens. *Journal of the American Medical Association, 264*, 3007–3012.

LaRosa, J. C., Grundy, S. M., Waters, D. D., for the Treating to New Targets (TNT) Investigators. (2005). Intensive lowering with atorvastatin in patients with stable coronary disease. *New England Journal of Medicine, 352*, 1425–1435.

Manuel, D. G., Wilson, S., & Maaten, S. (2008). The 2006 Canadian dyslipidemia guidelines will prevent more deaths while treating fewer people—but should they be further modified? *Canadian Journal of Cardiology, 24*(8), 617–620.

McPherson, R., Frohlich, J., Fodor, G., & Genest, J. (2006). Canadian Cardiovascular Society position statement—recommendations for the diagnosis and treatment of dyslipidemia and prevention of cardiovascular disease. *Canadian Journal of Cardiology, 22*(11), 913–927.

Nakou, E. S., Filippatos, T. D., Georgoula, M., Kiortsis, D. N., Tselepis, A. D., Mikhailidis, D. P., et al. (2008). The effect of orlistat and ezetimibe, alone or in combination, on serum LDL and small dense LDL cholesterol levels in overweight and obese patients with hypercholesterolaemia. *Current Medical Research and Opinion, 24*(7), 1919–1929.

Pedersen, T. R., Faergeman, O., Kastelein, J. P. P., Olsson, A. G., Tikkanen, M. J., Holme, I., et al. for the Incremental Decrease in End Points Through Aggressive Lipid Lowering (IDEAL) Study Group. (2005). High-dose atorvastatin vs. usual-dose simvastatin for secondary prevention after myocardial infarction—the IDEAL study: A randomized controlled trial. *Journal of the American Medical Association, 294*(19), 2437–2445.

Probstfield, J. L., & Rifkind, B. M. (1991). The Lipid Research Clinics Coronary Primary Prevention Trial: Design, results, and implications. *European Journal of Clinical Pharmacology, 40*(1), S69–S75.

Rossouw, J. E., Anderson, G. L., Prentice, R. L., LaCroix, A. Z., Kooperberg, C., Stefanick, M. L., et al., for the Writing Group for the Women's Health Initiative Investigators. (2002). Risks and benefits of estrogen plus progestin in healthy postmenopausal women: Principal results from the Women's Health Initiative randomized controlled trial. *Journal of the American Medical Association, 288*, 321–333.

Scandinavian Simvastatin Survival Study Group. (1994). Randomised trial of cholesterol lowering in 4444 patients with coronary heart disease: The Scandinavian Simvastatin Survival Study (4S). *Lancet, 344*, 1383–1389.

Sever, P., Dahlöf, B., Poulter, N., Wedel, H., Beevers, G., Caulfield, M., et al. (ASCOT investigators). (2003). Prevention of coronary and stroke events with atorvastatin in hypertensive patients who have average or lower-than-average cholesterol concentrations, in the Anglo-Scandinavian Cardiac Outcomes Trial—Lipid Lowering Arm (ASCOT-LLA): A multicentre randomised controlled trial. *Lancet, 361*, 1149–1158.

Shepherd, J., Cobbe, S. M., Ford, I., Isles, C. G., Lorimer, A. R., MacFarlane, P. W., et al. (1995). Prevention of coronary heart disease with pravastatin in men with hypercholesterolemia. West of Scotland Coronary Prevention Study Group. *New England Journal of Medicine, 333*(20), 1301–1307.

Staels, B., & Kuipers, F. (2007). Bile acid sequestrants and the treatment of type 2 diabetes mellitus. *Drugs, 67*(10), 1383–1392.

Tenkanen, L., Pietilä K., Manninen, V., & Mänttäri, M. (1994). The triglyceride issue revisited. Findings from the Helsinki Heart Study. *Archives of Internal Medicine, 154*(23), 2714–2720.

The Coronary Drug Project Research Group. (1973). The Coronary Drug Project. Findings leading to discontinuation of the 2.5-mg day estrogen group. *Journal of the American Medical Association, 226,* 652–657.

Ward, S., Lloyd Jones, M., Pandor, A., Holmes, M., Ara, R., Ryan, A., et al. (2007). A systematic review and economic evaluation of statins for the prevention of coronary events. *Health Technology Assessment, 11*(14), iii–iv, 1–160.

Chapter 30

Sam, S., & Frohman, L. A. (2008). Normal physiology of hypothalamic pituitary regulation. *Endocrinology & Metabolism Clinics of North America, 37*(1), 1–22.

Thomas, Z., & Fraser, G. L. (2007). An update on the diagnosis of adrenal insufficiency and the use of corticotherapy in critical illness. *Annals of Pharmacotherapy, 41*(9), 1456–1465.

Toogood, A. A., & Stewart, P. M. (2008). Hypopituitarism: Clinical features, diagnosis, and management. *Endocrinology & Metabolism Clinics of North America, 37*(1), 235–261.

Chapter 31

Brent, G. A. (2008). Graves' disease. *New England Journal of Medicine, 358*(24), 2594–2605.

Cooper, D. S. (2008). Thyroxine monotherapy after thyroidectomy: Coming full circle. *JAMA: Journal of the American Medical Association, 299*(7), 817–819.

Devdhar, M., Ousman, Y. H., & Burman, K. D. (2008). Hypothyroidism. *Endocrinology & Metabolism Clinics of North America, 36*(3), 595–615.

Chapter 32

Action to Control Cardiovascular Risk in Diabetes Study Group. (2008). Effects of intensive glucose lowering in type 2 diabetes. *New England Journal of Medicine, 358*(24), 2545–2559.

ADVANCE (Action in Diabetes and Vascular Disease: Preterax and Diamicron Modified Release Controlled Evaluation) Collaborative Group. (2008). Intensive blood glucose control and vascular outcomes in patients with type 2 diabetes. *New England Journal of Medicine, 358*(24), 2560–2572.

Bell, D. S. (2007). Insulin therapy in diabetes mellitus: How can the currently available injectable insulins be most prudently and efficaciously utilised? *Drugs, 67*(13), 1813–1827.

Bell, D. S. H., & Wyne, K. L. (2006). Symposium on diabetes. Treatment of type 2 diabetes: The addition of injection therapy. *Postgraduate Medicine, 119*(2), 15–20.

Browning, L. A., & Dumo, P. (2004). Sliding-scale insulin: An antiquated approach to glycemic control in hospitalized patients. *American Journal of Health-System Pharmacy, 61*(15), 1611–1614.

Campbell, R. K., & White, J. R. (2008). More choices than ever before. Emerging therapies for type 2 diabetes. *The Diabetes Educator, 34*(4), 518–534.

Canadian Diabetes Association Clinical Practice Guidelines Expert Committee. (2008). Canadian Diabetes Association 2008 clinical practice guidelines for the prevention and management of diabetes in Canada. *Canadian Journal of Diabetes, 32*(Suppl 1), S1–S201.

Chandra, S. T., Priya, G., Khurana, M. L., Jyotsna, V. P., Sreenivas, V., Dwivedi, S., et al. (2008). Comparison of gliclazide with insulin as initial treatment modality in newly diagnosed type 2 diabetes. *Diabetes Technology & Therapeutics, 10*(5), 363–368.

Cheng, A. Y. Y., & Fantus, I. G. (2005). Oral antihyperglycemic therapy for type 2 diabetes mellitus. *Canadian Medical Association Journal, 172*(2), 213–226.

Deeb, L. C. (2008). Diabetes technology during the past 30 years: A lot of changes and mostly for the better. *Diabetes Spectrum, 21*(2), 78–83.

Fain, J. A., & Miller, D. K. (2006). Pharmacologic interventions for type 1 and type 2 diabetes. *Nursing Clinics of North America, 41*(4), 589–604.

Fleury-Milfort, E. (2008). Practical strategies to improve treatment of type 2 diabetes. *Journal of the American Academy of Nurse Practitioners, 20*(6), 295–304.

Fonseca, V. (2006). Targeting the incretin system: Dipeptidyl peptidase IV inhibitors for the treatment of type 2 diabetes. *Medscape Diabetes & Endocrinology, 8*(2). Retrieved December 13, 2008, from http://www.medscape.com/viewarticle/541424_print

Funnell, M. M. (2007). Insulin detemir: A new option for the treatment of diabetes. *Journal of the American Academy of Nurse Practitioners, 19*(10), 508–515.

Holmkvist, J., Almgren, P., Lyssenko, V., Lindgren, C. M., Eriksson, K. F., Isomaa, B., et al. (2008). Common variants in maturity-onset diabetes of the young genes and future risk of type 2 diabetes. *Diabetes, 57*(6), 1738–1744.

Khanderia, U., Pop-Busui, R., & Eagle, K. A. (2008). Thiazolidinediones in type 2 diabetes: A cardiology perspective. *Annals of Pharmacotherapy, 42*(10), 1466–1474.

Kitabchi, A. E., & Nyenwe, E. (2007). Sliding-scale insulin: More evidence needed before final exit? *Diabetes Care, 30*(9), 2409–2410.

Kruger, D. F. (2008). Exploring the pharmocotherapeutic options for treating type 2 diabetes. *Diabetes Educator, 34*(Suppl 3), 60S–65S.

Levine, A., Brennan, A. P., & Seley, J. J. (2007). Diabetes under control. Rethinking sliding-scale insulin: One hospital's efforts in the ICU and elsewhere. *American Journal of Nursing, 107*(10), 74–79.

Martin, C. L. (2008). Beyond glycemic control: The effects of incretin hormones in type 2 diabetes. *Diabetes Educator, 34*(Suppl 3), 66S–74S.

Mathieu, C., & Bollaerts, K. (2007). Antihyperglycaemic therapy in elderly patients with type 2 diabetes: Potential role of incretin mimetics and DPP-4 inhibitors. *International Journal of Clinical Practice, 61*(Suppl 154), 29–37.

McIntosh, C. H. S. (2008). Incretin-based therapies for type 2 diabetes. *Canadian Journal of Diabetes, 32*(2), 131–139.

Morales, J. (2007). Defining the role of insulin detemir in basal insulin therapy. *Drugs, 67*(17), 2557–2584.

Odom, J., Williamson, B., & Carter, L. (2008). Rosiglitazone and pioglitazone in the treatment of diabetes mellitus. *American Journal of Health-System Pharmacy, 65*(19), 1846–1850.

Porcellati, F., Rossetti, P., Busciantella, N. R., Marzotti, S., Lucidi, P., Luzio, S., et al. (2007). Comparison of pharmacokinetics and dynamics of the long-acting insulin analogs glargine and detemir at steady state in type 1 diabetes: A double-blind, randomized, crossover study. *Diabetes Care, 30*(10), 2447–2452.

Riddle, M., Frias J., Zhang, B., Maier, H., Brown, C., Lutz, K., et al. (2007). Pramlintide improved glycemic control and reduced weight in patients with type 2 diabetes using basal insulin. *Diabetes Care, 30*(11), 2794–2799.

Sherman, F. T. (2008). Tight blood glucose control and cardiovascular disease in the elderly diabetic? *Geriatrics, 63*(8), 8–10.

Chapter 33

Salvatori, R. (2005). Adrenal insufficiency. *Journal of the American Medical Association, 294*(19), 2481–2488.

Chapter 34

Berger, C., Langsetmo, L., Joseph, L., Hanley, D. A., Davison, K. S., Josse, R., et al., and the Canadian Multicentre Osteoporosis Study Research Group. (2008). Change in bone mineral density as a function of age in women and men and association with the use of antiresorptive agents. *Canadian Medical Association Journal, 178*(13), 1660–1668.

Brown, J. B., Fortier, M., and the Osteoporosis Guidelines Committee. (2006). Canadian consensus conference on osteoporosis, 2006 update. *Journal of Obstetrics and Gynaecology Canada, 172,* S95–S112.

Cauley, J. A., Robbins, J., Chen, Z., Cummings, S. R., Jackson, R. D., LaCroix, A. Z., et al., for the Women's Health Initiative Investigators. (2003). Effects of estrogen plus progestin on risk of fracture and bone mineral density. *Journal of the American Medical Association, 290,* 1729–1738.

Cirigliano, M. (2007). Bioidentical hormone therapy: A review of the evidence. *Journal of Women's Health, 16*(5), 600–631.

Craney, A., Papaioannouu, A., Zytaruk, N., Hanley, D., Adachi, J., Goltzman, D., et al. (2006). Parathyroid hormone for the treatment of osteoporosis: A systematic review. *Canadian Medical Association Journal, 175*(1), 52–59.

Greneir, S. (2007). Vitamin D: Two indications for the price of one. *Canadian Pharmacists Journal, 140*(6), 390–394.

Hartman, T. J., Albert, P. S., Snyder, K., Slattery M. L., Caan, B., Paskett, E., et al. (2005). The association of calcium and vitamin D with risk of colorectal adenomas. *Journal of Nutrition, 135*(2), 252–259.

Hodsman, A., & Cranney, A. (2006). Clinical practice guidelines for the use of parathyroid hormone in the treatment of osteoporosis. *Canadian Medical Association Journal, 175*(1), 48–51.

Hsia, J., Heiss, G., Ren, H., Allison, M., Dolan, N. C., Greenland, P., et al. (2007). Calcium/vitamin D supplementation and cardiovascular events. *Circulation, 115*(7), 846–854.

Hui, D., Liu, G., Kavuma, E., Hewson, S. A., McKay, D., & Hannah, M. E. (2007). Preterm labour and birth: A survey of clinical practice regarding use of tocolytics, antenatal corticosteroids, and progesterone. *Journal of Obstetrics and Gynaecology Canada, 29*(2), 117–130.

Huncharek, M., Muscat, J., & Kupelnick, B. (2009). Colorectal cancer risk and dietary intake of calcium, vitamin D, and dairy products: A meta-analysis of 26,335 cases from 60 observational studies. *Nutrition and Cancer, 61*(1), 47–69.

IARC Working Group on Vitamin D. (2008). Vitamin D and cancer: A report of the IARC Working Group on Vitamin D. IARC Working Group Reports. Lyon, France: International Agency for Research on Cancer.

Jackson, R. J., LaCroix, A. Z., Gass, M., Wallace, R. B., Robbins, J., Lewis, C. E., et al., for the Women's Health Initiative Investigators. (2006). Calcium plus vitamin D supplementation and the risk of fractures. *New England Journal of Medicine, 354*(7), 669–683.

Kardsal, M. A., Henriksen, K., Arnold, M., & Christiansen, C. (2008). Calcitonin—a drug of the past or for the future? Physiologic inhibition of bone resorption while sustaining osteoclast numbers improves bone quality. *Biodrugs, 22*(3), 137–144.

Lappe, J. M., Travers-Gustafson, D., Davies, K. M., Recker, R. R., & Heaney, R. P. (2007). Vitamin D and calcium supplementation reduces cancer risk: Results of a randomized trial. *American Journal of Clinical Nutrition, 85*(6), 1586–1591.

Licata, A. A. (2007). Update on therapy for osteoporosis. *Orthopaedic Nursing, 26*(3), 162–168.

Manson, J. E., Hsia, J., Johnson, K. C., Rossouw, J. E., Assaf, A. R., Lasser, N. L., et al., for the Women's Health Initiative Investigators. (2003). Estrogen plus progestin and the risk of coronary heart disease. *The New England Journal of Medicine, 349*(6), 523–534.

McCullough, M. L., Robertson, A. S., Rodriguez, C., Jacobs, E. J., Chao, A., Carolyn, J., et al. (2003). Calcium, vitamin D, dairy products, and risk of colorectal cancer in the Cancer Prevention Study II Nutrition Cohort (United States). *Cancer Causes and Control, 14*(1), 1–12.

Reed, S. D., Newton, K. M., LaCroix, A. Z., Grothaus, L. C., Grieco, V. S., & Ehrlich, K. (2008). Vaginal, endometrial, and reproductive hormone findings: Randomized, placebo-controlled trial of black cohosh, multibotanical herbs, and dietary soy for vasomotor symptoms: the Herbal Alternatives for Menopause (HALT) Study. *Menopause, 15*(1), 51–58.

Reid, D. M., Hosking, D., Kendler, D., Brandi, M. L., Wark, J. D., Marques-Neto, J. F., et al. (2008). A comparison of the effect of alendronate and risedronate on bone mineral density in postmenopausal women with osteoporosis: 24-month results from FACTS-International. *International Journal of Clinical Practice, 62*(4), 575–584.

Roemheld-Hamm, B. (2005). Chasteberry. *American Family Physician, 72*(5), 821–824.

Rolnick, S. J., Jackson, J., Kopher, R., & Defor, T. A. (2007). Provider management of menopause after the findings of the Women's Health Initiative. *Menopause, 14*(3 Part 1), 441–449.

Sambrook, P., & Cooper, C. (2006). Osteoporosis. *Lancet, 367*(9257), 2010–2018.

Shumaker, S. A., Legault, C., Rapp, S. R., Thal, L., Wallace, R. B., Ockene, J. K., et al., for the WHIMS Investigators. (2003). Estrogen plus progestin and the incidence of dementia and mild cognitive impairment in postmenopausal women. *Journal of the American Medical Association, 289*(20), 2652–2662.

Simon, J. A. (2007). Hormone therapy in the 21st century: Clinical considerations for moving beyond oral therapy. Bringing clarity to current trial data. *Women's Health Care: A Practical Journal for Nurse Practitioners, 6*(2), 11–14, 16–17, 32–34.

Speroff, L. (2007). Transdermal versus oral postmenopausal hormone therapy: Is there a clinical difference? *Women's Health Care: A Practical Journal for Nurse Practitioners, 6*(2), 18, 21–24, 32–34.

Stroup, J., Kane, M. P., & Abu-Baker, A. M. (2008). Teriparatide in the treatment of osteoporosis. *American Journal of Health-System Pharmacy, 65*(6), 532–539.

Chapter 35

Edwards, J. L. (2008). Diagnosis and management of benign hyperplasia. *American Family Physician, 77*(10), 1403–1410.

Ellsworth, P., & Kirshenbaum, E. M. (2008). Current concepts in the evaluation and management of erectile dysfunction. *Urologic Nursing, 28*(5), 357–369.

Emberton, M., Cornel, E. B., Bassi, P. F., Fourcade, R. O., Gómez, J. M. F., & Castro, R. (2008). Benign prostatic hyperplasia as a progressive disease: A guide to the risk factors and options for medical management. *International Journal of Clinical Practice, 62*(7), 1076–1086.

Hatzimouratidis, K., & Hatzichristou, D. G. (2008). Looking to the future for erectile dysfunction therapies. *Drugs, 68*(2), 231–250.

Issa, M. M., & Kraft, K. H. (2007). 5-alpha-reductase inhibition for men with enlarged prostate. *Journal of the American Academy of Nurse Practitioners, 19*(8), 398–407.

Jewett, M. A. S., & Klotz, L. H. (2007). Advances in the medical management of benign prostatic hyperplasia. *Canadian Medical Association Journal, 176*(13), 1850–1851.

Keam, S. J., & Scott, L. J. (2008). Dutasteride: A review of its use in the management of prostate disorders. *Drugs, 68*(4), 463–485.

Lucia, M. S., Epstein, J. I., Goodman, P. J., Darke, A. K., Reuter, V. E., Civantos, F., et al. (2008). Finasteride and high-grade prostate cancer in the prostate cancer prevention trial. *Journal of the National Cancer Institute, 99*(18), 1375–1383.

Rich, K. T., & Safranek, S. (2008). FPIN's clinical inquiries. Medical treatment of benign prostatic hyperplasia. *American Family Physician, 77*(5), 665–666.

Turkoski, B. B. (2008). Drugs used to treat erectile dysfunction. *Orthopaedic Nursing, 27*(3), 201–206.

Chapter 36

Dicpinigaitis, P. V., & Gayle, Y. E. (2003). Effect of guaifenesin on cough reflex sensitivity. *CHEST, 124*(6), 2178–2181.

Kelley, L. K., Allen, P. J., & Allen, P. L. J. (2007). Primary care approaches. Managing acute cough in children: Evidence-based guidelines. *Pediatric Nursing, 33*(6), 515–524.

McElhaney, J. E., Goel, V., Toane, B., Hooten, J., & Shan, J. J. (2006). Efficacy of COLD-fX in the prevention of respiratory symptoms in community-dwelling adults: A randomized, double-blinded, placebo-controlled trial. *Journal of Alternative & Complementary Medicine, 12*(2), 153–157.

Pavord, I. D., & Chung, K. F. (2008). Management of chronic cough. *Lancet, 371*(9621), 1375–1384.

Predy, G. N., Goel, V., Lovlin, R., Donner, A., Stitt, A., & Basu, T. K. (2005). Efficacy of an extract of North American ginseng containing poly-furanosyl-pyranosyl-saccharides for preventing upper respiratory tract infections: A randomized controlled trial. *Canadian Medical Association Journal, 173*(9), 1043–1048.

Ryan, T., Brewer, M., & Small, L. (2008). Over-the-counter cough and cold medication use in young children. *Pediatric Nursing, 34*(2), 174–180, 184.

Schaefer, M. K., Shehab, N., Cohen, A. L., & Budnitz, D. S. (2008). Adverse events from cough and cold medications in children. *Pediatrics, 121*(4), 783–787.

Shah, S. S., Sander, S., White, C. M., Rinaldi, M., & Coleman, C. I. (2007). Evaluation of echinacea for the prevention and treatment of the common cold: A meta-analysis. *Lancet Infectious Diseases, 7*(7), 473–480.

Smith, S. M., Schroeder, K., & Fahey, T. (2008). Over-the-counter medications for acute cough in children and adults in ambulatory settings. *Cochrane Database of Systematic Reviews, 1*.

Woelkart, K., Linde, K., & Bauer, R. (2008). Echinacea for preventing and treating the common cold. *Planta Medica, 74*(6), 633–637.

Woo, T. (2008). Pharmacology of cough and cold medicines. *Journal of Pediatric Healthcare, 22*(2), 73–82.

Chapter 37

Aaron, S. D., Vandemheen, K. L., Boulet, L.-P., McIvor, R. A., FitzGerald, J. M., Hernandez, P., et al., for the Canadian Respiratory Clinical Research Consortium. (2008). Overdiagnosis of asthma in obese and nonobese adults. *Canadian Medical Association Journal, 179*(11), 1121–1131.

Asthma Guidelines Working Group of the Canadian Network for Asthma Care. (2005). Canadian pediatric asthma consensus guidelines, 2003 (updated December 2004). *Canadian Medical Association Journal, 173*(6), S1–S56.

Banasiak, N., & Bolster, A. (2008). Pediatric asthma. *RN, 71*(7), 26–32.

Bateman, E., Nelson, H., Bousquet, J., Kral, K., Sutton, L., Ortega, H., et al. (2008). Meta-analysis: Effects of adding salmeterol to inhaled corticosteroids on serious asthma-related events. *Annals of Internal Medicine, 149*(1), 33–42.

Belliveau, P. B., & Lahoz, M. R. (2007). Treating allergic asthma with omalizumab. *Disease Management & Health Outcomes, 15*(3), 165–179.

Bisgaard, H., Hermansen, M. N., Loland, L., Halkjaer, L. B., & Buchvald, H. (2006). Intermittent inhaled corticosteroids in infants with episodic wheezing. *New England Journal of Medicine, 354*(19), 1998–2005.

Cayley, W. E., Jr. (2008). Use of inhaled corticosteroids to treat stable COPD. *American Family Physician, 77*(11), 1532–1533.

Cornell, A., Shaker, M., & Woodmansee, D. P. (2008). Update on the pathogenesis and management of childhood asthma. *Current Opinion in Pediatrics, 20*(5), 597–604.

Global Initiative for Asthma (GINA). (2006). *Global strategy for asthma management and prevention 2007 update.* Retrieved December 21, 2008, from http://www.ginasthma.com/download.asp?intId=309

Guilbert, T. W., Morgan, W. J., Zeiger, R. S., Mauger, D. T., Boehmer, S. J., Szefler, S. J., et al. (2006). Long-term inhaled corticosteroids in preschool children at high risk for asthma. *New England Journal of Medicine, 354*(19), 1985–1997.

Hanania, N. A. (2008). Targeting airway inflammation in asthma: Current and future therapies. *CHEST, 133*(4), 989–998.

Hendeles, L., & Sorkness, C. A. (2007). Anti-immunoglobulin E therapy with omalizumab for asthma. *Annals of Pharmacotherapy, 41*(9), 1397–1410.

Janssens, H. M., Tiddnes, H. A. W. M. (2006). Aerosol therapy: The special needs of young children. Paediatric Respiratory Review, *75*, 583–585.

Lau, E. (2007). Pediatric considerations in asthma. *Canadian Pharmacists Journal, 140*(Suppl 3), S31–S32.

Nathan, R. A., Sorkness, C. A., Kosinski, M., Schatz, M., Li, J. T., Marcus, P., et al. (2004) Development of the asthma control test: A survey for assessing asthma control. *Journal of Allergy and Clinical Immunology, 113*(1), 59–65.

Randhawa, I., & Klaustermeyer, W. B. (2007). Oral corticosteroid-dependent asthma: A 30-year review. *Annals of Allergy, Asthma & Immunology, 99*(4), 291–302.

Seddon, P., Bara, A., Ducharme, F. M., & Lasserson, T. J. (2006). Oral xanthines as maintenance treatment for asthma in children. *Cochrane Database Systematic Review,* Art. No. CD002885.

Strunk, R. C., & Bloomberg, G. R. (2006). Omalizumab for asthma. *New England Journal of Medicine, 35*(25), 2689–2695.

World Health Organization. (2008) *Global initiative for chronic obstructive lung disease. Global strategy for the diagnosis, management, and prevention of chronic obstructive lung disease.* Retrieved December 21, 2008, from http://www.goldcopd.com/download.asp?intId=504

Chapter 38

American Academy of Pediatrics. (2006). The use of systemic fluoroquinolones. Policy statement. Committee on Infectious Diseases Pediatrics. *Pediatrics, 118*(3), 1287–1292.

Baldwin, C. M., Lyseng-Williamson, K. A., & Keam, S. J. (2008). Meropenem: A review of its use in the treatment of serious bacterial infections. *Drugs, 68*(6), 803–838.

Canadian Committee on Antibiotic Resistance (CCAR). (2004). Canadian Committee on Antibiotic Resistance report. *Canadian Journal of Infectious Diseases and Medical Microbiology, 15*(5), 257–260.

Dial, S., Kezouh, A., Dascal, A., Barkun, A., & Suissa, S. (2008). Patterns of antibiotic use and risk of hospital admission because of *Clostridium difficile* infection. *Canadian Medical Association Journal, 179*(8), 767–772.

Driscoll, J. A., Brody, S. L., & Kollef, M. H. (2007). The epidemiology, pathogenesis and treatment of *Pseudomonas aeruginosa* infections. *Drugs, 67*(3), 351–368.

Graham, D. Y., Lu, H., & Yamaoka, Y. (2008). Therapy for *Helicobacter pylori* infection can be improved: Sequential therapy and beyond. *Drugs, 68*(6), 725–736.

Hessen, M. T., & Kaye, D. (2004). Principles of use of antibacterial agents. *Infectious Diseases Clinics of North America, 18*, 435–450.

Lipsky, M. S. (2005). Ketolides in the treatment of community-acquired respiratory tract infections: A review. *Current Therapeutic Research, 66*(3), 139–153.

Noreddin, A. M., & Haynes, V. (2007). Use of pharmacodynamic principles to optimise dosage regimens for antibacterial agents in the elderly. *Drugs & Aging, 24*(4), 275–292.

Plouffe, J. F., & Martin, D. R. (2004). Re-evaluation of the therapy of severe pneumonia caused by *Streptococcus pneumonia*. *Infectious Diseases Clinics of North America, 18*, 963–974.

Stanley, I. M., & Kaye, K. M. (2004) Beta-lactam antibiotics: Newer formulations and newer agents. *Infectious Diseases Clinics of North America, 18*, 603–619.

Tenover, F. C. (2006). Mechanisms of antimicrobial resistance in bacteria. *American Journal of Infection Control, 34*(5), S3–S10, S75–S79.

Chapter 39

Burgess, D. S., & Rapp, R. P. (2008). Bugs versus drugs: Addressing the pharmacist's challenge. *American Journal of Health-System Pharmacy, 65*(9 Suppl 2), S4–S15.

Karageorgopoulos, D. E., Giannopoulou, K. P., Grammatikos, A. P., Dimopoulos, G., & Falagas, M. E. (2008). Fluoroquinolones compared with b-lactam antibiotics for the treatment of acute bacterial sinusitis: A meta-analysis of randomized controlled trials. *Canadian Medical Association Journal, 178*(7), 845–854.

Mehlhorn, A. J., & Brown, D. A. (2007). Safety concerns with fluoroquinolones. *Annals of Pharmacotherapy, 41*(11), 1859–1866.

Navarro, M. B., Huttner, B., & Harbarth, S. (2008). Methicillin-resistant *Staphylococcus aureus* control in the 21st century: Beyond the acute care hospital. *Current Opinion in Infectious Diseases, 21*(4), 372–379.

Roberts, J. A., Kruger, P., Paterson, D. L., & Lipman, J. (2008). Antibiotic resistance—what's dosing got to do with it? *Critical Care Medicine, 36*(8), 2433–2440.

Roe, V. A. (2008). Antibiotic resistance: A guide for effective prescribing in women's health. *Journal of Midwifery & Women's Health, 53*(3), 216–226.

van Zanten, A. R. H., Polderman, K. H., van Geijlswijk, I. M., van der Meer, G. Y. G., Schouten, M. A., & Girbes, A. R. J. (2008). Ciprofloxacin pharmacokinetics in critically ill patients: A prospective cohort study. *Journal of Critical Care, 23*(3), 422–430.

Volles, D. F., & Branan, T. N. (2008). Antibiotics in the intensive care unit: Focus on agents for resistant pathogens. *Emergency Medicine Clinics of North America, 26*(3), 813–834.

Chapter 40

Arvin, A. M. (2008). Humoral and cellular immunity to varicella-zoster virus: An overview. *Journal of Infectious Diseases, 197*(Suppl 2), S58–S60.

Carter, N. J., & Keating, G. M. (2007). Maraviroc. *Drugs, 67*(15), 2277–2288.

Casper, C., Krantz, E. M., Corey, L., Kuntz, S. R., Wang, J., Selke, S., et al. (2008). Valganciclovir for suppression of human herpesvirus-8 replication: A randomized, double blind, placebo-controlled, crossover trial. *Journal of Infectious Diseases, 198*(1), 23–30.

Celum, C., Wald, A., Hughes, J., Sanchez, J., Reid. S., Delany-Moretlwe, S., et al., for the HPTN 039 Protocol Team. (2008). Effect of aciclovir on HIV-1 acquisition in herpes simplex virus 2 seropositive women and men who have sex with men: A randomised, double-blind, placebo-controlled trial. *Lancet, 371*(9630), 2109–2019.

Centers for Disease Control and Prevention. (2009). *2009 H1N1 flu (swine flu).* Retrieved October 27, 2009, from http://www.cdc.gov/H1N1FLU/

Croxtall, J. D., Lyseng-Williamson, K. A., & Perry, C. M. (2008). Raltegravir. *Drugs, 68*(1), 131–138.

Dolin, R. (2008). A new class of anti-HIV therapy and new challenges. *New England Journal of Medicine, 359* (14), 1509–1511.

Government of Canada. (2007) *Avian influenza.* Retrieved December 28, 2008, from http://www.influenza.gc.ca/ai-ga_e.html

Hambleton, S., Steinberg, S. P., LaRussa, P. S., Shapiro, E. D., & Gershon, A. A. (2008). Risk of herpes zoster in adults immunized with varicella vaccine. *Journal of Infectious Diseases, 197*(Suppl 2), S196–S199.

Hatchette, T., Tipples, G. A., Peters, G., Alsuwaidi, A., Zhou, J., & Mailman, T. L. (2008). Foscarnet salvage therapy for acyclovir-resistant varicella zoster: Report of a novel thymidine kinase mutation and review of the literature. *Pediatric Infectious Disease Journal, 27*(1), 75–77.

Health Canada. (2008). *SARS.* Retrieved December 28, 2008, from http://www.hc-sc.gc.ca/dc-ma/sars-sras/index-eng.php

Lieberman-Blum, S. S., Fung, H. B., & Bandres, J. C. (2008). Maraviroc: A CCR5-receptor antagonist for the treatment of HIV-1 infection. *Clinical Therapeutics, 30*(7), 1228–1250.

Mell, H. K. (2008). Management of oral and genital herpes in the emergency department. *Emergency Medicine Clinics of North America, 26*(2), 457–473.

Mueller, N. H., Gilden, D. H., Cohrs, R. J., Mahalingam, R., & Nagel, M. A. (2008). Varicella zoster virus infection: Clinical features, molecular pathogenesis of disease, and latency. *Neurologic Clinics, 26*(3), 675–697.

Public Health Agency of Canada. (2006). *West Nile virus.* Retrieved December 28, 2008, from http://www.phac-aspc.gc.ca/wn-no/index-eng.php

Public Health Agency of Canada. (2009). *Get the facts on the H1N1 flu virus.* Retrieved October 27, 2009, from http://www.phac-aspc.gc.ca/alert-alerte/h1n1/index-eng.php

Reeves, J. D., & Piefer, A. J. (2005). Emerging drug targets for antiretroviral therapy. *Drugs, 65*(13), 1747–1766.

Simpson, D., & Lyseng-Williamson, K. A. (2006). Famciclovir: A review of its use in herpes zoster and genital and orolabial herpes. *Drugs, 66*(18), 2397–2416.

Steigbigel, R. T., Cooper, D. A., Kumar, P. N., Eron, J. E., Schechter, M., Markowitz, M., et al., for the BENCHMRK Study Teams. (2008). Raltegravir with optimized background therapy for resistant HIV-1 infection. *New England Journal of Medicine, 359*(4), 339–354.

Watson, B. (2008). Humoral and cell-mediated immune responses in children and adults after 1 and 2 doses of varicella vaccine. *Journal of Infectious Diseases, 197*(Suppl 2), S143–S146.

World Health Organization. (2009). *Pandemic (H1N1) 2009.* Retrieved October 27, 2009, from http://www.who.int/csr/disease/swineflu/en/

Yost, R., Pasquale, T. R., & Sahloff, E. G. (2009). Maraviroc: A coreceptor CCR5 antagonist for management of HIV infection. *American Journal of Health-System Pharmacy, 66*(8), 715–726.

Chapter 41

Canadian Lung Association. (2008). *Canada's role in fighting tuberculosis.* Retrieved December 29, 2008, from http://www.lung.ca/tb/index.html

Cox, H., & McDermid, C. (2008). XDR tuberculosis can be cured with aggressive treatment. *Lancet, 372*(9647), 1363–1365.

National Institute of Allergy and Infectious Diseases. (2008). *Tuberculosis.* Retrieved December 29, 2008, from http://www3.niaid.nih.gov/topics/tuberculosis/default.htm

Public Health Agency of Canada. (2007a). *BCG usage in Canada—current and historical.* Retrieved December 29, 2008, from http://www.phac-aspc.gc.ca/tbpc-latb/bcgvac_1206-eng.php

Public Health Agency of Canada. (2007b). *Canadian tuberculosis standards* (6th ed.). Retrieved December 28, 2008, from http://www.phac-aspc.gc.ca/tbpc-latb/pubs/tbstand07-eng.php

Public Health Agency of Canada. (2008). *Tuberculosis. Drug resistance in Canada—2007.* Retrieved December 28, 2008, from http://www.phac-aspc.gc.ca/tbpc-latb/pubs/tbdrc07/index-eng.php

Stewart, G. R., Robertson, B. D., & Young, D. B. (2003). Tuberculosis: A problem with persistence. *Nature Reviews Microbiology, 1*, 97–105.

Chapter 42

Canadian Paediatric Society. (2007). Antifungal agents for common paediatric infections. *Paediatrics & Child Health, 12*(10), 875–878.

Chowdhry, R., & Marshall, W. L. (2008). Antifungal therapies in the intensive care unit. *Journal of Intensive Care Medicine, 23*(3), 151–158.

Del Bono, V., Mikulska, M., & Viscoli, C. (2008). Invasive aspergillosis: Diagnosis, prophylaxis and treatment. *Current Opinion in Hematology, 15*(6), 586–593.

Hill, M. J. (2008). Dermatology nursing essentials: Core knowledge: Fungal infections. *Dermatology Nursing, 20*(2), 137–138.

Juang, P. (2007). Update on new antifungal therapy. *AACN Advanced Critical Care, 18*(3), 253–262.

Krishnan-Natesan, S., & Chandrasekar, P. H. (2008). Current and future therapeutic options in the management of invasive aspergillosis. *Drugs, 68*(3), 265–282.

Reboli, A. C., Rotstein, C., Pappas, P. G., Chapman, S. W., Kett, D. H., Kumar, D., et al., for the Anidulafungin Study Group. (2007). Anidulafungin versus fluconazole for invasive candidiasis. *New England Journal of Medicine, 356*(24), 2472–2482, 2557–2560.

Rüping, M. J. G., Vehreschild, J. J., & Cornely, O. A. (2008). Patients at high risk of invasive fungal infections: When and how to treat. *Drugs, 68*(14), 1941–1962.

Snow, M. (2008). Combating infection. Fighting fungal infections: Stopping tinea in its tracks. *Nursing, 38*(7), 62–63.

Thursky, K. A., Playford, E. G., Seymour, J. F., Sorrell, T. C., Ellis, D. H., et al. (2008). Recommendations for the treatment of established fungal infections. *Internal Medicine Journal, 38*(6), 496–520.

Chapter 43

Eziefula, A. C., & Brown, M. (2008). Intestinal nematodes: Disease burden, deworming and the potential importance of co-infection. *Current Opinion in Infectious Diseases, 21*(5), 516–522.

Greenwood, Z., Black, J., Weld, L., O'Brien, D., Leder, K., Von Sonnenburg, F., et al. (2008). Gastrointestinal infection among international travelers globally. *Journal of Travel Medicine, 15*(4), 221–228.

Kucik, C. J., Martin, G. L., Sortor, B. V., & Viera, A. J. (2004). Common intestinal parasites. *American Family Physician, 69*(5), 1161–1168, 1039–1041.

Public Health Agency of Canada. (2004). *Canadian recommendations for the prevention and treatment of malaria among international travellers.* Retrieved December 30, 2008, from http://www.phac-aspc.gc.ca/publicat/ccdr-rmtc/04vol30/30s1/index.html

Chapter 44

Pineau, L., Desbuquois, C., Marchetti, B., Luu, & Duc, D. (2008). Comparison of the fixative properties of five disinfectant solutions. *Journal of Hospital Infection, 68*(2), 171–177.

Public Health Agency of Health Canada. (2007). *Nosocomial infections.* Retrieved November 4, 2009, from http://www.phac-aspc.gc.ca/nois-sinp/index-eng.php

Chapter 45

American College of Rheumatology. Ad Hoc Group on Use of Selective and Nonselective Nonsteroidal Antiinflammatory Drugs. (2008). Recommendations for use of selective and nonselective nonsteroidal antiinflammatory drugs: An American College of Rheumatology white paper. *Arthritis & Rheumatism: Arthritis Care & Research, 59*(8), 1058–1073.

Dalessio, D. J. (2005). Caffeine as an analgesic adjuvant: Review of the evidence. *Headache: The Journal of Head and Face Pain, 34*(S1), 10–12.

Donahue, K. E., Gartlehner, G., Jonas, D. E., Lux, L. J., Thieda, P., Jonas, B. L., et al. (2008). Systematic review: Comparative effectiveness and harms of disease-modifying medications for rheumatoid arthritis. *Annals of Internal Medicine, 148*(2), 124–134.

Eggebeen, A. T. (2007). Gout: An update. *American Family Physician, 76*(6), 801–808.

Gaffo, A., Saag, K. G., & Curtis, J. R. (2006). Treatment of rheumatoid arthritis. *American Journal of Health-System Pharmacy, 63*(24), 2451–2465.

Harvey, W. F., & Hunter, D. J. (2008). The role of analgesics and intra-articular injections in disease management. *Rheumatic Disease Clinics of North America, 34*(3), 777–788.

Hoskison, K. T., & Wortmann, R. L. (2007). Management of gout in older adults: Barriers to optimal control. *Drugs & Aging, 24*(1), 21–36.

Kokebie, R., & Block, J. A. (2008). Managing osteoarthritis: Current and future directions. *Journal of Musculoskeletal Medicine, 25*(7), 346–352.

Millett, P., Gobezie, R., & Boykin, R. E. (2008). Shoulder osteoarthritis: Diagnosis and management. *American Family Physician, 78*(5), 605–611.

O'Mahony. R., & Oliver, S. (2008). Osteoarthritis: The NICE guideline. *Primary Health Care, 18*(6), 32–37.

Phillips, M. (2008). Salicylate poisoning. *Advanced Emergency Nursing Journal, 30*(1), 75–86.

Rice, S. (2003). Reye's syndrome isn't just child's play. *Nursing, 33*(9), 1–4.

Schett, G., Stach, C., Zwerina, J., Voll, R., & Manger, B. (2008). How antirheumatic drugs protect joints from damage in rheumatoid arthritis. *Arthritis & Rheumatism, 58*(10), 2936–2948.

Singh, H., & Torralba, K. D. (2008). Therapeutic challenges in the management of gout in the elderly. *Geriatrics, 63*(7), 13–18, 20.

Stamp, L. K., O'Donnell, J. L., & Chapman, P. T. (2007). Emerging therapies in the long-term management of hyperuricaemia and gout. *Internal Medicine Journal, 37*(4), 258–266.

Teng, G. G., Nair, R., & Saag, K. G. (2006). Pathophysiology, clinical presentation and treatment of gout. *Drugs, 66*(12), 1547–1563.

Chapter 46

Aliabadi, A. Z., Zuckermann, A. O., & Grimm, M. (2007). Immunosuppressive therapy in older cardiac transplant patients. *Drugs & Aging, 24*(11), 913–932.

Anderson, R. B., & Holman, J. R. (2007). Psoriasis: Update on therapeutic choices. *Consultant, 47*(5), 461–468.

Brugarolas, J., Lotan, Y., Watumull, L., & Kabbani, W. (2008). Sirolimus in metatastic [sic] renal cell carcinoma. *Journal of Clinical Oncology, 26*(20), 3457–3460.

Hampton, T. (2008). Clinical trials probe new therapies for some difficult-to-treat cancers. *JAMA: Journal of the American Medical Association, 300*(4), 384–385.

Kitahara, K., & Kawai, S. (2007). Cyclosporine and tacrolimus for the treatment of rheumatoid arthritis. *Current Opinion in Rheumatology, 19*(3), 238–245.

Knoll, G. (2008). Trends in kidney transplantation over the past decade. *Drugs, 68*(Suppl), 3–10.

Li, D., Lu, W., Zhu, J. Y., Gao, J., Lou, Y. Q., & Zhang, G. L. (2007). Population pharmacokinetics of tacrolimus and CYP3A5, MDR1 and IL-10 polymorphisms in adult liver transplant patients. *Journal of Clinical Pharmacy & Therapeutics, 32*(5), 505–515.

Mutch, K. (2008). Glatiramer acetate (Copaxone) and its use in the management of relapsing-remitting MS. *British Journal of Neuroscience Nursing, 4*(4), 186–1891.

Ollendorf, D. A., Castelli-Haley, J., & Oleen-Burkey, M. (2008). Impact of co-prescribed glatiramer acetate and antihistamine therapy on the likelihood of relapse among patients with multiple sclerosis. *Journal of Neuroscience Nursing, 40*(5), 281–290.

Snell, G. I., & Westall, G. P. (2007). Immunosuppression for lung transplantation: Evidence to date. *Drugs, 67*(11), 1531–1539.

Sun, Q., Liu, Z. H., Cheng, Z., Chen, J., Ji, S., Zeng, C., et al. (2007). Treatment of early mixed cellular and humoral renal allograft rejection with tacrolimus and mycophenolate mofetil. *Kidney International, 71*(1), 24–30.

Taylor, J. L., & Palmer, S. M. (2006). Critical care perspective on immunotherapy in lung transplantation. *Journal of Intensive Care Medicine, 21*(6), 327–344.

Chapter 47

Bader, M. S., & Hawboldt, J. (2008). Vaccinations for older adults. *Clinical Geriatrics, 16*(9), 38–46.

Baker, J. P. (2008). Mercury, vaccines, and autism: One controversy, three histories. *American Journal of Public Health, 98*(2), 244–253.

Capeding, M. R., Cadorna-Carlos, J., Book-Montellano, M., & Ortiz, E. (2008). Immunogenicity and safety of a DTaP-IPV//PRP approximately T combination vaccine given with hepatitis B vaccine: A randomized open-label trial. *Bulletin of the World Health Organization, 86*(6), 443–451.

Dawar, M., Deeks, S., &; Dobson, S. (2007). Human papillomavirus vaccines launch a new era in cervical cancer prevention. *Canadian Medical Association Journal, 177*(5), 456–461.

Fisher, R., Darrow, D. H., Tranter, M., & Williams, J. V. (2008). Human papillomavirus vaccine: Recommendations, issues and controversies. *Current Opinion in Pediatrics, 20*(4), 441–445.

Gold, R. (2006). *Your child's best shot* (3rd ed.). Ottawa, ON: Canadian Pediatric Society.

Harrison, L. H. (2008). A multivalent conjugate vaccine for prevention of meningococcal disease in infants. *Journal of the American Medical Association, 299*(2), 217–219.

Health Canada. (2006). *Canadian immunization guide* (7th ed.). Ottawa, ON: Canadian Medical Association.

Infectious Diseases and Immunization Committee, Adolescent Health Committee, Canadian Paediatric Society (CPS). (2007). Human papillomavirus vaccine for children and adolescents. *Paediatrics & Child Health, 12*(7), 599–603.

Merck Frosst. (2008). *Product monograph. RotaTeq.* Retrieved May 13, 2009, from http://www.merckfrosst.com/assets/en/pdf/products/RotaTeq_1129-a_3_08-E.pdf

Money, D. M., & Roy, M., for the HPV Consensus Guidelines Committee. (2007). Canadian consensus guidelines on human papillomavirus. *Journal of Obstetrics and Gynaecology Canada, 29*(8 Suppl 3), S1–S56.

Oxman, M. N., & Levin, M. J. (2008). Vaccination against herpes zoster and postherpetic neuralgia. *Journal of Infectious Diseases, 197*(Suppl 2), S228–S236.

Pace, D., & Pollard, A. J. (2007). Meningococcal A, C, Y and W-135 polysaccharide-protein conjugate vaccines. *Archives of Disease in Childhood, 92*(10), 909–915.

Parashar, U. D., & Glass, R. I. (2009). Rotavirus vaccines—early success, remaining questions. *New England Journal of Medicine, 360*(11), 1063–1065.

Pielak, K. L., McIntyre, C. C., Remple, V. P., Buxton, J. A., & Skowronski, D. M. (2008). One arm or two? Concurrent administration of meningococcal C conjugate and hepatitis B vaccines in pre-teens. *Canadian Journal of Public Health, 99*(1), 52–56.

Public Health Agency of Canada. (2008a). *Pandemic plan strengthened.* Retrieved January 6, 2009, from http://www.phac-aspc.gc.ca/cpip-pclcpi/20080905rev-eng.php

Public Health Agency of Canada. (2008b). *Vaccine safety. Canadian Adverse Events Following Immunization Surveillance System (CAEFISS).* Retrieved May 13, 2009, from http://www.phac-aspc.gc.ca/im/vs-sv/index.html

Public Health Agency of Canada. (2009a). *Key facts on H1N1 flu virus.* Retrieved November 19, 2009, from http://www.phac-aspc.gc.ca/alert-alerte/h1n1/fs-fr_h1n1-eng.php

Public Health Agency of Canada. (2009b). *The Canadian pandemic influenza plan* for the health sector. Retrieved January 6, 2009, from http://www.phac-aspc.gc.ca/cpip-pclcpi/

Schiffman, M., Castle, P. E., Jeronimo, J., Rodriguez, A. C., & Wacholder, S. (2007). Human papillomavirus and cervical cancer. *Lancet, 370*(9590), 890–907.

Siegrist, C. A. (2008). Blame vaccine interference, not neonatal immunization, for suboptimal responses after neonatal diphtheria, tetanus, and acellular pertussis immunization. *Journal of Pediatrics, 153*(3), 305–307.

Templeman-Kluit, A. (2008). No blame—no gain. *Canadian Medical Association Journal, 178*(2), 140–141.

Chapter 48

B.C. Cancer Agency. (2009). *Cancer drug manual.* Retrieved January 10, 2009, from www.bccancer.bc.ca

Blumel, S., Goodrich, A., Martin, C., & Dang, N. H. (2008). Bendamustine: A novel cytotoxic agent for hematologic malignancies. *Clinical Journal of Oncology Nursing, 12*(5), 799–806.

Di Leo, A., & Moretti, E. (2008). Anthracyclines: The first generation of cytotoxic targeted agents? A possible dream. *Journal of Clinical Oncology, 26*(31), 5011–5013.

Kaplow, R. (2005). Innovations in antineoplastic therapy. *Nursing Clinics of North America, 40*(1), 77–94.

Messersmith, W. A., & Ahnen, D. J. (2008). Targeting EGFR in colorectal cancer. *New England Journal of Medicine, 359*(17), 1834–1836.

Myers, J. S., Pierce, J., & Pazdernik, T. (2008). Neurotoxicology of chemotherapy in relation to cytokine release, the blood–brain barrier, and cognitive impairment. *Oncology Nursing Forum, 35*(6), 916–920.

Paoluzzi, L., Kitagawa, Y., Kalac, M., Zain, J., & O'Connor, O. A. (2008). New drugs for the treatment of lymphoma. *Hematology/Oncology Clinics of North America, 22*(5), 1007–1035.

Smith, M. R., & Boldt, D. H. (2008). Hematological malignancies: Current perspectives on diagnosis, prognosis, and treatment. *Oncology, 22*(10, Suppl 2), S9–S36.

Viale, P. H., & Moore, S. (2008). Postmarketing surveillance for oncology drugs. *Clinical Journal of Oncology Nursing, 12*(6), 877–886.

Weiss, P. A. (2008). Can chemotherapy dosing be individualized? *Clinical Journal of Oncology Nursing, 12*(6), 975–977.

Yancey, M. A., & Winkeljohn, D. L. (2008). Oncology drug development: What is changing? *Clinical Journal of Oncology Nursing, 12*(5), 713–715.

Chapter 49

Blumel, S., Goodrich, A., Martin, C., & Dang, N. H. (2008). Bendamustine: A novel cytotoxic agent for hematologic malignancies. *Clinical Journal of Oncology Nursing, 12*(5), 799–806.

Di Leo, A., & Moretti, E. (2008). Anthracyclines: The first generation of cytotoxic targeted agents? A possible dream. *Journal of Clinical Oncology, 26*(31), 5011–5013.

Messersmith, W. A., & Ahnen, D. J. (2008). Targeting EGFR in colorectal cancer. *New England Journal of Medicine, 359*(17), 1834–1836.

Myers, J. S., Pierce, J., & Pazdernik, T. (2008). Neurotoxicology of chemotherapy in relation to cytokine release, the blood–brain barrier, and cognitive impairment. *Oncology Nursing Forum, 35*(6), 916–920.

Paoluzzi, L., Kitagawa, Y., Kalac, M., Zain, J., & O'Connor, O. A. (2008). New drugs for the treatment of lymphoma. *Hematology/Oncology Clinics of North America, 22*(5), 1007–1035.

Smith, M. R., & Boldt, D. H. (2008). Hematological malignancies: Current perspectives on diagnosis, prognosis, and treatment. *Oncology, 22*(10, Suppl 2), S9–S36.

Viale, P. H., & Moore, S. (2008). Postmarketing surveillance for oncology drugs. *Clinical Journal of Oncology Nursing, 12*(6), 877–886.

Weiss, P. A. (2008). Can chemotherapy dosing be individualized? *Clinical Journal of Oncology Nursing, 12*(6), 975–977.

Yancey, M. A., & Winkeljohn, D. L. (2008). Oncology drug development: What is changing? *Clinical Journal of Oncology Nursing, 12*(5), 713–715.

Chapter 50

B.C. Cancer Agency. (2009). *Cancer drug manual.* Retrieved January 11, 2009, from www.bccancer.bc.ca

Blumel, S., Goodrich, A., Martin, C., & Dang, N. H. (2008). Bendamustine: A novel cytotoxic agent for hematologic malignancies. *Clinical Journal of Oncology Nursing, 12*(5), 799–806.

Di Leo, A., & Moretti, E. (2008). Anthracyclines: The first generation of cytotoxic targeted agents? A possible dream. *Journal of Clinical Oncology, 26*(31), 5011–5013.

Messersmith, W. A., & Ahnen, D. J. (2008). Targeting EGFR in colorectal cancer. *New England Journal of Medicine, 359*(17), 1834–1836.

Myers, J. S., Pierce, J., & Pazdernik, T. (2008). Neurotoxicology of chemotherapy in relation to cytokine release, the blood–brain barrier, and cognitive impairment. *Oncology Nursing Forum, 35*(6), 916–920.

Paoluzzi, L., Kitagawa, Y., Kalac, M., Zain, J., & O'Connor, O. A. (2008). New drugs for the treatment of lymphoma. *Hematology/Oncology Clinics of North America, 22*(5), 1007–1035.

Smith, M. R., & Boldt, D. H. (2008). Hematological malignancies: Current perspectives on diagnosis, prognosis, and treatment. *Oncology, 22*(10, Suppl 2), S9–S36.

Viale, P. H., & Moore, S. (2008). Postmarketing surveillance for oncology drugs. *Clinical Journal of Oncology Nursing, 12*(6), 877–886.

Weiss, P. A. (2008). Can chemotherapy dosing be individualized? *Clinical Journal of Oncology Nursing, 12*(6), 975–977.

Yancey, M. A., & Winkeljohn, D. L. (2008). Oncology drug development: What is changing? *Clinical Journal of Oncology Nursing, 12*(5), 713–715.

Chapter 51

Bray, J., Clarke, C., Brennan, G., & Muncey, T. (2008). Should we be 'pushing meds'? The implications of pharmacogenomics. *Journal of Psychiatric & Mental Health Nursing, 15*(5), 357–364.

Canadian Institutes of Health Research. (2009). *Institute of genetics.* Retrieved January 15, 2009, from http://www.cihr-irsc.gc.ca/e/13147.html

Canadian Institutes of Health Research, Natural Sciences and Engineering Research Council of Canada, and Social Sciences and Humanities Research Council of Canada. (1998 [with 2000, 2002 and 2005 amendments]). *Tri-Council policy statement: Ethical conduct for research involving humans.* Retrieved November 22, 2009, from http://reportal.jointcentreforbioethics.ca/document/view/id/17

Canadian Nurses Association. (2005). Nursing and genetics. Are you ready? *Nursing Now. Issues and Trends in Canadian Nursing, 20,* 1–6.

Court, M. H. (2007). A pharmacogenomics primer. *Journal of Clinical Pharmacology, 47*(9), 1087–1103.

Gibaldi, M. (2007a). Pharmacogenetics: Part I: Perspective. *Annals of Pharmacotherapy, 41*(12), 2042–2047.

Gibaldi, M. (2007b). Pharmacogenetics: Part II: Perspective. *Annals of Pharmacotherapy, 41*(12), 2048–2054.

Health Canada. (2005). *Gene therapy.* Retrieved January 15, 2009, from http://www.hc-sc.gc.ca/sr-sr/biotech/about-apropos/gen_therap-eng.php

Henry, N. L., Stearns, V., Flockhart, D. A., Hayes, D. F., & Riba, M. (2008). Drug interactions and pharmacogenomics in the treatment of breast cancer and depression. *American Journal of Psychiatry, 165*(10), 1251–1255.

Hines, R. N., & McCarver, D. G. (2006). Pharmacogenomics and the future of drug therapy. *Pediatric Clinics of North America, 53*(4), 591–619.

Kayser, S. R. (2007). Pharmacogenomics and the potential for personalized therapeutics in cardiovascular disease. *Progress in Cardiovascular Nursing, 22*(2), 104–107.

Lanfear, D. E., & McLeod, H. L. (2007). Pharmacogenetics: Using DNA to optimize drug therapy. *American Family Physician, 76*(8), 1179–1182.

Lobo, I. (2008). Same genetic mutation, different genetic disease phenotype. *Nature Education, 1*(1). Retrieved May 13, 2009, from http://www.nature.com/

McNamara, D. M. (2008). Emerging role of pharmacogenomics in heart failure. *Current Opinion in Cardiology, 23*(3), 261–268.

Nakamura, Y. (2008). Pharmacogenomics and drug toxicity. *New England Journal of Medicine, 359*(8), 856–858.

Paice, J. A. (2007). Pharmacokinetics, pharmacodynamics, and pharmacogenomics of opioids. *Pain Management Nursing, 8*(3, Suppl 1), S2–S5.

Public Health Agency of Canada. (2004). *The laboratory biosafety guidelines* (3rd ed.) Retrieved November 22, 2009, from http://www.phac-aspc.gc.ca/publicat/lbg-ldmbl-04/pdf/lbg_2004_e.pdf

Roden, D. M., Altman, R. B., Benowitz, N. L., Flockhart, D. A., Giacomini, K. M., Johnson, J.A., et al. (2006). Pharmacogenomics: Challenges and opportunities. *Annals of Internal Medicine, 145*(10), 749–757.

Shurin, S. B., & Nabel, E. G. (2008). Pharmacogenomics—ready for prime time? *New England Journal of Medicine, 358*(10), 1061–1063.

Streetman, D. S. (2007). Emergence and evolution of pharmaco-genetics and pharmacogenomics in clinical pharmacy over the past 40 years. *Annals of Pharmacotherapy, 41*(12), 2038–2041.

Vail, J. (2007). Pharmacogenomics: The end of trial-and-error medicine? *International Journal of Pharmaceutical Compounding, 11*(1), 59–65.

Chapter 52

Ables, A. Z., Simon, I., & Melton, E. R., (2007). Update on *Helicobacter pylori* treatment. *American Family Physician, 75*(3), 351–358.

Alberta Medical Association. (2007). *Guideline for treatment of* Helicobacter pylori *infection in adults.* Retrieved January 16, 2009, from http://topalbertadoctors.org/PDF/complete%20 set/Helicobactor%20Pylori/h_pylori_guideline.pdf

American Family Physician. (2007). Peptic ulcer disease. *American Family Physician, 76*(7), 1005–1012.

Chan, F. K. L. (2008). Proton-pump inhibitors in peptic ulcer disease. *Lancet, 372* (9645), 1198–1200.

Coron, E., Hatlebakk, J. G., & Galmiche, J. (2007). Medical therapy of gastroesophageal reflux disease. *Current Opinion in Gastroenterology, 23*(4), 434–439.

Fulco, P. P., Vora, U. B., & Bearman, G. M. (2006). Acid suppressive therapy and the effects on protease inhibitors. *Annals of Pharmacotherapy, 40*(11), 1974–1983.

Graham, D. Y, Lu, H., & Yamaoka, Y. (2008). Therapy for *Helicobacter pylori* infection can be improved: Sequential therapy and beyond. *Drugs, 68*(6), 725–736.

Gralnek, I. M., Barkun, A. N., & Bardou, M. (2008). Management of acute bleeding from a peptic ulcer. *New England Journal of Medicine, 359*(9), 928–937.

Jodlowski, T. Z., Lam, S., & Ashby, C. R., Jr. (2008). Emerging therapies for the treatment of *Helicobacter pylori* infections. *Annals of Pharmacotherapy, 42*(11), 1621–1639.

Kahrilas, P. J. (2008). Gastroesophageal reflux disease. *New England Journal of Medicine, 359*(16), 1700–1707.

Lanas, A., & Ferrandez, A. (2007). Inappropriate prevention of NSAID-induced gastrointestinal events among long-term users in the elderly. *Drugs & Aging, 24*(2), 121–131.

McKeage, K., Blick, S. K. A., Croxtall, J. D., Lyseng-Williamson, K. A., & Keating, G. M. (2008). Esomeprazole: A review of its use in the management of gastric acid–related diseases in adults. *Drugs, 68*(11), 1571–1607.

Singh, H., Houy, T. L., Singh, N., & Sekhon, S. (2008). Gastrointestinal prophylaxis in critically ill patients. *Critical Care Nursing Quarterly, 31*(4), 291–301.

Targownik, L. E., Lix, L. M., Metge, C. J., Prior, H. J., Leung, S., & Leslie, W. D. (2008). Use of proton pump inhibitors and risk of osteoporosis-related fractures. *Canadian Medical Association Journal, 179*(4), 319–326.

Vaira, D., Zullo, A., Vakil, N., Gatta, L., Ricci, C., Perna, F., et al. (2007). Sequential therapy versus standard triple-drug therapy for *Helicobacter pylori* eradication: A randomized trial. *Annals of Internal Medicine, 146*(8), 556–563.

Zullo, A., Hassan, C., Campo, S. M. A., & Morini, S. (2007). Bleeding peptic ulcer in the elderly: Risk factors and prevention strategies. *Drugs & Aging, 24*(10), 815–828.

Chapter 53

Anonymous. (2008). Controlling pain. Managing opioid-induced constipation. *Nursing, 38*(7), 55.

Burke, C. A., & Church, J. M. (2007). Enhancing the quality of colonoscopy: The importance of bowel purgatives. *Gastrointestinal Endoscopy, 66*(3), 565–573.

Dykes, C., & Cash, B. D. (2008). Key safety issues of bowel preparations for colonoscopy and importance of adequate hydration. *Gastroenterology Nursing, 31*(1), 30–37.

Ferrell, B. (2008). Polyethylene glycol laxative for chronic constipation. *Journal of Pain & Palliative Care Pharmacotherapy, 22*(2), 149–150.

Gallagher, P. F., O'Mahony, D., & Quigley, E. M. (2008). Management of chronic constipation in the elderly. *Drugs & Aging, 25*(10), 807–821.

Hawley, P. H., & Byeon, J. J. (2008). A comparison of sennosides-based bowel protocols with and without docusate in hospitalized patients with cancer. *Journal of Palliative Medicine, 11*(4), 575–581.

Ho, J., Kuhn, R. J., & Smith, K. M. (2008). Pharmacology update: Update on treatment options for constipation. *Orthopedics, 31*, 570.

Joanna Briggs Institute. (2008). Management of constipation in older adults. *Australian Nursing Journal, 16*(5), 32–35.

Kligler, B., & Cohrssen, A. (2008). Probiotics. *American Family Physician, 78*(9), 1073–1078.

Manzotti, M. E., Catalano, H. N., Serrano, A., Di stilio, G., Koch, F. M., & Guyatt, G. (2007). Prokinetic drug utility in the treatment of gastroesophageal reflux esophagitis: A systematic review of randomized controlled trials. *Open Medicine, 1*(3). Retrieved February 7, 2009, from http://www.open-medicine.ca/article/viewArticle/79/93

Montgomery, D. F., Navarro, F., Cromwell, P. F., & Yetman, R. J. (2008). Practice guidelines. Management of constipation and encopresis in children. *Journal of Pediatric Healthcare, 22*(3), 199–204.

Rao, S. S. (2007). Constipation: Evaluation and treatment of colonic and anorectal motility disorders. *Gastroenterology Clinics of North America, 36*(3), 687–711.

Thomson, M. A., Jenkins, H. R., Bisset, W. M., Heuschkel, R., Kalra, D. S., Green, M. R., et al. (2007). Polyethylene glycol 3350 plus electrolytes for chronic constipation in children: A double-blind, placebo-controlled, crossover study. *Archives of Disease in Childhood, 92*(11), 996–1000.

Videlock, E. J., & Chang, L. (2007). Irritable bowel syndrome: Current approach to symptoms, evaluation, and treatment. *Gastroenterology Clinics of North America, 36*(3), 665–685.

Chapter 54

Apfel, C. C., Malhotra, A., & Leslie, J. B. (2008). The role of neurokinin-1 receptor antagonists for the management of postoperative nausea and vomiting. *Current Opinion in Anaesthesiology, 21*(4), 427–432.

Dibble, S. L., Luce, J., Cooper, B. A., Israel, J., Cohen, M., Nussey, B., et al. (2007). Acupressure for chemotherapy-induced nausea and vomiting: A randomized clinical trial. *Oncology Nursing Forum, 34*(4), 813–820.

DiVall, M. V., & Cersosimo, R. J. (2007). Prevention and treatment of chemotherapy-induced nausea and vomiting: A review. *Formulary, 42*(6), 378–380.

Hawkins, R., & Grunberg, S. (2009). Chemotherapy-induced nausea and vomiting: Challenges and opportunities for improved patient outcomes. *Clinical Journal of Oncology Nursing, 13*(1), 54–64.

Hesketh, P. J. (2008). Chemotherapy-induced nausea and vomiting. *New England Journal of Medicine, 358*(23), 2482–2494.

Kapoor, R., Hola, E. T., Adamson, R. T., & Mathis, A. S. (2008). Comparison of two instruments for assessing risk of postoperative nausea and vomiting. *American Journal of Health-System Pharmacy, 65*(5), 448–453.

Kloth, D. D. (2009). New pharmacologic findings for the treatment of PONV and PDNV. *American Journal of Health-System Pharmacy, 66*(Suppl 1), S11–S18.

Lee, J., Dodd, M., Dibble, S., & Abrams, D. (2008). Review of acupressure studies for chemotherapy-induced nausea and vomiting control. *Journal of Pain & Symptom Management, 36*(5), 529–544.

Machado Rocha, F. C., Stefano, S. C., Haiek, R. C., Oliveira, L. M. Q., & Da Silveira, D. X. (2008). Therapeutic use of *Cannabis sativa* on chemotherapy-induced nausea and vomiting among cancer patients: Systematic review and meta-analysis. *European Journal of Cancer Care, 17*(5), 431–443.

Majumdar, A. K., Howard, L., Goldberg, M. R., Hickey, L., Constanzer, M., Rothenberg, P. L., et al. (2006). Pharmacokinetics of aprepitant after single and multiple oral doses in healthy volunteers. *Journal of Clinical Pharmacology, 46*(3), 291–300.

Naeim, A., Dy, S. M., Lorenz, K. A., Sanati, H., Walling, A., & Asch, S. M. (2008). Evidence-based recommendations for cancer nausea and vomiting. *Journal of Clinical Oncology, 26*(23), 3903–3910.

O'Brien, C. (2008). Nausea and vomiting. *Canadian Family Physician, 54*(6), 861–863.

Osorio-Sanchez, J. A. A., Karapetis, C., & Koczwara, B. (2007). Efficacy of aprepitant in management of chemotherapy-induced nausea and vomiting. *Internal Medicine Journal, 37*(4), 247–250.

Prommer, E. (2005). Aprepitant (EMEND): The role of substance P in nausea and vomiting. *Journal of Pain & Palliative Care Pharmacotherapy, 19*(3), 31–39.

Schwartzberg, L. S. (2007). Chemotherapy-induced nausea and vomiting: Which antiemetic for which therapy. *Oncology, 21*(8), 946–953.

Vrabel, M., & Steele, S. K. (2007). Evidence-based practice. Is ondansetron more effective than granisetron for chemotherapy-induced nausea and vomiting? A review of comparative trials. *Clinical Journal of Oncology Nursing, 11*(6), 809–813.

Vreeman, R. C., Finnell, S. M., Cernkovich, E. R., & Carroll, A. E. (2008). The effects of antiemetics for children with vomiting due to acute, moderate gastroenteritis. *Archives of Pediatrics & Adolescent Medicine, 162*(9), 866–869.

Chapter 55

Jones, N. E., & Heyland, D. K. (2008). Pharmaconutrition: A new emerging paradigm. *Current Opinion in Gastroenterology, 24*(2), 215–222.

Koretz, R. L. (2008). Parenteral nutrition and urban legends. *Current Opinion in Gastroenterology, 24*(2), 210–214.

Lochs, H., Dejong, C., Hammarqvist, F., Hebuterne, X., Leon-Sanz, M., Schütz, T., et al. (2006). ESPEN guidelines on enteral nutrition: Gastroenterology. *Clinical Nutrition, 25,* 260–274.

Siow, E. (2008). Enteral versus parenteral nutrition for acute pancreatitis. *Critical Care Nurse, 28*(4), 19–25, 27–32.

Ukleja, A. (2005). Dumping syndrome: Pathophysiology and treatment. *Nutrition in Clinical Practice, 20*(5), 517–525.

Wernerman, J. (2008). Role of glutamine supplementation in critically ill patients. *Current Opinion in Anaesthesiology, 21*(2), 155–159.

Wischmeyer, P. E. (2008). Glutamine: Role in critical illness and ongoing clinical trials. *Current Opinion in Gastroenterology, 24*(2), 190–197.

Chapter 56

Anonymous. (2008). Protect your patients from the ongoing threat of iron overload. *Journal of Infusion Nursing, 31*(3), 180–181.

Barton, J. C. (2008). Optimal management strategies for chronic iron overload. *Drugs, 67*(5), 685–700.

Clark, S. F. (2008). Iron deficiency anemia. *Nutrition in Clinical Practice, 23*(2). 128–141.

Coyer, S. M., & Lash, A. A. (2008). Pathophysiology of anemia and nursing care implications. *MEDSURG Nursing, 17*(2), 77–83, 91.

Dee, D. L., Sharma, A. J., Cogswell, M. E., Grummer-Strawn, L. M., Fein, S. B., & Scanlon, K. S. (2008). Sources of supplemental iron among breastfed infants during the first year of life. *Pediatrics, 122*(Suppl 2), S98–S104.

Fishbane, S., Larson, K., & VanBuskirk, S. (2008). Stabilizing hemoglobin levels: What's new in IV iron and anemia management? *Nephrology Nursing Journal, 35*(5), 493–502.

Lindsey, W. T., & Olin, B. R. (2007). Deferasirox for transfusion-related iron overload: A clinical review. *Clinical Therapeutics, 29*(10), 2154–2166.

Madore, F., White, C. T., Foley, R. N., Barrett, B. J., Moist, L. M., Klarenbach, S. W., et al. (2008). Clinical practice guidelines for assessment and management of iron deficiency. *Kidney International, 74*(Suppl 110), S7–S11.

Morin, K. H. (2008). The importance of iron. *American Journal of Maternal Child Nursing, 33*(5), 320.

Vichinsky, E. (2008). Oral iron chelators and the treatment of iron overload in pediatric patients with chronic anemia. *Pediatrics, 121*(6), 1253–1256.

Yang, L. P. H., Keam, S. J., & Keating, G. M. (2007). Deferasirox: A review of its use in the management of transfusional chronic iron overload. *Drugs, 67*(15), 2211–2230.

Chapter 57

Andresen, M. (2006). Accutane registry compulsory in US, but not Canada. *Canadian Medical Association Journal, 174*(12), 1701–1702.

Hampton, S. (2007). Bacteria and wound healing. *Journal of Community Nursing, 21*(10), 32, 34, 36.

Health Canada. (2005). *Questions for the Science Advisory Panel on isotretinoin to be held May 12th, 2005*. Retrieved January 23, 2009, from http://www.hc-sc.gc.ca/dhp-mps/prodpharma/activit/sci-consult/isotretinoin/sapi_rop_gcsi_crd_2005-05-12-eng.php

Hess, C. T. (2008). Wound and skin care. Assessing the total patient. *Nursing, 38*(11), 24.

Morin, R., & Tomaselli, N. (2008). Interactive dressings and topical agents. *Clinics in Plastic Surgery, 34*(4), 643–658.

Reddy, M. (2008). Skin and wound care: Important considerations in the older adult. *Advances in Skin & Wound Care, 21*(9), 424–438.

Sarvis, C. M. (2007). Wound and skin care. Using antiseptics to manage infected wounds. *Nursing, 37*(12), 20–21.

Thomas, G. W., Rael, L. T., Bar-Or, R., Shimonkevitz, R., Mains, C. W., Slone. D. S., Craun, M. L., & Bar-Or, D. (2009). Mechanisms of delayed wound healing by commonly used antiseptics. *Journal of Trauma, 66,* 82–90.

Chapter 58

Adis International Limited. (2008). Adverse effects in the eye may be caused by a wide range of drugs used to treat ocular and systemic disorders. *Drugs & Therapy Perspectives, 24*(10), 23–26.

Fiscella, R. G., Lewis, C. C., & Jensen, M. K. (2007). Topical ophthalmic fourth-generation fluoroquinolones: Appropriate use and cost considerations. *American Journal of Health-System Pharmacy, 64*(19), 2069–2073.

Latkany. R. (2008). Dry eyes: Etiology and management. *Current Opinion in Ophthalmology, 19*(4), 287–291.

Levy, Y., & Zadok, D. (2004). Systemic side effects of ophthalmic drops. *Clinical Pediatrics, 43*(1), 99–101.

Pekdemir, M., Yanturali, S., & Karakus, G. (2005). More than just an ocular solution. *Emergency Medicine Journal, 22*(10), 753–754.

Pugmire, B., & Borzadek, E. (2008). New ophthalmic antibiotics for bacterial conjunctivitis. *Evidence-Based Practice, 11*(10), 9–10.

Snow, M. (2007). Combating infection. Keeping an eye on infectious keratitis. *Nursing, 3*(11), 60–61.

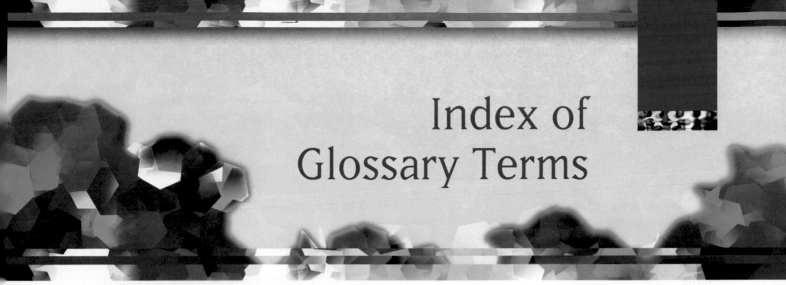

Index of Glossary Terms

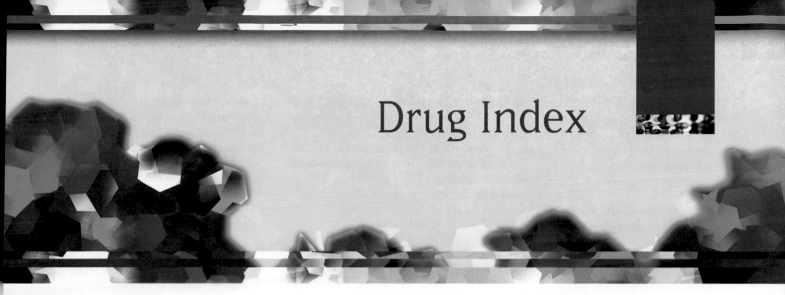

Drug Index

A

abacavir sulfate [Ziagen], 756t–757t, 772

abacavir/lamivudine [Kivexa], 773

abacavir/lamivudine/zidovudine [Trizivir], 773

abciximab [Reopro], 528t, 546

acarbose [Glucobay], 604, 606

acebutolol hydrochloride [Rhotrol, Sectral], 369–370, 427b, 427t, 429t

acetaminophen [Tylenol], 199t, 200, 204, 208

acetazolamide [Acetazolam], 492

acetylcholine chloride [Miochol E, Miogan PSW], 1056

acetylsalicylic acid [ASA, Aspirin], 533, 535t, 535–536, 547, 831, 837, 838b, 839

acetylsalicylic acid/butalbital/caffeine [Fiorinal, Trianal], 838b

acetylsalicylic acid/butalbital/ caffeine/codeine phosphate [Fiorinal C, Trianal C], 838b

acetylsalicylic acid/citric acid/sodium bicarbonate [Alka-Seltzer], 838b

acetylsalicylic acid/codeine phosphate/methocarbamol [Robaxisal C], 838b

acetylsalicylic acid/dipyridamole [Aggrenox], 838b

acetylsalicylic acid/nifedipine [Adalat XL Plus], 838b

acetylsalicylic acid/oxycodone hydrochloride [Percodan], 838b

acetylsalicylic acid/pravastatin sodium [PravAsa], 838b

acyclovir [Zovirax], 756t–758t, 759b, 761, 763

adalimumab [Humira], 942t, 943–944

adefovir dipivoxil [Hepsera], 756t–757t, 763

adenosine [Adenocard], 428t–429t, 435–436

albumin, 511t, 512, 519, 521

aldesleukin [Proleukin], 946, 948

alemtuzumab [MabCampath], 942t, 943–944

alendronate sodium [Fosamax], 639–640, 646, 648

alendronate/cholecalciferol [Fosavance], 640

alfacalcidol, 111t, 115b

alfentanil, 218t

aliskiren fumarate [Rasilez], 477–478

allopurinol [Alloprin, Zyloprim], 840–841, 890, 894, 916t

almotriptan maleate [Axert], 330

alprazolam [Xanax], 294–295, 315

alteplase [Activase, Cathflo], 540

altretamine [Hexalen], 915t, 919

aluminum hydroxide/magnesium hydroxide [Alumag, Gelusil, Maalox, Mylanta], 969

amantadine hydrochloride [Dom-Amantadine], 761–763, 776

amantadine [Symmetrel], 274–275, 276t, 277, 280, 758t, 759b

amifostine [Ethyol], 915t

amikacin sulfate, 736t, 738–739

amiloride hydrochloride [Midamor], 497

aminocaproic acid [Amicar], 528t

aminophylline [Phyllocontin], 692

amiodarone hydrochloride, 427b, 427t–430t, 434, 435t, 436, 438

amitriptyline [Elavil, Levate], 304–305

amlodipine besylate [Norvasc], 451t, 452

amoxicillin [Amoxil, Novamoxin], 717–718

amphetamine salts [Adderall XR], 330

amphotericin B [Fungizone], 795t–796t, 797–798, 800

amphotericin B lipid complex [ABCD, Abelcet, AmBisome, Amphotec], 798

ampicillin, 639, 718

anagrelide [Agrylin], 528t

anakinra [Kineret], 946

anastrozole [Arimidex], 916t

anidulafungin [Eraxis], 797

anthralin, 1041

antithrombin III [Thrombate], 528t, 529, 533

aprepitant [Emend], 1000

aprotinin [Trasylol], 528t, 537t

argatroban [Argatroban], 528t, 529, 531, 533

aripiprazole [Abilify], 313

artificial tears, 1069

asparaginase [Kidrolase], 884t, 898t, 899, 909, 911

atazanavir [Reyataz], 772

atenolol [Tenormin], 369–370, 433, 436, 450

atomoxetine hydrochloride [Strattera], 330

atorvastatin calcium [Lipitor], 558, 562

atovaquone [Mepron], 812t–813t, 814–815

atovaquone/proguanil hydrochloride [Malarone], 809

atropine sulfate, 391–393, 980t, 1068

attapulgite [Kaopectate], 981–982

auranofin [Ridaura], 842, 844

azathioprine sodium [Imuran], 852t–853t, 854–856

azatidine, 669t

azithromycin [Zithromax], 724–725

Page numbers followed by "*f*" denote figures, "*t*" denote tables, and "*b*" denote boxes

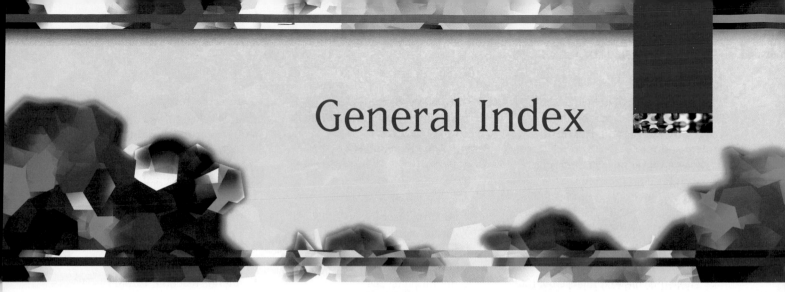

General Index

Page numbers followed by "f" denote figures, "t" denote tables, and "b" denote boxes

Potassium, 514–516, 522
Potassium-sparing diuretics, 495–497
Powders, 176–177, 1034*t*
Prebiotics, 94, 97
Precursor Control Regulations, 59, 61–62
Pregnancy
  angiotensin-converting enzyme inhibitor contraindications during, 471
  antiepileptic drug contraindications, 259
  drug therapy during, 44–45
  FDA drug safety categories, 44–45, 45*t*
  gestational diabetes, 589, 598
  human immunodeficiency virus in, 766
  teratogens, 39
  varicella-zoster virus exposure, 760
Premature ventricular contractions, 424*t*, 425
Premenstrual syndrome, 634
Preschoolers
  Erikson's description of, 87*b*
  medication administration in, 49*b*
Prescribing cascade, 48
Prescription
  abbreviations used in, 76*b*, 77*f*
  elements of, 10–11
Prescription drugs
  access to, 66*b*
  costs of, 66*b*
  handling of, 328
  reclassification as over-the-counter drugs, 95, 95*b*
Presynaptic drugs, 271, 275
Priapism, 655
Primary lesion, 880
Prinzmetal's angina, 444, 446
Priority Review of Drug Submission, 59, 65
PRN, 14
Probiotics, 94, 97
Proconvertin, 116
Prodrug, 20, 22, 460, 471
Progenitor cells, 936
Progesterone, 628
Progestins, 628, 634–635, 649
Prokinetic drugs, 997
Prolactin, 571*t*
Prophylactic antibiotic therapy, 708, 710

Prophylactic therapy, 36
Propionic acids, 837–838
Proprietary name. *See* Trade name
Prostaglandin(s), 831
Prostaglandin F$_{2\alpha}$ agonists, 1061–1062
Prostate cancer, 651, 654, 658
Prostate-specific antigen, 651, 655
Protease, 753
Protease inhibitors
  definition of, 753
  description of, 769
  nursing process for, 775–776
  types of, 772*t*
Protein synthesis, 955
Proteolytic enzyme, 539
Proteome, 955
Proteomics, 955
Prothrombin time, 541*t*
Protocol name, 62
Proton pump, 965
Proton pump inhibitors, 971–972, 974
Protozoal infections
  definition of, 805
  description of, 811
  drugs for. *See* Antiprotozoal drugs
  malaria. *See* Malaria
  transmission of, 811
  types of, 811*t*
Provitamin A carotenoids, 109
Proximal convoluted tubule, 490
Pruritus, 1032
Pseudomembranous colitis, 735, 742
Psoriasis, 1032, 1040
Psychoactive properties, 133, 136
Psychogenic pain, 186
Psychological dependence, 36, 133, 184, 193
Psychosis, 287, 288–289
Psychotherapeutic drugs
  antianxiety drugs. *See* Antianxiety drugs
  antidepressant drugs. *See* Antidepressant drugs
  antimanic drugs, 315–316, 322
  antipsychotic drugs. *See* Antipsychotic drugs
  in children, 315
  cultural considerations, 288
  definition of, 287
  nursing process for
    assessment, 314–318
    evaluation, 321
    implementation, 318–321

    nursing diagnoses, 318
    outcome criteria, 318
    planning, 318
  in older adults, 315
  patient education regarding, 322
Psychotropic, 287
Puberty, 628
Pulmonary embolus/embolism, 525, 528, 542
Pulse, apical, 149
Pupil, 1049, 1050
Purified protein derivative, 784
Purine antagonists, 890
Purkinje fibres, 420, 422
PURR, 1–5
Push medications, intravenous, 169–171, 170*f*–171*f*
Pustule, 1032
Pyrimidine antagonists, 890

Q

Quinolones. *See* Fluoroquinolones

R

Rabbit syndrome, 309
Race
  definition of, 68*b*
  drug responses affected by, 69
Radiation poisoning, 40
Radiopharmaceuticals, 924
RALES, 498
Randomized Aldactone Evaluation Study, 498
Randomized clinical trials, 41
Rapid eye movement sleep, 239–240
Rapid-acting insulin, 598, 600*t*
Rapid-sequence intubation, 228
Rational therapeutics, 22
Raves, 133, 136
Receptor(s)
  acetylcholine, 377
  adrenergic, 345–347, 347*t*, 362, 466
  definition of, 20, 22
  delta, 191*t*
  dopaminergic, 346
  drug interactions with, 35*t*
  interactions, 34, 35*t*
  muscarinic, 377, 466
  nicotinic, 377, 460, 466, 466*f*
  opioid, 191, 191*t*, 194
Receptor theory, 22
Recombinant, 861
Recombinant DNA, 868, 953, 956

SPECIAL FEATURES

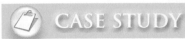

ETHNOCULTURAL IMPLICATIONS

EVIDENCE-INFORMED PRACTICE

SPECIAL FEATURES cont'd

 IN MY FAMILY

 LAB VALUES RELATED TO DRUG THERAPY

 LEGAL & ETHICAL PRINCIPLES

 NATURAL HEALTH PRODUCTS

 PREVENTING MEDICATION ERRORS